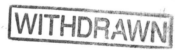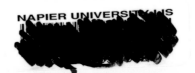

Current Techniques
in
Small Animal Surgery

FOURTH EDITION

Current Techniques in Small Animal Surgery

FOURTH EDITION

Edited by

M. Joseph Bojrab, DVM, MS, PhD

Diplomate, American College of Veterinary Surgery
Private Practice
Las Vegas, Nevada

Associate Editors

Gary W. Ellison, DVM, MS

Diplomate, American College of Veterinary Surgery
Professor of Small Animal Surgery
Department of Small Animal Clinical Sciences
University of Florida
College of Veterinary Medicine
Gainesville, Florida

Barclay Slocum, DVM

Slocum Veterinary Clinic
Private Practice
Eugene Oregon

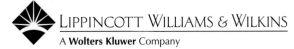

LIPPINCOTT WILLIAMS & WILKINS
A **Wolters Kluwer** Company
Philadelphia • Baltimore • New York • London
Buenos Aires • Hong Kong • Sydney • Tokyo

Editor: Susan Gay
Managing Editor: Paula Brown
Marketing Manager: Diane M. Harnish
Production Coordinator: Peter J. Carley
Project Editor: Jeffrey S. Myers
Designer: Elizabeth Sanders
Illustration Planner: Ray Lowman
Cover Designer: Elizabeth Sanders
Typesetter and Digitized Illustrations: Bi-Comp, Inc.
Printer/Binder: RR Donnelley & Sons Company

Copyright © 1998 Lippincott Williams & Wilkins

351 West Camden Street
Baltimore, Maryland 21201-2436 USA

530 Walnut Street
Philadelphia, Pennsylvania 19106-3621 USA

Accurate indications, adverse reactions and dosage schedules for drugs are provided in this book, but it is possible that they may change. The reader is urged to review the package information data of the manufacturers of the medications mentioned.

Printed in the United States of America

First Edition, 1975. Second Edition, 1983. Third Edition, 1990

Library of Congress Cataloging-in-Publication Data

Current techniques in small animal surgery / edited by M. Joseph
    Bojrab, consulting soft tissue editor, Gary W. Ellison, consulting
    bone and joint editor, Barclay Slocum. — 4th ed.
        p.   cm.
    Includes bibliographical references and index.
    ISBN 0-683-00890-0
    1. Dogs—Surgery.   2. Cats—Surgery.   3. Veterinary surgery.
I. Bojrab, M. Joseph.
SF991.C87   1997
636.089'7—dc21   97-22997
                                                    CIP

The publishers have made every effort to trace the copyright holders for borrowed material. If they have inadvertently overlooked any, they will be pleased to make the necessary arrangements at the first opportunity.

To purchase additional copies of this book, call our customer service department at **(800) 638-3030** or fax orders to **(301) 824-7390**. For other book services, including chapter reprints and large quantity sales, ask for the Special Sales Department. International customers should call **(301) 714-2324**.

Visit Lippincott Williams & Wilkins on the Internet: http://www.lww.com. Lippincott Williams & Wilkins customer service representatives are available from 8:30 am to 6:00 pm, EST.

                                                                    02 03
                                                    3 4 5 6 7 8 9 10

To my mother, Julia and in memory of my father, Joseph

━●━ PREFACE

Since the complexity of present day small animal surgery prevents the individual veterinarian from mastery of all operative procedures, we have designated this work to include the viewpoints and approaches of distinguished leaders in the various surgical fields. This concise, comprehensive, graphic text is a valuable reference as well as a review of the surgical procedures that the veterinary practitioner is called upon to perform. It is intended primarily for the practicing veterinarian and the veterinary student. It is designed to be simple accurate, and exemplary. Each author is challenged to present their procedure in a form that the practitioner and the student can easily understand and perform while being thorough and accurate.

This text is a must for every small animal practitioner since it outlines the current thinking of leaders in the field and gives the practitioner a solid base from which to make judgments, and to recommend and perform procedures. This is extremely important in this day and age when the public demands the best and latest for their pets.

We have continually tried to expand and keep this text on the cutting edge. This book reflects the efforts of many people. Our contributors have been extremely cooperative and to them we owe a debt of gratitude. The consulting editors, Drs. Gary Ellison and Barclay Slocum, did an outstanding job in their respective sections and to them I will ever be grateful. Finally, my deepest thanks go to Mr. Carroll Cann, Mrs. Susan Hunsberger, Mr. Peter Carley, and Mrs. Holly Lukens for their tremendous support and encouragement in the seemingly never-ending, and tedious task of text development.

MJ Bojrab

━●━ CONTRIBUTORS

John F. Amann, DVM, PhD
Associate Professor of Veterinary Anatomy
Department of Veterinary Biomedical Sciences
University of Missouri, Columbia
College of Veterinary Medicine
Columbia, Missouri

Mark A. Anderson, DVM, MS
Diplomate, ACVS
Veterinary Surgical Services, PC
Veterinary Specialty Services
Collinsville, Illinois

Steven P. Arnoczky, DVM
Diplomate, ACVS
Associate Professor of Surgery
Cornell University Medical School
New York, New York
Adjunct Associate Professor of Surgery
New York State College of Veterinary Medicine
Cornell University
Ithaca, New York
Director, Comparative Orthopedic Research Department
Michigan State University College of Veterinary
   Medicine
East Lansing, Michigan

Dennis N. Aron, DVM
Diplomate, ACVS
Associate Professor of Surgery
College of Veterinary Medicine
University of Georgia
Athens, Georgia

Michael G. Aronsohn, VMD
Diplomate, ACVS
Staff Surgeon, Veterinary Specialists of South Florida
Cooper City, Florida

James E. Bailey, DVM, MS
Diplomate, ACVA
Assistant Professor
Department of Anesthesiology
College of Veterinary Medicine
University of Florida
Gainesville, Florida

Kenneth E. Bartels, DVM, MS
McCasland Professor of Laser Surgery
Department of Medicine and Surgery
College of Veterinary Medicine
Oklahoma State University
Stillwater, Oklahoma

Joseph W. Bartges, DVM, PhD
Diplomate, ACVIM
Diplomate, ACVN
Assistant Professor
Department of Small Animal Medicine
College of Veterinary Medicine
University of Georgia
Athens, Georgia

Brian Beale, DVM
Diplomate, ACVS
Gulf Coast Veterinary Surgery
Houston, Texas

Trevor N. Bebchuk, DVM
Resident in Surgery
Department of Small Animal Clinical Sciences
Michigan State University, College of Veterinary
   Medicine
East Lansing Michigan

Neal L. Beeber, DVM
Diplomate, ABVP
Director, Rutherford Animal Hospital, PA
Rutherford, New Jersey

Jamie R. Bellah, DVM
Diplomate, ACVS
Associate Professor
Service Chief, Small Animal Surgery
Department of Small Animal Clinical Sciences
University of Florida, College of Veterinary Medicine
Gainesville, Florida

R. Avery Bennett, DVM, MS
Diplomate, ACVS
Assistant Professor, Zoo and Wildlife Medicine
Department of Small Animal Clinical Sciences
Wildlife and Zoological Medicine Service
University of Florida
College of Veterinary Medicine
Gainesville, Florida

John Berg, DVM, MS
Diplomate, ACVS
Associate Professor of Surgery
Department of Small Animal Surgery
Tufts University School of Veterinary Medicine
North Grafton, Massachusetts

James F. Biggart, III, DVM, MS
Diplomate, ACVS
Research Associate; Department of Orthopedics
University of California at San Francisco
President, Veterinary Surgery Service, Inc.
University Veterinary Hospital, Berkeley
Berkeley, California

Stephen J. Birchard, DVM, MS
Diplomate, ACVS
Associate Professor, Department of Veterinary Clinical
  Sciences
Head, Small Animal Surgery
The Ohio State University
Columbus, Ohio

Dale E. Bjorling, DVM, MS
Diplomate, ACVS
Professor and Chairman
Department of Surgical Science
School of Veterinary Medicine
University of Wisconsin
Madison, Wisconsin

Linda Blythe, DVM
Oregon State University
College of Veterinary Medicine
Corvallis, Oregon

Christopher M. Boemo, BVSc (hon), MRCVS
Keysborough Veterinary Practice
Keysborough, Victoria
Australia

M. Joseph Bojrab, DVM, MS, PhD
Diplomate, ACVS
Private Consulting Practice
Las Vegas, Nevada

David L. Bone, DVM
Diplomate, ACVS
Director and Staff Surgeon
Southwest University Surgical Service
Phoenix, Arizona

Harry W. Boothe, Jr., DVM, MS
Diplomate, ACVS
Professor of Surgery
Department of Veterinary Small Animal Medicine and
  Surgery
Texas A&M University
Chief, Small Animal Surgery
Texas Veterinary Medical Center
College Station, Texas

Randy Boudrieau, DVM
Diplomate, ACVS
Associate Professor of Surgery, Department of Surgery
Tufts University School of Veterinary Medicine
North Grafton, Massachusetts

Jim Boulay, DVM, MS
Diplomate, ACVS
Staff Surgeon
Angell Memorial Animal Hospital
Boston, Massachusetts

Terry Braden, DVM, MS
Veterinary Clinical Center
Michigan State University
College of Veterinary Medicine
East Lansing, Michigan

Eugene M. Breznock, DVM, MS, PhD
Diplomate, ACVS
Professor of Surgery
Chief, Small Animal Surgery
Veterinary Medical Teaching Hospital
Department of Veterinary Surgery and Radiology
University of California School of Veterinary Medicine
University of California, Davis
Davis, California

Ronald M. Bright, DVM, MS
Diplomate, ACVS
Professor, Department of Small Animal Clinical
  Sciences
General Surgeon, University of Tennessee Veterinary
  Teaching Hospital
University of Tennessee College of Veterinary Medicine
Knoxville, Tennessee

Jack Brinker, DVM
Brinker Veterinary Hospital
Lake Orion, Michigan

Wade O. Brinker, DVM, MS
Diplomate, ACVS
Professor Emeritus Michigan State University
East Lansing, Michigan

Kenneth A. Bruecker, DVM, MS
Diplomate, ACVS
Hospital Director
Veterinary Medical and Surgical Group
Ventura, California

Paul E. Cechner, DVM
Diplomate, ACVS
Los Alamitos, California
Staff Surgeon
Lakewood Animal Hospital
Bellflower, California

Joanna Chao, DVM
Intern in Small Animal Medicine and Surgery
Veterinary Teaching Hospital
Virginia-Maryland Regional College of Veterinary
  Medicine
Blacksburg, Virginia

Geoffrey N. Clark, DVM
Diplomate ACVS
Editor, Canine Sports Medicine Update
Staff Surgeon, Sea Coast Veterinary Associates
Dover, New Hampshire

Georghe M. Constantinescu, DVM, PhD, Dr.h.c.
American Association of Veterinary Anatomists
World Association of Veterinary Anatomists
European Association of Veterinary Anatomists
American Association Anatomists
Federation of American Societies for Experimental
    Biology (FASEB)
International Committee of Veterinary Gross
    Anatomical Nomenclature
National Computer Graphics Association
Professor of Veterinary Anatomy
University of Missouri - Columbia
College of Veterinary Medicine
Columbia, Missouri

Stephen W. Crane, DVM
Diplomate, ACVS
Director of Veterinary Affairs
Hill's Pet Nutrition
Topeka, Kansas

James E. Creed, DVM, MS
Assistant Dean for Service; Hospital Director
Oklahoma State University
College of Veterinary Medicine
Oklahoma State University Teaching Hospital
Stillwater, Oklahoma

Dennis T. Crowe, Jr., DVM
Diplomate, ACVS
Diplomate, ACVECC
Chief of Surgery
The Animal Emergency Center and Referral Services
Director of Research
The Veterinary Institute of Trauma, Emergency and
    Critical Care
Milwaukee, Wisconsin

William R. Daly, DVM
Diplomate ACVS
Houston Veterinary Referral Surgery Service
Houston, Texas

Jacqueline R. Davidson, DVM, MS
Diplomate, ACVS
Assistant Professor of Surgery
Department of Veterinary Clinical Sciences
Louisiana State University School of Veterinary
    Medicine
Baton Rouge, Louisiana

Paul W. Dean, DVM
Diplomate, ACVS
Veterinary Surgical Referral Center
Tulsa, Oklahoma

Jon Dee, DVM
Diplomate, ACVS
Head, Surgical Department
Hollywood Animal Hospital
Hollywood, Florida

Daniel A. Degner, DVM
Veterinary Surgeon
Michigan Veterinary Specialists
Southfield, Michigan

William S. Dernell, DVM, MS
Diplomate, ACVS
Assistant Professor, Surgical Oncology
Comparative Oncology, Colorado State University
College of Veterinary Medicine and Biomedical Sciences
Fort Collins, Colorado

Jennifer Devey, DVM
Diplomate, ACVECC
Director of Emergercy Services
Allpets Clinic
Boulder, Colorado

Chad Devitt, DVM, MS
Diplomate ACVS
Surgical Oncology Fellow
Comparative Oncology Unit
Colorado State University School of Veterinary
    Medicine
Fort Collins, Colorado

Bradford C. Dixon, DVM, MS
Staff Surgeon
Southwest Veterinary Surgical Service
Phoenix, Arizona

R. Tass Dueland, DVM, MS
Diplomate, ACVS
Professor of Orthopedic Surgery
School of Veterinary Medicine
University of Wisconsin-Madison
Madison, Wisconsin

Mary L. Dulisch, DVM, MS
Diplomate, ACVS
Veterinary Medical & Surgical Group
Ventura, California

Dianne Dunning, DVM, MS
Small Animal Surgery Resident
Colorado State University
Veterinary Teaching Hospital
Fort Collins, Colorado

Julie M. Duval, VMD
Diplomate, ACVS
Staff Surgeon
South Carolina Surgical Referral Service
Columbia, South Carolina

Thomas D. Earley, DVM, MS
Greater Altlanta Veterinary Referral Surgical Practice
Marietta, Georgia

Erick L. Egger, DVM
Diplomate, ACVS
Associate Professor of Surgery
Colorado State University
Veterinary Teaching Hospital
Fort Collins, Colorado

Nicole Ehrhart, VMD, MS
Diplomate, ACVS
Assistant Professor
University of Illinois
College of Veterinary Medicine
Urbana, Illinois

Gary W. Ellison, DVM, MS
Diplomate, ACVS
Professor of Surgery
Department of Small Animal Clinical Sciences
University of Florida
College of Veterinary Medicine
Gainesville, Florida

Mark H. Engen, DVM
Diplomate, ACVS
Chief of Staff
Puget Sound Animal Hospital for Surgery
Kirkland, Washington

Ron Fallon, DVM
Orthopedic Surgeon
Veterinary Referral Services
Gaithersburg, Maryland
Ambulatory Veterinary Surgery
Ellicott City, Maryland
Staff Surgeon
The Regional Veterinary Referral Center
Springfield, Virginia

Roger B. Fingland, DVM, MS
Diplomate, ACVS
Associate Professor of Surgery
Director, Veterinary Medical Teaching Hospital
College of Veterinary Medicine
University of Kansas
Manhattan, Kansas

Gretchen Flo, DVM, MS
Professor of Surgery, Department of Small Animal
  Clinical Sciences
Michigan State University, College of Veterinary
  Medicine
East Lansing, Michigan

Theresa W. Fossum, DVM, MS, PhD
Diplomate, ACVS
Associate Professor, Department of Small Animal
  Medicine and Surgery
College of Veterinary Medicine
Texas A & M University
College Station, Texas

David Fowler, DVM, MVSc
Diplomate, ACVS
Professor of Surgery
Department of Veterinary Anesthesiology, Radiology,
  and Surgery
University of Saskatchewan
Western College of Veterinary Medicine
Saskatoon, Saskatchewan, CANADA

Lynnetta J. Freeman, DVM, MS
Diplomate, ACVS
Principal Scientist, Surgical Research and Procedure
  Development
Ethicon Endo-Surgery, Inc.
Cincinnati, Ohio

Dean Gahring, DVM
Diplomate, ACVS
Head of Surgery
San Carlos Veterinary Hospital
Council Member, Association for Veterinary Orthopedic
  Research & Education
San Diego, California

Dougald R. Gilmore, BVSc
Diplomate, ACVS
Director of Surgery
Santa Cruz Veterinary Hospital
South Bay Veterinary
San Jose, California

Stephen D. Gilson, DVM
Diplomate, ACVS
Sonora Veterinary Surgery & Oncology
Scottsdale, Arizona

Cathy L. Greenfield, DVM, MS
Diplomate, ACVS
Assistant Professor, Soft Tissue Surgery
Department of Veterinary Clinical Medicine
University of Illinois, College of Veterinary Medicine
Urbana, Illinois

Clare R. Gregory, DVM
Diplomate, ACVS
Professor, Department of Surgical and Radiological
  Sciences
University of California School of Veterinary Medicine
Davis, California

Joseph Harari, DVM, MS
Diplomate, ACVS
Director of Surgery
Rowley Memorial Animal Hospital
Springfield, Massachusetts

Elizabeth M. Hardie, DVM, PhD
Diplomate, ACVS
Associate Professor, Small Animal Surgery
North Carolina State University, College of Veterinary
  Medicine
Raleigh, North Carolina

Robert J. Hardie, DVM
Diplomate, ACVS
Staff Surgeon
Bath-Brunswick Veterinary Associates
Brunswick, Maine

H. Jay Harvey, DVM
Diplomate, ACVS
Associate Professor of Surgery
Head, Companion Animal Hospital
Department Coordinator, Small Animal Surgery
Cornell University
New York State College of Veterinary Medicine
Ithaca, New York

Darryl Heard, BSc, BVMS, PhD
Diplomate, ACZM
Assistant Professor, Wildlife and Zoological Medicine
    Service
College of Veterinary Medicine
University of Florida
Gainesville, Florida

Cheryl S. Hedlund, DVM, MS
Diplomate, ACVS
Professor and Chief, Companion Animal Surgery and
    Anesthesia
Department of Veterinary Clinical Sciences
Louisiana State University
School of Veterinary Medicine
Baton Rouge, Louisiana

Ralph A. Henderson, DVM, MS
Diplomate, ACVS
Professor of Surgery
Department of Small Animal Surgery and Medicine
Auburn University
Auburn, Alabama

H. Phil Hobson, DVM, MS
Diplomate, ACVS
Professor, Small Animal Surgery
Department of Small Animal Surgery
Texas A & M University
College of Veterinary Medicine
College Station, Texas

**Peter E. Holt, B.V.M.S., Ph.D., C.Biol.,M.I.Biol.,
FRCVS**
Diplomate, ECVS
Senior Lecturer in Veterinary Surgery
University of Bristol
Department of Clinical Veterinary Science
Bristol, ENGLAND

David E. Holt, BVSc
Diplomate, ACVS
Assistant Professor of Surgery
VHUP-Department of Clinical Studies
University of Pennsylvania
School of Veterinary Medicine
Philadelphia, Pennsylvania

Andy Hopkins, BVSc, MVM, MRCVS
Diplomate, ACVIM (Neurology)
Diplomate, ECVN
Consultant; North Florida Neurology, PA
Orange Park, Florida

Giselle Hosgood, BVSc, FACVSc, MS
Diplomate, ACVS
Associate Professor
Department of Veterinary Clinical Sciences
Louisiana State University
School of Veterinary Medicine
Baton Rouge, Louisiana

Robert F. Hoyt, Jr., DVM, MS
Diplomate, ACLAM
National Institutes of Health
National Heart, Lung and Blood Institute
Bethesda, Maryland

Brian T. Huss, DVM, MS
Diplomate, ACVS
Owner, Veterinary Surgical Referrals
Sudbury, Massachusetts

Dennis A. Jackson, DVM, MS
Diplomate, ACVS
Staff Surgeon
Granville Island Veterinary Hospital
Vancouver, British Columbia, CANADA

William F. Jackson, DVM, DSc (Hon)
Diplomate, ACVO
Diplomate, ACVS
Diplomate, ABVP
World Small Animal Veterinary Association
Lakeland, Florida

Ann L. Johnson, DVM, MS
Diplomate, ACVS
Professor, Small Animal Orthopedics
Small Animal Clinic
University of Illinois School of Veterinary Medicine
Urbana, Illinois

Kenneth A. Johnson, MVSc, PhD, FACVSC
Diplomate, AVCS
Associate Professor of Orthopaedics
Department of Surgical Sciences
University of Wisconsin-Madison
Madison, Wisconsin

Robert E. Kaderly, DVM, PhD
Diplomate, ACVS
Staff Surgeon
Veterinary Referral Clinic
Cleveland, Ohio

Kyle K. Kerstetter, DVM
Chief Resident in Surgery
Department of Small Animal Clinical Sciences
University of Tennessee College of Veterinary Medicine
Knoxville, Tennessee

David W. Knapp, DVM
Diplomate, ACVS
Clinical Instructor of Small Animal Surgery
Staff Surgeon
Angell Memorial Animal Hospital
Boston, Massachusetts

Charles D. Knecht, VMD, MS
Diplomate, ACVS
Diplomate, ACVIM - Specialty, Neurology
Professor Emeritus, College of Veterinary Medicine
Auburn University Small Animal Clinic
Auburn, Alabama

Ronald J. Kolata, DVM, MS
Diplomate, ACVS
Ethicon Endo-Surgery, Inc.
Cincinnati, Ohio

D.J. Krahwinkel, Jr., DVM, MS
Diplomate ACVS
Diplomate, ACVA
Diplomate, ACVECC
Professor of Surgery
Department Head, Small Animal Clinical Sciences
University of Tennessee Veterinary Teaching Hospital
Knoxville, Tennessee

Karl Kraus, DVM, MS
Diplomate ACVS
Associate Professor of Surgery
Tufts University, School of Veterinary Medicine
Foster Hospital for Small Animals
North Grafton, Massachusetts

Andrew E. Kyles, BVMS, PhD, MRCVS
Clinical Instructor in Small Animal Surgery
General Surgery
University of Georgia, College of Veterinary Medicine
Department of Small Animal Medicine
Athens, Georgia

Thomas R. LaHue, DVM
Diplomate, ACVS
Small Animal Surgeon
Santa Cruz Veterinary Hospital
Santa Cruz, California

Douglas N. Lange, DVM
Assistant Professor
Department of Medicine and Surgery
Oklahoma State University College of Veterinary
    Medicine
Stillwater, Oklahoma

Gary Lantz, DVM
Diplomate, ACVS
Professor of Surgery
Department of Veterinary Clinical Sciences
Purdue University School of Veterinary Medicine
West Lafayette, Indiana

Otto Lanz, DVM
Resident, Department of Small Animal Clinical Sciences
University of Florida, College of Veterinary Medicine
Gainesville, Florida

Susan M. LaRue, DVM, PhD
Diplomate, ACVS
Diplomate, ACVR (Radiation Oncology)
Assistant Professor
Department of Radiological Health Sciences
Colorado State University School of Veterinary
    Medicine
Fort Collins, Colorado

Darien Lawrence, DVM, MS
Diplomate, ACVS
Lecturer of Small Animal Surgery
Honorary Clinical Associate
Department of Veterinary Clinical Sciences
University of Sydney
Sydney, Australia

Alice H. Lee, DVM, MS
Research Associate
Department of Physiology and Biophysics
University of Alabama, Birmingham
Birmingham, Alabama

Edward B. Leeds, DVM
Diplomate, ACVS
Surgical Group for Animals
Staff Surgeon, Century Veterinary Group
Los Angeles, California

Rose J. Lemaré, DVM
Resident, Small Animal Surgery
Department of Veterinary Clinical Sciences
School of Veterinary Medicine
Louisiana State University
Baton Rouge, Louisiana

Timothy Lenehan, DVM
Diplomate, ACVS
Staff Surgeon
Veterinary Surgical Specialists
San Diego, California

Arnold Lesser, VMD
Diplomate, ACVS
Surgeon/Owner
Veterinary Surgical Referral Service
Centerport, New York

Alan J. Lipowitz, DVM, MS
Diplomate, ACVS
Professor of Surgery, Department of Small Animal
    Clinical Sciences
University of Minnesota, College of Veterinary
    Medicine
St. Paul, Minnesota

Scott Lozier, DVM, MS
Diplomate, ACVS
Northwest Veterinary Specialists
Gresham, Oregon

Jody Lulich, DVM, PhD
Diplomate, ACVIM
Associate Professor
College of Veterinary Medicine
University of Minnesota
St. Paul, Minnesota

Douglas M. MacCoy, DVM
Diplomate, ACVS
Veterinary Surgical Associates, Inc.
Coral Springs, Florida

F.A. Mann, DVM, MS
Diplomate, ACVS
Diplomate, ACVECC
Associate Professor, Department of Veterinary Medicine
    and Surgery
University of Missouri-Columbia College of Veterinary
    Medicine
Columbia, Missouri

Sandra Manfra Marretta, DVM
Diplomate, ACVS
Diplomate, AVDC
Assistant Professor Small Animal Surgery and Dentistry
University of Illinois, College of Veterinary Medicine
Urbana, Illinois

Robert A. Martin, DVM
Diplomate, ACVS
Diplomate, ABVP
Professor, Small Animal Clinical Sciences
Hospital Director, Veterinary Teaching Hospital
Virginia/Maryland Regional College of Veterinary
    Medicine
Blacksburg, Virginia

John C. Meeks, DVM
Clinical Instructor, Neurology/Neurosurgery
Department of Companion Animal and Small Species
North Carolina State University, College of Veterinary
    Medicine
Raleigh, North Carolina

Michele Menard, DVM, MS, PhD
Diplomate, ACVP
Clinical Pathologist
Veterinary Cytopathology
Gresham, Oregon

Andrea Meyer-Lindenberg, DVM
Clinic of Small Animals
School of Veterinary Medicine
Hanover, GERMANY

Eric Monnet, DVM, MS, PhD
Diplomate, ACVS
Diplomate, ECVS
Assistant Professor of Surgery
Department of Clinical Sciences
Colorado State University Veterinary Teaching Hospital
Fort Collins, Colorado

James K. Morrisey, DVM
Senior Resident
Avian and Exotic Animal Medicine and Surgery Service
New York, New York

Holly S. Mullen, DVM
Diplomate, ACVS
Chief of Surgery, California Veterinary Surgical Practice
The Emergency Animal Hospital and Referral Center of
    San Diego
San Diego, California

Helen Newman-Gage, PhD, CTBS
Veterinary Tansplant Services, Inc.
Assistant Professor, Department of Aeorthopaedics
University of Washington School of Medicine
Seattle, Washington

Charles D. Newton, DVM, MS
Professor of Orthopedic Surgery
Associate Dean
University of Pennsylvania School of Veterinary
    Medicine
Philadelphia, Pennsylvania

Jenifer D. Newton, DVM
North Atlanta Veterinary Surgeons
Atlanta, Georgia

Matt G. Oakes, DVM
Diplomate, ACVS
Tampa Bay Veterinary Referral
Largo, Florida

Marvin Olmstead, DVM, MS
Diplomate, ACVS
Professor of Small Animal Orthopedics
The Ohio State University College of Veterinary
    Medicine
Columbus, Ohio

E. Christopher Orton, DVM, PhD
Diplomate, ACVS
Professor, Department of Clinical Sciences
Colorado State University, Veterinary Teaching Hospital
Fort Collins, Colorado

Carl A. Osborne, DVM, PhD
Diplomate, ACVIM
Professor, Department of Small Animal Clinical
    Sciences
College of Veterinary Medicine
University of Minnesota
St. Paul, Minnesota

Robert B. Parker, DVM
Diplomate, ACVS
Chairman, Department of Surgery
The Animal Medical Center
New York, New York

Michael M. Pavletic, DVM
Diplomate, ACVS
Professor of Surgery
Tufts University School of Veterinary Medicine
North Grafton, Massachusetts

Ghery D. Pettit, DVM
Diplomate, ACVS
Professor Emeritus
Washington State University School of Veterinary
    Medicine
Pullman, Washington

David Polzin, DVM, PhD
Diplomate, ACVIM
Professor of Internal Medicine
Department of Small Animal Clinical Sciences
College of Veterinary Medicine
University of Minnesota
St. Paul, Minnesota

Eric R. Pope, DVM, MS
Diplomate, ACVS
Associate Professor, Department of Veterinary
    Medicine & Surgery
University of Missouri
Columbia, Missouri

K. Ron Presnell, DVM, MSc
Diplomate, ACVS
Dundurn, Saskatchewan
CANADA

Wolff-Dieter Prieur, DVM
AO Veterinary Centre
Institut Straumann AG
Waldenberg, SWITZERLAND

Curtis W. Probst, DVM
Diplomate, ACVS
Professor and Chairperson
Department of Small Animal Clinical Sciences
Michigan State University
College of Veterinary Medicine
East Lansing, Michigan

Caroline Prymak, BVSc, Cert VR, MBA, DSAS
Diplomate ACVS,
Diplomate, ECVS
Diplomate, RCVS
Specialist in Small Animal Surgery
Head of Surgery Animal Health Trust
Newmarket, Suffolk, England

Charles M. Pullen, DVM, MS
Hospital Director, Cactus Animal Hospital and Surgical
    Center
Phoenix, Arizona

Clarence A. Rawlings, DVM, PhD
Diplomate, ACVS
Professor, Department of Small Animal Medicine and
Department of Physiology and Pharmacology
College of Veterinary Medicine
University of Georgia
Athens, Georgia

Jerome Reinke, DVM
Diplomate, ACVS
Madera Pet Hospital
Corte Madera, California

Walter C. Renberg, DVM
Department of Small Animal Clinical Sciences
VA-MD Regional College of Veterinary Medicine
Virginia Tech
Blacksburg, Virginia

Eberhard Rosin, DVM, PhD
Diplomate, ACVS
Professor of Surgery, Department of Surgical Sciences;
Chief of Staff, Small Animal Services
Veterinary Medical Teaching Hospital
University of Wisconsin School of Veterinary Medicine
Madison, Wisconsin

Robert G. Roy, DVM, MS
Diplomate, ACVS
Lighthouse Point, Florida

Jill E. Sackman, DVM, PhD
Diplomate, ACVS
Assistant Professor, Surgery
Department of Surgery and Small Animal Clinical
    Sciences
University of Tennessee College of Veterinary Medicine
Knoxville, Tennessee

M. Stacie Scardino, DVM
Research Associate
Scott-Ritchey Research Center
Auburn University College of Veterinary Medicine
Auburn University, Alabama

Thomas D. Scavelli, DVM
Diplomate, ACVS
Staff Surgeon
Veterinary Surgical Specialists
Tinton Falls, New Jersey

Susan L. Schaefer, DVM, MS
Resident in Small Animal Surgery
Department of Small Animal Clinical Sciences
Michigan State University College of Veterinary
    Medicine
East Lansing, Michigan

Kurt Schulz, DVM
Diplomate, ACVS
Lecturer, Department of Surgical and Radiologic
    Sciences
School of Veterinary Medicine
University of California - Davis
Davis, California

Peter D. Schwarz, DVM
Diplomate, ACVS
Associate Professor of Surgery
College of Veterinary Medicine/Clinical Sciences
Colorado State University
Ft. Collins, Colorado

Howard B. Seim III, DVM
Diplomate, ACVS
Associate Professor
Chief, Small Animal Surgery
Colorado State University
College of Veterinary Medicine
Fort Collins, Colorado

Peter K. Shires, BVSc, MS
Diplomate, ACVS
Professor, Department of Small Animal Clinical Services
Virginia - Maryland Regional College of Veterinary
    Medicine
Blacksburg, Virginia

Andy Shores, DVM, MS, PhD
Ridgeland, Mississippi

Stephen T. Simpson, DVM
Diplomate, ACVIM - Neurology
Associate Professor, Department of Small Animal
    Surgery and Medicine
Auburn University
Neurologist and Neurosurgeon
Small Animal Clinic, Auburn University
Auburn, Alabama

Kenneth R. Sinibaldi, DVM
Diplomate ACVS
Animal Surgical Clinic of Seattle
Seattle, Washington

Barclay Slocum, DVM
Slocum Veterinary Clinic
Private Practice
Eugene, Oregon

Theresa Devine Slocum, MS
Director, Animal Foundation, Inc.
Slocum Veterinary Clinic
Eugene, Oregon

Daniel D. Smeak, DVM
Diplomate ACVS
Professor, Head of Small Animal Surgery
Ohio State University College of Veterinary Medicine
Columbus, Ohio

Gail Smith, DVM
Professor and Chief of Surgery, Department of Clinical
    Studies
School of Veterinary Medicine
University of Pennsylvania
Philadelphia, Pennsylvania

Julie D. Smith, DVM, MS
Assistant Professor, Small Animal Surgery
Department of Clinical Sciences, College of Veterinary
    Medicine
Kansas State University
Manhattan, Kansas

Mark M. Smith, VMD
Diplomate, ACVS
Associate Professor, Department of Small Animal
    Clinical Sciences
VA-MD Regional College of Veterinary Medicine
Blacksburg, Virginia

Mary Lynn Stanton, DVM
Diplomate, ACVS
Staff Surgeon
Tampa Bay Veterinary Referral
Largo, Florida

Elizabeth Arnold Stone, DVM, MS
Diplomate, ACVS
Professor/Head of the Department of Companion
Animal and Special Species Medicine
College of Veterinary Medicine
North Carolina State University
Raleigh, North Carolina

Rodney C. Straw, BVSc, MS
Diplomate, ACVS
West Chemside Veterinary Clinic
Stafford Heights, Queensland
Australia

W. Preston Stubbs, DVM
Diplomate ACVS
Lecturer in Small Animal Surgery
Department of Veterinary Clinical Sciences
Massey University
Palmerston North, New Zealand

Richard P. Suess, Jr., DVM
Diplomate, ACVS
Staff Surgeon
The Veterinary Surgical Referral Practice of Northern
    Virginia, P.C.
Manassas, Virginia

Steven F. Swaim, DVM, MS
Professor, Small Animal Surgery
Department of Small Animal Surgery & Medicine
Scott-Ritchey Research Center
Auburn University College of Veterinary Medicine
Auburn, Alabama

Guy Tarvin, DVM
Diplomate, ACVS
Staff Surgeon
Veterinary Surgical Specialists
Garden Grove, California

Robert Taylor, DVM, MS
Diplomate, ACVS
Director, Bel Rea Institute of Animal Technology
Adjunct Associate Professor
University of Denver
Staff Surgeon
Alameda East Veterinary Hospital
Denver, Colorado

R. Jeffery Todoroff, DVM
Diplomate, ACVS
Veterinary Surgical Associates
Concord, California

James L. Tomlinson, Jr., DVM, MVSc
Diplomate ACVS
Associate Professor of Surgery
Department of Veterinary Medicine and Surgery
College of Veterinary Medicine
University of Missouri
Columbia, Missouri

Eric J. Trotter, DVM, MS
Diplomate, ACVS
Chief of Surgery
Orthopedic and Neurosurgery
Veterinary Medical Teaching Hospital
Cornell University College of Veterinary Medicine
Ithaca, New York

Thomas Turner, DVM
Assistant Professor
Department of Orthopedic Surgery
Rush-Presbyterian-St. Luke's Medical Center
Chicago, Illinois
Staff Surgeon
VCA Berwyn Animal Hospital
Berwyn, Illinois

Sharon Ullman, DVM, MS
Diplomate, ACVS
Veterinary Surgical Associates
Concord, California

Thomas Van Gundy, DVM, MS
Staff Surgeon
Animal Surgical Practice of Portland
Portland, Oregon

Philip Vasseur, DVM
Diplomate - ACVS
Professor, Department of Surgical and Radiological
  Sciences
University of California at Davis
School of Veterinary Medicine
Davis, California

James Vogt, DVM
Staff Surgeon
Akron Veterinary Referral Center
Akron, Ohio

Don R. Waldron, DVM
Diplomate, ACVS
Professor of Surgery
Section Chief, Small Animal Surgery and
  Anesthesiology
Department of Small Animal Clinical Sciences
VA-MD Regional College of Veterinary Medicine
Virginia Tech
Blacksburg, Virginia

Richard Walshaw, BVMS
Diplomate, ACVS
Professor, Small Animal Surgery
Michigan State University College of Veterinary
  Medicine
East Lansing, Michigan

Barbara J. Watrous, DVM
Diplomate, ACVR
Head of Radiology
Oregon State University, College of Veterinary
  Medicine
Corvallis, Oregon

Janet Welch, DVM
Assistant Professor of Surgery
Department of Small Animal Surgery and Medicine
Auburn University College of Veterinary Medicine
Auburn University, Alabama

Richard White, BvetMed, PhD, DSAS, DVR, FRCVS
Diplomate, ACVS
Diplomate, ECVS
Specialist in Small Animal Surgery
Department of Clinical Veterinary Medicine
University of Cambridge
Cambridge, ENGLAND

Wayne O. Whitney, DVM
Diplomate, ACVS
Specialist
Gulf Coast Veterinary Surgery
Houston, Texas

Randy Willer, DVM, MS
Diplomate, ACVS
Surgical Referral Services
Ft. Collins, Colorado

Stephen J. Withrow, DVM,
Diplomate, ACVS
Diplomate, ACVIM (Oncology)
Chief, Clinical Oncology/Comparative Oncology
Colorado State University
College of Veterinary Medicine and Biomedical Sciences
Fort Collins, Colorado

Daniel J. Yturraspe, DVM, MS, PhD
Diplomate, ACVS
Companion Animal Hospital
Belmont, California

⬤— CONTENTS

Part I

Soft Tissue

1

PAIN MANAGEMENT IN THE SMALL ANIMAL PATIENT

Elizabeth M. Hardie & Andrew E. Kyles

Earlier editions of this book do not contain a chapter on management of pain in small animal patients. Over the last 5 years, clinicians have become increasingly aware that pain control after surgery is an integral part of the management of the veterinary surgical patient. The benefits of pain control in human surgical patients include decreased morbidity and mortality, early return to normal behavior, early return to ambulation, and decreased need for hospitalization (1–4). Similar benefits are likely when pain control is practiced in veterinary patients, particularly patients with severe systemic disease and limited physiologic reserves. All surgeons are encouraged to become familiar with these techniques and to incorporate them into daily practice.

Philosophy

The International Society for the Study of Pain defines pain as "an unpleasant sensory and emotional experience associated with actual or potential tissue damage or described in terms of such damage" (5). Pain can be accurately scored only in verbal human patients; all scoring systems for pain in nonverbal humans and animals rely on interpreting or measuring the consequences of pain, such as limb withdrawal, vocalization, social withdrawal, increased heart rate, or increased cortisol concentration (6–9). Because of the difficulties in measuring pain in animals, the guideline used by institutional animal care and use committees is that if a surgical procedure causes pain in adult human pa-

tients, laboratory animals undergoing that procedure should be treated with analgesic therapy (10). When a similar philosophy is applied to daily veterinary practice and analgesic drugs are routinely used, the next question that arises is, "How does one know that adequate analgesia has been achieved?" The easiest answer is that if the animal can sleep comfortably after surgery, drug therapy is adequate. The more complex answer is that measuring the patient's response to analgesic therapy with certain variables (heart rate, respiratory rate, body posture, willingness to interact with the caregiver, vocalization, response to palpation or manipulation of the surgical site, willingness to move voluntarily) allows the clinician to assess drug efficacy.

A practice that should be avoided is forcing the animal to display behaviors associated with extreme pain or distress before providing analgesic therapy (11). Behaviors such as loud vocalization, growling, lifting of the lip, biting, maintaining an abnormal posture, displaying restlessness, or obvious social withdrawal occur when the animal has reached the limits of its coping mechanisms. Higher doses of analgesic and sedative drugs, with more side effects, are required to control pain and to reduce stress in such an animal.

In contrast, the clinician should assess the personality of the animal and the painfulness of the surgery or injury and should preempt expected pain by giving adequate doses of analgesic drugs before pain is present or early in its course (12–14). During surgical recovery, a baseline amount of analgesia drug is provided and additional drug is given if pain is poorly controlled. Clinicians should be aware that the response of individual animals to opioid therapy varies significantly, even among animals undergoing similar surgical procedures: individual drug titration is the rule, rather than the exception.

The length of time that animals require analgesics after surgery is controversial. The average human surgical patient requires pain control for 4 days after surgery (15). Analysis of the amounts of narcotics given to patients after surgery in the hospital intensive care unit of North Carolina State University in Raleigh suggests that pain in dogs and cats peaks approximately 24 hours after surgery and then tapers, unless ongoing injury is present. Patients typically requiring prolonged pain control include those undergoing median sternotomy or amputation, those with multiple injuries, burn patients, and patients with peritonitis or pancreatitis.

Local Analgesic Techniques

Drugs

Amide-type drugs, such as lidocaine and bupivacaine, block conduction in the peripheral nerves (Table 1.1) (16). They act by stabilizing the cell membrane, thus preventing depolarization of the nerve fiber. The sensitivity of the fibers depends on their size, with smaller nerves more sensitive. The small pain fibers are blocked by low doses of amide-type drugs. Large motor nerves are affected if a large enough dose of analgesic is given.

Lidocaine is a fast, short-acting drug (17). The onset of analgesia occurs in 5 to 10 minutes and lasts about 1.5 to 2 hours. Lidocaine is available as a 0.5%, 1%, 1.5%, or 2% solution, with or without epinephrine (1:100,000 or 1:200,000 dilution). The most com-monly used preparation is a 2% lidocaine solution with epinephrine (1:100,000). In high-risk patients, the more dilute epinephrine solution is used, or lidocaine without epinephrine is used. Dilute solutions may also be used when infusing lidocaine into large spaces, such as body cavities. The dose of lidocaine in the dog should not exceed 4.5 mg/kg of lidocaine, or 7 mg/kg of lidocaine with epinephrine, to give a wide margin of safety. The intravenous toxic dose of lidocaine in the dog is 20 mg/kg, and signs of toxicity include seizures, central nervous system depression, hypotension, and myocardial depression (18).

Bupivacaine has a slow onset of action (20 to 30 minutes), but it lasts up to 5 to 7 hours (17). Bupivacaine is available as a 0.25%, 0.5%, or 0.75% solution, with or without epinephrine (1:200,000 dilution). The most commonly used preparation is a 0.5% solution of bupivacaine with epinephrine (1:200,000). Bupivacaine without epinephrine is used in high-risk patients. The intravenous toxic dose of bupivacaine in the dog is 4 mg/kg; thus it is wise not to exceed a dose of 2 mg/kg, particularly when infusing the drug into a body cavity. Signs of toxicity are similar to those seen with lidocaine. High doses of bupivacaine, whether given intravenously or intratracheally, can cause cardiac arrhythmias (18).

Clinicians often recommend that the intravenous dose of lidocaine be decreased by a factor of 10 in the cat, which is more sensitive than the dog to the cardiovascular effects of these drugs. In rapid intravenous infusion studies, however, severe cardiovascular collapse in cats occurred only after infusion of 48 mg/kg lidocaine or 19 mg/kg bupivacaine (19). Healthy cats thus appear to be resistant to the toxic effects of amide-type drugs. However, occult heart disease is common in cats, and small doses of lidocaine or bupivacaine may rapidly result in toxic signs in these

Table 1.1.
Local Anesthetic Drugs Used to Prevent and Treat Surgical Pain

Drug	Dosage	Duration of Action	Major Toxicity
2% Lidocaine solution with epineph-rine (1:100,000)	Dog: 1–5 mL/site for direct nerve blocks, up to 7 mg/kg for infiltration techniques Cat: smallest dose possible, up to 2 mg/kg total dose	1.5–2 h	Seizures, central nervous system depression, hypotension, myocardial depression
0.5% Solution of bupivacaine with epinephrine (1:200,000)	Dog: 1–2 mL per site for diect nerve block, up to 4 mg/kg for infiltration techniques, 0.5 mL/kg in joint, 1.5 mg/kg intrapleurally: up to 8 mg/kg/d on first day and up to 4 mg/kg/d thereafter Cat: smallest dose possible, up to 2 mg/kg total dose	5–7 h	Seizures, central nervous system depression, hypotension, myocardial depression, cardiac arrhythmias
0.5% Bupivacaine		up to 4 h	See above; use in high-risk animals

animals. Caution is thus advisable when an animal's cardiac status is unknown.

In general, lidocaine and bupivacaine solutions with epinephrine are used when a local action of the drug is desired (17). The vasoconstriction caused by epinephrine prevents rapid systemic distribution of the drug, thereby decreasing toxicity and increasing efficacy. Solutions without epinephrine are used systemically or when epinephrine-induced cardiac arrhythmias would be catastrophic. The stinging sensation associated with lidocaine can be significantly reduced by mixing 1 part sodium bicarbonate (1 mEq/mL) with 9 parts of lidocaine (1 to 2% solution) just before injection.

Tissue Infiltration

Infiltration of the tissue surrounding the site of a surgical incision with lidocaine or bupivacaine is a technically simple and effective means of providing analgesia. This technique can be used with surgical procedures ranging from mass excisions to total ear canal ablations to laparotomies. In human patients, use of local anesthesia along an abdominal incision line aids in the control of pain associated with the movement of the abdominal muscles and makes overall movement more comfortable (20, 21). Placement of 0.5 mL/kg of a 0.5% bupivacaine solution in the stifle joint after cruciate surgery is an effective method of controlling postoperative pain in dogs (22). Many studies in human surgical patients have documented that the use of local anesthesia significantly reduces the need for systemic analgesic therapy after surgery (20, 23). That this effect lasts well beyond the time when the local anesthetic is effective suggests that blockade of the painful neural input to the spinal cord prevents the phenomenon of "cord wide-up," in which the spinal cord becomes hypersensitive to nociceptive input for days after surgery (23).

Specific Nerve Blocks

When large areas of the body are affected by the surgical procedure, or when the tissue involved in the operation does not lend itself to infiltration (tooth extraction), local anesthetics may be used to block the sensory nerves as they coalesce into larger, named nerves. These techniques require a working knowledge of peripheral neuroanatomy, but they are not difficult to master. Some of the most useful nerve block techniques for a small animal practitioner involve blocking the nerves to the teeth, the thoracic limb, and the chest wall (16, 24). Other specific nerve blocks are well described in handbooks of veterinary anesthesia (24).

MAXILLARY AND MANDIBULAR ALVEOLAR NERVE BLOCKS

The sensory nerves supplying the maxillary teeth are branches of the infraorbital nerve. The caudal maxillary alveolar nerve, which supplies the caudal maxillary teeth, branches off the infraorbital nerve just as the nerve enters the maxillary foramen. Within the infraorbital canal, the middle maxillary alveolar nerve branches off to supply the middle cheek teeth. Just before the infraorbital nerve exits the infraorbital foramen, the rostral maxillary alveolar nerve, which supplies the upper canine tooth and incisors, branches from it. The infraorbital artery and vein course through the infraorbital canal with the nerve.

The infraorbital foramen can be palpated through the buccal mucosa dorsal to the upper third premolar (Fig. 1.1). The nerve can be blocked at this site to provide analgesia for the canine and incisor teeth. The maxillary foramen is at the level of the ventral rim of the orbit, at the rostral end of the zygomatic arch. If the examiner places one finger on the animal's infraorbital foramen and one finger on the ventral rim of the orbit, the length of the infraorbital canal can be estimated. In large breed dogs, the canal may be several centimeters long. In small dogs, cats, and brachycephalic breeds, the infraorbital canal is short, often less than a centimeter in length. If a needle is inserted into the infraorbital canal, the middle and caudal maxillary alveolar nerves can be blocked, providing analgesia for the molars and premolars.

The average dog requires 1 to 2 mL of lidocaine or bupivacaine, preferably with epinephrine, for the infraorbital canal nerve block. The overall dose of the drug administered to block the nerves to all affected teeth should be checked to ensure that a toxic dose is not given. The required amount of drug is drawn into a syringe with a 25- to 22-gauge needle attached, de-

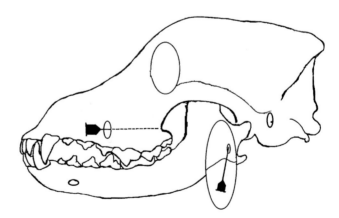

Fig. 1.1. Lateral view of a dog's skull demonstrating needle placement for maxillary and mandibular alveolar nerve blocks. The mandibular foramen (oval inset) is on the medial side of the right mandible.

pending on the length of the infraorbital canal. The clinician palpates dorsal to the third upper premolar until the infraorbital foramen is felt. The needle is inserted into the rostral aspect of the foramen by directing the needle caudally. The syringe is held parallel to the long axis of the jaw. The clinician draws back on the syringe, to ensure that the needle has not penetrated the infraorbital artery or the vein, and then slowly infuses the lidocaine or bupivacaine.

The mandibular alveolar nerve, which is the sensory nerve for the mandibular teeth, branches off the trigeminal nerve and enters the mandibular foramen on the medial side of the mandible. The nerve travels with the mandibular alveolar artery and vein in the mandibular canal, giving off sensory branches to the teeth.

The mandibular foramen is easiest to palpate inside the mouth, through the buccal mucosa, behind the last molar. The foramen is located about 1 to 1.5 cm rostral to the angle of the mandible on the medial aspect of the mandible. The opening is at the level of the body of the mandible; palpation high up on the ramus is too far dorsal. Often it is easiest to feel the nerve under the mucosa and then follow it to the foramen. Blocking the mandibular alveolar nerve at the level of the mandibular foramen provides analgesia for all the mandibular teeth.

The amounts of lidocaine and bupivacaine used for the mandibular nerve block are similar to those used for the infraorbital canal nerve block. A 25-gauge needle is used for small dogs and cats, whereas a 22-gauge needle is used for large dogs. An area of skin ventral to the angle of the mandible should be clipped and prepared for surgery. The clinician locates the mandibular foramen on the medial aspect of the mandible by palpating through the buccal mucosa and by keeping the hand that has located the foramen inside the animal's mouth. The needle is inserted through the prepared area of skin and is directed dorsally along the medial aspect of the mandible. When the tip of the needle can be palpated by the hand that is in the animal's mouth, and the tip is located at the mandibular foramen, the lidocaine or bupivacaine is infused slowly.

When animals regain feeling after nerve block, particularly in the mouth, they may experience unusual sensations. In some animals, mild tranquilization may be needed to relieve anxiety associated with these sensations.

BRACHIAL PLEXUS BLOCK

The brachial plexus block is used to provide analgesia from the elbow to the foot of the thoracic limb (Fig. 1.2). Affected nerves include the radial, median, ulnar, musculocutaneous, and axillary nerves. The nerves to be blocked are cranial to the first rib, medial to the

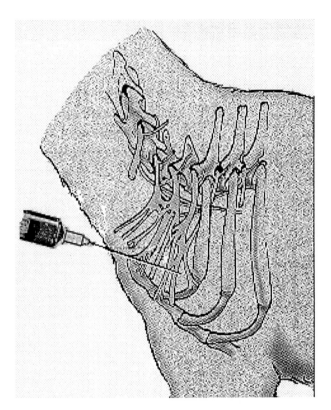

Fig. 1.2. Brachial plexus nerve block

shoulder. The skin cranial to the shoulder is clipped and prepared for surgery. A 3-inch, 22-gauge spinal needle is used, and 10 to 15 mL of lidocaine or bupivacaine solution are drawn into the syringe. If this amount of drug exceeds the maximum safe dose, the maximum safe dose is drawn up and saline or a sodium bicarbonate solution is used to dilute the drug to a final volume of 10 to 15 mL. The costochrondral junction of the second rib is palpated with one finger, while the needle is inserted medial to the point of the shoulder. The needle is advanced toward the finger on the second costochrondral junction, staying parallel to midline, medial to the shoulder, and lateral to the pleural cavity. When the needle is advanced to the level of the first rib, an aspiration is performed to ensure that no vessel has been entered. The needle is then slowly withdrawn while the drug is injected.

INTERCOSTAL NERVE BLOCK

The intercostal nerves are located on the medial surface of the internal intercostal muscles, caudal to the corresponding intercostal artery and vein. Numerous branches penetrate the muscles of the thoracic wall as the nerves course in a ventral direction. To obtain analgesia at the site of a lateral thoracotomy incision, the nerves must be blocked as dorsally as possible, just after they emerge from the intervertebral foramina.

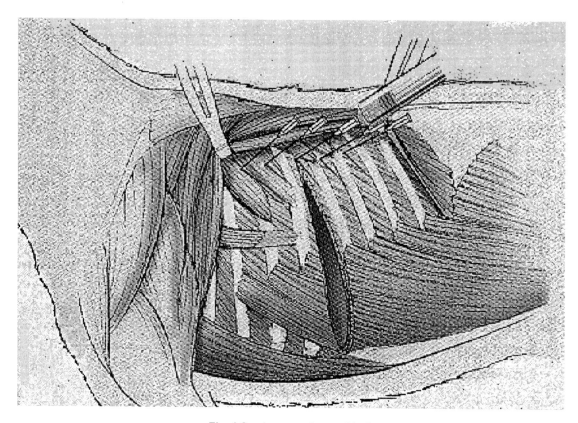

Fig. 1.3. Intercostal nerve block.

Blocking the nerves associated with several ribs cranial and caudal to the thoracotomy site ensures that sensations from nerve branches crossing intercostal spaces are blocked (Fig. 1.3).

The ribs are easily palpated on either side of a thoracotomy site. The clinician follows the rib dorsally until the head of the rib is located. Using a 22-gauge needle, 0.5 to 1 mL of 2% lidocaine or 0.5% bupivacaine, with epinephrine, is placed caudal to the head of the rib, just lateral to the vertebral column. Before injection, aspiration is performed to ensure that neither the intercostal artery nor the vein has been perforated. At least three ribs cranial to the surgical site and two ribs caudal to the surgical site are blocked. The adequacy of the nerve block is assessed in the awake dog, using hemostats to pinch the skin in the numbed area.

Infusions in Body Cavities

Infusion of bupivacaine through the thoracostomy tube into the chest cavity after thoracotomy provides significant analgesia. For maximum benefit, the infused drug must contact the thoracotomy site. The thoracostomy tube should be placed with this fact in mind. For 20 minutes after infusion of bupivacaine, the animal should be positioned in the appropriate recumbency to ensure contact between the incision and the bupivacaine. The starting dose of bupivacaine is 1.5 mg/kg (25). The drug is readministered every 4 to 6 hours, and the total daily dose on the first day should not exceed 8 mg/kg (26). On subsequent days, the total daily dose should not exceed 4 mg/kg (26). A more sophisticated system of drug delivery into the thoracic cavity involves the use of a narrow intrapleural catheter placed along the surgical incision and tunneled through the thoracic wall, similar to a thoracostomy tube (27). The catheter allows continuous delivery of local anesthetic to the surgical site. Bupivacaine administration into the pleural cavity should be avoided in animals undergoing pericardectomy because of the risk of cardiotoxicity.

Similar benefits are not seen when lidocaine or bupivacaine is infused into the abdomen (28), presumably because of rapid systemic absorption. As mentioned earlier, infiltration of local anesthetic along the abdominal incision helps to control abdominal wall pain. Visceral pain is best treated with other methods of pain control.

Epidural Analgesic Techniques

Drugs

The most commonly used drugs for the provision of epidural analgesia are morphine, bupivacaine, and lidocaine (Table 1.2) (16, 29). Drugs that are occasion-

Table 1.2.
Epidural Drugs Used in the Prevention and Treatment of Surgical Pain

Drug	Dosage	Major Toxicity	Duration of Action	Comments
Single injections				
Morphine (preservative-free)	Dog or cat: 0.1–0.2 mg/kg[a] Spinal: 0.05 mg/kg	Vomiting, urine retention, hyperesthesia, respiratory compromise	4–8 h	Cranial dispersion within 1 h
0.25–0.5% Bupivacaine with epinephrine	Dog: 1 mL/5 kg Spinal: 0.5–0.6 mL/kg	Respiratory compromise, hind leg weakness	4–6 h	Increase dose to 1 mL/3.5 kg to obtain abdominal analgesia; may be combined with morphine for additive effect
Oxymorphone	0.05 mg/kg	See morphine	2–4 h	
Medetomidine (not approved in the United States)	Cat: 10 μg/kg, diluted in 1 mL saline	Vomiting, sedation	4 h	Medetomidine alone: no analgesia in dog; analgesic effect more pronounced in caudal half of cat
Medetomidine and morphine	Dog: 5 μg/kg medetomidine and 0.1 mg/kg morphine	See morphine	13 h	
Catheter delivery				
Morphine (preservative-free)	Dog or cat: 0.1–0.2 mg/kg q8h or 0.3–0.5 mg/kg/d constant-rate infusion	See morphine		Observe closely for urine retention
Bupivacaine, 0.0625%–0.125% (preservative-free)	Dog: 1 mL/5 kg, followed by 0.1–0.4 mL/kg/h constant-rate infusion; do not exceed 4 mg/kg/d	Respiratory compromise, hind leg weakness		—
50:50 Mixture of morphine (1 mg/mL, preservative-free) and bupivacaine 0.25%	Dog: initial bolus dose of 0.1 mg/kg morphine, followed by a constant-rate infusion of the mixture at 0.6–1.0 mL/kg/d	See morphine and bupivacaine		Cat: catheter often spinal; bolus with 0.3 mL of the mixture and then constant-rate infusion of 0.1 mL/h
Buprenorphine (preservative-free)	Dog: 5–20 μg/kg q8h or 15–60 μg/kg/d constant-rate infusion	See morphine	4–8 h for intermittent injection	Lipophilic drug, administer by epidural catheter to site of desired spinal action
Fentanyl (preservative-free)	Dog: 5–20 μg/kg single injection or 1–5 μg/kg/h constant-rate infusion	Single injection: marked central effects, use under anesthesia for rapid analgesia	<0.5 h for single injection	Lipophilic drug, administer by catheter to site of desired spinal action

[a] All weights are lean body weight.

ally used are buprenorphine (30), oxymorphone (31), fentanyl (32), and medetomidine (33). In general, the preservative-free formulations of the drugs should be used, particularly if drug administration involves more than a single epidural injection. The drugs may be administered as a single injection, as multiple intermittent injections through a catheter, or as a constant-rate infusion through a catheter. Constant-rate infusions are recommended for cats with epidural catheters, because many of these catheters are actually spinal catheters, and intermittent dosing has adverse central side effects.

The actions of drugs in the epidural space depend on their potency and the distribution (34). In general, the more lipid soluble a drug is, the faster it binds to the active site and the less it distributes throughout the central nervous system. Fentanyl, an extremely lipid-soluble drug, has an almost immediate onset of action and a distribution that remains within several spinal cord segments of the site of injection. Fentanyl rapidly redistributes outside the central nervous system and has a short duration of action. Relatively lipid-soluble drugs, such as buprenorphine, oxymorphone, medetomidine, and the local anesthetics, have a predominately local effect and an onset of action of 10 to 20 minutes. The duration of action depends on the individual drug. Water-soluble drugs, such as morphine, distribute throughout the spinal canal when given as a lumbosacral epidural injection, providing analgesia to cranial body regions. The time to the peak analgesic effect of morphine can be as long as 90 minutes, but the duration of action may be up to 24 hours.

The opioid drugs (morphine, oxymorphone, buprenorphine, and fentanyl) act on the spinal cord by crossing the dura and binding to the opiate receptors in the dorsal horn of the affected spinal cord segments (33). This action occurs without major systemic side effects and without sensory, motor, or sympathetic blockade. The selective action of the opioids on the spinal opiate receptors renders their use safe. The major side effects of epidural opioids in dogs and cats are mild ataxia, urinary retention (seen mostly with repeated injections or infusions), vomiting (seen mainly with intermittent injections of morphine), and marked hyperesthesia (a rare complication of intrathecal or epidural morphine administration in dogs).

The local anesthetic drugs act at the epidural level by blocking nerve impulse conduction in the nerve roots of the spinal cord segments that directly contact the drug (16). If local anesthetics are given into the subarachnoid space, they have a direct spinal effect. Local anesthetics can block all types of nerve conduction, depending on the concentration of the drug that bathes the nerve root. Care must be taken with local anesthetics to avoid contact between high concentrations of drug and the spinal region supplying the muscles of respiration. Elevating the head and cranial torso, giving epidural injections slowly, and using dilute concentrations of drug help to avoid respiratory impairment. Sympathetic blockade can worsen hypotension, and local anesthetics should be avoided in hypotensive animals.

The α_2 agonists (xylazine, clonidine, detomidine, medetomidine, dexmedetomidine), given in the epidural space, cross the dura, bind to α_2 adrenoreceptors, and modify the same pain pathways in the dorsal horn of the spinal cord modified by opioids (34). One may see some species variation in the relative response to α_2 agonists and opiate agonists. In a study of cats, epidurally administered medetomidine had a more pronounced analgesic effect than epidurally administered fentanyl (32). In dogs, epidural morphine blocked the response to tail clamp, whereas epidural medetomidine did not (35). However, dexmedetomidine, a potent α_2 agonist, provided profound analgesia when given epidurally in dogs (36). When given with an opioid, medetomidine prolongs the analgesic action of the opioid in both cats and dogs. Side effects of medetomidine include vomiting and bradycardia (32, 37).

Single Injections

Single epidural injections are usually administered once the patient is heavily sedated or anesthetized (38). If the injection is given before surgery, the preemptive effect of controlling intraoperative pain may decrease the requirement for postoperative pain control drugs. The lumbosacral space is used to give the injection because it is a large space with recognizable landmarks. The dura usually ends cranial to this space in dogs, but it rarely does in cats. Most "epidural" injections in cats are thus subdural and enter the subarachnoid space immediately. Epidural injections are associated with fewer complications than subdural injections and are thus preferable, but drug doses can be adjusted to accommodate for the inevitable spinal injection.

The skin is first clipped over the dorsal midline from the dorsal spinous process of L4 to the midpelvis. The clip should extend laterally to the level of the greater trochanters. The following items are gathered: sterile surgical gloves; a 1- to 3-inch, 20- to 22-gauge spinal needle or an 18- to 20-gauge Tuohy needle (depending on the size of the animal); several 3-mL syringes without a Luer-Lok; and a syringe containing the drug to be administered. The animal is positioned in either sternal or lateral recumbency. If analgesia needs to be concentrated on one side of the animal, that side should be placed in the down position, to allow gravity to assist in distributing drug appropriately. The pelvic limbs are drawn forward, to enlarge the lumbosacral space. The clipped skin is prepared for surgery.

Wearing sterile gloves, the clinician palpates the dorsal aspect of the iliac wings and draws an imaginary line between these two points. The line should intersect the vertebral column just caudal to the dorsal spinous process of L6. The short dorsal spinous process of L7 is palpated caudal to the prominent dorsal spinous process of L6. The short fused dorsal spinous processes of the sacrum are then palpated. The lumbosacral space is under a depression just cranial to S1 and more caudal to L7.

The needle is directed at a 90° angle to the skin in the center of the lumbosacral depression, with the bevel facing the cranial aspect of the animal (Fig. 1.4). The needle is directed ventrally until it penetrates the dorsal spinal ligament (ligamentum flavum). During advancement, the clinician must keep the needle oriented on the dorsal midline. If bone is encountered, rather than ligament, the needle can be "walked" cranially or caudally into the lumbosacral space. The resistance of the dorsal spinal ligament alerts the clinician

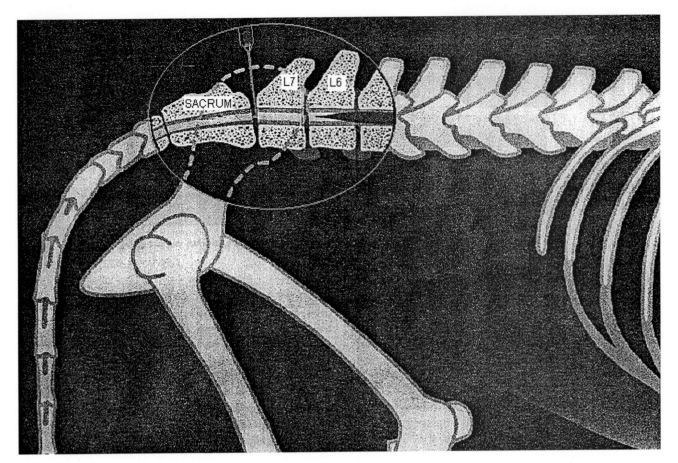

Fig. 1.4. Lumbosacral epidural injection.

that the spinal canal is near. The needle is advanced 2 to 4 mm further, until a loss of resistance is felt. The stylet is then removed, and the hub of the needle is inspected for the presence of cerebrospinal fluid (CSF) or blood. The presence of CSF indicates that the needle has penetrated the dura, and spinal doses of drugs, without epinephrine or preservative, should be used. The presence of blood usually indicates that the needle has deviated laterally and has entered a vein. The needle should be partially withdrawn and redirected.

The lack of fluid at the hub of the needle indicates probable correct placement of the needle. Placement in the epidural space is confirmed by one of several methods. First, 0.5 to 2 mL of air can be injected into the needle without any resistance, and often some of the air can be reaspirated. If the air cannot be injected, or if the air obviously goes into the subcutaneous space, then needle is incorrectly positioned. Second, a stethoscope is placed over the spine cranial to the needle while air is injected. If a "whoosh" sound is heard, needle placement is likely to be correct. If crepitus is heard, the needle is likely to be in the tissues around the spine.

If a Tuohy needle is used, two other techniques aid in determining correct placement. First, during the air injection, the needle and syringe are directed caudally, forcing the beveled tip of the needle cranially and dorsally. If the needle is in the epidural space, the dorsal spinal ligament acts as a fulcrum and the bevel moves cranially, encountering only epidural fat. One feels no resistance to the injection of air. If the beveled tip of the needle is paraspinal, the needle tip will compress the muscle and fascia. Marked resistance to air injection is noted. Second, the Tuohy needle is advanced until the dorsal spinal ligament is felt. The stylet is withdrawn, and the needle is filled with the drug to be injected. The needle is then advanced into the epidural space. As the needle enters the space, the negative pressure within the space causes the fluid to be aspirated.

Once the needle position is confirmed, the cranial direction of the bevel should be confirmed by observing the notch on the bevel side of the needle. The drug is injected slowly, preferably over at least 20 to 30 seconds. If large volumes of local anesthetic are injected, the injection should occur over 60 seconds.

Epidural Catheters

Commercial epidural catheters are inserted into the epidural space through a Tuohy needle (38). Commercial catheters can be used in dogs over 5 kg; recommended brands of catheters contain an imbedded spiral wire to prevent kinking. The type of catheter chosen depends on the surgical site. The Arrow Flex-Tip polyurethane catheter can routinely be advanced only 8 cm, whereas the stiffer Arrow Theracath catheter with a wire stylet can be advanced to the thoracolumbar junction. In small dogs and cats, an 8- to 12-inch, 22-gauge through-the-needle venous catheter can be used as an epidural catheter (38). The latter technique should only be attempted once the operator is thoroughly familiar with the single epidural injection technique. When a sharp venous needle is used for placement of an epidural catheter, the resistance usually felt at the dorsal spinal ligament is minimal. Dural puncture is common, particularly in cats, and approximately 50% of "epidural" catheters in cats are actually spinal catheters.

The animal is positioned and prepared as for a single epidural injection. The catheter is placed using routine sterile technique (drape, mask, gloves). In addition to the catheter and needle, the following equipment needs to be readily accessible: 3-mL syringes without a Luer-Lok; syringe containing the agent to be injected; in-line bacterial filter; small-volume extension sets; injection cap with a Luer-Lok fitting; 1-inch waterproof tape; 2-inch white tape; 2 × 2 gauze sponge; package of antiseptic ointment; 2-0 or 3-0 monofilament suture; needle holder; and scissors. If the animal is not anesthetized, the injection site to the level of the dorsal spinal ligament is anesthetized with an injection of 1 to 2% lidocaine. A spinal needle can be used for the injection, if needed. If the lidocaine is mixed with sodium bicarbonate, at a ratio of 9 parts lidocaine to 1 part bicarbonate, the sting of injection will be eliminated.

The technique for placement of a Tuohy needle is similar to that described for single epidural injection. Tuohy needles have a 90° bend at the tip, which causes the catheter to exit the needle at a right angle. The catheter is then parallel to the vertebral column, which aids in catheter advancement. To achieve a similar effect using an intravenous catheter needle, the needle is advanced into the epidural space at an acute angle. The skin is pulled tight caudally, over the first dorsal process of the sacrum. The needle is directed cranially into the lumbosacral space from this site, passing just over the edge of the cranial dorsal edge of the sacrum. The needle passes through the dorsal spinal ligament, and a slight loss of resistance is felt when the epidural space is entered. The plastic sleeve over the intravenous catheter is removed, a test injection of air is administered to assess correct placement, and the plastic sleeve is carefully replaced. The bevel of the needle must remain facing a cranial direction. The catheter is then slowly advanced. Pushing the hub of the needle in a caudoventral direction, bringing the long axis of the needle as close to parallel with the spinal canal as is possible, helps to direct the catheter correctly. Even with the Tuohy needle, it may be necessary to push the hub of the needle caudally to facilitate catheter advancement.

The catheter is advanced cranially, beyond the eventual site of placement. The catheter must not be forced and should advance with minimal resistance. Once the catheter is in place, the needle is withdrawn from the skin, while the operator takes care not to move the catheter. Depending on the design, the needle is either guarded or peeled away from the catheter. The stylet is removed and held along the catheter and vertebral column to assess the position of the catheter tip. The catheter is withdrawn until the tip is in the desired location.

The extension set, previously primed with the solution for injection, is connected to the catheter hub. The bacterial filter is attached to the end of the extension set; then an injection cap is attached. If a constant-rate infusion is planned, a second extension set and syringe are attached instead of the injection cap. A "butterfly" of the 1-inch waterproof white tape is directly attached to the epidural catheter at the skin exit site. The butterfly may be reinforced with several more pieces of overlaid tape. The proximal edge of the butterfly is sewn to the skin 3 to 5 mm on either side of the catheter. The skin exit site is covered with antiseptic ointment and a 2 × 2 gauze sponge. Every connection in the system is covered with waterproof tape to ensure that no breaks occur. The extension set is coiled, and both the epidural catheter and the extension set are taped to the skin with overlapping pieces of 2-inch white tape. Proper adherence between the tape and the skin is critical. Spraying the tape with medical adhesive or ether aids adherence.

Subsequent injections are made with a 22- to 25-gauge needle through the injection cap, which is first cleaned with alcohol. If a constant-rate infusion is used, large volumes of injectate should be drawn up, to ensure a minimal need to change syringes. The sterility of the system should be carefully maintained. The injection cap, filter, and extension sets are changed every 2 to 4 days, using aseptic technique. The skin exit site is observed regularly for evidence of inflammation or local pain. Epidural catheters have been maintained for up to 2 weeks in dogs and cats without complications. If a break in sterility occurs, or if the animal has obvious inflammation or pain, the catheter should be removed.

Amputations

Animals undergoing amputation should be protected against nervous system reactions that may result in chronic phantom limb pain (39, 40). A single epidural injection of morphine (thoracic limb amputations) or morphine and bupivacaine (pelvic limb amputations) helps to prevent sensitization of the spinal cord. Placement of an epidural catheter allows the clinician to provide effective pain control after surgery in addition to protecting the spinal cord during the procedure. In addition to providing epidural analgesia, the clinician should inject each named nerve with 1 to 2% lidocaine before sharp transaction with a scalpel. The combination of epidural analgesia and direct nerve block has reduced phantom limb pain substantially in human patients (39, 40).

Intravenous and Intramuscular Analgesic Drugs

Nonsteroidal Anti-Inflammatory Drugs

Injectable, centrally acting nonsteroidal anti-inflammatory drugs (NSAIDs) are routinely used to control postoperative pain in human patients (Table 1.3) (41). These drugs block the production of prostaglandins, which sensitize nociceptors at the surgical site. The NSAIDs are also likely to have a central effect on spinal pain pathways, because some NSAIDs are poor prostaglandin blockers but effective analgesic drugs (42).

Adverse side effects, such as gastrointestinal bleeding, gastrointestinal ulcers, and renal damage, limit the use of NSAIDs in dogs. Cats have limited quantities of the enzymes needed to metabolize NSAIDs and are at high risk of developing toxicity. Despite these problems, NSAIDs are effective analgesics for controlling postoperative pain in dogs. In particular, flunixin meglumine has been shown to be equivalent to morphine in relieving pain after surgery (43). Hypotension increases the risk of side effects, and the currently available drugs, such as flunixin meglumine and ketoprofen, should be used in dogs *after* anesthesia-induced hypotension has subsided. Carprofen, a potent NSAID with minimal toxicity, should be available for veterinary use soon, although initially only the oral form will be available. The injectable form of carprofen has been an effective analgesic during surgery and in the postoperative period in dogs (42, 44).

α_2-Agonist Drugs

The α_2-adrenergic agonist group includes drugs such as xylazine, detomidine, medetomidine, and clonidine. Medetomidine is likely to become the most widely used drug in this group in veterinary medicine, because it is highly lipophilic, has a high α_2:α_1 receptor selectivity, is more potent than other α_2 agonists, and is eliminated quickly from the body (45, 46). α_2 Agonists are potent analgesics and sedatives and can be used to induce anesthesia for short surgical proce-

Table 1.3.
Intravenous and Intramuscular Analgesic Drugs Used in the Prevention and Treatment of Surgical Pain

Drug	Dosage	Duration of Action	Major Toxicity
Nonsteroidal anti-inflammatory drugs			
Flunixin meglumine	1 mg/kg IV once	12–24 h	GI irritation, ulcers, kidney damage
Ketoprofen	2 mg/kg IV once	12–24 h	GI irritation, ulcers, kidney damage
Carprofen (awaiting FDA approval)	2 mg/kg IV q12h	12–24 h	None reported at therapeutic doses
Opioid agonist-antagonists			
Butorphanol	Dog: 0.2–0.8 mg/kg Cat: 0.1–0.4 mg/kg IV, IM, SC	Dog: 0.5–2 h Cat: 2–6 h	Dysphoria
Opioid partial agonists			
Buprenorphine	Dog: 0.005–0.02 mg/kg Cat: 0.005–0.01 mg/kg IV, IM	4–12 h	Respiratory depression
Opioid agonists			
Morphine	Dog: 0.1–0.5 mg/kg IV, 0.1–0.5 mg/kg/h continuous IV infusion	1–4 h	Respiratory depression, urinary retention, pruritus, vomiting
	Dog: 0.5–1.0 mg/kg IM, SC	2–6 h	
	Cat: 0.05–0.2 mg/kg IM, SC	2–6 h	
Oxymorphone	Dog: 0.02–0.1 mg/kg IV, 0.2–2.0 mg/kg IM, SC	2–4 h IV, 2–6 h IM, SC	Respiratory depression, nausea, sensitivity to noise
	Cat: 0.02–0.05 mg/kg IV, 0.05–0.1 mg/kg IM, SC	2–4 h IV, 2–6 h IM, SC	

dures. However, the cardiovascular side effects of these drugs can compromise older, sicker animals. Routine use of α_2 agonists should thus be restricted to young, healthy animals (47).

The exact role of systemically administered α_2 agonists in postoperative pain control remains to be determined (48). The cardiovascular side effects of these drugs may dictate that their best use is restricted to the epidural space (36). However, it is possible that judicious use of systemically administered medetomidine may prolong or enhance systemic opiate analgesia. Postoperative administration of xylazine has reduced the catecholamine response to declawing operations in cats (49).

Narcotic Agonist-Antagonist Drugs

Drugs in the narcotic agonist-antagonist group (butorphanol, pentazocine, nalbuphine) are useful for moderate pain (11, 50). These drugs are κ-receptor agonists and μ-receptor antagonists. Narcotic agonist-antagonists have an analgesia ceiling effect because of their μ-receptor antagonism. Giving higher than recommended doses does *not* result in more potent analgesia. It is also likely that the duration of analgesia differs between dogs and cats. In dogs, butorphanol has a short duration of action, producing analgesia for no longer than 0.5 to 2 hours (51, 52). In cats, analgesia may last as long as 6 hours (50). Plasma cortisol concentrations and systemic blood pressure are reduced when butorphanol is given to cats after ovariohysterectomy (53). Plasma cortisol concentrations are reduced in dogs treated with butorphanol after ovariohysterectomy (9).

Narcotic Partial Agonist Drugs

Buprenorphine is a partial opiate agonist that binds tightly to the μ receptor, even displacing any morphine present at the receptor (54). Buprenorphine is useful in situations in which animals are infrequently treated, because it has a long duration of action (possibly up to 12 hours). Rats treated with single doses of buprenorphine have shown a faster return to function after surgery (55). Buprenorphine should be used cautiously in animals with respiratory compromise because the avid binding of the drug to the μ receptor may require that larger than routine doses of naloxone be used to reverse respiratory depression.

Opioid Agonists

The opioid agonists, such as morphine and oxymorphone, activate the μ and κ opioid receptors. These agents are the most effective drugs for control of moderate to severe pain (11). Increasing the dose of the drug always increases analgesia; thus these drugs can be titrated as needed. Side effects associated with opioid agonists include respiratory depression, urine retention, dysphoria, pruritus, nausea, and vomiting. In contrast to human patients, respiratory depression is rarely a problem in the dog and cat. Urine retention may occur when morphine is administered as a constant-rate intravenous infusion. Dysphoria is most common in cats, and concurrent use of a sedative drug may be necessary. Dogs may display dysphoria and vocalization when opioid agonists are withdrawn. Pruritus is a rare but obvious side effect. Vomiting is mainly associated with intermittent dosing of morphine in young, healthy animals. Nausea can occur with any of the opioids, but it appears to be most common in healthy animals. Rapid intravenous administration of morphine may cause histamine release, resulting in hypotension.

Morphine is the least expensive of the three agonists and the most useful for routine postoperative pain control. If the animal is receiving intravenous fluids after surgery, morphine may be added to the fluids and administered as a constant-rate infusion, after the initial bolus dose of morphine is given. For the first 12 hours, an initial infusion rate of 0.5 mg/kg/hour is used for baseline pain control, and intermittent intravenous doses of morphine are given to provide additional analgesia as needed. After 12 hours, the infusion rate should be reduced to 0.25 mg/kg/hour or less.

Intermittent intravenous or intramuscular doses of morphine can be used if fluids are not given after surgery. Ideally, an intravenous catheter should be maintained, to avoid the pain associated with intramuscular injections. To determine the needed dose, morphine doses of 0.1 mg/kg are given intravenously every 2 to 3 minutes until the desired effect is obtained. The doses are summed and repeated at 3- to 4-hour intervals. Alternatively, a starting dose of 0.5 mg/kg can be used and adjusted to obtain the desired effect.

Oxymorphone is the only single-agent opioid agonist approved for use in the dog and cat in the United States. This drug causes less dysphoria than morphine in cats, making it the opioid of choice for this species. Dysphoria can occur with higher opioid doses, despite using oxymorphone, and it may be necessary to give cats small doses of sedatives such as diazepam or acepromazine. In dogs, oxymorphone is extremely expensive to use for postoperative pain control because of the high doses needed (0.02 to 0.2 mg/kg) and the short interval of effectiveness (2 to 4 hours).

Transdermally Administered Drugs

Transdermal administration is a method of delivering a drug from a patch applied to the skin, through an intact cutaneous surface, to the systemic circulation.

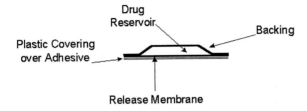

Fig. 1.5. Design of the transdermal fentanyl patch.

The drug is administered in a slow, continuous manner. This method results in constant drug plasma concentrations and thereby avoids the peaks and troughs in plasma concentrations (with the high probability of alternately overdosing and underdosing) associated with periodic systemic administration regimens. The transdermal patch consists of four basic layers: an adhesive layer, which attaches the patch to the skin; a release membrane that controls the rate of drug delivery; a drug reservoir; and a protective backing layer (Fig. 1.5).

The Duragesic patch is a transdermal fentanyl administration system licensed for the management of chronic cancer pain in human patients. Fentanyl is a μ-opioid agonist. The plasma concentration of fentanyl decreases rapidly after intravenous administration. Hence, intravenously administered fentanyl has limited application in postoperative analgesia, except when the drug is delivered by continuous infusion. However, fentanyl has a low molecular weight and high lipid solubility, making it an ideal drug for transdermal delivery. In human patients, transdermal fentanyl administration results in effective plasma opioid concentrations (56, 57) and is an efficacious and safe analgesic protocol (57, 58). In dogs and cats, transdermal fentanyl delivery produces plasma concentrations considered analgesic in human patients (59, 60). Transdermal fentanyl administration is an effective, well-tolerated, long-lasting, and relatively inexpensive postoperative analgesic regimen in dogs and cats.

Before patch placement, the animal's hair should be clipped, but not shaved. In dogs, the patch is placed on the skin on the dorsal aspect of the neck or thorax, and a bandage is applied to prevent inadvertent removal. In the cat, the patch adheres better to the lateral thorax or abdomen, and bandaging is not required (59). Care should be taken not to place the patch directly on a heating blanket, because heat may significantly increase the rate of drug delivery. The rate of release of fentanyl during transdermal administration is directly proportional to the patch surface area (2.5 μg/hour/cm²). The transdermal patch is available in four sizes (25, 50, 75, and 100 μg/hour), and the selected patch should deliver a dose rate of 2 to 4 μg/kg/hour. In cats and small dogs, part of the delivery

membrane can be covered to reduce the rate of drug delivery (59). After application of the transdermal delivery system, it takes 12 to 24 hours to reach effective plasma opioid concentrations (60). Hence, the patch should ideally be placed 12 to 24 hours preoperatively, to achieve an adequate plasma concentration during surgery and preempt the emergence of pain. Plasma fentanyl concentrations achieved after patch application vary, and patients should be monitored for signs of inadequate analgesia or adverse effects (60). Supplementary systemically administered narcotic drugs are used to treat breakthrough pain. The transdermal fentanyl patch is designed to deliver fentanyl at a constant rate for 72 hours. If further analgesia is required, a second patch may be placed on a different skin site. Alternatively, because considerable residual drug still remains in the patch after 72 hours, the original patch may be left in position longer.

Respiratory depression is the most serious potential side effect of transdermal fentanyl administration in human patients. However, no adverse effects were noted when transdermally administered fentanyl was used after surgery in over 100 dogs and cats in a teaching hospital (AE Kyles, unpublished data, 1996). In addition, the successful use of transdermal fentanyl patches in over 100 cats has been reported (59). If respiratory depression is observed, the patch should be removed and naloxone should be administered. Transdermal fentanyl patches are contraindicated in animals with bradyarrhythmias, respiratory compromise, and increased intracranial pressure. Transdermal fentanyl should not be used in animals with significant liver disease, because fentanyl is primarily metabolized in the liver. In addition, because increased body temperature can significantly increase transdermal drug delivery, patches should be avoided in animals with pyrexia.

Orally Administered Drugs

The NSAIDs are the most common orally administered analgesic agents in small animal practice (Table 1.4). In general, NSAIDs provide insufficient analgesia for the treatment of postoperative pain. These agents can be used alone for the management of mild to moderate acute pain, especially when associated with inflammation, and for diseases that produce chronic pain, such as osteoarthritis and cancer. For postoperative analgesia, NSAIDs are best combined with other types of analgesics, such as opioids. Combinations of NSAIDs and opioids produce additive, and perhaps synergistic, analgesic effects (61). In addition, oral NSAID administration can be used to taper, rather than abruptly discontinue, parenteral analgesic therapy. Severe postoperative pain can last for several days in some animals, and analgesics should not be stopped until the patient

Table 1.4.
Oral Drugs Used in the Treatment of Surgical Pain

Drug	Dosage	Major Toxicity
Nonsteroidal anti-inflammatory drugs (NSAIDs)		
Aspirin	10–25 mg/kg PO q12h in food (dog) 10 mg/kg PO q48–72h in food (cat)	GI irritation, ulcers, kidney damage
Piroxicam	0.3 mg/kg PO q24h, then q48h in food (dog)	GI irritation, ulcers, kidney damage
Phenylbutazone	22 mg/kg PO q8–12h (dog), maximum 800 mg/d	Bone marrow suppression, GI ulcers, kidney damage
Meclofenamic acid	0.5–1 mg/kg PO q24h, then q48h in food (dog)	GI irritation, ulcers, kidney damage
Carprofen (awaiting FDA approval)	2 mg/kg PO q12h, possibly q24h (dog)	None reported at therapeutic doses
NSAID/Opioid combinations		
Codeine 60 mg + aspirin 325 mg	1–2 mg/kg codeine PO q6–8h (dog)	GI irritation, ulcers, kidney damage
Codeine 60 mg + acetaminophen 300 mg	1–2 mg/kg codeine PO q6–8h (dog)	Acetaminophen is hepatotoxic; codeine toxicity is minimal at therapeutic doses
Codeine 2.4 mg/mL + acetaminophen 24 mg/mL	1–2 mg/kg codeine PO q6–8h (dog)	Acetaminophen is hepatotoxic; codeine toxicity is minimal at therapeutic doses
Opioid agonist-antagonists		
Butorphanol	0.5–1 mg/kg PO q6–8h (dog or cat)	Respiratory depression, decreased GI motility
Opioids		
Morphine	0.2–0.5 mg/kg PO q4h (dog)	Respiratory depression, decreased GI motility
Morphine, oral sustained release	1.5–3 mg/kg PO q12h (dog)	Respiratory depression, decreased GI motility
Morphine, rectal suppositories	0.2–0.5 mg/kg rectally q4h (dog)	Respiratory depression, decreased GI motility
Tricyclic antidepressants		
Amitriptyline	1–2 mg/kg PO q12–24h (dog) 2.5–12.5 mg/cat PO q24h	Sedation, psychosis, bone marrow depression, GI irritation
Imipramine	0.5–1 mg/kg PO q8h (dog) 2.5–5 mg/cat PO q12h	Sedation, bone marrow depression, GI irritation

shows reasonable evidence of an absence of distress (for example, normal sleeping, eating, drinking, and grooming patterns).

The NSAIDs that can be safely administered to dogs include aspirin, phenylbutazone, meclofenamic acid, and piroxicam. Naproxen and ibuprofen should be avoided because of the small safety margins, and tolmetin, indomethacin, and flubiprofen are unsafe in dogs. Newer NSAIDs with fewer adverse effects are being developed for both human and veterinary use. In dogs, carprofen has been shown to be efficacious, with few reported side effects (62), and it is being evaluated for approval by the United States Food and Drug Administration. Aspirin is the only NSAID recommended for use in cats.

Commonly used combinations of NSAIDs and opioids are acetaminophen and codeine and aspirin and codeine. These drugs are safe only in the dog. Fixed-dose preparations, such as acetaminophen 300 mg and codeine 60 mg, are convenient, but at high dose rates, the hepatotoxic effects of acetaminophen limit the analgesic effects of codeine. It is usually best to choose the preparation with the highest ratio of codeine to

NSAID. If more pain relief is needed, each component should be administered separately (63).

Until safer NSAIDs have been approved, these drugs should only be used after surgery. Irreversible cyclooxygenase inhibitors, such as aspirin, can cause bleeding problems by inhibiting platelet function. Renal ischemia, a side effect of vasodilatory prostaglandin inhibition, may be exacerbated by hypotension during anesthesia. Gastric and duodenal ulceration can be severe in dogs because of the extensive enterohepatic circulation of NSAIDs in this species. Perioperative use of acetaminophen may increase hepatotoxicity and should be delayed for 6 to 12 hours after anesthesia (64). These side effects are more common in patients that are already ill. Gastrointestinal complications can be reduced with NSAIDs, such as carprofen, that spare prostaglandin E, which is important in the maintenance of the gastric mucosal protective barrier. Alternatively, misoprostol, a synthetic prostaglandin E_1 analog, has prevented gastrointestinal ulceration in human patients undergoing NSAID therapy (65) and could be used in animals prone to gastrointestinal upset. NSAIDs have a low therapeutic ceiling; administering higher doses does not further increase analgesia, but rather it accelerates the incidence and severity of side effects.

Orally administered opioids can be useful as a follow-up to parenteral opioids in the management of severe, prolonged postoperative pain. Orally administered morphine is well established in the treatment of pain in human patients, and an empiric starting dose of 0.3 to 0.5 mg/kg every 4 hours can be recommended in dogs (66). Alternatively, 1.5 to 3 mg/kg of a sustained release oral morphine preparation can be given every 12 hours. The dose of oral morphine should be tapered over several days. Butorphanol tablets are also available and can be used in dogs or cats. A high dose is required because of the low bioavailability of oral butorphanol (0.5 to 1.0 mg/kg every 6 to 8 hours) (67).

Neuropathic pain can be severe after surgery for nerve root entrapment or nerve root tumor removal. In general, patients with neuropathic pain respond poorly to conventional pain control drugs. Tricyclic antidepressants have shown some benefits in controlling neuropathic pain (68).

References

1. Anand KJS, Sippell WG, Aynsley-Green A. Randomized trial of fentanyl anesthesia in preterm babies undergoing surgery: effects on the stress response. Lancet 1987;1:62–66.
2. Anand KJS, Phil D, Hickey PR. Halothane-morphine compared with high-dose sufentanil for anesthesia and postoperative analgesia in cardiac surgery. N Engl J Med 1992;326:1–9.
3. Kehlet H. Does analgesia benefit postinjury outcome? In: Parker MM, Shapiro MJ, Porembka DT, eds. Critical care state of the art. Anaheim, CA: Society of Critical Care Medicine, 1995;15:213–229.
4. Liu S, Carpenter RL, Neal JM. Epidural anesthesia and analgesia: their role in postoperative outcome. Anesthesiology 1995; 82:1474–1506.
5. Bonica JJ. Definitions and taxonomy of pain. In: Bonica JJ, ed. The management of pain. Philadelphia: Lea & Febiger, 1990:18–27.
6. McGrath PJ, Johnson G, Goodman JT, et al. CHEOPS: A behavioral scale for rating postoperative pain in children. In: Fields HL, ed. Advances in pain research and therapy. New York: Raven Press, 1985;9:395–401.
7. Conzemius MG, Brockman DJ, King LG, et al. Analgesia in dogs after intercostal thoracotomy: a clinical trial comparing intravenous buprenorphine and intrapleural bupivacaine. Vet Surg 1994;23:291–298.
8. Anand KJS, Hickey PR. Pain and its effects in the human neonate and fetus. N Engl J Med 1987;317:1321–1327.
9. Fox SM, Mellor DJ, Firth EC, et al. Changes in plasma cortisol concentrations before, during and after analgesia, anaesthesia, and anaesthesia plus ovariohysterectomy in bitches. Res Vet Sci 1994;5:110–118.
10. Howard-Jensen N, Cioms A. Ethical code for animal experimentation. WHO Chron 1985;39:51–56.
11. Hansen BD. Analgesic therapy. Compend Contin Educ Pract Vet 1994;16:868–875.
12. Abram SE, Yaksh TL. Morphine, but not inhalation anesthesia, blocks post-injury facilitation: the role of preemptive suppression of afferent transmission. Anesthesiology 1993;78:713–721.
13. McMahon SB, Lewin GR, Wall PD. Central hyperexcitability triggered by noxious inputs. Curr Opin Neurobiol 1993; 3:602–610.
14. Bullingham RE. Optimum management of postoperative pain. Drugs 1985;29:376–386.
15. Bonica JJ. Postoperative pain. In: Bonica JJ, ed. The management of pain. Philadelphia, Lea & Febiger, 1990:461–480.
16. Quandt JE, Rawlings CR. Reducing postoperative pain for dogs: local anesthetic and analgesic techniques. Compend Contin Educ Pract Vet 1996;18:101–111.
17. McEvoy GK, ed. American Hospital Formulary Service drug information. Bethesda, MD: American Society of Health-System Pharmacists, 1995:2228–2241.
18. Feldman HS, Arthur GR, Covino BG. Comparative systemic toxicity on convulsant and supraconvulsant doses of intravenous ropivicaine, bupivacaine, and lidocaine in the conscious dog. Anesth Analg 1989;69:794–801.
19. Chadwick HS. Toxicity and resuscitation in lidocaine- or bupivacaine-infused cats. Anesthesiology 1985;63:385–390.
20. Gibbs P, Purushotham A, Auld C, et al. Continuous wound perfusion with bupivacaine for postoperative wound pain. Br J Surg 1988;75:923–924.
21. Moss G, Regal ME, Lichtig L. Reducing postoperative pain, narcotics, and length of hospitalization. Surgery 1986;99:206–210.
22. Conzemius MG, Sammarco JL, Perkowski SZ, et al. Analgesic effect of intra-articular bupivacaine, morphine, or saline after cranial cruciate repair: a randomized, prospective, double-blind study. Vet Surg 1994;23:398.
23. Jebeles JA, Reilly JS, Gutierrez JF, et al. The effect of pre-incisional infiltration of tonsils with bupivacaine on the pain following tonsillectomy under gas anesthesia. Pain 1991; 47:305–308.
24. Muir WW, Hubbell JAE, Skarda RT, et al. Handbook of veterinary anesthesia. 2nd ed. St. Louis: CV Mosby, 1995.
25. Thompson SE, Johnson JM. Analgesia in dogs after intercostal thoracotomy: a comparison of morphine, selective intercostal nerve block, and interpleural regional analgesia with bupivacaine. Vet Surg 1991;20:73–77.
26. Mazoit JX, Lambert C, Berdeaux A, et al. Pharmacokinetics of bupivacaine after short and prolonged infusions in conscious dogs. Anesth Analg 1988;67:961–966.
27. Baker JW, Tribble CG. Pleural anesthestics given through an epidural catheter secured inside a chest tube. Ann Thorac Surg 1991;51:138–139.
28. Wallin G, Cassuto J, Hogstrom S, et al. Influence of intraperitoneal anesthesia on pain and the sympathoadrenal response to abdominal surgery. Acta Anaesthesiol Scand 1988;32:553–558.
29. Valverde A, Conlon PD, McDonnell WN, et al. Use of epidural morphine in the dog for pain relief. Vet Comp Orthop Trauma 1989;2:55–58.
30. Drenger B, Magora F. Urodynamic studies after intrathecal fentanyl and buprenorphine in the dog. Anesth Analg 1989; 69:348–353.
31. Popilskis S, Kohn D, Sanchez JA, et al. Epidural vs. intramuscular oxymorphone analgesia after thoracotomy in dogs. Vet Surg 1991;20:462–467.
32. Duke T, Komulainen Cox AM, Remedios AM, et al. The analgesic effects of administering fentanyl or medetomidine in the lumbosacral epidural space of cats. Vet Surg 1994;23:143–148.
33. Littrell RA. Epidural analgesia. Am J Hosp Pharm 1991; 48:2460–2474.
34. Lubenow TR, McCarthy RJ, Ivankovich AD. Management of acute postoperative pain. In: Barash PG, Cullen BF, Stoelting RK, eds. Clinical anesthesia. 2nd ed. Philadelphia: JB Lippincott, 1992:1547–1577.
35. Branson KR, Tranquilli WJ, Benson J, et al. Duration of analgesia induced by epidurally administered morphine and medetomidine in the dog. J Vet Pharmacol Ther 1993;16:369–372.
36. Sabbe MB, Penning JP, Ozaki GT, et al. Spinal and systemic action of the alpha 2 receptor agonist dexmedetomidine in dogs: antinociception and carbon dioxide response. Anesthesiology 1994;80:1057–1072.
37. Duke T, Cox AM, Remedios AM, et al. The cardiopulmonary effects of placing fentanyl or metetomidine in the lumbosacral epidural space of isoflurane-anesthetized cats. Vet Surg 1994;23:149–155.

38. Hansen B. Epidural anesthesia and analgesia. Proceedings of the Predictable Pain Management Symposium. Orlando, FL: North American Veterinary Conference, Pfizer, 1996:49–55.

39. Bach S, Noreng MF. Phantom limb pain in amputees during the first 6 months following limb amputation, after preoperative lumbar epidural blockade. Pain 1988;33:297–301.

40. Fisher A, Meller Y. Continuous postoperative regional analgesia by nerve sheath block for amputation surgery: a pilot study. Anesth Analg 1991;72:300–303.

41. Hopt HW, Weitz S. Postoperative pain management. Arch Surg 1994;129:128–132.

42. Lascelles BD, Butterworth SJ, Waterman AL. Postoperative analgesic and sedative effects of carprofen and pethidine in dogs. Vet Rec 1994;134:187–191.

43. Reid J, Nolan AM. A comparison of the postoperative effects of flunixin and papaveretum in the dog. J Small Anim Pract 1991;32:603–608.

44. Nolan A, Reid, J. Comparison of the postoperative analgesic and sedative effects of carprofen and paraveretum in the dog. Vet Rec 1993;133:240–242.

45. Scheinin M, MacDonald E. An introduction to the pharmacology of the alpha$_2$ adrenoceptors in the central nervous system. Acta Vet Scand 1989;85:11–19.

46. Vitranen R. Pharmacologic profiles of metedomidine and its antagonist atipamezole. Acta Vet Scand 1989;85:29–37.

47. Pettinger GR, Dyson DH. Comparison of medetomidine and fentanyl-droperidol in dogs: sedation, analgesia, arterial blood gases and lactate levels. Can J Vet Res 1993;57:99–105.

48. Maze M, Tranquilli WJ. Alpha$_2$ adrenoreceptor agonists: defining its role in clinical anesthesia. Anesthesiology 1991; 75:581–605.

49. Benson GJ, Wheaton LG, Thurmon JC, et al. Postoperative catecholamine response to onychectomy in isoflurane-anesthetized cats. Vet Surg 1991;20:222–225.

50. Sawyer DC, Rech RH. Analgesia and behavioral effects of butorphanol, nalbuphine, and pentazocine in the cat. J Am Anim Hosp Assoc 1987;23:438–446.

51. Houghton KJ, Rech RH, Sawyer DC, et al. Dose-response of intravenous butorphanol to increase visceral nociceptive threshold in dogs. Proc Soc Exp Biol Med 1991;197:290–296.

52. Raffe MR, Lipowitz AJ. Evaluation of butorphanol tartrate analgesia in the dog. In: Proceedings of the Second International Congress of Veterinary Anesthesiology, Chicago, IL. 1985:155.

53. Smith JD, Allen SW, Quandt JE, et al. Markers of postoperative pain and correlation with clinical criteria. In: Proceedings of the Fifth American College of Veterinary Surgeons Veterinary Symposium, Chicago, IL. 1995:21.

54. Lipman AG. Clinically relevant differences among the opioid analgesics. Am J Hosp Pharm 1990;47:S1–S13.

55. Liles JH, Flecknell PA. A comparison of of the effects of buprenorphine, carprofen, and flunxin following laparotomy in rats. J Vet Pharmacol Ther 1994;17:284–290.

56. Varvel JR, Shafer SL, Hwang SS, et al. Absorption characteristics of transdermally administered fentanyl. Anesthesiology 1989; 70:928–934.

57. Holley FO, Van Steennis C. Post-operative analgesia with fentanyl: pharmacokinetics and pharmacodynamics of constant rate IV and transdermal delivery. Br J Anaesth 1988; 60:608–613.

58. Gourlay GK, Kowlaski SR, Plummer JL, et al. The efficacy of transdermal fentanyl in the treatment of post-operative pain: a double-blinded comparison of fentanyl and placebo systems. Pain 1989;40:21–28.

59. Scherk-Nixon M. A study of the use of a transdermal fentanyl patch in cats. J Am Anim Hosp Assoc 1996;32:19–24.

60. Kyles AE, Papich M, Hardie EM. Disposition of transdermal fentanyl in dogs. Am J Vet Res 1996.

61. Dahl JB, Kehlet H. Non-steroidal anti-inflammatory drugs: rationale for use in severe postoperative pain. Br J Anaesth 1991;66:703–712.

62. Holtsinger RH, Parker RB, Beale BS, et al. The therapeutic efficacy of carprofen (Rimadyl-V^{TM}) in 209 clinical cases of canine degenerative joint disease. Vet Comp Orthop Trauma 1992;5:140–144.

63. Ashburn MA, Lipman AGH. Management of pain in the cancer patient. Anesth Analg 1993;76;402–416.

64. Cribbs PH. Precautions when using antiprostaglandins. Vet Clin North Am 1992;22:370–375.

65. Fenn GC, Robinson GC. Misoprostol: a logical therapeutic approach to gastroduodenal mucosal injury produced by non-steroidal anti-inflammatory drugs? J Clin Pharm Ther 1991;16:385–409.

66. Hardie EM, Kyles AE. Pharmacological management of pain and infection in the surgical oncological patient. Vet Clin North Am 1995;25:77–96.

67. Tranquilli WJ, Fikes LL, Raffe MR. Selecting the right analgesics: indications and dosage requirements. Vet Med 1989;84: 692–697.

68. McQuay HJ. Pharmacological treatment of neuralgic and neuropathic pain. Cancer Surv 1988;7:141–159.

—2—

SELECTION AND USE OF CURRENTLY AVAILABLE SUTURE MATERIALS AND NEEDLES

Daniel D. Smeak

Suture Classification and Definitions

Suture materials are classified in many ways to facilitate discussion of their characteristics and use, such as according to absorption properties, number of strands, capillary characteristics, and fiber origin.

Absorbable sutures undergo degradation and rapid loss in tensile strength within 60 days, whereas nonabsorbable sutures retain significant strength past 60 days. This definition can be misleading with respect to silk, cotton, linen, and multifilament nylon sutures because these materials are considered nonabsorbable, yet they can lose much of their tensile strength within 4 to 6 weeks after implantation.

Monofilament sutures are made of a single strand. Multifilament or braided sutures are woven or twisted from several smaller strands. In general, multifilament sutures are easier to handle than the monofilaments.

Capillary sutures are usually multifilament materials that can act as a wick, along which serum and bacteria can travel. These suture materials obviously are not recommended for penetration into contaminated or infected areas. Both chemical composition and coating of the suture influence capillarity. For example, coated caprolactam transports nearly twice as much fluid as uncoated polyester of the same suture size. Waxed silk is noncapillary, in contrast to the highly capillary nature of uncoated virgin silk.

Sutures are made of either natural or synthetic materials. Catgut, silk, linen, and cotton are naturally derived sutures; all other available suture materials are synthetic. Synthetic suture materials usually cause less tissue reaction and have more predictable absorption rates.

Suture Selection and Use

Many different suture materials are available to veterinary surgeons. No single suture is ideal for every surgical situation. Certain suture materials, however, are better suited for different wound environments and uses. When choosing a suture material, certain general principles should be considered.

Strength of Tissue

A suture should be at least as strong as the tissue through which it passes. A tissue's ability to hold sutures without tearing depends on its collagen content and on the orientation of collagen fibrils. This explains why ligaments, tendons, fascia, and skin are strongest, muscle is relatively weak, and fat is weakest. Muscle has little suture-holding capability across its fibers and even less in the direction of the fibers. Visceral tissue, in general, ranks between fat and muscle in strength. Bladder and colon are the weakest hollow organs of the body, and stomach and small intestine are among the strongest. Organ strength varies within the same organ and with the age and size of the animal.

Table 2.1.
Suture Material Sizes

Actual Size (mm)[a]	USP Size		Brown and Sharpe Wire Gauge
	Catgut	Synthetic	
0.02		10-0	
0.03		9-0	
0.04		8-0	
0.05	8-0	7-0	41
0.07	7-0	6-0	38–40
0.1	6-0	5-0	35
0.15	5-0	4-0	32–34
0.2	4-0	3-0	30
0.3	3-0	2-0	28
0.35	2-0	0	26
0.4	0	1	25
0.5	1	2	24
0.6	2	3;4	22
0.7	3	5	20
0.8	4	6	19
0.9		7	18

[a] To obtain metric gauge, multiply actual size (mm) by 10; for example, USP 0 catgut 0.4 mm in diameter is metric size 4.

The choice of suture size is based on the tensile strength of the tissue as well as of the suture material. Catgut and synthetic suture materials are sized according to either United States Pharmacopeia (USP) or metric gauge (Table 2.1). A larger numeric USP value means a larger-diameter suture; however, when the USP size is a number is followed by a (-0), a larger number denotes a smaller suture size (e.g., No. 2 polypropylene is larger than 0, and 2-0 is larger than 4-0). The metric gauge is the actual suture diameter expressed in millimeters multiplied by 10. Stainless steel wire can be sized by USP, metric gauge, or Brown and Sharpe wire gauge. Guidelines for suture usage and size for various tissues are summarized in Table 2.2. These guidelines are general and are based on currently available literature and my experience. Use of

the smallest suture size possible for wound closure results in less tissue trauma, allows smaller knots to be tied, and forces the surgeon to handle the sutures and tissue more carefully. Oversized sutures can actually weaken the wound through excessive tissue reaction and tissue strangulation. To maintain maximum suture strength once the suture is removed from the packet, certain suture handling rules are suggested (Table 2.3).

Loss of Suture Strength and Gain of Wound Strength

To use absorbable sutures safely, the loss of suture strength should be proportional to the anticipated gain in wound strength. The relative rates of suture strength loss and simultaneous wound strength gain are important. Fascia, tendons, and ligaments heal slowly (50% strength gain in 50 days) and are under constant tensile force. For these tissues, nonabsorbable sutures or the newer prolonged-degrading, synthetic absorbable sutures are indicated. Because visceral wounds heal relatively fast, often achieving most of their strength in 21 days, absorbable sutures are adequate. Monofilament nonabsorbable sutures are suggested for skin closure because they induce little foreign body response and the skin has a slower gain in healing strength when compared with visceral healing. General and local factors affecting wound healing must also be considered before an appropriate suture is selected. For example, catgut in the presence of infection or gastric enzymes placed in a catabolic patient can be degraded within days, rendering the wound closure susceptible to dehiscence.

Healing Considerations

Surgeons must consider how the suture alters the biologic processes in a healing wound environment. Tis-

Table 2.2.
General Suture Size and Usage Recommendations in Small Animal Surgery

Tissue	Suture Size (USP)	Suture Material: Classes
Skin	3-0 to 4-0	Monofilament nonabsorbable
Subcutaneous tissue	2-0 to 4-0	Absorbable
Fascia	1 to 3-0	Synthetic (prolonged degrading) absorbable, or synthetic nonabsorbable
Muscle	0 to 3-0	Skeletal: synthetic absorbable or nonabsorbable
		Cardiac: synthetic nonabsorbable
Parenchymal organ	2-0 to 4-0	Absorbable
Hollow viscus organ	2-0 to 5-0	Absorbable or monofilament nonabsorbable
Tendon, ligament	0 to 3-0	Monofilament nonabsorbable, synthetic (prolonged degrading) absorbable
Nerve	5-0 to 7-0	Monofilament nonabsorbable
Cornea	8-0 to 10-0	Synthetic absorbable, nonmetallic nonabsorbable
Vascular ligation	3-0 to 4-0	Absorbable
Vascular repair	5-0 to 7-0	Monofilament nonabsorbable

Table 2.3.
Suture Handling Suggestions

1. Protect all sutures from heat and moisture.
2. Never autoclave absorbable sutures.
3. Refrain from soaking absorbable sutures, particularly in hot water.
4. Use strands directly from the packet; avoid excessive handling of suture strands before use.
5. Avoid suture kinking or crushing suture with instruments.
6. Suture strands with "memory" may be straightened with a gentle tug.
7. Periodically check suture strands for evidence of fraying or defects, particularly when using a continuous suture pattern.

sues respond to sutures much as they do to other foreign material. The amount of reaction depends on the nature of the suture implanted (e.g., surgical gut versus inert, stainless steel), the amount or surface area of the suture, the type and location of tissue closed with sutures (intestinal viscera and skin react strongly to silk, whereas fascia reacts minimally to silk), the length of implantation (polyglycolic acid is moderately reactive early but within months is relatively inert), and the technique of suture placement (excessive suture tightening causes tissue strangulation). Excessive suture-induced tissue reaction increases the likelihood of suture cutout by softening surrounding tissues, and it delays the onset of fibroplasia. Sutures causing excessive tissue reaction are contraindicated in areas in which exuberant scar formation can cause a functional problem (e.g., for vascular repair or ureteral anastomosis) or a cosmetic problem (e.g., in skin). The surgeon should strive to inflict the least amount of trauma necessary for the operation, to reduce contamination, and to use sutures that cause the least tissue reaction to avoid excessive inflammation and delayed wound healing.

All suture materials are capable of increasing wound susceptibility to infection. The suture's filamentous nature, capillarity, chemical structure, bioinertness, and ability to adhere to bacteria all play a role in suture-related infection. In a classic experiment, a single silk suture reduced the total contaminating dose of Staphylococcus required to induce wound infection 10,000-fold. On the other hand, the byproducts of nylon and polyglycolic acid suture degradation in tissues have bactericidal effects. Sutures inducing the least foreign-body reaction in tissues, such as synthetic absorbable and monofilament nonabsorbable sutures, produce the lowest incidence of infection in contaminated wounds.

Multifilament nonabsorbable suture materials induce chronic sinus formation more often than absorbable or monofilament sutures. Multifilament nonab-

sorbable sutures harbor bacteria within the suture interstices, creating an effective barrier to phagocytosis.

Wound infection also affects suture integrity. If wound contamination is suspected, synthetic absorbable sutures should be chosen because these sutures are more stable and have predictable absorption rates in contaminated tissue. If long-term wound support is required of the suture material, a synthetic monofilament nonabsorbable or synthetic (prolonged degradation) absorbable suture such as polydioxanone or polyglyconate is indicated.

The presence of any suture material within the lumen of the biliary or urinary tract can induce calculus formation. Thus, absorbable sutures are recommended in these areas. Silk and polyester material, because of their documented calculogenic effects, should never remain in contact with urine or bile.

Mechanical Properties of Suture and Tissue

The mechanical properties or functions of the suture should be similar to those of the tissue being closed. For example, polybutester is most suitable for skin because of its elastic nature. Less elastic suture materials, such as those composed of polyester fibers, are more applicable for anchoring prosthetic materials or for joint imbrication.

The surgeon should consider these general suture principles and should choose the best suture, based on its physical and chemical characteristics, for the specific requirements of the tissues being closed (Table 2.4). Physical characteristics include durability, handling quality, knot security, and heat sterilization damage. Biologic characteristics include mode of absorption, tissue reactivity, predisposition to infection, sinus formation, and calculogenic potential. Subjective characteristics of each suture described in Table 2.4, such as handling quality and specific suture advantages or disadvantages, are based on the current literature and on my opinion.

Newly Developed Sutures
Fluorofil

A special dye was added to polypropylene to create Fluorofil, a suture material that glows pink when exposed to black light. It maintains the advantages of polypropylene (minimal tissue reaction, permanent, nonabsorbable, strength). Fluorofil was designed to compete against coated caprolactam for use primarily in skin closure. Although it does not handle as well as its competitors, it elicits far less tissue reaction when

Table 2.4.
General Characteristics of Suture Materials

Generic Name	Trade Name	Origin	Tensile Strength Loss	Completion of Absorption	Mode of Degradation	Tissue Foreign-Body Response
Chromic catgut	Catgut Softgut	Tanned intestinal sub-mucosa	A MU 33%–7 d 67%–28 d	60 d	Phagocyte and enzymatic degradation	Moderate to severe
Coated capro-lactam	Vetafil Supramide Braunamid	Polyamide polymer	N MU NA	NA	NA	Moderate[c]
Collagen	Collagen	Bovine flexor tendon filaments	A MU	60 d		
Poliglecaprone 25	Monocryl[d]	Copolymer glycolide and ε-caprolacton	A MO 50%–7 d 80%–14 d	91–119 d	Hydrolysis	Slight
Polyamide-nylon	MO-Dermalon Ethilon MU-Nurolon Surgilon	Extruded polyamide filament	N MO 30%–720 d MU 70–90%–180 d	NA	Chemical degradation	Minimal
Polybutester	Novafil	Copolymer polybutylene polytetramethylene	M NO NA	NA	NA	Minimal
Polydioxanone	PDS	Polydioxanone polymer	A MO 26%–14 d 42%–28 d	182 d	Hydrolysis	Slight
Polyester	UC Mersilene Dacron Ethibond C-Tevdek	Extruded synthetic resin polymers	N MU NA	NA	NA	Moderate
Polyethylene	Ticron Polyethylene	Polymerized ethylene	N MO slow loss over years	NA	Chemical degradation	Minimal
Polyglactin 910	UC Vicryl C Vicryl	Glycolic-lactic acid polymer C-calcium stearate	A MU 50%–14 d 80%–21 d	60–90 d	Hydrolysis	Slight
	C Vicryl Rapide[d]		A MU 50%–5 d 100%–10–14 d	42 d	Hydrolysis	Slight
Polyglycolic acid	UC-Dexon S C-Dexon Plus	Glycolic acid C-surfactant	A MU 37%–7 d 80%–14 d	120 d	Hydrolysis	Slight
Polyglyconate	Maxon	Polytrimethylene carbonate	A MO 19%–14 d 80%–28 d	180 d	Hydrolysis	Slight
Polypropylene	Prolene Surgilene Fluorofil[d]	Polymerized polyolefin hydrocarbons	N MO NA	NA	NA	Minimal
Silk	C-Perma-Hand Dermal UC-Virgin Silk	Silkworm cocoon fibers	N MU 30%–14 d 50%–365 d	>720 d	Mechanical fragmentation and breakage, phagocytosis	Moderate to severe
Stainless steel wire	MU-Flexon	Chromium nickel molybdenum alloy	N MO/NA MU	NA	NA	Almost inert
Stainless steel and tantalum clips	Hemoclip Versaclip	Malleable surgical-grade steel or tantalum	N MO NA	NA	NA	Almost inert
Surgical cotton	—	Cotton vegetable fibers	N MU 50%–180 d 70%–720 d	NA	NA	Moderate to severe
Surgical linen	—	Flax vegetable fibers	N MU 50%–180 d	NA	NA	Severe

A, absorbable; C, coated; MO, monofilament; MU multifilament; N, nonabsorbable; NA, not applicable; UC, uncoated.

[a] Monofilament nonabsorbable sutures have worse knot-holding capacity in large sizes; coating reduces knot security.

[b] Loss of suture strength with autoclaving: minimal—can withstand three autoclavings with little effect; moderate—significant loss of strength with autoclaving; severe—should not be resterilized with heat.

[c] If coating breaks.

[d] New suture materials.

Capillarity	Relative Knot Security[a]	Size-to-Tensile Strength Ratio	Overall Suture Handling Ease	Heat Sterilization Damage[b]	Comments
Minimal	Good when dry; poor to fair when wet	Poor to fair	Fair to good	Severe	Incites local inflammation and fibrosis; knots may loosen when wet; exhibits wide variability in strength loss; rapid strength loss in highly vascular or infected areas, in presence of stomach acid-pepsin, and in catabolic patients; occasional sensitivity reaction
+	Fair to good	Good	Good	Moderate	Coating tends to break, increasing capillary and tissue reaction; should not be buried or used in contaminated areas; dispensing reels do not provide sterile suture material
					Similar to chronic catgut in tissue reactivity and absorption
−	Good	Excellent	Very good	Severe	Best handling properties of monofilament absorbable sutures; can be used wherever braided absorbable sutures are recommended; should not be used where extended approximation of tissue under stress is required
−	Poor	Good	Fair	Minimal	Buried knot ends may cause frictional irritation, degradation products may be bactericidal; stable in contaminated wounds; requires 5 to 6 throws for knotting continuous lines
−	Fair to good	Good	Very good	Minimal	Much like monofilament nylon but better handling; less stiff; very elastic; excellent for plastic surgery
−	Fair to good	Excellent	Good	Severe	Tends to kink when used in a continuous pattern; minimal tissue drag; prolonged absorption; can be used wherever absorbable sutures are indicated, especially when prolonged strength is needed
UC +/C−	Poor	Excellent	Good	Minimal	Uncoated sutures cause excessive tissue drag; coating markedly reduces knot security—suggest 5 square throws; causes most tissue reaction of synthetic sutures; should not be used in contaminated areas
−	Poor	Fair to good	Fair	Severe	Loses excessive tensile strength when knotted; stable in contaminated wounds
UC minimal/ C−	Fair to good	Good	Good	Severe	Rapid hydrolysis in alkaline environment, moderate tissue drag, stable in contaminated wounds
C−	Fair to good	Fair	Good	Severe	Provides about 70% of initial strength of coated Vicryl; predictable rapid absorption; used as an alternative to gut suture; less reactive than gut; indicated for superficial closure of skin and mucosa
UC minimal/ C−	Fair to good	Good	Good	Severe	Degradation process may have antibacterial effects; rapid hydrolysis in alkaline environment and infected urine; excessive tissue drag; stable in contaminated wounds
−	Fair to good	Excellent	Good	Severe	Similar to polydioxanone; suture handling worse in large diameters; may lose strength faster than PDS
−	Fair to good	Good	Fair	Minimal	Greater knot security than most other monofilament, nonmetallic nonabsorbable sutures; least thrombogenic; stable in contaminated areas; Fluorafil has a pigment that glows pink under blacklight that helps to locate suture for removal
UC+/C−	Poor to fair	Fair	Excellent	Moderate	Potentiates infection; avoid in contaminated or infected wounds; calculogenic in biliary and urinary tract; standard for judging suture handling characteristics
−	Excellent	Excellent	Poor	Minimal	Knot end stiffness evokes inflammatory reaction; tends to fragment and migrate in tissue; tends to cut tissue; stable in contaminated wounds; standard for judging knot security and tissue reaction to suture materials
−	NA	NA	Excellent	Minimal	Clips allow easy and rapid ligation of vessels in poorly accessible areas; tantalum resists bending fatigue better than stainless steel but has less tensile strength
+	Good	Poor	Fair	Moderate	Potentiates infection; avoid in contaminated or infected wounds; electrostatic—clings to gloves and surgical linen; better sutures currently available
+	Good	Poor	Fair	Moderate	Similar to cotton

implanted in skin. Fluorescence of the dye assists in suture location in poorly exposed areas.

Coated Vicryl Rapide

This predictable, but very rapidly absorbable, suture material was created to model the performance characteristics of collagen or surgical gut suture. Rapide induces a tissue reaction similar to that elicited by the original coated Vicryl suture. Its initial strength is like nylon or gut suture, but it retains only 50% of its strength at 5 days. All the suture strength is lost by 10 to 14 days, and, when implanted beneath the skin, it is completely absorbed in about one-third the time (42 days) of the original coated Vicryl suture. Rapide is indicated only for use in superficial soft tissue approximation of the skin and mucosa, where only short-term wound support is necessary. Rapide sutures fall out within 7 to 10 days of percutaneous implantation. This property makes it an ideal suture for use in pediatric, exotic, or difficult-to-handle patients because suture removal is not required.

Monocryl

This new, rapidly absorbable suture material has the highest initial suture strength and is the most pliable of any monofilament corrected absorbable suture. Its smooth surface and reduced memory result in lower tissue drag than gut or braided absorbable sutures. Like the other synthetic absorbable suture materials, it is absorbed predictably even in the presence of infection, and it induces a minimal acute inflammatory reaction in tissues. This suture retains about 50% of its original strength at 7 days after implantation and 20% at 2 weeks. Monocryl is an excellent alternative to surgical gut or braided synthetic absorbable sutures for use in soft tissue approximation where prolonged suture strength is not required.

In conclusion, the final suture selection should be based on personal preference only after the suture material characteristics, the interaction between suture and tissue, and the biologic processes in a healing wound are fully understood (see the summary of suture use rules in Table 2.5). It is obvious that the choice of suture material for wound closure can determine the success or failure of a surgical procedure. The techniques of suture placement and tissue handling, however, remain even more important than suture selection for uncomplicated wound healing.

Suture Needles

Surgical needles are manufactured in a variety of sizes, shapes, and types. Needles are selected to ensure that the tissues being sutured are altered as little as possible

Table 2.5.
General Rules to Avoid Most
Suture-Related Complications

1. Avoid use of multifilament nonabsorbable suture material in contaminated or infected wounds. Multifilament suture harbors bacteria and may cause persistent sinus formation or local infection.
2. Avoid nonabsorbable suture exposure within the lumen of hollow organs, such as the urinary bladder or gallbladder, in which calculus formation at a suture nidus is possible.
3. Avoid burying nonabsorbable suture taken from a used open cassette. Consider all suture from an open cassette contaminated.
4. If continued suture strength is important, avoid use of chromic gut in inflamed or infected tissue and in wounds with delayed healing (catabolic conditions, radiation wounds). Gut in contact with proteolytic enzymes, such as in the stomach lumen or pancreas, loses most of its strength within days of implantation.
5. Avoid use of rapidly absorbable suture material in critical areas such as the abdominal fascia, tendons, or ligaments known to heal slowly and to be under continual tensile force.
6. Avoid using reactive suture materials in wounds predisposed to stricture (such as tracheostomies or urethrostomies) or excessive scar formation (such as the skin).
7. Avoid capillary suture material penetration through known contaminated areas such as the bowel lumen or skin. Bacteria are "wicked" or may be transported to adjacent sterile tissues to form microabscesses around sutures.

by the needle. The needle chosen should allow tissue passage without excessive force and without disruption of tissue architecture. In addition, the hole created by the needle should be just large enough to allow passage of the suture material.

Surgical needles have three basic components: the eye (or suture connection), the body (or shaft), and the point. Two types of needle eyes are commonly used in practice, the closed eye and swaged (eyeless). Needles permanently connected to suture (swaged needles) produce significantly less tissue trauma and are easier to handle than eyed needles; however, sutures supplied with needles are much more expensive.

The body or shaft of needles varies in shape and size. Some needle bodies are ribbed to prevent rotation of the needle in the jaws of needle holders. Easily accessible tissues such as the skin may be sutured by hand with straight needles, but most surgeons prefer curved needles because they are easier to use with instruments. Curved needles are supplied in one-quarter, three-eighths, one-half, and five-eighths circle shapes. Choice of length, width, and curvature of the needle depends on the size and depth of the area to be sutured (Table 2.6). Quarter-circle needles have limited use, primarily for eye surgery. Three-eighths circle needles are most commonly used in veterinary surgery and are suitable for most superficial wounds. Half-circle needles are preferred for deeper wounds and in body cavities. Five-eighths circle needles are

Table 2.6.
Principles of Suture Needle Use

1. Swaged needles are less traumatic and are always preferred.
2. The more superficial the tissue, the straighter the curve of the needle should be.
3. For general use, hold the needle one-third to half the way down from the eye to the point. Grasp the needle closer to the point if tissue is especially difficult to penetrate.
4. Hold needles in the narrow tips of the jaws of the needle holders.
5. Use taper needles wherever possible; they should not be used if it becomes difficult to pass through tissues.
6. Needles should be long enough to bite through both sides of the incision.

applicable for suturing wounds in confined areas such as the oral, nasal, and pelvic cavities.

Three general types of needle points are cutting, tapercut, and taper (or round point) (Fig. 2.1). Cutting needles provide edges that cut through dense connective tissue. They are most suitable for skin, tendon, and fascial closure. Like the conventional cutting needle, the reverse cutting needle has a triangular cross-sectional area; however, rather than possessing a sharp edge on the inner curvature that tends to cut tissue as the needle is passed, it has a flat inner curvature with an edge along the outer curvature of the needle point and shaft. A tapercut needle combines the cutting point with a round shaft. The cutting point readily penetrates tough tissue, but the shaft does not cut through or enlarge the needle hole when passed. This needle is indicated when ease of penetration is important or when a delicate tissue is sutured to a denser one, such as urethra to skin closure for a urethrostomy. Taper-point or round needles have no edges to cut through tissue. They are used for suturing easily penetrated tissues such as muscle, viscera, or subcutaneous tissue. Blunt-point taper needles have a rounded point and do not cut tissue. They are most useful for suturing soft parenchymal organs such as the liver or kidney.

Suggested Readings

Beardsley SL, Smeak DD, et al. Histologic evaluation of tissue reactivity and absorption in response to a new synthetic fluorescent pigmented polypropylene suture material in rats. Am J Vet Res 1995;56:1246–1251.

Bellenger CR. Sutures. Part 1. The purpose of sutures and available suture materials. Compend Contin Educ Pract Vet 1982; 4:507–515.

Bellenger CR. Sutures. Part 2. The use of sutures and alternative methods of closure. Compend Contin Educ Pract Vet 1982; 4:587–600.

Bezwada RS, et al. Monocryl, a new ultra-pliable absorbable monofilament suture. (In press)[3]

Boothe HW. Suture materials and tissue adhesives. In: Slatter DH, ed. Textbook of small animal surgery. Philadelphia: WB Saunders, 1985:334–344.

Bourne RB. In vivo comparison of four absorbable sutures: Vicryl, Dexon Plus, Maxon and PDS. Can J Surg 1988;31:43–45.

Canarelli JP, Ricard J, Collet LM, et al. Use of fast absorption material for skin closure in young children. Int Surg 1988;73:151–152.

Chu CC. Mechanical properties of suture materials: an important characterization. Ann Surg 1981;193:365–371.

Crane SW. Characteristics and selection of currently available suture materials. In: Bojrab MJ, ed. Current techniques in small animal surgery. 2nd ed. Philadelphia: Lea & Febiger, 1983:3–6.

Edlich RF, Panek PH, Rodeheaver GT, et al. Physical and chemical configuration of sutures in the development of surgical infection. Ann Surg 1973;177:679–687.

Katz AR, Mukherjee DP, Kaganov AL, et al. A new synthetic monofilament absorbable suture material from polytrimethylene carbonate. Surg Gynecol Obstet 1985;161:213–217.

Peacock EE. Wound repair. 3rd ed. Philadelphia: WB Saunders, 1984.

Ray JA, Doddi N, Regula D, et al. Polydioxanone (PDS), a novel monofilament synthetic absorbable suture. Surg Gynecol Obstet 1981;153:497–507.

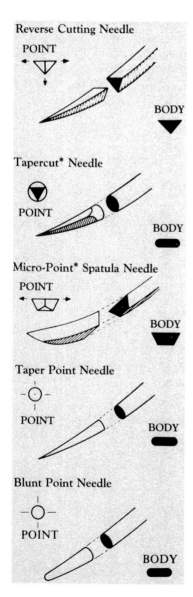

Reverse Cutting Needle
POINT
BODY

Tapercut* Needle
POINT
BODY

Micro-Point* Spatula Needle
POINT
BODY

Taper Point Needle
POINT
BODY

Blunt Point Needle
POINT
BODY

Fig. 2.1. Needle points. (From Jochen RF, ed. Veterinary surgical sutures. Washington Crossing, NJ: Pitman-Moore, no date.)

Smeak DD, Wendelberg KL. Choosing suture materials for use in contaminated or infected wounds. Compend Contin Educ Pract Vet 1989;11:467–478.

Stashak TS, Yturraspe DJ. Considerations for selection of suture materials. Vet Surg 1978;7:48–55.

Taylor, TL. Suture material: a comprehensive review of the literature. J Am Podiatr Assoc 1975;65:649–661.

Van Winkle W, Hastings JC. Considerations in the choice of suture material for various tissues. Surg Gynecol Obstet 1972;135:113–126.

⦁ 3 ⦁

BANDAGING AND DRAINAGE TECHNIQUES

Bandaging Open Wounds

M. Stacie Scardino & Steven F. Swaim

Wounds that are large, have extensive tissue damage, and are either contaminated or infected commonly are managed as open wounds until delayed primary or secondary closure can be performed. Other wounds of this type are managed as open wounds throughout their entire healing process. The proper use of bandages and medications helps to provide an optimal environment for development of tissue healthy enough to allow wound closure. These techniques also supply such an environment for rapid progression of contraction and epithelialization of wounds that will heal by second intention.

Bandage Components

A bandage consists of three layers, each of which has distinctive characteristics and functions (Fig. 3.1).

Primary (Contact) Layer

The primary (contact) layer of a bandage should be sterile and should remain in close contact with the wound surface while the animal is resting or moving. This layer should conform to all contours of a wound and, other than occlusive bandages, should allow fluid from draining wounds to pass through to the absorbent, secondary bandage layer. Depending on the wound type and stage of healing, the primary (contact) layer can function in debriding tissue, in delivering medication, in transmitting wound exudate, or in forming an occlusive seal over the wound. If it is necessary for the primary layer to adhere to the wound surface, this layer should be composed of a wide-mesh dressing material. If nonadherence to the wound is desired, a properly prepared narrow-mesh material or a commercial nonadherent or occlusive bandage is required to prevent granulation tissue and epithelium from invading this layer as healing occurs.

Secondary (Intermediate) Layer

Removal of bacteria, exudate, and debris from a wound by wound debridement, lavage, and chemotherapeutics greatly facilitates wound healing. Bandages can assist in this process by absorbing deleterious agents and removing them from a wound. Absorption of serum, blood, exudate, necrotic debris, and bacteria occurs within the secondary bandage layer. If a bandage allows evaporation of fluid (drying), then the exudate becomes concentrated, retarding bacterial growth.

The frequency of bandage changes depends on the volume of wound discharge and the storage capacity of the absorptive layer. Thus, wounds in the early stages of healing usually require more frequent bandage changes. It is important to change the bandage before the intermediate layer becomes completely saturated. If the outer bandage becomes wet, contamination by exogenous bacteria can occur. The secondary bandage layer (Sof-Band Bulky Bandage, Johnson & Johnson, New Brunswick, NJ; Kerlix rolls, Kendall Co., Mansfield, MA) should have a random pattern of fibers to provide maximum capillarity and absorption. The secondary layer should be applied thickly enough

27

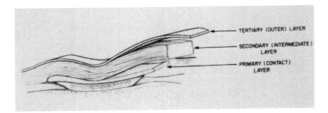

Fig. 3.1. The component layers of a bandage. (From Swaim SF, Wilhalf D. The physics, physiology, and chemistry of bandaging open wounds. Compend Contin Educ 1985;7:146.)

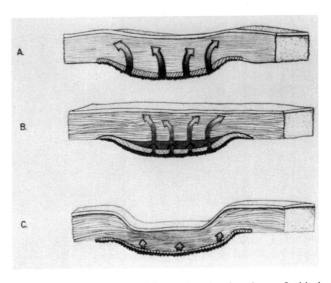

Fig. 3.2. Pressure exerted by tertiary bandage layer. **A.** Ideal pressure. All bandage layers are in contact with each other, and the best absorption takes place. **B.** Too loose. All bandage layers are not in contact with each other and the wound; fluid may accumulate. **C.** Too tight. All bandage layers are compressed, resulting in decreased absorption and possibly reduction in tissue blood supply and wound contraction. (From Swaim SF, Wilhalf D. The physics, physiology, and chemistry of bandaging open wounds. Compend Contin Educ Pract Vet 1985;7:146.)

to collect absorbed fluid as well as to pad and splint the wound.

Tertiary (Outer) Layer

The tertiary layer of a bandage serves primarily to hold other dressings in place and to immobilize the wounded area, especially when a splint is incorporated in the bandage. Surgical adhesive tape (porous, waterproof, or elastic) is commonly used for veterinary bandaging. Porous tape (Zonas porous tape, Johnson & Johnson, New Brunswick, NJ; Curity adhesive tape, KenVetAnimal Care Group, Ashland, OH) allows fluid evaporation, thus promoting dryness, but if the bandage becomes wet from exogenous fluid, surface bacteria can move inward by capillarity to contaminate the wound. Waterproof tape can protect a wound from exogenous fluid; however, if it is not properly applied, any fluid entering the bandage will be retained. Waterproof tape tends to create an occlusive bandage that may lead to tissue maceration; therefore, it is primarily indicated for wounds that are not producing large amounts of fluid. Elastic adhesive tape (Vetrap bandaging tape, 3M Co., St. Paul, MN; Conform stretch tape, KenVet Animal Care Group, Ashland, OH) provides pressure, conformation, and immobilization. We use porous adhesive tape more often than either elastic or waterproof tape.

If a wound has considerable drainage and absorption is the major function of the bandage, the tertiary layer of the bandage should be placed just tightly enough to hold all layers of the bandage in close contact with each other. An excessively loose bandage, with insufficient contact between the primary and secondary layers, allows fluid to accumulate over the wound, leading to tissue maceration. If the tertiary layer is applied too tightly, it may compress the intermediate layer and reduce absorption, impede tissue blood supply, and impair wound contraction (Fig. 3.2).

The tertiary bandage layer helps to ensure that a limb bandage remains in place. The final piece of adhesive tape is placed half on the bandage and half on the skin to prevent bandage slippage. To help adhere the tape to the skin, a hand is held over the tape for about a minute. The heat from the hand and from the animal's body will help to make the adhesive on the tape adhere better to the animal's skin.

Bandaging Materials and Techniques at Different Stages of Healing

Inflammatory Stage

Contaminated or infected wounds initially should be surgically debrided and lavaged with copious amounts of lavage solution. Debridement can be continued using adherent contact-layer dressings (dry-to-dry or wet-to-wet) or a calcium alginate felt-to-gel dressing (Curasorb, KenVet Animal Care Group, Ashland, OH). The larger interstices of wide-mesh, adherent gauze dressing pads facilitate the incorporation of loose debris, foreign bodies, and necrotic material into the pad; which are then removed when the bandage is changed. Cotton-filled gauze pads should not be used as adherent bandages because they may leave lint residue on tissue that could elicit a foreign body reaction within the healing tissues. Such pads do not effectively absorb tenacious exudates. In general, wounds that have a low-viscosity exudate should be bandaged with a dry-to-dry bandage, whereas wounds with a viscous exudate should be bandaged with a wet-to-dry bandage. Adherent bandages are generally used only during the first 3 to 5 days. After this time, most of the necrotic tissue and debris should have been removed. Staged surgical debridement can be used at each bandage change in conjunction with adherent bandages to remove any necrotic tissue. Felt-to-gel bandages work on a different principle. The gel formed in the wound helps to remove bacteria and debris. Staged debridement may also be used when the bandage is changed.

DRY-TO-DRY BANDAGES
Dry wide-mesh gauze pads are applied as the primary layer on wounds that have loose necrotic tissue, foreign matter, and copious amounts of low-viscosity exudate that does not aggregate. An absorbent secondary layer is placed over the contact layer. To allow for fluid evaporation, porous adhesive tape is placed over the secondary layer.

Necrotic tissue and foreign material adhere well to dry gauze bandages. The bandage should remain in place until both the contact layer and the absorbent secondary layer have absorbed fluid from the wound and the contact layer has subsequently dried and debris has adhered to it. The bandage is then removed (Fig. 3.3). If tissue debris remains physically attached to the wound surface, it should be surgically debrided.

The disadvantages of dry-to-dry dressings are that they may remove viable cells along with necrotic debris and they are painful to remove. Soaking the contact layer with warm saline facilitates bandage removal and reduces pain. Room temperature or body temperature 2% lidocaine without epinephrine may also be used to moisten the gauze in contact with the wound to make removal more comfortable. After waiting a minute or two, the gauze is removed. Sedation may be necessary for some bandage removals. If the bandage is left on a wound too long after the fluid has evaporated

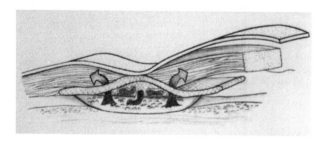

Fig. 3.3. With both dry-to-dry and wet-to-dry bandages, wound exudate is absorbed into the intermediate bandage layers (*arrows*). As exudate is absorbed and the bandage dries, necrotic tissue and foreign material adhere to the contact layer. Exudate, necrotic tissue, and foreign material are removed with the bandage. (From Swaim SF, Wilhalf D. The physics, physiology, and chemistry of bandaging open wounds. Compend Contin Educ Pract Vet 1985;7:146.)

from it, the dry environment may be detrimental to the healing tissue. These bandages should be changed every 24 hours.

WET-TO-DRY BANDAGES
Wide-mesh gauze pads moistened with sterile physiologic saline or an antiseptic solution (e.g., 1:40 chlorhexidine diacetate, Nolvasan-S, Ft. Dodge Co., Ft. Dodge, IA; ChlorhexiDerm Disinfectant, D.V.M. Pharmaceuticals, Miami, FL) are applied to wounds that have loose necrotic tissue, foreign matter, and a viscous exudate. Warming the wetting solution in a microwave oven makes bandage application more comfortable for the animal. An absorbent secondary layer is placed over the wet primary layer, and porous adhesive tape is placed over the secondary layer to allow fluid to evaporate.

The fluid in the primary bandage dilutes the viscous exudate, thus allowing it to be absorbed into the secondary layer. As the bandage dries, necrotic tissue and foreign material adhere to the gauze pad and are removed with the bandage (see Fig. 3.3).

As with dry-to-dry bandages, tissue damage and pain may be associated with removal of wet-to-dry dressings. Warm saline or lidocaine may also be used when changing wet-to-dry bandages. If a wet-to-dry bandage remains wet too long, bacterial growth is enhanced; a prolonged wet environment also macerates the wound tissues. A wet dressing allows bacteria to move peripherally by capillary action, but if a bandage is too wet and fluid reaches the outer layer of a porous bandage, environmental bacteria can move toward the wound.

When changing a dry-to-dry or wet-to-dry bandage, the contact layer does not have to be completely dry at removal to be effective in debridement. Some moisture can and should be present. Dryness is relative, compared with gauze that has just been wet with a wetting solution.

FELT-TO-GEL DRESSINGS
Calcium alginate dressing is a nonwoven, feltlike pad made from calcium alginate, a natural fiber derived from certain seaweed. When placed on a wound, it changes to gel form. It has strong hydrophilic properties and is indicated for moderately to heavily exudative or potentially exudative superficial wounds. When fluid from the wound is absorbed, calcium in the dressing is exchanged for sodium in the wound fluid to form a sodium alginate gel. This gel may entrap bacteria, which are lavaged away with the gel when the bandage is changed. The gel may enhance granulation tissue formation. Calcium alginate should not be used in wounds with exposed muscle, tendon, or bone. If this dressing is placed over a wound that is not pro-

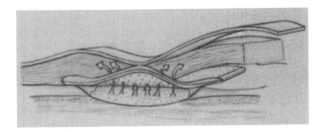

Fig. 3.4. With a nonadherent semiocculsive bandage, the primary layer allows absorption of enough excess fluid to prevent tissue maceration (*longer arrows* penetrating the primary layer) but retains sufficient moisture to prevent dehydration and promote healing (*shorter arrows*). (From Swaim SF, Wilhalf D. The physics, physiology, and chemistry of bandaging open wounds. Compend Contin Educ Pract Vet 1985;7:146.)

ducing sufficient fluid to convert the feltlike pad to a gel, a calcium-alginate eschar may form over the wound that can be more difficult to remove.

Reparative Stage

One technique for bandaging wounds in the reparative stage of healing is to use nonadherent semiocclusive primary bandages. These should be placed on partial-thickness wounds and on full-thickness wounds that are in the reparative stage of healing. This stage is characterized by a healthy bed of granulation tissue, development of epithelial tissue from the wound edges, and serosanguineous exudate. Semiocclusive bandages can keep the wound surface moist while allowing excess fluid to be absorbed into the secondary layer (Fig. 3.4). This helps to maintain an ideal environment for optimal wound healing. Because the bandage material does not adhere to the wound, newly formed reparative tissue is not disturbed when the bandage is changed. These bandages can be prepared from gauzes and medications. In addition, various types of nonadherent semiocclusive bandages are commercially available (Telfa adhesive pads, Kendall Co., Mansfield, MA; Release and Adaptic dressings, Johnson & Johnson, New Brunswick, NJ; Hydrasorb, KenVet Animal Care Group, Ashland, OH), with each manufacturer having a design for rendering the primary layer nonadherent.

Narrow-mesh gauze sponges lightly impregnated with petrolatum can serve as a semiocclusive nonadherent bandage. Such gauzes can be prepared by autoclaving gauze sponges covered with a layer of petrolatum. The petrolatum melts and impregnates the sponges as gravity pulls the petrolatum through the sponges. However, this procedure produces gauzes in which the top layer is lightly impregnated but the bottom layer is heavily impregnated (occlusive). In addition, although petrolatum renders gauzes nonadherent, it has been shown to impair epithelialization.

Impregnation with a bland, nontoxic, nonirritating, water-soluble, hydrophilic agent (e.g., polyethylene glycol) produces nonadherent bandages that do not interfere with epithelialization. In addition, because of their hydrophilic nature, these bandages are more effective than nonhydrophilic dressings in drawing wound fluids up through the contact layer, where they are absorbed into the secondary layer (Fig. 3.5). Polyethylene glycol is used as a base for dermatologic creams and lotions. A commonly used veterinary antibacterial wound management product with a polyethylene glycol base is a nitrofurazone product (EquiPhar, Vetco, St. Joseph, MO).

In addition to the commercially available nonadherent semiocclusive pads, a polyurethane foam sponge material is available as a highly absorbent nonadherent dressing. It absorbs large amounts of fluid while maintaining a moist wound environment. Because of its highly absorbent nature, bandages may not need changing as often, and also because of its high absorbency, this material can be saturated with liquid medications as a means of delivery to these wounds.

OCCLUSIVE DRESSINGS

Occlusive dressings may also be used to treat wounds in the reparative stage of healing. Occlusive hydrocolloid contact bandages are available; we use one particular dressing (Duodorm, Convatec-A, Bristol-Myers Squibb Co., Princeton, NJ). The hydrocolloid surface of the bandage over the wound reacts with the tissue fluid to produce a hydrocolloid gel. Although this gel is tenacious, the moist environment it creates enhances wound epithelialization. The hydrocolloid over the skin surrounding the wound adheres to the skin and thereby can reduce wound contraction. These bandages should be used on wounds in the reparative stage of healing when a good bed of granulation tissue is present and little wound fluid is produced. The bandage can be left in place for 2 to 3 days before it is changed. If the wound tissues or surrounding skin begin to show signs of maceration from retained moisture, this dressing should be discontinued and replaced with a nonadherent semiocclusive dressing.

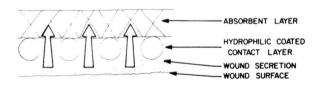

Fig. 3.5. Impregnating the primary layer with a hydrophilic agent increases its capillarity, which enhances transport of wound fluid through the primary layer into the overlying secondary layer. Fluids are not absorbed into the fibers of the primary layer because of its nonadherent character. (From Swaim SF, Wilhalf D. The physics, physiology, and chemistry of bandaging open wounds. Compend Contin Educ Pract Vet 1985;7:146.)

Hydrogel dressings are also available to help enhance epithelialization of wounds with a healthy bed of granulation tissue. One hydrogel dressing material is a thin composite of a hydrophilic polyethylene oxide polymer between two thin synthetic sheets (Bio Dres, Dermatologics in Veterinary Medicine, Miami, FL). Hydrogel absorbs the wound's fluids and turns into a gel without adhering to the surrounding skin. The gel remaining on the wound's surface tends to be less tenacious than the hydrocolloid gel and is easier to clean from the wound. Hydrogel has also been described for use over noninfected eschars to soften and aid in their removal.

PRESSURE BANDAGES

Although pressure bandages occasionally must be applied over open wounds to help control minor hemorrhage, they must be used with caution and for a short period of time. Pressure bandages can help to control wound edema, and they are more effective in controlling passive edema than inflammatory edema. Pressure bandages also help to prevent formation of excess granulation tissue, to obliterate dead space, and to immobilize an injured part.

Unless an elastic material is used to apply tension continuously, it is difficult to maintain pressure on a wound surface by using cotton or linen dressings. When cotton and similar materials are applied as a pressure bandage, they generally become compressed in a short time and thus no longer act as a pressure bandage. However, if cotton and linen do not compress sufficiently to relieve the constricting effect of tightly applied adhesive tape, the result may be circulatory embarrassment of the wound and bandaged structure.

A properly applied pressure bandage made with elastic material tends to keep some dynamic pressure on the wound as the patient moves. Even when an elastic material is used for a pressure bandage, excess pressure can impair arterial, venous, and lymphatic flow and can lead to tissue slough as well as impinging on nerves. Both the client and the veterinarian should observe the animal for swelling, hypothermia, cyanosis, dryness, loss of sensation, or odor in the area distal to a limb pressure bandage. If an animal licks or chews a pressure bandage, the bandage should be removed and the area should be examined.

Pressure caused by an elastic pressure bandage depends on the tension applied at the time of bandage application, the number of layers in the bandage, the degree of overlap among successive wraps, and the circumference of the bandaged body part. The smaller the circumference, the more pressure is applied, and the greater is the chance of circulatory compromise. Therefore, care should be taken when moving from an area of large circumference to one of smaller circumference while bandaging.

PRESSURE-RELIEF BANDAGES

The shape of the bandaged surface also has an effect on pressure exerted by the dressing on the tissue. The more convex the surface, the greater is the pressure exerted by the dressing on the tissue. Adding more gauze padding over a convex surface makes it even more convex. This can be detrimental when treating an open wound over a convex surface. Placing more padding over the wound in an attempt to protect it from pressure has the effect of increasing the pressure and impairing healing. Pressure-relief bandages are indicated for bandaging such areas.

Donut-shaped bandages may be used to relieve pressure over bony prominences. Donut-shaped bandages are made by rolling and taping some towels together and then forming them into a ring large enough to encircle the defect. The ring is then taped over the wound so the wound is within the "donut hole" (Fig. 3.6). These bandages are effective over bony prominences on the lower limbs.

Pipe insulation bandages can be used for wounds

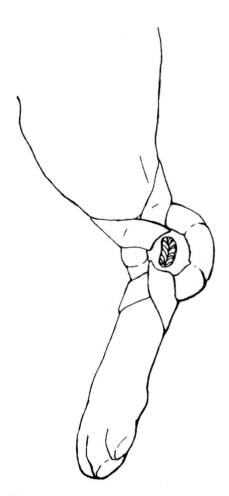

Fig. 3.6. Donut bandage placed over a lateral malleous pressure sore. The donut bandage is made from a rolled and taped towel made into a donut shape that is taped with the hole over the wound.

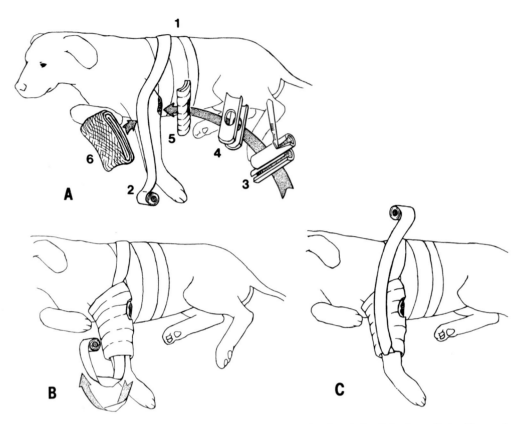

Fig. 3.7. **A.** Steps for putting on a pipe insulation bandage: 1) place a body bandage behind the front limbs; 2) transfer tape from the body bandage onto the limb; 3) split two pieces of pipe insulation; 4) cut holes in the pipe insulation to go over the elbow ulcer and stack the pipe insulation; 5) tape the pipe insulations together and place them over the olecranon wound; 6) put cast padding in front of the elbow area. **B.** Tape the pipe insulation and padding in place. Twist the tape on the limb (*arrow*) so the adhesive side is back against the bandage. **C.** Complete the tape stirrup back onto the body bandage.

over the olecranon. They are made by splitting two pieces of foam rubber pipe insulation lengthwise, cutting a hole large enough to go around the lesion in each piece, and then stacking and taping the pieces together. The cranial aspect of the radial–humeral area is *well* padded with cast padding before taping the pipe insulation bandage in place with the hole over the olecranon. Such padding helps to keep the dog from flexing the joint to position itself in sternal recumbency to place pressure on the olecranon area. It may be difficult to secure the bandage to keep it from slipping distally on the limb, especially on an obese dog that has a short segment of limb proximal to the radial–humeral articulation to which the bandage can be affixed. Affixing the pipe insulation bandage to a body bandage may be necessary to hold the pipe insulation bandage in place. A body bandage is placed just caudal to the forelimbs. A strip of 2-inch adhesive tape is placed, adhesive side down, on this bandage from the dorsal area well down onto the forelimb. The roll of tape is left on the strip. The padding and pipe insulation bandage are placed and taped over the radial–humeral area. The previously placed strip of adhesive tape is twisted at the base of this bandage so the adhe-

sive side faces outward. The tape is then placed adhesive side against the bandage and is taken back onto the body bandage over the animal's dorsum. This forms a "stirrup" to hold the pipe insulation bandage in place (Fig. 3.7). No pressure is on the wound, and medications can be applied to the wound through the holes in the pipe insulation.

Splints may also be used on the cranial surface of the forelimb to immobilize the radial–humeral joint in extension and to prevent pressure on wounds over the olecranon. A routine bandage wrap is placed around the radial–humeral area; then a section of aluminum splint rod is used to fashion a loop-type splint, which is incorporated into the front of the bandage (Fig. 3.8**A** and **B**). Another type of splint is a prefabricated padded fiberglass splint, which is placed and molded over the front of the limb. It extends from the midhumeral-level to below the carpus and is held in place with a secondary wrap and adhesive tape (Fig. 3.8**C**).

The pipe insulation bandage, splint rod loop bandage, and fiberglass splint bandage are also effective in keeping pressure off wounds on the sternum because they prevent elbow flexion and keep the animal

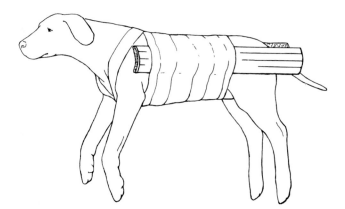

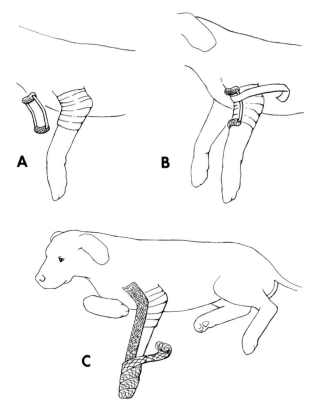

Fig. 3.8. **A** and **B.** Applying an aluminum rod loop-type splint in the front of an elbow bandage. **C.** Placing a splint in the cranial aspect of an elbow bandage to keep the elbow from bending, and wrapping the splint on front of limb with a secondary wrap.

Fig. 3.9. Aluminum-padded side splints are taped on either side of a body bandage. They extend behind the ischiatic area to keep a dog from attaining a sitting posture to put pressure on the ischiatic area.

out of sternal recumbency. A pressure-relief bandage for wounds (i.e., decubital ulcers) over the ischiatic tuberosities is composed of a body bandage with padded aluminum splints taped to either side of the bandage. These splints extend behind the dog and prevent it from attaining a sitting posture to place pressure on the ischiatic area (Fig. 3.9).

Mobilization Versus Immobilization

Whether a wound should be mobilized or immobilized during healing is controversial. The location and type of wound and the stage of wound healing are important factors in deciding whether to mobilize or immobilize a wound.

Maintaining mobility of wounds has been considered to minimize negative nitrogen balance of the tissues, to stimulate circulation, to help combat infection, and to allow movement that loosens adhesions. Mobility can also provide massage for better wound drainage and can prevent joint stiffness and osteoporosis.

Other arguments favor wound immobilization to enhance healing. An immobilizing bandage is needed for wounds with underlying orthopedic damage. In addition to providing orthopedic support, wound im-

mobilization may allow better healing over the olecranon, the calcaneal tuber, the flexor surface of the cubital and tarsal joints, and the popliteal area. Immobilization may also increase tissue resistance to bacterial growth and decrease the probability of infection and its spread by the lymphatics and tissue planes. Other factors favoring immobilization include patient comfort and support of the tissues during collagen synthesis. Wound immobilization also helps to prevent the dislodgment of fragile clots, ruptures of new capillaries, and disruption of new fibrin. In addition, immobilization prevents tension on repaired structures (e.g., muscle, tendons, and ligaments).

Pressure bandages help to immobilize wounds and casts; and splints also immobilize wounded limbs. Casts should be applied so swelling can be accommodated as well as controlled. Splitting a cast longitudinally on both sides allows for swelling and makes dressing changes possible. Application of half of the cast to the side of the limb opposite the wound can be used for immobilization. Such a half cast can act as a point of counterpressure when a pressure bandage is required. It can be applied so the dressing can be changed without affecting immobilization. Incorporating a Mason metasplint into a bandage placed on a lower limb is an example of this type of immobilization.

Wounds over extension surfaces and flexion surfaces of joints benefit from immobilization during healing. Because flexion of a joint tends to pull wound edges apart on the extensor surface of the joint, immobilization is indicated for such wounds. Large wounds over flexion surfaces of joints can benefit from early reconstructive surgery to help prevent wound contracture deformity of the joint. When large wounds over flexion surfaces are to be allowed to heal as open wounds, joint immobilization in extension is particularly important to help prevent contracture deformity. Another specific area where wound immobilization is indicated is the axillary region. Shearing and tension forces in this area as the forelimb moves interfere with wound healing. Reconstructive surgery and immobilization in a Velpeau bandage are needed for wound healing.

Suggested Readings

Bojrab MJ. Wound management. Mod Vet Pract 1982;63:867.

Bojrab MJ. A handbook on veterinary wound management. Ashland, OH: KenVet Prof Vet Co, 1994.

Lee AH, Swaim SF, McGuire JA. The effects of nonadherent bandage materials on the healing of open wounds in dogs. J Am Vet Med Assoc 1987;190:416.

Lee AH, Swaim SF, Yang ST. The effects of petrolatum, polyethylene glycol, nitrofurazone and a hydroactive dressing on open wound healing. J Am Anim Hosp Assoc 1986;22:443.

Morgan PW, Binnington AG, Miller CW, et al. The effect of occlusive and semiocclusive dressings on the healing of full-thickness skin wounds on the forelimbs of dogs. Vet Surg 1995;23:494.

Noe JM, Kalish S. Dressing materials and their selection. In: Rudolph R, Noe JM, eds. Chronic problem wounds. Boston: Little, Brown, 1983.

Ramsey DT, Pope ER, Wagner-Mann C, et al. Effects of three occlusive dressing materials on healing of full-thickness skin wounds in dogs. Am J Vet Res 1995;56:7.

Rudolph R, Noe JM. Initial treatment of the chronic wound. In: Rudolph R, Noe JM, eds. Chronic problem wounds. Boston: Little, Brown, 1983.

Swaim SF. Surgery of traumatized skin: management and reconstruction in the dog and cat. Philadelphia: WB Saunders, 1980.

Swaim SF. The effects of dressings and bandages on wound healing. Semin Vet Med Surg Sm Anim 1989;4:274.

Swaim SF. Bandages and topical agents. Vet Clin North Am 1990;20:47.

Swaim SF. Bandaging techniques. In: Bistner SI, Ford RB, eds. Handbook of veterinary procedures and emergency treatment. 6th ed. Philadelphia: WB Saunders, 1995.

Swaim SF, Henderson RA. Small animal wound management. 2nd ed. Baltimore: Williams & Wilkins, 1997.

Swaim SF, Wilhalf D. The physics, physiology, and chemistry of bandaging open wounds. Compend Contin Educ Pract Vet 1985;7:146.

Wound Drainage Techniques

M. Stacie Scardino, Steven F. Swaim &
Alice H. Lee

Indications

Although wounds drain best when left open, often they must be closed before they have drained completely. In general, wounds must be drained 1) when an abscess cavity exists, 2) when foreign material or tissue of questionable viability that cannot be excised is present, 3) when massive contamination is inevitable (e.g., wounds in the anal area), and 4) when it is necessary to obliterate dead space to prevent the accumulation of air, blood, exudate, or serum. More specifically,

wound drainage in veterinary surgery is used in the management of dog bite wounds with separation of the dermis from underlying tissue, lacerations with loose skin, mastectomy and lumpectomy sites, large excision wounds, seromas, auricular hematomas, elbow and ischial hygromas, and cat bite wounds.

Types of Drains and Drain Techniques

Materials used for wound drains should be relatively soft, nonreactive, and radiopaque. Flat drains such as Penrose drains are made of soft, thin latex rubber material shaped cylindrically. Tube drains are composed of rubber or plastic tubes or catheters with thicker walls that are not as easily collapsed as flat drains. Multilumen drains are a combination of drain tubes that allows fluid to drain from a wound through one lumen while allowing air or lavage fluids to enter the wound by another lumen.

Drains are classified as passive or active. Passive drains can be single-lumen flat drains, tubular drains, or multilumen drains. These drains function by pressure differentials, overflow, and gravity. Active wound drainage occurs when an external vacuum is applied to the end of a drain tube. Active drains may or may not be open to the atmosphere.

Passive Drains

FLAT DRAINS (PENROSE DRAINS)

Penrose drains are thin-walled rubber tubes available from $\frac{1}{4}$ to 2 inches in diameter and from 12 to 36 inches in length. The mechanical action of these drains depends on capillary action and gravity, because they provide a path of least resistance to the outside. Fenestrating a drain is not advised because drainage is related to surface area and fenestrating the drain reduces the surface area. Penrose drains allow egress of foreign material from the wound. Dead space is obliterated as fluid is drained and normal healing tissue fills the potential space.

Penrose drains are easily sterilized, are readily available, and cause little foreign body reaction. However, the latex causes the earlier formation of a fibrous tract in the tissue, a property that makes it good for draining abscesses because this tract between the abscess cavity and the skin is desirable for better drainage. Because they are soft and malleable, these drains do not exert undue pressure on adjacent blood vessels or other structures.

Single-Exit Drains

Penrose drains can be placed with one end of the drain emerging at the distal aspect of the wound. In preparation for placing such a drain, the hair around the area

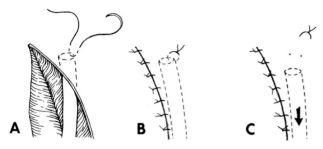

Fig. 3.10. Tacking a drain in the proximal aspect of a wound. **A.** The drain is placed off to one side of the wound, and a simple interrupted anchor suture is placed through skin, drain, and skin again. **B.** The wound is closed and the anchor suture is tied. **C.** When the drain is removed, the anchor suture is cut and the drain is pulled out.

where the drain will exit should be clipped liberally. The length of drain placed in a wound should be recorded for comparison with the length that is removed. The proximal end of the drain should be placed in the most proximal aspect of the wound and off to one side of the wound before wound closure. The preferred technique for fixing the drain in the proximal aspect of the wound is to pass a nonabsorbable suture through the skin and the drain and to tie it outside the skin. This suture is removed before the drain is removed (Fig. 3.10).

When the drain is placed in the wound, it should run as vertically as possible, and placement next to large vessels should be avoided. A drain should never emerge through the distal end of the suture line; instead, an incision is made in the skin ventral to the ventral aspect of the wound. A pair of hemostatic forceps can be used to make a tunnel just under the skin

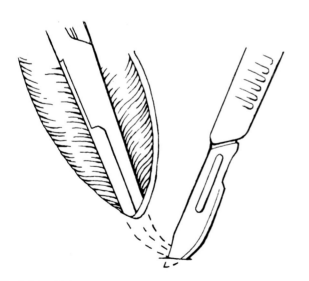

Fig. 3.11. Making a subcutaneous tunnel at the distal end of the wound with the tips of forceps. A scapel blade is used to incise the skin over the forceps tips to create a drain emergence site.

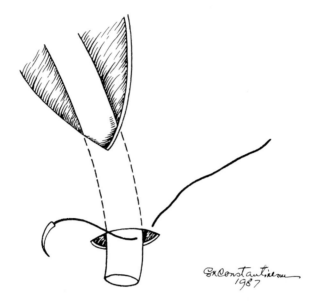

Fig. 3.12. Placing and anchoring a drain distally. The drain exits through a hole distal to the wound. The exit hole is large enough to allow drainage around the drain. A simple interrupted nonabsorbable suture is placed through the skin and drain at the drain's exit hole.

for the drain to exit at this incision (Fig. 3.11). The exit incision should be large enough to allow drainage around the drain, usually one and one-half to two-times the width of the drain. A tacking suture placed through the drain and skin where the drain emerges further secures the drain and prevents it from retracting into the wound (Fig. 3.12). As the wound is closed, contact between the drain and the skin suture line should be avoided. This goal can be accomplished by suturing subcutaneous tissue over the drain or directing the drain so it does not lie under the suture line. Care should be taken to avoid incorporating the drain into any sutures as they are placed. If the drain is incorporated into a skin suture, it cannot be removed until the sutures are removed. If a drain is incorporated into a subcuticular suture, its removal is definitely complicated.

When a wound that is already closed (e.g., an unruptured abscess) requires drainage, a long-bladed instrument, such as Doyen intestinal forceps, can be used to place the proximal end of the drain in the depths of the wound through a stab incision near the distal aspect of the wound. The tip of the forceps is used as a palpable landmark to pass a simple interrupted suture through the skin, into the drain, and back out through the skin. The suture is tied to anchor the drain in the proximal aspect of the wound.

Penrose drains can be used to drain deep wounds; however, care should be taken that an adequate pathway is created from the deep pocket to the skin surface to provide drainage. An open approach is usually made

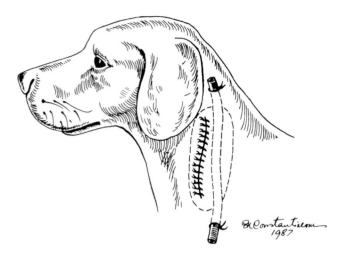

Fig. 3.13. A drain can exit at both proximal and distal aspects of a wound. The drain is anchored to the skin at both exit holes. (From Swaim SF. Surgery of traumatized skin: management and reconstruction in the dog and cat. Philadelphia: WB Saunders, 1980:159.)

to the deep wound to allow debridement, lavage, culture, and biopsy. Apposition of the tissues overlying the deep pocket is usually sufficient to hold the drain in place. The usual principles for exiting the drain distal to the open wound are followed.

Drains should be covered with sterile absorbent dressings to absorb wound fluid and to prevent external contamination. Bandages also help to prevent wound molestation. The bandage should be changed frequently to remove fluid from the wound area. The area around the exit drain should be cleaned at bandage change. Care should be taken that ointments and creams are not applied so thickly around the drain exit that drainage is obstructed. Inspection of the bandage reveals the nature and amount of drainage, to determine how long a drain should remain in place.

Double-Exit Drains
Penrose drains can also be placed with one end emerging above the proximal limit of the wound and the other end emerging below the distal end of the wound. Simple interrupted sutures are placed through the skin and drain at the points of emergence to prevent the drains from retracting into the wound (Fig. 3.13). Double-exit drains can be advantageous if the wound is to be flushed with an antibiotic or antiseptic. They are usually used in heavily contaminated or infected wounds. Lavaging the wound from the proximal tube emergence site exposes the wound tract to the solution, although the lavage solution may merely follow the path of least resistance, the drain tract, and not reach the crevices of the wound. Moreover, if pressure is applied to the lavage solution or if the distal drain

opening is occluded, the lavage solution can spread wound debris into normal tissue by hydrostatic pressure.

Another use for double-exit drains is when considerable subcutaneous dead space across the dorsum of an animal extends down along the sides of the trunk. A drain can be placed from the most dependent area of dead space on one side, across the dorsum of the animal to a like area on the opposite side. Thus, the drain passes subcutaneously across the animal's back with an exit on each side to provide drainage.

Cigarette Drains and Strip Drains
Cigarette drains are Penrose drains with gauze inside. The gauze increases capillary action and provides more bulk for faster and greater drainage. These drains are favored for rapid drainage of large abscesses. A thin strip of latex can be cut from a ¼-inch–diameter Penrose drain and used as a narrow flat drain to drain small wounds when an entire ¼-inch–diameter Penrose drain would be too large.

TUBE DRAINS
Rubber or plastic tubes and catheters of various diameters and designs can be used as tube drains. These cylindric tubes have a thicker wall than flat drains. They have a single lumen with or without small or large side holes. If the surgeon desires additional side holes, they should be cut in an oval and should be no more than one-third the diameter of the drain, to prevent kinking of the drain. The basic mechanism of action and the principle of application of tube drains are similar to those of flat drains.

Fenestrated tube drains can drain from both inside and outside the lumen, and they can be connected to a suction apparatus for use with a closed collection system. These tubes also allow irrigation through the drain. They are not expensive, and they are readily available. Plastic tube drains may cause less tissue reaction than rubber tube drains. One disadvantage of tube drains is that their stiffness can cause the patient postoperative discomfort. These drains may become obstructed by debris, necessitating flushing to clear them.

Active Drains

OPEN-SUCTION DRAINS
When a vacuum is applied to one lumen of a multilumen drain, fluid is removed from the wound as air enters the wound through another drain lumen as a sump drain. Although the procedure reduces the drainage time, we do not use it because the increased volume of environmental air drawn into the wound increases the chance of bacterial infection and can be traumatic to the tissues. Bacterial filters can be fitted to the air intake to help decrease contamination.

CLOSED-SUCTION DRAINS

Closed-suction drainage occurs when a vacuum is applied to a drainage tube that has no external air vent, thus creating a vacuum in the wound. This drainage system facilitates continuous flow and reduces the chance of drainage tube occlusion and the need for wound irrigation. Closed-suction drains do not depend on capillary action or gravity. Closed-suction drains have the same indications as passive drains; however, they work best when no foreign material or necrotic tissue is present, because these could plug the drain holes.

Numerous commercial portable closed-suction drainage systems are available. When taped to the animal in a bandage, these drains provide a portable, continuous, even-pressure, and aseptic closed-suction drainage system. In some of these systems, unless a one-way valve device is included, fluid may reflux back into the wound if the animal lies on or puts pressure on the evacuator. The location of the wound, the size of the animal, and the size of the commercial apparatus should be considered when choosing a commercial closed-suction system; for example, a large, bulky apparatus would not be indicated for use on a small animal.

An inexpensive and simple closed-suction drainage system can be made using a butterfly scalp needle with its extension tube as the drainage tube, and a 5- or 10-mL evacuated blood collection tube to provide suction. The syringe adapter of the butterfly scalp needle is cut off the tubing, and holes are cut into the sides of the tubing for a length a little shorter than the length of

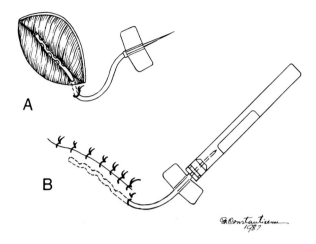

Fig. 3.15. Placement of a closed-suction drain in a wound. **A.** The fenestrated portion of the drain is inserted into the wound through a small opening near the distal end of the wound. The tube is secured to the skin with a simple interrupted nonabsorbable suture. **B.** The wound is closed. The needle on the tube is inserted into a 5- or 10-mL evacuated blood collection tube.

the wound (Fig. 3.14). The fenestrated portion of the tube is inserted through a small puncture wound near the site to be drained. The puncture wound should be the same diameter as the tube. The tubing is secured to the skin with a nonabsorbable pursestring suture. After the wound is closed, the needle on the free end of the tube is inserted into a standard 5- or 10-mL evacuated blood collection tube (Fig. 3.15). A light bandage into which the collection tube is incorporated is usually all that is necessary. For large wounds, two drain sets may be necessary.

If the drain is placed under a skin graft, the end of the drain should be placed under the skin at the edge of the graft. A simple interrupted tacking suture is placed through the skin, through the tube, and back out through the skin to anchor the end of the drain. This suture, along with the pursestring suture at the drain exit hole, secures the drain under the graft so it does not move to interfere with graft revascularization (Fig. 3.16).

A modification of this closed-suction apparatus involves the use of different sizes of plastic syringes. To prepare the drain tube, the butterfly needle is removed from the catheter, and the catheter is fenestrated. The Luer-Lok is left on the catheter (Fig. 3.17**A**). After the catheter has been placed in the wound and the wound has been closed, a plastic syringe is attached to the Luer-Lok. The plunger is withdrawn enough to create the desired negative pressure without collapsing the drain tubing, and a 16- or 18-gauge needle is used to hold the syringe plunger at the desired level within the syringe barrel (Fig. 3.17**B**). Fixation at different levels creates different negative pressures. A 30-mL

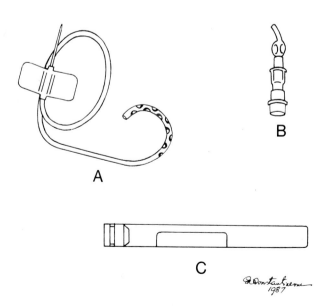

Fig. 3.14. Components of a simple closed-suction drain. **A.** A 19-gauge butterfly catheter with multiple fenestrations. **B.** Luer-Lok attachment that was removed from the catheter. **C.** A 10-mL evacuated glass tube.

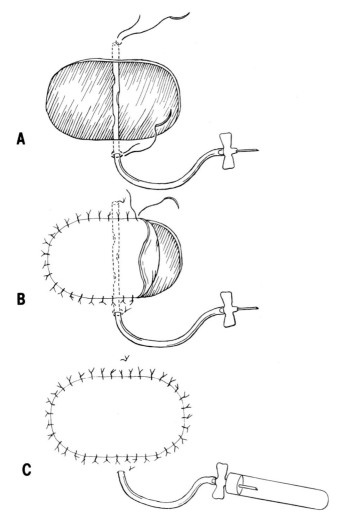

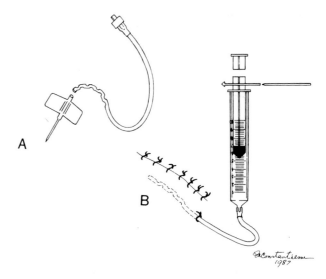

Fig. 3.17. Modified closed-suction drain. **A.** The butterfly needle is removed from the catheter and the catheter is fenestrated. The Luer-Lok is left on the catheter. **B.** A plastic syringe is attached to the Luer-Lok of the catheter. A metal pin is passed through the plunger just above the barrel after the plunger is withdrawn above the desired distance. The end of the plunger can be cut off.

Fig. 3.16. Placement of a closed-suction drain under a skin graft. **A.** A butterfly catheter with the Luer-Lok removed and the end fenestrated is placed across the wound bed before the graft is placed. The proximal end is secured with a simple interrupted suture placed through skin, catheter, and skin again. A pursestring suture is used to secure the distal end of the catheter to the skin. **B.** The graft is sutured into place over the drain. **C.** The needle on the catheter is inserted into a 5- or 10-mL evacuated blood collection tube. (From Swaim SF. Skin grafts. Vet Clin North Am Small Anim Pract 1990;20:147.)

syringe can be used when large amounts of fluid are to be removed.

Closed-suction drains allow wounds and dressings to be kept dry; they help to prevent bacterial ascension through or around the drain; they provide continuous drainage to decrease drainage time; they reduce the need for irrigation; and they have few complications. When used under skin grafts, these drains help to hold the graft in contact with the wound bed, allowing early revascularization and enhanced wound healing. Evacuated blood collection tubes can be changed as often as necessary, and fluid volume can be accurately measured and its nature studied to assess wound infection.

One disadvantage of closed-suction drainage is that high negative pressure can injure the tissue. In addition, although the 10-mL evacuated blood tubes are effective and not cumbersome to incorporate into a bandage, they may need to be changed several times each day in highly productive wounds.

Duration of Drainage

The times for drain removal vary depending on the type of wound drained. A drain should be removed as soon as possible, when the need for it no longer exists. Clinical judgment based on the amount and nature of drainage fluid is the most important factor in deciding when a drain should be removed. In general, a drain placed in a wound to prevent hematoma formation from capillary oozing can be removed within 24 hours. A drain used for an infection, such as an abscess, should be removed in 3 to 5 days, when the infection is controlled. For hygromas and large seromas, removal of the drain is in 10 to 14 days; for severe bite wounds, 4 to 6 days; and for mastectomies, 4 days.

Absorbent bandage material should be placed over a passive drain to give some indication of when the drain should be removed and to protect the wound and drain from being molested by the animal. The amount and nature of the drainage in the bandage can be observed at the time of daily dressing changes. The discharge should progress from exudative to more transudative, and it should diminish as healing progresses. Usually, when the discharge has decreased to a small amount and its nature and volume remain about the same from one bandage change to the next, the drain can be removed.

Complications and Failures

Failure to secure a drain to the skin or to protect it from molestation can result in removal of a drain before it has accomplished its purpose, slippage back into the wound, or breaking off in the wound. If strong adhesions form around a drain, the drain may break when being removed, leaving a portion in the wound. Use of drains can cause wound infection because of decreased local tissue resistance and infection ascending around the drain with bacterial proliferation in the area. Drains placed in some areas (e.g., axillary or inguinal areas) may allow air to be sucked into the wound as tissues move. This can result in subcutaneous emphysema. Surgeons should not rely on drains rather than good surgical technique to manage wounds, nor

should they give in to the temptation to close and drain areas that wound be better left open.

Suggested Readings

Fox JW, Golden GT. The use of drains in subcutaneous surgical procedures. Am J Surg 1976;132:673.

Hampel NL. Surgical drains. In: Harari J, ed. Surgical complications and wound healing in the small animal practice. Philadelphia: WB Saunders, 1993.

Hampel NL, Johnson RG. Principles of surgical drains and drainage. J Am Anim Hosp Assoc 1985;21:21.

Lee AH, Swaim SF, Henderson RA. Surgical drainage. Compend Contin Educ Pract Vet 1986;8:94.

Moss JP. Historical and current perspectives on surgical drainage. Surg Gynecol Obstet 1981;152:517.

Pope ER, Swaim SF. Wound drainage from under full-thickness skin grafts in dogs. Part I. Quantitative evaluation of four techniques. Vet Surg 1986;15:65.

Roush JK. Use and misuse of drains in surgical practice. Probl Vet Med 1990;2:482.

Swaim SF. Surgery of traumatized skin: management and reconstruction in the dog and cat. Philadelphia: WB Saunders, 1980:157–160.

Swaim SF, Henderson RA. Small animal wound management. 2nd ed. Baltimore: Williams & Wilkins, 1997.

4

ELECTROSURGERY AND LASER SURGERY

Electrosurgical Techniques

Robert B. Parker

Electrosurgical units are probably among the most frequently used and least understood surgical instruments. Little information is available in the veterinary literature concerning basic electronics, proper surgical techniques, and potential hazards. Judicious use of electrosurgery can be of great benefit to the veterinarian in maintaining a bloodless surgical field, but indiscriminate use can create serious complications. The following discussion describes available electrosurgical methods and apparatus and provides a guideline for their proper use.

Electrolysis

Electrolysis implies a unidirectional, direct-current flow that produces strong polarity in the anode and cathode (Fig. 4.1). The system is of low voltage and amperage. When the electrodes are inserted into the body, hydroxides are produced at the treatment cathode by the following formula:

$$2 \text{ NaCl} + 4 \text{ H}_2\text{O} \longrightarrow 2 \text{ NaOH} + 2 \text{ H}_2 \text{ (cathode)}$$
$$\searrow 2 \text{ HCl} + \text{O}_2 \text{ (anode)}$$

The hydroxides liquefy tissue, yet produce minimal discomfort.

Electroepilation has been used in ophthalmic surgery for treatment of ectopic cilia or distichiasis. The fine-cathode electrode is passed to the base of the cilia, where the current and hydroxides liquefy and destroy the ciliary root.

Electrocautery

The use of cautery to control hemorrhage dates back to ancient times, when a hot iron was used to cauterize wounds. More sophisticated microcautery is now available, but the technique of direct heat application is the same.

Low-voltage current is used to heat the treatment electrode, and therefore, electrical energy does not pass through the body (Fig. 4.2). The destructive effect is heat coagulation, and the temperature is proportional to the intensity of the current flowing through the resistance of the tip.

Advantages of this technique are that 1) the degree of tissue damage is apparent, 2) it coagulates well in a bloody field, and 3) it is inexpensive and simple. The disadvantages are that 1) tissue destruction can be extensive and 2) large lesions are slowly destroyed.

Electrocautery units are generally reserved for minor surgical procedures, such as dewclaw or tail removal in puppies. Disposable electrocautery units, frequently used in ophthalmic surgery, provide fine hemostasis by pinpoint heat application (Fig. 4.3).

High-Frequency Electrosurgery

Most electrosurgical units available today fall into this category. The unit is essentially a radio transmitter that produces an oscillating high-frequency electrical field of 500,000 to 100,000,000 hertz (cycles per second). Above 10,000 hertz, current can be passed through

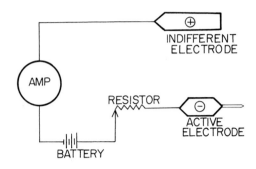

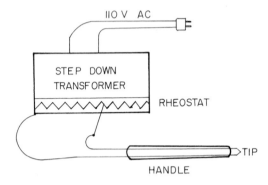

Fig. 4.1. Basic circuit diagram for an electrolysis unit.

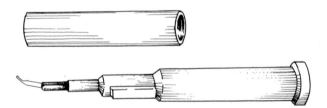

Fig. 4.2. Basic circuit diagram for a thermal electrocautery unit.

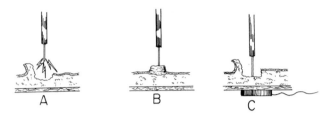

Fig. 4.4. Uniterminal techniques, electrofulguration (**A**) and electrodesiccation (**B**). Biterminal techniques, electrotomy and electrocoagulation (**C**).

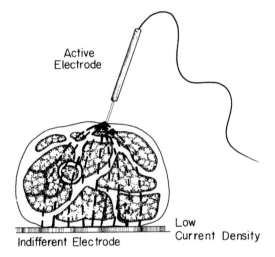

Fig. 4.5. High current density at the active electrode and low current density with a properly placed indifferent electrode.

Fig. 4.3. Disposable electrocautery unit.

the body without pain or muscle contraction. In contrast to electrocautery, the treatment electrode is not hot, but serves to deliver electrical energy at a concentrated area. The electrosurgical effect is determined by 1) the tissue resistance, 2) the mode of application, and 3) the amount and type of current. These factors can be modified to produce the desired surgical response.

Body tissue and fluids have a definite electrical impedance or resistance. Heat is produced by the resistance to current flow as electrical energy is absorbed and converted to thermal energy. Because resistance is inversely proportional to surface area, resistance decreases as the current spreads over the body.

The mode of application can be either uniterminal or biterminal. Biterminal application, used most frequently with cutting or coagulation, implies the use of an indifferent electrode or "ground plate" (Fig. 4.4). The indifferent electrode collects the current when it has passed through the body and dissipates it over a

large surface area to produce a low-current density. Because heat production is inversely proportional to the contact area, the large size of the indifferent electrode evenly distributes the heat to prevent burning. The active electrode concentrates the same energy at a small point and produces the surgical effect (Fig. 4.5).

With the uniterminal technique, the patient is not incorporated into the electrical circuit. An indifferent electrode is not used, and the electrical energy is absorbed by the patient and is radiated into the air. Thus, sparking is produced at the tip and is directly applied to the lesion to cause either fulguration or desiccation (see Fig. 4.4).

Most modern electrosurgical units provide different waveforms to bring about either cutting or coagulation. An undamped, continuous sine wave makes the most effective cutting current (Fig. 4.6). Little hemostasis is achieved with a pure sine wave. In older units, a triode vacuum tube was used to produce the sine wave, but newer solid-state units use electronic circuitry to yield a more refined current. A series of damped or interrupted waves achieve coagulation with limited cutting capability (Fig. 4.7). Blended currents are possible, and produce a combined cutting and coagulation mode (Fig. 4.8). The more expensive

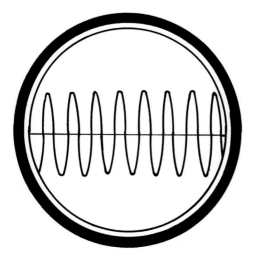

Fig. 4.6. Undamped, continuous sine (cutting) waves.

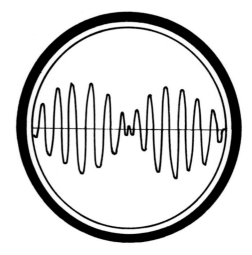

Fig. 4.8. Blended (combined cutting and coagulation) waves.

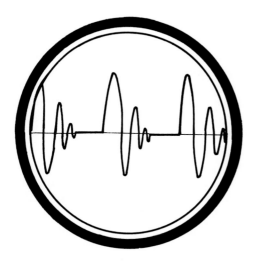

Fig. 4.7. Damped (coagulation) waves.

units are capable of varying the "on-to-off" time to accomplish degrees of cutting versus coagulation.

Surgical Techniques

These techniques include electrotomy, electrocoagulation, and electrofulguration and electrodesiccation.

Electrotomy

Electroincision of any tissue causes greater tissue damage than sharp incision; therefore, the veterinarian must weigh the advantages of reduced blood loss and operating time against the disadvantages of increased tissue destruction and healing time. Electroincision of the skin heals primarily, but a definite lag is seen in the ultimate healing of the wound. Healing does occur, however, and maximal breaking strength is achieved.

The primary indications for electroincision of the skin are in patients with clotting disorders or when anticoagulant treatment is anticipated, such as with cardiopulmonary bypass procedures. Because of the initial delay in wound healing, it is recommended that

skin sutures remain approximately 2 to 3 days longer with a skin incision made with an electrosurgical unit. The amount of coagulation and necrosis is proportional to the amount of heat produced and its duration of contact. Therefore, it is best to use a smooth, swift stroke when using an electrosurgical scalpel.

The high frequency electrosurgery units such as the Ellman Surgitron (Ellman International, Hewlett, NY) cause no more tissue destruction than traditional cold scalpel surgery if used in the pure cutting mode.

An electrosurgical scalpel has been used to cut virtually every type of tissue; its use in division of muscle or other highly vascular tissue is generally accepted procedure. By using blended currents, muscular tissue can be divided with less blood loss and in less operating time. The small blood vessels traversing muscular tissue can be effectively coagulated without the necessity of using ligatures that are difficult to place unless one includes significant amounts of normal tissue. With electrotomy of muscular tissues, particular attention should be made to large vessels; they can be incompletely coagulated, may retract, and may form a hematoma. If muscle twitching is a problem, one should tense the muscle between one's fingers to facilitate transection.

Although I do not routinely use them, electrosurgical scalpels and loops have been advocated for performing tonsillectomies, uvulectomies, ventriculocordectomies, anal sacculectomies, and skin tumor resections.

Electrocoagulation

The electrosurgical apparatus is extremely useful for coagulation of small bleeding vessels. A damped wave pattern provides the ultimate current for coagulation. Proper technique is required, and the technique of "frying tissue until it pops" is to be avoided. This practice is comparable to mass ligation of a bleeding point, and both lead to unnecessary tissue necrosis.

Vessels less than 1.5 mm in diameter can be sealed by pinpoint electrocoagulation. If larger vessels are coagulated by this method, delayed breakdown and hemorrhage may occur. Because fluids are current conductors, the field must be dry in the area surrounding the bleeding vessel. There are two ways to coagulate a bleeding vessel properly. The first is to apply the activated tip directly onto the vessel. The end point of coagulation is determined by tissue contraction and color change. A more precise method is to occlude the vessel initially with a hemostat or plain tissue thumb forceps. The active electrode is applied directly to the surgical instrument, which carries the current directly to the vessel. Care should be taken to prevent unwanted coagulation by not allowing the instrument to rest on normal tissue when the current is applied.

Electrofulguration and Electrodesiccation

These electrosurgical techniques cause dehydration and superficial destruction by a high-voltage, high-frequency current. These techniques are uniterminal; an indifferent electrode is not used. Electrofulguration damages tissue by electrical energy transmitted through an electrical arc or spark. Electrodesiccation is similar, although the electrode directly touches the lesion (see Fig. 4.4). Tissue damage is deeper than with fulguration and may be difficult to control. Electrofulguration of perianal fistulas after a sharp "deroofing" procedure has produced encouraging results. Electrodesiccation has been used for removal of superficial skin lesions.

Precautions

Accidental burns are probably the most frequently observed complication of electrosurgery. It is imperative that an adequate indifferent electrode ("ground plate") be incorporated in the system. Because of its large surface area, the indifferent electrode normally provides a low-current density to complete the electrosurgical circuit. If contact between patient and plate is inadequate, however, high-density electrical current can easily cause a burn (Fig. 4.9). Although the indifferent electrode is designed to be the preferential pathway for the current, a faulty connection between the plate and the unit can result in a burn where the patient touches the metal operating table or the attachment sites of electrical monitoring equipment. More expensive units have a 60-cycle monitoring current flowing through the "ground-plate" system. A break in the ground wire or in its ground-plate connection interrupts the monitoring current and sounds an alarm. Electrolyte jellies and a large area of contact with the patient are recommended to lower skin resis-

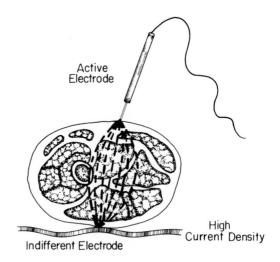

Fig. 4.9. High current density produced at the indifferent electrode with improper technique.

tance and to provide more intimate contact between the skin and the indifferent electrode.

Explosions and fire are potential hazards when inflammable anesthetics, such as ether, chloroform, and cyclopropane, and inflammable skin preparations, such as alcohol, are used.

Electrical channeling occurs when the treatment electrode is used on tissue that has a thin connection to the body. An example is the testicle mobilized out of the scrotum. If electrocoagulation is used, electric energy will be channeled or funneled along the spermatic cord and will cause heat damage.

Cardiac pacemakers are implanted with increasing frequency in veterinary medicine, and the veterinary surgeon should be aware that high-frequency electric energy may cause a cardiac arrest by interfering with the operation of the pacemaker.

Suggested Readings

Battig CG. Electrosurgical burn injuries and their prevention. JAMA 1968;204:91.

Fucci V, Elkins AD. Electrosurgery: principles and guidelines in veterinary medicine. Comp Contin Educ Pract Vet 1991;13:407.

Giddard DW, Jones WR, Wescott JW. Electrosurgical units: particular attention to tube, spark gap and solid state generated currents—their differences and similarities. J Urol 1972;107:1051.

Glover JL, Bendick PJ, Link WJ. The use of thermal knives in surgery: electrosurgery, lasers, plasma scalpel. Curr Probl Surg 1978;15:7.

Greene JA, Knecht CD. Electrosurgery: a review. Vet Surg 1980;9:27.

Greene JA, Knecht CD. Healing of sharp incisions and electroincisions in dogs: a comparative study. Vet Surg 1980;9:42.

Ormrod AN. Electrosurgery: its usefulness and limitations for the small animal surgeon. Vet Rec 1963;75:1095.

Swerdlow DB, et al. Electrosurgery: principles and use. Dis Colon Rectum 1974;17:482.

Wald AS, Mazzia VDB, Spencer FC. Accidental burns associated with electrocautery. JAMA 1971;217:916.

Laser Surgery

Kenneth E. Bartels

Light bulbs and lasers both generate *light*, which is the common name for electromagnetic energy that we can see. The electromagnetic spectrum extends from the very short wavelengths (γ radiation at 10^{-11} m) to radio waves (10^{-1} m). Laser wavelengths fall between the infrared and ultraviolet wavelengths of electromagnetic radiation, which include the invisible and visible light spectrum. The word "*LASER*" is an acronym that stands for *L*ight *A*mplification by the *S*timulated *E*mission of *R*adiation (1).

An extensive discussion of laser physics is not consistent with this general overview. In simpler terms, as a bow stores energy and releases it to propel an arrow, a laser stores energy in atoms, concentrates it, and then releases it in powerful waves of light energy. More specifically, an atom in its resting or ground state in a medium (solid crystal, liquid, or gas) is excited to a higher energy state by the absorption of thermal, electrical, or optical energy. After energy is absorbed, an atom spontaneously returns to its ground state and liberates that energy as a photon. This process is called *stimulated emission*. The resulting emission of photons resonates between mirrored ends of a laser chamber. These bouncing photons further excite other atoms in the laser medium. Momentum builds until a highly concentrated beam of light passes through a partially transmissive mirror at one end of the laser chamber.

Today's technology allows the manufacture of lasers producing wavelengths of light extending from the ultraviolet range to the far-infrared. Devices range in size from miniature diode lasers capable of being passed through the eye of a needle to a free electron laser that can cover an entire floor of a large building. However, each laser is composed of the same basic components and functions according to the medium stimulated to produce energy emission and light (Fig. 4.10).

Laser light can be thought of as periodic waves of energy traveling through space, indicated in units of length of nanometers or micrometers. By definition, 1 nanometer (nm) equals 10^{-9} m, or one-billionth of a meter. One micrometer (μm) is equal to 10^{-6} m or 1000 nm. More common medical laser wavelengths include 193 and 308 nm (ultraviolet or UV-excimer lasers); 532 and 630 nm (visible light lasers); 800 and 1064 nm (near-infrared lasers); 2100 nm or 2.1 μm (mid-infrared lasers); and 10,600 nm or 10.6 μm (far-infrared lasers). Only laser wavelengths between 400 and 700 nm are visible to the eye. Visible colors associated with certain medical lasers include the argon laser (blue: 488 nm), frequency-doubled yttrium aluminum

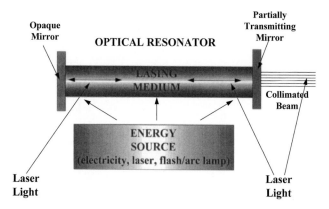

Fig. 4.10. Components of a laser.

garnet (YAG) laser, also known as the potassium titanyl phosphate laser or KTP laser (green: 532 nm), dye laser (yellow/orange/red: 577 to 665 nm), and the ruby laser (deep red: 694 nm). Tunable dye lasers represent a group that may have variable wavelengths but tend to be more complicated, large, expensive, and less user-friendly devices.

Types of Laser–Tissue Interactions

Laser radiation must be converted into another form of energy to produce therapeutic effects. Laser–tissue interactions are categorized according to whether laser energy is converted into heat (photothermal), chemical energy (photochemical), or acoustic energy (mechanical–photodisruptive). Photothermal interactions occur when laser light is absorbed by tissue and is converted into thermal energy or heat, which results in a rise in tissue temperature. When infrared laser wavelengths are used, the water component of tissue plays a predominant role in the absorption of laser energy. Water is heated directly with laser energy, and other molecules may then be indirectly heated by heat conduction. Other tissue components (hemoglobin, melanin, proteins) may also absorb energy at specific infrared wavelengths and play an important role in the tissue-heating process.

Visible laser wavelengths are poorly absorbed by water and usually rely on blood or other endogenous tissue pigments to absorb laser light and to convert it to heat. Naturally occurring molecules that absorb visible wavelengths include hemoglobin, xanthophyll, and melanin. Protein molecules, DNA, and RNA absorb UV wavelengths strongly and usually play a dominant role in converting UV light energy into heat. Figure 4.11 illustrates the water absorption curve, which is an essential component in understanding the concept of laser–tissue interaction (2).

Pulsed laser energy (holmium, erbium, or alexandrite lasers) can be converted into acoustic (mechani-

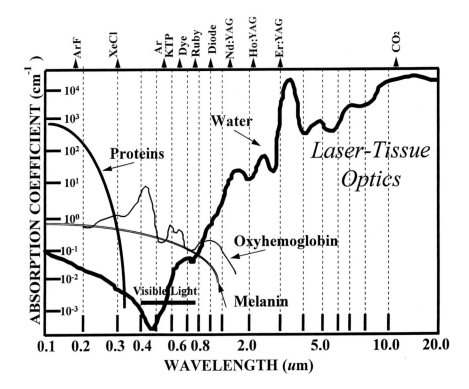

Fig. 4.11. Laser tissue optics: water absorption curve. This graph illustrates the varying degrees of absorption of a specific wavelength (color) of light by water compared to absorption in oxyhemoglobin, melanin, and tissue proteins including amino acids, DNA, and RNA. *Ar*, argon; *KTP*, potassium titanyl phosphate; *XeCl*, xenon chloride; *YAG*, yttrium aluminum garnet.

cal) energy in the form of a shock wave or high-pressure wave, which can disrupt the targeted tissue structure. Laser light can also be absorbed and converted into chemical energy that can break chemical bonds directly or can excite molecules into a biochemically reactive state. Laser wavelength is the critical factor in this process. Short UV wavelengths (e.g., 193 nm) are needed to maximize chemical bond-breaking processes while minimizing the photothermal process as observed with excimer laser energy (2).

Specific visible wavelengths can also induce photobiochemical reactions. This type of reaction can be related to photodynamic laser interaction. In general, photodynamic interactions use light-absorbing molecules (photosensitizers such as hematoporphyrin derivatives) to produce a biochemically reactive form of oxygen (singlet oxygen) in tissue when activated by light of a specific wavelength. Photodynamic interactions are considered a special type of photochemical interaction. Specific visible and near-infrared wavelengths (630 to 740 nm) can be used to control photodynamic interactions, depending on the specific light-absorbing molecules used to mediate the interaction. The therapeutic process is called photodynamic therapy (2).

Biostimulation is a process induced by low-power lasers that may relieve pain, stimulate wound healing, or alter other biologic processes. The entire concept is considered controversial partly because not all the physical, biochemical, and physiologic mechanisms are

understood. Many of the reported results are purely subjective and are difficult to quantify.

The effect of a laser on tissue depends on both wavelength and power. Power is usually expressed in watts. When time is also a factor, the term joule is used, which is defined as a watt per second. Focal spot size (size of the incident beam of the laser light) results in the concentration of energy within an area known as power density, expressed as joules per square centimeters. The advantage of a small spot size is that it results in more concentrated laser energy with less collateral damage, in which fewer cells are affected and destroyed at the margins of an incision. When a rapid, deep incision is required, a small spot size is advantageous in that it concentrates a high amount of energy into the tissue, leading to rapid vaporization. A larger spot size is less precise and enhances tissue coagulation rather than vaporization (2).

The tissue response to the application of laser energy is a dynamic process. Desiccation, followed by photochemical and thermal change, occurs initially. Changes in the local microcirculation influence the tissue reaction to additional laser energy. The generation of smoke, hemorrhage, and char can interfere with the incident laser beam by resulting in scatter, reflection, and absorption of the laser energy and possibly by uncontrolled effects on the target tissue or adjacent structures. The thermal effects produced by the laser beam are used for localized hyperthermia, coagulation, and vaporization. When the beam inter-

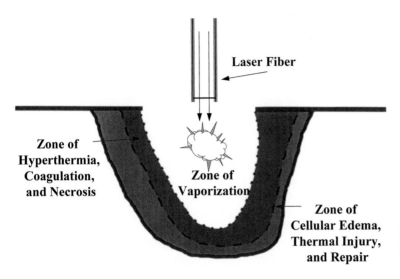

Laser Fiber

Zone of Hyperthermia, Coagulation, and Necrosis

Zone of Vaporization

Zone of Cellular Edema, Thermal Injury, and Repair

Fig. 4.12. Laser–tissue interaction. The generalized tissue response to the application of laser energy results in zones of vaporization, necrosis, and reversible thermal injury.

acts with tissue, the photothermal effect produces a characteristic lesion in living tissue. At the impact site, a crater may be formed when tissue has been vaporized from the region. Immediately surrounding the cavity is an area of hyperthermia, cellular coagulation, and eventually, necrosis. This zone is created by the diffusion of laser energy from the point of laser impact. Immediately adjacent to this zone is an area of cellular edema without evidence of alteration in the collagen stroma. The milder thermal injury to the tissue in this region may resolve within 48 to 72 hours. These phenomena are illustrated in Figure 4.12.

Laser vaporization is the process of removing solid tissue by converting it into a gaseous vapor or plume. This is usually in the form of steam or smoke, but laser plume may also contain noxious substances. Therefore, the use of smoke evacuation during laser surgery is deemed essential. Safety issues are discussed more specifically later in this chapter. The term "vaporization" is used as a synonym for tissue ablation.

Types of Medical Lasers

In medicine today, many different types of biomedical lasers are in use. Each instrument is usually acquired for a specific purpose, such as dermatologic or endoscopic applications. Overall, the use of laser energy can be an extremely precise method for tissue removal or cellular destruction. Medical lasers are expensive and require a dedication to proper use and objective evaluation. Lasers in common use today are the carbon dioxide (CO_2), neodymium YAG (Nd:YAG), argon (Ar), potassium titanyl phosphate (KTP) or frequency-doubled YAG, ruby, diode, holmium:YAG (Ho:YAG), and dye lasers. The following general descriptions are meant to be used as an overall guide to medical lasers. Changes in laser types, wavelength preference, and delivery devices are made frequently, since these in-

struments are closely aligned with changes in technologic advancements in computer hardware and software.

Carbon Dioxide Laser (10,600 nm)

The CO_2 laser was one of the first medical lasers used for tissue ablation. At 10.6 μm, the wavelength is ideal for cutting and vaporization because it is highly absorbed by water. It can cut tissue cleanly when the beam is focused onto tissue and can debulk tissue by photovaporization when defocused. At the tissue interface, blood vessels less than 0.6 mm in diameter can be coagulated and sealed, so use of the CO_2 laser is relatively hemostatic in most capillary beds and in the transection of small venules and veins. Lymphatics are also sealed, so postoperative edema may be minimized. Subjectively, less pain seems to be associated with laser incision and dissection. The reason for this observation could be that smaller nerves are sealed or even spared at some laser wavelengths. Microorganisms are also destroyed in the process of photothermal ablation, so tissues may be sterilized or disinfected during laser–tissue interaction. Because of the high absorption of water, CO_2 laser energy transmission requires a series of mirrors in an articulated arm, a requirement that makes it awkward for use in the abdomen or other areas. However, thermal injury from a given amount of energy is relatively superficial (50 to 100 μm in depth). The net surgical result with this type of laser can be expressed as "What you see is what you get" (2).

Nd:YAG Laser (Neodymium Yttrium Aluminum Garnet: 1064 nm)

The Nd:YAG or "YAG" laser differs from the CO_2 laser because the wavelength allows transmission through tissue in addition to surface absorption. High powers up to 100 W can be delivered through small-core optical fibers that can easily be inserted through the accessory channels of standard gastrointestinal endoscopes. Because the Nd:YAG laser has less specific absorption by water and hemoglobin than the CO_2 and argon lasers, the depth of thermal injury can exceed 3 mm in most tissues, a property that can be useful for coagulation of large volumes of tissue. Rapid tissue vaporization in noncontact mode is possible with a bare fiber, but collateral thermal injury may be substantial. Power levels approaching 100 W are usually needed for these soft tissue applications.

Continuous-wave Nd:YAG lasers can be used with "hot-tip" delivery systems to perform vaporization and cutting of soft tissue in a contact mode with surgical precision, little collateral thermal injury, and good hemostasis. Hot-tip fibers include sculpted quartz fibers, contact-tipped sapphire fibers, metal-capped fibers, temperature-controlled bare fibers, and dual-effect fibers. In principle, contact use of fibers for mechanical coaptation of tissue while it is being heated can be advantageous for hemostasis and controlled excision. Use of contact tips for endoscopic application is widely accepted, but some tips are too large to insert through flexible endoscopes (2).

Argon Laser (458 and 524 nm)

The blue–green argon laser is strongly absorbed by hemoglobin and is especially useful in nonbleeding vascular lesions when precision and minimal penetration (about 1 mm) are required. Although heavily absorbed by blood, argon laser energy can be readily transmitted through water, gastric fluid, aqueous or vitreous humor, or urine. As a result, this laser can be used precisely to cut, vaporize, and superficially coagulate soft tissue that is well perfused with blood. Treatment of hemoglobin-poor tissue generally relies on the production of char for efficient heating of tissue. Bare fibers can be used in contact or noncontact modes for cutting, vaporization, or coagulation. Whereas older versions of the argon laser often lacked enough power to vaporize target tissue, newer 15-W argon lasers are more efficient for vaporization and cutting applications (2, 3).

Frequency-Doubled YAG Laser (Potassium Titanyl Phosphate: 532 nm)

Frequency-doubled Nd:YAG lasers emit a visible green light and are basically equivalent to the argon lasers in many surgical and dermatologic applications. Present clinical applications use photothermal reactions to co-

agulate, vaporize, or cut soft tissue. Absorption of the 532-nm wavelength is negligible in water. The green laser beam passes through water and saline with virtually no absorption, a characteristic of extreme importance in a wet or flooded surgical field. The 532-nm wavelength is strongly absorbed by the oxyhemoglobin component of blood, so this wavelength can be used efficiently and precisely to heat blood-perfused soft tissue. Absorption depth at 532 nm in whole blood is about 0.5 mm. This strong absorption can actually be a problem if the target tissue is covered with blood, because the laser energy will be severely attenuated before it can reach the tissue's surface (2).

Currently manufactured frequency-doubled Nd:YAG lasers can provide either 532 or 1064 nm through the same optical fiber. The 532-nm wavelength is used for precise cutting and vaporization. By switching to the 1064-nm wavelength, the same laser and fiber delivery system can be used for deep tissue coagulation or rapid vaporization when only modest surgical precision is required. The laser is also used by one manufacturer as a dye laser pumping source to control photodynamic interactions (2, 3).

Ruby Laser (694 nm)

Although the ruby laser was first investigated for its medical potential by Maiman in 1961, it has not received widespread use (1). It was resurrected as a medical device in the late 1980s, when it was reintroduced as a device for removing tattoos and birthmarks. The 694-nm wavelength is absorbed strongly by dark pigments, such as melanin and the pigments used for making tattoos, but only weakly by hemoglobin. As a result, the visible ruby laser wavelength can penetrate several millimeters into skin without being severely attenuated by blood. This property allows the ruby laser to be used in the process called selective photothermolysis for procedures to remove tattoos (2, 3).

Diode Laser

Advancement of semiconductor diode laser development has progressed tremendously in concert with other aspects of medicine described previously. Engineering and commercial specifications have allowed development of devices with wavelengths varying from approximately 635 to 980 nm. Newer technologies may actually allow evolution of diode lasers capable of emitting wavelengths in the mid-infrared range (1.9 to 2.1 μm).

Therapeutic products that use semiconductor diode lasers were first approved for surgical use in this country in 1989. Diode lasers (1 to 4 W) are also used for photocoagulation of retinal and other ocular tissues, and they have had ophthalmologic applications since approximately 1984 (4, 5). Their compact size and high efficiency offer significant ergonomic and economic advantages. High-power semiconductor diode lasers appropriate for other surgical applications have been introduced for various uses. These lasers currently provide up to 25 to 60 W at 805 or 980 nm, wavelengths that can penetrate deeply into most types of soft tissue, and they produce tissue interactions comparable to those seen with the Nd:YAG laser (1064 nm) (6). Diode lasers can be used with bare-fiber delivery accessories in noncontact mode for deep coagulation or with hot-tip fibers for precise cutting or vaporization in contact mode. Surgical diode lasers offer considerable advantages compared with Nd:YAG lasers. They are smaller and lighter, require less maintenance, are extremely user-friendly, and can be more economical. Some clinicians predict that prices of diode lasers will eventually drop enough to become competitive with high-end electrosurgical equipment (7).

Additional applications for diode laser energy have been for chromophore-enhanced tissue ablation or coagulation, tissue fusion or laser welding, and photodynamic therapy. Sutureless tissue repair using laser energy has emerged over the last decade. Tissue welding or fusion has the potential to be one of the most important technical developments in surgery. In conjunction with laparoscopic as well as open procedures, laser energy used with biologic glue or "solder" reinforcement can provide a higher leakage pressure for vascular and alimentary tract structures than sutures alone. Preliminary investigations involving selective fusion of nerves, urethral tissue, skin, tracheal mucosa, and even bone fragments have also shown promise. Despite a decade of laboratory success in which the superiority of laser tissue welding has been demonstrated, clinical use of this technology is still uncommon (8).

The use of diode laser wavelengths of 805 to 810 nm has been reported for tissue welding investigations because applications have been centered around the peak absorption spectrum of indocyanine green (780 to 820 nm), the selective chromophore used in fibrinogen solder. Laser energy required for tissue fusion is significantly lower (300 mW to 9.6 W/cm^2) than for incisional or ablative procedures, because minimal thermal changes are required for noncovalent bonding between denatured collagen strands and for producing the weld (8). Diode laser (805 nm)–induced photothermolysis of tissue selectively stained with indocyanine green has also shown promise for selective coagulation and vaporization of tumors and contaminated wounds (9). The small, convenient size coupled with reliability and user friendliness has also focused extensive attention on diode laser development for applications in photodynamic therapy (10).

Holmium Lasers (2100 nm) and Erbium Lasers (2900 nm)

Clinical holmium lasers have been used for arthroscopic surgery, general surgery, laser angioplasty, and thermal sclerostomy. Additional applications have been laser discectomy, removal of sessile polyps in the gastrointestinal tract, and otorhinolaryngeal procedures. The main attraction of the holmium laser is its ability to cut and vaporize soft tissue like a CO$_2$ laser, with the added advantage that holmium energy can be delivered through flexible, low OH, quartz optical fibers. Good surgical precision and control can be obtained with a bare optical fiber. Unlike visible wavelength lasers, and again similar to the CO$_2$ laser, photothermal interactions with the holmium laser do not rely on hemoglobin or other pigments for efficient heating of tissue. The water component of tissue is responsible for absorbing holmium laser energy (2100 nm) and for converting it to heat. The depth of absorption is shallow at approximately 0.3 mm. When cutting or vaporizing tissue, actual zones of thermal injury vary from 0.1 to 1 mm, depending on exposure parameters and on the type of tissue. These small thermal necrosis zones provide better surgical precision and adequate hemostasis (2, 8).

Current holmium instruments are flashlamp-pumped systems. The active laser medium consists of a chromium-sensitized YAG host crystal doped with holmium and thulium ions. This active medium is referred to as Tm,Ho,Cr:YAG or THC:YAG and is common to all holmium laser medical devices. Unlike the CO$_2$ laser, higher-power holmium lasers cannot operate in a continuous-wave mode at room temperature. The relatively low pulse rates (10 to 20 Hz) available from most holmium lasers may be considered a disadvantage because cutting may be slow or may result in jagged tissue edges during incisional applications. In addition, at higher pulse energies (1 joule), considerable amounts of acoustical or mechanical energy are generated in tissue. An audible acoustical "pop" may be generated and actually heard during laser application. However, acoustical energy may be considered an advantage when using holmium energy for photodisruptive procedures such as lithotripsy of gallstones or urologic calculi (11).

Another mid-infrared, solid-state laser is the erbium laser. Its wavelength (2900 nm) is more highly absorbed in water. The erbium laser has the potential to be an excellent laser for orthopedic and dental applications, including hard tissue ablation and cutting. Hemostatic ability would be minimal, however, and lack of readily available delivery fibers has hindered its potential use (2, 8).

Dye Laser

Pulsed and continuous-wave dye lasers use an active laser medium that consists of an organic dye dissolved in an appropriate solvent. For the dye laser to work, the dye solution must be recirculated at high velocity through the laser resonator. Dye lasers are useful for medical applications because they can generate high-output powers and pulse energy at wavelengths throughout the visible wavelength spectrum (400 to 700 nm). They are usually pumped by argon lasers, flashlamps, or a frequency-doubled YAG laser. Dye lasers have been used for lithotripsy of biliary and urologic calculi (pulsed), activating photosensitizers for photodynamic therapy (continuous wave), ophthalmologic operations (pulsed or continuous wave), and dermatologic applications (pulsed and continuous wave) including treatment of birthmarks and removal of tattoos (2, 3).

Laser Safety

Laser instruments are probably safer to use than a scalpel or scissors in the hands of a trained operator. However, laser use by untrained personnel can be dangerous for both the operating team and the patient. Safety standards for medical laser applications have been issued that consider potential hazards and their control measures. The current consensus standard in the United States is through the American National Standards Institute's (ANSI) document entitled *Safe Use of Lasers in Health Care Facilities*. Application of surgical lasers in veterinary medicine must adhere to these regulations and guidelines to ensure operator and patient safety. Laser hazards depend on the laser, the environment, and the personnel involved with the laser operation. The laser hazard is defined by a hazard classification (I to IV). Surgical lasers are almost all classified as class IV laser products because they may represent a significant fire or skin hazard and may also produce hazardous diffuse reflections. Hazardous diffuse reflections are of concern because the probability of damaging retinal exposure is extreme without proper eye protection (12).

With the biomedical application of lasers, the safety concerns described in the next few paragraphs must be realized.

Inhalation of Smoke or Laser Plume

Laser surgery usually creates more smoke than electrosurgical procedures. Reports have mentioned that smoke products from lasers are really no different from those created by electrosurgery, although the quantity is most likely greater. Some studies have actually isolated viable tumor cells from smoke evacuation tubes, so the concept of uncontrolled viral or bacterial vaporization must also be taken into account (12). Because even sterile smoke can be an irritant, all products of combustion as a result of laser vaporization must be evacuated with a dedicated smoke evacuator. The filters and tubes on these devices require maintenance and periodic replacement, increasing the cost of laser surgical procedures.

Laser-Induced Combustion

Laser beams can cause fires. The obvious way to prevent laser-induced combustion is to make certain the beam is always directed toward the surgical site. In addition, the use of moistened sponges surrounding the surgical site decreases the chance of accidental ignition of drapes and other objects, especially when using wavelengths highly absorbed by water (CO_2). Polyvinyl chloride endotracheal tubes are especially prone to ignition. An endotracheal tube that is carrying oxygen literally becomes an airway blowtorch almost instantaneously after impact of the laser beam. In airway and oral surgery, endotracheal tubes should be of a type approved for laser surgery. These include specific laser-safe tubes and, less desirably, endotracheal tubes made of red rubber protected by an application of reflective metal tape.

Eye and Skin Burns

Prevention of laser energy burns to the eyes or skin of patients, operators, and assistants is of extreme importance. Safety glasses or goggles, *specified for each laser wavelength*, must be worn for every laser procedure. Moistened surgical sponges or even laser safety eyewear should be considered for protecting patients' eyes. In addition, window barriers, door interlocks, laser safety warning lights, use of an ebonized or dulled finish on surgical instruments to reduce reflection, and laser warning signs on doors are important safety features that should not be ignored. The potential for accidental burns and fires usually is related to accidental depression of the activating footswitch of the laser. All machines are equipped with a standby mode of operation in which the machine is running but laser energy cannot be activated. A major responsibility of the laser nurse or technician is to evaluate the progress of the laser operation and have the machine switched to standby whenever laser energy is not required. The phrase, "laser on," spoken by the operating laser surgeon is required before the laser is activated and the footswitch will operate, becomes as important as the use of safety glasses and smoke evacuators, or the engineering of the machine itself, in fostering safety. A team approach with the surgical laser technician, who basically runs the laser, and the surgeon is essential.

Ignition of methane from the rectum or rumen can also be an exciting occurrence; the gas should first be removed by suction or blocked by tamponade. Vaporization of iodine skin preparations into irritating fumes, ignition of alcohol, and ignition of any pure oxygen environment are also important concerns.

Miscellaneous Problems

Other hazards include electrical injury from the high-voltage power supply. Laser operation with newer devices is easy because they are extremely user-friendly and reliable, but machine maintenance, including the purchase of maintenance contracts, may be required to maximize use and to minimize safety concerns about mechanical, electrical, and optical failures. This aspect of medical laser usage must be recognized because maintenance contracts and laser repair can both be costly.

Clinical Applications

Many of the early reports involving the use of biomedical lasers concerned the endoscopic use of fiber-delivered devices (Nd:YAG) for treatment of laryngeal conditions and disorders of the upper respiratory system in the horse. Since that time, however, investigators have used lasers in the treatment of various surgical conditions in small animals (13–15).

Applications of both CO_2 and Nd:YAG lasers in general surgery have included conventional procedures in which precise dissection and control of hemorrhage is important. These procedures have included liver biopsy, resection of hepatic lobes, splenic biopsy, prostatic dissection and ablation, partial nephrectomy and nephrotomy, and excision or resection of various intra-abdominal, intrathoracic, cutaneous, and mammary neoplasms (14–16). Some reports have reviewed clinical uses of laser energy for ablation and palliation of a brain tumor (Nd:YAG), ablation, sterilization, and disinfection of neoplasms (CO_2, Nd:YAG), and treatment of eosinophilic granulomas (CO_2, Nd:YAG), perianal fistulas (Nd:YAG, CO_2), and acral lick dermatitis (Nd:YAG, CO_2) (14–19). With advantages of lower morbidity time for some conditions, fewer perceived signs of pain, and potential treatment regimens for conditions not amenable to conventional surgical or medical procedures, biomedical lasers have found use not only in the clinical small animal setting, but also in the realm of exotic animal practice. In addition, clinical use of the holmium:YAG laser for percutaneous prophylactic ablation of intervertebral discs in dogs

has recently been instituted and shows tremendous potential (20).

The use of biomedical lasers for veterinary ophthalmologic applications has been established, although this use has not become as common as it is in human medicine. The Q-switched or continuous-wave ophthalmic Nd:YAG, argon, and diode lasers have been used as funduscopic photocoagulators in retinopathies, for treatment of lens-induced pupillary opacification, and for transcleral laser cyclodestruction of the ciliary body for glaucoma therapy in dogs (4, 21). As experience and interest increase, and as lasers become more available to veterinary ophthalmologists, clinical applications will increase as treatment protocols are initiated and proved useful.

Photodynamic therapy has been used clinically in veterinary medicine by several investigators (22, 23). Certain initiatives have been reported using this technique for treatment of spontaneously occurring neoplasms in dogs and cats. This exciting treatment modality for selective destruction of neoplasms that uses the interaction of a photosensitizer with light in the presence of oxygen will undoubtedly play a much larger role in clinical veterinary medicine as protocols are established and as new photosensitizing drugs are manufactured and approved for use.

Use of biomedical lasers in small animal orthopedics has been more limited than similar applications in either human or equine surgery, primarily because of availability and limitation of equipment and limited accessibility or feasibility for arthroscopic surgical procedures in the dog and cat. The dog has been used as a model for biostimulation of articular cartilage and other research applications. Practical use of lasers for ablation of bone has not been effective, although laser ablation (CO_2) of methylmethacrylate during removal and revision of total hip prosthesis is possible (14, 15).

Future Innovations

The use of lasers in medicine is an exciting treatment modality that will continue to produce innovative methods for managing diseased tissue. Research focused on basic laser–tissue interaction and selective tissue destruction will become increasingly important. Selective tissue destruction of alimentary tract mucosa is possible using endoscopic application of holmium laser energy. The use of interstitial laser hyperthermia for treatment of malignant tumors will become an effective part of the veterinary oncologist's armamentarium, as will expanded and efficacious use of photodynamic therapy. Photothermolysis using appropriate chromophores for selective tissue destruction and sterilization or disinfection is currently proving effective in both clinical and laboratory settings. Minimally invasive urologic techniques for ablation of bladder, urethral, and prostatic pathologic conditions in small animals will become more common as technologically enhanced and smaller endoscopes are developed, as delivery systems are improved, and as new laser wavelengths are investigated. Laser lithotripsy is now possible using both visible and infrared wavelengths. This technology will eventually allow noninvasive removal of urologic and biliary calculi in animals. Tissue fusion or welding of blood vessels, alimentary tract, ureter or urethra, skin, and even bone will become clinically available in the near future. Application of lasers for micromanipulation of gametes and use of laser energy for improving fertilization and hatching rates during in vitro fertilization in domestic animals are close to becoming clinical realities. The use of lasers for soft tissue dental procedures is already feasible and, as investigations continue, laser energy techniques for hard tissue dental procedures will be possible.

References

1. Swaim CP, Mills TN. A history of lasers. In: Krasner N, ed. Lasers in gastroenterology. New York: Wiley-Liss, 1991:3–23.
2. JGM Associates, Inc. Therapeutic applications of advanced laser products, 1993. Vols I and II. 6 New England Executive Park, Suite 400, Burlington, MA 01803.
3. Wheeland RG. Clinical uses of lasers in dermatology. Lasers Surg Med 1995;16:2–23.
4. Sapienza JS, Miller TR, Gum GG, et al. Contact transcleral cyclophotocoagulation using a neodymium:yttrium aluminum garnet laser in normal dogs. Prog Vet Comp Ophthalmol 1993; 2:147–153.
5. Krauss JM, Puliafito CA. Lasers in ophthalmology. Lasers Surg Med 1995;17:102–159.
6. Judy MM, Matthews JL, Aronoff BL, et al. Soft tissue studies with 805 nm diode laser radiation: thermal effects with contact tips and comparison with effects of 1064 nm Nd:YAG laser radiation. Lasers Surg Med 1993;13:528–536.
7. Bartels KE, Zediker MS. Biomedical lasers at the cutting edge. Photonics Spectra 1993;27:92–97.
8. Treat MR, Oz MC, Bass LS. New technologies and future applications of surgical lasers: the right tool for the right job. Surg Clin North Am 1992;72:705–747.
9. Bartels KE, Morton RJ, Dickey DT, et al. Use of diode laser energy (808 nm) for selective photothermolysis of contaminated wounds. In: Progress in biomedical optics (SPIE proceedings series). Lasers in surgery: advanced characterization, therapeutics, and systems V. 1995;2395:602–606.
10. Wieman TJ, Fingar VH. Photodynamic therapy. Surg Clin North Am 1992;72:609–622.
11. Spindel ML, Moslem A, Bhatia KS, et al. Comparison of holmium and flashlamp pumped dye lasers for use in lithotripsy of biliary calculi. Lasers Surg Med 1992;12:482–489.
12. Sliney DH. Laser safety. Lasers Surg Med 1995;16:215–225.
13. Jako GJ. Laser biomedical engineering: clinical applications in otolaryngology. In: Goldman L, ed. The biomedical laser: technology and clinical applications. New York: Springer-Verlag, 1981:175–198.
14. Bartels KE. Lasers in veterinary medicine. In: Progress in biomedical optics (SPIE proceedings series). Lasers in orthopedic, dental, and veterinary medicine. 1994; 2128:538–543.
15. Bartels KE. Laser surgery for selected small animal soft tissue conditions. In: Progress in biomedical optics (SPIE proceedings series). Lasers in orthopedic, dental, and veterinary medicine. 1991;1424:164–170.
16. Hardie EM, Stone EA, Spaulding KA, et al. Subtotal canine prostatectomy with the neodymium:yttrium aluminum garnet laser. Vet Surg 1990;19:348–355.
17. Feder BM, Fry TR, Kostolich M, et al. Nd:YAG laser cytoreduction of an invasive intracranial meningioma in a dog. Prog Vet Neurol 1993;4:3–9.
18. Shelley BA, Bartels KE, Ely RW, et al. Use of the neodymium: yttrium aluminum garnet laser for treatment of squamous cell carcinoma of the nasal planum in a cat. J Am Vet Med Assoc 1992;201:756–758.
19. Ellison GW, Bellah JR, Stubbs WP, et al. Treatment of perianal fistulas with Nd:YAG laser: results in twenty cases. Vet Surg 1995;24:140–147.
20. Dickey DT, Bartels KE, Henry GA, et al. Use of the holmium yttrium aluminum garnet laser for percutaneous thoracolumbar intervertebral disk ablation in the dog. J Am Vet Med Assoc 1996.
21. Nasisse MP, Davidson MG, English RV, et al. Treatment of glaucoma by use of transcleral neodymium:yttrium aluminum garnet laser cyclocoagulation in dogs. J Am Vet Med Assoc 1990;97:350–353.
22. Peavy GH, Klein MK, Newman HC, et al. The use of chloraluminum sulfonated phthalocyanine as a photosensitizer in the treatment of malignant tumors in dogs and cats. In: Progress in biomedical optics (SPIE proceedings series). Lasers in orthopedic, dental, and veterinary medicine. 1991;1424:171–178.
23. Klein MK, Roberts WG. Recent advances in photodynamic therapy. Compend Contin Educ Small Anim Pract 1993;15:809–818.

5

RESTRAINT TECHNIQUES FOR PREVENTION OF SELF-TRAUMA

Howard B. Seim, III & James E. Creed

Numerous techniques to prevent self-trauma have been described, and even more have been used by practicing veterinarians. This chapter deals with an assortment of devices that we have learned about or have created to prevent self-trauma. We describe materials needed, methods of assembly, specific indications, contraindications, and complications of each device.

Self-trauma prevention techniques can be divided into two groups: chemical agents and mechanical devices. Those included are as follows:

Chemical Restraint Agents
Tranquilizers
Noxious-tasting agents
  Variton*
  Bitter apple
  Obtundia†
  Tabasco
  Stoma-nil‡
  Thumb-sucking preparations§

---

*Schering Corp., Kenilworth, NJ 07033.
†Otis Clapp & Sons, Inc., 143 Albany Street, Cambridge, MA 02139.
‡Dow B. Hickham, Inc., P.O. Box 35413, Houston, TX 77035.
§Thum, Num Specialty, Inc., P.O. Box 326, Murrysville, PA 15668.

Mechanical Restraint Devices
Elizabethan collar
Body brace
Side bar
Stockinette body bandage
Emergency ear laceration protector
Ear laceration protector
Taping ears to the head
Cast
Schroeder–Thomas splint with sheet aluminum
Soft padded bandage
Hobbles
  Hock, carpal, stifle-to-tail
Tail-tip protector

Chemical Restraint Agents

Tranquilizers have been advocated to restrain patients from inflicting self-trauma. These drugs must be used with caution, because they are often insufficient when used alone.

Noxious-tasting agents placed on body parts should also be used with discretion. Some patients endure the taste of a particular agent, so these substances are not always dependable. Many such agents are available; alternating them helps to prevent the patient from becoming accustomed to one.

The combined use of mechanical restraint devices and chemical agents has been helpful in controlling intractable patients.

Mechanical Restraint Devices

Elizabethan Collar

MATERIALS

Commercial
  Plastic collars*
  Cardboard collars†
Handmade
  Cardboard
  X-ray film
  Plastic bucket or waste basket

METHOD OF ASSEMBLY

Cardboard collars are best suited for dogs weighing 15 to 30 pounds. X-ray film can be used to construct collars for cats and small dogs (under 15 pounds). Regardless of the material selected, the method of assembly is the same. An appropriately sized circle is cut from material used. The collar's size depends on the size of dog and the purpose for which the collar is to be used. When completed, the collar should extend 1 to 2 inches beyond the patient's nose. A cut is then made from the edge of the circle to the center. A small circle, slightly larger than the patient's neck, is then cut from the center. Adhesive tape can be applied to the edge of the circular cut to protect the neck from any sharp edges. The collar is then placed around the patient's neck, and the edges are overlapped until the collar fits snugly. It should be tight enough to allow no more than one finger between the edge of the collar and the patient's neck. The collar is then secured by taping the overlapping edges (Fig. 5.1). The inside and outside edges should be taped to prevent trauma to the patient's face and to keep the edges from catching on objects. After application, rostral traction should be applied on the collar to make sure it will not slip off.

An alternative method for constructing an effective cardboard collar is to cut the center just large enough to allow it to be forced over the patient's head and ears. The resulting collar is flat instead of cone shaped. The advantages of this type of collar are comfort, acceptance, and better peripheral vision; disadvantages are ease with which the collar can slip off and greater width. In most cases, the patient's personality determines which collar should be used.

Cardboard and x-ray film collars should not be used on large dogs (over 30 pounds). Cardboard is not dura-

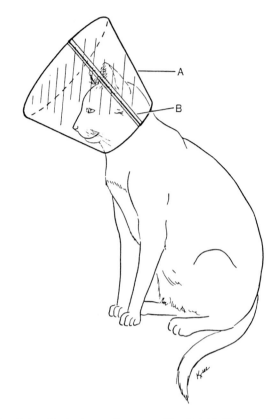

Fig. 5.1. Elizabethan collar: x-ray film (14 × 17 inch, A) and taped overlapped edge of film (B).

ble enough and x-ray film is not large enough to be effective. Instead, plastic buckets, waste baskets, or commercially available Elizabethan collars should be used.

Commercially available collars are similar in function to those previously described. The major difference is in their attachment to the patient. Plastic loops located around the inner edge of the Elizabethan collar are used to attach it to a leather or gauze collar placed around the patient's neck. The collar should be tight enough not to slip over the head. Such collars are durable and come in several sizes.

Plastic buckets or waste baskets of medium size can also be used for large dogs. They protect the animal's front legs more effectively than conventional Elizabethan collars. A circle is cut out of the bottom of the bucket just large enough to slip the bucket over the patient's head. Cloth tape or elastic adhesive tape (Elasticon Elastic Tape, Johnson & Johnson, New Brunswick, NJ 08903) bandage is placed over the sharp plastic edge to protect the patient's neck. Four or more holes are punched around the bottom of the bucket about 1 cm away from the cut edge. Gauze bandage is then placed through each hole and is tied

*Buster collar, Dr. Jorgensen Laboratories, P.O. Box 872, Loveland, CO 80537.
†Medicollar, Evsco Pharmaceutical Corp., P.O. Box 29, Harding Highway, Buena, NJ 08310.

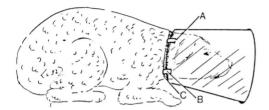

Fig. 5.2. Waste basket extending well beyond the dog's nose. Hole cut in the bottom of the basket 1 to 2 cm from the cut edge (A), gauze tied to form a loop (B), and leather collar or gauze tied around the neck (C).

to itself to form a loop. A leather or gauze collar is threaded through these loops and is secured around the dog's neck (Fig. 5.2). The only disadvantage of this variation of an Elizabethan collar is that the amount of material extending beyond the patient's muzzle can make eating and drinking difficult. Feeding and watering the patient on a slightly elevated surface help to eliminate this problem. In some patients, it may be necessary to remove the plastic bucket during feeding and watering.

INDICATIONS
Elizabethan collars are versatile, are widely accepted, and have few contraindications or complications. These collars prevent self-trauma if they are large enough to prevent the animal from licking, scratching, or chewing the affected area. They are especially useful for preventing self-trauma after surgical procedures and can also be used in conjunction with other mechanical restraint devices.

CONTRAINDICATIONS
Elizabethan collars are not effective in restraining patients from mutilating fore and hind extremities, unless long plastic waste baskets or large plastic cone-shaped collars are used.

COMPLICATIONS
The most devastating potential complication is from applying the collar too tightly, which can result in death of the patient by suffocation. This complication can be prevented by following these rules: 1) never place an Elizabethan collar on an anesthetized patient; 2) always secure the collar or roll gauze so one finger can easily be placed between the patient's neck and the collar; and 3) watch the patient for the first few minutes after application to assess respiratory function.

Body Brace

MATERIALS
Aluminum rod ($\frac{3}{16}$, $\frac{1}{4}$, $\frac{5}{16}$, or $\frac{3}{8}$-inch width; 6- and 12-foot length)
One-inch cloth tape
Splint bender

METHOD OF ASSEMBLY
The circumference of the base of the patient's neck is measured or is estimated using the thumb and forefinger of both hands; either method must allow for padding. With the aid of a splint bender or a round object, the mid-section of the rod is bent into an appropriately sized circle and a half. The rods on both sides of the ring are cut to a length equal to the distance from the base of the neck to the flank. Both rods are then bent at approximately 60° to the circle, so the ring will rest comfortably on the shoulders of the dog with the ends protruding caudally toward the flanks. The circle and tips of the rods are padded with cotton and tape for greater comfort.

The apparatus is placed with the padded ring resting against the shoulders and the rods along both sides of the thorax and abdomen (Fig. 5.3). Lateral rods are taped around the cranial abdomen with cloth tape to secure the rods to the patient's side and to help prevent dorsoventral movement. This device is comfortable for the patient and can be used for extended periods.

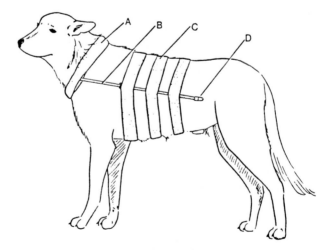

Fig. 5.3. Body brace: aluminum rod adjacent to each side of the trunk. Padded ring (A), lateral rod (B), tape encircling the trunk (C), and padded end of the rod (D).

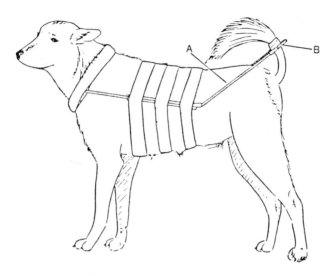

Fig. 5.4. Body brace with an angled aluminum rod added to keep the tail elevated. Angled rod taped to the lateral rod of the body brace (A) and tail taped to the apex of the tail lifter rod (B).

With a few simple additions, the body brace can be constructed to act as a tail lifter. An aluminum rod is bent back on itself to form a 30- to 45°-angled apex. Sufficient tail lifter rod is allowed to secure it with tape to each lateral rod of the body brace (Fig. 5.4). The triangular portion, located caudally, is bent upward about 45° at the flank, so the apex is situated 10 to 15 cm above the base of the tail. Once situated comfortably, the tail lifter rod is securely taped to the body brace; then the base of the tail is taped to the apex of the tail brace (see Fig. 5.4).

INDICATIONS

The body brace is indicated to protect the body caudal to the base of the neck, including the thorax, abdomen, anal region, and hind legs above the hocks. It is especially useful for patients that will not tolerate an Elizabethan collar.

With the tail lifter added, this device has been useful after surgical procedures for perianal fistulas and perianal neoplasms. Elevation of the tail facilitates ventilation, drainage, and local medication of the anal region.

CONTRAINDICATIONS

The head, neck, and forelegs are not adequately protected with this device, nor is it effective on the cat.

COMPLICATIONS

Lateral rods that are improperly padded or are too tightly taped may cause discomfort, skin irritation, and areas of necrosis. These problems are easily prevented by regular examination of the lateral rods, by application of padding as needed, and by not taping the trunk too tightly. The neck ring should be snug, but not compromising. If the patient exhibits respiratory dyspnea, the rods should be loosened.

Side Bar

MATERIALS

Aluminum rod
One-inch cloth tape
Leather collar

METHOD OF ASSEMBLY

Another useful device is a side bar. A leather or nylon collar is fixed around the patient's neck, and a smaller collar is placed around the hind leg just above the hock. A ring is formed in each end of a suitable length of adequately sized aluminum rod. The bar is attached to the collars by adhesive tape, leaving about 5 cm of slack at each attachment (Fig. 5.5). In giant breeds of dogs, two or three ⅜-inch aluminum rods should be taped together to provide sufficient strength. Advantages of this method are ease of application and minimal materials necessary for construction. Disadvantages include the awkward gait created by the device and the possibility that the animal may tangle its legs in the bar. The patient must be confined to a kennel or small room to avoid excessive trauma where the strap encircles the leg. This device is used infrequently, but it is helpful in selected cases.

INDICATIONS

A side bar prevents licking and chewing of the ipsilateral hind foot and hock.

CONTRAINDICATIONS

A side bar does not protect the contralateral side. It is not usually tolerated by cats.

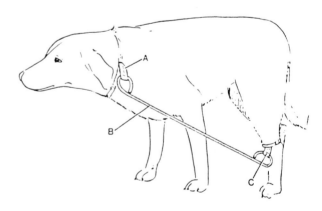

Fig. 5.5. Side bar. End of the bar taped to a collar (A) (collar can also be run through ring), aluminum bar (B) (additional rods can be added for increased strength), and end of the bar taped to a collar (C).

COMPLICATIONS
Some dogs may not tolerate a side bar because their feet can become tangled around the bar.

Stockinette Body Bandage
MATERIALS

Stockinette (2-, 3-, 4-, and 6-inch*)

METHOD OF ASSEMBLY
An appropriate size of stockinette is selected. A 3-inch size is used for cats and small dogs (under 15 pounds), and a 4- to 6-inch size is used for larger dogs. The length of stockinette is measured from the patient's head to the rump. Four small holes are cut in the stockinette to accommodate the legs. The stockinette is placed on the patient, with the legs protruding through the holes. In male dogs, a hole must be also be cut for the prepuce. If added bulkiness is desired, several layers of stockinette can be applied comfortably. If the stockinette rides up over the rump area, a hole can be cut in the dorsal midline of the stockinette and the tail placed through the hole.

INDICATIONS
A stockinette body bandage can be used to protect surgical wounds and lacerations of the thorax or abdomen. The bandage is comfortable and inexpensive and does not slip off.

CONTRAINDICATIONS
This bandage cannot be used for protecting the head, neck, legs, tail, or anal area.

COMPLICATIONS
Aggressive scratching, especially in cats, can cause a nail to be caught in the stockinette. This problem can be prevented by clipping the patient's nails when the bandage is applied.

Emergency Ear Laceration Protector
MATERIALS

Stockinette
or
Old sock

METHOD OF ASSEMBLY AND APPLICATION
A stockinette or a sock is cut to create an opening at both ends. The patient's ears are folded over the top of the head, and the sock or stockinette is slipped over

*Distributed by Whittaker General Medical, Richmond, VA 23228.

the patient's head to hold the ears in place. The edges of the sock or stockinette are taped to the patient's hair over the back of the neck and forehead to secure it to the head.

INDICATIONS
This quick, temporary immobilizing device prevents further trauma and bleeding of a lacerated ear. Clients can be instructed over the phone to use this bandage to protect a lacerated, bleeding ear for transport to the veterinarian. It can also be used as a final bandage cover for ears previously taped to the head.

CONTRAINDICATIONS
This bandage is not intended to be the only treatment for pinna lacerations.

COMPLICATIONS
The bandage is tolerated by most patients, but it is important to include enough hair in the tape to prevent slipping forward or backward. Patients not tolerating the bandage may require concurrent use of an Elizabethan collar.

Ear Laceration Protector
MATERIALS

One- and 2-inch cloth tape

METHOD OF ASSEMBLY AND APPLICATION
Once an ear laceration has been sutured, a gauze sponge is placed over the laceration to protect the suture line. The ear is then thoroughly dried. A strip of 2-inch cloth tape is placed on the lateral side of the pinna, over the gauze-covered laceration, and extended 4 to 6 cm beyond the tip of the ear. The tape is then doubled over on itself and is taped back to the medial side of the pinna. One-inch cloth tape is then used to encircle the ear gently, and the tape should extend beyond the pinna. Excessive tape distally is trimmed to be parallel to the ear tip (Fig. 5.6). A large area of adhesive tape must be in contact with the ear. Subsequent shaking of the head will result in whiplash of the tape instead of the tip of the ear.

INDICATIONS
This protector is used for lacerations of the ear involving the tip of the pinna.

CONTRAINDICATIONS
In patients with marginal auricular dermatitis, the adhesive can act as an irritant and can perpetuate the condition.

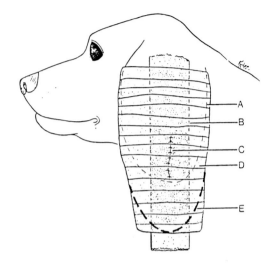

Fig. 5.6. Ear laceration protector. Edge of the pinna (A), 2-inch tape on both sides of the pinna (B), sutured laceration (C), 1-inch tape encircling the ear (D), and line for trimming off extra tape (E).

COMPLICATIONS

Some patients may find the device annoying and may try to scratch it off. If this occurs, an Elizabethan collar can be used in conjunction with the device.

Taping Ears to Head

MATERIALS

Two-inch cloth tape
Stockinette
Elastic adhesive tape
Sponge-rubber donuts

METHOD OF APPLICATION

The traumatized area or lesion is protected with a gauze sponge or nonadherent pad (Telfa Surgical Dressing, Kendall Co., 15 Hampshire St., Mansfield, MA 02048; Micropad Dressing, 3M Medical Products, 3M Center, St. Paul, MN 55101). A strip of 2-inch cloth tape is applied to the medial and lateral aspects of the pinna of both ears, so it extends 15 cm from the tip of the ear to form tape stirrups. The tape stirrups are then passed over the opposite side of the dog's head and around the neck. Care must be taken not to apply excessive tension. The stirrups are then extended by taping three or four added revolutions around the head. The external ear canal should remain exposed. A donut 7 to 10 cm in diameter cut from a soft rubber material can be placed over each ear canal. A stockinette is then placed over the patient's head and is taped to the bandage.

INDICATIONS

This is a good method for protecting the ears from continued shaking. Because the ear canals remain exposed to air, this apparatus can be used as an adjunct to medical or surgical management of otitis externa.

CONTRAINDICATIONS

The bandage should not be used in patients with severe dermatitis of the pinna because adhesive tape increases the irritation.

COMPLICATIONS

It is still possible for the patient to scratch the bandage and ear canal with a rear paw. This problem can be solved by concurrent use of an Elizabethan collar.

The bandage is removed by cutting the tape under the chin; the tips of the ears may inadvertently be cut if the bandage is removed by cutting tape on top of the head.

Cast

MATERIALS

Imex Veterinary Thermoplastic*
Cutter Cast 7 casting tape†
Plaster‡
Vetcast Plus casting tape§

METHOD OF ASSEMBLY

Routine application of a cast has been described (1, 2).

INDICATIONS

Casts protect a limb below the elbow and stifle and are especially useful for the initial protection of carpal and tarsal lick granulomas.

CONTRAINDICATIONS

This technique should not be used if draining wounds will be covered by the cast.

COMPLICATIONS

Improper application compromises the circulation to the toes, and dry gangrene can result. Some patients chew on a cast excessively.

---

*IMEX Veterinary, Inc., Longview, TX 75604.
†Cutter Biological, Division of Cutter Laboratories, Inc., 2200 Powell Street, Emeryville, CA 94608.
‡Zoroc, Johnson & Johnson, New Brunswick, NJ 08903.
§3M Animal Care Products, 3M Center, St. Paul, MN 55144.

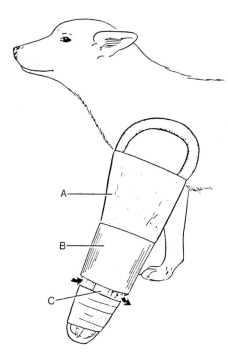

Fig. 5.7. Schroeder–Thomas splint with sheet aluminum secured to a splint. Tape covering the Schroeder-Thomas splint (A), sheet aluminum (B), and the leg left uncovered to provide ventilation (C).

Schroeder–Thomas Splint With Sheet Aluminum

MATERIALS

Aluminum rod
Cotton
Cloth tape
Splint bender
Sheet aluminum

METHOD OF ASSEMBLY

Construction of a Schroeder–Thomas splint has been described (2, 3). Once the splint has been secured to the patient's extremity, the area to be protected is covered with a light sheet of durable aluminum or tin (Fig. 5.7). The aluminum is taped securely to the vertical rods over the area requiring protection. Immediately distal to the aluminum sheet, the aluminum bars are not wrapped with tape, to ensure adequate ventilation of the protected area (see Fig. 5.7).

INDICATIONS

A regular Schroeder–Thomas splint is especially useful in hygroma of the elbow, where it is applied postoperatively to prevent trauma from lying on the elbow. It is also used to protect wounds and skin lesions of the legs adequately from licking and chewing. When all else fails, tin or aluminum can be applied around the splint. Aluminum can be used to adequately protect any part of the fore or hind extremity that is included in the Schroeder–Thomas splint. Generally speaking, this area is below the elbow and stifle.

CONTRAINDICATIONS

Protection is not offered above the distal humerus or femur.

COMPLICATIONS

The only complication of this device is from inappropriate application or construction of the splint, which can result in decubital sores, swollen toes, necrosis of toes, and stiff joints from prolonged immobilization.

Soft Padded Bandage

MATERIALS

Cloth tape
Cast padding* or cotton
Conforming gauze†
Elastic adhesive tape or conforming adhesive bandage‡

METHOD OF ASSEMBLY

Tape stirrups are placed on the medial and lateral aspects of the extremity, to extend 10 to 12 cm beyond the end of the limb. Cast padding or cotton is then wrapped up the limb, starting at the toes. Enough padding is used to cover the desired area adequately and to create the bulkiness necessary for protection. Conforming gauze is then applied up the extremity; one should apply enough pressure to conform the cotton snugly to the limb. The ends of the tape stirrups are then folded back and are taped to the outside of the bandage. An elastic tape or bandage is used to cover the gauze. This layer of material adds strength to the bandage, as well as additional protection to the area being covered.

INDICATIONS

This device is indicated for protection of extremities below the elbow and stifle.

---

*Specialist cast padding, Johnson & Johnson, New Brunswick, NJ 08903.
†Kling elastic gauze bandage, Johnson & Johnson, New Brunswick, NJ 08903.
‡Vet Wrap, Animal Care Products, 3M Co., 3M Center, St. Paul, MN 55144.

CONTRAINDICATIONS

Protection is not offered above the elbow or stifle. Extremely aggressive patients may need a combination of a soft padded bandage and a chemical restraint or an Elizabethan collar.

COMPLICATIONS

Complications arise from improperly applied bandages. If a bandage is too tight, the patient's circulation can be compromised; if it is too loose, pressure sores, decubital ulcers, or slippage will result. Experience helps to dictate the appropriate method of application.

Hobbles

MATERIALS

One-inch cloth tape

METHOD OF ASSEMBLY

When applying stifle-to-tail hobbles, encircling tape should be applied just distal to the stifle joint of both legs, and to the midportion of the tail (Fig. 5.8). Adequate hair-to-tape contact must be made to preclude slipping of tape down the leg or tail. The hobble should be long enough to allow normal defecation, but short enough to stop the damaging effect of continued tail wagging.

Tape hobbles can also be applied just proximal to each hock or carpus. The hobbles must be long enough to permit the dog to walk and short enough to be restrictive (Fig. 5.9).

INDICATIONS

Stifle-to-tail hobbles are used exclusively to prevent trauma to the tip of the tail resulting from constant wagging of the tail in a confined area.

Hock hobbles are used to prevent patients from scratching the head and forequarters. Such hobbles are also useful when a patient persists in scratching an Elizabethan collar or when such a collar allows the patient to lick or chew the perineal region. Carpal hobbles prevent a patient from removing an Elizabethan collar with the front feet.

CONTRAINDICATIONS

Hock or carpal hobbles should not be used on patients that cannot be confined to a cage or kennel. If allowed free run, a patient may continually stumble and fall.

COMPLICATIONS

The tape should be checked daily for evidence of skin irritation, slipping, or breaking. The patient's extremities should be examined for swelling, redness, and temperature. If problems develop, the device should be removed. If the patient chews at hobbles, an Elizabethan collar or body brace should be applied.

Tail-Tip Protectors

MATERIALS

Gauze sponges
Roll or conforming gauze

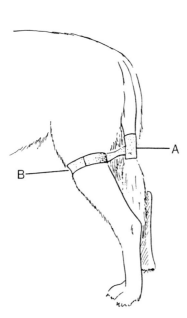

Fig. 5.8. Stifle-to-tail hobbles. Tape secured to the tail (A) and tape secured just distal to the stifle (B).

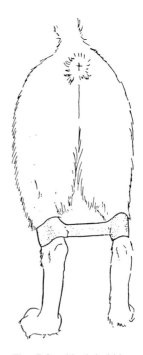

Fig. 5.9. Hock hobbles.

Conforming adhesive bandage or elastic adhesive
 tape
Hexalite, Light Cast, Cutter Cast 7, or Orthoplast

METHOD OF ASSEMBLY

The tip of the tail is wrapped with a gauze sponge and conforming gauze for initial padding. Cloth or elastic tape can be used to hold the padding in place. It is imperative to include 7 to 10 cm of hair in the tape cover to keep the apparatus from slipping off. Hexalite, Light Cast, Cutter Cast 7, or Orthoplast is molded to form a guard over the tip of the tail. A final cloth tape or elastic wrap is used to hold the cast in place.

INDICATIONS

Tail protectors are especially useful in large, long-tailed, short-haired breeds of dogs that have had recent tail amputations or trauma to the tip of the tail. Other indications are lacerations, abrasions, or crushing trauma requiring coaptation and prevention of further trauma.

CONTRAINDICATIONS

Patients with paresthesia from neurologic disorders, such as cauda equina syndrome, must have the underlying cause corrected for such a device to be helpful.

COMPLICATIONS

This coaptation device is not designed to protect the tail from constant licking or chewing. If that is a problem, concurrent use of an Elizabethan collar is indicated.

In conclusion, judicious use of devices and agents to prevent self-trauma often reduces morbidity from a surgical procedure or prevents a small lesion from becoming a major problem. The most frequent mistake is to wait too long to apply such a device or agent.

References

1. Hohn RB. Principles and applications of plaster cast. Vet Clin North Am 1975;5.
2. Knecht CD, et al. Fundamental techniques in veterinary surgery. Philadelphia: WB Saunders, 1975.
3. Leonard EP. Orthopedic surgery of the dog and cat. Philadelphia: WB Saunders, 1960.

6

TUMOR BIOPSY PRINCIPLES AND TECHNIQUES

Nicole Ehrhart, Stephen J. Withrow & Susan M. LaRue

The diagnosis of neoplastic and other pathologic conditions in animals depends on the procurement of an accurate biopsy specimen. Without an appropriate histologic diagnosis, it is impossible to plan appropriate therapy. Histopathologic results aid the clinician in providing an accurate prognosis and thereby guide the owner in the selection of various treatment options.

The ideal biopsy should procure enough tissue for specific pathologic diagnoses without jeopardizing the patient's well-being or the surgeon's ability to achieve local tumor control. Many biopsy techniques can be used on any given mass. The procedure used is determined by 1) the clinician's goals for the patient (i.e., diagnosis with no treatment versus diagnosis with treatment); 2) the skill and preference of the clinician; 3) the anatomic site of the mass; and 4) the general health status of the patient (1). Cytologic preparations obtained by fine-needle aspirate are often helpful in guiding the selection of the optimal biopsy technique.

General Considerations

Biopsies can be obtained before the initiation of definitive therapy (pretreatment biopsy), or histologic specimens may be evaluated after the mass is removed in its entirety. In most situations, pretreatment biopsy is the optimum route of action because it provides a diagnosis before the institution of invasive or aggressive therapeutics.

Pretreatment biopsy is warranted when the type of treatment would be significantly altered by knowing the tumor type. For example, if an animal presents with a mediastinal mass, the distinction between a thymoma (responsive to surgery) and lymphoma (responsive to chemotherapy), would be important to make before instituting treatment.

If the *extent* of treatment would be altered by knowing the tumor type, pretreatment biopsy should be performed. Certain cancer types (e.g., mast cell tumors and soft tissue sarcomas) have high local recurrence rates and therefore require removal with wider margins than benign or lower-grade malignant tumors. Many studies in both animals and human patients have shown that the best chance for surgical cure is to remove the lesion completely the first time. Clinicians who are tempted to "peel out" or "shell out" a lesion without knowing the histologic diagnosis are playing a dangerous game that may leave microscopic disease in the patient. If the lesion is malignant and incompletely excised, it will often grow back more quickly and invasively than the initial mass, thus potentially compromising further attempts at treatment.

Pretreatment biopsy should be considered when the tumor is in a difficult location for surgical reconstruction, such as a distal extremity, tail, or head and neck, or when the procedure could carry significant morbidity (e.g., maxillectomy or hemipelvectomy).

Finally, pretreatment biopsy is warranted when knowledge of the diagnosis would change the owner's willingness to treat the disease. An owner may be more willing to allow the veterinary surgeon to perform a thoracic wall resection for a low-grade soft tissue sarcoma (slow to metastasize) than for a high-grade osteosarcoma (metastasizes quickly).

In two situations, pretreatment biopsy is *not* indicated. The first is when knowledge of the tumor type would not change the surgical therapy. Examples of this are a splenectomy for a localized splenic mass or a lung lobectomy for a solitary lung mass. The second situation is when the biopsy procedure is as dangerous or as difficult as the definitive treatment (brain biopsy). In these cases, biopsy information is obtained after surgical removal of the lesion.

Soft Tissue Biopsy

Needle Core Biopsy

The most common use of the needle core biopsy is for externally palpable masses. This procedure can be done on an outpatient basis with local anesthesia and sedation. The method uses various types of needle core instruments (Tru-Cut [Tru-Cut biopsy needle, Travenol Laboratories, Inc., Deerfield, IL 60015] or A.B.C. Needles [A.B.C. Needles, Monoject, St. Louis, MO 63310]) to obtain a piece of tissue 1 to 2 mm in width and 1 to 1.5 cm long. The most commonly used size is a 14-gauge diameter needle; however, these needles are available in 16- and 18-gauge sizes as well. Any mass larger than 1 cm in diameter can be sampled using this instrument. These instruments can also be used for deep tissues, such as kidney, liver, and prostate, in a closed method or an open method at the

time of surgery. Despite the small sample size, the pathologist is usually able to discern tissue architecture and tumor type. With experience, the clinician can usually tell whether representative samples have been obtained. Fibrous and necrotic tumors may not yield diagnostic tissue cores. If the clinician believes that representative samples have not been obtained, an incisional biopsy is indicated.

The area to undergo biopsy is clipped and prepared as for minor surgery. Sensation in overlying skin and muscle can be blocked using a local anesthetic along the area that the needle will penetrate. The mass is fixed in place with one hand, and a 1-mm stab incision is made in the overlying skin. The needle biopsy instrument is introduced through the stab incision, and several needle cores are removed from different sites in the tumor through the same skin hole (Fig. 6.1). The tissue is then removed from the trough of the instrument with a hypodermic needle and is placed in formalin. Samples can be gently rolled on a glass slide for a cytologic preparation before fixation if desired. Skin sutures are usually not required. The biopsy tract, including the stab incision, should be removed at the time of definitive surgery.

Punch Biopsy

Another simple biopsy technique is the punch biopsy method (Fig. 6.2). This technique uses Baker's biopsy punch (Baker Cummons, Key Pharmaceuticals, Inc.,

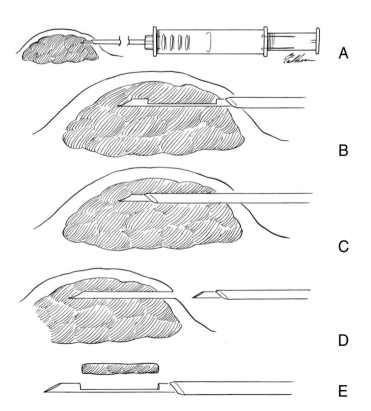

Fig. 6.1. Needle core biopsy technique. **A.** A stab incision is made, and the instrument is inserted through the tumor capsule with the outer sleeve closed over the inner cannula. **B.** The outer sleeve is held fixed while the inner cannula is thrust forward into the tumor. **C.** The outer sleeve is pushed forward to slice off the specimen, which is protruding into the trough. **D.** The instrument is removed closed. **E.** The inner cannula is exposed, revealing the tissue specimen in the trough. (Modified from Withrow SJ, MacEwen EC. Small animal clinical oncology. 2nd ed. Philadelphia: WB Saunders, 1996.)

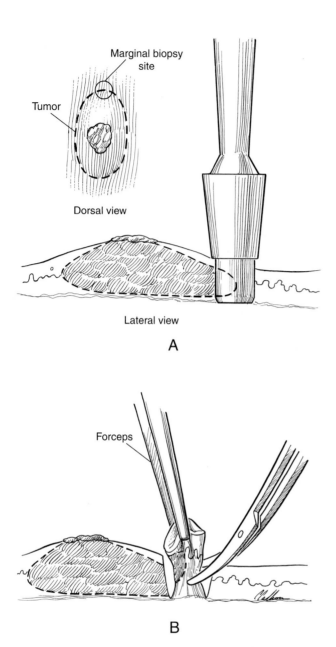

Fig. 6.2. Punch biopsy technique. **A.** Baker's punch biopsy instrument is applied directly to the mass, and downward pressure is exerted while the instrument is twisted. When the metal end is buried up to the plastic hub, the instrument is removed. **B.** Forceps are used to lift the biopsy specimen gently, and scissors are used to cut the base.

Miami, FL 33169) instrument to obtain the specimen. The skin is prepared for minor surgery, and the overlying skin is anesthetized with a local anesthetic. Baker's punch is applied to the mass in a manner that will yield a composite of normal and abnormal tissue. Pressure is applied as the instrument is twisted. The specimen is grasped and lifted with forceps while the operator uses scissors or a scalpel blade to cut the base. Care should be taken to not deform the tissue. Impression smears can be made for cytologic evaluation before placement in formalin. Multiple specimens may be taken from a single mass. A single skin suture per biopsy site is usually sufficient to close the defect and to control hemorrhage.

Incisional Biopsy

Incisional biopsy (Fig. 6.3) is used when neither cytologic examination nor needle core biopsy yields a diagnosis. As mentioned, incisional biopsy is preferred for ulcerated or necrotic tissue, because core biopsy rarely yields a diagnosis. Tumors are often poorly innervated, and as long as overlying skin is anesthetized, a wedge of tissue can often be removed without general anesthesia. Externally located tumors that are ulcerated may undergo biopsy without even the use of local anesthetics. The goal is to obtain a composite biopsy of abnormal tissue and adjacent normal tissue without compromising subsequent resection. The incisional biopsy tract always must be removed with a tumor at curative resection. Thus, the surgeon must not open uninvolved tissue planes that can become contaminated with tumor cells. In general, any normal tissue that the scalpel or surgical instruments have touched during an incisional biopsy is considered contaminated with tumor cells and is at risk for eventual tumor growth.

Excisional Biopsy

Excisional biopsy (see Fig. 6.3) can be both diagnostic and therapeutic. Excisional biopsy is best used when the treatment would not be altered by knowledge of the tumor type. Benign skin tumors and small malignant dermal lesions located in an area where reexcision (2- to 3-cm margins in all directions including deep) can be reasonably obtained are also amenable to excisional biopsy. All other masses should undergo biopsy before the curative surgical procedure. Additional uses of excisional biopsy are for solitary lung, splenic, and retained testicular masses.

Endoscopic Biopsy

Endoscopic biopsy is used most commonly in the gastrointestinal, respiratory, and urogenital systems. It is convenient, safe, and cost effective; however, it has several limitations. Visualization may be inadequate, resulting in nonrepresentative biopsy samples. Full-thickness biopsy specimens are often impossible to acquire in these organs, and therefore, inflamed tissue or normal tissue overlying a tumor may undergo biopsy, not the tumor itself. A histopathologic diagnosis of inflammation in an animal suspected of having neoplasia should be interpreted with caution.

Fig. 6.3. Excisional (top) and incisional (bottom) biopsy. The location of the top tumor would be amenable to wide excisional margins with an option to pursue a re-resection if needed. The location of the bottom tumor is less amenable to wide excisional margins. Attempts to excise this tumor with close margins may leave residual disease in this patient and may compromise the optimum surgical course of treatment. The bottom tumor should undergo biopsy before resection with curative intent. The axis of the biopsy incision is parallel to the long axis of the leg. (Modified from Withrow SJ, MacEwen EC. Small Animal clinical oncology. 2nd ed. Philadelphia: WB Saunders, 1996.)

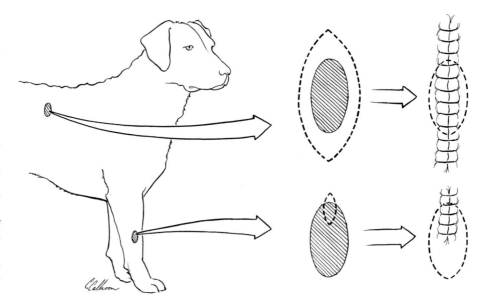

Laparoscopy and Thoracoscopic Biopsy

These techniques are best used when all staging and diagnostic procedures suggest inoperable and diffuse disease or when precise staging is indicated and an open procedure is not desired. Laparoscopic and thoracoscopic biopsy can yield important information regarding the extent of disease. Its disadvantages are that it can take as long as an exploratory laparotomy, it requires general anesthesia, and it does not give the clinician visualization as clear as that attained during open exploratory. In most cases, it cannot provide for excision. This procedure also carries some risk of hemorrhage and leakage of fluid from hollow organs and tumors. Animals staged by whatever means as having resectable disease are often best served by open exploratory laparotomy or thoracotomy, whereby resection with curative intent can be performed (1).

Image-Guided Biopsy

The use of fluoroscopy, computed tomography, and ultrasonography has greatly expanded the clinician's ability to stage and diagnose neoplasia. Image-guided biopsy may result in the avoidance of more invasive diagnostic procedures. A disadvantage of image-guided biopsy is that the technique requires specialized equipment and training. Biopsy in a closed space with limited visualization of the lesion carries some risk. As with laparoscopy and thoracoscopy, image-guided biopsy is best done when the clinician is fairly certain that an excisional attempt would be unsuccessful or when pretreatment biopsy results would change the owners' willingness to pursue more aggressive medical or surgical therapy.

Tissue Procurement and Fixation Guidelines

The concept that performing a biopsy releases tumor cells and leads to early metastasis and decreased survival has proved false. Although biopsy procedures do release tumor cells into the circulation, neoplastic cells are constantly shed into vessels and lymphatics on a day-to-day basis (1). No evidence in either human patients or animals indicates that a properly performed biopsy leads to a decrease in survival or early metastases. On the other hand, a poorly planned or improperly executed biopsy can result in significant alterations in the optimum treatment plan.

Biopsies should be planned so the tract may subsequently be removed with the entire mass. The ideal circumstance is when the biopsy is performed by the surgeon who will eventually perform the curative-intent procedure. Biopsies performed within a body cavity (either open or closed) should be done so tumor cells are not "spilled" into the cavity. This precaution prevents seeding of peritoneal or pleural cavities. The sample size of the specimen affects the accuracy of the diagnosis. Because tumors are not homogenous and often contain areas of necrosis and inflammation, larger samples or multiple samples from different areas in a mass are more likely to yield a diagnosis. The smaller the sample, the less representative it is of the whole tumor. Thus, if needle core biopsy specimens are obtained, several samples should be submitted. Biopsies should not be obtained with electrocautery because this technique will disturb and deform the tissue architecture. Likewise, the clinician should take care not to deform the sample with forceps, suction, or other handling methods. Cautery can be used after

bundles should be avoided. If evidence points toward primary bone tumor and if the clients are interested in pursuing limb-sparing surgery, referral for biopsy may be the best alternative. General anesthesia is usually necessary for bone biopsy. Selection of the anesthetic regimen depends on the general condition of the animal, on personal preference, and on experience. Because many of these patients are geriatric, complete blood count, serum biochemistry, and urinalysis are indicated. In some cases, particularly in animals with a lytic lesion, heavy sedation and local anesthesia may suffice.

Surgical Technique

The surgical site should be aseptically prepared and routinely draped. Adhesive drapes covering the biopsy site offer excellent protection allowing palpation and manipulation of the limb. A 1- to 2-mm stab incision in the skin is made at the desired location. The Jamshidi cannula, with the stylet locked in place, is gently pushed through the soft tissue structures. When bone is reached, the location of the cannula should be evaluated using the radiographs as reference (Fig. 6.5). The cannula can be shifted to a different location if desired. The stylet is removed. With a gentle twisting motion and the application of firm pressure, the cortex is penetrated. The cannula is advanced through the medullary cavity, taking care to avoid penetrating the opposite cortex (Fig. 6.6). After the instrument is removed,

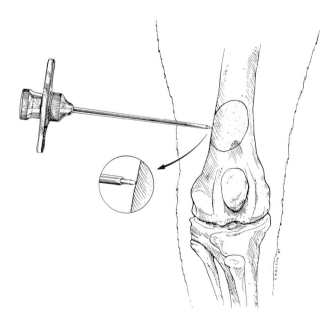

Fig. 6.5. With the stylet locked in place, the cannula is advanced through soft tissue structures until bone is reached. The cannula should point toward the center of the tumor.

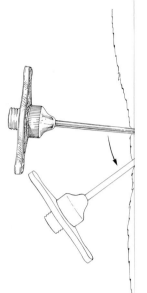

Fig. 6.6. After the stylet [...] motion and applying gentle pr[...] cannula is advanced until the [...] is withdrawn. The procedure [...] toward the periphery of the [...]

the specimen is pushed [...] base of the cannula with [...] (Fig. 6.7). The procedure [...] tissue tract previously es[...] be angled in different po[...] Two or three specimen[...] center of the lesion is so [...] be obtained, the cannu[...] the peripheral aspect of [...] erally not a problem wi[...] bleeding occurs, direct p[...] it. The Jamshidi instrum[...] is applied.

Damage to the cannu[...] biopsy of normal cortica[...] liferative and organized [...] cannot be inserted, its p[...] to ensure that the cann[...] bone. If the position ap[...] be indicated to obtain a[...] ture may be placed afte[...] of the lower extremities[...]

Biopsy specimens sh[...] tral-buffered formalin s[...] prevent desiccation. Sp[...] culture medium if desir[...]

blade removal of a specimen to control hemostasis if necessary.

The junction of normal and abnormal tissue is frequently the best area for sampling. This aids the histopathologist in comparing normal and abnormal tissue architecture. It is important to plan the incision so the normal tissue incised during the biopsy can easily be removed and is not necessary for reconstruction of the surgical defect. (The exception to the tissue junction rule is bone biopsies, discussed later in this chapter.) Biopsies performed on the legs or the tail should be done using an incision parallel to the long axis of the structure. This technique aids in resection of the biopsy scar if needed.

Excisional specimens submitted for biopsy should be evaluated for surgical margins. The surgeon should mark any areas of question or submit a margin from the patient in a separate container. It is good practice to mark all excisional margins routinely with ink. The pathologist samples tissue from several areas of the specimen. If tumor cells extend to the inked margin microscopically, the excision should be considered incomplete ("dirty"). Lateral and deep margins of an excised mass can be painted with India ink and allowed to dry before placement in formalin. Commercially available colored inks can be used to denote different sites on the tumor if desired (Davidson Marking System, Bloomington, MN).

Ultimately, the surgeon has the responsibility to communicate to the pathologist what is expected when evaluating margins on an excisional sample. Of course, incisional biopsies, needle core biopsies, and punch biopsies have incomplete margins by definition. Pathologists may not know whether the sample is intended to be excisional and do not always evaluate margins unless asked. Good communication between the pathologist and the clinician is vital to the care of the patient. Waiting until recurrence of the tumor to reoperate on a known malignancy that has been incompletely resected is a disservice to the client and the animal. Incomplete surgical resection of malignant disease is best dealt with early so further surgery or adjuvant therapy can be instituted immediately.

Tissues should be fixed in 10% neutral buffered formalin in a ratio of 1 part specimen to 10 parts fixative. Proper fixation is vital for accurate pathologic diagnosis. Tissue thicker than 1 cm does not fix deeply. Large masses can be sliced like a bread loaf, leaving one edge intact to allow for orientation. Alternatively, representative samples from the tumors can be sent while the larger portion of tumor is saved in formalin and further sections submitted if the pathologic diagnosis is in question. It is possible, especially in some large splenic masses, for only a small portion of the mass to be neoplastic and for the rest to consist of hematoma, necrosis, or fluid. This possibility empha-

sizes the need to submit several representative samples or, when possible, the entire mass. Tissue that is prefixed over 2 to 3 days in formalin can be mailed with a tissue-to-formalin ratio of 1:1.

For the pathologist to provide the most accurate diagnosis, each sample must be accompanied by a complete history. Whenever the histopathologic diagnosis does not concur with the history, clinical signs, or clinician's impression, a call to the pathologist is warranted. In some cases, a small but vital piece of information left out of the patient's history can drastically change the pathologist's impressions. Pathology is a combination of art and science, and diagnoses are only as accurate as the information provided by the clinician.

A veterinary-trained pathologist is always preferable to a pathologist trained in human disease. Although similarities exist across species lines, there are enough histologic differences to result in interpretive errors.

Frozen Sections

Frozen sections are becoming more common in the perioperative setting in veterinary medicine. This process provides a rapid means to a diagnosis at the time of surgery, as well as information on adequacy of tumor resection and the presence or absence of metastases. Although the use of this technique in veterinary medicine is limited to those institutions with specialized personnel and equipment, it is of potentially great value to the surgeon. Accuracy rates are high (93%) when results are compared with those from traditional paraffin-embedded tissues (2).

Bone Biopsy

Bone biopsy is essential in the diagnosis of proliferative and lytic bone lesions. Results of a bone biopsy often determine the course of treatment and may drastically change proposed operative intervention. As with all biopsies, the clinician must plan the biopsy with the intended curative treatment in mind. The most common instruments used for bone biopsies are the Michelle trephine (Michelle trephine, Kirschner Co., Timonium, MD) and the Jamshidi-type bone marrow biopsy needle (Jamshidi bone marrow/aspirate needle, American Pharmaseal, Valencia, CA 91335; Bone marrow biopsy needle, Sherwood Medical, St. Louis, MO 63130). When used properly, both instruments provide a suitable sample with minimal complications. The small size of the Jamshidi biopsy needle cannula is advantageous in that it requires a smaller skin approach (1-mm stab incision) and leaves a small-diameter bone defect, making biopsy-related fractures less likely than with a trephine. Trauma to soft tissue

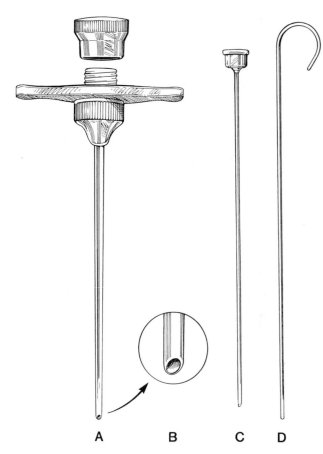

Fig. 6.4. Jamshidi-type biopsy device. **A.** Cannula and screw-on cap. **B.** Tapered point to "lock in" the biopsy specimen. **C.** Pointed stylet to advance the cannula through soft tissue structures. **D.** Probe to expel the specimen out of the cannula base. (From Powers BE, LaRue SM, Withrow SJ, et al. Jamshidi needle biopsy for diagnosis of bone lesions in small animals. J Am Vet Med Assoc [in press].)

structures and hemorrhage are minimal with the Jamshidi method.

Jamshidi needles are available in single-use and reusable models (3). The reusable model is "self-sharpening" and steam sterilizable. In our experience, the single-use model may be reused 10 to 15 times after gas sterilization. Jamshidi-type needles are available in various sizes, but the 8- and 11-gauge needles (4 inches long), are most commonly used. A Jamshidi-type needle features a pointed stylet that facilitates passage through the soft tissues (Fig. 6.4). The stylet is secured by a screw-on cap. The tip of the cannula is tapered, allowing the specimen to be locked into the cannula. This tapering eliminates the rocking motion necessary to break off and retrieve a tissue specimen when using a trephine. A small probe is also provided to assist in removing the specimen from the needle. The specimen must be pushed out the handle because

damage and compre[...] will occur if it is pus[...]

Indications and Pre[...]

Bone biopsies are mc[...] presence of a neopla[...] clinical evaluation. P[...] in dogs include osteo[...] sarcoma, and hema[...] eloma, and other rou[...] from bone. Metastat[...] mary tumors must a[...] bone can occur with[...] clinical and radiogra[...] static bone tumors c[...] ness of the affected li[...] tive when palpate[...] changes, which are[...] conditions that can r[...] and bacterial osteom[...] have generally travel[...] with bacterial osteor[...] drainage from the le[...] trauma or previous s[...]

Although history,[...] changes can aid in [...] the definitive diagno[...] only through histol[...] men. Radiographic e[...] clude two different [...] of the lesion. As pr[...] traditionally obtaine[...] normal tissue. Howe[...] plastic lesions is mos[...] (4). Bones surround[...] trauma, infection, a[...] Although biopsy spe[...] bone tumors often c[...] sue, tumor identific[...] quate sampling may [...] In these cases, the c[...] especially if the diag[...] the clinical picture. [...] measured on the r[...] nearby landmark, ge[...] diograph should be i[...] at the time of biops[...]

The skin incision [...] should be made wit[...] in mind (i.e., limb-s[...] preferred location o[...] referral institution t[...] surgery. In any case,[...] and dissection throu[...]

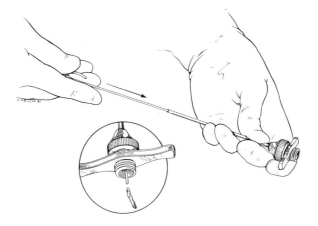

Fig. 6.7. The probe is inserted into the tip of the cannula, and the specimen is expelled through the cannula base (inset).

a pathologist and laboratory experienced in evaluating and processing bone specimens.

Nasal Biopsy

A nasal biopsy requires that the animal be anesthetized, with an endotracheal tube inserted. The cuff of the endotracheal tube should be inflated and checked periodically to prevent aspiration of blood during the procedure. Several procedures have been used to procure nasal biopsies. In our experience, the easiest and most successful procedure in dogs is the use of a rigid plastic tube, such as the outer sleeve of a Sovereign catheter (Sovereign indwelling catheter, Monoject, Division of Sherwood Medical, St. Louis, MO) or spinal needle (5). The actual catheter portion is discarded, and the metal stylet is cut off at the hub using bandage scissors. The catheter sleeve is slid over the remaining hub, and a 12-mL syringe is attached. The location of the tumor is visualized on radiographs, and the plastic sleeve is measured from the medial canthus of the eye to the tip of the nose. The sleeve can be marked or cut off so the clinician does not introduce the biopsy device further than this distance. This technique prevents disruption of the cribriform plate and invasion of the brain. The tube is introduced past the wing of the nostril using gentle pressure. It is then reamed in and out of the tumor repeatedly while suction is applied to the syringe. Hemorrhage is common but usually self-limiting and should not deter the clinician from being aggressive. The device is withdrawn from the nose, and the syringe is removed and filled with air. The specimen is then forced out by flushing the air through the tube using the syringe. Samples should be placed on a gauze sponge to allow blood to drain away. Tumor tissue is usually white to tan, although it may be hemorrhagic and mucoid. All tissues are

placed in 10% buffered formalin for evaluation. Smaller pieces can be placed on filter paper before placement in formalin to preserve architecture.

In cats, smaller dogs, and brachiocephalic breeds, a curette can be used followed by flushing the nose with saline. Care is taken to properly inflate the endotracheal tube cuff to prevent aspiration. The instrument should not be introduced further than the distance from the tip of the nose to the medial canthus. It is helpful to mark the instrument with a piece of tape at this distance. Sponges should be placed above the soft palate and at the external nares to catch bits of tissue. The curette is then introduced into the nasal cavity and a scooping action is used to dislodge tumor fragments. Cool saline is used to flush out specimen pieces using a pulsing action. All tissue is submitted for histopathologic evaluation.

Mild hemorrhage is noted for several hours after the biopsy. Sneezing after the biopsy can aggravate this hemorrhage. Patients should undergo recovery in a quiet area with supervision and should be kept for several hours or overnight after anesthetic recovery. These techniques are safe, they have minimal morbidity when compared to open biopsies, and they yield excellent specimens (5).

Interpretation of Results

The biopsy should be reviewed with respect to other data concerning the patient, such as clinical signs, history, and physical examination. A clinician should expect to receive the following information in a biopsy report: a determination of neoplasia versus no neoplasia; a diagnosis of benign versus malignant; a histologic type; grade of tumor if applicable; and margins if excisional. Interpretive errors can occur at any level of diagnosis. An estimated 10% of biopsy results may have some clinically significant inaccuracy. If the biopsy result is inconclusive or is inconsistent with the clinical findings, one of several actions should be taken. At the very least, the pathologist should be called and the concern expressed. This exchange should be looked on as welcome and helpful for both parties, not as an affront to the pathologist's expertise. In many cases, added information may lead to resectioning of the available paraffin tissue block, use of special stains for certain tumors, or a second opinion. Rebiopsy is also a possibility if the tumor is still present in the patient.

A properly performed biopsy and interpretation are the most important steps in the management of the cancer patient. The decision to submit a tissue specimen for histopathologic examination should not be left to the owner. If necessary, the charge for submission and interpretation of the biopsy should be included in the surgery fee. Mass excision without interpretation is no longer considered the standard of care. Because of increasing legal concerns, much more is at stake than the satisfaction of medical curiosity.

References

1. Withrow SJ, MacEwen EC. Small animal clinical oncology. 2nd ed. Philadelphia: WB Saunders, 1996.
2. Whitehair JG, Griffey SM, Olander HJ, et al. The accuracy of intraoperative diagnoses based on examination of frozen sections: a prospective comparison with paraffin embedded sections. Vet Surg 1993;22:255–259.
3. Jamshidi K, Swain WR. Bone marrow biopsy with unaltered architecture: a new biopsy device. J Lab Clin Med 1971;77:335.
4. Wykes PM, Withrow SJ, Powers BE, et al. Closed biopsy for diagnoses of long bone tumors: accuracy and results. J Am Anim Hosp Assoc 1985;21:489.
5. Withrow SJ, Susaneck SJ, Macy DW, et al. Aspiration and punch biopsy techniques for nasal tumors. J Am Anim Hosp Assoc 1985;21:551.

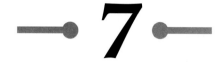

NERVOUS SYSTEM

Peripheral Nerve Injury and Repair

Andy Shores

The peripheral nervous system is comprised of the cranial nerves, the spinal nerves, and their branches. Injuries to the peripheral nervous system usually result from trauma, but peripheral nerve dysfunction can occur with other disorders represented in the DAMNIT (i.e., *d*egenerative, *a*utoimmune, *m*etabolic, *n*eoplastic, *i*schemic, *t*oxic) scheme of differential diagnoses. This section includes a brief review of peripheral nerve anatomy, physiology, and function and detailed discussions of the pathophysiology of injury to peripheral nerves and the surgical repair of peripheral nerve injuries.

Anatomy and Physiology of Peripheral Nerves

The cross-sectional anatomy of the peripheral nerve is illustrated in Figure 7.1. Axons are extensions of the nerve cell body and are the basic unit of the nerve. Each nerve contains multiple groups of axons (nerve fibers) arranged in fascicles. Surrounding the nerve fibers and their myelin sheaths is the endoneurium, the source of connective tissue support and nutrition for the fibers. The perineurium envelops each fascicle. Groups of fascicles are enclosed in the epineurium, which also surrounds the whole nerve, including the intraneural vessels. The fascicles and epineurium are important structures in the surgical repair of peripheral nerves (1, 2).

Motor (efferent) and sensory (afferent) fibers are present in most peripheral nerves. Most of the fibers are myelinated. Myelin is produced by Schwann cells, which surround the axons. Nodes of Ranvier are constrictions in the sheath along the axon and are the points at which nerve conduction occurs in myelinated fibers. The terminations of efferent peripheral nerves are at the myoneural junctions. The afferent fibers synapse in the dorsal root ganglia (1, 2).

The vascular supply to peripheral nerves originates from nearby large arteries and veins and from smaller adjacent muscular and periosteal vessels (3, 4). Branches of these vessels divide into ascending and descending branches when they reach the epineurium and anastomose with the intrinsic system. The intrinsic system is comprised of epineurial, perineurial, and endoneurial plexuses and their communicating vessels (4).

Nerve cells can be stimulated by electrical, chemical, or mechanical means. The threshold for excitation of nerve cells is low, and the resting membrane potential is approximately −85 mV. The membrane remains in a stable state until a sufficient threshold stimulus occurs. The threshold stimulus activates the cell membrane, allowing influx of sodium ions and depolarization of the membrane. When depolarization occurs, the impulse is transmitted the entire length of the nerve both proximal and distal to the stimulus. Once depolarization occurs, the entire membrane is obligated to depolarize (the "all-or-none" principle). Repolarization results from an efflux of potassium ions that reestablishes the resting membrane potential (2, 5).

The velocity of depolarization is determined by the degree of myelination of the nerve fibers, body tem-

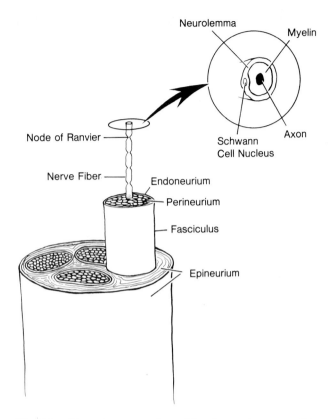

Fig. 7.1. Normal anatomy of a peripheral nerve in cross section.

perature, and fiber diameter. Heavy myelination, increased temperature, and large fiber diameter result in higher velocities. At the synaptic junctions, the nerve impulse results in an end-plate potential. Acetylcholine is liberated and occupies muscle receptor sites. Sarcolemmal depolarization occurs, and the muscle contracts. Acetylcholine esterase neutralizes the receptor site by degradation of the neurotransmitter (2).

Sensory nerve fibers are activated by peripheral receptors. Impulses are transmitted up the nerve (centrally) to the dorsal root and then result in a segmental reflex after integration at the level of the spinal gray matter. Further integration to higher centers is controlled by the internuncial neurons (2).

Nerve tissue is a poor, passive conductor and therefore requires an active, energy-expending process to conduct nerve impulses at the necessary velocities. Impulse transmission in myelinated axons is aided by *saltatory conduction* in which depolarization jumps from one node of Ranvier to the next. Because myelin is an excellent insulator and little current flows through it, conduction velocity would be much slower without saltatory conduction. Myelinated axons conduct impulses up to 50 times faster than unmyelinated axons (5).

Peripheral Nerve Injuries: Classification and Causes

Types of Injuries

Proper function of the peripheral nerve requires an anatomic and physiologic connection with the cell bodies in the central nervous system and a continuous and adequate supply of oxygen through the intraneural vascular system. Injuries to the peripheral nerves are traditionally categorized as follows:

Neuropraxia: Temporary loss of physiologic function without anatomic damage.
Axonotmesis: Loss of function with separation of the axons but with the endoneurium remaining intact.
Neurotmesis: Loss of function with complete division of the axons and connective tissue structures (severance of the nerve trunk) (1).

Neuropraxia can result from contusions or other disturbances in the blood supply to the nerve (e.g., application of a tourniquet for long periods during limb surgery). Ischemia of the nerve trunk produces rapid deterioration of peripheral nerve function (neuropraxia) after 30 to 90 minutes. It has been stated that 100% of peripheral nerve function will return if circulation is returned within a 6-hour period. Longer periods of ischemia result in epineural and endoneural edema with eventual axonotmesis (3). Recovery from neuropraxia usually requires 1 to 3 weeks (4).

Axonotmesis can occur in association with severe soft tissue injuries or can result from a stretch-type injury. If most of the axons within a nerve trunk remain intact, some function will remain in the limb, but this type of partial injury is uncommon. After disruption of the axons, the distal axon fragments undergo degeneration and are phagocytized. Return to function requires regrowth of the proximal axon segments distally to the end organ (e.g., muscles). The rate of axonal regeneration is 1 to 3 mm/day; complete regeneration may take 3 months to 1 year (1, 4).

After complete severance of the nerve trunk (neurotmesis), the flow of axoplasm is interrupted, and the distal segment undergoes degeneration of the axons and myelin (wallerian degeneration). Macrophages and Schwann cells remove the degenerated material; however, the connective tissue elements remain intact. Unless the nerve is repaired and the axons regrow, the connective tissue elements of the distal segment continually shrink. Electrophysiologic evidence of muscle denervation is evident in 5 to 7 days after injury (1). Axonal growth from the proximal segment begins approximately 21 days after injury. Unless the proximal and distal segments are connected, the axons lack direction and grow into the surrounding connective tissues, creating a neuroma. About 70 to 75% of the original function of the nerve may return after optimal surgical repair. Again, regrowth of the axons usually takes 3 months to 1 year (4).

Causes of Injuries

Trauma is the most frequent cause of peripheral nerve injury. Examples include deep lacerations, projectiles, bite wounds, and nerve damage from sharp fragments of long bone fractures. Brachial plexus avulsion occurs with extreme abduction of the forelimb and is usually a result of an automobile accident. Avulsion of the sacral nerve roots may occur in association with trauma to the pelvis and tail resulting from an automobile accident. Iatrogenic injuries can occur during orthopedic or soft tissue surgical procedures. Injuries to the cranial nerves are less common than those to the peripheral nerves of the forelimb and hindlimb. Intervertebral disc extrusions, spondylolisthesis, vertebral instability, fractures, and luxations in the lumbosacral area can also produce peripheral nerve injury. Primary neoplasms of the peripheral nerves (e.g., neurofibromas, schwannomas) also produce signs of peripheral nerve dysfunction. Metastatic tumors involving spinal nerves have been reported. Extramedullary tumors associated with the meninges or lymphoid tumors in the area of the lumbosacral intumescence can also produce peripheral nerve dysfunction. Surgical repair of peripheral nerve injuries is most applicable to injuries that result from trauma.

Diagnostic Methods

Complete physical and neurologic examinations should be performed on any animal with suspected peripheral nerve injuries. The neurologic assessment should include assessment of the cutaneous sensory function in all affected limbs. Figure 7.2 illustrates the cutaneous innervation pattern of the forelimb and hindlimb of the dog. A pinprick test over the areas shown in Figure 7.2 should reveal the pattern of peripheral nerve dysfunction in the limbs of most animals, but a more noxious stimulus may be required to evaluate sensory function adequately in a stoic dog.

Although electrodiagnostic testing is an important ancillary procedure in the diagnosis of peripheral nerve injuries, it is not commonly available in veterinary practice. Electromyography is performed using three electrodes placed percutaneously in the area to be studied (Fig. 7.3**A**). One electrode serves as the ground; the other two are the reference and recording electrodes. The electrical activity measured represents differences in the electrical potential between the reference and recording electrodes. From the recording electrode, the signal travels to a preamplifier and then to an amplifier. Visual and auditory representations of the signal are displayed on an oscilloscope and through a speaker, respectively.

A normal electromyogram produces a short burst of potentials when the recording electrode is inserted into the muscle (insertion potentials) followed by electrical silence. Denervation potentials consist of fibrillation and positive sharp waves (Fig. 7.3**B**). Electrodiagnostic evidence of denervation in selected skeletal muscle groups supports the diagnosis of a functional injury to the peripheral nerve that innervates the muscle group. Reinnervation of the affected muscle groups can also be monitored by electromyography, and early evidence of reinnervation may be represented by bizarre high-frequency waves.

Nerve conduction velocities also are used in the evaluation of peripheral nerve function. Both sensory and motor conduction velocities can be determined. Motor nerve conduction velocity is determined by stimulating a nerve at two separate points and recording an evoked response from each stimulation at a distal muscle innervated by that nerve (Fig. 7.4). The distance (in millimeters) between the two stimulation electrodes divided by the time difference in onset of the electromyographic response from each of the stimulations (in milliseconds) is the conduction velocity in meters/second.

Surgical Considerations and Techniques

The techniques used in peripheral nerve surgery within the spinal canal, such as in animals with the cauda equina syndrome, are discussed in other chapters. The material in this section pertains to the repair of peripheral nerves outside the spinal canal.

Exploratory Surgery and Assessment of Injury

After diagnosis of a traumatic peripheral nerve injury is made, exploratory surgery usually is indicated to assess the full extent of structural damage to the nerve. All areas of possible trauma to the nerve are assessed by visual inspection; this may require extensive exposure of the nerve trunk. Some caution should be exercised in preserving its blood supply, although the collateral circulation of the nerve trunk allows for a great margin of error. Experimental work has shown that loss of vascular supply over a length 45 times the

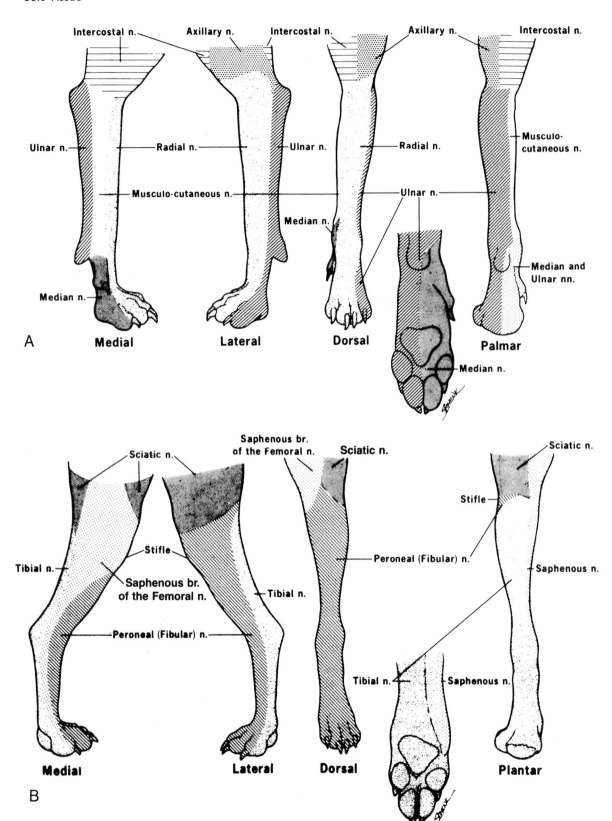

Fig. 7.2. Sensory regions of the forelimb (**A**) and of the hindlimb (**B**). (From Raffe MR. Peripheral nerve injuries in the dog. Part II. Compend Contin Educ Pract Vet 1979;1:269.)

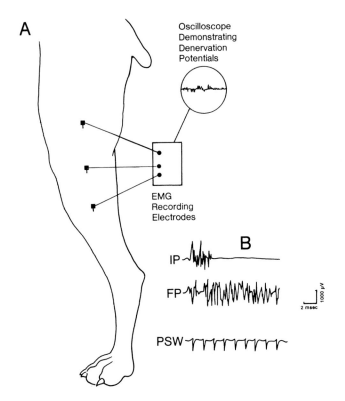

A

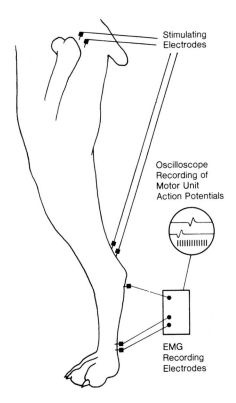

Fig. 7.3. **A.** Schematic representation of electromyography of the hindlimb. **B.** Electromyogram. Normal insertion potentials (IP), fibrillation potentials (FP), and positive sharp waves (PSW).

Fig. 7.4. Determination motor conduction velocity of the sciatic nerve. Motor nerve conduction velocity is calculated in meters per second from the formula (distance A to B)/(conduction time B − conduction time A).

diameter of the nerve (6 to 8 cm) does not impair circulation (6, 7).

If the area of injury appears relatively normal, it is likely that a neuropraxia has occurred, and additional surgical therapy is unnecessary. If the nerve trunk has undergone anatomic separation, then surgical repair obviously is indicated, the question being when to perform an anastomosis. Fresh injuries with little additional soft tissue trauma should be repaired immediately. When severe soft tissue trauma also is present, some surgeons prefer to delay nerve repair and recommend that the injured nerve segments be tagged with nonabsorbable, brightly colored suture material for later identification. The repair is attempted after the coexistent soft tissue inflammation has subsided (usually in about 21 days) (1, 6). However, I prefer primary neurorrhaphy even when the nerve endings are contused and bluntly divided. This retards retraction of the epineurium. If regrowth of the axons does not occur, resection and reanastomosis can be performed at a later date.

If the epineurium remains intact, the surgeon must determine whether the trunk should be incised for surgical repair. Neuroma formation indicates axonotmesis or neurotmesis. Several types or shapes of neuromas have been described. Fusiform neuromas, which can indicate axonotmesis or neurotmesis, result

from intraneural hemorrhage. The prognosis is better for axonal growth across the injury site without surgical intervention when the fusiform neuroma is soft. An indurated fusiform neuroma indicates intraneural scar formation. A firm, bulbous neuroma represents widespread neurotmesis, and surgical resection is indicated. A lateralized neuroma occurs with partial neurotmesis, which may be accompanied by preservation of some axons across the injury site. In general, if more than half the nerve diameter is severed, resection and anastomosis are required. A dumbbell-shaped neuroma indicates complete neural transection with the proximal and distal segments held together by a band of scar tissue (1, 6, 8).

After determining the site of injury, the area of interest is freed from surrounding tissues and the nerve is handled as atraumatically as possible, preferably only by the epineurium and with a nerve hook or fine 1 over 2 Adson-type thumb forceps. Only lint-free sponges should be used in the area (1, 6, 8).

Instrumentation

The use of an operating microscope and microsurgical instruments has become the rule rather than the exception for peripheral nerve repair in many veterinary colleges, but these expensive items are not necessary for a successful repair. The alternative is the use of ophthalmic surgical equipment including a magnification loupe (4×), jeweler's forceps (two pair), ophthalmic needle holder, small-toothed Adson forceps, and a No. 11 scalpel blade. Additional equipment includes lint-free sponges (Weck-Cel Sponges, Weck Co., Salvay Animal Health, Mendata Heights, MN 55120; Gelfoam, Upjohn Co., Kalamazoo, MI), a small square of blue nylon or latex for use as background material while suturing the nerve, and a right-angle vascular clamp. Sutures should be 5–0 to 7–0 in size with swaged-on atraumatic or reverse cutting needles. Polypropylene, nylon, or polydioxone are suture materials of choice because of their handling characteristics and lack of tissue drag. These are monofilament sutures and evoke minimal inflammatory response.

Preparation of a Nerve for Anastomosis

Exploration of the damaged nerve has been discussed. If a soft fusiform or lateral neuroma is identified, neurolysis may be indicated as an initial attempt to repair without resection and anastomosis. External neurolysis, which is indicated with soft fusiform neuromas, consists of gentle digital stroking of the injury site to "break up" any early attempts by the body to organize intraneural scar tissue. After external neurolysis, the injured site is freed from the surrounding scar tissue and is placed in a scar-free bed. Internal neurolysis requires an incision through the epineurium for removal of hematomas and perineural scar tissue. The integrity of the fascicles can be directly visualized at the same time, and the necessity for resection and anastomosis can be determined (1).

As noted earlier, the presence of a neuroma often indicates neurotmesis; in this case, resection is required. Before anastomosis of the nerve, the neuroma must be sectioned back to a level of functional nervous tissue (1). This is performed by first dividing the neuroma in half and then, starting at the distal end of the proximal segment, cutting serial 1-mm sections from the nerve ending with a No. 11 scalpel blade until normal, undamaged tissue is identified. This procedure is made easier by placing a piece of thin plastic or paper material around the circumference of the nerve stump and holding it in place with right-angle forceps (Fig. 7.5). The pressure produced by the wrapper allows the firmly held nerve to be sectioned easily with a No. 11 scalpel (9).

Fresh nerve injuries resulting from severance with a sharp object (e.g., glass or a knife) require little or no trimming, although the proximal segment undergoes retrograde traumatic degeneration for a distance of two or three nodes of Ranvier (1, 6).

It is important to have complete hemostasis of the nerve ending before suturing. This can be effected using lint-free sponges. If hemorrhage is extensive, the sponges can be soaked in a 1:100,000 epinephrine solution (1, 6, 8).

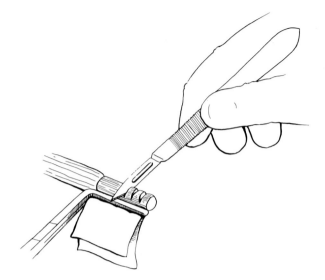

Fig. 7.5. Debridement of a nerve end is necessary when a nerve has been severely contused or a neuroma has formed. The nerve is wrapped circumferentially so a flush cut can be made. The proximal nerve segment is sectioned with a No. 11 scalpel blade in 1-mm sections until normal tissue is encountered. The clamp and plastic or paper wrap then are removed, and nerve repair is performed.

An important step in preparation of a nerve for anastomosis is to determine whether the nerve ends can be approximated without undue tension. The amount of tension at the anastomotic site is often the greatest factor in determining the success of surgery. If tension is excessive when nerve endings are approximated, the nerve should be gently freed from the surrounding tissue until the tension is sufficiently reduced. If this is not possible, the surgeon must consider the incorporation of nerve grafts (1).

When the foregoing steps have been completed, the adventitia should be stripped from the nerve endings because it represents connective tissue that would interfere with the growth of the axons through the anastomotic site. If the adventitia is not removed, this tissue will be carried through the epineurium with passage of the needle and suture. A small square of blue nylon or latex is placed under the site of the proposed anastomosis as a background visual aid.

Epineural Suture Neurorrhaphy

The most frequently used technique in veterinary peripheral nerve surgery is epineural suture neurorrhaphy. In this technique, four to six sutures are placed equidistantly around the nerve and through the epineurium (Fig. 7.6). An optical loupe is worn by the surgeon. Only the epineurium is handled, and this is done with jeweler's forceps. Before suturing, the nerve endings are lined up by visually matching fascicles. Locating the epineural blood vessels in the proximal and distal nerve segments may assist rotational orientation at the neurorrhaphy site (10). Polypropylene, nylon, or polydioxone (5–0 or 7–0) is used with an atraumatic or reverse cutting needle. The first sutures are placed at 3 o'clock and 9 o'clock if four sutures are to be used, or at 4 o'clock and 10 o'clock if six sutures are used. This placement assists in maintaining alignment. All sutures are first preplaced and are then tied to avoid excess tension at any one point. The 12-o'clock suture is placed next, followed by the 2-o'clock and 8-o'clock sutures if six sutures are used. The final suture is placed at 6 o'clock after gently rotating the nerve 90 to 180°. The ventral suture (6 o'clock) is tied first, followed by the dorsal suture and finally those on each side. When the anastomosis is completed, the site is inspected to ensure the absence of excessive tension or gaps in the anastomosis.

Fascicular Suture Neurorrhaphy

Although advances in microsurgery made fascicular suture neurorrhaphy feasible, this technique is not widely used in veterinary neurosurgery because there are relatively few fascicles in the animal nerves, the

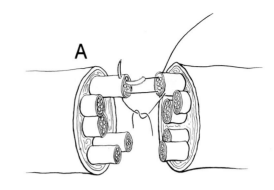

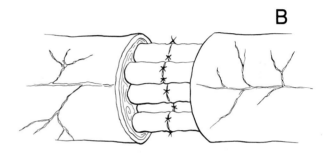

Fig. 7.7. Fascicular suture technique. See text for details.

equipment is expensive, microsurgical training is not standard in veterinary surgical training, and its advantages over the epineural technique have not been proved experimentally. The fascicular technique is important, however, when fascicular nerve grafting is required.

Fascicular suture neurorrhaphy produces exact alignment of the fascicles in the proximal and distal nerve segments. Sutures are placed in the perineurium. The same types of suture material are used as in the epineural techniques, but of a smaller size (9–0 or 10–0). Two to four sutures are placed in each fascicle (Fig. 7.7); additional sutures in the epineurium are optional. A major disadvantage of this technique is the presence of the suture in close proximity to the axons. The presence of any foreign material produces some inflammatory response and could result in scar formation at the anastomotic site.

Combined Epineural–Fascicular Neurorrhaphy

A third type of neurorrhaphy combines the fascicular and epineural techniques. In this procedure (Fig. 7.8), double-armed sutures are used and the initial sutures are placed in the perineurium outside the fascicles as guides for aligning the fascicles. These sutures are carried through the epineurium and later are brought through the skin and secured rather than tied (Fig.

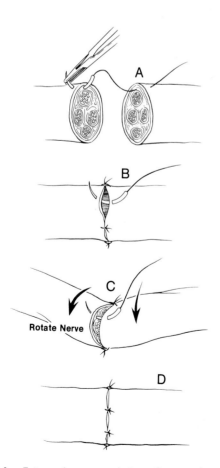

Fig. 7.6. Epineural suture technique. See text for details.

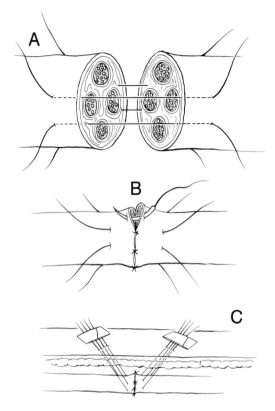

Fig. 7.8. Combined epineural and fascicular repair. Perineural sutures are placed with double-armed sutures, exit through the skin, and are secured with adhesive tape. These sutures are removed, as described in the text, after 7 days. (Adapted with permission from Smith JW, Newman FA. Current techniques in peripheral nerve repair. In: Rand RW, ed. Microneurosurgery. 3rd ed. St. Louis: CV Mosby, 1985.)

7.8**A** and **C**); this facilitates removal of the guide sutures after 7 days, thus limiting the intraneural inflammatory reaction. Epineural sutures also are placed at the time of anastomosis (Fig. 7.8**B**) and remain after removal of the perineural sutures. The guide sutures are removed by making a small skin incision, with the site under local anesthesia, cutting one end of the suture just under the skin, and gently pulling the sutures through the nerve and through the skin at the opposite end (9). The practical application of this technique in veterinary surgery has not been adequately explored.

Nerve Grafts

A nerve graft may be necessary when an animal has extensive loss of nerve tissue from the initial trauma, or when a large amount of tissue must be trimmed at the time of a delayed repair. Autogenous grafts are most acceptable because of the absence of a rejection factor; however, the use of allografts has been described. Xenografts are impractical because of the increased chance of rejection (1).

The caudal cutaneous sural nerve is usually used as

an *autogenous graft.* One to three fascicular segments from the donor nerve are used to span the distance between each recipient fascicle. The total cross-sectional area of each recipient fascicle is approximated with the donor fascicles. One fascicular graft is cut at a time and should be approximately 10% longer than the distance between the recipient segments, to avoid tension at the suture lines and to allow for shrinkage that occurs before the graft segment is revascularized (8).

The suture technique is the same as in perineural (fascicular) repair, and 9–0 or 10–0 sutures are used. This technique is most easily performed with the aid of an operating microscope. Two sutures are placed 180° apart to anastomose the proximal segment to the graft. The procedure is repeated until all proximal neurorrhaphies are completed. Next, the distal neurorrhaphies are completed, making sure that the correct proximal and distal fascicles are connected and that tension on the suture lines is not excessive. Finally, the graft segments are gently spread to allow as much contact as possible with the wound bed, thus avoiding a delay in the revascularization of the inner graft fascicles (10).

Peripheral nerve *allografts* may be more practical if an operating microscope is unavailable. The allograft is taken using sterile techniques from an animal of the same species and of a similar size. The graft should be 15 to 25% longer than the gap between the proximal and distal recipient segments. The proximal recipient fascicles and the graft fascicles are aligned, and the epineural neurorrhaphy technique is used (Fig. 7.9). The graft and distal segment sutures are then completed in a similar manner. The success or failure of the graft depends on proper neurorrhaphy technique and on the race between regeneration and rejection (1).

Postoperative Care and Assessment

The injection of triamcinolone (2.5 mg) around the anastomosis site has been advocated to enhance the quality of nerve regeneration by reducing fibroblastic infiltration, scar tissue formation, and the extraneural

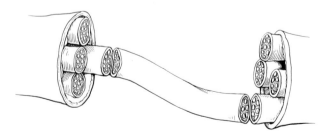

Fig. 7.9. Fascicular nerve allograft anastomosis. (Adapted with permission from Smith JW, Newman FA. Current techniques in peripheral nerve repair. In: Rand, RW, ed. Microneurosurgery. 3rd ed. St. Louis: CV Mosby, 1985.)

inflammatory reaction (1). After the surgical procedure has been completed, the limb is bandaged to reduce tension at the anastomotic site; this usually is accomplished by flexing the joint near the anastomosis. Additional bandaging may be necessary to prevent self-mutilation of the denervated distal limb. The bandage should immobilize the limb for at least 2 weeks, or longer if a nerve graft is used because two anastomotic sites must be crossed by the regenerating nerve. If a joint is bandaged in flexion, gradual extension of the joint is begun after the second week, and full extension is accomplished by the fifth week (1, 6, 8, 11).

The limb is evaluated daily until the patient is discharged from the hospital, then weekly or twice weekly. Physical examination should include sensitivity testing with a small hypodermic needle; the surgeon should remember that axonal growth averages 1 mm/day and that axons begin growth between 4 to 20 days after severance (1). Serial electrodiagnostic examinations are useful in evaluating the regrowth of the nerve.

References

1. Swaim SF. Peripheral nerve surgery. In: Oliver JE Jr, Hoerlein BF, Mayhew IG, eds. Veterinary neurology. Philadelphia: WB Saunders, 1987.
2. Raffe MR. Principles of peripheral nerve repair and regeneration. In: Newton CD, Nunamaker DM, eds. Textbook of small animal orthopaedics. Philadelphia: JB Lippincott, 1985.
3. Lundborg G. Structure and function of intraneural microvessels as related to trauma, edema formation, and nerve function. J Bone Joint Surg Am 1975;57A:938.
4. Raffe MR. Peripheral nerve injuries in the dog. Part I. Compend Contin Educ Pract Vet 1979;1:207.
5. Ganong WF. Physiology of nerve and muscle cells. In: Ganong WF, ed. Review of medical physiology. 11th ed. Los Altos, CA: Lange Medical Publications, 1983.
6. Raffe MR. Peripheral nerve injuries in the dog. Part II. Compend Contin Educ Pract Vet 1979;1:269.
7. van Beek A, Kleinert HE. Peripheral nerve injuries and repair. In: Rand RW, ed. Microneurosurgery. St. Louis: CV Mosby, 1978.
8. Simpson ST, Kornegay JN, Raffe MR. Surgical diseases of peripheral nerves. In: Slatter DH, ed. Textbook of small animal surgery. Philadelphia: WB Saunders, 1985.
9. Smith JW, Gillen FJ. Current techniques in peripheral nerve repair. In: Rand RW, ed. Microneurosurgery. St. Louis: CV Mosby, 1978.
10. Braun RM. Epineural nerve suture. Clin Orthop 1982;163:50.
11. Rodkey WG, Cabaud HE. Peripheral nerve injury and repair. In: Bojrab MJ, ed. Current techniques in veterinary surgery. 2nd ed. Philadelphia: Lea & Febiger, 1983.

Nerve Biopsy

Robert E. Kaderly

Diagnostic and prognostic information regarding peripheral neuropathies is obtainable by careful biopsy of an appropriate peripheral nerve. Biopsy of nerve and muscle tissue at the motor end plate should be considered when disorders of the neuromuscular junction (junctionopathies) or distal axonopathies are suspected. Fascicular nerve biopsy, rather than complete nerve transection and excision of a segment, is recommended to maintain the anatomic and electrophysiologic integrity of the parent nerve (1).

Several criteria for selecting a nerve for biopsy have been proposed (2). The selected nerve should be 1) affected by the neuropathy, as determined by a neurologic examination and electromyographic investigation; 2) consistent in its location, readily identifiable, and accessible for nerve conduction studies; 3) located away from vascular structures, tendons, and joints; 4) protected from areas of entrapment and trauma; and 5) one for which normal morphometric data are available. Mixed or purely motor or sensory nerves can be used for biopsy. The common peroneal nerve, as it passes over the lateral head of the gastrocnemius muscle near the stifle joint, and the ulnar nerve, as it courses parallel to the medial head of the triceps and superficial digital flexor muscles near the elbow, are commonly used (3).

A surgeon's loupe or operating microscope aids greatly in removing several nerve fascicles and in leaving the remaining parent nerve intact. The nerve sample should be less than 30% of the diameter of the parent nerve and 2 to 4 cm in length to provide individual portions for histologic, ultrastructural, biochemical, and teased-fiber studies. Before excision, the proximal end of the nerve sample is ligated using a length of 5–0 silk suture with a swaged-on atraumatic needle. Several nerve fascicles are selected, carefully separated from the parent nerve, and excised using sharp ophthalmic surgical scissors (Fig. 7.10). A 0.5- to 1.0-g weight is attached distally to provide slight tension on the tissue during fixing. Disposable muscle biopsy clamps (Heyer-Schulte Rayport muscle biopsy clamp, American Hospital Supply Corp., Chicago, IL) have been used to prevent shortening of the nerve sample, but they are not recommended. The longest length of usable nerve sample obtainable using a muscle biopsy clamp is 1.6 cm, and application of the clamp can easily cause excessive damage to the remaining nerve. The excised tissue is immediately suspended in 10% buffered formalin (3% glutaraldehyde is preferable if only ultrastructural studies are to be performed) (1). One portion may be embedded in paraffin for routine histologic sectioning. Alternatively, a portion may be embedded in epon, postfixed in 1% osmium tetroxide, sectioned (1 to 2 μm), and stained with paraphenylenediamine or toluidine blue for light microscopy (2). Ultrathin sections stained with uranyl acetate and lead citrate are used for electron microscopy (1). A teased-fiber sample should be prepared by postfixing in 1% osmium tetroxide and then passing the tissues through 66 and 100% glycerin (4). The individual fibers are carefully teased apart and are placed in a drop of glyc-

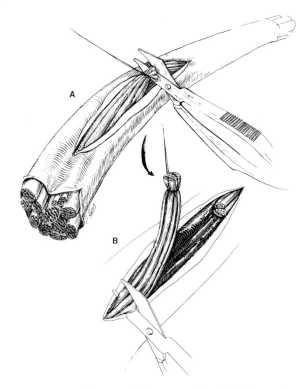

Fig. 7.10. A. Incision of the epineurium, isolation and mass ligation of several nerve fascicles, elevation of a bundle of fascicles from the parent nerve, and proximal transection using sharp ophthalmic scissors. **B.** Elevation of fascicular biopsy specimen by traction on the ligature and transection of the distal portion.

erin on a glass slide. Biochemical studies are performed on fresh nerve tissue that has been previously frozen in liquid nitrogen (3).

The nerve tissue is examined for the presence and number of inflammatory cells and for the number, size, density, and uniformity of nerve fibers. Teased-fiber preparations are examined for evidence of segmental demyelination (regions of nodal lengthening or absence of myelin between nodes) or axonal degeneration (long, linear rows of myelin ovoids or balls) (3). Successful axonal regeneration is characterized by uniformly short internodal lengths; variable internodal length with inappropriately thin myelin sheaths is characteristic of remyelination after segmental demyelination (3). Subtle changes may require quantitative morphometric analyses for accurate interpretation. Biopsy of nerve and muscle tissue at the motor end plate may demonstrate nerve terminal degeneration and regeneration, which would support a diagnosis of distal axonopathy.

References

1. Braund KG, Walker TL, Vandevelde M. Fascicular nerve biopsy in the dog. Am J Vet Res 1979;40:1025.
2. Dyck PJ, Lofgren EP. Nerve biopsy—choice of nerve, method, symptoms, and usefulness. Med Clin North Am 1968;52:885.
3. Shores A, Braund KG, Stockhan SL, et al. Diagnostic methods. In: Slatter DH, ed. Textbook of small animal surgery. Philadelphia: WB Saunders, 1985.
4. Braund KG, McGuire JA, Lincoln CE. Age-related changes in peripheral nerves of the dog. I. A morphologic and morphometric study of single-teased fibers. II. A morphologic and morphometric study of the cross-sectional nerve. Vet Pathol 1982;19:365.

Surgical Approaches and Techniques in the Management of Brain Tumors

Andrew L. Hopkins & John C. Meeks

Increased access to computed tomography (CT) and magnetic resonance imaging (MRI) over the last 10 years has provided for earlier recognition and accurate anatomic delineation of brain tumors and for a greater demand for their treatment. Treatment modalities used to manage brain tumors include varying combinations of surgery, radiation therapy, and chemotherapy, although the relative paucity of information in veterinary neuro-oncology often makes therapeutic decisions difficult. Veterinary experience with chemotherapy is currently limited to treatments extrapolated from the human literature on an empiric basis (1). Definite benefits, however, have been reported with varying combinations of surgical treatment and radiation therapy (Table 7.1), with clinicians achieving long-term survival rates of 1 to 3 years.

Although most studies have dealt with the treatment of brain tumors in general, the general consensus among neurologists and neurosurgeons is that the most successful treatment results have been achieved with meningiomas. This finding may be associated

Table 7.1.
Survival Times of Animals Treated With Surgery or Radiation Therapy

Therapy	Tumor Type	Survival time (reference)
Palliative therapy	Mixed	Means 59 days (22), 81 days (7)
	Meningioma	Median 6 days (6)
Surgery alone (dogs)	Meningioma	Mean 198 days (4) Median 143 days (17)
	Mixed	Median 212 days (4)
Surgery alone (cats)	Meningioma	Mean 485 days (4)
	Meningioma	Mean 780 days (11)
Radiation alone	Mixed	Median 322 days (7)
Surgery and radiation	Meningioma	147 days (6)
	Meningioma	27 days (signs ± ^{125}I) (6)
	Mixed	Median 345 days (5)

with the overall frequency and biologic characteristics of these tumors. Meningiomas are the most common brain tumor of dogs and cats. They typically have a superficial location (thereby allowing surgical access) and a tendency for slow growth, and they are often well demarcated from adjacent normal brain tissue (2). This is especially true of feline meningiomas, the physical characteristics of which make many of these lesions amenable to gross total resection with survival times in excess of 2 years after surgery alone (3, 4). Canine meningiomas, however, are softer, more friable, and more vascular, and they have less distinct boundaries with a greater tendency to show local invasion.

Much less is written about survival times of patients with other brain tumors. In one study, the median survival time for 10 animals with brain tumors of non-meningeal origin managed surgically was 414 days (4). Tumors included multilobulated osteochondrosarcoma, astrocytoma, metastatic carcinoma, choroid plexus carcinoma, glioma, lipofibrosarcoma, lymphosarcoma, osteoma, and pituitary carcinoma.

Preoperative Considerations

Intracranial surgery is a major surgical undertaking, and both surgeon and clients should be aware of the emotional commitments, potential treatment time, and the risks and costs. The likelihood of adjunctive, postoperative therapy should be considered from the beginning because radiation therapy often costs at least as much as the surgical treatment and may require 3 to 6 weeks for completion. The surgeon often has to weigh many factors in the discussion with the clients. These factors include the age of the animal (many animals with intracranial neoplasia are older), the existence of intercurrent disease, and the location (superficial or deep, nearby vital structures), size, and radiographic behavior of the tumor (invasion, definition from adjacent structures). Although primary brain tumors are more common than metastatic tumors, animals with intracranial masses should be evaluated for evidence of primary or metastatic neoplasia in other areas of the body.

Aims of Surgery

Surgery often plays an important role in the management of animals with brain tumors, but the surgeon must have definite and realistic goals and expectations of the surgical treatment. The goals in the surgical management of brain tumors include establishment of a definitive diagnosis, cytoreduction, and improvement of clinical signs and prolongation of life to permit further therapy.

Establishment of a Definitive Diagnosis

Although CT and MRI often allow an accurate determination of the tumor type, the number of instances where the tissue diagnosis is different and the need to have an accurate diagnosis for tailoring treatment to a specific histologic type require that a pathologic diagnosis be established. Histologic diagnosis may allow a more accurate determination of prognosis.

Cytoreduction (Debulking)

The process of debulking a mass reduces the tumor volume to be treated with adjunctive therapy. Gross, total resection is the surgeon's optimal goal, but with the exception of feline meningiomas, the firm texture of which frequently allows complete removal, surgical treatment of most brain tumors only permits gross subtotal resections. Stimulation of tumor growth is a common sequel to surgery necessitating adjunctive, postoperative therapy. The value of surgery in the management of aggressive human brain tumors, especially high-grade gliomas, is controversial. Stereotactic biopsy techniques, commonly used in human patients, circumvent the need for major surgery to obtain a tissue diagnosis and minimize surgical stimulation of the tumor. Although cytoreduction is practiced in some veterinary institutions, this field awaits further development in veterinary neurology.

Improvement of Clinical Signs and Prolongation of Life to Permit Further Therapy

Cytoreduction may alleviate the effects of local tissue distortion on the brain. Creation of a craniectomy "window" may alleviate or prevent development of intracranial hypertension because the cranial compartment is no longer closed. If tumor bulk is reduced, quiescent cells enter a more active phase of growth, making them more susceptible to radiation and chemotherapy. Probably the most frequently implemented and most beneficial adjunctive therapy to intracranial surgery is radiation therapy (5–7).

Anesthetic Considerations

Probably the most important considerations in anesthesia of animals with brain tumors is the existence of or susceptibility to increased intracranial pressure (intracranial hypertension) and its effects on cerebral blood flow and neural function. Many physiologic factors influence the dynamics of the intracranial compartment and must therefore be monitored in the anesthetized patient. These parameters include the arterial partial pressure of oxygen and carbon dioxide, temperature, blood pressure, and heart rate (Table

Table 7.2.
Intracranial Pressure: Anesthetic Goals

Factors Increasing Intracranial Pressure	Anesthetic Goals
Hypercapnia	Mild to moderate hypocapnea (25–30 mm Hg PaCO₂)
Hypoxia	Normoxia
Acidosis (systemic or local)	pH 7.4
Hyperthermia	Normothermia
Seizures	Seizure prophylaxis postoperatively
Systemic hypotension or hypertension	Blood pressure 100–140 mm Hg
Hypotonic fluids	Use of only isotonic fluids

7.2). Ideally, intracranial pressure is also monitored. A review of intracranial physiology is beyond the scope of this article and the reader is referred to reviews of pathophysiology of intracranial disease and anesthetic considerations (8, 9).

Methods for Reducing Intracranial Hypertension

MANNITOL

In animals with documented or intracranial hypertension or at high risk of having this condition (mass effect seen on CT or MRI), a mannitol infusion should be given either before or soon after anesthesia induction. Mannitol is infused at a dose of 1 g/kg over 5 minutes. This dose may be followed after 15 minutes with 0.7 mg/kg of furosemide to prolong the effect of the mannitol (10). Accurate use of mannitol requires measurement of intracranial pressure.

HYPERVENTILATION

Lowering of arterial carbon dioxide levels to 25 to 35 mm Hg is associated with lowering of intracranial pressure because of cerebral vasoconstriction. Peak reduction of intracranial pressure is achieved within 30 minutes. The effect is relatively short-lived (4 hours) because of adaptive buffering of the cerebrospinal fluid. Excessive hypocapnia (less than 25 mm Hg) may cause cerebral ischemia through excessive vasoconstriction.

Although the use and indications of methyl prednisolone sodium succinate are still shrouded in debate, some neurologists advocate the use of this agent immediately preoperatively in anticipation of the surgical injury and anesthesia to ameliorate development of vasogenic and cytotoxic edema. Although several experimental studies have demonstrated the benefits of steroids in neural injury, none has addressed the prophylactic use of these drugs in brain surgery (11). The dosage regimen used by many clinicians is based on that previously described for use in spinal injury, al-

though many clinicians have their own variations of the regimen, making interpretation of its value difficult. An initial intravenous dose of 30 mg/kg is given either before or soon after induction of anesthesia, with subsequent doses of 15 mg/kg at 2 and 6 hours and then 2.5 mg/kg every hour to a total of 48 hours (12).

Intracranial Pressure Monitoring

The treatment of intracranial hypertension is most rationally approached when intracranial pressure is directly monitored. Although use of such monitors is only sporadically reported in veterinary medicine, direct intracranial pressure monitoring provides the clinician with continuous, accurate intracranial pressure values that allow assessment of therapeutic manipulations and guide therapeutics decisions. A fiberoptic intraparenchymal catheter has been used in several veterinary institutions and is easy to work with although expensive (Fig. 7.11). When such a catheter is used in

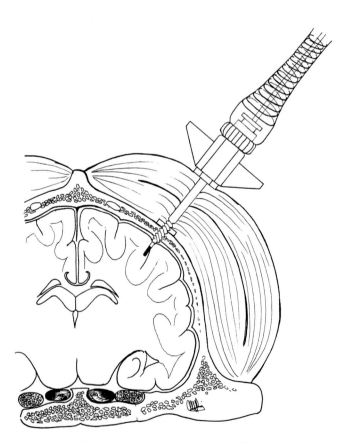

Fig. 7.11. Placement of an intraparenchymal fiberoptic catheter for measurement of intracranial pressure. A threaded bolt with compression screw secures the catheter in place. The information obtained is displayed continuously on a cageside monitor. The catheter should be placed on the side opposite the surgical site to avoid interference with the operation.

a surgical case, it is easier to put the catheter in at the beginning of the operation, after the surgical site has been draped. The surgeon should place the catheter such that it does not hinder the surgical procedure. Catheters may be kept in place for up to 4 days, to allow accurate postoperative evaluation of the intracranial compartment. The two main potential complications are hemorrhage from rupture of a meningeal or parenchymal vessel and infection. Prophylactic antibiotic therapy has not reduced the rate of catheter infections in human patients.

Intraoperative Monitoring

When operating on and around the brainstem, evaluation of intraoperative brainstem auditory evoked responses may allow early assessment of surgical damage to the brainstem pathways.

Instrumentation

Most brain surgery can be performed with routine neurosurgical equipment supplemented with some microsurgical instruments. Some procedures, however, may benefit from use of an operating microscope and intraoperative ultrasound. Ultrasound may be used to guide needle biopsy of intraparenchymal masses and to assess tumor resection. Ultrasonic aspirators and laser may facilitate the process of tumor reduction, but they do not reduce the need for adjunctive therapy. Instrumentation (with cost estimates) for intracranial surgery has been reviewed in the literature (13).

Patient Positioning

Positioning is an extremely important presurgical consideration. The surgeon should visualize the surgical approach and consequently the orientation of the head and brain to optimize access to the required site. Improper positioning can create extreme difficulty and frustration during surgical exposure. For dorsal cranial approaches, the animal should be placed in sternal recumbency with the head elevated. Lateral approaches may be helped with varying degrees of rotation of the animal's head and neck. Some surgeons favor the use of a head fixation apparatus (14, 15). The surgeon must ensure that the animal's jugular veins are not compressed because jugular vein occlusion compromises drainage of the cerebral circulation and raises intracranial pressure, and it may present problems with intraoperative bleeding. For these reasons, jugular catheters are probably best avoided in patients undergoing intracranial surgery. Care should be taken to ensure that the animal's tongue is not compressed during anesthesia because a swollen tongue in the recovery phase may compromise respiration.

Surgical Approaches

This section describes three common surgical approaches to the brain: 1) a lateral (parietal) approach; 2) a transfrontal approach (through the frontal sinus); and 3) a caudotentorial (suboccipital) approach. Each of the approaches can be modified and extended to suit the demands of the surgical procedure. We prefer craniectomy to craniotomy. This is because of the lack of necessity to replace the bone flap, the difficulty of wiring an ill-fitting bone flap back in place, and the concerns for creating a sequestrum. Several other texts are recommended to provide complete overviews of the topic (14–21).

Lateral (Parietal) Craniectomy

This approach is probably the most common, and it can be modified for access to a particular tumor. An inverted U-shaped incision is made from the dorsal to the lateral canthus, curving medially to the sagittal crest and then caudally and laterally to the caudal ear base. Subcutaneous tissue and facial muscles may be cut with scissors to expose the underlying temporalis muscle. Superficial nerves should be reflected to one side or other of the incision, although smaller branches may be cut with no detriment to the patient. The skin edges are reflected, and a secondary layer of surgical drapes is applied to the everted skin margins. The fascia of the temporalis muscle is incised parallel to (but 2 to 3 mm from) its attachment to the sagittal crest. This leaves a line of fascia for reapposition of the temporalis muscle during closure (Fig. 7.12). The temporalis muscle is reflected from the surface of the skull with a periosteal elevator. The surgeon should reflect as much as possible of the temporalis muscle at the beginning, to optimize exposure and allow for expansion of the operative site. Care should be taken to avoid damaging the occipital branch of the great auricular artery at the base of temporalis muscle. The temporalis muscle may be reflected completely from the occipital ridge and the back of the frontal sinus. Stay sutures may help to keep the temporalis muscle reflected.

The cranial vault may be perforated in various ways. Some surgeons prefer to create a square or circular bone flap using a nitrogen-powered drill and then lever out the resulting bone flap, which may or may not be replaced at the end of the surgical procedure. Careful use of the drill is required because tearing of the dura mater and meningeal artery is common using this technique. A craniotome can be used with a dural

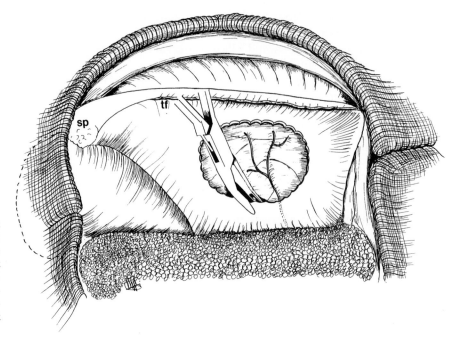

Fig. 7.12. Exposure of the cranial vault by parietal craniectomy. Rongeurs may be used to expand the initial bur hole. The middle meningeal artery is exposed intact within the dura. A thin strip of temporal fascia (tf) allows reapposition of the temporalis muscle during closure. The supraorbital process (sp) is the lateralmost extent of the frontal sinus.

guard to allow drilling of the calvarium without penetrating the dura. We prefer to create a 1.0- to 1.5-cm diameter bur hole at the center of the proposed craniectomy site with a nitrogen-powered drill, taking care not to penetrate the dura. The hole may then be expanded with rongeurs (see Fig. 7.12). This technique allows reflection of the dura mater away from the inner surface of the calvarial bone with the lower jaw of the rongeurs before removal of a bite of bone. Hemorrhage from the calvarial bone may be stemmed with bone wax. Continued expansion of the initial bur hole in this way allows preservation of an intact dura mater and visualization of the middle meningeal artery contained therein. Preservation of the integrity of the dura allows for its resuturing at closure. After exposure of the required area, the dura is incised. Whether the dura is left attached at one edge or whether it is removed completely, it should be kept stretched and moist to facilitate its resuturing during closure. If necessary, the middle meningeal artery may be cauterized. Using this technique of bone removal, the craniectomy may be extended over the midline because the dorsal sagittal sinus is contained in the dura and can also be reflected away from the parietal bone. One cannot extend the craniectomy caudally past the transverse sinus without destroying it because the transverse sinus is largely encased in a bony canal at the interface of the occipital bone and the parietal bone. However, the transverse sinus can be plugged unilaterally with gelatin sponge (Gelfoam, Upjohn Co., Kalamazoo, MI) and the craniectomy extended without adverse effects to the patient.

When removing or debulking a tumor, the surgeon should start at an edge and try to define a tumor capsule or plane of tissue separation between the tumor and the surrounding neuropil and should continue the separation along this plane. If no such plane is definable, the surgeon has the following options:

1. To remove as much of the tumor as possible, based on an estimate of the margins from the gross appearance and the accompanying CT or MRI. The margins the surgeon chooses are based on personal preference, location of the tumor, and tumor type. Intraoperative ultrasonography may aid in the delineation of the tumor margins. Histologic evaluation of the tumor at the time of the surgical procedure may also help with these determinations.

2. To remove a piece of tumor tissue sufficient to gain a histologic diagnosis. In both situations, residual tumor tissue is inevitable, and adjunctive therapy is required. The histologic diagnosis helps the clinician to determine subsequent therapy. Although large amounts of normal tissue may be removed, one often has a tradeoff between trying to remove every last piece of a poorly defined mass and inflicting surgical injury on the patient (21). This factor should be kept in mind when the surgeon is struggling for a total resection but is more than likely leaving residual tumor tissue. Biopsy may be performed with a scalpel, radiosurgery unit, or hand-held thermal cautery unit.

Before closure, the surgery site should be lavaged with saline, and as much debris as possible should be removed. The dura should be sutured back in place. A fascial graft taken from the outer surface of the temporalis muscle is frequently required to help cover the craniectomy defect.

Vascular compromise is an important consideration in any intracranial operation. However, no definitive guidelines are available about the value of different vascular structures, and most information is derived from practical experience. Surgeons generally accept that ablation of the rostral third to half of the dorsal sagittal sinus is not detrimental to the patient. Ablation of one transverse sinus is also well tolerated. Ablation of the whole dorsal saggital sinus (and hence the straight sinus draining the deep cerebral structures and potentially one or more transverse sinuses) results in venous infarction and necrosis of large areas of cerebrocortical tissue.

Frontal or Transfrontal Craniectomy

Access to frontal or paranasal tumors often requires penetration (and ablation) of the overlying frontal sinus. This approach is often used for access to canine olfactory or paranasal meningiomas. A skin incision is started dorsal to the medial canthus, is continued medially to the midline, and then is extended caudally to the nuchal crest. The temporalis muscle fascia is incised and reflected as previously described, although, depending on the anticipated size of craniectomy, the occipital ridge attachment may be left intact. The supraorbital process of the frontal bone is exposed, and the triangular outline of the frontal sinus is defined. Entry into the frontal sinus creates the potential risk of wound infection because of contiguity of the sinus with the nasal cavity. To enter and ablate the frontal sinus before penetrating the cranial vault is probably better. The frontal sinus may be penetrated using a trephine, rongeurs, or a nitrogen-powered drill. Every effort should be made to keep the instruments and bone fragments from this stage of the surgical procedure separate from the instruments used for the craniectomy. The hole into the sinus is enlarged, the dorsal and caudolateral walls are removed, and the sinus is ablated. The epithelial lining of the sinus should be stripped away with a periosteal elevator, and the sinus should be lavaged with sterile saline. The sinus ostium is then plugged with Gelfoam. The cranial vault may then be entered as previously described. The calvarium forming the floor of the frontal sinus is thin compared with the remainder of the skull.

Although ablation of the sinus and the supraorbital process does not result in any unattractive cosmetic abnormalities, closure can be difficult. We place a fascial graft over the ostium and a second one over the craniectomy defect. The grafts may be secured by suturing to holes drilled in the bony edges of the craniec-

tomy window. The surgeon should attempt to close the space left by the sinus ablation with temporalis muscle, although this can be difficult and an open pocket sometimes remains. With time, this pocket fills in with connective tissue.

Caudal (Occipital) Craniectomy

This approach may be used to gain access to the caudal cerebellum and caudal dorsal brainstem or, if extended laterally, to the caudal–dorsal cerebellopontine angle and caudolateral brainstem. As before, careful attention is required to patient positioning. The lateral approach is discussed here because it is more difficult and, if it is understood, the midline approach is easy. With the patient in sternal recumbency and the neck elevated, the head needs to be tilted with the nose downward. In the case of a lateral lesion, the animal's nose should be slightly rotated away from the side of the lesion. Care should be taken to avoid jugular vein occlusion. For a midline caudal cerebellar approach, the skin incision is made from the caudal aspect of the zygomatic arch on one side to the other along the occipital ridge. For a lateral approach, the skin incision should run from the caudal aspect of the zygomatic arch on the side of the lesion to the cranial, dorsal spinous process of C2. The caudal aspect of the temporalis muscle is reflected rostrally off the parietal bone. This may necessitate freeing the muscle from its caudal attachment to the interparietal bone and nuchal crest. The cervical musculature should be reflected from the occipital bone and retracted caudally. Leaving a small fibrous attachment may allow reapposition of the muscles at closure.

As with the other approaches, an initial bur hole may be made in the occipital bone with a nitrogen-powered drill and then extended with rongeurs allowing the dura mater to be kept intact over the caudal cerebellum (Fig. 7.13). Important structures that delineate this approach include the atlanto-occipital membrane, the basilar sinus running in the condyloid canal in the medial wall of the occipital condyle, and the transverse sinuses in the occipital bone. If breached, all the aforementioned sinuses can be plugged with Gelfoam, with little to no detriment to the patient on a unilateral basis. Hemostasis of the sinuses allows extension of the craniectomy beyond the boundaries created by the vessels. Extreme care is required while working around the brainstem. A fascial graft may be required to cover the craniectomy defect at closure. The dorsal cervical musculature should be sutured to the fibrous strip created during the approach or to the caudal aspect of the masticatory muscles.

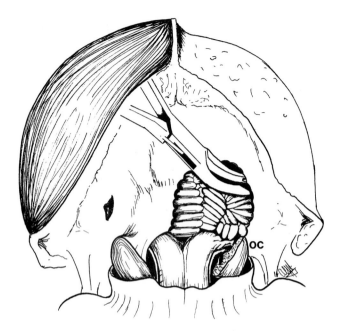

Fig. 7.13. Lateral, suboccipital craniectomy. Rongeurs may again be used to expand the initial bur hole. One-third to one-half of the medial dorsal aspect of the occipital condyle (oc) may be removed with a nitrogen-powered bur to improve exposure of the brainstem. The basilar sinus in the condyloid canal may be plugged with Gelfoam when breached.

Postoperative Care and Complications

Most intracranial surgery can be done with a surprisingly low degree of morbidity. In one study, radical cortical resection in anatomically normal dogs was associated with minimal patient morbidity. However, close postoperative monitoring of the patient is imperative because many physiologic processes may be altered by the neurosurgical procedure. As well as close monitoring of the patient's neurologic status, strict attention should be given to nutrition and to fluid and electrolyte balance. The following complications may occur:

1. Seizures. Anticonvulsant therapy is indicated in all animals undergoing brain surgery at least in the short term (4 to 6 months) and probably permanently in most animals.

2. Signs of severe neurologic disturbance within 24 hours of the operation (e.g., dementia, stupor, coma). This disturbance may be due to excessive removal or manipulation of normal neural tissue, vascular damage and ischemia, or progressive accumulation of blood or fluid at the surgery site causing intracranial hypertension.

3. Fluid and electrolyte imbalance. This disorder may result from use of mannitol and furosemide com-

bined with blood loss and altered hypothalamic secretion of vasopressin.

4. Cardiovascular disturbances (arrhythmia, hypotension, hypertension).

5. Respiratory disturbances (hyperventilation or hypoventilation).

6. Subcutaneous emphysema. Penetration and ablation of the frontal sinus are often associated with collection of air under the skin of the head. This complication may be avoided or minimized with preventive bandaging, but it usually resolves in 1 to 2 weeks.

7. Infections. The use of prophylactic, perioperative antibiotics is controversial; many studies fail to demonstrate any benefit. The choice is then largely personal. However, if fear of contamination of the operative site exists (e.g., frontal sinus penetration or a break-in surgical technique), then antibiotics are indicated. Broad-spectrum coverage should be instituted. We prefer a combination of enrofloxacin (5 mg/kg orally or intramuscularly every 12 hours) and cephalexin (22 mg/kg intravenously or orally every 8 hours). In cases of suspected or known contamination, it may be best to continue antibiotic coverage for 2 weeks.

Acknowledgments

We would like to thank David Hopkins, BVSc, for help with the illustrations.

References

1. Fulton LM, Steinberg HS. Preliminary study of lomustine in the treatment of intracranial masses in dogs following localization by imaging techniques. Semin Vet Med Surg 1990;5:241–245.
2. Lawson DC, Burk RL, Prata RG. Cerebral meningioma in the cat: diagnosis and surgical treatment of ten cases. J Am Anim Hosp Assoc 1984;20:333–342.
3. Gordon LE, Thacher C, Matthiesen DI, et al. Results of craniotomy for the treatment of cerebral meningioma in 42 cats. Vet Surg 1994;23:94–100.
4. Niebauer GW, Dayrell-Hart BL, Speciale J. Evaluation of craniotomy in dogs and cats. J Am Vet Med Assoc 1991;198:89–95.
5. Evans SM, Dayrell-Hart B, Powlis W, et al. Radiation therapy of canine brain masses. J Vet Intern Med 1993;7:216–219.
6. Heidner GL, Kornegay JN, Page RL, et al. Analysis of survival in a retrospective study of 86 dogs with brain tumors. J Vet Intern Med 1991;5:219–226.
7. Turrel JM, Fike JR, LeCouteur RA, et al. Radiotherapy of brain tumors in dogs. J Am Vet Med Assoc 1984;184:82–86.
8. Harvey RC, Paddleford RR. Anesthesia for the central nervous system and ophthalmic surgery. In: Slatter DH, ed. Textbook of small animal surgery. Philadelphia: WB Saunders, 1993:2271–2276.
9. Muir WM. Brain hypoperfusion post resuscitation. Vet Clin North Am 1989;19:1151–1166.
10. Roberts PA, Pollay M, Engels C, et al. Effect on intracranial pressure of furosemide with varying doses and administration rates of mannitol. J Neurosurg 1987;66:440–446.

11. Hall ED. The neuroprotective pharmacology of methylprednisolone. J Neurosurg 1992;76:13–22.
12. Braughler JM, Hall ED, Means ED, et al. Evaluation of an intensive methylprednisolone sodium succinate dosing regimen in experimental spinal cord injury. J Neurosurg 1987;67:102–105.
13. Shores A. Instrumentation for intracranial surgery. Prog Vet Neurol 1991;2:175–182.
14. Oliver JE. Surgical approaches to the canine brain. Am J Vet Res 1968;29:353–378.
15. Oliver JE, Hoerlein BF. Cranial surgery. In: Oliver JE, Hoerlein BF, Mayhew IG, eds. Veterinary neurology. Philadelphia: WB Saunders, 1987:470–492.
16. Knecht CD. Principles of neurosurgery. In: Oliver JE, Hoerlein F, Mayhew IG, eds. Veterinary neurology. Philadelphia: WB Saunders, 1987:408–415.
17. Kostolich M, Dulisch ML. A surgical approach to the canine olfactory bulb for meningioma removal. Vet Surg 1987;16:273–277.
18. Oliver JE. Principles of canine brain surgery. Anim Hosp 1966;2:73–88.
19. Parker AJ, Cunningham JG. Transfrontal craniotomy in the dog. Vet Rec 1972;90:622–624.
20. Shores A. Intracranial surgery. In: Slatter DH, ed. Textbook of small animal surgery. Philadelphia: WB Saunders 1993:1122–1135.
21. Sorjonen DC, Thomas WB, Myers LJ, et al. Radical cerebral cortical resection in dogs. Prog Vet Neurol 1991;2:225–236.
22. Foster ES, Carillo JM, Patnaik AK. Clinical signs of tumors affecting the rostral cerebrum in 43 dogs. J Vet Intern Med 1988;2:71–74.

⟞ 8 ⟝

TECHNIQUE OF SKELETAL MUSCLE BIOPSY

John F. Amann

When properly performed, skeletal muscle biopsy is an effective adjunct to the diagnosis of various neuromuscular diseases. Indications for muscle biopsy include atrophic or inflammatory myositis (especially of the muscles of mastication), polymyositis, muscle stiffness, muscle weakness, increased serum activity of muscle enzymes (particularly creatine kinase), and generalized or specific muscle atrophy (1–5). Muscle biopsy is especially indicated in inflammatory myositis because it can help to provide a rapid etiologic diagnosis on which treatment may be based. A consistent technique must be used in muscle biopsy and in sample handling after biopsy to avoid misleading artifacts (1–4, 7–10). When possible, the pathologist who will examine a biopsy sample should be consulted before the procedure; indeed, some pathologists require that a biopsy sample be obtained and processed in a specific way (9, 10). Only the most commonly accepted techniques of muscle biopsy and handling and an alternative method are discussed in this chapter. A newer method of percutaneous biopsy using a modified Baylor muscle biopsy set (Perfectum, Popper and Sons, New Hyde Park, NY) and suction has been reported by Reynolds and associates to produce suitable samples for muscle histochemical studies (11).

Selection of Biopsy Sites

Selection of the biopsy site—an important part of the procedure—is based on the patient's history and clinical signs. Easily accessible superficial muscles are obvi-

ous choices when other criteria do not prevail. If the history and clinical signs suggest a chronic problem, however, recently affected muscles should be included because chronically affected areas show purely reactive changes that are difficult to interpret in terms of primary pathologic process. Electromyography may be used to identify affected muscles to undergo biopsy, but the sites where electromyography needles are inserted should not be used for biopsy because they undergo artifactual changes. Data are available on the normal morphometric characteristics and fiber type distribution of several easily sampled muscles in the dog and cat, including the distal third of the biceps femoris and the long head of the triceps, and the proximal third of the superficial digital flexor (thoracic limb) and lateral gastrocnemius muscles (3, 7, 12–14).

Frequently, biopsy samples from two or more muscles are obtained from the same skin incision to provide information on the distribution of a disease; this approach minimizes sampling time and trauma. Biopsy of adjacent muscles innervated by different nerves can provide valuable information on the distribution of a neuromuscular disease. For example, the sciatic nerve–innervated biceps femoris muscle and the femoral nerve–innervated vastus lateralis muscle can be approached by a single skin incision on the lateral thigh. These nerves originate from different spinal cord segments and thus from different areas of the lumbosacral plexus, and they course over disparate routes to the muscles they innervate.

When a distal axonopathy is suspected, distal as

well as proximal muscles should undergo biopsy. The interosseus muscles along the abaxial side of the metacarpal or metatarsal bones of the second and the fifth digits are easily accessible. These muscles can be used if an analysis of neuromuscular end plates is intended because the muscle fibers are short and end plates are sure to be included in the biopsy sample without requiring tedious techniques of intravital staining or stimulation for motor zones. Intercostal muscles also are commonly sampled for biopsy when diseases affecting end plates (e.g., myasthenia gravis) are suspected.

Equipment

Specialized equipment is generally not required for muscle biopsy. The basic equipment is a No. 11 scalpel blade and 2–0 or 3–0 silk or synthetic suture. Special Y-shaped muscle biopsy clamps (Price muscle biopsy clamp, V. Mueller Instrument, Chicago, IL; see Fig. 8.6) are necessary for procedures that involve the immediate fixation of tissue in formalin or similar fixatives because of the immediate contraction of fresh muscle placed in fixative (15). The contraction of unclamped muscle can destroy the architecture of fiber relationships and can induce artifacts that could be interpreted as pathologic (9, 10). Some pathologists insist that clamps be used for all muscle biopsies, but this is not invariably the case (9). Surgeons often use clamps to facilitate handling a biopsy specimen atraumatically. Snap-freezing of muscle biopsy specimens (see later) is the most common tissue preparation technique and precludes the necessity for clamps (8, 11, 15, 16).

Surgical Procedure

Muscle biopsy is performed with the patient under general or local anesthesia, depending on the animal's physical condition and disposition. Deep infiltration with local anesthetics of muscle to undergo biopsy should be avoided. Preparation of the surgical site should be the same as for any sterile procedure.

The site of the biopsy should be exposed, and connective tissue and fat should be dissected away, so the direction of muscle fibers can be visualized. The muscle should be handled gently throughout the procedure, and care should be taken to avoid pinching the muscle with forceps. Stay sutures for manipulating the muscle are placed at each end of the muscle area to be sampled (1 to 2 cm apart) and at right angles to the long direction of the muscle fibers (Fig. 8.1). Both sutures should encompass the same cylinder of muscle fibers (approximately 0.5 cm in diameter) and should be tied loosely without compressing the muscle. Biopsy specimen can be manipulated atraumatically by means of these sutures.

Parallel incisions are made with a No. 11 scalpel

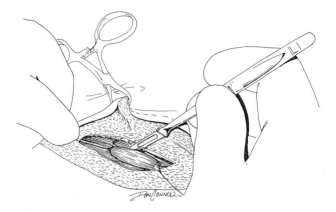

Fig. 8.1. After sutures have been placed at the ends of the area to be sampled for biopsy, incisions are made along each side of the biopsy specimen and parallel to the long axis of the muscle fibers.

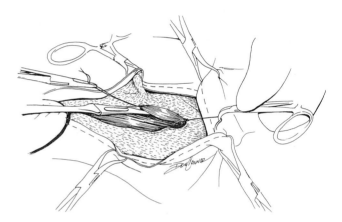

Fig. 8.2. After the parallel incisions have been made, the muscle is undermined by sharp dissection with a No. 11 scalpel blade.

blade along the sides of the biopsy specimen and are extended slightly beyond the sutures (see Fig. 8.1). While gentle traction is placed on the suture, the blade is used to undermine the specimen between these incisions (Fig. 8.2). Cleaning the blade with saline-soaked gauze to remove clotted blood and tissue residue after each incision facilitates the procedure and reduces tissue trauma. If multiple biopsy samples are taken, the blade should be replaced frequently. When the length of the biopsy specimen has been completely undermined, the ends of the specimen may be cut with a scalpel or sharp scissors (Fig. 8.3). A scalpel is preferred because it may compress the muscle less and therefore produce fewer artifacts. Hemorrhage can usually be controlled by moderate pressure after removal of the tissue. Occasionally, a large intramuscular artery is severed and requires ligation.

The biopsy specimen is placed in a gauze sponge lightly moistened with physiologic saline solution (Figs. 8.4 and 8.5). The muscle specimen contracts moderately when removed; however, it is not necessary to stretch the muscle unless special procedures

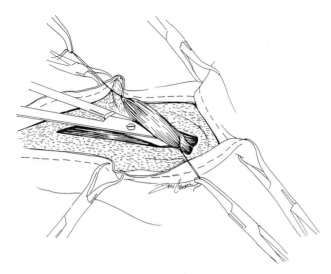

Fig. 8.3. When the specimen has been completely undermined, each free end is freed by cutting distal to the suture with sharp scissors or preferably a sharp scalpel blade.

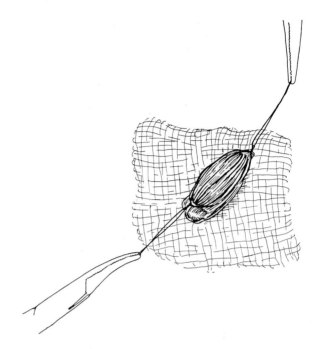

Fig. 8.5. The muscle biopsy specimen is removed with the sutures still attached and is placed on a gauze sponge that has been moistened lightly with physiologic saline.

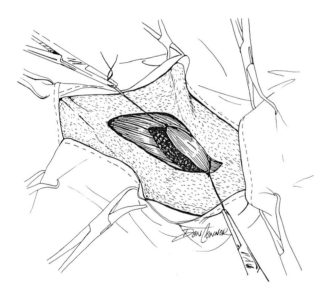

Fig. 8.4. The specimen is handled exclusively by means of the sutures on each end.

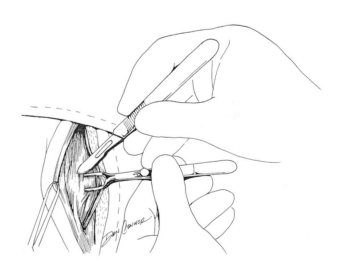

Fig. 8.6. An alternative surgical technique involves placing a Price muscle biopsy clamp on the muscle after parallel incisions have been made alongside the intended specimen.

Processing of Specimens

If kept cool (around 4°C) and moist, muscle intended for light microscopic examination remains useful for several hours (9, 15). Shipment to a pathology laboratory by overnight mail may be feasible if the specimen is loosely wrapped in a gauze sponge lightly dampened with physiologic saline, placed within a plastic container, and kept cold (0 to 4°C) but not allowed to freeze (15). The histochemical alterations that occur in a muscle specimen stored at 0°C over a 30-hour period have been reported and appear to be acceptable.

involving a definite sarcomere length are intended. In that case, a technique involving use of a muscle biopsy clamp (Fig. 8.6) is indicated. In this technique, parallel incisions are made as previously described, and the muscle specimen may or may not be fully undermined before placement of the clamp. Once the clamp is in place, the specimen is completely undermined by sharp dissection, and the ends of the biopsy specimen proximal and distal to the clamp are cut free of the muscle. The muscle may be left in the clamp while smaller sections are removed for processing. Once bleeding has been controlled, the surgical site is closed by simple continuous suture of subcutaneous tissue and simple interrupted sutures in the skin.

Frozen muscle biopsy sections can be stained by histochemical techniques to identify muscle cell fiber types (7, 16), which may be differentially affected in neuromuscular diseases (4, 8). In addition, the qualitative changes in muscle enzymes that occur in the metabolic myopathies can be assessed by histochemical techniques. Muscle fiber atrophy and inflammatory cell infiltrates may also be identified on frozen sections stained with hematoxylin and eosin. Paraffin-embedded and plastic-embedded, formalin-fixed tissue allows thinner histologic sections to be prepared in which inflammatory cell types or infectious agents may be more readily identified.

Electron microscopy of muscle biopsy specimens, although not routinely performed, may be required in special circumstances. If electron microscopy is anticipated before surgery, a combination of fixation and processing procedures can easily be performed on single or multiple biopsy samples to provide the most information.

The freezing procedure is the most crucial aspect of the processing of a muscle biopsy sample if artifacts are to be avoided (8). When possible, freezing of biopsy samples should be entrusted to an experienced laboratory. Improper freezing results in the formation of ice crystals in the muscle cells that distorts normal architecture (appearance) and may render the sample useless (9).

The sample must always be handled gently and never pinched or crushed. A new double-edged razor blade (cleaned with acetone) is used in a slicing motion to remove the suture and excess muscle at both ends and to subdivide the specimen. The portion to be frozen (approximately 0.5 cm in diameter and 1 cm long) is attached to a cork slice (approximately 1 cm in diameter and 1 cm long) by means of 10% gum tragacanth (Sigma Chemical Co., St. Louis) or OCT (Tissue Tek II, Miles Laboratories, Inc., Elkhart, IN) compound. The longitudinal axis of the muscle fibers is oriented at a right angle to the face of the cork so transverse sections ultimately can be cut. The cork with muscle attached is thrust for a few seconds into a container of 2-methylbutane (isopentane, Fisher Scientific, Pittsburgh, PA), which has previously been chilled to just above the freezing point ($-160°C$) by immersion in liquid nitrogen. Frozen muscle biopsy specimens should be transported on dry ice or in liquid nitrogen to prevent thawing and should be stored at -40 to $-70°C$ until histologic sections (10 mm) are cut on a cryostat ($-20°C$).

A portion (approximately 0.5 cm³) of the specimen that is not frozen should be placed in 10% buffered formalin (or alternate fixative) solution for subsequent paraffin or plastic embedding. Contraction artifacts caused by formalin fixation can be minimized if the time between biopsy sampling and fixation is extended to an hour (maximum 2 hours); during this period, the excitability of the tissue abates. Formalin-fixed tissue can be more useful for the identification of inflammatory cell infiltrates and infectious agents than frozen tissue because thinner sections can be prepared.

If a muscle specimen is to be prepared for electron microscopy, it should be stretched slightly or clamped before removal to prevent contraction artifacts. The sample should be fixed while still in the clamp by immersion in a suitable glutaraldehyde buffer solution as soon after sampling as possible because artifacts begin to appear in cellular organelles shortly after the blood supply is interrupted. The common electron microscopy fixatives penetrate tissue slowly; therefore, the thickness of the muscle biopsy should be limited to a few millimeters or preferably less.

If the proper technique is carefully followed, muscle biopsy can provide useful information about the pathologic processes occurring in muscle tissue in various neuromuscular diseases. Because this information may be necessary for a diagnosis, muscle biopsy is worth the required coordination of effort among surgeon, technician, and pathologist.

References

1. Bradley R. Skeletal muscle biopsy techniques in animals for histochemical and ultrastructural examination and especially for the diagnosis of myodegeneration in cattle. Br Vet J 1978;134:434.
2. Braund KG. Pediatric myopathies. Semin Vet Med Surg (Small Anim) 1994;9:99.
3. Braund KG. Skeletal muscle biopsy. Semin Vet Med Surg (Small Anim) 1989;4:108.
4. Cardinet GH, Holliday TA. Neuromuscular diseases of domestic animals: a summary of muscle biopsies from 159 cases. Ann NY Acad Sci 1979;317:290.
5. Cardinet GH. Neuromuscular diseases: the diagnosis and classification of muscle diseases in the dog. In: Proceedings of the 4th Kal Kan Symposium. 1980:1–10.
6. Braund KG, Amling KA. Muscle biopsy samples for histochemical processing: alterations induced by storage. Vet Pathol 1988;25:77.
7. Braund KG, McGuire JA, Lincoln CE. Observations on normal skeletal muscle of mature dogs: a cytochemical, histochemical, and morphometric study. Vet Pathol 1982;19:577.
8. Dubowitz V, Brooke MH. Muscle biopsy: a modern approach. London: WB Saunders, 1973.
9. McGavin MD. Muscle biopsy in veterinary practice. Vet Clin North Am Small Anim Pract 1983;13:135.
10. McGavin MD. Muscle biopsy: fruits and frustrations. In: Proceedings of the 4th Kal Kan Symposium. 1980:63–65.
11. Reynolds AJ, Fuhrer L, Valentine BA, et al. New approach to percutaneous muscle biopsy in dogs. Am J Vet Res 1995;56:982.
12. Armstrong RB, Saubert CW, Seeherman HJ, et al. Distribution of fiber types in locomotory muscles of dogs. Am J Anat 1982;163:87.
13. Braund KG, Amling KA, Mehta JR. Histochemical and morphometric study of fiber types in ten skeletal muscles of healthy young adult cats. Am J Vet Res 1995;56:349.
14. Braund KG, Mehta JR, Amling KA. Fibre type proportions of the buccinator muscle in clinically normal adult dogs. Res Vet Sci 1991;50:371.
15. Braund, KG. Clinical syndromes in veterinary neurology. Baltimore: Williams & Wilkins, 1986.
16. Braund KG, Hoff EJ, Richardson KEY. Histochemical identification of fiber types in canine skeletal muscle. Am J Vet Res 1978;39:561.

9

EAR

Pinna

Suture Technique for Repair of Aural Hematoma

Paul E. Cechner

Aural hematomas occur most frequently in dogs with pendulous ears and occasionally in dogs with erect ears and in cats. Hematomas are most apparent in the concave surface of the ear. The etiology is not clear, but the most accepted theory is that the lesion is self-inflicted from head shaking, scratching, and rubbing the ear.

The auricular cartilage is pierced by many foramina, a configuration that permits passage of numerous vessels from the great auricular artery. Shearing forces from trauma are believed to tear some of the vessels. Blood accumulates between the skin and the layers of cartilage of the pinna. Bleeding continues until the internal pressure equals the pressure of the feeder arteries.

The underlying causes for irritation to the ear should include all the external factors and diseases that predispose an animal to otitis externa, including immune-mediated diseases, food, and inhalant hypersensitivities.

Treatment Considerations

Hematomas should be treated immediately after diagnosis. Untreated hematomas usually cause various cosmetic alterations resulting from fibrous contracture. Some ears have a cauliflower-like appearance, which is a permanent alteration. Identification and treatment of the underlying cause are critical to long-term management of patients with aural hematoma.

Suture Technique

In my experience, incisional drainage combined with suturing has consistently been the most successful treatment for aural hematomas. The pinna is surgically prepared on both sides. Hematomas have been opened using longitudinal, S-shaped, and cruciate incisions, depending on the surgeon's preference. I prefer the longitudinal incision, and it is not necessary to remove additional skin to widen the incision.

The fibrin clot is removed, and the cavity is curetted and flushed with saline. The horizontal mattress sutures are placed in rows parallel to the skin incision (Fig. 9.1). The first row of sutures are placed at the outer edge of the hematoma cavity with each new row placed toward the skin incision. The spacing of sutures varies with the size and shape of the pinna and the size and location of the hematoma.

Mattress sutures are 5 to 10 mm wide, 5 to 10 mm apart in each row, and 5 to 10 mm between each row, and the last row of sutures is 2 to 5 mm from the skin incision. Usually, 2 to 5 rows of sutures are placed on each side of the incision. To promote wound drainage, the skin incision is not sutured. The same procedure is recommended for cats; however, the suture spacing is 2 to 4 mm apart. The sutures should not be placed perpendicular to the skin incision in either species (Fig. 9.2).

The sutures penetrate the full thickness of the pinna and are tied on the convex surface of the ear (Fig. 9.3). When placing the sutures, the surgeon should avoid the three main great auricular branches, which are visible on the convex surface of the pinna. Suture ten-

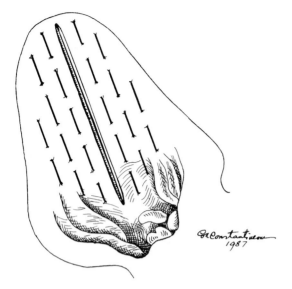

Fig. 9.1. Correct placement of sutures after removal of an aural hematoma.

sion is subjective. As a guideline, sutures should be placed with just enough tension to permit insertion of the needle holder tips to the level of the hinge.

Various suture materials have been used. My preference is 2–0, 3–0, or 4–0 nylon or polypropylene swaged onto a straight cutting needle. The use of stents or suturing through material, such as radiographic film, is usually not necessary if sutures are placed properly.

Postoperative Care

A light protective bandage is applied to protect and immobilize the ear. Pendulous ears are bandaged over the head or neck. Erect ears are bandaged to maintain a normal erect position. Ear bandages should not occlude the opening of the vertical canal. The bandage is changed in 3 days and is removed in 7 days. The sutures are removed in 3 weeks. An Elizabethan collar is recommended to prevent scratching of the unbandaged ear.

Complications

The most common complications of aural hematomas are cosmetic alterations and recurrence. Necrosis of the pinna has been reported from improper suture placement. Cosmetic alterations are usually the result of delayed treatment, improper suture placement, and excessive suture tension.

Aural hematomas can recur at the same site, but they are more likely to recur adjacent to the original hematoma. Recurrence of a hematoma is likely when inadequate numbers of sutures are used or inappropriately placed or when the underlying causes are not identified and treated appropriately. Necrosis of the pinna can be prevented by avoiding the ascending branches of the great auricular artery through the use of suture placement parallel, rather than perpendicular, to the incision.

Client Education

Communication with the animal's owner regarding all aspects of aural hematomas and their management will help to avoid misunderstandings, especially if complications occur. Owners should also understand

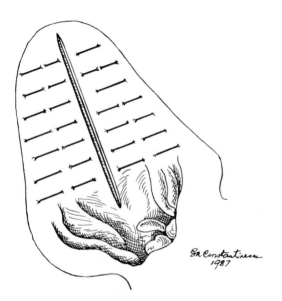

Fig. 9.2. Incorrect placement of sutures after removal of an aural hematoma.

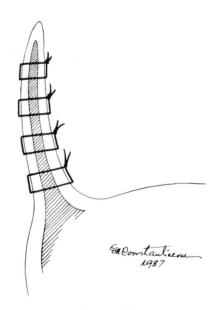

Fig. 9.3. After removal of an aural hematoma, sutures are placed through the full thickness of the ear and tied on the convex surface. See Figure 9.1 for correct placement of sutures.

that to treat the underlying causes properly, further investigation and expense will be required.

Suggested Readings

Angarano DW. Diseases of the pinna: Vet Clin North Am 1988;18:1.

Dubielzig RR, Wilson JW, Seireg AA. Pathogenesis of canine aural hematomas. J Am Vet Med Assoc 1984;185:873.

Harvey CE. Ear canal disease in the dog: medical and surgical management. J Am Vet Med Assoc 1980;177:136.

Henderson RA, Horne RD. The pinna. In: Slatter DH, ed. Textbook of small animal surgery. 2nd ed. Philadelphia: WB Saunders, 1993.

McKeever PJ. Otitis externa. Compend Contin Educ Pract Vet 1996;18:759.

McCarthy RJ. Surgery of head and neck. In: Lipowitz AL, Caywood DD, Newton CD, et al, eds. Complications in small animal surgery. Baltimore: Williams & Wilkins, 1996.

Sutureless Technique for Repair of Aural Hematoma

M. Joseph Bojrab &
Gheorghe M. Constantinescu

One disadvantage of suture techniques for repair of aural hematomas is the possibility that the treated ear

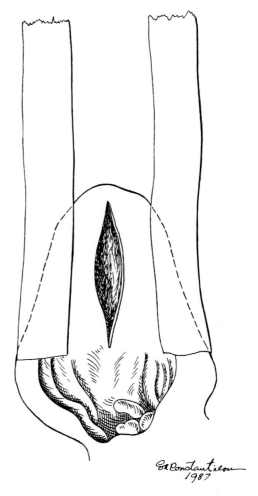

Fig. 9.5. Long pieces of tape are placed on the concave side of the rostral and caudal borders of the pinna. These tapes also extend beyond the ear border and contact the tape on the opposite side.

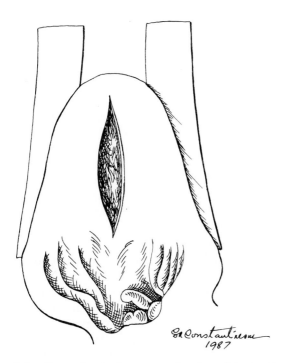

Fig. 9.4. Short pieces of tape are placed on the rostral and caudal borders of the convex side of the pinna. The tape extends beyond the ear border. The elliptic incision into the hematoma cavity is shown.

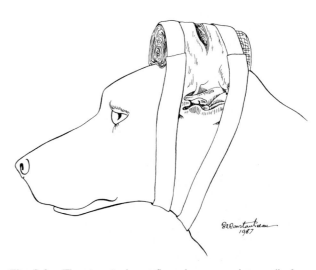

Fig. 9.6. The pinna is then reflected up over a large roll of cast padding, and the tape is brought around the neck, to secure the ear in place.

may thicken, wrinkle, and resemble a cauliflower. These unwanted changes do not occur with the sutureless technique described in this section.

After the pinna has been clipped, thoroughly cleaned, and prepared, an elliptic incision is made on the concave surface over the swelling. The incisions should expose the hematoma cavity from end to end. The cavity is thoroughly curetted and copiously irrigated. The ear is firmly taped so the incision is exposed (Figs. 9.4 and 9.5), and the pinna is then reflected over a large roll of cast padding and is taped in place (Fig. 9.6). A nonstick Telfa surgical dressing covered by a Tendersorb Wet Pruf (Ken Vet Animal Care Group, 100 Elm Street, Walpole, MA 02081) pad is applied to the incision surface and is changed as needed. Sutures are not used.

The ear is left firmly immobilized for 3 weeks. Healing is by second intention. The elimination of sutures helps to keep the pinna flat and prevents thickening, wrinkling, and cauliflowering.

External Ear

Treatment of Otitis Externa

M. Joseph Bojrab &
Gheorghe M. Constantinescu

Otitis externa is an inflammation of the epithelium of the external ear canal characterized by an increased production of ceruminous and sebaceous material, desquamation of epithelium, pruritus, and pain. The condition is caused by one or more etiologic agents including parasites, bacteria, and fungi. In addition, allergy and trauma may play a role in otitis externa.

The conformation of the ear canal and that of the pinna can predispose to development of acute and chronic otitis externa. For example, the high incidence of the disease in poodles and cocker spaniels indicates that the pendulous pinna and hair-filled external ear canal predispose to otitis externa. The high relative humidity of the external ear canal, in addition to the warmth, darkness, and enclosed nature of the ear canal of some breeds of dogs, provides an excellent environment for the growth of infective agents. Chronic otitis externa can permanently change the size and character of the external ear canal. The epithelium becomes thickened and fibrous and can become ulcerated. The ear canal can become stenotic if the epithelium becomes excessively scarred or undergoes metaplastic proliferation.

Diagnosis and Medical Treatment

A complete otoscopic examination of each ear, including visualization of the tympanum, is imperative for proper diagnosis and assessment of otitis externa. The initial treatment of this disease consists of irrigating and cleansing the external ear canal. Additional treatment consists of the use of ceruminolytic agents and, depending on the origin of the otitis, antibiotics (aqueous solutions) locally or parenterally, antifungal agents or parasiticides locally, and pH alteration. Bandaging the ears over the top of the animal's head allows better ventilation of the ear canal.

Culture and sensitivity tests in cases of severe or repeated occurrences of acute otitis externa may obviate a future ear canal operation by identifying the bacterial etiologic agent and thus the antibiotic that should effectively eliminate that agent. Chronic otitis externa must be treated more vigorously. Instillation of "swimmer's solution" (three parts 70% isopropyl alcohol and one part white vinegar) is useful for long-term treatment; it provides a cleaning–drying action and lowers the pH of the ear canal.

Surgical Treatment (Lateral Ear Canal Resection)

Indications

When otitis externa becomes unresponsive to medical therapy, a lateral ear canal operation is indicated. Lateral ear canal resection is also indicated for frequent recurrence of otitis externa, for chronic otitis externa resulting from inadequate treatment or lack of treatment, for external ear canal thickening that does not concurrently obstruct the horizontal portion of the external ear canal, and for exposure and removal of small tumors or polyps.

The purpose of lateral ear canal resection is to provide environmental alteration by means of ventilation so moisture, humidity, and temperature are decreased. Lateral ear canal resection also provides drainage for exudates and moisture in the ear canal.

Surgical Technique

The patient is placed in lateral recumbency and is draped so the pinna and external ear canal region are

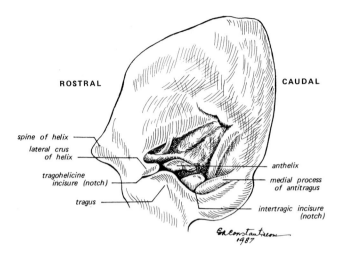

Fig. 9.7. Anatomic relationships of the ear.

left exposed and all anatomic relationships are identifiable (Fig. 9.7). The veterinary surgeon initially is positioned ventral to the patient. A probe is inserted into the ventral ear canal to determine the canal's depth. Two skin incisions are extended ventrally, parallel to each other, from the intertragic notch and the tragohelicene notch. These vertical incisions should be 1.5 times the length of the vertical ear canal. A transverse incision is made joining the vertical incisions ventrally (Fig. 9.8). The skin is reflected to its dorsal attachment on the dorsal rim of the vertical ear canal. An incision is made through the subcutaneous tissue of the lateral surface of the cartilaginous vertical canal. With scissors, the subcutaneous tissue is reflected rostrally and caudally off the vertical ear canal (Fig. 9.9). In similar fashion, the parotid salivary gland is reflected ventrally. The lateral aspect of the vertical ear canal should be exposed at this point.

The next portion of the surgical procedure is best performed from the dorsal aspect of the head. With scissors, two incisions are made in the cartilaginous vertical canal, one along the rostrolateral aspect of the canal and one along its caudolateral aspect. For the incisions to be made properly, the pinna and the skin flap must be pulled dorsally and the vertical portion of the ear canal visualized. One blade of the scissors is placed into the vertical canal (Fig. 9.10), which is then incised from the tragohelicene notch ventrally approximately half the length of the vertical ear canal. Both the rostral and caudal ear incisions should be alternately extended until the floor of the horizontal ear canal limits further advancement of the scissors. The lateral wall of the vertical ear canal is now reflected ventrally (Fig. 9.11). If the incisions have been made

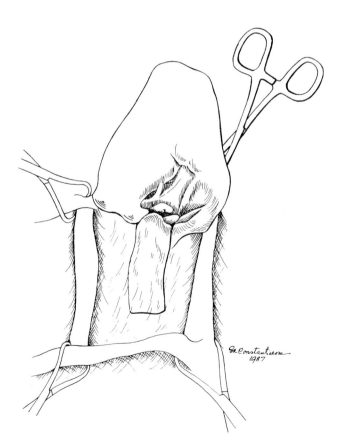

Fig. 9.8. The skin incisions are made to extend 1.5 times the length of the vertical canal.

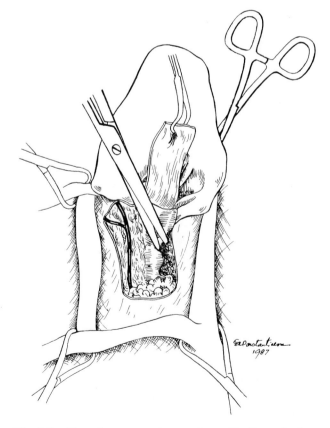

Fig. 9.9. The subcutaneous tissue and parotid salivary gland are reflected, exposing the cartilaginous canal.

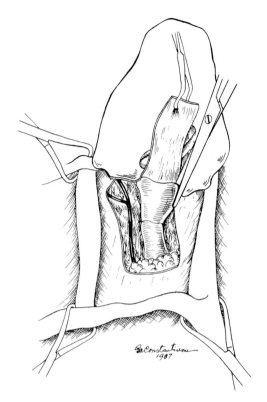

Fig. 9.10. After the subcutaneous tissue is reflected, the vertical ear canal is exposed and is ready for cutting with scissors.

properly, the lateral wall will have a base of attachment equal to the width of the floor of the horizontal ear canal. Next, the skin flap and all but the proximal 2 cm of the lateral wall are removed. This section is used as the "drain board" flap.

The lateral flap is pulled ventrally. Size 3–0 nonabsorbable, preferably swaged-on suture material is used to suture the lateral ear canal flap and the remaining vertical ear canal to the adjacent skin in a simple interrupted pattern (Fig. 9.12). The first suture is placed through the rostroventral edge of the epithelium and cartilage of the "drain board." This suture is angled rostroventrally and is sutured to the skin. Similarly, the second suture is placed through the caudoventral edge of the flap and is sutured caudoventrally to the skin. The skin is adjusted before placement of this suture, so no redundant skin persists between these two sutures. The next two sutures should anchor the skin to the rostral and caudal walls of the opening of the horizontal ear canal. Additional interrupted sutures are placed to join the lateral ear canal flap to the skin and the edges of the vertical ear canal to the skin in cosmetic fashion.

The ear is placed approximately in its normal position, and the ear canal is checked for possible obstruction to drainage and ventilation by the anthelicene tubercle or proliferative ridges of tissue. If these tissues

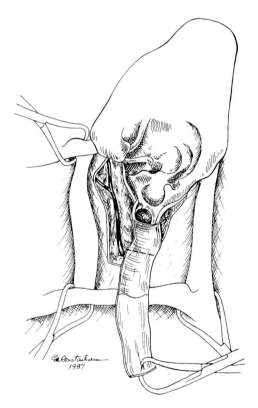

Fig. 9.11. The lateral wall of the vertical ear canal is reflected ventrally. The broken line indicates where the lateral cartilage flap is incised.

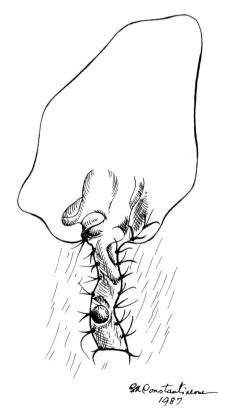

Fig. 9.12. The skin edges are sutured to the cartilage edges, creating a ventral "drain board."

cause obstruction, they should be excised, and the resultant wound should be allowed to heal by second intention.

After all incisions have been closed, the pinna needs to be anchored over the head of the dog to provide ventilation and to prevent damage from head shaking. A porous bandage may be placed over the surgical site to protect it from scratching. Paw pads may be fashioned, or the patient's legs may be hobbled as additional measures to protect the ear from self-trauma (see Chap. 5).

Postoperative Care

Postoperative care includes treatment with appropriate systemic antibiotics and management of self-trauma and ear movement. Coping with the prolonged healing time may be difficult. Healing time averages 10 to 14 days; if the suture line breaks down, healing may take longer. If lateral ear resection fails to control otitis externa, ear canal ablation needs to be considered. This procedure is discussed in the next section of this chapter.

Suggested Readings

Bojrab MJ, Dallman MJ. Lateral ear canal resection. In: Bojrab MJ, ed. Current techniques in small animal surgery. 2nd ed. Philadelphia: Lea & Febiger, 1983.

Coffey DJ. Observations on the surgical treatment of otitis externa in the dog. J Small Anim Pract 1970;11:265.

Fraser G. Factors predisposing to canine internal otitis. Vet Rec 1961;73:55.

Fraser G, Withers AR, Spruell JSA. Otitis externa in the dog. J Small Anim Pract 1961;2:32.

Fraser G. et al. Canine ear disease. J Small Anim Pract 1970;10:725.

Grono LR. Studies of the microclimate of the external auditory canal in the dog. Parts I, II, and III. Res Vet Sci 1970;11:307.

Grono LR. Otitis externa. In: Kirk RW, ed. Current veterinary therapy. Vol. 7. Philadelphia: WB Saunders, 1980.

Ott RL. Ears. In: Archibald J, ed. Canine surgery. 2nd ed. Santa Barbara, CA: American Veterinary Publications, 1974.

Singleton WB. Aural resection in the dog. In: Jones BV, ed. Advances in small animal practices. Vol. 2. Oxford: Pergamon Press, 1960.

Zepp CP. Surgical correction of diseases of the ear in the dog and cat. Vet Rec 1949;61:643.

Modified Ablation Technique

M. Joseph Bojrab &
Gheorghe M. Constantinescu

An alternative surgical technique for chronic otitis externa has been used when the entire vertical canal is grossly distorted or filled with hyperplastic mucosa.

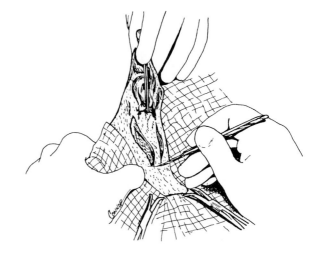

Fig. 9.13. Skin incisions for this modified ablation technique.

This technique combines the advantages of ablation (removal of the chronically infected vertical canal) with those of lateral ear canal resection (maintenance of drainage and hearing).

The preparation of the patient (Fig. 9.13), skin incision, and vertical canal isolation are the same as described for lateral ear canal resection in the previous section of this chapter. Isolation of the vertical canal is continued medially until the entire canal is isolated (Fig. 9.14). The auricular cartilage and skin are cut just dorsal to the opening of the vertical canal at the base of the pinna (Fig. 9.15). This method allows complete mobilization of the vertical canal, which remains attached only at the ventral end. The vertical canal is cut approximately 2 cm dorsal to the horizontal canal (Fig. 9.16) and is discarded. The remaining vertical canal is incised both rostrally and caudally down to the horizontal canal (see Fig. 9.16, *inset*), thus creating

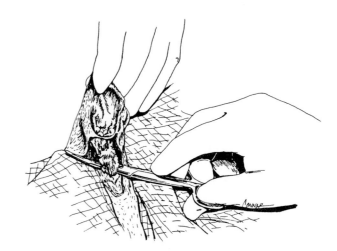

Fig. 9.14. Isolation of the vertical ear canal.

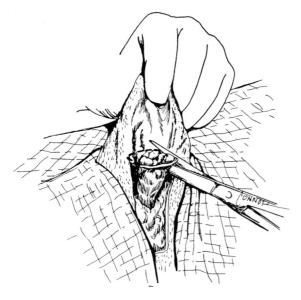

Fig. 9.15. The auricular cartilage and skin are cut dorsal to the opening of the vertical canal.

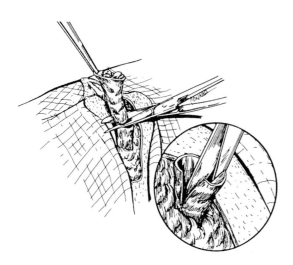

Fig. 9.16. The vertical canal is cut dorsal to the horizontal canal. *Inset,* incision of the remaining vertical canal, rostrally and caudally, down to the horizontal canal.

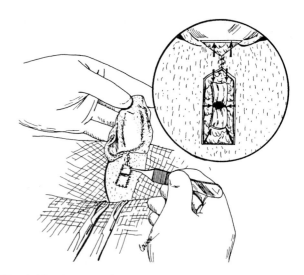

Fig. 9.17. Suturing of the dorsal and ventral rectangular flaps.

Total Ear Canal Ablation and Lateral Bulla Osteotomy

Daniel D. Smeak

two rectangular flaps, a dorsal flap and a ventral flap (Fig. 9.17). The ventral flap is sutured as described in the previous section of this chapter on treatment of otitis externa. The dorsal flap is sutured as depicted in Figure 9.17.

Aftercare consists of bandaging the patient's ear over the head for 1 week and administering systemic antibiotics as determined by culture and sensitivity tests.

Otitis externa is an insidious disease that is not debilitating, and the associated clinical signs are usually *controlled* until medical therapy is withdrawn. When multiple attempts at medical treatment fail, ear disease invariably progresses, and more extensive surgery is indicated to relieve the clinical signs permanently. Owners must understand that the frequency and severity of intraoperative and postoperative complications increase in proportion to the extensiveness of the surgery required. Thus, for the most part, *early* surgical intervention should be strongly advised when appropriate medical treatment for otitis externa fails or when the condition becomes recurrent. As the ear tissue damage becomes irreversible from chronic infection, drainage procedures fail, and removal of the entire horizontal and vertical ear canal is required. This salvage procedure is known as *total ear canal ablation (TECA).*

Secondary middle ear infection frequently develops in dogs with end-stage otitis externa. Variable results and high complication rates have been reported when TECA is performed without a means of middle ear exposure and drainage (bulla osteotomy and curettage). Because TECA eliminates a major pathway for exudate drainage, the external canal, recurrent deep infection occurs unless the middle ear is adequately drained and curetted. Inadequate removal of the secretory epithelium within the bulla or short osseous ear canal is responsible for such long-standing complications as persistent fistulation and abscessation. For these reasons, most surgeons routinely combine lateral bulla osteotomy (LBO) through the same approach used for TECA, if concurrent middle ear disease is suspected.

Indications

A TECA procedure is most often performed for irreversible inflammatory ear canal disease in dogs. Other less common indications include severe ear canal trauma, invasive neoplasia, and certain congenital malformations obstructing horizontal ear canal drainage. Irreversible inflammatory ear canal disease is present when one or a combination of the following is observed: hyperplasia of the epithelium occluding the horizontal ear canal; collapse or stenosis of the horizontal ear canal caused by infection within the cartilage or bone; or calcified periauricular tissue observed on skull radiographs.

Many dogs that present to the veterinarian for surgical treatment of inflammatory ear disease do not have a clinical picture that readily falls under the previous list of irreversible conditions or indications for TECA. If medically unmanageable otitis externa is related to an ongoing generalized skin condition such as atopy or hypothyroidism, treatment of the primary dermatologic disorder often helps to control the ear problem. Intercurrent skin disorders are common in dogs with otitis externa. Almost 80% of dogs undergoing TECA in one report had one or more primary dermatologic diseases including seborrhea, pyoderma, hypothyroidism, and atopy. When the related primary skin condition has been thoroughly diagnosed and appropriately treated but continues to be *unresponsive,* I prefer TECA for treatment of persistent otitis externa in these patients instead of surgical drainage procedures. As the skin disorder progresses, so does the ear disease in most circumstances, and a lateral ear resection will subsequently fail because of progressive inflammatory changes in the remaining canal. Similarly, if owners are incapable or unwilling to treat the skin or ear disease appropriately, TECA may be indicated *before* irreversible changes occur.

Although TECA combined with LBO is indicated for certain conditions in the dog, it is rarely performed on cats. Irreversible, proliferative inflammatory changes resulting from long-standing otitis externa do not appear to form as readily in cats as they do in dogs. Cats with otic tumors, such as ceruminous adenocarcinoma or basal cell carcinoma, or cats that have sustained severe trauma to the ear canal are potential candidates for TECA with or without bulla surgery, depending on the condition of the middle ear. Because the external ear canal disease is secondary and is rarely irreversible in cats, primary middle ear infection and ear polyps are treated by ventral bulla osteotomy alone; TECA is not usually required.

Owner Education

The animal's owner must be made fully aware of the purpose of TECA as well as the possible sequelae before contemplating surgery. The surgeon should remind owners that the principal aim of TECA is to make their pet more comfortable by removing the source of chronic infection. Elimination of further ear cleaning duties and discontinuance of the malodorous discharge are added benefits. Before surgery, however, owners seem to be concerned most about the appearance of their pet and about whether their animal will be deaf after surgery.

Generally, the appearance of floppy-eared dogs after TECA is unchanged. In erect-eared dogs, the extent of auricular and pinna cartilage removed determines whether the ear will stand after surgery. Removal of extensive proliferative tissue well up into the pinna causes the erect ear to fall, owing to lack of support at the ear base. The ear remains erect if more than the proximal third of the vertical canal cartilage is preserved; however, the surgeon must not limit the amount of canal resection because of pressure from owners who want to preserve ear carriage at all costs. Continued irritation and pain can be expected if proliferative ear canal tissue remains after TECA.

Because TECA obliterates the external aditus, most owners are skeptical about their pet's future hearing ability. Although the possibility of causing complete deafness exists, TECA combined with LBO should not be expected to affect hearing ability dramatically in most cases. Most complaints about hearing difficulty after TECA stem from inadequate owner evaluation or awareness of their pet's ability to hear beforehand. The surgeon should try to make owners aware of their dogs' hearing deficits before surgery to minimize this misunderstanding.

Owners must be prepared for serious and potentially long-standing problems resulting from TECA. If nystagmus, circling, and loss of balance are present before surgery, exacerbation of these signs is common afterward. These signs usually improve if middle ear infection is eliminated, but they may persist indefinitely. Transient, or more rarely, permanent facial nerve dysfunction may occur, causing drooling from ipsilateral lip paralysis. Hemifacial spasm or facial nerve deficits that are present before surgery usually indicate that the facial nerve is embedded in the horizontal canal or that serious secondary middle ear infection is present. More dissection and retraction of the nerve may be required to free it; this procedure increases the risk of iatrogenic facial nerve damage. Ocular problems from a diminished eye-blink response may be disastrous, particularly in exophthalmic dog breeds. Unresolved middle ear infection or any retained secretory tissue causes recurrent abscessation and fistulation, which may create conditions far worse for both owner and pet than the presenting otitis externa. The veterinary surgeon should prepare owners adequately for these potential problems before surgery.

Preoperative Considerations

A complete preoperative workup is essential to determine the extent and nature of the disease process and to predict possible surgical complications. After routine physical examination, the external ear is inspected and palpated. A sharp pain response elicited during deep palpation of the ear canal usually indicates middle ear infection. Thickened and firm (calcified) ear canal tissue is a manifestation of irreversible inflammatory change. The extent of distal ear canal resection is determined by the amount of scapha involvement. Evidence of a head tilt without other signs of inner ear disease (nystagmus, circling, loss of balance) usually indicates severe pain in the ear on the lower side. Neoplasia should be suspected if the ear drainage appears mostly as blood, as opposed to the more typical thick, foul-smelling exudate of primary otitis externa.

A complete neurologic examination should be performed to evaluate for facial nerve dysfunction (hemifacial spasm, poor palpebral reflex, lip droop) and inner ear involvement, especially in patients with chronic otitis externa. During the preoperative workup, approximately 15% of patients with end-stage otitis are found to have partial or total facial nerve deficits. The veterinary surgeon should identity patients with intercurrent otitis media because they more often develop complications such as cellulitis, persistent fistulation, or abscessation after TECA. In addition, their postoperative care is more demanding and costly. Any hearing deficits or other neurologic problems should be clearly noted in the medical record and brought to the owner's attention *before* TECA; otherwise, the owner may blame the surgeon if these deficits were first noticed after surgery.

If the ear problem is a possible manifestation of a systemic skin disorder, a complete dermatologic examination should be performed, and appropriate tests should also be completed. Postoperative head shaking and self-inflicted irritation to the remaining ear tissues may persist if the primary skin condition is neglected or inappropriately treated. This situation can be seen as a failure of the surgical procedure from the owner's point of view.

The remaining preoperative workup is best performed while the patient is anesthetized. Thorough ear cleaning must be accomplished to allow maximal visualization of the canal during otoscopic examination. Otoscopic examination of *both* canals is indicated even if one side superficially appears normal or if the condition of both ears is severely proliferative. Attention is directed at locating tumors or polyps because these are not infrequent in older patients with long-standing otitis externa. Otitis media is present if no tympanic membrane is found and the tympanic bulla is filled with debris. Samples of suspicious tissues are submitted to help diagnose occult neoplasia, which may drastically change the prognosis as well as the owner's consideration to allow surgery on the pet. If neoplasia is suspected, local lymph nodes are examined, and fine-needle aspirates are evaluated cytologically for tumor staging. Chest radiographs are evaluated for evidence of metastatic disease or other occult thoracic problems. Rather than culturing the exudate at otoscopic examination, a more reliable result may be obtained if deep wound tissue and middle ear exudates are sampled at the time of surgery.

Skull radiographs help to confirm the extent and severity of the ear canal disorder and may alert the clinician that otitis media or neoplasia is present. The ventrodorsal skull view may be used to help determine the horizontal canal patency and its diameter and to ascertain whether the canal walls have undergone irreversible change. Open-mouth views of the bulla are best to evaluate for subtle middle ear change. Oblique lateral views may help to demonstrate lytic neoplastic changes of the petrous temporal bone.

Radiography should not be regarded as a sensitive tool in the diagnosis of otitis media. Positive radiographic signs, such as thickening and calcification of the bulla, indicate the presence of middle ear disease, but false-negative radiographic results are common. The presence of predominately lytic changes in the ventrocranial aspect of the bulla on oblique lateral views most often is a result of chronic inflammation, in my experience. Conversely, evidence of bone lysis in other areas, particularly in the petrous temporal bone, suggests a neoplastic process. In summary, despite the lack of sensitivity, radiographic evaluation still is recommended to evaluate for the presence of neoplastic invasion of bone. Normal-appearing skull radiographs do not rule out otitis media or neoplasia.

Surgical Anatomy

The surgeon must be aware of certain important structures before surgery is contemplated (Figs. 9.18 and 9.19). Branches of the great auricular and superficial temporal vessels should be avoided when incising through and dissecting medial to the vertical ear canal cartilage. The V-shaped parotid gland overlies the lateral and ventral areas of the ear canal, and it may be

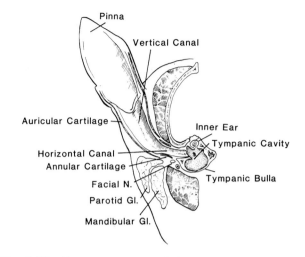

Fig. 9.18. Transverse section of the head showing ear canal, middle ear, and inner ear structures.

damaged if it is not retracted during horizontal ear canal exposure. Deep to the parotid gland are the facial nerve, internal maxillary vein, and branches of the external carotid artery. These structures are difficult

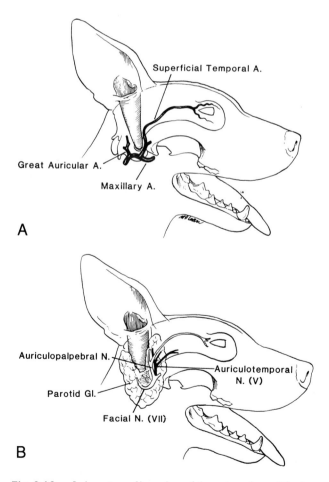

Fig. 9.19. **A.** Location of branches of the external carotid artery in relation to the ear canal. **B.** Location of the facial (VII) and auriculotemporal nerves (V) in relation to the ear canal.

to identify and to preserve when dissecting deeply around the horizontal ear canal and the tympanic bulla. The facial nerve emerges from the stylomastoid foramen, located just caudal to the osseous portion of the ear canal, and travels rostroventrally directly under the horizontal ear canal. Additionally, the terminal branches of the facial nerve and auriculotemporal branch of the mandibular portion of the trigeminal nerve should be avoided rostral to the ear canal. Careful retraction and meticulous dissection, staying close to the ear canal cartilage and osseous tympanic bulla, reduce the risk of iatrogenic damage to many of these vital structures.

The tympanic bulla contains the dorsally located auditory ossicles and, nearby, sensitive inner ear structures (see Fig. 9.19). Middle ear debris and exudate may be safely removed if curettage of the dorsal aspect of the tympanic cavity is avoided.

Surgical Technique

The ear canal is difficult to prepare aseptically, and contamination is inevitable during surgery. Therefore, a broad-spectrum, bactericidal, intravenous antibiotic is given before and during surgery, so adequate blood levels are maintained in tissues during dissection. These antibiotics are continued until the results of the intraoperative culture and susceptibility testing are available. The surgeon should use these susceptibility results to choose the appropriate drug for long-term therapy.

After anesthesia is induced, ample surrounding skin, ear canal, and pinna are routinely prepared for aseptic surgery. The patient is placed in lateral recumbency; the patient's head is elevated with a towel to a level parallel with the chest wall. A T-shaped skin incision is made; the horizontal incision is parallel and just below the upper edge of the tragus between the tragohelicine and intertragic notch; the vertical incision is created perpendicular to the midpoint of the horizontal incision to a point just ventral to the horizontal canal. Figure 9.20 illustrates the procedures for TECA and LBO. The surgeon undermines and retracts the two resulting skin flaps and exposes the lateral aspect of the vertical canal from the surrounding loose connective tissue. With curved Metzenbaum scissors, one bluntly dissects around the proximal and medial portion of the vertical canal, staying as close as possible to the cartilage. Starting from the rostral aspect, the surgeon cuts through the medial vertical canal wall with serrated Mayo scissors and continues cutting caudally until the ends of the original horizontal skin incision connect. One must avoid inadvertent damage to the branches of the great auricular vessels that travel in a dorsal direction just deep to the medial cartilage. Damage to these branches can lead to avascular necro-

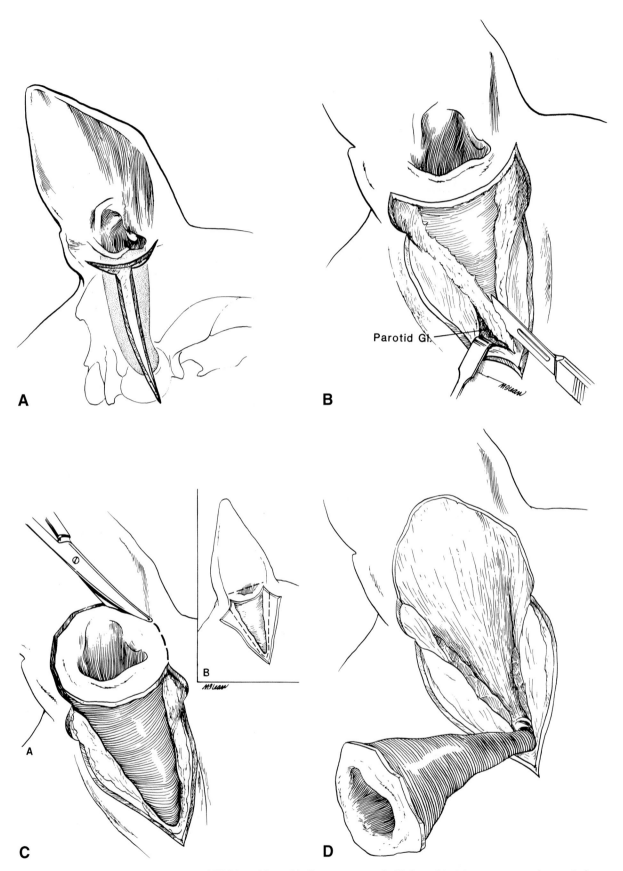

Fig. 9.20. Summary of surgical technique of TECA and lateral bulla osteotomy. **A.** T-shaped incision to expose the vertical ear canal. **B.** Loose connective tissue is incised and reflected from the vertical ear canal. The parotid gland is ventrally retracted to avoid damage during dissection of the ventral portion of the vertical ear canal. **C.** The dorsomedial aspect of the vertical canal is sharply incised with scissors connecting the ends of the original horizontal skin incision. **D.** The vertical and horizontal ear canal is isolated from surrounding soft tissues by blunt and sharp dissection. The facial nerve is isolated and gently retracted ventrally.

Parotid Gl.

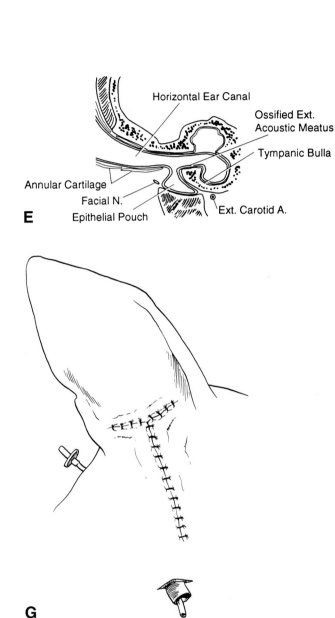

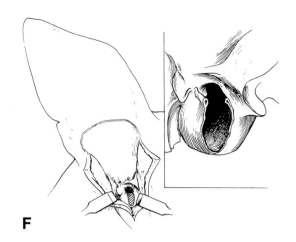

Horizontal Ear Canal

Ossified Ext.
Acoustic Meatus

Tympanic Bulla

Annular Cartilage
Facial N.
Epithelial Pouch
Ext. Carotid A.

E

F

G

Fig. 9.20 (continued). **E.** A pouch of secretory epithelium often forms between the tympanic bulla and the annular cartilage, extending into the external auditory meatus. This pouch should be completely excised. **F.** Soft tissues are bluntly dissected and are retracted to expose the entire lateral and ventral aspect of the tympanic bulla. The ventral and lateral aspect of the tympanic bulla is removed with rongeurs (cross-hatched area), and all epithelium and debris are curetted from the lumen. **G.** Subcutaneous and skin sutures are placed to form a T-shaped wound. A Penrose drain exits ventral to the incision.

sis of pinna skin, particularly in the area of the posterior incisure and cornu of the antitragus.

Starting at the dorsal and rostral aspect, the surgeon frees the remaining vertical canal of tissue connections and continues to dissect dorsally close to the horizontal canal cartilage down to the rim of the bony external auditory meatus. One avoids damage to the facial nerve and parotid gland by carefully retracting these structures away from the dissection plane at the *ventral* and *caudal* aspects of the horizontal canal. These aforementioned areas are approached last, so opposing soft tissues can be retracted sufficiently to allow maximal exposure during dissection. Occasionally, the facial nerve is entrapped and is hidden from view within extensively thickened and calcified horizontal canal

tissue. In such cases, I first search for peripheral small facial nerve branches (internal auricular nerves) that perforate the cartilage on the caudal and more superficial aspect of the horizontal canal; these branches lead to the seventh nerve trunk. Alternately, one may palpate for a small sharp bony protuberance, which is the rim separating the caudal bony ear canal from the stylomastoid foramen (origin of the facial nerve). Once this area is located, one follows the most proximal portion of the nerve as it courses directly lateral from the foramen. Entrapment is generally found just as the nerve begins its rostral course. The surgeon carefully dissects the remaining nerve from the canal. To avoid iatrogenic nerve trauma, one should always incise the horizontal canal attachment to the external auditory meatus with the honed edge of a No. 15 scalpel blade directed *away* from the nerve. Rongeurs or heavy scissors can be used if the ear canal is firmly attached to the external auditory meatus. Branches of the superficial temporal vessels originating from the retroglenoid vein (retroglenoid foramen) may be encountered during dissection of the rostral aspect of the canal from bone. Electrocoagulation or bone wax may be required to stop excessive hemorrhage. The entire canal should be removed and submitted for histologic examination. Rongeurs are usually required to excise remaining calcified attachments until the entire circumference of the external auditory meatus is seen as a white, glistening edge.

In severely affected ears, a greenish–brown epithelial pouch (similar to the shape of a sock) is present within the external auditory meatus and tympanic cavity extending lateral and ventral to the tympanic bulla. Removal of all secretory tissue is critical to the success of the surgery because chronic fistulation will occur if secretions form within this enclosed area. The surgeon should grasp the dorsal aspect of this pouch and, with traction, "tease out" the pouch in one piece if possible with a Freer elevator. A curette should be used to remove *any* remaining secretory tissue adherent to the walls of the bony meatus or separating into pieces during elevation; this tissue should be submitted for culture and susceptibility testing.

An LBO is performed to expose the tympanic cavity fully for location and removal of infected or secretory tissue. First, one should dissect all soft tissue bluntly from the ventral aspect of the bulla while taking care to avoid damaging the branches of the external carotid artery that travel just ventrally to the bulla. Hemostatic clips may be needed if these branches are inadvertently damaged. The surgeon should use rongeurs on the lateral and ventral aspect of the bulla, so the caudal aspect of the cavity (area usually hidden from view) can be reached with curettes. Use of air-driven burs helps to remove extensively thickened bone if rongeurs are not successful. Straight (Volkmann or Simon) curettes or ones with angled necks (e.g., Daubenspeck) are used to remove any remaining soft tissues. Curettage should not be attempted in the dorsal (epitympanic recess; housing the auditory ossicles) or dorsomedial area (promontory; housing inner ear structures) of the tympanic cavity. Copious irrigation of the wound is indicated to remove bone chips, exudate, or loose tissue. An ingress–egress drain or open wound management is chosen only when the bulla cannot be cleaned adequately or when extensive drainage is expected postoperatively. Otherwise, a tunnel should be bluntly dissected between fascial planes directly ventral to the bulla with large hemostatic forceps. The forceps should exit through a stab incision 4 to 6 cm ventral to the original vertical inci-

sion. The surgeon should pull a quarter-inch Penrose drain through this tunnel, insert the drain inside the tympanic cavity, and affix it with percutaneous sutures just deep to the proximal convex side of the pinna and at the ventral exit site. Routine closure of the subcutaneous tissue and skin in separate layers forms a T-shaped wound.

Postoperative Care

A loose, padded head bandage should cover the drain and surgical site until the drain is removed (usually within 2 to 5 days). Significant pharyngeal swelling can result if TECA and bulla osteotomy are performed bilaterally. In addition, bandages may further reduce pharyngeal airway size, and this can cause suffocation in the early postoperative period. Respiration should be monitored in these patients closely for the first 24 hours. An Elizabethan collar is used when needed to reduce self-trauma until sutures are removed (10 to 14 days). During bandage changing, wounds are examined for evidence of fluid accumulation or ensuing infection. If signs of acute postoperative infection occur, sutures in the vertical portion of the wound are removed, and the wound is opened fully to allow adequate drainage. Systemic antibiotics, based on intraoperative culture and susceptibility results, are administered for a minimum of 3 weeks. Open TECA wounds or those containing an ingress–egress system are irrigated locally twice daily with 20 mL lukewarm povidone–iodine and saline solution (1:10 dilution) or a tris-ethylenediaminetetra-acetic–antibiotic solution. Postoperative treatment should be continued for any underlying systemic skin disorder.

Complications and Treatment

Most complications related to the surgical procedure (wound infections and neurologic deficits) are short-lived and resolve within 2 weeks if treated appropriately. Extensive bacteria are present in occluded chronically infected ear canals even after proper aseptic preparation of the area. Acute postoperative wound infection is common after TECA because wound contamination is inevitable. Proper intraoperative wound irrigation, antibiotic administration, and drainage help to reduce this problem significantly. Evidence of avascular skin slough at the proximal caudal skin margin and acute cellulitis are managed with open wound management and debridement until the area reepithelializes. Those animals afflicted with inner ear signs before surgery may deteriorate immediately after anesthetic recovery, and these signs may persist indefinitely. Until proved otherwise, inner ear signs that first develop in a patient 1 week or more postoperatively are attributable to a fulminant abscess within the middle ear. Surgically induced Horner's syndrome tends to occur from middle ear curettage only in the cat. This disorder resolves within several weeks, provided middle ear infection has been eradicated.

Many dogs experience slow or incomplete eye-blink response and ear or lip droop immediately after surgery, owing to paresis of muscles innervated by the facial nerve. Artificial tears or ointments are used prophylactically until the affected eyes regain full function, usually within 5 days of the surgical procedure. If no evidence of eye blink is appreciable by 4 weeks postoperatively, permanent damage can be expected. Overall, about 10 to 15% of dogs have permanent facial nerve damage after TECA. This complication does not cause significant disability, in my experience, provided normal tear flow is present and the eye is not predisposed to exposure keratitis from exophthalmia. In summary, most facial nerve damage is iatrogenic and transient and is usually caused by overzealous retraction during ear canal dissection. Dissection of an entrapped facial nerve or en bloc resection of neoplasia often causes permanent damage.

Fistulation is considered the most serious complication because it can cause clinical disability far worse than the original chronic ear disease. Long-term antibiotic treatment and wound drainage rarely eliminate the problem, in my experience. Persistent infection usually requires wound reexploration for successful treatment, a costly and difficult procedure. Persistent wound drainage or fistulation forms anytime from 1 month to over 2 years after surgery in about 5 to 10% of patients undergoing TECA and LBO for chronic otitis. Persistent infection is most commonly attributed to a remnant of secretory tissue within the external auditory meatus or tympanic cavity. Isolation and removal of retained secretory epithelium with proper drainage of exudates permanently eliminate the problem. Ventral bulla osteotomy or LBO may be required, depending on the suspected source of the persistent infection. I prefer to use the lateral approach (through the original incision) if I believe retained horizontal ear canal tissue is the cause of fistulation. Ventral bulla osteotomy is the preferred route for exploration because it avoids dissection through the previous surgical site and allows maximal exposure of the tympanic cavity. Approximately 85% of patients that undergo surgical reexploration for persistent infection are cured. Despite the expense and potential for serious complications, most owners are satisfied with the procedure and with the improvement in their dog's demeanor.

References

1. Smeak D, DeHoff WD. Total ear canal ablation-clinical results in the dog and cat. Vet Surg 1986;16:161–170.
2. Mason LK, Harvey CE, Orsher RJ. Total ear canal ablation combined with lateral bulla osteotomy for end-stage otitis in dogs-results in thirty dogs. Vet Surg 1988;17:263–268.
3. Matthieson DT, Scavelli T. Total ear canal ablation and lateral bulla osteotomy in 38 dogs. J Am Anim Hosp Assoc 1990; 26:257–267.
4. Beckman SL, Henry WB, Cechner P. Total ear canal ablation combining osteotomy and curettage in dogs with chronic otitis externa and media. J Am Vet Med Assoc 1990;196:84–90.
5. Sharp NJH. Chronic otitis externa and otitis media treated by total ear canal ablation and ventral bulla osteotomy in thirteen dogs. Vet Surg 1990;19:162–166.
6. Nesbitt GH, Schmitz JA. Chronic bacterial dermatitis and otitis: a review of 195 cases. J Am Anim Hosp Assoc 1977;13:442–450.
7. Hitt ME. Ablation of the ear canal for treatment of chronic suppurative otitis externa in a cat. Vet Med Small Anim Clin 1980;75:1007–1009.
8. Krawinkle DJ. Effect of ear ablation on auditory function as determined by brainstem auditory evoked responses (BAER) and subjective evaluation. Presented at the 24th Annual Scientific Meeting of the American College of Veterinary Surgeons, 1989. Chicago, IL.
9. Smeak DD, Kerpsack SJ. Total ear canal ablation and lateral bulla osteotomy for management of end-stage otitis. Semin Vet Med Surg 1993;8:30–41.

Middle Ear

Ventral Bulla Osteotomy: Dog and Cat

Harry W. Booth, Jr.

A major indication for middle ear surgery is the treatment of otitis media that has responded inadequately to proper medical therapy or to less invasive surgical therapy. The main benefits of the bulla osteotomy procedure are that it provides a temporary path for continuous drainage of the tympanic cavity and it is a route for local treatment of the middle ear. Other indications for ventral bulla osteotomy include exploration of the tympanic cavity in animals with inflammatory polyps, neoplasia, or osteomyelitis of the tympanic bulla.

Surgical Anatomy

Knowledge of the anatomy of the middle ear is necessary to perform a bulla osteotomy properly. The middle ear consists of the tympanic cavity, tympanic membrane, and three auditory ossicles with their associated ligaments and muscles. The middle ear cavity (tympanic cavity) is connected to the pharynx by the audi-

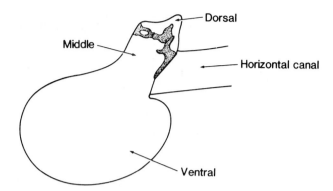

Fig. 9.21. Lateral view of the tympanic cavity showing the three divisions (ventral, middle, and dorsal), the horizontal ear canal, and the auditory ossicles (*stippled*). The ventral portion of the tympanic cavity is contained within the tympanic bulla.

tory tube. The tympanic cavity lies largely within the temporal bone (tympanic bulla) and is divided into three parts: ventral, middle, and dorsal (Fig. 9.21). The ventral portion is the largest division and is that portion contained within the tympanic bulla. In the dog and cat, the cavity is 8 to 10 mm in width and depth and about 15 mm in length. The tympanic cavity of the cat is divided into a larger ventromedial and smaller dorsolateral compartments by a nearly complete septum (Fig. 9.22).

The tympanic membrane is elliptic, with a concave external surface. The membrane is thicker peripherally. The auditory ossicles form a short chain across the dorsal part of the tympanic cavity. The malleus, the largest and most lateral of the ossicles, attaches to the tympanic membrane. The auditory tube, which extends from the rostral portion of the tympanic cavity to the nasal pharynx, equalizes air pressure and eliminates fluids from the middle ear.

Surgical Technique

Ventral bulla osteotomy provides better visualization and exposure of the ventral aspect of the tympanic cavity than the lateral approach. With the patient in dorsal recumbency, the surgeon incises the paramedian skin midway between the level of the angular process of the mandible and the level of the wings of the atlas (Fig. 9.23). Next, one bluntly dissects between the digastricus muscle and the hyoglossal and styloglossal muscles. The proper plane of dissection is verified by identification of the hypoglossal nerve on the lateral aspect of the hyoglossal muscle. Next is careful retraction of the hypoglossal nerve medially during this procedure with either hand-held or self-retaining retractors. The tympanic bulla is identified as a raised, rounded structure between the angular process of the mandible and the jugular (paracondylar) process of the skull. The thin jugulohyoideus muscle is incised over the canine tympanic bulla with scissors, and the muscle is reflected using a periosteal elevator. The surgeon penetrates the ventral aspect of the tympanic bulla using a Steinmann pin ($\frac{3}{32}$ inch) in a hand chuck (Fig. 9.24). One should proceed slowly to avoid damaging the dorsal aspect of the tympanic cavity with the pin. The opening into the tympanic cavity is enlarged

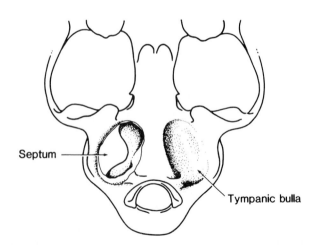

Fig. 9.22. The tympanic cavity of the cat is divided into two compartments by a nearly complete septum. Surgical entry through this septum is necessary to expose the entire tympanic cavity in the cat.

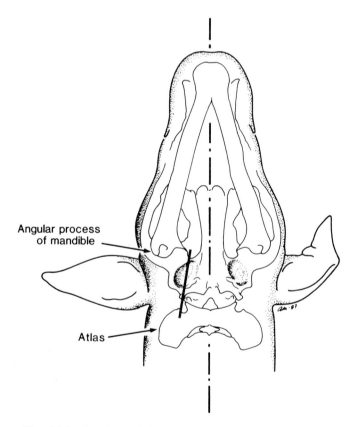

Fig. 9.23. Location of the paramedian skin incision (*solid line*) for performing a ventral bulla osteotomy is shown superimposed over the relevant osseous landmarks.

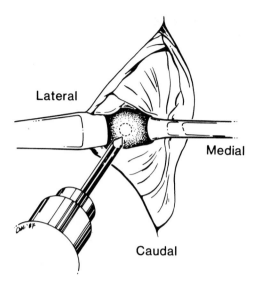

Fig. 9.24. Initial entry into the tympanic cavity is made using a Steinmann pin and a hand chuck. One must take care to avoid injury to the dorsal aspect of the tympanic cavity.

with rongeurs (Fig. 9.25). Infection of the tympanic cavity may cause thinning of the bone of the ventral tympanic bulla, leading to possible trauma to the middle ear during a ventral bulla osteotomy procedure. Presurgical radiographs of the bulla (oblique and open-mouth views) may help to visualize disease-induced changes in the tympanic bulla and may aid surgical planning.

The surgeon should obtain samples for culture and susceptibility testing and biopsy (if appropriate) once the tympanic cavity is reached. The tympanic cavity is irrigated with warm saline solution. Excessive curettage of the tympanic cavity should be avoided, because auditory function may be adversely affected. A Silastic

drain is placed from the tympanic cavity through the ventral cervical skin. The drain may be affixed to the lateral aspect of the tympanic bulla with an absorbable suture (e.g., surgical gut) by placing the suture through a small drill hole in the tympanic bulla. Alternatively, a fenestrated drain may be placed so it extends from the external ear canal, through the tympanic membrane, into the tympanic cavity, and through the ventral cervical skin. In the latter case, the surgeon should position the fenestrations within the tympanic cavity and affix the drain to the ear canal and the ventral cervical skin with sutures. Simple placement of the drain in the tympanic cavity to exit through the ventral cervical skin without suture usually results in premature dislodgment of the drain.

The subcutaneous tissue and skin are closed separately with absorbable and nonabsorbable sutures, respectively. If not done previously, a myringotomy (tympanotomy) should be performed at this time.

Follow-up Care and Postoperative Complications

The middle ear is flushed with warm saline solution either through the external ear canal or through the tubing. Antibiotic selection is based on susceptibility testing results and potential ototoxicity. Ototoxic symptoms are more likely when potentially ototoxic drugs are used topically in the middle ear than when they are used parenterally. The drain is removed in 5 to 10 days.

The efficacy of ventral bulla osteotomy for the treatment of otitis media depends partly on the duration of the disease. Ventral bulla osteotomy produces excellent long-term results in about 90% of reported cases, and it may have minimal deleterious effect on hearing. After ventral bulla osteotomy in normal dogs, the tympanic bulla rapidly re-forms, and hearing is preserved.

Possible complications of ventral bulla osteotomy include hypoglossal nerve damage, temporary sympathetic nerve irritation (ipsilateral Horner's syndrome), and damage to the parasympathetic nerve supply to the ipsilateral lacrimal glands (resulting in keratoconjunctivitis sicca).

Suggested Readings

Boothe HW Jr. Surgical management of otitis media and otitis interna. Vet Clin North Am (Small Anim Pract) 1988;18;901–911.

Faulkner JE, Budsberg SC. Results of ventral bulla osteotomy for treatment of middle ear polyps in cats. J Am Anim Hosp Assoc 1990;26:496–499.

Howard PE, Neer TM, Miller JS. Otitis media. Part II. Surgical considerations. Compend Contin Educ Pract Vet 1983;5:18–24.

Kapatkin AS, Mathiesen DT, Noone KE, et al. Results of surgery and long-term follow-up in 31 cats with nasopharyngeal polyps. J Am Anim Hosp Assoc 1990;26:387–392.

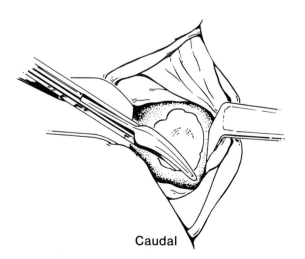

Fig. 9.25. The opening into the tympanic cavity is enlarged with rongeurs. After this step, the tympanic cavity can be visualized, and samples can be taken.

Little CJL, Lane JG. The surgical anatomy of the feline bulla tympanica. J Small Anim Pract 1986;27:371–378.

McAnulty JF, Hattel A, Harvey CE. Wound healing and brain stem auditory evoked potentials after experimental ventral tympanic bulla osteotomy in dogs. Vet Surg 1995;24:9–14.

Neer TM, Howard PE. Otitis media. Compend Contin Educ Pract Vet 1982;4:410–417.

Rosenzweig LJ. Anatomy of the cat: text and dissection guide. Dubuque, IA: Wm C Brown, 1990:26.

Seim HB III. Middle ear. In: Slatter DH, ed. Textbook of small animal surgery. 2nd ed. Philadelphia: WB Saunders, 1993:1568–1576.

Trevor PB, Martin RA. Tympanic bulla osteotomy for treatment of middle-ear disease in cats: 19 cases (1984–1991). J Am Vet Med Assoc 1993;202:123–128.

—•— *10* —•—

ORAL CAVITY

Repair of Cleft Palate

Eric R. Pope & Gheorghe M. Constantinescu

Congenital palate defects can affect the primary palate, secondary palate, or both. The primary palate extends from the lip to the caudal border of the premaxilla (incisive bone). The secondary palate includes the remainder of the hard palate and the soft palate. Incomplete fusion of these structures results in cleft of the primary palate (harelip), cleft of the secondary palate, or both. Clefts of the primary palate can involve the lip (cheiloschisis), the alveolar process (alveoloschisis), or both (cheiloalveoloschisis). Clefts of the secondary palate include midline defects of the hard or soft palate and unilateral or bilateral lateral clefts of the soft palate.

Most clefts are believed to be inherited as either recessive or irregularly dominant traits. Nutritional, hormonal, and mechanical factors have also been incriminated as causes, but these factors are more likely to affect the severity of the cleft in predisposed individuals rather than being a sole cause. Intrauterine infections and exposure to toxins at specific periods during gestation can also result in cleft palate. Cleft palate has been reported in many different breeds of dogs, but the brachycephalic breeds appear to be overrepresented. The Abyssinian, Siamese, and Manx breeds of cats seem to be at increased risk.

Clinical Signs

The clinical signs vary with the location and severity of the cleft. Clefts of the primary palate involving only the lip are primarily a cosmetic defect associated with few clinical signs. Primary clefts involving the lip and premaxilla may interfere with the ability to suckle and may allow milk to enter the nasal cavity resulting in rhinitis. Because the defect is readily apparent, the inability to nurse properly is likely to be recognized earlier by observant owners and hand rearing instituted. Clefts of the secondary palate may also interfere with the ability to nurse, but because these defects are less apparent, some neonates may die of malnutrition or aspiration pneumonia before other signs are recognized. Milk or food in the nasal cavity frequently causes sneezing or gagging. Milk may be seen running from the nose. The resulting rhinitis causes a serous to mucopurulent nasal discharge that may be malodorous. Aspiration of milk or food causes coughing, and aspiration pneumonia is a common sequela. Clefts involving only the distal half of the soft palate are unlikely to result in significant clinical signs.

Preoperative Patient Evaluation and Care

Animals with clefts of the primary palate that involve only the lip often need no special care. Except for their being "sloppy eaters," the defect is usually well tolerated. Tube feeding can be instituted if the defect prevents effective nursing. Repair of these defects can be delayed until the patient is older (3 months or more), when visualization is improved and tissue manipulations are easier. Animals with clefts involving the premaxilla are more likely to have difficulty in nursing and require tube feeding. Earlier repair (7 to 9 weeks of age) is recommended in these animals to reduce the severity of the rhinitis secondary to entrance of food into the nasal cavity if oral feeding is begun at weaning. Tube feeding is recommended for patients with clefts of the secondary palate to reduce the severity of the rhinitis associated with the passage of milk into the nasal cavity and to reduce the potential for aspiration pneumonia. Depending on the size of the patient, repair of clefts of the secondary palate is performed between 7 and 9 weeks of age when access to the oral cavity for tissue manipulation is better and when the tissues are less friable.

The diagnosis is generally obvious on physical examination. A complete examination is necessary to rule out other congenital defects. We routinely take thoracic radiographs of patients with clefts of the secondary palate before surgery to document the presence or absence of aspiration pneumonia. Aerobic and anaerobic bacterial cultures are performed on patients with purulent rhinitis, and appropriate antimicrobial therapy is initiated. Patients with minimal rhinitis are given a broad-spectrum antimicrobial perioperatively (administered when the intravenous catheter is placed before anesthesia induction and continued for up to 24 hours). Food is withheld the morning of surgery, but the operation should be performed as early in the day as possible to avoid hypoglycemia. Recently, we have been performing rhinoscopy on patients with purulent rhinitis immediately before the surgical procedure because some patients have had foreign bodies (typically plant material) that were not dislodged by flushing during surgical preparation and resulted in persistent rhinitis postoperatively.

Surgical Technique

A cuffed endotracheal tube is placed after induction of anesthesia and secured to the lower jaw. Access to the pharyngeal area can be improved by pharyngotracheal intubation, but it is generally unnecessary. Clefts of the primary palate are repaired with the patient placed in ventral recumbency and the head elevated on a cushion under the mandible. Elevating the head in this manner allows the lips to hang in a normal position and provides good surgical access. An oral speculum can be placed if the premaxilla is involved and better access to the oral cavity is needed. The hair on the muzzle is clipped, and the skin is prepared routinely. The oral cavity is prepared with dilute chlorhexidine or povidine–iodine solution.

Clefts of the secondary palate are repaired with the patient placed in dorsal recumbency (Fig. 10.1). The head is placed on a soft pad or beanbag, and the maxilla is immobilized with 1-inch tape placed over the incisors or canine teeth and secured to the operating table on each side. Access to the oral cavity is obtained by taping the animal's lower jaw, tongue, and endotracheal tube to an ether screen. A malleable retractor is also useful for retracting the tongue and endotracheal tube during repair of clefts of the soft palate. Pharyngotracheal intubation can be performed if greater access is needed. The nasal cavity should be liberally flushed

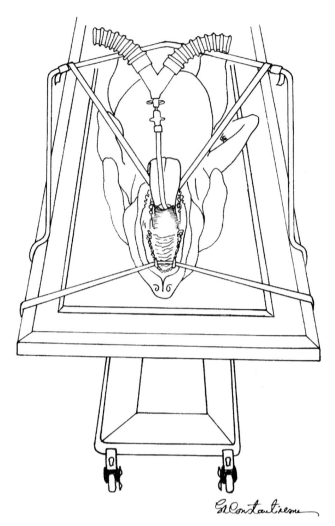

Fig. 10.1. Patient positioning for surgery of the hard or soft palate.

with saline to remove purulent exudate and possible foreign bodies before swabbing the oral cavity with dilute chlorhexidine or povidone–iodine solution.

Gentle tissue handling using skin hooks or bent hypodermic needles reduces tissue trauma. The use of electrosurgery should be minimized. Pinpoint cauterization of bleeders is acceptable, but use of the electroscalpel for making incisions and elevating flaps is not recommended. Two-layer closure in which suture lines on the nasal and oral cavity sides are offset is preferred. An airtight closure, free of tension, is mandatory. We prefer to use polyglactin 910 suture material in the oral cavity because the knot ends are not stiff and it is generally extruded by 14 to 21 days after surgery.

Cleft of the Primary Palate

The main objective in repairing a cleft of the primary palate is to establish the normal separation between the oral and nasal cavities. Clefts of the primary palate involving only the lip are easy to repair. Although complex flap techniques to reconstruct the nostril and columella accurately have been described, they are generally unnecessary because of the abundance of labial tissue in animals. The edges of the cleft defect are incised to a depth of 2 to 3 mm along the entire margin of the defect to create an inner mucosal layer and outer cutaneous layer (Fig. 10.2**A** and **B**). Beginning at the most dorsal point, the mucosal edges are apposed with interrupted 4–0 absorbable sutures (Fig. 10.2**C**). Accurate tissue apposition without tension is required. Skin closure should progress from the lip margin to avoid a step deformity using 3–0 to 4–0 monofilament nonabsorbable suture material in an interrupted pattern.

If the cleft also involves the premaxilla, closure is more difficult, but the objective is the same. The critical step is achieving closure of the oronasal communication. Careful preoperative planning is necessary to identify the best source and orientation of mucosal flaps to allow tension-free closure. Abnormal development of the premaxilla may necessitate extraction of teeth to facilitate the reconstruction. Mucosal flaps based on the nasal or oral mucosa are elevated from each side of the defect and are sutured together with fine (4–0 or 5–0) absorbable suture material. Although a two-layer closure is preferred, tissue may not be sufficient in all cases. If only a one-layer closure is performed, the nasal epithelial side should be reconstructed and the oral mucosal side allowed to heal by second intention. Finally, reconstruction of the lip is

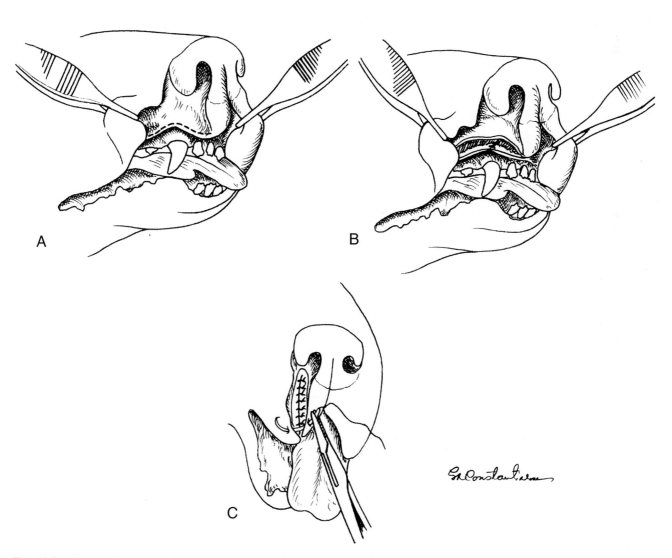

Fig. 10.2. Repair of a primary cleft palate. **A.** Incision along the cleft margin. **B.** Separation of the oral and nasal mucosa layers. **C.** The oral mucosa is closed first. Closure of the skin begins at the mucocutaneous junction to avoid step-deformity. (Redrawn from Krahwinkel DJ, Bone DL. Surgical management of specific skin disorders. In: Slatter DH, ed. Textbook of small animal surgery. Philadelphia: WB Saunders, 1985.)

performed as previously described. Potentially, all or part of the oral mucosal defect can be covered as the lip is reconstructed.

Cleft of the Secondary Palate

The technique for closing clefts of the secondary palate depends on the extent of the defect (i.e., hard and soft palate versus either individually), the width of the defect, and the availability of tissues to close the defect. In most cases, one of the following techniques can be successfully used. Key points to consider are: 1) two-layer closures that re-establish the nasal and oral epithelial surfaces are stronger and provide the potential for bony union across the defect; 2) tension on the suture line is probably the most common reason for failure and must be avoided; and 3) preserving the blood supply to the flap, whether from the palatine vessels (Fig. 10.3) in advancement flaps or the nasal cavity in "hinged" flaps, may limit the size or mobility of the flaps.

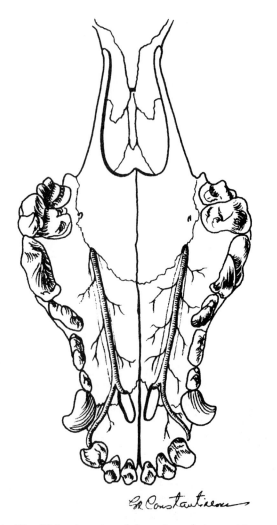

Fig. 10.3. Location of the major palatine arteries.

DOUBLE-LAYER MUCOPERIOSTEAL FLAP TECHNIQUE

This technique is most useful for clefts involving less than one-third of the width of the hard palate. The first step is to create unilateral or bilateral "hinged" flaps based on the edge of the cleft that are rolled back over the defect to create an epithelium-lined closure of the floor of the nasal cavity. A unilateral flap is preferred if the cleft is not too wide (approximately 10% of the width of the palate) because the suture lines from this layer and the bipedicle mucoperiosteal advancement flap of the second layer can be offset, potentiating an airtight closure. Bilateral flaps are used on wider clefts to reduce tension on the palatine arteries as the mucoperiosteal flaps are advanced to close the oral cavity side of the defect.

In the unilateral flap technique (Fig. 10.4), the hard palate mucosa is incised parallel to the cleft to create a flap that is slightly wider than the cleft. Perpendicular incisions are made at the rostral and caudal extents of the cleft to complete the flap. The flap is undermined with a periosteal elevator just to the edge of the bony defect, with care taken to preserve the blood supply coming from the nasal side. On the opposite side, the mucosa is incised along the edge of the defect to create a nasal side and an oral cavity side. The flap is rolled back toward the midline and is sutured to the nasal mucosa on the opposite side with preplaced 4–0 synthetic monofilament sutures using an interrupted pattern with the knots on the nasal side. The second layer of closure is started by making a releasing incision along the dental arcade on the side opposite the hinge flap to create a bipedicle flap. A periosteal elevator is used to undermine the flap beginning at the midline, with care taken to preserve the palatine arteries that enter the flap midway between the midline and the dental arcade approximately at the level of the caudal edge of the carnassial tooth (see Fig. 10.3). The flap is advanced over the fistula and is sutured to the cut edge of the mucoperiosteum on the first side. The donor site along the dental arcade heals by second intention.

When wider defects are present, "hinged" flaps are elevated bilaterally, rolled back, and sutured together over the middle of the defect (Fig. 10.5**A–C**). The second layer of the closure involves the development of bilateral, bipedicle mucoperiosteal flaps, which are advanced toward the midline and are sutured together. The hard palate mucosa is incised just medial (palatal) to the dental arcade, leaving the flap attached rostrally and caudally. The flaps are advanced toward the midline and are sutured together with 3–0 to 4–0 absorbable suture material.

The defects along the dental arcade can be allowed to heal by second intention, or they may be covered by buccal mucosal transposition flaps. Potential complications associated with allowing the defects to heal by second intention are shortening and narrowing of

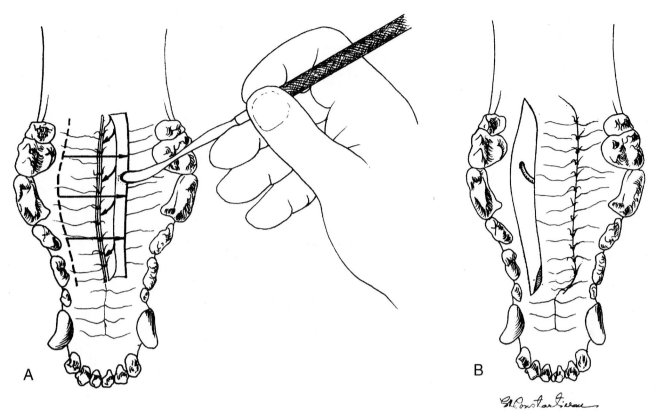

Fig. 10.4. Two-layer closure using a unilateral hinge flap. **A.** Incision is made along one side of the cleft separating the nasal and oral mucosa. A unilateral hinge flap is elevated from the opposite side, "rolled" back over the defect, and sutured to nasal mucosa. A releasing incision is made along the dental arcade creating a bipedicle mucoperiosteal flap. **B.** The flap is advanced over the first layer and is sutured to the mucoperiosteum on the opposite side.

the maxilla, but we have not found this to be a common clinical entity. Single-pedicle or double-pedicle buccal mucosal flaps can be mobilized to cover the palatal donor sites. The buccal mucosa donor sites usually can be easily closed with a simple continuous pattern. Two weeks later, the bases of the pedicle flaps are incised and sutured.

This technique may be difficult to perform without placing excessive tension on the suture lines or palatine vessels when wide defects are present. Although the technique can also be performed as a single tissue layer closure by creating bilateral, bipedicle mucoperiosteal flaps and advancing them to the midline, the suture line lies over the center of the defect, making it more difficult to achieve an airtight closure. Moreover, constant movement of the suture line with respiration and tongue movements predisposes to dehiscence. Therefore, when wide defects are present, the following technique is recommended.

HOWARD MUCOPERIOSTEAL HINGE FLAP

The hard palate mucosa is incised parallel to the edge of the defect so a mucoperiosteal flap slightly wider than the defect can be raised (Fig. 10.6). The flap is

undermined toward the midline, with care taken to maintain the blood supply from the nasal mucosa. The major palatine vessels are identified and ligated. The edge of the cleft on the opposite side is incised, and the oral mucosa is undermined for a depth of 2 to 3 mm. The mucoperiosteal hinge flap is rolled back over the defect. If it appears likely that tension will be present, a releasing incision is made along the dental arcade on the side opposite from the hinge flap. The bipedicle flap is undermined as previously described and is advanced toward the midline to eliminate the tension. The edge of the hinge flap is sutured to the underside of the mucoperiosteum on the opposite side with preplaced interrupted sutures using a mattress-type pattern. Overlapping the edges in this manner achieves an airtight closure and minimizes movement along the suture line. The donor sites are allowed to heal by second intention.

CLOSURE OF SOFT PALATE DEFECTS
Midline soft palate defects commonly accompany hard palate defects (see Fig. 10.5**D** and **E**). If possible, a two-layer overlapping technique is used. One flap is based on the nasal mucosa, and the second flap is

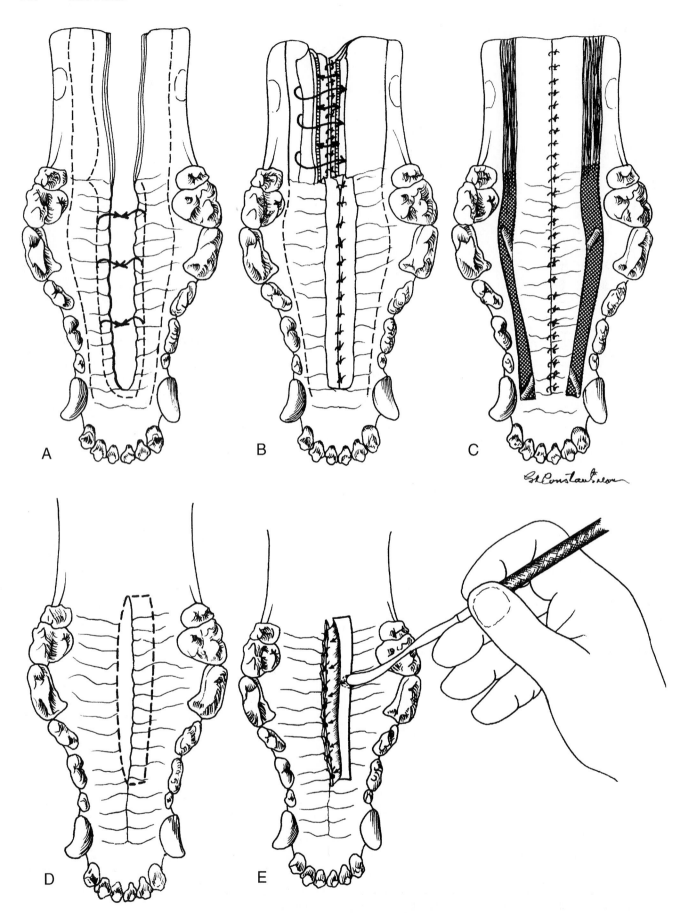

A

B

C

D

E

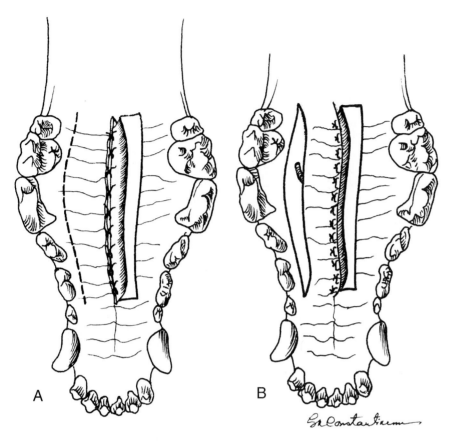

Fig. 10.6. Howard mucoperiosteal hinge flap. **A.** Mucoperiosteal flap based on the edge of the cleft is elevated. An incision is made along the edge of the cleft on the opposite side, and the mucoperiosteum is undermined for several millimeters. **B.** If the flap is wide enough, mattress-type sutures are preplaced to pull the edge of the hinge flap under the mucoperiosteum on the opposite side. If tension is present, a releasing incision is made along the dental arcade and the mucoperisoteum is undermined so it can slide toward the midline and relieve the tension.

based on the oral mucosa. The soft palate on one side is retracted laterally and rostrally to expose the nasal mucosa. The mucosa is incised the same distance from the edge as the width of the defect to create an orally based flap. On the opposite side, the oral mucosa is incised the same distance from the edge as the first flap to create a nasal mucosa–based flap. The flap based on the nasal side (i.e., side in which incision was made in the oral mucosa) is rolled back and is sutured to the lateral edge of the incision in the nasal mucosa on the other side of the defect. An attempt is made to suture the palatine muscles along the midline. The oral mucosa–based flap is moved across and is sutured to the oral mucosa incision on the opposite side. If any tension is present, releasing incisions are made in the oral mucosa laterally near the wall of the pharynx.

Postoperative Care

Intravenous fluids are continued until the patient recovers from anesthesia. Immature animals are given a liquid meal replacement diet or gruel after recovery from anesthesia. Placement of a pharyngostomy should be considered if tension exists on the suture line. Tube feeding is continued for at least 1 week until healing is confirmed. A soft diet is fed for a minimum of 1 month. Chew toys and other hard objects should also be withheld for a minimum of 1 month.

Dehiscence is the most common complication of cleft palate repair. The incidence can be minimized by performing tension-free closures and by gentle tissue handling. Repair of dehiscences should be delayed for 3 to 4 weeks to allow inflammation from the initial

Fig. 10.5. Two-layer reconstruction of a cleft of the hard palate using bilateral hinge flaps. **A.** Bilateral hinge flaps are elevated and "rolled" over the defect. The flaps are sutured together on the midline. **B.** Releasing incisions are made along the dental arcade creating bipedicle mucoperiosteal flaps. **C.** The bipedicle mucoperiosteal flaps are elevated, advanced over the first-layer closure, and sutured together on the midline. **D** and **E.** Soft palate reconstruction using an overlapping flap technique. **D.** Partial-thickness incision is made on the nasal surface of the soft palate on one side and the oral surface on the opposite side (*dotted line* closest to defect). The flaps are undermined to the midline. **E.** The oral mucosa–based flap is sutured to the nasal mucosa on the opposite side. Muscles are opposed if possible. The nasal mucosa–based flap is sutured to the oral mucosal on the opposite side to complete the repair. Releasing incisions are made along the pharyngeal wall, if necessary, to relieve tension. (Redrawn from Nelson AW. Upper respiratory system. In: Slatter DH, ed. Textbook of small animal surgery. 2nd ed. Philadelphia: WB Saunders, 1993.)

surgery to subside. Owners should be cautioned at the initial examination that more than one operation may be necessary to achieve complete closure of the defect.

Suggested Readings

Gunn C. Lips, oral cavity and salivary glands. In: Gourley IR, Vasseur PB, eds. General small animal surgery. Philadelphia: JB Lippincott, 1985.

Harvey CE. Palate defects in dogs and cats. Compend Contin Educ Pract Vet 1987;9:405–418.

Howard DR, et al. Mucoperiosteal flap technique for cleft palate repair in dogs. J Am Vet Med Assoc 1974;165:352.

Krahwinkel DJ, Bone DL. Surgical management of specific skin disorders. In: Slatter DH, ed. Textbook of small animal surgery. 2nd ed. Philadelphia: WB Saunders, 1985.

Nelson AW. Upper respiratory system. In: Slatter DH, ed. Textbook of small animal surgery. 2nd ed. Philadelphia: WB Saunders, 1993.

Salisbury SK. Surgery of the palate. In: Bojrab MJ, ed. Current techniques in small animal surgery. 3rd ed. Philadelphia: Lea & Febiger, 1990.

Repair of Oronasal Fistulas

Eric R. Pope & Gheorghe M. Constantinescu

Oronasal fistulas most commonly result from dental disease or its treatment (i.e., poor extraction technique), but they may also be caused by trauma, electrical burns, complications of maxillary fracture, and excision of nonneoplastic masses involving the hard palate, as well as by complications of surgery, radiation, or hyperthermia treatment of maxillary neoplasias. Common clinical signs of oronasal fistula include sneezing and serous, serosanguineous, or purulent nasal discharge. Food particles are occasionally seen in the nose. The diagnosis is often obvious during physical examination. Oronasal fistula due to periodontal disease or periapical infection is usually diagnosed by periodontal probing or radiography. The palatal surface of the maxillary canine teeth is a common site of oronasal fistula in small breeds of dogs.

Preoperative Evaluation

A complete physical examination and laboratory studies appropriate for the patient's anesthetic classification are indicated. Thoracic radiographs should be obtained when patients present with a cough or increased respiratory sounds (or history of either), to rule out aspiration pneumonia. Patients usually require anesthesia for thorough examination of the mouth and for skull radiography. The periodontal probe is useful for identifying small oronasal fistulas, particularly those associated with periodontal disease.

Intraoral radiographic techniques are helpful for identifying periodontal and periapical disease. Rhinoscopy should also be considered in patients with obvious oronasal fistula and purulent nasal discharge because foreign bodies may enter the nasal cavity through the fistula and may contribute to the rhinitis. Bacterial culture and sensitivity testing are performed on patients with severe purulent rhinitis or aspiration pneumonia. Culture samples are collected by transtracheal wash in patients with aspiration pneumonia. Alternatively, a broad-spectrum antimicrobial with efficacy against anaerobes can be given empirically. Treatment is continued for 10 to 14 days. In patients with minimal signs of infection, perioperative antimicrobials are administered intravenously when the catheter is placed before induction of anesthesia and are continued for 24 hours only.

Surgical Techniques

Successful repair of oronasal fistulas requires a well-supported, airtight closure that is free of tension. The options for surgical closure of oronasal fistulas are determined by the size, location, and chronicity of the fistula. Although many different techniques have been described, our preference is to perform a double-flap closure that reestablishes continuity of the nasal and oral mucosa whenever possible. Chronic fistulas, in which the nasal and oral mucosa have healed together, provide the option of creating "hinge" flaps based on the edge of the fistula similar to those described in the discussion of cleft palate repair in an earlier section of this chapter. These flaps receive their blood supply from vessels in the nasal mucosa that anastomose with vessels in the oral mucosa during the healing process.

Alveolar Ridge Fistulas

The technique used for repairing oronasal fistulas located along the dental alveolar ridge is determined primarily by the size and chronicity of the defect. Small fistulas resulting from advanced periodontal disease or tooth extraction are closed with a one-layer or two-layer technique, depending on whether the fistula is acute or chronic. Acute fistulas are corrected with single-pedicle advancement or transposition flaps from the buccal mucosa. Our preference is to excise a 2- to 3-mm–wide rim of mucosa from the palatal, rostral, and caudal edges of fistula so the suture line lies over bone. This technique helps to stabilize the flap against movement and aids in the formation of an airtight seal. Necrotic tissue and sharp bone edges are removed, and the wound is thoroughly lavaged. Single-pedicle advancement flaps are used unless they will restrict lip movement excessively (Fig. 10.7). Slightly diverging incisions are made in the gingival and labial mucosa

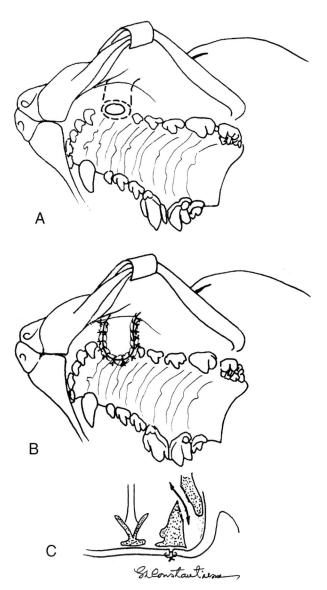

Fig. 10.7. Repair of an oronasal fistula with a single pedicle advancement. **A.** A 2- to 3-mm rim of mucosa is removed around the edge of the fistula. Slightly diverging incisions are made in the mucosa starting at the rostral and caudal borders of the defect. **B.** The flap is undermined, advanced over the defect, and sutured. **C.** Excising the rim of mucosa places the suture line over bone, providing better support.

starting at the rostral and caudal borders of the fistula and extending laterally. The labial mucosa and submucosa between the incisions is elevated by sharp and blunt dissection from the underlying bone. If a longer flap is needed, the dissection is continued toward the lip margin separating the layers of the lip. The flap should be sufficiently long that it can be advanced across the defect without tension. The flap is sutured with simple interrupted sutures using 3–0 to 4–0 synthetic absorbable suture material.

If the single-pedicle flap is likely to restrict movement of the lip, a transposition flap is used to repair the fistula (Fig. 10.8). Because of the abundance of cheek tissue in most breeds of dogs, we usually base transposition flaps on the rostral extent of the fistula and develop the flap caudally. The first incision is made beginning at the caudalmost point of the lateral border of the fistula and then continued caudally. The flap should be long enough to allow transposition of the flap over the flap without tension. A second incision is made parallel to the first one, so the width of the flap is equal to the width of the defect. The incisions are connected caudally. The flap is undermined by sharp and blunt dissection to make the flap as thick as possible. The flap is rotated over the fistula and is sutured as previously described. The donor site is closed with an interrupted or simple continuous pattern.

Chronic fistulas, in which the oral and nasal mucosa have healed together, can be repaired using a double-flap closure technique that provides a mucosal surface on both oral and nasal sides of the fistula. The first step is to create one or two "hinge" flaps based on the edge of the fistula that are rolled back over the fistula so the mucosal surface is on the nasal side (see Fig. 10.8**D**). If a single flap is used, it is usually raised from the hard palate. The alternative is to create opposing flaps from the hard palate and the labial (buccal) gingiva that are rolled back over the fistula. After the flaps have been created, the rostral and caudal edges of the fistula are incised to create nasal and oral sides. The hinge flaps are sutured to the nasal mucosa laterally or to each other at the center of the defect and to the rostral and caudal edges with interrupted sutures using 3–0 to 5–0 synthetic absorbable suture material. The second step is to create a flap from the buccal mucosa to cover the first layer of closure and the donor site on the hard palate completely. This step generally requires a transposition flap, as described earlier.

Large oronasal fistulas, as may result from the excision of neoplasms, are repaired with labial mucosa and submucosa advancement flaps (see the discussion of maxillectomy in the next section of this chapter). After completion of the maxillectomy, hemorrhage is controlled by packing the wound with gauze sponges. Diverging incisions are made in the labial (buccal) mucosa and submucosa extending toward the lip margin as far as necessary to allow closure of the defect without tension. The flap is created by undermining the mucosa and submucosa between the incisions by sharp and blunt dissection. The flap is sutured to the hard palate in two layers using synthetic absorbable suture material. The first layer apposes the submucosa of the labial flap with the mucoperiosteum of the hard palate. The sutures are placed so the knots lie in the nasal cavity. The second layer of sutures apposes the flap and hard palate mucosa with the knots in the oral cavity.

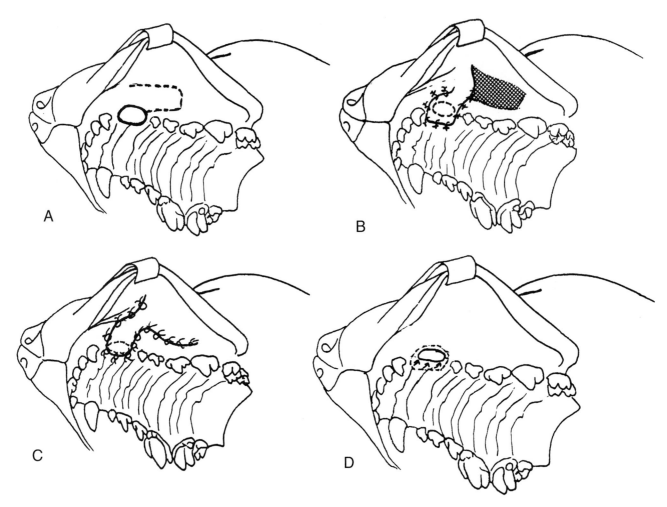

Fig. 10.8. Oronasal fistula repair using a transposition flap. **A.** Incisions for a rostrally based flap. **B.** The flap is undermined and transposed over the defect. **C.** Closure of the donor and recipient sites. **D.** When chronic fistulas are present, a hinge flap can be raised from the hard palate side of the defect and sutured laterally. A transposition flap is used to cover the flap and donor site.

Central Hard Palate Fistulas

Oronasal fistulas in the central portion of the hard palate are often more of a challenge given that reconstruction with labial (buccal) flaps is not an option because of the dental arcade. Oronasal fistulas rostral to the upper fourth premolar are amenable to closure with hard palate mucoperiosteal transposition flaps. Central hard palate oronasal fistulas at the level of the upper fourth premolar or more caudal can often be more easily closed with a partial-thickness transposition flap or a hinge flap from the soft palate.

The mucoperiosteal transposition flap is planned so one edge of the defect is incorporated into one side of the flap (Fig. 10.9**A**). Laterally, an incision is made parallel to the defect so the flap is 2 to 3 mm wider than the defect, if possible. The transverse diagonal (distance between the most lateral extent of the base of the flap and the rostral edge of the fistula) is measured to ensure creation of a flap of adequate length. Because the mucoperiosteum contains little elastic tissue, the pliability of these flaps is limited. Moreover, these flaps do not stretch, so the flap must be made long enough to avoid tension. Once the dimensions of the flap have been determined, the mucoperiosteum is incised. We make the side incisions first and the rostral incision last. By making alternating short incisions from the lateral and medial edges, the major palatine artery can usually be identified and clamped with hemostats before transection. Although some veterinary surgeons just sever the vessel as the rostral incision is made, retraction of the vessel rostrally may make grasping it for ligation difficult. The flap is elevated from bone with a periosteal elevator, with care taken not to injure the major palatine artery. The flap is transposed to cover the defect. In some instances,

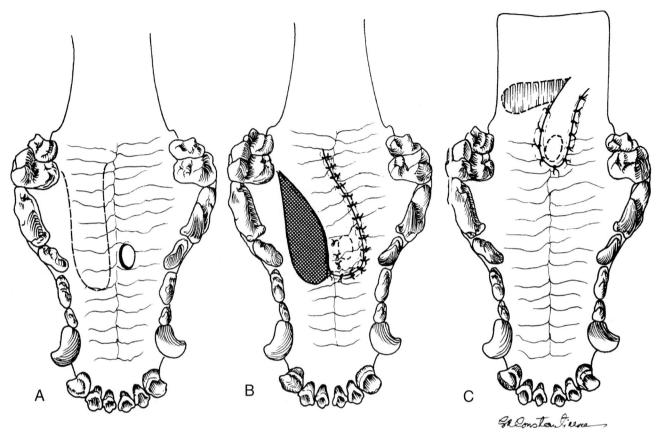

Fig. 10.9. Central palate fistulas can be closed with transposition flaps (**A** and **B**) from the hard palate mucoperiosteum or with partial-thickness flaps from the soft palate (**C**).

removing a triangular segment of mucoperiosteum from the caudal aspect of the fistula to the base of the flap is necessary to facilitate transposition of the flap over the defect. Because no soft tissue secures the flap to on one side of the fistula (the side adjacent to the donor site), holes can be drilled in the hard palate bone with a small K-wire to allow placement of sutures to secure the flap along the edge of the fistula (Fig. 10.9**B**). These sutures should be preplaced. The remainder of the flap is sutured in one or two layers with synthetic absorbable suture material. The exposed bone of the donor site is allowed to heal by second intention.

Fistulas located more caudally can be reconstructed using a partial-thickness flap from the soft palate. The transposition flap is designed to incorporate the edge of the defect into one side of the flap (Fig. 10.9**C**). The oral mucosa of the soft palate is incised, and a partial-thickness flap is elevated by sharp and blunt dissection. Again, one must elevate a flap of sufficient length to avoid tension on the closure. The flap is moved over the defect and is sutured with synthetic absorbable

suture material. The donor site is allowed to heal by second intention.

Postoperative Care

The pharyngeal area should be examined and any blood suctioned before extubation. Most patients are allowed nothing by mouth overnight. A soft diet is recommended for 3 to 4 weeks. Use of chew toys and other hard objects should also be avoided during this time. A pharyngostomy or esophagostomy tube can be placed if one desires to avoid oral feeding. In most instances, problems with healing become evident within the first week. If dehiscence occurs, the feeding tube can be maintained until another repair is attempted in 3 to 4 weeks. Tube feeding decreases the amount of material that can enter the nose and worsen the inflammatory response. Most complications can be avoided by gentle tissue handling, by achieving a tension-free closure, and by accurate suture placement. Although most fistulas can be successfully closed, instances of failure have been reported even after multiple attempts at surgical correction. Several different types of obturators have been used to create a barrier to movement of materials into the nasal cavity. A simple and successful technique is to use a nasal septal button to achieve obturation. The device is self-retaining but can be removed if necessary.

Suggested Readings

Ellison GW, Mulligan TW, Fagan DA, et al. A double reposition flap technique for repair of recurrent oronasal fistulas in dogs. J Am Anim Hosp Assoc 1986;22:803.

Gunn C. Lips, oral cavity and salivary glands. In: Gourley IR, Vasseur PB, eds. General small animal surgery. Philadelphia: JB Lippincott, 1985.

Harvey CE. Palate defects in dogs and cats. Compend Contin Educ Pract Vet 1987;9:405–418.

Nelson AW. Upper respiratory system. In: Slatter DH, ed. Textbook of small animal surgery. 2nd ed. Philadephia: WB Saunders, 1993.

Salisbury SK. Surgery of the palate. In: Bojrab MJ, ed. Current techniques in small animal surgery. 3rd ed. Philadelphia: Lea & Febiger, 1990.

Salisbury SK, Richardson DC. Partial maxillectomy for oronasal fistula repair in the dog. J Am Anim Hosp Assoc 1986;22:185.

Maxillectomy and Premaxillectomy

William S. Dernell, Peter D. Schwarz &
Stephen J. Withrow

Maxillectomy is the resection of variable portions of the maxillary, incisive, and palatine bones and closure of the resulting oronasal defect with a labial mucosal–submucosal flap. The remaining bony structure of the muzzle maintains adequate stability and contour, eliminating the need for bone replacement. Closure of the maxillectomy site is limited by the availability of normal labial and buccal mucosa. Tumors that extensively involve the labia or cross the midline of the hard palate may not be completely resectable because of the inability to close the defect. Appearance and function generally are good to excellent after maxillectomy.

Indications for partial maxillectomy and premaxillectomy are similar to those for mandibulectomy and include oral neoplasia, chronic osteomyelitis, and maxillary fractures with severe bone or soft tissue injury or loss. Another indication for maxillectomy is oronasal fistula (1–3). Partial maxillectomy and premaxillectomy are most often performed for local disease control of oral cancer (see the discussion of mandibulectomy in the next section of this chapter). Three basic techniques for partial maxillectomy and premax-

illectomy are available to the veterinary surgeon (1, 3): unilateral premaxillectomy, bilateral premaxillectomy, and hemimaxillectomy.

Preoperative Evaluation

The preoperative workup for maxillectomy is similar to that for mandibulectomy. The minimum database includes a complete blood count, biochemical profile, urinalysis, and thoracic radiographs for detection of distant metastasis. Regional lymph node aspirates should also be examined cytologically to detect nodal disease. Evidence of systemic disease or metabolic abnormalities may preclude or alter the mode of therapy and prognosis.

Radiographs of the skull and tumor site should be taken while the patient is under general anesthesia. Lateral, ventrodorsal, and oblique radiographs are recommended. High-quality radiographs, appropriate positioning, and an adequate number of views are essential for thorough evaluation of the skull. The radiographic assessment should include evaluation of cortical bone continuity, alterations in bone density, periosteal new bone formation, and involvement of adjacent soft tissues. Computed tomography or magnetic resonance imaging may assist in assessment of tissue involvement and surgical planning, especially for caudal maxillary tumors and those that involve various portions of the orbit, zygoma, and vertical mandibular ramus.

An incisional biopsy for accurate tissue identification is also important before definitive therapy is undertaken. The biopsy site should be selected so complete resection of the mass is not compromised (see Chap. 6). The preoperative database can be used to assign each patient a TNM (tumor, node, metastasis) classification and clinical stage (4).

General Surgical Considerations

Boundaries for partial maxillectomy or premaxillectomy for oral neoplasms with or without cortical bone penetration and destruction are determined by preoperative staging and oral examination. A 1-cm or larger, grossly visible, tumor-free margin should be obtained on all cut surfaces.

As a rule, an oronasal defect created after resection of tumors that cross the caudal midline is more difficult to close than a defect created from resection of tumors that do not cross the midline. Availability of normal labial, buccal, and palatal mucosa generally is the limiting factor. Immediately after resection, the excised tissue should be radiographed routinely to determine whether adequate bony disease-free surgical margins were obtained.

The pathologist must ascertain any extension of neoplasia to a cut edge. Margins of interest (osteotomy edges and closest soft tissue margin) should be identified with India ink or other suitable marking system, or margins should be submitted in separate containers. This technique aids the pathologist in determining the adequacy of mass removal (see Chap. 6). Specimens should be placed in 10% buffered formalin and submitted for histologic evaluation. Tumor extension to a cut margin generally implies the need for additional surgery or adjuvant therapy such as chemotherapy or, more commonly, irradiation.

Perioperative antibiotics are recommended. Antibiotic therapy for more than 24 hours is not indicated unless dictated by the situation. Although surgery of the oral cavity is considered contaminated or ''dirty,'' infection is rarely a postoperative complication. The antibiotic chosen should be effective against the bacterial flora normally found in the oral cavity, including gram-positive cocci (e.g., *Staphylococcus* sp. and *Streptococcus* sp.) and gram-negative rods (e.g., *Proteus* and *Pasteurella* spp.). The first-generation cephalosporins, penicillins, and synthetic penicillins are generally considered effective prophylactic oral antibiotics (5).

Polydioxanone (PDS, Ethicon, Inc., Somerville, NJ), polyglactin 910 (coated Vicryl, Ethicon, Inc.), polyglycolic acid (Dexon, Davis and Geek, Inc., American Cyanamid Co., Manati, PR), and polyglyconate (Maxon, Davis and Geek, Inc.) sutures (3–0 or 4–0) are recommended for wound closure after maxillectomy. These relatively nonreactive sutures minimize oral mucosal irritation and maintain adequate tensile strength during the critical early period of healing. Polydioxanone and polyglyconate have the advantages of being monofilament and absorbable. Their absorption is slow, however, and food can cling to the suture, or suture knots can be irritating, resulting in oral mucosal ulceration if the suture is not removed after healing. Although polyglactin 910 and polyglycolic acid are absorbable, they are braided suture materials and may increase the possibility of bacterial adherence or may result in a greater inflammatory response causing oral mucosal irritation. These latter two suture materials lose tensile strength sooner than polydioxanone or polyglyconate, a characteristic that should be considered if adjuvant radiation or chemotherapy may be administered postoperatively. These additional treatments may delay wound healing. Personal preference, cost, and availability should be considered when selecting a suture. A reverse-cutting swaged-on needle has been beneficial in suturing the tough, fibrous soft tissues of the oral cavity. This type of needle causes less surgical trauma when passed through tissues and provides better suture purchase into the soft tissues than other needle types (6). Use of electrocautery should be kept to a minimum. Incisions within the oral cavity made with electrocautery

are more likely to have delayed healing or to become dehiscent than incisions made with a scalpel (1, 7).

The choice of preanesthetic medication and induction agents is based on preoperative evaluation, personal preference, and expertise. The use of a narcotic is recommended for its analgesic effects. A fentanyl transdermal patch (Duragesic, Janssen Pharmaceutica, Titusville, NJ) can be placed on a shaved area over the dorsum of the neck and covered with a light bandage. Appropriate analgesic serum levels can take up to 12 hours to occur, so placement the night before the operation is helpful. Pharmacokinetic parameters have not been well established in the dog; however, we use a 25-μg/hour patch for dogs less than 25 kg, a 50-μg/hour patch for dogs between 25 and 50 kg, and two 50-μg/hour patches in dogs that weigh more than 50 kg. The use of these patches has subjectively resulted in decreased anesthetic needs and adequate postoperative analgesia for 2 to 3 days. Some dogs may need to be treated with additional narcotic agents, depending on pain response. Preoperative or intraoperative nerve blocks using a long-acting local anesthetic to the infraorbital nerve ventral to the zygoma may decrease anesthetic needs and postoperative pain.

After induction, general anesthesia should be maintained with a gas inhalant and oxygen. An endotracheal tube with an inflatable cuff is used to prevent aspiration of blood and fluid. The tube should be secured to the animal's lower jaw to minimize surgical interference. Because intraoperative hemorrhage can be profuse, a patent intravenous access catheter must be maintained at all times. A balanced electrolyte solution (10 mL/kg per hour) is started immediately after induction and is continued throughout the surgical procedure until the animal has recovered. Fluid levels may need to be increased, or whole blood, plasma, or colloids may need to be considered, depending on the degree of blood loss or hypotension. Depending on the extent of disease and the type of resection to be performed, clipping the patient's hair is either not necessary or minimally required.

Temporary unilateral or bilateral carotid artery occlusion has decreased blood volume loss and has improved visualization of the surgical field during maxillectomy, especially hemimaxillectomy and caudal maxillectomy (8). This procedure can be considered but is not routine. After removal of the tissue to be excised, and if carotid artery ligation was performed, blood flow is reestablished to allow maximum circulation to the surgical site. The blood flow to the nasal cavity and palatal mucosa originates from terminal branches of the maxillary artery, the main continuation of the external carotid artery. These branches include the sphenopalatine, major and minor palatine, infraorbital, and dorsal and lateral nasal arteries. Experimentally and clinically, the common carotid artery has been permanently occluded both unilaterally and bilaterally in dogs without causing neurologic or ischemic deficits (8, 9). This situation may not be true, however, in the cat (10).

Surgical Techniques

Positioning of the patient is critical, to visualize the entire surgical field. In our experience, placement of the animal in dorsal recumbency with the mouth taped open provides the greatest exposure. The lower jaw, tongue, and endotracheal tube are taped to an anesthesia screen. Movement of the head should be restricted by adhesive tape (Fig. 10.10).

The oral cavity is prepared by repeated flushing and swabbing with a 10% dilution of povidone–iodine solution (Betadine, Purdue Frederick Co., Norwalk, CT). The surgical site is draped, with drapes applied to the

mucocutaneous junction of the upper labia as well as to the lower jaw.

Unilateral Premaxillectomy

Unilateral premaxillectomy is indicated for lesions that are located rostral to the second premolar and do not come up to or cross the midline. The labial and gingival mucosa rostral and lateral to the tumor is incised at least 1 cm from the gross margins of the lesion. The incision is continued through the hard palate mucosa caudal and medial to the lesion (Fig. 10.11**A**). Hemorrhage from the hard palate mucosal incision generally is marked and requires ligation, electrocoagulation, and pressure to control. An oscillating bone saw or an osteotome and mallet may be used to cut the underlying bone following the mucosal incision lines. The sur-

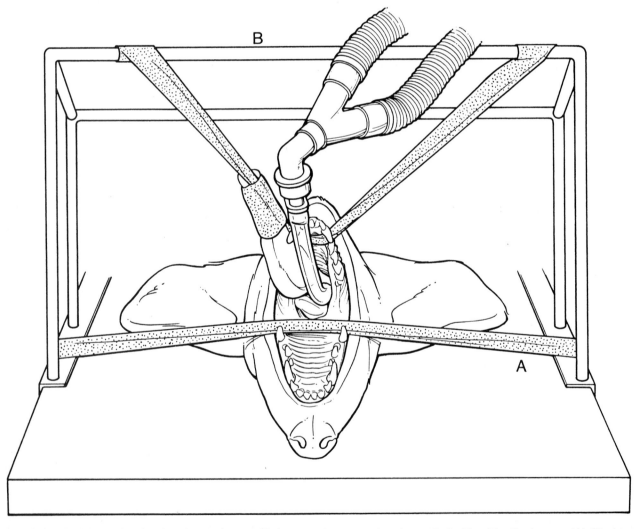

Fig. 10.10. The dog is placed in dorsal recumbency with the upper jaw secured to the surgical table with adhesive tape (A). The lower jaw, tongue, and endotracheal tube are suspended by tape from an anesthesia screen (B). A gauze sponge has been placed in the caudal oral pharynx to prevent passive aspiration.

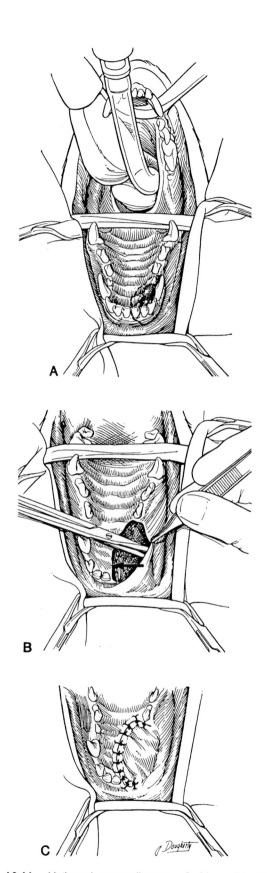

Fig. 10.11. Unilateral premaxillectomy. **A.** Mucosal incision is indicated by the dotted line. **B.** Undermining the labial mucosa-submucosa for a lip margin–based flap in which the mucosal surface faces the oral cavity. **C.** Simple interrupted or continuous closure of the mucosal flap.

geon should try to create curved bone margins, rather that square edges, to assist tissue apposition and healing. The incised segment of bone is freed of soft tissue attachments and is levered en bloc out of the surgical site. Branches of the major palatine artery may be visualized and ligated at this time. Hemorrhage is controlled with a combination of ligation, electrocautery, and pressure. Nasal turbinates should be visible at this time. If tumor has penetrated the bone or if the turbinates are traumatized during the resection, they should be excised with a scalpel or scissors. Before closure, the surgical site is copiously lavaged with sterile physiologic saline.

The oronasal defect created is covered with a labial mucosal–submucosal flap. The flap should be designed so sufficient tissue is obtained to cover the defect without tension. The flap should consist of mucosa, submucosa, and as much subcutaneous tissue as possible. The flap is elevated at the level of the dermis, is left attached at both ends, and is elevated only to the point that allows defect coverage without tension. The surgeon often can establish a tissue plane when undermining the labial mucosa and submucosa with Metzenbaum scissors (Fig. 10.11**B**). Blood supply is the critical factor for the survival of the mucosal–submucosal flap. The base of the pedicle must be of sufficient width to allow adequate vascularity to reach the tip of the flap.

The flap is sutured into position with a one-layer or two-layer closure. In two-layer closure, the first or deep layer consists of simple interrupted sutures placed through holes predrilled in the bony hard palate. This deep layer is especially important for patients that are anticipated to undergo adjuvant radiation or chemotherapy, because of the effects on wound healing. The second or superficial layer consists of simple interrupted or continuous sutures that appose the palatal mucosa to the labial mucosa (Fig. 10.11**C**). This superficial closure is used alone if a single-layer closure technique is chosen. Undermining the palatal mucosa 2 to 3 mm may help in tissue apposition in this closure (Fig. 10.12). If tension is encountered, vertical mattress sutures can be placed in addition to the primary sutures.

Bilateral Premaxillectomy

Bilateral premaxillectomy is indicated for lesions that come up to or cross the midline and are rostral to the second premolar. In essence, this procedure is similar to unilateral premaxillectomy, except the entire rostral bony floor of the nasal cavity is excised (Fig. 10.13**A**). This resection has been described in combination with nasal planum resection for tumors affecting both the premaxilla and the planum (11).

Closure is similar to that in the unilateral procedure,

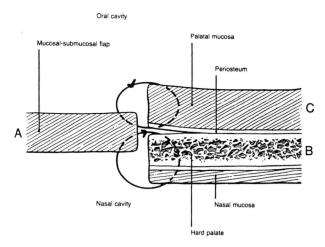

Oral cavity

Palatal mucosa

Mucosal-submucosal flap

Periosteum

A

C

B

Nasal cavity

Nasal mucosa

Hard palate

Fig. 10.12. A two-layer closure (A) is used to position the mucosal-submucosal flap over the defect created in a unilateral premaxillectomy. The first or deep layer (B) consists of simple interrupted sutures placed from the submucosa through predrilled bone holes in the bony hard palate. The second or superficial layer (C) consists of simple interrupted or continuous sutures opposing the labial mucosa to the mucoperiosteum of the hard palate.

only performed bilaterally. Half the flap is undermined from each side of the premaxillectomy defect (Fig. 10.13**B** and **C**). Submucosa can be attached to predrilled bone holes in the hard palate (Fig. 10.13**D–F**). The caudal half of each flap is sutured to the palatal mucosa from that side to the midline. The rostral halves are sutured together to form a T-shaped closure. The labial mucosa is sutured to the palatal mucosa and the opposing labial mucosa using simple interrupted or simple continuous sutures (Fig. 10.13**G**).

Hemimaxillectomy

The most aggressive of the maxillectomy procedures described here, hemimaxillectomy, is indicated for tumors that involve the majority of the hard palate on one side without crossing the midline. It involves removal of the oral mucosa, teeth, and portions of the incisive, maxillary, palatine, and zygomatic bones. The degree of resection is dictated by the size of the lesion, its location, the degree of tissue involvement, and the expected biologic behavior (of the tumor). Any portion of the maxilla can be excised unilaterally up to the entire hemimaxilla and still can result in normal function and adequate cosmetics. Caudal maxillary resections can be combined with resections of portions of the inferior orbit, zygoma, or vertical ramus of the mandible, depending on the degree of tissue involvement.

For tumors that have a large lateral or dorsal maxillary component, the dog can be placed in lateral or ipsilateral recumbency, and a dorsal incision can be made over the skin of the dorsolateral maxilla, to assist

dissection, in addition to the mucosal incision. The mucosal incision is begun rostrally at the labial–gingival junction dorsal to the middle incisors and is continued lateral and caudal to the level of the last molar tooth. Medially, the incision begins between the central incisors and extends along the midline of the hard palate. The two incisions are joined together just caudal to the last molar tooth at the junction of the hard and soft palate (Fig. 10.14**A**). Hemorrhage is often marked and is controlled with ligation, electrocautery, and pressure. An ostectomy is then performed along the incision lines with either an oscillating saw or an osteotome and mallet.

The caudal osseous incisions are at the rostral base of the zygomatic arch. The terminal branches of the maxillary artery are in this region and need to be identified and ligated. Major branches encountered include the infraorbital, sphenopalatine, and minor palatine vessels. Once the ostectomy incisions are complete, the tissue to be resected is levered loose, soft tissue attachments are excised, and the section is removed intact from the surgical site. Exposed or transected vessels can be identified and ligated at this time. Residual bleeding is controlled at this time. If temporary occlusion of the common carotid artery has been performed, blood flow should be reestablished to allow identification of cut vessels. When tumor penetrates the hard palate bone, the nasal turbinates, which overlie this area, should be excised with scissors or a scalpel and submitted for histopathologic examination. Turbinate hemorrhage can be controlled with a combination of ligation, electrocoagulation, and pressure.

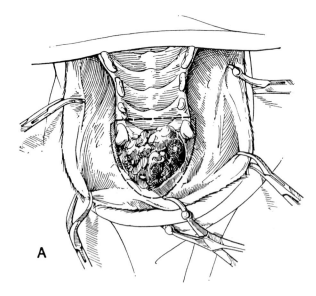

A

Fig. 10.13. Bilateral premaxillectomy. **A.** The dotted line indicates the area to be excised. (Reprinted with permission from Withrow SJ, Nelson AW, Manley PA, et al. Premaxillectomy in the dog. J Am Anim Hosp Assoc 1985;21:50.)

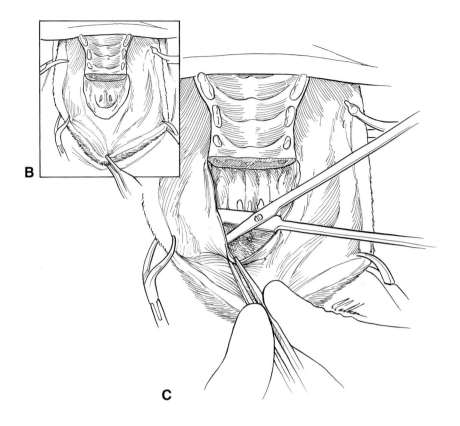

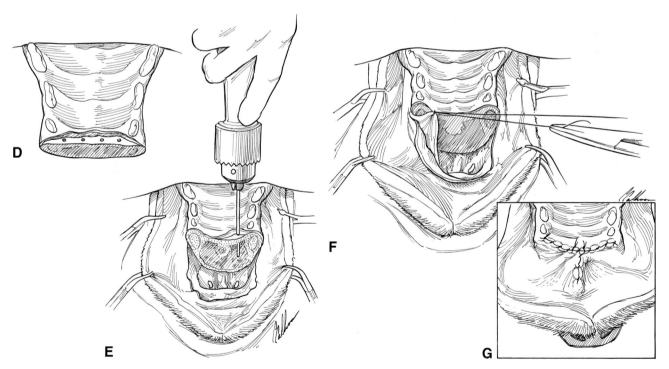

Fig. 10.13 (continued). **B.** The labial mucosa is incised perpendicular to the cut edge of the maxilla extending rostrally to the lip margin. **C.** Both sides of the labial mocosa are undermined deep to the submucosa and extending to the lip margins. **D** and **E.** Two to four bone holes can be placed in the rostral edge of the bony hard palate. **F.** Submucosa immediately under the mucosa is attached to the predrilled bone holes using preplaced simple interrupted sutures. **G.** Mucosal closure is completed by suturing half of the flap from each side to the mucoperiosteum of the hard palate and the remainder to the opposite side using simple interrupted or simple continuous sutures.

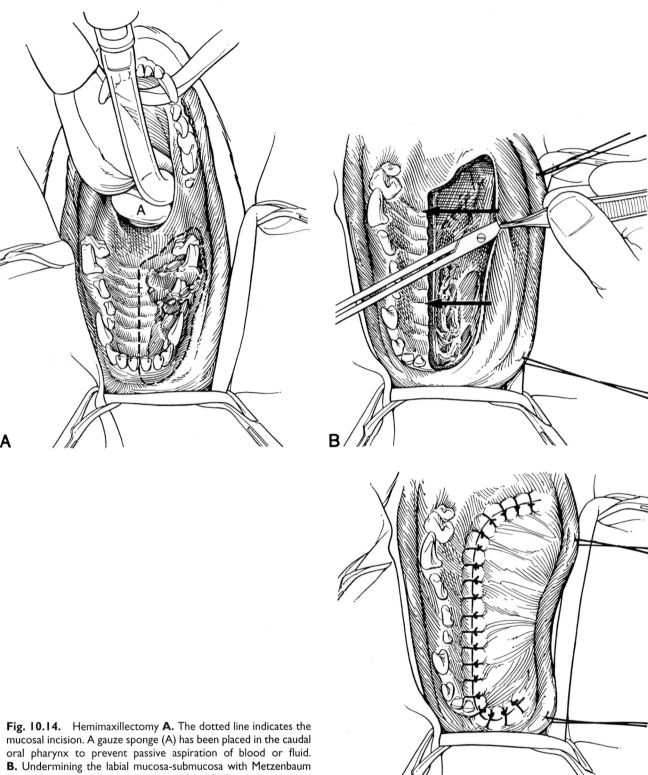

Fig. 10.14. Hemimaxillectomy **A.** The dotted line indicates the mucosal incision. A gauze sponge (A) has been placed in the caudal oral pharynx to prevent passive aspiration of blood or fluid. **B.** Undermining the labial mucosa-submucosa with Metzenbaum scissors for a lip margin–based labial flap. **C.** Simple interrupted or continuous suture closure of the mucosal flap.

A lip margin–based flap is created by undermining the labial mucosa and submucosa from the maxillectomy site toward the lip margin (Fig. 10.14**B**). The mucosa–submucosa flap must be of adequate size and sufficiently undermined so it can be brought into apposition with the mucoperiosteum of the hard palate without tension.

After thorough irrigation of the surgical site and

confirmation of complete hemostasis, the labial mucosal–submucosal flap is sutured to the subperiosteally elevated edge of the hard palate mucoperiosteum with simple interrupted or simple continuous sutures (Fig. 10.14**C**). If indicated, submucosal sutures can be placed through predrilled bone holes in the hard palate before closing the mucosal flap. The oropharynx is suctioned of blood before the animal is allowed to recover from anesthesia.

Postoperative Care and Sequelae

Because of the aggressiveness of maxillectomy procedures, the animal should be supported for the first 24 hours postoperatively with parenteral fluids and analgesics. Antibiotics given perioperatively generally are not indicated for more than 24 hours after the surgical procedure. An Elizabethan collar is often necessary to prevent self-induced trauma to the surgical site. The patient is allowed water after recovery from anesthesia, and soft foods are offered 24 to 48 hours after surgery. Pharyngostomy, esophagostomy, and gastrostomy tubes rarely are necessary.

The surgical site should be visualized for evidence of dehiscence and should be kept free of debris by flushing the mouth with water daily. Wound breakdown is the most significant postoperative complication after maxillectomy. Suture line tension, excessive use of electrocautery, ischemic necrosis of the mucosal–submucosal flap, and tumor recurrence are the major causes of dehiscence. Except for tumor recurrence, most problems result from technical error by the surgeon and can be eliminated by following proper case selection and technique and by minimizing surgical trauma. If the sutures holding the flap in place break down after surgery, the animal should be reanesthetized and the flap resutured. At the time of resuturing, rebiopsy of this surgical site is *always* indicated. What appears to be granulation tissue can easily be residual tumor. Up to 33% of maxillectomy patients have some degree of dehiscence during the postoperative period (10, 11). Not all cases of dehiscence, however, are of clinical significance. Dehiscence is most commonly noted after caudal maxillectomy or hemimaxillectomy, when tumors cross the midline, and whenever mucosa has been sutured next to a tooth on the occlusal margin of the ostectomy. Tension-free closure at the level of the occlusal ostectomy can be achieved by extracting an additional tooth, by elevating the palatal and labial gingiva, and by suturing the mucosal flaps over the alveolar bone.

Deformity of the muzzle contour can occur after partial maxillectomy and repair with a labial mucosal–submucosal flap. Such indentation generally results from an insufficient amount of normal labial tissues. It generally can be corrected by incising the base of the labial flap 3 weeks after surgery to allow the lip to return to its normal position. This procedure is rarely indicated because function is generally unaffected by the lip indentation.

In patients that undergo bilateral premaxillectomy, removal of the bony hard palate caudal to the canine teeth may shorten the nose. In some cases, the upper lip may actually be positioned caudal to the lower canines when the mouth is closed. Drooping of the nares and rostral muzzle also occurs when the mouth is open. Dogs that have undergone bilateral premaxillectomy seem to breathe through the nostrils in a normal fashion, however.

Follow-up

Maxillectomies performed for excision of tumor should be evaluated at 1 month and then every 3 months during the first postoperative year. Evaluations should include both visualization and palpation of the oral cavity, muzzle, and regional lymph nodes. Thoracic radiographs, depending on tumor type, may also be indicated for detection of distant metastasis. If gross evidence of local tumor recurrence or suspicious areas can be detected, an incisional biopsy should be made. Skull radiographs may be beneficial, but they are often difficult to evaluate, especially in the distinction of tumor and bony reactions resulting from surgical trauma. Complete surgical excision with adequate tumor-free margins generally is difficult to obtain after documentation of local tumor recurrence. Chemotherapy, hyperthermia, and radiation are alternative adjunctive therapies to consider in such cases.

Table 10.1 lists approximate reported local recurrence and median survival rates after maxillectomy for the major histopathologic tumor groups found in the dog (1, 3, 12–15). Not enough cases have been reported in the cat to draw any conclusions concerning survival rates.

Table 10.1.
Approximate Reported Local Recurrence and Survival Data for Oral Tumors Treated With Maxillectomy

Tumor Type	Number	Local Recurrence (%)	Median Survival (mo)
Acanthomatous epulis	10	10	26
Ameloblastoma	23	13	22
Malignant melanoma	40	40	8
Squamous cell carcinoma	16	31	18
Fibrosarcoma	35	46	12
Osteosarcoma	17	35	5

(Data from references 1, 3, and 12 to 15.)

References

1. Withrow SJ, Nelson AW, Manley PA, et al. Premaxillectomy in the dog. J Am Anim Hosp Assoc 1985;21:49–55.
2. Salisbury SK, Richardson DC. Partial maxillectomy for oronasal fistula repair in the dog. J Am Anim Hosp Assoc 1986; 22:185–192.
3. Salisbury SK, Richardson DC, Lantz GC. Partial maxillectomy and premaxillectomy in the treatment of oral neoplasia in the dog and cat. Vet Surg 1986;15:16–26.
4. Owen L, ed. TNM classification of tumors in domestic animals. Geneva: World Health Organization, 1980.
5. Prescott JF, Baggot JD. Principles of antimicrobial drug selection and use. In: Prescott JF and Baggot JD, eds. Antimicrobial therapy in veterinary medicine. Boston: Blackwell Scientific Publications, 1988:55–70.
6. Dernell WS, Harari J. Surgical devices and wound healing In: Harari J, ed. Surgical complications and wound healing in small animal practice. Philadelphia: WB Saunders, 1993:249–376.
7. Salisbury SK, et al. Partial maxillectomy: comparison of suture materials and closure techniques. Vet Surg 1985;14:265–276.
8. Hedlund CS, Tangner CH, Elkins AD, et al. Temporary bilateral carotid artery occlusion during surgical exploration of the nasal cavity of the dog. Vet Surg 1983;12:83–85.
9. Clendenin MA, Conrad MC. Collateral vessel development after chronic bilateral common carotid artery occlusion in the dog. Am J Vet Res 1979;40:1244–1248.
10. Gillian LA. Extra- and intracranial blood supply to brains in the dog and cat. Am J Anat 1976;146:237.
11. Kirpinsteijn J, Withrow SJ, Straw RC. Combined resection of the nasal planum and premaxilla in three dogs. Vet Surg 1994;23:341–346.
12. Schwarz PD, Withrow SJ, Curtis CR, et al. Partial maxillary resection as a treatment for oral cancer in 61 dogs. J Am Anim Hosp Assoc 1991;27:617–624.
13. Wallace J, Matthiesen DT, Patnaik AK. Hemimaxillectomy for the treatment of oral tumors in 69 dogs. Vet Surg 1992; 21:337–341.
14. White RAS. Mandibulectomy and maxillectomy in the dog: results of 75 cases. Presented at the 22nd Annual Meeting of the American College of Veterinary Surgeons, San Antonio, 1987.
15. White RAS, Gorman NT, Watkins SB, et al. The surgical management of bone-involved oral tumors in the dog. J Small Anim Pract 1985;26:693–708.

Mandibulectomy

*William S. Dernell, Peter D. Schwarz &
Stephen J. Withrow*

Mandibulectomy is the resection of variable sections of the mandible and closure of the surgical site with lingual, labial, and buccal mucosa and submucosa. No replacement of bone or stabilization is usually required. Appearance, owner acceptance, and function generally are excellent after mandibulectomy. Five mandibular removal procedures have been described (1, 2): 1) unilateral rostral body mandibulectomy (from the first or second premolar forward to the symphysis); 2) bilateral rostral body mandibulectomy (from the first or second premolar forward bilaterally); 3) total hemimandibulectomy (horizontal body with or without the vertical ramus on one side); 4) vertical ramus mandibulectomy (with or without temporomandibular joint removal); and 5) segmental horizontal body mandibulectomy. Variations and combinations of these are used, depending on lesion type and location.

Indications

Mandibulectomy is performed for local control of oral neoplasia, for treatment of chronic mandibular osteomyelitis, and for salvage of patients with mandibular fractures with severe bone or soft tissue injury. Removal of oral tumors is the most common indication for mandibular resections.

The oropharyngeal region is the fourth most common site of malignant neoplasia in the dog. The most common oropharyngeal neoplasms in the dog are malignant melanoma, squamous cell carcinoma, fibrosarcoma, and epulides or tumors arising from the periodontal ligament (3–6). In the cat, squamous cell carcinoma is the most common oropharyngeal cancer, followed by fibrosarcoma, undifferentiated sarcoma, hemangiosarcoma, lymphoma, and osteogenic sarcoma. Malignant melanoma and epulides occur rarely in the cat (6, 7). Odontogenic tumors, such as inductive fibroameloblastoma, are the most common benign oral tumors in the cat (8). Oropharyngeal tumors tend to be locally aggressive and slow to metastasize, except malignant melanoma, caudal tongue tumors (9), and pharyngeal and tonsillar squamous cell carcinoma (4–6). Morbidity and mortality often result from local disease rather than from distant metastasis. Many animals die or are euthanized because of signs of local disease, such as infection, dysphagia, and aspiration pneumonia, before metastases occur.

Control of local disease is the first goal of most surgical treatments for oral cancer. However, limited soft tissue excisions for attempted cure of oral tumors often fail because of recurrence of the tumor at the primary surgical site. Mandibulectomy accompanied by en bloc soft tissue resection for oral tumors has the potential for prolonged remission or cure in certain malignant diseases. If nothing else, the quality of life can be dramatically improved, even though distant metastasis may ultimately occur. Surgical resection should be considered as a first line of treatment for all oral neoplasms. Radiation therapy can be considered as primary treatment only for tumors that show consistent responses to radiation, such as lymphoma and acanthomatous epulis.

Preoperative Evaluation

Routine hematologic and biochemical profiles, as well as urinalysis, should be performed on all candidates for mandibulectomy for anesthetic considerations and to identify any coexisting medical problems. In cases of oral neoplasia, the tumor should be clinically staged according to the World Health Organization staging system, the TNM (tumor, node, metastasis) classification, before definitive treatment is selected (10). Staging requires a deep incisional biopsy while the patient is under general anesthesia for histopathologic analysis (see Chap. 6), as well as analysis of a regional lymph node aspirates and thoracic radiographs to detect regional and distant metastasis. Preoperative staging helps to determine the appropriate treatment and prognosis and also helps the client to decide whether to pursue therapy.

Radiographs of the mandible taken while the patient is under general anesthesia should be obtained preoperatively in all cases of oral cancer fixed to bone. These radiographs should include lateral, ventrodorsal, and oblique views, as well as an open-mouth view if the tumor involves the rostral horizontal ramus. Fine-detail screen with high-contrast film at low kilovolt potential is recommended. Advanced imaging modalities, such as computed tomography or magnetic resonance imaging, may be invaluable for evaluation of tissue involvement and for planning surgical margins, especially for caudal lesions that involve the vertical ramus and temporomandibular joint. Patients with tumors that are adherent or "fixed" to the underlying mandible without radiographic evidence of invasion are still candidates for mandibulectomy.

Boundaries for partial hemimandibulectomy for benign neoplasms with or without evidence of cortical bone penetration into the medullary cavity should be determined radiographically and by oral examination. Cortical bone penetration by malignant neoplasms with suspected bone marrow involvement is the main indication for total hemimandibulectomy versus partial hemimandibulectomy. If tumor cells follow the neurovascular bundle within the medullary cavity of the mandible, the entire hemimandible (minimally the mandibular body rostral to the vertical ramus) must be removed to excise the tumor completely. This is especially important in patients with malignant melanoma, fibrosarcoma, and osteosarcoma. Malignant disease without radiographic evidence of cortical bone penetration can be treated as though it were benign disease.

Mandibulectomy also is performed for treatment of chronic osteomyelitis or extensive bone or soft tissue injury. Often, these patients are presented in a debilitated condition. A gastrostomy tube can be placed to assist the anorectic preoperative and postoperative patient to maintain proper nutrition and hydration. Because most mandibular fractures are open fractures, broad-spectrum antibiotics are recommended. The duration of antibiotic therapy depends on the type and severity of infection.

General Surgical Considerations

When mandibulectomy is performed for treatment of an oral neoplasm, at least a 1-cm, grossly visible, tumor-free margin should be obtained on all cut surfaces. The removed mandible should be radiographed to aid in determining whether adequate bony disease-free surgical margins were obtained. Margins of interest (osteotomy edges and closest soft tissue margin) should be identified with India ink or other suitable marking system, or margins should be submitted in separate containers. This procedure aids the pathologist in determining the adequacy of mass removal (see Chap. 6). The entire specimen is then placed in 10% buffered formalin and is submitted for histologic evaluation. Tumor extension to the cut margins generally implies the need for additional surgery or adjuvant irradiation.

Mandibulectomy is considered a contaminated or "dirty" surgical procedure. Therefore, therapeutic levels of antibiotics are indicated at the time of surgery. Parenteral prophylactic antibiotic therapy begun preoperatively or intraoperatively and continued for a maximum of 24 hours is recommended when osteomyelitis is not already established. The antibiotic chosen should be effective against the bacterial flora normally found in the oral cavity, including gram-positive cocci (e.g., *Staphylococcus* sp. and *Streptococcus* sp.) and gram-negative rods (e.g., *Proteus* and *Pasteurella* spp.). The first-generation cephalosporins, penicillins, and synthetic penicillins are generally considered effective prophylactic oral antibiotics (11).

Polydioxanone (PDS, Ethicon, Inc., Somerville, NJ), polyglactin 910 (coated Vicryl, Ethicon, Inc.), polyglycolic acid (Dexon, Davis and Geek, Inc., American Cyanamid Co., Manati, PR), and polyglyconate (Maxon, Davis and Geek, Inc.) sutures (3–0 or 4–0) are recommended for wound closure after mandibulectomy. These relatively nonreactive sutures minimize oral mucosal irritation and maintain adequate tensile strength during the critical early period of healing. Polydioxanone and polyglyconate have the advantages of being monofilament and absorbable. Their absorption is slow, however, and food can cling to the suture, or suture knots and be irritating to the mucosa, resulting in ulceration if the suture is not removed after healing. Although polyglactin 910 and polyglycolic acid are absorbable, they are braided suture and may increase the possibility of bacterial adherence or may result in a greater inflammatory response causing oral mucosal irritation. These latter two sutures lose tensile strength sooner than polydioxanone or polyglycolate, a property that should be considered if adjuvant radiation or chemotherapy may be administered postoperatively, because these additional treatments may delay wound healing. Personal preference, cost, and availability should be considered when selecting a suture. A reverse-cutting swaged-on needle has been found beneficial in suturing the tough, fibrous soft tissues of the oral cavity. This type of needle causes less surgical trauma when passed through tissues and provides better suture purchase into the soft tissues than other needle types (12).

Surgical Techniques

The choice of preanesthetic medication is based on the preoperative evaluation and on personal preference. A narcotic is recommended for its analgesic effect. A fentanyl transdermal patch (Duragesic, Janssen Pharmaceutica, Titusville, NJ) can be placed on a shaved area over the dorsum of the neck and covered with a light bandage. Appropriate analgesic serum levels can take up to 12 hours to occur, so placement the night before the surgical procedure is helpful. Pharmacokinetic parameters have not been well established in the dog; however, we use a 25-μg/hour patch for dogs less than 25 kg, a 50-μg/hour patch for dogs between 25 and 50 kg, and two 50-μg/hour patches in dogs weighing more than 50 kg. The use of these patches has subjectively resulted in decreased anesthetic needs and adequate postoperative analgesics for 2 to 3 days. Some dogs may need to be treated with additional narcotic agents, depending on pain response. A local nerve block of the inferior alveolar nerve preoperatively or intraoperatively using a long-acting local anesthetic may also decrease postoperative pain and may lower anesthetic requirements.

After induction of anesthesia, an endotracheal tube should be inserted, and anesthesia should be maintained with a gas inhalant and oxygen. A cuffed endotracheal tube is mandatory to prevent passive aspiration of blood and fluid. The tube is anchored to the patient's muzzle to minimize its interference during surgery. Isotonic crystalloid fluid therapy is started immediately after induction at an initial dose of 10 mL/kg per hour. At times, hemorrhage is brisk, and the dose should be increased as dictated by the situation. Whole blood, plasma or colloids may be indicated, depending on the degree of blood loss. The patient is placed on a protected hot-water blanket and is monitored at all times with a continuous electrocardio-

gram and preferably with either direct or indirect blood pressure measurements. Before the surgical procedure is begun, the cuffed endotracheal tube should be checked to ensure that an airtight seal has been created with the trachea to prevent the aspiration of blood.

Depending on the type of mandibulectomy performed, the hair over the dorsal or ventral muzzle may or may not need to be clipped. Procedures done entirely through an intraoral approach usually do not require clipping. For procedures requiring caudal approaches, such as total hemimandibulectomy and vertical ramus mandibulectomy, hair should be clipped in the region of the commisure of the lip caudally to the base of the ear. Clipped regions are routinely prepared for aseptic surgery. The oral cavity should be swabbed with a 10% dilution of povidone–iodine solution (Betadine, Purdue Frederick Co., Norwalk, CT). A mouth speculum is placed between the teeth on the normal side to keep the mouth open. The surgical area is draped as aseptically as possible.

Unilateral Rostral Body Mandibulectomy

Tumors or injuries involving the incisors, lower canine, or first two premolars on one side are indications for unilateral rostral body mandibulectomy. The soft tissues medial to this region must be free of tumor to obtain a tumor-free margin and must have adequate soft tissues for closure (Fig. 10.15**A**). A bilateral rostral body mandibulectomy should be considered if the medial soft tissue structures are involved or if an adequate tumor-free margin cannot be obtained.

The animal is placed in lateral recumbency with the affected mandible placed dorsally. The labial mucosa is incised at a minimum of 1 cm outside the visible limits of the tumor (Fig. 10.15**B**). The dissection is continued around the body of the mandible to the sublingual mucosa until the symphysis and the caudal limit of the proposed ostectomy are exposed (Fig. 10.15**C**). The sublingual and mandibular salivary gland ducts open under the body of the tongue on the sublingual caruncle and are generally preserved. If excising this area is necessary, an attempt should be made to ligate these ducts.

After exposure of the symphysis, the tough fibrous

Fig. 10.15. Unilateral rostral body mandibulectomy. **A.** The shaded area represents the region of the mandible to be excised. **B.** The labial mucosa is incised and the rostral hemimandible is undermined to expose the symphysis and caudal limit of the proposed ostectomy. **C.** The sublingual attachments in the rostral intermandibular space are incised. **D.** An osteotome is used to split the symphysis. **E.** The dotted lines indicate the proposed osteotomy site for removal of the tumor adjacent to the symphysis. Note the eccentric osteotomy of the rostral mandible to include the symphysis and the tapered caudal osteotomy. **F.** Ostectomy site after unilateral rostral body mandibulectomy. No attempt is made to stabilize the two hemimandibles together. **G.** Single-layer simple interrupted or simple continuous closure of the ostectomy site. *T*, tongue. (Reprinted with permission from Withrow SJ, Holmberg DL. Mandibulectomy in the treatment of oral cancer. J Am Anim Hosp Assoc 1983;19:275–276.)

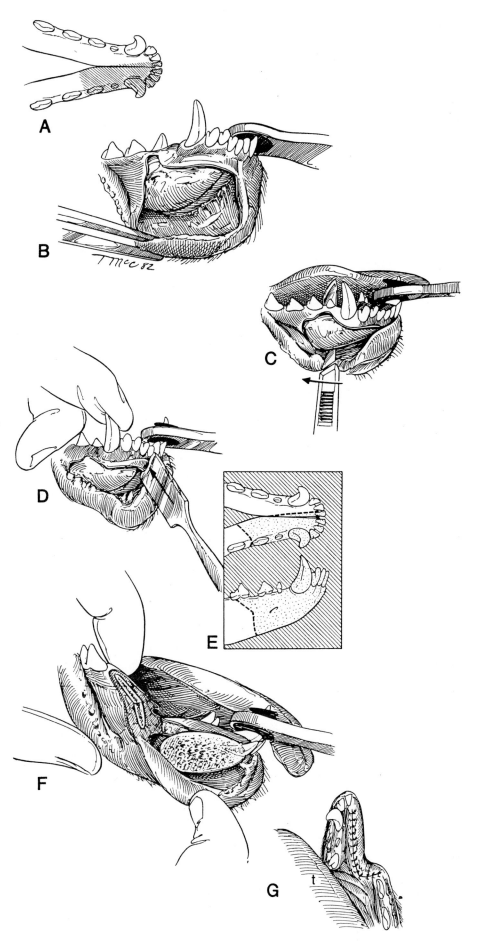

135

joint is split with an osteotome and mallet to separate the two hemimandibles (Fig. 10.15**D**). If the tumor has crossed over or is adjacent to the symphysis, the rostral osteotomy should be directed eccentrically between the incisors or canine tooth on the opposite hemimandible to excise the symphyseal joint completely. Because the body of the mandible is dense and brittle, an oscillating saw or Gigli wire is used to make the caudal osteotomy. Tapering the osteotomy at the occlusional margin decreases suture line tension on the mucosal closure (Fig. 10.15**E**). This may require the removal of an additional tooth. Hemorrhage from the mandibular medullary cavity is from the mental artery and vein and may be brisk. Bleeding is controlled with ligation, cautery, or bone wax. Portions of abnormal tooth roots remaining should be removed; however, normal roots need not be extracted. No attempt is made to stabilize the two hemimandibles together (Fig. 10.15**F**).

A one-layer simple interrupted or continuous suture closure of the sublingual mucosa to the labial mucosa attached to the skin is accomplished with 3–0 or 4–0 suture (Fig. 10.15**G**). The hair of the skin is partially in the mouth, but care should be taken to prevent inversion of the suture line. In some cases, tumor may adhere to the skin, thus requiring its excision. In these patients, effecting partial closure and allowing the defect to heal by second intention should result in a cosmetically acceptable appearance.

Bilateral Rostral Body Mandibulectomy

Bilateral rostral body mandibulectomy is indicated for tumors or injuries that cross the midline rostral to the second premolar (Fig. 10.16**A**). This procedure is commonly used in cancer patients because of the frequent soft tissue involvement of the opposite hemimandible. Even with unilateral disease, some patients function better with a bilateral resection. If the surgeon has any question about the extent of disease (crossing the midline or not), bilateral resection should be performed.

The patient can be placed in lateral, dorsal, or sternal recumbency. Dorsal recumbency affords the greatest exposure for dissection and osteotomy, whereas ventral recumbency affords the greatest exposure of the oral cavity for more difficult closures (Fig. 10.16**B**). This procedure is similar to unilateral rostral body mandibulectomy, except bilateral resection is performed. No attempt is made to stabilize the two hemimandibles together. The bodies are not pulled together but are allowed to remain in a normal anatomic position. In our experience, this procedure can be extended to the level of the first molar teeth bilaterally and still result in good function and adequate cosmetics.

Redundant skin may need to be removed before it is sutured to the sublingual mucosa during closure. This is easily accomplished by excising a V-shaped wedge of skin with the apex located ventrally. The excision can be performed at the most rostral tip of the exposed skin or just lateral to this point. The location

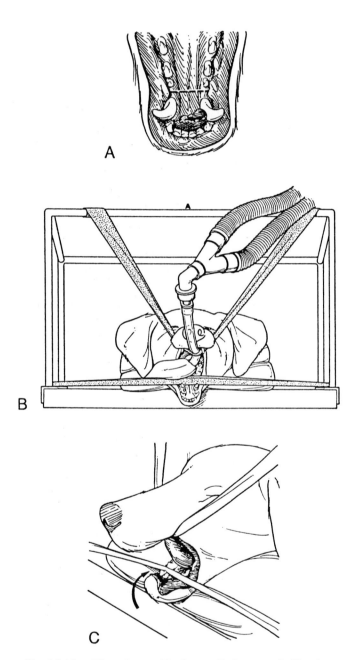

Fig. 10.16. Bilateral rostral body mandibulectomy. **A.** The dotted line indicates the proposed ostectomy site for tumor excision. **B.** With the dog in sternal recumbency, the rostral lower jaw overhangs the surgical table and is taped to the table with adhesive tape. The upper jaw is taped to an anesthesia screen (A) along with the endotracheal tube. **C.** A soft tissue ridge or "dam" is created to help keep saliva in the mouth.

Oral Cavity • 137

selected should be based first on location of the tumor and second on cosmetics. Any adherent skin overlying the tumor should be excised, to ensure a tumor-free margin. During suturing of the labial mucosa attached to skin to the sublingual mucosa, the surgeon should attempt to create a soft tissue ridge rostrally to help keep saliva in the mouth (Fig. 10.16**C**).

Total Hemimandibulectomy

Total hemimandibulectomy—the most aggressive form of mandibulectomy—entails total or subtotal removal of the hemimandible on one side. The procedure is indicated for patients with tumors or injuries involving a large segment of the mandible or for those with tumors (e.g., malignant melanoma, fibrosarcoma, osteosarcoma) that appear to have penetrated the medullary cavity.

The patient is placed in lateral or ipsilateral recumbency, with the involved mandible placed dorsally. The commissure of the lip is first incised at its midpoint, full thickness, to the rostral edge of the vertical ramus (Fig. 10.17**A**). The incision is then continued through the skin and the subcutaneous and fascial tissue to the level of the temporomandibular joint. Branches of the facial artery and vein are ligated or cauterized as necessary. The parotid duct is generally dorsal to this incision.

The labial and buccal mucosa are then incised, to ensure a visible 1-cm tumor-free margin, beginning at the symphysis and extending caudally to the angle of the mandible (Fig. 10.17**B**). The mandibular and sublingual ducts, if identifiable, are ligated at this time. The dissection is carried completely around the horizontal body of the mandible; the genioglossus, geniohyoideus, and mylohyoideus muscles are cut where they attach to the medial surface of the mandible. The sublingual mucosa is incised to free the lateral border of the tongue. As much mucosa as possible is saved to aid closure. Once the horizontal body is free of soft tissue attachments, the symphysis is cut with an osteotome and mallet (Fig. 10.17**C**). This technique allows free lateral movement of the affected mandible, enhancing visualization for caudal dissection.

For rostrally located masses with bone marrow involvement, the body of the mandible can be resected at the rostral edge of the masseter muscle (the marrow cavity ends at this level), and the vertical ramus and the temporomandibular joint can be left intact (Fig. 10.17**D**). If this is performed, the surgeon can then move to closure (see Fig. 10.18**B** and **C**).

If total hemimandibulectomy is performed, the masseter muscle is next sharply dissected off the ventrolateral surface and ventral margin of the ramus of the mandible and then is retracted dorsally and caudally (Fig. 10.17**E**). The digastricus muscle is then in-

cised at its insertion on the ventrocaudal border of the horizontal mandible (Fig. 10.17**F**). With lateral retraction of the mandibular body, the pterygoideus muscles are incised where they insert medially on the ventrocaudal surface of the angle of the mandible (Fig. 10.17**G**). Extreme care is necessary at this time to avoid accidental cutting of the mandibular alveolar artery, a branch of the maxillary artery, before its identification and ligation. This vessel passes across the lateral surface of the medial pterygoideus muscle before entering the mandibular canal. The mandibular foramen is located ventromedial and just rostral to the border that extends between the angular and coronoid processes of the mandible. After the capsule of the temporomandibular joint is visualized and incised both medially and laterally, the joint is luxated (Fig. 10.17**H**). This allows removal of the temporalis muscle as it inserts on the coronoid process of the mandible and of any remaining loose fascial attachments.

Closure is specific to each case, depending on the amount of soft tissue excised, but in all cases dead space must be closed, followed by mucosal apposition. A three-layer suture closure is recommended. The deep layer consists of opposing the pterygoideus, masseter, and temporalis muscles. If this does not close the dead space adequately, a negative drain may be placed to exit close to the incision. Exiting passive drains away from the surgical wound could potentially contaminate a larger area with tumor cells if the resection is microscopically incomplete. This could compromise adjuvant radiation therapy by enlarging the treatment field. The remaining closure sequence entails the stromal layer located below the mucosa followed by a mucosal layer. A continuous suture pattern works best in the mucosa to obtain a watertight seal.

In the caudal third of the incision, the oral mucosa lateral to the base of the tongue and oropharynx is sutured to the mucosa of the soft or hard palate. In the middle third of the incision, the upper buccal and labial mucosa is sutured to the sublingual mucosa remaining lateral to the tongue. This is continued to the rostral edge of the commissure incision. Because removal of the entire hemimandible results in loss of lateral support for the tongue, lateral drifting of the tongue often occurs. Closing the commissure of the lip farther rostrally can help to maintain the normal position of the tongue. To do this, the margin of the upper lip, where it previously met the lower lip to form the commissure, is incised at full thickness along its margin to the level of the first premolar or canine tooth (Fig. 10.18**A**). A three-layer suture closure consisting of mucosa, subcutaneous tissue, and skin is then performed (Fig. 10.18**B** and **C**). Because of excess tension at the rostral extent of the suture line when the mouth is opened, a vertical mattress suture with buttons or a rubber stent may be considered. To com-

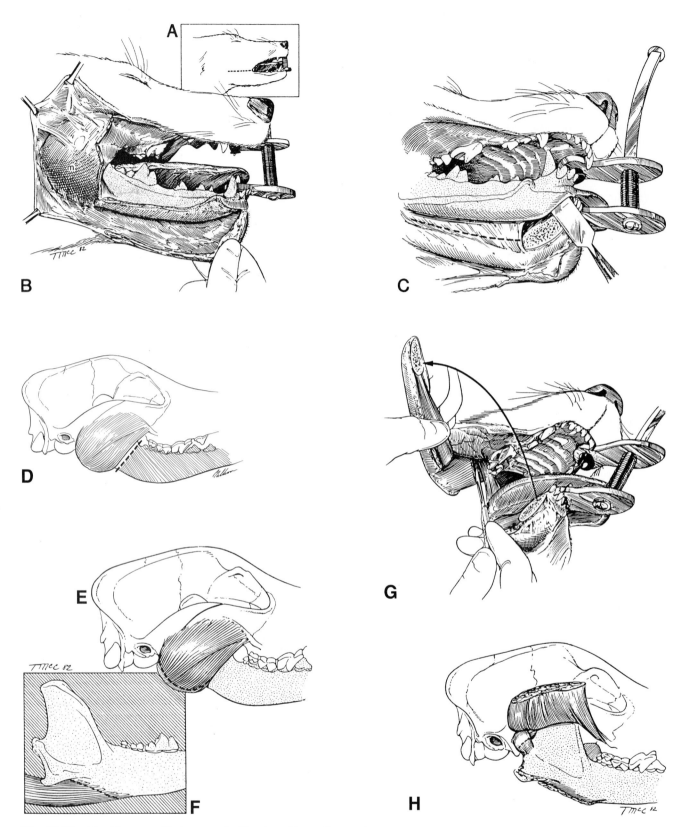

Fig. 10.17. Total hemimandibulectomy. **A.** The dotted line indicates the skin incision. **B.** The buccal and labial skin are dissected free from the masseter muscle (m) and mandible, respectively, after the labial mucosa has been incised. The dotted area represents the area on the mandible involved by tumor. **C.** The symphysis is split with an osteotome. The dotted line represents the incision level for removal of the intramandibular muscles. **D.** The dotted line represents the level of resection for rostrally located tumors that involve the mandibular medullary cavity. The cavity ends at the level of the rostral attachment of the masseter muscle. **E.** The dotted line represents the masseter muscle incision. **F.** The dotted line represents the line of incision on the digastricus muscle. **G.** The pterygoideus muscles are incised medially. Care must be taken to avoid cutting the mandibular alveolar artery before it is identified and ligated. **H.** The masseter muscle has been incised and elevated to expose the temporomandibular joint. The dotted line represents the joint capsule incision. (Reprinted with permission from Withrow SJ, Holmberg DL. Mandibulectomy in the treatment of oral cancer. J Am Anim Hosp Assoc 1983;19:277–278.)

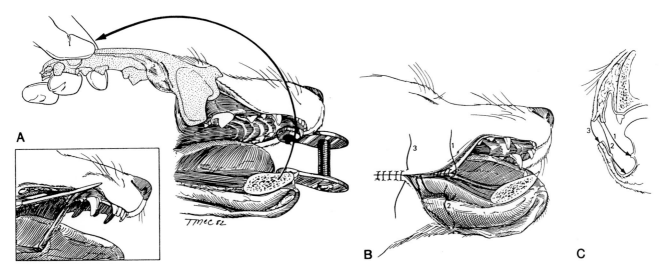

Fig. 10.18. Cheiloplasty, to prevent lateral drooping of the tongue, and closure after total hemimandibulectomy. **A.** Full-thickness incision of the upper lid margin to the level of the first premolar or canine tooth. **B** and **C.** Three-layer closure: *1*, oral mucosa; *2*, subcutaneous tissue; *3*, skin closure. (Reprinted with permission from Withrow SJ, Holmberg DL. Mandibulectomy in the treatment of oral cancer. J Am Anim Hosp Assoc 1983;19:279.)

plete the closure, the symphyseal oral mucosa is sutured to the lower labial mucosa, as described for a unilateral rostral body mandibulectomy.

Vertical Ramus Mandibulectomy

Vertical ramus mandibulectomy is indicated for tumors or injuries involving the angle, temporomandibular joint, or vertical ramus of the mandible. This procedure is versatile enough to allow preservation of the temporomandibular joint or excision of the entire hemimandible caudal to the last molar. This procedure can be combined with resection of the zygoma or inferior orbit for lesions with more extensive tissue involvement.

The animal is placed in lateral recumbency with the affected side placed dorsally. A curved skin incision is made over the length of the ventral aspect of the zygomatic arch (Fig. 10.19**A**). Multiple small vessels are encountered, and several thin superficial muscles are incised as they cross lateral to the zygomatic arch. The periosteum is incised over the lateral surface of the zygomatic arch. With a periosteal elevator, the temporalis and masseter muscles are subperiosteally elevated off the dorsal and medial aspect and the ventral aspect, respectively, of the zygomatic arch (Fig. 10.19**B**). Care should be taken not to injure the infraorbital artery, nerve, and vein as they course just medial to the zygomatic arch. Once the zygomatic arch is free of soft tissue attachments, it is cut with an oscillating saw or Gigli wire at its rostral and caudal margins (Fig. 10.19**C**); an osteotome should not be used because it tends to shatter the hard, brittle bone of the

zygomatic arch. Bleeding at the cut edges of the osteotomy site can be stopped with electrocautery or bone wax.

The masseter muscle is elevated ventrally off the lateral surface of the vertical ramus. The temporalis muscle is similarly elevated off the medial and rostral aspect of the mandibular ramus. Care should be taken as the medial dissection is continued ventrally to avoid the mandibular alveolar vessel. This vessel crosses the lateral surface of the medial pterygoideus muscle and enters the mandibular foramen located just rostral and ventral to the temporomandibular joint. If the temporomandibular joint is to be included in the excision, this vessel must be ligated and the medial pterygoideus muscle incised and elevated off the ventromedial aspect of the mandibular angle. The mandible is cut ventral and rostral to the involved bone with an oscillating saw or Gigli wire. Depending on the extent of the lesion to be removed, one may preserve the temporomandibular joint or include the joint in the excised bone (Fig. 10.19**D**). At this point, the ramus can be easily removed by incising any loosely attached muscle and fascia; the temporomandibular joint is dislocated if necessary.

After copious lavage with physiologic saline, the muscle groups at the angle of the mandible are closed together as well as possible to obliterate dead space. If drainage is necessary, a negative suction drain is placed, exiting close to the incision line. Replacing the osteotomized zygomatic arch is not necessary. The fascia of the masseter and temporalis muscles are then reattached to each other. Closure is completed with placement of subcutaneous and skin sutures.

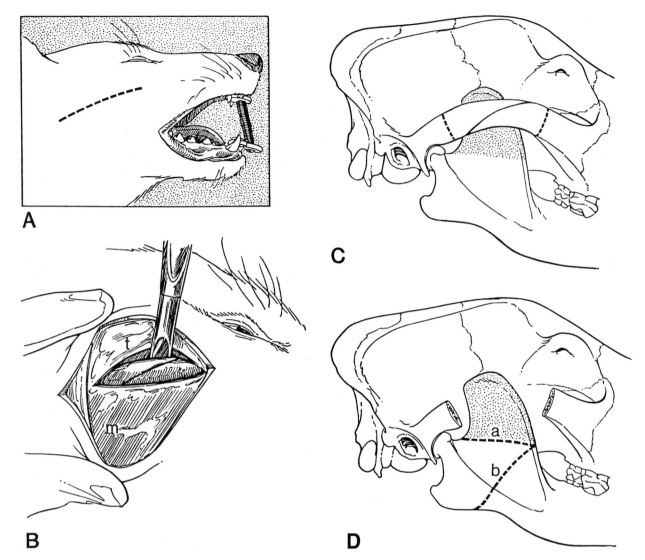

Fig. 10.19. Vertical ramus mandibulectomy. **A.** The dotted line represents the direction of the skin incision over the zygomatic arch. **B.** The temporalis (t) and masseter (m) muscles are elevated subperiosteally from the zygomatic arch. **C.** The dotted lines represent the rostral and caudal osteotomy sites on the zygomatic arch. The shaded area on the vertical ramus represents the proposed mandibular ostectomy. **D.** The dotted lines represent various ostectomy sites for tumor removal. The temporomandibular joint is preserved (a) or removed (b) depending on tumor involvement of the vertical ramus. (Reprinted with permission from Withrow SJ, Holmberg DL. Mandibulectomy in the treatment of oral cancer. J am Anim Hosp Assoc 1983;19:280–281.)

Segmental Horizontal Body Mandibulectomy

Segmental horizontal body mandibulectomy is indicated for benign disease processes and for malignant tumors that do not penetrate cortical bone and are confined to the horizontal body between the first premolar and the last molar.

The animal is placed in lateral recumbency with the affected side placed dorsally. The labial and lingual mucosa are incised 1 cm outside the visible limits of the tumor. Dissection is continued completely around the mandibular body until it is exposed for 360°. An oscillating saw or Gigli wire is then used to cut the mandibular body 1 cm rostral and caudal to the lesion. The dorsal aspect of the osteotomy should be angled away from the lesion (Fig. 10.20**A**). Bleeding from the exposed mandibular alveolar artery is controlled with ligation if possible. Cautery or bone wax can be used alternatively or in addition to ligation. A one-layer closure of sublingual mucosa to the remaining labial mucosa attached to the skin is accomplished with 3–0 or 4–0 suture material, similar to that used in unilateral rostral body mandibulectomy (Fig. 10.20**B**).

Postoperative Care and Complications

Analgesics generally are indicated for the first 24 hours postoperatively, particularly after the more aggressive

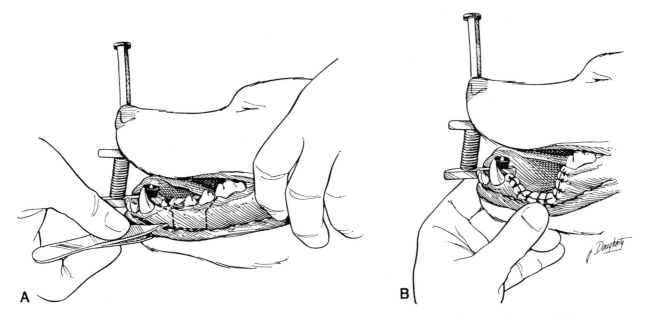

Fig. 10.20. Segmental horizontal mandibulectomy. **A.** The dotted line indicates the proposed area to be excised. The osteotomies should be tapered away from the lesion on the occlusal surface to minimize suture line tension. **B.** Simple interrupted or simple continuous closure of labial or oral mucosa.

procedures (i.e., total hemimandibulectomy). Oxymorphone, at a dosage of 0.11 to 0.22 mg/kg, can be used in addition to fentanyl patches if needed. A constant rate of infusion of fentanyl (2 to 4 µg/kg per hour) can also be considered. Maintenance parenteral fluids (20 mL/kg three times daily) also are recommended during this time. Antibiotics generally are not given for longer than 24 hours postoperatively. An Elizabethan collar should be placed on the patient as soon as it is sternally recumbent to prevent self-induced trauma at the surgical site. The collar should be kept on the animal for the first 7 to 10 days.

Patients may have water and soft foods on the day after surgery for all types of mandibulectomy. Most animals are able to maintain hydration and caloric intake by 24 to 48 hours postoperatively. Pharyngostomy, esophagostomy, or gastrostomy tubes are rarely necessary. The surgical site should be kept free of debris by flushing the mouth with water daily. After complete healing, return to the animal's normal diet is encouraged.

Complications are few after any type of mandibulectomy. Postoperative infection is rare unless a deep-seated infection was present at the time of surgery. The abundant blood supply to the oral cavity is a major reason for the low incidence of infection.

If dehiscence occurs at the surgery site, delaying closure for 7 to 10 days to allow better delineation of necrotic tissue and development of a healthy granulation bed is recommended. Dehiscence generally results from self-induced trauma by the animal, excessive use of electrocautery, premature feeding of hard foods be-

fore adequate healing, or excessive tension at the suture line. Overall dehiscence rates are reported to be less than 10% (13–15). Total hemimandibulectomy has the highest potential for dehiscence.

Excess tension is most often noted at the rostral extent of the cheiloplasty after total hemimandibulectomy or at the occlusal bone margin after horizontal body ostectomy as in unilateral and bilateral rostral body mandibulectomy and segmental horizontal body mandibulectomy. Tension-free closure of the mucosal suture line at the level of the ostectomy can be achieved by angling the dorsal (occlusal) bone margin away from the lesion and by suturing the mucosa over the tapered bone. Often, this requires extraction of an additional tooth. Drooping of the tongue to one side of the mouth can occur after total hemimandibulectomy if cheiloplasty is not performed or if the wound dehisces. Prehensile function of the tongue generally is normal, however.

If ostectomy is performed caudal to the second premolar bilaterally, prehensile function and drooping of the tongue may occur after bilateral rostral body mandibulectomy. This complication is a result of loss of support to the base of the tongue. In our experience, most animals regain complete control of tongue function in time. The owners and veterinarian must be willing to hand feed these animals during the recovery period. Different types of food should be tried (i.e., soft or hard), and a patient and persistent owner is required. Oral feeding should be encouraged to allow the animal to adapt and develop a "new" prehensile function of the tongue.

After total hemimandibulectomy, edema or a "false" ranula may develop at the lateral base of the tongue on the surgically treated side. This condition is self-limiting and generally disappears within 7 days. Removal of the sublingual and mandibular salivary glands is not necessary for resolution of this condition. Ligation or surgical trauma and inflammation with occlusion of the ducts of these glands at the time of surgery lead to atrophy of the glands.

The only long-term common complication of mandibulectomy is shifting of the lower jaw toward the operated side. This shift results from loss of a portion of the mandibular support at either the temporomandibular joint or the symphyseal region. The malocclusion that results generally is clinically insignificant. Occasionally, filing down the top 20% of the remaining lower canine tooth may be necessary because of chronic irritation and ulceration of the hard palate mucosa. Mandibular drift can be more of a problem in cats. If drift is anticipated after extensive resections, the remaining intact mandible can be immobilized to the maxilla by wiring the upper and lower canine teeth together. The teeth are etched, and a figure-of-eight wire is placed between the upper and lower canine teeth and is secured with dental acrylic. Enough of a gap between the mandible and the maxilla is left to allow the cat to lap water and a gruel diet. Within 2 to 4 weeks, soft tissue contraction is usually complete, resulting in more normal stability and alignment and allowing removal of the wire.

Follow-up

When mandibulectomy is performed for tumor excision, periodic checks should be performed at 1, 3, 6, 9, and 12 months. The animal should be evaluated for local tumor recurrence, nodal metastasis, and distant metastasis. When the surgical margins of either the histologic sections or the postoperative radiographs are questionable, more frequent rechecks are recommended. Less frequent rechecks are required when

mandibulectomy is performed for treatment of chronic mandibular osteomyelitis or mandibular fractures.

Table 10.2 lists approximate recurrence and median survival rates reported for dogs undergoing mandibulectomy for oral tumors (13–21). The reported 1-year survival rate for cats with squamous cell carcinoma treated by mandibulectomy alone is 20% (5 cats: local recurrence, 4; metastatic disease, 3) (2).

References

1. Withrow SJ, Holmberg DL. Mandibulectomy in the treatment of oral cancer. J Am Anim Hosp Assoc 1983;19:273–286.
2. Bradley RL, MacEwen EG, Loar AS. Mandibular resection for removal of oral tumors in 30 dogs and 6 cats. J Am Vet Med Assoc 1984;184:460–463.
3. Dorn CR, et al. Survey of animal neoplasms in Alameda and Contra Costa Counties, California. I. Methodology and description of cases. J Natl Cancer Inst 1968;40:295.
4. Theilen GH, Madewell BR. Tumors of the digestive tract. In: Theilen GH, Madewell BR, eds. Veterinary cancer medicine. Philadelphia: Lea & Febiger, 1987:499–534.
5. Head KW. Tumors of the alimentary tract. In: Molten JE, ed. Tumors in domestic animals. 3rd ed. Berkeley, University of California Press, 1990:347–428.
6. Norris AM, Withrow SJ, Dubielzig RR. Oropharyngeal neoplasms. In: Harvey CE, ed. Veterinary dentistry. Philadelphia: WB Saunders, 1985:123–139.
7. Cotter SM. Oral pharyngeal neoplasms in the cat. J Am Anim Hosp Assoc 1981;17:917–920.
8. Dernell WS, Hullinger GH. Surgical management of amelioblastic fibroma in the cat. J Small Anim Pract 1994;35:35–38.
9. Carpenter LG, Withrow SJ, Powers BE, et al. Squamous cell carcinoma of the tongue in ten dogs. J Am Anim Hosp Assoc 1993;29:17–24.
10. Owen L, ed. TNM classification of tumors in domestic animals. Geneva: World Health Organization, 1980.
11. Prescott JF, Baggot JD. Principles of antimicrobial drug selection and use. In: Prescott JF, Baggot JD, eds. Antimicrobial therapy in veterinary medicine. Boston: Blackwell Scientific Publications, 1988:55–70.
12. Dernell WS, Harari J. Surgical devices and wound healing. In: Harari J, ed. Surgical complications and wound healing in small animal practice. Philadelphia: WB Saunders, 1993:349–376.
13. Salisbury SK, Lantz GC. Long-term results of partial mandibulectomy for the treatment of oral tumors in dogs. J Am Anim Hosp Assoc 1988;24:285–294.
14. Kosovsky JK, Matthiesen DT, Manfra Marretta S, et al. Results of partial mandibulectomy for the treatment of oral tumors in 142 dogs. Vet Surg 1991;20:397–401.
15. Schwarz PD, Withrow SJ, Curtis CR, et al. Mandibular resection as a treatment for oral cancer in 81 dogs. J Am Anim Hosp Assoc 1991;27:601–610.
16. White RAS, Gorman NT. Wide local excision of acanthomatous epulides in the dog. Vet Surg 1989;18:12–14.
17. White RAS. Mandibulectomy and maxillectomy in the dog: results of 75 cases. Presented at the 22nd Annual Meeting of the American College of Veterinary Surgeons, San Antonio, 1987.
18. Vernon FF, Helphrey M. Rostral mandibulectomy: 3 case reports in dogs. Vet Surg 1983;12:26–29.
19. Penwick RC, Nunamaker DM. Rostral mandibulectomy: a treatment for oral neoplasia in the dog and cat. J Am Anim Hosp Assoc 1987;23:19–25.
20. White RAS, Gorman NT, Watkins SB, et al. The surgical management of bone-involved oral tumor in the dog. J Small Anim Pract 1985;26:693–708.
21. Bjorling DE, Chambers IN, Mahaffey EA. Surgical treatment of epulides in dogs: 25 cases (1974–1984). J Am Vet Med Assoc 1987;190:1315–1318.

Table 10.2.
Approximate Reported Local Recurrence and Survival Data for Oral Tumors Treated by Mandibulectomy

Tumor Type	Number	Local Recurrence (%)	Median Survival (mo)
Acanthomatous epulis	47	0	28
Ameloblastoma	44	22	19
Malignant melanoma	75	13	8
Squamous cell carcinoma	73	7	9
Fibrosarcoma	53	34	11
Osteosarcoma	32	5	7

(Data from references 12 to 14 and 16 to 21.)

11

PHARYNX

Surgery for Elongated Soft Palate (Staphlectomy)

Ronald M. Bright

Elongation of the soft palate may occur occasionally in any breed, but it is most often seen in the brachycephalic breeds as part of the "brachycephalic syndrome." In addition to the soft palate abnormality, this syndrome may include stenotic nares, everted laryngeal saccules, enlarged tonsils, edema of the pharyngeal mucosa, hypoplastic trachea, and various degrees of laryngeal collapse, the last seen most often in older animals.

Clinical signs of elongated soft palate include gagging, emesis, stertorous "gurgling" breathing sounds, and, occasionally, dyspnea. Syncope with or without cyanosis may be seen because of the additive effects of other nasolaryngeal structural abnormalities.

Intromission of the tip of the elongated soft palate into the laryngeal opening during inspiration interferes with the movement of air into the trachea (Fig. 11.1). When stenotic nares is a concomitant problem, the severity of the dyspnea is greater because the resistance of air movement caused by the stenotic nares causes the tip of the soft palate to be drawn deeper into the larynx, thereby increasing the amount of obstruction to air flow. The excessive movement of the soft palate during the inspiratory effort contributes to the inflammatory and edematous appearance of the soft palate and surrounding laryngeal structures that is sometimes observed during examination of the laryngeal area.

Preoperative Considerations

Common postoperative problems after staphlectomy include swelling and edema of the pharyngeal structures that could interfere with the smooth recovery of the animal. To counter these potential problems, I encourage the careful handling of the soft palate, the minimal use of crushing forceps, and the avoidance of electrocautery. In addition, the animal should be given a corticosteroid intravenously during anesthetic induction.

If additional procedures are done to correct other abnormalities seen with the brachycephalic syndrome, visualization is improved when endotracheal intubation is accomplished through a left-sided pharyngotomy or a tracheostomy. A tracheostomy helps to minimize the adverse effects of the surgically induced edema postoperatively as well.

Surgical Technique

The patient is placed in sternal recumbency. Some type of oral speculum is used to open the mouth widely. Allis tissue forceps grasp the tip of the soft palate. The soft palate is allowed to return to its normal position. The line of amputation is along an imaginary line at the level of the midpoint of each tonsil (Fig. 11.2**A**). The tip of the soft palate is now drawn forward, and stay sutures using 3–0 or 4–0 polyglactin 910 (Vicryl, Ethicon, Inc., Somerville, NJ) are placed and tied in the lateral margins of the soft palate just cranial to the proposed incision line. Excellent visualization of the soft palate and of the line of incision is provided by the forceps, which pull the tip forward, and the stay sutures, which pull the soft palate laterally.

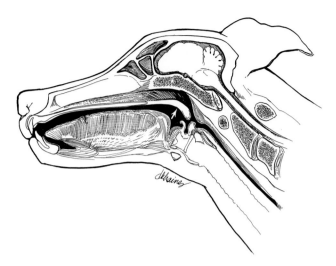

Fig. 11.1. The elongated soft palate (*arrow*) is more likely to be "sucked" into the laryngeal opening on inspiration.

A scalpel blade or a sharp pair of curved Metzenbaum scissors is used to incise half the width of the soft palate (Fig. 11.2**B**). The cut edges of the nasal and oral mucosa are gently apposed in a continuous pattern with the other length of the stay suture, which has the needle attached. The nasal mucosa tends to retract cranially, so care must be taken to include it in the suture line. The remaining palate is incised, and the suturing is continued to the opposite margin (Fig. 11.2**C**). It is then tied to one end of the opposite stay suture.

The soft palate is allowed to return to its normal position so the length can be evaluated. Adequate palate length ensures the closure of the nasopharyngeal opening during deglutition and prevents nasal regurgitation of food and water. If the length is adequate, the ends of the sutures are trimmed close to the knots.

Suggested Readings

Bright RM, Wheaton LG. A modified technique for elongated soft palate in dogs. J Am Anim Hosp Assoc 1983;19:288–292.
Knecht CD. Upper airway obstruction in brachycephalic dogs. Compend Contin Educ Pract Vet 1971;1:25–31.
Orsher RJ. Brachycephalic airway disease. In: Bojrab MJ, ed. Disease mechanisms in small animal surgery. Philadelphia: Lea & Febiger, 1993:369–370.

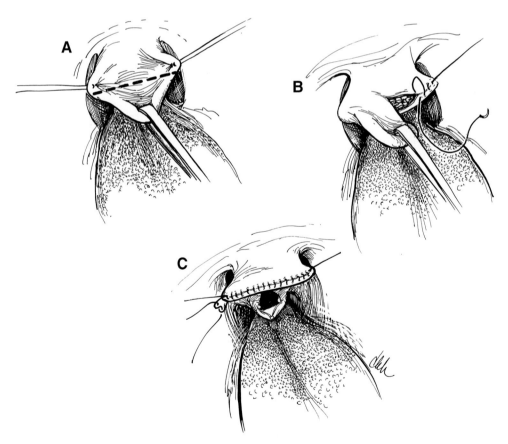

Fig. 11.2. **A.** The tip of the soft palate is grasped with Allis tissue forceps. After noting the length of soft palate to be amputated, stay sutures are placed just cranial to the proposed line of resection. **B.** The full thickness of the soft palate is incised with a surgical blade approximately half the width of the soft palate. A length of the "stay" suture with the needle attached is used to appose the edges of the cut surface while one takes care to incorporate both the pharyngeal and nasal mucosa. **C.** After completing mucosal apposition, the suture is tied to a length of suture being used as a "stay" suture on the opposite side.

Cricopharyngeal Dysphagia

Eberhard Rosin

Cricopharyngeal dysphagia, although an uncommon condition, is considered in the differential diagnosis of persistent dysphagia of young dogs. This condition is characterized by inadequate or asynchronous relaxation of the cricopharyngeal sphincter that prevents the normal movement of food from caudal portions of the pharynx into the cranial esophagus. The etiologic basis of this failure of reflex relaxation has not been established. Dogs with cricopharyngeal dysphagia usually have a history of dysphagia persisting since weaning. Attempts to swallow solid food result in anxiety, gagging, and expulsion of food from the mouth by forward movements of the tongue. After repeated ingestion of the masticated food, the entire meal passes into the stomach.

Diagnosis

Except for slight nasal exudate and occasional coughing, physical examination reveals no abnormality. Examination of the pharynx reveals no inflammatory or obstructive lesions. While the patient is under anesthesia, an esophagoscope can be passed into the stomach without difficulty. The resting pressure provided by the closed sphincter, as encountered by passage of the endoscope and as measured by manometry, is normal.

Radiographs of a barium swallow study reveal contrast material remaining in the pharynx. In some dogs, barium is aspirated into the lungs. Fluoroscopic examination of a barium swallow demonstrates normal movement of the barium bolus into the oropharynx by elevation of the tongue and contraction of the pharyngeal musculature. Despite the presence of sufficient force to distend the caudal pharyngeal wall, inadequate or asynchronous relaxation of the cricopharyngeal sphincter prevents normal movement of the bar-

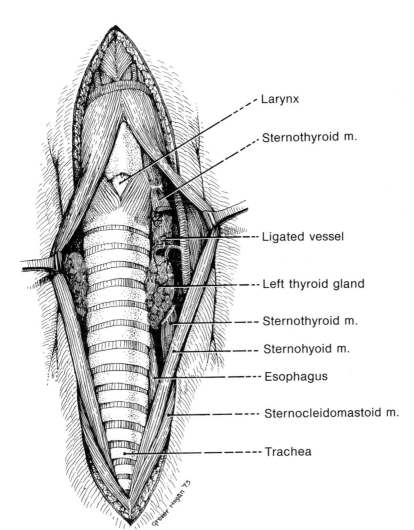

Larynx

Sternothyroid m.

Ligated vessel

Left thyroid gland

Sternothyroid m.

Sternohyoid m.

Esophagus

Sternocleidomastoid m.

Trachea

Fig. 11.3. Mobilization of the left side of the trachea and the cranial esophagus.

ium bolus into the proximal esophagus. The thin stream of barium that passes through the sphincter moves into the stomach with no evidence of failure of reflex relaxation of the gastroesophageal sphincter. This cycle is repeated in rapid succession until all the barium is swallowed. As the epiglottis, which closes the glottis in normal fashion during swallowing attempts, opens during inspiration, the residual barium filling the caudal pharyngeal region may be aspirated into the trachea and discharged by coughing.

Immediate relief of the dysphagia is achieved by cricopharyngeal myectomy. Complete division of muscle fibers of the cricopharyngeal muscle is essential for permanent elimination of the condition.

Technique for Cricopharyngeal Myectomy

The dog is anesthetized, intubated, and placed in dorsal recumbency. A midline incision is made from the cranial aspect of the larynx to the thoracic inlet. Exposure of the trachea and esophagus is by midline dissection of the ventral neck musculature. Partial incision of the insertion of fibers of the sternohyoid muscle on the basihyoid bone may be necessary. The bisected sternohyoid muscle is retracted to expose the trachea. Dissection is continued to the left of the trachea by transection of the insertion of the left sternothyroid muscle to the lateral surface of the thyroid lamina. The left thyroid gland is exposed between the trachea and the sternothyroid muscle. Several small branches of the cranial thyroid artery that supply the upper aspect of the left thyroid gland are ligated and transected (Fig. 11.3). The left recurrent laryngeal nerve should be preserved.

The cricopharyngeal muscle and dorsal proximal esophagus can be exposed by grasping the larynx and rotating it. The cricopharyngeal muscle can be identified as a bundle of transverse muscle fibers converging on the dorsal midline and blending into the longitudinal muscle fibers of the cranial esophagus. Two parallel incisions, approximately 2 mm apart, are made on the dorsal midline through the cricopharyngeal muscle and onto the cranial esophageal musculature (Fig. 11.4). The esophageal mucosa is not incised. The in-

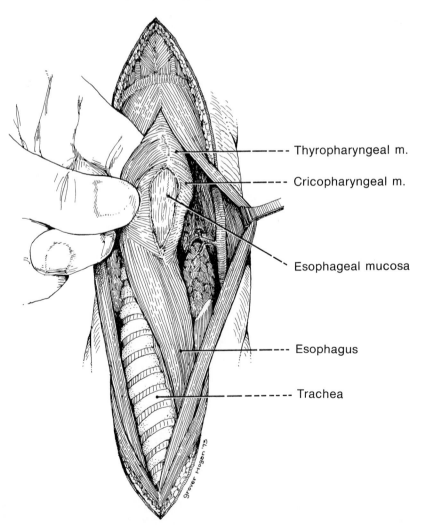

Thyropharyngeal m.

Cricopharyngeal m.

Esophageal mucosa

Esophagus

Trachea

Fig. 11.4. Myectomy through the length and thickness of the cricopharyngeal and the cranial esophageal musculature. The esophageal mucosa is not incised.

cised muscle fibers are separated from the mucosa and are excised. Bleeding is controlled by use of gauze and pressure; the myectomy is not sutured.

Closure of the incision is initiated by apposition of the sternohyoid muscle with simple interrupted 3–0 absorbable sutures. Suturing the transected insertion of the sternothyroid muscle is not necessary. The subcutaneous tissue and skin are sutured routinely. Although other tissue planes that were separated for exposure are not sutured, seroma formation is uncommon.

Postoperative Care

No special postoperative care is required. Patients tolerate solid food the day after the operation. Recurrence of dysphagia because of fibrosis and constriction at the myectomy site is prevented by adequate removal of sphincter muscle fibers during the original surgical procedure.

Suggested Readings

Hurwitz A L, Duranceau A. Upper esophageal sphincter dysfunction: pathogenesis and treatment. Am J Digest Dis 1978;23:275.

Lund WS. The functions of the cricopharyngeal sphincter during swallowing. Acta Otolaryngol (Stockh) 1965;59:497.

Pearson H. The differential diagnosis of persistent vomiting in the young dog. J Small Anim Pract 1970;11:403.

Rosin E, Hanlon GF. Canine cricopharyngeal achalasia. J Am Vet Med Assoc 1972;160:1496.

Seaman WB. Functional disorders of the pharyngoesophageal junction. Radiol Clin North Am 1969;11:113.

Sokolovsky V. Cricopharyngeal achalasia in a dog. J Am Vet Med Assoc 1967;150:281.

Suter PF, Watrous BJ. Oropharyngeal dysphagias in the dog: a cinefluorographic analysis of experimentally induced and spontaneously occurring swallowing disorders. I. Oral stage and pharyngeal stage dysphagias. Vet Radiol 1980;21:24.

Otopharyngeal Polyps

Jacqueline R. Davidson

Otopharyngeal polyps, also termed nasopharyngeal polyps or inflammatory polyps, are benign pedunculated growths that arise from the otopharyngeal mucous membranes in cats. The polyp stalk may originate from the nasopharynx, the auditory canal, or the tympanic cavity (1, 2). The polyp may grow into the nasopharynx or tympanic cavity or both. The mucosal lining from the nasopharynx to the tympanic cavity is continuous and histologically similar, so identifying the origin of polyps is difficult. Polyps are composed of variable amounts of submucosal lymphocytic plasmacytic cellular infiltration with fibroplasia, and the epithelium ranges from stratified squamous to ciliated columnar cells (2, 3).

The exact cause of otopharyngeal polyps is unknown. The presence of submucosal inflammatory cells suggests that polyps may arise from inflammation or from chronic inflammation. Polyps are also associated with rhinitis or otitis media, suggesting a viral or bacterial origin. However, whether the inflammation and infection are primary or secondary conditions is unclear. Because polyps have been identified in young kittens, a congenital origin has also been suggested (4, 5).

Otopharyngeal polyps occur in cats of any age, although these animals are often less than 2 years old and may be as young as 4 weeks of age (1, 4, 6, 7). No apparent sex or breed predisposition has been noted. Polyps have also been reported in the dog (8). Although polyps are most commonly unilateral, they can be bilateral.

Clinical signs may be present for weeks to years before a polyp is diagnosed, and the signs vary depending on location (3, 9). Polyps in the nasopharyngeal region may cause obstruction resulting in respiratory stridor, dyspnea, dysphagia, or voice changes. Respiratory distress, cyanosis, and syncopal episodes may also occur. Nasopharyngeal polyps may cause signs of upper respiratory tract infection such as sneezing, coughing, and nasal or ocular discharge. The respiratory signs may be mildly responsive to symptomatic treatment if a secondary bacterial infection is present. Polyps in the external or middle ear may be associated with infection or may cause signs that mimic otitis externa, otitis media, or otitis interna. These signs include head shaking, ear scratching, head tilt, Horner's syndrome, and nystagmus. Any cat with chronic upper respiratory tract disease should be evaluated for polyps. The differential diagnosis includes upper respiratory tract infections, such as with feline calicivirus and feline rhinotracheitis virus, nasal foreign bodies, and nasopharyngeal masses such as cryptococcal granuloma and neoplasms.

Preoperative Considerations

A thorough physical examination should be performed, including complete otoscopic and oropharyngeal evaluations. Polyps may rupture through the tympanic membrane and may appear in the external ear canal. Examination of the external ear canal may reveal signs of otitis externa with a visible pink or gray, smooth, spheric mass occluding the canal. If the history and physical findings suggest a pharyngeal mass, sedation or general anesthesia may be necessary to perform a thorough oral examination. Inspection of the oral cavity may reveal ventral displacement of the soft palate. The nasopharynx can be evaluated by retracting the caudal edge of the soft palate rostrally using a spay hook or stay suture. The nasopharynx can also be visualized by use of a flexible fiberoptic bronchoscope.

Skull radiographs should be obtained, with particular attention paid to the nasal cavity and middle ear. A soft tissue density may be seen in the nasopharynx on the lateral radiographic view. Radiographic examination of the osseous and tympanic bulla and petrous temporal bones is recommended. Thickening or sclerosis of the osseous bulla and sclerosis of the petrous–temporal bone indicate middle ear involvement. The tympanic bulla may be best evaluated for increased soft tissue density using open-mouth and oblique radiographic views of the skull. Increased soft tissue density may also be seen within the external canal if a polyp is located there. Most cats with polyps have radiographic changes compatible with middle ear infection. However, radiographic evaluation is not a sensitive method to diagnose otitis media, so the disorder should be suspected in cats with otopharyngeal polyps even in the absence of radiographic evidence (2, 10).

Surgical Technique

Polyp removal with a ventral bulla osteotomy performed on the side associated with the polyp is the treatment of choice. Regardless of whether the polyp is in the external ear canal or the nasopharynx, a ventral bulla osteotomy should be performed before removing the polyp, to facilitate removal of inflammatory tissue and detachment of the pedicle. This procedure may reduce the chance of recurrence. A bulla osteotomy should be considered even with no radiographic evidence of otitis media.

To perform a ventral bulla osteotomy, the cat is placed in dorsal recumbency with the head and neck extended. The ventral wall of the tympanic bulla can usually be palpated between the angular process of the mandible and the larynx. A paramedian skin incision is made over the bulla beginning near the angle of the mandible and extending about 6 cm caudally, where the linguofacial vein may be identified. The incision is continued through the subcutaneous tissues and cutaneous muscles. Blunt dissection between the digastric muscle laterally and the hyoglossal and styloglossal muscles medially exposes the bulla, which is palpable cranial to the hyoid apparatus. The hypoglossal nerve and the lingual artery and vein may be identified on the hyoglossal muscle, and they are retracted medially. The ventral branch of the external carotid artery is located lateral to the bulla. Self-retaining retractors may be used to maintain exposure, with care taken to avoid the hypoglossal nerve and the vessels. Connective tissue and periosteum is bluntly dissected off the ventral aspect of the bulla using a periosteal elevator.

A Steinmann pin is used to create a hole in the ventral bulla. The hole should be large enough to accommodate one jaw of small rongeurs. The ventral aspect of the bulla is then removed with the rongeurs.

The middle ear of the cat contains a septum that divides the bulla into small dorsolateral and larger ventromedial compartments (11, 12). This septum must be removed to gain access to the dorsolateral compartment of the bulla, where the external auditory meatus and the auditory os of the eustachian tube are located (Fig. 11.5). The septum can be removed as described for removal of the ventral bulla. Both compartments of the bulla should be cultured. The bulla should undergo careful inspection and gentle curettage to remove the epithelial lining and any granulation tissue. Aggressive curettage or direct suctioning of the dorsomedial aspect of the bulla should be avoided to reduce the risk of damaging the postganglionic sympathetic nerve fibers, auditory ossicles, semicircular canals, and cochlea. Damage to these structures can result in Horner's syndrome and otitis interna. Any tissue removed from the bulla should be

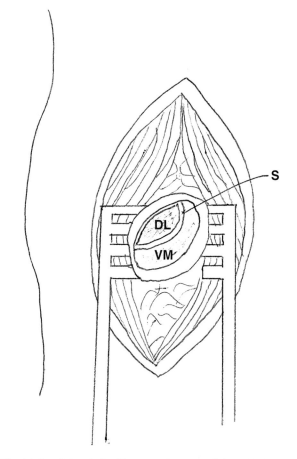

Fig. 11.5. Feline bulla. The ventral aspect of the bulla has been removed to gain access to the large ventromedial compartment (VM). The ventral aspect of the septum (S) has also been removed to gain access to the dorsolateral compartment (DL).

submitted for histologic evaluation. Before closing, the bulla is lavaged with sterile saline, and a drain is placed to exit through a separate stab incision. A closed-suction drain may be constructed by cutting the end from a butterfly infusion set (E-Z Set, Becton Dickinsin, Sandy, UT) and creating several fenestrations in the tubing. Once the drain has been placed in the bulla and the wound has been closed, the needle is inserted into a Vacutainer tube to provide suction. This system is preferable to a Penrose drain because the quantity and character of the drainage can be easily monitored. The cutaneous muscles and subcutaneous tissues are sutured with 3–0 or 4–0 absorbable suture material in a simple continuous pattern. The skin may be closed using 4–0 absorbable suture material in a simple continuous intradermal pattern or using 4–0 nylon as external skin sutures. The drain should be sutured to the skin to prevent premature removal, and a bandage is placed around the head to stabilize the vacutainer tube. The vacutainer should be replaced twice daily to ensure that it is providing negative pressure. The drain is removed when the drainage is minimal, usually within 3 to 7 days. If a Penrose drain is used, it must be covered with a bandage that is changed daily to monitor any drainage. The skin sutures may be removed 7 to 10 days postoperatively.

Simple traction using Allis tissue forceps or alligator forceps is usually sufficient to remove the polyp. If the polyp is visible in the external canal, a lateral ear canal resection may be required for adequate exposure. Nasopharyngeal polyps can be removed through an oral approach, and retraction of the soft palate rostrally usually provides adequate exposure. If necessary, exposure may be increased by making a longitudinal incision on the midline of the soft palate (Fig. 11.6). Stay sutures may be used to retract the palate while the polyp is being removed. A three-layer closure is performed on the palate by suturing the nasal mucosa,

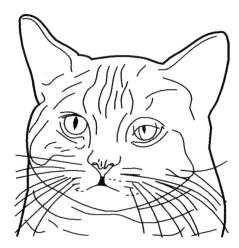

Fig. 11.7. A cat with Horner's syndrome after ventral bulla osteotomy. Miosis, ptosis, enophthalmos, and prolapse of the third eyelid are present.

submucosal tissue, and oral mucosa separately using 4–0 or 5–0 absorbable suture material in a simple continuous pattern. The polyp should be submitted for histopathologic evaluation.

Surgical complications are related to the ventral bulla osteotomy, and the most common is damage to the postganglionic sympathetic resulting in Horner's syndrome, which is characterized by miosis, ptosis, enophthalmos, and prolapse of the third eyelid (Fig. 11.7). It usually resolves within 1 month, although it may be permanent (2, 7). Signs of otitis interna including head tilt, ataxia, and nystagmus may be present postoperatively. Nystagmus usually resolves within 24 hours, but head tilt or ataxia may persist (11, 13). Damage to the hypoglossal nerve results in deficits of swallowing, prehension, and mastication. Facial nerve paralysis has also been reported (2, 3).

Prognosis is good with complete excision, but the polyp may recur months to years postoperatively (3, 9). Recurrence is less common when surgical removal is combined with bulla osteotomy (2, 11, 13).

References

1. Bradley RL, Noone KE, Saunders GK, et al. Nasopharyngeal and middle ear polypoid masses in five cats. Vet Surg 1985;14:141.
2. Kapatkin AS, Matthiesen DT, Noone KE, et al. Results of surgery and long-term follow-up in 31 cats with nasopharyngeal polyps. J Am Anim Hosp Assoc 1990;26:387.
3. Lane JG, Orr CM, Lucke VM, et al. Nasopharygeal polyps arising in the middle ear of the cat. J Small Anim Pract 1981;22:511.
4. Brownlie SE, Bedford PGC. Nasopharyngeal polyp in a kitten. Vet Rec 1985;117:668–669.
5. Stanton ME, Wheaton LG, Render JA, et al. Pharyngeal polyps in two siblings. J Am Vet Med Assoc 1985;186:1311–1313.
6. Parker NR, Binnington AG. Nasopharyngeal polyps in cats: three case reports and a review of the literature. J Am Anim Hosp Assoc 1985;21:473–478.
7. Trevor PB, Martin RA. Tympanic bulla osteotomy for treatment of middle-ear disease in cats: 19 cases (1984–1991). J Am Vet Med Assoc 1993;202:123–128.

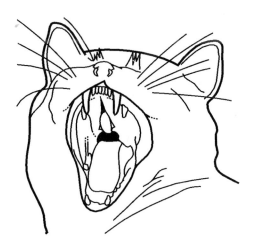

Fig. 11.6. A midline incision has been made in the soft palate to improve exposure of a feline nasopharyngeal polyp.

8. Fingland RB, Gratzek A, Vorhies MW, et al. Nasopharyngeal polyp in a dog. J Am Anim Hosp Assoc 1993;29:311–314.
9. Harvey CE, Goldschmidt MH. Inflammatory polypoid growths in the ear canal of cats. J Small Anim Pract 1978;19:669.
10. Remedios AM, Fowler JD, Pharr JW. A comparison of radiographic versus surgical diagnosis of otitis media. J Am Anim Hosp Assoc 1991;27:183–188.
11. Ader PL, Boothe HW. Ventral bulla osteotomy in the cat. J Am Anim Hosp Assoc 1979;15:757–762.
12. Little CJL, Lane JG. The surgical anatomy of the feline bulla tympanica. J Small Anim Pract 1986;27:371–378.
13. Faulkner JE, Budsberg SC. Results of ventral bulla osteotomy for treatment of middle ear polyps in cats. J Am Anim Hosp Assoc 1990;26:496–499.

12

SUPPLEMENTAL OXYGEN DELIVERY AND FEEDING TUBE TECHNIQUES

Nasal, Nasopharyngeal, Nasotracheal, Nasoesophageal, Nasogastric, and Nasoenteric Tubes: Insertion and Use

Dennis T. Crowe & Jennifer J. Devey

Indwelling tubes that enter the nose and stop in the ventral nasal meatus (nasal), pharynx (nasopharyngeal), or trachea (nasotracheal) are effective for the delivery of supplemental oxygen (O_2). Those that continue on through the ventral nasal meatus and pharynx and stop in the caudal thoracic esophagus (nasoesophageal [NEO]) are useful for the delivery of fluids and nutritional supplements or for the aspiration of air and fluids to provide decompression of the esophagus in conditions causing megaesophagus. Tubes that continue on into the stomach and either stop there (nasogastric [NG]) or continue into the duodenum or jejunum (nasoenteric [NET]) are useful for delivery of fluids and nutrients or for removal of accumulated air and fluids. All these tubes are placed initially into the nasal passage and are passed into the ventral meatus using the same technique. The type of tube selected depends on its intended use. Placement of each of the types of tube is simple to perform. In rare instances, placement under fluoroscopic guidance may be required (i.e., placing an NG tube past an esophageal stricture or placing an NET tube). After insertion, all indwelling tubes are generally well tolerated by most patients, even patients that are completely alert. On occasion, an Elizabethan collar is recommended to prevent the patient from dislodging the tube. Sedation is not necessary in most patients. The nose generally accommodates up to three to four types of tubes at the same time. When more than one type of tube is placed in the nose, the tubes must be labeled appropriately to avoid complications.

Oxygen Administration

Nasal Tubes

INDICATIONS

Supplemental oxygen (O_2) should be provided as a first line of treatment to dogs and cats in shock (septic, traumatic, cardiogenic) and cardiac failure and those with respiratory compromise. This supplementation is also a useful treatment in postoperative critically ill patients during the anesthetic recovery period and in anemic animals.

The use of O_2 cages has been helpful in providing an O_2-enriched atmosphere for animals. However, these cages are expensive, and available sizes often cannot house large to giant breed dogs adequately. They also are inefficient to operate because a considerable amount of O_2 is dissipated into the room each time the door is opened. Furthermore, once a patient is placed into an O_2 cage, careful evaluation, continued monitoring, and treatment are difficult in the "forced" isolation that this form of O_2 therapy requires. Much time is also required to generate the higher levels of O_2 recommended in patients placed in O_2 cages. The law of displacement dictates the time required. The cubic volume of commercial O_2 cages varies from 300 to 500 L. If O_2 is provided at a flow rate of 20 L/minute into the cage, and no leakage occurs, it will take a

151

minimum of 12 minutes to achieve the O_2 concentration of near 100% that is recommended in patients suffering from life-threatening conditions. O_2 cages are also inefficient at providing sustained concentrations of O_2 higher than 50% because of unavoidable leaks. In investigations with one O_2 cage, the O_2 concentration could not be held above 40%.

Other available means of providing supplemental O_2 therapy include the use of face masks, O_2 hoods, bilateral human nasal cannulas, and transtracheal catheters. Difficulties with the use of a mask in nervous and apprehensive animals are all too familiar. O_2 hoods are well tolerated and provide up to 80% O_2 concentrations, but access to the face is restricted, and the animal is unable to drink or eat (Fig. 12.1). These collars can, however, be used in conjunction with nasal catheters or short nasal cannulas to increase tracheal O_2 concentration.

Short human nasal cannulas are inserted into the nares and are secured around the neck using a drawstring. These devices are well tolerated, but they frequently dislodge if the patient is active. Complications with transtracheal catheters have been reported. Nasal O_2 administration is an efficient and effective means of providing high inhalational concentrations of O_2 (up to 85 to 95%). *The deeper the placement of the end of the tube in the respiratory tract, the more efficient the device is in elevating the concentration of O_2.* Nasal tubes are not as effective as nasopharyngeal tubes in raising the inhaled tracheal O_2 concentration. The highest concentrations of O_2 are achieved with the use of nasotracheal tubes.

INSERTION TECHNIQUE
The animal's head is held gently restrained upward, and 1 mL of 2% lidocaine (dogs) (Animal Health Asso-

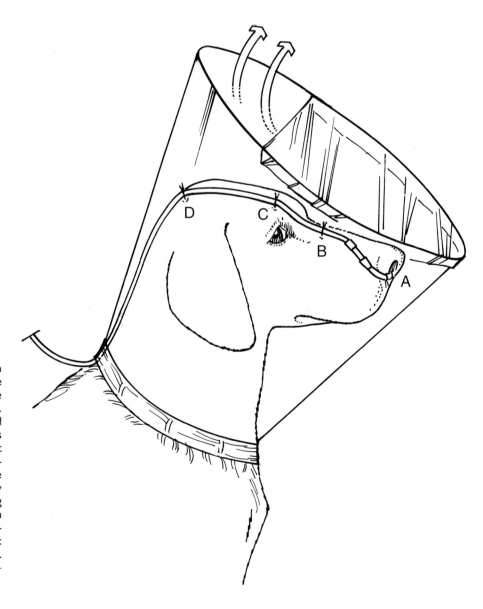

Fig. 12.1. Nasal oxygen tube in place and fixated with a skin suture close to the external nares. The tube is also secured with other skin sutures. The tube could also be secured ventral to the eye and ear. Elizabethan collars with clear plastic wrap over the front can be used to increase oxygen concentrations if required. This "Crowe collar" can also be used independently to provide a rapid means of increasing inspired oxygen levels. (Modified from Fitzpatrick RK, Crowe DT. Nasal oxygen administration in dogs and cats: experimental and clinical investigation. J Am Anim Hosp Assoc 1986;22:293–297.)

ciates, Kansas City, MO) or 5 drops of 0.5% proparacaine ophthalmic solution (dogs and cats) (Ophthaine, ER Squibb & Sons, Princeton, NJ) are administered into either nostril. The right nostril generally is preferred for right-handed operators and the left nostril for left-handed operators. The local anesthetic solution is allowed to run down the nasal passage. This procedure is repeated after 10 to 20 seconds. After another short waiting period to allow for desensitization, the tip of the selected catheter is lubricated on its outer surface with a commercial water-soluble lubricant (Xylocaine Jelly 2%, Astra Pharmaceutical Products, Inc., Worcester MA). The catheter can be a 3.5- to 8-French red rubber (Sovereign, Sherwood Medical Products, St. Louis, MO) or polyvinyl chloride (Cook Critical Care, Bloomington, IN) tube, or for extremely small patients, a long flexible 17-gauge polyethylene intravenous catheter. The addition of small side holes helps to disperse the stream of O_2 more evenly within the nasal passage; however, these holes are not usually required.

For nasal O_2 tube placement, the tube is premeasured alongside the patient's face so the tube's tip, after placement, extends into the nasal cavity to the level

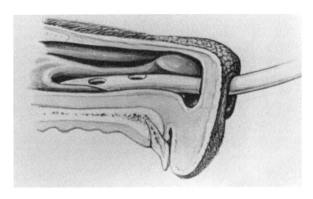

Fig. 12.3. Parasagittal section showing completion of the insertion of a nasal tube to be used for oxygen delivery. The tube stops in the ventral nasal meatus just before the level of the maxillary turbinate. (From Crowe DT. Clinical use of an indwelling nasogastric tube for enteral nutrition and fluid therapy in the dog and cat. J Am Anim Hosp Assoc 1986;22:675–678.)

of the first or second premolar. This facilitates flow through the ventral nasal meatus. This tube can be measured alongside the animal's teeth or by measuring from the tip of the nose to the medial canthus of the eye. After premeasuring, the tube is introduced into the nasal orifice while the patient's head is held firmly. Cats have a straight nasal passage, and the tubes generally pass easily. In the dog, pushing the tip of the nose upward allows the tube to be passed more easily into the ventral meatus. The tip is directed ventromedially (Fig. 12.2). In the cat, the tube can be simply inserted straight in most cases. After this initial introduction, the tip, in both the dog and the cat, is directed ventromedially until the desired length has been inserted (Fig. 12.3). Most animals object to the initial passage of the tube by sneezing and trying to shake their heads, but then they remain quiet after tube passage has been completed. If an animal objects to the insertion of the tube, slight sedation is recommended using low doses of intravenous neuroleptanalgesia (e.g., butorphanol [Torbugesic], 0.1 to 0.4 mg/kg, and diazepam [Valium], 0.05 to 0.2 mg/kg, or acepromazine .02 to .04 mg/kg).

After insertion to the level required, the tube is fixed to the skin using 3–0 or 2–0 silk suture with a swaged-on cutting needle. The most critical area requiring initial fixation is the first 0.5 cm after the tube exits from the nostril. This suture is usually *preplaced* to facilitate securing the tube immediately after it is placed. Several sutures are used to secure the tube (Fig. 12.4). Each suture is placed through the skin in a "quick-pass" fashion without hair clipping, aseptic preparation, or local anesthesia. After a loose simple interrupted suture is tied, the ends are wrapped around the tube and are tied again. An alternative fixation method is to apply a few drops of cyanoacrylate glue to the tube and tufts of hair on the nose and

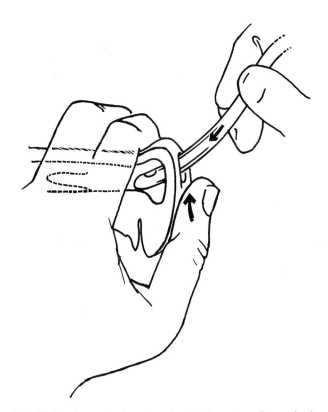

Fig. 12.2. Parasagittal section showing insertion of a nasal tube through the nares. Note the ventral protuberance at the base of the nostril and the ventral direction of the tube after it passes over the small ventral protuberance. (Modified from Crowe DT. Clinical use of an indwelling nasogastric tube for enteral nutrition and fluid therapy in the dog and cat. J Am Anim Hosp Assoc 1986;22:675–678.)

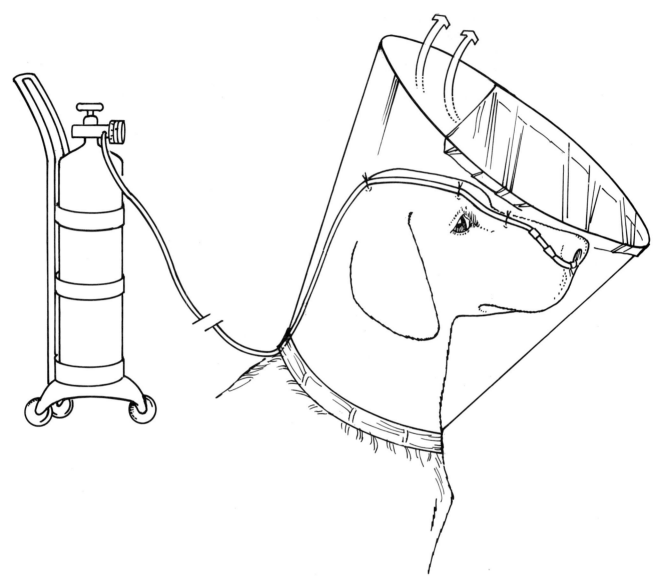

Fig. 12.4. Detailed drawing showing suture at: the base of the nose in the skin, then going around the tube and tied tightly (*A*); the mid-dorsal region of the nose in the skin, then going around the tube and tied tightly (*B*); eye level on the dorsum of the head in the skin, then going around the tube and tied tightly (*C*); ear level on the dorsum of the head in the skin, then going around the tube and tied tightly (*D*). The tube is then brought behind the neck and is secured with a section of tape around the neck (*inset*). A section of oxygen tubing or intravenous administration tubing is used to connect the tube to the oxygen source with a regulator. For animals that are extremely active, a section of tape can also be placed around the chest and the tube secured to this tape.

along the face, or skin staples can be used to secure the tube. Elizabethan collars are only required in patients objecting to the tube.

OXYGEN DELIVERY PROTOCOL
Tubing for O_2 administration (Tomac, American Hospital Supply Corp., Chicago) or an intravenous administration set is connected to the external end of the tube. The other end, in turn, is attached to the O_2 source with a standard O_2 flow meter. If O_2 supplementation for more than 24 hours is anticipated, use of a commercial humidification chamber is recommended. Al-

ternatively, a homemade humidifier can be fashioned using a crated intravenous fluid infusion bottle. The O_2 source is attached to the vent hole, and O_2 is bubbled through warm water. Additional tubing, as necessary, is used between the patient and the humidifying unit to allow the animal freedom to move without fear of tube disconnection. The homemade humidification chamber full of water must not tip over, because this would result in rapid delivery of water into the patient's nasal passage.

For patients being resuscitated, flow rates that generate at least 60 to 80% O_2 concentrations are recommended. In patients that have hemodynamic and pulmonary stability, flow rates are decreased 50% to provide approximately 40% inspired O_2. The flow rate to provide 60 to 80% O_2 concentrations is approximately 50 mL/kg body weight per minute in small dogs and cats and approximately 100 mL/kg body weight per minute in large dogs when delivering O_2 using properly placed nasal catheters. A proportionally greater amount probably is required in large breed dogs because of a concomitant increased amount of anatomic dead space in larger animals.

After O_2 administration is begun, the patient should be observed carefully to determine the response to therapy and to identify adverse effects, which are rare. Clinical signs such as decreased anxiety and decreased respiratory rate and effort indicate an improvement in response to the O_2. Pulse oximetry can also be used to assess oxygenation. O_2 supplementation is indicated whenever O_2 saturation is below 92%. Accurate measurements are, however, sometimes difficult to obtain in the awake patient because of probe placement difficulties. In the critically ill patient, arterial blood gases should be monitored whenever possible. Partial O_2 pressures considered sufficient should be at least 60 to 65 mm Hg. If hypercapnia exists (PCO_2 greater than 50 mm Hg), mechanical ventilation rather than simple O_2 supplementation should be performed. Provided sufficient volume exchange is taking place to prevent hypercapnia, the O_2 flow rate can be increased to provide greater inspiratory O_2 concentrations if no favorable clinical response is observed or arterial PO_2 values remain below 65 mm Hg. Permissible flow rates and the corresponding O_2 percentages in the inspired air are given in Table 12.1. If after increasing the flow

Table 12.1.
Oxygen Flow Rates and Estimated Corresponding Inspired Oxygen Concentrations

Flow Rate (mL/min/kg)	Inspiratory O_2 Conc. (%)
Animals weighing under 25 kg:	
50	30–40
100	40–50
150	50–60
*200	60–70
*250	70–80
*300	80–90
Animals weighing 25 kg or more:	
100	30–40
150	40–50
200	50–60
*250	60–70
*300	70–75
*350	75–80
*400	80–90

* Flow rates over 200 mL/min/kg may result in gastric distension. Therefore, at high flow rates, patients should be watched for distension and the condition treated by decompression if it occurs.

rates arterial O_2 values do not increase above 70 mm Hg, intermittent positive pressure ventilation (IPPV) with positive end-expiratory pressure should be instituted. *If the patient's work of breathing does not improve with the high concentration of O_2, then control of breathing with IPPV should be provided. The use of mechanical ventilation in these patients is important; otherwise, ventilatory failure and death will ensue.*

COMPLICATIONS

Complications with the use of nasal O_2 administration are uncommon. O_2 is dry and cool; therefore, prolonged use (more than 3 to 5 days) may cause rhinitis and sinusitis. When these complications do occur, they usually are mild and become evident as a persistent serous nasal discharge. The discharge usually clears within several days after the nasal tube is removed. The use of nasal O_2 in patients with nasal bone fractures may lead to subcutaneous emphysema. If blood is present in the nose, nasal O_2 administration is not recommended because bubble formation and foam may interfere with air exchange. In these patients, nasotracheal or transtracheal O_2 is recommended.

Tube dislodgment is an infrequent complication if the catheter is placed in the nose for a sufficient distance and if fixation of the tube is performed correctly. Persistent sneezing and continued irritation are rare and necessitate the use of repeated local anesthetic instillation, an Elizabethan collar, or light intravenous chemical sedation (e.g., oxymorphone at 0.02 mg/kg or diazepam at 0.1 mg/kg). Mild epistaxis caused by misdirection of the tube into the maxillary or ethmoid turbinates during placement may occur, but in our experience this occurs rarely and is not severe enough to warrant discontinuation of a tube's insertion or use.

CONTRAINDICATIONS

Patients with severe tracheobronchial froth or fluid accumulation, as observed in animals with severe pulmonary edema, should receive nasotracheal or transtracheal O_2 rather than nasal O_2. Nasal tubes should be avoided in those patients with severe epistaxis or mucopurulent nasal discharge, suspicion of maxillary or cranial vault fracture after head injury, or head injury or any condition in which elevation of intracranial pressures secondary to sneezing or struggling is contraindicated. Ineffective ventilation requiring other primary care (intubation and positive-pressure ventilation) is also a contraindication to the placement of nasal O_2 tubes.

Nasopharyngeal Tubes

Nasopharyngeal tubes allow delivery of O_2 into the nasopharynx. This method can provide high concentrations of O_2 and, if flows are high enough, some level of continuous positive airway pressure (CPAP). CPAP is even more effective if bilateral nasopharyngeal tubes are placed. As the patient exhales, it exhales against some force created by the flow of the O_2 in a caudal laryngeal direction. The goal is to create an increase in the patient's functional residual volume. This can be done with CPAP.

A nasopharyngeal tube is placed in a fashion similar to that of a nasal catheter, but the lubricated tip of the tube is continued through the ventral meatus past the maxillary turbinate. The tube is held alongside the face and neck and is premeasured from the external naris to just proximal to the larynx. In dogs, some resistance may be encountered at the maxillary turbinate region because of a narrowing of the ventral meatus in a dorsoventral direction. If the tube cannot be passed farther than the level of the eyes in dogs or cats, the tube is assumed to be in the dorsal meatus with its tip in the ethmoid turbinate. The tube must be withdrawn and redirected ventrally if this occurs. After the tip is past the maxillary turbinate in the ventral meatus, resistance to the tube's passage decreases, and the tube

can be passed into the nasal pharynx and pharyngeal isthmus. The ideal location is just dorsal to the rima glottis (Fig. 12.5).

High O_2 flow rates (greater than 200 mL/kg per minute) should be administered carefully when providing O_2 through nasopharyngeal tubes. Rarely, gastric distension occurs if flow rates are exceedingly high (greater than 200 mL/kg per minute) or if the nasopharyngeal catheter migrates into the esophagus. Bradycardia, believed to be vagally mediated, can also occur.

Nasotracheal Tubes

Nasotracheal tubes provide an effective means of providing O_2 to the patient that has laryngeal palsy or a collapsing cervical trachea. These catheters also generate some degree of CPAP when high flow rates are used. Patient tolerance is usually good, with little coughing. In animals that do not tolerate the tubes, mild sedation may be required.

Before placement of a nasotracheal tube, the tube

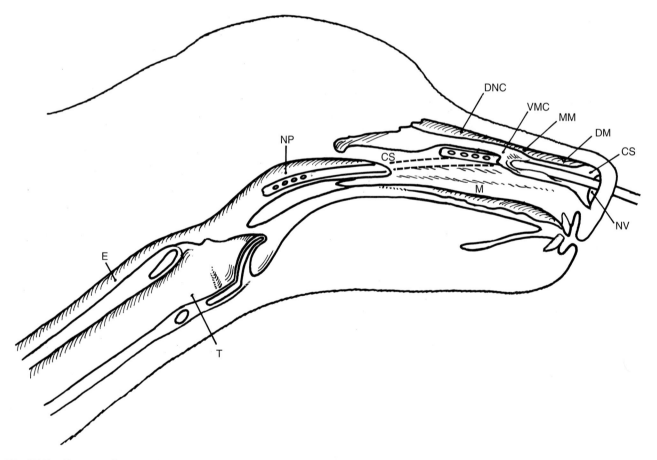

Fig. 12.5. Parasagittal section showing the insertion of a nasopharyngeal oxygen tube through the nasal passage and into the nasopharynx. Structures identified include the nasal vestibule (*NV*), cartilaginous septum (*CS*), maxilla (*M*), dorsal meatus (*DM*), middle meatus (*MM*), ventral nasal concha (*VNC*), dorsal nasal concha (*DNC*), and nasopharynx (*NP*). (Modified from Crowe DT. Clinical use of an indwelling nasogastric tube for enteral nutrition and fluid therapy in the dog and cat. J Am Anim Hosp Assoc 1986;22:675–678.)

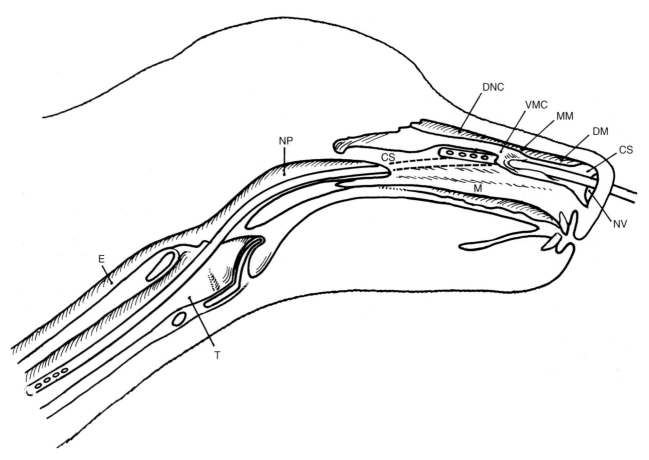

Fig. 12.6. Parasagittal section showing the insertion of a nasotracheal oxygen tube through the nasal passage and into the trachea. Structures identified include the nasal vestibule (*NV*), cartilaginous septum (*CS*), maxilla (*M*), dorsal meatus (*DM*), middle meatus (*MM*), ventral nasal concha (*VNC*), dorsal nasal concha (*DNC*), nasopharynx (*NP*), esophagus (*E*), and trachea (*T*). (Modified from Crowe DT. Clinical use of an indwelling nasogastric tube for enteral nutrition and fluid therapy in the dog and cat. J Am Anim Hosp Assoc 1986;22:675–678.)

should be premeasured such that the tip will rest at the level of the tracheal bifurcation or fifth intercostal space. A 3.5- to 8-French feeding tube is generally used. The tube is placed in a fashion similar to that of a nasopharyngeal catheter. The tube is passed blindly into the trachea through the larynx by hyperextending the patient's head and neck and advancing the tube (Fig. 12.6). If coughing is noted, another 0.33 mL of local anesthetic is infused through the tubing, with the tubing in the mid-distal pharynx. Once the membranes around the larynx are anesthetized, the tube is advanced as inhalation occurs. If the tube does not pass after several attempts, a short-acting neurolepto-analgesic can be administered to the patient, and the tube can be placed by direct visualization using a laryngoscope and something to grasp the tip of the tube and direct it through the rima glottis into the trachea.

The position of the tube should be confirmed with a radiograph or by aspiration using a 60-mL syringe. If the tube is in the trachea, air should continue to be aspirated easily. If the catheter is in the esophagus, air may be initially aspirated, but it should stop.

The nasotracheal tube is used in a fashion similar to that of nasal and nasopharyngeal tubes. For nasotracheal catheters, flow rates are decreased by 50% from those recommended for nasal O_2 tubes to provide equivalent O_2 concentrations. Humidification of the O_2 is essential with the use of nasotracheal tubes, to prevent mucosal drying and dysfunction of the mucociliary apparatus, which can lead to an inability to clear secretions and possible pneumonia. Infusion of saline through the nasotracheal tube can be used to help loosen secretions in patients with dysfunction of the mucociliary apparatus or pneumonia.

Tubes for Gastrointestinal Access

Indications

NEO, NG, and NET tubes can be used for decompression and feeding. Smaller-bore NEO, NG, and NET tubes are useful for the administration of water, electrolytes, and liquid enteral support diets. Because dehydration and protein–energy malnutrition frequently are encountered in seriously ill or injured animals, the use of these indwelling tubes for rehydration and nutritional support often is a key component in successful overall patient management. Contraindications to use of NEO or NG fluid and nutritional therapy support include persistent vomiting and high gastric residual volumes. The presence of stupor or coma is a relative contraindication to NEO and NG feeding, particularly if bolus feeding is provided. If slow, continuous-rate infusions result in minimal residual volumes, then the risk of regurgitation and aspiration is low enough that NEO or NG feeding can be used.

Decompression of a dilated esophagus, stomach, or intestinal tract can be accomplished by use of large-bore single-lumen or double-lumen (sump) NEO, NG, or NET tubes. Decompression of the esophagus alleviates some of the risk of aspiration in the patient with megaesophagus and actively decreases the stretch in the skeletal muscle that results in dilatation. In the stuporous or comatose patient, or in the patient receiving mechanical ventilation, active decompression helps to prevent aspiration. In the patient having difficulty ventilating, decompression of the stomach improves ventilation because of reduced impedance to diaphragmatic excursions. This is particularly helpful in cats and small dogs because they breathe primarily using the diaphragm. Clinically, NG decompression has been helpful in the temporary management of gastric dilation–volvulus syndrome when the gastric distension has been due primarily to air and fluid. Decompression of the stomach after abdominal surgery helps to decrease the time to return to normal gastric motility. After placement, the NG tube is periodically aspirated (e.g., once every 1 to 2 hours). The tube is left in place until bowel sounds return or the patient is believed to be out of danger of postoperative redistension. Antral dilation is a strong stimulus for vomiting. The use of NG tubes decreases the incidence of vomiting in the patient with gastrointestinal or pancreatic disease and is especially useful in the patient with canine parvovirus infection.

Tube Selection and Insertion

The techniques for inserting an NEO, NG, or NET tube for decompression or feeding are the same. Polyvinyl chloride (Argyle nasogastric feeding tube, Sherwood Medical Products), polyurethane (Cook Critical Care), or red rubber tubes from 3.5 French (cats and small dogs) to 12 French (medium to large dogs) are used. Specially designed tubes that are weighted on their proximal ends with either tungsten or mercury are useful to ensure that the tube will stay in the stomach lumen (Travasorb dualport feeding tube, Baxter Health Care Corp., Deerfield, IL). The smaller the tube, the more difficult it is to use for decompression. A nylon stylet that accompanies commercial polyurethane tubes provides added stiffness necessary for insertion. With smaller polyvinyl chloride tubes, a woven angiographic wire stylet (Wire guide, Cook Critical) is used to provide added stiffness. One or two milliliters of vegetable or mineral oil is injected into the lumen of a tube to facilitate ease of insertion and withdrawal of the woven wire through the lumen.

After selection of the tube and placement of the stylet, the length necessary to reach the distal thoracic esophagus (NEO) or the stomach (NG) is determined by measuring alongside the patient's neck and body from the tip of the nose to the eighth or ninth rib for NEO tubes or to the thirteenth rib for NG tubes (Fig. 12.7). For NET tubes, length is added to ensure that the tip of the proximal end of the tube will reach the area of the bowel lumen selected. Most often, the tube for enteral feeding is a nasoduodenal tube with a tip that ends near the pelvic flexure of the duodenum. The tube in these cases is premeasured to extend from the nose to the wing of the ilium (see Fig. 12.7).

The lubricated tip of the tube is introduced into the patient's nostril in the same manner as described for nasopharyngeal tubes. After the tip is past the maxillary turbinate in the ventral meatus, resistance to the tube's passage decreases, and the tube can be passed into the nasal pharynx and pharyngeal isthmus. At this point, the patient's head must be kept in a neutral position, with the neck gently flexed to facilitate passage of the tube into the esophagus (Fig. 12.8). If the neck is hyperextended, the tube may enter the larynx and trachea. With continued advancement of the tube, the patient is often observed to swallow several times. Once the tip of the tube has been advanced into the caudal thoracic esophagus (NEO tube) or into the proximal portion of the stomach (NG tube), the lubricated stylet is withdrawn. The use of a stylet also helps to facilitate the passage of the tube into the stomach through the cardia.

Air is injected into the tube while auscultation of the left chest wall and left paralumbar fossa is performed; the presence of gargling sounds during this procedure indicates that the tube is in the distal esophagus or stomach, respectively. In most cases, a lack of coughing during injection of 5 to 10 mL of sterile saline down the tube indicates that the tube is not in the trachea. However, the result of this test may vary with the individual animal, and the position of all tubes should be radiographically confirmed if they are to be used for infusion of fluids or liquid diets.

Special tubes or manipulations are required for placement of NET tubes into the duodenum or jejunum. The tube can be guided by peristaltic action into the duodenum, but this is often difficult to accomplish. The tubes can be guided through the pylorus using endoscopy or fluoroscopy. NET tubes have been most successfully placed at the time of abdominal surgery by the surgeon guiding the tip of the tube, which is palpated and guided through the stomach and intestine into the portion of the bowel intended. Weighted tungsten or mercury tubes have been used to help in guiding tubes through the stomach into the intestine (Travasorb dualport feeding tube, Baxter Health Care Corp.). The weighted tip also may help to ensure that the tube will stay in the bowel lumen and not curl or kick back into the stomach. Passage of the tube into the small intestine through the action of peristalsis has been unreliable, particularly in sick patients with at least some degree of gastroparesis. Metoclopramide, 0.4 mg/kg per day intravenously, has been used to help stimulate gastric motility to facilitate the tube's passage into the duodenum.

Once the tip of the tube has been placed in the desired location, the tube is secured with several sutures placed at the base of the nostril and around the tube, or with glue as described previously for nasal O_2 tubes. If the tube demonstrates a tendency to back out of the nose, 1 to 2 cm of coated copper wire (18-gauge telephone wire) can be used to support the bend in the tube as it exits from the nose. On occasion, the tube may back out of the intestine, or the dog or cat may vomit the tubes into the mouth. In this case, the tube must be removed. A narrow-gauge flexible wire can sometimes be left in the tube to help prevent tube migration. Specially designed catheters are also available that allow the delivery of nutrients while the wire is left inside the catheter lumen.

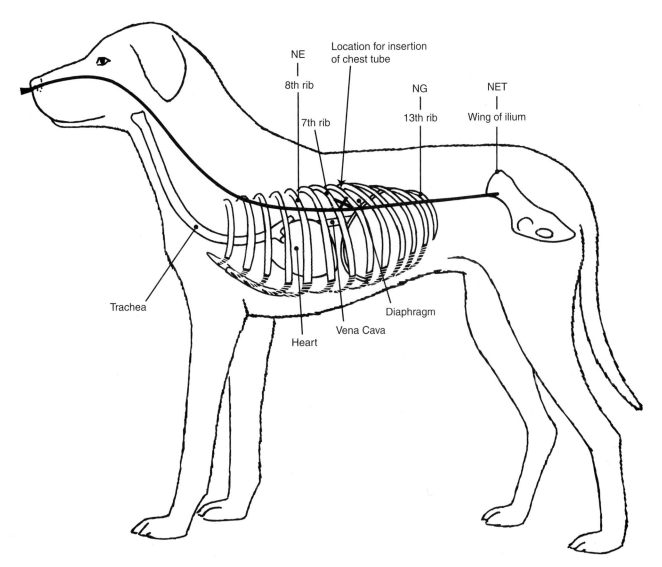

Fig. 12.7. Drawing depicting landmarks used to premeasured the various feeding or decompression tubes. The tube should be premeasured from the tip of the nose of the animal to the eighth rib for nasoesophageal (NE) tubes, to the thirteenth rib for nasogastric (NG) tubes, and at least to the wing of the ilium for nasoenteric (NET) tubes.

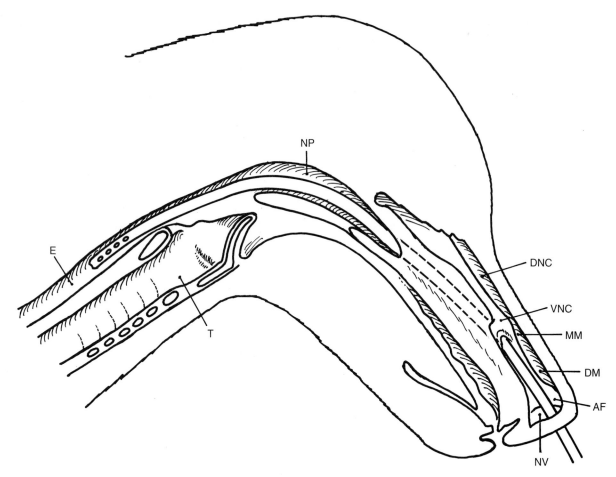

Fig. 12.8. Parasagittal section showing the insertion of a nasogastric tube through the nasal passage and into the esophagus. The head is bent to help the tube follow the dorsum of the wall of the pharynx and then course dorsally into the esophagus. Structures identified include the nasal vestibule (*NV*), cartilaginous septum (*CS*), dorsal meatus (*DM*), middle meatus (*MM*), ventral nasal concha (*VNC*), dorsal nasal concha (*DNC*), alar fold (*AF*), nasopharynx (*NP*), esophagus (*E*), and trachea (*T*). (Modified from Crowe DT. Clinical use of an indwelling nasogastric tube for enteral nutrition and fluid therapy in the dog and cat. J Am Anim Hosp Assoc 1986;22:675–678.)

The remaining length of the tube or an attached extension tube (intravenous administration extension set) is secured to the top of the patient's head or the side of the face. An Elizabethan collar can be applied if necessary. The end of the tube is capped to prevent air from entering the gastrointestinal tract by diaphragmatic movement until its use is required.

Protocol for Using Tubes for Decompression

A 60-mL syringe is attached to the end of the tube, and aspiration is done as often as required to keep a slight amount of negative pressure on the hollow viscus aspirated. For prevention of recurrence of gastric dilation or for decompression of the small intestine, aspiration generally is performed every 1 to 2 hours until a negative pressure is reached each time. If the fluid aspirated is viscous, dilution with sterile water or saline may be required. The tube should be flushed with a small amount of saline or water each time the tube is used, and then the tube should be capped. Holding the column of water in the tube helps to prevent clogging. Maintenance of decompression usually is required only for 24 to 48 hours because most intestinal ileus or gastroparesis is resolved by then.

The efficiency of gastrointestinal decompression achievable with a simple single-lumen tube (Argyle stomach tube (Levine Type), Sherwood Medical Products) and intermittent aspiration with a syringe can be improved by the use of a double-lumen sump tube (Salem sump tube, Sherwood Medical Products) with continuous 20- to 30-mm Hg suction or intermittent mechanical 80- to 90-mm Hg suction. This type of suction requires the use of specially designed equipment. Automatic intermittent suction, for example, is often best performed with the use of a thermotic drainage pump that is electronically driven (Thermotic drainage pump, GOMCO, Allied Healthcare Inc., Buffalo, NY). Fortunately, in most clinical patients, this type of special equipment is not necessary, and simple intermittent syringe decompression is sufficient.

Protocol for Using Tubes for Feeding

For the administration of fluids and liquid enteral diets, a syringe is used for slow bolus delivery. Slow bolus delivery of fluids and liquid enteral diets can be done safely through NEO and NG tubes in animals that are conscious. However, bolus feeding is not recommended in unconscious or semiconscious patients because of the higher risk of pulmonary aspiration. Bolus feeding should not be done through an NET tube initially because of the high occurrence of vomiting and diarrhea, which can be caused by the acute overload of hyperosmolar nutrients in the small intestine. Drip infusion is the preferred method of the delivery in these circumstances. A pediatric intravenous fluid administration set and bottle are used for the delivery of enteral diets. The use of an enteral or intravenous infusion pump or a syringe facilitates the delivery of these enteral liquid diets.

Initially, an electrolyte and glucose mixture is administered at a rate of 0.25 to 0.5 mL/kg per hour. This rate can be used in all patients including those that have had gastrointestinal surgery; however, it may be too fast for those patients that have undergone massive bowel resections or have pancreatitis. In such patients, the initial rate infused should be no greater than 0.1 to 0.2 mL/kg per hour. The drip rate is steadily increased until caloric requirements are met. Rates higher than 4 mL/kg per hour are usually associated with severe, osmotically induced diarrhea; therefore, the maximum rate usually used for constant rate infusions is 2.0 to 3.0 mL/kg per hour.

Many monomeric and polymeric liquid diets are available for tube feeding. Monomeric or elemental diets are composed of amino acids (Vivonex, Sandoz Nutrition, Minneapolis MN; Alitraq, Ross Laboratories, Columbus, OH) or dipeptides and tripeptides (Peptamen, Clintec Nutrition Co., Deerfield, IL) and require no digestion before absorption. The amino acid–based diets tend to be hyperosmotic and may require dilution initially to a 50% concentration. They usually are more expensive than polymeric diets, but they may be useful in patients with decreased digestive ability. The dipeptide- and tripeptide-based diets tend to be isosmolar and can generally be given initially at full strength concentration. Polymeric diets (Impact, Sandoz Nutrition; Jevity, Ross Laboratories) are made of complex carbohydrates and proteins and require digestion before absorption, but they are usually isosmotic unless they are flavored. Special polymeric diets designed specifically for cats and dogs (CliniCare and RenalCare, Pet-Ag Inc., Hampshire, IL) have been de-

veloped and have been clinically effective in providing nutritional support to critically ill or injured dogs and cats. Polymeric diets are usually administered either full strength if plasma proteins are normal and anorexia has not been present for longer than 3 days. If plasma protein levels are below normal or anorexia has been present for longer than 3 days the diets should be initially diluted to a 50% concentration with water. The monomeric diets may require dilution to 25% concentration for initial administration. After the rate of administration is stabilized at 2 to 3 mL/kg per hour and the diet is found to be tolerable (no abdominal pain, vomiting, or diarrhea), the concentration of the diet can be gradually increased.

Complications

Complications with feeding and decompression tubes are primarily associated with tube migration, especially dislodgment. Dislodgment is usually caused by vomiting or by the animal's pawing at the tube or rubbing its face.

When concern exists about the location of the tip of the tube, a radiograph should be taken to ensure that the location is correct. Disaster can occur if a tube is displaced into the trachea and food is administered.

Suggested Readings

Crowe DT. Clinical use of an indwelling nasogastric tube for enteral nutrition and fluid therapy in the dog and cat. J Am Anim Hosp Assoc 1986;22:675–678.

Crowe DT. Use of a nasogastric tube for gastric and esophageal decompression in the dog and cat. J Am Vet Med Assoc 1986; 188:1178–1182.

Crowe DT. Enteral nutrition for critically ill or injured patients. Part I. Compend Contin Educ Pract Vet 1986;8:603.

Crowe DT. Enteral nutrition for critically ill or injured patients. Part II. Compend Contin Educ Pract Vet 1986;8:826.

Fitzpatrick Rl, Crowe DT. Nasal oxygen administration in dogs and cats: experimental and clinical investigations. J Am Anim Hosp Assoc 1986;22:293–297.

Esophagostomy Tube Placement and Use for Feeding and Decompression

Dennis T. Crowe & Jennifer J. Devey

Esophagostomy tubes provide a simple and effective means of administering fluid and nutritional support to the small animal patient. The tubes can also be used for esophageal or gastric decompression (1). Esophagostomy tubes can be rapidly placed (generally within 5 minutes) and require minimal surgical equipment (a scalpel blade, a pair of curved forceps, and nonabsorbable suture material). Simple red rubber feeding tubes are most frequently used. Patients have been fed for up to 2 years using these tubes. No cases of esophageal stricture or permanent esophagocutaneous fistula have been observed.

Indications

Esophagostomy tubes are indicated whenever nutritional support is required and the stomach is functional but the patient is unwilling or unable to ingest food or water. Esophagostomy tubes can also be used to keep the stomach and esophagus decompressed because aspiration of these tubes helps to prevent air or fluid from accumulating. This may be useful in the management of patients with megaesophagus or those that have undergone surgical correction of gastric dilatation–volvulus.

Esophagostomy tubes were developed and first used in clinical veterinary medicine by Crowe (2). They were developed and used to avoid the airway difficulties associated with pharyngostomy tubes (Fig. 12.9) (3). With pharyngostomy tubes, a portion of the tube can interfere with laryngeal function, even after careful placement using modified techniques. The surgical approach for placement of the esophagostomy tube is simpler than that of the pharyngostomy tube, with less likelihood of damage to vital vascular and neurologic structures. Percutaneous gastrostomy tubes require special feeding tubes and because of penetration of the stomach and peritoneal cavity, the risk of leakage and subsequent development of peritonitis always exists. From our experience, the patient does not need to be subjected to these risks, and, whenever possible, an esophagostomy tube should be selected over a gastrostomy tube. Most conditions for which clinicians use percutaneous gastrostomy tubes for feeding can be also managed with esophagostomy tubes. Esophagostomy tubes can be used in patients that have had esophageal surgery; however, care should be taken to ensure that a smaller-bore flexible feeding tube is used and that

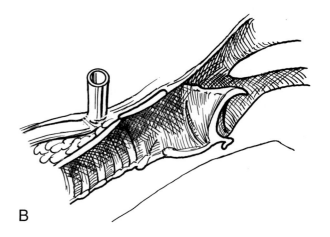

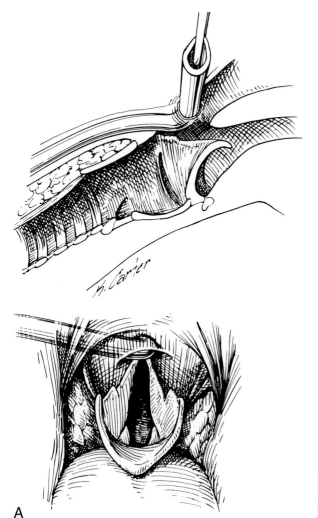

Fig. 12.9. **A.** Lateral view of placement of a pharyngostomy tube (*inset* reveals the open-mouth view). **B.** Lateral view of placement of an esophagostomy tube. (No part of the esophagostomy tube is visible in the open-mouth view.)

the end of the tube is not rubbing against a wound site or surgical incision.

Contraindications

In general, esophagostomy tubes should not be used for feeding or decompression if the patient 1) is vomiting, 2) has cervical or thoracic esophageal disease that will be worsened by the placement of a tube passing through the affected area, and 3) has an infection involving the cervical region close to the tube exit site. Because placement of esophagostomy tubes requires light general anesthesia, the risks of anesthesia should be weighed against the benefits of the placement of esophagostomy tubes in critically ill animals.

Tube Selection

The type and length of tube selected depends on the intended use of the tube. Esophagostomy tubes used for feeding or for esophageal decompression (i.e., for long-term management of megaesophagus) should end in the distal thoracic esophagus. Tubes that pass through the lower esophageal sphincter increase the risk of gastroesophageal reflux in some patients. For gastric decompression or feeding, whenever the esophagus needs to be bypassed, an esophagogastric tube is placed with the tip of the tube resting in the midfundic region of the stomach. An esophagoenteral tube can also be placed at the time of abdominal surgery if the stomach needs to be bypassed. The proximal end of the tube should be shortened as required, so only sufficient tubing protrudes from the skin to permit attachment to a syringe for feeding or decompression. Excessive tube length protruding from the skin may be annoying to the animal and may catch on objects.

Esophagostomy tubes used for feeding or decompression should be flexible and in general of as large a bore as possible. This provides less chance for kinking and occlusion. The actual size of each tube selected depends on the size of the animal and on the intended purpose for the tube (Table 12.2). Generally, no tube smaller than 10 French should be used for decompression or if a canned or gruel diet is to be used for feeding. For small cats and dogs, a 10- to 12-French tube is used. For medium-sized dogs, a 12- to 18-French tube is used, and for large to giant breed dogs, an 18- to 30-French tube is inserted. When using the tube only for the delivery of liquids, smaller-diameter tubes can be used. Tubes should be flexible yet stiff enough to resist kinking. Commonly, tubes made of red rubber (Sovereign, Sherwood Medical Products, St. Louis, MO), polyvinyl chloride (Argyle feeding catheter, Sherwood Medical Products; Cook Critical Care, Bloomington, IN), polyurethane (Cook Critical Care),

Table 12.2.
Guidelines for Esophagostomy Tube Size Selection*

Body Weight (kg)	Decompression Gastric or Esophageal	Feeding Gruel	Feeding Liquids Only
<1	8–10	10	3.5–6
1–3	10	10	6
3–5	10–12	10–12	6
5–10	12–18	12–18	8
10–20	14–20	14–20	8
20–30	20–26	20–26	10
30–40	26–28	26–28	10
>40	28–30	28–30	12

* All tube sizes are in French.

Teflon (Cook Critical Care), and silicone (Baxter Health Care Corp., Deerfield, IN) are used. Tubes made of polyurethane or silicone resist the hardening caused by gastric fluids and are recommended if one anticipates that the tube will be used for longer than 1 week. Commercially available tubes frequently require the addition of three to five side holes. These holes can be made carefully using curved scissors. The diameter of the holes should not exceed approximately 20% of the tube's circumference.

Surgical Technique

Tube Esophagostomy

Light general anesthesia is induced and is maintained throughout the procedure. The airway is protected with a cuffed endotracheal tube. The entire lateral cervical region from the ventral midline to near the dorsal midline is clipped and is aseptically prepared for surgery. Usually, the left side is chosen; however, both sides can be used. The procedure is illustrated in Figure 12.10. Curved forceps are inserted into the pharynx and then into the proximal cervical esophagus. Curved Kelly forceps are recommended for use in cats and small dogs. In larger dogs, longer curved Carmalt, Mixter, or Schnidt forceps are recommended. The tips of the forceps are turned laterally, and pressure is applied in an outward direction, thereby tenting up the tissues so the tips can be seen and palpated (Fig. 12.10**A**). A small skin incision (just large enough to accommodate the tube) is made over the tips of the forceps using a scalpel blade, and the tips of the forceps are bluntly forced to the outside (Fig. 12.10**B**). In larger animals, as continued pressure is applied, the scalpel blade is used to cut through the thicker esophagus and to allow passage of the forceps.

The selected tube is premeasured and marked using the landmarks listed in Table 12.3. Esophagostomy tubes are usually measured to the level of the xiphoid or ninth intercostal space. Esophagogastrostomy tubes are measured to the thirteenth rib.

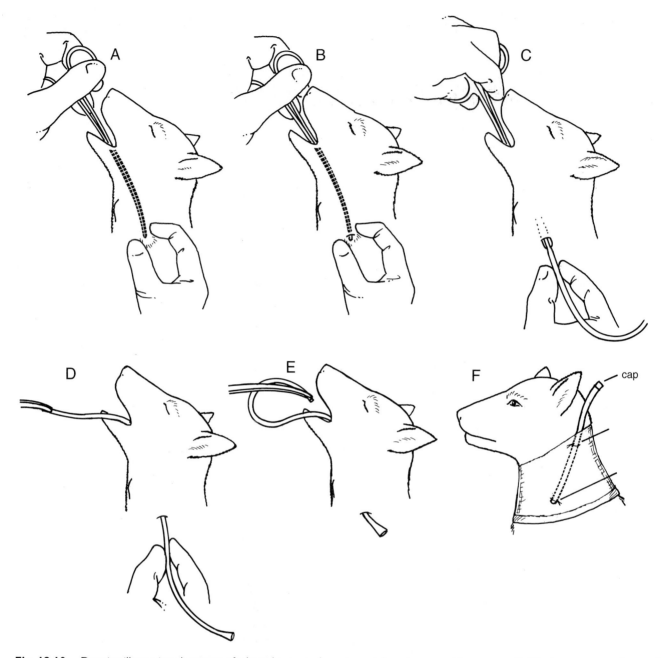

Fig. 12.10. Drawing illustrating placement of a large-bore esophagostomy tube using curved hemostats. **A.** The hemostats are inserted into the oral cavity, oropharynx, and proximal esophagus; then the tips are pushed laterally. **B.** A skin incision is made, and the tips of the hemostats are pushed through the wall of the esophagus and the subcutaneous tissues. **C.** The flexible feeding tube is grasped with the tips of the hemostats. **D.** The tube is pulled out through the mouth with the hemostats. **E.** The tube's tip is regrasped with the hemostats and is guided down the pharynx and esophagus. **F.** The tube is pulled gently to straighten the curve in the tube, and after it is advanced so the tip is in the midthoracic esophagus, it is anchored with a suture that enters the fascia and periosteum around the wing of the atlas.

The tip of the tube is grasped by the forceps (Fig. 12.10**C**) and is pulled into the esophagus and out through the mouth (Fig. 12.10**D**). The aboral tip of the tube is turned around and is redirected into the esophagus. The tube is then pushed into the esophagus with the aid of the forceps (Fig. 12.10**E**) By retracting the external end of the tube 2 to 4 cm, the tube is felt to "straighten," and then it passes more easily. The tube is then passed to the premeasured mark. The oropharynx is visually examined to confirm location of the tube in the esophagus. Ideally, the location of the tip should be confirmed with a lateral radiograph in patients with megaesophagus, esophageal stricture, or any other unusual condition involving the esophagus.

Table 12.3.
Premeasured Landmarks Where Distal End of Tube Should Reach

Type of Tube	Landmark
Esophagoesophagostomy for decompression	Slightly caudal to point of maximum intensity of heart tones (ninth ICS)
Esophagoesophagostomy for feeding	Point of maximum intensity of heart tones (6th ICS)
Esophagogastrostomy for decompression	Thirteenth rib corresponding to midgastric region
Esophagogastrostomy for feeding	Thirteenth rib corresponding to midgastric region
Esophagoenterostomy for feeding	Wing of ilium (or whatever is necessary for surgeon manipulating the tube)

ICS, intercostal space.

An alternative method of confirming appropriate location of the tube in the distal esophagus involves passing the tube into the stomach. Placement is checked by infusing 30 mL or more of air (using a syringe) and ausculting for bubbles over the stomach region. Once bubbles are heard, the tube is retracted to locate the tip in the distal esophagus. If bubbles are not ausculted in the desired location, a chest radiograph should always be taken to confirm appropriate location.

The tube is secured to the periosteum of the wing of the atlas or deep fascia using nonabsorbable suture (Fig. 12.10**F**). The suture is secured to the tube by using several wraps of the suture around the tube. The tube should also be secured to the skin where the tube exits. Care should be taken not to tighten the suture to the point that it binds the skin to the tube because this may cause irritation and necrosis.

Percutaneous Esophagostomy Tube Placement

An alternative technique for placement of smaller-bore esophagostomy tubes that are only used for administration of water and other liquids involves percutaneous insertion of a long 10- to 14-gauge venous catheter (Intracath, Becton Dickinson, Sandy, UT) into the esophagus (4). This "needle" esophagostomy tube can be inserted under sedation without passage of an endotracheal tube. Curved Kelly forceps are passed into the pharynx and proximal esophagus similar to the procedure described for surgical esophagostomy tube placement. The tips of the forceps are then turned outward and are opened slightly so they can be palpated. The needle is inserted through the skin into the target location between the tips of the forceps. Once a popping sensation is felt, indicating puncture of the esophagus, the catheter, with the stylet backed out slightly, can be passed through the needle and down to the premeasured location in the distal third of the esophagus. The catheter is sutured to the cervical fascia and skin in a manner similar to that described for surgical esophagostomy tubes. Sterile saline is then injected through the catheter to ensure good fluid flow. If one has any question about the location of the catheter, a lateral radiograph should be taken.

Bandaging

A 4 × 4 gauze dressing containing chlorhexidine, povidone–iodine, or triple antibiotic ointment is placed over the tube's exit site in the skin, and a light circumferential wrap is placed. The end of the tube should be capped to prevent spontaneous air or fluid movement through the tube. Commercial feeding tubes are supplied with caps. For most noncommercial tubes, the cap to a hypodermic needle makes a tight fit and easily can be removed.

Care of the Tube

A "trap door" is made in the bandage to allow inspection, cleaning, and 4 × 4 gauze dressing changes (Fig. 12.11). The ostomy site should be inspected on a daily basis for the first 5 days after insertion, then every other day for 10 days, then every 3 days thereafter. The ostomy site should be cleaned of exudate with a dilute bactericidal solution suitable for using on wounds or a 50:50 mixture of 3% hydrogen peroxide and sterile saline. Triple antibiotic ointment is then applied, and the 4 × 4 gauze dressing is replaced.

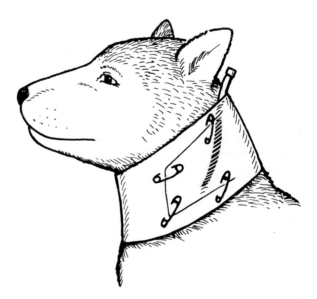

Fig. 12.11. Drawing illustrating the cervical dressing covering the esophagostomy tube. A trap door over the tube's exit site at the skin is made and is held closed with four safety pins when it is not needed.

Procedure for Administration of Fluids and Liquids

Fluids (crystalloids, oral rehydrating solutions, water) and liquid diets can be infused as a constant-rate infusion using an administration set and pump similar to that used for intravenous crystalloids. Rates should be set at 1 mL/kg per hour initially. The infusion can be gradually increased by 1 mL/kg per hour until the desired infusion rate is achieved. The infusion rate should not exceed 6 mL/kg per hour.

Fluids, liquid medications, and liquid diets can also be infused slowly using a syringe. The esophagostomy tube should be flushed with water (5 to 60 mL, depending on the size of the tube and patient) after every bolus feeding or every 6 hours in patients fed by constant-rate infusions.

Procedure for Administration of Gruel Diets

Gruel diets should be blenderized to ensure that no large particles that may cause an obstruction are infused. If one has any doubt about whether the gruel is liquid enough to pass through the tube, the gruel should be infused through a tube of equivalent diameter first. Boluses should be limited to less than 5 mL/kg initially. Rates can be slowly increased based on patient tolerance. The feeding should be stopped if one sees evidence of salivation, regurgitation, or vomiting or if the animal appears nauseated or uncomfortable. Boluses should not be larger than 25 mL/kg at one time. A bolus should not be given rapidly, and extremely hot or cold materials should not be infused. Immediately after the conclusion of the bolus feeding, the tube should be flushed with water. This helps to prevent the gruel from remaining in the tube where, over time, it may become inspissated and cause an obstruction. A plastic shield or plastic wrap should be used to cover the bandage when infusions are administered, to prevent soiling of the dressing.

Procedure for Use for Decompression

Esophagostomy tubes ending in the esophagus can be used to keep the esophagus decompressed in the patient that has poor esophageal motility. Patients with chronic megaesophagus, persistent right aortic arch, or acute megaesophagus are at increased risk for pulmonary aspiration and may benefit from esophageal decompression (2). Decompression is performed by aspirating the tube periodically until all the retained air, fluid, and other material is removed. Esophagostomy tubes ending in the esophagus or stomach can also be used to prevent the recurrence of gastric dilatation in patients recovering from surgery to correct gastric dilatation–volvulus. Studies in human patients have shown that, by preventing passage of air into the stomach, patients return to full oral feeding much more rapidly (5). This finding is assumed, but not proved, to be true in dogs and cats. The tube can be hand suctioned as frequently as needed or connected to a continuous suction device (GOMCO, Allied Healthcare, Buffalo, NY). If viscous or tenacious fluids are suctioned, small volumes of saline or water should be infused into the tube to prevent tube obstruction. An esophagogastric tube can be used for gastric decompression. If gastric secretions are tenacious, saline can be infused initially to break up the secretions before aspiration.

Removal of the Tube

As opposed to gastrostomy tubes, which must remain in place at least several days before removal to allow for a good seal to form between the stomach and the abdominal wall, esophagostomy tubes can be safely removed the same day they are placed. The dressing and the sutures are removed while the tube is held in place. The tube is then occluded and pulled out. The ostomy site should be cleaned, bactericidal ointment should be applied, and a light bandage should be placed around the patient's neck. The bandage should be removed in 24 hours and the wound inspected. If the ostomy site has not sealed yet, the bandage should be replaced. In patients requiring a new bandage, changes are done every 1 to 2 days until the ostomy site has sealed. This generally takes only a few days.

Long-Term Feeding

On occasion, animals require the use of an esophagostomy feeding tube for weeks or months. A fistula usually develops after a few weeks. If the feeding tube needs to be replaced, it is generally a simple procedure because the old tube is removed and a new one is directly fed into the fistula. This usually only requires a local anesthetic block for suture placement. Once these tubes are no longer needed, they are removed as described previously. The fistula closes quickly (within a maximum of a few days), but it may take a week or more to completely heal.

Complications

Most complications relate to skin irritation and inflammation. These problems usually can be prevented by ensuring that the skin sutures are not placed too tightly and that the skin is not pinched or folded during suture placement. If the tube is not secured to the periosteum or deep fascia, the tube will retract and move as the animal moves around, leading to possible inadvertent tube removal and significant skin irritation. If mild dermatitis is present, it will usually resolve with time and regular wound cleaning. On occasion, the dermatitis may not resolve until the tube is removed.

By pushing the forceps out in a lateral direction, the esophagus is approximated to the skin. If this maneuver is not performed adequately, the surgeon risks lacerating the external jugular vein as well as creating additional tissue trauma. This complication is rare when proper technique is used. Bleeding from a lacerated jugular vein has occurred in one known patient; this bleeding was controlled easily and definitively using direct pressure.

In extremely debilitated animals, care must be taken to adhere closely to the technique described. Serious complications can result, with dissection of the tube alongside the esophagus, if the tube is not brought out into the patient's mouth after grasping of the tip of the tube with the forceps. Because the surrounding soft tissues are more easily penetrated, the tube can then course alongside the esophagus instead of in the esophageal lumen. Because the clinician may not be aware of this situation, the tube must be brought out into the patient's mouth before being passed back into the esophagus.

Comments

The use of esophagostomy tubes for both feeding and decompression is both a practical and a life-saving procedure. More than 500 of these tubes are estimated to have been used to feed dogs and cats since 1988, with beneficial results. The technique has also been used in other mammalian species including the rat, ferret, and monkey. Esophagostomy tubes can also be used effectively in the nutritional support of birds. When comparing the technique with percutaneous gastrostomy tube placement, the use of esophagostomy tubes is less costly, it requires no special equipment or special tubes, it takes less operative and anesthetic time, it is easier to perform, and it is associated with fewer complications. No threat of peritonitis exists, and the tube can be removed safely at any time.

References

1. Crowe DT. Use of a nasogastric tube for gastric and esophageal decompression in the dog and cat. J Am Vet Med Assoc 1986;188:1178–1182.
2. Crowe DT. Feeding the sick patient. In: Proceedings of the Eastern States Veterinary Conference. Orlando, FL. 1988;3:95–96.
3. Crowe DT, Downs MO. Pharyngostomy complications in dogs and cats and recommended technical modifications: experimental and clinical investigations. J Am Anim Hosp Assoc 1986; 22:493–496.
4. Crowe DT. Nutritional support for the hospitalized patient: an introduction to tube feeding. Compend Contin Educ Pract Vet 1990;12:1711–1721.
5. Moss G. Maintenance of gastrointestinal function after bowel surgery and immediate enteral full nutrition. II. Clinical experience, with objective demonstration of intestinal absorption and motility. JPEN J Parenter Enteral Nutr 1981;5:215–220.

Esophagostomy Tube Placement: Alternate Technique

Clarence A. Rawlings & Joseph W. Bartges

An esophagostomy tube is placed percutaneously in the midcervical region of the esophagus (1). Although general anesthesia is required, the equipment is simple, and only a short skin incision is needed. The tube is large enough to permit bolus administration of a gruel made from canned dog or cat food. The tube can be withdrawn within a few days or left in for weeks, depending on when the animal regains the ability to feed itself.

Tube feeding is commonly indicated in dogs and cats that are ill or have recently undergone surgery (2–4). These patients commonly have energy–protein malnutrition, thus requiring supplemental nutrition to return to health. Typical surgical candidates include those after trauma, surgery for sepsis, orofacial surgery, subtotal colectomy, and major urinary surgery. Patients that are debilitated, dehydrated, or anorectic are frequently candidates for nutritional support. The gastrointestinal tract should be used when it is intact and other feeding options have either failed or are unlikely to work. Tube feeding became popular when Bohning and associates described the pharyngostomy tube technique (2). Problems with upper airway obstruction and aspiration were encountered, resulting in a recommendation for more caudal placement of the tube (5). In a review of 125 pharyngostomy tube uses, Crowe and Downs reported 18 dogs and cats with respiratory problems induced by pharyngostomy tubes (6). Because placing a pharyngostomy tube into the stomach through the esophageal hiatus can result in gastroesophageal reflux, the distal end of the feeding is left in the caudal area of the esophagus (7). We have discontinued use of the pharyngostomy tube in favor of an esophagostomy tube.

Other enteral tube placements are options when considering selection of the esophagostomy tube. In the severely depressed animal with chronic disease, anesthesia may be contraindicated. A nasogastric tube can be placed with less stress and without general anesthesia (8, 9). Because these patients should have their nutritional replacement started gradually, the low volume and speed of administration through the small-diameter esophagostomy tube is not a major disadvantage. Diets usually consist of special convalescence diets, which are calorically dense and may be administered with an infusion pump. Both esophagostomy and gastrostomy tubes require a functional stomach. Jejunostomy tubes are used in those few animals with gastric disease. The choice between esophagostomy and percutaneously placed gastrostomy tubes is usually personal, but each has some advantages. The esophagostomy tube is well tolerated, avoids concern for peritonitis, and can be withdrawn at any time. A gastrostomy tube, especially a surgically placed tube, can be used for feeding for years in diseases such as megaesophagus. Most clinicians prefer to remove gastrostomy tubes only after 1 week has elapsed, in the hope that adhesions will reduce the likelihood of peritonitis. Although we have used esophagostomy tubes to feed dogs with decreased esophageal motility and mild esophageal dilation, a gastrostomy tube is preferred when dilated esophagus is diagnosed before tube placement.

Surgical Technique

At least three techniques have been described to place the esophagostomy tube into the esophagus midway between the larynx and the thoracic inlet. The esophagostomy tube is the widely available polyvinyl chloride feeding and urethral catheter (Monoject, Sherwood Medical Products, St. Louis, MO) of at least 14-French diameter in mature dogs and cats. Our initial technique used a stiff polyvinyl chloride tube and an 18-gauge over-the-needle-catheter (1). This is described step by step, but currently most esophagostomy tubes are placed using an ELD percutaneous gastrostomy feeding tube applicator (Jorgensen Laboratories, Inc., Loveland, CO). The ELD tube applicator, which is designed for percutaneous placement of gastrostomy tubes without an endoscope (10), requires fewer manipulations than the published technique for esophagostomy tube placement.

The patient is anesthetized, and trachea is intubated. The ELD tube applicator is passed through the oral cavity until the blunt cannula end is midway between the larynx and the thoracic inlet. It is rotated so the tip deflects the esophagus above the normal contour of the neck. The projection of the tip should be just ventral to the external jugular vein, which should be distended by compression at the thoracic inlet. The cutting stylet is thrust through the skin. To avoid injury, the stylet can be directed into a syringe case. A surgical blade is used to extend the incision started by the stylet so the entire tube applicator can be projected through the skin. The end of the feeding tube is cut at right angles so there is a single end hole that, when finally positioned, is at the eighth to tenth thoracic space. A suture is passed through the wall of the tube 1 cm from the end, through the eye of the stylet, and then through the opposite wall of the tube. The suture is tied such that the tube is secured over the stylet and the feeding tube is flush with the applicator. The applicator is withdrawn from the patient's mouth to pull the tube out the mouth. A malleable stylet, as used to stiffen endotracheal tubes, is passed through the flared end of the feeding tube. The end of the rod should be 1 to 2 cm from the end of the feeding tube. The tube as stiffened by the malleable stylet is retracted while the rod is used to force the tubes end against the right side of the esophagus. When the tube is perpendicular to the esophagus, the tube is directed caudally and is advanced. The tube should pass easily even as the malleable rod is withdrawn. The flared end of the tube is secured by suture to the neck skin near the tube exit (Fig. 12.12).

The third esophagostomy tube placement technique is used in cats and smaller dogs. Long, sharp, curved forceps, such as Mixter forceps, are passed through the patient's mouth to the same site as described previously. The tip of the forceps is projected toward the left side of the neck, and the skin is incised sufficiently to expose the tips. The tube is prepared, is inserted into the tips of the forceps, is withdrawn to the patient's mouth, and then is positioned as described previously.

Postoperative Care

A light bandage to encircle the neck is usually placed over the tube exit. The exit is cleaned daily, and an antibacterial ointment is placed over the wound. Some animals require an Elizabethan collar to reduce self-trauma. When the animal has regained the ability to feed itself and is in a positive nutritional plane, the tube is withdrawn. The animal's appetite can be tested with the tube in place because ingesta can easily pass around the tube. After the tube is removed, the exit site should be cleansed at least daily; the wound normally heals by second intention.

Larger feeding tubes, regardless of placement site and technique, permit administration of pureed specialty diets as a bolus. This feature is ideal in the busy practice and for the owner because feeding can be done rapidly, and the diet and feeding interval more closely resemble the animal's normal feeding habits. Initially, a small amount of water is given to ensure that the tube will function without problems. The quantity of food is calculated using energy requirements for the animal's weight, age, activity, and disease condition. Daily volume and feeding schedules

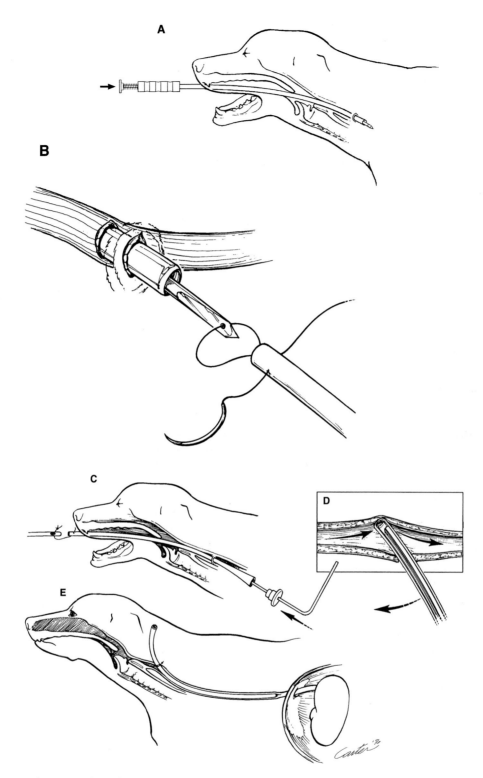

Fig. 12.12. Steps in placement of esophagostomy tube. **A.** The ELD (Jorgensen Laboratories, Inc., Loveland, CO) tube applicator is passed through the oral cavity until the blunt cannula end is midway between the larynx and the thoracic inlet. It is rotated so the tip deflects the esophagus above the normal contour of the neck. The cutting stylet is thrust through the skin, and the incision is extended with a surgical blade until the entire applicator is passed through the incision. In small animals, the ELD tube applicator may be replaced by Mixter forceps. **B.** The end of the feeding tube is cut at right angles so there is a single end-hole that, when finally positioned, will be at the eighth to tenth thoracic space. A suture is passed through the wall of the tube 1 cm from the end, through the eye of the stylet, and then through the opposite wall of the tube. The suture is tied so the tube is secured over the stylet and the feeding tube is flush with the applicator. The applicator is withdrawn from the patient's mouth to pull the tube out the mouth. **C.** A malleable stylet, which is typically used to increase the stiffness of endotracheal tubes, is passed within the tube to within 1 to 2 cm of the tube. **D.** The tube with intraluminal stylet is slowly withdrawn while applying lateral pressure on the tip forcing it toward the right side. When the tube is perpendicular to the surface of the skin, the tube is then directed caudally within the esophagus. The stylet is then withdrawn. The tube should pass easily. **E.** Retention sutures (such as 0 nylon) are used to secure the tube to the skin just dorsal to the catheter exit. The suture should be tied securely enough to the tube to indent the tube. Then the same suture is attached loosely to the skin. The proper position for the caudal end of the tube is just cranial to the esophageal hiatus.

are based on the amount of water required to make a gruel that is liquid enough to be injected through the tube. Surgical patients that had an adequate nutritional plane before surgery are normally started at or above their caloric maintenance. Patients with chronic disease and malnutrition must be started at a fraction of their calculated maintenance. Feeding volumes and total calories are increased to the desired level over a few days. Generally, no more than 20 mL/kg per feeding is given at intervals of at least 4 hours. When full feeding is achieved, many animals tolerate 50 to 75 mL/kg of food administered three to four times per day. Preparation of gruel from prescription diets provides a readily available formula with nutrients deemed best for specific diseases. Food can be pureed and stored in the refrigerator. The appropriate aliquot can be microwaved to decrease the gruel's viscosity. Care should be taken to heat and mix the food properly before feeding, to prevent thermal burns to the esophagus.

Patients that are sick enough to require supplemental feeding must be monitored closely, especially those that have had their tube placed to correct their malnutrition. The patient must be weighed and hydration status checked daily. Body temperature, attitude, and urine production and other fluid loss should be monitored regularly. Hematocrit, total solids, albumin, glucose, and serum electrolytes should be measured frequently. Septic patients should have regular complete blood counts determined. Debilitated patients frequently require intravenous fluids, including potassium supplementation, in addition to tube feedings. Patients with decreased gastrointestinal motility should be treated with metoclopramide hydrochloride (Reglan) at 0.2 to 0.4 mg/kg orally every 6 to 8 hours (11). Patients with potential aspiration should monitored for respiratory effort and by thoracic radiography, if necessary.

Acknowledgment

The illustrations by Kip Carter are appreciated.

References

1. Rawlings CA. Percutaneous placement of a midcervical esophagostomy tube: new technique and representative cases. J Am Anim Hosp Assoc 1993;29:526–530.
2. Bohning RH Jr, DeHoff WD, McElhinney A, et al. Pharyngostomy for maintenance of the anorectic animal. J Am Vet Med Assoc 1970;156:611–615.
3. Crowe DT. Nutritional support for the hospitalized patient: an introduction to tube feeding. Compend Contin Educ Pract Vet 1990;12:1711–1721.
4. Morris ML. Nutrition and diet in small animal medicine. Denver: Mark Morris Associates, 1960:84–85.
5. Rawlings CA. Pharyngostomy. In: Wingfield WE, Rawlings CA, eds. Small animal surgery: an atlas of operative techniques. Philadelphia: WB Saunders, 1979:65–67.
6. Crowe DT, Downs MO. Pharyngostomy complications in dogs and cats and recommended technical modifications: experimental and clinical investigations. J Am Anim Hosp Assoc 1986;22:493–503.
7. Lantz GC. Pharyngostomy tube induced esophagitis in the dog: an experimental study. J Am Anim Hosp Assoc 1983;19:207–212.
8. Ford RB. Nasogastric intubation in the cat Compend Contin Educ Pract Vet 1980;1:29–33.
9. Forenbacher S. Passing the stomach tube through the nose of the cat. Vet Med 1950;45:407–410.
10. ELD gastrostomy tube applicator (brochure). Loveland, CO: Jorgensen Laboratories, Inc., no date.
11. Graves GM, Becht JL, Rawlings CA. Metoclopramide reversal of decreased gastrointestinal myoelectric and contractile activity in a model of canine postoperative ileus. Vet Surg 1989;18:27–33.

Use of Percutaneous Gastrostomy Tubes and Low-Profile Feeding Devices

Ronald M. Bright

Maximal health and activity of companion animals are maintained when nutritional support is adequate. When an animal becomes anorectic as a result of a debilitating disease, injury, or surgery, the malnourished state likely intensifies the effects of these challenges. Within 3 to 5 days of anorexia, animals have a decreased ability to respond to stressful situations. Wound healing and fracture healing are delayed, and susceptibility to the effects of shock and of septicemia is increased. Restoration of an adequate plane of nutrition in many chronically ill or critical care patients is often pivotal in ensuring complete recovery.

In human patients, morbidity and mortality rates are higher in poorly nourished individuals owing to a high incidence of nosocomial infections (1). Similarly, animals given inadequate nutrition are more likely to succumb to a septic challenge (2).

In one study, human patients undergoing a major operation had higher rates of complications when they suffered from protein–energy undernutrition. A preoperative weight loss of more than 20% of normal body weight was associated with a 10-fold increase in mortality when compared with patients with less weight loss and the same disease (3).

The prevalence of malnutrition in hospitalized animals was not a major concern in veterinary medicine until recently. The frequency of this problem is probably relatively constant despite population differences among veterinary hospitals or the nature of the illnesses. In my own hospital, the trend toward earlier intervention to support the nutritional needs of patients has played an important role in decreasing the incidence of complications in patients with chronic disease or those in need of critical care.

When feasible, gastrointestinal feedings provide the most effective and appropriate route for nutritional supplementation (3). Advantages over the parenteral route of feeding include maintenance of more physiologic metabolism, preservation of gastrointestinal structure and function, greater economy, and the avoidance of intravenous catheter complications.

The introduction of percutaneous endoscopic gastrostomy (PEG) in human patients in 1980 allowed the establishment of permanent or temporary enteral access without the need for a deep surgical plane of anesthesia or a laparotomy (4, 5).

PEG became popular in veterinary medicine in the mid-1980s after the successful experimental and clinical work by Bright (6, 7) and Matthews (8). Data collected on clinical patients suggested that PEG has the same advantages in veterinary patients as in human patients (9, 10).

The original PEG required the use of endoscopy. The PEG technique has become more practical, however, with the use of "blind placement" techniques (11, 12).

Anesthetic Considerations

Anorectic and severely debilitated animals are prone to cardiac and respiratory complications while under the effects of sedatives or general anesthesia. Multiple orogastric or nasogastric feedings or continuous total parenteral nutrition may be prudent before placing the PEG tube.

Regardless of the method of chemical restraint, the animal should have sufficient jaw relaxation. When using the endoscopy-assisted technique, an endotracheal tube must be in place to assist ventilatory movements during a brief period of stomach distension.

A balanced electrolyte solution is used to support the patient's circulatory volume. In patients under 6 months of age, dextrose is added to the solution.

Anatomic Considerations

At rest, the stomach extends caudally to the border of the last rib. It makes contact with the abdominal wall in this position. The transverse colon and spleen lie close to the greater curvature of the stomach. Insufflation of the stomach using the endoscopy-assisted technique pushes these two structures caudally. The stomach distended with air "tents" the abdominal wall when the animal is in right lateral recumbency. This causes the stomach and abdominal walls to be pushed together and to be under slight tension while the liver, spleen, and colon are pushed caudally out of the way.

This maneuver allows a large unobstructed area of the greater curvature of the stomach to be used for PEG placement. "Blind" techniques also take advantage of the relationship between the stomach and the abdominal wall.

Indications

Any animal that has been anorectic for 3 to 5 days, is severely debilitated on the initial presentation to the veterinarian, or is expected to be incapable of eating by the oral route after oropharyngeal or esophageal surgery is a candidate for a PEG. Placement of a PEG has been used to support many different conditions in veterinary patients. Oronasal trauma or neoplasia, esophageal disorders, and liver disorders appear to be the most frequent indications for PEG. The use of this technique is limited to animals with an intact and unobstructed gastrointestinal tract. Although PEG is used primarily for medium-term or long-term support of nutritional needs, its simplicity also encourages its use for short periods.

Tube Placement (Endoscopically Assisted)

The animal is placed in right lateral recumbency with the mouth kept open by a partially used roll of tape or a mouth gag. A small area of skin (3 × 3 cm square) 2 cm behind the last rib and halfway between the dorsal and ventral midlines is clipped and is surgically prepared with an antiseptic solution. A 3-mm incision through the skin is made in the middle of this square. A fiberoptic gastroscope is placed into the stomach. The stomach is insufflated with air until it causes the skin to stretch and become "tented" and tense. An 18-gauge sheathed catheter (Sherwood Medical Industries, St. Louis, MO) is placed in the 3-mm incision and is thrust abruptly into the lumen of the stomach (an 18-gauge 1.5-inch hypodermic needle can be substituted) (Fig. 12.13). The stylet is withdrawn as the catheter sheath is gently pushed inward to prevent its displacement (Fig. 12.14). Air from the stomach is allowed to escape through the sheath. A length of 1–0 suture is placed through the sheath and into the stomach, where a basket snare or biopsy forceps can be used to grasp the end of the suture (Fig. 12.15). The gastroscope and suture within the grasp of the snare or forceps are then slowly withdrawn from the stomach and allowed to exit the oral cavity. The catheter sheath is removed from the stomach.

The end of the suture exiting the oral cavity is passed in retrograde fashion through a sheath catheter or a similarly sized plastic laboratory pipette. A 20-French Pezzer mushroom-tip catheter (Bard Urological

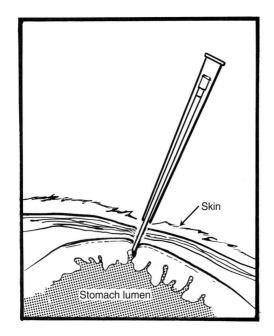

Fig. 12.13. A sheath-type catheter is thrust percutaneously through a 3-mm length skin incision after the endoscope is in place and the stomach is expanded with air.

Division, CR Bard, Inc., Murray Hill, NJ; Cook Veterinary Products, Spencer, IN) is modified by removing a V-shaped piece from the end of the catheter opposite the mushroom tip (Fig. 12.16**A**). This forms a pointed and narrow tip of the feeding tube that will eventually be placed into the flared end of the sheath catheter or pipette (Fig. 12.16**D**). The end of the suture exiting the oral cavity is then passed in retrograde fashion through an 18-gauge hypodermic needle placed transversely through the feeding tube just below the modified tip of the feeding tube (Fig. 12.16**B**). The suture is then tied in a square knot (Fig. 12.16**C**). The narrow and pointed end of the feeding tube is then inserted into the flared end of the catheter sheath or a 2-inch 200 μl laboratory pipette (Pipette tips, Costar, Cambridge, PA; Pipet tips, Baxter Diagnostics, Inc., McGaw Park, IL). If a catheter sheath is used, a 3–0 nylon suture with a straight needle is passed transversely through the sheath catheter and the feeding tube and is tied back to itself. This helps to prevent the pointed tip of the feeding tube from becoming separated from the sheath. An additional length of suture is looped through the holes in the mushroom tip, so if the tube

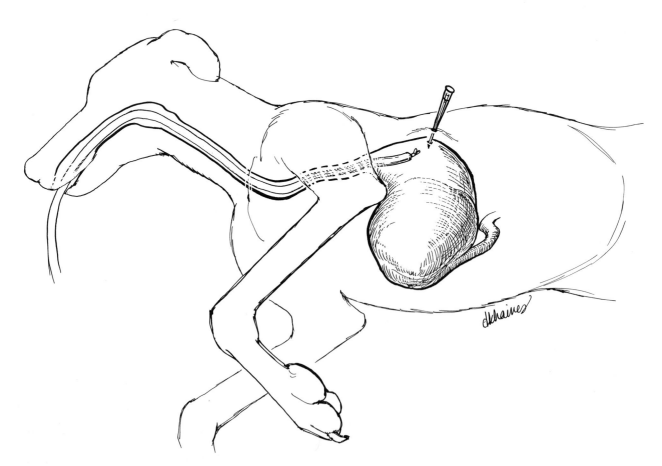

Fig. 12.14. After the stylet is removed, the sheath is pushed into the lumen to hold it securely in place.

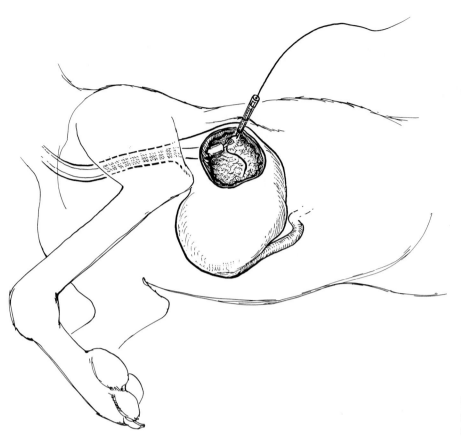

Fig. 12.15. A length of suture is passed through the sheath and is grasped by endoscopic forceps.

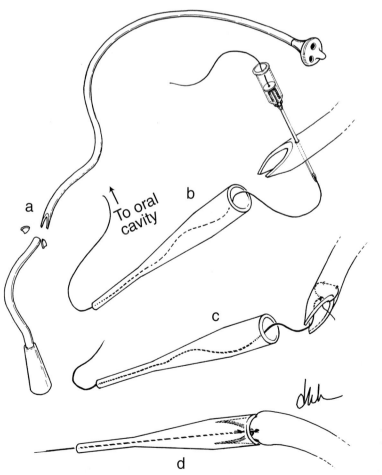

a

b

c

d

To oral cavity

Fig. 12.16. **A.** The flared end of the mushroom-tip catheter is cut, and the remaining tip is modified into a V shape to fit snugly into the flared end of a pipette or catheter sheath. **B** and **C.** A catheter sheath or pipette has been placed on the length of suture exiting from the oral cavity. The modified end of the gastrostomy tube has a suture passed transversely below the V-shaped defect using an 18-gauge hypodermic needle. The suture is tied (**C**) until the knot lies within the modified tip of the catheter. **D.** The tip is directed into the flared end of the pipette or catheter sheath.

173

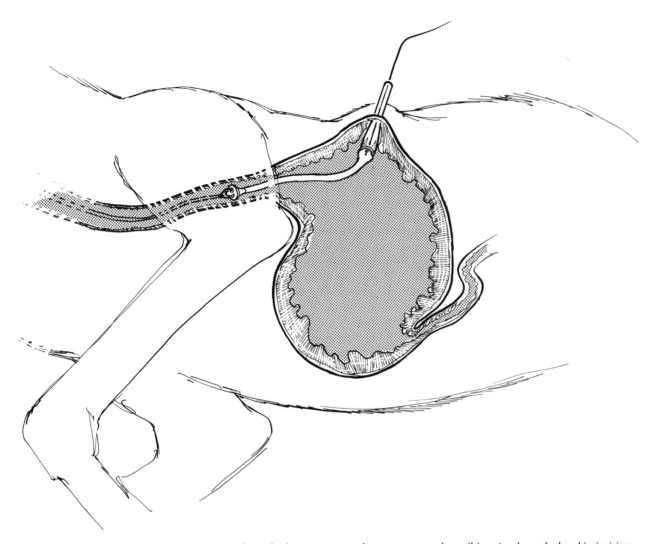

Fig. 12.17. An assistant pulls the suture and attached gastrostomy tube percutaneously until it exits through the skin incision.

becomes dislodged when attempting to pass it transabdominally, it can be recovered (Fig. 12.17). Water-soluble lubricating jelly is applied liberally to the surface of the sheath catheter and feeding tube.

An assistant applies traction on the suture exiting the stomach wall. The sheath or pipette, acting as a dilator, pulls the feeding tube transabdominally until it emerges through the skin incision (see Fig. 12.17). The feeding tube is advanced until the mushroom tip is felt to lie gently against the gastric mucosa.

The tube is marked at the level of the skin with a permanent marking pen. This allows the position of the tube to be monitored closely for any inward movement into the stomach that, if the tube is lodged in the pylorus, could cause vomiting.

Antiseptic or antibiotic ointment is applied to the skin at the tube exit site. A small gauze sponge and a light bandage are then placed over the area. An orthopedic stockinette or an infant's T-shirt can be modified and used in lieu of the bandage material. An Elizabethan collar may be necessary for the first 3 to 5 days to discourage licking and possible dislodgment of the tube.

Nonendoscopic or Blind Percutaneous Gastrotomy Technique

The animal is prepared as previously described for the PEG technique (11, 12). A vinyl tube (outside diameter 1.5 to 2.0 cm) is placed in a low-temperature environment (less than 25° F) for 10 minutes. This stiffens the slightly curved end of the tube that will be passed into the stomach. A length of aluminum orthopedic tubing slightly longer than the vinyl tube is placed within the tube to act as a stylet. This eases the passage of the tube through the cardia. The tube is coated liberally with water-soluble jelly and is passed into the stomach. The tip of the tube is directed so it lies just under the surgically prepared area of skin. The tube is advanced until an outward bulge is seen. The tip and overlying tissue are grasped between the surgeon's thumb and forefinger. A 1.5-inch 14-gauge hypodermic needle is directed into the lumen of the tube (Fig. 12.18). The hub of the needle is moved laterally back and forth, so the inside of the tube can be felt. The aluminum tubing (rod) is removed.

The loop end of a 0.020- to 0.024-inch diameter (LW 20, 22 or 24) banjo wire (GHS Strings, Battle Creek, MI) is flattened to allow its passage through the hypodermic needle and into the vinyl tube. The wire is advanced through the vinyl tube until it exits the oral cavity (see Fig. 12.18). The hypodermic needle is removed. A small 3-mm incision in the skin is made contiguous with the hole in the skin where the wire is emerging. A size 0 or 1 nonabsorbable suture is threaded through the flattened loop of the banjo wire and is tied in a square knot. The wire with attached

suture has traction applied to it until the suture exits the skin. The suture is clamped with a hemostat while the mushroom-tip tube is attached to the other end, as previously described. The final placement of the feeding tube is similar to the PEG technique (Figs. 12.16 and 12.17).

The foregoing technique can be repeated using a special tube placement device (11) (Percutaneous non-endoscopic gastrostomy tube placement device, Veterinary Products Laboratories, Phoenix, AZ). The length of this device limits its use to small dogs or cats.

Low-Profile Feeding Devices

Occasionally, it may be desirable to replace the standard PEG tube with a low-profile gastrostomy device (LPGD). This device is ideal when long-term enteral feeding is necessary (13). The LPGD can be inserted easily through the gastrocutaneous fistula created by

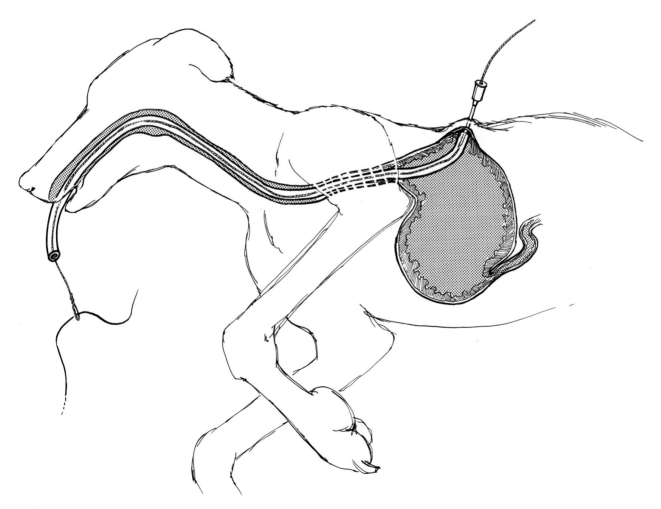

Fig. 12.18. Blind percutaneous technique. A polyvinyl tube is placed into the stomach, and the tip is directed laterally to "tent" the skin and abdominal wall overlying the stomach. A 14- or 16-gauge hypodermic needle is directed into the end of the tube that is palpated with the opposite hand. A banjo wire is directed through the lumen of the needle and is passed cranially within the tube until it exits the oral cavity. A length of suture is the loop on the end of the wire and is pulled in the opposite direction until it exits the skin. The steps shown in Figure 12.16 are followed to complete the gastrostomy tube placement.

the original gastrostomy tube (see earlier). Replacing the PEG tube with an LPGD should not be done until a mature gastrocutaneous fistula forms (3 to 4 weeks). Insertion of the LPGD can be done without fluoroscopy or endoscopy and can usually be accomplished in the awake or lightly sedated animal.

Several LPGDs are available, but I prefer either the Bard Button (Bard Interventional Products, CR Bard, Jewksbury, MA) or the Surgitek Button (Surgitek, Cabot Medical Company, Racine, WI). The "button" is simply designed and comes in various lengths and diameters. The button used to replace the PEG tube should fit snugly to prevent its removal, leakage of gastric juices, and excessive to-and-fro movement. As a general rule, a size of 2- to 4-French diameter larger than that of the PEG tube it is replacing is likely to be correct.

A stoma-measuring device is inserted into the fistula after the PEG is removed. The curved tip of the stoma-measuring device is retracted until it comes in contact with the gastric mucosa (Fig. 12.19). The length of the button needed is determined by noting which of three premeasured marks located on the shaft of the stoma-measuring device approximates the distance between the gastric mucosa and the level of the skin. As mentioned previously, the diameter of the button required is generally a little larger than the diameter of the PEG tube.

An obturator is placed into the lumen of the button and is advanced into the tip with enough force to cause its flattening and elongation (Fig. 12.20). This maneuver allows easy advancement of the button into the

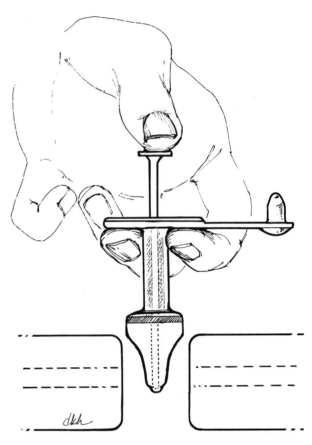

Fig. 12.20. An appropriate length and diameter of a low-profile gastrostomy device is placed into the lumen with the aid of an obturator that elongates and flattens the mushroom tip for easier placement.

stomach through the fistula. The obturator is removed, allowing the mushroom tip of the button to regain its original shape (Fig. 12.21). An attached plug is used to cap the opening between feedings. The device can be affixed to the skin with two simple interrupted sutures, but this is usually not necessary.

A right-angle or straight adapter tube is available to

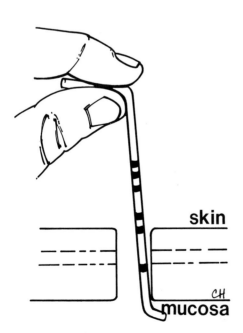

Fig. 12.19. The depth of the gastrocutaneous fistula is measured with a stoma-measuring device.

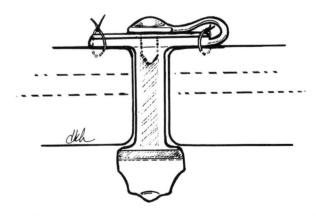

Fig. 12.21. The device is sutured to the skin and is capped between feedings.

attach to the opening of the button during feedings. A light bandage, stockinette, or modified infant's T-shirt can be used to cover the button between feedings.

One potential complication related to the placement of any LPGD is disruption of the gastrocutaneous fistula. If this happens, a device with a larger diameter may need to be substituted.

The most important advantages of any LPGD are its practicality and the decreased potential that it will become dislodged. Pets have greater freedom of movement because of the low-profile design.

References

1. Scrimshaw NS. Effect of infection on nutrient requirements. JPEN J Parenter Enteral Nutr 1991;15:589–597.
2. Russell JR, Brokman M, Norris F. Percutaneous gastrostomy: a new simplified and cost effective technique. Am J Surg 1984;148:132–137.
3. Studley HO. Percentage of weight loss: a basic indicator of surgical risk. JAMA 1936;106:458–464.
4. Gauderer MWL, Ponsky JL. A simplified technique for constructing a tube feeding gastrostomy. Surg Gynecol Obstet 1981;152:83–86.
5. Gauderer MWL, Ponsky JL, Izant RJ. Gastrostomy without laparotomy: a percutaneous endoscopic technique. J Pediatr Surg 1980;15:872–875.
6. Bright RM. Percutaneous tube gastrostomy with and without endoscopy. In: Proceedings of the fourth annual veterinary medical forum. Washington, DC. 1986;65–68.
7. Bright RM, Burrows CF. Percutaneous endoscopic tube gastrostomy in dogs. Am J Vet Res 1988;49:629–633.
8. Mathews KA, Binnington AG. Percutaneous incisionless placement of gastrostomy tube utilizing a gastroscope: preliminary observations. J Am Anim Hosp Assoc 1986;22:601–610.
9. Armstrong PJ, Hardie EM. Percutaneous endoscopic gastrostomy: a retrospective study of 54 clinical cases in dogs and cats. J Vet Intern Med 1990;4:202–206.
10. Bright RM, Okrasinski EB, Pardo AD, et al. Percutaneous tube gastrostomy for enteral alimentation in small animals. Compend Contin Educ Pract Vet 1991;13:15–21.
11. Mauterer JV, Abood SK, Buffington CA, et al. New technique and management guidelines for percutaneous nonendoscopic tube gastrostomy. J Am Vet Med Assoc 1994;205:574–579.
12. Fulton RB, Dennis JS. Blind percutaneous placement of a gastrostomy tube for nutritional support in dogs and cats. J Am Vet Med Assoc 1992;201:697–703.
13. Bright RM, DeNovo RC, Jones JB. Use of a low-profile gastrostomy device for administering nutrients in two dogs. J Am Vet Med Assoc 1995;207:1184–1186.

Use of Jejunostomy and Enterostomy Tubes

Chad M. Devitt & Howard B. Seim III

Metabolic support is becoming an integral part of surgical critical care in veterinary medicine (1). Jejunostomy or enterostomy tubes are methods of nutritional supplementation in patients after abdominal surgery. Small animal patients undergoing abdominal surgical procedures are often compromised and are likely in need of nutritional support.

Nutritional support is indicated in patients that are unable to meet nutritional demands by oral consumption of food. Malnutrition can be defined by one or more of the following criteria: anorexia for longer than 5 days, weight loss of more than 10% body weight, increased nutrient loss (i.e., vomiting, diarrhea, protein-losing nephropathy), low albumin, and increased nutrient demands (i.e., surgical stress, sepsis, cancer, chronic infections).

A basic premise "if the gut works, use it" may seem an oversimplification of the benefits of providing nutritional support by physiologic routes (i.e., the gastrointestinal tract versus parenteral administration). In general, the more orad nutrients are placed in the gastrointestinal tract, the better patients are able to assimilate complex diets into essential nutrients. Conversely, bypassing a functional segment of the gastrointestinal tract (i.e., stomach) results in necessary alteration of the dietary composition to accommodate for the loss of the portion of gastrointestinal tract.

General Considerations

Whenever a surgeon enters the abdominal cavity, one question should be answered: Could this patient benefit from a feeding tube? Surgically placed feeding tubes carry little additional operative risk, are economical, and are simple to place and manage; therefore, they pose little risk to the patient while providing a large potential benefit. Special equipment is not required for placement of enteral feeding tubes. The tubes used are 3.5- to 5-French infant feeding tubes at least 36 inches in length. If intestinal surgery is performed, the catheter is placed aboral to the site of surgery. Appropriate diets include commercially available polymeric and monomeric diets. The preferred mode of administration is by slow, continuous-rate infusion; however, small frequent boluses can suffice.

Indications

Placement of an enterostomy feeding tube may be indicated in any patient undergoing an abdominal operation. The major criteria are a functional small intestine and the need for nutritional support (2, 3). Choosing the appropriate method and determining the need for nutritional support are based on applying the least invasive technique that carries the greatest likelihood of success with the least amount of morbidity.

Feeding through an enterostomy tube has induced pancreatic secretion and therefore was previously contraindicated in patients with pancreatitis (4, 5). Acute pancreatitis induces a hypermetabolic state with increased caloric and nitrogen demands and at the same time renders the gastrointestinal tract unable to meet these increased needs (4, 5). Because the exocrine function of the pancreas is stimulated by the vagus nerve and by release of gastrointestinal hormones in response to food, one can reasonably expect that if the diet is administered into the jejunum, thereby bypassing the cephalic, gastric, and duodenal source of pancreatic stimulation, no significant increase will occur in the exocrine activity of the pancreas (6). Patients with pancreatitis experience modulation of bacterial flora within the intestinal tract and increased bacterial translocation, and they suffer from a negative energy balance. Early alimentation through an enterostomy tube in human patients with pancreatitis results in improved immune status and fewer complications (4, 6, 7). A jejunostomy tube may allow aggressive nutritional support at an earlier time in the postoperative period. Although these issues are controversial, enteral nutrition is considered an integral part of aggressive treatment of acute pancreatitis in human patients (4, 6, 7).

Contraindications

The major contraindication to the use of a jejunostomy tube is any disorder causing a nonfunctional gastrointestinal tract (i.e., ileus or neoplastic obstruction of the intestine) (2, 3).

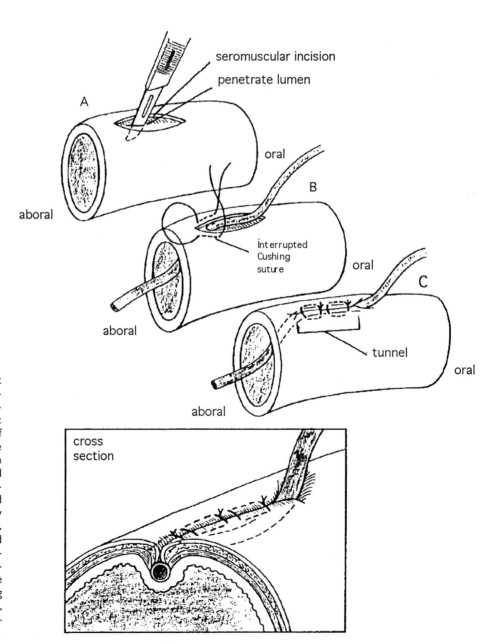

Fig. 12.22. Steps in the placement of a jejunostomy tube. **A.** A 2- to 3-cm longitudinal seromuscular incision is made in the antimesenteric border of the isolated segment of jejunum. At the aboral end of the seromuscular incision, a stab incision is made through the submucosa and mucosa into the lumen of the jejunum. **B.** The feeding tube is directed through the stab incision aborally into the lumen of the jejunum. **C.** The seromuscular incision is closed with 3–0 or 4–0 monofilament synthetic absorbable suture in an interrupted Cushing pattern. *Inset.* The incision is closed to bury the feeding tube in the submucosa of the incision, thereby effectively creating a submucosal tunnel.

Operative Technique

From a midline laparotomy incision, a segment of proximal jejunum that is easily approximated to the ventrolateral body wall is isolated. The direction of ingesta flow (orad to aborad) is determined by tracing the bowel segment from a known anatomic landmark (i.e., stomach or duodenum). A 2- to 3-cm longitudinal seromuscular incision is made in the antimesenteric border of the isolated segment of jejunum. At the aboral end of the seromuscular incision, a stab incision is made through the submucosa and mucosa into the lumen of the jejunum (Fig.12.22**A**). A 5-French Argyle feeding tube (Sherwood Medical Products, St. Louis, MO) is directed through the stab incision aborally into the lumen of the jejunum. Approximately 20 cm of feeding tube is threaded aborally into the small intestine (Fig. 12.22**B**). The seromuscular incision is closed with 3–0 or 4–0 monofilament synthetic absorbable suture in an interrupted Cushing pattern (Fig.12.22**C**). The surgeon should close this incision in such a manner that the feeding tube is buried in the submucosa of the incision, effectively creating a submucosal tunnel (Fig. 12.22, *inset*). The remaining catheter is exteriorized through a small stab incision in the ventrolateral body wall. Care is taken to select a site that will not result in excessive tension or radial directional changes of the bowel. The enterostomy site is sutured to the peritoneal surface of the adjacent body wall (Fig. 12.23). Care is taken to create a watertight jejunopexy on all sides of the enterostomy. The catheter is secured to the skin of the adjacent body wall with a Chinese finger trap friction suture. Abdominal wall closure is routine. A protective bandage is placed on the patient after the procedure, and an Elizabethan collar is used to prevent premature removal of the jejunostomy tube.

Diet Selection, Dose, and Administration

The ideal enteral diet formulation is isotonic, has a caloric density of 1 kcal/mL, a protein content of 4.0 g/100 kcal (16% of total calories), and approximately 30% of calories as fat. Commercially available diets designed for humans are the best diets for small animal patients. Liquid enteral diets can be categorized as polymeric diets or monomeric diets. Polymeric diets contain large molecular weight proteins, carbohydrates, and fats. They require normal intestinal digestion. Most are relatively isotonic, contain about 1 kcal/mL, and are readily available. Monomeric diets are composed of crystalline amino acids as the protein source, glucose and oligosaccharides as the carbohydrate source, and safflower oil as the essential fatty acid source. They are hyperosmolar and expensive. A summary of polymeric and monomeric diets is included in Table 12.4.

For patients with impaired digestive or absorptive function (pancreatitis, enteritis, hepatic disease) or suspected food allergy, a commercial polymeric, enteral liquid diet may be indicated. Patients should be closely monitored for formula intolerance. Jevity (Ross Laboratories, Columbus, OH) is the initial formula of choice, owing to the potential benefits of its fiber content. If the patient becomes intolerant to Jevity, Osmolite HN (Ross Laboratories) should be used. The protein sources of many human products may not provide adequate arginine and sulfur-containing amino acids for cats, and additional protein supplementation is required for long-term use.

Monomeric diets are indicated for patients with exocrine pancreatic insufficiency, short bowel syndrome, or inflammatory bowel disease or when polymeric diets are not tolerated. Monomeric diets pro-

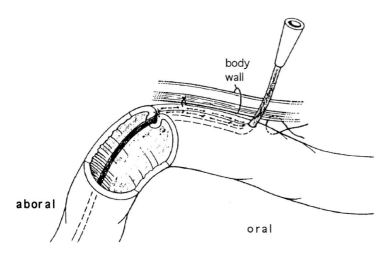

Fig. 12.23. The remaining catheter is exteriorized through a small stab incision in the ventrolateral body wall. Care is taken to select a site that will not result in excessive tension or radial directional changes of the bowel. The enterostomy site is sutured to the peritoneal surface of the adjacent body wall. The catheter is secured to the skin of the adjacent body wall with a Chinese finger trap friction suture. Abdominal wall closure is routine. A protective bandage is placed on the patient after the surgical procedure, and an Elizabethan collar is used to prevent premature removal of the jejunostomy tube.

Table 12.4.
Commercially Available Polymeric and Monomeric Diets and Their Composition

Diet	Calorie content (kcal/mL)	Protein (g/100 kcal)	Protein (g/mL)	Fat g/100 kcal	Osmolality (mOsm/kg)
Polymeric					
Jevity	1.06	4.20	0.045	3.48	310
Osmolite HN	1.06	4.44	0.047	3.68	310
Impact	1.00	5.50	0.055	2.80	375
Clincare feline	0.92	7.0	0.064	4.60	368
Clincare canine	0.99	5.0	0.050	6.10	340
Monomeric					
Vivonex HN	1.00	4.60	0.042	0.90	810
Vital HN	1.00	4.17	.046	1.08	460

mote maximal nutrient absorption and minimal digestive and absorptive work. In addition, monomeric diets are less stimulatory for exocrine pancreatic secretion and may have a role in nutritional support of pancreatitis patients (8). To match the caloric density of polymeric formulas, their osmolality must be two to three times higher, a feature that can create disorders of gut motility or fluid balance. Their cost is about seven times more per calorie compared with polymeric formulas. In most cases, a polymeric diet may be tried first, owing to the decreased cost, ease of preparation, and physiologic benefits to enterocyte function.

To determine the dosage of diet to feed, one must first calculate the basal energy requirement (BER, resting energy requirement) based on body weight. The BER is calculated from the following formulas for dogs weighing less than 2 kg:

$$BER \ (kcal/day) = 70(wt_{kg}0.75)$$

The following formula is used for dogs weighing more than 2 kg:

$$BER \ (kcal/day) = 30(wt_{kg}) + 70$$

After determination of the BER, additional factors can be multiplied depending on the condition of the animal:

$$ER \ (kcal/day) = BER \times 1.25 \ to \ 1.5$$

Table 12.5.
Recommended Enterostomy Feeding Schedule

Day	Fraction of Calculated Volume*	Dosing Interval
>1	$\frac{1}{4}$	qid
2	$\frac{1}{2}$	qid
3	$\frac{3}{4}$	qid
4	full dose	qid

* Calculated dose is diluted to the full volume with tap water.

Protein supplementation should be considered in patients with significant negative nitrogen balance. Commercially available polymeric and monomeric enteral diets are designed for human patients and have significantly lower protein levels. ProMod (Ross Laboratories) is a readily available protein supplement and contains approximately 75% high-quality protein (5 g/6.6 g scoop). The guideline for dietary protein requirements in dogs is 5 to 7.5 g/100 kcal, the guideline for cats is 6 to 9 g/100 kcal. Patients with renal or hepatic insufficiency should be reduced to less than 3 g/100 kcal in dogs and less than 4 g/100 kcal in cats.

Feeding can begin immediately in patients with good peristalsis noted at surgery, a secure jejunopexy, and an adequate submucosal tunnel of the feeding tube. However, if uncertainty exists, waiting 18 to 24 hours after placement allows a fibrin seal to form at the jejunostomy site and gut motility to normalize. The calculated volume of diet is gradually administered over 4 days (Table 12.5). These are only guidelines, however, and each patient requires a feeding regimen tailored to fit individual needs.

Complications

Complications of jejunostomy tubes include leakage of intestinal contents or diet and are rare; however, they can be devastating (2, 3). Therefore, critical placement and monitoring of the tubes in the early postoperative period are imperative. Peritonitis can result from leakage of intestinal contents from the jejunostomy site or from tube displacement into the peritoneal cavity. Clinical signs of peritonitis include vomiting, tachycardia, pyrexia, and abdominal pain. Patients in which a leak is suspected should be evaluated and treated immediately, because progression of clinical signs can be rapid.

Abdominal discomfort, nausea, vomiting, and diarrhea can occur if the diet is infused too rapidly, if a large dose is given, or if the formula is not tolerated by the patient. Decreasing the amount, rate, or concentration of diet infused may alleviate these problems. If gastrointestinal upset persists, one should consider changing the diet or method of nutritional support.

Metabolic complications can occur and include transient hyperglycemia as a result of the insulin resistance present in many critically ill patients. Occasionally, these patients require additional insulin supplementation. Hypophosphatemia has been reported to develop subsequent to enteral alimentation in severely debilitated cats (9). Complications associated with hypophosphatemia include hemolytic anemia and neurologic signs. Investigators have hypothesized that cats in a state of chronic malnutrition have phosphorus depletion despite normal serum phosphorus levels. The institution of enteral alimentation stimulates insulin secretion and cellular uptake of phosphorus and glucose for glycolysis. Phosphorylation of adenosine diphosphate to adenosine triphosphate results in further phosphorus depletion and severe hypophosphatemia. This condition is referred to as the refeeding phenomenon in humans and was first described in World War II victims. One should begin feeding cautiously in debilitated, hypophosphatemic patients.

References

1. Carnevale JM, et al. Nutritional assessment: guidelines to selecting patients for nutritional support. Compend Contin Educ Pract Vet 1991;13:255–261.
2. Orton EC. Needle catheter jejunostomy. In: Bojrab MJ, ed. Current techniques of small animal surgery. Philadelphia: Lea & Febiger, 1990:257.
3. Moore EE, Moore FA. Immediate enteral nutrition following multisystemic trauma: a decade perspective. J Am Coll Nutr 1995;10:633–648.
4. Marulenda S, Kirby DF. Nutrition support in pancreatitis. Nutr Clin Pract 1995;10:45–53.
5. Freeman LM, et al. Nutritional support in pancreatitis: a retrospective study. J Vet Emerg Crit Care 1995;5:32–41.
6. Bodoky G, et al. Effect of enteral nutrition on exocrine pancreatic function. Am J Surg 1991;161:144–148.
7. Simpson WG, Marsino L, Gates L. Enteral nutritional support in acute alcoholic pancreatitis. J Am Coll Nutr 1995;14:662–665.
8. Guan D, Ohta H, Green GM. Rat pancreatic secretory response to intraduodenal infusion of elemental vs. polymeric defined formula diet. JPEN J Parenter Enteral Nutr 1994;18:335–339.
9. Justin RB, Hohenhaus AE. Hypophosphotemia associated with enteral alimentation in cats. J Vet Intern Med 1995;9:228–233.

— • 13 • —

SALIVARY GLANDS

Sialoceles and Other Salivary Gland Disorders

Charles D. Knecht

Salivary glands and ducts can be affected by inflammation, neoplasia, calculus formation, and rupture. Sialoadenitis is uncommon in mandibular and sublingual glands in the absence of duct rupture, but it is common with rupture of the duct and secondary mucocele. Inflammation of the zygomatic salivary gland, however, is often the result of nonspecific bacterial infection and is one of the causes of retrobulbar abscess. Signs of zygomatic sialoadenitis include tearing, divergent strabismus, and exophthalmos. Drainage of a zygomatic abscess is accomplished through incision of the inflamed mucosa caudolateral to the upper fifth cheek tooth.

Salivary gland tumors are uncommon in small animals. Adenocarcinomas are reported to be more frequent in the mandibular than in the parotid salivary gland and are easier to remove. Tumors of the mandibular gland are associated with a better prognosis if metastasis has not occurred.

Fistulas of the mandibular, sublingual, and zygomatic glands are rare. Fistulation of the parotid gland can result from penetrating wounds or surgical trauma. Fistulas rarely respond to conservative treatment. Complete excision of the gland, closure around a drain, and appropriate antibiotics are required. Fistulas that result from a wound severing the salivary duct can be treated effectively by ligation of the duct proximal to the point of rupture and local excision of the track.

Obstruction of the salivary duct causes transient swelling followed by atrophy of the respective gland. Rupture generally results in accumulation of saliva in the adjacent tissues as a sialocele (mucocele) and in secondary sialoadenitis. According to the usual definitions, cervical sialoceles are located caudal to the mandible in the rostral ventral neck, and sublingual sialoceles (ranulas) are found adjacent to the base of the tongue in the oral cavity. Sialoceles usually are either cervical or sublingual, but they may be both. Pharyngeal sialoceles are less common.

Diagnosis of Salivary Gland Disorders

Neoplasms of the salivary glands generally are characterized by progressive, unilateral enlargement and slow metastasis, with the probable exception of early metastasis of tumors of the parotid salivary gland. Adenocarcinoma of the zygomatic salivary gland causes swelling, exophthalmos, divergent strabismus, and soft tissue swelling adjacent to the globe. The oral mucosa at the duct openings generally is not inflamed. Erosion of the bony orbit is possible and aids in diagnosis. Fine-needle aspiration also may aid in diagnosis.

Although poodles and German shepherds are reported to be most commonly affected with cervical mucoceles, no breed is immune to the disorder. Physical location is helpful in the diagnosis of salivary mucoceles. In the cervical region, onset is marked by a firm, painful swelling medial and caudal to the angle of the mandible. As inflammation subsides, a soft, fluctuant, nonpainful mass gradually enlarges in the neck. Large cervical mucoceles may appear to cross the midline and expand into the pharyngeal area, mimicking branchial cleft cysts. Ranulas appear as elongated fluid accumulations adjacent to the tongue.

Sialography with injection of aqueous contrast medium into the sublingual and mandibular duct openings adjacent to the frenulum of the tongue is an excellent method to define which duct is ruptured, but the procedure is technically difficult and rarely necessary. Aspiration of clear, viscid saliva with an 18-gauge needle is usually diagnostic. The side involved can be defined by careful palpation and observation with slight pressure applied. Observation and palpation may be repeated with the animal in standing and in dorsal recumbent positions.

Surgical Treatment of Sialoceles

Cervical Sialocele

Although incision and drainage of a cervical sialocele occasionally result in cessation of fluid accumulation,

definitive treatment consists of removal of the mandibular and sublingual glands on the affected side. The dog is placed in slight dorsolateral recumbency, with the neck extended over a sandbag or towel and the head rotated so the mandibular salivary gland, located in the confluence of the maxillary and linguofacial veins to form the jugular vein, is dorsal. The skin, subcutaneous tissue, and platysma and depressor auriculae muscles are incised over the glands from the origin of the jugular vein rostrally, medial to the mandible (Fig. 13.1**A**). The capsule of the glands is incised longitudinally to expose the mandibular and the caudal bundle of the sublingual gland (Fig. 13.1**B**). Small veins and one artery deep to the glands may be clamped and not ligated. The glands are elevated to expose the mandibular and sublingual ducts. A combination of blunt and sharp dissection is used to elevate these and the adjacent rostral lobes of the sublingual

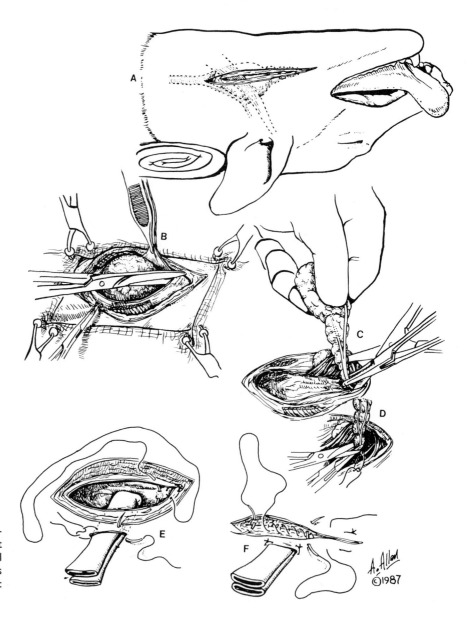

Fig. 13.1. A–F. Cervical sialoadenectomy. See text for details. (From Knecht CD, et al. Selected small animal surgical procedures. In: Fundamental techniques in veterinary surgery. 3rd ed. Philadelphia: WB Saunders, 1987.)

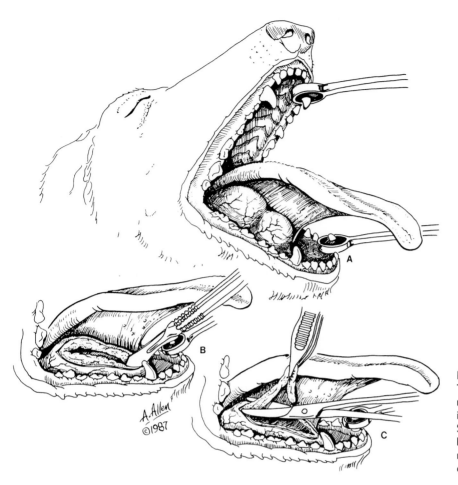

Fig. 13.2. Marsupialization of a ranula. **A.** The mouth is fixed open and prepared with noncaustic surgical scrubs. **B.** A longitudinal incision is made along the dorsal sialocele. Separations between compartments should be excised. **C.** The redundant mucous membrane and granulation tissue are excised around the entire perimeter.

glands to and beneath the mylohyoid muscle (Fig. 13.1**C**). This muscle may be incised to obtain greater exposure of the rostral portion of the ducts. The ducts are ligated with absorbable suture rostral to all glands and then are incised caudal to the ligation and removed with the accompanying glands (Fig. 13.1**D**). The folded center of a Penrose drain is inserted into the sialocele through a small incision made adjacent and parallel to the existing incision; the Penrose drain is fixed with simple interrupted sutures (Fig. 13.1**E**). The mylohyoid muscle, subcutaneous tissue, and platysma are apposed with simple interrupted or simple continuous absorbable sutures, and the skin is closed routinely (Fig. 13.1**F**).

Sublingual Sialocele

Sublingual sialoceles are best treated by marsupialization and partial excision (Fig. 13.2). The animal's mouth is fixed open with a speculum, and the oral cavity is flushed with a suitable noncaustic surgical scrub. The sialocele is incised and bluntly dissected to ensure a single cavity. The redundant mucous membrane and attached granulation tissue lining are excised with scissors. Sutures are not needed.

Zygomatic Sialocele

The zygomatic salivary gland can be approached dorsally or laterally. The lateral approach is more commonly used and is described here. The animal is placed in lateral recumbency, and the affected side of the head, including the eyelids, is prepared for aseptic surgery (Fig. 13.3**A**).

An incision is made through the skin and subcutaneous tissue along the dorsal rim of the zygomatic arch (Fig. 13.3**B**). The palpebral fascia is incised in the same plane, and the periosteum of the zygomatic arch is reflected ventrally. The dorsal half of the zygomatic arch is removed with rongeurs, and the palpebral fascia is retracted dorsally (Fig. 13.3**C**). The globe is retracted dorsally, and orbital fat is bluntly dissected to reveal the zygomatic salivary gland (Fig. 13.3**D**). The gland is lifted dorsally, and the branch of the malar artery to the gland is isolated, clamped, and ligated. The gland is removed if necessary. Then the palpebral fascia is sutured to the periosteum of the zygomatic arch with absorbable suture material (Fig. 13.3**E**). If the retractor anguli muscle has been incised, the cut ends should be reapposed. Subcutaneous tissue and skin are apposed routinely (Fig. 13.3**F**).

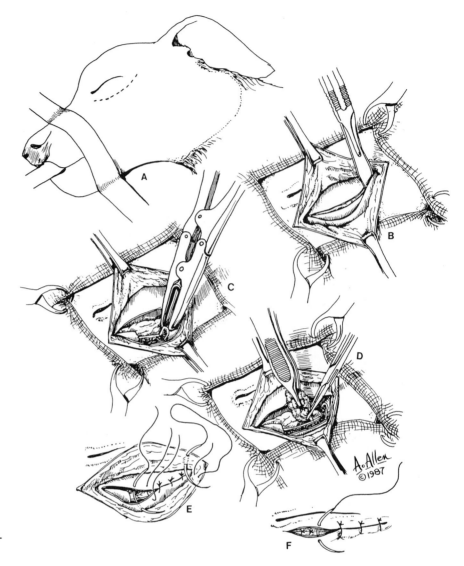

Fig. 13.3. A–F. Zygomatic sialoadenectomy. See text for details.

Suggested Readings

Grandage J, et al. The salivary glands In: Slatter DH, ed. Textbook of small animal surgery. Philadelphia: WB Saunders, 1985.

Harvey CE, et al. Oral, dental, pharyngeal and salivary gland disorders. In: Ettinger SS, ed. Textbook of veterinary internal medicine. 2nd ed. Philadelphia: WB Saunders, 1983.

Knecht CD. Treatment of diseases of the zygomatic salivary gland. J Am Anim Hosp Assoc 1970;6:13.

Knecht CD. Diseases of the salivary glands of the dog. Compend Contin Educ Pract Vet 1980;2:932.

Lammerding JJ. Salivary glands. In: Bojrab MJ, ed. Current techniques in small animal surgery. 2nd ed. Philadelphia: Lea & Febiger, 1983.

Smith MM. Surgery of the canine salivary system. Compend Contin Educ Pract Vet 1985;7:457.

14

ESOPHAGUS

Surgical Approaches to the Esophagus

Walter Renberg & Donald R. Waldron

Surgical Anatomy

The esophagus connects the pharynx and stomach and traverses most of the neck and all of the thorax. In the cranial cervical region, the esophagus is located dorsolateral to the left side of the trachea. The esophagus assumes a left lateral position as it courses caudally in the cervical area. As the esophagus enters the cranial mediastinum at the thoracic inlet, it returns to a more dorsal location by traversing the left lateral trachea at the level of the third thoracic vertebra. At the level of the tracheal bifurcation, the esophagus is dorsal to the trachea and courses along the base of the heart to the right of the aorta. Caudal to the heart, the esophagus lies ventral to the aorta and just to the right of midline; the esophagus and aorta diverge caudally. The esophagus penetrates the diaphragm at the esophageal hiatus, and the gastroesophageal junction normally lies within the abdominal cavity. In the caudal thorax, both right and left vagal nerves course over the lateral esophagus before dividing into dorsal and ventral trunks.

Cervical Esophagus

The patient should be positioned in dorsal recumbency with the head and neck extended and the forelimbs extended caudally and secured. A rolled towel is placed dorsal to the animal's neck in the surgical region, to enhance exposure. Care is taken to ensure that the patient is straight, and tape is used to secure the animal's thorax and head in position.

A skin incision is made on the ventral midline from the level of the larynx to the manubrium, and the subcutaneous fascia is incised to expose the sternohyoideus muscle. The midline is marked by the thin median raphe of the sternohyoideus muscle, which is incised to expose the ventral trachea. Exposure is enhanced by retracting the paired muscle bellies with hand-held or self-retaining Balfour or Rigby retractors (Fig. 14.1). Moistened laparotomy pads are placed to protect the retracted trachea and soft tissues. Branches of the prominent thyroidea ima vein on the ventral surface of the trachea are cauterized or ligated, and the trachea and right carotid sheath are retracted to the right. Care is taken to protect the left recurrent laryngeal nerve, which is closely associated with the left dorsolateral aspect of the trachea. Placement of an esophageal tube aids in identification and manipulation of the esophagus. The esophagus is then packed off with moist laparotomy pads. The surgeon should strive to minimize exposure of the esophagus, to prevent excessive disruption of vasculature.

Approach to the cranial cervical esophagus in animals with cricopharyngeal achalasia is enhanced by placing stay sutures in the thyroid cartilage of the larynx and rotating the larynx to expose the cricopharyngeus and thyropharyngeus muscles. The caudal cervical and cranial thoracic esophagus may be approached (Fig. 14.2) in the manner described, with the following exceptions. The sternocephalicus muscle should be elevated from its insertion on the manubrium and retracted laterally. Gentle cranial traction is applied to the esophagus with stay sutures to gain exposure to the thoracic inlet. If necessary, the manubrium and second sternebra may be divided with bone cutters or an osteotome to increase exposure of the thoracic esophagus.

If extensive tissue dissection is performed, or if esophageal perforation has occurred, a Penrose drain

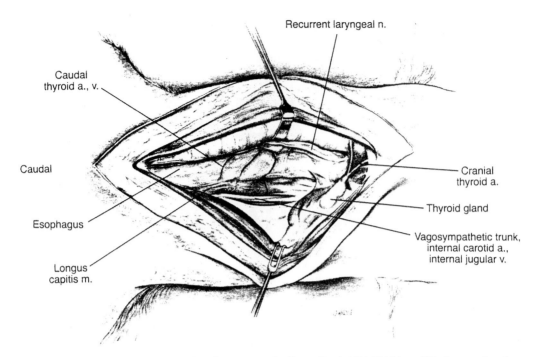

Fig. 14.1. Cervical trachea as seen from a ventral midline approach. (From Smith MM, Waldron DR. Approaches for general surgery of the dog and cat. Philadelphia: WB Saunders, 1993.)

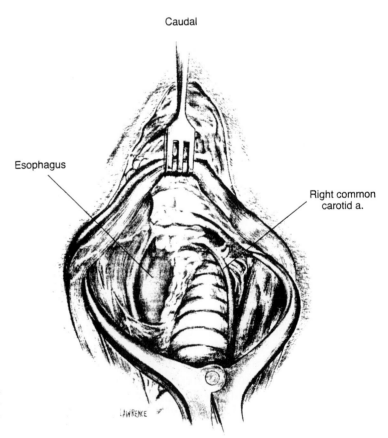

Fig. 14.2. Cranial thoracic esophagus as seen from a cervical approach. (From Smith MM, Waldron DR. Approaches for general surgery of the dog and cat. Philadelphia: WB Saunders, 1993.)

or closed-suction drain should be placed in the peri-esophageal area to decrease postoperative fluid accumulation. The sternohyoideus and sternocephalicus muscles are apposed with absorbable suture. If the sternebrae are incised, they should be apposed with orthopedic wire or nonabsorbable suture. The subcutaneous tissue and skin are closed in a routine manner.

Thoracic Esophagus

Cranial Thoracic Esophagus Through a Left Third Intercostal Thoracotomy

The patient is positioned in right lateral recumbency with a rolled towel placed parallel to the ribs between the patient and the operating table to elevate the surgical field. The clip should extend from past the dorsal and ventral midlines and from the point of the shoulder cranially to the thirteenth rib caudally. Many surgeons prefer a right thoracotomy in this area; however, we believe that the presence of the trachea on the right side makes exposure of the esophagus more difficult.

The skin incision is made just caudal to the caudal border of the scapula (Fig. 14.3). The correct intercostal space can be definitively identified after the latissimus dorsi muscle is incised. The skin incision should extend from the angle of the rib dorsally to the level of the costochondral junction ventrally. The subcutaneous tissues, cutaneous trunci muscle, and latissimus dorsi muscle are incised in the same line. Prominent

bleeding vessels are encountered when transecting the latissimus dorsi muscle and should be cauterized or ligated. Alternatively, the latissimus muscle may be retracted by an assistant; however, we bellieve that this technique is cumbersome. The third intercostal space should be repalpated to verify the location of the incision. An incision is continued ventrally through the scalenus muscle, which inserts on the fifth rib, and then dorsally to parallel the fibers of the serratus ventralis muscle. The intercostal muscles and parietal pleura are gently incised in turn along a line centered between the third and fourth ribs. Moistened laparotomy pads are placed to protect the ribs and soft tissues, and self-retaining Finochietto retractors are used to maintain exposure (Fig. 14.4).

To visualize the esophagus, the cranial lung lobe is packed off caudally with a laparotomy pad moistened with saline. If necessary, an esophageal tube may be placed to aid in identification of the esophagus. The left subclavian artery and vagus nerve should be identified and retracted ventrally (Fig. 14.5). The esophagus is exposed by blunt and sharp dissection of the mediastinal pleura and packed off with moistened laparotomy pads. In the cranial mediastinum, the costocervical vein is seen crossing the esophagus and may be ligated and transected if necessary.

Before closure, a thoracostomy tube is placed to allow evacuation of air from the thorax in the postoperative period. The ribs are loosely apposed using preplaced heavy suture material. The scalenus and serra-

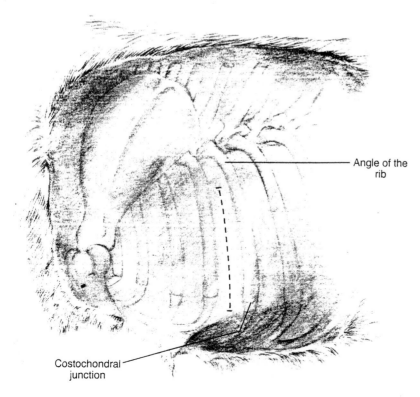

Angle of the rib

Costochondral junction

Fig. 14.3. Location of incision for a left lateral thoracotomy at the fourth intercostal space. (From Smith, Waldron DR. Approaches for general surgery of the dog and cat. Philadelphia: WB Saunders, 1993.)

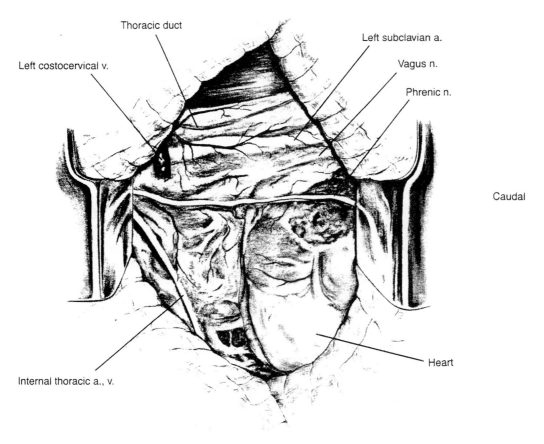

Fig. 14.4. Left cranial thorax seen from the third intercostal space. (From Smith MM, Waldron DR. Approaches for general surgery of the dog and cat. Philadelphia: WB Saunders, 1993.)

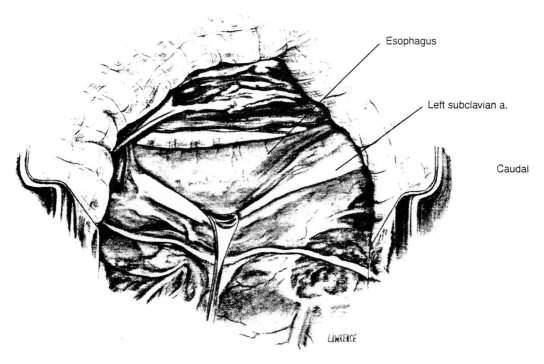

Fig. 14.5. Thoracic esophagus seen from the left third intercostal space. (From Smith MM, Waldron DR. Approaches for general surgery of the dog and cat. Philadelphia: WB Saunders, 1993.)

tus ventralis muscles are apposed, followed by the latissimus dorsi and cutaneous trunci. Finally, the subcutaneous tissues and skin are closed routinely. The thorax should be evacuated, and a bandage should be applied to protect the chest tube. We prefer to administer intrapleural analgesia (1.5 mg/kg bupivacaine in 10 to 20 mL saline given through the thoracotomy tube) to manage postoperative discomfort. When using this technique, the patient must remain in lateral recumbency with the operated side down for approximately 5 minutes after drug administration before anesthesia is concluded.

Midthoracic Esophagus Through a Right Fifth Intercostal Thoracotomy

The patient is positioned in left lateral recumbency with a rolled towel placed parallel to the ribs between the patient and the operating table to elevate the surgical field. The clip should extend from past the dorsal and ventral midlines and from the point of the shoulder cranially to the thirteenth rib caudally.

The skin incision is centered over the fifth intercostal space. This space can be definitively palpated after the latissimus dorsi muscle is incised. The skin incision is made 5 cm caudal to the caudal border of the scapula and extends from the angle of the rib dorsally to just below the level of the costochondral junction ventrally. The subcutaneous tissues, cutaneous trunci muscle, and latissimus dorsi muscle are incised in the same line. The location of the fifth intercostal space

should be reconfirmed by palpation. The scalenus muscle arises from the fifth rib and extends cranially, while the external abdominal oblique muscle arises from the same rib but extends caudally. The external oblique muscle should be elevated from the rib, so the intercostal muscles and parietal pleura may be incised. The rib space is opened with self-retaining retractors after placement of moist laparotomy pads to protect soft tissues.

The lung lobes are packed off caudally using additional moist laparotomy pads. The esophagus is identified with the aid of an esophageal tube. The azygous vein is identified and isolated as it crosses the esophagus at the base of the heart (Fig. 14.6). It may be retracted craniodorsally or doubly ligated and transected. The esophagus is bluntly dissected free of the mediastinal pleura while caution is exercised to prevent damage to the vagus nerve or nearby vessels.

A thoracostomy tube should be placed to allow evacuation of air from the thorax postoperatively, and the ribs are loosely apposed using preplaced heavy nonabsorbable suture material. The latissimus dorsi and cutaneous trunci muscles are apposed after the external abdominal oblique muscle is sutured to the fifth rib, and the latissimus dorsi and cutaneous trunci muscles are apposed with absorbable suture. Finally, the subcutaneous tissues and skin are closed routinely. The thorax should be evacuated, and a bandage should be applied to protect the chest tube. We prefer to administer intrapleural analgesia, as described previously, to manage postoperative pain.

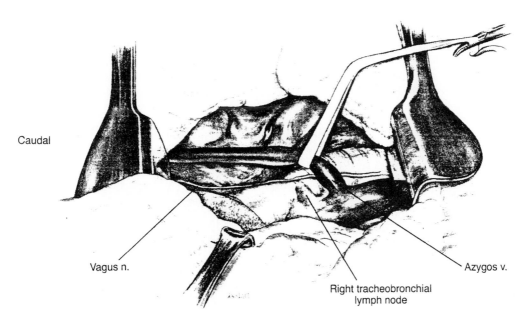

Caudal

Vagus n.

Right tracheobronchial lymph node

Azygos v.

Fig. 14.6. Midthoracic esophagus (base of heart) seen from the right fifth intercostal space. (From Smith MM, Waldron DR. Approaches for general surgery of the dog and cat. Philadelphia: WB Saunders, 1993.)

Caudal Thoracic Esophagus Through a Left Eighth Intercostal Thoracotomy

The patient should be positioned in right lateral recumbency with a rolled towel placed parallel to the ribs between the patient and the operating table to elevate the surgical field. The clip should extend from past the dorsal and ventral midlines and from the point of the shoulder cranially to caudal to the thirteenth rib.

The skin incision is centered over the eighth intercostal space. This space can be definitively palpated after the initial skin and muscle layer incisions. The skin incision should extend from the angle of the rib dorsally to just below the level of the costochondral junction ventrally. The subcutaneous tissues and cutaneous trunci muscle are incised along the same line. The latissimus dorsi muscle can be incised or retracted dorsally. The eighth intercostal space should be repalpated, and the intercostal muscles and parietal pleura should be incised individually along the middle of the intercostal space. Moistened laparotomy pads are placed along the incision to protect the tissue, and the rib space is opened with self-retaining Finochietto retractors.

The left caudal lung lobe is packed off cranially using a moistened laparotomy pad. This technique necessitates transecting the avascular pulmonary ligament, which tethers the lung lobe to the mediastinal pleura. The esophagus is identified, if necessary with the aid of an esophageal tube. Care must be taken to identify the vagal branches, which are bluntly isolated and retracted with umbilical tape (Fig. 14.7). The esophagus is isolated with moist laparotomy pads after blunt dissection of the mediastinum.

A thoracostomy tube should be placed to allow evacuation of air from the thorax, and the ribs are loosely apposed using heavy nonabsorbable suture material. The latissimus dorsi and cutaneous trunci muscles are apposed with absorbable suture, and the subcutaneous tissues and skin are closed routinely. The thorax should be evacuated, and a bandage should be applied to protect the chest tube. We prefer to administer intrapleural analgesia, as described earlier, to manage postoperative pain.

Caudal Thoracic Esophagus Through a Transdiaphragmatic Approach After a Left Eighth Intercostal Thoracotomy

This approach allows removal of distal esophageal foreign bodies through a gastrotomy, thereby avoiding an esophagotomy but allowing visualization of the esophagus (1). The initial approach is identical to that described previously up to and including identification and isolation of the esophagus.

If the surgeon determines that the foreign body is best removed by gastrotomy, the diaphragm is stabilized with stay sutures and an incision is made through the central tendinous portion of the diaphragm. The stomach is identified and is brought into the diaphragmatic incision with additional stay sutures. A gastrotomy incision is made, and care is taken to avoid spillage of gastric contents. Forceps can then be introduced into the distal esophagus from the stomach to remove the foreign body.

The stomach is closed in two layers by first apposing the mucosa in a continuous pattern with an absorbable suture. The remaining layers are closed in an inverting pattern (Cushing or Lembert) with absorbable suture material. The diaphragm is sutured using a continuous pattern of nonabsorbable suture. The thorax is closed as described earlier.

A thoracotomy tube should be placed to allow evacuation of air from the thorax, and the ribs are loosely apposed using preplaced heavy nonabsorbable suture material. The latissimus dorsi and cutaneous trunci muscles are apposed using absorbable suture. Finally, the subcutaneous tissues and skin are closed routinely.

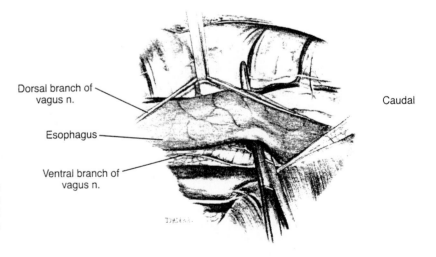

Dorsal branch of vagus n.

Esophagus

Ventral branch of vagus n.

Caudal

Fig. 14.7. Caudal thoracic esophagus seen from the left eighth intercostal space. (From Smith MM, Waldron DR. Approaches for general surgery of the dog and cat. Philadelphia: WB Saunders, 1993.)

The thorax should be evacuated, and a bandage should applied to protect the chest tube. We prefer to administer intrapleural analgesia, as described earlier, to manage postoperative pain.

Abdominal Esophagus (Hiatal Herniorraphy)

The patient is placed in dorsal recumbency and is clipped from cranial to the xiphoid process to the inguinal area caudally. If the surgeon is considering placement of a gastrostomy tube, the preoperative preparation must extend farther dorsolaterally on the left side than normal.

A ventral midline approach to the abdomen is made from the xiphoid process extending caudally to the umbilicus as determined by the conformation of the patient. Moistened laparotomy pads are placed to protect the tissues, and a self-retaining retractor is used to increase exposure to the abdomen. A systematic abdominal exploration is performed, and biopsy samples are taken if indicated.

To expose the hiatal region of the esophagus, the left medial and lateral lobes of the liver are retracted medially (Fig. 14.8). A small incision can be made in the diaphragm to eliminate thoracic negative pressure and thereby to increase mobility of the liver. Stay sutures placed in the diaphragm also assist in caudal retraction and can aid in hiatal exposure. The stomach is retracted caudally with stay sutures, and the ventral and dorsal branches of the vagus nerve are identified. To expose the esophagus fully, the phrenicoesophageal ligament must be incised. This procedure creates a pneumothorax if one has not already been created by incising the diaphragm, so positive-pressure ventila-

tion is required. Care must be taken during closure to seal the thoracic cavity and evacuate air in the chest.

Exposure of the distal esophageal lumen through a gastrotomy is performed with a similar ventral midline abdominal incision. The stomach is stabilized with stay sutures and is packed off with moist laparotomy sponges. A stab incision is made through all layers of the stomach in a minimally vascular area between the lesser and greater curvatures. This incision is extended as needed to obtain visualization of the cardia. The stomach is closed in two layers by first apposing the mucosa in a continuous pattern with an absorbable suture. The remaining layers are closed in an inverting pattern with absorbable suture material. The abdomen is closed using a routine three-layer closure.

Reference

1. Taylor RA. Transdiaphragmatic approach to distal esophageal foreign bodies. J Am Anim Hosp Assoc 1982;18:749–752.

Esophagotomy and Esophageal Anastomosis

Rose J. Lemarié & Giselle Hosgood

Anatomy and Blood Supply

The esophagus can be divided into cervical, thoracic, and abdominal portions. The cervical portion extends from the caudal pharynx to the thoracic inlet and courses slightly to the left of midline. The thoracic portion extends from the thoracic inlet to the esophageal hiatus of the diaphragm. Cranial to the heart, the thoracic esophagus lies to the left of the trachea within the mediastinum. At the level of the carina, the esophagus courses dorsally and to the right to continue ventral to the longus colli muscles along the midline. The dorsal branches of the right and left vagus nerves course along the dorsolateral esophagus and combine to form the dorsal vagal trunk approximately 2 to 4 cm cranial to the esophageal hiatus. The abdominal portion of the esophagus is a short segment that is ventrally apposed to the caudate lobe of the liver (1).

Histologically, the esophagus is divided into four layers consisting of the adventitia, muscularis, submucosa, and mucosa. The thoracic esophagus is partially covered by pleura; the abdominal esophagus is partially covered by peritoneum. The muscular layer of the esophagus consists essentially of two oblique layers of striated muscle fibers. In the caudal esophagus, the fibers of the inner muscle layer become more transverse, whereas those of the outer muscular layer be-

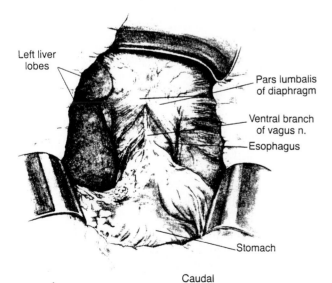

Fig. 14.8. Esophageal hiatus seen from the abdomen. (From Smith MM, Waldron DR. Approaches for general surgery of the dog and cat. Philadelphia: WB Saunders, 1993.)

Left liver lobes

Pars lumbalis of diaphragm

Ventral branch of vagus n.

Esophagus

Stomach

Caudal

come more longitudinal. The striated muscle of the esophagus gradually blends with the smooth muscle of the stomach in the dog (1). In the cat, smooth muscle extends into the thoracic esophagus for approximately one-third of its length and gradually blends with the esophageal striated muscle (2). The submucosa is the connective tissue layer between the mucosa and the muscularis that contains blood vessels, nerves, and glands. It is considered to be the holding layer of the esophagus (3). The esophageal mucosa is composed of superficially cornified stratified squamous epithelium (1).

The arterial blood supply to the cervical esophagus is mainly from branches of the cranial and caudal thyroid arteries. The bronchoesophageal artery is believed to supply the cranial two-thirds of the thoracic esophagus, whereas the esophageal branches of the aorta and the dorsal intercostal arteries are responsible for the blood supply to the remaining thoracic and abdominal esophagus. Venous drainage is through the external jugular veins in the cervical region and through the azygous vein in the thorax. Innervation of the esophagus is through the paired pharyngoesophageal and recurrent laryngeal nerves as well as the dorsal and ventral vagal trunks caudally. Innervation from the sympathetic trunk may also be present. A myenteric plexus is located between the two muscle layers (1).

Indications for Esophagotomy or Resection and Anastomosis

Indications for esophagotomy or esophageal resection and anastomosis include the presence of a foreign body, esophageal perforation, esophageal fistula, esophageal diverticula, and neoplasia. Esophageal foreign body is a common problem in dogs and can be life-threatening. Four areas of the esophagus are predisposed to lodging of foreign bodies because of narrowing: pharyngeal esophagus, thoracic inlet, base of the heart, and diaphragmatic hiatus (4). The diaphragmatic hiatus is the most common site of foreign bodies (4, 5). The most commonly ingested foreign bodies in dogs are bones. Subsequent esophageal perforation can occur as a direct result of ingestion of a sharp, pointed object or from ischemic necrosis due to pressure on the esophageal wall. For this reason, esophageal foreign bodies should be removed as soon as possible. Because of the increased morbidity associated with esophageal surgery, nonsurgical removal with an endoscope or rigid proctoscope may be attempted before surgery if the equipment is available (6). If removal with an endoscope is unsuccessful, it may be possible to push a foreign body from the distal thoracic esophagus into the stomach, to allow removal by gastrotomy, thus avoiding a thoracotomy. In some cases, the for-

eign body may be pulled through the cardia from the distal esophagus through a gastrotomy incision. These techniques for removal should be performed with care if the foreign body has been present for longer than 36 to 48 hours because of the increased risk of perforation through devitalized tissue.

Esophageal perforation may be caused by a foreign body, as noted previously, or it may occur secondary to ingestion of caustic substances, penetrating external trauma, such as bite wounds, incisional dehiscence, traumatic endoscopy, intraluminal stricture dilatation, or esophageal neoplasia. Prolonged clinical signs of esophageal disease and evidence of increased numbers of immature neutrophils on a hemogram may indicate esophageal perforation, and further diagnostic tests should be performed (5). Esophagography and esophagoscopy are the most helpful diagnostic tools in diagnosing esophageal perforation; however, false-negative results can occur with both tests (5). Depending on the length of time the perforation has been present, subcutaneous emphysema, pneumomediastinum, cellulitis, mediastinal abscessation, pleuritis, and pyothorax may result. An untreated esophageal perforation may develop into an esophageal fistula (5, 7).

Esophageal fistulas can be congenital or acquired and may communicate with the trachea, bronchus, or lung parenchyma. Congenital fistulas are probably due to failure of separation of the gastrointestinal and respiratory tracts during embryogenesis (8). Acquired esophageal fistulas are most commonly associated with foreign body ingestion and are most commonly located between the esophagus and the right caudal lung lobe in dogs and between the esophagus and the accessory lobe and left caudal lung lobe in cats (9).

Esophageal diverticuli are congenital defects that result from inherent weakness in the esophageal wall or incomplete separation of the respiratory and gastrointestinal tracts during embryogenesis (9). Diverticuli may be classified as either pulsion or traction. A pulsion diverticulum is defined as an outpouching of mucosa and submucosa between muscular layers and results from intraluminal forces. A traction diverticulum is defined as an outpouching of all layers of the esophagus and usually results from extraluminal forces. Both types of diverticuli are rare in small animals. A normal developmental redundancy of the esophagus may be seen in brachycephalic breeds and shar–peis and should not be confused with a congenital diverticulum (2, 10).

Esophageal neoplasia is rare in small animals in the United States. The most common metastatic esophageal neoplasms are thyroid carcinoma and pulmonary tumors. Reported primary esophageal neoplasms in dogs and cats include squamous cell carcinoma, undifferentiated carcinoma, leiomyoma, osteosarcoma, fibrosarcoma, and scirrhous carcinoma. Sarcoma formation may be more common in locations where *Spirocerca lupi* is found (10).

Clinical Signs

Common clinical signs of esophageal disorders include dysphagia, regurgitation, ptyalism, and repeated attempts to swallow. Depending on the disease and its duration, the animal may appear otherwise healthy. If perforation or fistula formation is present, the animal may appear lethargic and may be febrile. Coughing is a common finding if aspiration pneumonia, esophageal perforation, or bronchoesophageal fistula is present.

Diagnostic Plan

If esophageal disease is indicated from the history and physical examination, thoracic radiography is essential. Because most foreign bodies in dogs are bones, plain radiography may be satisfactory to make the diagnosis. Other radiographic findings associated with esophageal disease include pneumomediastinum, aspiration pneumonia, gaseous dilation of the esophagus, and a mediastinal mass (10).

If thoracic radiographs are nondiagnostic, a positive-contrast esophagram or esophagoscopy is indicated. The most commonly used contrast agent is barium paste or liquid barium. If a perforation is suspected and a positive-contrast esophagram is performed, an organic iodine contrast medium should be used instead of barium until a perforation can be ruled out. The normal canine esophagus has linear mucosal striations throughout its length, whereas the distal feline esophagus usually has circular mucosal folds that form a herringbone pattern with positive contrast (10).

Esophagoscopy has the advantage of enabling one to visualize the mucosal surface of the esophagus and to evaluate the damage. A foreign body may be grasped with forceps and removed with the endoscope. If a mass is present, endoscopy can be used to obtain a biopsy sample without the need for surgery. Complications of esophagoscopy include perforation of a compromised esophagus and inability to evaluate the structures surrounding the esophagus completely for evidence of perforation that is not visible from the mucosal surface.

Surgical Technique

General Principles

The esophagus has several inherent characteristics that make it predisposed to postoperative complications such as dehiscence. These characteristics include its segmental blood supply, lack of a serosal covering, and lack of the omentum to provide an initial seal in the thoracic cavity. The esophagus is also constantly moving and exposed to luminal irritation and distension by ingesta and saliva. If a section of esophagus is removed, tension on the suture line can result in failure (7, 11). For these reasons, tissues must be handled carefully and atraumatically. Tension along the suture line should be avoided (7).

Esophagotomy

Stay sutures are placed in the esophagus for atraumatic immobilization, and the affected segment is isolated from the rest of the thorax using moistened laparotomy sponges. A stomach tube or esophageal stethoscope may help to facilitate identification of the esophagus as well as to provide support while incising the esophagus. The esophagus should be packed off from surrounding tissues using moistened sponges or laparotomy pads. The esophageal incision is made longitudinally in a healthy portion of the esophagus. If a foreign body is present, the esophagus is incised just distal to it, and the foreign body is grasped with an instrument and removed with gentle traction and manipulation. The tissues are inspected for damage and viability. The surgeon must explore the surrounding mediastinum and thorax for damage or additional foreign bodies. If nonviable esophageal tissue is suspected, various patching techniques or resection and anastomosis should be considered. The wound is lavaged thoroughly before closure.

Closure of the esophagus is best performed using a two-layer, simple interrupted suture pattern. This pattern results in the greatest immediate wound strength and the best tissue apposition and healing when compared with single-layer techniques (Fig. 14.9) (11). The first layer should incorporate the mucosa and submucosa, with the knots tied in the lumen of the esophagus. The second layer should incorporate the muscularis and adventitia, and the knots should be tied externally. Sutures should be placed carefully and should be approximately 2 mm apart. The holding layer of the esophagus has been shown to be the submucosa; therefore, the first layer is the most important (3). An absorbable, monofilament, minimally reactive suture material (3–0 or 4–0), such as polydioxanone (PDS, Ethicon, Inc., Somerville, NJ) or poliglecaprone 25 (Monocryl, Ethicon, Inc.), with a swaged-on taper or reverse-cutting needle is recommended for esophageal surgery (7).

Esophageal Resection and Anastomosis

Because of the complications associated with esophageal healing and excessive tension, resection of the esophagus should be considered only if necessary.

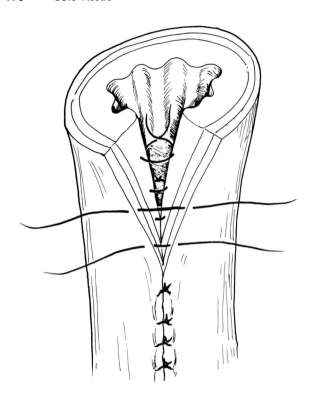

Fig. 14.9. The mucosa and submucosa are closed using simple interrupted sutures with the knots placed in the lumen. The muscularis is closed over the mucosa and submucosa in a separate layer using simple interrupted sutures with the knots on the outside.

Small perforations should be debrided and closed primarily in two layers if possible (5, 7). Tension has been reported to be present when only 2 cm of the esophagus is removed. If a larger segment of esophagus needs to be removed, an esophageal reconstruction technique may be attempted. The desired esophageal segment to be resected is isolated as described previously and is held with stay sutures. The esophageal lumen is occluded with atraumatic intestinal clamps, such as Doyen or Péan clamps, and the desired tissue segment is resected along the outside edge of the clamps.

The esophageal lumen is closed in a two-layer, interrupted pattern as described for esophagotomy closure. The first layer should incorporate the mucosa and submucosa, and the knots should be tied intraluminally as described for esophagotomy (Fig. 14.10). The first suture should be placed on the far side between the dorsal and the ventral stay sutures, and subsequent sutures should be placed on either side in alternating fashion until closure is complete. The final sutures placed in the inner layer may be preplaced to facilitate tying of the knots in the lumen. The second layer is placed in the muscularis and adventitia and is also placed in an interrupted pattern with external knots.

Fig. 14.10. Anastomosis of the esophagus using simple interrupted sutures in the mucosa and submucos, with the knots placed in the lumen. Note the stay sutures. The muscularis would be closed over the mucosa and submucosa in a separate layer using simple interrupted sutures with the knots on the outside. (From Bojrab MJ, ed. Current techniques in small animal surgery. 2nd ed. Philadelphia: Lea & Febiger, 1983:138.)

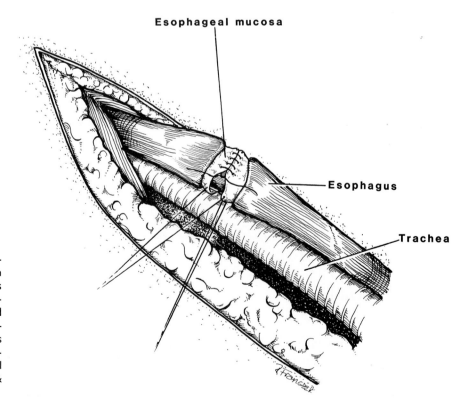

Esophageal mucosa

Esophagus

Trachea

To minimize tension at the anastomotic site, several procedures have been attempted. Esophageal immobilization by dissection from surrounding structures provides minimal advancement and may risk damage to the segmental blood supply. A circular myotomy of the outer muscular layer of the esophagus while preserving the inner muscular layer may relieve tension in some cases. This can be performed at a site proximal and distal to the anastomosis (7, 12). After closure of the intrathoracic esophagus, a section of omentum may be pulled through an incision in the diaphragm or a subcutaneous tunnel and placed over the esophageal incision to provide a seal and to enhance blood supply to the area (7, 13).

Postoperative Care and Complications

Postoperative care should be aimed at decreasing mechanical trauma to the esophageal incision while providing nutritional support to the patient. Feeding tubes have been advocated to reduce mechanical trauma caused by food and peristaltic activity. Gastrostomy tubes are superior to pharyngostomy tubes because the physical presence of a pharyngostomy tube across the esophageal incision can delay healing (5, 7). If a feeding tube is not placed at surgery, soft food should be fed for 7 days beginning 24 hours postoperatively (7). Esophageal stricture has been reported after esophageal surgery and may be due to tissue damage by a foreign body, excessive surgical trauma, or reflux esophagitis. Esophageal inflammation may decrease the effectiveness of esophageal peristaltic activity and may diminish lower esophageal sphincter tone, resulting in continued gastroesophageal reflux and esophagitis (4). The H_2-receptor blocking agents, such as cimetidine or ranitidine, should be used to control esophagitis by decreasing reflux of gastric acid into the esophagus. Esophageal wounds are also predisposed to infection; therefore, perioperative and postoperative antibiotics are indicated (4, 5, 7).

References

1. Evans HE, Christensen GC, eds. Miller's anatomy of the dog. 2nd ed. Philadelphia: WB Saunders, 1979.
2. Twedt DC. Diseases of the esophagus. In: Ettinger SJ, Feldman EC, eds. Textbook of veterinary internal medicine. Philadelphia: WB Saunders, 1995:1124–1142.
3. Dallman MJ. Functional suture-holding layer of the esophagus in the dog. J Am Vet Med Assoc 1988;192:638–640.
4. Spielman BL, Shaker EH, Garvey MS. Esophageal foreign body in dogs: a retrospective study of 23 cases. J Am Anim Hosp Assoc 1992;28:570–574.
5. Parker NR, Walter PA, Gay J. Diagnosis and surgical management of esophageal perforation. J Am Anim Hosp Assoc 1989;25:587–594.
6. Tams TR. Endoscopic removal of gastrointestinal foreign bodies. In: Small animal endoscopy. St. Louis: CV Mosby, 1990:245–255.
7. Flanders JA. Problems and complications associated with esophageal surgery. Probl Vet Med 1989;1:183–194.
8. Basher AWP, Hogan PM, Hanna PE, et al. Surgical treatment of a congenital bronchoesophageal fistula in a dog. J Am Vet Med Assoc 1991;199:479–482.
9. Fingeroth JM. Surgical diseases of the esophagus. In: Slatter D, ed. Textbook of small animal surgery. Philadelphia: WB Saunders, 1993:534–548.
10. Stickle RL, Love NE. Radiographic diagnosis of esophageal diseases in dogs and cats. Semin Vet Med Surg (Small Anim) 1989;4:179–187.
11. Oakes MG, Hosgood G, Snider TG, et al. Esophagotomy closure in the dog: a comparison of a double-layer appositional and two single-layer appositional techniques. Vet Surg 1993;22:451–456.
12. Attum AA, Hankins JR, Ngangana J, et al. Circular myotomy as an aid to resection and end-to-end anastomosis of the esophagus. Ann Thorac Surg 1979;28:126–132.
13. Hosgood G. The omentum—the forgotten organ: pathophysiology and potential surgical applications in dogs and cats. Compend Contin Educ Pract Vet 1990;12:45–50.

Esophageal Hiatal Hernia Repair

Caroline Prymak

An esophageal hiatal hernia is defined as the protrusion of abdominal contents through the esophageal hiatus of the diaphragm into the thorax. Of the two types of hiatal hernia recognized in the dog and cat, a sliding hiatal hernia, in which the abdominal part of the esophagus and part of the stomach are displaced cranially through the esophageal hiatus, is the most common type (1–15). A paraesophageal hiatal hernia, in which the abdominal part of the esophagus and lower esophageal sphincter remain in a fixed position but a portion of the stomach herniates into the mediastinum alongside the thoracic esophagus, has also been reported (16, 17).

Esophageal hiatal hernias are also classified as congenital or acquired (2, 14). Investigators have proposed that congenital hiatal hernia results from an inherent weakness of the phrenoesophageal suspensory apparatus. Acquired hiatal hernias are usually associated with a history of blunt abdominal trauma with sudden increases in intra-abdominal pressure and degenerative or traumatic weakening of the diaphragmatic structures forming the esophageal hiatus. Most cases of esophageal hiatal hernia have been reported in animals younger than 1 year of age and are congenital. The most commonly affected breed is the Chinese shar–pei (1, 2).

Diagnosis

CLINICAL SIGNS AND PHYSICAL FINDINGS

The clinical signs associated with hiatal hernia vary in severity from occasional episodes of anorexia, dysphagia, hypersalivation, and regurgitation to vomiting, hematemesis, and dyspnea. Cardiac arrest may occur when large hernias affect the cardiopulmonary system. Hiatal hernias may also be asymptomatic and have been reported as incidental findings during thoracic or abdominal radiography or on postmortem examination. Clinical signs are usually more severe with congenital lesions than with acquired lesions.

Physical examination is often nonremarkable in mild cases, but signs can include fever, dehydration, hypersalivation, and pulmonary wheezes and crackles. In most cases, the results of laboratory tests are not significant, although hemoconcentration and mature neutrophilia may occur.

RADIOGRAPHY AND OTHER DIAGNOSTIC PROCEDURES

Most cases of congenital hiatal hernia can be diagnosed on survey radiographs by the presence of a caudodorsal gas-filled intrathoracic soft tissue opacity and by varying degrees of megaesophagus. In patients with sliding hiatal hernia in which the esophagus and stomach are displaced only intermittently, positive pressure applied to the abdomen may be necessary to induce cranial displacement of the distal esophagus and stomach. The diagnosis of acquired hiatal hernia may be more difficult and can require repeated barium esophagram studies. Barium esophagrams have been recommended to examine the caudal esophageal sphincter, esophageal hiatus, and cardia. When contrast studies are performed under fluoroscopy, results can be used to assess esophageal motility, diameter, and, to a lesser extent, caudal esophageal sphincter function by the extent of gastroesophageal reflux. Survey radiographs of the chest should be evaluated for dependent alveolar consolidation consistent with aspiration pneumonia.

In patients with paraesophageal hiatal hernia, definitive diagnosis generally is made by fluoroscopic detection of the gastric herniation after special studies such as esophagography and gastrography. With paraesophageal hiatal hernia, various degrees of displacement of the stomach have been seen on serial radiographs (16).

Endoscopic examination may provide additional evidence of a sliding hiatal hernia. Distal reflux esophagitis and an open lower esophageal sphincter have been identified (8). In one case, manometry has been used to record a loss of the caudal esophageal sphincter pressure (7).

Esophageal acid–clearing tests, 24-hour pH monitoring for reflux, and manometry are routinely used in human patients to help characterize esophageal hiatal hernia so proper therapy can be selected. The usefulness of many of these tests is limited in veterinary medicine.

Pathophysiology

In the absence of known causative factors, an inherent weakness of the phrenoesophageal suspensory apparatus is believed to be responsible for the development of esophageal hiatal hernia (18). A hiatal hernia rarely causes clinical signs itself unless a large hernia impairs cardiopulmonary function. Of more significance is the role of hiatal hernia in the development of gastroesophageal reflux and esophagitis causing secondary megaesophagus and esophageal hypomotility. The role of hiatal hernia in the pathophysiology of gastroesophageal reflux disease has not been fully elucidated in dogs and cats. To complicate the situation further, gastroesophageal reflux has been documented as a normal physiologic occurrence in the dog (20). Furthermore, one report documented radiographic evidence of primary segmental or generalized esophageal hypomotility in clinically normal Chinese shar–pei pups (21). This breed has a high incidence of hiatal hernia. Important factors in the occurrence and severity of reflux esophagitis with hiatal hernia are the age of the animal and the composition of the refluxed material (22–24). The occurrence of gastroesophageal reflux is significantly increased in young animals because of developmental immaturity of the caudal esophageal sphincter.

The pathogenesis of gastroesophageal reflux disease is multifactorial: the caudal esophageal sphincter, esophageal peristalsis, esophageal clearance, and gastric function are important factors (25). Evidence suggests that the caudal esophageal sphincter and diaphragmatic crura work together to form a sphincter in which the muscle of the caudal esophageal sphincter coordinates with the striated muscle of the diaphragm to protect the esophagus against reflux (26). By altering this anatomic relationship, a hiatal hernia could contribute to incompetence at the gastroesophageal junction. In a study in human patients with gastroesophageal reflux disease, those with a small hiatal hernia and those with no hiatal hernia had similar abnormalities of lower esophageal sphincter function and acid clearance. In patients with larger hiatal hernias (larger than 3 cm), the lower esophageal sphincter was shorter and weaker, the amount of reflux was greater, and acid clearance was less efficient. The degree of esophagitis was worse in patients with a large hiatal hernia (27).

With paraesophageal hiatal hernia, a portion of the stomach is displaced into the mediastinum alongside the adjacent esophagus. The caudal esophageal sphincter is usually considered to remain functional because it is maintained in a normal intra-abdominal position. Reflux esophagitis is therefore less commonly associated with this condition. Clinical signs are generally those associated with caudal esophageal obstruction and gastric strangulation.

Medical Therapy

The rationale for medical therapy is based on the assumption that reflux esophagitis contributes to the clinical signs of hiatal hernia. Neutralization or suppression of gastric acid secretion can be achieved by the use of antacids or H_2-receptor antagonists. Antacids also work by increasing the caudal esophageal sphincter pressure secondary to the elevation of the pH of the gastric contents. Metoclopramide is a prokinetic drug that decreases reflux esophagitis by increasing the caudal esophageal sphincter pressure. It can also reduce intragastric pressure by its positive effect on gastric emptying. Sucralfate has also been recommended to provide a diffusion barrier to peptic mucosal digestion. Dietary management is also important. A low-fat, liquid diet enhances gastric emptying and thereby may reduce the incidence of gastroesophageal reflux. Several small daily feedings are recommended. Patients with megesophagus and esophageal hypomotility should be fed from a height.

Conservative therapy has been most effective in patients with small hiatal hernias and mild to moderate clinical signs. Symptomatic animals with congenital hiatal hernia generally have responded less well to medical therapy than those with acquired hiatal hernia (2). In general, symptomatic animals with large hiatal hernias or permanent displacement of the herniated stomach and those that do not respond to conservative management are surgical candidates. Animals with paraesophageal hiatal hernia should be treated surgically.

Preoperative Evaluation

The patient should be evaluated for fluid and electrolyte imbalances, which must be corrected before surgery. Clinical or radiographic signs of aspiration pneumonia should be treated aggressively with antimicrobial therapy.

Surgical Techniques

SLIDING ESOPHAGEAL HIATAL HERNIA

The aims of surgical treatment are to reposition the cardia and terminal esophagus below the diaphragm, to narrow the hiatus if enlarged, and to fix the stomach and caudal esophageal sphincter caudal to the diaphragm. In animals with a primary incompetence of

the caudal esophageal sphincter, an antireflux procedure is indicated.

The patient is placed in dorsal recumbency with the operating table tilted so the animal's head and neck are slightly elevated relative to the abdomen. A ventral midline celiotomy is performed from the xiphoid to the umbilicus. The hepatogastric ligament is transected, and the left lateral and medial lobes of the liver are retracted medially to expose the esophageal hiatus. If the stomach is partially herniated, it is reduced manually together with any other abdominal organs contained in the hernia sac (Fig. 14.11). A ventral 180° circumferential incision is made in the phrenoesophageal ligament (comprising the parietal peritoneum and the transversalis fascia), with care taken to avoid damage to the ventral vagal trunk (Fig. 14.12). This allows the caudal 2 to 3 cm of the distal esophagus containing the caudal esophageal sphincter to be retracted into the abdomen. The right and left crura of the diaphragm are identified and are approximated to reduce the hiatus to a diameter of 1 to 2 cm. Four to five 2–0 polypropylene or polydioxanone sutures are closely placed in a simple interrupted pattern. The abdominal esophagus is anchored in the abdomen by placing two to four simple interrupted sutures of 3–0 polydioxanone through the surrounding diaphragm and into the tunica muscularis of the esophagus as it passes through the esophageal hiatus (esophagopexy) (Fig. 14.13). A fundic gastropexy to the left body wall is performed using either tube or incisional gastropexy technique. A tube gastropexy has the added advantage of minimizing the problem of "gas bloat syndrome" that has been reported when using antireflux procedures. It also provides a route for enteral nutrition if the patient has severe preexisting esophageal dysfunction or if anorexia occurs postoperatively.

After hiatal plication, a catheter can be inserted through the diaphragm and air evacuated from the pleural cavity until negative pressure is established. If evacuation of the pleural cavity is inadequate, a temporary chest tube can be inserted through a lateral thoracotomy stab incision at the sixth or seventh intercostal space.

PARAESOPHAGEAL HIATAL HERNIA

Surgical repair includes reduction of herniated contents, plication of the diaphragmatic crura, esophagopexy, and gastropexy.

ANTIREFLUX PROCEDURES

Antireflux procedures are indicated when primary incompetence of the caudal esophageal sphincter causes gastroesophageal reflux disease. These techniques have been developed to create an intra-abdominal high-pressure zone. In animals with hiatal hernia, primary incompetence of the caudal esophageal sphincter

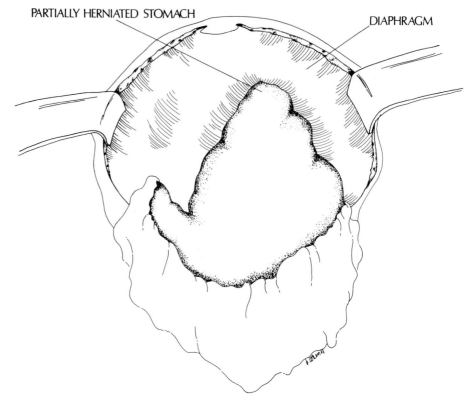

PARTIALLY HERNIATED STOMACH

DIAPHRAGM

Fig. 14.11. Cranial displacement of the stomach through the esophageal hiatus of the diaphragm. (From Prymak C, Saunders HM, Washabau RJ. Hiatal hernia repair by restoration and stabilisation of normal anatomy: an evaluation in four dogs and one cat. Vet Surg 1989;18:386–391.)

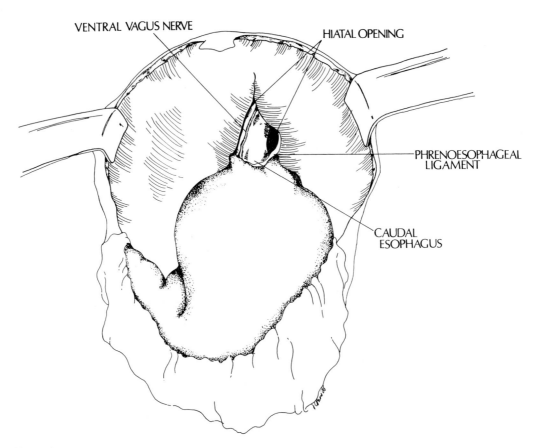

VENTRAL VAGUS NERVE

HIATAL OPENING

PHRENOESOPHAGEAL LIGAMENT

CAUDAL ESOPHAGUS

Fig. 14.12. Ventral incision in the phrenoesophageal ligament for retraction of the esophagus into the abdomen. (From Prymak C, Saunders HM, Washabau RJ. Hiatal hernia repair by restoration and stabilisation of normal anatomy: an evaluation in four dogs and one cat. Vet Surg 1989;18:386–391.)

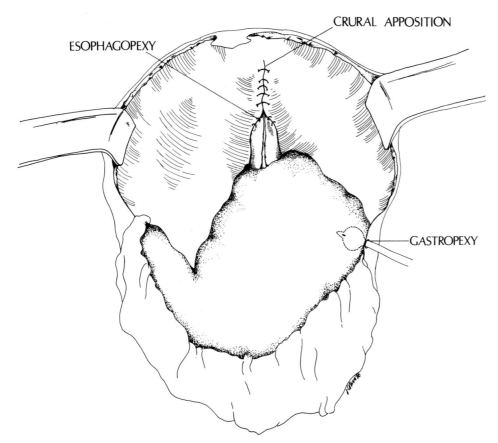

ESOPHAGOPEXY

CRURAL APPOSITION

GASTROPEXY

Fig. 14.13. Diaphragmatic crural apposition, esophagopexy, and gastropexy for reduction in size of the esophageal hiatus and fixation of the esophagus and stomach within the abdomen. (From Prymak C, Saunders HM, Washabau RJ. Hiatal hernia repair by restoration and stabilisation of normal anatomy: an evaluation in four dogs and one cat. Vet Surg 1989;18:386–391.)

has not been routinely documented because of the difficulty in performing manometric studies. Success has been reported with and without the use of antireflux procedures in the surgical management of hiatal hernia (1–3, 14). The two antireflux techniques reported in small animals are Nissen fundoplication (3, 5, 11, 12, 14) and Belsey fundoplication (7, 17). The Nissen technique is the simplest procedure and is most commonly used in small animals.

NISSEN FUNDOPLICATION

Before the procedure, the patient's stomach is intubated with a large stomach tube (28 to 32 French) to act as a stent. The esophagus below the diaphragm is drawn caudally into the abdomen with a loop of umbilical tape or Penrose drain (Fig. 14.14). The cranial wall of the fundus is passed with one or two fingers underneath the esophagus toward the right side of the abdomen (Fig. 14.15). The fundus of the stomach is sutured back to itself using a simple interrupted partial-thickness suture pattern. Each suture incorporates the tunica muscularis of the esophagus. About four sutures of 2–0 or 3–0 nonabsorbable material are used to hold the cuff in place (Fig. 14.16). The fundus of the stomach should comfortably form a cuff around

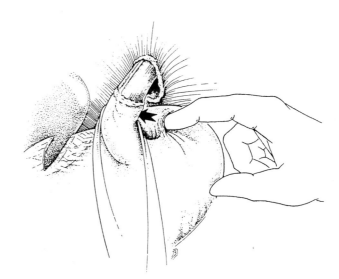

Fig. 14.14. Nissen fundoplication. The fundus of the stomach is passed underneath the retracted esophagus. The ventral vagal nerve is visible at the displaced thoracic part of the esophagus.

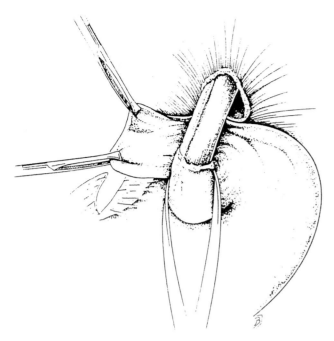

Fig. 14.15. Nissen fundoplication. The displaced fundus of the stomach is held in position with tissue forceps. The ventral vagal nerve is visible at the displaced thoracic part of the esophagus.

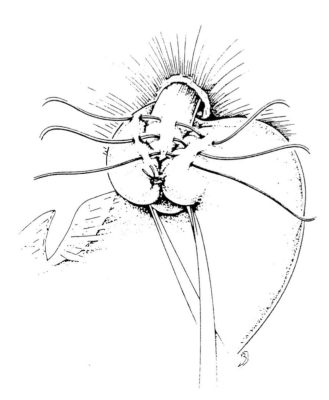

Fig. 14.16. Nissen fundoplication. Seromuscular sutures are passed through the stomach and esophagus. Retraction is maintained until the first two sutures have been tied.

the lower 3 to 4 cm of the esophagus without excess tension on the displaced stomach wall.

Postoperative Care and Complications

Medical therapy with antibiotics, antacids, and prokinetic agents is recommended postoperatively, depending on the clinical course and radiographic assessment of lobar pneumonia, esophageal size, and motility. Resolution of megaesophagus and improved esophageal motility have been documented as early as 7 days postoperatively, but patients should be individually monitored until esophageal function returns to normal (1). Patients with severe esophagitis should have oral food withheld, but they can be fed through a gastrostomy tube if gastric function is normal. When oral feeding is commenced, patients should be fed from a height if they have esophageal dysfunction. Small quantities of low-fat, liquid diets are initially recommended.

The most commonly reported postoperative complications are death from aspiration pneumonia and persistent vomiting and or regurgitation (1, 2, 7, 11, 13, 14, 17) These signs have been attributed to chronic gastric dilation and delayed gastric emptying of solids. Gastroparesis may occur secondary to interference with gastric vagal innervation, or it may be caused by temporary disruption of the gastric pacemaker in the gastric body by the gastropexy technique. In the Chinese shar–pei, investigators have also suggested that hiatal hernia may be one manifestation of a more diffuse gastrointestinal motility disorder (28).

The gas bloat syndrome has been reported as a specific complication of a fundoplication technique (11) This may occur because of a combined effect of difficult eructation resulting from fundoplication and gastroparesis. Careful surgical technique is required to minimize this complication. Pneumothorax has also been reported as a complication of hiatal hernia repair, but it is a logical consequence of severing the phrenoesophageal membrane and should be managed accordingly during the surgical procedure (5, 11).

References

1. Prymak C, Saunders HM, Washabau RJ. Hiatal hernia repair by restoration and stabilisation of normal anatomy: an evaluation in four dogs and one cat. Vet Surg 1989;18:386–391.
2. Callan MB, Washabau RJ, Saunders HM, et al. Congenital esophageal hiatal hernia in the Chinese Shar-Pei dog. J Vet Intern Med 1993;7:210–215.
3. Ellison GW, Lewis DD, Phillips L, et al. Literature review of hiatal hernia in small animals. J Am Anim Hosp Assoc 1987;23:391–399.
4. Waldron DR, Moon M, Leib MS, et al. Esophageal hiatal hernia in two cats. J Small Anim Pract 1990;31:259–253.
5. Peterson SL. Esophageal hiatal hernia in a cat. J Am Vet Med Assoc 1983;183:325–326.

6. Ackerman NA. Esophageal hiatal hernia in a dog. J Am Vet Radiol Soc 1982;23:107–108.

7. Dhein CRM, Rawlings CA, Rosin E, et al. Esophageal hiatal hernia and eventration of the diaphragm with resultant gastroesophageal reflux. J Am Anim Hosp Assoc 1980;16:517–522.

8. Robotham GR. Congenital hiatal hernia in a cat. Feline Pract 1979;9:37–39.

9. Iwasaki M, De Martin BW, Alvarage J, et al. Congenital hiatal hernia in a dog. Mod Vet Pract 1977;58:1018–1019.

10. Alexander JW, Hoffer RE, MacDonald JM, et al. Hiatal hernia in the dog: a case report and review of the literature. J Am Anim Hosp Assoc 1975;11:793–797.

11. Gaskell CJ, Gibbs C, Pearson H. Sliding hiatal hernia with reflux esophagitis in two dogs. J Small Anim Pract 1974;15:503–509.

12. Frye FL. Hiatal diaphragmatic hernia and tricholithiasis in a golden cat. Vet Med Small Anim Clinician 1972;67:391–392.

13. Kluth GA, Kennea TL. A case of hiatus hernia in a boxer dog. Vet Rec 1964;76:501–502.

14. Bright RM, Sackman JE, DeNovo C, et al. Hiatal hernia in the dog and cat: a retrospective study of 16 cases. J Small Anim Pract 1990;31:244–250.

15. Twedt DC. Endoscopy case of the month: regurgitation in a puppy. Vet Med 1993;88:830–835.

16. Miles KG, Pope ER, Jergens AE. Paraesophageal hiatal hernia and pyloric obstruction in the dog. J Am Vet Med Assoc 1988;193:1437–1439.

17. Teunissen GHB, Happe RP, Van Toorenburg J, et al. Esophageal hiatal hernia. Tijdschr Diergeneeskd 1978;103:742–749.

18. Eliska O. Phrenoesophageal membrane and its role in the development of hiatal hernia. Acta Anat 1973;86:137–150.

19. Baue AE, Hoffer RE. The effects of experimental hiatal hernia and histamine stimulation on the intrinsic esophageal sphincter. Surg Gynecol Obstet 1967;125:791–799.

20. Patrikios J, Martin CJ, Dent J. Relationship of transient lower esophageal sphincter relaxation to postprandial gastroesophageal reflux and belching in dogs. Gastroenterology 1986; 90:545–551.

21. Stickle R, Sparschu G, Love N, et al. Radiographic evaluation of esophageal function in Chinese Shar Pei pups. J Am Vet Med Assoc 1992;201:81–84.

22. Hillimeier C, Gryboski J, McCallum R, et al. Developmental characteristics of the lower esophageal sphincter in the kitten. Gastroenterology 1985;89:760–766.

23. Cohen S. Developmental characteristics of lower esophageal sphincter function. Gastroenterology 1974;67:252–258.

24. Evander A, Little AG, Riddell RH, et al. Composition of the refluxed material determines the degree of reflux esophagitis in the dog. Gastroenterology 1987;93:280–286.

25. Kahrilas PJ, Dodds WJ, Hogan WJ. Effects of peristaltic dysfunction on esophageal volume clearance. Gastroenterology 1988;94:73–80.

26. Boyle JT, Altschuler SM, Nixon TE, et al. Role of the diaphragm in the genesis of lower esophageal sphincter pressure in the cat. Gastroenterology 1985;88:723–730.

27. Patti MG, Goldberg HI, Arcerito M, et al. Hiatal hernia size affects lower esophageal sphincter function, esophageal acid exposure, and the degree of mucosal injury. Am J Surg 1996;171:182–186.

28. Knowles KE, O'Brien DP, Amann JF. Congenital idiopathic megaesophagus in a litter of Chinese shar peis: clinical, electrodiagnostic, and pathological findings. J Am Anim Hosp Assoc 1990;26:313–318.

15

STOMACH

Gastrotomy

Mary L. Dulisch

The most common indications for gastrotomy are to remove foreign bodies, to inspect the gastric mucosa for ulcers, neoplasms, or hypertrophy, and to obtain a biopsy specimen. Before the surgical procedure, the entire gastrointestinal tract should be examined thoroughly by physical examination and radiography to determine whether additional lesions are present. The patient should be evaluated for fluid and electrolyte imbalances; these should be corrected before the operation.

Surgical Technique

The patient is placed in dorsal recumbency, and a ventral midline incision is made extending from the xiphoid to just caudal to the umbilicus. Moistened laparotomy pads are placed on either side of the incision and are folded over the cut edges. A Balfour retractor is used to retract the abdominal wall, and a complete abdominal exploratory operation is performed. The stomach is grossly inspected and then is elevated from the abdomen with the use of Babcock forceps (Fig. 15.1A) or stay sutures. The forceps or sutures are placed in the least vascular area of the body of the stomach approximately 10 cm apart. The surrounding abdominal structures are packed off with moistened laparotomy pads. The gastrotomy incision is made in the hypovascular area on the ventral aspect of the stomach between the lesser and greater curvatures. Using a No. 10 Bard–Parker scalpel blade with the cutting edge up, a stab incision is made into the lumen of the stomach (Fig. 15.1B). This incision is extended with Metzenbaum scissors toward the forceps (Fig. 15.1C and D). The length of the incision depends on the reason for the gastrotomy. Suction is used to evacuate the stomach and to prevent spillage of gastric contents. After inspection of the lumen, the stomach is closed in a two-layer inverting seromuscular pattern using 2–0 or 3–0 synthetic absorbable suture. The first layer consists of a Cushing pattern. The sutures begin at the serosal surface and penetrate to, but not through, the mucosa (Fig. 15.1E and F). The second layer consists of a Lembert pattern using 2–0 or 3–0 synthetic absorbable, polypropylene or nylon suture (Fig. 15.1G). After closure, the area should be gently cleansed or lavaged with warm, sterile saline solution. Omentum may be placed over the incision if desired. Two simple interrupted sutures of 3–0 absorbable suture material are sufficient for local omental attachment.

Postoperative Care

No food, water, or medication is given for 24 hours. Maintenance fluid requirements are sustained with intravenous fluids. Water can be offered 24 hours after the operation. Once the patient has started to drink on its own, the intravenous fluids are gradually discontinued. A soft diet consisting of small amounts of baby food or a soft dog food gruel can be started if water is not vomited. This diet can be fed several times a day, and the consistency of the food can be thickened with each succeeding day. If vomiting occurs, oral intake is discontinued, and injectable metoclopramide can be given at a dosage of 0.2 to 0.4 mg/kg every 8 hours. Once vomiting is controlled, food can be offered again. Oral metoclopramide may be continued as needed.

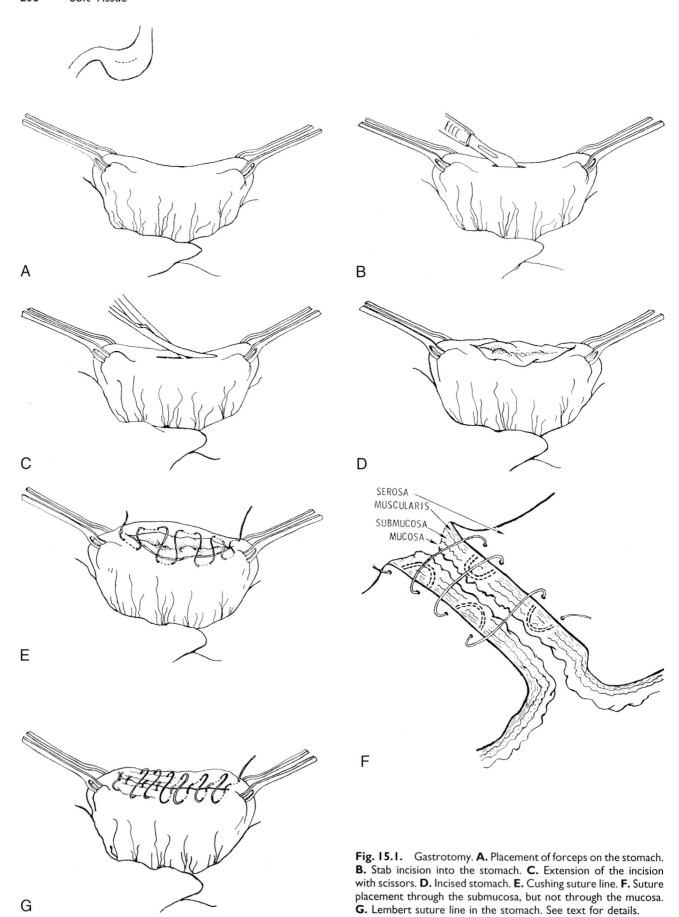

A

B

C

D

E

SEROSA
MUSCULARIS
SUBMUCOSA
MUCOSA

F

G

Fig. 15.1. Gastrotomy. **A.** Placement of forceps on the stomach. **B.** Stab incision into the stomach. **C.** Extension of the incision with scissors. **D.** Incised stomach. **E.** Cushing suture line. **F.** Suture placement through the submucosa, but not through the mucosa. **G.** Lembert suture line in the stomach. See text for details.

Pyloromyotomy, Pyloroplasty, and Pyloric Resection

Mary L. Dulisch

Pyloric disease or obstruction is characterized by intermittent projectile vomiting after eating. Antral polyps, neoplasia, and pyloric stenosis can cause obstructions in this area. Pyloric stenosis, either acquired or congenital, usually results from hypertrophy of the pyloric sphincter muscle or hypertrophied mucosal folds after chronic gastritis.

Pyloromyotomy (Fredet–Ramstedt) and pyloroplasty (Heineke–Mikulicz) are two surgical procedures used to increase the diameter of the pyloric lumen (1), with a resulting decrease in gastric emptying time. Pyloroplasty is a permanent technique, whereas a pyloromyotomy may scar over, thus allowing the clinical problem to recur. These procedures are indicated in patients with a diagnosis of pyloric stenosis.

Gastric outflow obstruction resulting from excessive hypertrophy of the mucosa may not be adequately alleviated by a pyloromyotomy or pyloroplasty. In these patients, a submucosal resection is preferred. If the pyloric muscular layers are excessively hypertrophied or if pyloric neoplasms or ulcers are present, excision of the pylorus and a gastroduodenal anastomosis (Billroth I) should be done (2).

Preoperative Considerations

Before any pyloric procedures are attempted, the entire gastrointestinal tract should be examined thoroughly by physical examination and radiography to determine whether additional lesions are present. The patient should be evaluated for fluid and electrolyte imbalances; if present, these should be corrected before surgery.

Surgical Techniques

The patient is placed in dorsal recumbency, and a ventral midline incision is made extending from the xiphoid to caudal to the umbilicus. Moistened laparotomy pads are placed on both sides of the incision and are folded over the cut edges. A Balfour retractor is used to retract the body wall, and a complete exploratory operation of the abdominal structures is performed. The stomach and pylorus are then elevated from the abdomen. It may be useful to transect the gastrohepatic ligament to increase pyloric mobilization (Fig. 15.2). The gastrohepatic ligament is a thin band

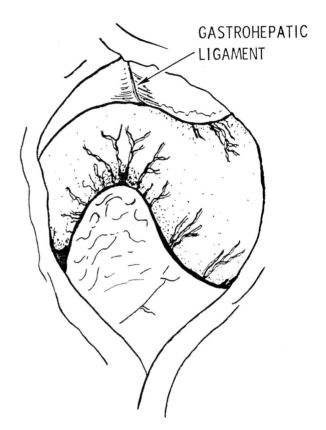

Fig. 15.2. Relation of the gastrohepatic ligament to the pylorus.

of tissue extending from the pyloric region to the hilus of the liver. Care is taken not to cut the common bile duct, which is cranial and dorsal to the ligament, or the hepatic arteries. The abdominal structures are packed off with moistened laparotomy pads, so the stomach, pylorus, and descending duodenum are the only structures visible.

Pyloromyotomy

During pyloromyotomy, the pylorus can be elevated into view by an assistant, Babcock forceps, or stay sutures (Fig. 15.3**A**). An incision approximately 4 cm long is made into the least vascular area of the pyloric canal, pylorus, and proximal duodenum (Fig. 15.3**B**). The pylorus is the midpoint of the incision. The incision extends through the tunica serosa and the muscle layer. The muscle layer is cut and separated by sharp and blunt dissection with Metzenbaum scissors (Fig. 15.3**C**). All muscular bands should be identified and severed. Care is taken not to cut through the tunica mucosa.

If a small hole is made in the tunica mucosa, it can be closed with a single, simple interrupted or pursestring suture of 3–0 synthetic absorbable material. If a larger hole has been made, the incision should be converted into a pyloroplasty. When the muscle

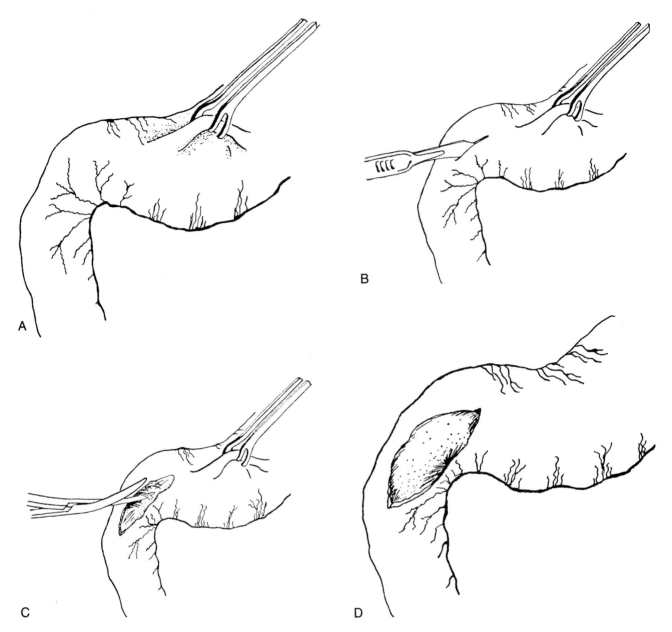

Fig. 15.3. Pyloromyotomy. **A.** Placement of Babcock forceps on the stomach. **B.** Incision through the tunica serosa of the pyloric region. **C.** Dissection of the muscle from the pyloric region. **D.** Bulging of the tunica mucosa through the incision line. See text for details.

bands have been completely severed, the tunica mucosa bulges out of the incision site (Fig. 15.3**D**).

Pyloroplasty

When a pyloroplasty is performed, temporary stay sutures of 3–0 chromic catgut or monofilament suture are placed in the least vascular portions of the ventral stomach and the proximal duodenum (Fig. 15.4**A**).

These sutures are approximately 10 cm apart, with the pylorus as the midpoint. Using a No. 10 or 15 Bard–Parker scalpel blade with the cutting edge up, a stab incision is made into the lumen and is extended with scissors to span a distance of 1 to 2 cm on either side of the pylorus (Fig. 15.4**B–D**). The longitudinal incision is closed transversely (Fig. 15.4**E**) with 3–0 synthetic absorbable, polypropylene, or nylon suture in a simple interrupted appositional or Gambee suture

Fig. 15.4. Pyloroplasty. **A.** Stay suture in the least vascular area of the stomach. **B.** Incision into the pyloric region. **C.** Extension of the incision with Metzenbaum scissors. **D.** Completed pyloric incision. **E.** Transverse suturing of pyloric incision. **F.** Completed closure. See text for details.

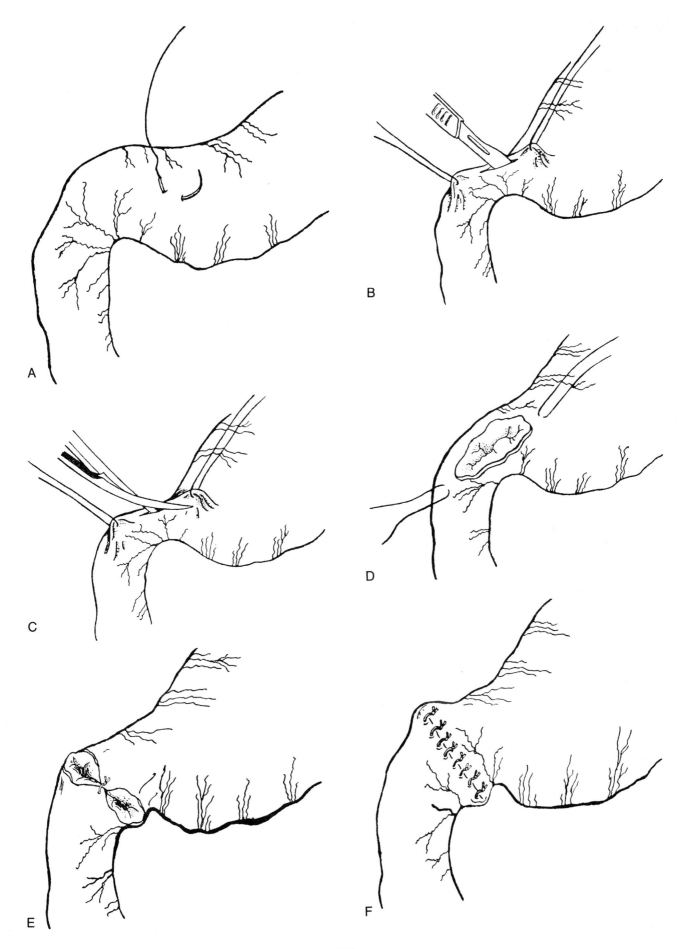

pattern (Fig. 15.4**F**). Omentum is placed over the incision area to act as a seal and may be tacked down with one or two simple interrupted sutures of 3–0 absorbable material. Abdominal closure is performed in a routine manner.

Pyloric Submucosal Resection

The pyloric region is isolated and incised as for a Heineke–Mikulicz pyloroplasty (see Fig. 15.4**B–D**).

Traction sutures of 3–0 chromic catgut or monofilament suture are placed on either side of the incision at the midpoint to expose the mucosa. Starting at the duodenal end of the incision, a transverse incision is made through the mucosa and submucosa (Fig. 15.5**A**). Submucosal dissection is started and continued orally to an area just beyond the hypertrophied pyloric mucosa (Fig. 15.5**B**). Usually, this area is no more than 3 cm from the pyloric sphincter. With a 3–0 synthetic absorbable suture placed in a Cushing or

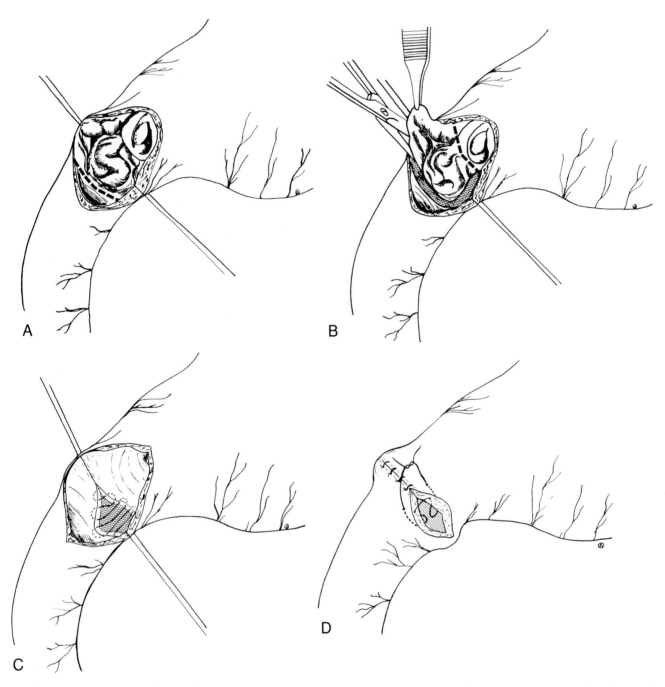

Fig. 15.5. Pyloric submucosal resection. **A.** Transverse incision (*broken line*) through the duodenal mucosa and submucosa. **B.** Submucosal dissection of hypertrophied mucosa. **C.** Gastric submucosa apposed to duodenal submucosa. **D.** Transverse closure of pyloric incision. See text for details.

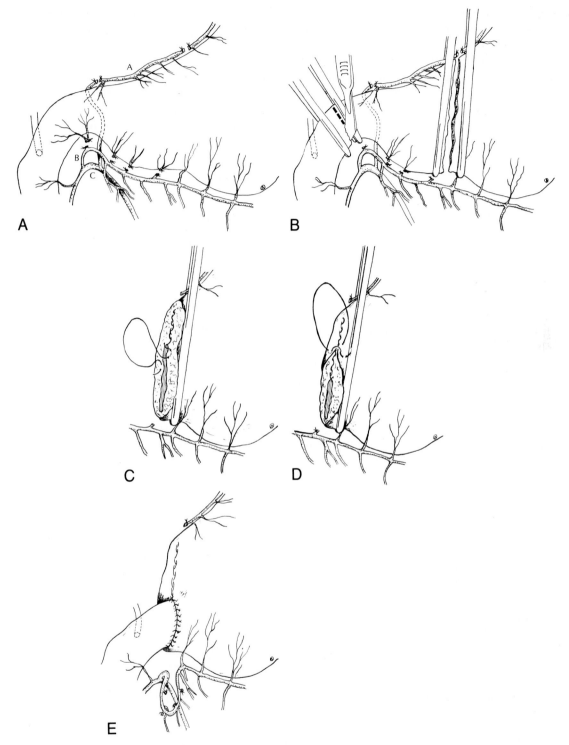

Fig. 15.6. Gastroduodenostomy (Billroth I). **A.** Arteries to be ligated are right gastric (A) and right gastroepiploic (B); avoid the gastroduodenal artery (C). **B.** Excision of pyloric sphincter and canal. **C.** Apposition of gastric submucosa in Cushing suture pattern. **D.** Apposition of gastric seromuscular layers in Lembert suture pattern. **E.** Completed anastomosis between stomach and duodenum. See text for details.

buried continuous pattern, the duodenal submucosa is apposed to the gastric submucosa (Fig. 15.5**C**). The initial longitudinal pyloric incision is closed transversely as for a pyloroplasty with 3–0 synthetic absorbable, polypropylene, or nylon suture in a simple interrupted appositional or Gambee suture pattern (Fig. 15.5**D**).

Gastroduodenostomy (Billroth I)

Before a gastroduodenostomy is begun, the extent of the diseased tissue should be determined by palpation or by direct visualization of the mucosal surface through a pyloric incision. The right gastric artery and vein are isolated by blunt dissection through the lesser omentum. These vessels are ligated near the pylorus and on the lesser curvature of the stomach just oral to the tissue to be excised. Injury to the gastroduodenal vessels should be avoided. Similarly, the right gastroepiploic vessels are isolated on the medial surface of the duodenum, while care is taken not to injure the pancreas; the pyloric and gastric branches supplying the area to be resected are ligated (Fig. 15.6**A**) Two straight atraumatic intestinal clamps are placed 1.5 cm apart across the pyloric antrum, and another two are placed across the proximal duodenum just distal to the pylorus and avoiding the common bile duct. The pyloric sphincter and canal are excised by transecting the stomach with a blade between the clamps but close to the distal clamp and then transecting the duodenum in a like manner close to the proximal clamp (Fig. 15.6**B**).

The gastric mucosa is apposed with 3–0 synthetic absorbable suture in a Cushing pattern starting from the lesser curvature and continuing toward the greater curvature. The suture line is continued until the opening of the stomach is equal in size to the duodenal diameter (Fig. 15.6**C**). The gastric seromuscular layers are similarly apposed with 3–0 synthetic absorbable, polypropylene, or nylon suture in a Lembert pattern (Fig. 15.6**D**). The duodenum is then anastomosed to the stomach with 3–0 synthetic absorbable, polypropylene, or nylon suture in a simple interrupted appositional or Gambee suture pattern (Fig. 15.6**E**) starting from the dorsal surface. The stumps must be rotated to facilitate the anastomosis.

Postoperative Care

Postoperative care is the same for all procedures described. No food, water, or oral medication is given for 24 hours. Maintenance fluid requirements are sustained with intravenous fluids. Water can be offered 24 hours after the operation. Once the patient has started to drink on its own, the intravenous fluids are gradually discontinued. A soft diet consisting of small amounts of baby food or a soft dog food gruel can be started if water is not vomited. This diet can be fed several times a day, and the consistency of the food can be thickened with each succeeding day. If vomiting occurs, oral intake is discontinued and injectable metoclopramide can be given at a dosage of 0.2 to 0.4 mg/kg every 8 hours. Once vomiting is controlled, food can be offered again. Oral metoclopramide may be continued as needed.

References

1. Twedt DC. Disorders of gastric retention. In: Kirk RW, ed. Current veterinary therapy. Vol 8. Philadelphia: WB Saunders, 1983.
2. Sikes RI, Birchard S, Patnaik A, et al. Chronic hypertrophic pyloric gastropathy: a review of 16 cases. J Am Anim Hosp Assoc 1986;22:99.

Y–U Antral Flap Pyloroplasty

Ronald M. Bright

Most animals undergoing surgery on the distal stomach have vomiting as a cardinal sign. The vomiting may be sporadic and infrequent and of little consequence to the metabolic state of the animal. However, frequent vomiting can result in serious metabolic changes such as hypochloremia, hypokalemia, metabolic alkalosis, and dehydration. Hypoalbuminemia and hypoglycemia must be monitored more closely in the pediatric patient. These abnormalities must be corrected before attempting pyloric surgery. Treatment should be directed toward correction of electrolyte and fluid imbalances, to minimize the anesthetic risk to these patients.

Preoperative Considerations

Preoperative preparation of animals with gastric retention should always include decompression of the stomach with a stomach tube shortly after anesthetic induction. Suction should be used to ensure the quick and efficient emptying of the fluid that has been retained in the stomach. Evacuation of the stomach lessens the likelihood of aspiration pneumonia. In addition, less spillage occurs when the pylorus is entered during the pyloroplasty procedure.

Pyloroplasty procedures are intended to increase the diameter of the pylorus. In human patients, pyloroplasty techniques were first used to relieve obstruction and symptoms caused by duodenal ulcers (1). In veterinary medicine, pyloroplasty techniques have been used successfully as treatment of acquired antral pyloric hypertrophy (3) and ulcer disease and as palliation for neoplasia involving the pyloric canal and antrum.

Surgical Technique

The Y–U pyloroplasty technique (1, 2) has been met with good clinical success and is my preferred method when pyloroplasty is indicated (4, 5). This procedure involves the plastic surgery technique that converts a "Y"-shaped incision into a "U"-shaped closure (Fig. 15.7). Each limb of the "Y" incision should be 3 to 5 cm in length, depending on the size of the animal. The base of the "Y" should always extend a small distance into the proximal duodenum (Fig. 15.7A).

The Y–U pyloroplasty gives excellent exposure to lesions in the distal stomach. If the lesion appears to be consistent with acquired antral pyloric hypertrophy, a submucosal resection of mucosa and submucosa above and below the pyloric ring can be done before closure

of the pyloroplasty (Fig. 15.7B) (6). After the removal of this rectangular piece of tissue, the two exposed edges of the duodenal and gastric mucosa and submucosa are apposed with a continuous layer of 3–0 synthetic absorbable suture material. I rarely do this pyloroplasty technique without including the submucosal resection procedure.

Once the submucosal resection is completed, the tip of the "V"-shaped antral flap is trimmed to a "U" shape. This tissue and that removed during the submucosal resection are included as part of the tissue submitted for histopathologic evaluation.

Closure of the Y–U pyloroplasty is begun by bringing the tip of the "U"-shaped antral flap distally into apposition with the center of the duodenal incision using 3–0 or 4–0 synthetic absorbable suture and a full-thickness approximating suture pattern (Fig. 15.7B and C). The closure of the lesser curvature is followed by closure of the greater curvature side.

Postoperative Care

Postoperative management depends on the physical condition of the animal before the surgical procedure. In all animals, I continue fluid therapy until the first postoperative day. Animals with significant preoperative electrolyte and fluid imbalances should be monitored for 2 or 3 days, with laboratory confirmation of their status. Fluid and electrolyte therapy may have to continue in these patients for 48 to 72 hours.

Feeding is usually begun the day after surgery using a low-fat diet to enhance gastric emptying. Occasionally, a patient continues to vomit after a pyloric surgical procedure. Oral intake is discontinued for 12 hours, and the animal is placed on subcutaneous or intravenous metoclopramide at a dose of 0.2 to 0.4 mg/kg every 8 hours. The patient is weaned off the metoclopramide over the next 24 to 48 hours. Attempts to feed the animals begin about 12 hours after the initiation of metoclopramide.

Persistent vomiting persists and the presence of bile in the emesis suggest the possibility of reflux alkaline gastritis secondary to duodenogastric reflux. This condition usually responds to a 2- to 3-week course of metoclopramide (oral form), systemic antacids (H_2 blockers) and sucralfate. If the disease treated with the Y–U pyloroplasty is benign, the prognosis is good.

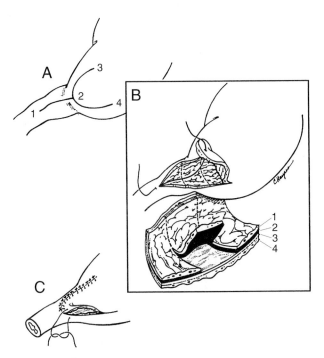

Fig. 15.7. A. The base of the "Y" incision extends slightly onto the stomach side of the pyloric ring (1–2). Each limb of the "Y" (1–2, 2–3, and 3–4) is approximately 3 to 5 cm in length. **B.** Once the stomach lumen is exposed, two parallel incisions are made through the mucosa and submucosa above and below the pylorus, taking care to incorporate the mucosal lesions. Submucosal dissection proceeds from one side to the other until a rectangular piece can be lifted from the underlying muscle layer. The edges of the mucosa and submucosa above and below the remaining defect are apposed with a continuous suture pattern using synthetic absorbable suture material. **C.** The pyloroplasty incision is closed by opposing the leading edge of the "U"-shaped stomach flap and to the middle of the incision extending into the duodenum (see **B**). The remaining portions of the flap are apposed using a simple continuous or interrupted approximating suture pattern.

References

1. Randolph JG. Y–U advancement pyloroplasty. Ann Surg 1975; 181:586–590.
2. Moschel DM, Walske BR, Neumayer F. A new technique of pyloroplasty. Surgery 1958;46:813–816.
3. Walter MC, Matthiesen DT. Acquired antral pyloric hypertrophy in the dog. Vet Clin North Am Small Anim Pract 1993;23: 547–552.

4. Bright RM, Richardson DC, Stanton ME. Y–U antral flap pyloroplasty in the dog. Compend Contin Educ Pract Vet 1988; 10:139–141.
5. Stanton ME, Bright RM, Toal R, et al. Effects of the Y–U pyloroplasty on gastric emptying and duodenogastric reflux in the dog. Vet Surg 1987;16:392–397.
6. Bright RM. New techniques in gastrointestinal surgery. In: Proceedings of the 17th Waltham/Ohio State University Symposium. Columbus, OH. 1993:7–12.

Surgery for Gastric Neoplasia

Janet A. Welch & Ralph A. Henderson

Gastric tumors account for fewer than 1% of all malignancies in dogs and cats. The most common type of gastric tumor diagnosed in dogs is adenocarcinoma, and in cats it is lymphoma. In humans, geographic origin, occupation, family history, and diets high in smoked, salt-cured, or pickled foods have been identified as risk factors for the development of gastric cancer. Strong familial and dietary correlations have not been identified in dogs. A breed incidence of gastric adenocarcinoma has been reported in Belgian shepherds, the rough collie, and the Staffordshire bull terrier. The average age of dogs with gastric adenocarcinoma is 8 years. A sex predilection for males has been documented, with a reported ratio of 2.4:1. The prognosis for patients with gastric adenocarcinoma is poor, with survival estimates of less than 3 months after the onset of clinical signs in untreated dogs and less than 6 months after tumor excision in operated dogs. Chemotherapy that has been used most extensively in human patients includes 5-fluorouracil, doxorubicin, and mitomycin-C. The addition of methotrexate to this combination has shown encouraging results in several human trials. No successful regimens have been reported in canine patients.

Leiomyosarcoma is the second most common malignant tumor of the stomach in dogs. Gastric leiomyosarcoma has a lower metastatic rate than adenocarcinoma and is often amenable to resection, with a survival time of 1 year or more postoperatively. In one study, however, severe ulceration and hemorrhage were typical features of gastric leiomyosarcomas, and patients required intensive perioperative therapy. Leiomyomas are the most common benign gastric tumors in dogs. They occur in older dogs, with an average age of 15 years, in the region of the gastroesophageal junction. Leiomyomas have also been detected in other regions, such as the gastric antrum. This tumor may cause obstruction if it reaches a large size.

Gastric lymphoma occurs primarily in older cats that test negative for feline leukemia virus. Gastric lymphoma may present as a localized process or as diffuse organ infiltration and is treated with chemotherapy. Significant improvement in survival times with surgical excision of localized lymphoma before chemotherapy has not been documented.

Clinical Signs and Diagnosis

The presence of neoplasia causes clinical signs by obstructing gastric outflow, interfering with normal peristalsis, or creating ulceration and inflammation of the gastric mucosa. Clinical signs include vomiting, with or without blood, weight loss, anorexia, evidence of abdominal pain, and occasionally melena and anemia. Vomiting is generally not related to feeding. Gastric carcinomas are frequently advanced at the time of detection, possibly because of empiric management of gastrointestinal disturbances and delay in definitive diagnosis. Large gastric masses may occasionally be palpated on physical examination. Radiographic signs are usually subtle and suggest a mass in the gastric region, thickening of the gastric wall, or absence of a normal rugal pattern. Contrast radiography (13 mL/kg of barium orally) enhances radiographic detail and permits visualization of filling defects, ulcers, and delayed gastric emptying. Up to 30% of dogs have visible pulmonary metastasis when initially presented. Regional lymph node metastasis (up to 75% of cases) and metastasis to other abdominal organs such as the liver (20 to 30% of cases) may be detected using abdominal ultrasound.

Endoscopy is highly effective in obtaining a diagnosis. Adenocarcinoma usually appears as an ulcerated bleeding crater located at the lesser curvature or pyloric region of the stomach, but it may also appear as a broad-based mass or as diffuse gastric infiltration. The tumor may be accompanied by a thick, plaquelike lesion of the gastric wall. Although usually accurate, endoscopic biopsies may fail to diagnose the tumor if only the deeper layers, and not the mucosa, are involved. The histologic appearance of gastric adenocarcinoma is classified as either intestinal or diffuse, using the descriptive scheme of Lauren. The intestinal classification denotes well-polarized epithelial cells organized in tubular structures without marked infiltration of the gastric wall. The diffuse type is composed of anaplastic cells with a highly infiltrative growth pattern. Most dogs (65.3%) have diffuse adenocarcinoma, which is associated with shorter survival.

Surgical Therapy
Definitions and Indications

The term gastrectomy refers to the removal of any portion of the stomach. An antrectomy involves removing the distal 30 to 40% of the stomach, and a partial gastrectomy, the distal 40 to 70%. A subtotal gastrectomy involves removing the distal 70 to 90%

of the stomach. After antrectomy, reconstruction is accomplished with either a gastroduodenostomy (Billroth I) or a gastrojejunostomy (Billroth II). A Billroth I reconstruction is preferred because it is more physiologic. However, a gastroduodenostomy is considered to be only a short-term palliative procedure for gastric adenocarcinoma. The poor long-term prognosis may be due to failure to obtain adequate margins with this procedure, or it may result from the highly metastatic nature of this tumor precluding a surgical cure without early detection. A gastroduodenostomy should be performed if this will result in 1) a minimum of 2 cm tumor-free margins on the gastric and duodenal sides and 2) a tension-free anastomosis.

A Billroth II should be performed if a more radical gastrectomy is required, if there is excessive duodenal involvement, or both. The Billroth II has been associated with the disadvantages of duodenal stump leakage, afferent limb obstruction, anastomotic ulceration, and alkaline reflux gastritis. Frozen sections obtained during surgery aid in determining the optimal extent of the excision. Recommendations for margins in the resection of distal gastric tumors in human patients specify 1 to 3 cm of duodenum distally and at least 5 cm of normal stomach proximal to the gross margin of the tumor for intestinal types of adenocarcinoma. A proximal gastric margin of 8 cm is recommended for diffuse types of adenocarcinoma. Whether obtaining more aggressive margins in canine gastric neoplasia will result in improved survival times is unknown.

Factors determining a more favorable outcome in human gastric cancer include the following:

1. Early cancer with the lesion confined to the mucosa and submucosa.
2. Pyloric antral involvement versus the proximal two-thirds of the stomach.
3. Metastasis in four or fewer lymph nodes.

Lymphadenectomy is recommended, although it has not been shown to improve survival in human patients in the United States. Lymphadenectomy or lymph node biopsy is helpful in tumor staging. The regional lymph nodes draining the gastric region in the dog are found dorsal and cranial to the lesser curvature, roughly following the long axis of the stomach. One to two pancreaticoduodenal lymph nodes and three to five splenic lymph nodes are found caudal to the greater curvature of the stomach. A recommendation for the management of lymph nodes in oncologic surgery is to perform nondestructive biopsies of grossly normal nodes and complete excision of grossly abnormal nodes if possible.

Approach for Gastric Surgery

The patient is placed in dorsal recumbency, and a ventral midline incision is made that begins at the xiphoid and ends cranial to the pubis. Moistened laparotomy pads are placed on both sides of the incision and are folded over the cut edges. A Balfour retractor is used to retract the body wall, and a complete exploratory operation of the abdomen is performed to look for lymph node or abdominal organ metastasis. The stomach and pylorus are then elevated from the abdomen. Transection of the hepatogastric ligament near its pyloric attachment increases the caudoventral mobility of the stomach. The hepatogastric ligament is a section of the lesser omentum and appears as a thin band of tissue extending from the pyloric region to the hilus of the liver. Care is taken not to damage the common bile duct, which is dorsal and lateral to this ligament, or the hepatic arteries, during transection of the ligament. The abdominal structures are packed off with moistened laparotomy pads, so the stomach pylorus, omentum, and descending duodenum are the only structures visible.

Throughout the surgical procedure, care must be taken to avoid injury to the duodenum, bile duct, portal vein, pancreas, spleen, and hepatic artery. Accurate dissection, gentle tissue manipulation and precise suture placement are necessary to avoid trauma to these structures. The principal postoperative complications to avoid are those common to all hollow organ surgery including luminal obstruction, dehiscence or infection, and hemorrhage.

Antrectomy for Neoplasms Involving the Pylorus

The borders of the diseased tissue are determined by visual inspection and palpation. An appropriate surgical margin is added to the area of resection. The right gastric artery and vein are isolated by blunt dissection through the lesser omentum. These vessels are ligated near the pylorus and on the lesser curvature of the stomach just proximal to the intended area of resection. The right gastroepiploic vessels are isolated along the duodenum and the greater curvature of the stomach and are ligated. Care is taken to avoid injury to the gastroduodenal vessels or the pancreas. Two Doyen tissue forceps are placed 1.5 cm apart, just proximal to the pyloric antrum, at an oblique angle toward the lesser curvature. Similarly, two forceps are placed across the duodenum just distal to the pylorus. The resection is begun at the distal end, so the portal vein and celiac artery arborization may be visualized and protected. The lumen of the resected specimen must be kept closed in an attempt to avoid exposure of the abdomen to exfoliating neoplastic cells. The omentum is resected in conjunction with the resected specimen, except for that portion associated with the pancreas. Concomitant resections of the spleen and left pancreas

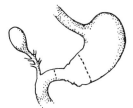

Fig. 15.8. Resection for antrectomy is performed proximal to the pyloric antrum and distal to the pylorus. A 5-mm margin of normal tissue must separate the common bile duct's entrance into the duodenum.

are performed if needed with more extensive lesions. A 5-mm margin of normal tissue must separate the common bile duct's entrance into the duodenum from the line of resection. If extensive duodenal lesions necessitate transection of the common bile duct, a biliary redirection procedure by means of cholecystoenterostomy will be required (see Chap. 17). The stomach is transected between the forceps using a scalpel. Sufficient tissue must remain above the remaining clamp for suturing. The duodenum is transected in a similar manner (Fig. 15.8).

The gastric incision is closed. Any closure technique that properly apposes "like tissue" engages the submucosa, provides a watertight seal, and uses suture material of sufficient strength, is appropriate. We recommend a simple continuous or interrupted pattern through all four layers of the gastric wall using 2–0 or 3–0 absorbable suture, followed by a simple continuous or inverting (Cushing or Lembert) pattern in the seromuscular layer. Reconstruction is then accomplished with gastroduodenostomy or gastrojejunostomy.

Gastroduodenostomy (Billroth I)

After closure of the gastric body, the duodenum is anastomosed to the stomach. Most descriptions of this surgical procedure depict the anastomosis of the duodenum and stomach in the same gastric oversew suture line near the greater curvature. Although the operation is generally successful, suture line leakage has been a reported complication. The inverted Y configuration of the resulting three suture lines can be avoided by anastomosing the duodenum as a separate site midway between the lesser and greater curvatures on the visceral surface of the stomach. A simple interrupted appositional pattern is performed using 3–0 monofilament suture (Figs. 15.9 and 15.10). Laparotomy pads are removed, and gloves are changed. A jejunostomy tube is placed. The abdomen is lavaged and closed routinely.

Intravenous fluids are supplemented with increasing amounts of enteral nutrition. H_2 receptor blockers are given during the postoperative period. Metoclopramide may be given every 6 to 8 hours, or as a continuous drip, if vomiting or evidence of gastric hypotonia is present. Serum potassium levels should be monitored and supplemented if necessary.

Gastrojejunostomy (Billroth II)

The duodenal segment is closed in a simple interrupted appositional pattern using 3–0 monofilament suture. Two stay sutures are used to attach the jejunum to the gastric stump, with the jejunal segment positioned parallel and 2.5 to 3.0 cm away from the gastric incision. The point of attachment of the jejunum to the greater curvature of the stomach determines the length of the afferent loop of the duodenum, which

Fig. 15.9. Gastroduodenostomy (Billroth I). **A** and **B.** After closure of the gastric body, the stay sutures are retracted toward the left side of the patient to facilitate the gastroduodenostomy. The duodenum is anastomosed to the visceral surface of the stomach. This surface of the stomach faces the liver when the patient is in dorsal recumbency. The anastomosis is performed midway between the lesser and greater curvatures using a simple interrupted pattern with monofilament suture.

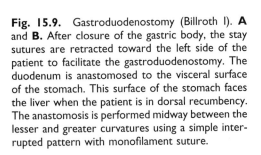
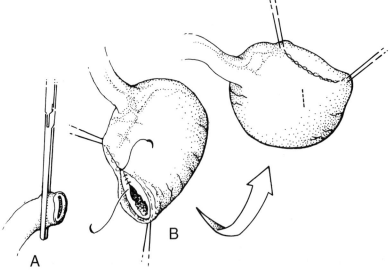

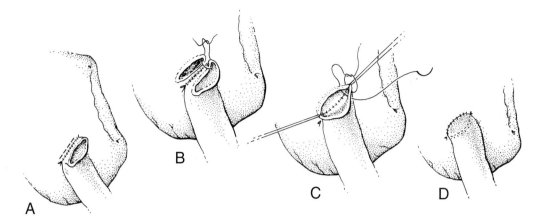

Fig. 15.10. A–D. Demonstration of the correct positioning for a gastroduodenostomy. The duodenum is sutured to the visceral surface of the stomach.

should be as short as possible without resulting in tension. The maximum length of the afferent loop should be 25 cm. The antimesenteric border of the jejunum is sutured to the gastric wall, midway between the greater and lesser curvatures, in a simple continuous seromuscular suture pattern. A full-thickness longitudinal incision is made into the stomach and jejunum. Incisions are made to result in a stoma size equal to or slightly greater than the bowel lumen diameter. A full-thickness closure of the stomach and jejunum is performed using a simple continuous or interrupted pattern. Each half of the stoma is sutured separately if a continuous suture is used to prevent "pursestring" narrowing of the closure (Fig. 15.11). A jejunostomy tube is placed. The abdomen is lavaged and closed

routinely. Intravenous fluid therapy, enteral therapy, and postoperative medication are similar to those with gastroduodenostomy.

Stapling Technique for Gastroduodenostomy (Billroth I)

A Billroth I procedure can be performed using end-to-end anastomosis (EEA) and thoracoabdominal (TA) staplers. The TA 55-mm or TA 90-mm cartridge (United States Surgical Corporation [USSC], Norwalk, CT) with 4.8-mm staples (green cartridge) is generally used to close the gastric pouch. The jaws of the instrument are placed around the greater curvature of the stomach, closed, and fired. Before removing the sta-

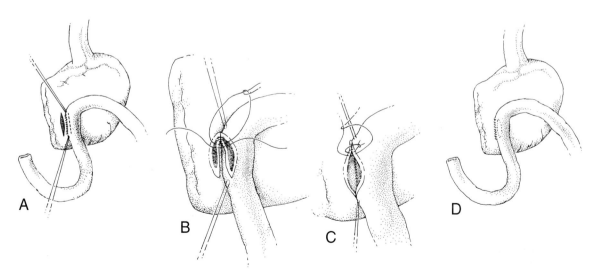

Fig. 15.11. Gastrojejunostomy (Billroth II). **A–D.** After closure of the gastric body, the duodenal segment is closed in a simple interrupted appositional pattern. The antimesenteric border of the jejunum is positioned parallel and 2.5 to 3.0 cm away from the gastric incision, midway between the greater and lesser curvatures of the stomach. Full-thickness incisions are made in the stomach and jejunum, and the gastrojejunal anastomosis is performed using a simple interrupted appositional pattern with monofilament suture.

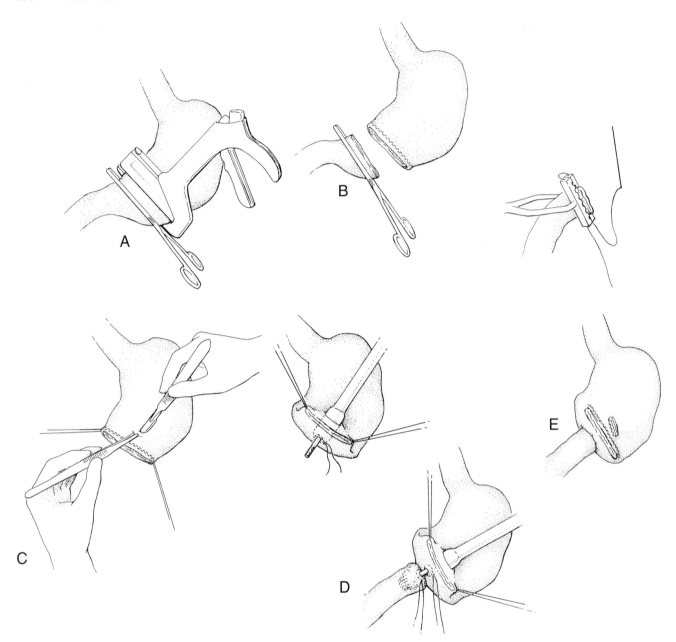

Fig. 15.12. **A.** Stapling technique for gastroduodenostomy (Billroth I). After ligation and division of omental vessels, the gastric pouch is closed using a thoracoabdominal 90-mm (TA 90) instrument. The instrument is placed proximal (oral) to the mass, leaving appropriate margins of grossly normal tissue. Tissue forceps are placed adjacent to the mass, and the stomach is transected with a scalpel blade, using the TA 90 instrument edge as a cutting guide. **B.** The pursestring instrument (Furniss clamp) is placed around the duodenum, distal (aboral) to the mass, leaving appropriate margins of grossly normal tissue. Monofilament 3–0 suture is passed through the superior jaw of the pursestring instrument and returned through the inferior jaw. Tissue forceps are placed adjacent to the mass, and the duodenum is transected using the pursestring instrument edge as a cutting guide. **C.** The pursestring instrument is removed and the appropriately sized end-to-end anastomosis (EEA) cartridge is chosen on the basis of the luminal diameter of the proximal duodenum. A stab incision is made in an avascular portion of the ventral aspect of the stomach, approximately 3 cm away from the edge of the staple line. Stay sutures aid in the retraction of the stomach. **D.** The EEA instrument is introduced, without the anvil, through the stab wound on the ventral surface of the stomach. The center rod of the instrument is exited through a small stab incision in the center of a pursestring suture that has been placed on the dorsal surface of the stomach. The pursestring suture is tied on the stomach side, and the anvil is placed on the central rod. The anvil is introduced into the duodenal lumen and the pursestring suture is tied. The EEA instrument is then closed and fired. A circular, double-staggered row of staples joins the organs, and the circular blade in the instrument cuts a stoma. **E.** Completion of the gastroduodenostomy. The EEA instrument has been gently removed from the entry site on the ventral surface of the stomach and the staple line inspected for hemostasis. The gastrotomy incision has been closed with a TA 55 instrument. The completed anastomosis consists of two linear staple closures on the stomach and a circular stapled anastomosis forming the gastroduodenostomy.

pler, a clamp is placed on the specimen side, and the stomach is transected using the TA instrument as a cutting guide. The duodenum is transected, and the gastroduodenostomy is performed by introducing the EEA instrument through a stab incision in the stomach and into the duodenum. The EEA delivers a circular, double-staggered row of staples to join the stomach and duodenum. The gastrotomy access hole is closed with a TA 55-mm instrument (Fig. 15.12). Identical precautions are needed to protect surrounding structures as with the hand-sewn method.

Stapling Technique for Gastrojejunostomy (Billroth II)

A Billroth II procedure can be performed using TA and gastrointestinal anastomosis (GIA) instruments. The duodenum is stapled using the TA 55-mm cartridge (or 30-mm cartridge in smaller patients) and then is transected proximal to the stapler, which may be used as a cutting template. Either the TA 90-mm or the TA 55-mm stapler is used for division of the stomach at the level of the incisura angularis or higher. As with

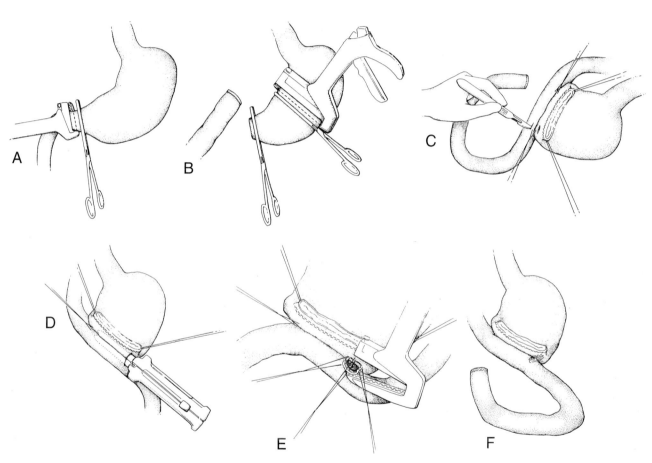

Fig. 15.13. **A.** Stapling technique for a gastrojejunostomy (Billroth II). The borders of the gastrectomy are chosen, and the corresponding omental vessels have been ligated and transected. The duodenal side is closed with a thoracoabdominal 55-mm (TA 55) instrument. Before removing the instrument, tissue forceps are placed proximal (oral) to the staple line, and the duodenum is transected, using the edge of the TA instrument as a cutting guide. **B.** The gastric pouch is closed using the TA 90 instrument. Before removal of the instrument, tissue forceps are placed distal (aboral) to the staple line, and the stomach is transected using the TA 90 instrument edge as a cutting guide. **C.** Stay sutures are used to retract the gastric stump and allow attachment of a segment of jejunum to the visceral surface of the stomach. This surface of the stomach faces the liver when the patient is in dorsal recumbency. Using stay sutures near the greater and lesser surfaces of the stomach, the jejunum is positioned parallel to and 2.5 to 3.0 cm away from the staple line. Stab wounds are made for introduction of the two jaws of the gastrointestinal anastomosis (GIA) instrument. **D.** The jaws of the GIA-50 instrument are inserted into the gastric and jejunal lumens. The instrument is closed and fired. Two double-staggered rows of staples join the organs, and simultaneously, the knife blade in the instrument cuts between the two double staple lines to create a stoma. The GIA instrument is opened slightly and is gently removed. **E.** The anastomotic staple lines are inspected for hemostasis before closing the now-common stab wound with the TA 55 instrument. Everting traction sutures are placed around the stab wound, and the jaws of the TA 55 instrument are slipped around the tissue. The instrument is closed and fired, and before its removal, excess tissue is excised using the instrument edge as a guide. **F.** The completed appearance of the gastrojejunostomy. The completed anastomosis consists of a single linear staple closure of the stomach, two parallel linear staple closures forming the gastrojejunal anastomosis, and a single linear staple closure of the gastric and jejunal stab incision.

the Billroth I technique, 4.8-mm staples are generally used for gastric tissue. The jejunum is anastomosed to the stomach wall in a side-to-side fashion using a GIA 50-mm stapling instrument. The length of the afferent loop of jejunum should be a maximum of 25 cm from the blind end to the anastomotic site. The GIA instrument places two double-staggered rows of staples and creates a division between to produce a stoma. The entry incision for the GIA is closed using a TA 55-mm staple (Fig. 15.13). Identical precautions are needed to protect surrounding structures as with the hand-sewn method.

Potential Complications of Billroth I and Billroth II Procedures

POTENTIAL SHORT-TERM COMPLICATIONS

In one report, the most prominent complication of a Billroth II procedure was vomiting. The incidence of vomiting was significantly higher in those dogs who had large stomal diameters. Stomal diameters larger than 3.0 cm have been associated with vomiting, which may be a reflection of the "dumping syndrome." Investigators have speculated that large stomal diameters result from gastric distension in the postoperative period that results in stretching of the stoma. Because of this possibility, enteral feeding through a jejunostomy tube and immediate gastric decompression, if necessary, are recommended after this surgical procedure.

POTENTIAL LONG-TERM COMPLICATIONS

Pathophysiologic complications that may occur after antrectomy or partial gastrectomy procedures include the dumping syndrome, alkaline reflux gastritis, stomal ulceration, and the afferent loop syndrome. In general, these are more common with gastrojejunal reconstructions (Fig. 15.14).

The dumping syndrome results from the sudden emptying of hyperosmolar substances into the duodenum and jejunum. It is characterized by postprandial vomiting, diarrhea, faintness, and pallor. The transient fall in serum potassium noted may be associated with alterations in the electrocardiogram. Episodes of the dumping syndrome occur in 20 to 25% of human patients who undergo gastric resection. Symptoms are pronounced in approximately 1% of human patients and result in considerable weight loss, anemia, and malnutrition. Symptoms suggestive of the dumping syndrome have been observed in dogs. Surgical treatment in human patients includes implantation of a single short reversed jejunal segment between the gastric remnant and duodenum or conversion to a Roux-en-Y to bypass duodenal and proximal jejunal pacemakers and slow peristalsis in the efferent jejunal limb. Clinical use of these procedures has not been reported in dogs.

Alkaline reflux gastritis is another cause of vomiting that results from the reflux of bile into the gastric remnant. This is the most frequently encountered postgastrectomy disorder requiring remedial surgery in human patients and is more likely to occur after gastrojejunostomy than after gastroduodenostomy. Medical treatment involves H_2-receptor blockers, sucralfate, or metoclopramide. Operative treatment in human patients is a Roux-en-Y procedure to divert duodenal content away from the gastric remnant.

Anastomotic ulcers can be a source of vomiting and melena. They may result from any procedure that approximates gastric and jejunal mucosa. Ulceration is more liable to occur after a gastrojejunostomy, because the intestinal segment is not bathed with alkaline duodenal secretions. Anastomotic ulcers have also been attributed to incomplete resection of the gastric antrum or to incorporation of antral tissue in the closure of the duodenal stump. Gastrin-secreting cells retained in the duodenal stump are continually bathed in an alkaline media. This bypasses the negative feedback normally provided by hydrochloric acid secretion and leads to chronic elevations of gastrin. Therefore, antral tissue must be excised completely.

Acute and chronic afferent loop syndromes are postoperative complications of the Billroth II technique that result from mechanical obstruction of the afferent jejunal limb. Increased pressure in the afferent loop develops because of the accumulation of bile and pancreatic juice. This is evidenced by epigastric discomfort, nausea, and bilious vomiting that can occur weeks to months postoperatively. An affected limb can distend and rupture, thus risking fatal peritonitis. The creation of an afferent limb that is as short as possible (without tension) may avoid this problem.

Resection of Midbody or Fundic Lesions

Leiomyomas, leiomyosarcomas, adenocarcinomas, and occasionally granulomatous lesions involving the

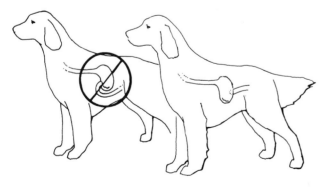

Fig. 15.14. The position of the gastrojejunostomy in a standing patient.

midportion of the stomach can be removed by resecting the midportion and performing an EEA of the remaining segments (Fig 15.15). If the tumor occupies the fundic region only, a focal resection can be performed in this area using a technique analogous to resection of necrotic stomach secondary to gastric dilatation and volvulus (Fig. 15.16). The dorsal and ventral vagal trunks pass through the esophageal hiatus and send branches to the lesser curvature of the stomach. The dorsal vagal trunk also sends branches to the ventral wall of the stomach. In human patients with injury to the vagal nerves, pylorospasm or functional closure of the pyloric canal is a reported complication. For this reason, we perform pyloromyotomy as an adjunctive procedure whenever the gastric vagal nerves are transected.

END-TO-END ANASTOMOSIS OF THE STOMACH

The surgical approach to the stomach is performed. The intended area of resection is determined by visual inspection and palpation. Stay sutures or Babcock forceps are placed in normal gastric tissue to aid in manipulation and to avoid spillage. Doyen clamps are placed on the left and right sides of the tumor, leaving at least 2 cm of healthy tissue between the tumor and the line of resection. Branches of the right and left gastric and gastroepiploic vessels supplying the section of stomach to be removed are ligated along the gastric wall. Care is taken not to damage the main gastric or gastroepiploic vessels. Greater and lesser omental attachments to the section of stomach to be removed are excised. If dispar-

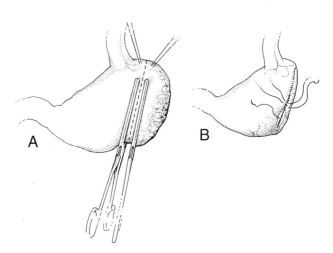

Fig. 15.16. Resection of a mass in the fundic region of the stomach. **A.** Stay sutures, Doyen tissue forceps, or both, are placed on either side of the lesion to aid in manipulation of the stomach and avoid spillage. **B.** The gastrectomy is closed using a simple continuous or interrupted pattern through all four layers of the gastric wall, followed by an inverting pattern (Cushing or Lembert) in the seromuscular layers.

ity exists between the two remaining ends of the stomach, the smaller-diameter section of stomach can be cut at an angle to increase its size. If too much disparity exists for this technique to be effective, then the section of stomach with the greater luminal diameter can be partially oversewn using two layers of 2–0 or 3–0 absorbable suture in a simple continuous pattern, followed by an inverting pattern. We recommend apposing the mucosa and submucosa in a simple interrupted or continuous pattern, using 2–0 or 3–0 absorbable suture. The seromuscular layer is closed in a simple continuous or inverting pattern. The dorsal aspect of the anastomosis is sutured first, followed by the ventral aspect (see Fig. 15.15). The abdomen is lavaged, and a jejunostomy tube is placed. Abdominal closure is routine. Postoperative care is similar to that for Billroth I procedures.

Resection of Leiomyomas and other Benign Masses from the Cardiac Region

The immobility of the gastroesophageal region of the stomach complicates surgery in this area. The inability to visualize the dorsal aspect of the cardia can result in inadvertent laceration of the left gastric artery and vein, and closure of this region may compromise the lumen of the cardia. The cardiac region may be approached by a left thoracoabdominal intercostal incision or by a midline abdominal incision. Benign masses such as leiomyomas are often located in this area and may be excised without penetration of the serosal aspect of the cardia. This procedure, described here, involves a gastrotomy with submucosal resection of the

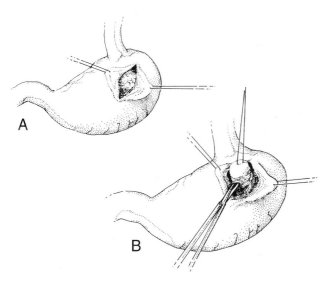

Fig. 15.15. Resection of a midbody lesion of the stomach. **A.** Stay sutures are placed on either side of the lesion to aid in manipulation of the stomach and to avoid spillage. **B.** The involved region is transected. An end-to-end anastomosis is performed by apposing the mucosa and submucosa in a simple interrupted or continuous pattern and closing the seromuscular layer in a simple continuous or inverting pattern.

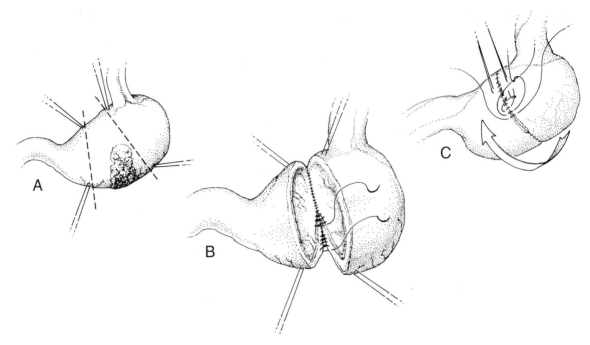

Fig. 15.17. Resection of a benign mass from the cardiac region of the stomach. **A.** A gastrotomy incision is made directly opposite the mass, midway between the lesser and greater curvatures. Stay sutures are placed on either side of the incision. A stay suture is placed in the mass and traction is applied. **B** and **C.** Resection is performed through the mucosal and submucosal layers without penetrating the outer muscular or serosal layers. See text for details.

mass and is approached by the ventral midline. If the serosal surface of the stomach is invaded by tumor, this technique should not be performed.

SURGICAL TECHNIQUE

The greater curvature of the stomach is elevated with Babcock forceps or stay sutures. The gastrotomy incision is performed in the body and fundus of the stomach, midway between the lesser and greater curvatures, and directly opposite from the tumor. The mass is located within the gastric lumen, and a stay suture is placed in the mass. Traction of the stay suture advances the mass toward the gastrotomy incision. The resection is begun at the aboral border of the mass, using Metzenbaum scissors to incise through the mucosa and submucosa. The pedunculated attachment to the muscularis is severed with sharp dissection. Avoid penetration of the outer muscular layer and serosa. The closure of the mucosa is begun using 3–0 or 4–0 absorbable suture in a simple continuous pattern before the mass is completely excised. Excision is completed, followed by closure of the remaining mucosal defect. Care is taken not to compromise the esophageal lumen. The gastrotomy is closed in two layers with 2–0 or 3–0 absorbable suture in a simple continuous pattern, followed by a simple continuous or inverting pattern (Fig. 15.17). The abdomen is lavaged and closed routinely. A gastrotomy or jejunostomy tube is placed if needed.

POSTOPERATIVE CARE

Patients are maintained on balanced intravenous fluids for the next 24 to 48 hours, and small amounts of food and water may be offered beginning 12 hours postoperatively. Oral or intravenous H_2-receptor blockers are administered during the postoperative period.

Resection of Malignant Masses from the Cardiac Region

The incidence of gastric adenocarcinoma of the cardiac region is increasing in human patients in the United States. Tumor excision has been managed satisfactorily with the use of ablative techniques such as complete gastrectomy with a Roux-en-Y procedure. These procedures have not been investigated in dogs and cannot be recommended at this time.

Suggested Readings

Magne ML. Oncologic applications of endoscopy. Vet Clin North Am Small Anim Pract 1995;25:69.

Gilson SD. Clinical management of the regional lymph node. Vet Clin North Am Small Anim Pract 1995;25:149.

Kepsack SJ, Birchard SJ. Removal of leiomyomas and other noninvasive masses from the cardiac region of the canine stomach. J Am Anim Hosp Assoc 1994;30:500.

Ahmadu-suka F, Withrow ST, Nelson AW, et al. Billroth II gastrojejunostomy in the dog: stapling technique and postoperative complications. Vet Surg 1988;17:211.

Suggested Readings

Clark GN. Gastric surgery with surgical stapling instruments. Vet Clin North Am Small Anim Pract 1994;24:279.

Fonda D, Gualtieri M, Scanziani E. Gastric carcinoma in the dog: a clinicopathological study of 11 cases. J Small Anim Pract 1989;30:353.

Lynwood Herrington J Jr. Remedial operations for postgastrectomy and postvagotomy syndromes. In: Cameron JL, ed. Current surgical therapy. 4th ed. St. Louis: Mosby–Year Book, 1992.

Matthiesen DT. Indications and techniques of partial gastrectomy in the dog. Semin Vet Med Surg 1987;2:248.

Patnaik AK, Hurvitz AI, Johnson GF. Canine gastric adenocarcinoma. Vet Pathol 1978;15:600.

Sullivan M, Lee R, Fisher EW, et al. A study of 31 cases of gastric carcinoma in dogs. Vet Rec 1987;120:79.

Walter MC, Matthiesen DT, Stone EA. Pylorectomy and gastroduodenostomy in the dog: technique and clinical results in 28 cases. J Am Vet Med Assoc 1985;187:909.

Willard MD. Diseases of the stomach. In: Ettinger SJ, Feldman EC, eds. Textbook of veterinary internal medicine. 4th ed. Philadelphia: WB Saunders, 1995.

Treatment of Gastric Dilatation–Volvulus

Gary C. Lantz

Gastric dilatation–volvulus (GDV) most commonly occurs in large and giant canine breeds, although smaller breeds are also affected. It is life-threatening and requires immediate treatment consisting of therapy for shock, surgical repositioning and evaluation of the stomach, and prevention of recurrence. The causes of GDV are not well understood. Multiple environmental and hereditary factors are most likely involved. Overeating, pica, postprandial activity, diet, and delayed gastric emptying are some factors that have been implicated. The disease occurs most commonly in middle-aged dogs and is evenly distributed between males and females.

Diagnosis

Clinical Signs and Physical Findings

Clinical signs of GDV include restlessness, pacing, and acute onset of cranial abdominal distension, rapid shallow breathing, and nonproductive vomiting. Profuse salivation may indicate pain. Rapid deterioration results in signs of shock including prolonged capillary refill time, pallor, weak femoral pulses, and tachycardia. The patient's condition at presentation varies. The patient can be alert and ambulatory or comatose, in severe shock, and near death. All patients with these signs require prompt, aggressive treatment. Gastric distension without rotation can cause identical clinical findings. A history of these signs followed by a decrease in abdominal distension should alert the clinician to a possible gastric perforation.

Radiography

Radiographs are obtained during or after the initiation of shock therapy. Radiography is necessary to differentiate simple gastric distension from GDV and is performed before surgery. The right lateral recumbent survey abdominal radiograph is the best radiographic view to confirm the diagnosis of GDV. Ventrodorsal radiographs usually are not needed, and this position adds to the patient's stress. The radiographic signs of GDV include a large, distended stomach, the pylorus located cranial or dorsal to the stomach, a tissue-density line dividing the gas-filled stomach into compartments, splenomegaly, and splenic malposition. The most significant finding is a gas-filled pylorus located dorsal to the fundus of the stomach. In a ventrodorsal radiograph, the pylorus is near or to the left of the midline. If gastric perforation has occurred, pneumoperitoneum is present.

Pathophysiology Overview

Investigators have postulated that gastric rotation occurs after dilatation. Aerophagia is the probable major source of intragastric gas. Gastric luminal fluid is from gastric secretions and transudate is from venous obstruction. Ingested material is often found in the stomach lumen. Gastric distension alters the gastroesophageal angle and impairs eructation. Rotation of the distended stomach further impairs expulsion of gastric contents through the esophagus and compresses the duodenum to prevent gastric emptying. The distended stomach decreases venous return to the heart by compressing the caudal vena cava and portal vein. Therefore, cardiac output is reduced, resulting in decreased systemic tissue perfusion and shock. Bacterial toxins probably are released by the ischemic bowel, and the resultant endotoxemia produces further hypotension. Diaphragmatic excursions are limited by gastric distension, and thus ventilation is reduced. The respiratory rate increases, and the tidal volume decreases. Cardiac arrhythmias are attributed to acid-base and electrolyte disturbances, myocardial ischemia, and autonomic nervous system imbalance. Rotation of the stomach interferes mainly with its venous drainage. This venous outflow obstruction and the increased intragastric pressure result in gastric wall edema and anoxia. The degree and duration of stomach rotation and distension determine the extent of damage to the stomach. Mucosal ulcerations, hemorrhage, and necrosis often occur. The stomach wall may become necrotic, with the left aspect of the greater curvature and fundus most commonly affected.

Experiments indicate that reperfusion injury may play a role in GDV. The decreased tissue perfusion from the reduced cardiac output contributes to tissue hypoxia. When perfusion is increased subsequent to shock therapy, molecular oxygen is reintroduced to these tissues. The oxygen combines with products of anaerobic metabolism, resulting in production of various oxygen radicals. The effect of the radicals is lipid peroxidation and cellular death. The importance of reperfusion injury in the overall complex pathophysiology of GDV is unknown. Definitive clinical treatment has not yet been established.

Preoperative Care

Aggressive therapy must be undertaken immediately when a dog with the signs of GDV enters the hospital. The initial treatment is gastric decompression and therapy for shock to increase venous return to the heart, which increases cardiac output and tissue perfusion. Ideally, both treatments should be started at the same time. However, if lack of personnel precludes simultaneous initiation of both treatments, gastric decompression should be performed first.

Gastric Decompression

Gastric decompression can be accomplished by several methods. A rapid way to remove intragastric gas is needle trocarization. A large-bore needle (18 gauge) is thrust percutaneously through the patients' right or left abdominal wall, at the point of greatest distension, and into the stomach lumen. The stomach wall is against the body wall, and other viscera have been displaced; therefore, the risk of injuring other tissues is minimal. Two to four needles may be inserted. This technique relieves some of the gas component of distension; however, particulate matter or fluid may obstruct the needles and prevent the escape of gas. A small risk of leakage of gastric fluid from these needle holes exists, particularly if an area of compromised stomach wall was perforated.

If the abdominal distension is not visibly and rapidly reduced by trocarization, a stomach tube should be passed. A mouth gag is inserted, and a lubricated stomach tube is passed down the esophagus and into the stois marked, so the operator knows where the end of the tube is located. The tube is gently advanced to avoid esophageal or gastric perforation. If resistance is encountered in the region of the gastroesophageal junction, the tube is rotated and advanced. Removal of some intragastric gas by trocarization, if not previously attempted, may allow some correction of the gastroesophageal angle and easier stomach tube passage. Passage of the tube into the stomach lumen does not mean gastric rotation is absent. Similarly, inability to pass the tube does not confirm rotation. Once the gastric contents are draining through the tube, the tube is not advanced further because of the risk of perforating a compromised area of stomach wall. The tube is withdrawn after decompression. Stomach tube passage should not be attempted if undue resistance from the patient occurs. Narcotic sedation can be used.

If adequate decompression cannot be achieved and the patient is not ready for exploratory surgery, a temporary gastrostomy is constructed. This method removes all stomach contents. This procedure is indicated when needle trocarization or stomach tube passage is unsuccessful or for decompression of the moribund patient that is too great a risk for early anesthesia and surgery. Temporary gastrostomy can be the initial method of decompression, or it can follow one of the previous methods. The gastrostomy is performed in the right paracostal area, which is clipped and prepared for surgery. After an inverted L line block using 2% lidocaine is placed in the skin and muscle, a 10-cm paracostal skin incision is made (Fig. 15.18**A**), followed by a grid incision through the abdominal wall (Fig. 15.18**B**). After entry into the peritoneal cavity, the stomach is identified and is initially attached to the skin with two stay sutures (Fig. 15.18**C**); it is then sutured to the margins of the skin with 2–0 monofilament nonabsorbable suture material in a continuous pattern (Fig. 15.18**D**). The stomach wall is incised, and its contents are removed. Although this procedure results in decompression of the stomach, the organ still may be abnormally rotated. Scalding of surrounding skin by gastric contents is prevented by the application of a petroleum-based ointment. Volvulus is confirmed radiographically. When the patient is taken to surgery to correct the volvulus, the peritoneal cavity is entered through the midline incision, and the temporary gastrostomy is released. The stomach incision is repaired by a two-layer continuous inverting closure; necrotic gastric tissue, if present, is excised by a partial gastrectomy, as described later. The paracostal incision is repaired with 2–0 monofilament nonabsorbable material in the muscle and routine closure of subcutaneous tissue and skin.

Therapy for Shock

Shock therapy consists of intravenous fluids, glucocorticoids, and antibiotics. An isotonic balanced electrolyte solution is administered at 90 mL/kg per hour for the first hour and then is adjusted according to the patient's vital signs. In certain patients, colloids or hypertonic solutions may be required for shock resuscitation. In severe shock, two large-bore catheters can be placed in the cephalic or jugular veins for rapid volume expansion. A urinary catheter is placed, and urine production is monitored as an indicator of tissue perfu-

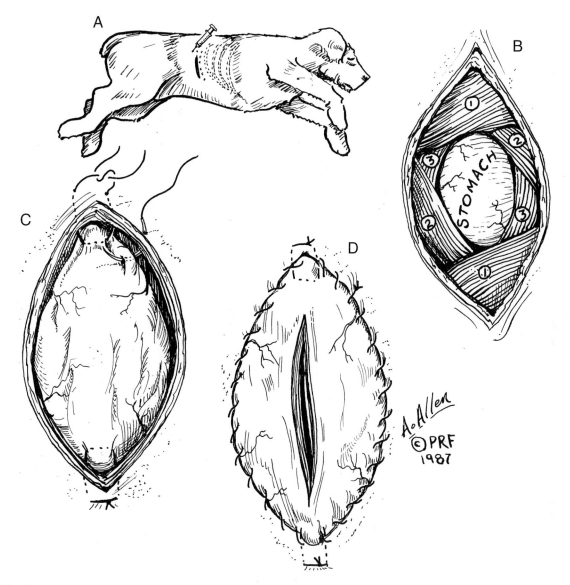

Fig. 15.18. Temporary gastrostomy is performed by placing an inverted L line block and right paracostal skin incision (**A**), by exposing the stomach by grid incision (**B**), by securing the stomach to the skin margins (**C** and **D**), and, finally, by incising the stomach wall (**D**). In **B**: *1,* external abdominal oblique muscle; *2,* internal abdominal oblique muscle; *3,* transversalis muscle.

sion. Urine production of at least 2.0 mL/kg per hour should be obtained. A central venous catheter can be placed for the monitoring of volume overload. Prednisolone sodium succinate (50 mg/kg) and a bactericidal antibiotic such as ampicillin (10 to 20 mg/kg) or a cephalosporin such as cephalothin sodium (20 mg/ kg) are administered intravenously. Cardiac monitoring is started by electrocardiogram to detect GDV associated arrhythmias. Approximately 25% of arrhythmias are present during initial examination. Patients that do not resist a face mask may benefit from oxygen. Acid-base imbalances vary among patients, and specific treatment must be based on a blood gas analysis. Imbalances cannot be determined by physical examination. In the absence of blood gas analysis, acid-base

imbalances are treated indirectly by improving tissue perfusion and ventilation.

Surgical Correction of Volvulus

The timing of surgery depends on the initial patient evaluation, the response to preoperative treatment, and the radiographic confirmation of gastric rotation. The surgeon's experience and judgment are important in the final decision. Most clinicians support exploratory surgery as soon as the patient is a reasonable anesthetic risk (within 2 to 6 hours of presentation). The clinician must always remember that gastric necrosis may be present, and the prognosis worsens as surgery is delayed. Moreover, decompression does not always result in normal gastric position. The venous congestion and ischemia occurring in the stomach as a result of rotation may potentiate gastric necrosis. The radiographic demonstration of pneumoperitoneum or hydropneumoperitoneum warrants rapid surgical intervention. If one has any question about stomach wall integrity and possible leakage, abdominal paracentesis or peritoneal lavage is performed. Dogs that are ambulatory and show minimal signs of shock may be taken directly to surgery after decompression and when treatment for shock has been started. Dogs that are more severely compromised may benefit from decompression and volume expansion for 1 to 2 hours. Improvement in capillary refill time, mucous membrane color, pulse character, respiratory rate, and general attitude signifies a patient that can be taken to surgery. The patient in severe shock should undergo decompression and should be treated for shock until improvement in vital signs is noted. Surgery usually can be performed by 4 to 6 hours after presentation. Occasionally, a longer stabilization period is needed. If necessary, decompression can be maintained with a pharyngostomy tube, esophagostomy tube, or temporary gastrostomy. Poor decompression or gastric necrosis contributes to a patient's continued deterioration and warrants immediate surgical treatment.

Neuroleptanalgesics or narcotics are preferred for anesthesia induction, and anesthesia is maintained with isoflurane or halothane. Isoflurane is recommended over halothane because it is less cardiodepressive and does not sensitize the heart to catecholamines that can produce arrhythmias. An occasional patient may tolerate mask induction. Nitrous oxide contributes to further gastrointestinal distension and should not be used. Because of cardiac and respiratory depression and arrhythmogenicity, ultrashort-acting barbiturates should be avoided. The clinician should be aware of the depressive effects of specific agents.

The dog is placed in dorsal recumbency, and the ventral abdomen is prepared routinely for aseptic surgery. A standard midline abdominal incision is made from the xiphoid to caudal to the umbilicus. The incision is lengthened as necessary. Balfour abdominal retractors are helpful for exposure.

Surgical Anatomy and Degree of Rotation

In this description, the dog is assumed to be lying on an operating table in dorsal recumbency. Clockwise rotation of the stomach is most commonly found. The normal position of the stomach is shown in Figure 15.19**A.** In an animal with GDV, the stomach is rotated about the distal esophagus and is tilted cranially. Various degrees of rotation are possible. A 90° rotation moves the pylorus cranially (Fig. 15.19**B**). With a 180° rotation, the pylorus is located ventral to the esopha-

gus (Fig. 15.19**C**); with a 270° rotation, it is dorsal to the stomach (Fig. 15.19**D**). A full 360° rotation moves the pylorus to near its original position (Fig. 15.19**E**). Most rotations are between 180 and 270°. Occasionally, a counterclockwise rotation up to 90° is present.

As illustrated in Figure 15.19, the duodenum follows the pylorus and passes immediately ventral to the esophagus and then dorsal to the stomach as the degree of rotation increases. The fundus moves from left to right and ventrally, so the greater curvature is found along the ventral abdominal wall with increasing rotation. As a result, the stomach is covered with greater omentum, and the gastroepiploic vessels nearly parallel the abdominal midline. The spleen passively follows the displacement of the left side of the stomach because of the ligamentous and vascular connections between the two structures. The spleen may be found at various locations in the cranial abdomen and is usually dramatically congested and may be torsed on its own vascular pedicle contained in the gastrosplenic ligament.

Repositioning of the Stomach

The first structure the surgeon sees is the omentum covering the stomach. If possible, it is manipulated so the surgeon can directly touch the stomach and decrease the chance of creating omental tears. The surgeon's hand is placed between the stomach and the liver, and the stomach is withdrawn caudally to eliminate the cranial tilt. The stomach is then grasped to elevate the pylorus (toward the ventral abdominal wall incision) and to depress the fundus (toward the spine). The stomach is gently twisted in a counterclockwise direction until it is returned to normal position. Movement of the spleen is manually assisted during this manuver to avoid possible injury or avulsion of stomach and splenic vascular connections.

Complete derotation is determined by palpating and visualizing the cardia and intra-abdominal esophagus. Passage of a stomach tube can serve as a reference to aid palpation. Easy passage of the tube and lack of tissue folds at the gastroesophageal junction indicate complete derotation. The presence of corkscrew folds in this region indicates incomplete derotation. After positioning of the stomach, the gastrosplenic ligament is examined and derotated if necessary.

Intraoperative Gastric Decompression

Preoperative stomach decompression is often incomplete, and the remaining contents can be evacuated during the surgical procedure by passing a stomach tube, usually after stomach repositioning. If intraoperative decompression is necessary before stomach repo-

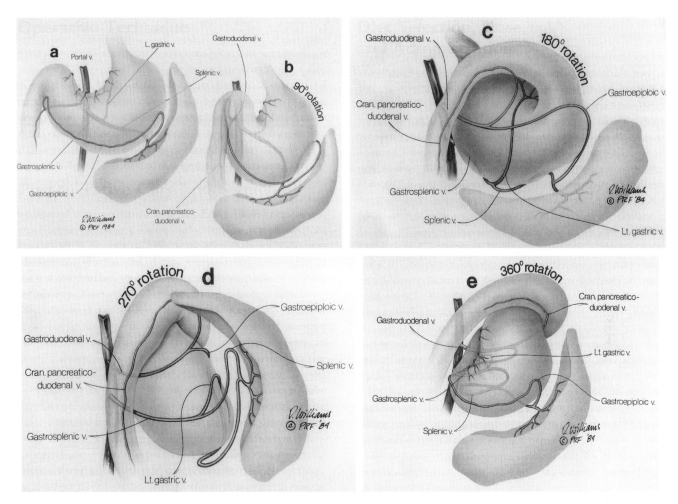

Fig. 15.19. **A.** Normal stomach position when viewed in a ventrodorsal position. **B–E.** In gastric dilatation–volvulus, the stomach is rotated about the esophagus in a clockwise direction causing malposition of the pylorus, fundus, and spleen. For illustrative purposes, the gastric dilatation has not been pictured. Vessels are included for orientation.

sitioning, removal of gas can also be accomplished by suction. A large-bore needle attached to a suction unit tube is inserted through an area of relatively normal-appearing stomach wall and into the stomach lumen to withdraw the gas. Removal of bulk material, which may be difficult, can be done after the stomach is placed in normal position. If food is present and can be compressed by palpation of the stomach, its dilution and suction removal through an orogastric tube or an orogastric tube combined with a temporary gastrostomy tube should be attempted before gastrotomy. To remove lesser amounts of material, tap water is passed into the stomach through the orogastric tube, the stomach contents are "kneaded" by hand, and suction is applied to the tube to remove stomach contents. For removal of a larger volume of solid material, when a larger volume of water may be necessary to liquefy ingesta, a stomach tube is passed to evacuate remaining gas and liquid. A normal-appearing area of

stomach wall is identified, and a pursestring suture of 2–0 synthetic absorbable material is placed. An incision is made in the center of the pursestring, through the stomach wall. One end of a large-bore tube is placed into the stomach lumen; the other end is attached to a suction unit. Tap water is introduced into the stomach through the stomach tube, and the stomach is gently kneaded by hand to mix the water with the stomach contents. The dilute material is suctioned off through the gastrostomy tube. Once the stomach is empty, the gastrostomy tube is withdrawn, the pursestring is tightened, and two Lembert (inverting) sutures are placed at the incision site. The presence of material that cannot be broken apart (i.e., foreign bodies) necessitates removal through gastrotomy. Gastrotomy should be avoided whenever possible. In addition to the risk of spillage, healing may be delayed, resulting in greater stomach suture line leakage potential.

Determination of Stomach Viability

Approximately 10% of GDV patients have gastric necrosis. After repositioning of the stomach, gastric viability is assessed, and devitalized areas are excised by partial gastrectomy. Clinical criteria to evaluate for gastric necrosis are usually, but not consistently, accurate. Serosal color, thickness of the stomach wall as determined by palpation, and vascular patency are assessed. The greater curvature of the stomach is most severely damaged from vascular compromise. This results primarily from obstruction of venous outflow and subsequent ischemia. The stomach wall is initially palpably thicker than normal from congestion with blood and edema. Thrombosis or avulsion of the short gastric and epiploic branches of the left gastroepiploic vessels may be found. Vessel avulsion results in hemoperitoneum.

Diffuse petechial or ecchymotic stomach serosal hemorrhage indicates vascular damage, but tissue resection is not necessary. Diffuse dark red or red–purple hemorrhagic areas indicate more severe compromise, but these areas usually do not require resection. Once the stomach is repositioned, thereby relieving venous outflow obstruction, the appearance of the serosa can greatly improve in 5 to 10 minutes; this finding indicates intact intramural circulation. In blue–black or black areas, tissue may survive once the vascular compromise is relieved by stomach repositioning. Small serosal incisions are made in these areas; the appearance of arterial blood indicates probable survival. Extensive stomach wall collateral circulation contributes to tissue survival. If arterial blood is not seen, severe hypoxic damage and tissue necrosis are present, and the segment is excised. Gray or green serosal discoloration indicates severe vascular damage and tissue necrosis; such areas must be excised. Necrotic segments are thin when palpated, compared with adjacent areas of stomach wall. All areas of thin gastric wall that are associated with abnormal-appearing serosa or serosal tearing are considered devitalized and are resected.

Partial gastrectomy removes necrotic tissue at the left aspect of the stomach body and fundus (Fig. 15.20). The technique is performed with or without atraumatic clamps applied to viable stomach tissue adjacent to the necrotic area. The local area is packed off to contain potential spillage. The use of clamps minimizes the risk of spillage. Monofilament nonabsorbable (polypropylene) or synthetic absorbable (polydioxanone or polyglyconate) suture material is used as a two-layer inverting suture pattern that penetrates all layers of the stomach. Alternatively, the stomach lumen may be closed with staples. In selected patients with a smaller area of necrosis, invagination of the tissues may be performed instead of resection (see the discussion in a later section of this chapter).

When a partial gastrectomy or decompression gastrotomy is performed, the surgeon commonly finds large areas of infarcted gastric mucosa. Such areas need not be resected, because the mucosa regenerates quickly. Because subjective criteria are used to assess stomach viability, an unnecessary partial gastrectomy occasionally is performed, or a necrotic area is left in place when it should have been excised. If any question exists about the viability of an area, that area should be excised. Intravenous fluorescein dye is not a reliably accurate indicator of gastric viability and can contribute to hypotension.

Evaluation of Other Abdominal Organs

The spleen is engorged with blood in the patient with GDV and is found in various locations in the cranial abdomen. Thrombosis of the splenic vessels and vessel avulsion resulting in splenic necrosis require splenectomy; however, in most patients with GDV, the spleen is viable. The spleen is returned to normal position, and areas of questionable parenchyma are reevaluated later in the surgical procedure. Torsion of the splenic pedicle is corrected if present. However, if splenic torsion is present with splenic necrosis, splenectomy is performed without correcting the torsion to prevent toxin release. Removal of the spleen does not prevent recurrence of GDV.

The pancreas and intestine are often edematous because of obstruction of venous drainage through the portal vein. Pyloromyotomy or pyloroplasty has been advocated to speed gastric emptying to help prevent recurrence of GDV. However, because no conclusive evidence indicates that a primary pyloric abnormality is involved in GDV, pyloric surgery cannot be recommended. In addition, these procedures do not significantly alter gastric emptying time or lumen diameter. Pyloroplasty enlarges the outflow diameter if obstruction is present. The pyloric region is always palpated, and any unusual thickening should be investigated by pyloroplasty and biopsy.

Gastropexy

Gastropexy techniques with the goal of creating a permanent adhesion between the stomach and body wall greatly decrease the rate of GDV recurrence. Without gastropexy, recurrence rates of up to 80% have been reported. Therefore, all affected dogs should have a gastropexy. The pyloric antral region is fixed to the adjacent right abdominal wall. The common procedures for accomplishing gastropexy are right-sided tube gastrostomy (tube gastropexy), circumcostal gastropexy, belt loop gastropexy, and incisional gastropexy (discussed in a later section of this chapter). A gastropexy is always performed on the right side of

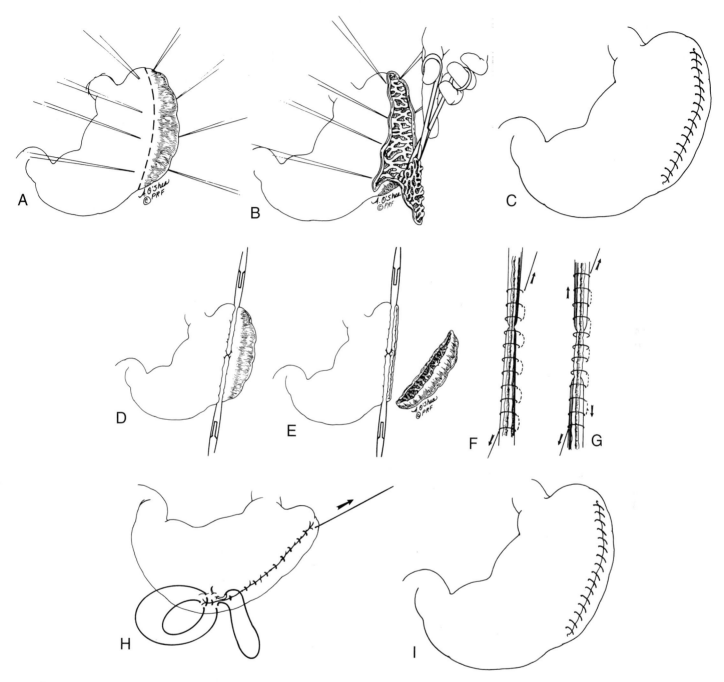

Fig. 15.20. Two variations of partial gastrectomy are shown. In **A–C,** stay sutures are placed to elevate the stomach and to minimize leakage. Necrotic tissue is excised with a rim of viable tissue (*dotted line*). A two-layer inverting closure is used. In **D–I,** atraumatic clamps are placed across viable tissue, and the necrotic tissue is excised. The stomach body is subsequently closed with a Parker–Kerr suture line. The first inverting layer of suture is placed over the clamps. The clamps are subsequently removed as the suture line is pulled tight to invert the suture line. A second inverting suture line completes the closure. (Redrawn in part from Matthiesen DT. Gastric dilatation–volvulus syndrome. In: Slatter DH, ed. Textbook of small animal surgery. Philadelphia: WB Saunders, 1995:580–593.)

the stomach because some rotation can still occur if it is performed between the left gastric wall and the left abdominal wall.

Postoperative Care and Complications

Routine intensive care monitoring and nursing care are indicated. Intravenous fluids, supplemented with potassium (Table 15.1), are continued, and electrolyte levels are monitored postoperatively. Hypokalemia is the most common electrolyte abnormality. It may contribute to generalized weakness, gastrointestinal atony, and augmentation or development of cardiac arrhythmias and poor response to antiarrhythmic therapy. Remaining fluid deficits are estimated and are administered in addition to the maintenance requirements of 60 mL/kg per day. Because of the gastritis caused by GDV, nothing is offered per mouth for 48 hours. Patients are gradually returned to their normal diet, as described later. Continued accumulation of intragastric gas suggests decreased gastric motility. Gas is removed easily through the gastrostomy tube if tube gastropexy was performed. Nasogastric tube placement or orogastric tube passage is required for gastric decompression if another gastropexy technique was performed. Gastric atony is secondary to stomach hypoxia or hypokalemia. The potassium supplementation added to the daily intravenous fluid requirements and subcutaneous metoclopramide (0.2 to 0.4 mg/kg three or four times daily) are used to treat gastric atony. When gastric motility returns, usually within 2 to 3 days, water or broth is offered. Food of gruel consistency can be offered on the next day in small, frequent feedings. The normal diet is provided in 4 to 5 days. This schedule can be accelerated if the stomach appeared relatively healthy during surgery and if gastrointestinal motility is present as determined by auscultation of borborygmus. Antibiotics are continued for 7 to 10 days. Melena, secondary to gastric mucosal necrosis and hemorrhage, may be seen for several days. Gastritis, which may result in persistent vomiting, is treated by providing intravenous fluid support, nothing by mouth, subcutaneous metoclopramide or other antiemetics such as chlorpromazine, and intramuscular cimetidine (5 to 10 mg/kg three or four times daily) to reduce gastric acid production.

Postoperative shock may develop secondary to hypovolemia from inadequate resusitation and surgical hypotension and blood loss. Moreover, bacterial toxin absorption through injured gastric mucosa, bowel mucosa, or peritoneum, if gastric necrosis and perforation are present, also potentiates shock.

Cardiac arrhythmias can occur preoperatively, intraoperatively, or, most commonly, postoperatively. The occurrence rate is approximately 40 to 50%. Onset may not occur for 12 to 72 hours after hospital admission. The most common arrhythmias are ventricular (e.g., premature depolarization, tachycardias, multifocal rhythms). Indications for antiarrhythmic drug therapy include ventricular premature depolarizations (more than 20 per minute) and continuous or paroxysmal ventricular tachycardia and signs of inadequate cardiac output such as weak femoral pulses, pale mucous membranes, and decreased refill time. Optimal treatment also includes maintenance of normal hydration, acid-base balance, and serum electrolyte concentrations. Lidocaine, at 1 to 2 mg/kg as an intravenous bolus, is given until normal sinus rhythm appears, or a total dose of 8 mg/kg is administered; a maintenance infusion rate of 0.04 to 0.08 mg/kg per minute is then started. Vomiting is the principal sign of lidocaine toxicity at lower dosages, whereas muscle tremors and convulsions may occur at higher levels. Lidocaine is stopped if signs of toxicity are observed. Procainamide or quinidine is given as a supplement or alternative to lidocaine in refractory cases. Intravenous procainamide is given (0.5 mg/kg) until a total of 6 mg/kg is administered; the subsequent maintenance dose is 6 to 8 mg/kg intramuscularly every 6 hours or 0.04 mg/kg per minute intravenously. Quinidine is given at 6 to 8 mg/kg intravenously every 6 hours. Not all arrhythmias are converted by drug therapy, but their frequency usually is reduced. Most arrhythmias resolve by 5 or 6 days after surgery.

Most deaths occur within 96 hours after the surgical procedure. Overall mortality is approximately 30 to 60%. However, aggressive intervention and advances in shock treatment and intensive care can reduce mortality to about 15%. Mortality in the presence of gastric necrosis is 63 to 80%. This underscores the need for rapid intervention and intensive postoperative care. Other complications include pancreatitis, disseminated intravascular coagulation, and local or diffuse peritonitis from leakage through an area of devitalized stomach wall along the greater curvature.

Delayed leakage can occur from areas judged by the surgeon as viable during the initial surgery that were

Table 15.1.
Intravenous Potassium Supplementation Guidelines

Serum Potassium[a] (meq/L)	meq Potassium Chloride to Add to 250 mL Fluid	Maximal Fluid Infusion Rate[b] (mL/kg/h)
<2.0	20	6
2.1–2.5	15	8
2.6–3.0	10	12
3.1–3.5	7	16

[a] If serum potassium is not available, add potassium to a total concentration of 20 meq/L.
[b] Do not exceed 0.5 meq/kg/h.
(Courtesy of RC Scott, D.V.M., Animal Medical Center, New York.)

either actually devitalized at that time or became necrotic later, secondary to vascular compromise and irreversible damage. Clinical signs of peritonitis can be seen approximately 2 to 5 days after surgery and include vomiting, lethargy, anorexia, fever, and abdominal tenderness. Survey abdominal radiographs reveal pneumoperitoneum from the initial surgery. Loss of radiographic contrast from intra-abdominal fluid may be seen. A diagnosis of peritonitis can be made based on finding a leukocytosis with a left shift on a complete blood count and evidence of septic peritonitis on examination of peritoneal fluid. A gastric mucosal filling defect or leakage in the area of the greater curvature may be revealed on a positive-contrast gastrogram using water-soluble contrast media. Endoscopic examination may not confirm leakage because a small stomach wall hole can be hidden by rugal folds. Suspected leakage requires exploratory surgery. Partial gastrectomy and excision of adhered omentum are required. All tissue debris is removed from the peritoneal cavity by copious irrigation with warm isotonic fluid. Samples for bacterial culture are obtained. If diffuse peritonitis is present, open peritoneal drainage may be required. Similar clinical signs and management are required for leakage from a partial gastrectomy suture line.

Prevention

Because the causes of GDV are unknown, specific measures in patient management to prevent recurrence cannot be given. Postprandial gastric distension can be reduced by premoistening dry foods, dividing the daily ration into two or three smaller meals, and limiting activity before and after eating and drinking to reduce aerophagia.

Recurrence of dilatation is possible, but the development of rotation is greatly reduced with gastropexy. Dilatation can be as serious as dilatation–rotation. Owner education concerning the clinical signs of dilatation and the prompt need for medical attention is important.

Suggested Readings

Brockman DJ, Washabau RJ, Drobatz KJ. Canine gastric dilatation-volvulus syndrome in a veterinary critical care unit: 295 cases (1986–1992). J Am Vet Med Assoc 1995;207:460–464.

Eggertsdottir AV, Moe L. A retrospective study of conservative treatment of gastric dilatation–volvulus in the dog. Acta Vet Scand 1995;36:175–184.

Ellison GW. Gastric dilatation volvulus surgical prevention. Vet Clin North Am 1993;23:513–530.

Glickman LT, Glickman NW, Perez CM, et al. Analysis of risk factors for gastric dilatation and dilatation–volvulus in dogs. J Am Vet Med Assoc 1994;204:1465–1471.

Harvey RC. Anesthetic management for canine gastric dilatation volvulus. Semin Vet Med Surg 1986;1:230–237.

Hathcock JT. Radiographic view of choice for the diagnosis of gastric volvulus: the right lateral recumbent view. J Am Anim Hosp Assoc 1984;20:967–969.

Hosgood G. Gastric dilatation–volvulus in dogs. J Am Vet Med Assoc 1994;204:1742–1747.

Jennings PB, Mathey WS, Ehler WJ. Intermittent gastric dilatation after gastropexy in a dog. J Am Vet Med Assoc 1992;200:1707–1708.

Lantz GC, Badylak SF, Hiles MC, et al. Treatment of reperfusion injury in dogs with experimentally induced gastric dilatation–volvulus. Am J Vet Res 1992;53:1594–1598.

Lantz GC, Bottoms GD, Carlton WW, et al. The effect of 360° gastric volvulus on the blood supply of the nondistended normal dog stomach. Vet Surg 1984;13:189–196.

Matthiesen DT. The gastric dilatation–volvulus complex: medical and surgical considerations. J Am Anim Hosp Assoc 1983;9:925–932.

Matthiesen DT. Partial gastrectomy as treatment of gastric volvulus, results in 30 dogs. Vet Surg 1985;14:185–193.

Meyer-Lindenberg A, Harder A, Fehr M, et al. Treatment of gastric dilatation–volvulus and a rapid method for prevention of relapse in dogs: 134 cases (1988–1991). J Am Vet Med Assoc 1993;203:1303–1307.

Muir WW. Acid-base and electrolyte disturbances in dogs with gastric dilatation–volvulus. J Am Vet Med Assoc 1982;181:229–231.

Muir WW, Bonagura JD. Treatment of cardiac arrhythmias in dogs with gastric distention–volvulus. J Am Vet Med Assoc 1984;184:1366–1371.

Orton EC, Muir WW. Hemodynamics during experimental gastric dilatation–volvulus in dogs. Am J Vet Res 1983;44:1512–1515.

Walshaw R, Johnston DE. Treatment of gastric dilatation–volvulus by gastric decompression and patient stabilization before major surgery. J Am Anim Hosp Assoc 1976;12:162–167.

Wheaton LG, Thacker HL, Caldwell S. Intravenous fluorescein as an indicator of gastric viability in gastric dilatation–volvulus. J Am Anim Hosp Assoc 1986;22:197–204.

Chronic Gastric Rotation

Gary C. Lantz

Chronic gastric rotation is a condition in the dog in which the stomach rotates, usually 90 to 120°, and is not associated with an acute onset of gastric dilatation or the other usual signs of gastric dilatation–volvulus. It is not an acute, life-threatening condition. Although chronic gastric rotation has been reported only infrequently, in my experience, large and giant dogs of variable ages can be affected by this condition. Common clinical signs of chronic gastric rotation include chronic vomiting, lethargy, anorexia, and weight loss. Chronic vomiting is the most common owner complaint. Signs can be intermittent and may occur over 1 to 4 weeks before presentation to the veterinarian. Historical evidence of mild abdominal distension may be confirmed by the owners.

Differential diagnosis should include other causes of chronic vomiting such as gastric outflow obstruction, ulcer disease, or gastritis; hepatic, pancreatic, or renal disease; hypoadrenocorticism; and primary splenic torsion. A definitive diagnosis of gastric rotation is made from radiographic demonstration of a malpositioned stomach. Positive-contrast radiography may aid in defining the stomach position and in determining the presence of an outflow obstruction.

Surgical Technique

Fluid and electrolyte imbalances are corrected before surgery. After induction of general anesthesia, a standard ventral midline abdominal incision is made from the xiphoid cartilage to caudal to the umbilicus.

The stomach may have returned to normal position; however, it is usually covered with greater omentum (as a result of gastric rotation and subsequent omental displacement) and is minimally distended with gas. The stomach and spleen are grasped and derotated as described for acute gastric dilatation–volvulus. A complete abdominal exploratory operation is performed. The stomach wall is usually flaccid on palpation, an indication of chronic distension. The empty stomach is often larger than expected for the dog. The stomach is mobile, indicating probable laxity of the gastric ligaments. The pyloric region is examined visually and by palpation to determine whether an outflow obstruction is present. If one has any question of outflow obstruction, a pyloroplasty is performed to inspect the gastric tissues at this level and to obtain samples for histopathologic examination.

A gastropexy of the surgeon's preference is created before abdominal closure. Because postoperative gastric distension usually is not a problem with this condition, a tube gastropexy for postoperative decompression is not strongly recommended.

Postoperative Care

Maintenance intravenous fluids are administered until normal oral intake is resumed. Free-choice water and a bland diet fed two or three times daily are started 24 hours postoperatively. Cranial abdominal discomfort or distension often indicates gastric atony. Gastric atony causing clinical signs is usually not apparent in these dogs. However, if clinical signs occur, treatment is by orogastric or nasogastric intubation for decompression if needed. In addition, gastric prokinetic agents such as cisapride or metoclopramide are administered for 5 to 7 days. The normal diet and feeding schedule is started 2 to 5 days after the surgical procedure.

Suggested Readings

Booth HW, Ackerman N. Partial gastric torsion in two dogs. J Am Anim Hosp Assoc 1976;12:27–30.

Frendin J, Funkquist B, Stavenborn M. Gastric displacement in dogs without clinical signs of acute dilation. J Small Anim Pract 1988;29:775–779.

Lieb MS, Monroe WE, Martin RA. Suspected chronic gastric volvulus in a dog with normal gastric emptying of liquids. J Am Vet Med Assoc 1987;191:699–700.

Partial Invagination of the Canine Stomach for Treatment of Infarction of the Gastric Wall

Douglas M. MacCoy

Infarction of a portion of the gastric fundus and cardia is most commonly associated with gastric volvulus in the dog. Immediate surgical management is indicated to prevent perforation and peritonitis. The traditional partial gastrectomy not only adds to the length of the surgical procedure, but also creates the potential for contamination of the abdomen with gastric contents. Dehiscence of the gastrectomy closure may be a further complication of surgery. As a general surgical principle, operative time should be minimized, to limit surgical and anesthetic stress on the patient (1, 2). Invagination of the compromised portion of the stomach wall into the lumen of the stomach is easily and quickly performed (5 to 10 minutes), has little risk of intraoperative contamination of the abdomen because the gastric lumen is not opened, and has a low potential for complications (3).

Surgical Technique

The surgical approach for the gastric wall invagination is the same as that for reduction of gastric volvulus, and this operation is usually done in conjunction with that procedure. Once the area of stomach to be invaginated has been identified (Fig. 15.21**A**), any torn or thrombosed vessels leading to it are ligated (Fig. 15.21**B**).

A continuous Lembert pattern suture using 1–0 polypropylene is started beyond the damaged tissue and is advanced in the normal tissue to either side of the thrombosed area. This suture line is ended in the normal tissue beyond the suspect area. A second layer of Lembert sutures using the same material is placed to cover the first line of sutures completely, providing two layers of serosal seal between the gastric lumen and the peritoneal cavity (Fig. 15.21**C**).

Any additional procedures such as tube gastrostomy or one of the varieties of gastropexy are performed after the invagination procedure is completed. The abdomen is closed in three layers using polypropylene for the rectus muscle closure.

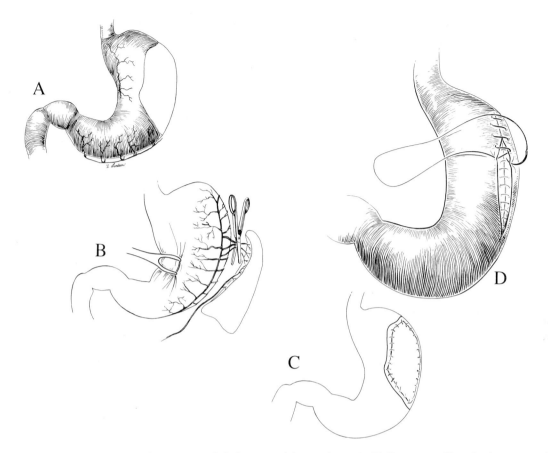

Fig. 15.21. **A.** Area of the stomach to be invaginated. **B.** Ligation of damaged vessels. **C.** Placement of invaginating sutures. **D.** Closure with simple continuous suture technique. (From MacCoy DM, Kneller SK, Sundberg JP, et al. Partial invagination of the canine stomach for treatment of infarction of the gastric wall. Vet Surg 1986;15:237–245.)

Postoperative Care

The sloughing of the invaginated tissue leaves what is essentially a gastric ulcer. Cimetidine or one of the other H_2 antagonists should be started immediately and maintained for 4 weeks. Sucralfate may be mixed with water and placed through a gastrostomy tube if one is present, or it may be started as soon as oral intake is allowed. Sucralfate should be given for 4 weeks to coat the sloughing area during healing. Clinically, melena may occur for several days after the procedure. The dog's stomach has the ability to rapidly dilate despite extreme reductions in diameter (4), and no loss of size has been seen experimentally (3) or clinically.

References

1. Feigal DW, Blaisdell FW. The estimation of surgical risk. Med Clin North Am 1979;63:1131–1143.
2. Cooper P, ed. The craft of surgery. Boston: Little, Brown, 1964:4–5.
3. MacCoy DM, Kneller SK, Sundberg JP, et al. Partial invagination of the canine stomach for treatment of infarction of the gastric wall. Vet Surg 1986;15:237–245.
4. Eskind SD, Massie JD, Born ML, et al. Experimental study of double staple lines in gastric partitions. Surg Gynecol Obstet 1981;152:751–756.

Tube Gastropexy

Gary C. Lantz

Tube gastropexy is one of several gastropexy methods that may be used to create a permanent adhesion between the pyloric antrum and the adjacent right abdominal body wall in dogs with gastric dilatation–volvulus (GDV). Right-sided gastropexy techniques that have the goal of creating permanent adhesions reduce the recurrence rate of GDV.

Tube gastropexy is technically easy to perform and can be constructed more rapidly than some other techniques. It has the advantage of providing rapid, easy access to the gastric lumen for the administration of medications or nutrients. Most important, episodes of postoperative gastric distension are simply relieved, thereby avoiding the need for orogastric tube passage and the accompanying stress to the patient. This gastropexy technique is highly recommended for patients requiring partial gastrectomy for the removal of necrotic gastric tissue. In these patients, gastric decompression must be maintained to minimize tension on the gastric suture or staple line that is opposing edematous, friable gastric tissues.

Disadvantages of tube gastropexy include potential leakage of gastric contents because of entry into the gastric lumen, premature removal of the tube that may result in gastric leakage, and management of the tube length that is exterior to the skin. Failure to develop a permanent adhesion occurs in 5 to 29% of patients, with resulting recurrence of GDV. Lower recurrence rates in recent reports make these rates more comparable with those associated with other gastropexy techniques.

Surgical Technique

The tube is actually a larger-gauge Foley catheter (20 to 30 Fr for large to giant breed dogs) with a balloon

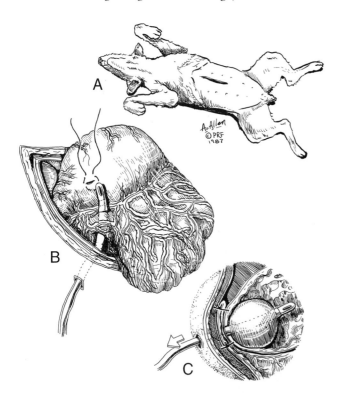

Fig. 15.22. Tube gastropexy. **A** and **B.** The Foley catheter is placed into the abdominal cavity through a small stab incision in the body wall. It is bluntly passed through omentum and into the stomach lumen through a small incision encircled by a pursestring suture. The stomach lumen entry site is the junction of stomach body and pyloric antrum. **C.** The cross section shows the inflated Foley catheter balloon within the stomach lumen and sutures holding the stomach wall to the body wall with interposed omentum. Gentle traction is applied to the Foley catheter, which is then secured to the skin with sutures.

capacity of 20 to 30 mL of fluid. The balloon integrity is tested by distension before the catheter is placed.

The tube placement technique is illustrated in Figure 15.22. The procedure is performed just before closure of the midline abdominal incision. The ventral surface of the pyloric antrum is manually apposed to the peritoneal surface of the adjacent right body wall in a location dorsolateral to the abdominal incision and caudal to the last rib, resulting in the least amount of displacement of the pyloric antrum. At this predetermined level of the abdominal body wall, a small skin incision is made to allow passage of the Foley catheter. Underlying fascia and muscle are similarly incised, and the catheter is passed through the body wall. A pursestring suture (2–0 polypropylene), passing through all layers of the stomach, is placed at the junction of the gastric body and pyloric antrum and is centered between the greater and lesser curvatures. The catheter end is bluntly passed through omentum and into the gastric lumen through an incision in the center of the pursestring suture. Four horizontal mattress sutures (2–0 polypropylene) are placed circumferentially around the catheter stomas between the gastric wall and the body wall to appose these tissues with the omentum interposed. These sutures pass through all layers of the stomach, the omentum, and the transversalis fascia. All sutures are preplaced and then tied. (Alternatively, the catheter is not passed through the omentum. The gastric wall and body wall are sutured together, and the omentum then is wrapped around this suture line and is secured in position by two or three simple interrupted sutures.) The catheter balloon is distended, and the catheter is placed under traction to appose the catheter balloon gently to the gastric mucosa. The catheter is then secured to the skin with sutures. The abdominal incision is closed routinely.

Patient Management and Tube Removal

The catheter lumen is capped to prevent spillage of gastric contents, and the tube length is secured to the skin by a light circumferential body wrap. The catheter is left in position for 7 days. (Some surgeons recommend up to 10 days.) The wrap is changed as needed, and the skin around the catheter is kept clean and dry. Minor serous drainage is found during this time. The patient may be sent home with the tube in position and returned for periodic rechecks. When the catheter is removed, a gastrocutaneous fistula remains. This heals by second intention in 7 to 10 days. The skin should not be sutured because this may promote development of a body wall abscess. Again, minor serous drainage is normal, and the surrounding skin is kept clean and dry. Excessive drainage may contain gastric juices that scald the skin. The skin is then protected with zinc oxide or petroleum gel.

On rare occasion, a permanent stoma develops and must be closed. An incision is made across the stoma, and tissues are retracted. Dissection is continued until gastric mucosa is visualized. Everted mucosa is excised, and the gastric lumen is sutured closed. The incision is sutured to the original stoma size. Second-intention healing is complete in 7 to 10 days.

The purpose of the distended catheter balloon is to decrease the potential of gastric fluid leakage. Gentle traction of the catheter is used to appose all tissue layers and the balloon. The sutures between the stomach and the body wall maintain the tissue apposition. Excessive tube traction may result in pressure necrosis of the gastric wall and subsequent leakage. The balloon should be distended with 15 to 20 mL of saline; however, this is relative to the patient's size. Balloon inflation results in partial compromise of gastric outflow, and the surgeon must decide during the surgical procedure how much distension can be tolerated without causing a clinical obstruction. Placing the catheter entry site at the junction of the gastric body and pyloric antrum minimizes the potential for obstruction. Minimal balloon distension (i.e., 5 mL in a large dog) may result in premature dislodgment of the catheter or inadequate "sealing" of the catheter track. Premature catheter removal or an inadequate seal may result in peritonitis or cellulitis as gastric fluid dissects along the muscle or fascia of the abdominal wall. The use of omentum by either of the foregoing methods helps to minimize leakage risk. Omentum develops a watertight fibrin seal within 4 to 6 hours when it is wrapped around various intra-abdominal drains. The balloon is eroded by gastric acid and may rupture as early as 5 to 7 days after placement. Early connective tissue deposition has resulted in a well-isolated tract lumen by this time. The fibrous tissue adhesion development is apparently the inflammatory response to the combination of serosal injury, the presence of foreign material, and probable minimum gastric fluid contamination of the local site.

Suggested Readings

Flanders JA, Harvey HJ. Results of tube gastrostomy as treatment for gastric volvulus in the dog. J Am Vet Med Assoc 1984;185:74–77.

Fox SM, Ellison GW, Miller GJ, et al. Observations on the mechanical failure of three gastropexy techniques. J Am Anim Hosp Assoc 1985;21:729–734.

Fox SM, McCoy CP, Cooper RC, et al. Circumcostal gastropexy versus tube gastrostomy: histological comparison of gastropexy adhesions. J Am Anim Hosp Assoc 1987;24:273–279.

Johnson RG, Barrus J, Greene RW. Gastric dilatation–volvulus: recurrence rate following tube gastrostomy. J Am Anim Hosp Assoc 1982;20:33–37.

Levine SH, Caywood DD. Biomechanical evaluation of gastropexy techniques in the dog. Vet Surg 1983;12:166–169.

Parks JL, Greene RW. Tube gastrostomy for the treatment of gastric volvulus. J Am Anim Hosp Assoc 1976;12:168–172.

Incisional Gastropexy

Douglas M. MacCoy

Gastric volvulus is a serious, often fatal problem that occurs primarily in large, deep-chested dogs. Gastropexy (1, 2), gastroplasty (3), tube gastrostomy (4), and gastrocolopexy (5) have all been used in an attempt to fix the stomach to the body wall permanently and to prevent recurrent volvulus. The incisional gastropexy (1) offers a method of producing a permanent gastropexy without the potential complications and aftercare associated with tube gastrostomy. It may be used as an alternative to a tube gastrostomy when postoperative decompression will be provided by pharyngostomy tube or is not thought necessary, but a permanent gastropexy is still desired (6). The same low potential for complications also makes it suitable as a prophylactic procedure in high-risk patients.

Surgical Technique

The cranial abdomen is approached by a ventral midline laparotomy. The pyloric antrum is identified and is held in the surgical field by thumb forceps, Babcock forceps, or stay sutures. Using a scalpel, the surgeon makes an incision equal in length to the diameter of the duodenum through the gastric serosa and into but not through the muscularis over the parietal surface of the pyloric antrum equidistant from the attachments of the greater and lesser omenta (Fig. 15.23**A**). The incision should be at least one duodenal diameter away from the pylorus, to avoid distortion of the pylorus. A second incision of the same length is made through the peritoneum and internal fascia of the rectus abdominis muscle or transversus abdominis muscle of the ventrolateral abdominal wall adjacent to the incision on the pyloric antrum (Fig. 15.23**B**).

The edges of the abdominal wall incision are sutured to the edges of the pyloric incision using 2–0 or 1–0 monofilament nylon or polypropylene in a simple continuous pattern, creating an imperforate, circular stoma (Fig. 15.23**C**). The abdominal incision is closed in a routine fashion.

Postoperative Care

Exercise is restricted for a minimum of 3 weeks to allow healing of the abdominal incision. No dietary restrictions are needed.

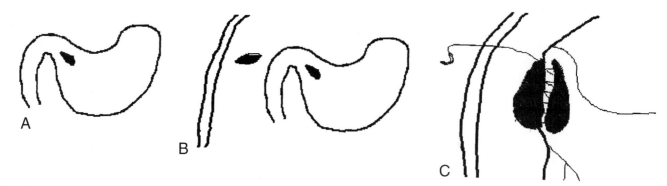

Fig. 15.23. **A.** Initial pyloric antrum incision. **B.** Matching incision on body wall. **C.** Suturing of body wall and pyloric antrum.

References

1. MacCoy DM, Sykes GP, Hoffer RE, et al. A gastropexy technique for permanent fixation of the pyloric antrum. J Am Anim Hosp Assoc 1982;18:763–768.
2. Woolfson JM, Kostolich M. Circumcostal gastropexy: clinical use of the technique in 34 dogs with gastric dilation–volvulus. J Am Anim Hosp Assoc 1986;22:825–830.
3. Matthiesen DT. Partial gastrectomy as treatment of gastric volvulus; results in 30 dogs. Vet Surg 1985;14:185–193.
4. Parks JL, Greene RW. Tube gastrostomy for the treatment of gastric volvulus. J Am Anim Hosp Assoc 1976;12:168–172.
5. Christie TR, Smith CW. Gastrocolopexy for prevention of recurrent gastric volvulus. J Am Anim Hosp Assoc 1976;12:173–176.
6. Lindgren WG, Mullen HS, Marino DJ, et al. Long-term follow-up and clinical results of incisional gastropexy for repair of gastric dilation–volvulus syndrome. In: Proceedings of the Fifth American College of Veterinary Surgeons Veterinary Symposium. American College of Veterinary Surgeons. Chicago, IL. 1995:11.

Circumcostal Gastropexy

Gary W. Ellison

The circumcostal gastropexy technique (1) has become popular with many small animal surgeons because it forms a stronger adhesion than the tube gastrostomy or incisional gastropexy technique (2). Other potential advantages of this technique include a viable muscle flap adhesion and a more proper anatomic placement of the stomach (1). Potential disadvantages of the circumcostal gastropexy technique include possible rib fracture or creation of pneumothorax when the operation is performed by surgeons who are inexperienced with the technique (3). This procedure is also reported to be more technically demanding and time-consuming to perform than other gastropexy techniques, but I disagree with this statement.

Surgical Technique

To perform the circumcostal gastropexy, two 1 × 4 cm partial-thickness gastric flaps are created and are wrapped around either the eleventh or twelfth costal cartilage. Initially, 2–0 polypropylene stay sutures are placed 2 and 8 cm proximal to the pylorus, respectively. A transverse nick incision is then made 3 cm distal to the pylorus with Metzenbaum scissors. A second transverse nick incision is made at the other end 4 cm proximal to the first. To avoid penetrating the gastric lumen when making these incisions, the serosa and muscularis are first grasped between the surgeon's thumb and forefinger. This maneuver separates these layers from the underlying submucosa. The two transverse incisions are then connected with a scalpel or scissors. The seromuscular layer is then separated from the submucosa with scissors on both sides, thereby creating two 1.0 × 4 cm seromuscular pedicle flaps (Fig. 15.24). The chondral portion of the right eleventh or twelfth rib is encircled with towel clamps from the abdominal surface, and the peritoneum and transverse

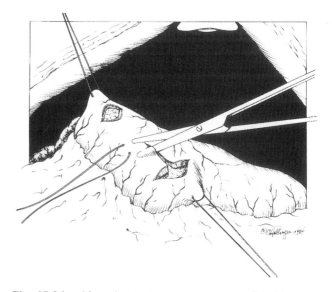

Fig. 15.24. After placing stay sutures, two small incisions are made through the seromuscular layer of the pyloric antrum and are connected with scissors. The flaps are undermined for a distance of 1 cm. (From Ellison GW. Gastric dilatation volvulus: surgical prevention. Vet Clin North Am Small Anim Pract 1993;23:524.)

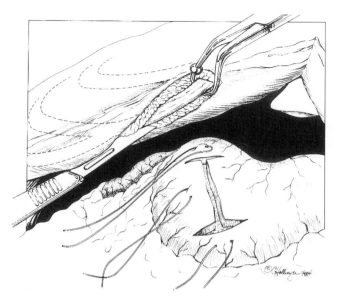

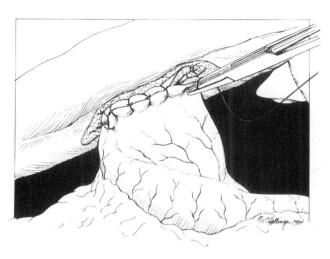

Fig. 15.25. The eleventh or twelfth rib is then grasped with towel clamps from the abdominal surface, and the peritoneum and transverse abdominal muscle are incised with a No. 10 blade. (From Ellison GW. Gastric dilatation volvulus: surgical prevention. Vet Clin North Am Small Anim Pract 1993;23:524.)

abdominal muscle are incised with a No. 10 blade (Fig. 15.25). A tunnel is then made around the medial aspect of the rib using Metzenbaum scissors. If the eleventh or twelfth rib is used, the incision is caudal to all diaphragmatic attachments, and the thoracic cavity is not entered. The caudal arm of each stay suture is then passed through the rib tunnel, and the stomach is pulled up against the right abdominal wall. The caudal

Fig. 15.27. The two flaps are then apposed with simple interrupted sutures. (From Ellison GW. Gastric dilatation volvulus: surgical prevention. Vet Clin North Am Small Anim Pract 1993;23:524.)

muscular flap is passed around the lateral aspect of the rib with a stay suture or grasping forces, and the two stay sutures are tied around the rib (Fig. 15.26). The caudal muscular flap is then apposed to the cranial muscular flap with simple interrupted sutures of 2–0 polypropylene (Fig. 15.27). A second layer of simple interrupted sutures of 3–0 polypropylene is used to appose gastric serosa to the incised transversus muscle (Fig. 15.28). The ventral midline is then closed routinely. Postoperative care is similar to that for other gastropexy techniques.

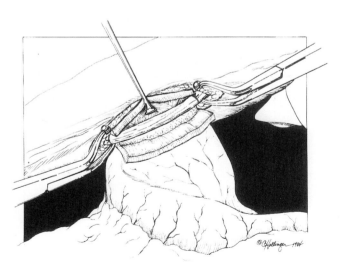

Fig. 15.26. After dissecting lateral to the rib, the caudal flap is brought around, and the two stay sutures are tied. (From Ellison GW. Gastric dilatation volvulus: surgical prevention. Vet Clin North Am Small Anim Pract 1993;23:524.)

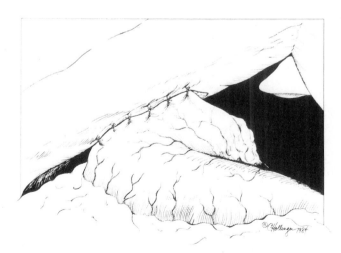

Fig. 15.28. A second layer of simple interrupted sutures apposes the stomach wall with the incised transverse abdominal muscle and completes the procedure. (From Ellison GW. Gastric dilatation volvulus: surgical prevention. Vet Clin North Am Small Anim Pract 1993;23:524.

Results

In one study, 30 patients with GDV were followed-up for an average of 12.7 months after circumcostal gastropexy with contrast studies or necropsy (4). Of the animals that survived, just 1 dog (3.3%) suffered a clinical recurrence of gastric dilatation. In another study, 34 dogs were followed-up after circumcostal gastropexy, with a mean follow-up of 11.3 months. One patient developed peritonitis as a result of inadvertent penetration of the gastric wall during flap formation. The overall mortality was 8.8%, and suspected recurrence occurred in 2 patients (6.9%) because of a second episode of gastric distension (5). Neither of these recurrences was documented with radiographs or necropsy as due to gastropexy failure.

References

1. Fallah AM, Lumb WV, Nelson AW, et al. Circumcostal gastropexy in the dog: a preliminary study. Vet Surg 1982;11:19–22.
2. Fox SM, Ellison GW, Miller GJ. Observations on the mechanical failure of three gastropexy techniques. J Am Anim Hosp Assoc 1985;21:739–734.
3. Leib MS, Blass CE. Gastric dilatation–volvulus in dogs: an update. Compend Contin Educ Pract Vet 1984;6:961–967.
4. Leib MS, Konde LJ, Wingfield WE, et al. Circumcostal gastropexy for preventing recurrence of gastric dilatation–volvulus in the dog: an evaluation of 30 cases. J Am Vet Med Assoc 1985; 187:245–248.
5. Woolfson JM, Kostolich M. Circumcostal gastropexy: clinical use of the tech nique in 34 dogs with gastric dilatation–volvulus. J Am Anim Hosp Assoc 1986;22:825–830.

Belt Loop Gastropexy

Wayne O. Whitney

Belt loop gastropexy is a modification of the circumcostal gastropexy. The technique differs from the circumcostal gastropexy in two main respects: 1) the seromuscular stomach flap is created in the shape of a tongue or "belt," instead of an "I," to eliminate corners and to simplify flap passage and suturing; and 2) the seromuscular stomach flap is passed around a "belt loop" of transverse abdominous muscle located just caudal to the last rib rather than around the rib itself. This eliminates the possibility of iatrogenic rib fracture and pneumothorax, which are occasionally seen with circumcostal gastropexy in the early stages of the learning curve.

Indications

Belt loop gastropexy can be performed for most cases requiring prophylactic gastropexy. Although it is pri-

marily used in patients with GDV, it has been performed successfully in the management of gastroesophageal intussusception (1) and as a supplement to hiatal herniorrhaphy. I use the technique in con-

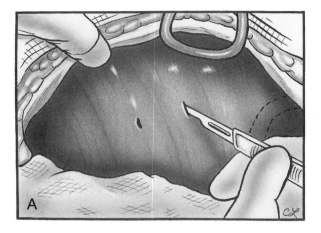

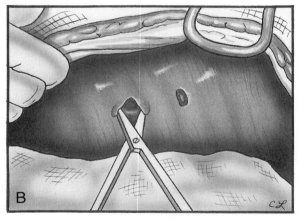

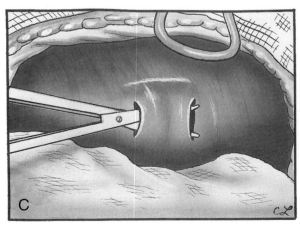

Fig. 15.29. Creation of the "belt loop." **A.** Two small stab incisions are made through the transverse abdominal muscle just caudally to the right costal arch. **B.** The muscle fibers are bluntly dissected longitudinally. **C.** Care is taken to develop the natural plane only directly beneath the 2.5 × 2.5 cm flap.

junction with gastrointestinal anastomosis–assisted gastric resection in stomachs that appear to have good motility and are not severely stretched, but more often I use tube gastropexy when gastric resection is required or if marked gastric atony is anticipated.

Surgical Technique

The technique is essentially performed as it was originally described in 1989 (2) (Figs. 15.29 to 15.31). The fibers of the transverse abdominous muscle are located

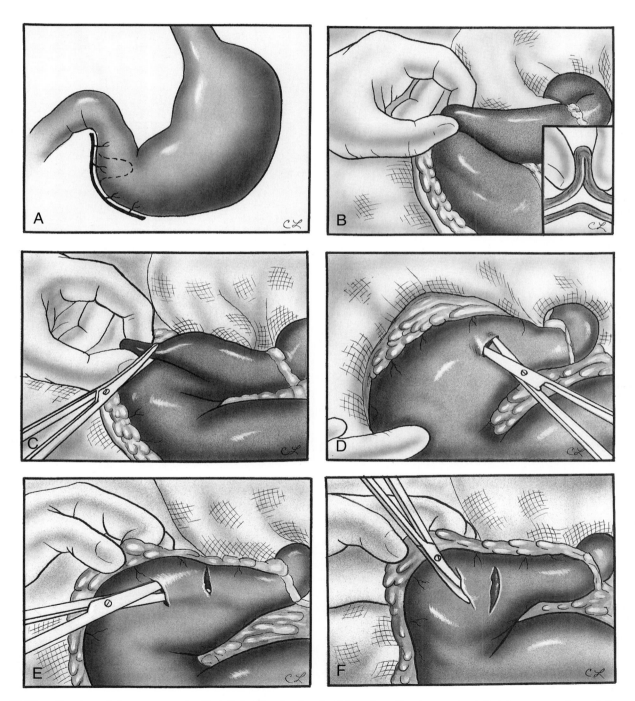

Fig. 15.30. Creation of the seromuscular "belt." **A.** The site for the 2.5 × 4 cm flap is conceived. **B.** The proper plane of dissection between the seromuscular layer and the mucosal layer is identified by allowing the mucosa to slip between the thumb and finger while the seromuscular layer is held. **C–F.** An incision is made through the seromuscular layer with Metzenbaum scissors, then bluntly developed directly beneath the planned flap. After the layers have been separated, the tongue-shaped seromuscular incision is fashioned accordingly.

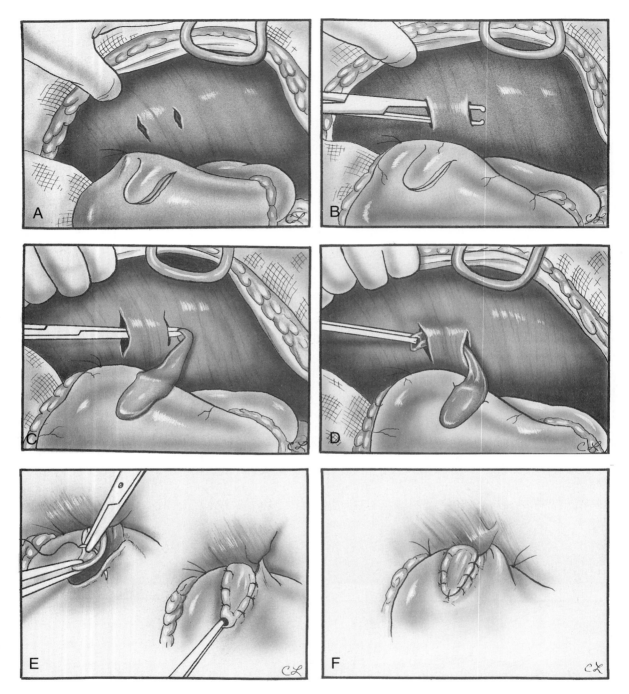

Fig. 15.31. Flap passage and reattachment. **A.** The greater curvature at the base of the flap is sutured to the abdominal wall to facilitate flap passage. **B–D.** Allis tissue forceps are passed caudally to cranially through the belt loop. The tip of the seromuscular flap is grasped and gently pulled through the belt loop. **E and F.** The forceps are used to reposition the flap over its original location while it is reattached.

just caudal to the right costal arch. The "belt loop" flap should be centered approximately 3 to 4 cm caudal to the costal arch and approximately one-third of the distance from the ventral to the dorsal midline. Two small parallel stab incisions 2.5 cm apart are made through parietal peritoneum and fascia of the transverse abdominal muscle. The transverse abdominal

muscle fibers are separated bluntly 2.5 cm longitudinally with Metzenbaum scissors. Care is taken to undermine only in the natural plane directly beneath the completed 2.5 × 2.5 cm "belt loop" flap. The site for a 2.5 × 4.5 cm tongue-shaped seromuscular stomach flap is conceived in the pyloric antrum. Care is taken to center a branch of the right gastroepiploic artery in the base of the flap. The seromuscular layer of the stomach is identified by gently grasping the stomach wall between the thumb and index finger and allowing the mucosa to slip between the thumb and finger while the seromuscular muscular layer is held. An incision is made through the seromuscular layer with Metzenbaum scissors, and the plane between the seromuscular layer and the mucosa is developed carefully with blunt dissection beneath the previously conceived flap. A similar technique is used to incise the opposite border of the seromuscular flap and to complete undermining of the flap. The tongue-shaped flap is then completed with sharp scissor dissection of the seromuscular layer. The flap should be flared slightly at its base. The greater curvature of the stomach is sutured to the abdominal wall with a single 0 polydioxanone suture to hold the stomach in place, a technique that facilitates passage of the stomach flap. Allis tissue forceps are passed caudally to cranially through the ''belt loop'' flap, and the tip of the stomach flap is grasped with forceps and gently pulled through the ''belt loop.'' Care is taken to prevent twisting of the flap during this part of the procedure. Using the forceps, the flap is repositioned over its original anatomic location and is held in position with forceps while it is reattached with simple interrupted 0 polydioxanone sutures. It is not necessary to amputate the small tip of the flap held by the forceps. The stomach is tacked to the abdominal wall anterior and posterior to the surgical site with additional 0 polydioxanone sutures to relieve tension on the flap while it heals.

Complications

The most common complication of belt loop gastropexy is accidental perforation of the gastric mucosa during development of the seromuscular flap. This is uncommon and can be most easily prevented by careful palpation of the two distinct stomach layers before incising the seromuscular layer. By gently grasping the stomach wall between the thumb and index finger and then allowing the mucosa to slip away while the seromuscular layer is held, the surgeon can identify the proper plane of dissection. If the gastric lumen is inadvertently violated, one should simply close the mucosa with simple interrupted sutures and continue with the technique after the proper plane has been reestablished.

Postoperative gastric atony has been uncommon in my experience, but it is troublesome when it occurs. If it is unresponsive to medical management and if gastric dilatation persists, percutaneous endoscopic tube gastrostomy can be used after belt loop gastropexy to maintain decompression. Rarely, the pyloric antrum is so edematous that seromuscular flap techniques should be avoided, and tube gastropexy is then indicated. I have not experienced a nonviable gastric mucosa beneath a viable seromuscular layer in association with GDV.

References

1. Clark G. Belt loop gastropexy in the management of gastroesophageal intussusception in a pup. J Am Vet Med Assoc 1992; 201:739–742.
2. Whitney WO, et al: Belt-loop gastropexy: technique and results of surgery in 20 dogs. J Am Anim Hosp Assoc 1989;25:75.

Ventral Midline Gastropexy

Andrea Meyer-Lindenberg

Gastric dilatation–volvulus is an acute, potentially fatal disease with a high mortality rate. Even after successful treatment, relapse is observed in some dogs, despite surgical intervention. Intraoperative fixation of the stomach is important for the prevention of relapse in gastric dilatation–volvulus in dogs. Because of disturbed hemodynamics in the course of disease, it is critical for the patient's survival that duration of surgery, including gastropexy, and anesthesia be kept as short as possible. Several surgical techniques have been described for prevention of recurrence. The ventral midline gastropexy is technically simple and easily learned. The method is rapid, does not prolong the surgical time, and keeps duration of anesthesia as short as possible.

Surgical Technique

The patient is placed in dorsal recumbency. Celiotomy is performed along the linea alba, beginning at the level of the xiphoid cartilage and extended between the umbilicus and the pubis.

After decompression of the bloated stomach with a suction trocar, the stomach is moved back into its physiologic position, and the remaining stomach contents are removed through a gastric tube. For this purpose, a large plastic (polyvinyl chloride) tube has proved most suitable, because it allows the removal of large particles (e.g., potatoes, pieces of bone) without gastrotomy. The ventral midline gastropexy is performed with the closure of the abdominal cavity. After excision of the falciform fat, the gastric wall in the area of the pyloric antrum (Fig.15.32) is grasped by the surgical assistant between the thumb and index finger and is held into the cranial part of the celiotomy incision. A continuous suture pattern of slowly absorbable atraumatic synthetic suture material, 0–0 or 1–0 polyglactin 910 (Vicryl, Ethicon, Inc., Somerville, NJ)

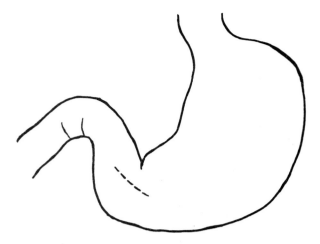

Fig. 15.32. The location of the gastropexy site in the area of the pyloric antrum.

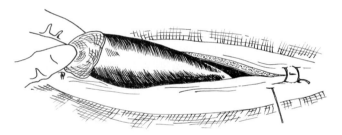

Fig. 15.33. The seromuscular layer of the gastric wall at the pyloric antrum is grasped with the thumb and index finger and is held into the cranial laparotomy wound. The closure of the abdominal cavity is started at the caudal end of the laparotomy incision in a simple continuous pattern using absorbable suture material (polyglactin 910: Vicryl, Ethicon, Inc., Somerville, NJ).

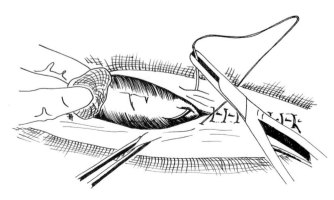

Fig. 15.34. Seromuscular layers of the gastric wall included in the continuous suture pattern.

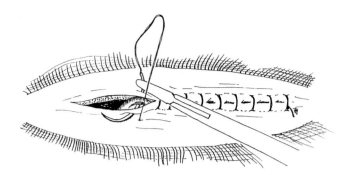

Fig. 15.35. The pattern is extended cranially including approximately 5 cm of gastric wall.

is started at the caudal end of the laparotomy incision (Fig. 15.33). The gastric wall is fixed by incorporating it into the cranial part of the main suture of the linea alba over a length for approximately 5 cm (Figs. 15.34 to 15.36). This suture line includes the muscularis of the stomach, without penetrating into the stomach lumen. The subcutaneous tissues and the skin are closed routinely. Editor's note: The editor suggests the use of monofilament non-absorbable suture material such as polypropylene sutures (Prolene, Ethicon, Somerville, N.J.) for this technique.

Postoperative Considerations

After the surgical procedure, the cardiovascular functions as well as electrolyte and acid-base status are monitored closely. Patients are not fed orally for 2 to 3 days; during this time, they receive a balanced electrolyte solution intravenously, at a rate of 60 to 120 mL/kg per day. Oral feeding is instituted after 2 to 3 days with small portions of food offered five times daily, initially as a soup and later as a paste. Antiarrhythmic medication is given intravenously until the dogs begin eating. From then on, antiarrhythmic drugs can be given orally.

Because the gastropexy site is located cranially, it does not interfere with subsequent celiotomies (e.g., for ovariohysterectomy, enterotomy, or cystotomy). However, the cranial location may require paracostal incision in dogs with diaphragmatic hernia or for hepatic surgery. Thus, the owners of these dogs must

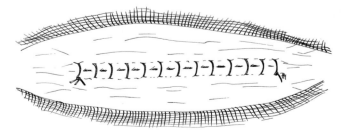

Fig. 15.36. Final closure of the laparotomy wound.

be advised to inform the surgeon about the type of gastropexy performed previously when a second celiotomy is necessary.

Suggested Readings

Betts CW, et al. "Permanent" gastropexy as a prophylactic measure against gastric volvulus. J Am Anim Hosp Assoc 1976;12:177.

Fallah AM, et al. Circumcostal gastropexy in the dog: a preliminary study. Vet Surg 1982;11:9.

Fox SM. Gastric dilatation–volvulus: results from 31 surgical cases circumcostal gastropexy vs. tube gastrotomy. Calif Vet 1985; 39:8.

Fox SM, et al. Observations on the mechanical failure of three gastropexy techniques. J Am Anim Hosp Assoc 1985;21:729.

Frendin J, Funquist B. Fundic gastropexy for prevention of recurrence of gastric volvulus. J Small Anim Pract 1990;31:78.

Funkquist B. Gastric torsion in the dog. III. Fundic gastropexy as a relapse-preventing procedure. J Small Anim Pract 1979;20:103.

Leib MS, Blass CF. Gastric dilatation–volvulus in dogs. Compend Contin Educ Pract Vet 1984;6:961.

Meyer-Lindenberg A, et al. Treatment of gastric dilatation–volvulus and a rapid method for prevention of relapse in dogs: 134 cases (1988–1991). J Am Vet Med Assoc 1993;203:1303.

Parks JL, Greene RW. Tube gastrotomy for the treatment of gastric volvulus. J Am Anim Hosp Assoc 1976;2:168.

Schulmann AJ, et al. Muscular flap gastropexy: a new surgical technique to prevent recurrence of gastric dilation–volvulus syndrome. J Am Anim Hosp Assoc 1986;22:339.

Van Sluijs FJ, Happe RP. The gastric dilatation–torsion syndrome. In: Slatter DH, ed. Textbook of small animal surgery. Philadelphia: WB Saunders, 1985.

Whitney WO, et al. Belt-loop gastropexy: technique and surgical results in 20 dogs. J Am Anim Hosp Assoc 1989;25:75.

Wingfield WE, et al. Operative techniques and recurrence rates associated with gastric volvulus in the dog. J Small Anim Pract 1975;6:427.

— 16 —

INTESTINES

Enterotomy

Gary W. Ellison

Indications

The most common indication for enterotomy in small animals is intraluminal intestinal foreign bodies that cause obstruction. Foreign bodies can be present in animals of any age, but they are most common in puppies or kittens because of indiscriminate eating habits. Common intestinal foreign bodies in dogs include bones, balls, corncobs, and cellophane wrappers. Cats commonly ingest sharp foreign bodies (e.g., straight pins and needles) and linear foreign bodies (e.g., yarn, tinsel, fishing line, and string meat wrappings). Enterotomy also is performed to examine the intestinal lumen for evidence of mucosal ulceration, strictures, or neoplasia. Superficial ulcerations or intestinal polyps sometimes can be resected by enterotomy, but most intramural lesions require intestinal resection and anastomosis.

Pathophysiology and Preoperative Treatment of Intestinal Obstructions

Animals with incomplete intestinal obstructions caused by intraluminal foreign bodies or neoplasia usually vomit sporadically or are anorectic. Surprisingly, sharp foreign bodies such as nails, straight pins, and bones often pass spontaneously through the entire gastrointestinal tract without causing a perforation. Conversely, complete intraluminal obstructions usually cause acute bowel distension and unrelenting clinical signs. With proximal (duodenal) obstructions,

vomiting may be projectile. With distal jejunal or ileal obstructions, vomiting may be seen early in the course of the disease, but anorexia and bowel distension follow. After experimental obstruction of the midjejunum in dogs, vomiting decreases to once a day after 24 to 36 hours, and the dogs can live for as long as 3 weeks if free-choice water is available.

Most intestinal obstructions are distal to the bile and pancreatic ducts, resulting in loss of highly alkaline duodenal, pancreatic, and biliary secretions. Metabolic acidosis usually occurs from loss of these bicarbonate-rich duodenal contents. Dehydration is corrected and maintenance fluid needs usually are met with a balanced electrolyte solution such as lactated Ringer's solution. Sodium bicarbonate and potassium chloride supplementation often are indicated, depending on the patient's acid-base status and serum potassium level. With obstructions at the pylorus or proximal duodenum, gastric fluids rich in potassium, sodium, hydrogen ion, and chloride are vomited, and metabolic alkalosis with hypochloremia, hyponatremia, and hypokalemia may result. Maintenance fluid requirements are met and dehydration is corrected with intravenous 0.9% sodium chloride solution supplemented with potassium chloride depending on the patient's preoperative serum potassium level.

The level of obstruction, the metabolic status of the animal, and the amount of contamination determine whether antibiotic therapy is necessary. The bacterial population of the small intestine is lowest in the proximal duodenum and highest in the distal ileum. Uncomplicated enterotomies of the proximal small bowel may not require antibiotic therapy. However, when spillage occurs or when an enterotomy is performed on the distal small bowel, parenteral antibiotics are initiated before surgery and are continued for 24 to 48 hours postoperatively. Broad-spectrum bactericidal agents such as intravenous cephalothin, at 10 mg/kg four times daily, in combination with enrofloxacin, 7.5 mg/kg twice daily, provide good prophylaxis against most gram-negative enteric organisms. Intravenous metronidizole, at 15 mg/kg four times daily, is also effective against anaerobic organisms.

Surgical Technique

A ventral midline laparotomy incision is made from the xiphoid to the pubis. Moistened laparotomy sponges are applied to the wound edges, and an abdominal retractor is applied. The affected bowel segment is isolated from the remainder of the viscera with saline-soaked laparotomy sponges. In patients with a complete obstruction, intestinal distension proximal to the obstruction is often profound, and the distended loops of bowel usually take on a congested or cyanotic appearance (Fig. 16.1**A**).

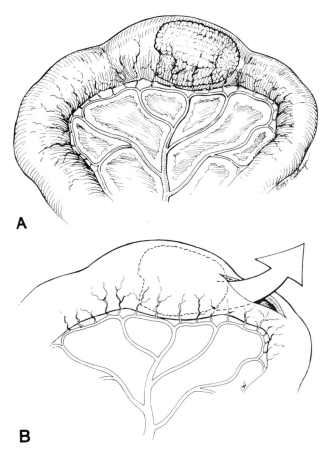

Fig. 16.1. **A.** Complete intestinal obstruction caused by a luminal foreign body such as a corncob causes fluid and gaseous distension. Congestion or cyanotic appearance of the bowel wall occurs proximal to the obstruction. **B.** An enterotomy is made in the antimesenteric surface of viable bowel just distal to the foreign body. The length of the incision approximates the diameter of the foreign body. The foreign body is delivered through the incision with gentle manual pressure.

Intestinal viability is best evaluated after decompression of fluid and gas from dilated loops of intestine. Decompression is performed with a 20-gauge needle and suction apparatus or a 60-mL syringe with a three-way stopcock. If intestinal wall ischemia and necrosis are present, resection and anastomosis must be performed. In most cases of simple mechanical obstruction, however, bowel viability is maintained, and the gross appearance of dark, distended loops of bowel improves rapidly after decompression and removal of the obstruction.

After remaining intestinal contents are milked 10 cm to either side of the foreign body, the bowel is held between an assistant's fingers or with Doyen intestinal forceps. With a No. 15 scalpel blade, a full-thickness longitudinal incision is made in the antimesenteric border of the intestine in the viable tissue immediately distal to the foreign body. The length of the enterotomy approximates the diameter of the foreign body. Continuous suction is used to reduce spillage, and the surgeon pushes the foreign body gently through the enterotomy, taking care not to tear the incision margins (Fig. 16.1**B**). The bowel lumen is examined for evidence of perforations or strictures before closure.

Linear foreign bodies such as string, fishing line, meat wrappers, and sewing yarn present a difficult surgical problem. The trailing end of a linear foreign body usually catches over the base of the tongue or in the pyloric antrum and acts as an anchor. Intestinal peristalsis attempts to move the foreign body distally, but because it remains fixed proximally, the bowel plicates itself along the length of the foreign body, which often cuts through the intestinal wall on the mesenteric surface, resulting in local peritonitis.

Linear foreign bodies should be managed by identifying the glossal anchor point initially and releasing it before laparotomy. Commonly, a gastrotomy is also necessary to free wadded string or fishing line from a gastropyloric anchor. Multiple enterotomies usually are required to facilitate complete removal of the foreign body (Fig. 16.2). If too few enterotomies are made with too much traction placed on the foreign body, the mesenteric border may be perforated in an area that is difficult to explore and suture. Occasionally, the intestinal foreign body perforates at several locations before surgery, and local peritonitis is evident. Sometimes, in patients with long-standing cases, enough fibrosis has occurred around the foreign body so, even after its removal, the bowel retains its plicated conformation. In these patients, intestinal resection and anastomosis may be necessary.

Closure of the enterotomy incision usually is made with a simple interrupted suture pattern in side-to-side longitudinal fashion (Fig. 16.3). Single-layer closures are recommended because double-layer closures may cause excessive compromise of the lumen diame-

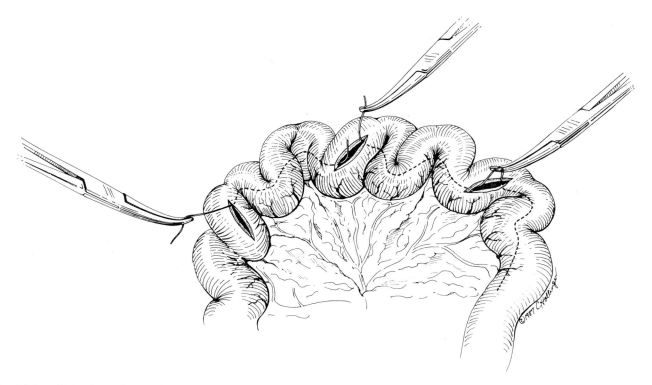

Fig. 16.2. With a linear foreign body (e.g., a piece of string), multiple enterotomies usually are required. Mosquito hemostats are used to locate and grasp a loop of the string at each enterotomy site. The string is then sequentially cut and withdrawn through the nearest proximal enterotomy site. See text for details.

ter. Various suture patterns are acceptable, but with all techniques, the collagen-rich submucosa must be incorporated in the sutures. Single-layer appositional techniques such as the simple interrupted appositional or crushing techniques may be used (see Fig. 16.7). I prefer a modified Gambee suture, which incorporates the serosa, muscularis, and submucosa but excludes the mucosa and is helpful in reducing mucosal eversion (see Fig. 16.8). Sutures are placed 3 to 4 mm apart and 2 to 3 mm from the cut edge, taking care to incorporate all layers of the intestinal wall.

The enterotomy also can be closed using a simple continuous approximating pattern (Fig. 16.4). Suture bites are taken perpendicular to the bowel wall 2 to 3 mm from the cut edge and 3 mm apart. The suture line is advanced outside the bowel lumen. Sutures are pulled snugly enough to appose the wound edges gently. Pulling the suture line too tightly may cause strangulation of the wound edge and may lead to dehiscence. Enterotomy leakage is more likely to occur in hypoproteinemic and chronically debilitated animals, whose wound healing capacities are impaired. In such

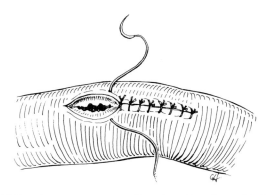

Fig. 16.3. An enterotomy usually is closed in side-to-side fashion with a simple interrupted suture pattern. Appositional, crushing, or modified Gambee sutures can be used.

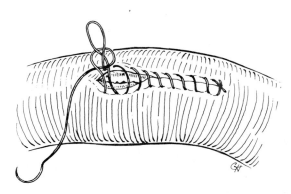

Fig. 16.4. An enterotomy also can be closed with a simple continuous appositional pattern.

patients, a continuous inverting Cushing pattern gives good serosa-to-serosa apposition and luminal bursting strengths that exceed those of the interrupted approximating patterns. Suture bites are placed 2 to 3 mm from the wound edge to minimize the amount of inversion (Fig. 16.5). The tough submucosal layer is secured with each pass of the needle.

If the enterotomy is in a small-diameter loop of bowel, longitudinal closure is likely to cause luminal constriction. To prevent this constriction, the ends of the enterotomy can be closed in transverse fashion. A simple interrupted suture is used to approximate the proximal and distal ends of the longitudinal incision. Additional sutures are then placed 3 to 4 mm apart to appose the remaining bowel wall, resulting in a widened lumen diameter (Fig. 16.6).

Enterotomies are sutured with 3–0 to 4–0 synthetic polyglactin 910 (Vicryl, Ethicon, Inc., Somerville, NJ), polyglycolic acid (Dexon, Davis and Geck, Pearl River, NY), or polydioxanone (PDS, Ethicon, Inc.) on a narrow-taper, taper-cut, or small reverse-cutting needle. Nonabsorbable monofilament materials such as nylon (Ethilon, Ethicon, Inc.) or polypropylene (Prolene, Ethicon, Inc.) also may be used. Chromic surgical gut has been used with clinical success, but it is not recommended because it loses tensile strength rapidly in the presence of collagenase and is quickly phagocytized in an infected environment. After the enterotomy closure is complete, it is rinsed with saline and covered with omentum, as described in the next section of this chapter.

Postoperative Care

Replacement intravenous fluids and electrolyte therapy are continued in the postoperative period until dehydration and acid-base and electrolyte abnormalities are resolved. Prophylactic parenteral antibiotics, if indicated, are continued for 24 to 48 hours. In the absence of vomiting, a small amount of a bland com-

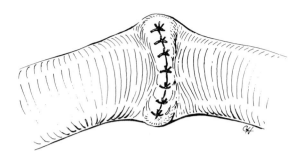

Fig. 16.6. In a small-diameter loop of bowel, the longitudinal incision can be closed transversely to prevent luminal stenosis. A simple interrupted pattern is used.

mercial starter diet (Ensure, Ross Laboratories, Columbus, OH) is offered three times on the day after the operation. Early introduction of food stimulates bowel contraction, reduces the likelihood of postoperative ileus or adhesion formation, and also serves as a valuable source of fluid and electrolytes. Persistent vomiting, fever, and leukocytosis in the presence of abdominal tenderness may indicate peritonitis resulting from leakage from the enterotomy. Abdominal paracentesis or diagnostic lavage should be performed. If a septic exudate is present, early exploration of the abdomen is indicated, and resection and anastomosis or one of the serosal patching techniques may be performed.

Suggested Readings

Enquist IF, Bauman FG, Rehder E. Changes in body fluid spaces in dogs with intestinal obstruction. Surg Gynecol Obstet 1968; 127:17.

Krahwinkel DJ, Richardson DC. Surgery of the small intestine. In: Bojrab MJ, ed. Current techniques in small animal surgery. 2nd ed. Philadelphia: Lea & Febiger, 1983.

Lipowitz AJ. Intestinal obstruction in the dog. Calif Vet 1980;3:8.

Mishra NK, Appert HE, Howard JM. The effects of distention and obstruction on the accumulation of fluid in the lumen of small bowel of dogs. Ann Surg 1974;180:791.

Randall HT. Fluid, electrolyte and acid-base balance. Surg Clin North Am 1976;56:1019.

Rosin E. Principles of intestinal surgery. In: Slatter DH, ed. Textbook of small animal surgery. Philadelphia: WB Saunders, 1985.

Intestinal Resection and Anastomosis

Gary W. Ellison

Indications

Intestinal resection and anastomosis commonly are performed for various lesions in small animals. Me-

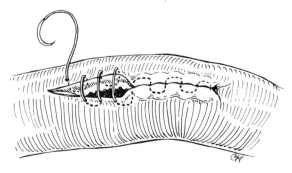

Fig. 16.5. A continuous inverting Cushing suture pattern may be chosen for chronically debilitated animals who have a higher than normal risk of enterotomy leakage.

chanical obstructions, whether luminal, intramural, or extramural, often require intestinal resection and anastomosis. Lodged intraluminal foreign bodies often cause local bowel wall necrosis or perforation, which may necessitate intestinal resection. Intramural lesions caused by strictures, neoplasms, or fungal granulomas such as phycomycosis must be removed by resection of the affected section of bowel. Occasionally, extramural lesions caused by adhesions secondary to previous surgery, regional peritonitis, or abdominal abscesses require resection of the obstructed segment of intestine.

Strangulated (ischemic) obstructions resulting from mesenteric arterial and venous occlusion or thrombosis often require emergency resection and anastomosis. Strangulated loops of bowel may be associated with diaphragmatic, ventral, inguinal, perineal, or femoral triangle hernias. Animals with intestinal volvulus have peracute mesenteric vascular pedicle obstruction, and secondary bowel wall ischemia often requires massive resection and anastomosis. With intussusception, the invaginated segment of bowel undergoes early venous congestion and becomes edematous. Intussusceptions become rapidly irreducible as a result of venous congestion and outpouring of fibrinous exudate from the invaginated serosal surface. If arterial thrombosis occurs, the invaginated bowel will become ischemic and necrotic. In either case, resection and anastomosis of the affected section of bowel often are necessary.

Determining Intestinal Viability

Standard clinical criteria for establishing intestinal viability are color, arterial pulsations, and the presence of peristalsis. Of these three parameters, peristalsis is the most dependable criterion of viability. The "pinch test" should be performed on questionable areas of bowel to determine whether smooth muscle contraction and peristalsis can be initiated. If clinical criteria are inadequate to determine viability, intravenous fluorescein dye can be used. A 10% fluorescein solution (Fundescein-10, Cooper Laboratories, San Germain, PR) is given at a dosage of 1 mL/5 kg intravenously through any peripheral vein. After 2 minutes, the tissues are subjected to long-wave ultraviolet light (Wood's lamp). Areas of bowel are considered viable if they have a bright green glow with a smooth uniform fluorescence or a fine granular fluorescent pattern in which areas of nonfluorescence do not exceed 3 mm. Areas of bowel are not viable if they have a patchy density with areas of nonfluorescence exceeding 3 mm, have only perivascular fluorescence, or are completely nonfluorescent.

Pulse oximetry may also be a reliable method of determining tissue viability. Recent studies have shown this method to be more accurate than either clinical criterion or intravenous dyes.

Selecting Suture Pattern and Suture Material

Although numerous suture techniques have been used for end-to-end intestinal anastomosis in small animals, approximating patterns are recommended at present. Properly performed approximating techniques create an increased lumen diameter, result in rapid and precise primary intestinal healing, and minimize the potential for postoperative adhesion formation. Everting techniques (e.g., horizontal mattress pattern) initially create a larger lumen diameter, but ultimately they cause narrowing and stenosis of the lumen. Everting anastomoses are not recommended because they have a greater tendency to leak and because of delayed mucosal healing, prolonged inflammatory response, and increased adhesion formation compared with approximating anastomoses. Inverting anastomoses using Cushing or Connell patterns provide a more leak-resistant serosa-to-serosa approximation but they create an internal cuff of tissue, which may cause luminal stenosis. Inflammation is more severe and healing time is slower with inverting patterns than with approximating techniques. Despite these dangers, inverting techniques should be considered in patients with a high risk of leakage or for use in colonic resection and anastomosis; in the latter situation, the high bacterial content of feces makes leakage of the anastomosis extremely dangerous.

Approximating end-to-end intestinal anastomoses can be created with various simple interrupted suture patterns or with a simple continuous suture pattern. Interrupted patterns generally are easier to perform, but the simple continuous pattern minimizes mucosal eversion and therefore provides better serosal apposition and primary intestinal healing. Regardless of the suture technique used, proper incorporation of the tough submucosa and reduction of mucosal eversion are vital in performing consistently successful intestinal anastomosis.

A simple interrupted appositional suture incorporates all tissue layers and gently apposes the wound edges (Fig. 16.7**A**). A crushing suture is pulled tightly and cuts through the serosa, muscularis, and mucosa and engages only the tough submucosal layer of the bowel wall (Fig. 16.7**B**). A crushing suture creates more tissue ischemia directly at the suture line, but its bursting strength is equal to that of an appositional technique. With both the appositional and crushing techniques, mucosal eversion tends to occur between sutures. I prefer a modified Gambee suture pattern because it reduces mucosal eversion. In this technique, the needle is passed through the serosa, muscularis, and submucosa, but the mucosal layer is not incorporated in the suture (Fig. 16.8**A**). The suture is tied snugly enough to approximate all layers of the intesti-

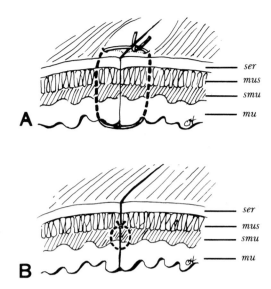

Fig. 16.7. **A.** Simple interrupted appositional suture. **B.** Crushing suture. *mu*, mucosa; *smu*, submucosa; *mus*, muscularis; *ser*, serosa.

nal wall gently. The mucosa tends to be pushed into the intestinal lumen and does not evert between sutures (Fig. 16.8**B**).

A taper-cut, narrow-taper, or small reverse-cutting needle with 3–0 or 4–0 swaged-on suture material is suitable for most anastomoses. Braided, nonabsorbable materials such as silk or braided polyesters should be avoided. Chromic surgical gut has been used successfully, but it loses significant tensile strength within 1 week. Synthetic, braided, absorbable suture materials such as polyglactin 910 (Vicryl, Ethicon, Inc., Somerville, NJ) or polyglycolic acid (Dexon, Davis and Geck, Pearl River, NY) are acceptable, but they have significant tissue drag. Polydioxanone (PDS, Ethicon, Inc.) and polyglyconate (Maxon, Davis and Geck), which are monofilament absorbable sutures with little tissue drag, have been used successfully for intestinal anastomoses. Nonabsorbable monofilament sutures such as nylon (Ethilon, Ethicon, Inc.) or polypropylene (Prolene, Ethicon, Inc.) also are acceptable for simple interrupted anastomoses, but they should not be used for simple continuous anastomoses.

Surgical Technique

A standard midline laparotomy is performed, as well as a thorough examination of the intestinal tract. The area to be resected is packed away from the abdomen with moistened laparotomy sponges. Intestinal contents are milked proximally and distally, and the bowel is held between an assistant's index fingers or with Doyen intestinal forceps 4 to 5 cm from the proposed resection site. A 1- to 2-cm margin of normal viable intestine is included in the proximal and distal bound-

aries of the area to be resected, which is clamped off with Carmalt or Doyen forceps. If luminal disparity is present, the forceps are placed at a 75 to 90° angle on the dilated proximal segment (Fig. 16.9**A**) and at a 45 to 60° angle on the contracted distal segment of bowel (Fig. 16.9**B**). Branches of the mesenteric artery and veins supplying the devitalized bowel are isolated with curved mosquito forceps and are double-ligated with 3–0 silk. The arcadial vessels located within the mesenteric fat are double-ligated at the area of proposed resection. A scalpel blade is used to excise the bowel along the outside of the intestinal forceps (see Fig. 16.9, *dashed lines*). With dissecting scissors, the vessels are divided, the mesentery is transected (see Fig. 16.9, *dotted lines*), and the excised bowel is removed from the surgical field. After resection, the small intestinal mucosa has a tendency to evert and can be trimmed back with Metzenbaum scissors (Fig. 16.10).

If angling of the intestinal incision does not adequately correct for luminal disparity, the smaller stoma can be enlarged by incising the bowel section for a distance of 1 to 2 cm along the antimesenteric surface and then trimming off two triangular flaps (Fig. 16.11). This procedure creates an ovoid larger stoma, which can be anastomosed to the larger-diameter section of the bowel.

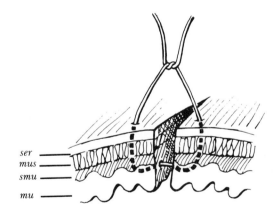

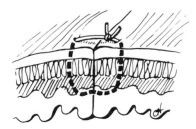

Fig. 16.8. Modified Gambee suture. When tied, this suture gently approximates all tissue layers and slightly inverts the mucosa, thereby minimizing mucosal eversion between sutures (*bottom*). *mu*, mucosa; *smu*, submucosa; *mus*, muscularis; *ser*, serosa.

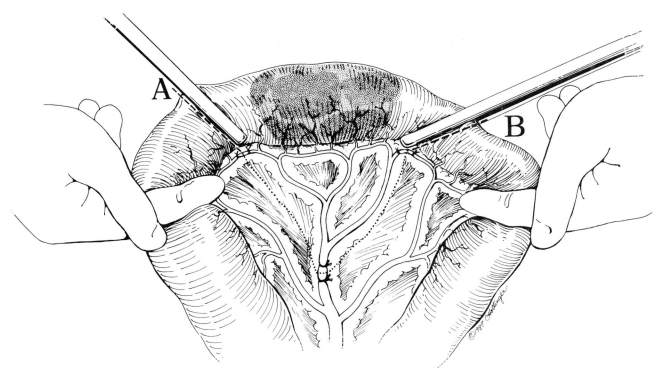

Fig. 16.9. Proximal (**A**) and distal (**B**) forceps are placed around the area to be resected. Mesenteric and arcadial vessels are double-ligated as shown. The bowel is transected with a scalpel blade outside of the clamps (*dashed lines*), and the mesentery is incised with dissecting scissors (*dotted lines*). See text for details.

When the anastomosis is formed with a simple interrupted suture technique, the first suture is placed at the mesenteric border because the presence of fat in this area makes suture placement most difficult, and this is where leakage is most likely to occur. The second suture is placed on the antimesenteric border, and the third and fourth sutures are placed laterally at the 90° quadrants (Fig. 16.12**A**). Two to three more sutures are placed between each of the quadrant sutures (Fig. 16.12**B**). All sutures are placed 3 to 4 mm apart and 2 to 3 mm from the wound edge. Suture bites on

the dilated side of the anastomosis are placed farther apart than on the contracted side of the anastomosis to correct for luminal disparity. Once one side of the anastomosis is sutured, the bowel is flipped over, and the opposite side is completed. From 12 to 16 sutures are used to complete the anastomosis. After the anastomosis has been completed, it is checked for leakage by infusing saline under low pressure into the bowel lumen and massaging the fluid past the anastomosis. This test is subjective because all anastomes can be made to leak if enough pressure is applied. The anasto-

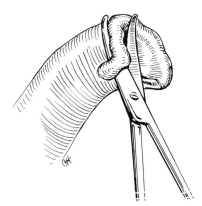

Fig. 16.10. Everted mucosa can be trimmed back before anastomosis is formed.

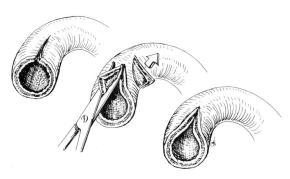

Fig. 16.11. Enlargement of bowel section with a smaller diameter may be necessary to form anastomosis. See text for details.

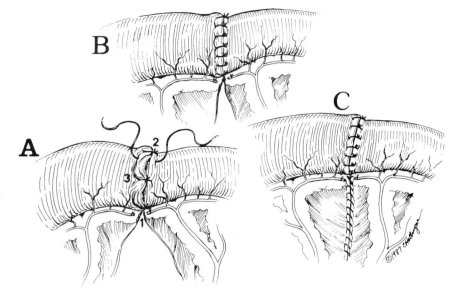

Fig. 16.12. Closing anastomosis with simple interrupted suture pattern. **A.** Placement of first (1), second (2), and third (3) sutures; the fourth suture is placed on the lateral bowel wall opposite to the third suture. **B.** Additional sutures are placed between each of the original four. **C.** Final step is closure of the mesenteric defect with simple continuous sutures. See text for details.

mosis can also be checked by gently probing the spaces between sutures with mosquito hemostats for areas likely to leak. The surgeon then closes the mesenteric defect with a simple continuous pattern, taking care not to include any mesenteric vessels within the suture line (Fig. 16.12**C**).

Occasionally, the small-diameter loop of bowel cannot be enlarged enough to be anastomosed to the larger one. In this case, the large-diameter stoma is reduced by initially angling the cut at 45°. The antimesenteric portion of the incision is then apposed with simple interrupted sutures in side-to-side fashion until the remaining opening is an appropriate width to anastomose to the smaller-diameter loop of bowel (Fig. 16.13).

Alternatively, a simple continuous approximating technique can be used to form the anastomosis. This is performed with two lengths of suture or with a double swaged-on suture. The first knot is tied at the mesenteric border (Fig. 16.14**A**). The sutures are then ad-

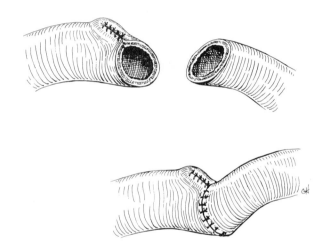

Fig. 16.13. Lumen diameter of larger stoma can be reduced to equal that of smaller diameter (*top*), so anastomosis can be completed (*bottom*). See text for details.

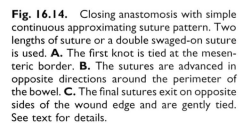

Fig. 16.14. Closing anastomosis with simple continuous approximating suture pattern. Two lengths of suture or a double swaged-on suture is used. **A.** The first knot is tied at the mesenteric border. **B.** The sutures are advanced in opposite directions around the perimeter of the bowel. **C.** The final sutures exit on opposite sides of the wound edge and are gently tied. See text for details.

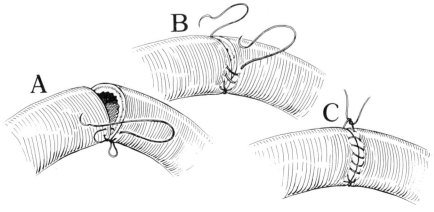

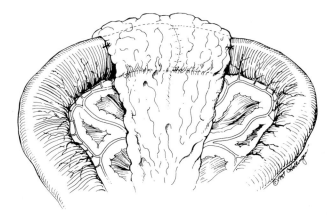

Fig. 16.15. A pedicle of greater omentum is wrapped around the anastomotic suture line and is tacked to the serosa with two simple interrupted sutures.

vanced around the perimeter approximately 3 mm apart and 2 to 3 mm from the cut edge (Fig. 16.14**B**), with the wound edges gently approximated. The needles are advanced in opposite directions, so the final sutures exit on opposite sides of the wound edge at the antimesenteric border. The final knot is tied gently on the antimesenteric border (Fig. 16.14**C**). If the knot is tied too tightly, a pursestring effect will be produced, and stenosis of the anastomosis may occur. The completed anastomosis is tested for leakage, and the mesenteric defect is closed, as described already.

On completion of any intestinal anastomosis, a pedicle of greater omentum is wrapped around the suture line. The omentum is tacked to the serosa with two simple interrupted sutures of 3–0 surgical gut placed on each side of the bowel wall (Fig. 16.15). The omentum is critical to the successful healing of intestinal wounds because it can seal small anastomotic leaks and can prevent peritonitis. Dogs with the greater omentum removed have significant morbidity and mortality associated with intestinal anastomosis, whereas most dogs survive and do well when the omentum is retained.

Postoperative Care

Fluid and electrolyte deficits are corrected and antibiotic therapy is continued in the postoperative period. Feeding with an elemental diet such as Ensure (Ross Laboratories, Columbus, OH) or baby food should be started after 24 hours in the absence of vomiting. In uncomplicated cases, reasonable appetite usually resumes within 48 hours. Anorexia or vomiting in the presence of fever, abdominal tenderness, and leukocytosis suggests that anastomotic leakage and peritonitis may have occurred.

If anastomotic dehiscence is suspected, abdominocentesis and/or diagnostic peritoneal lavage should be performed. If toxic neutrophils with engulfed bacteria or free peritoneal bacteria are present, early reexploration of the abdomen is warranted. Further resection and reanastomosis or use of one of the serosal patching techniques described later in this chapter may be required. Aggressive treatment of generalized peritonitis may be needed to salvage the patient.

Effects of Massive Resection

The propensity for short-bowel syndrome after intestinal resection depends on the amount of tissue excised, the location of the resection, and the time allowed for adaptation. Resection of up to 80% of the small intestine in puppies may allow for normal weight gain, whereas resection of 90% produces morbidity and mortality. After resection of large portions of small intestine, maldigestion, malabsorption, diarrhea induced by fatty acids or bile salts, bacterial overgrowth, and gastric hypersecretion may occur. Location of the resection is important. High resection of the duodenum and upper jejunum may decrease pancreatic enzyme secretion because pancreatic-stimulating hormones such as secretin and cholecystokinin are produced in the mucosa of these sections. These reductions in release of pancreatic enzymes contribute to maldigestion. Maldigestion of protein, carbohydrate, and fat leads to catabolism, negative nitrogen balance, and steatorrhea. Unabsorbed sugars also may cause osmotic diarrhea. If the ileocecal valve is resected, bacteria may ascend, overgrow in the small bowel, and contribute to diarrhea.

After massive resection, the remaining small intestine adapts by increasing lumen diameter, enlarging microvilli size, and increasing mucosal cell number. These compensatory changes may take several weeks; during this period, parenteral fluids, electrolytes, and hyperalimentation may be necessary for the survival of the animal. During this time, the animal ideally will be able to maintain weight even with diarrhea. If diarrhea does not ultimately resolve, medical management must be attempted. Medical treatments for unresponsive diarrhea after massive resection include frequent small meals, low-fat diets such as intestinal diet (I/D Hills, Topeka, KS) elemental diet supplements, medium-chain triglyceride oils, pancreatic enzyme supplements, B vitamins, kaolin antidiarrheals, and poorly absorbed oral antibiotics such as neomycin.

Suggested Readings

Bone DL, Duckett KE, Patton CS, et al. Evaluation of anastomosis of small intestine in dogs: crushing versus noncrushing suturing techniques. Am J Vet Res 1983;44:2043.

Chatworthy HW, Saleby R, Lovingood C. Extensive small bowel resection in young dogs: its effect on growth and development. Surgery 1952;32:341.

Crowe DT. Diagnostic abdominal paracentesis techniques: clinical evaluation in 129 dogs and cats. J Am Anim Hosp Assoc 1984;20:223.

Ellison GW. End to end intestinal anastomosis in the dog: a comparison of techniques. Compend Contin Educ Small Anim Pract 1981;3:486.

Ellison GW, Jokinen MC, Park RD. End to end intestinal anastomosis in the dog: a comparative fluorescein dye, angiographic and histopathologic evaluation. J Am Anim Hosp Assoc 1982; 18:729.

Krahwinkel DJ, Richardson DC. Intestines. In: Bojrab MJ, ed. Current techniques in small animal surgery. 2nd ed. Philadelphia: Lea & Febiger, 1983.

McLackin AD. Omental protection of intestinal anastomosis. Am J Surg 1973;125:134.

Rosin E. The intestines. In: Slatter DH, ed. Textbook of small animal surgery. Philadelphia: WB Saunders, 1985.

Wheaton LB, Strandberg JD, Hamilton SR, et al. A comparison of three techniques for intraoperative prediction of small intestinal injury. J Am Anim Hosp Assoc 1983;19:897.

Enteroplication to Prevent Recurrent Intestinal Intussusception

Matt G. Oakes

Intestinal intussusception is a surgically treatable problem seen occasionally in dogs and cats. Puppies and kittens have a higher incidence than adult animals. Most intussusceptions are considered idiopathic, but predisposing factors may include intestinal parasitism, nonspecific gastroenteritis, linear foreign bodies, virally induced enteritis, intraluminal intestinal masses, and recent surgery. Celiotomy and manual reduction or resection of the involved segment are the most common treatments for intussusceptions. Recurrence may follow surgical correction in as many as 25% of dogs treated. The recurrent intussusception is often located at a different site from the initial lesion.

Pharmacologic prevention of intussusceptions has been investigated, but results are inconsistent. Although several surgical procedures have been attempted for the prevention of recurrent intussusceptions in dogs, enteroplication is the one most often recommended. Enteroplication is a modification of a procedure described by Noble to prevent obstructive adhesion formation after abdominal surgery in human patients. The procedure involves the surgical plication of the entire jejunum and ileum. A retrospective study of this procedure in dogs showed that it is safe and effective in preventing recurrent intussusceptions. Re-

current intussusceptions frequently form at distant sites from the initial lesion. Therefore, plication of only the intestinal segments adjacent to the initial lesion may not be effective.

Surgical Technique

A midline celiotomy is performed, and the intussusception is treated by either manual reduction or resection and anastomosis. The involved intestinal segment and abdomen are then lavaged with warm saline. Starting at the duodenocolic ligament, the small bowel is arranged in a series of gentle loops by laying adjoining segments side to side. Adjacent loops of intestine are sutured to each other with 3–0 or 4–0 absorbable or nonabsorbable sutures, placed midway between the mesenteric and antimesenteric borders (Fig. 16.16). The sutures may be placed in a simple interrupted or simple continuous pattern and should penetrate the submucosal layer of the intestine. The plication should start at the duodenocolic ligament and end at the ileocecocolic junction. Abdominal closure is routine, and normal postoperative care for intestinal surgery should be provided.

Suggested Readings

Lewis DD, Ellison GW. Intussusception in dogs and cats. Compend Contin Educ Pract Vet 1987;9:523.

Oakes MG, Lewis DD, Hosgood G, et al. Enteroplication for the prevention of recurrent intussusceptions in dogs. J Am Vet Med Assoc 1994;205:72.

Management of Rectal Prolapse

Mark H. Engen

Although rectal prolapse can occur with any condition that causes prolonged tenesmus, it is most common in heavily parasitized animals that have severe diarrhea and tenesmus. Other causes of straining resulting in rectal prolapse are dystocia, urolithiasis, intestinal neoplasms and foreign bodies, prostatic disease, perineal hernia, constipation congenital defects, and postoperative tenesmus after anal or perineal surgery.

Diagnosis

The diagnosis of rectal prolapse is made by visual observation of a tubelike mass, of varying length, pro-

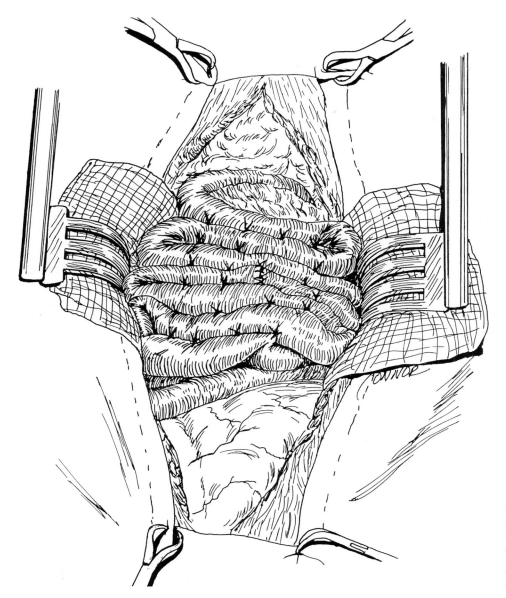

Fig. 16.16. After resection and anastomosis, the small intestine is arranged in a series of gentle loops. Adjacent loops are sutured to each other with sutures placed midway between the mesenteric and antimesenteric borders.

truding from the anus. If rectal prolapse is diagnosed early, the protruding tissue may be short, and the prolapsed mucosa will appear bright red and nonulcerated. In patients with rectal prolapse of long duration, the protrusion is longer, and the mucosa appears red or black and is either ulcerated or necrotic.

True rectal prolapse must be differentiated from prolapsed intussusception of the intestine or colon. These conditions can be differentiated by passing a probe between the anus and the prolapsed mass. The probe can be passed if an intussusception is present, but it cannot be passed if a rectal prolapse has occurred. To achieve a permanent cure for rectal prolapse, the underlying cause of tenesmus must be diagnosed and treated.

Nonsurgical Treatment

Treatment to correct a rectal prolapse depends on the viability of the exposed tissue and the size of the prolapse. A small prolapse with viable-appearing mucosa usually can be replaced by using a finger or bougie to reposition the bowel. Topical application of hypertonic sugar solution for 20 to 30 minutes may be helpful in relieving edema, so the prolapse can be reduced more easily. When the prolapse has been reduced, an anal pursestring suture is used to prevent recurrence. General anesthesia or epidural analgesia is used in some patients to facilitate reduction of the prolapse and placement of the anal pursestring suture (Fig. 16.17).

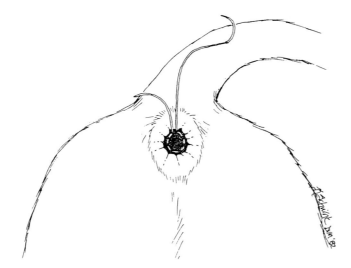

Fig. 16.17. Placement of anal pursestring suture after reduction of rectal prolapse by manipulation.

After reduction of the prolapse, epidural analgesia prevents straining for several hours. Periodic rectal application of a local anesthetic ointment (1% dibucaine [Nupercainal ointment, Ciba Pharmaceutical, Ciba–Geigy, Summit, NJ]) may be done initially and after removal of the anal pursestring suture to prevent further straining. The anal pursestring suture is left in place for a minimum of 24 to 48 hours, and the animal is given only fluids orally during this time.

Surgical Treatment

When a rectal prolapse cannot be reduced by manipulation and the lack of tissue viability contraindicates reduction, rectal resection and anastomosis are performed. This procedure is performed under general anesthesia or epidural analgesia. The patient is positioned and draped (Fig. 16.18**A** and **B**). A test tube or a saline-soaked sponge is placed into the lumen of the bowel to prevent fecal contamination. Three stay sutures are placed through the full thickness of both layers of the prolapse to form a triangle (Fig. 16.18**C** and **D**). The prolapse is then resected 1 to 2 cm from the anus. The anastomosis is performed with a single-layer closure using a simple interrupted suture pattern (Fig. 16.18**E**). Synthetic absorbable or chromic gut suture (3–0 or 4–0) is preferred. The sutures are placed through the full thickness of the incised ends of the bowel. The sutures must pass through the submucosa to ensure proper holding strength. The stay sutures are then removed, and the anastomosis is reduced manually inside the anus.

When the rectal prolapse cannot be reduced by external manipulation, but the rectal tissue is still viable, a celiotomy is performed, and the prolapse is manually reduced by gentle traction on the colon (Fig. 16.19**A**). A colopexy is performed after reduction of the prolapse to prevent recurrence using synthetic absorbable or chromic catgut suture (2–0 or 3–0) (Fig. 16.19**B** and **C**). A colopexy may also be performed in cases of recurrent rectal prolapse that can be reduced by external manipulation. Such a colopexy is rarely needed, however, if the cause of straining has been diagnosed and eliminated.

Postoperative Care

Topical anesthetic (1% dibucaine) ointment is instilled rectally after correction of any rectal prolapse to prevent further tenesmus. The patient may be fed on the day after the operation. A diet of soft food and a fecal softener (dioctyl sodium sulfosuccinate) also may be administered for 1 week postoperatively. Diarrhea should be treated with neomycin, intestinal coating agents, and anticholinergic drugs. Feces should be examined, and antihelminthic agents should be administered, based on results of fecal examinations for parasitic ova.

In conclusion, once a rectal prolapse has been corrected by surgical or nonsurgical means, recurrence is rare if the cause of the tenesmus has been diagnosed and resolved (e.g., removal of intestinal parasites by worming).

Suggested Readings

Annis JR, Allen AR. An atlas of canine surgery. Philadelphia: Lea & Febiger, 1967.

Archibald J. Canine surgery. 2nd ed. Santa Barbara, CA: American Veterinary Publications, 1974.

Evans HE, DeLahunta A. Miller's guide to the dissection of the dog. Philadelphia: WB Saunders, 1971.

Greiner T, Christi T. The cecum, colon, rectum, and anus. In: Bojrab MJ, ed. Current techniques in small animal surgery. Philadelphia: Lea & Febiger, 1975.

LeRoux PH. Dilation of the cecum in dogs. J S Afr Vet Med Assoc 1962;33:73.

Markowtiz J, Archibald J, Downie HG. Experimental surgery. 5th ed. Baltimore: Williams & Wilkins, 1964.

Sabiston DC. Davis–Christopher textbook of surgery. 12th ed. Philadelphia: WB Saunders, 1982.

Schiller AG, Helper LC, Knecht CD. Repair of rectocutaneous fistulas in the dog. J Am Vet Med Assoc 1967;50:758.

Stockman V, Stockman MRJ. Cecal impaction in the dog. Vet Rec 1961;73:337.

Swenson O, Bill AH. Resection of rectum and rectosigmoid with preservation of the sphincter for benign spastic lesions producing megacolon. In: Surgery 24. St. Louis, CV Mosby, 1948.

Walshaw R, Harvey CE. The rectum and anus. In: Bojrab MJ, ed. Pathophysiology in small animal surgery. Philadelphia: Lea & Febiger, 1981.

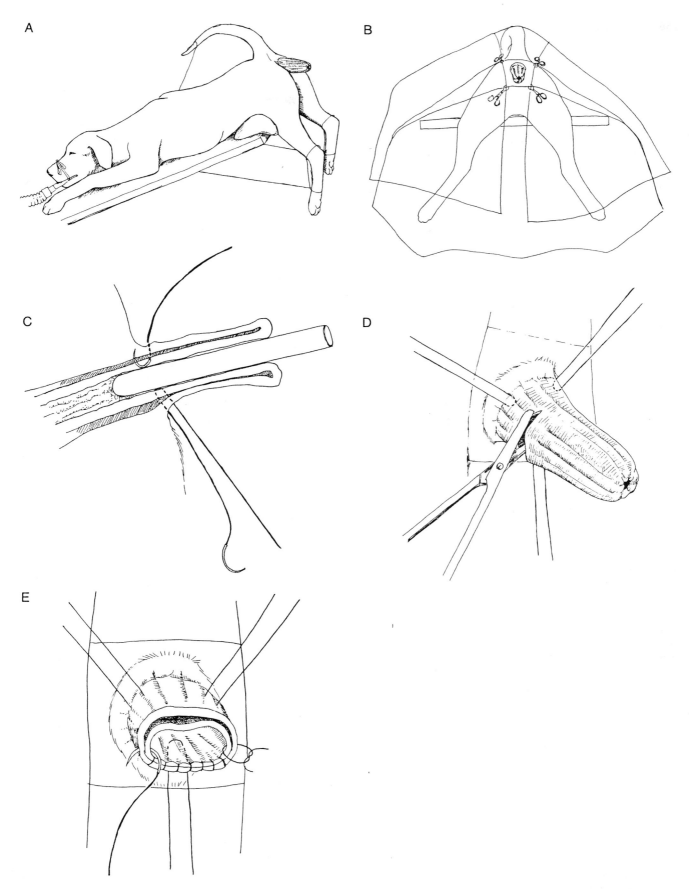

Fig. 16.18. Rectal resection and anastomosis to correct prolapse. **A.** Positioning of patient on a perineal stand. **B.** Sterile draping of the prolapse. **C.** Insertion of test tube into rectum and placement of stay sutures. **D.** Excision of the prolapsed mass. **E.** Full-thickness anastomosis of the rectal lumen.

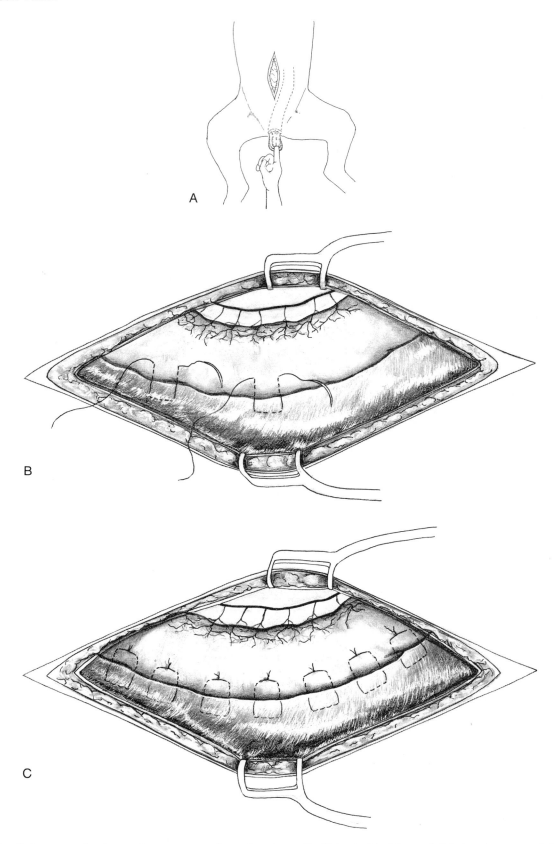

Fig. 16.19. Celiotomy and colopexy for treatment of rectal prolapse. **A.** Abdominal incision and digital replacement of the prolapsed tissue. **B.** Placement of colopexy mattress sutures. **C.** Six to eight mattress sutures are placed to complete the colopexy.

Surgery of the Colon and Rectum

Brian T. Huss

Colorectal surgery has classically been feared as fraught with operative and postoperative complications. However, the use of modern techniques and materials has resulted in surgical success rates comparable with those of other gastrointestinal operations.

The large intestine of the dog and cat is shorter than the small intestine, ranging from approximately 20 to 35 cm in length (1, 2). As a general rule, the large intestine is approximately the length of the trunk in dogs and cats, with the small intestine measuring about four times the length of the trunk. Because of its shorter mesentery, the large intestine does not vary as much in length or position as the small intestine. The large intestine is, however, considerably larger in internal diameter than the small intestine and has neither the taeniae (longitudinal bands) nor the haustra (sacculations) seen in other species. Classically, the large intestine has been divided into the cecum, colon (ascending, transverse, and descending), and rectum (Fig. 16.20).

Microscopically, the colon is composed of five layers. From the inner surface outward, the layers of the colon are 1) mucosa, 2) submucosa, 3) circular muscle layer, 4) longitudinal muscle layer, and 5) serosa. The mucosa consists of columnar epithelial lining cells, mucus-secreting goblet cells, and enteroendocrine cells. Intestinal villi are absent in the colonic mucosa; however, intestinal crypts (crypts of Lieberkühn) remain. Intestinal crypts are elongated and straight, opening onto the luminal surface of the colon. The submucosa is composed of collagen and elastin fibers arranged in an orderly honeycomb pattern, with submucosal glands and lymphoid tissue dispersed throughout this layer. The submucosa's high collagen and elastin content makes it the important suture-holding layer of the intestine. Tunica muscularis is the term commonly given the combined smooth muscle layers of the intestine. Contraction of this group of muscles is responsible for intestinal motility. Finally, the tunica serosa consists of loose connective tissue covered with a layer of squamous mesothelial cells.

The large intestine is anchored to the sublumbar region by the mesocolon, which arises from the left side of the mesentery and is divided into the same parts as the colon that it suspends. The blood supply to the colon and rectum arises from the cranial and caudal mesenteric arteries supported in the mesocolon (see Fig. 16.20). The cranial mesenteric artery supplies the cecum and the ascending, transverse, and part of

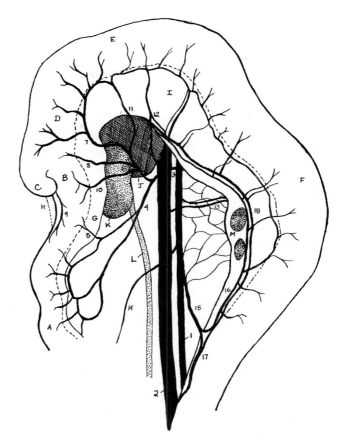

Fig. 16.20. Surgical anatomy of the feline large intestine, ventral view. *A,* jejunum; *B,* ileum; *C,* cecum; *D,* ascending colon; *E,* transverse colon; *F,* descending colon; *G,* mesentery; *H,* ileocecal fold; *I,* mesocolon; *J,* caudate process of liver; *K,* right kidney; *L,* right ureter; *M,* caudal mesenteric lymph nodes; *1,* abdominal aorta; *2,* caudal vena cava; *3,* cranial mesenteric artery; *4,* jejunal artery; *5,* ileal artery; *6,* ileocolic artery; *7,* colic branch; *8,* cecal artery; *9,* antimesenteric ileal branch; *10,* ileal mesenteric branch; *11,* right colic artery; *12,* middle colic artery; *13,* left renal vessels; *14,* testicular artery; *15,* caudal mesenteric artery; *16,* left colic artery; *17,* cranial rectal artery; *18,* middle colic vein.

the descending colon. The caudal mesenteric artery supplies the remainder of the descending colon as well as the rectum (1–4). Numerous perpendicular branches (vasa recta) split from the colic arteries, anastomosing with each other along the lesser curvature of the colon. Most of the large intestine is drained by the portal system through the ileocolic and caudal mesenteric veins (1–4). The caudal rectal vein drains the anal canal and empties directly into the caudal vena cava (1–4).

Indications for Surgery

The need for colonic surgery in small animals is not common, usually requiring primary closure of defects, resection and anastomosis, or biopsy techniques. Trauma to the colon can result from intraluminal or extraluminal sources. Intraluminal causes of injury are rare, but such injury can result from ingested sharp foreign bodies or improper use of transanal instruments. Colonic foreign bodies can often be gently milked through the colon to a point at which they can be grasped by an assistant using transanal forceps. Rarely, a colotomy must be performed to retrieve a foreign body. Extraluminal sources of trauma are more common and include gunshot and knife wounds and, less commonly, penetrating bone fragments from pelvic fractures. Indirect or blunt trauma to the colon can also result in contusions, vessel thrombosis, or even avulsions of the colon. Penetrating wounds of the colon require immediate treatment. Primary repair of clean lacerations, debridement and primary closure of more severe wounds, or resection and anastomosis of devitalized segments may be required to close colonic defects. In one study of dogs with rectal tears resulting from pelvic fractures, only dogs with tears repaired within 24 hours of trauma survived (5).

Neoplasia of the colon is less common than in other parts of the alimentary system. Benign tumors of the colon commonly include leiomyomas, papillary adenomas, and adenomatous polyps. Adenomatous polyps can convert to malignant carcinomas; however, data are currently insufficient to consider polyps precancerous in small animals. Malignant tumors of the colon commonly include lymphosarcomas, carcinomas, and adenocarcinomas. Metastasis of colonic tumors occurs most commonly to the regional lymph nodes and the liver.

Intussusception of the large intestine occurs most frequently at the ileocecocolic junction. Intussusception of the body of the colon is rare. Intussusceptions of the large intestine are treated in the same way as those occurring in the small intestine.

Colectomy, either partial or complete, may be the treatment of choice for patients with unresponsive megacolon, severe unresponsive inflammatory bowel disease, colonic ulcerations, colonic strictures, and pelvic canal stenosis resulting from pelvic fracture malunion. Removal of the cecocolic valve has been advocated in the case of megacolon caused by pelvic fracture malunion, to create a soft stool. Most surgeons, however, recommend leaving the cecocolic valve in the treatment of other colonic diseases.

Surgical biopsy of the colon may be the diagnostic method of choice in some colonic diseases. Direct visualization of the entire colon, the ability to safely obtain multiple full-thickness samples of colonic wall and regional lymph nodes, and readily available instrumentation make open colonic biopsy a viable diagnostic method.

Diagnostic Methods

Plain abdominal and pelvic radiographs are recommended in all patients with suspected large intestinal disease. Radiographs can give indications of luminal contents, including the degree of colonic filling and the overall density of the luminal contents. Radiographs can also help to diagnose intraluminal or extraluminal foreign bodies, or space-occupying lesions, and they give a rough estimate of intestinal wall thickness, as well as of plication or intusscuseptions of the intestine. Poor abdominal detail or a "ground-glass" appearane and free gas in the abdomen indicate a gastrointestinal perforation. Positive-contrast enemas may be helpful diagnostic tools in selected cases; however, they are contraindicated when perforations or weakened intestinal walls are suspected.

Other diagnostic methods that may be of benefit in large intestinal diseases are proctoscopy and ultrasonography. Proctoscopy should be performed with care if weakened intestinal walls are suspected, and it is contraindicated when large intestinal perforations are suspected. Ultrasonography can be a useful tool in some intestinal diseases and is rapidly becoming the diagnostic method of choice for intussusuceptions.

Preoperative Preparation

Bacterial populations in the normal gastrointestinal tract increase dramatically from oral to aboral, changing from predominately aerobic to predominately anaerobic. A gram of feces from the colon contains up to 10^9 organisms (6). Aerobic bacteria in the large intestine normally include the gram-positive genera *Streptococcus*, *Staphylococcus*, *Bacillus*, and *Corynebacterium* and gram-negative members of the family Enterobacteriaceae, especially *Escherichia coli*, *Enterobacter*, *Klebsiella*, *Pseudomonas*, *Neisseria*, and *Moraxella* (6). Up to 90% of the bacteria in the large intestine are anaerobes, including members of the gram-positive genera *Clostridium*, *Lactobacillus*, *Propionibacterium*, and *Bifidobacterium*; the gram-negative anaerobic bacteria include *Bacteroides*, *Fusobacterium*, and *Veillonella* (6). The importance of anaerobic bacteria as pathogens in small animals, especially *Bacteroides fragilis*, has been demonstrated (7, 8).

Mechanical cleansing of the bowel decreases the risk of intraoperative bacterial contamination by decreasing the quantity of feces in the intestine while the lumen is opened. Mechanical cleansing, however, does not decrease the concentration of bacteria per gram of feces, only the quantity of feces present. The current veterinary regimen of choice for mechanical bowel cleansing is the technique used for colonoscopy preparation (9, 10). The lavage solutions Colyte

(Reed & Carnrick, Piscataway, NJ) or GoLytely (Braintree Laboratories, Inc., Braintree, MA), at 80 mg/kg, are administered orally in two divided doses 4 to 6 hours apart 18 to 24 hours before the procedure. These lavage solutions produce osmotic diarrhea that cleanses the entire gastrointestinal tract. Potential problems with using mechanical cleansing are poor cleansing of the proximal colon when using enemas only and watery intestinal contents, which are more difficult to control once the intestinal tract is open. One human study comparing mechanical preparation alone before colorectal surgery demonstrated an overall postoperative infection rate of up to 45% compared with mechanical preparation with some form of antibiotic solution at 18% (11). To reduce infection rates to an acceptable level after colorectal surgery, some form of antibiotic prophylaxis is also recommended.

Oral antibiotics used for prophylaxis in colorectal surgery are generally those that are poorly absorbed from the intestinal lumen. The purpose of oral antibiotics is to lower the concentration of bacteria within the intestine. To be effective, oral antibiotics should be active against the organisms most commonly found in the large intestine. Most oral antibiotic regimens include an aminoglycoside, such as neomycin or kanamycin, in combination with an antibiotic effective against anaerobic bacteria, such as metronidazole, erythromycin, tetracycline, lincomycin, or clindamycin (6, 11–16). Neomycin used alone has actually been incriminated in higher postoperative infection rates (16). When combined with mechanical bowel cleansing, oral antibiotic prophylaxis reduces postoperative infection rates to 5 to 18% in human patients undergoing colorectal surgery (11, 14, 15). Oral antibiotic regimens should not be administered earlier than 24 hours before surgery to prevent possible resistant bacterial overgrowth.

Systemic antibiotics have been used alone or in combination with mechanical or oral antibiotic bowel preparation for surgical prophylaxis. The rationale for systemic antibiotics is to obtain blood and tissue levels of antibiotic higher than the minimum inhibitory concentration of potential pathogens at the time of maximum tissue contamination. In cases of emergency gastrointestinal surgery, systemic antibiotics are the only feasible method of preoperative prophylaxis. Controversy and conflicting research exist in the human literature over whether oral or systemic antimicrobial prophylaxis, or a combination of the two, is best (13, 15–17).

Systemic antibiotic prophylaxis must be effective against both the aerobic and the anaerobic bacteria found in the large intestine. Mixed aerobic–anaerobic infections result in a biphasic infection pattern, with an acute phase resulting in mortality from endotoxin-bearing gram-negative aerobic bacteria and a chronic phase resulting in abscess formation as a result of anaerobic bacteria (18). Studies have found that the use of antibiotics effective only against aerobic bacteria (i.e., aminoglycosides) dramatically decreases mortality associated with gram-negative sepsis; however, these drugs do not decrease postoperative abscess or adhesion formation (6, 8). Conversely, the use of antibiotics effective primarily against anaerobic bacteria decreases the incidence of abscess formation, but the mortality from gram-negative sepsis is high (6, 8).

General recommendations for systemic antibiotic prophylaxis in colorectal surgery include using a drug, or drugs, that can be administered by a bolus intravenous injection that can rapidly achieve peak serum levels. Bactericidal antibiotics with the narrowest effective spectrum, the lowest cost, the least toxic side effects, and the easiest administration regimen should be used. Drugs should be given preoperatively to obtain effective target-tissue concentrations at the time of potential primary bacterial invasion; generally, these drugs are administered approximately 30 minutes before the start of surgery. Antibiotics should be readministered approximately every two half-lives during the surgical procedure to maintain effective tissue levels. Finally, prophylactic antibiotics should be discontinued after surgery, with 24 hours being the maximum accepted duration (12). Continued postoperative antibiotic administration, or administration of systemic antibiotics for extended periods preoperatively, can result in bacterial antibiotic resistance and superinfections.

Systemic antibiotic prophylaxis for colorectal surgery can be broken into combination therapy regimens and monotherapy regimens. The most commonly used combination antibiotic regimens for human colorectal surgery are aminoglycosides, such as gentamicin, kanamycin, amikacin, or tobramycin along with lincomycin, clindamycin, or metronidazole (14, 18). Effective monotherapy drugs used for antimicrobial prophylaxis in colorectal surgery include cefoxitin, several third-generation cephalosporins, and ampicillin/sulbactam (8, 14, 19). Cefoxitin is currently recommended by several authors as the systemic prophylactic antibiotic of choice for colorectal surgery in veterinary medicine (20–22). The drug is a single agent intravenous antibiotic that has low toxicity, is relatively inexpensive, and has good bactericidal effects against the primary bacterial pathogens. Cefoxitin dosage recommendations in small animals range from 6 to 30 mg/kg intramuscularly or intravenously given every 8 hours (21, 23) With a half-life of 41 to 59 minutes, cefoxitin should be readministered every 1.5 to 2 hours as surgical prophylaxis. A newer third-generation cephalosporin, cefotetan, has recently been demonstrated in the laboratory to have pharmacokinetic properties superior to those of cefoxitin in the dog (24). Cefotetan dosage recommendations in dogs are 30 mg/kg intravenously every 8 hours or subcutaneously every 12 hours.

Surgical Techniques

Colonic Healing

The colon follows the same stages of healing as skin and other soft tissue: inflammation, debridement, repair, and maturation (25). A unique property of colonic healing, however, involves the balance of collagen synthesis and degradation. During the first 3 to 5 days after wounding, collagen synthesis is competing with collagenolysis (25–29). This is important, because the collagen content of a wound has been directly correlated with wound strength (27). There is an especially high turnover rate of collagen in the wounded colon (25–28). Earlier work suggests that as much as 40% of the rat colon's original collagen content, throughout the entire colon, is lost to collagenolysis during the first 4 to 6 days after wounding (28). However, early studies have overemphasized the drop in collagen content in colonic wounds. With the use of more advanced techniques in measuring the collagen content of a wound, researchers have found that the drop in collagen content is not as dramatic as originally thought (29). Rapid gain occurs in colonic tensile strength between the third and seventh days after wounding (29). Local factors in the colon can, however, shift a wound toward increased collagen lysis. Traumatic handling of colonic tissue, bacterial contamination, foreign material, and certain suture patterns used for intestinal anastomoses all increase the amount of collagenase produced locally in colonic tissue.

Methods of Colonic Anastomosis

After intestinal resection, the continuity of the intestinal tract can be reconstructed using three basic anastomotic techniques: end-to-end, side-to-side, and end-to-side. When hand suturing is used, the end-to-end intestinal anastomosis is the easiest and quickest technique to perform and results in a more physiologic reconstruction. Side-to-side and end-to-side anastomosis of the intestine have also been incriminated, with formation of blind pouches where bacterial overgrowth and resulting malabsorption can occur.

When a disparity of luminal diameters is present, especially as seen with ileocolic anastomoses, several techniques are available to aid in end-to-end anastomoses. A funneled closure is the simplest anastomosis if minor disparities of luminal diameters exist. Sutures are placed equidistant around the circumference of the lumen ends. This stretches the smaller luminal opening and constricts the larger luminal opening (Fig. 16.21**A**). With larger luminal disparities, the smaller-diameter intestine can be cut at an angle, with more tissue removed from the antimesenteric border (Fig. 16.21**B**). If a luminal disparity still exists, the antimesenteric border of the smaller-diameter intestine can be further incised 1 to 2 cm. Two triangular flaps of intestinal wall can then be cut off each side of the incision, leaving an ovoid stoma that can be anastomosed to the larger-diameter intestine (Fig. 16.21**C**). Finally, if the smaller-diameter intestinal lumen cannot be opened widely enough, the larger-diameter intestine can be partially sutured closed until the luminal diameters are equal (Fig. 16.21**D**).

Two-layer anastomotic closures of the colon are still advocated by some surgeons. Several studies, however, have demonstrated no increase in intestinal dehiscence and actually an increased healing rate, using a single-layer closure versus two-layer closure (30, 31). In fact, two-layer anastomotic closures have been demonstrated to have significantly greater incidences of dehiscence and stricture formation in the rectum because of avascular necrosis of the tissue incorporated in the inner suture pattern (32). Leakage at the anastomosis site is not a problem if the omentum is healthy and intact. A fibrin seal forms at the anastomosis site within about 3 hours in most patients (32).

Numerous intestinal anastomosis studies have been performed comparing simple continuous, simple interrupted, inverting, everting, or appositional suture techniques. The anastomosis techniques that are the easiest to perform, with the least leakage, the least adhesion formation, and the best histologic healing, have been the single-layer simple interrupted approximating techniques. In 1968, Poth and Gold described the crushing appositional anastomosis technique in human patients (33). This technique involved a through-and-through suture, which was then tightened to cut through all the layers of the intestine except the tough submucosa (Fig. 16.22**A**). This technique kept the suture from exposure to the luminal surface, where it could become infected, and from exposure to the abdominal lumen and serosal surface, where adhesions could form. At about the same time the crushing technique was developed, DeHoff and associates investigated the use of a simple interrupted approximating technique for intestinal anastomosis in dogs (Fig. 16.22**B**) (34). Both appositional techniques maintain luminal diameter, diminish adhesion formation, and allow for rapid primary healing of the intestinal anastomosis. Some eversion commonly occurs with both these appositional techniques, resulting in adhesions and some altered healing (32). The Gambee suture pattern is favored by some surgeons to help

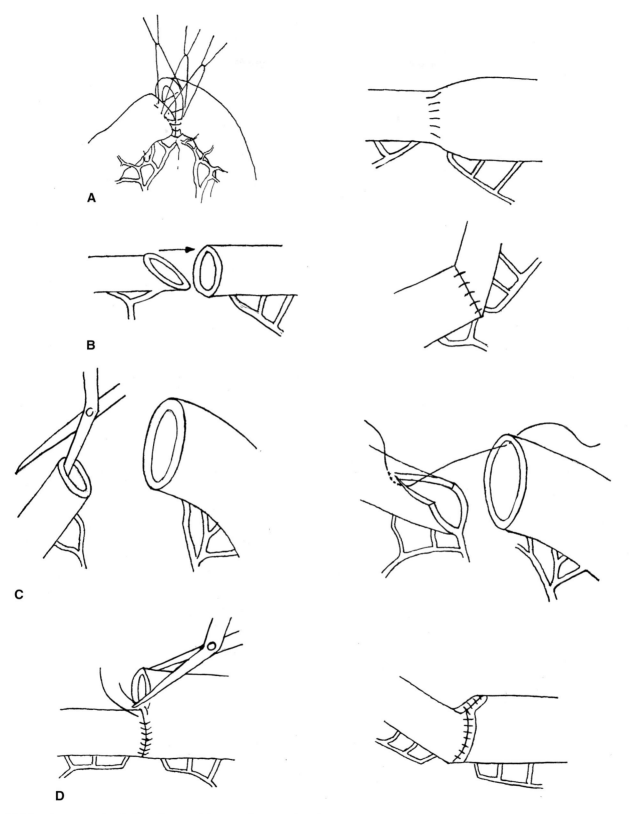

Fig. 16.21. Anastomosis of dissimilar sized lumens. See text for details. **A.** Funneled closure. **B.** Oblique transection of the smaller lumen. **C.** Spatulated closure. **D.** Partial oversew.

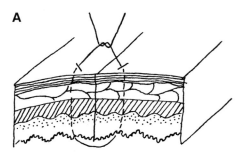

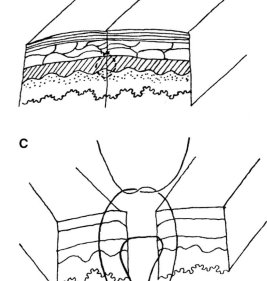

Fig. 16.22. **A.** The simple interrupted appositional suture pattern. **B.** The Poth and Gold crushing suture pattern. Notice the suture crushes through all of the tissue layers to hold just the submucosa. **C.** The Gambee suture pattern. Notice the suture passes through the mucosa and causes slight tissue inversion.

eliminate the slight eversion caused by the simple appositional suture patterns (Fig. 16.22**C**).

Various suture materials are used successfully for intestinal anastomosis, including monofilament and braided absorbable and nonabsorbable sutures. The monofilament absorbable sutures polydioxanone and polyglyconate are closest to the ideal suture material available for intestinal anastomosis today. Nonabsorbable monofilament suture material such as nylon or polypropylene may be useful in patients that are expected to have delayed tissue healing. Braided nonabsorbable suture such as silk was used for intestinal anastomosis for many years. However, with our current knowledge of the increased likelihood of infection forming around braided suture in contaminated surgery, nonabsorbable braided sutures are not recommended for colonic anastomosis. The braided absorbable sutures polyglycolic acid and polyglactin 910 are absorbed in a short period of time. These sutures have a constant absorption rate that is not affected by infection, so infected suture tracts and granulomas are of little concern. The biggest problem with absorbable braided sutures is the tissue trauma (drag or chatter) as they are pulled through tissue. The surface characteristics of braided sutures have been shown by electron microscopy to increase trauma to the tissue they have been pulled through, as opposed to smooth monofilament suture material (35). In small animal colonic surgery, a size 3–0 to 4–0 suture should have sufficient tensile strength to hold intestinal tissue.

A swaged-on reverse cutting or taper-cut suture needle is recommended for colonic surgery. These suture needles facilitate penetration of the intestine's tough submucosa with the least effort and tissue trauma. Taper-point or narrow-taper needles have been suggested by some surgeons, because less intestinal leakage occurs around the suture tract. The increased trauma of passing the taper needle through the submucosa must be balanced with this minor benefit.

The number of sutures placed to form an anastomosis should be the minimum needed to prevent leakage of the anastomosis. Most intestinal anastomosis techniques describe placing sutures 2 to 4 mm from the cut serosal surface and 3 to 4 mm apart. This averages approximately 12 to 16 simple interrupted sutures evenly spaced around the anastomosis. The first suture is normally placed at the mesenteric border because this is the most difficult to see, and this area has the highest incidence of leakage and dehiscence (Fig. 16.23**A**). The second suture is normally placed at the antimesenteric border, with the remaining sutures filling in the area between the first two sutures (Fig. 16.23**B**). The anastomosis can be tested by filling the segment of intestine with saline under slight pressure or by milking luminal contents across the anastomosis and looking for leaks. Any anastomosis will leak if too much pressure is applied. Too many sutures decrease anastomosis healing by interfering with blood supply to the intestinal edges. Some authors recommend wrapping or even suturing the omentum around the anastomosis site. This is normally not necessary because the omentum naturally moves to cover any leaks in an intestinal anastomosis.

Surgical stapling is another method of intestinal anastomosis that has become increasingly popular. The device commonly used in colonic resection and anas-

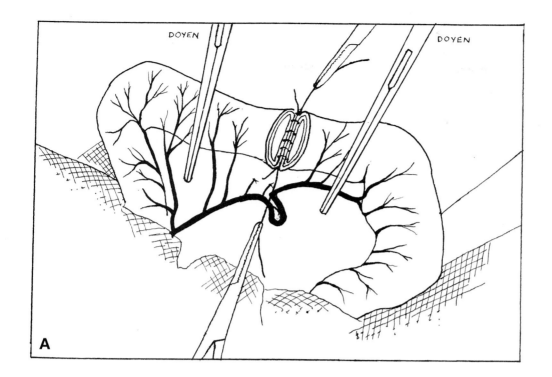

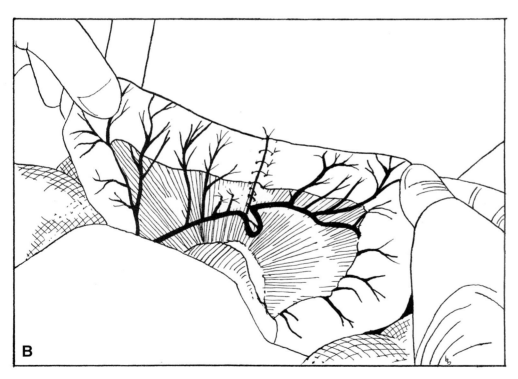

Fig. 16.23. Technique for colonic anastomosis. **A.** The two colonic segments are held together with the aid of the atraumatic forceps as a mesenteric, and then antimesenteric suture is placed to start the anastomosis. These first two sutures can be used as stay sutures to handle the bowel. **B.** The anastomosis is completed with a single-layer appositional suture pattern filling in the sutures between the stay sutures. The mesentery is closed with a simple continuous suture pattern.

tomosis is the circular stapler manufactured by Ethicon (Proximate ILS, Ethicon, Inc., Somerville, NJ) or United States Surgical (EEA, United States Surgical Corp., Norwalk, CT). The circular stapler inverts the intestinal ends and places two circumferential rows of staggered B-shaped sutures. The device then cuts out a donut-shaped section of the inverted tissue from the ends of the intestine being joined. The circular stapler can be inserted through the anus or through an access incision in the intestine. A modified Furness clamp is used to place a pursestring suture around the ends of the intestinal segments to be joined. One intestinal end is then slipped over the cartridge, and the other intestinal segment is placed over the anvil. The pursestring sutures are then tied to the movable metal shaft between the cartridge and anvil. The shaft is shortened, compressing the cartridge to the anvil with the intestinal ends in between. The stapler is then fired, forming the anastomosis and cutting out the pursestring along with the tissue in the middle of the lumen (Fig. 16.24). The circular stapler forms a true inverting anastomosis. Occasionally, the result is the same problem caused by a hand-sutured inverting anastomosis, that is, luminal strictures. The circular stapler is a technically demanding stapler to use. Improper usage of the stapler, or poor surgical technique, may result in anastomotic stricture or dehiscence. In experienced hands, the stapled anastomosis line has been demonstrated to leak less, to be better aligned, and to heal better than single-layer hand-sutured anastomoses (36). Various other sutureless intestinal anastomosis techniques have been studied through the years, from cyanoacrylate adhesives and fibrin glue, to laser welding and anastomosis rings.

The Valtrac biofragmentable anastomosis ring (BAR, Davis and Geck, Danbury, CT) is an implant that is easy to use and results in safe, reproducible anastomoses (37). Composed of a plastic polymer of polyglycolic acid and barium sulfate, the device fragments by 11 to 17 days in dogs and by 10 to 13 days in cats. The anastomosis ring is currently available in four external diameters sizes ranging from 25 to 34 mm. The Valtrac is made of two identical segments that interdigitate. Using a method similar to that used for the circular staplers, the two intestinal ends are secured over the BAR with pursestring sutures. When pushed together, the two BAR segments lock in place, leaving a specified gap between the two segments. The inner scalloped edges of the Valtrac prevent compromise of the intramural blood supply to the ends of the intestine.

Approaches

The colon and rectum can be approached through a ventral midline celiotomy, through a partial or complete pubic (ischial–pubic) osteotomy, by prolapsing the distal rectal mucosa, by a rectal pull-through, or by a dorsal approach.

A caudal ventral midline celiotomy from 2 to 3 cm cranial to the umbilicus extending to the pubic rim permits access to the entire colon and the colorectal junction. The patient should be clipped and aseptically prepared from midthorax to beyond the caudal edge of the pubis. Laterally, the skin preparation should extend slightly beyond the flank folds. The prepuce of male dogs should be flushed with a dilute chlorhexidine or povidone–iodine solution.

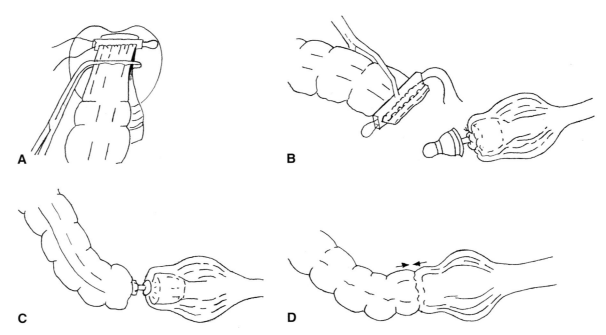

Fig. 16.24. Distal colorectal anastomosis with a circular stapler. See text for details. **A.** A modified Furness clamp is used to place a pursestring suture on the aboral intestinal segment (*top*). The affected orad segment is isolated and resected. **B.** A transrectal circular stapler is placed to the level of the aboral pursestring suture. The pursestring is then tied around the center anvil of the stapler. **C.** A pursestring suture around the orad intestinal segment is used to secure the segment to the circular stapler anvil cranial to the aboral segment. **D.** The circular stapler is then compressed and fired to form the anastomosis.

Exposure to the proximal and middle rectum can be made by extending the caudal midline celiotomy through a partial or complete pubic osteotomy, respectively. The skin incision is extended caudally over the pubis. For a partial pubic osteotomy, the aponeurosis of the gracilis and adductor muscles are incised on the midline and subperiostally are reflected laterally (Fig. 16.25A) (38). The obturator nerve and vessels lie at

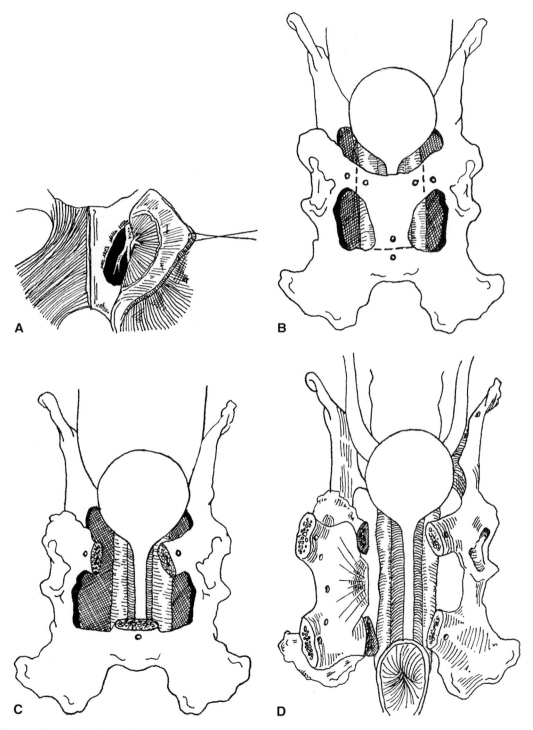

Fig. 16.25. Approach to the colon and rectum through a pubic osteotomy. See text for details. **A.** The aponeurosis of the gracili and adductor muscles is incised on the midline and reflected laterally. Note the obturator nerve and vessels at the cranial lateral edge of the obturator foramina. **B.** Osteotomy sites and drill holes for a partial pubic osteotomy. **C.** After reflecting the pubic floor segment caudally, the rectum is visible under the urinary tract. **D.** Reflecting the pubic floor laterally after a complete osteotomy, the entire ventral rectum can be visualized.

the cranial lateral edge of each obturator foramina and must be protected. Drill holes are made on each side of the osteotomies to facilitate later repair of the defect (Fig. 16.25**B**). Guarding the soft tissue, the pubis is then cut on both sides with a sagittal saw, Gigli wire, osteotome, or bone cutter. The cut should be made 2 to 3 mm medial to the lateral edge of each obturator foramen. Leaving the periosteum and soft tissue attached caudally to the floor of the pelvis, a third osteotomy is made, joining the caudal edges of the obturator foramina. The pubis is then hinged caudally as a caudally attached flap (Fig. 16.25**C**). The flap is reattached with two orthopedic wires through the predrilled holes. Approach to the rectum through a complete pubic osteotomy is performed in a similar manner; however, the caudal osteotomies are made from the obturator foramina transversely through the caudal ischii (39). The ischial–pubic flap is then hinged to one side (Fig. 16.25**D**). Before the osteotomies, drill holes are made on each side of each osteotomy to facilitate repair of the flap. Drill holes craniocaudally along one side of the pubic symphysis have been recommended to aid in reattachment of the muscle aponeuroses.

Distal rectal masses that are small and noninvasive can be approached by prolapsing the tissue through the anus. This procedure can be performed digitally or by placing a stay suture or sutures proximal to the mass.

Approaches to the middle and distal thirds of the rectum can be made through various pull-through techniques. These techniques can involve prolapsing tissue, extensive tissue dissection, or a combination of the two. A simpler approach to the middle and distal rectum is through a dorsal approach to the rectum.

Resection and Anastomosis

Resection and anastomosis of the colon are performed in a manner similar to that in the small intestine. After making an approach to the affected segment, a complete exploration of the area is performed. Regional lymph nodes, adjacent organs, and, in the abdomen, the liver are thoroughly examined to determine the extent of the disease process. Examination for unrelated but potentially complicating disease processes should also be performed.

The area to be resected should be carefully isolated with laparotomy sponges moistened with warm isotonic saline (Fig. 16.26**A**). The exposed tissue should be kept moist at all times to prevent desiccation and trauma. Two to three layers of laparotomy sponges or 4 × 4 sponges allow for removal of contaminated material with minimal chance for further contamination. Contaminated material should be removed from the sterile field as soon as possible to prevent further spread of contamination. An area for contaminated surgical instruments on the sterile field can be made with a dry lap sponge. As soon as the instruments are no longer needed, they should be removed from the operating table.

Once the affected colonic segment is isolated, the luminal contents should be milked orally and aborally from the area that will be resected. The blood supply to the affected segment should then be double-ligated using 3–0 to 4–0 suture material or ligation staples (Fig. 16.26**B**). For short segments, only the vasa recta perpendicular to the colon need to be ligated, preserving the vessels running parallel to the colon. Resection of longer segments necessitates ligation of the main blood supply running parallel to the colon. Once the blood supply has been ligated, delineation between vascular and avascular segments of colon can be easily observed.

Carmalt forceps can be placed at the edges of the colonic segment to be resected. Approximately 1 to 2 cm of healthy vascularized tissue should be included within the segment to be resected. Carmalt forceps can be placed perpendicularly across the colon, or they can be back cut on the antimesenteric side to create a larger anastomotic diameter. Atraumatic clamps (Doyen forceps, bobby pins, or an assistant's fingertips) are placed 4 to 5 cm to the outside of the Carmalt forceps. The atraumatic forceps keep luminal contents from leaking from the cut ends of the colon, as well as assisting in manipulation of the cut ends of the colon. Any remaining mesocolon is then resected as far from any vessels as possible. The affected colon segment can then be resected with a scalpel, using the outside edge of the Carmalt forceps as a guide. Colonic mucosa commonly everts over the cut edge of the intestine. It is easier to anastomose the colon if the mucosa is resected level to the cut edge of the outer colonic wall. This procedure is easily performed using Metzenbaum scissors. The colonic segments are then anastomosed using one of the previously mentioned techniques.

After performing and testing the colonic anastomosis, the anastomotic site is flushed with saline. Layers of laparotomy sponges can be removed in between flushing the anastomosis. Surgical gloves, instruments, and other contaminated equipment should be changed at this time. A sterile fenestrated drape can be placed over the surgical site. If the patient has no obvious contamination of the abdomen, abdominal lavage is not necessary. Otherwise, the abdomen should be lavaged with warm isotonic saline until the effluent is clear. The mesocolon should be closed with a continuous suture pattern of 3–0 or 4–0 absorbable material. Care should be taken not to damage the adjacent blood supply to the colon. The surgical approach is then closed in a routine manner.

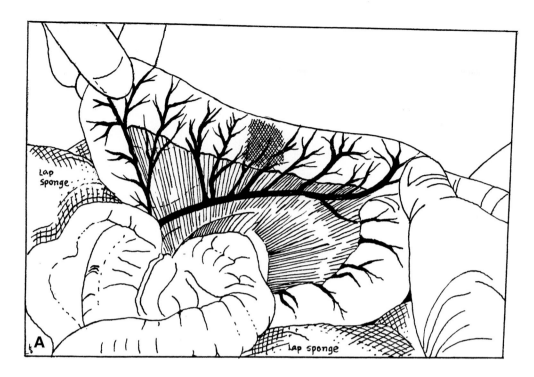

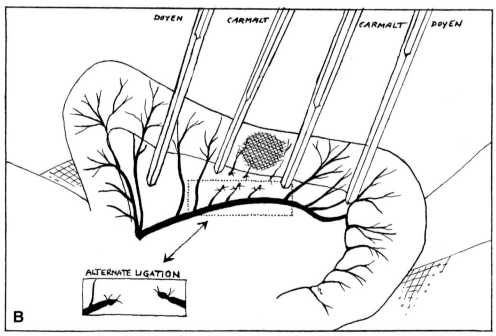

Fig. 16.26. Preparation for colonic resection and anastomosis. **A.** Moistened laparotomy sponges are placed under the Balfour retractor and wrapped around the base of the mesentery to isolate the affected colonic segment. **B.** The blood supply to the affected segment is double-ligated. For short colonic segments, individual vasa recta should be ligated, preserving the longitudinal mesenteric vessels. For longer colonic segments, the longitudinal mesenteric vessels can be ligated. Carmalt forceps are placed oral and aboral to the segment of colon to be resected, making certain to include all of the avascular bowel. Atraumatic forceps are then placed outside the carmalt forceps. The affected colonic segment is now transected using the outside of the Carmalt forceps as a guide.

Biopsy

Full-thickness biopsy techniques of the colon are similar to those in the small intestine. Luminal contents are milked from the biopsy site, and the site is isolated with a moistened laparotomy sponge. A full-thickness longitudinal incision approximately 1 to 2 cm long is made in the antimesenteric colonic wall. A full-thickness segment approximately 2 to 3 mm wide is cut from the side of the incision. Care should be taken not to crush the sample with forceps. The colonic defect is then closed transversely using simple interrupted sutures (Fig. 16.27).

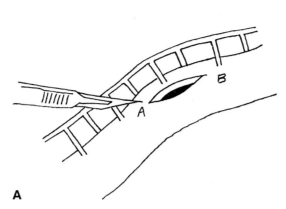

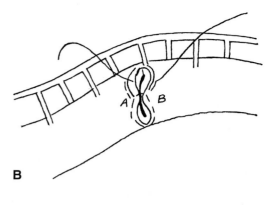

Fig. 16.27. Longitudinal incisions in bowel (**A**) can be closed transversely (**B**) to prevent reduction of the luminal diameter.

Postoperative Care and Complications

Immediate Postoperative Care

Patients undergoing major colorectal surgery often require significant postoperative care. Intravenous fluids should be continued postoperatively until the patient is taking food and water by mouth and the patient's temperature is below approximately 103.6°F. Rectal thermometers should be used with care. The newer infrared ear thermometers are preferred in animals that have undergone rectal surgery. Patients should be observed for signs of peritonitis for the first 3 to 5 days after surgery. These signs include fever, depression, anorexia, abdominal pain, vomiting, and shock. Postoperative antibiotics are generally not recommended unless intraoperative signs of established infection are present. Inappropriate use of antibiotics can mask signs of peritonitis and can result in superinfections. I routinely give one dose of narcotic analgesics immediately after extubation and administer further doses as needed. Clinically, the use of analgesics does not normally appear necessary beyond 12 to 24 hours after surgery. Patients can be offered water once they are fully awake from anesthesia. A low-residue diet can be offered within 12 to 24 hours after surgery. This diet should be continued for the first 2 to 3 weeks, after which the animal's normal diet can be gradually introduced. Stool consistency, color, and presence of blood should be carefully monitored. The patient's first bowel movement commonly contains a large amount of soft to liquid, dark stool with whole blood. Stool softeners can be administered as necessary to maintain a semifirm consistency. Patients that recover without complications are usually discharged on the third postoperative day.

Early Complications

The most serious early postoperative complications of colorectal surgery are infection and fecal incontinence. In a review of intestinal surgery in dogs and cats, patients with peritonitis had a morality rate of 31% (40). Infection after colorectal surgery can result from preoperative trauma, interoperative contamination of the abdomen, and intestinal dehiscence. Although rare, pelvic fractures resulting in rectal perforation can be successfully treated if diagnosed before significant contamination of surrounding tissue occurs. In one small study of patients with rectal perforations caused by pelvic fractures, definitive treatment within 24 hours of occurrence resulted in no mortality (5). Patients with delayed diagnosis or treatment had universally fatal outcomes. Postoperative intestinal dehiscence is one of the most common causes of infection. In one study, dehiscence resulted in a mortality rate of 80% (40). This same study found no significant difference between small and large intestinal dehiscence rates, with an average of 7%. Many factors can result in colorectal dehiscence, including poor surgical technique, traumatic tissue handling, disrupted blood supply, poor suture placement, tension on the anastomosis, improper use of drains, delayed healing, and inappropriate postoperative care.

The clinical signs of peritonitis are described previously. Diagnostic procedures for postoperative peritonitis and dehiscence may include abdominocentesis or peritoneal lavage, gentle rectal palpation, complete blood count, plain abdominal and pelvic radiographs, and abdominal ultrasonography. Contrast radiographs or proctoscopic examinations are contraindicated and may result in further abdominal contamination.

If signs of peritonitis or intestinal dehiscence are present, the animal should be supported with appropriate intravenous fluids and started on an appropriate therapeutic regimen of antibiotics based on culture and sensitivity testing. The surgeon should not hesitate to perform a "second-look" operation if indicated. These patients generally do not stabilize without adequate abdominal drainage and, if necessary, repair of leaking intestine. Open abdominal drainage is one successful method of surgical drainage that also allows serial evaluation of the affected colorectal segment. For recurrent dehiscence, or for areas of questionable vascularity, the use of omental flaps, jejunal patch grafts, and peritoneal muscle flaps has been commonly reported in the veterinary literature. The use of diversional colostomies has been reported in the human and equine literature. This technique has been reported in a dog, and it may become a viable treatment option in selected small animal cases (41).

Fecal incontinence, although not in itself fatal, often results in euthanasia of house pets. Fecal incontinence can be divided into reservoir and sphincter incontinence (42). Patients with reservoir incontinence generally have a conscious, but frequent, need to defecate. This condition is in contrast to unconscious anal dribbling found in patients with sphincter incontinence. Reservoir incontinence can be caused by colorectal irritability, decreased rectal capacity or compliance, increased propulsive motility, and increased fecal volume. One author suggests that fecal continence is retained if less than 4 cm of rectum is resected or if more than 1.5 cm of distal rectum is retained in the dog (43). Treatment for surgically induced reservoir incontinence includes anti-inflammatory drugs, drugs that slow intestinal transit time, dietary manipulation to decrease fecal volume, and surgical techniques that increase rectal capacity. Some animals, over time, may develop ileoanal continence. This is where the ileum distends, taking over the reservoir function of the colon and rectum. The causes of sphincter incontinence are not fully understood, but they include neurologic and muscular trauma or disease. Along with the external anal sphincter, studies have demonstrated that the muscles of the pelvic girdle, especially the levator ani, play an important role in fecal continence. Treatment for surgically induced sphincter incontinence may include the same medical treatments used for reservoir incontinence. Surgical treatments for sphincter incontinence include reconstruction of the pelvic girdle and external anal sphincter, sphincteroplasty, replacing muscles of continence with muscle flaps or synthetic material, and ileal J-pouch anal anastomoses.

Late Complications

The most common late complication of colorectal surgery is luminal stricture. Most intestinal anastomoses result in some degree of luminal stricture. Single-layer and double-layer inverting suture patterns have been reported to result in 39 and 54% luminal stricture, respectively. These results were compared with 4% luminal stricture using an approximating Gambee pattern closure (44). In another study, colonic anastomoses created with a 25-mm circular stapler resulted in an average 32% decrease in luminal diameter at the anastomosis (45). Too much tissue inversion, suture patterns that restrict the luminal diameter, tension at the anastomosis, and extraluminal adhesions can result in excessive luminal stricture. Diagnosis of colorectal stricture include clinical signs, rectal or abdominal palpation, contrast radiographs, and proctoscopy. Most commonly, colorectal strictures can be treated medically with diet change and stool softeners. Treatment of severe colorectal strictures may require resection and anastomosis of the strictured segment, or, less commonly, mechanical dilation may be attempted. Mechanical dilation can be achieved digitally, by bougienage, or with balloon catheters. Care should be taken not to perforate the intestinal lumen using dilation techniques.

References

1. Taylor WT, Weber RJ. Functional mammalian anatomy (with special reference to the cat). Toronto: D. Van Nostrand, 1951.
2. Evans HE, Christensen GC. Miller's anatomy of the dog. 2nd ed. Philadelphia: WB Saunders, 1979.
3. Schaller O, Constantinescu GM. Illustrated veterinary anatomical nomenclature. 1992.
4. Goldsmid SE, Bellenger CR, Hopwood PR, et al. Colorectal blood supply in dogs. Am J Vet Res 1993;54:1948–1953.
5. Lewis DD, Beale BS, Pechman RD, et al. Rectal perforations associated with pelvic fractures and sacroiliac fracture-separations in four dogs. J Am Anim Hosp Assoc 1992;28:175–181.
6. Greene CE. Infectious diseases of the dog and cat. Philadelphia: WB Saunders, 1990.
7. Boothe DM. Anaerobic infections in small animals. Probl Vet Med 1990;2:330–347.
8. Dow SW. Management of anaerobic infections. Vet Clin North Am Small Anim Pract 1988;18:1167–1182.
9. Burrows CF. Evaluation of a colonic lavage solution to prepare the colon of the dog for colonoscopy. J Am Vet Med Assoc 1989;195:1719–1721.
10. Richter KP, Cleveland MvB. Comparison of an orally administered gastrointestinal lavage solution with traditional enema administration as preparation for colonoscopy in dogs. J Am Vet Med Assoc 1989;195:1727–1731.
11. Peck JJ, Fuchs PC, Gustafson ME. Antimicrobial prophylaxis in elective colon surgery: experience of 1,035 operations in a community hospital. Am J Surg 1984;147:633–637.
12. Miles AA, Miles EM, Burke J. The value and duration of defence reactions of the skin to the primary lodgement of bacteria. Br J Exp Pathol 1957;38:79–96.
13. Penwick RC. Perioperative antimicrobial chemoprophylaxis in gastrointestinal surgery. J Am Anim Hosp Assoc 1988;24:133–145.
14. Burnakis TG. Surgical antimicrobial prophylaxis: principles and guidelines. Pharmacotherapy 1984;4:248–271.
15. Condon RE, Bartlett JG, Greenlee H, et al. Efficacy of oral and systemic antibiotic prophylaxis in colorectal operations. Arch Surg 1983;118:496–502.
16. Washington JA II, Dearing WH, Judd ES, et al. Effect of preoperative antibiotic regimen on development of infection after intes-

tinal surgery: prospective, randomized, double-blind study. Ann Surg 1974;180:567–572.

17. Baum ML, Anish DS, Chalmers TC, et al. A survey of clinical trials of antibiotic prophylaxis in colon surgery: evidence against further use of no-treatment controls. N Eng J Med 1981; 305:795–799.

18. Onderdonk AB, Bartlett JG, Louie T, et al. Microbial synergy in experimental intraabdominal abscess. Infect Immun 1976; 13:22–26.

19. De La Hunt MN, Karran SJ, Chir M. Sulbactam/ampicillin compared with cefoxitin for chemoprophylaxis in elective colorectal surgery. Dis Colon Rectum 1986;29:157–159.

20. Bright RM. Treatment of feline colonic obstruction (megacolon). In: Bojrab MJ, ed. Current techniques in small animal surgery. 3rd ed. Philadelphia: Lea & Febiger, 1990:263–265.

21. Rosin E, Dow S, Daly WR, et al. Surgical wound infection and use of antibiotics. In: Slatter DH, ed. Textbook of small animal surgery. 2nd ed. Philadelphia: WB Saunders, 1993:84–95.

22. Huss BT, Payne JT, Wagner-Mann CC, et al. Pharmacokinetic disposition of cefoxitin in serum and tissue during colorectal surgery in cats (unpublished data).

23. Plumb DC. Veterinary drug handbook. 3rd ed. White Bear Lake, MN: PharmaVet, 1995:117–118.

24. Petersen SW, Rosin E. In vitro antibacterial activity of cefoxitin and cefotetan and pharmacokinetics in dogs. Am J Vet Res 1993;54:1496–1499.

25. Ravo B. Colorectal anastomotic healing and intracolonic bypass procedure. Surg Clin North Am Small Anim Pract 1988; 68:1267–1294.

26. Ellison GW. Wound healing in the gastrointestinal tract. Semin Vet Med Surg (Small Anim) 1989;4:287–293.

27. Ballantyne GH. Intestinal suturing: review of the experimental foundations for traditional doctrines. Dis Colon Rectum 1983;26:836–843.

28. Cronin K, Jackson DS, Dunphy JE. Changing bursting strength and collagen content of the healing colon. Surg Gynecol Obstet 1968;126:747–753.

29. Irvin TT, Hunt TK. Reappraisal of the healing process of anastomosis of the colon. Surg Gynecol Obstet 1974;138:741–746.

30. Everett WG. A comparison of one layer and two layer techniques for colorectal anastomosis. Br J Surg 1975;62:135–140.

31. Ballantyne GH. The experimental basis of intestinal suturing: effect of surgical technique, inflammation, and infection on enteric wound healing. Dis Colon Rectum 1984;27:61–71.

32. Ellison GW. End-to-end anastomosis in the dog: a comparison of techniques. Compend Contin Educ Pract Vet 1981;3: 486–494.

33. Poth EJ, Gold D. Intestinal anastomosis: a unique technic. Am J Surg 1968;116:643–647.

34. DeHoff WD, Nelson,W, Lumb WV. Simple interrupted approximating technique for intestinal anastomosis. J Am Anim Hosp Assoc 1973;9:483–489.

35. Lord MG, Broughton AC, Williams HTG. A morphologic study on the effect of suturing the submucosa of the large intestine. Surg Gynecol Obstet 1978;146:211–216.

36. Stoloff D, Snider TG III, Crawford MP, et al. End-to-end colonic anastomosis: a comparison of techniques in normal dogs. Vet Surg 1984;13:76–82.

37. Huss BT, Payne JT, Johnson GC, et al. Comparison of a biofragmentable intestinal anastomosis ring with appositional suturing for subtotal colectomy in normal cats. Vet Surg 1994;23: 466–474.

38. Walshaw R. Removal of rectoanal neoplasms. In: Bojrab MJ, ed. Current techniques in small animal surgery. 3rd ed. Philadelphia, Lea & Febiger, 1990:274–290.

39. Allen SW, Crowell WA. Ventral approach to the pelvic canal in the female dog. Vet Surg 1991;20:118–121.

40. Wylie KB, Hosgood G. Mortality and morbidity of small and large intestinal surgery in dogs and cats: 74 cases (1980–1992). J Am Anim Hosp Assoc 1994;30:469–474.

41. Swalec-Tobias KM. Rectal perforation, rectocutaneous fistula formation, and enterocutaneous fistula formation after pelvic trauma in a dog. J Am Vet Med Assoc 1994;205:1292–1296.

42. Guilford WG. Fecal incontinence in dogs and cats. Compend Contin Educ Pract Vet 1990;12:313–326.

43. Holt D, Johnston DE, Orsher R, et al. Clinical use of a dorsal surgical approach to the rectum. Compend Contin Educ Pract Vet 1991;13:1519–1528.

44. Hamilton JE. Reappraisal of open intestinal anastomoses, Ann Surg 1967;165:917.

45. Yamane T, Takahashi T, Okuzumi J, et al. Anastomotic stricture with the EEA stapler after colorectal operation in the dog. Surg Gynecol Obstet 1992;174:41–45.

Subtotal Colectomy in the Cat

Ronald M. Bright

Constipation is not a disease; rather, it is a sign of many diseases. It is defined as infrequent and difficult passage of feces with the retention of hard feces in the colon and rectum. Prolonged retention of feces in the colon leads to increased absorption of water. Two distinct groups of feline patients have been recognized: those with colonic inertia (idiopathic megacolon) and those with outlet obstruction. *Obstipation* is an intractable form of constipation, in which fecal impaction is severe and defecation is impossible. *Megacolon* is defined as distension of the large intestine. In the cat, this condition is primarily an acquired disorder affecting adults. Mechanical obstruction from foreign bodies, intramural or extramural tumor masses, pelvic fracture malunion, or neurologic deficits can result in secondary megacolon.

Normally, cats can retain feces in the colon for several days without harm. Mechanical obstruction to the passage of feces can lead to prolonged retention of feces and possible formation of concretions. These hard and impacted feces are difficult to pass and, if not removed, may cause the colon to become distended. If the distension is chronic, irreversible colonic hypomotility can result. The duration and degree of colonic distension needed to produce this change are unknown. Results of one limited study suggest that sufficient motility may return if mechanical obstruction caused by a pelvic malunion is corrected within 6 months (1). Beyond 6 months, intramural myoneural changes secondary to chronic distension prevent return to normal function even after the obstruction is relieved (2–4).

Lumbosacral spinal cord disease can result in a chronically constipated cat by causing disruption of the innervation of the colon. The hypomotility that results can lead to retention of feces with severe impaction and megacolon. Manx cats with partial or complete absence of the sacral and caudal spinal cord may have megacolon with concurrent urinary or fecal incontinence (3).

Another neurologic condition associated with constipation in cats is dysautonomia (Key–Gaskell syndrome). This progressive polyneuropathy of the autonomic nervous system is seen in older cats (5).

Megacolon resulting from unknown causes (idiopathic megacolon) is probably the most common form of acquired megacolon in cats that leads to intractable constipation. The likely cause may be an abnormality in either the intrinsic or extrinsic nerve supply to colonic smooth muscle or a functional abnormality of the anorectal area that results in a partial obstruction and retention of feces. This may be similar to Hirschsprung's disease in humans, a congenital form of megacolon caused by aganglionosis of a segment of colon that leads to a functional obstruction.

History and Clinical Signs

Cats with a history of trauma may have a constipation disorder related to either a pelvic fracture or lumbosacral disease. Cats without any known form of trauma probably suffer from the idiopathic form of megacolon. These cats have recurring signs of constipation, which progresses to obstipation over time.

Idiopathic megacolon occurs mostly in mature cats. Many of these cats have had nonspecific and subtle signs related to fecal impaction. They may go several days without defecating, but they do not have constipation severe enough to warrant treatment.

Systemic signs may be present, depending on the duration of the constipation. Physical examination findings in a cat with simple constipation of short duration may be unrewarding. In cases of long-standing constipation or obstipation, the cat may be anorectic, depressed, emaciated, dehydrated, and anemic. Some cats appear to be unthrifty and have perineal soiling. Abdominal palpation sometimes elicits discomfort and reveals a distended colon filled with hard fecal material. Rectal palpation should be done to evaluate for a narrowed pelvic canal resulting from previous trauma or a stricture of the rectum or anus. A rectal examination also helps in defining the presence of a perineal hernia, which in some cats may be the sole cause of the constipation (6).

Diagnosis

The diagnosis of megacolon is based on the history of tenesmus and of unproductive attempts at passing stool, physical examination findings of a large, feces-filled colon, and abdominal and pelvic radiographs that confirm megacolon and possibly uncover any predisposing causes such as pelvic canal stenosis, soft tissue masses, or foreign material in the colon or lumbosacral spinal lesions.

Barium enema radiography can be done after digital removal of the impaction and multiple enemas. This test may help to define any strictures or neoplasia. Endoscopy of the emptied colon may reveal inflammatory or neoplastic disease while allowing biopsy of grossly abnormal tissue.

Conservative Treatment

Cats with chronic constipation should be treated conservatively to relieve signs. Those with severe constipation that do not show improvement with dietary and laxative treatment may be candidates for surgical treatment. When an underlying disorder can be identified (e.g., pelvic fracture malunion), correction of the primary problem may alleviate the problem (1).

Cisapride (Propulsid, Janssen-Pharmaceutica, Inc., Titusville, NJ) has been used to stimulate colonic motility, and in some instances it has delayed or obviated the need for surgery. The dose is 0.25 mg/kg or 2.5 mg every 8 to 12 hours for smaller cats and 5 to 10 mg every 8 to 12 hours for larger cats or for those that do not respond to lower doses (7). Ideally, this agent should be given concurrently with lactolose. The therapeutic index of safety is high with cisapride, so increasing the dose is usually not associated with any adverse effects.

Surgical Palliation

If fecal impaction is associated with a perineal hernia and an associated megacolon has not been a long-standing problem, then correction of the hernia generally alleviates the constipation (6).

When surgical intervention is necessary, a subtotal colectomy is recommended. Removal of most (95%) of the colon is done with or without preservation of the ileocolic valve (8–11).

Subtotal colectomies have been performed successfully in cats over the past decade. Before a cat is subjected to this procedure, however, it should be systematically evaluated for concurrent problems. Performing a subtotal colectomy in cats with loss of anal sphincter tone may not give satisfactory results. Owners of a cat with decreased anal tone should be thoroughly cautioned about the likelihood of incontinence, which is a more serious problem in the cat after subtotal colectomy.

Similarly, cats may have a rectal emptying problem that can result from decreased rectal sensitivity and increased rectal tolerance. Cats so affected generally have a megarectum, and a large, flaccid rectum is felt on rectal palpation. Defecography may show that the cat is unable to empty the rectum of contrast material. Owners should be advised about the poor prognosis in these cases if a subtotal colectomy is done.

The antibiotic I prefer for perioperative antibiotherapy is a second-generation cephalosporin that targets gram-negative enteric microbes and anaerobes. I prefer to give the antibiotic cefoxitin (Mefoxin, Merck & Co., West Point, PA), 20 to 30 minutes before surgery begins. It is given at a dose of 30 mg/kg and is given intravenously and intramuscularly concomitantly for a total of 60 mg/kg. A dose of 30 mg/kg intravenously is repeated 1.5 to 2 hours later.

Surgery for megacolon is approached through a ventral midline caudal abdominal incision. The colon is exteriorized, and the appropriate colic and caudal mesenteric vessels are ligated (Fig. 16.28).

Surgeons disagree about whether the ileocolic valve should be preserved. At present, the surgeon's discretion determines the fate of this valve. However, some evidence now suggests that preserving it is preferable (11).

I prefer to leave the ileocolic valve intact and restore bowel continuity with a colocolostomy (Fig. 16.29). A 1- or 2-cm segment of the ascending colon just distal to the valve is retained and is anastomosed to a 1- to 2-cm segment of the descending colon or proximal rectum just cranial to the pubis. Luminal disparity can be corrected by enlarging the lumen of the smaller segment of bowel, by transecting it at an angle, or by oversewing the larger segment to coincide with the smaller diameter of the bowel (Fig. 16.30).

Restoration of bowel continuity with an end-to-end

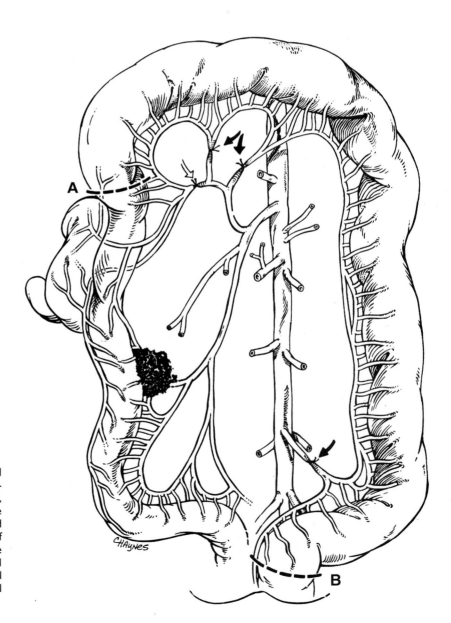

Fig. 16.28. The appropriate colic and caudal mesenteric vessels (*arrows*) are ligated before division of the colon. If the ileocolic valve is removed, the ileocecocolic vessels (*open arrow*) need to be ligated as well. With the ileocolic valve preserved (my preference), a small length (1 to 2 cm) of ascending colon remains after transecting the bowel (A). Likewise, when transecting the distal colon (B), a small remnant of colon or cranial rectum is left to anastomose to the proximal segment.

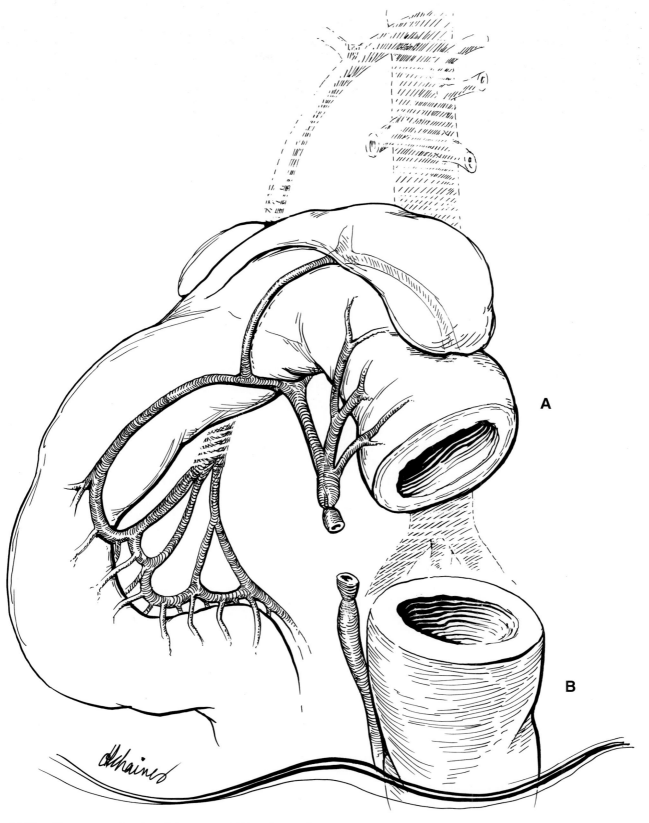

Fig. 16.29. The mesenteric sides of the proximal (A) and distal (B) bowel segments are aligned before proceeding with the anastomosis.

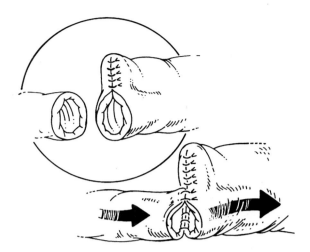

Fig. 16.30. When lumen disparity exists between the two segments to be anastomosed, the larger lumen is sutured closed until the remaining lumen approximates the size of the opposite segment.

anastomosis and an intact ileocolic valve is enhanced by adhering to the following guidelines:

1. Gently place most of the small bowel outside of the abdominal cavity and to the right of the midline incision and cover it with lap sponges moistened with warm saline.

2. Use straight intestinal clamps (Doyen) to hold the segments of bowel while performing the anastomosis.

3. Keep the urinary bladder evacuated of urine so it will not interfere with the operation.

4. Use a simple interrupted or continuous appositional suture pattern, being careful to incorporate the serosal layer, which tends to slip under the intestinal clamps. I prefer to use 3–0 or 4–0 polypropylene suture or 4–0 polydiaxonone (Prolene and PDS, Ethicon, Inc., Somerville, NJ).

Applying these principles allows the surgery to progress with relative ease while allowing the reestablishment of a tension-free anastomosis. At no time should the surgeon be tempted to resect only that portion of the colon that grossly appears abnormal. Partial or segmental colectomies have resulted in recurrence of constipation.

For 5 to 7 days postoperatively, tenesmus may be observed. Occasionally, hematochezia may be seen, but this generally resolves within 2 weeks. A liquid or semisolid stool eventually forms over 7 to 14 days. Usually, cats increase their frequency of defecation, and anal sphincter tone remains normal.

Some cats may develop signs of constipation after a subtotal colectomy. This may be a single event relieved with enemas and digital removal of the feces, followed by the use of short-term stool softeners. Occasionally, these patients need to be given a stool softener or a laxative indefinitely.

When medical management cannot alleviate the recurrence of constipation, the length of colon removed may have been insufficient. A second surgical procedure for removal of the remaining colonic segment may be necessary for palliation.

Recurrence of tenesmus can be related to a stricture at the site of anastomosis. Balloon dilation and the use of laxatives have been successful in relieving this problem in some cases (10).

References

1. Schrader SC. Pelvic osteotomy as a treatment for obstipation in cats with acquired stenosis of the pelvic canal: six cases (1978–1989). J Am Anim Hosp Assoc 1992;28:208–213.
2. Bright RM. Treatment of feline colonic obstruction (megacolon). In: Bojrab MJ, ed. Current techniques in small animal surgery. 3rd ed. Philadelphia: Lea & Febiger, 1990:263–265.
3. Bertoy RW. Megacolon. In: Bojrab MJ, ed. Disease mechanisms in small animal surgery. 2nd ed. Philadelphia: Lea & Febiger, 1993:262–265.
4. DeNovo RC, Bright RM. Chronic feline constipation/obstipation. In: Kirk RW, Bonagura JD, eds. Current veterinary therapy XI. Philadelphia: WB Saunders, 1992:619–626.
5. Hoskins JD. Management of fecal impaction. Compend Contin Educ Pract Vet 1990;12:1579–1584.
6. Welches CD, Scavelli TD, Aronsohn MG, et al. Perineal hernia in the cat: a retrospective study of 40 cases. J Am Anim Hosp Assoc 1992;28:431–438.
7. Tams TR. Cisapride: clinical experience with the newest GI prokinetic drug. In: Proceedings of the 12th annual veterinary medical forum. San Diego, CA. 1994:100–101.
8. Matthiesen DT, Scavelli TD, Whitney WO. Subtotal colectomy for the treatment of obstipation secondary to pelvic fracture malunion in cats. Vet Surg 1991;20:113–117.
9. Bright RM, Burrows CF, Goring R, et al. Subtotal colectomy for treatment of acquired megacolon in the dog and cat. J Am Vet Med Assoc 1986;12:1412–1416.
10. Rosin E, Walshaw R, Mehlhaff C, et al. Subtotal colectomy for treatment of chronic constipation associated with idiopathic megacolon in cats: 38 cases (1979–1985). J Am Vet Med Assoc 1988;193:850–853.
11. Sweet DC, Hardie EM, Stone EA. Preservation versus excision of the ileocolic junction during colectomy for megacolon: a study of 22 cats. Vet Surg. In press.

Deroofing, Fulguration, and Excision of Perianal Fistulas in the Dog

Clare R. Gregory

Perianal fistula disease is a chronic suppurative condition involving the perianal and perirectal tissue of dogs (1). Lesions can be focal, multifocal, or diffuse (Fig. 16.31). Secondary involvement of the anal sacs is common. Clinical signs include tenesmus, constipation, rectal bleeding, mucopurulent discharge, and licking at the perianal area. German shepherd dogs are af-

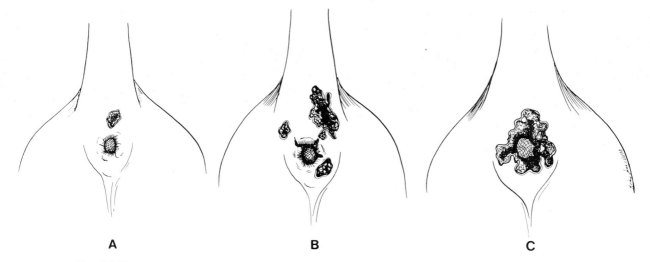

Fig. 16.31. Perianal fistula disease can present with focal (**A**), multifocal (**B**), and diffuse (**C**) lesions.

fected most commonly, although the disease is found in numerous other breeds.

The cause of perianal fistula disease remains obscure, and current treatment is directed at the lesion and not the underlying cause. Tail amputation to reduce fecal contamination and to promote a clean perianal environment is being studied as a means of prophylaxis in conjunction with surgical excision of existing lesions (2). Several studies have described various techniques for surgical excision of perianal fistulas (3–7). Despite differences among these techniques, the underlying goal of surgical treatment is the complete removal or destruction of all affected tissues. Presurgical rectal examination performed with the patient under general anesthesia is essential to assess the depth and extent of the lesions, including the possible presence of anal or rectal strictures. Owners must be made aware of the frequent occurrence of postoperative complications, which include recurrence of the fistulas, fecal incontinence, flatulence, and anal stricture formation.

Preoperative Preparation

Physical examination and appropriate laboratory assays are performed. Enemas are avoided because the resulting loose fecal material contributes to excessive contamination at the time of surgery. Antibiotics (ampicillin, 25 mg/kg intravenously) are administered only during the immediate perioperative period.

A wide region surrounding the perianal region and tail is aseptically prepared for surgery. Gauze sponges are inserted into the rectum to reduce fecal contamination. The dog is positioned in ventral recumbency on a padded perineal stand or on a padded table with the hind legs hung over the edge.

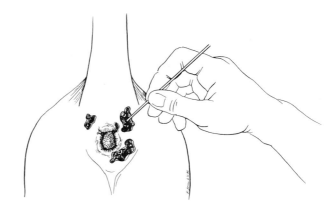

Fig. 16.32. Each tract is probed to determine the direction and extent of the lesions and any communications with the rectum and anus.

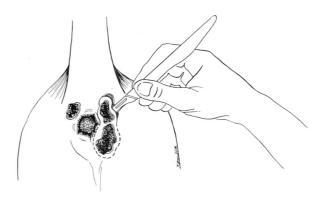

Fig. 16.33. The skin over the affected area is incised.

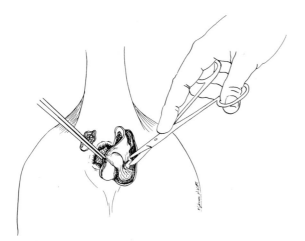

Fig. 16.34. Sharp dissection is used to remove all granulation and scar tissue.

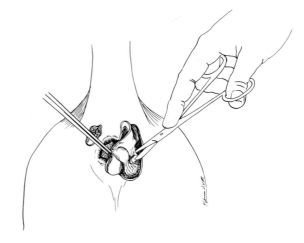

Fig. 16.35. The remaining thin lining of superficial lesions is destroyed by electrofulguration.

Surgical Technique

The technique described here to ablate the affected tissues combines deroofing and fulguration of more superficial lesions with radical excision of deeper fistulas that enter the rectum (8). Concern for the continuity of the external anal sphincter is justified, but it should not limit removal of all diseased tissue (1, 4).

Anal sacculectomy is performed in all cases by incising the lateral wall of each anal sac and dissecting the sac free from the underlying external anal sphincter.

All tracts are explored with a probe to determine the extent and direction of the lesions and communications with the anus and rectum (Fig. 16.32). The overlying skin is incised (Fig. 16.33), and sharp dissection is used to remove all granulation and scar tissue

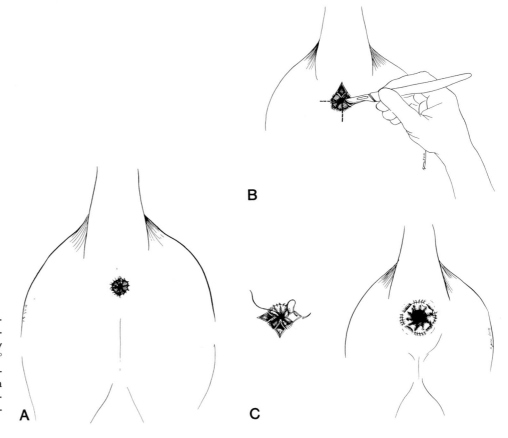

Fig. 16.36. Superficial anal strictures (**A**) sometimes occur after fistula surgery. They are relieved by making releasing incisions every 90° through the scar tissue at the mucocutaneous junction (**B**). The mucosa and skin are reapposed with absorbable suture material in a simple interrupted pattern (**C**).

(Fig. 16.34). Fistulas into the anus and rectum are excised with the wall of the anus or rectum that surrounds the opening. Hemorrhage is controlled by electrocauterization. The wound bed is then carefully probed and palpated for further lesions that may have been overlooked. The remaining thin lining of more superficial tracts is destroyed by electrofulguration (Fig. 16.35). The surgical wounds are left open to heal by second intention. At the end of the procedure, the gauze sponges are removed from the patient's rectum.

Postoperative Care and Complications

Elizabethan collars or side braces generally are not used after perianal fistula surgery. The perineum is cleansed daily, if necessary, with warm water and mild soap. Patients are discharged to clients 48 to 72 hours postoperatively with instructions to continue cleansing the perineal area as necessary. Special handling is needed for patients that have been rendered incontinent by the procedure. If appropriate, clients should be warned of the possibility of myiasis. The wounds generally heal in 3 to 6 weeks.

Of the previously mentioned postoperative complications, recurrence and anal stricture are managed surgically. Recurrence requires exploration and excision of the tracts, with or without fulguration. Superficial anal strictures can be relieved by multiple releasing incisions (Fig. 16.36). If stricture formation becomes extensive, it may be necessary to resect a portion of the rectal or anal canals using a rectal pull-through procedure.

Fecal incontinence is a potential complication when extensive, bilateral destruction of the external anal sphincter occurs. If the feces are firm, incontinence may present a problem only when the dog becomes stressed or excited (e.g., "doorbell" incontinence). Dogs unable to retain their feces for suitable periods of time and dogs with more liquid feces are not suitable house pets. These animals must be housed outdoors or in kennels.

References

1. Vasseur PB. Results of surgical excision of perianal fistulas in dogs. J Am Vet Med Assoc 1981;185:60.
2. van Ee RT, Palminteri A. Tail amputation for treatment of perianal fistulas in dogs. J Am Anim Hosp Assoc 1987;23:95.
3. Goring RL, Bright RM, Stoncil ML. Perianal fistulas in the dog; retrospective evaluation of surgical treatment by deroofing and fulguration. Vet Surg 1986;15:392.
4. Harvey CE. Perianal fistula in the dog. Vet Rec 1972;91:25.
5. Lane JG, Burch DG. The cryosurgical treatment of canine anal furunculosis. J Small Anim Pract 1975;16:387.
6. Budsberg SC, Robinelle JD, Farrell RK. Results of cryotherapy on perianal fistulas. Vet Med Small Anim Clin 1981;76:667.
7. Vasseur PB. Perianal fistulae in dogs: a retrospective analysis of surgical techniques. J Am Anim Hosp Assoc 1981;17:177.
8. Johnston DE. Rectum and anus; surgical diseases. In:Slatter DH, ed. Textbook of small animal surgery. Philadelphia: WB Saunders, 1985.

Excisional Techniques for Perianal Fistulas

Gary W. Ellison

Prescribing treatment for perianal fistulas is difficult because the exact etiology remains obscure. Low tail carriage peculiar to the German shepherd breed may allow moisture and bacteria from feces, rectal mucus, or anal sac secretion to accumulate in the perianal region, with resultant inflammation of the anal skin and adnexa. Other proposed causes of perianal fistulas include impaction and infection of the anal sinuses or anal crypts, inflammation and necrosis of the apocrine glands, infection of circumanal glands or hair follicles, and anal sac infection or abscessation. In a study of 106 dogs with perianal fistulas, 52 dogs had hidradenitis or folliculitis, 30 had fistulas of the anal sinuses, 66 had ruptured anal sacs, and 30 had submucosal fistulas in the rectum or various combinations of the foregoing (1, 2). The presence of concomitant inflammatory bowel disease and recent success of medical treatment using immunosuppressive drugs such as prednisolone (3) and cyclosporine (4) lend support to the hypothesis that perianal fistulas may be an immune-mediated condition. Nevertheless, most cases of perianal fistulas require some type of surgical therapy.

Indications

Surgical excision with anal sacculectomy is most often indicated for patients with moderate to severe cases of perianal fistula involving a large percentage of the anal circumference and causing tenesmus or dyschezia with obstipation caused by anal stenosis. Potential limitations of excision include the inability to excise all the tracts if they extend too far peripherally and the danger of creating incontinence if the tracts deeply invade the external anal sphincter (5). However, if an anal stricture is present because of deep-seated invasion of the external anal sphincter by the fistulas, then excision of the areas of fibrosis is usually necessary for release of the constriction and for relief of painful defecation.

Preoperative Medical Treatment

Removal of all perianal hair and twice-daily cleansing of the perianal region with local antiseptics such as

0.5% chlorhexidine gluconate may be useful in reducing suppurative inflammation. Elevation of the tail with an aluminum brace may allow for better aeration of the perianal region and may result in healing of superficial ulcerations. Short-term topical or systemic antibiotic therapy may help to reduce the effects of secondary bacterial infection by diminishing the local inflammatory pyogranulomatous reaction. However, long-term administration of antibiotics is of questionable value. The use of high doses of prednisolone at 2 mg/kg of body weight, once daily for 2 weeks, and 1.0 mg/kg, once daily for an additional 4 weeks, may be an effective treatment for perianal fistulas in dogs concomitantly affected with infiltrative bowel disease. Nine of 30 German shepherd dogs with inflammatory bowel disease had coexisting perianal fistulas completely resolve after this treatment. Eleven dogs had improvement in the severity of their fistulas; the remaining 10 dogs did not improve during administration of prednisolone (3). More recently, 20 dogs were treated with cyclosporine over 4 weeks, with a 75% reduction in mean surface area and a 60% reduction in depth of fistulas when compared with placebo-treated dogs (4). This latter therapy shows promise, but the cost of the medication and the need to perform serum cyclosporine trough levels make this treatment more expensive than most forms of surgical therapy.

Surgical Technique

A thorough rectal examination should be performed while the patient is under general anesthesia to determine how much of the circumference is involved, whether anal sphincter involvement or stricture formation is present, and how far the tracts extend peripherally. The fecal contents are evacuated digitally. Enemas are usually not administered preoperatively unless significant fecal impaction is present. Culture of the fistulous tracts usually is not warranted because a mixed culture of gram-positive cocci and gram-negative coliform bacteria is usually isolated. The animal can be positioned in ventral or dorsal recumbency with the tail pulled over the back or below the operating table, respectively. The rectum is packed with

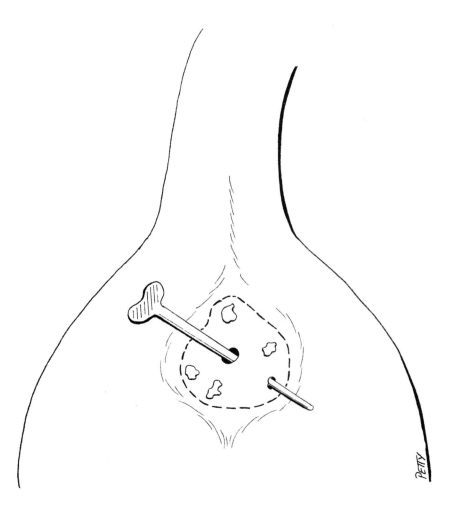

Fig. 16.37. A groove director is used to probe the fistulous tracts and also to check for patency of the anal sacs. An incision is made around the perimeter of the tracts with a No. 10 scalpel or with a needle-tipped electrosurgical unit.

chlorhexidine-soaked sponges, and routine surgical preparation of the perianal region is performed.

The fistulas and anal sacs are carefully probed with a groove director to determine their extent and depth. When the anal sacs are not diseased, they are removed before fistulectomy (see the next section of this chapter). More commonly, the anal sacs are ruptured or abscessed, and they are best excised concurrently with the fistulous tracts. A circular incision is made around the periphery of the fistulas using a No. 10 blade or a needle-tipped electrosurgical unit (Fig. 16.37). A plane is established deep to the fistulas, and dissection is carried medially toward the anal canal. Care must be taken to stay as close to the fistulas as possible to preserve the external anal sphincter, but the surgeon must dissect deep to the fibrous tracts (Fig. 16.38). Hemorrhage is moderate and is controlled with electrocoagulation. The wall of any remaining anal sac is carefully dissected from the surrounding fibers of the external anal sphincter with mosquito hemostats

or fine dissection scissors (see Fig. 16.38, *inset*). The entire secretory lining of the anal sac must be removed, or sinus tracts may develop postoperatively. The dissection is carried medially to the anal canal, and a circular incision is made in healthy rectal mucosa cranial to any rectal or anal sinuses (Fig. 16.39). The excised fistulous tracts and a portion of rectal mucosa should be submitted for histopathologic examination to rule out neoplasia or to check for evidence of inflammatory bowel disease. Eight to ten simple interrupted sutures of 3–0 synthetic monofilament absorbable suture material are used to appose the rectal submucosa to the subcutis. The rectal mucosa is then sutured to the skin with simple interrupted 3–0 monofilament nylon or polypropylene sutures (Fig. 16.40). Often, the fistulas in some areas extend so far peripherally that direct skin to mucosal apposition is not possible. In these cases, the adjacent areas of skin can be apposed, or the area can be left open to heal by granulation.

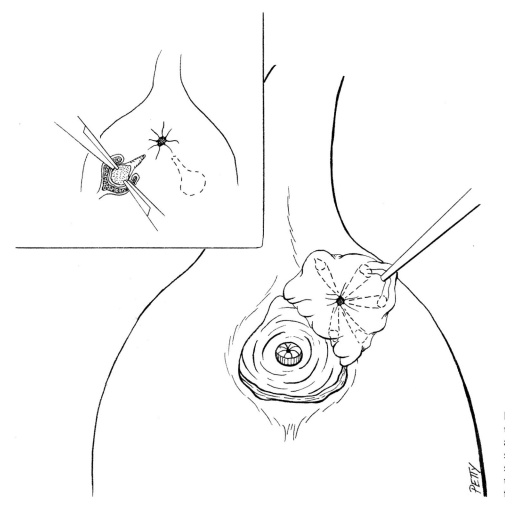

Fig. 16.38. The dissection is continued deep to the tracts, with efforts at preserving as much of the anal sphincter. Residual anal sac lining should be removed by blunt dissection using mosquito hemostats or fine-tipped scissors (*inset*).

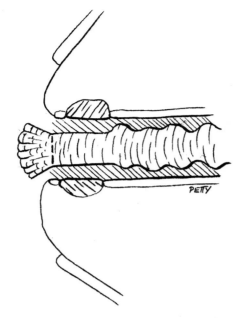

Fig. 16.39. Cross section of the anus and rectum showing dissection of the fistulas with preservation of the external anal sphincter. The fistulas are transected through the rectal mucosa cranial to the anocutaneous junction.

Laser Excision

A neodymium: yttrium–aluminum–garnet contact-tip laser has also been used successfully to treat perianal fistulas (6). A frosted, synthetic sapphire tip and a continuous impulse of 13 to 15 watts was used to excise the fistulas, and the wound was closed primarily. Anal tone was reduced and flatulence was increased in 60% of the dogs, and 20% of the dogs developed fecal incontinence. However, fecal incontinence, when present, was effectively managed by means of diet modification. The overall success rate for resolution of fistulas was 95% during a mean follow-up time of 22.9 months. The treatment was particularly effective in relieving pain in those dogs with preexisting anal stenosis (6).

Postoperative Care and Complications

Dogs may experience significant postoperative pain the evening of surgery, and parenteral morphine or

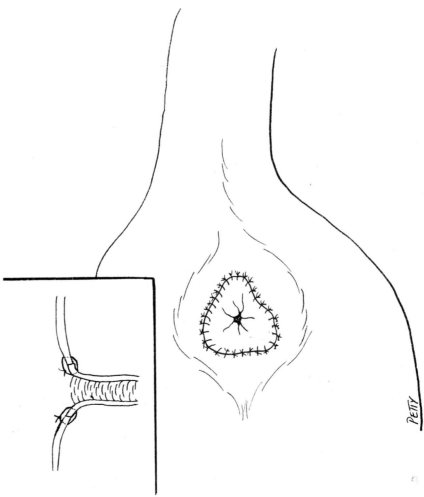

Fig. 16.40. After apposing the deep subcutaneous tissues with simple interrupted sutures, the rectal mucosa is apposed to the skin with simple interrupted sutures. The surgeon must approximate the rectal mucosa closely with the skin (*inset*).

oxymorphone or morphine epidural analgesia is often prescribed (see Chap. 1). Pain seems to resolve rapidly, and often within 48 hours animals are in less pain than they were preoperatively. Drainage of serosanguineous fluid from the wound edge is expected for 2 to 3 days. Perioperative antibiotics may be indicated because fecal contamination commonly occurs during surgery. Intravenous cephazolin (10 mg/kg intravenously three times daily) in combination with metronidazole (15 mg/kg intravenously three times daily) is initiated preoperatively and is continued for 24 hours. Oral cephalexin (10 mg/kg twice daily) and metronidazole (15 mg/kg twice daily) is then continued for 5 days postoperatively. The area is gently cleaned twice daily, and sutures are removed in 10 days. Mild wound dehiscence is not uncommon. When it occurs, it is managed by local wound flushes and parenteral antibiotics as needed. Most open areas heal by second intention in 2 to 3 weeks. Stool softeners are only used if preoperative constipation was present. Periodic clipping and daily cleaning of the perianal region should be performed by the owners during the remainder of the dog's life. All dogs should undergo reexaminations every 2 months to look for early signs of recurrence. Various degrees of fecal incontinence or flatulence may occur after the procedure. Fecal incontinence is usually less common with first-time procedures, but it has occurred more commonly when other procedures have been performed previously (6, 7). When present, fecal incontinence is often successfully managed by feeding the animal a diet with high digestibility. Postoperative anal strictures are rare with this technique. The reported long-term success rates of excision techniques vary from 46 to 95% (4, 7). However, many animals undergoing this procedure have had other procedures performed before the excision technique.

References

1. Johnston DE. Rectum and anus. In: Slatter DH, ed. Textbook of small animal surgery. Philadelphia: WB Saunders, 1985: 777–785.
2. Day MJ, Weaver BMQ. Pathology of surgically resected tissue from 305 cases of anal furunculosis in the dog. J Small Anim Pract 1992;33:583–589.
3. Harkin KR, Walshaw RW, Mullaney TP. Association of perianal fistula and colitis in the German shepherd dog: response to high dose prednisone and dietary therapy. J Am Anim Hosp Assoc 1996;35:515–520.
4. Mathews KA, Sukiana HR. Cyclosporine treatment of canine perianal fistulas: a prospective randomized double blind controlled study. Abstracts of the 31st Annual American College of Veterinary Surgeons Scientific Meeting, San Francisco, CA. 1996:15–16.
5. Vasseur PB. Results of surgical excision of perianal fistulas in dogs. J Am Vet Med Assoc 1984;185:60–62.
6. Ellison GW, Bellah JR, Stubbs WP. Treatment of perianal fistulas with ND/YAG laser: results of 20 cases. Vet Surg 1995;24: 140–147.
7. Ellison GW. Treatment of perianal fistulas in dogs. J Am Vet Med Assoc 1995;206:1680–1682.

Anal Sac Disease and Removal

Sandra Manfra Marretta

Anal sac disease occurs frequently in small breed dogs, less frequently in large breed dogs, and infrequently in cats. The most common indications for anal sacculectomy are chronic and recurrent episodes of anal sac impaction or infection and as an adjunctive surgical treatment of perianal fistulas. Anal sac adenocarcinomas are treated by anal sacculectomy.

Preoperative Care

Before anal sacculectomy, animals with anal sac impaction or infection should be treated medically. Failure to resolve any inflammatory reaction associated with anal sac disease before anal sacculectomy increases the potential for postoperative complications.

Medical management includes expression of anal sacs and instillation of an oil-based antibiotic and corticosteroid-containing ointment injected through the ducts into the sacs. Broad-spectrum antibiotics are recommended in patients with severe infection or abscess formation. Hot compresses applied to the perineal region help to keep the area clean and to promote drainage. Preoperatively, animals suspected of having anal sac adenocarcinoma must be evaluated for hypercalcemia and distant metastatic disease.

Surgical Technique

Several techniques have been used in the removal of anal sacs. The two basic techniques are the closed and open techniques. When using the closed technique, the surgeon may elect to fill the anal sacs with a self-hardening gel or resin that can be injected into the anal sac through the duct. The closed technique is used in animals suspected of having an anal sac adenocarcinoma.

The surgical procedure described here is the open technique, which is preferred by some surgeons because of the ease and speed with which it can be performed. An additional advantage of this technique is that the secretory lining of the anal sac is visualized, which helps to ensure complete removal of the anal sac. The open technique also permits removal of the anal sac duct and orifice.

After anesthetic induction, the anal sacs are emptied and flushed with a dilute antiseptic such as chlorhexidine or povidone–iodine solution. The animal is positioned in a perineal stand (Fig. 16.41). Several gauze

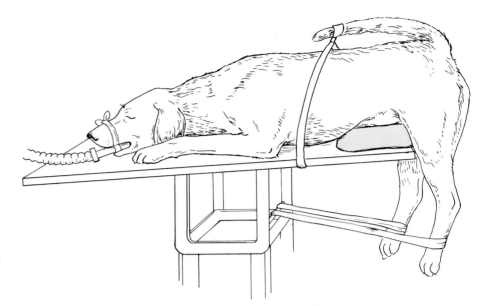

Fig. 16.41. A routine perineal stand involves placing the animal in ventral recumbency with the table slightly tilted forward. Adequate padding should be placed beneath the abdomen and at the caudal edge of the surgery table. The animal's legs and tail are loosely tied to the surgery table.

sponges are placed in the animal's rectum, and the perineal region is clipped and surgically scrubbed in a routine manner. The perineal region is surgically draped to expose the surgical site.

The anal sacs are located between the fibers of the internal and external anal sphincter at approximately the 4 o'clock and 8 o'clock positions. The orifice of the anal sac duct in dogs opens into the lateral margins of the anus at the anocutaneous junction, whereas the orifice of the anal sac duct in cats opens on a pyramidal prominence 0.25 cm lateral to the anus and not at the mucocutaneous junction. After localization of the anal sac orifice, a grooved director is placed through the orifice into the sac. The tip of the grooved director is then placed at the ventralmost aspect of the anal sac (Fig. 16.42). The tip of the grooved director is then pointed toward the surface of the skin while still at the most ventral aspect of the anal sac. An incision is made over the grooved director with a No. 10 Bard–Parker scalpel blade starting at the anal sac orifice and extending down the full length of the gland while maintaining the tip of the grooved director in a caudal direction so the grooved director can be palpated beneath the skin (Fig. 16.43). The depth of the incision is slowly increased from the orifice of the anal sac duct toward the ventral aspect of the gland, to expose the gray mucosal lining of the anal sac while directing the tip of the grooved director in a caudal direction.

In small dogs and cats, Allis tissue forceps are placed on the most ventral aspect of anal sac mucosa, and gentle traction is applied to the anal sac. Blunt dissection with small Metzenbaum scissors or with Stevens tenotomy scissors is used to free the anal sac gently from its attachments. This is accomplished by inserting the tips of the scissors in a closed position between

the external anal sphincter and the anal sac and then opening them with the tips of the scissors in position, thereby separating the sphincter from the sac. The scissors are repositioned between these structures in a closed position with the tips located a little deeper and then are opened again. This process is repeated, starting at the most ventral aspect of the anal sac and progressing toward the anal sac duct and orifice. Care should be taken during dissection to stay as close to the anal sac as possible, thereby minimizing trauma to the external anal sphincter. The caudal rectal nerve, artery, and vein lie at the cranial pole of the anal sac,

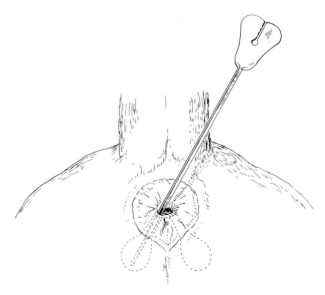

Fig. 16.42. A grooved director is placed through the anal sac duct to the ventralmost aspect of the anal sac.

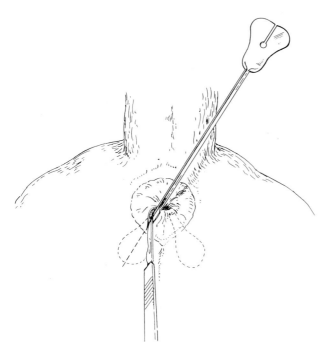

Fig. 16.43. The anal sac duct and anal sac are incised over the caudally directed grooved director tip.

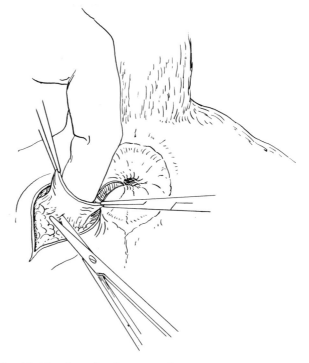

Fig. 16.44. An index finger may be placed in the opened anal sac in medium to large breed dogs to assist in blunt dissection of the anal sac from the external anal sphincter.

making careful blunt dissection in this area mandatory.

In medium and large breed dogs, the left index finger of a right-handed surgeon can be placed in the animal's anal sac after the exposure of the lining of the anal sac as previously described. Blunt dissection is the same as for small dogs, except dissection is easier because the anal sac is more clearly defined with the surgeon's finger inside the sac. Blunt dissection is continued around the animal's anal sac and the surgeon's index finger beginning at the most ventral aspect of the anal sac and progressing toward the anal sac duct and orifice (Fig. 16.44).

Once the entire anal sac is bluntly dissected from the surrounding tissues, the surgical procedure is continued in a similar manner for all animals. Blunt dissection is continued around the duct to the orifice (Fig. 16.45**A**). A circular incision is made around the previously incised anal sac orifice to permit the entire removal of the anal sac, duct, and orifice. The anal sac should be carefully inspected after removal to ensure complete excision of the entire sac. The surgical site is lavaged with warm sterile saline. The muscle fibers are apposed with a few simple interrupted sutures with 3–0 synthetic absorbable suture material (Fig. 16.45**B**). The subcutaneous tissue and subcuticular layers are closed in a similar manner. If skin sutures are used to close the incision, a soft suture material such as polyglactin 910 (Vicryl, Ethicon, Inc., Somer-

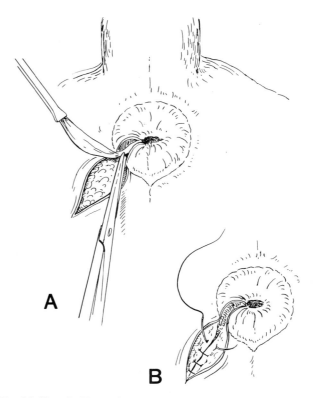

Fig. 16.45. **A.** The anal sac is retracted to allow blunt dissection of the anal sac duct from the underlying tissues. **B.** The external anal sphincter and subcutaneous tissues are apposed with simple interrupted absorbable sutures. A subcuticular suture pattern or skin sutures can be used to appose the skin edges.

ville, NJ) is recommended. If a stiff suture such as nylon is used in the skin, the ends of the sutures may cause unnecessary discomfort before suture removal.

Postoperative Care

The anal sacs should be submitted for histopathologic examination. An Elizabethan collar is placed on the animal. Broad-spectrum antibiotic therapy should be continued for 1 week postoperatively. Hot compresses should be applied to the perineal region twice daily. This procedure helps to keep the incision line clean and also forces the owner to observe the incision regularly so any postoperative complications can be reported early. The skin sutures are removed in 10 to 14 days.

Complications

Short-term postoperative complications of anal sacculectomy include hemorrhage, wound infection, and tenesmus or dyschezia. Postoperative hemorrhage can be minimized with meticulous intraoperative hemostasis. If postoperative hemorrhage occurs, it can usually be controlled with cold compresses and sedation with acepromazine. Tenesmus or dyschezia may be associated with local inflammation or infection. Wound infection usually becomes apparent 48 to 72 hours postsurgically. The ventralmost sutures are removed, and the surgical site is flushed with sterile saline or a dilute disinfectant such as povidone–iodine or chlorhexidine solution. Systemic broad-spectrum antibiotics are administered.

Long-term postoperative complications of anal sacculectomy include fecal incontinence, chronic fistula formation, and anal stricture. All these complications can be minimized with careful intraoperative surgical technique. Fecal incontinence associated with anal sacculectomies may result from excessive surgical trauma to the external anal sphincter or damage to the caudal rectal branch of the pudendal nerve. Unless the damage is severe and bilateral, the fecal incontinence usually can be controlled with dietary management. Chronic fistula formation usually appears several weeks after surgery and is caused by incomplete resection of the anal sacs. Surgical exploration and removal of residual anal sac tissue are curative. Anal stricture occurs infrequently after anal sacculectomy. Anal stricture may cause difficult defecation several weeks after surgery. Stool softeners and periodic bougienage may be curative. If stenosis is severe, surgical correction may be necessary.

Suggested Readings

Lipowitz A. Perineal surgery. In: Lipowitz AJ, Caywood DD, Newton CD, et al, eds. Complications in small animal surgery. Baltimore: Williams & Wilkins, 1996:527–540.

Manfra Marretta S, Matthiesen DT. Problems associated with the surgical treatment of diseases involving the perineal region. Probl Vet Med 1989;1:215–242.

Matthiesen DT, Manfra Marretta S. Diseases of the anus and rectum. In: Slatter DH, ed. Textbook of small animal surgery. 2nd ed. Philadelphia: WB Saunders, 1993:627–645.

Niebauer GW. Rectum, anus, and perianal and perineal regions. In: Harvey CE, Newton CD, Schwartz A, eds. Small animal surgery. Philadelphia: JB Lippincott, 1990:381–402.

van Sluijs FJ. Anal sacculectomy. In: van Sluijs FJ, ed. Atlas of small animal surgery. New York: Churchill Livingstone, 1992: 114–115.

17

LIVER AND BILIARY SYSTEM

Partial Hepatectomy and Hepatic Biopsy

Dale E. Bjorling

Surgical Anatomy

In dogs and cats, the liver is divided into six distinct lobes: left medial, left lateral, right medial, right lateral, quadrate, and caudate (Fig. 17.1). Although in the cat, the caudate lobe appears to be a projection or process of the right medial lobe, it is usually considered a separate lobe. The lobes are further subdivided into three divisions: left, central, and right. The left division (left medial and lateral lobes) constitutes about 40% of the total mass of the liver, and the other two divisions contribute approximately 30% each (1). The liver lobes are clearly separate near the periphery, but at the hilus, the hepatic parenchyma becomes confluent. The caudate and right lateral and medial lobes envelope the caudal vena cava as it passes the liver, and these lobes are joined to the remainder of the liver over a broad area.

The common hepatic artery arises from the celiac artery and separates into one to five (usually three) proper hepatic arteries before continuing as the gastroduodenal artery (Fig. 17.1**A**) (2). The distribution of the portal vein is much more predictable, consisting of a right branch that supplies the right division and a larger left branch that continues to the central and left divisions. The hepatic veins vary in number and location. They are a common source of hemorrhage after hepatic lobectomy, especially those veins draining the right division. The hepatic veins tend to be short and broad and often are not easily secured by an encircling ligature.

The gallbladder lies in a depression between the quadrate and right medial lobes. Usually, four major ducts drain bile from the liver: one from both the right and left divisions and two from the central division (Fig. 17.1**B**). The two ducts from the central division join the short cystic duct near the gallbladder to form the common bile duct, which passes to the duodenum within the hepatogastric ligament.

The hepatogastric and hepatoduodenal ligaments are components of the lesser omentum, within which lie the common bile duct, hepatic artery, and portal vein. The epiploic foramen is limited ventrally by the portal vein, and the common hepatic artery lies in a reflection of the hepatoduodenal ligament near the epiploic foramen. This arrangement allows the surgeon temporarily to obstruct the common bile duct, portal vein, and common hepatic artery by inserting an index finger, or one jaw of atraumatic forceps, into the epiploic foramen and applying pressure across these three structures (Pringle maneuver).

Preoperative Care

Liver disease can result in hypoproteinemia (primarily hypoalbuminemia), ascites, fasting hypoglycemia, abnormalities of clotting, or other nonspecific symptoms of gastrointestinal disease (vomiting, diarrhea). Increased concentrations of hepatic enzymes or bilirubin in the peripheral blood reflect obstruction of the biliary tract or leakage of intracellular enzymes, but they are not accurate indicators of hepatic function.

Functional hepatic mass is best estimated by the results of sulfobromophthalein (BSP) or indocyanine green clearance from peripheral blood after intravenous injection or by ammonia tolerance after oral administration of ammonium chloride. Because most tranquilizers and injectable anesthetic agents are metabolized by the liver, when liver function is decreased

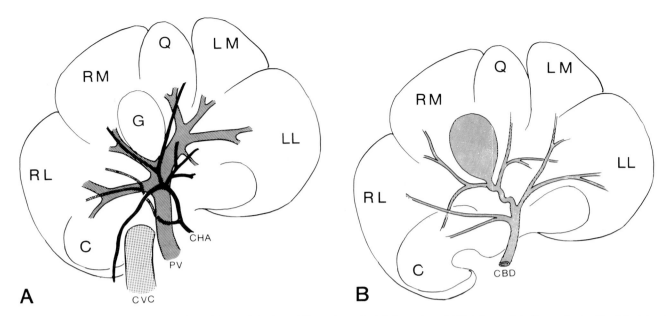

Fig. 17.1. Anatomic relationship of the lobes of the liver (*C*, caudate; *LL*, left lateral; and *LM*, left medial; *Q*, quadrate; *RL*, right lateral; *RM*, right medial) and gallbladder (*G*) as viewed from the caudoventral perspective. **A.** Afferent vascular supply of the liver (*CHA*, common hepatic artery; *CVC*, caudal vena cava; *PV*, portal vein). **B.** Biliary system (*CBD*, common bile duct).

the effects of these compounds can be prolonged. Hypotension during anesthesia results in decreased arterial perfusion of the liver. Hypoxemia of the liver in conjunction with the toxic effects of anesthetics or other drugs can contribute to the development of centrilobular necrosis. Anesthesia and perioperative fluid administration should be planned to minimize the occurrence and duration of hepatic ischemia. Although lactated Ringer's solution is usually a satisfactory choice for fluid therapy, infusion of 5% dextrose in water may be preferable in the presence of hypoglycemia.

Impaired protein synthesis by the liver can result in decreased peripheral concentrations of albumin and clotting factors. Because hypoproteinemia increases the unbound (and therefore active) fraction of circulating anesthetic, the dosage and rate of administration should be decreased accordingly. Plasma oncotic pressure is determined primarily by albumin concentration, and low albumin concentrations predispose the animal to edema (peripheral and pulmonary). Low plasma protein concentrations also can delay healing. Hepatic disease can cause abnormal results of coagulation tests (3), but hemorrhage associated with open hepatic biopsy or lobectomy is most often due to ligature failure.

Surgical Techniques

Biopsy of the liver is indicated to establish definitively the presence and cause of liver disease, to determine an appropriate course of therapy, and to enable the clinician to offer a prognosis. Biopsy of the liver performed during the course of celiotomy has several advantages over closed or percutaneous hepatic biopsy: the potential for injury to the biliary system is greatly reduced, a focal disease process is not missed, post-biopsy hemorrhage can be more easily controlled, and the liver and biliary system can be examined directly.

Hepatic abscessation or necrosis, neoplasia, cysts, ongoing hemorrhage, or intralobar arteriovenous fistulas may necessitate partial hepatectomy. Up to 80% of the liver can be removed, provided the hepatic remnant is functionally normal (1, 4). Liver mass is restored to normal in a matter of weeks by compensatory hypertrophy of the remaining tissue.

Hepatic Biopsy

Regardless of the technique used to perform biopsy of the liver, the sample should be handled gently to avoid causing artifactual changes. If biopsy samples are to be submitted for special stains or tests (such as copper content), the laboratory performing the analysis should be contacted before submission, to ensure that an adequate amount of tissue is obtained and that the biopsy is placed in the proper fixative or transport medium. Samples collected for microbial culturing should be obtained as soon after opening the abdomen as possible, especially if anaerobic culturing is to be performed.

Small samples of hepatic tissue can be obtained using a biopsy needle or cutaneous biopsy punch. Biopsy needles (Menghini or Tru-Cut [Baxter Laboratories, Morton Grove, IL]) allow the surgeon to perform biopsy on any area of the liver and to procure small amounts of tissue without creating a large defect. A cutaneous biopsy punch (Baker or Keyes) allows the surgeon to obtain a larger sample of any area of the liver. After the site for biopsy is determined, a biopsy punch of appropriate size is advanced to the desired depth by applying pressure while rotating the punch back and forth. The remaining attachment of the biopsy sample to the liver is severed by placing the biopsy punch at an oblique angle to the direction in which it was inserted and advancing it a short distance. With the punch held at this oblique angle, the punch and biopsy sample are withdrawn from the liver. Hemorrhage is controlled by placing one or two mattress sutures of absorbable suture material deeply through the tissues to draw the apposing sides of the defect together. Alternatively, hemorrhage can be controlled by inserting a piece of absorbable hemostatic sponge rolled to fit the diameter of the defect. Omentum can also be used to fill the defect. The omentum should be lightly tacked to the liver with absorbable suture material.

Biopsy samples are easily obtained from the tips of narrow lobes by placing a loop of absorbable suture material around the lobe proximal to the tissue to be sampled. The loop is then tightened and tied, strangulating the tissue and occluding the vasculature and bile canaliculi. The tissue should be sharply incised a sufficient distance distal from the ligature to prevent slippage of the ligature, but an excessive amount of devitalized tissue should not be left within the abdomen.

Larger biopsy samples or biopsies from rounded liver lobes can be taken by placing interlocking sutures or mattress sutures of absorbable material across the lobe or around the lesion to isolate a wedge of tissue (Fig. 17.2). The number of sutures required to isolate the biopsy sample depends on the shape of the lobe and the desired size of the biopsy. Interlocking mattress sutures often provide a degree of hemostasis that could not be achieved with a single strangulating suture. Interlocking sutures should be preplaced before tightening to ensure that they actually interlock and that the hepatic parenchyma proximal to the biopsy sample is completely included within sutures (Fig. 17.2). The sutures are then tightened and tied, and the biopsy sample is removed. The exposed surface of hepatic parenchyma should be examined for hemorrhage, and vessels should be cauterized or ligated with fine-gauge absorbable suture material. The raw surface of the liver is usually not covered or closed. Omentum can be placed over the incised tissue or lightly tacked to the liver with absorbable suture to control capillary

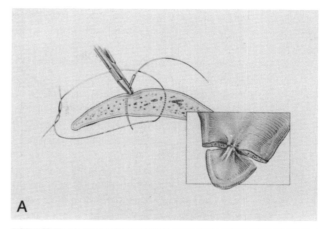

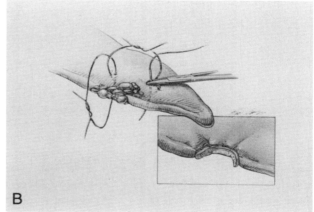

Fig. 17.2. Interlocking sutures of an absorbable material are preplaced to isolate the proposed biopsy site. Although two sutures are often adequate for biopsies obtained from the tip of the liver lobe (**A**), multiple sutures may be needed for other areas (**B**). The sutures are tightened and tied, and the biopsy sample is removed by sharply incising the tissue a few millimeters from the suture line.

hemorrhage. Minor hemorrhage after liver biopsy in dogs has also been controlled by application of fibrin glue (5).

Partial Hepatectomy

Larger biopsy samples or entire lobes can be removed using a parenchymal crushing or "finger fracture" technique. The area to be removed is identified, and the capsule of the liver is sharply incised at the proximal extent of the tissue to be excised (Fig. 17.3). The parenchyma is separated along this line using digital pressure or a forceps to compress the tissue, leaving the vessels and biliary ducts intact. These structures are grasped with forceps, severed, and ligated. Continued capillary hemorrhage can usually be controlled by pressure or by securing the greater omentum to the hepatic bed with 3–0 or 4–0 plain catgut. In the dog, partial hepatectomy with the "finger fracture" technique in one study resulted in fewer complications

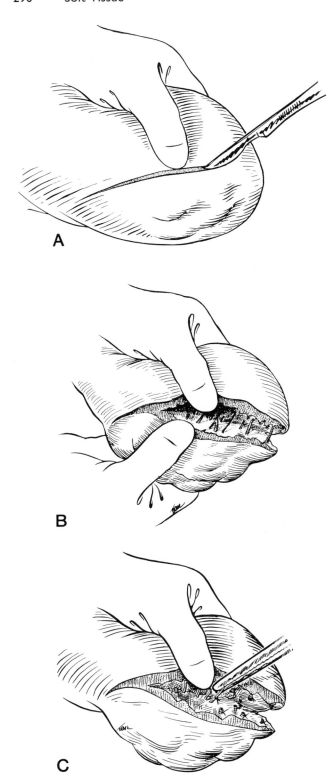

and better healing of the hepatic remnant than when partial hepatectomy was performed using mattress sutures or a specially designed hepatic clamp (6). Partial hepatectomy can also be performed using stapling equipment or ultrasonic dissection–suction devices (7, 8). If staples are to be applied across the liver parenchyma, including vessels and bile canaliculi, staples 3.5 mm (if tissue can be compressed to 1.5 mm) or 4.8 mm in length should be used (9). To minimize the potential for postoperative hemorrhage, it may be preferable to use staples specifically designed for application to vascular structures if large hepatic veins are included in the tissue across which staples are applied. Ultrasonic dissection–suction devices have been used to remove parenchyma along the proposed line of resection, exposing or "skeletonizing" vessels that are then occluded with sutures or vascular clips (8). Investigators have suggested that the use of stapling devices may decrease hemorrhage associated with partial hepatectomy (7); however, studies comparing various techniques for partial hepatectomy have observed that only the ultrasonic dissection and suction devices result in less blood loss and tissue necrosis than other techniques (10, 11). The use of stapling equipment or ultrasonic dissection–suction devices definitely decreases operative time and may decrease subsequent complications; however, these alternatives require specialized equipment.

Although investigators have reported that, in the dog, individual lobes of the liver can be excised after a single encircling ligature is placed near the hilus (1), this technique is dangerous and can result in severe postoperative hemorrhage if the ligature is dislodged. Severing the liver lobe a sufficient distance from the ligature to maintain security of the ligature is difficult. Excision of the liver lobe near the hilus requires careful identification of the vessels and biliary ducts to ensure that those structures associated with the remaining hepatic tissue are left intact. The hepatic veins (especially those associated with the right division of the liver) are short and broad and should be grasped with a vascular forceps and oversewn with 5–0 polypropylene suture. The surgeon should be particularly aware of the location of the caudal vena cava when operating on the right and central divisions of the liver, because inadvertent damage to this structure results in profuse hemorrhage that is difficult to control. Removal of an entire liver lobe can be facilitated by use of stapling equipment or an ultrasonic dissection–suction device, but particular attention must be paid to achieving effective occlusion of large vessels near the hilus.

Hemorrhage during partial hepatectomy can be minimized using temporary vascular occlusion (6). In preparation for temporary occlusion of the vascular supply to the liver, the phrenicoabdominal veins are

Fig. 17.3. **A.** Partial lobectomy of the liver begins by lightly incising the capsule of the liver with a scalpel along the proposed line of excision. **B.** The parenchyma of the liver is separated with digital pressure, isolating the vasculature and larger intralobar bile ducts. **C.** The blood vessels and intralobar bile ducts are grasped with forceps and are ligated.

ligated, and Rumel tourniquets (loops of umbilical tape passing through rubber tubing) are placed around the thoracic caudal vena cava near the diaphragm, the portal vein near the hilus of the liver, and the abdominal caudal vena cava between the renal veins and the liver. The celiac and cranial mesenteric arteries are identified and isolated near the aorta. Hepatic vascular occlusion is achieved by tightening the Rumel tourniquets and applying vascular clamps to the celiac and cranial mesenteric arteries. Under normothermic conditions, the duration of hepatic vascular occlusion should be limited to 15 to 20 minutes (7). This limit can be extended if hypothermia has been induced, a maneuver not often practical. The surgeon should be prepared to proceed with dissection of the liver lobes as rapidly as possible once vascular occlusion is initiated. If hemorrhage is observed when vascular occlusion is discontinued, pressure should be applied to the hepatic bed using laparotomy pads. Blood flow to and from the liver should be allowed to continue undisturbed for at least 5 minutes unless hemorrhage becomes life-threatening. Vascular occlusion can be reinstituted after a brief period of normal circulation by again tightening the Rumel tourniquets and applying the vascular forceps to the arteries. The duration of this period of vascular occlusion should be as short as possible, and additional periods of vascular occlusion are not advisable (12, 13). Investigators have suggested that the hepatic artery can be permanently ligated to decrease hemorrhage during treatment of neoplastic or traumatic disorders of the liver in dogs with few untoward effects (14), and selective angiographic embolization of branches of the hepatic artery has been reported to decrease blood loss during hepatic resection in humans (15). However, these techniques have not gained widespread use in clinical veterinary practice.

Postoperative Care

Postoperative hemorrhage most often results from dislodgment of ligatures and is rarely the result of derangements of the clotting mechanism. The abdomen should be surgically explored to identify and treat the cause of hemorrhage. Hypoglycemia commonly occurs after partial hepatectomy in dogs (8, 9) and becomes more severe as increasing amounts of liver are removed. Isotonic (5%) dextrose in water should be given during and after partial hepatectomy to prevent hypoglycemia. Hypoproteinemia is rarely a problem if the animal's nutritional requirements are met (10, 11).

Plasma bilirubin is slightly increased, and serum alkaline phosphatase and serum alanine aminotransferase can be greatly increased during the first week after partial hepatectomy (10, 11). Serum alkaline phosphatase and serum alanine aminotransferase can remain slightly increased up to 6 weeks after surgery. Prolonged significant increases in bilirubin or hepatic enzymes indicate the presence of biliary obstruction or hepatic inflammation or necrosis.

Antibiotic therapy is best determined by the results of microbial culturing and sensitivity testing. Broad-spectrum antibiotics are a good empiric choice for prophylactic use during hepatic surgery. The combination of penicillin and an aminoglycoside has been used successfully (12), but metronidazole, which should be used in combination with other antibiotics, has greater activity against anaerobic organisms. The cephalosporins and chloramphenicol reach the liver in high concentrations and have satisfactory spectrums of activity for use in conjunction with hepatic surgery (14–16).

References

1. Francavilla A, et al. Liver regeneration in dogs: morphologic and chemical changes. J Surg Res 1978;25:409–419.
2. Sleight DR, Thomford NR. Gross anatomy of the blood supply and biliary drainage of the canine liver. Anat Rec 1970;166:153–160.
3. Badylak SF, Dodds J, Van Vleet JF. Plasma coagulation factor abnormalities in dogs with naturally occurring hepatic disease. Am J Vet Res 1983;44:2336–2340.
4. Islami AH, et al. Regenerative hyperplasia following major hepatectomy: chemical analysis of the regenerated liver and comparative nuclear counts. Ann Surg 1959;140:85–89.
5. Wheaton LG, Greenshields R, Meyers K, et al. Fibrin glue: a topical hemostatic agent to control hemorrhage after liver biopsy. Vet Surg 1992;21:409–410.
6. Tsuzuki T, et al. Repair of the resected liver stump: an experimental study. Surgery 1972;72:395–400.
7. Lewis DD, Bellenger CR, Lewis DT, et al. Hepatic lobectomy in the dog. a comparison of stapling and ligation techniques. Vet Surg 1990;19:221–225.
8. Millat B, Hay JM, et al. Prospective evaluation of ultrasonic surgical dissectors in hepatic resection: a cooperative multicenter study. HPB Surg 1992;5:135–144.
9. Bellah JR. Surgical stapling of the spleen, pancreas, liver, and urogenital tract. Vet Clin North Am Small Anim Pract 1994;24:375–394.
10. Tranberg KG, Rigotti P, Brackett KS, et al. Liver resection. a comparison using the Nd:YAG laser, an ultrasonic surgical aspirator, or blunt dissection. Am J Surg 1986;151:368–373.
11. Ottow RT, Barbieri SA, Surarbaker PH, et al. Liver transection: a controlled study of four different techniques in pigs. Surgery 1985;95:596–601.
12. Whiting PG, et al. Partial hepatectomy with temporary occlusion in dogs with hepatic arteriovenous fistulas. Vet Surg 1986;15:171–180.
13. Raffucci FL, Wangensteen OH. Tolerance of dogs to occlusion of entire afferent vascular inflow to the liver. Surg Forum 1951;1:191–193.
14. Gunn C, Gourley IM, Koblik PD. Hepatic dearterialization in the dog. Am J Vet Res 1986;47:170–175.
15. Robinette DR, Gardner CC Jr, Thomas HA. Selective hepatic arterial embolization as an adjunct to hepatic resection. South Med J 1987;80:1302–1304.
16. Caruana JA, Gage AA. Increased uptake of insulin and glucagon by the liver as a signal for regeneration. Surg Gynecol Obstet 1980;150:390–394.

Portosystemic Shunts

Robert A. Martin, Richard P. Suess &
Joanna Chao

Portosystemic shunts (PSS) are abnormal vascular communications between the portal venous and systemic circulation. Shunts may be acquired or congenital, single or multiple, macrovascular or microvascular, and intrahepatic or extrahepatic. Acquired shunts result from a sustained increase in portal vascular resistance, usually associated with primary hepatic disease, and are multiple, macrovascular, and extrahepatic. Congenital shunts are those most frequently seen in young dogs and cats presented with related neurologic, digestive, or urologic signs (Table 17.1). Congenital shunts are usually single but may rarely be double, are macrovascular, and are either intrahepatic or extrahepatic. Macrovascular shunt location, whether intrahepatic or extrahepatic, is the major determining factor in the ease of surgical isolation. Microvascular shunting of portal blood within the liver has been described as a nonsurgical congenital vascular anomaly that may occur concurrently with a congenital macrovascular shunt (1, 2).

Diagnosis

Diagnosis of PSS is suspected based on history, signalment, physical findings, laboratory abnormalities,

Table 17.1.
Abnormalities Related to Portosystemic Shunts by System Affected

Nervous System	
Aggression	Hysteria
Ataxia	Mydriasis
Behavioral change	Pacing
Blindness	Seizures
Circling	Stunted growth
Deafness	Stupor and coma
Dementia	Tremors
Disorientation	Weakness
Head pressing	
Digestive System	
Anorexia	Pica
Ascites	Polydipsia
Depression	Ptyalism
Diarrhea	Vomiting
Lethargy	Weight loss
Nausea	
Genitourinary System	
Cryptorchidism	Polyuria
Dysuria	Stranguria
Hematuria	Urethral obstruction
Pollakiuria	Urolithiasis
Cardiovascular System	
Heart murmur (cats)	
Portosystemic shunt	

Table 17.2.
Common Laboratory Abnormalities

Hematologic	Biochemical
Anemia	Hyperammonemia
Hypochromasia	Hypocholesterolemia
Microcytosis	Hypoproteinemia
Neutrophilic leukocytosis	Increased ALP (mild)
Poikilocytosis	Increased ALT (mild)
Target-cell formation	Low BUN
Urinalysis	Electrolyte
Ammonium biurate crystalluria	Hyperchloremia
Low specific gravity	Hypernatremia
	Hypokalemia

Liver Function Tests
High sulfobromophthalein retention
High resting and postprandial serum bile acid concentrations
Hyperammonemia after ammonia tolerance test

Coagulation
Hypofibrinogenemia
Increased partial thromboplastin time

and survey abdominal radiography. The historical and physical abnormalities are primarily related to the neurologic, digestive, and urinary systems. Common laboratory abnormalities are listed in Table 17.2. Abdominal radiography may reveal a small liver characterized by cranial displacement of the gastric shadow (the gastric shadow becomes more vertical on a lateral projection) and enlarged renal silhouettes. Demonstration of fasting serum bile acid concentrations above normal or hyperammonemia or abnormal liver function tests (elevated 2-hour postprandial serum bile acid concentrations or abnormal ammonia tolerance test) are more specific indicators of PSS. A suspected diagnosis is confirmed by abdominal ultrasonography, scintigraphy, portography, direct intraoperative visualization, and histopathologic evaluation of the liver.

Surgical Considerations

Congenital PSS is a surgical disease. The goals of surgery are to identify and occlude the shunting vessel, thereby establishing normal hepatic portal blood flow while maintaining safe pressure changes within the portal system. Extrahepatic shunts are usually found in small breed dogs and cats, whereas intrahepatic shunts are more frequently found in large breed dogs. This generalization is not consistent, in that large breed dogs with extrahepatic shunts and small breed dogs and cats with intrahepatic shunts are occasionally seen. Preoperative ultrasonography is useful in both locating PSS (extrahepatic versus intrahepatic [left, central, or right]) and characterizing morphology of intrahepatic shunts, guiding the surgeon's intraoperative approach to shunt management (3–5). Operative portography is also useful when intraoperative shunt identification cannot be made. The identification of extrahepatic shunts can be made by the experienced surgeon in nearly all cases intraoperatively. Opening the omental sac and observing the confluence of the splenic vein and left gastric vein frequently reveal the location of an extrahepatic portocaval or portoazygos shunt at the level of the epiploic foramen (Fig. 17.4) (6). Careful liver lobe palpation also frequently results in identification of intrahepatic shunt location, recognized as a soft, fluctuant aneurysmal dilatation easily compressible and with accompanying elevation in portal pressure values.

Ease of surgical isolation of the shunt is largely influenced by its location. An extrahepatic shunt should be isolated as near to its entry into the systemic circulation as possible. Selection of intrahepatic shunt isolation is based on the surgeon's experience and preference and on the location of the shunt within the liver. Extravascular and intravascular approaches are described (7–11). Left hepatic division shunts may be occluded by extravascular isolation of the left hepatic vein draining the shunt on the diaphragmatic surface of the liver (posthepatic) or by isolation of the shunt entering the left hepatic vein at that site. Left, central, and right division shunts may also be approached by extravascular isolation by way of posthepatic parenchymal dissection or dissection of the main portal branch at the portal hilus (prehepatic). An ultrasonic aspirator improves hepatic parenchymal dissection over blunt dissection by removing hepatic parenchyma without damaging vascular structures (9). Intravascular shunt occlusion of intrahepatic shunts can be approached from a prehepatic portal venotomy or a posthepatic thoracic vena cava venotomy after total occlusion of the hepatic vascular supply and drainage (celiac, cranial and caudal mesenteric arteries, portal vein, and thoracic and abdominal caudal vena cava). The shunt window into its respective hepatic vein or the abdominal vena cava (prehepatic portal venotomy approach) or the opening of the hepatic vein draining the shunt into the abdominal vena cava (vena caval venotomy) can be directly occluded by suturing. Transvenous embolization of an intrahepatic shunt using Teflon-coated coils has also been described (12).

Variability among patients in the potential for portal vascular regeneration after shunt occlusion influences the resolution of clinical signs in the long term. Some animals tolerate complete shunt occlusion and develop normal hepatic portal blood flow. Long-term resolution of clinical signs results. Other animals do not tolerate any shunt occlusion because of complete portal atresia. Most patients tolerate at least partial shunt occlusion with temporary or long-term improvement. In these patients, the partially occluded shunt may remain patent indefinitely or may occlude over time. Acquired multiple extrahepatic shunts may or may not develop, and hepatic portal blood flow usually improves to varying degrees. The clinical outcome therefore depends on the degree of an individual animal's portal vascular response to shunt occlusion.

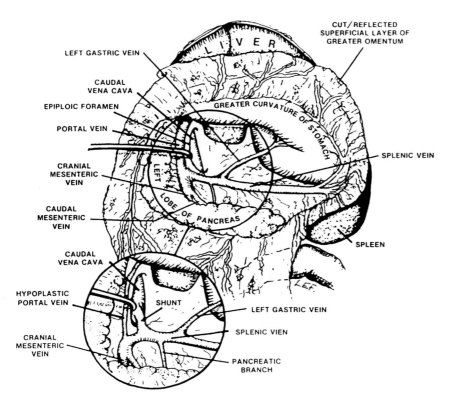

Fig. 17.4. Ventral view into the omental bursa. Note the normal topographic relationships between the splenic, left gastric, and portal vein and compare with a typical single extrahepatic portocaval shunt diagram (*inset*). (From Martin RA. Identification and surgical management of portosystemic shunts in the dog and cat. Semin Vet Med Surg (Small Anim) 1987;2:304.)

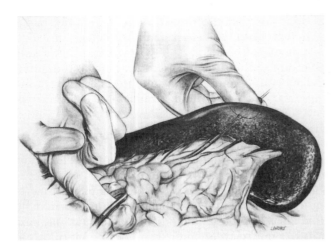

Fig. 17.5. A transsplenic through-the-needle catheter has been placed through the parenchyma and into the splenic vein. The catheter may be used for photography or portal pressure measurements. (From Schultz KS, Martin RA, Henderson RA. Transsplenic portal catheterization: surgical technique and use in two dogs with portosystemic shunts. Vet Surg 1993;22:365.)

Intraoperative measurements of portal pressure, peripheral arterial pressure, central venous pressure and observations of intestinal motility and arterial pulsation and of pancreatic and small bowel congestion help the surgeon to judge the tolerable limits of shunt ligation. I prefer placing a transsplenic portal catheter for measurement of intraoperative portal pressures during shunt occlusion and for routine postoperative portography (Fig. 17.5). Advantages include ease of large-bore catheter placement and noninvasive removal (13). Postoperative portography verifies the location of shunt occlusion, rules out the presence of a second shunt, and demonstrates the hepatic portal circulation present immediately after shunt occlusion.

Surgical Techniques

When the surgeon is confident that complete shunt occlusion can be achieved, total ligation is performed. When partial occlusion is performed, short-term follow-up (4 to 6 weeks) should be done to assess continued patency of the shunt. The sensitivity of transcolonic scintigraphy is the noninvasive procedure of choice for determining the continued presence of portosystemic shunting after surgery (14). A dose of [^{99m}]technetium is placed in the distal colon, and the absorption and distribution of radioactivity are visualized with a gamma camera. In normal dogs, the portal vein is seen first, followed by the appearance of activity in the liver. Seconds later, the heart is visualized. In dogs with PSS, one notes simultaneous visualization of the portal vein and caudal vena cava, with activity in the heart preceding activity in the liver. Shunt fraction values can be calculated (normal, less than 15%). Scintigraphy cannot be used to distinguish between continued patency of the attenuated shunt and development of acquired shunts.

When partial occlusion of a shunt with suture has been performed and scintigraphy indicates continued shunting, ultrasonography may help to distinguish between continued congenital shunt patency and development of acquired shunts. A second surgical procedure is indicated to attempt total occlusion of the congenital shunt when multiple acquired shunts have not developed. Operative portography best demonstrates the current state of portal blood flow. Extrahepatic shunts are usually technically simple to reisolate and ligate, whereas reisolation of intrahepatic shunts may induce additional risks to the patient. We have preplaced monofilament nonabsorbable suture (Prolene) around attenuated intrahepatic shunts at the initial surgical procedure, tying the ends to the diaphragm for easy identification at a second operation. The suture ends can be freed from the diaphragm and tied to occlude the shunt partially or completely without additional hepatic parenchymal dissection. One report indicated successful identification of the attenuating suture after a prehepatic intravascular approach to intrahepatic shunts when further occlusion was performed (10).

Alternatively, a surgical material known to occlude the shunt gradually but totally over the short term (28 to 35 days) may be used without the need for monitoring intraoperative portal pressures; this material is associated with a lower risk of perioperative complications of portal hypertension and with no need for a second operation to occlude a partially ligated shunt (15). Improved hepatic portal blood flow or acquired shunts will result, but, in either case, the goals of total shunt occlusion while maintaining safe portal pressures will have been achieved, leaving the patient's outcome dependent on the variability of the individual's hepatic portal system to respond to increased pressure and blood flow. The rate of gradual occlusion may affect the development of acquired shunts, as opposed to complete hepatic vascular regeneration (15).

Long-term success favors patients with complete shunt ligation. Improved surgical materials capable of producing total vascular occlusion over a longer range of time (60 to 90 days) and improved intravascular and extravascular isolation and manipulation of intrahepatic shunts will likely continue to advance the surgical management of PSS in the near future.

Surgical complications are listed in Table 17.3. Reported surgical mortality rates are from 5 to 21% (15).

Table 17.3.
Potential Complications Resulting From Surgery for Portosystemic Shunts

Acquired shunt formation
Death
Failure to resolve clinical signs
Hemorrhage
Portal hypertension
Portal vein thrombosis
Seizures

Even higher success rates can be expected with continued surgical advancements in the management of PSS.

References

1. Phillips L, Tappe J, Lymon R. Hepatic microvascular dysplasia without demonstrable macroscopic shunts (Abstract). In: Proceedings of the 11th American College of Veterinary Internal Medicine Forum, San Diego, CA. 1993:438–439.
2. Schermerhorn T, Center SA, Rowland PJ, et al. Characterization of inherited portovascular dysplasia in cairn terriers (Abstract). In: Proceedings of the 11th American College of Veterinary Internal Medicine Forum, Washington, DC. 1993:949.
3. Lamb CR. Ultrasonographic diagnosis of congenital portosystemic shunts in dogs: results of a prospective study. Vet Radiol Ultrasound 1996;37:281–288.
4. Lamb CR, Forster-van Hijfte MA, White RN, et al. Ultrasonographic diagnosis of congenital portosystemic shunt in 14 cats. J Small Anim Pract 1996;37:205–209.
5. Lamb CR, White RN. Morphology of congenital intrahepatic portocaval shunts in dogs and cats. Vet Rec (in press).
6. Martin RA, Freeman LE. Identification and surgical management of portosystemic shunts in the dog and cat. Semin Vet Med Surg (Small Anim) 1987;2:302–306.
7. Breznock EM, Berger B, Pendray D, et al. Surgical manipulation of intrahepatic portocaval shunts in dogs. J Am Vet Med Assoc 1983;182:798–805.
8. Martin RA, August JR, Barber DL, et al. Left hepatic vein attenuation for treatment of patent ductus venosus in a dog. J Am Vet Med Assoc 1986;189:1465–1468.
9. Tobias KMS, Rawlings CA. Surgical techniques for extravascular occlusion of intrahepatic shunts. Compend Contin Educ Small Anim Prac 1996;18:745–754.
10. Hunt GB, Bellenger CR, Pearson MRB. Transportal approach for attenuating intrahepatic portosystemic shunts in dogs. Vet Surg 1996;25:300–308.
11. White RN, Trower ND, McEvoy FJ, et al. A method for controlling portal pressure after attenuation of intrahepatic portacaval shunts. Vet Surg 1996;25:407–413.
12. Partington BP, Partington CR, Biller DS, et al. Transvenous coil embolization for treatment of a patent ductus venosus in a dog. J Am Vet Med Assoc 1993;202:281–284.
13. Schulz KS, Martin RA, Henderson RA. Transsplenic portal catheterization: surgical technique and use in two dogs with portosystemic shunts. Vet Surg 1993;22:363–369.
14. Koblik PD, Hornof WJ. Transcolonic sodium pertechnetate Tc 99m scintigraphy for diagnosis of macrovascular portosystemic shunts in dogs, cats, and potbellied pigs: 176 cases (1988–1992). J Am Vet Med Assoc 1995;207:729–733.
15. Vogt JC, Krahwinkel DJ, Bright RM, et al. Gradual occlusion of portosystemic shunts in dogs and cats using the Ameroid constrictor. Vet Surg 1996;25:495–502.

Gradual Occlusion of Single, Extrahepatic Portosystemic Shunts Using the Ameroid Constrictor

James C. Vogt & D. J. Krahwinkel, Jr.

Pathophysiology

Congenital single, extrahepatic portosystemic shunts are the most frequently observed type of portovascular anomaly in dogs and cats (1–4). The treatment of choice is surgical ligation of the primary shunting vessel (4–11). Signalment, clinical signs, pathophysiology, and recommendations for medical and surgical management are reviewed in the previous section of this chapter. Recommendations for partial rather than total ligation of the shunting vessel have been made to prevent portal hypertension, based on resting and total occlusion portal pressures, central venous pressure, and gross observations of abdominal viscera (7–9, 12). This treatment, however, has led to mortality rates from 5 to 21% (6–8). Death occurs in the intraoperative or early postoperative period from anesthetic complications, portal hypertension, portal vein thrombosis, and status epilepticus (4–15).

Gradual occlusion of the portosystemic shunt should allow time for normal hepatic architecture to develop in response to the increased blood flow or should permit the development of collateral circulation, thereby avoiding fatal portal hypertension (16, 17). Case reports have been published of gradual occlusion of portosystemic shunts using cellophane tape and a transvenous coil (18, 19).

Gradual occlusion of single, extrahepatic portosystemic shunts using the Ameroid constrictor (Research Instruments & Mfg, Corvallis, OR) in 12 dogs and 2 cats was evaluated in a prospective clinical trial (20). The Ameroid constrictor is a gradual vascular occlusion device that has been used experimentally since the 1950s to create canine models of coronary arterial stenosis, esophageal varices, and a condition resembling Budd–Chiari syndrome (21–24). Ameroid is hygroscopic, compressed casein that expands when immersed in fluid. An early rapid phase of expansion during the first 14 days is followed by 2 months of slow expansion. Size, shape, and encasement of the Ameroid and type and temperature of the surrounding fluid modify but do not change its typical expansion pattern (22). The Ameroid constrictor is a cylinder of Ameroid in a stainless steel collar. An Ameroid constrictor was placed on the shunting vessel of 12 dogs and 2 cats with single, extrahepatic portosystemic shunts whose total occlusion portal pressures exceeded current recommendations for total ligation (20). The Ameroid constrictors used in the clinical trial had inside luminal diameters of 3.5 and 5.0 mm and weighed approximately 1.5 and 2.3 g, respectively.

Surgical Technique

A ventral celiotomy incision is made from the xiphoid extending caudally past the umbilicus. The liver is examined, and a liver biopsy specimen is taken. The descending duodenum is first retracted to examine the portal vein. Hypoplasia or atresia of the portal vein at the entry into the liver suggests an extrahepatic portosystemic shunt. The caudal vena cava is next examined. Any vessel entering the vena cava cranial to the phrenicoabdominal vein is presumed to be anomalous. Commonly found sites of portosystemic shunts are mentioned in the previous section of this chapter. Each site should be examined meticulously. The experienced surgeon can usually identify the portosystemic shunt by direct examination in most cases; however, it may be necessary to perform a mesenteric portogram if the shunt is not obvious. An intravenous catheter with an attached extension set is placed in a jejunal vein and is secured with 2–0 silk ligatures. The extension set is exteriorized, and the abdomen is closed. A positive-contrast mesenteric portogram is then performed using iothalamate sodium (Conray 400, Mallinckrodt, St Louis, MO) (25).

Once the anomalous vessel is identified, either by direct examination or by mesenteric portogram, the jejunal vein catheter and extension set may be used to measure portal pressures with a water manometer (Baxter Healthcare Corp., General Healthcare Div., Deerfield, IL). Measuring portal pressures, which may be a tedious and time-consuming exercise, does not appear to be necessary when using the Ameroid constrictor. Excessively high total occlusion portal pressures did not influence the outcome of gradual occlusion of portosystemic shunts using the Ameroid constrictor. Measuring portal pressures, however, may benefit the surgeon by identifying the shunting vessel at times.

The shunting vessel is minimally dissected near the level of the caudal vena cava in cases of portocaval shunts or at the crus of the diaphragm for portoazygous shunts. The shunting vessel is elevated with curved forceps. Opening the blades of the forceps flattens the vessel and thus allows placement of the Ameroid constrictor. An Ameroid constrictor with either a 3.5- or 5.0-mm lumen is applied to the shunting vessel, allowing minimal initial occlusion (less than 25%). To prevent dislodgment from the vessel, the Ameroid

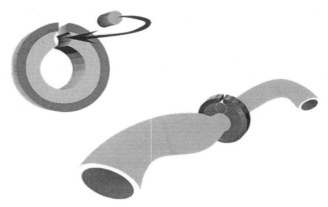

dkh ©1996 University of Tennessee College of Veterinary Medicine

Fig. 17.6. After the application of the Ameroid constrictor to the portosystemic shunt, the unit is locked with a key to prevent dislodgment.

constrictor is secured with the key (Fig. 17.6). The small intestine and pancreas are then observed for 5 minutes for development of cyanosis indicating portal hypertension. If cyanosis is observed, a larger-lumen Ameroid constrictor is required. The abdomen is then lavaged with warm saline, and a three-layered abdominal closure is performed.

Postoperative Care

Each animal is monitored for 2 days postoperatively for signs of portal hypertension (increasing abdominal tenderness, ascites, bloody diarrhea, and seizures). Blood glucose and body temperature should be critically evaluated initially, because these animals may develop hypoglycemia or hypothermia postoperatively. Five percent dextrose in water (4 mL/kg per 24 hours) and ampicillin (20 mg/kg every 8 hours) are given intravenously during the postoperative period until the animal is eating and drinking on its own. Pain is treated in the postoperative period with butorphanol (0.4 mg/kg intravenously every 4 hours) as necessary.

Most animals are discharged from the hospital by the third postoperative day. All animals should be placed on a low-protein diet (Hill's K/D) until total portosystemic shunt occlusion has occurred. Amoxicillin (20 mg/kg orally twice a day) and lactulose (1 mL/ 4.5 kg orally three times daily) may be required for those animals with neurologic signs for 3 weeks postoperatively. Suture removal and physical examination should be scheduled for the second week postoperatively. Assessment of shunt occlusion is recommended at 8 weeks postoperatively and should include rectally administered [99m]technetium per technetate portal scintigraphy (if available) (20, 26). A shunt fraction of

pensated hepatic dysfunction may limit the degree and time of hepatic ischemia from interruption of hepatic arterial flow.

Cholecystotomy and Extrahepatic Exploration of the Biliary System

The most frequent indication for cholecystotomy in the dog and cat is for decompression of the biliary tract and tube exploration of the extrahepatic biliary tree. Inspissated bile is frequently observed in the geriatric or anorectic dog or cat. If the patient's condition indicates biliary stasis from inspissated bile, exploration and flushing of the extrahepatic biliary system are usually indicated. Although cholecystotomy is indicated for biliary flukes in cats and cholelithiasis, the rarity of these conditions limits the frequency of this procedure for such conditions.

If the gallbladder appears normal, before cholecystotomy, I apply moderate increasing pressure to the gallbladder to evaluate patency of the extrahepatic biliary system. Care should be taken to avoid excessive compression and rupture of the gallbladder wall. Stay sutures or noncrushing forceps are placed over the fundus of the gallbladder. I prefer curved, vascular,

partially occluding forceps as traction instruments on the gallbladder. The incision in the gallbladder can be made, the forceps removed, and the bile aspirated. Once the bile has been removed, tube exploration of the extrahepatic binary tract is undertaken. Appropriately sized soft latex or polyvinyl tubing ($3\frac{1}{2}$-Fr infant feeding tube for cats and small dogs) can be used for evaluation of the extrahepatic biliary system. If the collecting ducts or cystic duct arise at an acute angle and preclude passage of the exploring tube, an angiographic flexible-tipped guidewire can be first passed around the sharp angle, followed by the exploring catheters passage over the guidewire. The extrahepatic binary system can be visually inspected for attenuation or disruption by the injection of 5 to 8 mL of dilute patent blue violet dye. Needle aspiration through the duodenal wall confirms the patency of the common bile duct. If attenuation of the common bile duct is suspected as it courses within the duodenal wall or at its entry into the intestinal lumen, a 50% dextrose solution may be injected through the catheter to estimate flow resistance. Elevated resistance to flow without visually apparent biliary tract disease is an indication for enterotomy and exploration of the common bile duct hillock within the duodenum. The gallbladder is closed in two layers with 3–0 or 4–0 monofila-

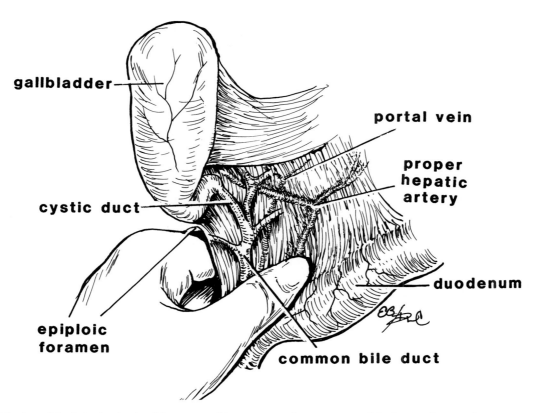

Fig. 17.8. Palpation of the hepaticoduodenal ligament and intimate portal vein, common bile duct, and proper hepatic arteries. (Redrawn from Nora PF, ed. Operative surgery. Philadelphia: Lea & Febiger, 1972.)

ment, absorbable or nonabsorbable suture. The first layer is a continuous approximating pattern and the second a continuous inverting Lembert pattern.

Cholecystostomy Tube

A cholecystostomy tube can be placed to decompress the intrahepatic and extrahepatic binary system after surgical manipulations of the extrahepatic system, when the system is temporarily obstructed as in acute pancreatitis, as a palliative, rapid procedure in the geriatric, decompensated patient, or as a method to treat intrahepatic and extrahepatic biliary cholestasis. In addition, such a tube can be used for contrast radiographic studies of the extrahepatic biliary system. I have used the cholecystostomy tube to flush the biliary tree in dogs and cats with intrahepatic and extrahepatic biliary cholestasis. The flush solution has been warm, sterile saline containing an appropriate antibiotic. Additionally, the patient may be administered an anticholestatic drug to facilitate a more normal bile consistency and flow. Usually, placement of a polyvinyl chloride or latex (Foley) catheter within the gallbladder does not require mobilization of the gallbladder from its hepatic fossa. As a rule, the tube is left in place a minimum of 5 days or until resolution of the problem. The diverted bile should be placed in gelatin capsules and administered orally at the time of feeding of the patient if the cholecystostomy tube is to remain longer than 7 to 10 days.

Cholecystectomy

Tumors, trauma, cholecystitis, and gallstones are potential indications for excision of the gallbladder. In my experience, the most common indication for cholecystectomy is gangrenous cholecystitis. A median epigastric incision extending to the xiphoid process is preferred. In deep-chested dogs, exposure of the gallbladder can be improved by extending the incision paracostally to the right side. To palpate the structures in the hepaticoduodenal ligament, the veterinarian's

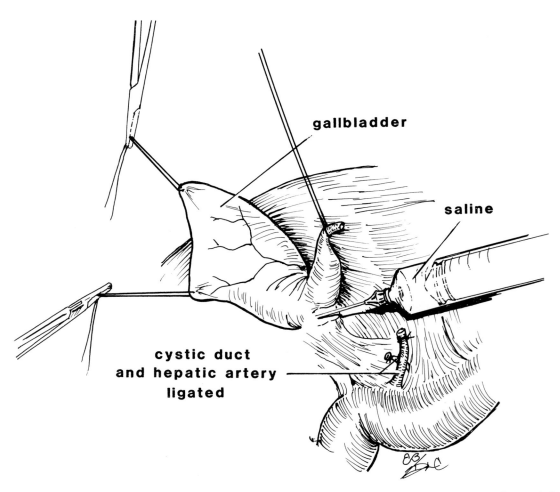

Fig. 17.9. Saline solution injected subserosally, where the gallbladder adheres to the liver, aids in dissection during cholecystectomy. (Redrawn from Nora PF, ed. Operative surgery. Philadelphia: Lea & Febiger, 1972.)

left index and middle fingers are passed through the epiploic foramen into the left lesser omental cavity; with the aid of the left thumb, one may palpate the common bile duct, the portal vein, and the common and proper hepatic arteries (Fig. 17.8). If the gallbladder is overly distended, bile should be expressed or aspirated. Complete decompression of the gallbladder, however, limits visualization of the cleavage plane between liver and gallbladder fossa. To allow better development of the surgical plane between the gallbladder and the hepatic fossa, saline solution can be injected subserosally (Fig. 17.9). The injection of saline subserosally may leave serosa attached to the liver and thus may prevent a raw liver surface. By sharp and blunt dissection, peritoneal attachments of the gallbladder to the liver are divided, with cautious observation of anatomic relationships and arterial and ductal anomalies (Fig. 17.10). Any anomalous vascular or ductal structures should be individually ligated. Depending on the disease encountered and the exposure, the gallbladder may be removed by identifying the cystic duct and artery with the initial dissection and working toward the fundus or by starting the dissection at the fundus and moving toward the bladder

neck (Fig. 17.11). I prefer the former method whenever visualization of important vascular structures is obvious. The cystic artery is identified, skeletonized, and ligated near the gallbladder. The junction of the cystic and common bile duct is identified. At this time, the surgeon may wish to slip a catheter into the cystic duct near the junction of the common bile duct to identify it and to determine patency of the extrahepatic biliary system.

In the dog, extrahepatic ducts dilate after removal of the gallbladder. The intramural portion of the common bile duct is surrounded by a double layer of smoother muscle, and the discharge of bile depends to a large extent on the activity of the duodenum. After cholecystectomy, the intraductal tension increases until it overcomes the powerful sphincter mechanism at the intramural portion of the common bile duct.

Choledochotomy and Choledochostomy

Open exploration of the common bile or collateral biliary ducts in companion animals is infrequently performed because of the small size of these patients and

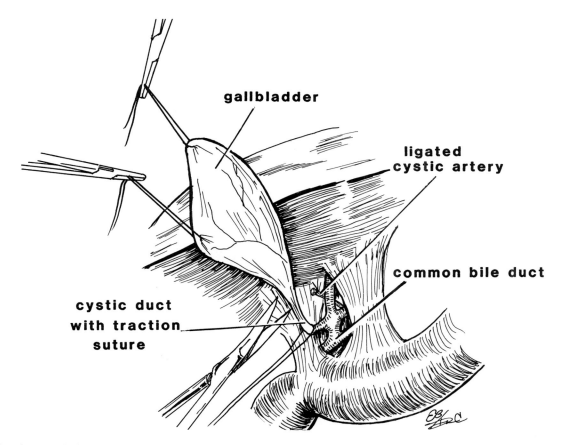

Fig. 17.10. Sharp and blunt dissection isolates the cystic duct with traction sutures; the cystic artery is doubly ligated and transected between ligatures. (Redrawn from Nora PF, ed. Operative surgery. Philadelphia: Lea & Febiger, 1972.)

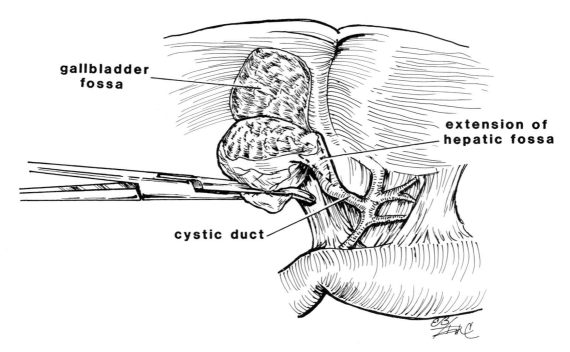

Fig. 17.11. Tissue clamp is placed on the fundus of the gallbladder, and dissection from fundus to neck begins. (Redrawn from Nora PF, ed. Operative surgery. Philadelphia: Lea & Febiger, 1972.)

the potential for stricture formation. However, obstruction usually results in marked dilation of the extrahepatic binary system allowing surgical exploration of this system. Choledochotomy is usually only performed on patients with a dilated bile duct greater than 4 to 5 mm in diameter (Figs. 17.12 and 17.13). I prefer tube exploration through a cholecystotomy. If tube exploration of the extrahepatic biliary tree indicates an abnormal resistance, the cause of which cannot

be visualized, a duodenotomy is performed, and the common bile duct hillock is explored (Fig. 17.14). Noncrushing intestinal or vascular forceps may be applied to the proximal and distal duodenum to minimize intestinal spillage. Locating the bile duct hillock in small dogs and cats can be difficult. Placing a choledochal tube into the duodenum aids in locating the hillock and, if necessary, in performing reconstructive manipulations of the bile duct sphincter (i.e., sphinc-

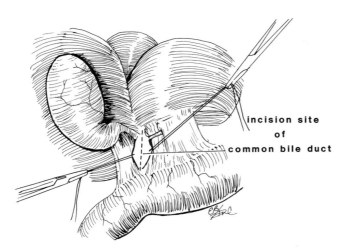

Fig. 17.12. The common bile duct is isolated below the cystic duct. Two traction sutures stabilize the common duct before incision (*dashed line*). (Redrawn from Nora PF, ed. Operative surgery. Philadelphia: Lea & Febiger, 1972.)

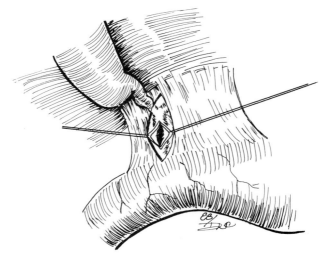

Fig. 17.13. The common bile duct is incised for intraluminal exploration. (Redrawn from Nora PF, ed. Operative surgery. Philadelphia: Lea & Febiger, 1972.)

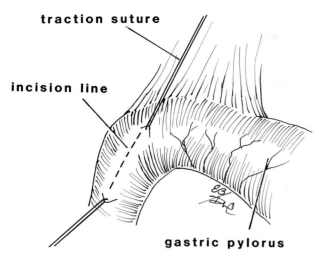

traction suture

incision line

gastric pylorus

Fig. 17.14. Duodenotomy site is just distal to the pylorus of the stomach. (Redrawn from Nora PF, ed. Operative surgery. Philadelphia: Lea & Febiger, 1972.)

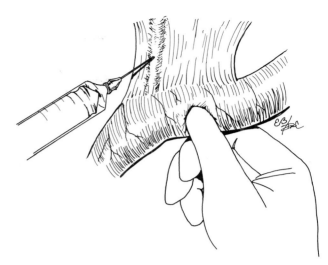

Fig. 17.16. Syringe aspiration identifies the common bile duct if fibrosis of the hepaticoduodenal ligament prevents easy identification. (Redrawn from Nora PF, ed. Operative surgery. Philadelphia: Lea & Febiger, 1972.)

terotomy, sphincterectomy, sphincteroplasty) (Fig. 17.15). Frequently, gastric or intestinal carcinomas, pancreatitis, and other inflammatory diseases can result in significant tissue reaction, fibrosis, and adhesions, which make identification of the common bile duct and collateral ducts difficult. A sterile syringe and a 25-gauge needle may be used to aspirate the structure in question. If bile is inspissated, aspiration through a 25-gauge needle may be difficult (Fig. 17.16). If the bile is viscous and cannot be aspirated, saline may be injected into the structure. If saline flows smoothly, dilute blue violet dye may be injected to identify the vessel, its course, and branches. Polypropylene traction sutures can be used to support the duct during incisional exploration.

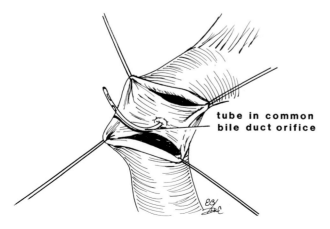

tube in common bile duct orifice

Fig. 17.15. The duodenal incision is opened with four traction sutures. A choledochal tube passed into the duodenum identifies the common duct orifice.

After choledochotomy, a choledochal tube (T-tube) may be placed within the incision of the common duct to act as a stent to support the sutured incision (see discussion following on reconstruction of the biliary tract). If decompression is required or is determined to be advantageous at the time of the operation, a temporary cholecystotomy tube is placed and is brought to the exterior through a small abdominal incision (Fig. 17.17). The tube cholecystopexy is performed with 4–0 polypropylene suture material. If exploration of the common bile duct determines that an obstruction exists at the common duct sphincter or as the common duct courses intramurally within the duodenum, an enterotomy incision is made, and depending on the nature of the disease and the size of the hillock and common duct, a sphincterotomy, sphincterectomy, or sphincteroplasty may be required to alleviate the obstruction (Fig. 17.18). More frequently, however, because of small duct size, poor accessibility, and the potential for stricture, a biliary–intestinal (i.e., cholecystointestinal) bypass procedure is performed to alleviate the obstruction.

Unless the extrahepatic common duct, collateral duct, or bile duct ostium is larger than 3 to 4 mm, I prefer a bypass procedure such as a cholecystogastrointestinal or choledochointestinal anastomosis for bile duct obstruction. However, a biliary–intestinal anastomosis is only efficacious in patients with obstructive bile duct disease distal to where the cystic duct joins the common bile duct. Treatment of tumors in this area depends on the extent, location, infiltration, and kind of tumor. A biopsy is usually in order to determine whether a simple excision or a bypass procedure is to be performed. Because of the severe

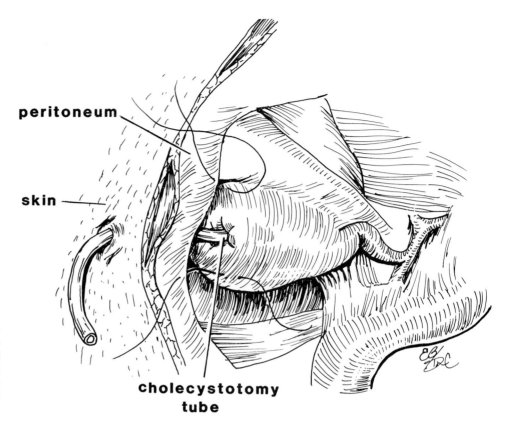

peritoneum

skin

cholecystotomy tube

Fig. 17.17. A cholecystostomy tube is maintained in the gallbladder with a pursestring suture. Two (of five or six) chromic catgut sutures are placed through the serosa of the gallbladder and peritoneum at the place of exit through the skin.

complications, rarely is radical pancreaticoduodenectomy performed.

Sphincterotomy can be safely performed by placing a tube or groove directly through the gallbladder into the intraluminal common duct, and the incision is made through the sphincter onto the preplaced guide. Sphincteroplasty requires the excision of a wall of duodenum and intramural common bile duct; the edges of the incised tissue are sutured in a simple interrupted pattern with 5–0 or 6–0 polypropylene or absorbable suture. Because the common bile duct can run intramurally for 2 to 3 cm in large dogs, excision of the intramural intestine and bile duct usually does not result in bile leakage.

The major pancreatic duct empties into the duodenal hillock with the common bile duct in approximately 50% of dogs and in nearly all cats. The accessory pancreatic duct usually enters the duodenum some distance from the bile duct hillock and usually intercommunicates with the major pancreatic duct. Iatrogenic obstruction of the major pancreatic duct during surgical manipulations of the common bile duct ostium in most instances does not result in pancreatic insufficiency. However, because the surgeon cannot assume that intercommunications exist, in performing sphincterotomy, sphincterectomy, or sphincteroplasty, care should be taken to identify and avoid the pancreatic ducts.

Biliary–Intestinal Anastomosis

Malignant or benign obstructions of the biliary tract, trauma, the patient's size, and other conditions may necessitate biliary bypass procedures. Bile stasis, fibrosis of the common bile duct, erosion of the common bile duct with peritonitis and fibrosis of surrounding tissues, tumors involving the common bile duct, or traumatic injuries may require some type of biliary bypass. Biliary–intestinal diversion procedures include cholecystogastrostomy, cholecystoduodenostomy, cholecystojejunostomy, choledochoduodenostomy, and choledochojejunostomy. Although anastomoses involving the gallbladder are less complicated procedures than those involving the common duct, if the common duct is notably dilated, the difference is minimal.

The surgical technique is similar for all three types of gallbladder–gastrointestinal anastomoses. The fundus of the gallbladder is grasped with noncrushing intestinal or vascular clamps or is retained by traction sutures. If mobility of the gallbladder is minimal, the fundus can be dissected and partially freed as described for cholecystectomy. The serosa of the intestinal tract (jejunum or duodenum) is approximated to the serosa of the gallbladder by a continuous Lembert 4–0 or 5–0 polypropylene suture. Noncrushing intestinal or vascular clamps should be applied to the proximal and distal jejunum (not needed for the duodenum or stomach) to minimize intestinal spillage. An incision is made in both the gallbladder and the intestine close to the previously placed serosal suture line (Fig. 17.19). The incision length depends on the size of the patient and is approximately one and one-half times the diameter of the duodenum. The gallbladder–intestine anastomosis is approximated with a continuous mucosal and submucosal 5–0 polypropylene suture pattern. The remaining serosal layer is further approximated with the continuous Lembert 4–0 or 5–0 polypropylene suture pattern. Intestinal reflux has

not been a recognized problem after biliary–intestinal bypass procedures. However, after a gastrobiliary bypass procedure, normal enterohepatic biliary function may be altered because of a changed pH environment. In addition, gastric acid reflux into the gallbladder may predispose to a metaplastic cellular reaction resulting in neoplasia or ulceration in the long term.

Choledochoenterostomy can be performed if the common bile duct is large enough to permit such an anastomosis (commonly observed after chronic bile duct obstruction) (Fig. 17.20). An oblique or longitudinal incision is made in the common duct for purposes

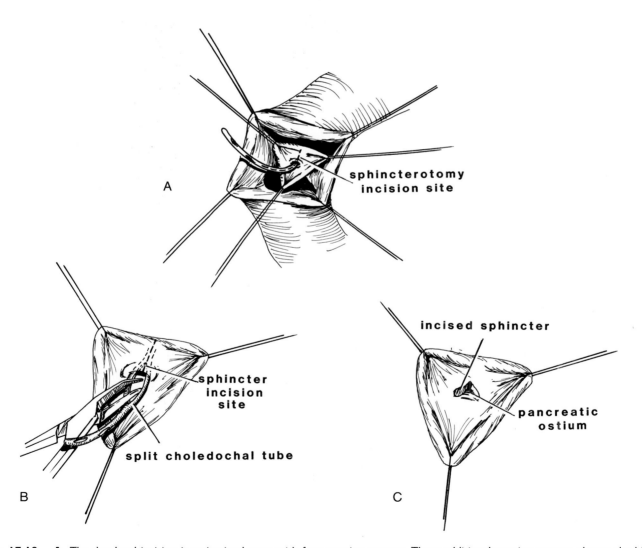

Fig. 17.18.   **A.** The duodenal incision is maintained open with four traction sutures. Three additional traction sutures elevate the bile duct hillock containing a choledochal tube in the bile duct orifice. *Dashed lines* on the hillock and tube indicate incision lines. **B.** The choledochal tube is split and retracted into the common bile duct. Mosquito forceps spread the split tube in and out of the common duct. Sphincterotomy can be easily performed along the split tube (*dashed line*). **C.** Sphincterotomy is complete. The ventral pancreatic duct may be present within the common bile duct hillock.

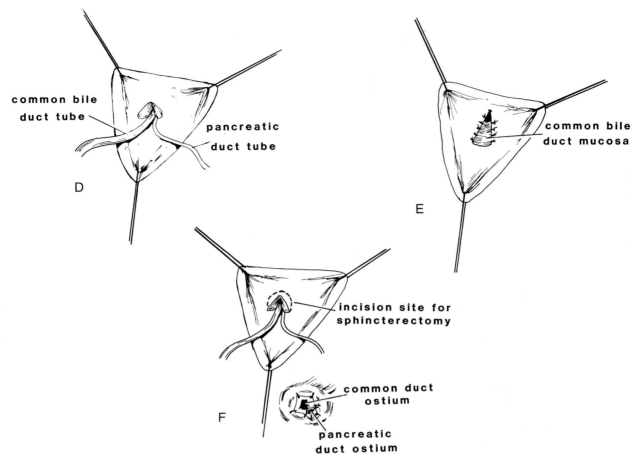

Fig. 17.18 (continued). **D.** After sphincterotomy of the common bile duct, the surgeon should cannulate the pancreatic duct for identification during other manipulative techniques. **E.** Sphincteroplasty is completed with simple interrupted fine catgut sutures. (Redrawn from Nora PF, ed. Operative surgery. Philadelphia: Lea & Febiger, 1972.) **F.** Sphincterectomy (*dashed line*) after sphincterotomy can be performed after identification of the pancreatic ostium in the common bile duct hillock. Two ostia (common and pancreatic ducts) may need to be constructed after excision of the bile duct sphincter.

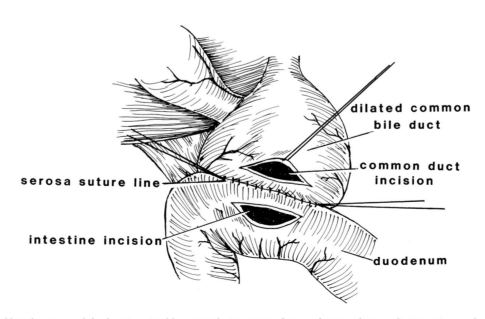

Fig. 17.19. The dilated common bile duct is united by a simple interrupted serosal suture line to the intestine, and a gallbladder incision and enterotomy are made close to the serosal suture line. (Redrawn from Nora PF, ed. Operative surgery. Philadelphia: Lea & Febiger, 1972.)

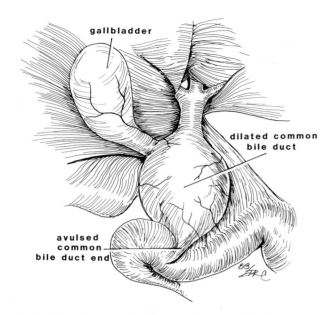

Fig. 17.20. An avulsed and scarred common bile duct has occurred in a common bile duct and collecting ducts.

of exploration and anastomosis. Assuming that the bypass procedure is for a benign condition with a dilated common bile duct, the adjacent intestinal serosa and common bile duct serosa are approximated by a continuous 5–0 polypropylene suture pattern. A parallel incision is made in the dilated common duct and intestine 1 or 2 mm adjacent to the preplaced continuous serosal stitch. The length of the incisions should be one and one-half times the diameter of the duodenum. The mucosa of the common bile duct and that of the intestine are approximated with a continuous polypropylene suture started on the back half of the midline and continued toward the surgeon. The near aspect of the mucosal anastomosis is reinforced with a continuous 5–0 polypropylene suture by a Cushing stitch through the serosa (Fig. l7.21).

Reconstruction of the Biliary Tract

The biliary tree may be injured by trauma or by iatrogenic surgical errors. Because of interlobular communications of the biliary tree, small intrahepatic or extrahepatic duct lacerations may be best ligated, usually without consequence. An attempt should be made to salvage large ducts of the extrahepatic biliary tree, however. The identification of lacerations or transections of major bile ducts may be difficult, especially in patients with bile peritonitis. Cholecystotomy tube exploration and dye infusions aid in identifying ductal trauma and bile leakage in all divisions of the bile excretory system. If the cystic duct is not patent, or if extensive obliteration of the common bile duct has

taken place, conversion must be made to a transduodenal entry into the common bile duct to see whether it is salvageable.

After identification of trauma, leakage, stricture, or fibrosis, serial sectioning of the junction of normal and pathologic tissue is used to isolate viable, patent duct tissue. Normal duct tissue is essential for the anastomosis to succeed. The length of the bile duct is usually not important because the distal common duct with duodenum may be moved to the hiatus of the liver to accept the anastomosis and may be anchored to the stomach. The effects on the reconstructive outcome, of suture type, of the manner in which the suture is placed, and of the number of layers used are equivocal at this time. The surgical goal, however, should always be a technically accurate mucosal repair using fine, well-spaced sutures with no tension on the suture line.

The effect of choledochal tubes (T-tubes) as supportive stents within the anastomosis is controversial. Although clinical data indicate less scar contraction with long-term as opposed to short-term placement of supportive stents, laboratory studies indicate that such stents act as a stimulus for fibrosis and delay healing. Appropriately sized stents decompress the anastomosis, and their use remains a matter of judgment. If bile is drained externally during convalescence, bile salt replacement tablets or encapsulated biliary fluid will be necessary.

Maturation of any scar follows an exponential curve and is most pronounced during the first phase of heal-

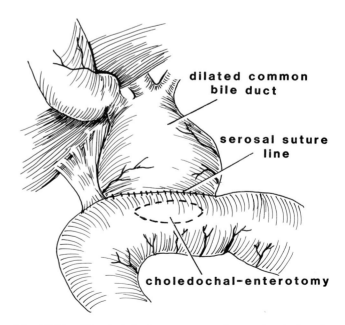

Fig. 17.21. The choledochoenterostomy is completed when the initial serosal suture line is extended completely around the enterotomy suture line. (Redrawn from Nora PF, ed. Operative surgery. Philadelphia: Lea & Febiger, 1972.)

ing. A duct that is anastomosed with a larger diameter shows less chance for recurring stricture. Thus, certain plastic procedures may be used to increase the diameter of the proximal duct before anastomosis (Fig. 17.22).

Although the lumen size of the postoperative biliary duct affects bile transit, bile flow may be retarded in a visually patent bile duct. Fibroblastic proliferation surrounding the anastomosis may render a segment of the bile duct rigid and thus may impair the transit of bile to the intestine and result in extrahepatic bile duct dilation.

Lacerations located in the common duct proximal to the cystic duct may be anastomosed to the gallbladder more easily than to a smaller portion of the duct itself. If the common duct is available for anastomosis only above the cystic duct, the situation becomes difficult. The best option is probably a choledochojejunostomy into a 12-inch Roux loop of jejunum. Because reflux is not harmful, a simple loop of jejunum, with or without an enteroenterostomy at its base, is satisfactory for the biliary drainage in the course of biliary tract reconstruction (Fig. 17.23).

In most instances, the use of autologous tissues (i.e., vein small bowel, pericardial constructed vessel) for reconstruction of the biliary tract has no real clinical application because the marked degree of mobilization of the extrahepatic biliary tree precludes their use. The use of autologous tissues requires one suture line to be replaced by two suture lines. Such a maneuver increases the risk of failure from fibroblastic contraction or dehiscence and bile leakage. Although alternatives are available to the veterinary surgeon for reconstruction of a diseased biliary tract in companion animals, the size of the patient often precludes the use of certain

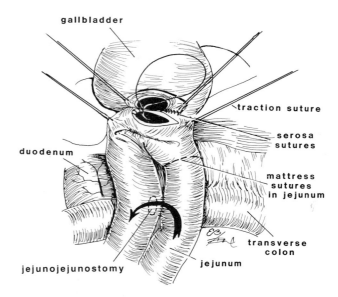

Fig. 17.23. A serosal suture line joins the gallbladder to the jejunum. The mucosa of the gallbladder and the jejunum are united with a simple continuous suture line. Traction sutures maintain apposition of the organs during cholecystoduodenostomy. Mattress sutures across the ascending limb of the jejunum together with a jejunojejunostomy prevent reflex of intestinal content into the biliary system. (Redrawn from Nora PF, ed. Operative surgery. Philadelphia: Lea & Febiger, 1972.)

techniques without microsurgical equipment and supplies.

Suggested Readings

Breznock EM. Surgery of hepatic parenchymal and binary tissues. In: Bojrab MJ, ed. Current techniques in small animal surgery. 2nd ed. Philadelphia: Lea & Febiger, 1983:216–225.

Drazner FR. The liver and biliary tract. In: Gourley G, Vasseur P, eds. General small animal surgery. Philadelphia: JB Lippincott, 1985:413–436.

Martin RA. Liver and binary system. In: Slatter DH, ed. Textbook of small animal surgery. Philadelphia: WB Saunders, 1993: 645–660.

Martin RA. Biliary obstruction and stones. In: Bojrab MJ, ed. Disease mechanisms in small animal surgery. 2nd ed. Philadelphia: Lea & Febiger, 1993:306–310.

Tangner CH. Biliary surgery. In: Bojrab MJ, ed. Current techniques in small animal surgery. 3rd ed. Philadelphia: Lea & Febiger, 1990:299–303.

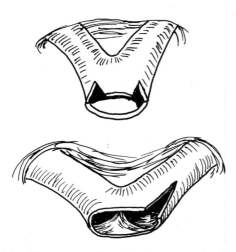

Fig. 17.22. Plastic procedures for increasing the diameter of vessels or ducts before anastomosis. (Redrawn from Nora PF, ed. Operative surgery. Philadelphia: Lea & Febiger, 1972.)

Percutaneous Biliary Drainage (Cholecystostomy)

Darien Lawrence

Extrahepatic bile duct obstruction (EHBDO) may be caused by the presence of stones (choleliths or choledocholiths), inspissated bile, inflammatory processes (cholecystitis, cholangitis), pancreatitis, neoplasia, and parasitic gallbladder disease (1, 2). Obstruction may be partial or complete and may be intermittent. Clinical signs of obstructive diseases depend on the cause, but they include icterus, cranial abdominal pain, vomiting, anorexia, depression, fever, acholic feces, and progressive weight loss (1–3). Because the clinical signs are nonspecific, biliary tract disorders are often overlooked, and frequently the disease has been present for several weeks before diagnosis. Animals are frequently debilitated when presented (1–3).

The PC technique is widely used in human medicine for temporary or definitive treatment of certain biliary conditions, including cholelithiasis, acute cholecystitis, and benign common bile duct obstruction, or as palliative treatment for malignant biliary tract obstruction (4–6). In human patients, this technique is performed with ultrasound guidance, with the patient under sedation or light gaseous anesthesia, and often on an emergency basis. This method is especially useful in high-risk patients (7, 8).

The goals of PC are to provide rapid preoperative relief of jaundice, to allow control of biliary sepsis, and to improve the nutritional status of the patient before definitive surgery (7). In a study in cats with experimental bile duct obstruction, PC resulted in rapid clinical improvement. Within 24 to 48 hours, the general attitude and appetite of the cats improved, and serum bilirubin, fasting serum bile acid values, alanine aminotransferase and aspartate aminotransferase all decreased significantly in the first 72 hours (9). Results of studies in dogs suggest that the major benefit of temporary bile diversion may be the result of other factors not directly related to biliary drainage (e.g., nutrition and antibiotics) (10–11).

Two main indications for PC are recognized. PC can be used for biliary decompression when the bile duct is temporarily obstructed but is expected to remain functional after the primary inflammatory process is resolved (12). Cholecystostomy tubes have been placed in two dogs at surgery for temporary relief of common bile duct obstruction secondary to pancreatitis (13). Positive contrast cholangiography can be easily performed to determine patency of the bile duct before tube removal (12).

Veterinarians can also use PC in severely ill patients requiring biliary decompression as a temporary procedure before definitive surgical treatment of bile duct obstruction (9, 12, 14, 15). Not all animals with EHBDO are candidates for PC. High bilirubin levels, renal insufficiency, sepsis, poor nutritional condition, and other systemic diseases that require treatment or stabilization before definitive surgery for the biliary tract problem are indications for PC in humans (7, 8, 16).

Although specific indications have not been evaluated for veterinary patients, they are likely to be similar.

Preoperative Considerations

The patient should be evaluated carefully preoperatively, with a biochemistry panel, complete blood count, prothrombin time (PT), and partial thromboplastin time (PTT), or proteins induced by vitamin K absence (PIVKA), abdominal radiographs, and abdominal ultrasound. Evidence of a ruptured gallbladder is a contraindication for PC.

The consequences of EHBDO are well documented and include impaired function of the reticuloendothelial system, increased absorption of endotoxins into the portal and peripheral circulations, depletion of coagulation factors, acquired platelet dysfunction, and an increased incidence of postoperative renal failure (17). The surgeon should be aware of these consequences and should take steps to correct or counteract them before PC.

Vitamin K$_1$ Deficiency

Within 2 weeks of EHBDO, bleeding tendencies that are responsive to vitamin K$_1$ administration can develop (1, 3). Bile salts enhance absorption of the fat-soluble vitamins A, D, E, and K, and biliary obstruction can contribute to a clinically important decrease in the vitamin K–dependent coagulation factors II, VII, IX, and X, resulting in a prolongation of PT and PTT. Because factor VII has the shortest half-life (1.2 to 6 hours), PT usually is prolonged before PTT (18).

Before PC, coagulation studies should be done (platelet count, PT, PTT, or PIVKA). The test for PIVKA evaluates the occurrence of both depleted vitamin K–dependent coagulation factors and buildup of PIVKA. PIVKA are circulating nonfunctional precursor forms of vitamin K–dependent proteins that are synthesized and normally stored in the liver microsomal system but accumulate and spill over into the circulation when a relative to absolute vitamin K deficiency occurs (14). If coagulation time or PIVKA time is prolonged, vitamin K$_1$ (AquaMEPHYTON, Merck Sharpe and Dohme, Div. of Merck and Co., West Point, PA) should be administered at a daily dose of 1 to 2 mg/kg divided every 8 hours and given subcutaneously every 12 hours for 24 to 48 hours (14). In most instances, coagulation normalizes within 3 to 12 hours of the initial administration. If bleeding tendencies persist or if abnormal coagulation times fail to correct with vitamin K$_1$ therapy (because of underlying primary hepatocellular disease), a fresh blood or plasma transfusion is indicated before PC.

Antibiotics

Appropriate antibiotic coverage should be instituted before attempting PC, even in patients without clinical evidence of infection. Organisms commonly found in obstructive biliary disease are *Escherichia coli*, *Klebsiella*, *Pseudomonas*, *Streptococcus*, *Clostridium spp.*, and *Proteus* (14). Antibiotics not reliant on hepatic biotransformation or excretion are preferable. Cephalosporins are broad-spectrum antibiotics concentrated in bile. These antibiotics have minimal side effects in patients with impaired liver function and may be used orally or parenterally. Cefazolin, 22 mg/kg intravenously, should be given before PC. Once culture and sensitivity results are available on aspirated bile, the antibiotic may be changed if indicated.

Chloramphenicol, chlortetracycline, oxytetracycline, erythromycin, hetacillin, lincomycin, streptomycin, and sulfonamides are not recommended in the management of hepatobiliary disease (3, 19). These drugs are inactivated by the liver, require hepatic metabolism, or are capable of causing hepatic damage.

Fluid Therapy

Renal function may be impaired by dehydration and endotoxemia. Endotoxemia is one of the most common causes of complications and multiple organ failure before and after surgery with biliary obstruction. Up to 50% of human patients with obstructive jaundice have endotoxemia, probably because of increased endotoxin release from the gastrointestinal tract together with impaired hepatic clearance (20). Aggressive fluid therapy may help to prevent the renal vasoconstriction and redistribution of intrarenal blood flow away from the renal cortex that is seen with endotoxemia. Similarly, if the patient is septic, aggressive fluid therapy and glucose supplementation should be provided.

Surgical Technique

The cholecystostomy catheter can be placed either percutaneously with a needle-guide system or by using a small paracostal incision. These procedures may be performed while the patient is under heavy sedation and local anesthetic or inhalation anesthesia. Drugs metabolized by the liver should be avoided.

Anatomy

The gallbladder lies in a depression on the visceral surface of the liver between the quadrate and right medial liver lobes, at the level of the eighth to tenth intercostal spaces. The hepatic ducts (three to five in number) enter the cystic duct, which in turn drains into the gallbladder. Distal to the junction with the first hepatic duct, the cystic duct becomes the common bile duct and empties into the duodenum (1.5 to 6.0 cm) distal to the pylorus at the major duodenal papilla (2). The cystic artery, which supplies blood to the gallbladder, originates from the left branch of the proper hepatic artery (1).

Percutaneous Technique With Ultrasound Guidance

The Hawkins needle-guide system consists of a long, 22-gauge cannulated needle with stylet and a guidewire (Cook, Inc., Bloomington, IN). A 6.5-Fr polytetrafluoroethylene self-retaining accordion catheter, with 14 side holes for drainage, is preloaded onto the needle (Fig. 17.24). The gallbladder can be penetrated either at its free wall or at the attached gallbladder wall (with the needle and catheter passing through the liver) (5). The needle is advanced into the gallbladder under ultrasound guidance, the stylet is removed, and a small amount of bile aspirated to confirm the position. The guidewire is threaded into the gallbladder, and the accordion catheter is advanced into the gallbladder over the guidewire. A mark on the needle-guide cannula indicates when the most proximal side holes are beyond the tip of the needle and inside the gallbladder. The catheter is accordioned by retracting the attached monofilament suture and securing it to a Tuohy-Borst fitting (9, 21). Because the catheter is self-retaining, it does not need to be attached to the skin, provided it is bandaged well to prevent mutilation by the patient.

Keyhole Incision With Gallbladder Visualization

With this method, either the Hawkins needle-guide system with a self-retaining catheter or a small Foley catheter (7 to 14 Fr) can be used. The former is preferred because of a decreased incidence of catheter dislodgment (4, 22). A small right paracostal incision (or a small ventral midline incision, if preferred) is made, and the gallbladder is visualized and immobilized gently, either digitally or with Babcock forceps. The cholecystostomy tube is introduced through the right ventral body wall just caudal to the costal arch and through several layers of omentum. If a Foley catheter is used, a pursestring suture is placed into the fundus of the gallbladder with 3–0 or 4–0 absorbable suture material without mobilizing the gallbladder. A stab incision is made through the gallbladder fundus inside the pursestring suture, and the Foley catheter is introduced. Care should be taken to avoid peritoneal contamination with bile by packing the area with moist laparotomy sponges or by aspirating gallbladder contents with a needle and syringe before incising the

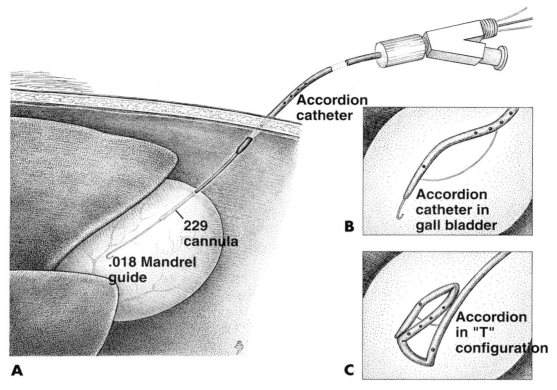

Fig. 17.24. **A.** The accordion catheter is preloaded over a Hawkins needle guide before placement. Under ultrasound guidance or by keyhole laparotomy, the needle guide is inserted into the gallbladder and a mandrel guide 0.46 mm (0.018 in) in diameter is advanced through the guide. **B.** The accordion catheter is advanced over the guide into the gallbladder. **C.** The guide is removed, and the monofilament line is tightened. (Modified from Pearse DM, Hawkins IF, Shaver R, et al. Percutaneous cholecystostomy in acute cholecystitis and common duct obstruction. Radiology 1984;152:365–367.)

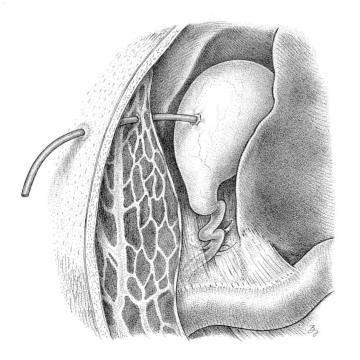

fundus. The pursestring suture is tied, and the balloon of the Foley catheter is inflated with saline (12). The tube is sutured to the skin as it exits (Fig. 17.25). If the Hawkins needle-guide system and self-retaining catheter are used, neither a pursestring suture in the gallbladder nor suture attachment of the catheter to the skin is needed (9).

Postoperative Care

The optimal duration of PC in veterinary patients is unknown. PC tubes placed at surgery for temporary

Fig. 17.25. A small paracostal incision is made, and the Foley catheter is introduced through the right ventral body wall just caudal to the costal arch and through several layers of omentum. The catheter is inserted into the fundus of the gallbladder through a pursestring suture, and the balloon is inflated with saline. The gallbladder is not mobilized from its fossa. The Foley catheter is sutured to the skin with a Chinese finger trap pattern as it exits. (Modified from Breznock EM. Surgery of the biliary tract. In: Bojrab MJ, ed. Current techniques in small animal surgery. 2nd ed. Philadelphia: Lea & Febiger, 1983:212–236.)

bile diversion in two dogs with acute distal obstruction of the biliary tract resulting from pancreatic disease were maintained for 2 weeks and 10 days, respectively, without significant problems developing (13). In most cases, only a few days are necessary to allow bilirubin and liver enzyme levels to decrease, nutrition and renal function to improve, and sepsis to be controlled, making the patient a better candidate for a longer anesthetic and more complicated surgical procedure to treat the underlying disease definitively.

Although many human patients with malignant disease have catheters maintained for months with minimal morbidity, this would not be an option for most veterinary patients because of poor patient compliance, the risk of ascending infection, and the poor prognosis associated with underlying malignant disease.

Patient Management

A bile sample should be collected and submitted for cytologic examination and for culture and sensitivity at the time of PC, and the antibiotics should be changed if indicated. Antibiotic therapy, started before PC, should be continued while the catheter is in place. A common complication in humans with PC is cholangitis (1.6 to 47%), with the highest rates evident in patients with malignant disease (2, 22–24). Three of four cats with experimental EHBDO and PC developed positive bile cultures by the fourth day of bile diversion; this high rate was probably because these cats were not given prophylactic antibiotics at the time of catheter placement (9).

Fluid and electrolyte therapy should also be continued while the catheter is in place. High-volume bile output is an infrequent complication that occurs within the first few days of PC—it is temporary, and its pathophysiology is unknown. Aggressive replacement fluid therapy can occasionally be required. The mean daily volume of bile collected in cats with experimental EHBDO and PC ranged from 58 ± 9 to 224 ± 20 mL. Electrolytes should be monitored regularly because approximately 5% of human patients develop severe electrolyte imbalances within 6 days of drainage (25). Daily bile losses can be replaced with an equal volume of oral solution with the same electrolyte composition of bile (25). Hemobilia may be evident after catheter placement. It is usually mild and resolves spontaneously (9, 22).

Catheter Management

The catheter is bandaged and connected to a sterile collection system that is emptied daily. Gravity drainage is adequate. In the postoperative period, the catheter should be flushed regularly with sterile saline, infection should be prevented around the skin entry point, and the catheter should be watched carefully for signs of obstruction, dislodgment, and infection (4, 22, 26). All removable external components should be changed at least twice weekly. The addition of povidone–iodine to the collecting bag reduces the incidence of exogenous infection and cross-contamination (25).

Catheter Removal

In most instances, the catheter is removed at the time of definitive surgery to correct the bile duct obstruction. A catheter placed to provide temporary relief for reversible bile duct obstruction (e.g., pancreatitis) can be safely removed after 5 to 10 days (once a fibrous tract has formed around the catheter), with minimal risk of bile leakage once the obstruction has resolved (12).

References

1. Blass CE. Surgery of the extrahepatic biliary tract. Compend Contin Educ Pract Vet 1983;5:801–809.
2. Neer TM. A review of disorders of the gallbladder and extrahepatic biliary tract disorders in the dog and cat. J Vet Intern Med 1992;6:186–192.
3. Center SA. Feline liver disorders and their management. Compend Contin Educ Pract Vet 1986;8:889–901.
4. Günther RW, Schild H, Thelen M. Review article. Percutaneous transhepatic biliary drainage: experience with 311 procedures. Cardiovasc Intervent Radiol 1988;11:65–71.
5. Shaver RW, Hawkins IF Jr, Soong J. Percutaneous cholecystostomy. Am J Radiol 1982;138:1133–1136.
6. vanSonnenberg E, D'Agostino H, Casola G. Interventional gallbladder procedures. Radiol Clin North Am 1990;28:1185–1190.
7. Lu DSK, Ho CS, King M. Percutaneous transhepatic biliary drainage for malignant biliary obstruction: a report of two cases with five year survival. Clin Radiol 1991;44:329–331.
8. Klimberg S, Hawkins I, Vogel SB. Percutaneous cholecystostomy for acute cholecystitis in high-risk patients. Am J Surg 1987;153:125–129.
9. Lawrence D, Bellah JR, Meyer DJ, et al. Temporary bile diversion in cats with experimental extrahepatic bile duct obstruction. Vet Surg 1992;21:446–451.
10. Fraser IA, Schaffer P, Tuttle SV, et al. Hepatic recovery after biliary decompression of experimental obstructive jaundice. Am J Surg 1989;158:423–427.
11. Koyama K, Takagi Y, Ito K, et al. Experimental and clinical studies on the effect of biliary drainage in obstructive jaundice. Am J Surg 1981;142:293–299.
12. Martin RA. Liver and biliary system. In: Slatter DJ, ed. Textbook of small animal surgery. 2nd ed. Philadelphia: WB Saunders, 1993:645–677.
13. Martin RA, MacCoy DM, Harvey HJ. Surgical management of extrahepatic biliary tract disease: a report of eleven cases. J Am Anim Hosp Assoc 1986;22:301–307.
14. Martin RA. Biliary obstruction/stones. In: Bojrab MJ, ed. Disease mechanisms in small animal surgery. 2nd ed. Philadelphia: Lea & Febiger, 1993:306–310.
15. Tangner CH. Biliary surgery. In: Bojrab MJ, ed. Current techniques in small animal surgery. 3rd ed. Philadelphia: Lea & Febiger, 1990:299–303.

16. Gobien RP, Stanley JH, Soucek CD, et al. Routine preoperative biliary drainage: effect on management of obstructive jaundice. Radiology 1984;152:353–356.

17. O'Connor MJ. Mechanical biliary obstruction: a review of the multisystemic consequences of obstructive jaundice and their impact on perioperative morbidity and mortality. The Am Surg 1985;51:245–251.

18. Center SA. Pathophysiology and laboratory diagnosis of liver disease. In: Ettinger SJ, ed. Textbook of veterinary internal medicine. 3rd ed. Philadelphia: WB Saunders, 1989:1421–1478.

19. Tams TR. Liver disease: surgical considerations. In: Bojrab MJ, ed. Current techniques in small animal surgery. 3rd ed. Philadelphia: Lea & Febiger, 1990:292–297.

20. Hunt DR, Allison MEM, Prentice CRM, et al. Endotoxemia, disturbance of coagulation, and obstructive jaundice. Am J Surg 1982;144(3):325–329.

21. Caridi JG, Hawkins IF Jr, Hawkins MC. Single-step placement of a self-retaining "accordion" catheter. Am J Radiol 1984;143:337–340.

22. Gazzaniga GM, Faggioni A, Bagarolo C, et al. Percutaneous transhepatic biliary drainage: twelve years' experience. Hepatogastroenterology 1991;38:154–159.

23. Carrasco CH, Zornoza J, Bechtel WJ. Malignant biliary obstruction: complications of percutaneous biliary drainage. Radiology 1984;152:343–346.

24. Mueller PR, vanSonnenberg E, Ferrucci JT Jr. Percutaneous biliary drainage: technical and catheter-related problems in 200 procedures. Am J Radiol 1982;138:17–23.

25. McPherson GAD, Benjamin IS, Habib NA, et al. Percutaneous transhepatic drainage in obstructive jaundice: advantages and problems. Br J Surg 1982;69:261–264.

26. Barth KH. Percutaneous biliary drainage for high obstruction. Radiol Clin North Am 1990;28(6):1223–1235.

18

DIAPHRAGM

Traumatic Diaphragmatic Hernia

Jamie R. Bellah

In small animals, diaphragmatic injury may occur by direct or indirect trauma (1, 2). Indirect injury to the diaphragm is the most common cause of diaphragmatic hernia and originates from blunt trauma to the abdominal cavity (1). Pleuroperitoneal pressure gradients vary from 7 to 20 cm H_2O during quiet inspiration and can increase to over 100 cm H_2O during maximal inspiration (3). Blunt trauma results in a sudden increase in abdominal pressure, and if it is concomitant with an open glottis, the resultant pleuroperitoneal pressure gradient increases dramatically and domes and tears the diaphragm (1, 2). Prolapse of abdominal viscera is expected to occur simultaneously with the tear. Direct injury to the diaphragm is rare, but it may be inflicted by gunshot, bite, or stab wounds (4, 5). Iatrogenic injury to the diaphragm may occur by inappropriate abdominal incision cranial to the xiphoid process or inappropriate placement of a chest drain (5).

Loss of continuity of the diaphragm does not necessarily result in severe respiratory distress (6). The cause of respiratory impairment associated with diaphragmatic hernia is multifactorial (6). Hypovolemic shock, chest wall trauma, pleural fluid or air, pulmonary contusions, and cardiac dysfunction all contribute to hypoventilation (6). Rib fractures and an associated flail chest cause mechanical dysfunction. Pulmonary compliance is decreased by pleural fluid, by the presence of abdominal organs in the thorax, or by pneumothorax. Pulmonary hemorrhage, edema, and atelectasis reduce total lung capacity, vital capacity, and functional resid-

ual capacity. Myocardial contusion may decrease cardiac output and, in conjunction with impaired ventilation, may result in tissue hypoxia. Pain resulting from chest and abdominal contusion and accompanying injuries causes voluntary restriction of motion (thoracic excursion) (6).

Diagnosis

Thoracic injury occurs in 39% of small animals with musculoskeletal trauma, and 2% have diaphragmatic hernia (7). Therefore, animals examined for blunt traumatic injury must be evaluated for diaphragmatic injury. The average length of time between traumatic injury and the diagnosis of diaphragmatic hernia is several weeks, but it ranges from hours to 6 years (8–10). Young male dogs have the highest incidence of diaphragmatic hernia (8, 10). Clinical signs of diaphragmatic hernia vary from no overt signs to severe respiratory compromise and shock (8, 11–13). Dyspnea is the most common clinical sign and relates multifactorily to the presence of shock, chest wall dysfunction, the presence of air, fluid, or viscera in the pleural space, decreased pulmonary compliance, edema, and cardiovascular dysfunction (8, 11–13). Cardiac arrhythmias are present in 12% of small animals with diaphragmatic hernia (8). Other common clinical signs include muffled heart and lung sounds, thoracic borborygmi, a strong apex beat ausculted on one side of the chest because of shifting of the apex to one side, and an asymmetric decreased caudoventral resonance when the thoracic cavity is percussed (5). A "tucked up" abdomen is a rare finding (5, 14).

Lateral radiographs of the thorax show an incomplete diaphragmatic silhouette in 97% of animals with a diaphragm tear (15). In 61% of these animals, air-filled small intestinal loops are identified on the thoracic side of the diaphragm (15). Hydrothorax, which may be pleural effusion or hemothorax depending on the chronicity of the hernia, may be identified and may obscure the diaphragm. Repeated radiography after thoracocentesis is advisable, but it may not show a diaphragmatic hernia definitively (15). Ultrasonographic evaluation is useful to identify abdominal viscera on the thoracic side of the diaphragm, especially in the presence of pleural fluid because it enhances sonographic evaluation (16). Ultrasound can show abdominal organs, can differentiate organs such as the spleen or liver from pleural fluid, and can sometimes demonstrate the defect in the diaphragm (16). Cytologic evaluation of pleural fluid in patients with acute hernias usually reveals hemorrhage, whereas in a chronic diaphragmatic hernia, a modified serosanguineous transudate is identified (5).

Alternative techniques to attempt to confirm the presence or absence of a diaphragmatic hernia include barium administration (1.0 mL/kg) to verify herniation of a portion of the gastrointestinal tract, pneumoperitoneography, and positive-contrast peritoneography (using 1 to 2 mL/kg of an aqueous tri-iodidinated contrast agent) (17, 18). These techniques are done only if, in the clinician's judgment, the patient can tolerate the stress of such a procedure and if plain radiographs and ultrasonography are nondiagnostic (15). Moreover, when viscera or omentum plugs the diaphragm defect, a false-negative evaluation is made (19, 20).

Ventilation can be evaluated by arterial blood gas analysis and noninvasive pulse oximetry (21, 22). These techniques may identify ventilation–perfusion inequalities (alveolar–arterial oxygen difference) (14) and physiologic shunting (estimated shunt equation) (14). Impaired ventilation (hemoglobin saturation) can be determined using pulse oximeter probes attached to the lip in the awake dog (23). The ear, tail, and toe may also be used effectively in awake dogs if good contact is maintained across the vascular beds (23).

Timing of Surgical Intervention

The timing of anesthesia and surgical correction of diaphragmatic injury has a profound effect on the outcome of treatment (5, 14). Approximately 15% of small animals with diaphragmatic hernia die before surgery (5). Animals with diaphragmatic herniorrhaphy performed within the first 24 hours after injury have the highest mortality rate (33%) (8). When surgery must be done depends on the extent of the initial cardiopulmonary dysfunction, the presence or absence of organ entrapment, and the degree of compromised pulmonary function (14). Diaphragmatic herniorrhaphy may become an emergency procedure if aggres-

sive supportive care cannot stabilize respiratory function (9). Acute dilatation of a herniated stomach and strangulated bowel are situations in which emergency surgery may be indicated (9). Gastric outflow obstruction, metabolic alkalosis, and hypokalemia have been reported in a dog with diaphragmatic hernia (24). A herniated stomach can rapidly distend from aerophagia, decreasing pulmonary compliance, and can compress the caudal vena cava, decreasing venous return, resulting in a vicious cycle that can be rapidly fatal (5). A herniated parenchymal organ such as the spleen may tear as it passes through the diaphragm; the result may be acute hemothorax and a patient that may deteriorate rapidly after an initial response to shock therapy. Most small animals with diaphragmatic hernia can be stabilized over 24 to 72 hours because the mere presence of a diaphragmatic hernia is not an indication for emergency surgery (8). For example, thoracic injuries such as pulmonary contusion improve dramatically in 24 to 48 hours, and pneumothorax may be managed by thoracostomy tube insertion. The goal of initial management is to improve the cardiorespiratory status of the patient, to improve its capability of tolerating the stress of anesthesia and surgery.

Anesthesia

Anesthesia in the patient with diaphragmatic hernia is induced with as little stress as possible. Intravenous catheterization, appropriate intravenous fluid administration (crystalloid or colloid), and cardiorespiratory monitoring are important. Premedication with a phenothiazine or a narcoleptic combination may relieve apprehension, but care is taken not to use cardiorespiratory depressing drugs when possible if the decompensation of the patient's status is predictable (8). Mask induction of anesthesia is avoided because it is stressful and does not allow control of respiration or provide the ability to assist ventilation (8). An ultrashort-acting barbiturate or propofol is used because it allows rapid induction of anesthesia, quick intubation, and near-immediate control of ventilation with assistance or by a mechanical ventilator (25). Isoflurane is preferred for maintenance of anesthesia because a surgical plane of anesthesia is attained more quickly, it is associated with decreased recovery time, it subjects the patient to less cardiac depression, and it does not sensitize the myocardium to arrhythmias (8). Halothane is also acceptable. Nitrous oxide is avoided because it may diffuse rapidly into an air-filled pleural space or into gas-filled loops of bowel and thereby potentially may worsen hypoxemia. Nitrous oxide also may cause diffusion hypoxia during recovery if care is not used when anesthetic agents are discontinued (8).

Ventilation assistance is important as soon as anesthesia is induced because of decreased pulmonary compliance secondary to the presence of air, fluid, or abdominal viscera within the pleural space (5, 14). Assisted ventilation should not exceed 20 cm H$_2$O, to limit potential barotrauma from pulmonary hyperinflation (8). Overinflation of the lungs during surgery may result in rupture of pulmonary parenchyma, intrapulmonary hemorrhage, plumonary edema, and, rarely, pneumothorax (26). Intraoperative elimination of atelectic areas subjects chronically atelectic lungs to mechanical and reperfusion injury (8, 26). In this situation, reperfusion of these collapsed vascular channels disrupts capillary integrity and causes fluid to leak into the interstitium; reexpansion pulmonary edema may result within several hours after surgery (5, 8, 27) Atelectic areas that do not inflate with 20 cm H$_2$O gradually reexpand over several hours with a continual negative pleural pressure of 10 cm H$_2$O (28). Preoperative treatment with glucocorticoids and antihistamines has been recommended (based on experimental evidence) to inhibit the effects of mediators of pulmonary vascular permeability that are activated by lung injury in patients with chronic diaphragmatic hernia, but care is advised because antihistamines may potentiate hypotension (6, 8).

Surgical Approach

A ventral midline celiotomy extending from the xiphoid process to a point caudal to the umbilicus is used to provide initial exposure for diaphragmatic herniorrhaphy. The incision should be large enough to allow exploration of the abdominal cavity. This exposure allows access to all regions of the diaphragm. Most diaphragmatic tears are muscular and are located ventrally and may favor either the right (12) or left side (10, 29). The liver, small intestine, and pancreas are most commonly prolapsed into the thoracic cavity when the diaphragm defect is on the right side, whereas the stomach, spleen, and small intestine prolapse on the left side (5). The surgeon must examine the entire diaphragm because more than one tear may occur (14). Exploration of the abdominal cavity is indicated because injury to other abdominal organs may be present and treatable concomitantly. Should additional exposure be required to retrieve abdominal viscera adhered to structures within the thoracic cavity, surgical exposure can be improved by enlargement of the rent in the diaphragm, by paracostal extension of the celiotomy, and by caudal midline sternotomy (Fig. 18.1). Lateral thoracotomy is not a practical or appropriate method to expose a diaphragmatic tear because it requires preoperative knowledge of the extent and side of the hernia, and the approach does not allow exploration of the abdomen (8, 14). Lateral thoracostomy also decreases thoracic compliance from pain and thus may contribute to hypoventilation (8).

Strangulated viscera found within the thoracic cavity should be resected in situ without reestablishing circulation if possible (8). By doing so, prevention of toxemia from bacterial endotoxins and exotoxins and the by-products of tissue autolysis is possible (8). Viscera may be incarcerated, strangulated, or obstructed after passing through a diaphragmatic hernia and the systemic effects such as gastrointestinal obstruction or extrahepatic bile duct obstruction may occur acutely or chronically (5, 14, 30). Chronic strangulation of a liver lobe results in a modified serosanguinous transudate approximately 30% of the time (5).

Before closing the diaphragm defect, a chest drain is placed from a paramedian stab incision, it is tunneled subcutaneously, and it is inserted intercostally into the pleural space (Fig. 18.2). The advantages of placing the chest drain early are that the drain can be placed accurately with direct visualization and, after herniorrhaphy, control of the pleural space is obtained for the duration necessary. The diaphragm closure need not be airtight because the chest drain provides control. Should an inadvertent tear in the lung parenchyma occur during herniorrhaphy, the presence of the tube will detect it and allow simple management. The chest drain is managed for a short time, usually 8 to 12 hours, or until the volume of air or fluid is 2 to 3 mL/kg per day or less. Air can be aspirated from the pleural space as the last suture is tied, but if a parenchymal tear is leaking air or if the herniorrhaphy is not airtight, hypoventilation may result.

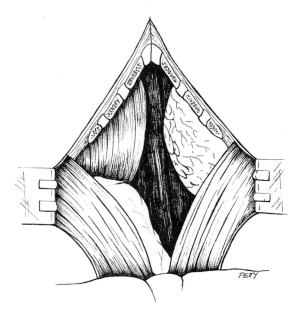

Fig. 18.1. In this view, the midline celiotomy has been extended to expose the caudal thorax by caudal midline sternotomy. The diaphragm is incised to the hernia defect to allow blunt and sharp dissection to release abdominal viscera from restriction thoracic adhesions.

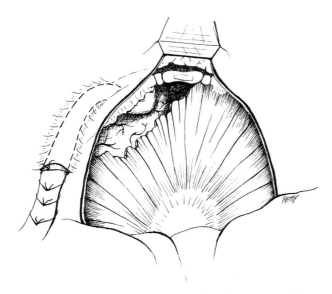

Fig. 18.2. In this view, a chest drain has been inserted from a paramedian incision, tunneled over the costal arch, and placed within the pleural space under direct visualization before closing the diaphragmatic hernia.

Assessment of the wound margin of the diaphragm is important after viscera have been replaced into the abdominal cavity. Debridement of the wound margins is usually not necessary, but sutures should be placed through portions of the torn edge of the diaphragm that has an intact fascial surface to afford good suture holding strength. Chronic hernias that have produced scar tissue and collagen at the wound margins have good suture-holding strength, but the scar restricts the normal elasticity of the diaphragm. Paracostal incisions are usually sufficient to release the maturing scar tissue and to allow the elastic portions of the diaphragm to be advanced to close the defect.

The suture material and pattern used to appose the diaphragm depend largely on the surgeon's preference. Radial tears are apposed with simple continuous patterns or a combination of a horizontal mattress pattern oversewn with a simple continuous pattern. A single-layer simple continuous pattern is quickly completed, but it is susceptible to reherniation should the implant break. The surgeon should suture from the deepest portion of the tear toward the more superficial regions. Large tears or combined radial and paracostal tears may be apposed with several interrupted sutures to arrange apposition of the wound margins to minimize tension. Closure follows, using a simple continuous pattern (Fig. 18.3). Polypropylene, monofilament nylon, poliglecaprone Monocryl (Ethicon, Inc., Somerville, NJ), polydioxanone, and polyglyconate are sutures materials acceptable for herniorrhaphy. Paracostal tears are sutured using simple continuous patterns by suturing the diaphragmatic wound edge to paracos-

tal fascia or encircling the ribs. Mattress patterns that encircle the costal arch or paracostal muscle fascia may also be used. Preplacing sutures sometimes facilitates closure of chronic diaphragmatic defects. Use of 3–0 and 2–0 suture for small cats and dogs and 2–0 and 1–0 for larger dogs is recommended. Larger sizes are appropriate for giant breeds.

Closure of large diaphragm defects sometimes requires mobilization of the diaphragm or other tissues (5, 9, 14). Paracostal incisions may be made to release the diaphragm from restrictive scar tissue, and the diaphragm may be advanced cranially to allow apposition ventrally (Fig. 18.4) (5, 14). Muscle flaps originating from the transversus abdominis muscle have been used to close diaphragm defects (31, 32). In chronic hernias, the liver capsule may be thickened in response to incarceration, and if the liver lobe is viable and can be oriented to cover the defect in the diaphragm partially without tension, it can be used to close or partially close the defect (33). Autologous fascia and omentum has also been used to close large diaphragm defects or small defects that remain after mobilization of the diaphragm (34, 35). Synthetic materials, such as polypropylene mesh or silicone rubber sheeting, may also be used (32, 36, 37). If a rough synthetic material such as polypropylene mesh is used, it is advisable to mobilize omentum to create an "omental envelope" that provides angiogenesis to aid incorporation of the prosthetic material and to protect the adjacent soft tissues from the mesh surfaces (Fig. 18.5). Sometimes, the time and trauma required to mobilize muscular pedicles, especially in small kittens and puppies, result in significant hemorrhage and can jeopardize the life of the patient. Prosthetic materials may be a better option if the potential to use autologous tissue may injure the patient.

Abdominal closure is accomplished routinely in patients with acute hernias. In those with chronic her-

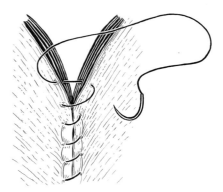

Fig. 18.3. A simple continuous pattern may be used to appose edges of the diaphragm. A fascial layer is included to ensure that encircling tissue is strong enough to hold sutures.

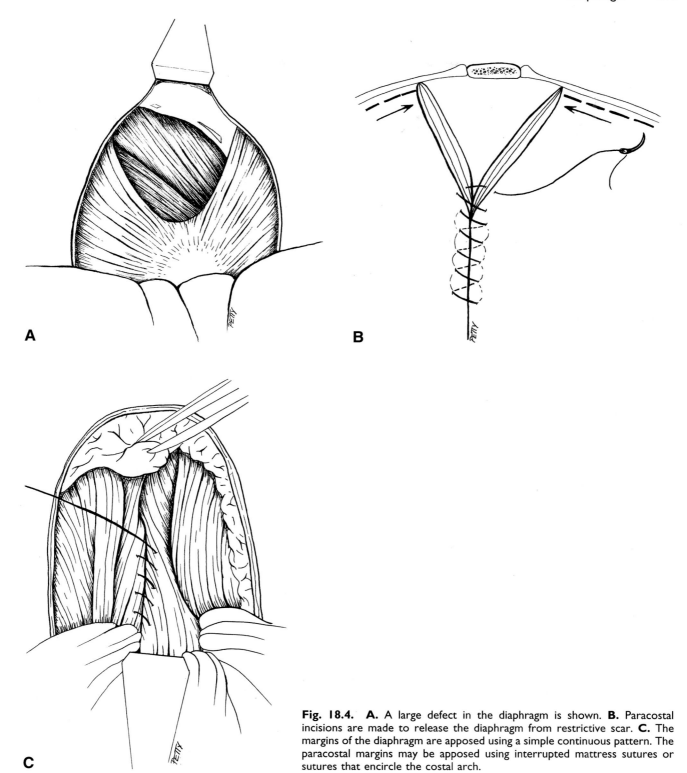

A

B

C

Fig. 18.4. A. A large defect in the diaphragm is shown. **B.** Paracostal incisions are made to release the diaphragm from restrictive scar. **C.** The margins of the diaphragm are apposed using a simple continuous pattern. The paracostal margins may be apposed using interrupted mattress sutures or sutures that encircle the costal arch.

nias, accommodation of the viscera within the peritoneal cavity may be difficult because of the contracted abdominal musculature. The abdominal musculature relaxes over time (14). Increased intraperitoneal pres-sure may occur. If intra-abdominal pressure increases over 13 cm H_2O, hepatic and portal venous flow may decrease (39). Intra-abdominal pressure (30 cm H_2O) in one dog necessitated surgical decompression (39).

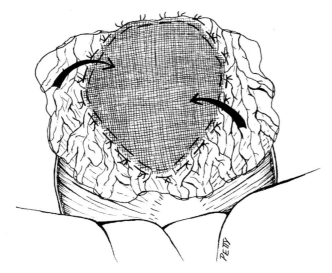

Fig. 18.5. In this view, a large defect in the diaphragm is covered with an omental flap intitially. Polypropylene mesh is placed over the omentum and is secured to the margins of the diaphragm defect with mattress sutures. The remainder of the omental pedicle is sutured over the abdominal side of the mesh.

Postoperative Care

Evacuation of air from the pleural space should be done carefully in patients with atelectasis that does not reinflate with inflation pressures of 20 cm H_2O, such as may occur with chronic hernias. Air may be evacuated in these patients slowly over a 12-hour period by using periodic evacuations or by using a Pleurivac (water seal) with no greater than a negative pleural pressure of 10 cm H_2O.

Oxygen supplementation can be administered during recovery by mask, nasal insufflation or by placing the patient in an oxygen cage (40% oxygen) (8). Nasal insufflation allows the same degree of oxygen supplementation, but it offers the advantage of allowing frequent and close access to the patient should it be required. Heart rate, capillary refill time, mucous membrane color, pulse strength and character, and respiratory rate should be monitored. Direct or indirect blood pressure monitoring, blood gas analysis, and pulse oximetry may also be done.

Analgesics are administered to comfort the patient and to ease apprehension during recovery. Morphine, 0.1 to 0.2 mg/kg, may be used subcutaneously without significant respiratory depression (5). If a caudal median sternotomy is performed, intrapleural bupivicane may be administered for short-term local analgesia.

Prognosis

Death from diaphragmatic hernia is usually attributed to hypoventilation resulting from lung compression, shock, cardiac dysrrhythmias, and multiorgan failure (5). The survival rate in dogs varies from 52 to 88% (8–10, 40, 41). Approximately 1 in 3 dogs undergoing repair within the first 24 hours after trauma dies, as opposed to 1 in 10 dogs in which repair is delayed for 1 to 3 weeks (5). In dogs that had chronic diaphragmatic hernias repaired more than 1 year after trauma, 73% of the deaths were attributed to a problem unrelated to the hernia (5).

References

1. Dronen SC. Disorders of the chest wall and diaphragm. Emerg Med Clin North Am 1983;1:449.
2. Ticer JW, Brown SG. Thoracic trauma. In: Ettinger SJ, ed. Veterinary internal medicine. Philadelphia: WB Saunders, 1975.
3. Marchand P. A study of the forces productive of gastro-oesophageal regurgitation and herniation through the diaphragmatic hiatus. Thorax 1957;12:189.
4. Bellenger CR, et al. Bile pleuritis in a dog. J Small Anim Pract 1975;16:575.
5. Johnson KA. Diaphragmatic, pericardial, and hiatal hernia. In: Slatter DH, ed. Textbook of small animal surgery. 2nd ed. Philadelphia: WB Saunders, 1985:485.
6. Altura BM, Lefer AM, Schumer W. Handbook of shock and trauma. New York: Raven Press, 1983.
7. Spackman CJA, et al. Thoracic wall and pulmonary trauma in dogs sustaining fractures as a result of motor vehicle accidents. J Am Vet Med Assoc 1984;185:975.
8. Boudrieau RJ, Muir WE. Pathophysiology of traumatic diaphragmatic hernia in dogs. Compend Contin Educ Pract Vet 1987;9:379–385.
9. Bjorling DE. Management of thoracic trauma. In: Birchard S, Sherding S, eds. Saunders manual of small animal practice. Philadelphia: WB Saunders, 1994:593–599.
10. Stokhof AA. Diagnosis and treatment of acquired diaphragmatic hernia by thoracotomy in 49 dogs and 72 cats. Vet Q 1986; 8:177.
11. Wilson GP, Muir WW. Diaphragmatic hernia. In: Bojrab MJ, ed. Current techniques in small animal surgery. 2nd ed. Philadelphia: Lea & Febiger, 1983.
12. Wilson GP, Hayes HM. Diaphragmatic hernia in the dog and cat: a 25-year overview. Semin Vet Med Surg (Small Anim) 1986;1:318–326.
13. Wilson GP, Newton CD, Burt JK. A review of 116 diaphragmatic hernias in dogs and cats. J Am Vet Med Assoc 1971;159:1142–1145.
14. Boudrieau RJ. Traumatic diaphragmatic hernia. In: Bojrab MJ, ed. Current techniques in small animal surgery. 3rd ed. Philadelphia: Lea & Febiger, 1990:309–314.
15. Sullivan M, Lee R. Radiological features of 80 cases of diaphragmatic rupture. J Small Anim Pract 1989;30:561.
16. Stowater JL, Lamb CR. Ultrasonography of noncardiac thoracic diseases in small animals. J Am Vet Med Assoc 1989;195:514.
17. Myer W. Diagnostic imaging of the respiratory system. In: Birchard S, Sherding S, eds. Saunders manual of small animal practice. Philadelphia: WB Saunders, 1994:534–535.
18. Punch PI, Slatter DH. Diaphragmatic hernias. In: Slatter DH, ed. Textbook of small animal surgery. Philadelphia: WB Saunders, 1985.
19. Evans SM, Biery DN. Congenital peritoneopericardial diaphragmatic hernia in the dog and cat: a literature review and 17 additional case histories. Vet Radiol 1980;21:108.
20. Stickle RL. Positive-contrast celiography (peritoneography) for the diagnosis of diaphragmatic hernia in dogs and cats. J Am Vet Med Assoc 1984;185:295.
21. Kolata RJ, Kraut NH, Johnston DE. Patterns of trauma in urban dogs and cats: a study of 1000 cases. J Am Vet Med Assoc 1974;164:499–502.
22. Shapiro BA, Harrison RA, Walton JR. Clinical application of

blood gases. 3rd ed. Chicago: New York Medical Publishers, 1982.

23. Huss BT, Anderson MA, Branson KR, et al. Evaluation of pulse oximeter probes and probe placement in healthy dogs. J Am Anim Hosp Assoc 1995;31:9–14.

24. Roe SC, Smith CW, Stowater JL. Diaphragmatic hernia producing gastric outflow obstruction, metabolic alkalosis, and hypokalemia in a dog. Compend Contin Educ Pract Vet 1986:12:943.

25. Bednarski RM. Diaphragmatic hernia: anesthetic considerations. Semin Vet Med Surg (Small Anim) 1986;1:256–258.

26. Baeza OR, et al. Pulmonary hyperinflation: a form of barotrauma during mechanical ventilation. J Thorac Cardovasc Surg 1975;70:790.

27. Sewell RW, et al. Experimental evaluation of reexpansion pulmonary edema. Ann Thorac Surg 1978;26:126.

28. Lenaghan R, et al. Hemodynamic alterations associated with expansion rupture of the lung. Arch Surg 1969;99:339.

29. Al-Nakeeb SM. Canine and feline traumatic diaphragmatic hernias. J Am Vet Med Assoc 1971;159:1422.

30. Donald CL, et al. Diaphragmatic rupture and biliary tract damage in a dog. J Small Anim Pract 1985;26:61.

31. Carb A. Diaphragmatic hernia in the dog and cat. Vet Clin North Am 1975;5:477–484.

32. Helphrey ML. Abdominal flap graft for repair of chronic diaphragmatic hernia in the dog. J Am Vet Med Assoc 1982; 181:791–793.

33. Neville WE, Clowes GHA. Congenital absence of hemidiaphragm and use of a lobe of liver in its surgical correction. Arch Surg 1954;69:282.

34. Schairer BE, Keeley JL. Experimental use of homologous fascia lata to repair diaphragmatic defects in dogs. Surg Gynecol Obstet 1957;105:565.

35. Bright RM, Thatcher HL. The formation of an omental pedicle flap and its experimental use in the repair of a diaphragmatic rent in the dog. J Am Anim Hosp Assoc 1982;18:283–289.

36. Rosenkrantz JG, Cotton EK. Replacement of left hemidiaphragm by a pedicled abdominal muscular flap. J Thorac Cardiovasc Surg 1964;48:912.

37. Touloukian RJ. A "new" diaphragm following prosthetic repair of experimental hemidiaphragmatic defects in the pup. Ann Surg 1978;187:47.

38. Reed JH, Pennock PW. Concurrent ventral and pericardial diaphragmatic hernias in 2 dogs. Mod Vet Pract 1971;52:47–49.

39. Conzemius MG, Sammarco JL, Holt DE, et al. Clinical determination of preoperative and postoperative intra-abdominal pressures in dogs. Vet Surg 1995;24;195.

40. Downs MC, Bjorling DE. Traumatic diaphragmatic hernias: a review of 1674 cases. Vet Surg 1987;16:87.

41. Wilson GP, et al. A review of 116 diaphragmatic hernias in dogs and cats. J Am Vet Med Assoc 1971;159:1142.

Congenital Diaphragmatic Hernia

Jamie R. Bellah

About 5 to 10% of diaphragmatic hernias are congenital (1–3). Congenital pleuroperitoneal hernia (4–7) and congenital peritoneopericardial diaphragmatic hernia (8–14) have been reported in puppies and kittens. Pleuroperitoneal hernias are thought to develop when the pleuroperitoneal membrane fails to fuse with the pleuroperitoneal canal during development of the diaphragm. This defect is proposed to be heritable by an autosomal recessive mechanism (6, 15). Congenital peritoneopericardial diaphragmatic hernias are thought to be the result of a uterine accident during embryogenesis and are not heritable (11, 16, 17). The ventral diaphragmatic defect is believed to result from faulty development of the septum transversum (16). Because congenital peritoneopericardial diaphragmatic hernia may or may not be associated with cranioventral abdominal defects, some of these hernias are not easily identified at birth and some are obvious (11).

Clinical Signs

Clinical signs of congenital diaphragmatic hernia may be identified at any age. Overt structural defects such as cranioventral abdominal hernia result in an earlier diagnosis, often before 2 years of age. The diagnosis may be incidentally noted while radiographing the thorax for another reason, or it may be found at necropsy (10, 11, 13). Respiratory signs including dyspnea, tachypnea, coughing, and wheezing are common, but many nonspecific signs such as vomiting and diarrhea may be identified (18). Auscultation of the thorax may reveal muffled heart sounds, a heart murmur, and abnormal position of the apex beat (11, 18). An electrocardiogram may reveal electrical alternans or may be normal (18). Radiographs of the thorax usually reveal an ovoid cardiac silhouette that joins the ventral diaphragm ventrally. Gas-filled loops of bowel may be seen over the cardiac silhouette (13, 18). Other diagnostic procedures that may be used include administration of contrast material into the upper gastrointestinal tract, pneumoperitoneography or contrast peritoneography, and ultrasonography (9). Ultrasonography from the right fifth intercostal space may reveal cardiac tamponade if liver lobes herniate into the pericardial sac and produce an effusion (9, 18).

Congenital Diaphragmatic Hernia With Cranioventral Abdominal Defects

Congenital cranioventral abdominal wall defects in puppies occur cranial to the umbilicus, but they may extend caudally toward and to the umbilicus (Fig. 18.6). The cranial extent of the defect is often in the area of the commonly absent xiphoid process. Although cranioventral abdominal hernias are not frequently encountered in small animal practice, the clinician must recognize that the abnormality differs from the much more common umbilical hernia. Cranioventral abdominal hernias are commonly associated with four other defects, which are recognized as a syndrome in humans and which have been reported in dogs (11, 12). Cranioventral abdominal hernia, failure of caudal sternal fusion, intracardiac defects (most

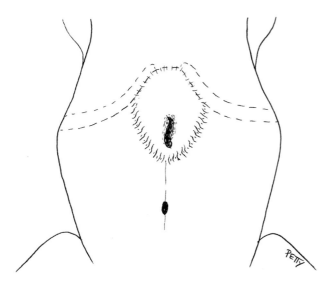

Fig. 18.6. Drawing of the cranial abdominal region of a male puppy with a cranioventral abdominal hernia. The position of the hernia is cranial to the umbilicus and is centered in the region of the xiphoid process.

commonly ventricular septal defect) and caudoventral pericardial defect may commonly accompany a congenital diaphragmatic hernia (11, 12). These defects may occur in varying degrees, depending on the individual dog, and they do not always appear together. Commonly, the heart has no apparent abnormality.

This pentalogy of defects has been noted in several breeds, including cocker spaniels, Weimaraners, dachshunds, and collies, and I have seen it in two kittens. This syndrome is similar in some respects to thoracoabdominal ectopia cordis in human infants and has been termed peritoneopericardial diaphragmatic hernia in small animals (13, 16). Peritoneopericardial diaphragmatic hernias are not always associated with cranioventral abdominal wall defects or intracardiac defects, and they are often difficult to detect unless clinical signs are obvious (usually exercise intolerance or a restrictive breathing pattern).

The sternum normally fuses from cranial to caudal in dogs, and the abdominal wall fuses from caudal to cranial. The ventral portion of the diaphragm is

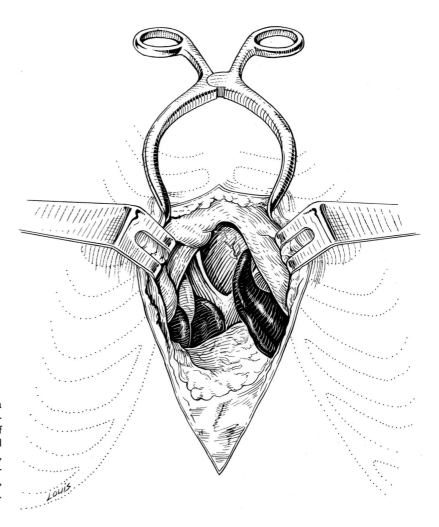

Fig. 18.7. Drawing of the surgeon's view of a congenital diaphragmatic hernia before surgical correction. Notice the flared costal arches, absence of a xiphiod process, and a smooth-bordered V-shaped diaphragmatic defect. (From Bellah JR, Whitton DL, Ellison GW, et al. Surgical correction of concomitant cranioventral abdominal wall, caudal sternal, diaphragmatic, and pericardial defects in young dogs. J Am Vet Med Assoc 1989;195:1722.)

thought to originate from the septum transversum, which develops at the same time as cardiac septation; therefore, it seems reasonable that disruption of fetal development at this particular time could cause defects in both regions. Dogs do not have a communication between the pericardial cavity and the peritoneal cavity, so if such a communication is present congenitally, it is due to a defect in development. The pericardium normally attaches to the ventral diaphragm by the sternopericardial ligament and visceral mediastinum. Communication of the peritoneal and pericardial cavities is not always obvious in this defect.

In human beings, these defects are attributed to a uterine accident and are not considered heritable. Parents with children affected with thoracoabdominal ectopia cordis have gone on to have anatomically normal children thereafter. No data support heritability of the defects in dogs or cats.

Surgical Correction

Surgical repair of the cranioventral abdominal defect and the diaphragmatic defect can be done early (I have performed such operations on animals as young as 7

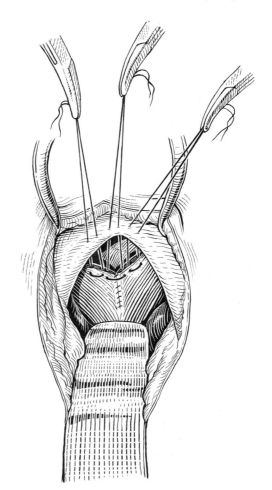

Fig. 18.9. When placement of the continuous suture is complete, three horizontal mattress sutures are placed to close the remaining defect between the diaphragm and the costal arch. (From Bellah JR, Whitton DL, Ellison GW, et al. Surgical correction of concomitant cranioventral abdominal wall, caudal sternal, diaphragmatic, and pericardial defects in young dogs. J Am Vet Med Assoc 1989;195:1722.)

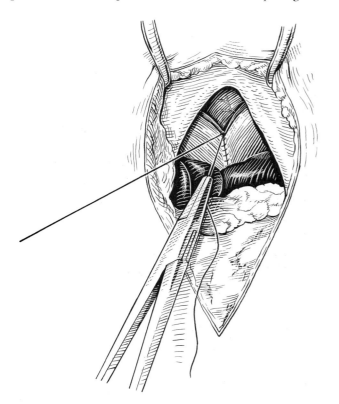

Fig. 18.8. After incising the fascia on the abdominal side of the diaphragmatic defect, a simple continuous suture pattern of 3–0 polypropylene is used to appose the crura of the diaphragm. (From Bellah JR, Whitton DL, Ellison GW, et al. Surgical correction of concomitant cranioventral abdominal wall, caudal sternal, diaphragmatic, and pericardial defects in young dogs. J Am Vet Med Assoc 1989;195:1722.)

weeks of age), usually between 8 and 12 weeks of age. The puppies are usually masked with isoflurane to induce and maintain general anesthesia unless they have significant respiratory restriction. In the latter example, anesthesia may be induced with propofol with prompt intubation, so ventilation may be carefully assisted. All puppies with these defects benefit by some assistance with ventilation because of the space-occupying abdominal viscera within their caudal mediastinum and/or pericardial sac (12, 19).

Surgical correction of the defects follows a midline abdominal incision that allows identification of the triangular diaphragmatic defect, the pericardial defect, and the flared, unfused caudal sternebrae (Figs. 18.7 to 8.10). In most puppies, the diaphragm defect can be closed by using a simple continuous pattern from the dorsalmost aspect of the defect and continuing in a ventral direction (toward the sternal defect). When

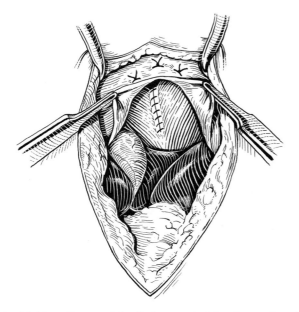

Fig. 18.10. Closure of the diaphragmatic defect is complete after the mattress sutures are tied. (From Bellah JR, Whitton DL, Ellison GW, et al. Surgical correction of concomitant cranioventral abdominal wall, caudal sternal, diaphragmatic, and pericardial defects in young dogs. J Am Vet Med Assoc 1989;195:1722.)

the diaphragm apposition becomes tense, the suture can be tied, and mattress sutures can be preplaced from the diaphragm to the costal arch to complete the separation of the thoracic and abdominal cavities. The pleural cavity does not have to be invaded or opened when this defect is closed. Accidental opening of the pleural cavity by dissection or by needle penetration is possible while suturing. After the mattress sutures are tied, the abdominal defect can usually be apposed with simple interrupted nonabsorbable suture, followed by routine subcutaneous and skin apposition. When closure of the defects as described is routine, young puppies and kittens recover quickly and often do not require specialized postoperative care, other than that appropriate for pediatric patients.

Sometimes, the diaphragmatic defect is too wide to appose without excessive tension. Three methods can be used to alleviate this problem. First, the caudal sternal costal arch can be apposed by encircling with nonabsorbable suture. This can effectively decrease the distance between right and left edges of the diaphragm and therefore can reduce the tension on the closure. The pliability of the unfused costal arch in the young puppies and kittens makes this maneuver possible. If caudal sternal apposition does not narrow the defect to a size that can be apposed without tension, the pericardium can be incised cranial to the diaphragm and flaps can be created to close the defect (20). A free graft of pericardium may also be used to close the defect (20). The third method is insertion of polypropylene mesh to separate the body cavities. Omentum

can be mobilized and sutured to each side of the implant to cover its surface.

Congenital diaphragmatic hernias that are not associated with ventral abdominal wall defects and that lack obvious clinical signs may not be diagnosed until much later in the pet's life, often when the animal is radiographed for another reason. Correction of all congenital diaphragmatic hernias may not be necessary, especially hernias diagnosed in old animals with no clinical signs of abdominal viscera (usually omentum) in the caudal mediastinum or the pericardial sac. However, dogs or cats with clinical signs of congenital diaphragmatic hernia that are adults when the diagnosis is made are much more likely to have intrathoracic adhesions that prevent simple replacement of abdominal viscera into the abdominal cavity. These adhesions may require extension of the diaphragmatic defect or a caudal midline sternotomy to provide enough exposure for safe dissection within the caudal thorax. Closure of the diaphragmatic defect often requires releasing incisions from the paracostal arch to use the inherent elasticity of the diaphragm to facilitate apposition. Entrance into the pleural space is inevitable in most situations and requires assisted ventilation during surgery, chest drain insertion, and intensive postoperative management for 24 to 48 hours.

Postoperative management of pain in dogs that have undergone caudal midline sternotomy usually require analgesia. Morphine sulfate (0.1 to 0.5 mg/kg, administered subcutaneously every 4 to 6 hours) or butorphanol (0.1 to 0.5 mg/kg, administered subcutaneously every 4 to 6 hours) is used most frequently at our teaching hospital. Chest drains, when necessary, are usually removed 12 to 24 hours postoperatively.

References

1. Boudrieau SJ, Muir WW. Pathophysiology of traumatic diaphragmatic hernia in dogs. Compend Contin Educ Pract Vet 1987;9:379.
2. Wilson GP, Hayes HM. Diaphragmatic hernia in the dog and cat: a 25-year overview. Semin Vet Med Surg (Small Anim) 1986;1:318–326.
3. Wilson GP, Newton CD, Burt JK. A review of 116 diaphragmatic hernias in dogs and cats. J Am Vet Med Assoc 1971;159:1142–1145.
4. Noden DM, De Lahunta A. The embryology of domestic animals: developmental mechanisms and malformations. Baltimore: Williams & Wilkins, 1985.
5. Pass MA. Small intestines. In: Slatter DH, ed. Textbook of small animal surgery. Philadelphia: WB Saunders, 1985.
6. Feldman DB, et al. Congenital diaphragmatic hernia in neonatal dogs. J Am Vet Med Assoc 1968;153:942.
7. Keep JM. Congenital diaphragmatic hernia in a cat. Aust Vet J 1950;26:193.
8. Frye FL, Taylor DON. Pericardial and diaphragmatic defects in a cat. J Am Vet Med Assoc 1968;152:1507.
9. Hay WH, et al. Clinical, echocardiographic, and radiographic findings of peritoneopericardial diaphragmatic hernia in two dogs and a cat. J Am Vet Med Assoc 1989;195:1245.
10. Punch PI, Slatter DH. Diaphragmatic hernias. In Slatter DH, ed.

Textbook of small animal surgery. Philadelphia: WB Saunders, 1985.

11. Bellah JR, Spencer CP, Brown DJ, et al. Congenital cranioventral abdominal wall, caudal sternal, diaphragmatic, and pericardial, and intracardiac defects in cocker spaniel littermates. J Am Vet Med Assoc 1989;194:1741.

12. Bellah JR, Whitton DL, Ellison GW, et al. Surgical correction of concomitant cranioventral abdominal wall, caudal sternal, diaphragmatic, and pericardial defects in young dogs. J Am Vet Med Assoc 1989;195:1722.

13. Evans SM, Beiry DN. Congenital peritoneopericardial diaphragmatic hernia in the dog and cat: a literature review and 17 additional case histories. Vet Radiol 1980;21:108.

14. Eyster GJ, et al. Congenital pericardial diaphragmatic hernia and multiple cardiac defects in a litter of collies. J Am Vet Med Assoc 1977;170:516.

15. Valentine BA, et al. Canine congenital diaphragmatic hernia. J Vet Intern Med 1988;2:109.

16. Kaplan LC, et al. Ectopia cordis and cleft sternum: evidence for mechanical teratogenesis following rupture of the chorion or yolk sac. Am J Med Genet 1985;21:187.

17. Noden DM, De Lahunta A. The embryology of domestic animals: developmental mechanisms and malformations. Baltimore: Williams & Wilkins, 1985.

18. Thomas WP. Pericardial disorders. In: Ettinger SJ, ed. Textbook of veterinary internal medicine: diseases of the dog and cat. 3rd ed. Philadelphia: WB Saunders, 1989.

19. Bednarski RM. Diaphragmatic hernia: anesthetic considerations. Semin Vet Med Surg (Small Anim) 1986;1:256–258.

20. Johnson KA. Diaphragmatic, pericardial, and hiatal hernia. In: Slatter DH, ed. Textbook of small animal surgery. 2nd ed. Philadelphia: WB Saunders, 1985:485.

— 19 —

PERITONEUM AND ABDOMINAL WALL

Closure of Abdominal Incisions

Eberhard Rosin

The most common surgical procedure in small animal practice is incision and closure of the abdominal cavity. Although use of simple interrupted sutures to appose the peritoneum and all fascial layers is the traditional method to close an abdominal incision, a simple continuous suture pattern for a single-layer closure of the rectus fascia, without concern for the peritoneum, is a faster and safe alternative. In paralumbar grid incisions, a layered simple continuous closure is used if the patient's musculature is well developed.

Surgical Anatomy

The external leaf of the rectus sheath is composed of the aponeurosis of the external abdominal oblique muscle, most of the aponeurosis of the internal abdominal oblique muscle, and, near the pubis, a portion of the aponeurosis of the transversus abdominis muscle. The internal leaf of the rectus sheath consists of a portion of the aponeurosis of the internal abdominal oblique muscle, the aponeurosis of the transversus abdominis muscle, and the transversalis fascia. In the caudal third of the abdominal wall the internal leaf disappears. The aponeurosis of the internal abdominal oblique muscle joins the external leaf, and the rectus abdominis muscle is covered only by a thin continuation of the transversalis fascia and peritoneum (Fig. 19.1) (1).

Healing of the Peritoneum

The peritoneum is a layer of flat cells, cemented edge to edge at their intercellular margins. This mesothelial layer is supported by an underlying layer of areolar tissue that blends with the connective tissue of the transversalis fascia. Within the peritoneal cavity, a small amount of serous fluid contains freely floating cells including macrophages, desquamated mesothelial cells, and small lymphocytes (2).

During the first 2 days after wounding, the peritoneal defect is red, with a glistening, slightly irregular surface. During the next 5 or 6 days, the color fades gradually, the surface becomes smoother, and the defect develops a homogeneous, transparent gray sheen. Abdominal tissues slide readily over the defect. Gradually, this gray sheen becomes more opaque until, after 2 or 3 weeks, the area usually is indistinguishable from normal peritoneum. Milky streaks beneath the wound area, apparently resulting from scar formation, may remain. These changes occur simultaneously throughout the entire defect. Large wounds heal as rapidly as small wounds (2–4).

Microscopically, defects in the peritoneum are covered rapidly by macrophages, which are present in large number in the peritoneal fluid bathing the wound surface. The wound also is invaded by monocytes and histiocytes from blood and underlying exposed tissues. Cells from peritoneal fluid, blood, or underlying tissues differentiate to form fibroblasts, and the superficially located cells undergo metaplasia, gradually forming mesothelial cells. At the same time, intact mesothelial cells at the perimeter of the wound help in the repair by proliferation and migration. Small defects in the peritoneum are healed by proliferation of adjacent mesothelial cells, whereas large defects are

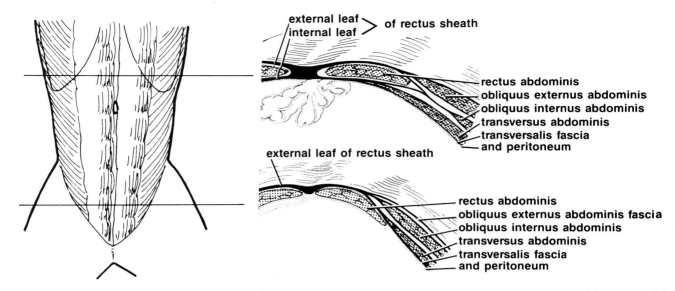

Fig. 19.1. Cross sections showing the anatomy of the sheath of the rectus abdominis muscle in the cranial and caudal portions of the abdominal wall.

covered by undifferentiated cells that then become mesothelial cells (2–4).

Peritoneal defects that are sutured have a higher incidence of adhesions than defects that are left open to heal. The stimulus for adhesion formation is not the peritoneal defect itself, but rather the ischemic tissue that results when edges of the defect are brought together by sutures.

No evidence, experimental or clinical, supports the contention that closure of the peritoneum is necessary for wound strength, to minimize postoperative dehiscence or hernia formation, or to minimize the development of adhesions. On the contrary, experimental and clinical studies in dogs, horses, and human patients indicate that suturing the peritoneum should be avoided to minimize the incidence of postoperative intra-abdominal adhesions (3–7).

Closure Alternatives

Closure of the Internal and External Leaves of the Rectus Sheath Versus Closure of the External Leaf Only

Closure of the paramedian abdominal incision by apposition of the internal and external leaves of the rectus sheath is traditional and has proved successful for years of clinical experience. However, closure of the internal leaf takes time and requires that the abdominal wall be manipulated to expose the internal leaf, which frequently retracts after incision. Studies have refuted the admonition that closing only the external leaf of the rectus sheath provides insufficient strength to the incision. In a biomechanical study of healing abdominal incisions in the dog, the strength of incisions closed by suturing the internal and external leaves of the rectus sheath and the strength of incisions closed by suturing the external leaf only were similar (8).

Simple Interrupted Versus Simple Continuous Suture Pattern

The traditional method to close an abdominal incision is simple interrupted sutures. The same incision can be closed more quickly using a simple continuous pattern, with no difference in wound healing. In a randomized prospective trial of 3135 human patients comparing continuous and interrupted abdominal midline incision closure, no difference was found in the incidence of wound dehiscence (9). In clinical use of simple continuous closure of abdominal incisions in over 5000 dogs and cats, the incidence of dehiscence is negligible.

Closure Techniques

Midline Incision

With an incision through the linea alba in the cranial two-thirds of the abdominal hall, fibers of the rectus abdominis muscle are not exposed, and the linea alba, including the peritoneum, can be apposed accurately by full-thickness sutures. An adequate portion of fascia must be included with each suture, and the falciform ligament must not be interspersed between the edges of the linea alba (Fig. 19.2). Although the traditional suture pattern is simple interrupted, a simple continuous pattern is a safe and faster alternative.

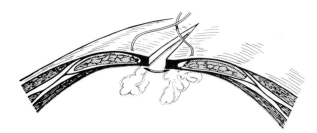

Fig. 19.2. Linea alba incision in the cranial two-thirds of the abdominal wall closed by a full-thickness suture placed carefully to avoid the falciform ligament.

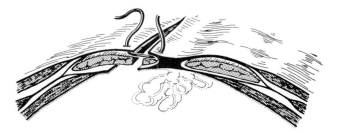

Fig. 19.4. Single-layer closure of only the external leaf of the rectus sheath. Care is taken to avoid interspersing rectus muscle between the edges of the rectus sheath.

In the caudal third of the abdominal wall, the width of the linea alba decreases. An incision here frequently exposes the rectus abdominis muscle. Because fibers of the rectus abdominis muscle have little holding power, sutures are not full thickness. Instead, sutures are placed to include an adequate portion of the external leaf of the rectus sheath on each side of the incision and to appose this fascia accurately without interspersion of rectus abdominis muscle (Fig. 19.3). The transversalis fascia and the peritoneum are not included in the sutures. Sutures traditionally are simple interrupted, but a simple continuous pattern is a satisfactory alternative.

Paramedian Incision

If the incision is paramedian in the cranial two-thirds of the abdominal wall, the linea alba will be on one side and the external and internal leaves of the rectus sheath and rectus abdominis muscle will be exposed on the other side, or on both sides of the incision, the internal and external leaves of the rectus sheath and rectus abdominis muscle will be exposed. The external leaf of rectus sheath is closed with a simple interrupted or continuous pattern. The internal leaf of the rectus sheath and the peritoneum are left unsutured (Fig. 19.4).

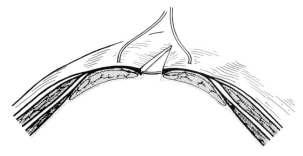

Fig. 19.3. Midline incision in the caudal third of the abdominal wall closed by a suture placed to appose the external leaf of the rectus sheath accurately.

A paramedian incision in the caudal third of the abdominal cavity is closed by suturing the rectus fascia in a simple interrupted or continuous pattern. The transversalis fascia and peritoneum have little strength and are not sutured.

Simple Continuous Suture Technique

Acceptable suture materials include polyglycolic acid, polyglactin 910, polydioxanone, polyglyconate, polypropylene, and nylon. Surgical gut, stainless wire, and multifilament nonabsorbable suture materials should not be used. Suture size is based on patient size: 3–0 suture material should be used for cats and small breed dogs, 2–0 for medium-sized dogs, 0 for large dogs, and 1 for giant breed dogs.

For a simple continuous suture pattern used in long incisions, more than one strand of suture material is used. Sutures are placed through the linea alba or through the external leaf of the rectus sheath, depending on patient size, and, include a 3- to 10-mm width of fascia on each side of the incision. Sutures are placed 5 to 10 mm apart, depending on the size of the animal. Care is taken to ensure edge-to-edge apposition of the fascia without interspersion of muscle. The internal leaf of the rectus sheath and the peritoneum are not included in the suture pattern.

All knots are placed with care. The first throw is tied with appositional tension only to ensure that tissue is not strangulated. Five additional square, flat throws are placed (10). After each throw is made, the ends of the suture are pulled tight to make the knot secure. The ends of the suture are cut 4 mm from the knot. As the continuous suture is placed, the rectus fascia must be loosely approximated, not apposed with tension. Wound strength is adversely affected if fascia is closed tightly (11).

Subcutaneous tissues are closed with the same suture materials, usually a smaller size, placed in simple continuous pattern. Care is taken to avoid cutting the rectus fascia suture during closure of the subcutaneous tissue. Skin is closed with 3–0 nonabsorbable suture placed in a simple interrupted or cruciate pattern, or skin staples are used.

References

1. Evans HE, Christensen GC. Miller's anatomy of the dog. 2nd ed. Philadelphia: WB Saunders, 1979.
2. Ellis H, Ashby EC, Mott TJ. Studies in peritoneal healing: a review. J Abdom Surg 1969;11:110.
3. Hubbard TB, et al. The pathology of peritoneal repair: its relation to the formation of adhesions. Ann Surg 1967;165:908.
4. Ellis H. The cause and prevention of postoperative intraperitoneal adhesions. Surg Gynecol Obstet 1971;133:497.
5. Karipineni RC, Wilk PJ, Danese CA. The role of the peritoneum in the healing of abdominal incisions. Surg Gynecol Obstet 1976;142:729.
6. Swanwick RA, Milne FJ. The non-suturing of parietal peritoneum in abdominal surgery of the horse. Vet Rec 1973;93:328.
7. Ellis H, Heddle R. Does the peritoneum need to be closed at laparotomy? Br J Surg 1977;64:733.
8. Rosin E, Richardson S. Effect of fascial closure technique on strength of healing abdominal incisions in the dog: a biomechanical study. Vet Surg 1987;16:269.
9. Fagniez P, Hay JM, Lacaine F, et al. Abdominal midline incision closure: a multicentric randomized prospective trial of 3,135 patients, comparing continuous vs interrupted polyglycolic acid sutures. Arch Surg 1985;120:1351.
10. Rosin E, Robinson GM. Knot security of suture materials. Vet Surg 1989;18:269.
11. Stone KI, vonFraunhofer JA, Masterson BJ. The biochemical effects of tight suture closure upon fascia. Surg Gynecol Obstet 1986;163:448.

Open Peritoneal Drainage for Peritonitis

Cathy L. Greenfield

Septic peritonitis is a condition of peritoneal inflammation associated with the presence of virulent bacteria. It is usually caused by rupture of one or more hollow visceral organs within the peritoneal cavity or by a wound that penetrates the abdominal body wall. When septic peritonitis is present, the peritoneal cavity essentially becomes an abscess cavity with no means of drainage to the outside. Septic peritonitis is diagnosed by performing a peritoneal tap or lavage and finding increased numbers of degenerative neutrophils with intracellular bacteria in the peritoneal fluid.

Septic peritonitis is a serious condition with mortality rates as high as 67% in small animal patients (1). Many methods of treatment have been tried, some with better results than others (2–14). Open peritoneal drainage, a technique that allows continued drainage of peritoneal exudates during the resolution of active septic peritonitis, has been successful in small animal patients (12–14).

Indications

Open peritoneal drainage is indicated in the treatment of generalized septic peritonitis, in which large amounts of peritoneal fluid are expected to be produced in response to the peritoneal inflammation. By leaving the peritoneal cavity open, peritoneal exudates can freely drain out of the peritoneal cavity during the resolution of the peritonitis. Common conditions for which open peritoneal drainage is indicated include, but are not limited to, leakage of gastrointestinal contents into the peritoneal cavity (secondary to foreign body perforation, ruptured stomach in gastric dilatation–volvulus syndrome, and traumatic wounds that have penetrated the gastrointestinal tract), postsurgical complications (such as leakage from surgical incisions into the gastrointestinal tract, dehiscence of body wall incisions with subsequent evisceration, and dehiscence of cystotomy or gallbladder incisions in animals that have urinary or biliary tract infections, respectively), and penetrating wounds with damage to intra-abdominal organs (caused by traumatic events such as gunshot wounds and bite wounds).

Open peritoneal drainage is usually not necessary in cases with sterile, chemical peritonitis, such as that caused by biliary tract rupture in an animal with sterile bile or urinary tract rupture in an animal with sterile urine. In these cases, correction of the underlying cause of the peritonitis, followed by copious peritoneal lavage before closure of the peritoneal cavity, is usually adequate. Peritoneal exudation is usually minimal after correcting the underlying cause in these types of peritonitis, and continued postoperative peritoneal drainage is usually not necessary for successful treatment of the patient.

Principles of Open Peritoneal Drainage

The basic principle of open peritoneal drainage is to treat the infected peritoneal cavity in the same manner as if it were an abscess in any other location of the body, by allowing the exudates to drain from the animal. The underlying problem responsible for the development of the septic peritonitis is surgically corrected. The peritoneal cavity is then left open to drain to the outside while the peritoneal infection resolves. Additionally, the patient is given appropriate antibiotic therapy. Once the peritonitis has resolved, the peritoneal cavity is routinely closed. Open peritoneal drainage is more effective than simple placement of drains in the peritoneal cavity because the omentum walls off all types of drains in a short time, preventing adequate drainage of peritoneal exudates (15).

Surgical Technique and Bandaging

Once the diagnosis of generalized septic peritonitis is made, the patient should be stabilized as necessary to make it the best anesthetic candidate possible. Stabilization should consist of treatment for shock as well as administration of one or more broad-spectrum intravenous antibiotics. A good initial choice of antibiotics before culture and susceptibility results are available is a combination of gentamicin and ampicillin, or gentamicin and cephalexin or cephaloridine. Many of the intravenously administered antibiotics are nephrotoxic if given to a dehydrated patient. Consequently, in an animal that is volume depleted and in shock, rehydration should be started before administering antibiotics that may temporarily or permanently compromise renal function. After the patient is as hemodynamically stable as possible, it is taken to surgery for exploration of the peritoneal cavity.

A ventral midline incision is made from the xiphoid process to the pubis for an exploratory celiotomy. All abdominal organs should be carefully examined to ensure that all sources of peritoneal contamination are identified. Multiple sites of leakage are frequently found in cases of peritonitis caused by trauma such as gunshot wounds or foreign body ingestion. The causes of the peritoneal contamination are surgically corrected. The falciform ligament may be removed to prevent it from obstructing drainage from the cranial portion of the incision, if necessary.

The peritoneal cavity is thoroughly lavaged with warm (approximately 39°C) sterile saline (0.9% NaCl) to remove all gross contaminants. Several liters of saline are usually needed, and lavaging should continue until all evidence of gross contamination is removed. Aerobic and anaerobic bacterial cultures are taken after completion of lavaging. The abdominal viscera are replaced into their normal anatomic locations, and omentum is draped over the ventral surface of the abdomen.

Two strands of monofilament nonabsorbable suture material are used to close the linea alba loosely (Fig. 19.5). Monofilament nylon (Ethilon, Ethicon, Inc., Somerville, NJ) and polypropylene (Prolene, Ethicon, Inc.) are good suture choices. One strand of suture material is tied at the cranial end of the incision, and a simple continuous suture pattern is placed working from the tied end toward the middle of the incision, leaving a gap between the edges of the incision. A second strand of suture material is tied at the caudal end of the incision, and a simple continuous suture pattern is again placed working from the knot toward the middle of the incision while leaving the same gap between the edges of the incision. The untied ends of the two strands of suture material are tied to each

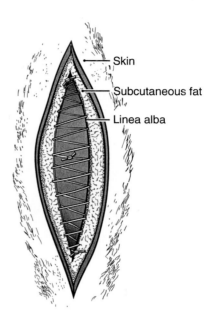

Fig. 19.5. Simple continuous suture pattern used to close the linea alba loosely during open peritoneal drainage. Two strands of suture material are used. Knots are tied at the cranial and caudal ends of the incision and the two strands of suture material are tied to each other in the middle of the incision.

other in the middle of the incision (see Fig. 19.5). Each bite of the continuous suture pattern must be placed close to the adjacent bite. The risk of postoperative herniation of abdominal viscera or omentum is increased if too much space is left between the suture bites.

A gap of 1 to 4 cm is left between the edges of the linea alba to facilitate postoperative drainage from the peritoneal cavity through the incision. The size of the gap that is left is proportional to the size of the patient. A 1-cm gap is appropriate for a cat or small dog, whereas a 4-cm, or larger, gap is appropriate for a large or giant breed dog.

The subcutaneous tissue and skin are not closed at this time. The incision is covered with sterile bandage material to keep the peritoneal cavity clean, to collect drainage from the peritoneal cavity, and to prevent evisceration of abdominal contents. Sterile gloves must be worn whenever the bandaging material is handled. If the patient is a male dog, a urinary catheter must be placed in sterile fashion, and a sterile closed collection system is attached to the catheter before the application of any bandaging materials. Alternately, some surgeons routinely elect to close the caudal portion of the incision to the level of the front of the prepuce to preclude the need for a urinary catheter during the open drainage period. However, I believe that the benefits of leaving the entire incision open for drainage

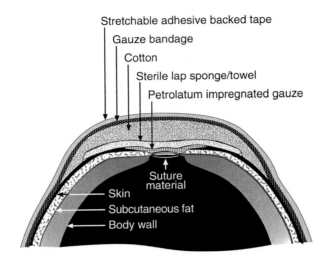

Stretchable adhesive backed tape
Gauze bandage
Cotton
Sterile lap sponge/towel
Petrolatum impregnated gauze

Suture material

Skin
Subcutaneous fat
Body wall

Fig. 19.6. Cross section of the body wall and bandaging materials used on a dog during open peritoneal drainage. The actual layers of bandaging materials used for absorption of peritoneal exudates (demonstrated here with laparotomy sponges and sterile roll cotton) may vary depending on the size of the patient and the amount of drainage expected before the next bandage change.

outweigh the risks of urinary catheterization for the duration of the open drainage period.

The first layer of bandage material that is applied directly over the open incision is petroleum-impregnated gauze (Adaptic nonadhering dressing, Johnson & Johnson Medical Inc., Arlington, TX) (Fig. 19.6). This material allows fluid to drain through it while preventing the other layers of bandaging materials from sticking to the abdominal incision or from entering the abdominal cavity. Several layers of sterile materials are then placed to absorb the peritoneal fluid as it drains from the peritoneal cavity. Sterile laparotomy sponges or 4 × 4-inch gauze pads are the next layer placed. Sterile hand towels are placed on the outside of the laparotomy sponges or gauze pads. The layered bandage is secured to the dog with stretchable roll gauze (Kling conforming gauze bandage, Johnson & Johnson Medical Inc.) covered by stretchable adhesive backed tape (Elasticon elastic tape, Johnson & Johnson Medical Inc.), or stretchable bandaging tape (Vetrap bandaging tape, 3M Animal Care Products, St. Paul, MN). In some animals, the outer securing bandage needs to be wrapped around the front or rear legs in a figure-of-eight pattern to prevent the bandage from slipping, thus allowing the incision to become exposed. If additional bandaging material is needed for added absorbency, sterile roll cotton can be used on the outside of the sterile hand towels. Alternately, on a small patient in which hand towels may be too bulky, an additional layer of laparotomy sponges or gauze pads can be used in place of the hand towels.

Care During the Open Drainage Period

During open drainage period, the patient must be kept in a facility with 24-hour monitoring capabilities. Patients with septic peritonitis are critically ill and must be closely monitored during the postoperative period. The actual monitoring necessary varies from patient to patient.

The peritoneal cavity should be left open as long as necessary to allow the peritonitis to resolve. Red blood cells and plasma proteins are lost with the peritoneal fluid that is draining out of the body, and some patients may need one or more transfusions with red blood cells, plasma, or whole blood. The patient's packed cell volume and total protein (or albumin) should be monitored on a daily basis so transfusions may be given if necessary.

Intravenous fluid therapy should be continued until the animal is eating and drinking adequately and is able to maintain its own hydration without supplementation. Initially, fluid requirements are high because of the losses from peritoneal exudation and drainage of the fluid out of the peritoneal cavity. Fluid rates three to five times the maintenance requirements are sometimes needed during the first 1 to 2 days of open drainage. Requirements usually drop back toward maintenance amounts after the initial period, when the largest losses occur. Oral alimentation should be reinstituted as soon as possible. However, the exact timing depends on the individual patient and on the surgical procedures performed to correct the cause of the peritonitis.

Antibiotic therapy should be continued at least until the peritoneal cavity is closed. Antibiotic selection should be altered, if necessary, once culture and susceptibility results are available from the initial samples. When oral alimentation is reinstituted, the route of antibiotic administration may be changed if an appropriate oral antibiotic is available.

The bandage should be changed a minimum of once daily, or more frequently if needed. The bandage should be changed immediately if it becomes wet or soiled (with urine, feces, or any other substance), if peritoneal fluid soaks through from the inside to the outside, or if the bandage slips forward or backward, exposing a portion of the incision. Bandages may need to be changed more often than once daily during the first 1 to 2 days of open drainage because large volumes of fluid are lost from the peritoneal cavity until the peritonitis starts to resolve.

After the animal has recovered from anesthesia, all subsequent bandage changes are done with the animal standing or held in a standing position. Before the soiled or wet bandage is removed, the sterile portion of the new bandage is preassembled by a person wearing sterile gloves, working from the outer layer to the inner layer. The patient is then restrained in a standing position, and the soiled bandage is removed. A sample of peritoneal fluid can be collected for cytologic analysis at this time by catching fluid as it drips out of the incision into a tube containing ethylenediaminetetraacetic acid (EDTA). The preassembled, sterile portion of the bandage is placed over the incision by a person wearing sterile gloves. The bandage is then secured to the body as previously described. Care should be taken to apply the bandage snugly, but not so tightly as to compromise respiration, whenever the bandage is secured to the patient's body.

Several criteria are used to determine when it is time to close the peritoneal cavity. Within a few days of correcting the cause of the peritonitis and leaving the peritoneal cavity open to drain, the patient's overall condition should start to improve. The animal's attitude should return to normal, and body temperature should stay in the normal range. In most cases, the patient starts to show interest in food and water. When these changes occur, the surgeon should begin to think about closing the abdomen. The amount of drainage from the peritoneal cavity should decrease dramatically, and bandage changing should be required no more than once daily when the decision to close the abdomen is made.

Peritoneal fluid should be evaluated cytologically every 1 to 2 days during the open drainage period. In patients with resolving peritonitis, the fluid should be clear and pale yellow or reddish yellow. When the peritoneal cavity is ready to be closed, the peritoneal tap should indicate active inflammation without any evidence of sepsis. One sees more than the normal number of neutrophils in the fluid than in a peritoneal tap from a healthy animal that has not undergone abdominal surgery, but the neutrophils should not have degenerative changes or intracellular bacteria.

In two retrospective studies of small animal patients with peritonitis treated with open peritoneal drainage, the average duration of open peritoneal drainage was 4.4 days, with a range of 2 to 9 days (13, 14). Some patients do not improve adequately in the first few postoperative days and may need to have their peritoneal cavity reexplored to determine whether complications have developed. Indications for reexploration of the peritoneal cavity include the following: 1) the patient's overall condition fails to improve; 2) the volume of fluid draining from the peritoneal cavity does not dramatically decrease after 4 to 5 days of open peritoneal drainage, or it actually increases; 3) the character of the fluid suddenly changes in color or from clear to turbid; or 4) gross contaminants are seen in the peritoneal fluid. If complications occur, the source of persistent contamination should be corrected, and the peritoneal cavity should be copiously lavaged. The open peritoneal drainage procedure should be repeated as previously described if the remaining peritonitis is severe and if large amounts of peritoneal drainage are expected. In our hospital, some patients with generalized septic peritonitis treated with open peritoneal drainage have survived after having the peritoneal cavity open for up to 14 days and undergoing up to three surgical explorations of the peritoneal cavity.

Closing the Peritoneal Cavity

Once the decision is made to close the peritoneal cavity, the patient is routinely anesthetized and placed in dorsal recumbency. The bandage is removed from the abdomen, and sterile laparotomy sponges are packed along the incision to prevent surgical scrub from entering the open peritoneal cavity. The surgical field is routinely prepared for aseptic surgery. After completion of the final surgical scrub, the laparotomy sponges are removed. If a spray, such as povidone–iodine solution, is routinely used in preparing the patient for surgery, the entire surgical field (including the incision line) can be sprayed with it.

When present, granulation tissue overlying the linea alba sutures is removed using sharp dissection. The middle knot attaching the cranial and caudal strands of suture material is located and removed, opening the linea alba. If the patient's recovery has been uncomplicated, the peritoneal cavity is not routinely reexplored. Samples for aerobic and anaerobic bacterial cultures and susceptibility testing are obtained from within the peritoneal cavity. The previously placed continuous linea alba sutures are tightened by working from the proximal and distal ends of the incision toward the middle of the incision until the edges of the linea alba are apposed. The ends of the suture material in the middle of the incision are tied to each other, and excess suture material is removed. The subcutaneous tissue and skin edges are debrided if necessary and are routinely closed.

Systemic antibiotics are continued until closure culture results are available. If no organisms grow on the closure cultures, antibiotics are discontinued. If the closure cultures are positive for bacterial growth, appropriate antibiotics are continued for an additional 10 to 14 days.

If the patient has had complications warranting reexploration of the abdomen, the previously placed continuous linea alba sutures are removed. All abdominal organs are thoroughly examined, and the source of the problem is located and corrected. The peritoneal cavity is lavaged, and the abdomen is either routinely closed or open peritoneal drainage is performed again, depending on the situation.

Complications

Several complications can occur during open peritoneal drainage. One is failure to correct the underlying problem adequately, with recurrence or continuation of the septic peritonitis. This can be avoided in most cases by carefully evaluating all intra-abdominal organs at the time of the initial exploratory celiotomy and surgically correcting all sources of peritoneal contamination. In some cases, recurrent leakage of contaminants may not be avoidable, such as the dehiscence of an intestinal wall suture line, and a second attempt at resolving the leakage is necessary.

Large amounts of fluid are lost from the peritoneal cavity, especially early in the open drainage period. Plasma proteins and red blood cells, which would normally be at least partially resorbed from peritoneal fluid if left in the peritoneal cavity, are lost to the outside. Hypoproteinemia, hypoalbuminemia, and anemia have all been reported as complications of open peritoneal drainage. Peripheral edema has been reported in some hypoalbuminemic patients that have been treated with open peritoneal drainage, but it has not been a clinical problem in others. If clinical signs relating to hypoalbuminemia are present and the patient's albumin level is below 1.5 g/dL, a plasma transfusion should be considered. Multiple plasma transfusions may be necessary to elevate the albumin toward the normal range in larger dogs. Alternately, if the albumin is between 1.0 and 1.5 g/dL and no clinical signs relating to hypoalbuminemia are present, I do not usually give plasma to the patient.

Anemia is another potential complication that may develop because of the loss of red blood cells through the irritated peritoneal surfaces into the peritoneal fluid, which then drains to the outside through the opened peritoneal cavity. Packed cell volume should be evaluated on a daily basis during the open drainage period, and a complete blood count should be obtained periodically to keep track of this variable. Packed red blood cells, or whole blood, should be administered to the patient as necessary.

Care must be taken during the open drainage period to ensure that the patient does not become dehydrated because fluid losses from the peritoneal cavity are large during the resolution of the peritonitis. Large volumes of intravenous fluids may need to be administered initially during the open drainage period, until the peritonitis starts to resolve and oral alimentation is reinstituted. The normal clinical parameters used to evaluate hydration should be monitored, and fluid administration should be adjusted to ensure adequate hydration and adequate urine output.

Cultures taken at the time of definitive closure of the peritoneal cavity frequently reveal growth of bacterial organisms. In two retrospective studies, positive closure cultures were reported in 80 to 100% of the cases that were cultured, although fewer than 50% of the animals in either of these studies had cultures taken at the time of closure of the peritoneal cavity (13, 14). In some cases, the organisms cultured at closure were the same as those cultured at the initial surgery; whereas in others, different organisms were cultured. When different organisms were cultured during the two surgical procedures, the organisms cultured at closure were thought to represent nosocomial infections with organisms that entered the peritoneal cavity during the period of open peritoneal drainage. However, the authors of both studies concluded that the presence of positive bacterial cultures at the time of closure was not associated with death in the patients in their study (13, 14). Consequently, the significance of this finding is unknown.

Because it takes 2 to 3 days to determine whether bacteria will grow from the closure cultures, the way that I handle a patient with a positive closure culture is as follows. If the patient meets the foregoing criteria for peritoneal cavity closure, the peritoneal cavity is routinely closed. If the closure cultures are positive, the patient is given an appropriate antibiotic (based on susceptibility testing) for 10 to 14 days, and the owner closely monitors the patient for any recurrence of clinical signs during this period. If any clinical signs recur, the patient is returned to the hospital, closely examined, and a decision is made about appropriate treatment on a case-by-case basis. If the closure cultures are negative, antibiotics are discontinued as soon as culture results are available.

The mortality rate from generalized septic peritonitis in small animal patients has been reported to be as high as 67% (1). Open peritoneal drainage is a good procedure to allow exudates to drain from the peritoneal cavity, enabling the peritonitis to successfully resolve. Mortality rates in two retrospective studies of clinical cases of septic peritonitis in small animal patients treated with open peritoneal drainage were 20.8 and 48% (13, 14). Although this surgical procedure does appear to save the lives of many patients with septic peritonitis, all patients with septic peritonitis are in critical condition, and some of these animals die, regardless of the treatment provided.

Open peritoneal drainage is a time-consuming treatment technique that is also expensive. At least two surgical procedures are required before the animal is released from the hospital. Large quantities of bandaging materials are used, contributing significantly to the cost, and the animal must be kept in a facility where it can be monitored at all times. Typical bills for patients treated with open peritoneal drainage in our hospital range between $1500 and $3000, and the length of hospitalization from the time of diagnosis to release from the hospital ranges from 4 to 16 days.

Although this procedure is effective for the treatment of this complicated disease, many owners may not be able to afford it, and open peritoneal drainage should be used only in properly selected cases.

References

1. Hardie EM, Rawlings CA, Calvert CA. Severe sepsis in selected small animal patients. J Am Anim Hosp Assoc 1986;22:23–41.
2. Schumer W, Lee DK, Jones B. Peritoneal lavage in postoperative therapy of late peritoneal sepsis: preliminary report. Surgery 1964;55:841–845.
3. McKenna JP, MacDonald JA, Mahoney LJ, et al. The use of continuous postoperative peritoneal lavage in the management of diffuse peritonitis. Surg Gynecol Obstet 1970;130:254–258.
4. Stephen M, Lowenthal J. Continuing peritoneal lavage in high-risk peritonitis. Surgery 1979;85:603–606.
5. Hoffer RE, Prange JR, O'Neil JG, et al. Treatment of acute peritonitis in dogs by intermittent peritoneal lavage. J Am Anim Hosp Assoc 1970;6:182–193.
6. Hanna EA. Efficiency of peritoneal drainage. Surg Gynecol Obstet 1970;131:983–985.
7. Hudspeth AS. Radical surgical debridement in the treatment of advanced generalized bacterial peritonitis. Arch Surg 1975;110:1233–1236.
8. Steinberg D. On leaving the peritoneal cavity open in acute generalized suppurative peritonitis. Am J Surg 1979;137:216–220.
9. Duff JH, Moffat J. Abdominal sepsis managed by leaving abdomen open. Surgery 1981;90:774–778.
10. Maetani S, Tobe T. Open peritoneal drainage as effective treatment of advanced peritonitis. Surgery 1981;90:804–809.
11. Parks J, Gahring D, Greene RW. Peritoneal lavage for peritonitis and pancreatitis in twenty-two dogs. J Am Anim Hosp Assoc 1973;9:442–446.
12. Greenfield CL, Walshaw R. Open peritoneal drainage for treatment of contaminated peritoneal cavity and septic peritonitis in dogs and cats: 24 cases (1980–1986). J Am Vet Med Assoc 1987;191:100–105.
13. Woolfson JM, Dulish ML. Open abdominal drainage in the treatment of generalized peritonitis in 25 dogs and cats. Vet Surg 1986;15:27–32.
14. Orsher RJ, Rosin E. Open peritoneal drainage in experimental peritonitis in dogs. Vet Surg 1984;13:222–226.
15. Crowe DT Jr., Bjorling DE. Peritoneum and peritoneal cavity. In: Slatter DH, ed. Textbook of small animal surgery. Vol 1, 2nd ed. Philadelphia: WB Saunders, 1993:407–430.

Closed Peritoneal Drainage

Giselle Hosgood

Indications

The use of drains to remove fluid, pus, or contaminated material from the peritoneal cavity is hereby referred to as closed peritoneal drainage. The use of drains in the peritoneal cavity is primarily indicated in the treatment of peritonitis (1, 2). Other indications include diagnostic peritoneal lavage (3), peritoneal dialysis (4), and drainage of specific organs within the peritoneal cavity such as the prostate and pancreas (5–8). Placement of drains after routine abdominal procedures is discouraged, and the use of drains should not replace meticulous surgical technique. The use of drains can be associated with multiple complications, and drainage is not a reliable indicator of wound or body cavity events; the absence of drainage does not always imply the absence of fluid (1). However, in the event of serious contamination of the peritoneal cavity during surgery, the placement of drains may be indicated. Complete drainage of the peritoneal cavity is difficult, and the most efficient means may be open peritoneal drainage (9–11).

Physiology

Passive Drainage

The abdomen can be compared with a fluid-filled, flexible container with two separate pressure zones. Positive atmospheric pressure exists within the gastrointestinal tract, whereas the peritoneal cavity has an extraluminal subatmospheric pressure between -5 and -8 cm water; the pressure is most negative in the cranial abdomen near the diaphragm (12). Passive drainage of fluid from the peritoneal cavity requires an air vent to break the vacuum and to create a positive atmospheric pressure within the peritoneal cavity (12).

Passive peritoneal drainage relies on a pressure differential between the peritoneal cavity and the environment and functions primarily by overflow. In addition is some capillary action along the drain. Passive drainage is gravity dependent, and the drain provides a tract of least resistance along which excess fluid flows. Positive pressure occurs after celiotomy, and postoperative pneumoperitoneum is responsible for the onset of passive peritoneal drainage. The air is normally resorbed after several days, but it can be maintained in the peritoneal cavity with appropriate drain modifications (2, 12).

Active Drainage

Active drainage requires an external vacuum to create negative pressure within the peritoneal cavity. This allows drainage to occur independent of gravity and the physiologic properties of the peritoneal cavity. The vacuum is achieved by connection of the drain to a compressible container or a constant, low-pressure, motor-driven suction device (Fig. 19.7) (1, 2). Some commercial collection systems have one-way valves to prevent fluid reflux from the collection system into the peritoneal cavity. Suction should be applied to the drain before complete abdominal closure to prevent occlusion of the drain by intraluminal blood clot formation or tissue debris. The optimal level of suction is

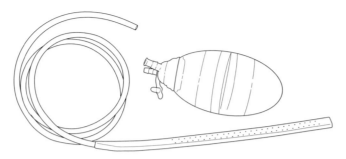

Fig. 19.7. A silicone wound drain and compressible collection canister that can be connected together and used for active peritoneal drainage. Note the one-way valve on the canister.

unclear. Low-level suction is effective, but higher levels are not harmful and may remove more fluid. Suction levels between −9 mm Hg (−12 cm water) (13) and −15 mm Hg (−20 cm water) (14) are typically used in human wound drainage, although higher levels of suction, −80 mm Hg (−112 cm water) (15) and −150 mm Hg (−200 cm water) (16), have been used successfully. These drains are effective in removing large volumes of fluid; however, as the volume of intraperitoneal fluid decreases, active drainage causes suction of tissue, viscera, omentum, or abdominal wall toward the drain, resulting in occlusion (1, 17). Tissue debris may also occlude the lumen. High-level suction may promote obstruction.

An active drain is always connected to a collection system. Connecting a passive drain to a collection system has several advantages, and this technique is strongly recommended. An inexpensive and easily accessible collection system is through an intravenous administration set into a bag. Although passive drains are gravity dependent (1), the level of the drain and the collection bag proportionally affect the gravitational force and the rate of drainage. Increasing this distance may promote obstruction of the drain by omentum or intestinal loops.

A collection system, whether by passive or active drainage, reduces the risk of ascending infection along the lumen of the drain. Ascending infection is one of the most common complications of peritoneal drainage, a function of both bacterial load migrating up the drain and decreased local tissue resistance because of the presence of the drain (18). Although bacteria can also migrate along the outside of the drain (19), a closed system greatly reduces the bacterial load. Protection of the drain by a sterile bandage can reduce bacterial migration along the outside of the wound. Additional benefits from a closed system include only requiring a small exit wound that may minimize the risk of ascending infection (18) and tissue or organ evisceration (1).

Collection systems also eliminate the chance of saturating the bandage covering the drain. A wet bandage over a freely draining passive drain provides an additional source of contamination by bacterial strike-through from the environment. Collection systems also allow accurate assessment of fluid character and volume.

Drains Suitable for Peritoneal Drainage

Three basic types of drains are suitable for use in the peritoneal cavity: the simple tube drain, the sump drain, and the disc catheter. Modifications of these drains are also used, including the peritoneal dialysis catheter, a modified simple tube drain. All these drains can be used to drain freely into a bandage covering the wound, or preferably they can be connected to a collection system.

Although a Penrose drain is an effective passive drain in certain situations, it is not recommended for use in the peritoneal cavity because it cannot counteract the negative atmospheric pressure in the abdomen and therefore does not actively drain an area, but provides a tract of least resistance along which excess fluid can flow (1). In addition, it cannot be connected to a collection system. The Penrose drain can, however, be used specifically for drainage of pancreatic masses (5, 6) and prostatic abscesses (7, 8). The Penrose drain is placed into the mass or abscess and exits through the ventral abdominal wall in a dependent position. A tract forms along the drain, allowing fluid to flow along the tract but remain isolated from the peritoneal cavity. Alternate techniques of open peritoneal drainage for the management of pancreatic masses (5) and marsupialization for the management of prostatic abscesses (8) may be more effective.

Simple Tube Drain

The simple tube or single-lumen drain acts primarily by gravity-dependent intraluminal flow, with some extraluminal capillary flow (Fig. 19.8) (20). Because most of the drainage is intraluminal, fenestration improves drainage efficiency (21). However, fenestration reduces the tensile strength of the drain and may predispose to tearing on removal (22). Prefenestrated commercial drains can be used, or fenestrations can be made by hand in a solid drain. Fenestrations should be oval and less than one-third the diameter of the drain, to prevent kinking and tearing (18). Fenestration using oval-tipped bone rongeurs rather than scissors may give a more precise, controlled cut with easy and safe removal of the fragment in the instrument's jaws (23). Silicone drains are preferred over plastic (polyvinyl chloride) or rubber drains because silicone

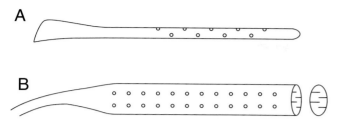

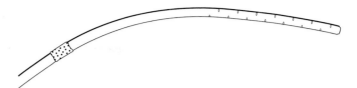

Fig. 19.8. Simple, fenestrated tube drain (**A**) and a silicone wound drain (**B**). (Modified from Crowe DT, Bjorling DE. Peritoneum and peritoneal cavity. In: Slatter DH, ed. Textbook of small animal surgery. Philadelphia: WB Saunders, 1985:587.)

Fig. 19.9. A commercial, multifenestrated, peritoneal dialysis catheter. Note the Dacron cuff toward the end of the drain and the radiopaque ridge on top of the drain.

is relatively inert (24). Silicone drains used in the contaminated peritoneal cavity of dogs have remained patent for at least 7 days postoperatively (25), and this has been my experience using silicone wound drains (Closed Wound Drainage System, Sil-Med, Sil-Med Corporation, Taunton, MA). Silicone drains have less tensile strength than polyvinyl chloride drains, and care is required on removal to prevent tearing (22).

Simple tube drains are relatively inefficient (20, 21). A study of peritoneal drainage in dogs showed similar drainage efficiency for Penrose drains (40%) and simple tube drains (38%) (21). Soft tube drains may collapse under strong suction; however, rigid drains may cause tissue damage (17, 26). The use of gauze inside drains (known as cigarette drains) to increase the capillary action (27) is not recommended because the gauze and remaining gauze particles incite an intense foreign body reaction (28). A safer alternative may be the placement of a Penrose drain inside a simple tube drain, the end of the Penrose protruding from the tip of the tube drain (15). This may avoid occlusion of the lumen of the tube drain, protect the tip of the tube drain, and increase fluid flow through the lumen of the tube drain. Excellent clinical results have been reported using this configuration in human patients; however, the study did not include control subjects (15).

Peritoneal Dialysis Catheter

A modification of the simple tube drain is the multifenestrated peritoneal dialysis catheter (Tenckhoff Peritoneal Catheter, Quinton Instrument Co., Seattle, WA; Impersol, Abbott Laboratories, Abbott Park, IL; Trocath, McGraw Laboratories, Glendale, CA; Parker DiaLavage, CPA Vet Inc., Davis, CA) (Fig. 19.9). Some catheters have a Dacron cuff around the tubing that is sutured to the body wall and subcutaneous tissue to stimulate a fibroblastic reaction and to prevent subcutaneous fluid leakage. These catheters are rigid and should be used for short-term drainage only. In addition to their use for peritoneal dialysis, these catheters

have been used for diagnostic peritoneal lavage (3) and for the treatment of peritonitis by intermittent postoperative peritoneal lavage (4). They are particularly useful for diagnostic peritoneal lavage and peritoneal dialysis because they can be inserted through a small abdominal incision using local anesthesia in a sedated animal (3). Softer, silicone wound drains are preferred over the peritoneal dialysis catheter for long-term drainage.

Sump Drain

Multilumen (sump) drains best conform to the physics of peritoneal cavity drainage. Multilumen drains are more efficient than simple tube drains (58% versus 38%) (21). Double-lumen sump drainage is two to four times more efficient than active drainage through a simple tube drain or passive Penrose drainage of the peritoneal cavity (21, 30, 31). Drainage is primarily by intraluminal flow through the large lumen, assisted by gravity. Fenestration of the large lumen improves drainage efficiency (21). The small sump lumen allows passive ingress of air into the peritoneal cavity, displacing fluid into the larger drainage lumen (Fig. 19.10). The air in peritoneal cavity keeps tissue from obstructing the drain and prevents the main lumen from collapsing (1, 2). Because air is drawn into the peritoneal cavity, the potential exists for bacteria to enter with the environmental air, particularly with the high air flows (20 L/minute) of suction (32). Airborne bacteria can be reduced by the use of bacterial filters (33). Rigid drains resist collapse when suction is applied, but they may cause tissue damage (17, 26). Enclosure of the sump drain by a fenestrated Penrose drain provides a

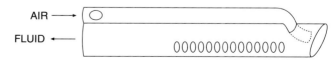

AIR →

FLUID ←

OOOOOOOOOOOOOOO

Fig. 19.10. A commercial sump drain. Air enters the small lumen to displace fluid within the peritoneal cavity that drains out the larger lumen. (Modified from Crowe DT, Bjorling DE. Peritoneum and peritoneal cavity. In: Slatter DH, ed. Textbook of small animal surgery. Philadelphia: WB Saunders, 1985:587.)

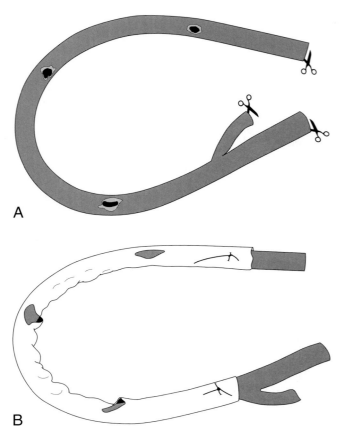

A

B

Fig. 19.11. A noncommercial sump Penrose drain constructed from a modified Foley catheter with the balloon, connector, and injection ports cut off (**A**) and placed inside a fenestrated Penrose drain (**B**).

cushion to reduce adjacent soft tissue damage (17) and improves drainage efficiency (21). The Penrose drain is fenestrated to allow fluid access to the inner sump drain (27).

Commercial double-lumen and triple-lumen sump drains are available (Argyle sump drain, Sherwood Medical Industries, St Louis, MO; Shirley wound drain, HW Anderson Products, Chapel Hill, NC; Percuflex sump drain, Medi-Tech, Westwood, MA). Noncommercial drains can be prepared from cheaper, readily available drains manufactured in multiple sizes. A sump–Penrose drain can be fashioned from a Foley catheter (Norta Foley Catheter, Beiersdorf, Inc., Norwalk, CT; Foley Catheter, American Latex Corporation, Sullivan, IN), enclosed in a Penrose drain (Penrose drain tubing, Davol, Inc., Cranston, RI) (2, 18). The Foley catheter is prepared by removing the bulb and the syringe adapter of the injection port and fenestrating the distal third (Fig. 19.11). The modified Foley catheter is then placed inside a fenestrated Penrose drain and is transfixed to the Penrose drain with a proximal and distal suture.

Disc Catheter

The disc catheter (Lifecath, Quinton, AH Robbins Co., Seattle, WA) was intended for long-term peritoneal dialysis drainage (34), but it is also effective for long-term drainage such as required for the treatment of peritonitis (Fig. 19.12). It is an expensive catheter, and the cost (approximately $200 compared with $40 for a fenestrated peritoneal dialysis catheter) may be prohibitive in some cases. The silicone catheter has large holes in a firm, circular base that creates low-pressure

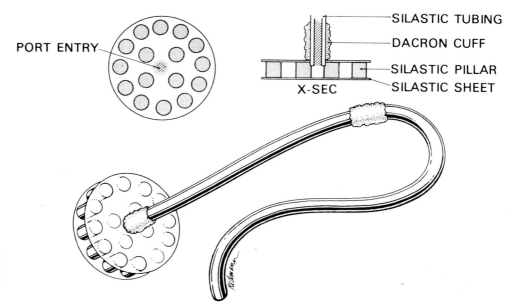

PORT ENTRY

SILASTIC TUBING
DACRON CUFF
SILASTIC PILLAR
SILASTIC SHEET
X-SEC

Fig. 19.12. A column disc peritoneal dialysis catheter. (From Bojrab MJ. Current techniques in small animal surgery. 2nd ed. Philadelphia: Lea & Febiger, 1983:244.)

drainage, which lessens the likelihood of occlusion of the catheter by blood clots, omentum, and other tissue (34).

Drain Placement

Efficient peritoneal drainage is difficult because of the convoluted nature of the peritoneal cavity, the sometimes intense fibrinous and fibrous reactions encountered during peritonitis, and the persistence of the omentum's attempt to isolate the drain from the peritoneal cavity. Normal forces associated with movement of the diaphragm, abdominal wall, and intestine affect the intraperitoneal circulation of fluid and cause fluid to pool beneath the diaphragm (9, 35, 36) and in the peritoneal reflections near the distal colon. In addition to normal forces, fluid can become isolated by peritoneal adhesions (9). Drain placement is extremely important to maximize drainage.

Drains are usually placed during celiotomy. Alternately, in acute situations such as diagnostic peritoneal lavage, emergency drainage of fluid from the abdomen (uroabdomen), or for establishment of peritoneal dialysis, a stab incision in the skin of the ventral midline is made, and the drain is "punched" through the body wall. Commercial, simple, peritoneal dialysis catheters and some tube drains come with a stylet–trocar for this purpose. Insertion of these drains in an emergency can often be performed under local anesthesia and sedation.

To drain the peritoneal cavity effectively, two tubular drains may be required, one directed cranially along the ventral abdominal wall toward the diaphragm and the other caudally along the ventral abdominal wall to the peritoneal reflections near the distal colon (9). The drains should exit close to the midline, in a dependent position, usually between the umbilicus and the xiphoid. The exit incision through the abdominal wall and skin should be only as large as the diameter of the drain. A large incision is not required with tube drains because drainage is mostly luminal (unlike a Penrose drain). A small exit incision reduces subcutaneous fluid leakage and subsequent cellulitis and possible incisional herniation. The exit incision should not so small as to obstruct the drain. The epigastric vessels, which run through the middle of the mammary chains, should be avoided. If the exit incision is small, it can be made between the epigastric vessel and the midline (incision) without weakening the midline celiotomy incision. Exiting lateral to the epigastric vessels moves away from a dependent exit site and may promote subcutaneous fluid leakage and cellulitis.

If celiotomy is performed, tacking the omentum to the stomach may help to prevent it from enveloping the drains. The omentum should not be excised unless it is obviously compromised. Excising excessive falci-

form fat may help to reduce tissue obstruction of the drains.

Insertion of disc catheters is best performed during celiotomy because this allows assessment of the kidneys (if for peritoneal dialysis) and tacking of the omentum away from the drain. The circular base is pulled against the abdominal wall (27), and the flexible draining tube exits through a stab incision in a dependent area of the ventral abdominal wall, close to the midline. Alternately, the catheter can be placed through a single right or left paramedian incision to exit through a stab incision in the ventral midline, rather than the paramedian region, to reduce subcutaneous fluid leakage (37). Dacron cuffs around the tubing are sutured to the body wall and subcutaneous tissue to stimulate a fibroblastic reaction and to prevent subcutaneous fluid leakage (34, 37). The exit tubing can be connected to a collection system, to function by passive drainage or low-pressure suction (40 to 60 mm Hg) (34).

All drains should be sutured to the skin using a secure suture such as the Chinese finger trap suture (38). Suction is applied as soon as the drain is placed, to prevent intraoperative obstruction of the drain with blood clots or tissue debris. All drains should be covered with a sterile bandage on completion of the surgical procedure. Multilayered, thick, absorbent bandage material is indicated, especially if a collection system is not used. Sterile cloth towels and disposable diapers (sterilized with ethylene oxide) make useful absorbent bandage layers.

Postoperative Management

The bandage should be changed as often as required to prevent complete soaking by exudate and possible strikethrough of bacteria from the environment. The frequency of bandage changes is reduced for drains using a collection system, but some leakage can occur through the exit site around the drain. Contamination of the bandage from the environment (urine, feces) can also occur. Use of an indwelling urinary catheter, particularly in male dogs, may help to prevent urine contamination. This is especially useful if the animal is recumbent. Using a waterproof outer covering on the bandage may help to reduce environmental contamination. Bandaging also helps to prevent self-mutilation of the drainage area and premature removal or damage to the drain by the animal.

The volume and nature of the fluid should be monitored closely, at least three to four times a day or more if profuse. The collection system should be changed using sterile technique when it is full or the vacuum has been lost. The vacuum may be lost before the collection system is completely full. Without vacuum and fluid flow, the risk of obstruction of the drain by tissue debris or fibrin and blood clots is increased. In addition, fluid that remains in the collection system for a prolonged period may promote bacterial growth.

The drain is removed once the volume of fluid becomes significantly reduced and the fluid becomes serosanguineous. The presence of a drain incites an inflammatory reaction and some fluid production, hence drainage usually does not cease. If drainage ceases suddenly, it may represent drain obstruction rather than resolution of the disease. Fluid may continue to drain for 2 to 3 days after drain removal, and a bandage should remain in place during this time to collect drainage and to prevent contamination of the exit site.

All drains become contaminated by the time of removal. If one is concerned that this contamination may have caused drainage tract infection, the tip of the drain should be submitted for bacterial culture and sensitivity testing, and appropriate antimicrobial medication should be initiated.

Complications

The most common complications of abdominal drains are obstruction and ascending infection. In a classic study by Yates in 1905 (28), passive gauze and rubber drains placed in the peritoneal cavity of dogs were sealed from the rest of the peritoneal cavity as early as 6 hours after placement. A later study in healthy dogs showed that omentum completely plugged the drain entry site and incompletely surrounded the Penrose drain by 24 hours. At 48 hours, the Penrose drain was completely surrounded by fibrin and omentum and was isolated from the peritoneal cavity (29). More recent studies in dogs (9) and human patients (31) suggest that, whereas the omentum does surround the intraperitoneal drain, the apparent occlusion may not be completely functional. Drainage continued readily for 48 hours in dogs with intraperitoneal sump–Penrose drains (9) and for up to 3 to 6 days in human patients with intraperitoneal sump drains (31). I have observed peritoneal drainage using silicone wound drains connected to a passive collection device for as long as 10 days.

Nosocomial bacterial contamination of the drain and drainage site is a common complication of any drain. In one study in healthy dogs, nosocomial contamination of the drain did not necessarily indicate intraperitoneal infection (40). This does not obviate the need for conscientious drain management to prevent overwhelming contamination that may lead to infection.

Retraction of the drain may occur once the animal begins to move and stand. This tends to occur with drains that are not connected to a collection system and that are cut short at the exit site. Leaving several inches of drain beyond the exit site is recommended, although leaving excessive length may make it more difficult to prevent contamination, especially during bandage changes. Suturing the drain securely, at several sites, is also important.

Exit site and drain tract cellulitis may occur. This complication is not serious and usually resolves once the drain is removed. Subcutaneous fluid leakage is more common when peritoneal lavage is used. Subcutaneous fluid leakage and cellulitis can be reduced by using a short subcutaneous tunnel between the skin and the abdominal wall exit site for the drain and by having the exit site in a dependent position. The Dacron cuffs on the peritoneal dialysis catheter and disc catheter also help to reduce this complication. Applying a water-repellent ointment to the skin around the exit site (petroleum jelly) may help to prevent skin irritation from drainage fluid.

Hypoproteinemia and hypoalbuminemia are significant complications of peritonitis (10, 11) and drainage, but they are not really complications of drainage per se (40). Close monitoring of plasma protein concentrations in animals with peritonitis is imperative, and intravenous plasma or colloid infusion may be required.

References

1. Donner GS, Ellison GW. The use and misuse of abdominal drains in small animal surgery. Compend Contin Educ Pract Vet 1986;8:705–715.
2. Hosgood G. Drainage of the peritoneal cavity. Compend Contin Educ Pract Vet 1993;15:1605–1617.
3. Hunt CA. Diagnostic peritoneal paracentesis and lavage. Compend Contin Ed Pract Vet 1980;11:449–453.
4. Willauer CC, Gregory CR, Parker HH. Treatment of peritonitis with the Parker dialysis catheter. J Am Anim Hosp Assoc 1988;24:546–550.
5. Edwards DF, Bauer MS, Walker MA, et al. Pancreatic masses in seven dogs following acute pancreatitis. J Am Anim Hosp Assoc 1991;26:189–198.
6. Rutgers C, Herring DS, Orton EC. Pancreatic pseudocyst associated with acute pancreatitis in a dog: ultrasonographic diagnosis. J Am Anim Hosp Assoc 1985;21:411–416.
7. Mullen HS, Matthiesen DT, Scavelli TD. Results of surgery and postoperative complications in 92 dogs treated for prostatic abscessation by a multiple Penrose drain technique. J Am Anim Hosp Assoc 1990;26:369–379.
8. Salisbury SK, Lantz GC, Kazacos EA. Pancreatic abscess in dogs: six cases (1978–1986). J Am Vet Med Assoc 1988;193:1104–1108.
9. Hosgood G, Salisbury SK, Cantwell HD, et al. Intraperitoneal circulation and drainage in the dog. Vet Surg 1989;18:261–268.
10. Woolfson JM, Dulisch ML. Open abdominal drainage in the treatment of generalized peritonitis in 25 dogs and cats. Vet Surg 1986;15:27–32.
11. Greenfield CL, Walshaw R. Open peritoneal drainage for treatment of contaminated peritoneal cavity and septic peritonitis in dogs and cats: 24 cases (1980–1986). J Am Vet Med Assoc 1987;191:100–105.
12. Gold E. The physics of the abdominal cavity and the problem of peritoneal drainage. Am J Surg 1956;91:415–416.
13. Tenta LT, Maddalozzo, Friedman CD, et al. Suction drainage of wounds of the head and neck. Surg Gynecol Obstet 1989;169:558.
14. Kern KA. Technique for high volume drainage beneath large tissue flaps. Surg Gynecol Obstet 1990;170:70.

15. Garcia-Rinaldi R, Defore WW, Green ZD, et al. Improving the efficiency of wound drainage catheters. Am J Surg 1975;130:372–373.

16. Moss JP. Historical and current perspectives on surgical drainage. Surg Gynecol Obstet 1981;152:517–527.

17. Formeister JF, Elias EG. Safe intra-abdominal and efficient wound drainage. Surg Gynecol Obstet 1976;142;415–416.

18. Hampel NL, Johnson RG. Principles of surgical drains and drainage. J Am Anim Hosp Assoc 1985;21:21–28.

19. Raves JJ, Slitkin M, Diamond DL. A bacteriologic study comparing closed suction and simple conduit drainage. Am J Surg 1984;148:618–620.

20. Withrow SJ, Black AP. Generalized peritonitis in small animals. Vet Clin North Am Small Anim Pract 1979;9:363–379.

21. Hanna EA. Efficiency of peritoneal drainage. Surg Gynecol Obstet 1970;131:983–985.

22. Paton RW, Powell ES. Which drain? A comparison of the tensile strengths of vacuum drainage tubes. J R Coll Surg Edinb 1988;33:127–129.

23. Arnstein PM. Custom tube drains. Lancet 1988;1:215.

24. Baker BH, Brochardt KA. Sump drains and airborne bacteria as a cause of wound infection. J Surg Res 1974;17:407–410.

25. Santos OA, Hastings FW, Mohamad KM. Effectiveness of silicone as an abdominal drain. Arch Surg 1962;84:63–65.

26. Vercoutere AL, Humphrey R. Improved method for intraabdominal drainage. Surg Gynecol Obstet 1984;158:587–588.

27. Lee AH, Swaim SF, Henderson RA. Surgical drainage. Compend Contin Educ Pract Vet 1986;8:94–103.

28. Crowson WN, Wilson CS. An experimental study of the effects of drains on colon anastomoses. Am Surg 1973;39:597–601.

29. Okudaira Y, Sugimachi K, Matsumata T. Combined Penrose and silicone drains provide excellent drainage. Surg Gynecol Obstet 1987;165:449–450.

30. Golden GT, Roberts TL III, Rodeheaver G, et al. A new filtered sump tube for wound drainage. Am J Surg 1975;129:716–717.

31. Robbs JV, MacIntyre IM. The efficacy of intraperitoneal drains: an experimental study. S Afr J Surg 1979;17:191–197.

32. Baker MS, Borchardt KA, Baker BH, et al. Sump tube drainage as a source of bacterial contamination. Am J Surg 1977;133:617–618.

33. Spengler MD, Rodeheaver GT, Edlich RF. Performance of filtered sump wound drainage tubes. Surg Gynecol Obstet 1982;154:333–336.

34. Thornhill JA. Adjunct to intraperitoneal drainage. In: Bojrab MJ, ed. Current techniques in small animal surgery. 2nd ed. Philadelphia: Lea & Febiger, 1983:571–591.

35. Meyers MA. Peritoneography: normal and pathologic anatomy. Am J Res 1973;117:353–365.

36. Autio V. The spread of intraperitoneal infection. Acta Chir Scand Suppl 1964;321:1–31.

37. Birchard SJ, Chew DJ, Crisp MS, et al. Modified technique for placement of a column disc peritoneal dialysis catheter. J Am Anim Hosp Assoc 1988;24:663–666.

38. Smeak DD. The Chinese finger trap suture technique for fastening tubes and catheters. J Am Anim Hosp Assoc 1990;26:215–218.

39. Yates JL. An experimental study of the local effects of peritoneal drainage. Surg Gynecol Obstet 1905;1:473–492.

40. Hosgood G, Salisbury SK, DeNicola DB. Open peritoneal drainage versus sump-Penrose drainage: clinico-pathological effects in normal dogs. J Am Anim Hosp Assoc 1991;27:116–121.

— 20 —

NASAL CAVITY

Resection of the Nasal Planum

Rodney C. Straw

Cats with unpigmented skin of the nasal planum may, over several years, develop squamous cell carcinoma with prolonged exposure to ultraviolet (UV-B) irradiation (1). Older, white cats or those with lightly pigmented noses and that live in sunny climates are at risk. Lesions progress slowly through early solar damage with crusting and erythema to carcinoma in situ to invasive squamous cell carcinoma (2). Invasive squamous cell carcinoma initially is confined to the nasal planum, but it slowly becomes more extensive, affecting deep and adjacent tissues late in the course of the disease. Lymph node or lung metastases are rare (2). Cutaneous hemangiosarcoma of the nasal planum also occurs and is also thought to be associated with solar irradiation (3, 4). Basal cell tumor has been reported to occur on the nose of cats (5). Cancer involving the nasal planum or premaxilla is uncommon in dogs, but such tumors include squamous cell carcinoma, fibrosarcoma, melanoma, mast cell tumor, and osteosarcoma (6). Biopsy with histopathologic examination is necessary to diagnose cancer of the nasal planum and is important to rule out nonneoplastic causes of nasal ulceration.

Indications

Various methods have been described to treat cats with squamous cell carcinoma of the nasal planum including radiation therapy, hyperthermia, intratumoral administration of carboplatin, cryosurgery, conservative (marginal or intralesional) surgery, and photodynamic therapy (7–11). Unfortunately, with most of these treatments, the tumor margins cannot be evaluated to ensure that an adequate volume of tissue is treated. Each of these modes of therapy has other disadvantages, including the need for special equipment and facilities for some techniques, high rates of tumor recurrence, and reported control rates for deeply infiltrating lesions of up to 55% at 1 year. Most of these techniques may work for early, small lesions or carcinoma in situ, but the most cost-effective, reliable treatment for selected patients with invasive squamous cell carcinoma is nasal planum resection. Fifteen of 20 cats with invasive squamous cell carcinoma treated with nasal planum resection were free of recurrent disease at 1 year (5). Nasal planum resection can also be effectively used to treat other invasive neoplasms in dogs and cats. Although the cosmetic results in cats are generally good and acceptable to most owners, dogs are more noticeably deformed by the surgery. Function is usually excellent.

Nasal Planum Resection

The animal, maintained under general anesthesia and intubated with a cuffed endotracheal tube, is positioned in sternal recumbency with the head slightly elevated. The surgical area is carefully palpated to try to estimate tumor extension into adjacent tissue. A small area of hair is clipped, but the tactile vibrissae are avoided, and the site is prepared for aseptic surgery. A drape with a circular hole is placed over the prepared site. The nasal planum is completely removed with a 360° skin incision made with a No. 15 scalpel blade (Fig. 20.1). The incision is made so it transects the underlying turbinates. If the tumor does not extend to the lip margin, then a thin strip of skin and buccal

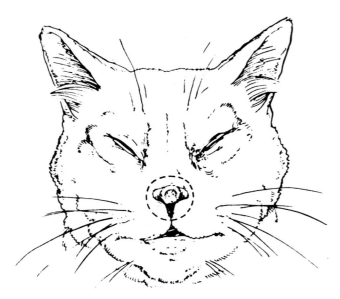

Fig. 20.1. The 360° incision around the nasal planum is indicated by the dotted line. If possible, a strip of skin is left ventrally so the lips are left attached at the midline. (From Withrow SJ, Straw RC. Resection of the nasal planum in nine cats and five dogs. J Am Anim Hosp Assoc 1990;26:219–222.)

mucous membrane is preserved at the rostral lip margins on the midline. If tumor has extended into this region, then the lip margin must be removed, resulting in a closure involving rostral advancement of the lips. This may leave the incisor teeth slightly exposed. The cartilage of the nasal planum and the turbinates are cut with an incision angled at about 45° to the hard palate (Fig. 20.2). Bleeding is usually brisk. Hemorrhage is controlled by direct pressure with a sponge. Electrocautery should only be used sparingly to avoid thermal necrosis, which delays healing

Once the nasal planum is removed, the skin edges retract and the nasal conchae are exposed. A pursestring suture of 3–0 monofilament nonabsorbable suture material is placed through the skin around the incision. The surgeon does not need to place any deep sutures into the cartilage or nasal mucosa. It is only necessary to tighten the pursestring suture lightly; for cats, the new nasal orifice is closed to approximately 1 cm in diameter (Fig. 20.3). The entire excised nasal planum is submitted for histopathologic examination, with a request for the pathologist to examine the surgical margins carefully. India ink or other tissue marking ink may be painted on the cut edges of the specimen to delineate the surgical margins. Analgesics are used, and patients are usually sent home within 24 hours. Owners are advised not to try to clean the surgical site and are warned that the patient may sneeze blood for several days. Patients should be tempted with favored food, but they may be reluctant to eat for a few days after surgery. Older animals with compromised renal function need fluid support until water intake becomes adequate. Elizabethan collars are usually not necessary. Sutures are removed ap-

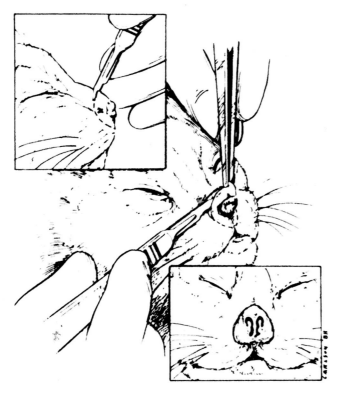

Fig. 20.2. The angle of the deep incision as seen from the lateral side is angled at approximately 45°. The turbinates are sharply divided. Skin retracts after removal of the nasal planum, exposing the nasal cavity. (From Withrow SJ, Straw RC. Resection of the nasal planum in nine cats and five dogs. J Am Anim Hosp Assoc 1990;26:219–222.)

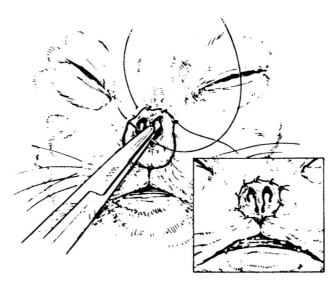

Fig. 20.3. A continuous pursestring suture is used to reduce the nasal orifice to about 1 cm diameter. No sutures are placed in cartilage. (From Withrow SJ, Straw RC. Resection of the nasal planum in nine cats and five dogs. J Am Anim Hosp Assoc 1990;26:219–222.)

proximately 10 days after surgery, and sedation or a short course of anesthesia may be required.

Combined Resection of the Nasal Planum and Premaxilla

For extensive neoplasms of the nasal planum and pre-maxilla, nasal planum resection or premaxillectomy alone may be inadequate. Wide surgical margins can be attained using combined resection of the nasal pla-num and premaxilla (6). This technique offers a surgi-cal treatment for large tumors in dogs that obviates the need for adjuvant or primary radiation therapy. Cosmetic results are considered acceptable by most owners.

The dog, maintained under general anesthesia and intubated with a cuffed endotracheal tube, is posi-tioned in sternal recumbency with the mouth slightly open. The skin overlying the maxilla and upper lip is clipped and prepared for aseptic surgery. The oral mucosa of the lips and hard palate is prepared with a disinfectant such as a dilute povidone–iodine solution. The area is draped, allowing access to the oral cavity (Fig. 20.4A). The upper lip is incised from the skin

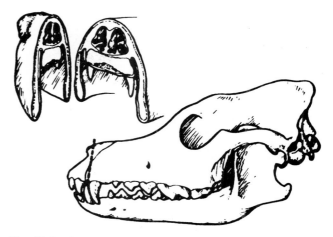

Fig. 20.5. The nasal cartilages are incised perpendicular to the long axis of the skull down to the floor of the nasal cavity. The mucosa of the hard palate is transversely incised at a level just rostral to the canine teeth (or caudal to the canine teeth, depending on the extent of tumor invasion) down to bone. An oscillating saw is used to cut the bone of the hard palate and lateral bodies of the maxilla. (From Kirpensteijn J, Withrow SJ, Straw RC. Combined resection of the nasal planum and premaxilla in three dogs. Vet Surg 1994;23:341–346.)

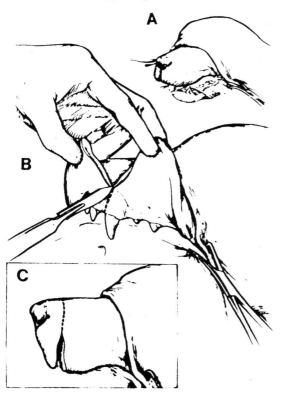

Fig. 20.4. A. The dog is placed in sternal recumbency and is draped after preparation for aseptic surgery. The mouth is open, and the lower drape is within the mouth. **B.** The upper lip is incised full thickness on each side of the nasal planum. **C.** The two incisions are united on the dorsal midline of the nose caudal to the nasal planum. (From Kirpensteijn J, Withrow SJ, Straw RC. Combined resection of the nasal planum and premaxilla in three dogs. Vet Surg 1994;23:341–346.)

through the mucosa on each side of the nasal planum (Fig. 20.4B). The two incisions are connected at the dorsal midline of the nose caudal to the nasal planum (Fig. 20.4C). The nasal cartilages are incised to the palatal region of the maxillary bone. At the level just either rostral to or caudal to the canine teeth, de-pending on the extent of invasion of the tumor, the mucosa of the hard palate is incised transversely with a scalpel blade down to bone. An oscillating saw is used to cut the palatal and maxillary or incisive bone (Fig. 20.5). The excised specimen is submitted for his-topathologic examination, with emphasis on evalua-tion of margins for completeness of resection. Hemor-rhage is controlled by a combination of direct pressure, electrocautery, and vessel ligation. Four or five small holes are drilled 2 to 3 mm from the cut edge of the hard palate. The submucosa of the incised lip is sutured through the holes in the hard palate with 2–0 mono-filament absorbable suture material. The lip is joined on the midline of the palate with sutures that are placed approximately in the middle of each lip incision (Fig. 20.6A). The mucous membrane of the lip is su-tured to the mucous membrane of the hard palate, and the contralateral lip is sutured with 3–0 monofilament absorbable suture material in a continuous or inter-rupted pattern. This technique results in closure of the oral cavity in the form of a "T" (Fig. 20.6B). The skin of the lips is closed on the midline with 2–0 or 3–0 monofilament nonabsorbable suture material. As with closure after nasal planum resection alone, the diame-ter of the nasal opening is reduced using a pursestring suture of monofilament nonabsorbable suture mate-rial (Fig. 20.6C). The nasal opening is reduced to a size

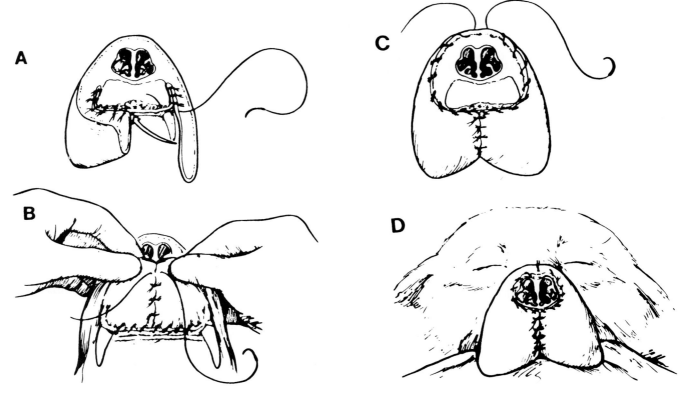

Fig. 20.6. **A.** The submucosa and mucosa of the lip is sutured through drill holes in the hard palate and to the contralateral lip. **B.** This results in closure of the oral cavity from the nasal cavity in the form of a "T." **C.** The nasal orifice is reduced in diameter by placing a simple continuous pursestring suture. **D.** View from the front of the dog after surgery. The new nasal orifice is approximately the diameter of the resected nasal planum. (From Kirpensteijn J, Withrow SJ, Straw RC. Combined resection of the nasal planum and premaxilla in three dogs. Vet Surg 1994;23:341–346.)

corresponding to the diameter of the nasal planum removed (Fig. 20.6**D**).

Analgesia is provided using narcotics as necessary. An Elizabethan collar may be needed to prevent mutilation of the wounds. Dogs are allowed to drink water on recovery and are offered food 24 hours after surgery. Antibiotics can be given during the immediate perioperative period, but they are usually not necessary. Dogs are sent home within 2 to 3 days, and sutures are removed 10 days postoperatively.

Mild postoperative bleeding may occur and resolves within a day or so. Lip dehiscence can be avoided if the closure is tension free. Stenosis of the new nares can occur if the pursestring suture is too tight. Crusting of the nasal orifice is possible and resolves after suture removal; however, serous nasal discharge can persist.

References

1. Hargis AM. A review of solar-induced lesions in domestic animals. Compend Contin Educ Pract Vet 1981;3:287–293.
2. Withrow SJ. Tumors of the respiratory system. In: Withrow SJ, MacEwen EG, eds. Veterinary oncology. 2nd ed. Philadelphia: WB Saunders, 1996:268–286.
3. Hargis AM, Ihrke PJ, Spangler WL, et al. A retrospective clinicopathological study of 212 dogs with cutaneous hemangiomas and hemangiosarcomas. Vet Pathol 1992;29:316–328.
4. Miller MA, Ramos JA, Kreeger JM. Cutaneous vascular neopla-
sia in 15 cats: clinical, morphologic, and immunohistochemical studies. Vet Pathol 1992;29:329–336.
5. Withrow SJ, Straw RC. Resection of the nasal planum in nine cats and five dogs. J Am Anim Hosp Assoc 1990;26:219–222.
6. Kirpensteijn J, Withrow SJ, Straw RC. Combined resection of the nasal planum and premaxilla in three dogs. Vet Surg 1994;23:341–346.
7. Carlisle CH, Gould S. Response of squamous cell carcinoma of the nose of the cat to treatment with X rays. Vet Radiol 1982;5:186–192.
8. VanVechten MK, Théon AP. Strontium-90 plesiotherapy for treatment of early squamous cell carcinomas of the nasal planum in 30 cats. In: Proceedings of the 13th Annual Conference of the Veterinary Cancer Society, Columbus, OH 1993: 107–108.
9. Théon AP, Madewell BR, Shearn VI, et al. Prognostic factors associated with radiotherapy of squamous cell carcinoma of the nasal plane in cats. J Am Vet Med Assoc 1995;206:991–996.
10. Théon AP, VanVechten MK, Madewell BR. Intratumoral administration of carboplatin for treatment of squamous cell carcinomas of the nasal plane in cats. Am J Vet Res 1996; 57:205–210.
11. Peaston AE, Leach MW, Higgins RJ. Photodynamic therapy for nasal and aural squamous cell carcinoma in cats. J Am Vet Med Assoc 1993;202:1261–1265.

Rhinotomy Techniques

Cheryl S. Hedlund

Dogs and cats with chronic nasal and paranasal sinus disease may require rhinotomy (surgical exploration of the nasal cavity) if other diagnostic techniques fail to provide a definitive diagnosis or as part of a therapeutic protocol. Potential candidates for rhinotomy have symptoms that may include nasal discharge, epistaxis, sneezing, gagging, stertorous breathing, dyspnea, fetid breath, nasal discomfort, or nasal deformity. Causes of diseases of the nasal cavity and paranasal sinus can be difficult to identify, but these disorders are most commonly infectious or neoplastic. Other inciting causes include trauma, parasites (*Pneumonyssoides caninum, Linguatula serrata*), dental disease, and congenital anomalies (1).

Diagnostic Procedures

A standard protocol of evaluation should be used for all dogs and cats presenting with chronic nasal disease. The protocol should include a thorough history and physical examination. In addition, a complete blood count, serum chemistry profile, coagulation profile, radiographs, computed tomography, serology, rhinoscopy, and nasal biopsy may be required for accurate diagnosis and prognosis (2). The clinical history provides important diagnostic clues. A destructive process is suspected if the discharge changes from unilateral to bilateral. Sneezing suggests involvement of the rostral or middle nasal chambers, and gagging suggests nasopharyngeal involvement. A history of trauma or dental disease may suggest an oronasal fistula.

Physical examination findings are as follows: Epistaxis may indicate a systemic disease, an acute nasal disease, or an ulcerative, destructive disease. A mucopurulent discharge with or without epistaxis suggests chronic rhinitis. Obstruction of nasal airflow through one or both nostrils suggests a unilateral or bilateral condition. Facial or palatal deformity suggests neoplasia. Mouth breathing may indicate nasopharyngeal obstruction. Labored breathing suggests possible pulmonary involvement with a fungal or neoplastic condition. An ocular discharge may indicate nasolacrimal duct erosion. General debility suggests systemic disease.

A complete blood count, serum chemistry panel, and urinalysis should be obtained to assess the patient's overall status. A coagulation profile is indicated if exploratory rhinotomy is planned or if epistaxis is a major clinical sign. Serologic evaluation for *Aspergillus* and *Penicillium* species can be beneficial when fungal disease is suspected. Serologic evaluation for *Ehrlichia canis* may be beneficial if epistaxis is the predominant clinical sign. Nasal swabs for culture or cytologic evaluation are of limited value, but they may be helpful in identifying parasites, cryptococcal organisms, and single bacterial infections. Positive fungal cultures can be obtained in 40% of normal dogs.

Radiographs of the thorax and skull are taken to demonstrate the extent of disease involvement. Radiographs of the thorax are taken in the awake patient to evaluate for evidence of cardiac or pulmonary disease (metastasis or infection). Skull radiographs require general anesthesia to allow accurate evaluation of the nasal cavity and paranasal sinuses. Skull radiographs are performed before any rhinoscopic, flush, or biopsy procedures to avoid iatrogenic fluid densities within the cavities. Skull radiographs should include lateral, ventrodorsal, rostrocaudal, and rostroventral–caudodorsal open-mouth or occlusal views. The two most useful radiographic views are the ventrodorsal view of the maxilla made using intraoral radiographic film and the rostrocaudal projection highlighting the frontal sinuses. Skull radiographs are examined for evidence of increased or decreased tissue densities, distortion or loss of turbinates and bone, and symmetry between right and left sides of the nasal cavity and sinuses. Computed tomography localizes lesions better than radiography.

Rhinoscopy is useful because it allows visual recognition of lesions and acquisition of material for examination. Rhinoscopy is performed on an anesthetized patient in sternal recumbency after skull radiography. The nasal mucosa is sensitive to manipulation; it bleeds easily, and this may obscure visualization. Therefore, gentleness, suction, and lavage are advantageous during this procedure. The rostral aspect of the nasal cavity may be visualized with an otoscope and an appropriate speculum. A flexible pediatric bronchoscope (less than 1 cm diameter) or a rigid scope (bronchoscope or arthroscope, 2 to 5 mm diameter) facilitates visualization of the entire cavity. Both normograde and retrograde rhinoscopy should be performed. During rhinoscopy, suitable biopsy forceps are used to collect tissue for culture and histologic evaluation.

Lesions that are not accessible to biopsy during rhinoscopy may be sampled by nasal flushing or coring procedures. These procedures are performed in the anesthetized patient. Gentle flushing of the nasal cavity with saline does not usually dislodge tissue for evaluation. Nasal coring, punch biopsy, and needle biopsy are more effective biopsy techniques. To prevent aspiration, the endotracheal tube cuff is inflated, gauze sponges are placed in the nasopharynx, and the nose is tilted ventrally during sampling. To prevent penetration of the cribriform plate, biopsy instruments should be marked and not advanced further than the distance from the external nares to the medial canthus of the eyes. One technique for nasal coring uses a stiff plastic tube inserted through the nares and vigorously moved in and out of the nasal passages while flushing saline and aspirating tissue. The collected lavage fluid, debris, and tubing are examined for tissue fragments.

Patients whose disease has not been diagnosed by the foregoing procedures are candidates for exploratory surgery. Rhinotomy may also be included in treatment protocols for fungal diseases, tumors, and foreign bodies. Rhinotomy can be performed using dorsal or ventral approaches. The approach chosen depends on the location and extent of the lesion. The objectives of rhinotomy include the following: 1) to obtain sufficient samples from the nasal cavity or sinuses to achieve a definitive diagnosis; 2) to eliminate or debulk a lesion; 3) to facilitate administration or effectiveness of adjuvant therapy; 4) to minimize patient morbidity; 5) to maintain a cosmetically acceptable appearance.

In addition to a standard surgical pack, equipment that may be needed for rhinotomy includes a periosteal elevator, Gelpi retractor, oscillating saw, air drill, pins and pin chuck, osteotome and mallet, bone curette, rasp, bur, rongeur, trephine, fenestrated tubes, and synthetic mesh. If temporary carotid artery occlusion is performed in conjunction with rhinotomy, vascular occlusion is accomplished with umbilical tape, vascular tape (Vas-Tie, Sil-Med Corp., Taunton, MA), or bulldog vascular clamps.

Surgical Anatomy

The nasal cavity is bound by the nasal bones dorsally, the maxilla laterally, and the hard palate ventrally. The orbit contributes to the lateral boundary of the nasal cavity and frontal sinuses. The nasal cavity is separated into two fossae by the nasal septum. The maxilloturbinates fill the rostral portion of each fossa, and the ethmoturbinates extend caudally to the cribriform plate and frontal sinus (Fig. 20.7). When dividing the dorsoventral nasal height at the medial canthi of the eyes, the nasofrontal opening occupies the dorsal third, the cribriform plate the middle third, and the sphenoidal sinus recess and caudal nasal meatus (internal nares or choanae) the ventral third. The paranasal sinuses are hollow, membrane lined, air-filled diverticula from the nasal cavity that invaginate into adjacent bones. They are not fully developed at birth and continue to grow as the animal matures. The limits of the frontal sinus vary with the age, breed, and head shape of the patient. Dogs have a frontal sinus divided into three compartments and a maxillary sinus (recess). Cats have an undivided frontal sinus, and in addition to the maxillary sinus, they have a sphenoid sinus. Communication between the frontal sinus and the nasal cavity occurs through small ostia in the ethmoid region. Mucous membrane swelling reduces the size of these openings and can obstruct drainage, leading to sinus mucocele formation. The blood supply to the nasal cavity is extensive and originates from the branches of the maxillary artery, a terminal vessel of the external carotid artery.

Surgical Techniques

Temporary Carotid Artery Occlusion for Rhinotomy

Occluding the common carotid arteries reduces blood loss during exploration of the nasal cavity, improves visualization during surgery, facilitates exploration, and obviates blood transfusions in most patients (3). Although hemorrhage (50 to 100 mL/25 kg body weight) occurs during removal of the turbinates and nasal mucosa, it diminishes within a few minutes. Suction is advantageous but not necessary for visualization. Release of the carotid arteries at the conclusion of the operation does not result in clinically significant hemorrhage, and nasal packing is not necessary. The common carotid arteries can be occluded for 2 to 3 hours with no evidence of neurologic or ischemic damage.

Temporary carotid artery ligation is performed after positioning the patient in dorsal recumbency with the front legs secured caudally along the chest and the neck dorsiflexed by positioning it over a pad. The skin is incised along the ventral cervical midline from the larynx to the midtrachea. The paired sternohyoideus muscles are separated and retracted to expose the trachea. To locate the carotid sheath, the surgeon palpates the carotid pulse dorsolateral to the trachea, then bluntly dissects the adjacent loose connective tissue and exteriorizes the carotid sheath. The surgeon carefully incises the carotid sheath and separates the external carotid artery from the vagosympathetic trunk and internal jugular vein. The carotid artery is occluded with a vascular tie (Vascular Ties, Sil-Med Corp.), umbilical tape, or a vascular clamp (Fig. 20.8). The procedure is repeated on the opposite carotid artery, the skin incision is closed with a continuous suture pattern

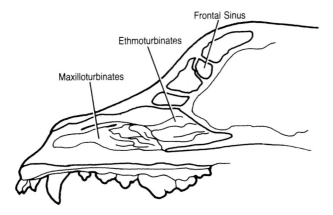

Fig. 20.7. The nasal fossae are filled with maxilloturbinates in the rostral portion and ethmoturbinates in the caudal portion. The ethmoturbinates extend caudally to the cribriform plate and frontal sinus.

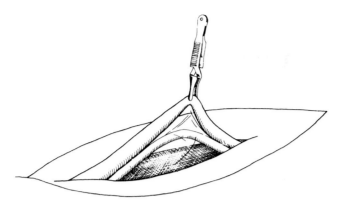

Fig. 20.8. The common carotid artery is occluded with a bulldog clamp after being separated from the vagosympathetic trunk and internal jugular vein.

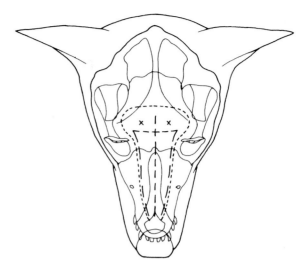

Fig. 20.9. The *outer dotted line* outlines the approximate extent of the nasal cavity and frontal sinus. The *inner dashed lines* outline the bone flap for a unilateral or bilateral rhinotomy. The *Xs* over the frontal sinuses indicate the site for insertion of a drain.

or staples. Immediately after rhinotomy, the surgeon exchanges contaminated instruments and gloves and positions the patient to allow reexposure of the carotid arteries. The ventral midline incision is opened, the carotid arteries are exposed, and the vascular clamps or ties are removed. The surgeon lavages the area thoroughly and apposes sternohyoid muscles, subcutaneous tissue, and skin in separate layers.

Dorsal Rhinotomy

Dorsal rhinotomy allows access to the entire nasal cavity and the frontal sinuses (4). After the anesthetized animal is intubated, the endotracheal tube cuff is inflated, and the pharynx is packed with gauze sponges to prevent drainage of fluids into the distal trachea. The patient is positioned in ventral recumbency, then the dorsum of the head is clipped and is prepared aseptically for surgery.

The surgeon begins the rhinotomy by making a midline skin incision over the nasal cavity and frontal sinus that extends caudal to the orbits (Fig. 20.9). The dense fascia and periosteum overlying the bone are incised, elevated, and retracted laterally. The bone is scored with a scalpel blade, and a unilateral or bilateral bone flap is created, depending on the extent of the disease and the exposure necessary (Fig. 20.10). The flap is made using an oscillating saw, drill, osteotome and mallet, or trephine and rongeurs. The margins of the bone are beveled inward if bone flap replacement is anticipated. The bone flap is elevated from the underlying turbinates with an osteotome or periosteal elevator. The bone flap is reflected rostrally, leaving it attached to the dorsal parietal cartilage of the rhinarium by the nasal ligaments if flap replacement is planned (Fig. 20.11). After exposing the nasal cavity and frontal sinus, the surgeon suctions secretions or exudate and explores the area. The lesion and involved

turbinates are removed or sampled for biopsy with forceps, a bone curette, and Metzenbaum scissors (Fig. 20.12). Total turbinectomy is often necessary to eliminate extensive areas of nasal mucosa with chronic irreversible hyperplasia. One should avoid traumatizing or perforating the cribriform plate during turbinectomy. Identifiable bleeding vessels are ligated. When external carotids are not occluded, it may be necessary to control hemorrhage with cautery, iced saline, or pressure. Tissues are submitted for histologic and culture evaluation. During a unilateral rhinotomy, if the nasal septum has been perforated or eroded by the disease pro-

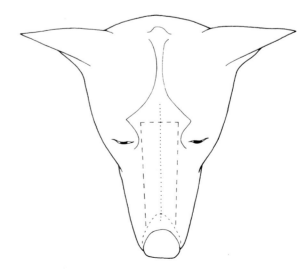

Fig. 20.10. The *dashed line* represents bone scoring for a bilateral bone flap. The *dotted line* represents the location of the nasal septum, which divides the nasal cavity into two fossae.

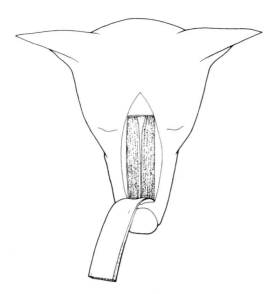

Fig. 20.11. The bone flap is reflected rostrally and remains attached to the dorsal parietal cartilages.

cess, the other fossa is explored and curetted through the septal defect or by creating a second bone flap. When mucoid secretions fill the frontal sinuses, the surgeon enlarges the ostia and breaks down the septa to facilitate drainage. The caudal nasal meatus (internal nares and choanae) is probed with a hemostat to verify patency. The nasal cavity and sinuses are lavaged with saline or lactated Ringer's solution before closure to remove debris and blood clots. Fenestrated indwelling tubes are placed if necessary for adjuvant therapy. These drains are placed through a trephine hole into the frontal sinus and extend into the nasal fossa.

The bone flap is replaced or discarded, depending on the extent of disease and the surgeon's preference. The flap is discarded if it is involved in the disease process or if fragmentation occurs during removal. If the flap is being replaced, the surgeon drills three or four holes in the flap and the adjacent margins of the defect. The surgeon then preplaces nonabsorbable sutures (nylon, polypropylene) through the holes, positions the flap, and ties the sutures to secure the flap (Fig. 20.13). One should not use wire to secure the bone flap if radiation therapy is planned. Occasionally, when the defect is large, the flap is discarded, and cosmetics are critical, a bone graft or synthetic mesh is stretched across the bony defect and secured. Potential risks with the use of such implants include sequestration and infection. Soft tissues are apposed in three layers (fascial–periosteal layer, subcutaneous tissues, and skin) using continuous suture patterns. Air leakage from the rhinotomy site and subcutaneous emphysema may be controlled by suturing a stent over the surgical site, placing a drain in the frontal sinus and nasal cavity, or leaving a small gap between tissue edges during closure.

Technique variations may be necessary, depending on the disease type and extent. Postoperative nasal flushing, prevention of emphysema, and brachytherapy for tumors are facilitated by placing a drain in the frontal sinus and nasal cavity through a trephine hole (Fig. 20.14). An incision is made through the soft tissues and a hole in the bone is drilled or trephined just lateral to the midline on a line connecting the rostral margins of the supraorbital processes. Biopsy and culture specimens may be collected through this hole if not previously obtained. A fenestrated tube is inserted into the sinus, advanced into the nasal cavity, and

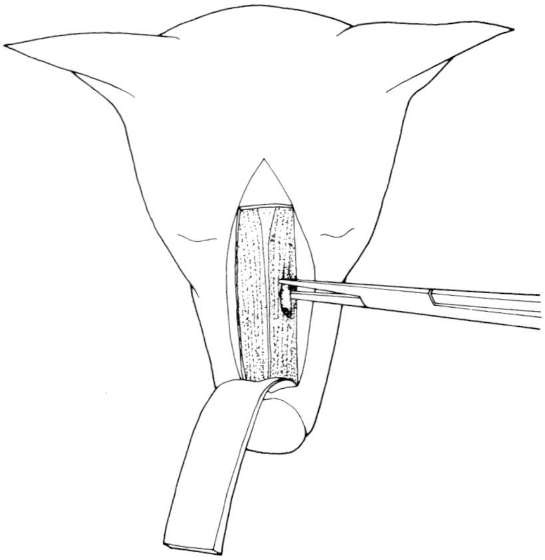

Fig. 20.12. Turbinectomy begins by removal of the diseased turbinates with forceps.

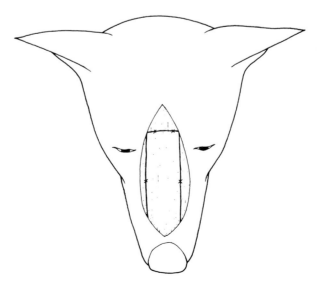

Fig. 20.13. The bone flap is replaced by placing sutures through holes drilled in the flap and margins of the defect.

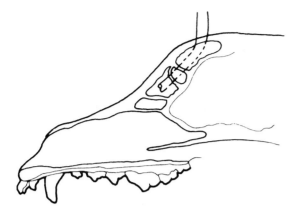

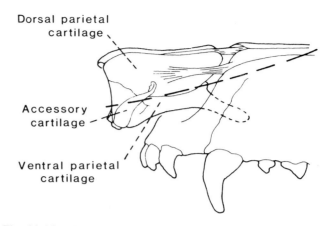

Fig. 20.14. A drain can be positioned in the frontal sinus for adjuvant therapy or to reduce subcutaneous emphysema.

Fig. 20.16. The lateral rhinotomy incision is directed between the dorsal and ventral parietal cartilages, but it transects the accessory cartilage.

secured to the skin. The hole is allowed to heal by second intention after tube removal. Protocols for treatment of nasal fungal diseases may include packing the nasal cavity with mediated gauze or creating a stoma. Stomas are created by securing the skin edges directly to the margins of the bony defect (5). Creation of a stoma facilitates topical therapy postoperatively. If the stoma is small, it may heal by second intention; otherwise, at the conclusion of medical therapy, the skin edges are debrided, undermined, and apposed. Removal of lesions in the rostral nasal cavity may be facilitated by extending the incision through the rhinarium lateral to the nasal septum.

Lateral Rhinotomy

Lateral rhinotomy is occasionally used to approach lesions in the rostral one-fourth to one-third of the nasal passages. The surgeon directs the incision dorsocaudally from the angle of the rhinarium toward the nasomaxillary notch between the dorsal and ventral parietal cartilage (Figs. 20.15 and 20.16). The accessory cartilage is invariably transected. The edges of the inci-

sion are retracted with stay sutures to expose the rostral nasal passages. The incision is closed in three layers (nasal mucosa, cartilage or subcutaneous tissue, and skin).

Ventral Rhinotomy

Ventral rhinotomy allows exploration of the nasal cavity and nasopharynx (4). Evaluation and evacuation of the frontal sinuses are limited to the rostral half with ventral rhinotomy. Concurrent mandibulotomy may be advantageous to improve access to the caudal nasal cavity and nasopharynx. Although most surgeons prefer dorsal rhinotomy, advantages of ventral rhinotomy may include improved cosmesis and less risk of subcutaneous emphysema. Disadvantages include incomplete access to the frontal sinuses and the potential for oronasal fistula formation.

The patient is positioned in dorsal recumbency with the oral cavity maximally exposed by hanging and securing the mandible in a wide, open-mouth position. One should use mild antiseptic solutions (0.05% chlorhexidine or 0.1 or 1% povidone–iodine) to cleanse the oral cavity.

Cranial Ventral Rhinotomy

The mucoperiosteum of the hard palate is incised on the midline from the level of the canine teeth to the fourth premolar to expose lesions restricted to the rostral nasal cavity. Alternatively, the nasal cavity may also be exposed using a U-shaped mucoperiosteal incision parallel to the dental arcade (Fig. 20.17). After incision, the surgeon elevates and retracts the mucoperiosteum to expose the hard palate while preserving the major palatine arteries during incision and dissection. The major palatine arteries emerge from the ma-

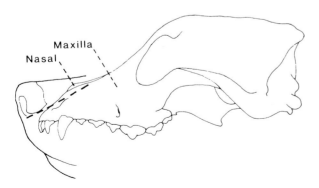

Fig. 20.15. The incision for a lateral rhinotomy is directed dorsocaudally from the angle of the rhinarium toward the nasomaxillary notch.

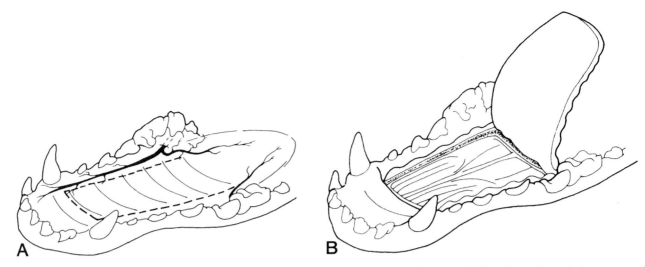

Fig. 20.17. **A.** The *dashed line* represents a U-shaped mucoperiosteal incision made just medial to the major palatine artery when performing a ventral approach to the rostral aspect of the nasal cavity. **B.** A rectangular palatine bone flap of similar size is created and is removed to expose the nasal turbinates.

jor palatine foramen at the caudal edge of the fourth upper premolar and course rostrally, midway between the midline and dental arcade. A rectangular palatine bone flap is removed with an oscillating saw, air drill, or osteotome (see Fig. 20.17). The lesion and involved turbinates are removed with forceps and curettage. The surgeon lavages and suctions the area before replacing or discarding the bone flap as with dorsal rhinotomy (Fig. 20.18). The mucoperiosteum is apposed using a one-layer or two-layer closure with simple interrupted sutures (3–0 or 4–0 polydioxanone, polypropylene).

Caudal Ventral Rhinotomy

Caudal ventral rhinotomy is selected for exposure of lesions in the caudal nasal passages and nasopharynx.

A midline cranial ventral rhinotomy incision can be extended to expose the nasopharynx when necessary. A midline soft palate incision is made, beginning 5 to 10 mm rostral to the tip of the soft palate and extending through the mucoperiosteum of the hard palate as far as necessary to expose the lesion adequately (Fig. 20.19). Stay sutures are placed in the incised edges of the soft palate to facilitate retraction and to minimize trauma. The mucoperiosteum is elevated, and the hard palate is rongeured as far rostrally as necessary for exposure. The surgeon explores, removes the lesion, and lavages the area. The soft palate is apposed in two (nasal and pharyngeal mucosa) or three layers (nasal mucosa, muscle and connective tissue, and pharyngeal mucosa) with simple interrupted or continuous monofilament sutures (4–0 polydioxanone, polypropylene) (Fig. 20.20). The mucoperiosteum is apposed with one or two layers of simple interrupted sutures.

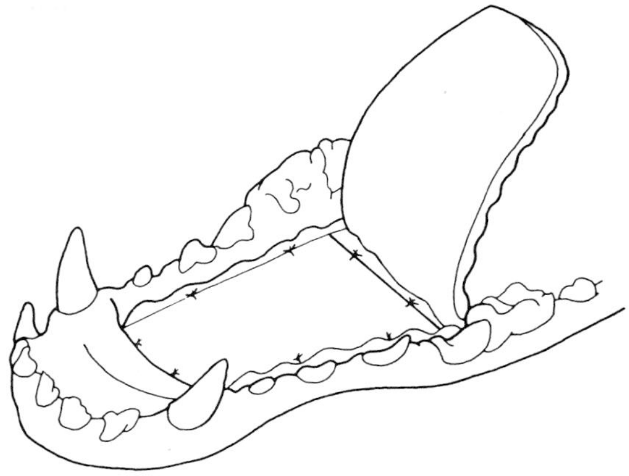

Fig. 20.18. The palatine bone flap is replaced by sutures secured through holes drilled in the flap and bone margins.

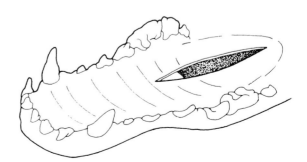

Fig. 20.19. The caudal aspect of the nasal cavity and nasopharynx is approached ventrally by incising the soft and hard palates for varying distances.

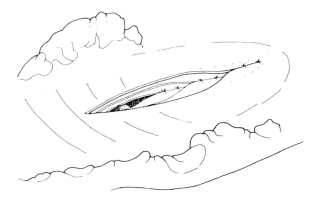

Fig. 20.20. The soft palate incision is closed with two or three layers of sutures to allow adequate apposition of the nasal and oral mucosae.

Postoperative Management

After surgical procedures involving the nasal cavity and sinuses, the patient is recovered in a slightly head-down position, and the endotracheal tube is removed with the cuff slightly inflated to prevent tracheal aspiration of fluid and debris. Analgesics are given for 3 to 5 days as needed. Good analgesia is expected with butorphanol (0.2 to 0.4 mg/kg intravenously or intramuscularly) or oxymorphone (0.05 to 0.1 mg/kg intravenously or intramuscularly). The patient's vital signs are monitored carefully, and supportive care is administered as needed. Sneezing and mild epistaxis are expected for several days. A serous to serosanguineous discharge occurs for several days to weeks, depending on the primary disease condition and the effectiveness of adjuvant therapy. Breathing sounds are harsh and resonant. Inward and outward movement of the skin flap is expected if the bone flap is discarded. Appetite may be depressed for several days. Cats tolerate rhinotomy poorly and may not readily resume eating. Diazepam or oxazepam may be given to stimulate their appetite. Chewing on hard objects is forbidden if the hard palate bone flap is discarded. Patients are discharged from the hospital within 2 to 3 days after the operation unless complications or adjuvant therapies dictate longer hospitalization.

Complications

Complications of rhinotomy include hemorrhage, entrance into the cranium, pain, emphysema, airway obstruction, nasal discharge, and disease recurrence. Intraoperative hemorrhage is minimized by temporary occlusion of the external carotid arteries and adequate intraoperative hemostasis. Packing the nasal cavity is discouraged because it may lead to hyperventilation

and subcutaneous emphysema; in addition, removal of the packing material 2 to 3 days after surgery is painful. Although postoperative hemorrhage is rare, blood transfusions are sometimes necessary to replace lost volume.

Disease erosion of the cribriform plate or curettage may result in exposure of the brain and subsequent cerebral edema. Tumor extension into the cranium should be suspected when the animal exhibits neurologic signs or when defects in the cribriform plate are identified with computed tomography. Animals with brain edema should be treated with rapid-acting water-soluble intravenous corticosteroids, osmotic agents (mannitol) hyperventilation, hyperbaric oxygen, calcium channel blockers, and antioxidants.

Subcutaneous emphysema occurs when air leaks from the nasal cavity into the subcutaneous tissues at the surgical site and is usually associated with violent sneezing or obstruction to nasal airflow. Airflow may be obstructed by nasal packing, occlusion of the nares with crusted blood and secretions, or severe mucosal edema. Subcutaneous emphysema is usually self-limiting and resolves within 1 to 2 weeks. It may be prevented by suturing a stent over the surgical site, inserting a drain, or creating a stoma and avoiding obstruction of the nasal passages. Subcutaneous emphysema is primarily a cosmetic concern, although it can facilitate the spread of infection. The animal's level of comfort may improve if the subcutaneous air is aspirated and a drain placed into the nasal cavity to reduce recurrence.

Rhinotomy is a painful procedure. Analgesics should be given at the conclusion of the operation and as needed for 3 to 5 days. Anorexia is expected after surgery and may be due to pain or a diminished sense of smell. Anorexia is worse in cats than in dogs because cats depend on their ethmoturbinates for olfaction and appetite stimulation. Cats are given diazepam or oxazepam to stimulate their appetite if necessary. Dogs usually require no treatment and have a normal appetite within a few days. After ventral rhinotomy, animals should not be allowed to chew on hard objects. Oronasal fistulas develop if dehiscence occurs or when soft tissues are perforated by hard, sharp objects.

Although airway obstruction is uncommon, it may occur in animals after rhinotomy. Animals should be monitored closely during recovery. Obstruction may be due to failure to breathe through the mouth, mucosal edema, and anxiety. These animals should be sedated and provided with supplemental oxygen in a quiet, cool environment. Corticosteroids should be given to reduce mucosal edema. An endotracheal or tracheostomy tube is indicated if dyspnea is severe.

A serosanguineous nasal discharge is expected after rhinotomy. The discharge diminishes and becomes more serous as denuded bone is covered with epithelium. If the primary disease has been eliminated, the discharge remains minimal and serous. If the disease progresses or the area becomes infected, the discharge increases and becomes mucopurulent or hemorrhagic. Chronic infections are treated with antibiotics selected on the basis of culture and sensitivity tests.

Recurrence of most diseases is expected after rhinotomy unless appropriate adjuvant therapy is instituted. Rhinotomy for foreign body removal may be an exception if irreversible chronic rhinitis and osteomyelitis have been avoided. Rhinotomy for fungal disease should be followed with administration of with antifungal agents, and rhinotomy for neoplasia should be followed by radiation therapy, to extend the animal's disease-free period.

References

1. Gartrell CL, O'Handley PA, Perry RL. Canine nasal disease. Part I. Compend Contin Educ Pract Vet 1995;17:323–328.
2. Gartrell CL, O'Handley PA, Perry RL. Canine nasal disease. Part II. Compend Contin Educ Pract Vet 1995;17:539–547.
3. Hedlund CS, Tangner CH, Elkins AD, et al. Temporary bilateral carotid artery occlusion during surgical exploration of the nasal cavity of the dog. Vet Surg 1983;12:83–85.
4. Hedlund CS. Rhinotomy techniques. In: Bojrab MJ, ed. Current techniques in small animal surgery. 3rd ed. Philadelphia: Lea & Febiger, 1990:321–326.
5. Pavletic MM, Clark GN. Open nasal cavity and frontal sinus treatment of chronic canine aspergillosis. Vet Surg 1991;20:43–48.

Frontal Sinus Drainage Techniques

David E. Holt

Surgical Anatomy and Indications

The frontal sinus is located between the internal and external tables of the frontal bones. The left and right frontal sinuses are separated by a midline septum. In the dog, each frontal sinus is divided into lateral, rostral, and medial compartments. Each compartment communicates with the nasal passages through separate nasofrontal openings. Cats have no further division of the left and right frontal sinuses. A single narrow opening connects each frontal sinus with the ethmoid region of the nasal cavity in the cat. Indications for surgery of the frontal sinus include fungal disease, chronic rhinitis or sinusitis, neoplastic disease, trauma, and the need for biopsy and culture samples to provide a definitive diagnosis.

Treatment of Aspergillosis

Aspergillosis often involves the nasal passages and frontal sinuses. Currently, the most successful reported treatment involves topical administration of antifungal drugs through tubes placed in the frontal sinuses and nasal passages. The animal is placed in sternal recumbency. A transverse incision is made between the zygomatic processes of the frontal bone. The subcutaneous tissue is dissected on the same line. Incisions are made through the periosteum over the left and right frontal sinuses midway between the zygomatic process of the frontal bone and the midline. The periosteum is elevated, and a Steinmann pin, trephine, or air-driven drill is used to create an opening into each frontal sinus. If necessary, the opening can be enlarged with rongeurs. The frontal sinuses are inspected, and fungal material is removed and submitted for culture and biopsy. The nasofrontal openings are enlarged if necessary. In many cases, the infection has eroded the thin bony plates among the lateral, rostral, and medial frontal sinuses. A second small hole is drilled in the caudal aspect of each sinus. A fenestrated intravenous extension set tube is placed through the skin and into each frontal sinus through this hole. The tube is positioned to lie in the frontal sinus, nasofrontal opening, and caudal nasal passage on each side (Fig. 20.21). Treatment of both sides is vital, even if the disease appears to be unilateral. One must ensure that the portion of the tube in each frontal sinus contains several fenestrations, and that a fenestrated part of the tube is not positioned subcutaneously. The periosteum over the larger frontal sinus openings is sutured closed. The skin and subcutaneous tissue are closed, and the tubes are secured to the skin of the patient's head using sutured tape butterflies or Chinese finger trap sutures.

Treatment involves twice-daily flushing with enilconazole (10 mg/kg total dose for both sides each treatment) for 7 to 10 days. The medication is diluted with an equal volume of warm saline or water, equal volumes are flushed into each tube, and the tube is

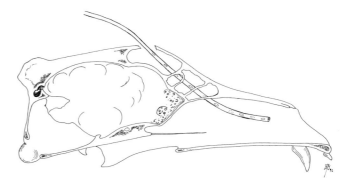

Fig. 20.21. Placement of tubes for treatment of nasal aspergillosis with enilconazole.

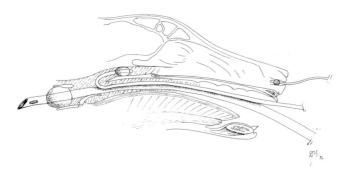

Fig. 20.22. Placement of the Foley catheter dorsal to the soft palate and in the external nares for single dose clotrimazole treatment of nasal aspergillosis.

flushed with air at the end of each treatment. Complications are usually limited to premature removal of the tubes. Occasionally, dogs become anorectic and vomit; these signs resolve when the medication is discontinued. Unfortunately, enilconazole is not widely available in the United States.

A less invasive treatment protocol has been described. Dogs are placed in dorsal recumbency, a Foley catheter is placed dorsal to the soft palate at the junction of the hard and soft palates, and the balloon is inflated. Sponges are placed in the oropharynx, and the cuff on the endotracheal tube is checked to prevent aspiration. Polypropylene catheters are advanced into each nostril, the nostrils are occluded with two additional Foley catheters, and clotrimazole (1 g for each dog) is slowly infused into each nostril (Fig. 20.22). The excess medication is allowed to drain from the nostrils. The medication remains in the nasal passages and sinuses for 1 hour. The Foley catheters are removed from the nostrils and above the palate, and the pharynx is cleared before anesthetic recovery. Initial studies indicate excellent distribution of the medication, even in animals with severe fungal disease.

Treatment of Chronic Rhinitis or Sinusitis

Chronic rhinitis or sinusitis is most commonly seen in cats as a sequel to viral respiratory infection or, rarely, as the result of chronic obstruction of nasal drainage by nasopharyngeal polyps. Chronic rhinitis or sinusitis is also occasionally seen in dogs. Several surgical treatments have been described, including frontal sinus flushing, drainage, obliteration, and rhinotomy combined with frontal sinus curettage. However, precise indications for each technique and the benefits of one technique over another are unclear.

Surgery is performed in cases of chronic rhinitis or sinusitis that fail to respond to appropriate medical therapy. A single transverse incision from one supraor-

bital process to the other is used to access both sinuses. A longitudinal midline incision is used if curettage of the entire nasal cavity is contemplated. The periosteum is elevated from the site of the sinus incision. The sinus is opened with a trephine, Steinmann pin, or air-powered drill. For sinus flushing in kittens, the hole is made just lateral to the midline, midway between the zygomatic process of the frontal bone and the medial canthus of the eye; in mature cats, the hole is made just lateral to the midline and rostral to a line connecting the zygomatic process of the frontal bone on each side. Samples are immediately taken for biopsy and culture. Diseased tissue and debris are removed, and the sinuses are flushed. At this point, the surgeon must choose among sinus flushing, sinus obliteration, or complete curettage of the nasal cavity and sinuses.

To flush the sinuses, fenestrated tubing is placed through each hole into the sinuses. The sinonasal opening is inspected on each side for patency. The opening is gently enlarged if necessary. Silicone sheeting has been recommended to reestablish patency of blocked sinonasal openings in dogs. The tubes are secured to the skin using tape butterflies or Chinese finger trap sutures (Fig. 20.23). The midline incision is closed routinely. Postoperatively, systemic antibiotics are administered based on results of culture and sensitivity testing. Tubes are flushed with a trypsin solution (one part trypsin powder to two parts water), 0.5 to

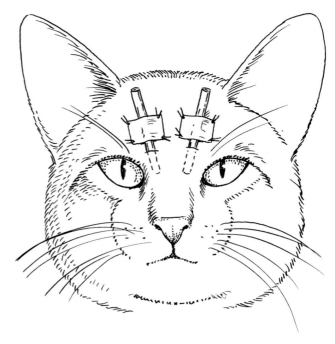

Fig. 20.23. Placement of tubes in the frontal sinuses for irrigation. (Redrawn from Slatter D. Textbook of small animal surgery, 2nd ed. Philadelphia: WB Saunders, 1993;752.)

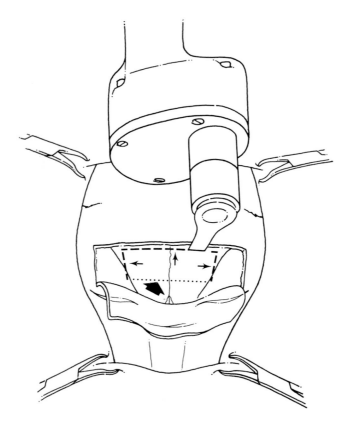

Fig. 20.24. Creating a bone flap for greater exposure of the frontal sinus. The periosteum is reflected from the proposed incision lines, and an oscillating saw or osteotome is used to cut a full-thickness flap (*dashed lines*). The rostral edge is scored only (*dotted lines*). (From Bright RM. Surgical treatment of chronic sinusitis in the cat using autogenous fat implants. In: Bojrab MJ, ed. Current techniques in small animal surgery. 2nd ed. Philadelphia: Lea & Febiger, 1983:259.)

1.5 mL per sinus in cats. Once the tubes are removed, granulation tissue and epithelium rapidly close the openings.

To obliterate the sinuses in cats, the surgical exposure is increased either with rongeurs or by creating a bone flap (Fig. 20.24). The mucosal lining of the sinuses is meticulously removed. A small piece of temporalis muscle fascia is harvested and is placed in each sinus to occlude each nasofrontal ostium. Fat previously harvested from the ventral abdomen is placed into each sinus, and the periosteum is closed or the bone flap replaced.

Treatment of Neoplasms

In cases of neoplasia, exposure of the frontal sinus is simply a caudal extension of the bone flap created for nasal exploration, because most tumors involve both the frontal sinus and the nasal passages. The caudal margin of the bone flap should be just caudal to the zygomatic process of the frontal bone. Once curettage is completed, a small hole is drilled in the dorsal roof of the caudal frontal sinus with a Steinmann pin. A fenestrated plastic tube is placed through the hole and is passed through the nasofrontal opening. Once the incision is closed, this tube acts as a "pop-off" valve during expiration and prevents the development of subcutaneous emphysema. Surgical treatment alone does not benefit animals with nasal and frontal sinus neoplasia. Surgical treatment is considered only when subsequent orthovoltage radiation treatment is planned; it does not prolong survival in animals subsequently treated with cobalt irradiation.

Acknowledgment

I wish to acknowledge the original artwork of Daniel Brockman, BVSc.

Suggested Reading

Anderson GI. The treatment of chronic sinusitis in six cats by ethmoid conchal curettage and autogenous fat graft sinus ablation. Vet Surg 1987;16:131.

Birchard SJ, Bradley RL. Surgery of the respiratory tract and thorax. In: Sherding RG, ed. The cat: diseases and clinical management. 2nd ed. New York: Churchill Livingstone, 1994.

Bright RM. Surgical treatment of chronic sinusitis in the cat using autogenous fat implants. In: Bojrab MJ. Current techniques in small animal surgery. 2nd ed. Philadelphia: Lea & Febiger, 1983.

Evans SM, Goldschmidt M, McKee LJ, et al. Prognostic factors and survival after radiotherapy for intranasal neoplasms in dogs: 70 cases (1974–1985). J Am Vet Med Assoc 1989;194:1460.

Grandage J, Richardson K. Functional anatomy. In: Slatter DH, ed. Textbook of small animal surgery. 2nd ed. Philadelphia: WB Saunders, 1993.

Matthews KG, Richardson EF, Koblik AP, et al. Computed tomographic evaluation of intranasal infusions in dogs with fungal rhinitis. Vet Surg 1995;24:432.

Nelson AW. Upper respiratory system. In Slatter DH, ed. Textbook of small animal surgery. 2nd ed. Philadelphia: WB Saunders, 1993.

Sharp NJH, Harvey CE, Sullivan M. Canine nasal aspergillosis and penicilliosis. Compend Contin Educ Pract Vet 1991;13:41.

Sharp NJH, Sullivan M, Harvey CE, et al. Treatment of canine aspergillosis with enilconazole. J Vet Intern Med 1993;7:40.

Theon AP, Madewell BR, Harb MF, et al. Megavoltage irradiation of neoplasms of the nasal and paranasal cavities in 77 dogs. J Am Vet Med Assoc 1993;202:1469.

Todoroff RJ. Soft tissue surgery. In: Holzworth J, ed. Diseases of the cat: medicine and surgery. Philadelphia: WB Saunders, 1987.

21

LARYNX

Brachycephalic Syndrome

Cheryl S. Hedlund

Brachycephalic animals (especially English bulldogs, Boston terriers, Chinese pugs, Pekingese, shar-pei dogs, and Himalayan and Persian cats) often exhibit signs of upper airway obstruction resulting from anatomic and functional abnormalities. Brachycephalic animals are characterized by having a compressed face with poorly developed nares and a distorted nasopharynx. Their head shape is the result of an inherited developmental defect in the bones of the base of the skull. These bones grow to normal width but reduced length. The soft tissues of the head are not proportionally reduced and often appear redundant. These anatomic exaggerations result in increased airflow resistance and increased inspiratory effort that lead to functional airway abnormalities. Brachycephalic animals with these anatomic exaggerations and clinical signs are diagnosed as having the "brachycephalic syndrome."

The major components of the brachycephalic syndrome are stenotic nares, elongated soft palate, and eversion of the laryngeal saccules. Most dyspneic brachycephalic animals have more than one and often all components of the syndrome. Some animals, especially English bulldogs, also have tracheal hypoplasia. These abnormalities may restrict airflow so severely that the condition progresses to include laryngeal and pharyngeal inflammation and edema, tonsil eversion from their crypts, and epiglottic, laryngeal, or tracheal collapse.

Affected brachycephalic animals exhibit mild to se-

vere signs of respiratory distress, depending on the degree and location of the obstruction. Signs of upper airway obstruction include exercise intolerance, stertorous breathing, mouth breathing, gagging, restless sleep ("sleep-disordered breathing"), cyanosis, and collapse. Other signs may include restlessness, tachypnea, dysphagia, fever, and an abnormal posture. Excitement, stress, and increased heat and humidity frequently make clinical signs worse. Dogs present for stridorous breathing and exercise intolerance, gagging, or episodes of cyanosis and collapse.

Clinical evaluation of patients with severe respiratory distress should be conducted in a manner that does not upset the animal, to avoid exacerbating its condition. The animal should be allowed to maintain a position of comfort and should be restrained minimally during the initial evaluation. Before a more thorough evaluation and workup, patients with severe respiratory distress are provided emergency therapy. Emergency treatment includes controlling the environment to keep the animal cool and to minimize stress, providing supplemental oxygen and a patent airway, and administering corticosteroids, sedatives, and other drugs as needed to stabilize the patient. Further diagnostic tests and treatment follow stabilization of the patient.

A tentative diagnosis of the patient's upper respiratory tract obstruction is usually achieved by obtaining a complete history, thorough physical examination, and results of clinical pathologic examination. These diagnostic measures are followed by lateral neck and routine thoracic radiographs, endoscopic respiratory tract examination, and sample collection for bacterial culture and biopsy as needed. Additional diagnostic measures may include blood gas analysis and respiratory function testing.

Components of the Syndrome

Stenotic Nares

Stenotic nares are congenital malformations of the nasal cartilages that are commonly seen in brachycephalic breeds. The nasal cartilages of animals with stenotic nares lack normal rigidity and collapse medially, causing occlusion of the external nares. Airflow into the nares is restricted, and greater inspiratory effort is necessary, causing mild to severe dyspnea. Stenotic nares are diagnosed on physical examination when the orifice of the external nares is restricted or compressed by this collapsed tissue. Severe inspiratory dyspnea results if airflow obstruction is marked. Marked occlusion of the nares results in open-mouthed breathing and can interfere with olfaction and air warming, moisturizing, and filtering.

Elongated Soft Palate

The normal soft palate just touches or slightly overlies (1 to 3 mm) the tip of the epiglottis. Congenital soft palate elongation is the most commonly recognized component of the brachycephalic syndrome. The elongated soft palate extends more than 1 to 3 mm caudal to the tip of the epiglottis, is often thickened, and obstructs the dorsal aspect of the glottis (Fig. 21.1). The elongated palate is pulled caudally during inspiration and is sometimes pulled between the corniculate processes of the arytenoids. Increased inspiratory effort is required and more turbulent airflow. The arytenoids and palate become inflamed and irritated by the movement of the palate against the arytenoids and airflow turbulence. Diagnosis of soft palate elongation is made

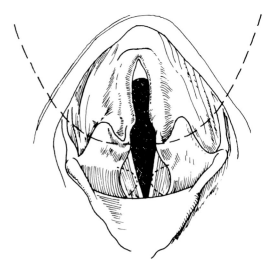

Fig. 21.1. The dorsal dashed line represents the position of an elongated soft palate obstructing the dorsal aspect of the larynx. Everted laryngeal saccules (*ventral dashed line*) protrude from their crypts cranial to and partially obscure the vocal folds.

during endoscopic examination of the nasopharynx and larynx.

Laryngeal Saccule Eversion

Laryngeal saccule eversion or prolapse of the mucosa lining the laryngeal crypts is the first stage of laryngeal collapse. In their normal position between the vocal cords and the ventricular bands (false vocal cords), the laryngeal saccules are not visualized. Increased airflow resistance and increased negative pressure generated to move air past obstructed areas because of stenotic nares and soft palate elongation pull the saccules from their crypts and cause them to swell. Everted and edematous saccules obstruct the ventral aspect of the glottis, further restricting airflow (see Fig. 21.1). Diagnosis of laryngeal saccule eversion is made during endoscopic examination. The everted saccules are recognized as edematous or fleshy soft tissue masses immediately rostral to and often obscuring the vocal folds. Acutely everted saccules are whitish and glistening. Chronically everted saccules are pink and fleshy. It is difficult to visualize and evaluate the laryngeal saccules and larynx thoroughly before soft palate resection because the soft palate obscures the other structures and the severely affected patient may become cyanotic. For these reasons, laryngeal saccule eversion is diagnosed less often than elongated soft palate or stenotic nares.

Advanced Laryngeal Collapse

Advanced laryngeal collapse is caused by chronic upper airway obstruction that results in increased inspiratory efforts and causes the cartilages to fatigue and lose their rigidity. Stage 2 and 3 laryngeal collapse may be recognized during endoscopic evaluation of animals with the brachycephalic syndrome. In stage 2 collapse or collapse of the aryepiglottic fold, the cuneiform process of the arytenoid cartilage and the fold of tissue connecting it to the epiglottis weaken and deviate medially (Fig. 21.2). Medial deviation of this aryepiglottic fold causes further obstruction of the ventral aspect of the glottis. In stage 3 collapse or collapse of the corniculate processes of the arytenoid cartilages, the corniculate processes lose their rigidity and deviate medially, obstructing the dorsal aspect of the glottis (see Fig. 21.2). The normal glottic diameter at rest is narrowed, and widening of the glottis during inspiratory abduction of the corniculate processes is reduced.

After definitive diagnosis, the condition is treated with the goal of achieving long-term relief from respiratory distress and preventing progression of the disease. Partial resection of the nares, soft palate, and laryngeal saccules is recommended for all patients with brachycephalic abnormalities. Patients with advanced

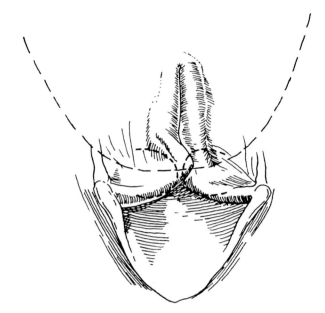

Fig. 21.2. Severe collapse of the arytenoid cartilages in conjunction with an elongated soft palate (*dorsal dashed line*) and eversion of the laryngeal saccules (*ventral dashed lines*). The aryepiglottic folds and cuneiform cartilage collapse medially, obstructing the ventral aspect of the glottis in stage 2 laryngeal collapse. The corniculate processes of the arytenoid cartilages collapse medially, narrowing the dorsal glottis with stage 3 laryngeal collapse.

laryngeal collapse that do not improve adequately after resection or those that improve and then later relapse with severe signs of respiratory distress often benefit from a permanent tracheostomy, which allows airflow to bypass the upper airway. In addition to surgery, medical management may be beneficial. A weight-reduction program is instituted for obese animals. Exercise restriction and elimination of precipitating causes may be beneficial.

Before surgical evaluation and treatment, special precautions must be taken because brachycephalic animals with respiratory distress are at extreme risk, especially during anesthetic induction and recovery. Sedatives and anesthetics agents relax the upper airway–dilating muscles and relax muscles used by brachycephalic animals to facilitate breathing. This relaxation allows the upper airway to collapse and reduces respiratory drive. Risks of complete airway obstruction at induction can be minimized by preoxygenating, rapidly inducing anesthesia with an injectable agent, and then quickly intubating the patient. Risks of complete airway obstruction during recovery are minimized by intensive monitoring and prevention of nasopharyngeal and laryngeal edema. The patient should receive anti-inflammatory doses of corticosteroids (dexamethasone, 0.5 to 2 mg/kg subcutaneously or intramuscularly) immediately before or after induction of anesthesia to reduce swelling and edema during

and after the surgical procedure. Corticosteroid administration should be repeated as needed after surgery to reduce airway obstruction.

Nasopharyngeal and laryngeal inflammation and edema are also minimized by using atraumatic examination and surgical techniques. The patient should be sedated as anesthetic recovery begins, to allow a slow, smooth recovery with the endotracheal tube in place for as long as possible. Administration of oxygen through a nasal catheter facilitates a slow, smooth recovery and minimizes anxiety due to hypoxia. Alternatively, a tracheostomy tube is placed at the beginning of surgery and is removed when the animal is fully recovered from anesthesia and shows minimal signs of respiratory distress.

Various surgical techniques have been described to resect portions of the nares, soft palate, and laryngeal saccules. Resections should be performed early in the animal's life (often before 1 year of age) to prevent progressive deterioration of airway function. I prefer resection using sharp incisions with a scalpel or scissors rather than using electrosurgical or laser instruments. Preoperatively, the patient should be positioned for optimal visualization and lighting (Fig. 21.3). The patient should be in ventral recumbency with the neck extended and the maxilla suspended from an overhead rod. The mandible is pulled ventrally with tape to open the mouth maximally, and the tongue is pulled rostrally. The cheeks are pulled laterally for further visualization. The surgical procedure is begun by resecting the elongated soft palate (see later). This allows subsequent resection of the laryngeal saccules with a less obstructed view. Finally, reposition the head so the chin rests symmetrically on the table and resect the nares.

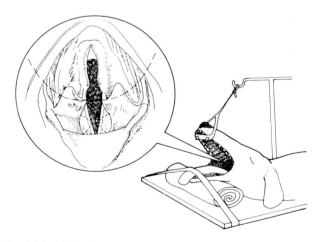

Fig. 21.3. The dog is positioned in ventral recumbency with its maxilla suspended to allow an oral approach to the soft palate and laryngeal ventricles.

Surgical Techniques

Laryngeal Saccule Resection

The stay sutures are left on the edges of the soft palate after resection to facilitate retraction of the palate and to improve visualization of the everted laryngeal saccules. Blood and mucus are aspirated from the field. The endotracheal tube is elevated dorsally and is deviated to one side to allow access to the laryngeal saccule on the opposite side. Alternatively, the endotracheal tube may be temporarily removed to allow less restricted access to the laryngeal saccules; this technique, however, increases the intraoperative risks of aspiration and hypoxia. The everted saccule is grasped with Allis tissue forceps and gently is retracted rostrally and medially to allow positioning of long-handled, curved Metzenbaum scissors across the base of the saccule (Fig. 21.4). The everted tissue is amputated. Amputation may also be accomplished using laryngeal cup forceps or similar biopsy instruments. Hemorrhage is usually mild, but some surgeons twist the saccule after it is grasped to reduce hemorrhage. More severe hemorrhage is controlled with direct pressure. One must be careful not to inadvertently resect the vocal fold, which lies immediately caudal to the everted saccule. The procedure is repeated to remove the opposite laryngeal saccule. The resection sites are allowed to heal by second intention.

Stenotic Nares Wedge Resection

The patient is positioned in sternal recumbency, with the head taped to the table to avoid rotation. The obstructing portion of the nares is grasped with Brown–Adson thumb forceps to delineate and stabilize the segment of nares to be resected. Maintaining this grip,

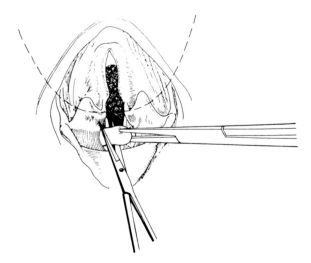

Fig. 21.4. The laryngeal saccule is grasped with tissue forceps and is amputated at its base.

the surgeon makes a V-shaped incision around the forceps with a No. 11 scalpel blade. First is a medial incision angled in a caudolateral direction. Then a second incision is made from the lateral aspect of the nares in a caudomedial direction to meet the first incision at the vortex of the wedge (Fig. 21.5). The wedge of nasal planum and cartilage is removed. Hemorrhage is controlled by applying pressure and apposing the cut edges. Occasionally, identified vessels may be occluded with hemostats or electrocoagulation. The ventral margin of the nares and mucocutaneous junction are aligned, and the incised edges are apposed with three or four simple interrupted sutures using a monofilament absorbable suture (4–0 polydioxanone). The procedure is repeated by removing a similar wedge of tissue from the opposite naris and apposing the edges.

Aryepiglottic Fold Resection

Aryepiglottic fold resection is occasionally performed in patients with aryepiglottic fold collapse. It is performed when other resection techniques have not adequately alleviated the patient's respiratory distress or concurrently with resection of palate, nares, and saccules if respiratory distress is extreme and permanent tracheostomy is not acceptable to the client. Aryepiglottic fold resection is performed unilaterally through an oral approach. The surgeon grasps and stabilizes the fold with forceps and then transects the fold and cuneiform process with Mayo scissors or uterine biopsy forceps. Healing is by second intention.

The nasopharynx and larynx are aspirated, and a nasal catheter is placed for oxygen administration after surgical resections. The catheter is advanced to the end of the soft palate if possible. The surgeon sutures or glues the catheter to the skin and fits the animal with an appropriately sized Elizabethan collar to prevent the patient from removing the catheter. The animal is kept quiet and sedated to allow a slow, quiet recovery with the endotracheal tube in place for as long as possible. The tube is removed with the cuff slightly inflated to withdraw any blood clots that may have entered the trachea. Supplemental oxygen is instituted through the nasal catheter (50 mL/kg per minute) just before or after the endotracheal tube is removed. Nasal oxygen administration is continued until the patient is fully recovered from anesthesia and breathing with minimal or no distress. The patient is monitored continuously during recovery and postoperatively for 24 to 72 hours because inflammation and edema may result in airway obstruction. The surgeon must be prepared to reanesthetize and reintubate or perform a tube tracheostomy in patients with severe dyspnea. Additional doses of corticosteroids may also be necessary. A weight-reduction program should be instituted for obese animals.

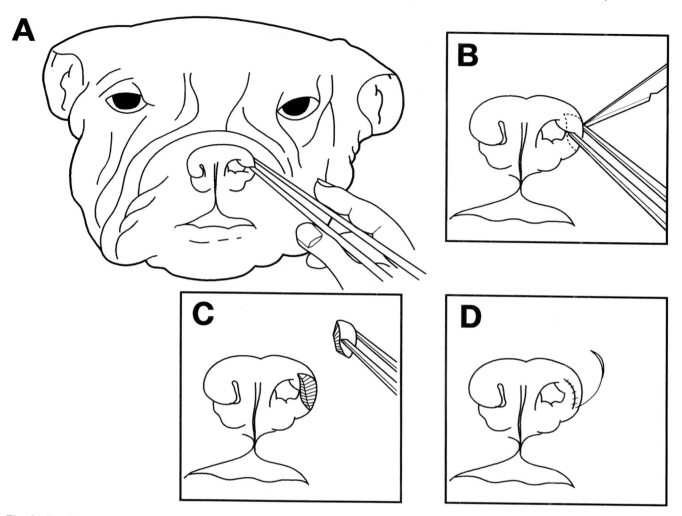

Fig. 21.5. Stenotic nares resection. **A.** Resection of the nares begins by grasping the movable margin of the nares to outline the wedge to be removed and to stabilize the tissue. **B.** Using a No. 11 scalpel blade, medial and lateral incisions are made adjacent to the tips of the forceps. **C.** The wedge is removed and discarded. **D.** The external nares are then widened by placing appositional sutures to appose the incised edges.

Serious surgical complications include death due to glottic obstruction from inflammation and edema and nasal regurgitation and rhinitis or sinusitis due to excessive soft palate resection. Inadequate resection of tissue results in persistent signs of upper airway obstruction. Excessive glottic manipulation may cause vagally induced bradycardia. Hemorrhage, gagging, and coughing may also occur in the early postoperative period. Dehiscence of the nares may occur if the patient frequently licks or rubs its nose. Healing then occurs by second intention and may cause a pink scar. Scarring or stenosis after laryngeal saccule or aryepiglottic resection causes voice change, loss of bark, respiratory noise, or progressive signs of upper airway obstruction.

Prognosis depends on the severity of the condition at the time of operation. Partial resection of the soft palate, laryngeal saccules, and nares is expected to relieve moderate to severe signs of respiratory distress in patients that do not have laryngeal collapse. Patients breathe with less effort and noise and are more tolerant of exercise and excitement. Some patients that initially respond well to resection sometimes deteriorate and again show signs of severe respiratory distress. Laryngeal collapse often is severe in these patients. Patients with advanced laryngeal collapse at the time of diagnosis and resection may respond unsatisfactorily to resection and require permanent tracheostomy to relieve their respiratory distress.

References

Bright RM, Wheaton LG. A modified surgical technique for elongated soft palate surgery. J Am Anim Hosp Assoc 1983;19: 288–292.

Clark GN, Sinibaldi KR. Use of a carbon dioxide laser for treatment of elongated soft palate in dogs. J Am Anim Hosp Assoc 1994;204: 1779–1785.

Harvey CE. Upper airway obstruction surgery. Part 1. Stenotic nares surgery in brachycephalic dogs. J Am Anim Hosp Assoc 1982; 18:535–537.

Harvey CE. Upper airway obstruction surgery. Part 2. Soft palate resection in brachycephalic dogs. J Am Anim Hosp Assoc 1982;18:538–544.

Harvey CE. Upper airway obstruction surgery. Part 3. Everted laryngeal saccule surgery in brachycephalic dogs. J Am Anim Hosp Assoc 1982;18:545–547.

Harvey CE. Upper airway obstruction surgery. Part 4. Partial laryngectomy in brachycephalic dogs. J Am Anim Hosp Assoc 1982;18:548–550.

Hendricks JC. Brachycephalic airway syndrome. Vet Clin North Am Small Anim Pract 1992;22:1145–1153.

Wykes PM. Brachycephalic airway obstructive syndrome. Probl Vet Med 1991;3:188–197.

Treatment of Laryngeal Paralysis by Bilateral Ventriculocordectomy

David E. Holt

Laryngeal paralysis occurs when the normal innervation of the laryngeal muscles is interrupted. Hereditary defects, trauma or masses involving the recurrent laryngeal nerves, central nervous system lesions, generalized polyneuropathy, and hypothyroidism have been associated with laryngeal paralysis; however, most cases are idiopathic. The paired arytenoid cartilages and vocal folds do not abduct during inspiration because of denervation atrophy of the dorsal cricoarytenoideus muscles. Clinical signs associated with this condition include respiratory stridor, bark change, exercise intolerance, and respiratory distress. Coughing

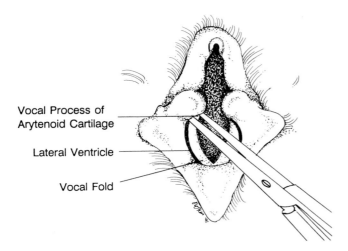

Fig. 21.6. Vocal fold resection, oral approach. Dorsal incision of the vocal process, vocal fold, and vocalis muscle.

Vocal Process of Arytenoid Cartilage

Lateral Ventricle

Vocal Fold

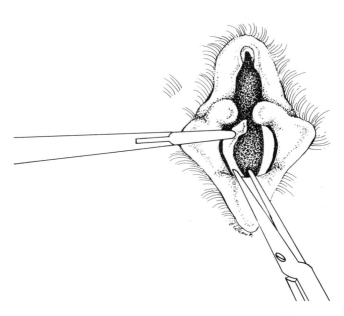

Fig. 21.7. Vocal fold resection, oral approach. Ventral incision of the vocal fold and vocalis muscle.

may indicate aspiration pneumonia, which occurs because adduction of the arytenoid cartilages and vocal folds during swallowing is compromised.

The diagnosis is based on the clinical signs and evaluation of the larynx while the animal is under short-acting barbiturate anesthesia. Animals should be under a light enough plane of anesthesia to gag intermittently during laryngeal examination. In a normal animal, the arytenoid cartilages and vocal folds should abduct during inspiration. In an animal with laryngeal paralysis, the arytenoids remain motionless or can be pulled medially by the negative airway pressure generated during inspiration. The larynx should be inspected carefully for any evidence of collapse. In my opinion, ventriculocordectomy is not a suitable procedure for animals with concurrent laryngeal collapse.

Surgical Techniques

Vocal fold resection is a straightforward surgical alternative to more technically demanding laryngeal procedures, and it can be performed using either an oral or a ventral cervical approach.

Oral Approach

The animal is placed in sternal recumbency with the endotracheal tube placed through a tracheostomy. The epiglottis is depressed, and a vocal fold is grasped gently with a long needle holder or forceps. One scissor blade is placed as far dorsally as possible in the lateral ventricle, the scissor angled dorsally, and a cut is made through the vocal process, the dorsal extent of the

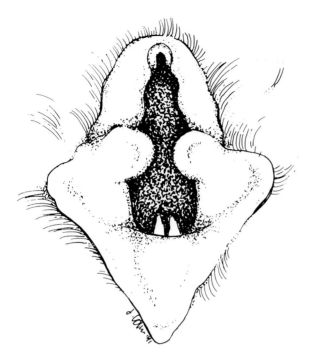

Fig. 21.8. Vocal fold resection, oral approach. Completed vocal fold resection, illustrating the remaining 3 to 5 mm of ventral vocal fold on the midline to prevent scarring.

vocal fold, and the vocalis muscle (Fig. 21.6). The vocal fold is then cut ventrally (Fig. 21.7). It is important to cut parallel to the floor of the larynx ventrally and to leave approximately 3 to 5 mm of each vocal fold ventrally (Fig. 21.8), to prevent ventral scar formation. The vocal fold is then excised by a caudal cut. The procedure is repeated on the opposite vocal fold. The larynx is inspected for residual tags of mucosa and for hemorrhage before anesthetic recovery. In my opinion, all dogs should be recovered with a temporary double-lumen tracheostomy tube in place. The inner canula of the tube is removed and cleaned frequently, and the dog is nebulized at the tracheostomy site. The tube is removed when the animal can comfortably breathe around it, usually 12 to 24 hours postoperatively.

Ventral Approach

The animal is intubated with a cuffed endotracheal tube one or two sizes smaller than would normally be used. This allows more room for vocal fold removal in the larynx. The animal is placed in dorsal recumbency, and the entire ventral mouth and neck are prepared for aseptic surgery. The large, ringlike cricoid cartilage is palpated at the caudal aspect of the larynx. An incision is made in the skin and subcutaneous tissue centered over the cricoid cartilage, and the paired sterno-

hyoid muscles are separated on the midline to reveal the thyroid, cricoid, and cranial tracheal cartilages (Fig. 21.9). The hyoid venous arch at the cranial extent of the larynx is identified and avoided. The cricothyroid ligament is palpated between the cricoid cartilage caudally and the thyroid cartilage cranially. This ligament and the thyroid cartilage are sharply incised along the ventral midline. The edges of the laryngeal incision are gently separated using self-retaining retractors, and the vocal folds are visualized (Fig. 21.10**A**). One vocal fold is grasped and excised with scissors (Fig. 21.10**B** and **C**). The vocal process of the arytenoid is included in the excised tissue. The process is repeated for the second vocal fold, and the mucosal defects are closed using interrupted 4–0 or 5–0 absorbable sutures. Mucosa is apposed over the edges of the remnants of the vocal processes. The thyroid cartilage is closed using interrupted 3–0 absorbable suture. Subcutaneous tissue and skin are closed in routine fashion.

Postoperative Care

All animals are monitored continuously for signs of respiratory difficulty. When aspiration pneumonia is

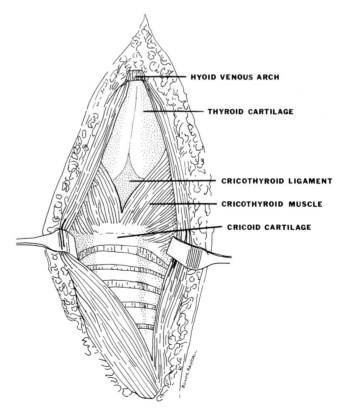

HYOID VENOUS ARCH

THYROID CARTILAGE

CRICOTHYROID LIGAMENT

CRICOTHYROID MUSCLE

CRICOID CARTILAGE

Fig. 21.9. Ventral approach to the larynx. (From Kagan KG. Ventriculocordectomy. In: Bojrab MJ, ed. Current techniques in small animal surgery. 3rd ed. Philadelphia: Lea & Febiger, 1990: 332–335.

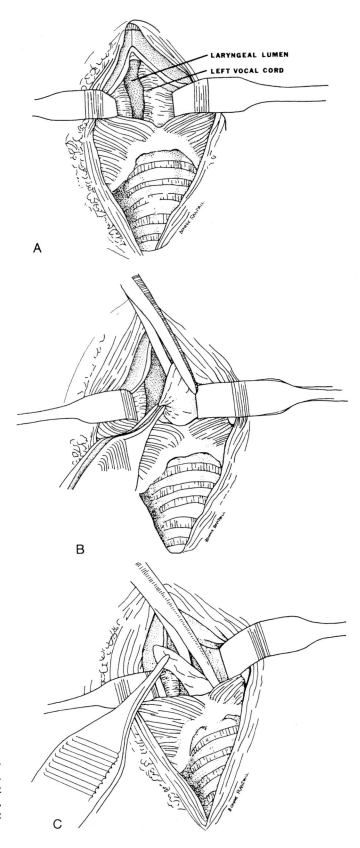

LARYNGEAL LUMEN

LEFT VOCAL CORD

A

B

C

Fig. 21.10. A. Ventral approach to the larynx, incising the crico-thyroid ligament and the caudal half of the thyroid cartilage. **B.** Traction applied to the left vocal fold. **C.** Excision of the left vocal fold. (From Kagan KG. Ventriculocordectomy. In: Bojrab MJ, ed. Current techniques in small animal surgery. 3rd ed. Philadelphia: Lea & Febiger, 1990:332–335.)

absent, corticosteroids are given to minimize swelling of airway tissues and subsequent respiratory distress. Animals are maintained on intravenous fluids until they resume drinking and eating without difficulty. Animals receive small amounts of water and soft food under supervision 12 to 24 hours after the surgical procedure.

Possible Complications

Complications of this procedure include ventral scarring or "webbing" and aspiration pneumonia. Scarring occurred in 14% of animals in one study in which oral ventriculocordectomy was used to treat dogs with laryngeal paralysis. A prednisolone regimen with a high initial dose (2 mg/kg per day) and a tapering course has been recommended to inhibit scar formation as the larynx epithelializes. Scarring is treated by scar excision, mucosal flap coverage of the defect, and placement of a silicone intraluminal stent.

Aspiration can occur before, during, or after the surgical procedure. During swallowing, the protective adductive function of the larynx is lost, predisposing animals to aspiration and subsequent pneumonia. Animals with aspiration pneumonia should be treated with antibiotics based on the results of culture and sensitivity.

Acknowledgment

I wish to acknowledge the original artwork of Jane Cohen, AHT.

Suggested Readings

Braund KG, Steinberg S, Shores A, et al. Laryngeal paralysis in immature and mature dogs as one more sign of a more diffuse polyneuropathy. J Am Vet Med Assoc 1989;194:1735–1740.

Gaber CE, Amis TX, LeCouteur RA. Laryngeal paralysis in dogs: a review of 23 cases. J Am Vet Med Assoc 1985;186:377–380.

Grandage J, Richardson K. Functional anatomy. In: Slatter DH, ed. Textbook of small animal surgery. 2nd ed. Philadelphia: WB Saunders, 1992:698–790.

Holt DE, Brockman DJ. Diagnosis and management of laryngeal disease in the dog and the cat. Vet Clin North Am 1994;24:855–871.

Holt DE, Harvey CE. Idiopathic laryngeal paralysis: results of treatment by bilateral vocal fold resection in 40 dogs. J Am Anim Hosp Assoc 1994;30:389–395.

Matushek KJ, Bjorling DE. A mucosal flap technique for correction of laryngeal webbing: results in four dogs. Vet Surg 1988;17:318–320.

Nelson AW. Upper respiratory system. In: Slatter DH, ed. Textbook of small animal surgery. 2nd ed. Philadelphia: WB Saunders, 1992:753–768.

Peterson SL, Smith MM, Senders CW. Evaluation of a stented laryngoplasty for correction of cranial glottic stenosis in four dogs. J Am Vet Med Assoc 1987;192:1582–1584.

Venker-van Haagen AJ. Diseases of the larynx. Vet Clin North Am 1992;22:1155–1172.

Treatment of Laryngeal Paralysis with Arytenothyroid Lateralization

Stephen D. Gilson

Laryngeal paralysis occurs predominantly in older male large and giant breed dogs, but it can affect any dog (1). It can be associated with generalized neuromuscular disease syndromes, hypothyroidism, and trauma, or it can occur as an inherited anomaly (2). In most dogs, however, the cause of paralysis is undetermined (1). Laryngeal paralysis has also been described in four cats (3, 4). The cause was not determined for three young adult domestic shorthaired cats, although feline leukemia virus infection was suspected in one cat (3). The fourth cat was an 11-year-old domestic shorthair with lymphosarcoma involving the right vagus nerve (4).

Common clinical signs of laryngeal paralysis are respiratory distress, gagging and coughing, exercise intolerance, and stridor. When paralysis is severe, cyanosis, hyperthermia, and collapse can occur. Neurologic examination often reveals signs of generalized neurologic disease. Common signs in cats are difficulty in swallowing and coughing and gagging. Working dogs can be symptomatic, with unilateral paralysis; house pets have usually clinical signs apparent only with bilateral paralysis (5).

Definitive diagnosis is made by laryngeal examination while the patient is under light anesthesia. Paralyzed arytenoid cartilages and vocal folds lie in a paramedian position and, on inspiration, normal abduction of these structures is not seen. Because of decreased intraluminal glottic pressure during inspiration, the arytenoid cartilages and vocal fold can be drawn into a more median position or may oscillate, giving the visual appearance of normal motion. Arytenoid motion *must* be carefully associated with phase of respiration. Concurrent edema and inflammation of the pharynx and larynx are seen frequently. When examining cats, the clinician must be careful to differentiate laryngeal paralysis from laryngospasm; laryngospasm is an active closure of the glottis by tight adduction of the vocal folds and, if severe, the arytenoid cartilages and vestibular folds (3). Other diagnostic tests include radiography and xeroradiography of the neck to detect laryngeal and pharyngeal masses and thoracic radiography to evaluate for aspiration pneumonia. For cases difficult to diagnose, denervation can be confirmed with laryngeal electromyography (1).

Several surgical techniques are described for treatment of laryngeal paralysis including ventriculocordectomy and partial arytenoidectomy from an oral (6) or ventral laryngotomy (7) approach, castellated laryngofissure and vocal fold resection (8), neuromuscular pedicle grafts to reinnervate the dorsal cricoarytenoideus muscle (9), and arytenoid cartilage lateralization from a lateral (10) or paramedian approach (6, 11). The procedure described here is a modification of other techniques (6, 11) and is recommended for larger animals. I find this technique difficult to perform in small animals and prefer partial arytenoidectomy or permanent tracheostomy when animals weigh less than 2 to 3 kg.

Surgical Technique

Dexamethasone (0.1 mg/kg body weight, intramuscularly) is given preoperatively and 12 hours postoperatively to help control edema. The dog is anesthetized, placed in dorsal recumbency, and prepared for surgery. Anesthesia is maintained with inhalant anesthetic ad-

ministered by a cuffed endotracheal tube. Placement of a tracheostomy tube is not necessary in large breed dogs, although doing so may be beneficial in small breed dogs and cats or when undue surgical trauma or other complications associated with increased edema are anticipated after surgery. The tracheotomy tube can generally be removed within 24 hours of the surgical procedure.

A ventral midline skin incision is made over the larynx, extending from the hyoid apparatus to the fifth tracheal ring. Subcutaneous tissues are incised to expose the underlying sternohyoideus muscles. The midline raphe of these muscles is divided to expose the larynx and proximal trachea (Fig. 21.11**A**). The dorsal edge of the thyroid cartilage is grasped through the thyropharyngeus muscle and is rotated ventrally (Fig. 21.11**B**). The thyropharyngeus muscle and its underlying fascial sheath are incised along the edge of the thyroid cartilage (Fig. 21.12). The cricothyroid articulation can be transected if needed, to allow further lateral displacement of the thyroid cartilage and expo-

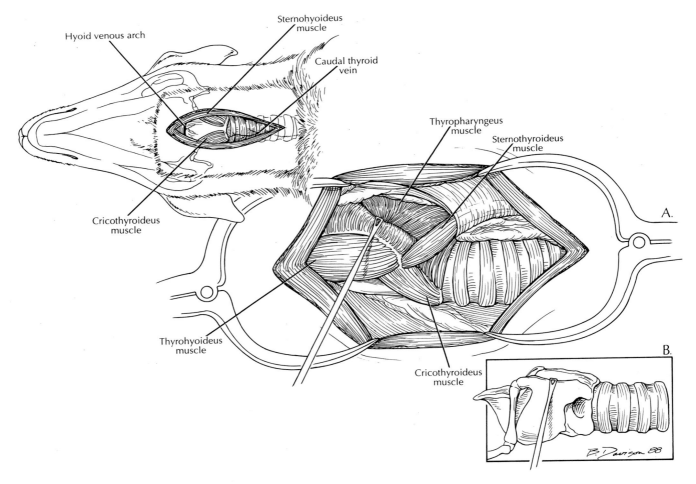

Fig. 21.11. **A.** Ventral approach to the larynx. Rotation of the thyroid cartilage ventrally. **B.** Schematic diagram showing placement of retractor.

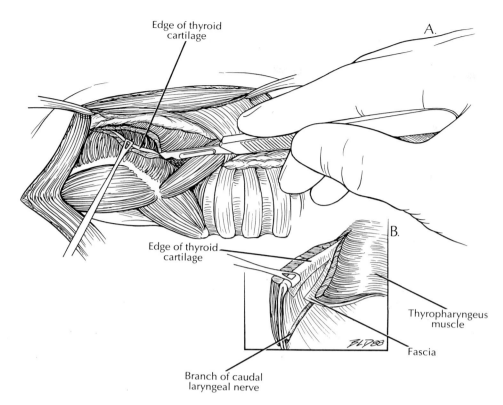

Edge of thyroid
cartilage

Edge of thyroid
cartilage

B.

Thyropharyngeus
muscle

Fascia

Branch of caudal
laryngeal nerve

Fig. 21.12. **A.** Incision of the thyropharyngeus muscle. **B.** Inset showing relationship of the thyroid cartilage, thyropharyngeus muscle, and branch of the caudal laryngeal nerve.

sure of the intrinsic muscles of the larynx (Fig. 21.13). If exposure is adequate, disarticulation is best not performed; it disrupts lateral support of the larynx and can cause vertical collapse when combined with cricoarytenoid lateralization, especially when the procedure is performed bilaterally (12). The dorsal cricoarytenoideus muscle is isolated and transected, with care

taken not to damage the adjacent branch of the caudal laryngeal nerve (Fig. 21.14). The arytenoid remnant of this muscle is retracted rostrally to facilitate disarticulation of the cricoarytenoid joint (Fig. 21.15). Rostral retraction is maintained to expose the shiny cricoarytenoid articular surface. The arytenoid–arytenoid articulation can be transected by advancing the scissor

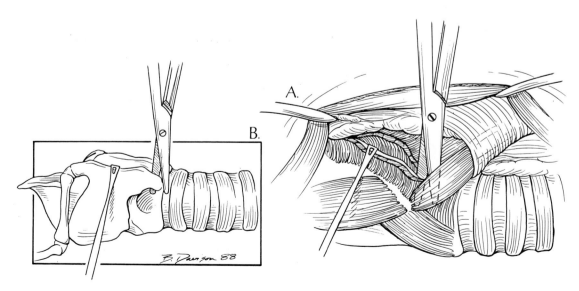

Fig. 21.13. **A.** Transection of the cricothyroid articulation is performed if further lateral displacement of the thyroid cartilage is needed for adequate exposure. **B.** Schematic diagram showing transection of cricothyroid articulation.

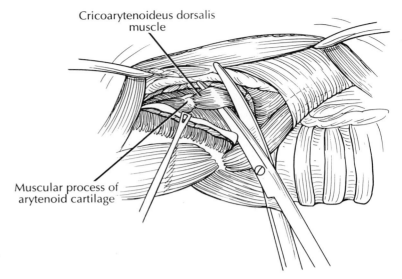

Fig. 21.14. Transection of the cricoarytenoideus dorsalis muscle.

tips over the cricoarytenoid articulation toward the dorsal midline of the larynx (Fig. 21.16). The need for this step remains controversial, but its use can be considered if the surgeon believes that arytenoid abduction is inadequate otherwise. An 18- or 19-gauge hypodermic needle is bored through the muscular process of the arytenoid cartilage so it exits in the center of the cricoarytenoid articular surface, and nonabsorbable monofilament suture (0 or 2–0) is passed through the needle. The needle is withdrawn, leaving the suture in place. The suture must be well placed in the arytenoid cartilage to prevent it from pulling out. The other end of the suture is placed through the caudodorsal border of the thyroid or cricoid cartilage using

the same technique (Fig. 21.17). The suture is tightened and tied to abduct the arytenoid cartilage maximally (Fig. 21.18). An assistant can temporarily remove the endotracheal tube and confirm by laryngoscopy that the arytenoid cartilage is abducted. The thyropharyngeus muscle is repaired using a simple continuous suture pattern with 4–0 absorbable suture material (Fig. 21.19). If the arytenoid is inadequately abducted (as occasionally occurs because of fibrosis and mechanical fixation of the arytenoids near midline), the procedure can be immediately performed on the contralateral side. The sternohyoideus muscles are reapposed using a simple continuous suture pattern with 3–0 absorbable material, and the subcutaneous

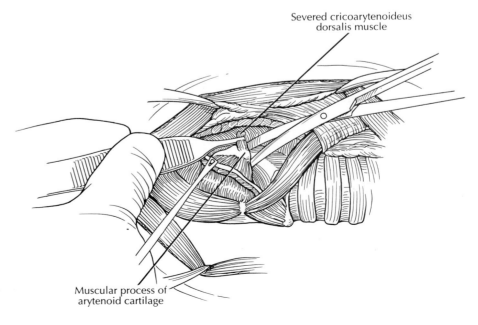

Fig. 21.15. Transection of the cricoarytenoid articulation.

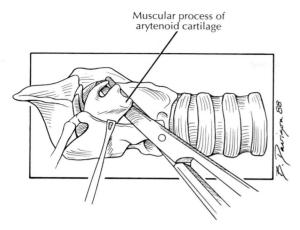

Muscular process of
arytenoid cartilage

Fig. 21.16. Schematic diagram showing transection of the aryte-noid–arytenoid articulation. Controversy remains over the benefit of this step.

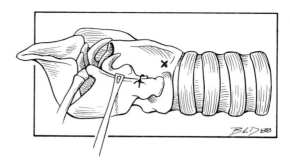

Fig. 21.18. Schematic diagram showing the completed suture maximally adducting the arytenoid cartilage. Alternatively, the ary-tenoid can be sutured to the cricoid cartilage at the site marked with an "X."

tissues and skin are closed in a routine manner (Fig. 21.20).

Postoperative Care

The animal should be closely monitored during recovery from anesthesia. With effective lateralization, obstruction is relieved immediately, and signs of respiratory distress are significantly reduced in the early postoperative period. Oral intake is resumed 12 to 24 hours postoperatively beginning with water and followed by food when the animal shows no signs of coughing or gagging. The animal should always be fed from a low, head-down position for the rest of their life.

The significant advantages of this procedure include less intraoperative hemorrhage, less postoperative edema, and no intralaryngeal adhesions because invasion of the airway is not required. The animal's voice is less impaired because the vocal folds are not resected, and most often no tracheotomy tube is needed, further reducing surgical morbidity. Disadvantages are that the glottal opening is more cumbersome to visualize during surgery than with an intraoral procedure. Complete lateralization may not be possible if the arytenoids are chronically fixed on midline, and success is poor if the animal has concurrent laryngeal collapse. As with all other described procedures (except the

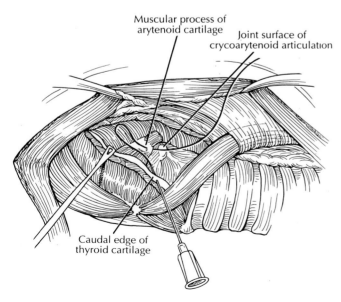

Muscular process of
arytenoid cartilage
Joint surface of
crycoarytenoid articulation

Caudal edge of
thyroid cartilage

Fig. 21.17. Suture placement through the muscular process of the arytenoid cartilage and the caudal edge of the thyroid cartilage.

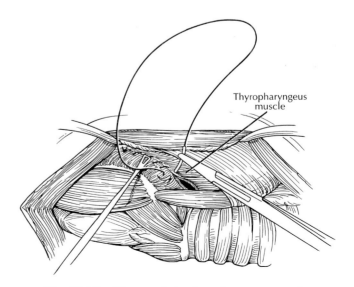

Thyropharyngeus
muscle

Fig. 21.19. Closure of the thyropharyngeus muscle.

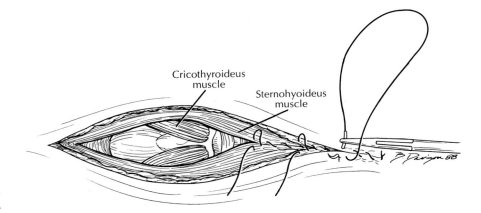

Fig. 21.20. Closure of the sternothyroideus muscles, subcutaneous tissue, and skin.

neurovascular pedicle graft technique), the animal has a permanently enlarged laryngeal opening and is therefore predisposed to aspiration of fluids and food.

Controversy remains over whether cricoarytenoid lateralization (provides more anatomic abduction) is better than thyroarytenoid lateralization (suturing is easier and more accurately placed) and over the need for transection of the interarytenoid ligament. Most studies have focused on the degree of rima glottidis enlargement and have used cadaver specimens (12, 13). The limitation of these studies is that the ideal amount of enlargement is not known (both too much and too little can be detrimental), and anatomic analysis of a cadaver specimen may not correlate with clinical function and success. Clinical trials comparing the techniques are needed to determine whether any significant difference in outcome and incidence of complications exists; in clinical use, I have not perceived notable differences between the techniques.

References

1. Gaber CE, Amis TC, LeCouteur RA. Laryngeal paralysis in dogs: a review of 23 cases. J Am Vet Med Assoc 1985;186:377–380.
2. Venker-van Haagen AJ, Hartman W, Goedegebuure SA. Spontaneous laryngeal paralysis in young bouviers. J Am Anim Hosp Assoc 1978;14:714–720.
3. Hardie, EM, et al. Laryngeal paralysis in three cats. J Am Vet Med Assoc 1979;179:879–882.
4. Schaer M, Zaki FA, Harvey HJ. Laryngeal hemiplegia due to neoplasia of the vagus nerve in a cat. J Am Vet Med Assoc 1979;174:513–515.
5. O'Brien JA, et al. Neurogenic atrophy of the laryngeal muscles of the dog. J Small Anim Pract 1973;14:521–532.
6. Harvey CE, Venker-van Haagen AJ. Surgical management of pharyngeal and laryngeal airway obstruction in the dog. Vet Clin North Am 1975;5:515–535.
7. Baker GJ. Surgery of the canine pharynx and larynx. J Small Anim Pract 1972;13:505–513.
8. Gourley IM, Paul H, Gregory C. Castellated layrngofissure and vocal fold resection for the treatment of laryngeal paralysis in the dog. J Am Vet Med Assoc 1983;182:1084–1086.
9. Greenfield CL, et al. Neuromuscular pedicle graft for restoration of arytenoid abductor function in dogs with experimentally induced laryngeal hemiplegia. Am J Vet Res 1988;49:1360–1366.
10. Lane JG. ENT and oral surgery of the dog and cat. Bristol, England: Wright, 1982:113–118.
11. Rosin E, Greenwood KG. Bilateral arytenoid cartilage lateralization for laryngeal paralysis in the dog. J Am Vet Med Assoc 1982;180:515–518.
12. Lozier S, Pope E. Effects of arytenoid abduction and modified castellated laryngofissure on the rima glottidis in canine cadavers. Vet Surg 1992;21:195–200.
13. Lussier B, Flanders JA, Erb HN. The effect of unilateral arytenoid lateralization on rima glottidis area in canine cadaver larynges. Vet Surg 1996;25:121–126.

Treatment of Laryngeal Paralysis With Unilateral Cricoarytenoid Laryngoplasty

Thomas R. LaHue

Bilateral laryngeal paralysis is a common cause of upper airway obstruction in older dogs. Clinical signs include inspiratory stridor, exercise intolerance, respiratory distress, and, in severe cases, cyanosis and collapse. Other signs include voice change and coughing or gagging. The long-term prognosis with medical therapy alone is poor. Surgery is considered the best method of treatment for dogs with laryngeal paralysis. The goal of surgery is to provide complete relief of the upper airway obstruction while minimizing discomfort and postoperative complications. The prognosis for laryngeal paralysis with proper surgical treatment is good.

The technique described here is a form of arytenoid lateralization called unilateral cricoarytenoid laryngoplasty. This procedure and other forms of unilateral arytenoid lateralization have been used successfully by many surgeons to obtain consistently good results in the treatment of laryngeal paralysis.

Diagnosis

Thoracic and cervical radiographs should be obtained to rule out other causes of respiratory compromise and to document concurrent disease. In addition to a complete blood count and chemistry profile, thyroid status is evaluated (thyroxine or thyroid-stimulating hormone stimulation). The incidence of hypothyroidism is increased in dogs with laryngeal paralysis, although no cause-and-effect relationship has been proved. Hypothyroidism, like acquired laryngeal paralysis, tends to be a disease of older dogs. Hypothyroidism has been reported as a cause of generalized polyneuropathies (1). Supplementation with thyroxine does not reverse the laryngeal paralysis, but it may help to prevent or slow the progression of hypothyroid-induced generalized neuromuscular disease.

Definitive diagnosis of laryngeal paralysis is made with laryngoscopy while the patient is under light anesthesia. Although light anesthesia using barbiturates has been the standard protocol for many years, I have used propofol (Diprivan) (2 to 6 mg/kg, intravenously) in the past 3 to 4 years with excellent results (2). The arytenoid cartilages fail to abduct during inspiration in lightly anesthetized dogs with laryngeal paralysis. The arytenoid cartilages also fail to abduct if the level of anesthesia is too deep. To make an accurate diagnosis, the patient must be under as light a plane of anesthesia as possible, and the evaluation must be of adequate duration to be sure that no effective arytenoid abduction occurs during inspiration (at least 5 to 10 minutes). Some patients actually have paradoxic movement of the arytenoid cartilages in which these cartilages are drawn medially because of the negative pressure created during inspiration (3). The surgeon must correlate any laryngeal movement with the phase of respiration. Laryngoscopy often reveals laryngeal edema and inflammation, which may worsen the signs of laryngeal paralysis and may change the character of dyspnea from primarily inspiratory to both inspiratory and expiratory (3).

Treatment

The recommended emergency medical treatment for an acute respiratory crisis resulting from laryngeal paralysis is sedation and endotracheal intubation, followed by gradual wakening (2). These severely affected patients should be observed continuously and may need emergency surgery to relieve the upper airway obstruction. It is best to perform a definitive corrective procedure rather than a tracheotomy.

Alleviation of the upper airway obstruction caused by laryngeal paralysis can be best achieved with surgery (4). Medical therapy, including the use of corticosteroids, tranquilizers, and oxygen, may be helpful in management of severely affected patients preoperatively. Patients with preexisting aspiration pneumonia should be treated before the surgical procedure, and they may be more likely to develop postoperative aspiration pneumonia. Patients with laryngeal paralysis and megaesophagus have a poor prognosis because of the probability of developing severe aspiration pneumonia after surgery.

The goal of surgery is to provide complete relief of upper airway obstruction while minimizing discomfort and postoperative complications. After the operation, patients should be able to breathe comfortably and have a normal activity level for their age.

Unilateral arytenoid lateralization in some form (cricoarytenoid laryngoplasty is described here) has been used successfully to achieve these goals in treating laryngeal paralysis and is the procedure of choice of many surgeons (2–13). Other reported surgical techniques include partial laryngectomy (partial arytenoidectomy with vocal fold resection) using either an oral or ventral laryngotomy approach (14, 15) and modified castellated laryngofissure with vocal fold resection (16, 17).

Surgical Technique

Several variations of unilateral arytenoid lateralization have been reported. The procedure described here, cricoarytenoid laryngoplasty (2, 3), involves the placement of two sutures in the same location as the cricoarytenoideus dorsalis muscle, from the caudal dorsolateral aspect of the cricoid cartilage to the muscular process of the arytenoid cartilage. Arytenoid lateralization has been used as a general term or to describe the procedure in which sutures are placed from the caudal border of the thyroid cartilage to the muscular process of the arytenoid cartilage (4, 6, 7, 12, 13). Regardless of the technique used, the surgeon must become familiar with the anatomy of the laryngeal region and the surgical procedure. The surgeon should observe the technique before performing it if possible.

Routine endotracheal intubation is performed after laryngoscopy. The unilateral cricoarytenoid laryngoplasty can be performed on either side. I perform the procedure on the left side for consistency only. The patient is placed in right lateral recumbency with a slight rotation toward dorsal recumbency. A ventrolateral approach to the larynx is made, beginning with an 8- to 10-cm long skin incision starting near the angle of the mandible and extending caudally just ventral to the external jugular vein (Fig. 21.21). Palpation of the caudal border of the cricoid cartilage as a landmark is helpful during the approach. Dissection is continued to the lateral and dorsal aspects of the larynx through the subcutaneous tissue and the superficial

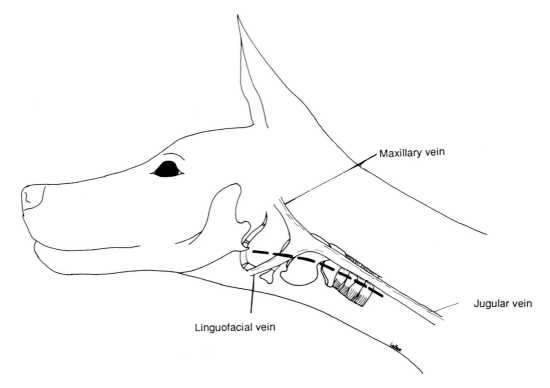

Fig. 21.21. The site of the skin incision is shown by the *dotted line*. A ventrolateral approach to the larynx is made, beginning with an 8- to 10-cm long skin incision starting near the angle of the mandible and extending caudally just ventral to the external jugular vein. It is helpful to palpate the caudal border of the cricoid cartilage as a landmark during the approach.

muscles of the neck, being careful to avoid the external jugular, linguofacial, and maxillary veins.

The dorsal margin of the wing of the thyroid cartilage is palpated and retracted laterally. The thyropharyngeus muscle is incised along the dorsal rim of the thyroid cartilage (Fig. 21.22). Lateral retraction is important, to avoid the esophagus. A layer of connective tissue is incised just medial and parallel to the rim of the thyroid cartilage and is separated bluntly. The

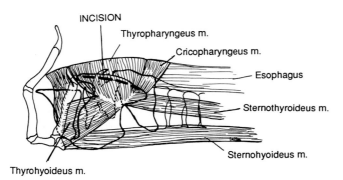

Fig. 21.22. The dorsal margin of the wing of the thyroid cartilage is palpated and retracted laterally. The thyropharyngeus muscle is incised along that margin (*dotted line*).

cricothyroid articulation at the caudal edge of the thyroid cartilage is separated with scissors or a Freer septum elevator (Fig. 21.23**A**). This disarticulation is necessary to provide adequate exposure. The cricoarytenoideus dorsalis muscle and muscular process of the arytenoid cartilage are identified. The cricoarytenoideus dorsalis muscle is undermined and incised close to the muscular process, leaving enough muscle on the muscular process to attach mosquito forceps to facilitate gentle manipulation (Fig. 21.23**B**). The cricoarytenoid articulation is separated using blunt dissection with a Freer elevator; one must be careful not to damage the muscular process or penetrate the laryngeal mucosa (Fig. 21.23**C**). The rostral aspect of the cricoarytenoid joint capsule is left intact as long this allows mobility of the arytenoid cartilage to be attained. The purpose of cricoarytenoid joint disarticulation is to gain mobility of the arytenoid cartilage in relation to the cricoid cartilage so the arytenoid cartilage can be abducted adequately. Laryngoplasty procedures have been described in which cricoarytenoid disarticulation is not done (10). However, some patients have significant fibrosis and ankylosis of this joint. If disarticulation is not performed in these patients, adequate abduction of the arytenoid cartilage will not be achieved.

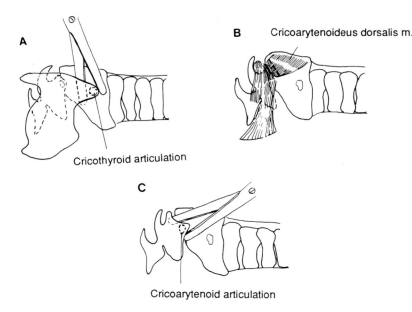

A. Cricothyroid articulation

B. Cricoarytenoideus dorsalis m.

C. Cricoarytenoid articulation

Fig. 21.23. **A.** The cricothyroid articulation at the caudal edge of the thyroid cartilage is separated with scissors or a Freer septum elevator. **B.** The cricoarytenoideus muscle and muscular process of the arytenoid cartilage are identified. The muscle is undermined and is incised close to the muscular process, leaving enough muscle on the muscular process to attach mosquito forceps for use in gentle manipulation. **C.** The cricoarytenoid articulation is separated using blunt dissection with fine scissors or a Freer elevator, with care taken not to damage the muscular process or penetrate the laryngeal mucosa. The rostral aspect of the cricoarytenoid joint capsule is left intact as long as this allows mobility of the arytenoid cartilage to be attained. Thyroid cartilage is not pictured in **B** and **C**. It would be retracted laterally during these stages of the procedure.

When performing this procedure, I no longer routinely include separation of the sesamoid band that connects the two arytenoid cartilages as long as mobilization of the arytenoid cartilage and optimal abduction can be achieved without it.

The disarticulated left arytenoid cartilage is now movable in relation to the cricoid cartilage. Two sutures of monofilament nylon or polypropylene (0 in large dogs, 2–0 in medium dogs) are passed over the caudal edge of the cricoid cartilage and are directed cranially to penetrate the cartilage on the dorsolateral aspect (approximately 5 to 8 mm from the caudal edge), with care taken not to penetrate laryngeal mucosa (Fig. 21.24A). These sutures are passed from me-

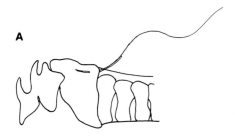

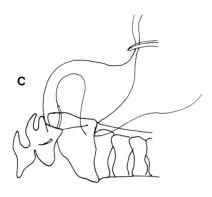

Muscular process (arytenoid cartilage)

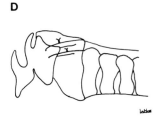

Fig. 21.24. **A.** The first of two sutures is passed over the caudal edge of the cricoid cartilage and is directed cranially to penetrate through the cartilage on the dorsolateral aspect (approximately 5 to 8 mm from the caudal edge), with care taken not to penetrate laryngeal mucosa. **B.** Suture is then passed from medial to lateral through the articular surface or muscular process of the arytenoid cartilage at least 2 to 3 mm from the cartilage edge. **C.** The second suture is passed in a similar manner. **D.** Each suture is tied separately. The intact rostral portion of the cricoarytenoid joint capsule helps to prevent overabduction of the arytenoid cartilage. Thyroid cartilage is not pictured. It would be retracted laterally during these stages of the procedure.

dial to lateral through the articular surface or muscular process of the arytenoid cartilage at least 2 to 3 mm from the cartilage edge (Fig. 21.24**B** and **C**). The sutures are tied separately (Fig. 21.24**D**). The intact rostral portion of the cricoarytenoid joint capsule helps to prevent overabduction of the arytenoid cartilage. The dog is extubated briefly while laryngoscopy is performed to confirm adequate abduction of the left arytenoid cartilage. The endotracheal tube is replaced. Closure of the thyropharyngeus muscle is completed using fine (3–0 or 4–0) absorbable suture material in a simple continuous pattern. Subcutaneous tissues and skin are closed routinely.

Postoperative Management

Postoperative care includes continuous (24-hour) monitoring, intravenous fluid therapy, and withholding of food and water for 12 to 24 hours. Cefazolin (20 mg/kg, intravenously) is given at the time of anesthetic induction and is repeated 2 hours later. Antibiotic therapy (ampicillin 20 mg/kg, orally three times daily) is continued for an additional 5 days if the laryngeal mucosa is penetrated. Patients most often do well postoperatively and go home within 1 to 2 days of the operation. A soft, canned-food diet with no excess gravy or crumbs is recommended to minimize the risk of aspiration pneumonia. A voice change (like that of a debarked dog) is expected after cricoarytenoid laryngoplasty and other techniques. Occasional coughing after drinking water occurs commonly in the postoperative period, but usually it lessens after a short period of adaptation (6).

Unilateral cricoarytenoid laryngoplasty or some form of unilateral arytenoid lateralization has been shown to relieve signs of upper airway obstruction, such as stridor, dyspnea, and exercise intolerance in 82 to 100% of patients (3, 5, 7–9, 12, 13). Lane reported a 97% overall success rate in surgical treatment of 167 cases of laryngeal paralysis using several modifications of arytenoid cartilage lateralization (7). My success rate with unilateral cricoarytenoid laryngoplasty in over 200 dogs has been consistent with these results. White reported alleviation of exercise intolerance or stridor after arytenoid lateralization (with attachment of arytenoid cartilage to cricoid or thyroid cartilage) in 82% of dogs with laryngeal paralysis (12). Greenfield and Harvey and Venker van Haagen reported alleviation of clinical signs of upper airway obstruction in 89 and 95%, respectively, with unilateral arytenoid lateralization (4, 8). Payne and associates reported results of abductor muscle prosthesis in 11 dogs, in which placement of the sutures from cricoid cartilage to muscular process of the arytenoid cartilage was done without cricoarytenoid disarticulation (10). When the procedure was done bilaterally, 3 of 7 dogs

died of aspiration pneumonia. No cases of aspiration pneumonia were reported with unilateral procedures.

Acknowledgments

I wish to thank J.G. Lane, who first showed me the technique of arytenoid lateralization at a veterinary conference in Amsterdam in 1985, and Lawrence E. Stickles, who helped me immensely with the diagnostic evaluation of patients with laryngeal disease during my internship and residency at Santa Cruz (California) Veterinary Hospital.

References

1. Harvey HJ, Irby NL, Watrous BJ. Laryngeal paralysis in hypothyroid dogs. In: Kirk RW, ed. Current veterinary therapy VIII. Small animal practice. Philadelphia: WB Saunders, 1983:694–697.
2. LaHue TR. Laryngeal surgery: lateralization techniques. In: Scientific proceedings of the 22nd annual surgical forum. Washington, DC: American College of Veterinary Surgeons, 1994:255–257.
3. LaHue TR. Treatment of laryngeal paralysis in dogs by unilateral cricoarytenoid laryngoplasty. J Am Anim Hosp Assoc 1989;25:317–324.
4. Harvey CE, Venker van Haagen AJ. Surgical management of pharyngeal and laryngeal airway obstruction in the dog. Vet Clin North Am Small Anim Pract 1975;5:515–535.
5. Gaber CE, Amis TC, LeCouteur RA. Laryngeal paralysis in dogs: a review of 23 cases. J Am Vet Med Assoc 1985;186:377–380.
6. Lane JG. ENT and oral surgery of the dog and cat. Bristol, England: Wright, 1982:113–118.
7. Lane JG. Diseases and surgery of the larynx. In: Scientific proceedings of the 53rd annual meeting of the American Animal Hospital Association. Denver: American Animal Hospital Association, 1986:620–623.
8. Greenfield CL. Canine laryngeal paralysis. Compend Contin Educ Pract Vet 1987;9:1011–1020.
9. Peterson SW, Rosin E, Bjorling DE. Surgical options for laryngeal paralysis in dogs: a consideration of partial laryngectomy. Compend Contin Educ Pract Vet 1991;13:1531–1540.
10. Payne JT, Martin RA, Rigg DL. Abductor muscle prosthesis for correction of laryngeal paralysis in 10 dogs and one cat. J Am Anim Hosp Assoc 1990;26:599–604.
11. Lozier S, Pope E. Effects of arytenoid abduction and modified castellated laryngofissure on the rima glottidis in canine cadavers. Vet Surg 1992;21:195–200.
12. White RAS. Unilateral lateralization: an assessment of technique and long term results in 62 dogs with laryngeal paralysis. J Small Anim Pract 1989;30:543–549.
13. Venker van Haagen AJ. Laryngeal diseases of dogs and cats. In: Kirk RW, ed. Current veterinary therapy IX. Small animal practice. Philadelphia: WB Saunders, 1986:265–269.
14. Harvey CE, O'Brien JA. Treatment of laryngeal paralysis in dogs by partial laryngectomy. J Am Anim Hosp Assoc 1982;18:551–556.
15. Ross JT, Matthiesen DT, Noone KE, et al. Complications and long-term results after partial laryngectomy for the treatment of idiopathic laryngeal paralysis in 45 dogs. Vet Surg 1991;20:169–173.
16. Gourley IM, Paul H, Gregory C. Castellated laryngofissure and vocal fold resection for the treatment of laryngeal paralysis in the dog. J Am Vet Med Assoc 1983;182:1084–1086.
17. Smith MM, Gourley IM, Kurperschoek MS, et al. Evaluation of a modified castellated laryngofissure for alleviation of upper airway obstruction in dogs with laryngeal paralysis. J Am Vet Med Assoc 1986;188:1279–1283.

Treatment of Laryngeal Paralysis With Modified Castellated Laryngofissure

Mark M. Smith

Spontaneous paralysis of laryngeal muscles occurs predominantly in aging large or giant breed dogs. This disease is heritable in bouvier des Flandres and Siberian huskies (or husky cross-breeds), with clinical signs manifested in young members of these breeds. The primary component of the upper airway obstruction is medial displacement of the vocal folds during inspiration. All surgical procedures for this disease address the vocal folds as a major component of the surgical procedure. Modified castellated laryngofissure is a laryngoplasty with three components: castellated laryngofissure, bilateral vocal chordectomy, and bilateral arytenoid cartilage lateralization.

The patient is positioned in dorsal recumbency with the neck extended. The neck is positioned over an elevated, padded area (rolled towel) and is stabilized by taping the maxilla to the operating table. A ventral midline skin incision is made over the thyroid cartilage beginning rostral to the basihyoid bone and extending caudally to the proximal tracheal area. Inhalation anesthesia for the procedure should be administered by tracheostomy tube placed at the third and fourth tracheal rings. Dissecting scissors are used to incise subcutaneous tissues and to divide the paired sternohyoideus muscles to expose the ventral laryngeal area. The hyoid venous arch is cranial to the laryngofissure

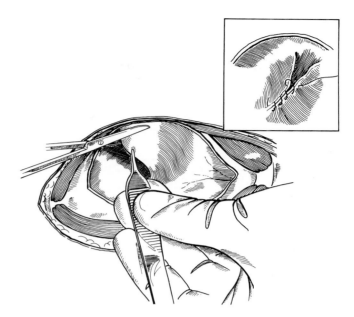

Fig. 21.26. Dissecting scissors resect the vocalis muscle from the vocal process of the arytenoid cartilage and dorsocaudal attachment to the thyroid cartilage. *Inset,* Continuous appositional suture.

site and should not require ligation. However, if present, the laryngeal impar should be ligated and divided before laryngofissure.

The ventral midline castellated laryngofissure is performed in stepwise fashion (Fig. 21.25). A No. 15 blade is used to incise flaps A, B, C in the thyroid cartilage (see Fig. 21.25, *dotted line*). Each flap is equal to one-third the distance (approximately 1 cm) of the ventral thyroid cartilage. The incision for flap B is angled caudally, paralleling the caudal direction of the thyroid lamina. The cricothyroid ligament is incised to complete the laryngofissure (see Fig 21.25, *solid line*). Vocal chordectomy may be performed by using dissecting scissors to resect the vocalis muscle from the palpable vocal process of the arytenoid cartilage and dorsocaudal attachment to the thyroid cartilage (Fig 21.26). The mucosal defect left after vocal chordectomy is repaired by a simple continuous appositional suture using fine chromic gut or synthetic absorbable suture (see Fig 21.26, *inset*). Intraglottic arytenoid lateralization is performed by placement of a single horizontal mattress suture of nonabsorbable material through the vocal process of the arytenoid cartilage and lamina of the thyroid cartilage traversing the recess of the lateral ventricle (Fig. 21.27). The vocal process is covered by mucosa and is the most prominent medial component of the arytenoid cartilage. The suture is tied on the lateral aspect of the thyroid lamina (extraglottic).

The rostral aspect of flap B is repositioned using 2–0 or 3–0 synthetic nonabsorbable suture in a simple interrupted pattern around the basihyoid bone. Flaps

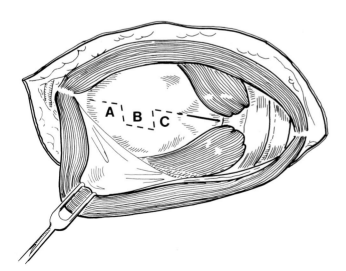

Figure 21.25. Cricothyroid ligament is incised to complete the laryngofissure.

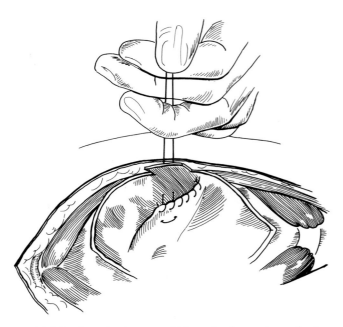

Fig. 21.27. Intraglottic arytenoid lateralization performed using one horizontal mattress suture.

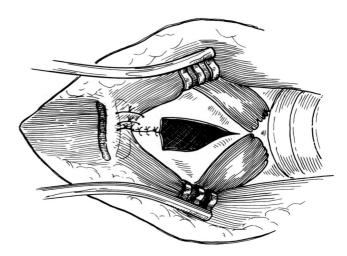

Fig. 21.28. Apposition and closure of flaps.

A and B are apposed using 3–0 or 4–0 synthetic nonabsorbable suture in a simple interrupted pattern (Fig. 21.28). Flap C is resected to avoid displacement into the glottic lumen. The L-shaped laryngofissure is not sutured and heals by epithelialization over granulation tissue. The paired sternohyoideus muscles are apposed using synthetic absorbable suture in a simple interrupted pattern. Subcutaneous tissues are apposed in a second layer followed by skin apposition using synthetic nonabsorbable suture in a simple interrupted pattern.

Disruption of the ventral commissure of the vocalis muscles may heal with excessive granulation tissue leading to laryngeal stenosis (web). Apposition of the intralaryngeal mucosa after vocal chordectomy establishes apposition of epithelialized tissue that may prevent laryngeal stenosis. Bilateral arytenoid cartilage lateralization is generally not recommended because of the common complication of aspiration pneumonia. However, using this technique, the ventrally located vocal processes are lateralized. This maneuver, combined with the castellated laryngofissure, increases the glottic lumen aperture, especially in a ventral location. Bilateral arytenoid cartilage lateralization suturing of the muscular process increases the glottic lumen aperture dorsally, an area less likely to be covered by the epiglottis during deglutition.

The tracheostomy tube may be removed after the patient's recovery from anesthesia. The tracheostomy wound requires superficial cleansing for 7 days postoperatively during the period of second-intention healing. A broad-spectrum antimicrobial is administered during this period. Corticosteroids are not administered preoperatively or postoperatively because the patient preferentially breathes through the tracheotomy while any excessive laryngeal edema is resolving.

Mucosal apposition after vocal chordectomy should avoid the complication of laryngeal stenosis (web) related to disruption of the ventral commissure. The patient may gag while drinking water during the first few postoperative days. This clinical sign is secondary to laryngeal irritation and should be transient. As with other laryngoplasty techniques for laryngeal paralysis, aspiration pneumonia may be a complication of the surgery or the disease.

Modified castellated laryngofissure is not recommended for dogs with laryngeal collapse because cartilage integrity and shape are abnormal. Finally, this procedure may be used when vocal chordectomy or unilateral arytenoid cartilage lateralization has failed to alleviate clinical signs of upper airway obstruction.

Suggested Reading

Smith MM, Gourley IM, Amis TC, et al. Evaluation of a modified castellated laryngofissure for alleviation of upper airway obstruction in dogs with laryngeal paralysis. J Am Vet Med Assoc 1986;188:1279–1283.

22

TRACHEA

Treatment of Tracheal Collapse: Spiral Ring Technique

Roger B. Fingland

Polypropylene spiral prostheses (PSP), 6 cm in length, are made from 3-mL syringe cases (1). Prostheses are aerated for a minimum of 12 hours mechanically and a minimum of 24 hours in room air after ethylene oxide sterilization.

Anesthesia is maintained with an inhalation agent vaporized in 100% O_2 through a semiclosed rebreathing system through a high-volume, low-pressure, cuffed endotracheal tube. The cuff pressure is maintained between 15 and 20 cm H_2O. The endotracheal tube should be long enough to reach the thoracic inlet and should be positioned distal to the segment of trachea where prostheses will be applied. Preparations should be made for intraoperative deflation and reinflation of the endotracheal tube cuff and repositioning of the endotracheal tube.

Surgical Technique

The patient is positioned in dorsal recumbency with the neck hyperextended over a rolled towel. The ventral cervical area is prepared for aseptic surgery. A ventral cervical midline incision is made from the larynx to a point 1 cm caudal to the manubrium. The sternocephalicus muscles are separated at the cranial border of the manubrium, and the sternohyoideus muscles are separated on the midline from the larynx to the manubrium. The left recurrent laryngeal nerve is identified and preserved. The left lateral pedicle, including the segmental blood supply, is dissected from the trachea (Fig. 22.1). A 3-mm fenestration is made in the right lateral pedicle, adjacent to the trachea, 5 mm caudal to the thyroid gland (Fig. 22.2). One end of the PSP is grasped with right-angled forceps and is directed through the fenestration. The PSP is applied to the trachea in a spiraling manner by rotating the free end of the prosthesis around the trachea (Fig. 22.3). The right lateral pedicle is fenestrated approximately every 6 mm along its length where the PSP passes around the right lateral aspect of the trachea. The PSP is spiraled onto the trachea as far proximally (aboral) as the exposure allows or as far as necessary to provide support to the collapsed segment of the cervical trachea. If the endotracheal tube cuff is positioned in the segment of trachea covered by the PSP, the cuff is deflated, and the endotracheal tube is positioned distal (oral) to the prosthesis before suturing begins.

Prostheses are sutured to the trachea with 4–0 polypropylene suture material placed in a simple interrupted pattern (Fig. 22.4). Sutures are placed along the right and left lateral and ventral aspects of the trachea, incorporating each turn of the PSP and the underlying tracheal cartilage. Tagging the left lateral sutures facilitates rotation of the trachea for exposure of the dorsal tracheal membrane. The dorsal tracheal membrane is sutured to the PSP (Fig. 22.5). All sutures enter the tracheal lumen.

The endotracheal tube cuff is deflated and repositioned to ensure that a suture has not been placed through the cuff. The endotracheal tube cuff is reinflated, and the incision is closed routinely.

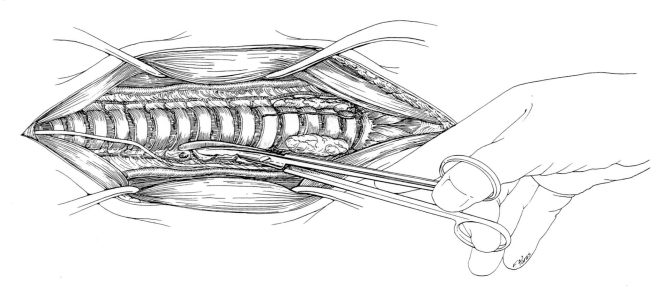

Fig. 22.1. The lateral pedicles are dissected from the left lateral aspect of the trachea. The left recurrent laryngeal nerve is identified and preserved.

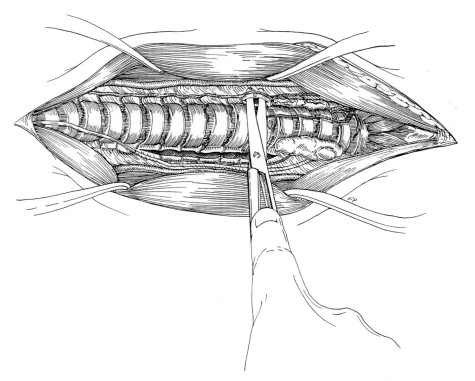

Fig. 22.2. A 3-mm window is made between the right lateral pedicle and the trachea.

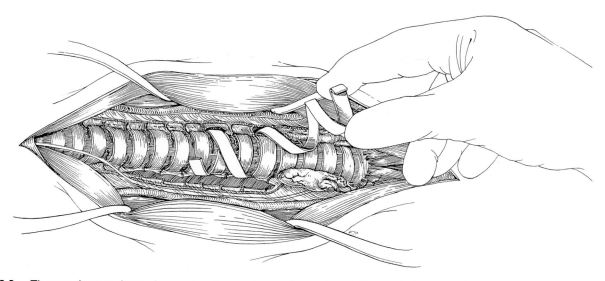

Fig. 22.3. The prosthesis is directed around and rotated onto the trachea. A 3-mm window is made in the right lateral pedicle where the prosthesis passes around the right lateral aspect of the trachea.

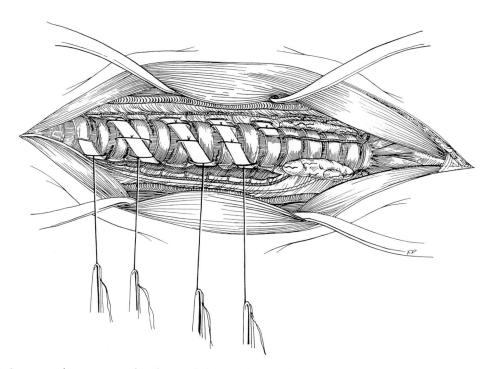

Fig. 22.4. Simple interrupted sutures are placed around the prosthesis and individual cartilage rings on the ventral and lateral aspects of the trachea.

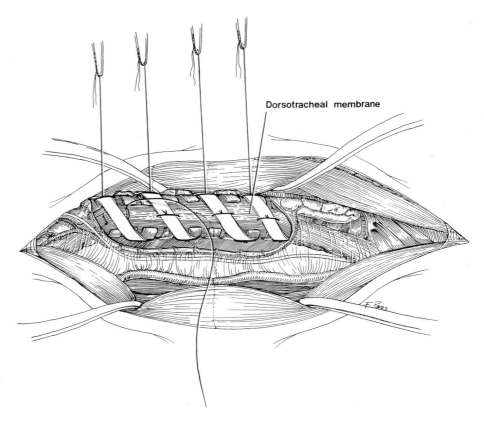

Dorsotracheal membrane

Fig. 22.5. The tagged left lateral sutures are retracted to the right to expose the dorsal tracheal membrane for suturing.

Reference

1. Fingland RB, DeHoff WD, Birchard SJ. Surgical management of cervical and thoracic tracheal collapse in dogs using extraluminal spiral prostheses. J Am Anim Hosp Assoc 1987;23:163.

Treatment of Tracheal Collapse: Ring Prosthesis Technique

H. Phil Hobson

The normal trachea is a dynamic organ composed of multiple hyaline cartilaginous rings, joined together laterally by fibroelastic annular ligaments, and across the tips of the cartilaginous rings dorsally by the tracheal membrane consisting of the trachealis muscle covered medially by ciliated epithelial mucosa. The fibroelastic annular ligaments allow for the flexion in any direction, whereas the trachealis muscle allows for expansion and contraction of the circumference and thus the diameter of the trachea and the volume of air that can move along the airway. Classic tracheal collapse occurs in a dorsoventral direction and results in presenting symptoms varying in degree of severity from mild cough to total respiratory collapse. The patient is usually a middle-aged toy breed dog, but the age may vary, in my experience, from less than 1 year to 16 years.

Pathophysiology

The cause of tracheal collapse is unknown, but it is generally accepted to be a congenitally predisposed, probably inherited, condition. Respiratory allergies, including tobacco smoke allergy, obesity, chronic infections, trauma from collars, and endotracheal tube placement from general anesthesia have been reported to exacerbate the clinical signs. Lack of adequate innervation to the trachealis muscle is considered to be a possible cause. In a few cases, Dallman demonstrated an irregular hypocellular condition of the cartilage rings with less calcium and chondroitin sulfate present. In some cases, the tracheal cartilage is softer than normal, with considerable loss of rigidity. However, occasionally the cartilage is more rigid than normal, resulting in difficulty in recontouring the cartilage during ring placement. The cartilage rings may be shorter than normal, especially at the thoracic inlet.

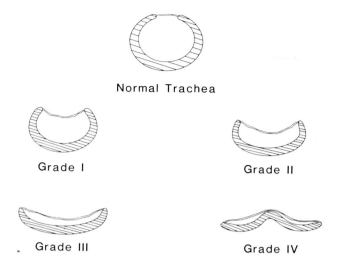

Normal Trachea

Grade I

Grade II

Grade III

Grade IV

Fig. 22.6. Classification of collapsed trachea. Grade I: The trachea is nearly normal. The trachealis muscle is slightly pendulous, and the tracheal cartilages maintain a circular shape. The tracheal lumen is reduced by approximately 25%. Grade II: The trachealis muscle is widened and pendulous. The tracheal cartilages are partially flattened, and the tracheal lumen is reduced by approximately 50%. Grade III: The trachealis muscle is almost in contact with the dorsal surface of the tracheal cartilages. The tracheal cartilages are nearly flat, and the ends may be palpated on physical examination. The tracheal lumen is reduced by approximately 75%. Grade IV: The trachealis muscle is lying on the dorsal surface of the tracheal cartilages. The tracheal cartilages are flattened and may invert dorsally. The tracheal lumen is essentially obliterated. (From Tangner CH, Hobson HP. A retrospective study of 20 surgically managed cases of collapsed trachea. Vet Surg 1982;11:146.)

Usually, the ends of the tracheal rings become progressively further apart (Fig. 22.6), allowing the tracheal membrane to sag into the tracheal lumen. Resonant vibration of the redundant tracheal membrane results in the classic honking cough. Increased negative pressure within the tracheal lumen during inhalation collapses the cervical trachea further and may balloon the thoracic trachea. Exhalation results in compression of the thoracic trachea and often ballooning of the cervical trachea. Stenosis of the airway results in either event, especially on inhalation.

Tracheal collapse may extend into the mainstem bronchi, especially the left bronchus. This may be accentuated by compression by an enlarged left atrium. Heart enlargement, especially right ventricular hypertrophy, is common. Tracheal mucosal erosion or metaplasia may be seen as a result of chronic inflammation as well as from alveolar emphysema and mineralization.

Lateral collapse of the trachea or ventral collapse with minimal widening of the dorsal membrane associated with loss of cartilage rigidity is seen infrequently. Collapse from pressure from external masses is rare. Laryngeal function may be less than optimal.

Diagnosis

A presumptive diagnosis is often made on the presentation of a toy breed dog exhibiting a honking cough, with a history of chronic respiratory infections. Yorkshire terriers, toy poodles, Pomeranians, Chihuahuas, and Maltese are most commonly affected. The condition has also been seen rarely in mixed or larger breeds of dogs, cats, and miniature horses. The disorder has no sex predilection.

Most patients respond to medical therapy consisting of antibiotics, cough suppressants, and corticosteroids, perhaps including bronchodilators and atropine, and these animals are not considered surgical candidates. Patients that fail to respond to conservative therapy should be evaluated thoroughly.

Collapsed tracheas can often be palpated readily in the dog with a long, thin neck, but palpation is difficult in the obese dog with a short, stocky neck. Lateral radiographs, although helpful, may yield false-negative results from ballooning of the trachea or false-positive results because of the esophagus and other tissues overlying the trachea. In the awake patient, fluoroscopic examination of the trachea provides the best evaluation of the airway, including the mainstem bronchi. However, I have seen a false-negative result. Patients in respiratory distress must be handled with care, with oxygen administered as needed. Diagnostic procedures can be life-threatening.

Undoubtedly, the best evaluation of the trachea is accomplished by direct visualization, tracheoscopically. This evaluation requires general anesthesia and should be performed on those patients whose owners have agreed to allow surgical treament if recommended, before the administration of the general anesthesia, or whose owners are available for consultation while the patients are still under anesthesia. Recovery of patients with severe collapse from anesthesia may be difficult, if surgical treatment is not performed.

Preoperative Considerations

The client should be well informed of the prognosis and possible complications at the outset. Dogs with less than a 50% collapse of the trachea are not considered surgical candidates. The clinical signs are not usually a result of inadequate airway and are better managed medically. Early surgical intervention undoubtedly has advantages, but the degree of collapse may remain static in many patients over a prolonged period. Periodic reevaluation is considered the best approach for these patients.

Patients with a 50% or greater collapse of the trachea are likely to experience respiratory distress, especially during times of excitement, when oxygen demands are high or when respiratory infections are present. These patients are considered far less likely to respond to, or already have not responded to, conservative therapy, and thus surgery should be considered.

Postoperative infection with swelling of the mucosal lining, dorsal membrane, and surrounding tissue is always of concern, because the sutures are likely to penetrate the unsterile lumen of the trachea. If infections are to occur, they are most likely during the first 2 weeks after the operation. Abscessation around a prosthetic ring when antibiotics are administered is rare. The mortality rate is in the range of 3 to 5% and is likely to be associated with impairment of air movement during the postsurgical recovery period.

The greatest concern of the surgical procedure is injury to the recurrent laryngeal nerves with resulting laryngeal paralysis. The nerves lie in close approximation to the ventral lateral aspect of the trachea just caudal to the larynx, to a more ventral medial position at the thoracic inlet. The nerves are 1 mm or less in diameter in the toy breeds of dogs and are subject to injury during dissection of the trachea, tissue handling, prosthetic ring placement, or possibly even from the prosthetic ring itself if not placed properly.

Owners should be alerted to the need to perform a tracheostomy should laryngeal paralysis result. The patient should be checked before leaving the operating room, and a tracheostomy should be performed if needed. A permanent tracheostomy is considered preferable to laryngeal tie-backs or arytenoid cartilage resection in toy breeds of dogs with laryngeal paralysis.

Laryngeal function should be evaluated while the patient is under a light plane of anesthesia as part of the preoperative examination. Drugs with analgesic properties administered as preanesthetic agents make evaluation of laryngeal function on stimulation of the larynx more difficult and should be avoided when possible. Anaerobic cultures should be taken directly from the trachea, avoiding the pharyngeal area. Tracheoscopy should follow, with the patient under a surgical plane of anesthesia. Oxygen can be administered directly through the bronchoscope. Brush biopsies for cytologic evaluation should be taken of the caudal trachea at the completion of the visual examination. With proper preparation, the examination, culture, and biopsy can be completed expeditiously, thus keeping the use of intravenous anesthetic induction agents to a minimum.

Radiographs of the lungs should follow, with the intubated patient under general gaseous anesthesia. Compression of the rebreathing bag provides for deep inspiratory radiographs to be made and thus for optimal evaluation of the lungs by the radiologist. Most concurrent lung disease can be ruled in or out by these techniques. The final decision whether or not to proceed with surgery is made at this time.

When surgical treatment is to follow, antibiotics should be administered. A broad-spectrum bactericidal antibiotic, especially one such as enrofloxacin that is effective against the gram-negative organisms, should be used until the results of culture and sensitivity testing are available. The appropriate antibiotic should be continued for 2 weeks postoperatively.

Surgical Management

Various surgical techniques have been proposed. Everting plication of the dorsal tracheal membrane has been effective in moderately affected animals with rigid cartilage rings. Chondrotomy of the ventral aspect of every other tracheal ring has also been effective in some moderately affected patients with rigid cartilage rings. Resection and anastomosis are effective when few rings are collapsed, usually by trauma. Intraluminal prosthetic dilators have been useful for the short term, but they can erode the tracheal wall, stimulate granuloma formation, or interfere with mucus clearance over the longer term. Intraluminal vascular stints have been used in research animals and may prove effective in the future, especially when tracheal collapse is primarily within the thorax and for collapsing mainstem bronchi. Problems experienced with the stents include collapse when subjected to too much flexion, failure to anchor well, resulting in expulsion when coughing, pulmonary edema, availability of inappropriate sizes, and uneven contact between the stent and the airway wall.

Currently, the surgical techniques most universally accepted are those that support the trachea, including the dorsal tracheal membrane, with extraluminal prosthetic devices to which the trachea is sutured. Earlier use of long sections of extraluminal prosthetic devices restricted needed flexion of the trachea, and shorter sections applied only to the ventral aspect of the trachea failed to support the sagging dorsal membrane. Current prosthetic devices provide that support. Support is reinforced by connective tissue proliferation around the prosthesis and through the holes in the prosthesis when individual ring prostheses are used. The individual ring technique consists of the placement of four to seven individual prosthetic rings around the trachea with spacing between the rings, whereas the spiral technique is essentially a continuous spiral prosthesis (see the first section of this chapter).

Total Ring Prosthesis

Prosthetic rings are made from 3-mL polypropylene syringe cases by cutting the syringe case into 7- to 10-mm sections with a pipe cutter over a wood dowel rod or by sawing the syringe case into sections and drilling approximately 3-mm diameter holes with either a hand drill or with a No. 11 Bard–Parker scalpel blade. Five holes are usually drilled, with the syringe case ring cut at the location of the sixth equally spaced hole. Angled serrated wire-cutting scissors work well for cutting the ring to facilitate placement of the ring around the trachea. The ends of the ring are rounded and smoothed, as are the edges of the ring and the edges of the holes, to minimize irritation after placement. The polypropylene rings can be autoclaved or sterilized by other methods. The rings can be made larger if necessary by simply spreading the ends of the rings before suturing them to the trachea. Conversely, they can be made smaller by trimming the ends of the rings, squeezing the rings, and placing a figure-of-eight suture across the cut ends of the rings through the adjacent holes after placement, but before suturing to the trachea. Polypropylene rings break if too much pressure is applied in either expansion or compression to alter the size for surgery.

The patient is positioned in dorsal recumbency with the forelegs secured caudally. A towel roll is positioned under the neck near the shoulders. A ventral midline incision is made from the larynx to just caudal to the manubrium (Fig. 22.7). The sternohyoideus and sternocephalicus muscles are separated to expose the trachea; the surgeon should avoid the thyroid vein as much as possible. The thyroid vein lies between the sternocephalicus muscles. The trachea is surrounded by loose areolar tissue and receives its primary blood supply segmentally from the thyroid arteries and its nerve supply segmentally from the recurrent laryngeal nerves. Preservation of as much of the blood supply and innervation to the trachea as possible is desirable. The recurrent laryngeal nerves lie in close approximation to the ventral lateral aspect of the trachea near

the larynx coursing more medially as the thoracic inlet is approached. These nerves must be handled carefully during dissection and ring placement. No tissue should be cut without knowing that the nerves are out of the way. The nerves should be retracted gently by grasping adjacent tissue, not the nerve itself, during dissection.

Curved hemostats are used to dissect bluntly a tunnel dorsally around the trachea (Fig. 22.8). Care is taken to dissect between the recurrent laryngeal nerves and the trachea and gently to retract them as one end of the ring is grasped with the tip of the curved hemostat and gently is delivered through the tunnel around the trachea. The cut end of the ring is positioned ventrally. The prosthetic ring is sutured in place with 3–0 or 4–0 polydioxanone sutures passed around a tracheal ring, up through a hole in the prosthesis, and tied. The prosthesis is grasped with forceps, and the trachea is rotated in either direction to facilitate placement of the more dorsal sutures, including at least one in the dorsal tracheal membrane.

In the occasional severe case, multiple small chondrotomies must be made through the rigid cartilage to facilitate recontouring the tracheal rings. These tracheal cartilages may be in the shape of an opened W. Care should be exercised to cut only the cartilage and not the tracheal mucosa.

Placement of the rings is begun just caudal to the larynx and is continued caudally with approximately the width of the prosthetic ring left between each ring placed. The neurovascular supply to the trachea is carefully left intact between the rings. Movement of the endotracheal tube during surgery is essential to prevent suture from passing through the cuff of the endotracheal tube.

Rings can be placed around the trachea deep within the thoracic inlet by gentle but strong rostral traction on the trachea. This is facilitated by grasping a prosthetic ring that has been sutured to the trachea (see Fig. 22.8). Lateral ventral retraction of the tissue from the trachea at the thoracic inlet, including the recurrent laryngeal nerves, vagosympathetic trunk, and carotid arteries, aids in placement of these rings. With some effort, these rings can be placed far enough into the thoracic inlet that, when the patient is standing in a normal upright position after surgery, the caudal ring will be located at the second intercostal space.

Severe tracheal collapse within the thoracic cavity can be approached, preferably through a right third intercostal space, for further ring placement. This is rarely done, however, because only about one additional ring can be applied rostral to the carina. No external support can be applied to a collapsed mainstem bronchus.

When the rings can be placed as far caudally as the second intercostal space, even in patients with severe intrathoracic tracheal collapse, inspiratory efforts

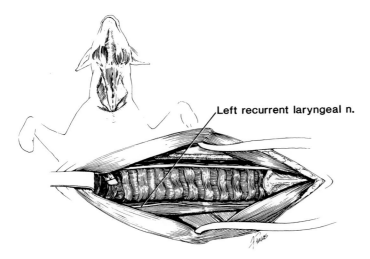

Left recurrent laryngeal n.

Fig. 22.7. Ventral cervical midline approach to the cervical trachea. The skin incision extends from the larynx to the manubrium.

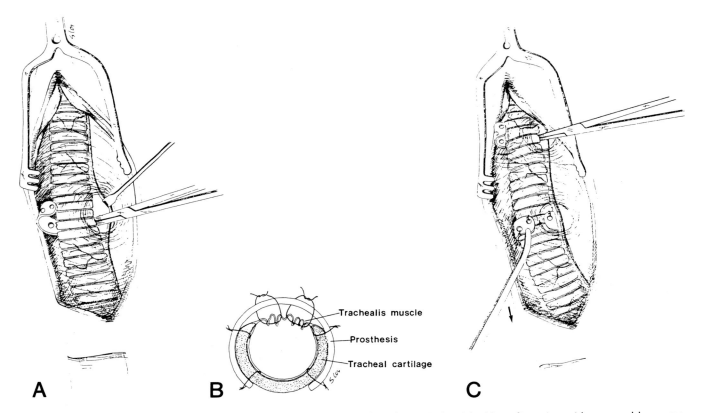

A **B** **C**

Trachealis muscle
Prosthesis
Tracheal cartilage

Fig. 22.8. Implantation of total ring prosthesis. **A.** A small section of trachea is isolated by blunt dissection with a curved hemostat. The hemostat is then used to direct the prosthesis around the trachea. The recurrent laryngeal nerves are carefully retracted. **B.** Suture placement. **C.** Cranial retraction on the cervical trachea facilitates placement of total ring prostheses to the thoracic inlet portion of the trachea. (From Walker TL, Hobson HP. Tracheal collapse. In: Bojrab MJ, ed. Current techniques in small animal surgery. 2nd ed. Philadelphia: Lea & Febiger, 1983.)

should result in adequate air movement to maintain normal oxygenation as the thoracic airways balloon on inspiration. The patient, however, may still cough, even to the point of exhibiting the honking cough, and is predisposed to infections and secondary changes because of the narrow airway.

Postoperative Considerations

Laryngeal function is of prime concern. It is usually evaluated before removal of the patient from the operating room. A tracheostomy is performed if deemed necessary.

Most patients do not require further surgery, nor do they require postoperative oxygen. Most are recovered in the postoperative recovery room. Analgesics are administered as indicated. Prednisolone is often given at the end of the operation to minimize effects of irritation to the airway and the recurrent laryngeal nerves. Appropriate antibiotics are continued for 2 weeks postoperatively. Antitussives and bronchial dilators are given rarely, but they are administered if deemed necessary. Any concurrent medical problems

are treated as indicated because many of these patients are older dogs with other maladies.

Suggested Readings

Anderson GR. Surgical correction of tracheal collapse using Teflon rings. Okla Vet 1971;23:6.

Buback JL, Boothe HW, Hobson HP. Surgical treatment of tracheal collapse in dogs: 90 cases (1983–1993). J Am Vet Med Assoc 1996;208:308.

Dallman MJ, Brown EM. Structural considerations in tracheal disease. Am J Vet Res 1979;40:555.

Dallman MJ, McClure RC, Brown EM. Histochemical study of normal and collapsed trachea in dogs. Am J Vet Res 1988;49:2117.

Delehanty DD, Georgi JR. A tracheal deformity in a pony. J Am Vet Med Assoc 1954;125:42.

Fingland RB, Dettoff WD, Birchard SJ. Surgical management of cervical and thoracic tracheal collapse in dogs using extraluminal spiral prosthesis: results in seven cases. J Am Anim Hosp Assoc 1987;23:163.

Hobson HP. Total ring prosthesis for the surgical correction of collapsed trachea. J Am Anim Hosp Assoc 1976;12:822

Knowles RP, Snyder CC. Chondrotomy for congenital tracheal stenosis. In: Proceedings of the American Animal Hospital Association. 1967:246.

Leonard HC. Surgical correction of collapsed trachea in dogs. J Am Vet Med Assoc 1971;158:598.

Leonard HC, Wright JJ. An intraluminal prosthetic dilator for tracheal collapse in the dog. J Am Anim Hosp Assoc 1978;14:464.

Radlinsky MG, Fossum TW, Walken MA. Evaluation of Palmaz stents in the trachea and bronchi of normal dogs. In: Proceedings of the American College of Veterinary Surgery. Chicago, IL 1995:19.

Rubin GJ, Neal TM, Bojrab MJ. Surgical reconstruction for collapsed tracheal rings. J Sm Anim Pract 1973;14:607.

Schiller AG, Helper LC, Small E. Treatment of tracheal collapse in the dog. J Am Vet Med Assoc 1964;145:669.

Slatter DH. A surgical method for correction of collapsed trachea in the dog. Aust Vet 1974;50:41.

Tangner CH, Hobson HP. A retrospective study of 20 surgically managed cases of collapsed trachea. Vet Surg 1982;11:146.

Permanent Tracheostomy

Cheryl S. Hedlund

A permanent tracheostomy is a stoma in the ventral tracheal wall created by suturing tracheal mucosa to skin. Tracheostomy tubes are not needed to maintain lumen patency after this procedure. Tracheostomas are maintained for life or until the stoma is surgically closed. Permanent tracheostomies are recommended for animals with upper respiratory obstructions causing moderate to severe respiratory distress that cannot be successfully managed by other methods. Dogs and cats with cyanosis or severe dyspnea at rest or on minimal exertion are candidates. Respiratory distress is commonly associated with laryngeal dysfunction secondary to laryngeal collapse or neoplasia, and sometimes nasopharyngeal or proximal tracheal obstruction. Before creating a tracheostoma, the clinician must establish the client's willingness and ability to provide postoperative care. Although most patients requiring a permanent tracheostomy function much better after surgery, some clients refuse the procedure and elect less beneficial surgical procedures or euthanasia.

Surgical Technique

A permanent tracheostomy is performed with the anesthetized patient in dorsal recumbency. The skin of the ventral and lateral neck is clipped and aseptically prepared for surgery. On the operating table, the patient's forelegs are positioned caudally along the chest, and then the animal's neck is elevated and extended with a dorsal cervical pad. The proximal cervical trachea is exposed with a ventral cervical midline incision beginning at the distal larynx and extending caudally 8 to 10 cm. The paired sternohyoid muscles are separated and are retracted laterally to visualize the trachea. The endotracheal tube cuff distal is advanced to the proposed tracheostomy site. The surgeon creates a tunnel dorsal to the trachea from the third to sixth tracheal cartilages and, using this tunnel, apposes the sternohyoid muscles dorsal to the trachea with hori-

zontal mattress sutures to create a muscle sling (Fig. 22.9). The muscle sling serves to deviate the trachea ventrally, reducing tension on the mucosa-to-skin sutures. Beginning with the second or third tracheal cartilages, a rectangular segment of tracheal wall three to four cartilage widths long and one-third the circumference of the trachea in width is outlined (see Fig. 22.9). Using a No. 11 scalpel blade, the cartilage and annular ligaments are incised to the depth of the tracheal mucosa. The surgeon elevates a cartilage edge with thumb forceps and dissects the cartilage segment from the mucosa using the blunt edge of the scalpel blade. If tracheal cartilages show any weakness or tendency to collapse, one or two prosthetic tracheal rings should be placed cranial and caudal to the stoma. A similar segment of skin adjacent is excised to the stoma. If the patient has loose skinfolds or abundant subcutaneous fat, larger segments of skin are excised to help prevent skinfold occlusion of the stoma. Excess fat is excised in obese patients to allow direct contact of the skin and peritracheal fascia. The surgeon sutures the skin directly to the peritracheal fascia laterally and the annular ligaments proximal and distal to the stoma with a series of interrupted intradermal sutures (3–0 or 4–0 polydioxanone), without entering the tracheal lumen with the skin–peritracheal sutures. These sutures promote adhesion of the skin to the trachea and are important in reducing postoperative skinfold problems, seroma formation, and tension on the stomal sutures. An I-shaped or H-shaped incision is made in the mucosa. The mucosa is folded over the cartilage edges and is sutured to the edges of the skin with approximating sutures (4–0 polypropylene) (Fig. 22.10). Simple interrupted sutures are placed at the corners and a simple continuous pattern is used along the sides of the stoma. Sutures are spaced approximately 2 mm apart. Precise apposition is important to minimize tracheostomal stenosis, but it not always possible. Precise apposition is not possible if the tracheal mucosa is disrupted during dissection or previous tube tracheostomy or if it is of poor quality because of disease. If the patient

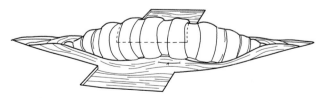

Fig. 22.9. The trachea is deviated ventrally by apposing the sternohyoid muscles dorsally to create a muscle sling. A rectangular segment of ventral tracheal wall, approximately one-third the tracheal circumference and three to four cartilages long, is excised without penetrating the mucosa. Loose skin adjacent to the tracheal incisions is excised. (From Hedlund CS. Tracheostomies in the management of canine and feline upper respiratory disease. Vet Clin North Am Small Anim Pract 1994;24:873–886.)

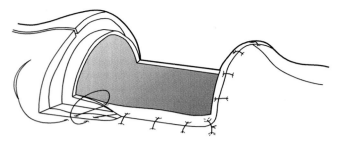

Fig. 22.10. After placing skin–peritracheal fascial sutures and incising the tracheal mucosa, the mucosa is rolled over the cartilage edges and is apposed to the skin edges. Simple interrupted sutures are placed in the corners, and apposition is completed with a simple continuous pattern. (From Hedlund CS. Tracheostomies in the management of canine and feline upper respiratory disease. Vet Clin North Am Small Anim Pract 1994;24:873–886.)

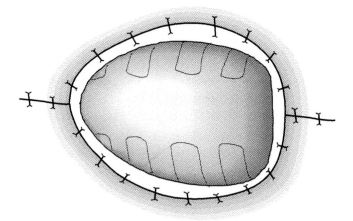

Fig. 22.12. The dorsal tracheal membrane is apposed to the proximal skin edges with simple interrupted sutures. The tracheostoma is completed by apposing skin to mucosa with a simple continuous pattern. (From Hedlund CS. Tracheostomies in the management of canine and feline upper respiratory disease. Vet Clin North Am Small Anim Pract 1994;24:873–886.)

does not have enough mucosa to cover the incised cartilage edges and annular ligaments, the surgeon should appose as much mucosa to the skin as possible and allow the exposed areas to heal by second intention. If necessary, sutures are passed around or through adjacent cartilages or annular ligaments. Skin edges are apposed proximal and distal to the stoma with simple interrupted or cruciate sutures. Blood and mucus are suctioned from the stoma before the animal recovers from anesthesia.

Permanent tracheostomy following total laryngectomy requires the creation of a tracheostoma after the transected end of the trachea is closed or deviated to the skin. Closure of the transected trachea is accomplished by preserving a flap of dorsal tracheal membrane from the more proximal trachea that can be folded over the exposed lumen of the distal trachea and then sutured. Alternatively, the transected distal trachea is closed by placing a series of interrupted horizontal mattress sutures to appose the dorsal tracheal membrane to the cartilage. After using either of these closure techniques, a permanent tracheostomy is performed as described previously.

Another option after total laryngectomy is to incorporate the distal tracheal end in the tracheostoma. This is accomplished by apposing the sternohyoid muscles dorsal to the distal tracheal end. Then, beginning at the distal tracheal transection site, the surgeon removes segments of four to six tracheal cartilages from the ventral aspect of the tracheal wall, while preserving as much mucosa as possible (Fig. 22.11). At the most proximal aspect of the proposed stoma, the dorsal tracheal membrane is apposed directly to the skin with simple interrupted sutures. Excess skin is excised as necessary to prevent skinfolds at the site, and then the skin is sutured directly to the peritracheal fascia and annular ligaments with intradermal sutures. The tracheostoma is completed by apposing the tracheal mucosa at the lateral and distal cartilage margins to the skin with simple continuous sutures (Fig. 22.12).

Postoperative Care

Patients that have undergone permanent tracheostomy are monitored in the intensive care unit for 24 to 48 hours after surgery to observe for dyspnea and to care for the tracheostoma. Obstruction of the tracheostoma can result in death by asphyxiation. The stoma is inspected every 1 to 3 hours. The stoma is cleaned aseptically when mucus begins to occlude the tracheostoma or when respiratory effort increases. Mucus accumulating around the tracheostoma is removed with moistened gauze sponges. Mucus accumulating in the tracheal lumen is removed with a moistened sterile cotton swab or suction tip. Cleaning must be performed carefully to avoid disrupting the

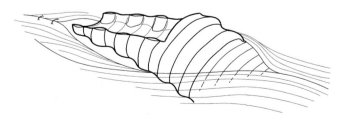

Fig. 22.11. Permanent tracheostomy after complete laryngectomy can be accomplished by apposing the sternohyoid muscles dorsal to the trachea and then removing a segment of tracheal wall four to six cartilages long. The mucosa is preserved as with the standard permanent tracheostomy technique. (From Hedlund CS. Tracheostomies in the management of canine and feline upper respiratory disease. Vet Clin North Am Small Anim Pract 1994;24:873–886.)

suture line or irritating the tracheal mucosa. A water-impermeable ointment (petrolatum or boric acid ointment) is applied around the tracheostoma to discourage tracheal secretions from adhering and crusting. Low humidity during the first 4 to 6 days seems to reduce the amount of exudation and also promotes healing.

Initially, most animals secrete a moderate amount of mucus, with cleaning needed every 1 to 3 hours, but the interval gradually increases to every 4 to 6 hours by 7 days and twice daily by 30 days postoperatively. Patients are usually ready for discharge within 7 days of surgery; at this time, the stomas should be inspected every 4 to 6 hours and mucus removed as needed. Animals with severe tracheal irritation, secretory diseases, or those exposed to mucosal irritants may require more frequent cleaning. Most animals learn to expel mucus forcefully from the stoma in a self-cleaning manner. Hair is clipped from around the tracheostoma once or twice a month to prevent matting with mucus. Exercise and housing should be limited to clean areas free of smoke and unnecessary fragrances. Swimming is prohibited, and the stoma should be protected when sprays are used near the pet.

Owners are usually satisfied with their pet's response after permanent tracheostomy. Most pets have improved breathing, less noisy breathing, and increased activity. Approximately 60% of dogs and cats with permanent tracheostomy (without laryngectomy) lose their ability to vocalize normally.

Complications of permanent tracheostomy include stomal occlusion by skinfolds or mucus, dehiscence, and stenosis. Skinfold occlusion is the most common long-term complication. It may be intermittent, related to the animal's posture, or continuous. Skinfold problems can be minimized by carefully assessing and excising larger amounts of skin in animals with loose skinfolds during permanent tracheostomy. Adhesions created by skin–peritracheal sutures are important in preventing skinfold problems. When skinfolds do interfere with tracheostomal airflow, skin lateral and dorsal to the stoma is excised without disturbing the mucosa-to-skin junction. Obstruction of the stoma by mucus is prevented by diligent observation and management. Dehiscence occurs if tension or irritation is present at the mucosa-to-skin junction. It is prevented by using good surgical and management techniques. Dehiscence leads to a greater degree of stomal stenosis. Some stenosis occurs at all tracheostomal sites, but it may progress to nearly complete stomal obstruction with dehiscence or trauma. If dyspnea recurs secondary to stenosis, it may be necessary to revise the tracheostoma surgically. Defense mechanisms in the bronchi, bronchioles, and lungs are adequate in most cases to prevent pulmonary infections in animals with permanent tracheostomies.

Suggested Readings

Dalgard DW, Marshall PM, Fitzgerald GH, et al. Surgical technique for permanent tracheostomy in beagle dogs. Lab Anim Sci 1979;29:367–370.

Hedlund CS. Tracheostomies in the management of canine and feline upper respiratory disease.Vet Clin North Am Small Anim Pract 1994;24:873–886.

Hedlund CS, Tangner CH, Montgomery DL, et al. A procedure for permanent tracheostomy and its effects on tracheal mucosa. Vet Surg 1982;11:13–17.

Hedlund CS, Tangner CH, Waldron DR, et al. Permanent tracheostomy: perioperative and long-term data from 34 cases. J Am Anim Hosp Assoc 1988;24:585–591.

Tracheal Resection and Anastomosis

Roger B. Fingland

Tracheal anastomosis is indicated for management of benign and malignant tracheal stenoses, traumatic tracheal disruption, and segmental tracheomalacia. Important preoperative considerations include localization of the lesion, determination of the proximal and distal margins of the lesion, and, in the case of malignant lesions, evaluation of the animal for distant metastases. Plain film radiography, tracheoscopy, and computed tomography are helpful in localization of tracheal lesions.

Tracheal anastomosis in veterinary patients typically is accomplished by apposition of circumferentially divided tracheal cartilages with sutures placed in simple interrupted fashion (split-ring technique) (1). Alternative techniques such as overriding segments, creation of mucosal flaps, and apposition of annular ligaments are less desirable because these techniques are technically more difficult or result in critical anastomotic stenosis (1, 2). In one study, simple continuous and simple interrupted suture techniques for tracheal anastomosis after large-segment tracheal resection were compared in dogs. Differences in surgical time and anastomotic stenosis were not clinically significant (3).

Tension has a profound effect on anastomotic healing and is the major factor limiting the extent of tracheal resection. Tracheal anastomoses consistently are successful in mature dogs when tension on the anastomosis is less than 1750 g (4). Unfortunately, attempts to correlate grams of tension with number of tracheal cartilages have produced widely disparate results (5). In general, 25% of the trachea (8 to 10 tracheal cartilages) can be resected in a mature dog with consistently satisfactory results. In young animals and in animals with primary tracheal disease, this number may be significantly lower (6).

Surgical Techniques

Cervical Trachea

Preoperative planning is imperative. An endotracheal tube with a high-volume, low-pressure cuff should be used. Ideally, the endotracheal tube should be positioned proximal to the affected tracheal segment, and the entire procedure should be performed "over" the endotracheal tube. In patients with significant luminal compromise, the endotracheal tube should be positioned distal (orad) to the lesion for the surgical approach and the initial tracheal dissection. Tracheal anastomosis necessitates intraoperative manipulation of the endotracheal tube and, on occasion, direct intubation of the distal segment of the trachea. A sterile endotracheal tube should be available for intraoperative intubation of the distal segment of the trachea. The endotracheal tube cuff must be deflated when the tube is repositioned within the trachea and then reinflated before the procedure continues. Prophylactic administration of a broad-spectrum antibiotic is recommended.

The patient is positioned in dorsal recumbency, and the ventral cervical region is prepared for aseptic surgery. The skin and subcutaneous tissues are incised from the larynx to the manubrium. The trachea is exposed by midline separation of the paired sternocephalicus and sternohyoideus muscles. The segment of trachea to be resected is determined based on preoperative evaluation and intraoperative inspection and palpation. The lateral pedicles are dissected from the trachea along a segment that includes two cartilage rings proximal and two cartilage rings distal to the proposed margins of the excision. Carrying the lateral pedicle dissection beyond the proposed margins of excision facilitates manipulation of the proximal and distal tracheal segments and placement of primary anastomotic and tension sutures. Traction sutures (3–0 polydioxanone, SH-1 taper needle, 70 cm) are placed around the right and left lateral aspects of the second tracheal cartilage proximal to the cartilage to be incised. The swaged-on needle is left in place, and the suture is looped but not tied. These traction sutures facilitate manipulation of the proximal tracheal segment and are used as tension sutures after the primary anastomosis is completed.

The segment of trachea is excised by circumferentially incising one tracheal cartilage at each end of the segment (Fig. 22.13). Care is taken to incise the tracheal cartilages circumferentially in two equal halves. If the endotracheal tube was initially positioned distal to the lesion, the cuff is deflated, the endotracheal tube

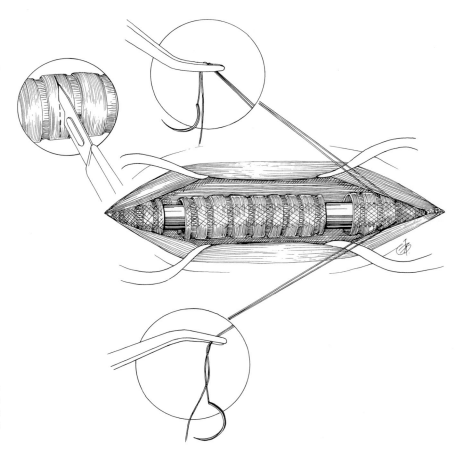

Fig. 22.13. Ventral view of the exposed cervical trachea showing placement of traction sutures. The segment to be removed has been excised by circumferentially incising (*inset*) the proximal and distal tracheal cartilages.

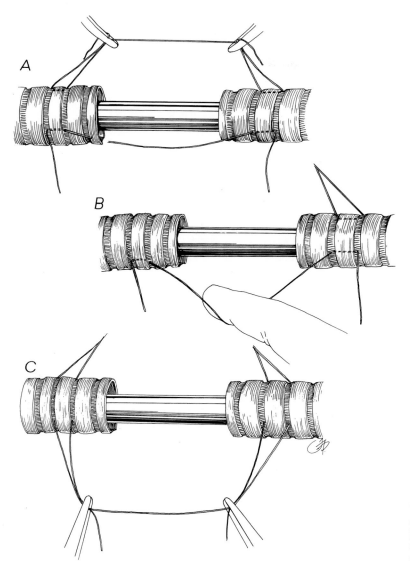

Fig. 22.14. The tracheal segment has been excised. **A.** The proximal and distal segments of the trachea are joined by tension sutures. The tension sutures are drawn through the tracheal wall (**B**) and are tagged to facilitate manipulation of the trachea for primary anastomosis.

is directed into the proximal tracheal segment, and the endotracheal tube cuff is reinflated. On both sides of the trachea, the swaged-on arm of the lateral traction suture is passed around the second complete tracheal cartilage distal to the incised tracheal cartilage. These sutures are used to approximate and maintain apposition of tracheal segments and to facilitate rotation of the trachea for placement of primary anastomotic sutures (Fig. 22.14).

The proximal and distal circumferentially incised tracheal cartilages are approximated using the preplaced lateral tension sutures (Fig. 22.15). Accurate alignment of the two split cartilages is important. The primary anastomosis is created using 4–0 polydioxanone suture placed in a simple interrupted pattern approximately 3 mm apart (Fig. 22.16). Each suture incorporates the split proximal and distal tracheal cartilages. All sutures enter the lumen of the trachea.

The dorsal tracheal membrane is exposed by rotating the trachea with the preplaced lateral tension sutures (Fig. 22.17). Anastomotic sutures are placed in the dorsal tracheal membrane in a manner that ensures accurate apposition and an airtight seal.

The lateral tension sutures are tied after the primary anastomosis is complete (Fig. 22.18). A third tension suture is placed on the ventral aspect of the trachea. The tension sutures should be tight enough to relieve tension from the primary anastomotic sutures, but they should not cause deviation or overlapping of the apposed ends of the proximal and distal segments of the trachea.

Thoracic Trachea

The thoracic segment of the trachea is approached through a right third intercostal thoracotomy. The

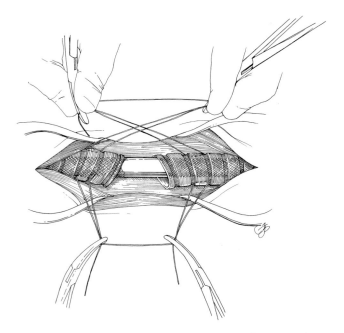

Fig. 22.15. The tagged tension sutures are used to approximate the proximal and distal segments of the trachea for primary anastomosis.

technique for resection and anastomosis of the thoracic segment is similar to the technique described for the cervical segment of the trachea. Direct intubation of the proximal segment of the trachea intraoperatively usually is necessary. Direct intubation of an isolated primary bronchus may be necessary to maintain ventilation. Preoperative planning and technical expertise are necessary to ensure success.

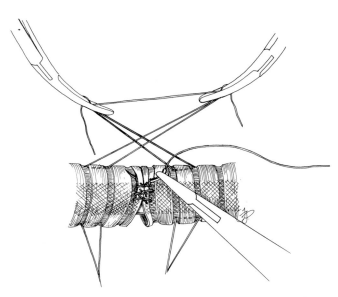

Fig. 22.16. The primary anastomosis begins on the ventral aspect of the trachea by placing simple interrupted sutures around the split proximal and distal tracheal cartilages.

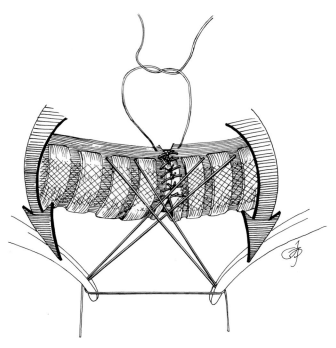

Fig. 22.17. A tagged tension suture is used to rotate the trachea for exposure of the left lateral and dorsal aspects. Simple interrupted anastomotic sutures are placed approximately 3 mm apart.

Postoperative Considerations

Brief, atraumatic tracheal suctioning after extubation is helpful to remove clotted blood from the lumen of the trachea. The patient should be observed closely for

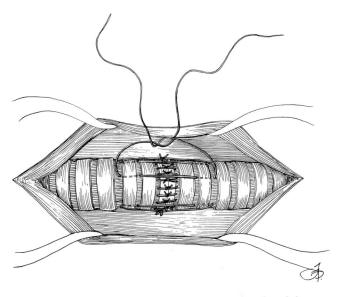

Fig. 22.18. The primary anastomosis is completed, and the tension sutures are knotted. A third tension suture is placed on the ventral aspect of the trachea. The tension sutures should relieve tension from the primary anastomosis, but they should not result in deviation or overlapping of the tracheal segments.

respiratory distress for 12 to 24 hours after surgery. Postoperative respiratory distress can result from laryngeal or pharyngeal edema, occlusion of the tracheal lumen at the anastomotic site, or iatrogenic laryngeal paralysis from intraoperative recurrent laryngeal nerve injury. Antitussives and glucocorticoids are administered as needed to reduce inflammation and to suppress coughing.

The nature of tracheal wound healing ensures some degree of anastomotic stenosis. Periodic endoscopic examination of the trachea after anastomosis is helpful to evaluate wound healing and anastomotic stenosis. Anastomotic stenosis usually is not clinically significant in sedentary patients until the tracheal lumen is compromised by 50 to 75% (7). Meticulous, atraumatic surgical technique and elimination of tension on the anastomosis usually result in a successful outcome.

References

1. Hedlund CS. Tracheal anastomosis in the dog: comparison of two end-to-end techniques. Vet Surg 1984;13:135.
2. Lau RE, Schwartz A, Buergelt CD. Tracheal resection and anastomosis in dogs. J Am Vet Med Assoc 1980;176:134.
3. Fingland RB, Layton CE, Kennedy GA, et al. A comparison of simple continuous versus simple interrupted suture patterns for tracheal anastomosis after large-segment tracheal resection in dogs. Vet Surg 1995;24:320.
4. Cantrell JR, Folse JR. The repair of circumferential defects of the trachea by direct anastomosis: experimental evaluation. J Thorac Cardiovasc Surg 1961;42:589.
5. Vasseur PB, Morgan JP. The trachea. In: Gourley IM, Vasseur PB, eds. General small animal surgery. Philadelphia: JB Lippincott, 1985.
6. Maeda M, Grillo HC. Effects of tension on tracheal growth after resection and anastomosis in puppies. J Thorac Cardiovasc Surg 1973;65:658.
7. McKeown PP, Tsuboi H, Togo T, et al. Growth of tracheal anastomoses: advantages of absorbable interrupted sutures. Ann Thorac Surg 1991;51:636.

─ ● 23 ● ─

LUNG AND THORACIC CAVITY

Thoracic Approaches

Dianne Dunning & E. Christopher Orton

Intercostal thoracotomy and median sternotomy are the most commonly used thoracic approaches in small animals. The choice of a thoracic approach depends mostly on the type of access to the thoracic cavity that is needed. Intercostal thoracotomy is easy to perform and does not require special surgical instrumentation, but it allows only limited access within the thoracic cavity. Median sternotomy provides wide access to the thoracic cavity, except for structures in the dorsal mediastinum such as the esophagus and bronchial hilus. However, median sternotomy requires access to an oscillating saw or sternal splitter. Nevertheless, median sternotomy is the thoracic approach that allows the most complete exploration of the thoracic cavity.

Surgical Technique

Intercostal Thoracotomy

Intercostal thoracotomy is chosen to provide access to a defined area of interest within one hemisphere of the thoracic cavity. Approximately one-third of one side of the thoracic cavity and its associated mediastinal structures are visible with this approach. The intercostal space chosen depends on the thoracic structures of interest. In general, the cardiac structures are approached best through the fourth or fifth intercostal

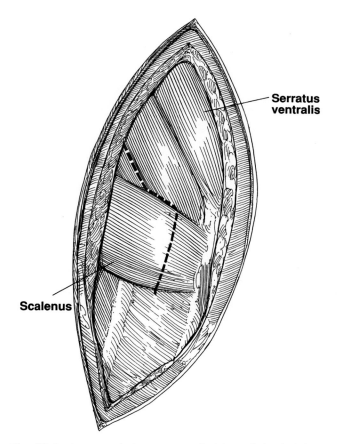

Serratus ventralis

Scalenus

Fig. 23.1 Intercostal thoracotomy. Incision of the latissimus dorsi muscle. The fifth rib is identified as the caudal insertion of the scalenus muscle and the cranial origin of the external abdominal oblique muscle. (From Orton EC. Small animal thoracic surgery. Baltimore: Williams & Wilkins, 1995:57.)

space. The cranial lung lobes are accessed through the fourth or fifth intercostal space, whereas the caudal lung lobes are best accessed through the fifth or sixth intercostal space. The right middle lung lobe is accessed through the right fifth intercostal space. The cranial esophagus can be accessed from either the third or the fourth intercostal space on the right or left side. The caudal esophagus is accessed on either the right or left side between the seventh and eighth intercostal spaces. The thoracic duct in the dog is best accessed between the eight and tenth intercostal spaces on the right side. Access to the caudal vena cava can be gained from the right side between the seventh and tenth spaces. Thoracic radiographs also should be reviewed before the surgical procedure to help identify the most appropriate intercostal space.

To perform an intercostal thoracotomy, an incision is made with a scalpel through the skin, subcutaneous tissues, and cutaneus trunci muscle. The latissimus dorsi and pectoralis muscles are incised parallel to the skin incision. The fifth rib is easily identified as the caudal insertion of the scalenus muscle and the cranial origin of the external abdominal oblique muscle (Fig.

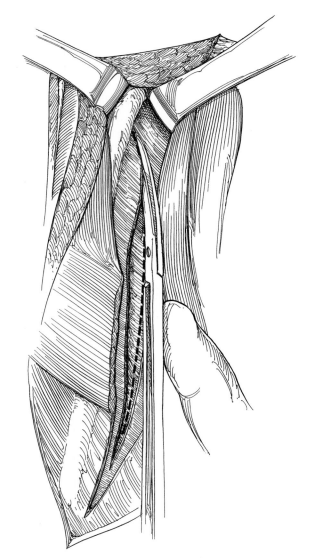

Fig. 23.3. Intercostal thoracotomy. Incision of the intercostal muscles midway between the ribs to avoid damaging the intercostal vessels. (From Orton EC. Small animal thoracic surgery. Baltimore: Williams & Wilkins, 1995:58.)

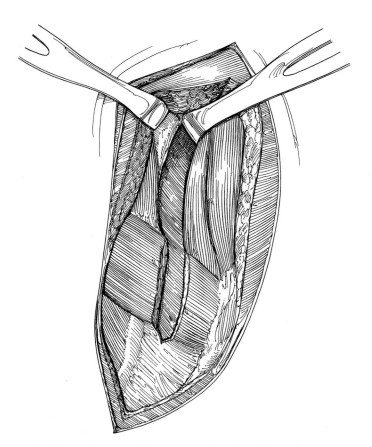

Fig. 23.2. Intercostal thoracotomy. Incision of the scalenus muscle and the serratus ventralis muscle. (From Orton EC. Small animal thoracic surgery. Baltimore: Williams & Wilkins, 1995:57.)

23.1). Depending on the intercostal space entered, either the scalenus or the external abdominal oblique muscle is incised. The serratus ventralis muscle is separated to expose the desired intercostal space (Fig. 23.2). The intercostal muscles are incised midway between the ribs to avoid lacerating the intercostal vessels, coursing on the caudal aspect of each rib (Fig. 23.3). The pleura is punctured, and the incision is extended with scissors dorsally to the tubercle of the rib and ventrally past the costochondral arch to the internal thoracic vessels. A Finochietto retractor is used to expose the thoracic structures.

Just before closure of the thoracotomy, a thoracostomy tube is placed through the caudodorsal thoracic

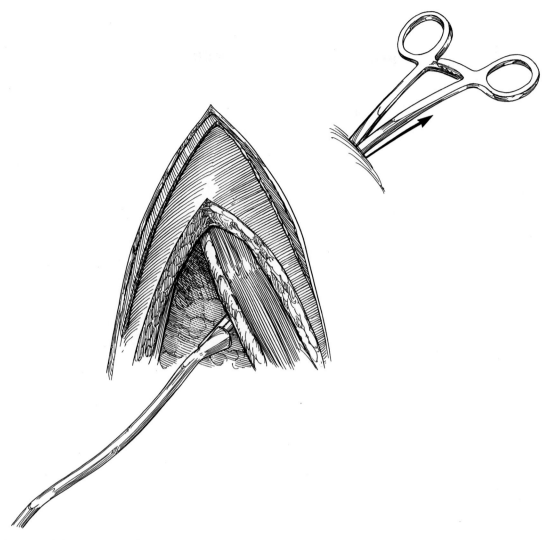

Fig. 23.4. Intercostal thoracotomy. Placement of a thoracostomy tube in the caudodorsal thorax before closure. (From Orton EC. Small animal thoracic surgery. Baltimore: Williams & Wilkins, 1995:60.)

wall (Fig. 23.4). The thoracostomy tube should remain open to the atmosphere during closure of the thoracotomy site to prevent inadvertent tension pneumothorax. After the closure is airtight, the pleural space is evacuated, and the thoracostomy tube is closed. Before thoracotomy closure, a selective intercostal nerve block of the adjacent intercostal spaces with 0.75% bupivacaine may be administered to decrease postoperative pain and to improve ventilation.

The thoracotomy is closed by preplacing five to eight heavy-gauge sutures around the adjacent ribs. The preplaced circumcostal sutures are used by an assistant to approximate the ribs while the surgeon ties each suture (Fig. 23.5). The serratus ventralis or external abdominal oblique and scalenus muscles are closed in a single layer with a simple continuous suture pattern. The latissimus dorsi muscle, cutaneus trunci muscle, subcutaneous tissues, and skin are closed in separate layers with a simple continuous suture pattern (Fig. 23.6).

Median Sternotomy

Median sternotomy is indicated when exploratory surgery of the thoracic cavity is necessary. Median sternotomy should not be avoided because of a belief that it is associated with higher postoperative pain and complication rates than intercostal thoracotomy. Complication rates associated with median sternotomy are no higher than those associated with thoracotomy.

Median sternotomy is performed with the animal in dorsal recumbency. The skin and subcutaneous tissues are incised with a scalpel over the midline on the sternum (Fig. 23.7). The pectoral musculature is

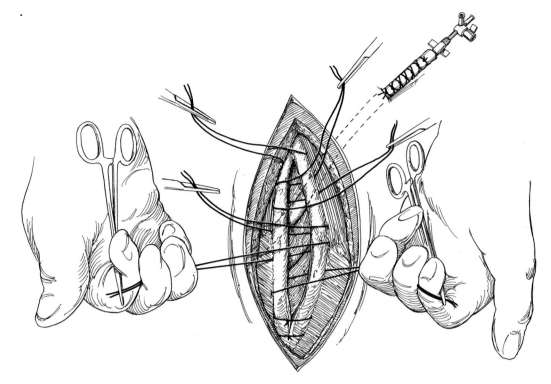

Fig. 23.5. Intercostal thoracotomy closure. Approximation of the ribs by an assistant using the preplaced circumcostal sutures while the surgeon ties each suture. (From Orton EC. Small animal thoracic surgery. Baltimore: Williams & Wilkins, 1995:61.)

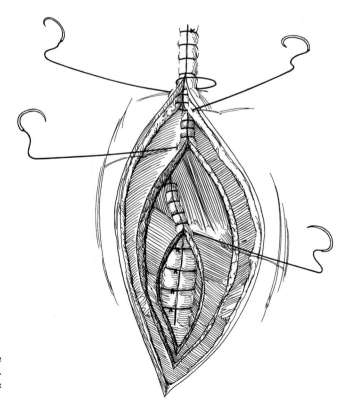

Fig. 23.6. Intercostal thoracotomy closure. Closure of the muscle and skin in separate layers with a simple continuous suture pattern. (From Orton EC. Small animal thoracic surgery. Baltimore: Williams & Wilkins, 1995:62.)

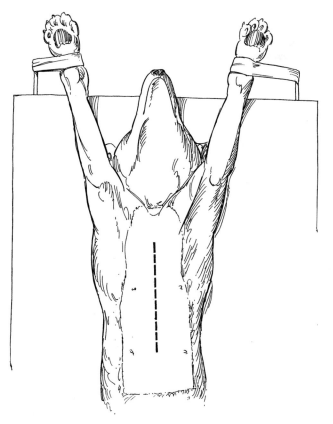

Fig. 23.7. Median sternotomy. Median sternotomy is performed with the animal in dorsal recumbency. (From Orton EC. Small animal thoracic surgery. Baltimore: Williams & Wilkins, 1995:65.)

incised and is elevated from the sternebrae with electrocautery. The sternum is then cut on its midline with an oscillating saw or sternal splitter (Fig. 23.8). Care is taken to limit the penetration of the saw or osteotome to avoid injury to internal thoracic structures. Either the manubrium or the xiphoid is left intact to achieve a stable closure of the sternum. Finochietto retractors are used to expose thoracic structures. A caudal median sternotomy can be combined with a ventral midline celiotomy to gain further exposure of caudal thoracic and cranial abdominal structures (Fig. 23.9). A partial incision of the diaphragm can be made to facilitate wider retraction. A midline cervical incision can be combined with a sternotomy through the manubrium to expose the structures of the thoracic inlet.

Before closure, a thoracostomy tube is placed subcostally and lateral to the midline (Fig. 23.10). The sternotomy is closed with alternating figure-of-eight 20- to 22-gauge orthopedic wires (Fig. 23.11). The pectoralis muscles, subcutaneous tissues, and skin are closed in separate layers with a simple continuous suture pattern.

Postoperative Care

Hypoventilation, hypoxemia, hypothermia, acid-base imbalance, hypotension, and hemorrhage are among the problems that may arise in the first 12 to 24 hours after thoracotomy. Median sternotomy and intercostal thoracotomy are both associated with alterations in pulmonary function that may be attributed to several factors including pain. These changes may inhibit deep inspiration and may promote small airways collapse, resulting in ventilation–perfusion mismatch. Measurement of arterial blood gases after surgery provides information about ventilation and pulmonary gas exchange. Additional postoperative monitoring should include frequent assessment of drainage from the thoracic cavity, temperature, pulse rate, respiratory rate, and mucous membrane color.

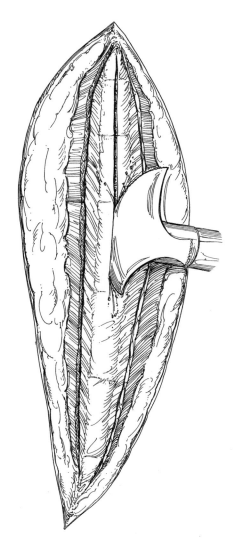

Fig. 23.8. Median sternotomy. The sternum is cut on midline with an oscillating saw. (From Orton EC. Small animal thoracic surgery. Baltimore: Williams & Wilkins, 1995:66.)

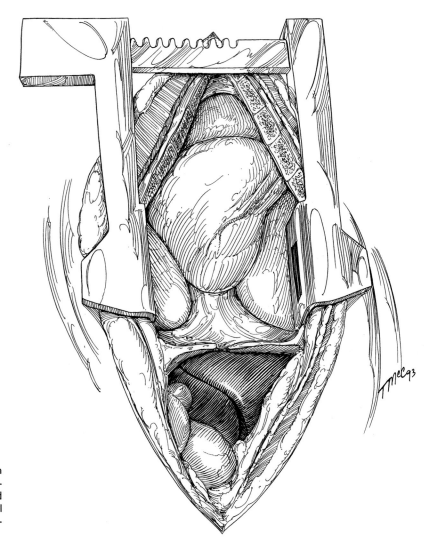

Fig. 23.9. Median sternotomy. A caudal median sternotomy combined with a ventral midline celiotomy to gain exposure to the caudal thoracic and cranial abdominal organs. (From Orton EC. Small animal thoracic surgery. Baltimore: Williams & Wilkins, 1995:67.)

Table 23.1.
Commonly Used Drugs for Postoperative Calming and Alleviation of Postoperative Pain[a]

Drug	Route	Dose (mg/kg)	Duration (h)
Morphine	SQ, IM	0.2–0.8	3–6
Morphine	Epidural	0.1	1–12
Oxymorphone	SQ, IM, IV	0.05–0.1	1.5–3
Butorphanol	SQ, IM, IV	0.2–0.8	1.5–3
Buprenophine	SQ, IM, IV	0.01–0.04	4–12
Lidocaine	Intrapleural	1	0.5–1.0
Bupivacaine	Intrapleural	1.5–3.0	3–12
Acepromazine	SQ, IM, IV	0.02–0.1	1.5–6
Diazepam[b]	IM, IV	0.2	0.5–2

[a] When using any of these drugs intravenously, the lower end of the dose range should be administered, and then repeated if necessary.

[b] Diazepam should be administered in conjuction with an opioid, but it may still cause excitement. If excitement occurs, antagonism with flumazenl (0.1 mg/animal, IV) should be administered.

(From Orton EC. Small animal thoracic surgery. Baltimore: Williams & Wilkins; 1995:39.)

Analgesia is indicated in all animals after thoracotomy. Parenteral opioids, epidural morphine, intrapleural anesthetics, or selective intercostal nerve blocks using 0.75% bupivacaine may be used alone or in combination to provide postoperative analgesia (Table 23.1).

Suggested Readings

Bright RM, McIntosh J, Richardson DR, et al. Clinical and radiographic evaluation of median sternotomy in the dog. Vet Surg 1983;12:13–19.

Dhokarikar P, Caywood DD, Stobie D, et al. Effects of intramuscular or interpleural administration of morphine and interpleural administration of bupivacaine on pulmonary function in dogs that have undergone median sternotomy. Am J Vet Res 1996; 57:375–380.

Orton EC. Small animal thoracic surgery. Baltimore: Williams & Wilkins, 1995.

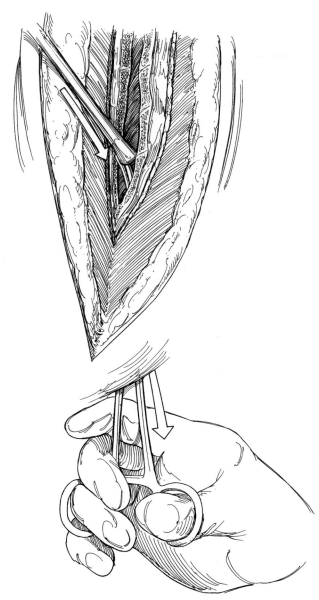

Fig. 23.10. Median sternotomy. Placement of a thoracostomy tube paramedially and subcostally before closure. (From Orton EC. Small animal thoracic surgery. Baltimore: Williams & Wilkins, 1995:69.)

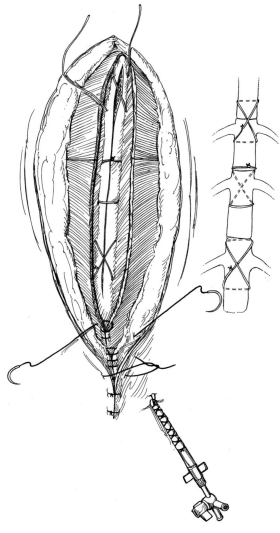

Fig. 23.11. Median sternotomy closure. Stable closure of the sternotomy is achieved by preplaced alternating figure-of-eight orthopedic wire around each sternebra. The muscle, subcutaneous tissues, and skin are closed in separate layers in a simple continuous suture pattern. (From Orton EC. Small animal thoracic surgery. Baltimore: Williams & Wilkins, 1995:69.)

Ringwald RJ, Birchard SJ. Complications of median sternotomy in the dog and literature review. J Am Anim Hosp Assoc 1989; 25:430–434.

Stobie D, Caywood DD, Rozanski EA, et al. Evaluation of pulmonary function and analgesia in dogs after intercostal thoracotomy and use of morphine administered intramuscularly or intrapleurally and bupivacaine administered intrapleurally. Am J Vet Res 1995;56:1098–1109.

Thompson SE, Johnson JM. Analgesia in dogs after intercostal thoracotomy: a comparison of morphine, selective intercostal nerve block, and interpleural regional analgesia with bupivacaine. Vet Surg 1991;2073–2077.

Williams JM, White RAS. Median sternotomy in the dog: an evaluation of the technique in 18 cases. Vet Surg 1993;22:246.

Pulmonary Surgical Techniques

Dianne Dunning & E. Christopher Orton

Partial and complete lung lobectomies are occasionally indicated in small animal practice. Although the surgical techniques are not difficult, they do require a familiarity with thoracic anatomy and pulmonary physiology, as well as a support staff to monitor the animal

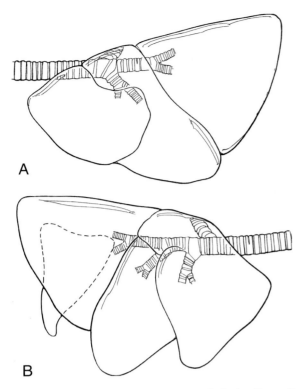

Fig. 23.12. Lung lobe anatomy. **A.** Left. **B.** Right. (From Orton EC. Small animal thoracic surgery. Baltimore: Williams & Wilkins, 1995:162.)

Surgical Anatomy

The trachea of dogs and cats divides into two principal bronchi, which in turn subdivide into lobar bronchi that supply each lung lobe (Fig. 23.12). The left and right lungs are separated by a thin but complete mediastinum. The left lung is divided into cranial and caudal lobes by a deep fissure. The left cranial lung lobe is further divided by an incomplete fissure into cranial and caudal parts, but they share a common lobar bronchus. The right lung is divided into cranial, middle, caudal, and accessory lobes. The accessory lobe passes dorsal to the caudal vena cava and lies medial to the plica vena cava, a fold of pleura that extends around the caudal vena cava. These structures should be identified during manipulation of the right caudal and accessory lung lobes. The pulmonary vessels closely follow the lobar distribution of the bronchi. Pulmonary arteries are located on the craniodorsal aspect of each bronchi, whereas pulmonary veins are located on the caudoventral aspect. Partial or complete lung lobectomy may be performed through a standard intercostal thoracotomy in the fourth through sixth intercostal space or through a median sternotomy.

Surgical Techniques

Partial Lung Lobectomy

Partial lung lobectomy is used to obtain a biopsy or to excise localized marginal lesions of the distal two-thirds of the lung. Partial lung lobectomy may be performed by freehand suturing or with a stapling device. To perform a partial lobectomy by hand, the lung is clamped with noncrushing vascular or intestinal clamps proximal to the isolated lesion (Fig. 23.13). The lung is excised distal to the clamps. A continuous horizontal mattress pattern of 4–0 monofilament suture is placed proximal to the clamps (Fig. 23.14). Delicate swaged-on taper-point needles should be used. Smooth fluid movements that follow the curvature of the needle should be used when driving the needle through the tissue to minimize air leaks at the suture line. The ends of the suture are tied and "tagged" with hemostatic forceps to facilitate manipulation of the lung. The clamps are removed, and the lung incision is oversewn in a simple continuous pattern (Fig. 23.15). The incision is then checked for air leaks by submerging the lung in saline during positive-pressure ventilation of 20 to 30 cm of H_2O. Additional sutures both during and after surgery to ensure a successful outcome.

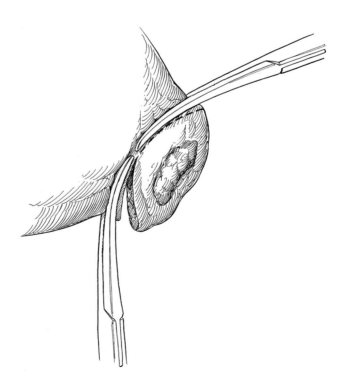

Fig. 23.13. Partial lung lobectomy. The lung is clamped proximal to the isolated lesion. (From Orton EC. Small animal thoracic surgery. Baltimore: Williams & Wilkins, 1995:165.)

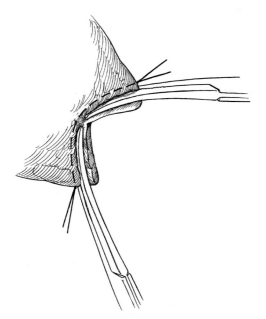

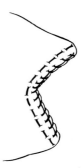

Fig. 23.14. Partial lung lobectomy. A continuous horizontal mattress pattern is placed proximal to the clamps. (From Orton EC. Small animal thoracic surgery. Baltimore: Williams & Wilkins, 1995:165.)

Fig. 23.15. Partial lung lobectomy. The clamps are removed, and the incision is oversewn with a simple continuous pattern. (From Orton EC. Small animal thoracic surgery. Baltimore: Williams & Wilkins, 1995:165.)

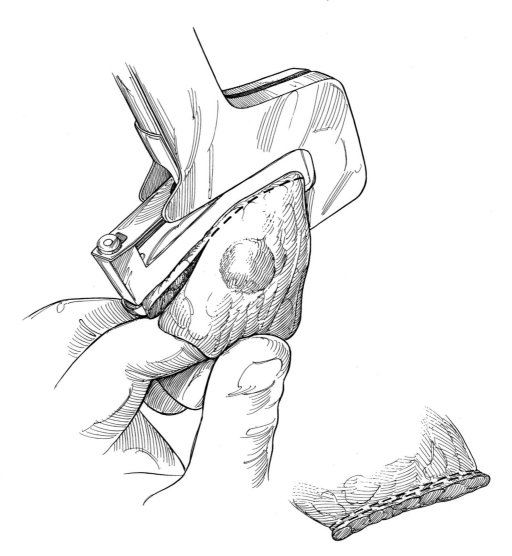

Fig. 23.16. Partial lung lobectomy with staples. The stapler is placed across the lung and is clamped proximal to the lesion. (From Orton EC. Small animal thoracic surgery. Baltimore: Williams & Wilkins, 1995:166.)

may be placed as necessary. Some leakage of air after this technique may be expected, but this usually resolves within a few hours after surgery.

Stapling devices are now commonly available to veterinary surgeons. The advantages of stapling equipment for partial lobectomy are shortened surgical and anesthetic time, decreased blood loss, and reduction in the incidence of bronchopleural fistulas after lung lobe resection. The most useful device for pulmonary procedures is the thoracoabdominal (TA) stapler. This instrument has two staggered rows of stainless steel staples that form a B shape when compressed. The 3.5-mm (blue) or the 2.5-mm (white, V or V3) staple cartridges may be used for pulmonary procedures. A gastrointestinal anastomosis stapler also may be used for longer staple lines. The stapler is placed across the lung and is clamped proximal to the lesion (Fig. 23.16). The staple device is fired and the lung is transected utilizing the edge of the TA stapling device as a cutting edge. After the removal of the stapling device, the lung is checked for air leaks in the manner described previously.

Complete Lung Lobectomy

Excision of an entire lung lobe is indicated for severe trauma, neoplasia, lobe torsion, abscesses, or refractory infections. The affected lung lobes should be manipulated gently to minimize embolization of neoplastic cells or extrusion of purulent material into adjacent airways. Dogs and cats can survive removal of up to 50% of lung lobe mass. Removal of more than 75% of the lung is invariable fatal. Because the right lung

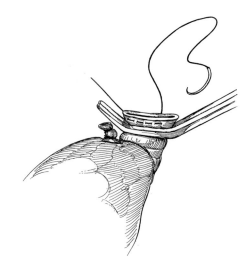

Fig. 23.18. Complete lung lobectomy. The lobar bronchus is clamped and divided, and the bronchial stump is closed in a continuous mattress pattern. (From Orton EC. Small animal thoracic surgery. Baltimore: Williams & Wilkins, 1995:164.)

constitutes more than 50% of the lung capacity, removal of the entire right lung is contraindicated. Excision of the entire left lung is tolerated in the dog, assuming the right lung is normal.

Lung lobectomy should follow the anatomic distribution of the bronchi. The left cranial and caudal lung lobes may be removed individually. The cranial, middle, and caudal right lobes may be removed individually because they each have separate bronchi. The accessory lung lobe usually is removed with the left caudal lung lobe. Before removal of the caudal and accessory lobes, the pulmonary ligaments must be divided from the mediastinum with Metzenbaum scissors.

The pulmonary artery is accessed first by ventral and caudal retraction of the lung lobe. The lobe may be grasped gently with a dry gauze sponge. The artery is isolated by blunt dissection with right-angle forceps parallel to the long axis of the vessel (Fig. 23.17). The artery is triple ligated and is divided between the middle and distal ligature. The pulmonary vein is accessed by dorsal and cranial retraction of the lung lobe. The vein is isolated, ligated, and divided in a similar manner to the artery. The lobar bronchus is then clamped with a noncrushing tangential clamp and is divided 3 mm distal to the clamp. The bronchial stump is closed with 4–0 suture in a continuous mattress pattern (Fig. 23.18). The tangential clamp is removed, and the bronchial stump is oversewn with a continuous pattern (Fig. 23.19). The bronchus is then checked for air leaks by saline immersion.

En bloc stapling of the hilus may be used to remove large lung lobe abscesses or tumors when minimal handling of the affected lung is desired. When using

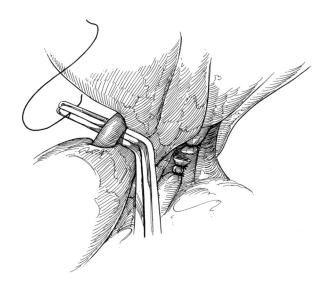

Fig. 23.17. Complete lung lobectomy. Dissection of the ligatures around the pulmonary vessels is accomplished with right-angle forceps parallel to the long axis of the vessel. (From Orton EC. Small animal thoracic surgery. Baltimore: Williams & Wilkins, 1995:164.)

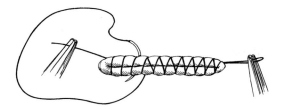

Fig. 23.19. Complete lung lobectomy. The bronchial stump is oversewn with a continuous pattern. (From Orton EC. Small animal thoracic surgery. Baltimore: Williams & Wilkins, 1995:164.)

2.5-mm staples (TA 30 V or V3, white), it is rarely necessary to separately ligate and divide the pulmonary vessels. Dissection of the lung lobe from the mediastinum is performed if needed to exteriorize the lobe. The stapler is placed across the hilus of the lobe and is clamped. A clamp is placed distal to the TA stapler across the lobe to prevent spillage of material from the lobe. The staple device is fired, and the lobe is transected, using the edge of the TA stapling device as a cutting edge. After the removal of the stapling device, the hilus is inspected for leaks in the same manner as described previously.

Postoperative Care

Placement of a thoracostomy tube is always recommended before closure of the thoracotomy. If the thoracostomy tube is nonproductive, it may be removed soon after the surgical procedure (see the earlier section of this chapter on thoracic approaches). Animals should be monitored frequently for pneumothorax or hemorrhage after pulmonary surgery. Pneumothorax usually resolves spontaneously after pulmonary surgery. High-volume air leaks can be managed by continuous underwater suction until they resolve.

Suggested Readings

Orton EC. Small animal thoracic surgery. Baltimore: Williams & Wilkins, 1995:161.
Walshaw R. Stapling techniques in pulmonary surgery. Vet Clin North Am 1994;24:335–366.

Thoracic Drainage

Dennis T. Crowe & Jennifer J. Devey

The ability to recognize and manage the dog or cat with various types of fluid (blood, chylous effusion, suppurative effusion, transudate) or air accumulation in the pleural cavity is vital. Although small accumulations of fluid or air in the pleural space may be easily tolerated and hence go undetected, larger amounts prevent normal lung expansion during the inspiratory phase of the ventilatory cycle and can cause a significant increase in ventilatory effort. If significant air or fluid accumulations are present, the animal may display signs of respiratory distress, orthopnea, polypnea, and poor tolerance for exercise or stress. Immediate thoracentesis of fluid or air can be accomplished with a minimal stress to the patient and may provide enough drainage to be lifesaving. Although mild conditions may require treatment only by thoracentesis, more severe conditions require the placement of a chest tube (tube thoracostomy) and either intermittent or continuous pleural evacuation. If suppurative or infected fluids are retained in the pleural space, the patient is at an increased risk of systemic infection or sepsis. Retention of chylous effusions can lead to fibrosing pleuritis and atelectasis. This discussion reviews the common methods of pleural drainage used in small animal practice.

Needle Thoracentesis

Procedure

If the patient has any evidence of respiratory distress, oxygen should be provided immediately. This can be administered by flow-by oxygen at high flow rates (10 to 15 L/minute), oxygen mask, human nasal cannulas, nasal oxygen tubes, or oxygen hoods. Oxygen cages are not recommended because of the inability to monitor and treat the patient (see Chap. 12).

Before performing needle thoracentesis in the conscious and aware patient, a local anesthetic block is recommended. Using a 22- to 25-gauge needle 1% lidocaine is infiltrated into all layers from the skin down to and including the pleura, with a small amount of anesthetic deposited into the pleural space. The lidocaine should be buffered with sodium bicarbonate. A suggested ratio is two-thirds 1% lidocaine to one-third sodium bicarbonate. Systemic analgesia is not generally required for needle thoracentesis; however, when the patient is in pain, parenteral analgesics may also be used.

Emergency and diagnostic needle thoracentesis can be performed with various needles and catheters, including an 18- to 20-gauge hypodermic needle, a short plastic intravenous catheter, or a bovine teat cannula (Fig. 23.20). In extremely small patients, an 18- to 20-gauge butterfly catheter can also be used. A three-way stopcock and a 35- or 60-mL syringe are attached to the needle either directly or by a 20-inch section of intravenous extension tubing. The intravenous tubing, three-way stopcock, syringe should be assembled and capped to maintain sterility and stored in a crash cart for emergencies. A second section of tubing, attached

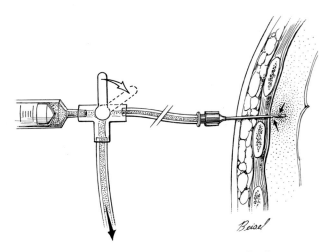

Fig. 23.20. Apparatus for thoracentesis: an indwelling intravenous catheter or a bovine teat cannula, a three-way stopcock, a large syringe, and tubing from an intravenous administration set. Plastic catheters and blunt teat cannulas can remain perpendicular to the chest wall because of the low likelihood of causing lung injury. (From Bojrab MJ, ed. Current techniques in small animal surgery. 2nd ed. Philadelphia: Lea & Febiger, 1983.)

to the sidearm of the stopcock, is useful in directing aspirated fluids into a collection jar. This assembled apparatus can be operated by one person.

Thoracentesis is usually performed at the seventh or eighth intercostal space (Fig. 23.21). The animal should be allowed to rest in the position providing the least stress. Usually, this is standing, sitting, or in sternal recumbency. The lateral recumbent position is only acceptable if the patient is unconscious, intubated, and being ventilated. The dorsoventral location of the puncture site within the intercostal space is influenced by whether air or fluid is to be aspirated. If air is to be aspirated, the midthoracic region is preferred, with the animal in lateral recumbency. If the animal is standing or is in sternal recumbency, air is aspirated at the junction of the dorsal and middle thirds. Fluid is best removed from the middle third of the seventh intercostal space, when the animal is standing or is in sternal recumbency. More caudal placement of a needle may

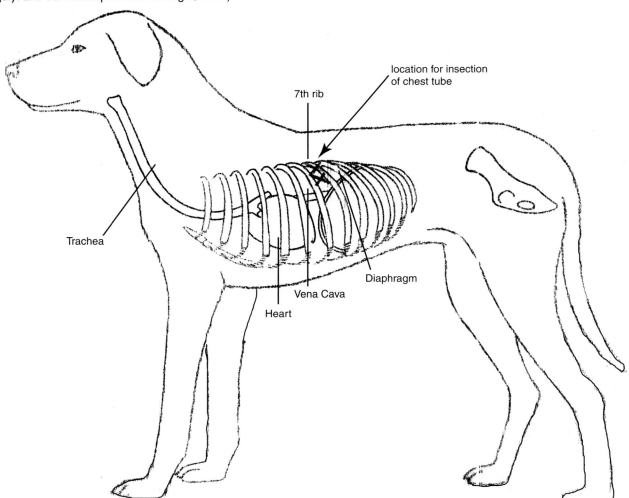

Fig. 23.21. The seventh intercostal space is the ideal location for thoracentesis and chest tube insertion in most patients because of safety. Here at the junction of the dorsal third and ventral third of the space is the least danger of causing injury to vascular structures, the large airway, and the diaphragm.

lead to penetration of the dome of the diaphragm and or liver injury.

Inadvertent injury to the lung parenchyma with the tip of the needle may lead to pneumothorax, particularly if the lung is lacerated in the process. This complication can be avoided by the use of the following technique: An 18- or 20-gauge needle is placed through the skin with the bevel facing caudally. A drop of saline is placed on the needle hub, and the needle is then slowly advanced into the pleural space (Fig. 23.22**A**). Once the pleural space is entered, the negative pressure within the thorax causes the fluid in the hub to be pulled into the chest. In cases of tension pneumothorax, the pressure causes the fluid to be pushed out of the needle hub (Fig. 23.22**B**). The surgeon must stop advancing the needle at this point, to avoid lung injury. The needle is then tilted in a caudal direction. At this time, the bevel of the needle should be directed parallel to the chest wall, with the opening directed away from the chest wall (Fig. 23.22**C**).

Indications

Thoracentesis used as a diagnostic procedure can provide a fluid sample for laboratory evaluation. Thoracentesis is ideal for the initial treatment of acute pneumothorax and pleural effusions and as a method of intermittent drainage of the pleural cavity for treatment of slow accumulations of fluid or air. The surgical placement of a chest drainage tube (tube thoracostomy), however, is preferred for the removal of large volumes of fluid or continuing accumulation of air in the pleural space. Clinical experience has also suggested that it is impossible to drain the pleural space adequately with simple thoracenteses when accumulations of blood, chylous effusion, or pus are present.

Complications

Inadvertent trauma to the lung from overpenetration and movement of the needle leading to lung laceration is the most common complication. This is best prevented using the foregoing technique. The intercostal vessels can be lacerated during the procedure if the needle is introduced immediately adjacent to the ribs. A minor laceration is likely to be self-limiting; however, if an expanding hematoma is noted over the thoracentesis site, this area should be surgically explored and the vessel ligated or cauterized. Rarely, tangential laceration of an intercostal artery can cause serious hemothorax.

Minithoracostomy

Indications and Tube Selection

Various commercial thoracentesis and minithoracostomy tube kits are available (Argyle Turkel Safety Tho-

racentesis System, Sherwood Medical Products, St. Louis, MO; Pneumothorax Sets, Cook Critical Care, Bloomington, IN). These kits contain a medium-bore multiholed catheter (8 to 10 French) for pleural drainage. These catheters can be used for temporary drainage and may be valuable for short-term indwelling chest tubes for cats and small dogs.

Procedure

If a minithoracostomy tube is selected for insertion, the lateral chest wall at the level of the seventh to ninth intercostal spaces is aseptically prepared. A local anesthetic block using 1 to 2% lidocaine is placed. On rare occasions, the animal may require minor sedation or short-acting neuroleptanalgesia. If sedation or neuroleptanalgesia is required, it should be provided intravenously to effect, and ventilation should be monitored. A small skin incision (large enough to allow passage of the thoracostomy tube) is made. The needle and catheter system are slowly introduced into the pleural space, and suction is applied. If an indwelling system is required, the catheter assembly is advanced, the needle assembly is removed, and the tube is secured. Some systems (Argyle Turkel Safety Thoracentesis System, Sherwood Medical Products) have color indicators to detect when the pleural space has been entered. After placement, the catheter is fixed in place by suturing the tube to the fascia, and a bandage is applied. A radiograph is taken to assess tube location.

Complications

The short length of these minithoracostomy catheters may lead to dislodgment, particularly in larger dogs (A Mann, unpublished data). The catheter may also be too small to achieve adequate pleural drainage in big dogs or in those animals with rapid reaccumulations of fluid or air. Kinking can also be a problem with these catheters.

Tube Thoracostomy

Tube Selection

Tube thoracostomy involves the surgical placement of flexible sterile red rubber (Sovereign, Sherwood Medical Products), polyvinyl chloride (Argyle Straight Thoracic Catheter, Sherwood Medical Products; Cook Critical Care), or silicone (Cook Critical Care) tube into the pleural space. Sterile endotracheal tubes can also be used if they are modified by knotting the cuff inflation mechanism, cutting the valve off, and removing the cuff. The tubing should be flexible, but not collapsible. The internal diameter of the tube should be at least one-half to two-thirds the width of one of the larger intercostal spaces (approximate diameter of a

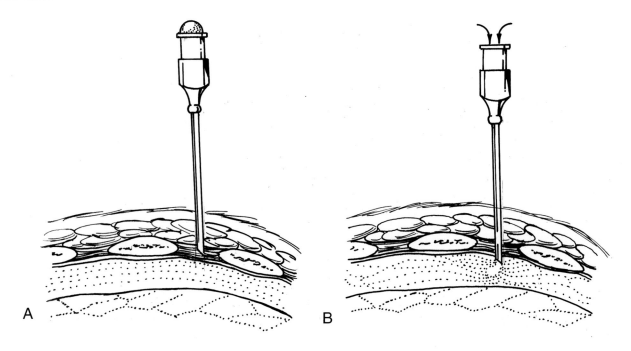

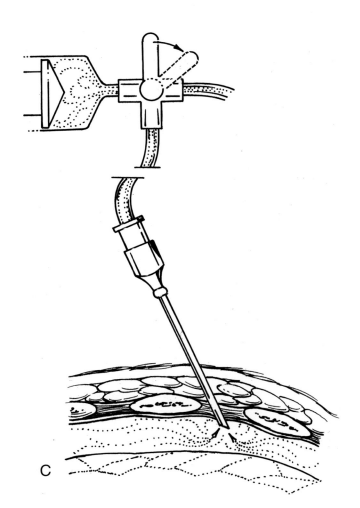

Fig. 23.22. A–C. A hypodermic needle is used to evacuate air or fluid from the pleural space. A drop of saline added to the hub of the needle is used to indicate when the tip of the needle is in the pleural space. The drop of fluid is aspirated into the pleural space if the fluid is still under negative pressure. If it is under positive pressure, the fluid moves outward; if it moves outward under force, a tension pneumothorax is present. The needle is then angled to allow the bevel of the needle to face the open pleural space and is held there while aspiration is performed. (The syringe depicted in the drawing is too small for the job.)

mainstem bronchus). This is important if tension pneumothorax is being treated and to help prevent occlusion by clots or viscous fluids.

The number and size of the holes placed in the catheter also influence the flow rate and effectiveness of the tube. Experimental flow studies on catheters indicate that, when three side holes are present, each additional hole increases the flow rate by only 6%. Most commercially available chest tubes contain an end hole and five or six side holes. If a noncommercial tube is used, side holes can be created using a pair of scissors or a No. 15 scalpel blade. The recommended size of the hole is approximately one-fourth the circumference of the tube. Diameters exceeding one-third the circumference of the tube cause considerable weakness and predispose the tube to kinking.

Commercially available chest tubes contain a marker strip throughout their length to allow radiographic confirmation of placement. The end of a chest tube should be placed on the ventral floor of the patient's thorax and cranial to or adjacent to the heart. In this location, both air and fluid can be drained efficiently from the pleural cavity where the tube is located. All holes must be located within the chest cavity. This placement can be verified radiographically with tubes that have a "sentinel eye," that is, an interruption in the radiopaque marker where the last hole is located. For best function, the tube should be placed no farther cranially than the level of the second rib; more cranial placement may obstruct the flow of air or fluid and may cause phrenic nerve irritation and dysfunction (Fig. 23.23). In tubes where holes have been created, the last hole should be placed through the radiopaque marker for identification purposes. In some cases, because the mediastinum is intact, two chest tubes are required, one for each side of the pleural space.

Chest Tube Placement During Thoracotomy

To place a chest tube at the time of a thoracotomy, the tip of a curved hemostat is bluntly forced through intercostal muscle and parietal pleura at the seventh or eighth intercostal space or two spaces caudal to the thoracotomy incision. A subcutaneous tunnel is made in a caudal direction from the inside of the thorax to the outside for a distance of two to three intercostal spaces. A small skin incision is made at the ninth or tenth intercostal space over the tips of the hemostats. The proximal part of the chest tube is grasped, and the tube is pulled into the thoracic cavity and positioned. The tube can also be placed by advancing a curved hemostat through the incision into the pleural cavity, by grasping the distal part of the tube and pulling the tube out of the chest cavity in a reverse fashion (Fig. 23.24). Cutting the distal part of the tube on an oblique angle creates a pointed end that facilitates its movement through the thoracic wall if it is placed in a reverse fashion. The tip of the tube is positioned cranial and ventral. In all cases, radiographs should be taken after the tube is placed to ensure that the tube is in a proper location and is not kinked or twisted (Fig. 23.25).

Anchoring the Chest Tube

The tube is secured by passing a heavy suture on a taper needle through the skin next to the tube and into the periosteum of the rib adjacent to the tube. A hinge is created by tying 6 to 10 knots and then the

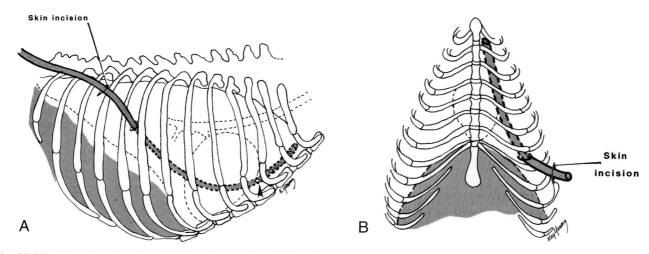

Fig. 23.23. Drawings from lateral (**A**) and ventrodorsal (**B**) radiographs demonstrate proper intrathoracic location of the chest drain. The *arrowhead* in **A** indicates the location of the last side hole in the catheter as seen on the radiograph (where the radiopaque line is interrupted). (For best function, the tube should be placed no farther cranially than the level of the second rib; more cranial placement may obstruct the flow of air or fluid.) (From Bojrab MJ, ed. Current techniques in small animal surgery. 2nd ed. Philadelphia: Lea & Febiger, 1983.)

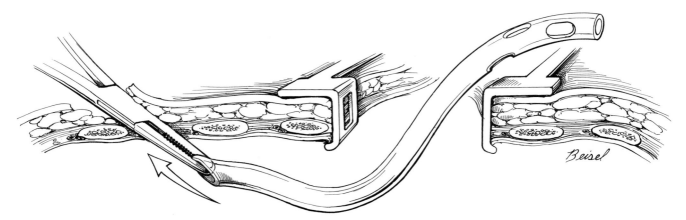

Fig. 23.24. In pulling the chest drain out through the seventh or eighth intercostal space, cutting the end of the tube on an oblique angle facilitates its movement through the thoracic wall. (From Bojrab MJ, ed. Current techniques in small animal surgery. 2nd ed. Philadelphia: Lea & Febiger, 1983.)

suture is passed around the tube in a simple criss-cross fashion and tied with 2 knots. This criss-cross "friction knot" is repeated 2 to 3 times, and then 3 to 5 more knots are tied (Fig. 23.26). The use of this friction knot avoids the need for tape, which is not sterile and can slip. A second hinge is created on the other side of the tube with the same suture, and the suture is anchored again through the skin and into the periosteum. In small patients, the suture can be passed around the rib. If this is done, care is taken to ensure that the needle does not lacerate the lung. If the suture is not anchored to the periosteum, the tube may migrate as the patient breathes and moves, and the tip may exit the pleural space. The thoracotomy is then closed.

Chest Tube Placement With the Chest Closed

A "closed" tube thoracostomy is performed outside the operating room with the patient in a sitting or standing position or whichever position causes the

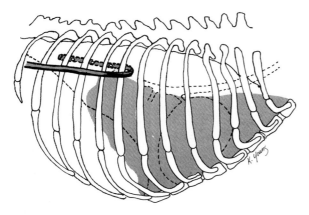

Fig. 23.25. Line drawing of a lateral radiograph demonstrates improper placement and kinking of the chest drain. (From Bojrab MJ, ed. Current techniques in small animal surgery. 2nd ed. Philadelphia: Lea & Febiger, 1983.)

least distress to the animal. This factor is particularly important in patients showing any signs of respiratory distress. Anxiety and struggling may be dangerous to the animal with compromised ventilation, and restraint should be kept to a minimum, especially in cats. A small amount of a sedation can be given intravenously to effect (e.g., butorphanol [Torbugesic], 0.1 to 0.4 mg/kg, and diazepam [Valium], 0.05 to 0.2 mg/kg or acepromazine, .02 to .05 mg/kg). If the patient continues to struggle despite the sedation, the chest tube should be placed while the patient is under general anesthesia. Rapid induction is essential to gain rapid control of the airway. A cuffed endotracheal tube is placed, and positive-pressure ventilation is instituted. Ventilation is closely monitored because peak airway pressures greater than 30 cm H_2O can cause significant decreases in cardiac output. Because of the underlying disorder, delivery of normal tidal volumes may not be possible. In these patients, smaller tidal volumes with a more rapid ventilatory rate should be used.

The skin is clipped over the entire lateral chest wall and cranial flank region and is aseptically prepared for surgery. Local anesthetic is infiltrated into the proposed site of tube insertion at the seventh intercostal space as previously described. This should include the nearby pleura and intercostal nerve. The skin over the lateral chest wall is pulled cranially by an assistant such that the skin over the ninth or tenth intercostal space overlies the seventh or eighth intercostal space. The skin should be pulled at least the same distance as two rib spaces (Fig. 23.27**A**).

Using aseptic technique, a small skin incision is made in the middle of the seventh intercostal space (Fig. 23.27**B**). Curved Kelly forceps are then used to separate the intercostal muscles in a controlled fashion (Fig. 23.27**C**). The tips of the forceps are inserted into the incision, and mild pressure is exerted in a medial

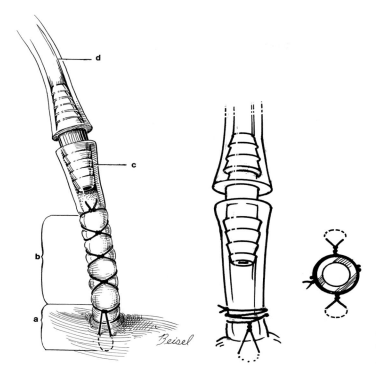

Fig. 23.26. Securing the drain tube using a Chinese finger trap friction suture. First, the suture is tied without tension to prevent irritation of the skin (*a*); then, in a criss-cross fashion, multiple surgeon's knots are tied around the tube (*b*), chest catheter (*c*), and gum-rubber tubing (*d*). Although the drawing depicts a finger trap, all that is really required are several "friction knots" tied in criss-cross fashion and wrapped around the tube (*inset*). (From Bojrab MJ, ed. Current techniques in small animal surgery. 2nd ed. Philadelphia: Lea & Febiger, 1983.)

direction; the tips are then opened to spread the tissues, and then the forceps are removed (Fig. 23.27**D**). This dissecting action is used to create a small defect in the pleural space (Fig. 23.27**E**). A small amount of air is intentionally allowed to move into the pleural space, to cause the lung to retract away from the pari-

etal pleura as the tips of the forceps penetrate the pleural space. This maneuver permits the chest tube to be inserted without injuring the lung. The hemostat is left in place to allow continued identification of the thoracotomy site. A stylet is used in the tube to help guide it into the appropriate position. The tip of the

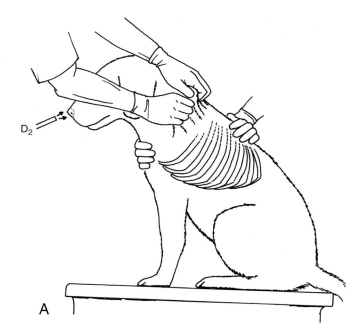

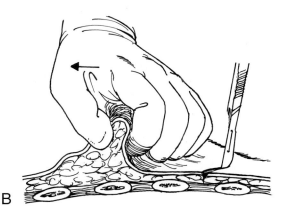

Fig. 23.27. **A–F.** Placement of a chest tube with the skin pulled as far forward as possible that creates a flap when the tube is inserted and the skin is released.

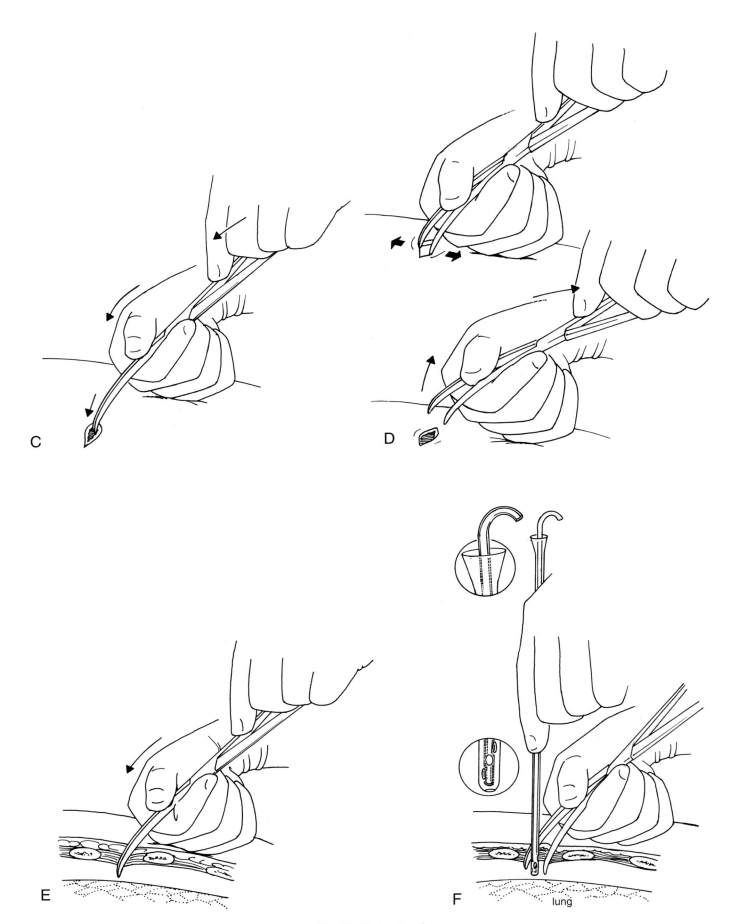

C

D

E

F

lung

Fig. 23.27 (continued)

stylet should not protrude beyond the end of the tube. The tube tip is then passed into the chest cavity through intercostal musculature previously separated by the tip of the hemostat and is gently guided (without undue force) into the cranioventral thorax (Fig. 23.27**F**). The stylet is removed, and the tube is rotated to ensure that it is not kinked. The assistant releases the skin so the skin returns to its original position, thus creating a subcutaneous tunnel for the tube (Fig. 23.28). The tube is then anchored as described previously. If an assistant is not available, the skin incision should be made over the tenth or eleventh intercostal space, and a curved hemostat should be used bluntly to create a tunnel cranial to the seventh or eighth intercostal space. The catheter tip is then grasped in the jaws of stout hemostatic clamps, is passed down the subcutaneous tunnel, and is forced into the chest cavity through intercostal musculature previously separated by the tip of the hemostat. This maneuver is difficult and must be closely controlled to prevent overpenetration. Practice with a cadaver is recommended. Placing a tube using local anesthetic alone can be more easily accomplished using the former technique.

Placement of a thoracostomy tube can also be accomplished using a commercially available tube and trocar stylet unit, which is pushed through the chest wall. This procedure is strongly discouraged because of the high likelihood of iatrogenic injury to intrathoracic structures and the high degree of tolerance of the first procedure described earlier. The skin over the tenth to eleventh intercostal space is pulled cranially by an assistant to overlie the eighth to ninth intercostal space. The trocar-pointed stylet is then forced through the intercostal space with a controlled thrust. As soon as the tip of the tube enters the chest, the metal stylet is retracted to just inside the cannula. The rigidity of the stylet aids in manipulating the tube into the correct cranioventral position. The assistant then allows the patient's skin to retract caudally to its normal position. Once released, the skin and subcutaneous tissue form a seal over the hole.

Bandaging the Chest Tube

An occlusive dressing is placed using sterile antibiotic ointment or petrolatum over the ostomy site. The exiting catheter and torso are then wrapped gently but securely with gauze and tape for further protection. A stockinette can also be used to cover the entire area. The end of the catheter should be exposed near the dorsum of the animal's back, and the rest of the cathe-

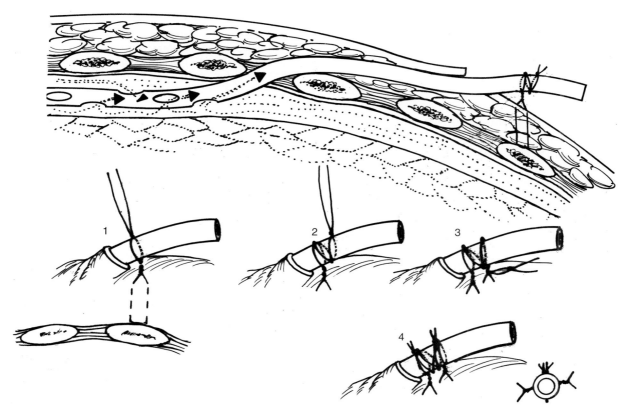

Fig. 23.28. When the skin is allowed to return to normal position, a tunnel is created that helps to prevent air from migrating into the pleural space. Note the position of some of the side holes in the tube that allow air and fluid to drain from the pleural space as the lung reexpands (*1* to *4*).

ter should be covered to prevent its being damaged or dislodged.

Methods of Pleural Space Evacuation

The open end of the tube must be attached to one of the following: 1) a Heimlich valve (Bard–Parker, Rutherford, NJ) or another one-way egress valve; 2) a three-way stopcock; 3) an underwater seal; 4) an underwater seal with controlled continuous, low-vacuum suction drainage (high-volume or low-volume types depend on the rate of air or fluid–blood accumulation); 5) an underwater seal with controlled, intermittent low-vacuum suction drainage; or 6) under emergency conditions, a regular suction unit with a side hole cut into the connective tubing to control the suction pressure. The choice of device depends on the size of the patient, the size of the air leak, the nature of the pleural fluid, and the patient's tractability. All attachments to the chest tube should be secured with tape placed in a criss-cross fashion. This allows the inside of the tubing or attachment to be visualized. If the attachment is inadvertently pulled, the tape will tighten and prevent loosening or detachment.

Heimlich Valve

The Heimlich valve consists of a rubber one-way flutter valve that is enclosed in a clear plastic tube open at each end (Fig. 23.29). The end of the chest tube is attached to the wide end of the flutter valve and is an excellent device for evacuating air. It is a good temporary device for evacuating blood and other fluids; however, the valve should be replaced frequently during drainage of blood or other tenacious fluids because the rubber valve becomes sticky and does not open freely. The end of a Heimlich valve has a fitting that accommodates a syringe in case manual suction is required. Although the valve has been used with success in animals weighing less than 15 kg, some smaller patients may not be able to generate sufficient increases in intrapleural pressure during expiration to open the valve and to allow evacuation. One-way valves are especially useful in the initial management of tension pneumothorax in patients weighing more than 15 kg if an underwater seal and suction system is not immediately available.

Stopcock

A stopcock attached to the end of a catheter prevents air or fluid from moving either in or out without manual operation. Its use is recommended in animals weighing less than 15 kg and in animals that are not accumulating air or fluid rapidly in their pleural cavity. The rate of fluid or air evacuation is determined by

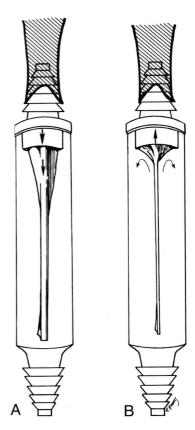

Fig. 23.29. These diagrams demonstrate the function of the Heimlich flutter valves. **A.** During inspiration, the valve stays closed, and no air can enter the thoracic cavity. **B.** During expiration, as intrapleural pressure increases, the air or fluid is forced out of the pleural space through the chest tube and one-way valve. (From Bojrab MJ, ed. Current techniques in small animal surgery. 2nd ed. Philadelphia: Lea & Febiger, 1983.)

the size of the stopcock because the stopcock is of a smaller diameter than the chest tube. A large syringe is used for periodic aspiration by opening and closing the valve as needed to accomplish thoracentesis. The syringe plunger should be pulled back gently with only sufficient pressure applied to evacuate the fluid. Excessive pressure (greater than 30 cm H_2O) can lead to lung injury or ineffective evacuation caused by the aspiration of mediastinal tissue.

Temporary Emergency Underwater Seal and Suction System

A disposable plastic intravenous administration set can be used to facilitate emergency drainage of large quantities of pleural effusion. The male end of the plastic tubing is fitted to the side arm of the stopcock, and the drip chamber is cut from the other end and is placed underwater. When the side arm tubing is filled and the stopcock is opened, drainage of the pleural

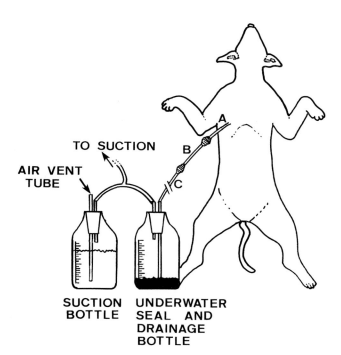

Fig. 23.30. Two-bottle suction drainage: A, Distal end of the chest tube exiting from the bandaged thorax: B, gum-rubber tubing (approximately half an inch in diameter) to allow "stripping" of the chest tube, about 3 feet long (see text): C, polyvinyl chloride "bubble" tubing. (From Bojrab MJ, ed. Current techniques in small animal surgery. 2nd ed. Philadelphia: Lea & Febiger, 1983.)

space to a collecting vessel is possible by siphon action. To make and use an underwater seal, a length of tubing connected to the chest catheter is placed 1 to 2 cm below the fluid's surface in a bowl or bottle containing 2 to 3 cm of sterile saline solution. This useful, quickly

made underwater seal and one-way valve are recommended as a temporary measure when no other instruments or one-way valves are available and when time does not permit delayed action. The device can also be used for patients that need a vent if pleural fluid or air accumulates. When using this technique, care is taken to make sure that the tube stays submerged because, if the seal is broken, pneumothorax rapidly develops. Constant observation of this temporary device is mandatory.

Underwater Seal and Suction Drainage

Underwater seal and suction drainage of the pleura can be easily accomplished using several systems. Both two-bottle (Fig. 23.30) and three-bottle (Fig. 23.31) systems are adaptable to veterinary practice, and the equipment is unsophisticated and reusable. With a two-bottle suction drainage system, the chest catheter is connected to a 500- to 2000-mL sterile glass bottle containing enough sterile saline solution to fill it to a level of 2 to 3 cm from the bottom. The tube within the bottle is placed 1 to 2 cm below the surface of the saline solution. The bottle acts as both a collection reservoir and an underwater seal system to prevent air from being aspirated into the pleural space. A second bottle is partially filled with sterile saline solution and is connected to the first. A rigid plastic vent tube is open to room air, so it permits air to be aspirated into the bottle as vacuum is applied. Thus, by raising or lowering the tube in the second bottle, the amount of vacuum applied to the catheter extending into the patient's chest can be controlled. If the vacuum regula-

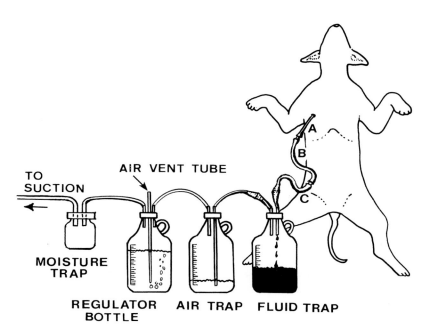

Fig. 23.31. Three-bottle suction drainage: A, Distal end of the chest tube exiting from the bandaged thorax; B, gum-rubber tubing (approximately half an inch in diameter) to allow "stripping" of the tube, about 3 feet in length (see text); C, polyvinyl chloride "bubble" tubing. (From Bojrab MJ, ed. Current techniques in small animal surgery. 2nd ed. Philadelphia: Lea & Febiger, 1983.)

tion tube is submerged to 10 cm, the patient will not experience more than 20 cm water transpleural suction pressure.

Experimental and clinical studies have shown that a continuous 15 to 20 cm negative pressure effectively aspirates tension pneumothorax and allows pulmonary visceral and parietal pleural surfaces to be approximated and to remain approximated. This pressure has proved to be key to the successful, spontaneous sealing of large defects in the lungs of human and animal patients. With the use of suction drainage, many pneumothoraces close, and the need for thoracotomy is thus obviated. This finding is in contrast to drainage without suction, experimental and clinical studies of which have shown that large leaks either do not seal or seal slowly.

With a three-bottle suction drainage system, the first bottle is connected to the chest catheter and acts as a fluid trap. Such a system is particularly useful if hemorrhage or hydrothorax is voluminous. If traumatic hemorrhage is severe, autotransfusion may be considered from this vessel. In this case, approximately 50 to 75 mL anticoagulant solution is initially added to the bottle. When 500 to 1000 mL blood has been aspirated, a second fluid-trap bottle containing anticoagulant is substituted for the first bottle, and autotransfusion is begun. The second bottle of the three-bottle system is connected to the first bottle and acts as the underwater seal. Its function and filling are similar to those of the first bottle of a two-bottle system. The third bottle is connected to the second and again acts as suction regulator.

For the underwater seal and suction drainage system, at least the first 3 feet of the tubing leading from the chest catheter to the underwater seal should be made of gum rubber (Tomac amber latex intravenous tubing, American Hospital Supply Corp., McGaw Park, IL). Any animal whose chest catheter is connected to an underwater seal device by a tube must be watched carefully because knocking over of the bottles and detachment or chewing of the tubing can lead to massive pneumothorax. This possibility is the major drawback of the use of bottle suction systems in many small animal practices in which staff coverage is not available on a 24-hour basis. If an intensive care unit, hospital with 24-hour staff coverage, or emergency practice is available, however, continuous suction and drainage may be accomplished and continued for as long as necessary.

With several alternatives available, selection of a drainage system depends on the following criteria: 1) the patient's size; 2) the type of material drained and its rate of accumulation within the pleural space; 3) the facilities and staff available for monitoring; and 4) economic considerations. Without question, the underwater seal and suction drainage system is the most effective. A three-bottle system is no longer available, but one may buy a two-bottle and a one-bottle system and combine them (American Hospital Supply Corp.). The Pleur-evac chest drainage unit (Deknatel, Inc., Fall River, MA) is a commercially available underwater seal system that is in essence a three-bottle system. This also has an autotransfusion system that can be attached for collecting blood for autotransfusion. The Pleur-evac does require the use of a suction unit to generate the vacuum powering the system. The AN50 Thorovac (H. W. Andersen Products, Inc., Haw River, NC) is a commercial example of a two-bottle system. This is an electrically driven underwater seal suction system. Up to 20 cm of water pressure can be generated; however, in patients with large leaks, the unit may not be able to evacuate rapidly enough. It is generally useful if the air leak from a pneumothorax is less than 500 mL per hour.

Troubleshooting and Tube Stripping

When using any form of continuous underwater suction system, the chest tube should be intermittently stripped and, in some cases, hand suctioned using a stopcock and syringe to ensure that the system is working adequately. The best way to hand suction using a stopcock is to attach a "Y" connector (Abbott Laboratories, Chicago) to the chest tube. A red rubber tube (Sovereign, Sherwood Medical Products) is used to connect the stopcock to the Y connector. The other end of the Y connector is attached to the suction tubing (Fig. 23.32). A clamp is placed across the section of tubing not being used. This method allows either continuous suctioning or syringe aspiration without disruption of the connections.

With continuous-suction systems, leaks and generation of inadequate suction pressure are the two most common complications. Leaks can occur anywhere along the system from the ostomy site to the suction unit. If the tube was not tunneled at least two spaces, the tube may start to leak at the ostomy site. This is more likely to occur the longer the tube is in place because the skin edges retract around the ostomy site, thereby creating a larger hole. If the tube backs out of the chest, holes in the tube may communicate with the environment.

The pressure generated at the chest tube should be checked periodically. This can be done by placing a manometer near the chest tube and monitoring the pressure as the suction is applied. A commercial manometer (Vital Signs Inc., Totawa, NJ) can be used for this purpose, or tubing can be placed in a bottle of sterile saline. A column of saline pulled upward into the tubing should be between 15 and 20 cm above the surface of the saline. The pressure indicated at the suction unit itself is always less than the pressure gen-

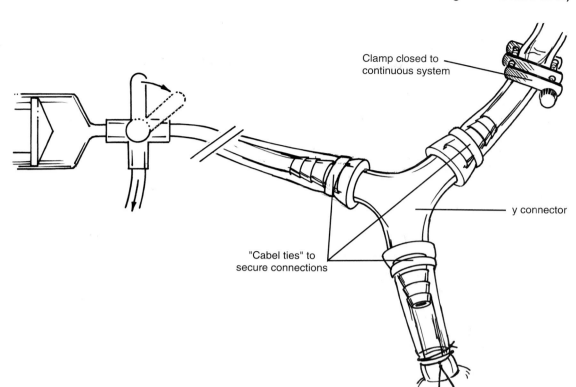

Fig. 23.32. Y connecter attached to a chest tube to allow a continuous-suction system to be connected as well as a stopcock to aspirate intermittently, to ensure function of the continuous system and to act as a "fail safe" for evacuation of the pleural space if the system stops working properly.

erated at the chest tube because of resistance within the tubing. This problem worsens in proportion to the length and collapsibility of the tubing.

Fluid accumulations within the suction tubing also interfere with operation of the system. Stripping is re-quired to keep the fluid from accumulating. By grasp-ing the tubing as near to the patient as possible and by pinching it closed, a stripping motion (a sliding motion, with the tube pinched off) is applied along the length of the tube for 20 to 40 cm (Fig. 23.33). The stripping

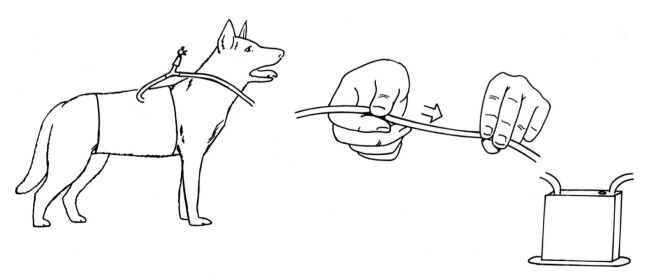

Fig. 23.33. Chest tube stripping done by a nurse every 6 to 8 hours to keep the tubing and the tube patent. The left hand pinches the tubing (made of gum rubber) shut, and the right hand is used to strip the tube, by pinching and then sliding using the thumb and index finger, which are lubricated with water or petroleum jelly. When the right hand meets the left, the tube in the left hand is allowed to snap open, creating a sudden popping of air.

action creates a sudden, high negative pressure inside the tube past the area where the tube has been pinched closed. At the end of each stripping action, the pinch is released, and a surge of negative pressure is transferred to the thoracic catheter. The high negative pressure generated also loosens and evacuates fibrin clots and debris inside the catheter. This stripping should be done every hour when a significant amount of blood or other viscous or sticky fluid is encountered. The frequency of stripping may be decreased as the amount of fluid removed decreases. Generally, by the second day, stripping is only necessary every 4 to 8 hours.

Special Considerations for the Rapid Accumulation of Fluid or Air

Currently, an underwater seal and suction drainage system attached to the chest tube is the recommended method of treatment for trauma or disease conditions involving the continuous or rapid accumulation of air or fluid in the pleural space. In these situations, a Heimlich valve should only be used as a temporary means of evacuating the chest if the patient's weight exceeds 15 kg, such as when transporting the patient from the emergency treatment area to the intensive care unit. For patients under 15 kg, use of a three-way stopcock and syringe is the only method recommended for the drainage of rapid accumulation of air or fluid other than underwater seal and suction systems.

Under emergency conditions, if an underwater seal and suction system is not immediately available, a regular suction unit can be used. The vacuum is reduced to 20 to 30 cm H_2O by one of three methods: 1) cutting a small hole in the side of the tubing; 2) partially clamping the tubing; and, 3) opening the "escape" valve or using the control valve on the suction unit.

Analgesia

The presence of chest tubes can be painful for the patient, and analgesia should be administered on a regular basis as required. Intercostal nerve blocks can be provided with 0.25 to 1.0 mL of 0.25% bupivacaine through intermittent injections or with the use of an indwelling catheter. Intrapleural analgesia is best provided with 0.25 to 0.5% bupivacaine (up to 2 mg/kg) administered into the chest tube. The addition of sodium bicarbonate (one-third sodium bicarbonate to two-thirds bupivacaine) to the local anesthetic helps to decrease the irritation from the acidity of the drug. Warming the medication to body temperature and administering the drugs slowly also provide less discomfort. Systemic administration of a neuroleptanalgesic

is also recommended in combination with local analgesia.

Tube Removal

The chest drain should be removed whenever it is no longer needed. This time may range from the immediate postoperative period to more than a week. Suction should be continued until no air has been removed for 12 to 24 hours or until fluid accumulations are less than 1 to 2 mL/kg per day. If any question exists concerning the safe removal of the chest tube, it should be clamped for 24 hours. The patient should be closely monitored during this time, and the tube should be suctioned if the patient has any evidence of respiratory compromise. The tube is aspirated after the 24-hour period, and radiographs are then taken to determine whether any intrapleural accumulation of air or fluid is present. If no accumulation is present, the tube may be safely removed.

When the surgeon determines that the tube is no longer needed, the bandage and sutures are removed, and the tube is quickly removed using traction. The hole is covered with a gauze dressing impregnated with an antibiotic ointment. The gauze is held in place with a torso bandage. Complete sealing of the wound generally occurs in 2 or 3 days. Until then, the dressing is changed as required to maintain a clean, dry, and occlusive (with ointment) environment.

Complications

As previously mentioned, whenever the patient must be left unattended, the entire chest catheter and attached apparatus must be covered completely under a well-secured dressing to prevent disturbance or dislodgment. If disconnection occurs in the patient with a large-bore chest tube, death can occur within 5 to 10 minutes because of the effects of a progressive pneumothorax.

An occasional problem is the accumulation of fibrin clots, especially when a small-lumen-diameter catheter (smaller than 20 French) is used or when a large amount of fibrin, blood, or other proteinaceous material is drained. Blockage is prevented by frequent stripping of the tubing. When using a three-way stopcock on the end of the chest catheter, a small amount of sterile heparinized saline solution can be infused every few hours; when using the Heimlich valve or other one-way rubber valve, it may be necessary to change the valve frequently.

Reexpansion pulmonary edema has been occasionally reported in patients with chronic cases of atelectasis when the lung is reinflated rapidly after rapid removal of pleural fluid or air. In general, this complication is not seen until the lungs have been atelectatic for longer than 3 days.

Another reported complication is subcutaneous emphysema as the result of a large hole in the chest wall that is not completely occluded by the presence of the drainage tube. An occlusive dressing applied around the exit site helps to minimize this problem. Lung tissue entrapment and subsequent infarction by vigorous chest suction have been reported. This complication may be considered whenever a radiographic pulmonary infiltrate appears near a side or end hole of the chest tube. Unregulated, high vacuum levels, as in operating room or portable suction units (80 to 120 mm Hg), should not be used. All active suction must be regulated by a two- or three-bottle system, the emergency system mentioned earlier, or, if one is aspirating with a syringe, it should be done gently.

Although infection can occur whenever any indwelling catheter is used, this problem is minimized by careful tube placement and care. In a randomized study of 120 human patients with indwelling chest drains, half were treated with prophylactic antibiotics, and the other half were given a placebo. Those patients given antibiotics had the higher infection rate. Our clinical results with the use of chest drains in dogs and cats also seem to indicate similar conclusions. Proper wound care at the site where the drainage catheter enters the chest and strict attention to aseptic technique and suction drainage remain the most important factors in preventing serious infection of the pleural cavity and subcutaneous tissue. If any concerns exists, the evacuated fluid should undergo periodic cytologic assessment, and Gram staining and culture should be performed as indicated. Culture of tips of the tubes on removal should be considered in any tubes that have been in place for an extended period.

A rare complication of chest tubes is phrenic nerve irritation and palsy. This problem may be severe enough to cause diaphragmatic paresis. If the tube rubs the pericardium or the heart after pericardiectomy, arrhythmias may occur. These are generally self-limiting.

If the tube has been in place for several days, adhesions may have formed, and mild intrathoracic bleeding may occur when the tube is removed. Rarely, bleeding may persist to the point that surgical exploration and vessel ligation are required.

Comments

Often, animals suffering from multiple injuries, including fractures, have a pneumothorax. Mild pneumo-

thoraces do not cause respiratory distress, but they are readily diagnosed by chest radiographs. If anesthesia is necessary for fracture repair, a chest tube should be inserted to aid resolution of the pneumothorax, to help in lung healing, and to allow earlier and safer use of anesthesia. Positive-pressure ventilation during anesthesia may predispose the healing lung or bronchus to rupture. Without a chest tube in place, a tension pneumothorax can rapidly develop and can prove fatal. The placement of prophylactic chest tubes is also indicated in patients with lung injury that require positive-pressure ventilation.

Bilateral chest tubes may be required to permit adequate evacuation of the pleural space. In many trauma patients, the mediastinum ruptures, thus allowing both sides of the thorax to be evacuated with a unilateral tube. However, the mediastinum may seal, and a second tube may be required. In many patients with bilateral fluid accumulations, chest tubes may be required on both sides of the thorax to provide effective drainage because the mediastinum is intact and is often thicker than normal.

Chest tubes can be used as a method of core rewarming of the severely hypothermic patient. In such cases, through-and-through lavage is done with warm sterile saline. Instillation of sterile saline or lactated Ringer's solution into the pleural cavity using chest tubes can also be used for the treatment of uremia, similar to peritoneal dialysis.

Suggested Readings

Brandstetter RD, Cohen RP. Hypoxemia after thoracentesis. JAMA 1979;242:1060.

Butler WB. Use of a flutter valve in treatment of pneumothorax dogs and cats. J Am Vet Med Assoc 1969;155:1997.

Crowe DT. Help for the patient with thoracic hemorrhage. Vet Med 1988:83:578–588.

Graham JM, Mattox KL, Beall AC. Penetrating trauma of the lung. J. Trauma 1979;19:665.

Griffith GL, et al. Acute traumatic hemothorax. Ann Thorac Surg 1978;26:204.

Harrah JD, Wangensteen SL. A simple emergency closed thoracostomy set. Surgery 1970;68:583.

Holtsinger RH, Beale BS, Bellah JR, et al. Spontaneous pneumothorax in the dog: a retrospective analysis of 21 cases 1993; 29:195–210.

Richards W. Tube thoracostomy. J Fam Pract 1978;6:629.

Sauer BW. Valve drainage of the pleural cavity of the dog. J Am Vet Med Assoc 1969;155:1977.

Turner WD, Breznock EM. Continuous suction drainage for management of canine pyothorax: a retrospective study. J Am Anim Hosp Assoc 1988;24:485–494.

Withrow SJ, Fenner WR, Wilkins RJ. Closed chest drainage and lavage for treatment of pyothorax in the cat. J Am Anim Hosp Assoc 1975;11:90.

Zimmerman JE, Dunbar BS, Klingenmaier CH. Management of subcutaneous emphysema, pneumomediastinum, and pneumothorax during respirator therapy. Crit Care Med 1975;3:69.

＊ 24 ＊

THORACIC WALL

Diaphragmatic Advancement for Reconstruction of the Caudal Thoracic Wall

Michael G. Aronsohn

Reconstruction of the canine caudal thoracic wall by advancement of the diaphragm has been advocated as a way to reestablish the integrity of the thorax after trauma and tumor resection. Osteosarcoma and chondrosarcoma, the most common thoracic wall tumors, usually occur at the costochondral junction. This procedure also can be used in the management of congenital malformations of the rib cage and deep soft tissue infections or osteomyelitis with draining fistulas that are unresponsive to medical therapy. Diaphragmatic advancement is indicated for reconstruction of the thoracic wall supported by the eighth through thirteenth ribs.

The advantages of diaphragmatic advancement are that it is a technically uncomplicated procedure; no foreign material or graft is needed to close a defect, thus eliminating rejection problems; and it gives a good functional result with a good cosmetic appearance. Disadvantages include a reduction in the size of the thoracic cavity with associated decreased tidal volume and inspiratory capacity, some loss of protection of underlying structures, and limitation to use of the eighth through thirteenth ribs.

Surgical Anatomy and Physiology

Two aspects of canine anatomy permit use of this procedure in the dog. First, although recesses present between the diaphragm and caudal thoracic wall allow for the expansion of the lungs during inspiration (Fig. 24.1), even in forced inspiration, the lungs do not completely fill these spaces. Thus, a reduction in the size of the thoracic cavity can occur without significantly compromising lung expansion. Second, the first eight pairs of ribs, which articulate directly with the sternum, constitute the most stable portion of the canine rib cage. The ninth through thirteenth ribs are known as asternal ribs because they attach to the costal cartilage of the immediately preceding rib and not directly to the sternum. The thirteenth pair of ribs does not attach to the sternum; these are called floating ribs. Because the most rigid portion of the rib cage is not compromised by this procedure, vital underlying structures including the heart, lungs, and great vessels remain protected.

The thoracic cavity is reduced in size, and tidal volume and inspiratory capacity also may be reduced, thus creating an area of lung with a ventilation–perfusion inequality resulting from underinflation. This condition is not considered significant in nonathletic patients.

Preoperative Considerations

Dorsoventral and lateral radiographs should be obtained to define the extent of thoracic involvement, because diaphragmatic advancement is indicated only for lesions of the eighth through thirteenth ribs. Thoracic radiographs also are obtained to determine whether tumors of the thoracic wall have metastasized or to diagnose concurrent conditions such as pneumothorax or pulmonary contusion in trauma patients.

Anesthetic management is tailored to the patient. Because hypoventilation may lead to respiratory acidosis and hypoxemia, drugs that potentiate hypoventilation, such as narcotics, should be avoided. Controlled

419

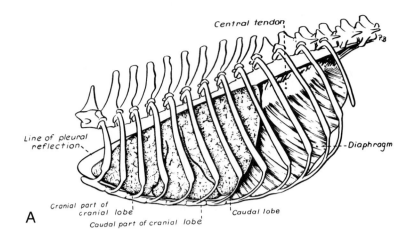

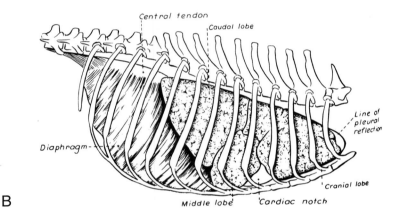

Fig. 24.1. Left (**A**) and right (**B**) lateral views of the canine thorax showing the relation of the lungs, diaphragm, and ribs. (From Evans HE, Christensen GC. Miller's anatomy of the dog. 2nd ed. Philadelphia: WB Saunders, 1979.)

or assisted ventilation, by use of a respirator, is recommended; however, positive-pressure ventilation by an assistant can be used.

Surgical Technique

Resection of Lesion

When approaching a body wall tumor, the skin incision is made over the mass and through the subcutaneous tissues. The extent of the mass becomes more evident at this point. Primary bone tumors of the costochondral junction usually involve adjacent ribs and soft tissue by extension, necessitating resection of a significant amount of thoracic wall. First-intention closure usually can be performed if no more than two ribs are involved. Care is taken to preserve large, flat muscles such as the external abdominal oblique and rectus abdominis, if possible. These muscles may be used later to protect and reinforce the primary suture line. Any attached skin, subcutaneous tissue, fascia, muscle, or pleura should be removed en bloc with the tumor. Multiple-action bone-cutting forceps are used

to transect ribs and cartilage dorsally and ventrally to the lesion. Incisions are made through the intercostal muscle and pleura to free the mass from surrounding tissue. Intercostal arteries are ligated. Involvement of lung tissue or diaphragm by direct extension may also occur. Metastatic lung disease that was not diagnosed by thoracic radiographs may be visualized at this time.

In patients with thoracic wall trauma, a skin incision is made directly over the defect, and the chest wall and thoracic cavity are examined. Devitalized muscle and rib are resected, so only viable tissue remains. Sharp edges of fractured ribs are resected with bone-cutting forceps or a rongeur. Intercostal muscle caudal to the last intact rib is preserved if possible. The intercostal artery, located near the caudal edge of each rib, is ligated if necessary.

Advancement of Diaphragm

Once the tumor or devitalized tissue has been resected, advancement of the diaphragm and closure of the defect can proceed. A chest tube is placed, under visual-

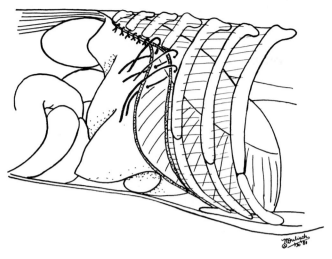

Fig. 24.2. The diaphragm has been incised and sutured to the epaxial musculature. Placement of sutures between the diaphragm and muscles of the ninth intercostal space is underway. (From Aronsohn M. Diaphragmatic advancement for defects of the caudal thoracic wall in the dog. Vet Surg 1984;13:26.)

ization, two or three intercostal spaces cranial to the last intact rib. An incision is made through the diaphragm near its lateral attachment to the body wall. Care is taken to avoid injury to underlying structures in the abdominal cavity. The diaphragm is advanced and is sutured to the superficial epaxial muscles (longissimus and iliocostalis muscles) and the intercostal muscles caudal to the last intact rib (Fig. 24.2).

Sutures may be placed around ribs or through holes drilled in ribs, if adequate muscle is not available. Care is taken to avoid ligating uninvolved intercostal arteries. The diaphragm may be incised a little at a time and advanced and sutured so an excessive amount of diaphragm is not inadvertently detached. Simple interrupted sutures of a monofilament nonabsorbable material are preferred. The last few sutures may be preplaced to ensure an airtight closure. Muscle tissue is mobilized to protect and reinforce the suture line. Subcutaneous tissue and skin are closed routinely. Penrose or sump drains may be needed if dead space or infection is present.

Postoperative Care

After free air and fluid are aspirated, a noncompressing bandage is placed to protect the chest tube. Aspirated fluid and air are recorded and generally diminish significantly or stop during the first 24 hours. If chest radiographs taken 24 to 48 hours postoperatively show no free air or fluid, the chest tube is removed. Activity is restricted to leash walking during the first 2 weeks after surgery and is gradually increased to normal during the next 4 weeks.

Suggested Readings

Aronsohn MG. Diaphragmatic advancement for defects of the caudal thoracic wall in the dog. Vet Surg 1984;13:26.
Bonath KA. Thoracic wall closure. In: Lipowitz AJ, Caywood DD, Newton CD, et al, eds. Complications in small animal surgery. Baltimore: Williams & Wilkins, 1996.
Brasmer TH. Thoracic wall reconstruction in dogs. J Am Vet Med Assoc 1971;159:1758.
Fevney DA, et al. Malignant neoplasia of canine ribs: clinical radiographic, and pathologic findings. J Am Vet Med Assoc 1982;180:927.

Surgical Management of Flail Chest

Dale E. Bjorling

Flail chest by definition is the fracture or dislocation, both proximal and distal, of two or more adjacent ribs. This condition creates an isolated segment of the thoracic wall that fails to move in concert with the rest of the thoracic wall. Because the affected area (flail segment) is no longer attached to the thoracic wall, it actually moves in a paradoxic manner relative to the thoracic wall (i.e., during inspiration, when the thoracic wall moves in an outward direction, the flail segment moves inward, and during expiration, the flail segment moves outward while the chest wall moves inward). Although flail chest is usually the result of a traumatic injury, structural or metabolic abnormalities, particularly in young or old animals, occasionally result in decreased stiffness of the ribs, allowing paradoxic movement of a segment of the chest wall after fracture or dislocation of only the proximal aspect of two or more adjacent ribs.

Injuries of the chest wall and lungs may not be detected initially in animals sustaining blunt trauma, and as many as 79% of dogs with reported skeletal injuries may have undetected thoracic trauma (1). The primary traumatic insult may damage the lungs, or contact with the fractured ends of the ribs may lacerate the lungs, resulting in persistent pneumothorax or hemothorax. Trauma that results in flail chest may also cause myocardial contusions, and animals should be monitored for development of traumatically induced cardiac arrhythmias.

For many years, it was assumed that paradoxic movement of the flail segment during the respiratory cycle decreased tidal volume, thereby impairing ventilation (2, 3). Experimental studies have demonstrated that flail segments involving several ribs have little effect on pulmonary function in dogs with normal or contused lungs (4). Normal animals compensate for limited abnormalities of the thoracic wall by flattening the diaphragm or taking deeper breaths to expand the normal chest wall further. The primary cause of respiratory dysfunction is damage of the lungs and underlying parenchyma (lacerations and pulmonary contusions), which occurs when the ribs are fractured (5).

A pulmonary contusion is analogous to a bruise, with disruption of the tissues and capillaries resulting in extravasation of blood and accumulation of fluid within the pulmonary parenchyma. Thoracic radiographs made within 1 to 2 hours of injury may not accurately reflect the severity of pulmonary damage, and radiographic signs of pulmonary contusion may be progressive for up to 36 hours after injury as hemorrhage and fluid accumulation within the lungs continues (6, 7). Pulmonary contusions commonly require 10 days or more to resolve, and the radiographic appearance may change little during this time (8). Pulmonary dysfunction associated with severe pulmonary contusions appears to be due to functional shunting of blood within the lungs, because blood flowing through the pulmonary capillaries within contused areas is exposed to alveoli that may be collapsed or filled with fluid, and the contusion reduces compliance of adjacent normal alveoli (9).

The effects of flail chest injury on respiratory function are cumulative. Although parenchymal injuries appear to be the primary determinant of the severity of respiratory dysfunction, paradoxic movement of the flail segment may contribute to decreased tidal volume, and pain associated with rib fractures or other injuries may cause animals with traumatically induced flail chest to breathe more shallowly. Accumulation of air and fluid within the pleural space may cause a further decrease in tidal volume.

Medical Treatment

Treatment of animals with flail chest injuries should be directed toward improving respiratory function and preventing continued injury. It may be necessary to place a thoracostomy tube to drain air and blood from the pleural space. Consideration should also be given to administration of supplemental oxygen by face mask, nasal catheter, or other means. However, administration of supplemental oxygen alone does not improve hypoxemia resulting from severe pulmonary contusions. Positive-pressure mechanical ventilation, possibly incorporating the use of positive end-expiratory pressure, may be required to ventilate animals with severe pulmonary contusions satisfactorily (10).

Aggressive fluid therapy may result in fluid accumulation within the lungs. This is most likely the result of decreased plasma oncotic pressure. Intravenous infusion of greater than 30 mL/kg of crystalloid fluids over the course of 1 hour increases the size of experimentally created pulmonary contusions in dogs (8, 11). Transfusions of plasma or whole blood help to maintain plasma oncotic pressure. Alternatively, dextrans or hetastarch may be used. The administration of methylprednisolone sodium succinate (30 mg/kg) within 30 minutes of injury may help to limit the size of pulmonary contusions (12). Investigators have suggested that diuretics should be given to remove excess water and to limit the size of contusions (8); however, diuretics may reduce total body fluid at a time when volume expansion is critical to resuscitate the animal.

Antibiotics should be given to animals with pulmonary contusions to minimize the potential for development of bacterial pneumonia. Antibiotics should initially be given intravenously to establish satisfactory tissue concentrations. This can be followed by oral administration. Prophylactic antibiotic treatment for pulmonary injuries should provide broad-spectrum antibacterial activity. A satisfactory combination is cefazolin (20 mg/kg three times daily) and gentamicin (2 to 4 mg/kg twice daily or 4 to 8 mg/kg once daily). Alternatively, cefatetin (30 mg/kg intravenously three times daily) may be used, but this drug is expensive in animals weighing more than 10 kg. Orally, the combination of amoxicillin and clavulanic acid (20 mg/kg three times daily) is usually effective.

Stabilization of Rib Fractures and Flail Chest

The decision to stabilize the flail segment is based on the following criteria: continued leakage of blood or air into the pleural space because of repeated trauma to the lungs by the jagged, displaced ends of fractured ribs; failure to respond to other supportive measures; pain associated with movement of the fractured ribs (pain may prevent the animal from generating an adequate tidal volume); and unacceptable cosmetic deformity.

Most rib fractures in dogs and cats do not require stabilization. As mentioned previously, stabilization is required when a gross deformity has occurred, when displacement of the fragments results in ongoing damage to the underlying viscera, or when displacement or instability of the fragments interferes with ventilation. Rib fractures may be stabilized by open fixation using pins and wires. This is often not a viable option in animals with flail chest. Alternatively, the ribs may be secured to an external frame or device by percutaneous placement of sutures around the ribs. This technique requires minimal or no sedation and works well in animals with flail chest. A frame or brace made of malleable rodding (13) or stiff plastic splinting material (14) used to construct splints may be contoured to the normal curvature of the thoracic wall. The bars or

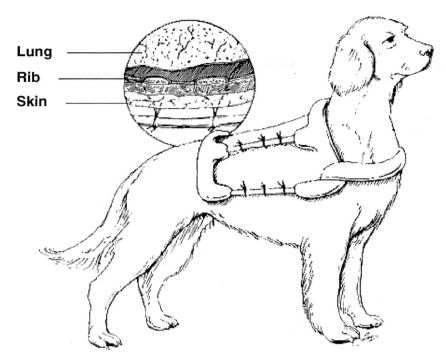

Lung

Rib

Skin

Fig. 24.3. Schematic illustration of application of external brace to stabilize flail chest. Sutures are passed around the proximal and distal aspects of ribs within the flail segment and are secured to the external brace. (From Bjorling DE. Management of thoracic trauma. In: Scherding RG, Birchard SJ, eds. Saunders manual of small animal practice. Philadelphia: WB Saunders, 1994:598.)

brace should pass over the dorsal and ventral aspect of the flail segment and should rest on the unaffected chest wall. At least two sutures are placed around the ribs of the flail segment both dorsally and ventrally and are tied to the frame to displace the flail segment in a lateral or outward direction (Fig. 24.3). Damage to the underlying lung tissue usually does not occur during passage of the needle around the rib because of the presence of pneumothorax. The potential for injury to the underlying lungs can also be minimized by grasping the ribs with towel forceps and retracting them laterally.

Alternatively, a single suture can be passed percutaneously around the midpoint of each rib of the flail segment and tied to a tongue depressor or piece of stiff plastic aligned along the dorsoventral axis of the ribs (15). Additional tongue depressors or plastic splints are placed beneath and perpendicular to the dorsal and ventral ends of the vertically oriented splints that have been attached to the ribs. Cotton padding is placed between the splints secured to the ribs and the horizontally oriented splints to draw the flail segment outward and to prevent oscillation of the flail segment during the respiratory cycle by creating a pivot point at the single suture passed around each rib. The advantage of this technique is that only one suture must be placed around each rib, and the materials required may be more readily available; however, either technique works satisfactorily.

The splint should remain in place for at least 3 weeks. Stabilization of rib fractures by application of a tight bandage should be avoided, because this displaces the ribs medially, resulting in continued damage to the underlying viscera and healing of the ribs in such a position that lung volume is permanently decreased.

References

1. Selcer BA, Buttrick M, Barstad R. The incidence of thoracic trauma in dogs with skeletal injury. J Small Anim Pract 1987;28:21–27.
2. Jones TB, Richardson EP. Traction on the sternum in the treatment of multiple fractured ribs. Surg Gynecol Obstet 1926;52:283–285.
3. Avery EE, Morch ET, Benson DW. Critically crushed chests: a new method of treatment with continuous mechanical hyperventilation to produce alkalotic apnea and internal pneumatic stabilization. J Thorac Surg 1956;32:291–311.
4. Craven KD, Oppenheimer L, Wood LDH. Effects of contusion and flail chest on pulmonary perfusion and oxygen exchange. J Appl Physiol 1979;47:729–737.
5. Schaal MA, Fischer RP, Perry JF. The unchanged mortality of flail chest injuries. J Trauma 1979;19:492–495.
6. Blair E, Topuzlu C, Ravis JH. Delayed or missed diagnosis in blunt chest trauma. J Trauma 1971;11:129–145.
7. Erickson DR, Shinozaki T, Beekman E, et al. Relationship of arterial blood gases and pulmonary radiographs to the degree of pulmonary damage in experimental pulmonary contusion. J Trauma 1971;11:689–694.
8. Trinkle JK, Furman RW, Hinshaw MA, et al. Pulmonary contusion: pathogenesis and effect of various resuscitative measures. Ann Thorac Surg 1973;16:568–573.
9. Oppenheimer L, Craven KD, Forkert L, et al. Pathophysiology of pulmonary contusion in dogs. J Appl Physiol 1979;47:718–728.

10. King LG, Hendricks JC. Positive pressure ventilation in dogs and cats: 41 cases (July 1990–January 1992). J Am Vet Med Assoc 1994:204:1045–1052.
11. Fulton RL, Peter ET. Physiologic effects of fluid therapy after pulmonary contusion. Am J Surg 1973;126:773–777.
12. Franz JL, Richardson JD, Grover FL, et al. Effect of methylprednisolone sodium succinate and experimental pulmonary contusion. J Thorac Cardiovasc Surg 1974;68:842–844.
13. Bjorling DE, Kolata RJ, DeNovo RC. Flail chest: review, clinical experience, and new method of stabilization. J Am Anim Hosp Assoc 1982;18:269–276.
14. Fossum TW. Thoracic wall and sternum: diseases, disruptions, and deformities. In: Bojrab M, ed. Disease mechanisms in small animal surgery. 2nd ed. Philadelphia: Lea & Febiger, 1993: 411–416.
15. McAnulty JF. A simplified method for stablization of flail chest injuries in small animals. J Am Anim Hosp Assoc 1995; 31:137–141.

Surgical Management of Pectus Excavatum

Theresa W. Fossum

Etiology

Pectus excavatum (PE) is a deformity of the sternum and costocartilages that results in a dorsal to ventral narrowing of the thorax. Pectus carinatum is a protrusion of the sternum that occurs much less frequently than PE. Synonyms include funnel chest, chondrosternal depression, chonechondrosternon, koilosternia, and trichterbrust.

The cause of the PE in animals is unknown. Theories proposed include shortening of the central tendon of the diaphragm, intrauterine pressure abnormalities, and congenital deficiency of the musculature in the cranial portion of the diaphragm. Abnormal respiratory gradients appear to play a role in the development of this disease in some animals because brachycephalic dogs are most commonly affected, many of which have concurrent hypoplastic tracheas. Pectus excavatum may be associated with "swimmer's syndrome," which is a poorly characterized disease of neonatal dogs in which the limbs tend to splay laterally, impairing ambulation. Abnormalities of the joints of the limbs and the long bones may also occur.

Patients with PE may have abnormalities of both respiratory and cardiovascular function. Circulatory disorders in animals with PE may be caused by abnormal cardiac positioning resulting in kinking of the large veins and disturbance of venous return, compression of the heart predisposing to arrhythmias (particularly the atrea), restriction of ventricular capacity, and decreased respiratory reserve. Cardiac abnormalities are also common (see later under differential diagnosis).

Diagnosis
Signalment

Pectus excavatum is a congenital abnormality in dogs and cats. In symptomatic animals, the onset of clinical signs is usually at birth, or shortly thereafter. PE may occur in any breed, but brachycephalic dogs appear to be predisposed to the condition. A sex predisposition has not been identified.

History

Many animals with PE are asymptomatic; however, the defect is often palpable, and this may prompt owners to seek veterinary care, despite lack of obvious clinical signs. Symptomatic animals may present for evaluation of exercise intolerance, weight loss, hyperpnea, recurrent pulmonary infections, cyanosis, vomiting, persistent and productive coughing, inappetence, or mild episodes of upper respiratory disease. A correlation between severity of clinical signs and severity of anatomic or physiologic abnormalities has not been observed.

Physical Examination Findings

The sternal deformity is usually palpable. Other physical findings may include cardiac murmurs and harsh lung sounds. Dyspnea is variable, but rapid, shallow respirations may be noted.

Radiography

Thoracic radiographs show abnormal elevation of the sternum in the caudal thorax. Objective assessment of the deformity may be determined by measuring the frontosagittal and vertebral indices on thoracic radiographs (Table 24.1). The frontosagittal index is calculated as the ratio of the width of the chest at the tenth thoracic vertebra, measured on a dorsoventral or ventrodorsal radiograph, and the distance between the center of the ventral surface of the tenth thoracic vertebra and the nearest point on the sternum (Fig. 24.4). The vertebral index is calculated as the ratio of the distance between the center of the dorsal surface of the selected vertebral body to the nearest point on the

Table 24.1.
Normal Frontosagittal and Vertebral Indices

	Frontosagittal	Vertebral
Nonbrachycephalic dogs	0.8–1.4	11.8–19.6
Brachycephalic dogs	1.0–1.5	12.5–16.5
Cats	0.7–1.3	12.6–18.8

(From Fossum TW, Boudrieau RJ, Hobson HP. Pectus excavatum in 8 dogs and 6 cats. J Am Anim Hosp Assoc 1989;25:595.)

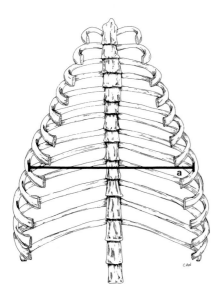 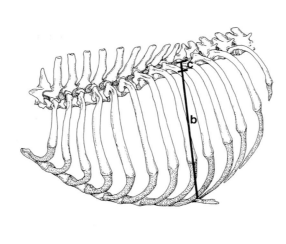

Fig. 24.4. Diagram of the thoracic skeleton. The frontosagittal index is the ratio between the width of the chest at the tenth thoracic vertebra (a) and the distance between the center of the ventral surface of the tenth thoracic vertebral body and the nearest point on the sternum (b). The vertebral index is the ratio between the distance from the center of the dorsal surface of the tenth vertebral body to the nearest point on the sternum (b+c) and the dorsoventral diameter of the vertebral body at the same level (c). (From Fossum TW, Boudrieau RJ, Hobson HP. Pectus excavatum in 8 dogs and 6 cats. J Am Anim Hosp Assoc 1989; 25:595.)

sternum and the dorsoventral diameter of the center of the same vertebral body (see Fig. 24.4). Investigators have proposed that the severity of PE be characterized as mild, moderate, or severe, based on the frontosagittal index and the vertebral index (Table 24.2). Such determination may aid in the objective assessment of improvement of thoracic diameters after surgical treatment.

Thoracic radiographs should be evaluated for the evidence of concurrent abnormalities (i.e., tracheal hypoplasia, cardiac abnormalities, pneumonia). Most animals with PE have abnormally positioned hearts that may appear enlarged radiographically; thus, true cardiac enlargement should always be distinguished from apparent enlargement resulting from abnormal heart position.

Differential Diagnosis

Diagnosis of pectus excavatum is straightforward; however, associated abnormalities may be more difficult to diagnose. Cardiac murmurs are common in patients with PE and appear to be associated with cardiac malpositioning. These murmurs often disappear after surgical correction of the defect or a change in the

patient's position. Systolic murmurs in some patients appear to be related to kinking of the pulmonary artery or to exaggeration of its normal vibrations because of its proximity to the chest wall. Animals with PE and innocent systolic murmurs must be differentiated from those that have underlying cardiac defects, such as pulmonic stenosis or atrial septal defects.

Medical Management

Animals with merely a "flat" chest may contour to a normal or near-normal configuration without surgical intervention. However, owners should be encouraged to perform medial-to-lateral compression of the chest regularly on these young animals. Animals with severe elevation of the sternum do not benefit from this technique or from splintage that simply provides medial-to-lateral compression and does not correct the malpositioned sternum. Other medical management includes treatment of respiratory tract infections and, if the animal is severely dyspneic, oxygen therapy.

Surgical Treatment

Application of an external splint to the ventral aspect of the thorax is the most common technique used to correct this defect in animals. Definitive treatment of PE using external splintage is possible because of the young age of affected patients at the time of diagnosis. The costal cartilages and sternum are pliable in these young animals, and the thorax can be reshaped by applying traction to the sternum using sutures placed around the sternum and through a rigid splint. Soft tissues that may be abnormal and play a role in the development of this deformity are probably stretched

Table 24.2.
Characterization of Pectus Excavatum (PE) in Dogs and Cats Based on Frontosagittal and Vertebral Indices

Severity of PE	Index Frontosagittal	Vertebral
Mild	≤2	>9
Moderate	2–3	6–8.99
Severe	>3	<6

(From Fossum TW, Boudrieau RJ, Hobson PH. Pectus excavatum in 8 dogs and 6 cats. J Am Anim Hosp Assoc 1989;25:595.)

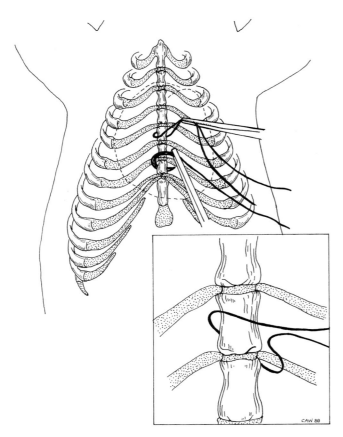

Fig. 24.5. Diagram showing placement of sutures around the sternum for correction of pectus excavatum. (From Fossum TW, Boudrieau RJ, Hobson HP, et al. Surgical correction of pectus excavatum using external splintage in two dogs and a cat. J Am Vet Med Assoc 1989;195:91.)

a small Steinmann pin. The holes are positioned so the distance between adjacent holes is slightly greater than the width of the sternum. The selected suture (see later) is passed around the sternum by maneuvering the needle blindly off the lateral edge of the sternum. Alternately, the needle is passed around the sternebra at a 45° angle to incorporate the costocartilage and possibly to decrease the chance of the suture pulling through the soft sternebral bone (Fig. 24.5). Sutures must be placed around the sternum and not subcutaneously. Additionally, sutures must be placed in the area of the greatest concavity. If the sutures are placed proximal to the area with the greatest depression, the sternum cannot be pulled into a normal position, resulting in less than optimal correction of the defect. The needle is kept as close to the dorsal aspect of the sternum as possible, to avoid piercing the heart or lungs. The suture ends are left long and are tagged. When all sutures have been placed, the ends are passed through the predrilled holes in the splint and are tied securely on its ventral aspect (Fig. 24.6). Two sutures may be placed and tied to themselves and then these sutures may be tied together, so the splint can be adjusted without replacement of sutures or the use of anesthesia.

or torn when the sternum is pulled ventrally. Whether surgical correction of the defect should be performed in asymptomatic patients with moderate or severe PE is unknown. Symptomatic patients that do not have associated cardiac abnormalities benefit from surgery.

Respiratory infections should be treated preoperatively. If the animal is severely dyspneic, oxygen should be provided by nasal insufflation or an oxygen cage until the surgical procedure is performed. Prophylactic antibiotic therapy may be given; however, antibiotics are unlikely to prevent skin infections around the splint. Development of intrathoracic infection associated with surgery is uncommon.

The patient is placed in dorsal recumbency and the ventral thorax is prepared for aseptic surgery. A rectangular piece of moldable splinting material is fashioned into a U-shape and is molded to fit the ventral aspect of the thorax. A small amount of adhesive padding is applied to the cranial border and inner surface of the splint, or alternately, the splint is padded with cast padding after it has been positioned. Two parallel rows of four to six holes are placed in the splint with

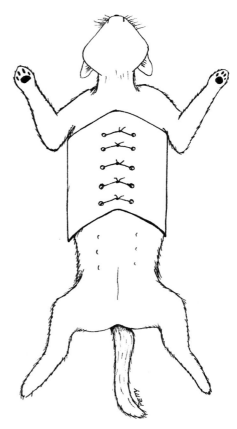

Fig. 24.6. Illustration showing the appearance of a splint in a cat with pectus excavatum.

A taper-point needle is recommended; if suture material with a large, swaged-on needle is not available, a large-eyed taper-point needle should be selected (to prevent bending and possible breakage as it is passed around the sternum). Large (i.e., 0 to 2), monofilament absorbable or nonabsorbable suture material is recommended (i.e., polydioxanone, polyglyconate, or nylon suture).

Postoperative Care and Assessment

The animal should be evaluated in the early postoperative period for intrathoracic hemorrhage because piercing of the heart, lung, or internal thoracic vessels is possible as the needle is passed around the sternum. Positioning the animal in dorsal recumbency, paying close attention to the phase of respiration, and keeping the needle as close to the sternum as possible help to prevent such complications. The splint should be left in place for 10 to 21 days. Suture abscesses, mild superficial dermatitis, and skin abrasions are common, but these are usually minor and heal quickly after splint removal. Adequate padding of the splint may help to prevent abrasions.

Prognosis

The prognosis is excellent for animals without underlying disease that undergo the operation at a young age. Older animals with a less pliable sternum may not respond as favorably to external splintage. Partial sternectomy may benefit such animals.

Suggested Readings

Boudrieau RJ, Fossum TW, Hartsfield SM, et al. Pectus excavatum in dogs and cats. Compend Contin Educ Pract Vet 1990;12:341.

Fossum TW, Boudrieau RJ, Hobson HP. Pectus excavatum in 8 dogs and 6 cats. J Am Anim Hosp Assoc 1989;25:595.

Fossum TW, Boudrieau RJ, Hobson HP, et al. Surgical correction of pectus excavatum using external splintage in two dogs and a cat. J Am Vet Med Assoc 1989;195:91.

Grenn HH, Lindo DE. Pectus excavatum (funnel chest) in a feline. Can Vet J 1968;9:279.

Pearson JL. Pectus excavatum in the dog. Vet Med Small Anim Clin 1973;68:125.

Shires PK, Waldon DR, Payne J. Pectus excavatum in three kittens. J Am Anim Hosp Assoc 1988;24:203.

Smallwood JE, Beaver BV. Congenital chondrosternal depression (pectus excavatum) in the cat. J Am Vet Radiol Soc 1977;18:141.

Soderstrom MJ, Gilson SD, Gulbas N. Fatal reexpansion pulmonary edema in a kitten following surgical correction of pectus excavatum. J Am Anim Hosp Assoc 1995;31:133.

— 25 —

KIDNEY

Nephrectomy

Eberhard Rosin

Nephrectomy may be indicated by the following unilateral conditions: 1) solitary renal cysts causing serious renal dysfunction; 2) hydronephrosis; 3) polycystic disease of the kidney complicated by pyelonephritis refractive to medical treatment; 4) infestation by *Dioctophyma renale* with severe degenerative changes; 5) neoplasms of the kidney if metastasis has not occurred; 6) traumatic destruction of most of the renal parenchyma; 7) avulsion of the renal pedicle or uncontrolled hemorrhage; and 8) abnormal kidney drained by an ectopic ureter. The diagnosis of these conditions and assessment of adequate function of the contralateral kidney are described elsewhere (1).

Nephrectomy is seldom performed when the architecture and vascular supply of the kidney are normal. In certain chronic pathologic states, the kidney is frequently enlarged and is extensively supplied by neovascularization. The normal renal artery and vein can be present or nonexistent. Surgical technique for nephrectomy in such instances is improvised by the veterinary surgeon and may approximate the dissection required to remove any abdominal mass. The operative technique described in the following paragraphs is based on the removal of a kidney in which the gross anatomic structure is recognizable.

Surgical Technique

The patient is anesthetized and is placed in dorsal recumbency. The abdomen is prepared for an aseptic surgical procedure. A midline abdominal incision is made from the xiphoid process through the umbilicus. The edges of the incision are protected with moist laparotomy pack, and a Balfour retractor is inserted.

The right kidney is exposed by lifting the descending portion of the duodenum and by positioning the other loops of intestine to the left of the mesoduodenum. The left kidney is similarly exposed by using the mesentery of the descending colon as a retractor to displace bowel loops to the right (Fig. 25.1). The viscera are covered with moist laparotomy packs.

To mobilize the kidney to be removed, first the peritoneum over the caudal pole of the kidney is grasped with tissue forceps and is incised with scissors. The surgeon inserts a finger into the opening and gently peels the peritoneum from the kidney. Occasionally, the peritoneum adheres firmly to the kidney surface at scattered points; these attachments are severed with scissors. Bleeding generated by this reflection of the peritoneum is controlled by electrocautery. Perirenal fat is reflected from the ventromedial surface of the renal hilus to expose the renal vein and ureter. The ureter is further mobilized by dissection through the retroperitoneum, to permit ligation as close to the urinary bladder as feasible. The ureter is divided between 2–0 absorbable ligatures (Fig. 25.2).

The kidney is lifted from its bed and is retracted medially to expose the perirenal fat on the dorsolateral surface of the renal hilus (see Fig. 25.2). Reflection of this fat exposes the renal artery. Care must be taken to avoid transection of *one or more branches* of the renal artery that may be present.

The exposed renal artery and vein are separated and are independently ligated with 3–0 suture material (Fig. 25.3). The artery and vein are transected distal to each ligature, and the kidney is removed. A separate suture ligature of 4–0 suture material is passed through the lumen of the renal artery and vein, distal

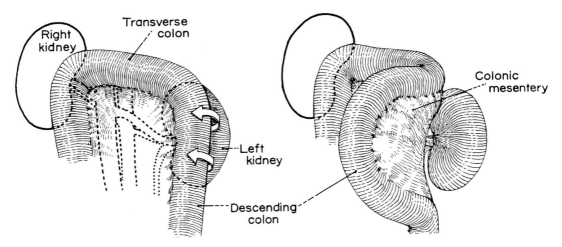

Fig. 25.1. The left kidney is exposed by using the mesentery of the descending colon as a retractor for the small intestine.

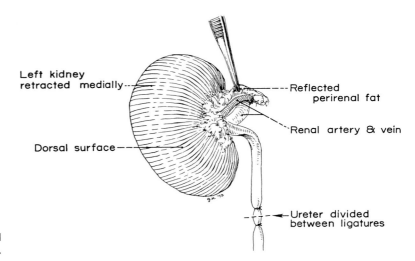

Fig. 25.2. Reflection of the perirenal fat on the dorsal lateral surface of the renal hilus exposes the renal artery.

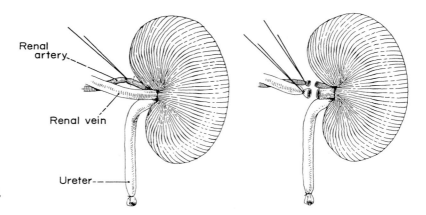

Fig. 25.3. The renal artery and vein are separated, ligated individually, and transected.

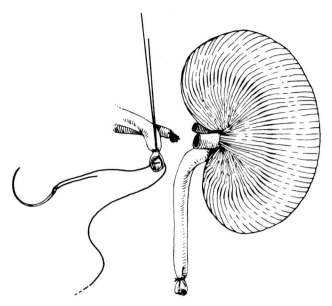

Fig. 25.4. A second ligature is passed through the lumen of the renal artery and vein distal to the first ligature.

to the first ligature, to transfix the distal ligature and to prevent retraction of the vessel from the ligature (Fig. 25.4).

The intestines are returned to normal position, the greater omentum is repositioned over the small intestine, and the abdomen is closed in a standard manner.

Reference

1. Osborne CA, Finco DR, eds. Canine and feline nephrology and urology. Baltimore: Williams & Wilkins, 1995.

Removal of Nephroliths

Andrew E. Kyles & Elizabeth Arnold Stone

Surgical removal of nephroliths is indicated in patients with obstruction of the renal pelvis, uncontrollable infection, enlargement of the calculus, or deterioration of renal function. Nephroliths may progressively destroy the renal parenchyma and may cause persistence of infection. Nephrectomy is indicated when the affected kidney is nonfunctional and the contralateral kidney is functional. Nephrotomy or pyelolithotomy is performed to remove nephroliths and to preserve remaining renal function. After removal of nephroliths, compensatory hypertrophy and improved renal function are possible, even in a diseased kidney.

In the dog and cat, the undilated renal pelvis is completely surrounded by renal parenchyma and is not accessible by pyelolithotomy. Thus, bisection nephrotomy is performed to remove nephroliths from a normal-sized renal pelvis. Nephrotomy is also indicated to examine the renal pelvis for polyps, tumors, or causes of renal hematuria. Bisection nephrotomy has been reported to reduce renal function in the operated kidney temporarily by 30 to 50% (1, 2). Pyelolithotomy can be used to remove nephroliths from a dilated renal pelvis. The dilated renal pelvis protrudes beyond the renal parenchyma, permitting direct incision into the relatively avascular renal pelvis. Pyelolithotomy causes less parenchymal damage and hemorrhage than bisection nephrotomy.

Bilateral nephroliths can be removed in one or two operations. The safest approach is to allow the patient 4 to 6 weeks to recover from the first surgical procedure before operating on the second kidney. However, in a nonazotemic animal, if the expense of two operations discourages an owner from pursuing treatment, the nephroliths can be removed from both kidneys during one surgical procedure.

Preoperative Management

Renal function is evaluated preoperatively using blood urea nitrogen and serum creatinine concentrations. In a nonazotemic dog, 24-hour endogenous creatinine clearance or subcutaneous exogenous creatinine clearance can be used to measure glomerular filtration rate (GFR) of the entire renal mass. Renal scintigraphy using [99m]technetium dimercaptosuccinic acid can be used to determine single kidney GFR and the relative contribution of each kidney.

Plain and contrast radiographs and ultrasonographic examination are used to determine the number and position of all calculi in the urinary tract and to demonstrate any obstruction of the urinary tract.

Urine is collected by cystocentesis, and bacteriologic culture is used to diagnose urinary tract infection. Antibiotic therapy, based on antimicrobial sensitivity testing, is initiated before surgery to establish adequate parenchymal and urine antibiotic concentrations.

Fluid and electrolyte imbalances are corrected before anesthesia is induced. A urinary catheter connected to a closed collection system is used to monitor urine output. Osmotic diuresis is initiated preoperatively to increase GFR, renal blood flow, and urine output and to help preserve renal function during surgery. An infusion of mannitol (0.25 to 0.5 g/kg intravenously) is administered as a 20% solution over 3 to 5 minutes. Once diuresis is established, a maintenance infusion (5 to 10% mannitol in a balanced electrolyte solution) can be continued for 12 to 24 hours.

Surgical Techniques

Bisection Nephrotomy

The kidney can be approached with either a midline abdominal incision or a paracostal incision. A midline laparotomy permits examination of both kidneys, ureters, and the urinary bladder. After a midline incision, the peritoneum overlying the cranial pole of the affected kidney is incised. The cranial pole is elevated, and additional peritoneal and fascial attachments are incised as needed to expose the renal vessels. Complete mobilization of the kidney is not usually necessary, and the caudal pole can remain within its peritoneal covering. A paracostal incision is used if only one kidney requires surgery and abdominal exploration is unnecessary. The kidney is exposed without entering the peritoneal cavity, and the cranial pole is elevated from the incision using umbilical tape.

A moist gauze sponge is used to remove the fat gently around the vessels. The renal artery is located craniodorsal to the vein. A small mosquito hemostat or right-angled forceps should be used to isolate the renal artery. A vascular clamp or tourniquet is placed on the renal artery. Occlusion of the renal artery, and not the renal vein, allows venous drainage of the kidney and increases the pliability of the kidney. Alternatively, the surgical assistant can manually occlude the renal vessels and immobilize the kidney. Hemostats should not be used for temporary vascular occlusion as they damage the vessel. Double or triple arteries are reported in 12% of left and 0.5% of right renal arteries (3, 4) and should be clamped separately. In addition, the renal artery divides into dorsal and ventral branches at varying distances from the aorta and these branches may require separate clamping. The duration

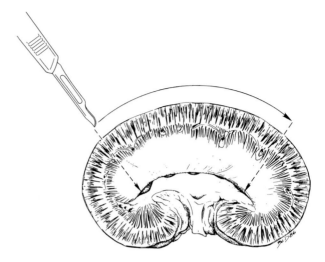

Fig. 25.6. Dog kidney sectioned longitudinally through both renal poles and hilus. The nephrotomy incision is made over the renal pelvis and should not extend over the cortical areas of the cranial and caudal poles of the kidney. (From Stone EA. Canine nephrotomy. Compend Contin Educ Pract Vet 1987;9:883.)

of ischemia in the normothermic kidney should not exceed 20 minutes (5).

The kidney is isolated with moistened laparotomy sponges and immobilized between the thumb and forefinger. The renal capsule is incised sharply with a scalpel on midline for about two thirds of the length of the kidney (Fig. 25.5). Extending the incision into the cranial and caudal poles does not increase exposure, but does increase parenchymal damage and therefore should be avoided (Fig. 25.6). The renal parenchyma is bluntly separated with a scalpel handle or blunt osteotome (see Fig. 25.5). Blunt separation is preferable to sharp incision because it reduces the damage to small blood vessels and the renal hilus. The cut edges are retracted with hemostats. Arcuate or interlobar vessels within the incision are ligated and severed (Fig. 25.7).

Large calculi are removed from the renal pelvis with forceps, with care taken not to fragment the calculi. Urine or tissue can be taken for bacteriologic culture. Each renal diverticulum should be systematically explored with small mosquito forceps and flushed with warm saline using a small (3.5-French gauge) soft catheter and syringe (Fig. 25.8). The catheter is passed down the ureter to check for obstruction and to flush small fragments through the ureter.

The two sides of the incision are apposed with digital pressure from the thumb and forefinger, while a synthetic absorbable suture material is placed in a simple continuous suture pattern in the renal capsule and a small amount of renal parenchyma. Monofilament suture is less likely to tear tissue. Mattress sutures through the renal parenchyma are unnecessary and

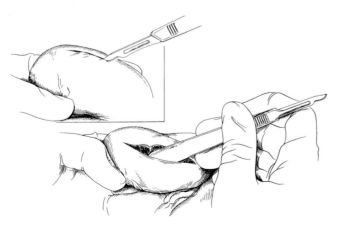

Fig. 25.5. Nephrotomy incision. The renal capsule is incised sharply with a scalpel blade (*inset*). The renal parenchyma is then separated bluntly with a scalpel handle or blunt osteotome. (From Stone EA. Canine nephrotomy. Compend Contin Educ Pract Vet 1987;9:883.)

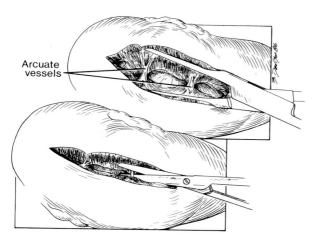

Fig. 25.7. Exposure of the renal parenchyma after nephrotomy incision. The cut edges of the kidney are retracted with forceps *(top)*. Arcuate and interlobar vessels within the incision are ligated and are severed with scissors *(bottom)*. (From Stone EA. Canine nephrotomy. Compend Contin Educ Pract Vet 1987;9:883.)

cause additional destruction of nephrons. The vascular clamp or tourniquet is removed, and the source of any hemorrhage from the kidney is identified. A bleeding collateral or capsular vessel can be controlled with ligation, or additional capsular sutures can be placed. Parenchymal bleeding can usually be controlled by digital compression of the kidney. Occasionally, interlobar arterial bleeding may require reclamping of the renal

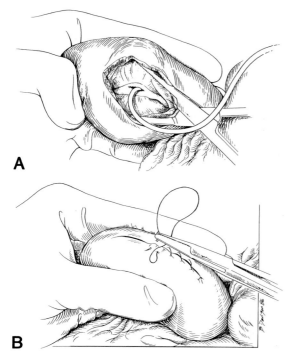

Fig. 25.8. **A.** After removal of the calculi, a 3.5-French gauge soft catheter is passed down the ureter. **B.** The renal parenchyma is sutured with a simple continuous suture pattern. (From Stone EA. Canine nephrotomy. Compend Contin Educ Pract Vet 1987;9:883.)

artery and digital compression of the kidney for an additional 5 to 10 minutes.

The kidney is returned to its original position. Care is taken to ensure that the kidney has not been rotated through 180°. If the kidney is excessively mobile, tacking sutures should be placed between the renal capsule and the abdominal wall to prevent rotation and possible strangulation of the renal vein postoperatively. Abdominal closure is routine.

Pyelolithotomy

Pyelolithotomy can be performed from a midline or paracostal incision. With a midline laparotomy, the ventral aspect of the renal hilus is visible. The ventral aspect of the renal pelvis is, however, obscured by the renal vessels (Fig. 25.9**A**). Therefore, the kidney is mobilized by incising the overlying peritoneum and rotating the kidney toward midline to expose the dorsal surface of the renal pelvis. From a paracostal incision, the kidney is retracted ventrally, with umbilical tape, to expose the dorsal surface of the renal pelvis. A moist gauze sponge is used gently to remove the fat and to expose the dilated renal pelvis. The surgeon should ensure that the renal pelvis and proximal ureter are sufficiently dilated to allow removal of the nephrolith. If it is not possible to remove the calculus without tearing the parenchyma or fragmenting the calculus, a bisection nephrotomy should be performed.

The dilated renal pelvis and proximal ureter are incised longitudinally (Fig. 25.9**B**). Occlusion of the renal artery is not necessary because the pelvis is relatively avascular. The nephrolith is gently removed with forceps (Fig. 25.9**C**), and the renal diverticula and renal pelvis are flushed with warm saline using a small (3.5-French gauge) soft catheter and syringe (Fig. 25.9**D**). The catheter is passed into the ureter, and the ureter is flushed (Fig. 25.9**E**). The pyelotomy incision is closed with 5–0 synthetic absorbable suture in a simple continuous pattern. Retention of the ureteral catheter initially assists the surgeon in beginning the closure (Fig. 25.9**F** and **G**). An attempt should be made to avoid placing the suture material into the lumen of the renal pelvis and ureter. However, unless the wall of the pelvis and ureter is thickened, it is usually necessary to penetrate the lumen to obtain an adequate seal. Magnification, in the form of optical loupes or an operating microscope, aids in the accuracy of closure. Tacking sutures should be placed between the renal capsule and the abdominal wall to prevent rotation of the kidney in the early postoperative period.

Postoperative Care

Intravenous fluid therapy is continued until the patient can maintain hydration. Urination should be

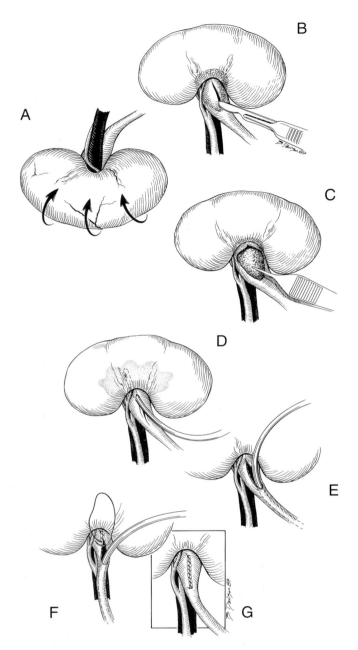

Fig. 25.9. Pyelolithotomy. **A.** The right kidney from a midline incision. The renal vessels lie ventral to the ureter. **B.** The kidney is reflected medially to expose the dorsolateral surface of the renal pelvis. A longitudinal incision is made in the dilated renal pelvis and proximal ureter. **C.** The calculus is gently removed with forceps. **D.** A small catheter is used to flush the renal pelvis and diverticuli. **E.** Catheter is passed down the ureter to check for ureteral obstruction. **F.** Catheter is left in place as the simple continuous closure is started. **G.** Complete closure. (From Stone EA, Barsanti JA. Surgical therapy for urolithiasis. In: Stone EA, Barsanti JA, eds. Urologic surgery of the dog and cat. Philadelphia: Lea & Febiger, 1992:174.)

monitored, and if one has any doubt about urine production, a urine catheter and closed urine collection system should be used to monitor urine output. Postoperative radiographic or ultrasonographic examination is performed to document the removal of all calculi. The calculi are submitted for quantitative mineral analysis, and appropriate medical management is initiated to help prevent recurrence. Antibiotic therapy, based on the results of bacteriologic culture and antimicrobial sensitivity testing, is continued for 3 to 4 weeks postoperatively. One week after completion of antibiotic therapy, the urine culture should be repeated. Occasionally, long-term antibiotic therapy may be needed to suppress bacterial growth in a damaged kidney.

References

1. Fitzpatrick JM, et al. Intrarenal access: effects on renal function and morphology. Br J Urol 1980;52:409.
2. Gahring DR, et al. Comparative renal function studies of nephrotomy closure with and without sutures in dogs. J Am Vet Med Assoc 1977;171:537.
3. Reis RH, Tepe P. Variations in the pattern of renal vessels and their relation to the type of posterior vena cava in the dog (*Canis familiaris*). Am J Anat 1956;99:1.
4. Shively MJ. Origin and branching of renal arteries in the dog. J Am Vet Med Assoc 1978;173:986.
5. Selkurt EE. The changes in renal clearance following complete ischemia of the kidney. Am J Phys 1945;144:395.

Suggested Readings

Greenwood KM, Rawlings CA. Removal of canine renal calculi by pyelolithotomy. Vet Surg 1981;10:12.
Stone EA, Barsanti JA. Surgical therapy for urolithiasis. In: Stone EA, Barsanti JA, eds. Urologic surgery of the dog and cat. Philadelphia: Lea & Febiger, 1992:174.

Renal Transplantation

Clare R. Gregory

Three major factors have led to the successful performance of renal transplantation in veterinary practice: 1) the introduction of new and effective immunosuppressive agents; 2) a better understanding of the immune response to foreign organs and tissue (rejection); and 3) the development of microsurgical techniques. The introduction of the immunosuppressive agent cyclosporine started a new era in successful immunotherapy for organ transplantation in cats (1–3).

The recognition of foreign tissue antigens by sensitized cells or antibodies marks the beginning of the active effort of rejection by the recipient's immune system. The primary mechanism of destruction is by generation of T lymphocytes that are cytotoxic for the allograft. Graft cell lysis is accomplished through the direct action of T-cytotoxic cells and by the activation of cascading enzyme systems, including the complement, clotting, and probably the kinin pathways. Other cellular mediators, such as B lymphocytes, plasma cells, macrophages, platelets, and polymorphonuclear leukocytes, play both direct and indirect roles in allograft rejection (4).

Three overlapping "types" of organ rejection are recognized clinically (4). Hyperacute rejection is an accelerated form of rejection associated with preformed circulatory antibody in the serum of the recipient that reacts with donor cells, particularly the endothelium of vessel walls. Polymorphonuclear leukocytes line the capillary walls, and most capillaries and arterioles are blocked by microthrombi, resulting in tissue necrosis. In hyperacute rejection, the recipient has been sensitized to the allograft antigens by previous blood transfusions, pregnancy, or transplantation. Fortunately, I have not experienced this type of rejection in a clinical patient (1). Most recipients have not borne litters or received a transplanted organ.

Acute rejection occurs typically 7 to 21 days after transplantation or when effective immunosuppression is terminated. Pathologic studies of the rejected organ reveal a predominant pattern of mononuclear leukocyte infiltration in the tissue (4). Chronic rejection is characterized by gradual loss of organ function over months to years, often without any clear-cut clinical rejection episode.

Without the use of immunosuppressive agents, matching the donor and recipient for similar or identical cell surface histocompatibility antigens prolongs allograft survival (4). Approximately half of the genetic information that codes for cell surface histocompatibility antigens is inherited from each parent. Therefore, siblings may be matched (25%), partially matched (50%), or mismatched (25%). For canine transplant recipients, therefore, siblings and parents constitute the best source of donor organs, but many are incompatible. If related canine organ donors can be found, an estimate of histocompatibility between the donor and recipient can be made using a microcytotoxicity assay or a mixed lymphocyte response assay, and by indirect DNA typing (4). Although these tests are performed only at major hospitals or university laboratories, blood samples can be shipped, using special handling techniques, over long distances.

Initially, investigators hoped that the immunosuppressive effects of cyclosporine would allow organ transplantation across major histocompatibility barriers, that is, between unrelated canine pairs. However, I performed renal allograft transplantation on three dogs using unrelated donors. Cyclosporine and pred-

nisolone were used to immunosuppress the host immune response. The average survival time before loss of the grafts to rejection was approximately 70 days (5). Combination daily and alternate-day treatment using cyclosporine and azathioprine has been studied in dogs receiving kidneys from unrelated donors. Seventy-seven percent of the dogs survived less than 275 days (6). Combination cyclosporine and azathioprine does provide excellent immunosuppression for canine recipients of matched renal allografts. Other combination therapies using antilymphocyte sera, donor-specific bone marrow transfusions, cyclosporine, and azathioprine are under investigation for canine recipients of a nonmatched renal allograft. A new immunosuppressive agent, leflunomide, when combined with cyclosporine, appears to prevent renal allograft rejection in nonmatched dogs. Successful research trials using this combination have stimulated clinical trials (7).

Using cyclosporine and prednisolone as immunosuppressant agents, cats tolerate renal allografts from unrelated donors (1). Renal allograft rejection has occurred in cats receiving cyclosporine under the following circumstances: 1) clients did not administer the correct dose or adequate dose of the drug; 2) the cat had concurrent lymphocytic or plasmacytic bowel disease; and 3) the cat became infected with, or expressed a latent infection with, the feline leukemia virus.

Clinical Renal Transplantation in the Cat

Selection of a Recipient

Renal transplantation is one method of treatment for renal insufficiency (1, 2). It cannot be regarded as an emergency treatment or "last-ditch" effort to save the life of a critically ill, malnourished patient. Surgical intervention does not replace failed medical management.

I consider body weight an important indication of the status of the renal transplant candidate. If a cat has been in compensated renal failure and starts to lose body weight, or if it presents in renal failure with a history of chronic weight loss, renal transplantation should be considered as an option before further weight loss occurs. My previous attempts to alter the course of physical deterioration resulting from decompensated renal failure by enteral or parenteral alimentation before renal transplantation failed. Age, plasma creatinine, blood urea nitrogen, and other clinical pathologic assessments of renal function cannot in themselves enable one to select a suitable patient for transplantation. Animals in poor physical condition or in which standard methods of medical therapy have failed should not be considered good candidates for renal transplantation.

Candidates for renal transplantation should be free of bacterial urinary tract infection (UTI). If the candidate has had several negative urine cultures but has a past history of UTI, a renal biopsy should be considered. In my experience, dogs or cats with a previous history of UTI become bacteriuric after renal transplantation and immunosuppression. Bacterial UTIs in the transplant recipient cause direct morbidity and mortality because of the infection itself, and these infections may also activate the rejection process. If the history of the patient is uncertain, cyclosporine can be administered for 2 or 3 weeks before renal transplantation. Urinalysis with bacterial culture can then be performed.

Feline candidates for renal transplantation should be free of feline leukemia virus infection and lymphocytic, plasmacytic enterocolitis. Both diseases in the cat appear to stimulate T-cell responses and stimulate a rejection response despite cyclosporine therapy. Renal insufficiency can also produce systemic hypertension in the feline patient leading to congestive heart failure. Cats in renal failure often have systolic murmurs secondary to anemia that may not represent significant cardiac disease. Cardiac enlargement determined by ultrasonographic examination, gallop rhythms, and electrocardiographic abnormalities are all indications to decline a candidate for renal transplantation.

The feline renal donor–recipient pair does not have to be related or tissue matched, but these animals must be blood cross matched. The antigens present on red blood cells are also found on the endothelium of the graft blood vessels. Preformed antibodies to these antigens cause clotting of the graft vessels and infarcts of the organ at the time of surgery.

The feline renal recipient must also be blood cross matched to 2 to 3 units of blood or blood donor cats. The primary reason for this is the anemia that accompanies chronic renal failure. After preoperative rehydration of a patient, packed red blood cell volumes may fall as low as 12 to 15%. From 180 to 250 mL of whole blood may be required to attain a packed red blood cell volume of 30% in the renal recipient preoperatively. In addition, in my experience, some cats in chronic renal failure are not transfusable; that is, all cross-match assays show agglutination of donor red cells even though they share the same blood type. This consideration is important if the transplant recipient is traveling a great distance to the transplant clinic. Cross matching should be done locally to ensure that transfusions can be given before the surgical procedure.

Selection of a Donor

The renal donor should be in excellent health and should have no evidence of renal insufficiency based on clinical pathologic testing, complete blood count, serum chemistry panel, and urinalysis. Intravenous pyelography is performed to ensure that the donor has two, normally shaped, well-vascularized kidneys. The feline donor should be free of feline leukemia virus infection and should be blood cross-match compatible with the recipient. The donor cat should be as large as possible, and not more than 0.5 kg smaller than the recipient. The renal donor should have a normal life expectancy after unilateral nephrectomy (8).

Preoperative Preparation of the Recipient

Once a candidate for renal transplantation is identified, if the hematocrit is below 30%, the administration of erythropoietin should be started at least 3 to 4 weeks before the surgical procedure. Erythropoietin stimulates the hematopoietic stem cells in the bone marrow to produce red blood cells. The dose is 100 IU subcutaneously every third day until the target hematocrit is achieved, approximately 35% (9). Then the dose is decreased to once or twice a week, as needed to keep the hematocrit between 35 and 40%. Increasing the hematocrit by the use of erythropoietin negates the need for blood transfusions and makes the patient a better anesthetic risk. Moreover, once the hematocrit returns to normal, most cats have an increased appetite, and chronic weight loss usually subsides. Elevation of the hematocrit should be achieved gradually, however, because a rapid increase in hematocrit may produce systemic hypertension and other complications.

If necessary, gastrostomy tubes should be placed to aid in feeding the transplant candidate. Again, supplemental feedings should begin as soon as possible before the surgical procedure is scheduled.

Before the operation, the renal recipient is given balanced electrolyte solutions subcutaneously or intravenously at one and one-half times to twice the daily maintenance requirements. Whole blood transfusions are administered, if needed, until a packed red cell volume of 30% is achieved. Twenty-four to 48 hours before the surgical procedure, cyclosporine oral solution is administered at a dose of 5 mg/kg every 12 hours. The cyclosporine oral solution should be placed in gelatin capsules before administration. Capsule sizes 0 or 1 work well for most cats. Cyclosporine oral solution has an unpleasant taste that causes some cats to salivate profusely, resulting in partial loss of the dose (1).

The morning of the operation, a blood sample is taken from the recipient 12 hours after the last oral dose of cyclosporine. This sample gives a 12-hour trough blood level. I follow whole blood levels of cyclosporine assayed by high-pressure liquid chromatography. In cats, a level of 500 ng/mL is maintained for the first 30 to 180 postoperative days, reducing to 350 ng/mL by 3 months after transplantation. Prednisolone, 0.25 mg/kg per 12 hours orally, is also started the morning of surgery and is reduced to 0.25 mg/kg per 24 hours by 1 month postoperatively.

Surgical Technique

If possible, two teams perform renal transplantation; one team harvests the donor kidney and closes the abdominal wound, and one team prepares the recipient vessels and receives the kidney. The two-team approach minimizes the warm ischemia time of the donor kidney, which should be kept to less than 60 minutes. I have not used perfusion solutions or ice baths to maintain the kidney before revascularization.

Anesthesia protocols vary with each patient. In general, the recipient receives atropine (0.03 mg/kg) and oxymorphone (0.05 mg/kg) subcutaneously before induction. Anesthesia in the cat is induced by mask or box, and it is maintained using isoflurane inhalant anesthesia and oxygen. During the procedure, balanced electrolyte solutions and whole blood are administered intravenously. Systemic arterial pressure is monitored by direct arterial catheterization or by indirect measurement using Doppler ultrasonography. If arterial catheterization is used, the hind limb should not be used to measure systemic arterial pressure. If the iliac vessels selected for transplantation are on the same side as the rear leg used for arterial catheterization, there will be interference with collateral perfusion of the leg postoperatively. A large, 18- to 20-gauge catheter is placed in a jugular vein and is sutured in place. The jugular catheter is used to collect blood samples postoperatively; this greatly reduces the stress of repeated venipuncture.

Both cats receive broad-spectrum antibiotics administered intravenously just before the surgical procedure. During the anesthetic induction and preparation for surgery, the recipient must be kept as warm as possible. Heating pads are placed over the recipient whenever possible.

The donor nephrectomy is performed through a ventral midline celiotomy (Fig. 25.10). Magnifying loops providing 2 to 3× magnification are recommended for the vascular dissection. The vascular pedicle of the donor kidney can contain only one artery. Renal arteries may bifurcate close to the aorta. A length of 0.5 cm or more is required for arterial anastomosis. If two or more veins are present, the largest is saved for venous anastomosis. The vascular pedicle should contain the longest vein possible, so the left kidney is explored first.

Once the kidney to be harvested is selected, the recipient team should be informed so they can prepare the recipient vessels. For ease of anastomosis, a left

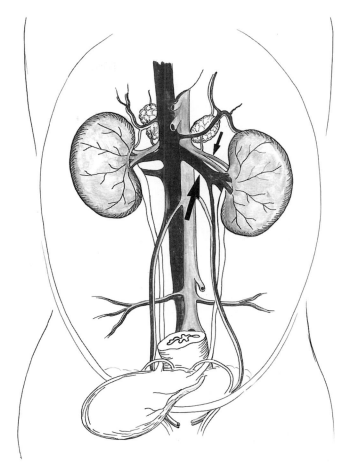

Fig. 25.10. Normal renal anatomic structures of a cat used as a donor for renal transplantation. As it joins the vena cava, the renal vein (*large arrow*) lies ventral to the renal artery. The gonadal veins are ligated. The left renal artery (*small arrow*) often bifurcates close to the aorta, making it unsuitable for transplantation. (From Gregory C, Gourley IM, Kochin EJ, et al. Renal transplantation for treatment of end stage renal failure in cats. J Am Vet Med Assoc 1992;201:285–291.)

donor kidney is placed in the right iliac fossa of the recipient, and vice versa. If necessary, a donor kidney can be placed in the ipsilateral iliac fossa of the recipient; however, the arterial anastomosis is more difficult to perform. The donor renal artery and vein must be cleaned of as much fat and adventitia as possible. The large fat pad in the renal pelvis should be removed, being careful not to damage the ureter. Removal of the fat and adventitia from the vessels before nephrectomy reduces warm ischemia time. The ureter is isolated to the bladder.

Donor nephrectomy is performed when the recipient is prepared to receive the kidney. Fifteen to 20 minutes before nephrectomy, mannitol (1 to 2 g/kg) is administered intravenously to the donor cat. Mannitol significantly reduces the incidence and duration of acute tubular necrosis associated with warm ischemia.

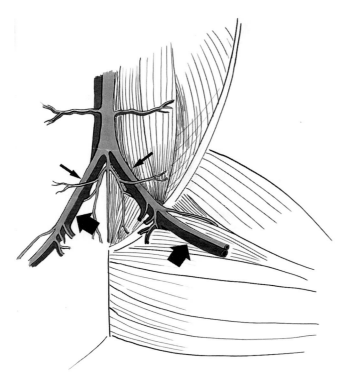

Fig. 25.11. Normal anatomic features of the external iliac and femoral arteries (*small arrows*) and veins (*large arrows*) of the cat. For ease of anastomosis, a right donor kidney is placed in the left iliac fossa, and vice versa. (From Gregory C, Gourley IM, Kochin EJ, et al. Renal transplantation for treatment of end stage renal failure in cats. J Am Vet Med Assoc 1992;201:285–291.)

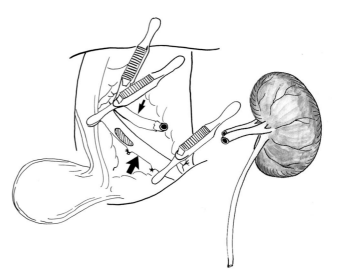

Fig. 25.12. Preparation of the left external iliac vessels for renal transplantation. The renal artery is anastomosed from end to end with the external iliac artery (*small arrow*). The renal vein is anastomosed from end to side with the external iliac vein (*large arrow*). Between the occluding clamps, the external iliac vein may have one or more tributary veins that must be ligated. A "window" is created in the external iliac vein that is slightly larger than the renal vein. (From Gregory C, Gourley IM, Kochin EJ, et al. Renal transplantation for treatment of end stage renal failure in cats. J Am Vet Med Assoc 1992;201:285–291.)

Anastomosis of the renal vessels and the ureter in the small dog and cat requires 3 to 10× magnification. High magnification is necessary to anastomose the ureter to the bladder. The chosen iliac fossa is prepared for end-to-end anastomosis of the renal artery to the iliac artery and end-to-side anastomosis of the renal vein to the iliac vein (Fig. 25.11). The iliac artery is isolated, and a bulldog or other vascular clamp is used to occlude it near the aortic bifurcation. The iliac artery is then ligated distally, near the femoral ring, and is severed. The free length of the artery is flushed clean of blood using heparinized saline solution. The end of the artery is gently dilated, and the adventitia is ex-

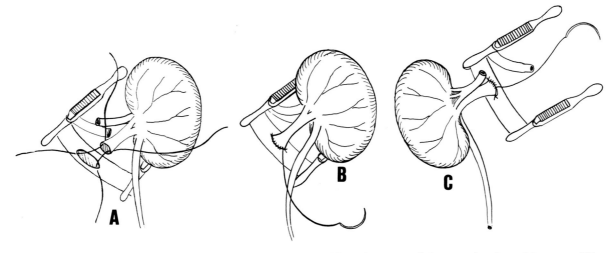

Fig. 25.13. Anastomosis of the renal vein to the external iliac vein. After placement of the cranial and caudal sutures (**A**), a simple continuous suture pattern is used on each side of the vessel (**B** and **C**). Careful attention is needed to avoid including the opposite wall in the suture. (From Gregory C, Gourley IM, Kochin EJ, et al. Renal transplantation for treatment of end stage renal failure in cats. J Am Vet Med Assoc 1992;201:285–291.)

cised from the proximal 0.25 to 1 mm (Fig. 25.12). The iliac vein lies deep to the artery in fat and adventitia (see Fig. 25.11). It is isolated over the same area as the artery, gaining as much free length as possible. The iliac vein has multiple tributary veins in this region that must be ligated. Careful inspection dorsal and caudal to the vein reveals these branches. Once the tributary veins have been ligated, two vascular clamps are placed on the iliac vein as far apart as possible. The first is placed distally, and the second proximately. A section of the wall is excised from the iliac vein that is slightly larger than the diameter of the donor renal vein. The surgeon must create a defect in the vein wall and not just a slit (see Fig. 25.12). The vein is flushed clean of blood using heparinized saline solution.

Two 7–0 sutures of silk are placed at each end of the defect in the vein wall. Each suture is subsequently placed at the cranial or caudal aspect of the renal vein and is tied. The renal vein is then anastomosed to the iliac vein using a simple continuous pattern on both the medial and lateral sides of the vessels (Fig. 25.13).

On completion of the venous anastomosis, the renal artery and iliac artery are isolated near the midline of the recipient. The arteries are anastomosed using 8–0 nylon in a simple interrupted pattern (Figs. 25.14 and 25.15). Once the arterial anastomosis is complete, the vascular clamps are removed from the vein and then from the artery. Some hemorrhage is expected, can be controlled with light pressure, and should stop within a few minutes. Large defects in the arterial anastomosis must be controlled by placement of additional sutures.

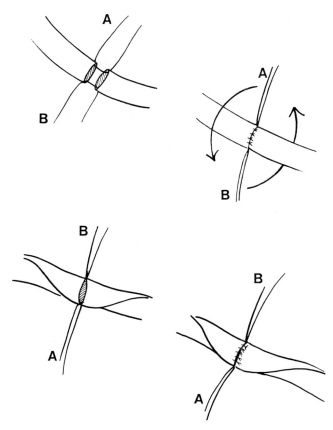

Fig. 25.15. After the front walls of the arteries have been sutured (**A** and **B**), they are turned 180° (**C**), and the back walls are sutured (**D**). All occluding clamps are released after the arterial anastomosis; venous followed by arterial. (From Gregory C, Gourley IM, Kochin EJ, et al. Renal transplantation for treatment of end stage renal failure in cats. J Am Vet Med Assoc 1992;201:285–291.)

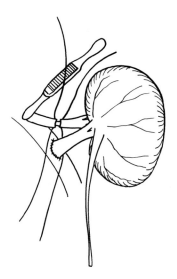

Fig. 25.14. Anastomosis of the renal artery to the external iliac artery. Simple interrupted sutures placed cranially and caudally are used to facilitate suture placement (vascular clamps occluding the iliac vein have been omitted for clarity). (From Gregory C, Gourley IM, Kochin EJ, et al. Renal transplantation for treatment of end stage renal failure in cats. J Am Vet Med Assoc 1992;201:285–291.)

Once all hemorrhage is controlled, the recipient receives mannitol (1 to 2 g/kg) intravenously.

Ureteroneocystostomy is then performed (10). A cystotomy incision is performed through the ventral wall of the bladder. The ureter is tunneled through the dorsal bladder wall using fine mosquito vascular forceps (Fig. 25.16). The crushed end of the ureter is excised, and the periureteral fat is removed from the distal 1 cm. The ureteral artery is isolated and ligated if possible. Fine scissors are used to make a 0.75-cm longitudinal cut in the ureter (Fig. 25.17). The cut ureteral mucosa is then sutured to the torn bladder mucosa using simple interrupted sutures of 8–0 nylon (Fig. 25.18). The first stitch is placed from the proximal end of the ureteral incision to the adjacent bladder mucosa. The remaining sutures serve to fan out the ureteral mucosa. The ureter should be easily catheterized after the sutures are tied.

Unless the patient has evidence of bacterial nephritis or extremely large polycystic kidneys, I do not remove the recipient's native kidneys at the time of transplantation. These kidneys are available to provide

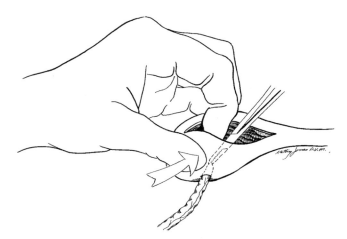

Fig. 25.16. A cystotomy is performed on the ventral surface of the bladder. The ureter is tunneled directly through the bladder wall, and using the thumb and index finger, the bladder is everted so the interior of the dorsal wall becomes convex. (From Gregory C, Lirtzman RA, Kochin EJ, et al. A mucosal apposition technique for ureteroneocystostomy after renal transplantation in cats. Vet Surg 1996;25:13–17.)

some support if the transplanted organ should fail and can be removed at a later date if indicated.

If not already in place, a gastrostomy tube is placed to supplement feeding and to give medications to fractious patients. Finally, to prevent rotation around the vascular pedicle, the transplanted kidney is fixed to the lateral body wall with two mattress sutures using 3–0 polypropylene suture material. The sutures should just penetrate the renal capsule and should be placed so no tension exists on the renal vein.

Postoperative Care of the Recipient

In the early postoperative period, the three major dangers for the renal transplant patient are anemia, hypothermia, and hypotension. As soon as the procedure is completed, the recipient's skin and coat are dried, and the recipient is wrapped in towels and heating pads. Hypothermia and shock result in poor perfusion of the transplanted kidney and possible delayed function or failure of graft.

For the first 24 hours after the operation or until the patient's condition is stable, the recipient is monitored for hypothermia, central nervous system disturbances (seizures, depression, coma), acid-base and electrolyte disturbances, and anemia. The recipient receives balanced electrolyte solutions intravenously at a daily maintenance rate until eating and drinking resumes. If the patient is not eating by 24 hours postoperatively, a complete liquid diet is administered through the gastrostomy tube. Cyclosporine is administered at levels necessary to achieve trough whole blood levels of 500 ng/mL. Prednisolone is administered at 0.25 mg/kg per 12 hours orally and is tapered to 0.25 mg/kg per 24 hours by 4 weeks postoperatively.

Urine specific gravity is followed twice daily by free catch of the urine. Urine specific gravity is usually greater than 1.020 by the third postoperative day. Approximately every second day, packed blood cell volume, total plasma protein level, and the plasma creatinine level are assessed. During the early postoperative period, needless venipuncture, blood sampling, and patient handling should be avoided. If the surgery is a technical success, the urine specific gravity will be increased, and the plasma creatinine will be decreased by the third postoperative day. The recipient looks

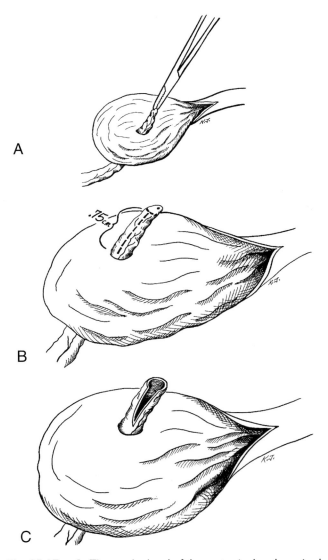

Fig. 25.17. **A.** The crushed end of the ureter is sharply excised, and the fat is removed from the distal 0.75 cm. **B.** The ureteral artery is isolated and ligated if possible. **C.** Using fine dissecting scissors, a longitudinal incision is made in the distal ureter, exposing the mucosal surface. (From Gregory C, Lirtzman RA, Kochin EJ, et al. A mucosal apposition technique for ureteroneocystostomy after renal transplantation in cats. Vet Surg 1996;25:13–17.)

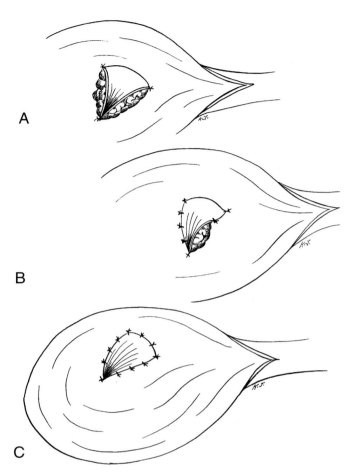

Fig. 25.18. The ureteral mucosa is apposed to the torn edge of the bladder mucosa using simple interrupted sutures of 8–0 monofilament nylon. **A.** The first suture enters the ureteral lumen at the proximal end of the longitudinal cut; the adjacent edge of the bladder mucosa is identified, included in the suture and the suture is tied. **B.** Additional sutures are placed to evenly appose the ureteral mucosa to the torn edge of the bladder mucosa. **C.** The periureteral fat that bulges into the bladder lumen is tucked adjacent to the bladder submucosa, or is excised. (From Gregory C, Lirtzman RA, Kochin EJ, et al. A mucosal apposition technique for ureteroneocystostomy after renal transplantation in cats. Vet Surg 1996;25:13–17.)

clinically improved, and normal appetite usually returns by postoperative day 3 to 5. If the graft has failed, the recipient will be depressed and anoretic. The urine remains isosthenuric.

If kidney function is not improving by 3 to 5 days after the operation, an ultrasonographic examination of the transplanted kidney and ureter can be performed for evidence of ischemia or hydronephrosis or hydroureter secondary to obstruction. Obstruction of the ureter is usually accompanied by a urine specific gravity of 1.015 or less. When all signs indicate that the graft is functioning well and caloric and water intake are adequate, the recipient is discharged from the hospital.

Long-Term Management of the Recipient

Management of the transplant patient must be coordinated with the client, the local veterinarian, and the transplant center (1). Examinations are initially performed weekly by the local veterinarian. Packed blood cell volume, total serum protein level, plasma creatinine, whole blood cyclosporine level, and urinalysis are performed. Periods between examinations are gradually extended to 3 or 4 weeks. I recommend that a complete blood count be performed bimonthly, and a serum chemistry panel and cardiac consultation be obtained two to three times a year.

Clinical Renal Transplantation in the Dog

Only a few differences exist in the technical aspects of renal transplantation between the dog and the cat (2). Most dogs, because of their size, do not require magnification for anastomosis of the vessels, although 2 to 3× magnifying loupes are helpful. Ureteroneocystostomy is technically much simpler in the dog. For venous anastomosis in a 20- to 25-kg dog, I use 4–0 silk in a continuous pattern. For arterial anastomosis, I use 5–0 polypropylene in a simple interrupted pattern.

The primary difference in transplantation between dogs and cats is selection of the donor. Using cyclosporine, azathioprine, and prednisolone to achieve immunosuppression, I use only mixed lymphocyte response–matched, or DNA-matched, related donors.

Complications of Renal Transplantation

In the first hours after renal transplantation, shock and hypothermia can lead to loss of graft function or death (1, 2). Seizures, depression, and coma can result from, or produce, fatal cerebral edema. Periodic monitoring of pupillary light reflexes, peripheral pain sensation, gag reflex, cerebral oculomotor reflexes, and general awareness should be performed during the first 24 to 48 hours postoperatively. Loss of these reflexes may indicate the progression of cerebral edema that must be treated aggressively. I administer mannitol, 0.5 to 1 g/kg intravenously every 30 to 60 minutes, until improvement is seen in central nervous system reflexes. Early postoperative mortality can be decreased by careful patient selection. Severely debilitated patients are much more likely to suffer postsurgical complications.

Technical failure of the graft because of thrombosis of the renal artery or vein can occur up to 72 hours postoperatively. Before use of the previously described method of ureteroneocystostomy, ureteral obstruction was common (10). Falling urine specific gravity and rising creatinine levels caused by ureteral obstruction may be confused with graft rejection. Diagnosis of ureteral obstruction is made by ultrasonographic examination of the ureter and kidney or by exploratory laparotomy. Obstruction usually occurs distal to the junction of the ureter and the bladder wall. The ureter is freed from the bladder, and the stenotic section is excised. Ureteroneocystostomy is then performed at a new site. Often mucosa-to-mucosa anastomosis between the bladder and the ureter can be achieved by dilation of the ureter. Despite what may appear to be severe hydronephrosis, the kidney can return to normal function.

The most common form of bacterial infection affecting human renal transplant recipients is UTI (1, 2). Treatment should be based on proper antibiotic sensitivity testing and a knowledge of the antibiotics that can be toxic when administered with cyclosporine. All aminoglycoside antibiotics should be avoided. Trimethoprim alone or combined with sulfamethoxazole may produce nephrotoxicity. I have used cephalosporin and fluoroquinolone antibiotics to treat UTI successfully in renal transplant recipients.

Two feline renal transplant recipients died at 5 and 11 months after renal transplantation of systemic bacterial infections caused by an *Actinobacillus* species and an *Actinomyces* species (1). Despite a lower reported incidence of posttransplantation infections, cyclosporine and prednisolone immunosuppression can permit the development of lethal bacterial and fungal infections. However, both these cats were maintained with at least twice the currently recommended trough whole blood levels of cyclosporine. Further experience in clinical transplantation will better define the minimum trough whole blood levels of cyclosporine necessary to maintain renal allografts in the cat; however, any level below 150 ng/mL should be corrected as soon as possible.

Acute renal rejection can occur at any time, but it is most common within the first 30 days after transplantation (4). In the dog, clinical signs of malaise, vomiting, and severe depression ("hang-dog look") precede elevations in serum creatinine and blood urea nitrogen. However, the cat may suffer severe graft damage without exhibiting any clinical signs. If acute allograft rejection is suspected, it must be treated aggressively. Delay in treatment may result in loss of the graft. To treat acute allograft rejection, cyclosporine intravenous solution is administered at 6 to 8 mg/kg over a 4- to 6-hour period daily. Initially, prednisolone is administered at 10 mg/kg per 12 hours intravenously until creatinine levels begin to normalize. Parenteral administration of cyclosporine and prednisolone are continued until oral intake of food and water is tolerated by the patient or until graft function normalizes. Oral administration of cyclosporine is then resumed at a level that achieves higher trough whole blood levels than those present before the rejection episode. Acute renal rejection is rare in the cat but has been encountered in cats whose owners did not administer the cyclosporine correctly or gave an insufficient dose of cyclosporine, in cats with lymphocytic plasmacytic enterocolitis, and in cats that had a latent infection with or became infected with the feline leukemia virus.

Three feline renal transplant recipients developed signs of mild to severe congestive heart failure after the transplantation procedure (1). Ultrasonographic evaluation of the heart in two cases revealed mild hypertrophic enlargement of the left ventricle. Two of the cats responded to symptomatic treatment with diuretics, and one died of congestive heart failure 22 months after renal transplantation. Heart failure in these cats could have been a primary problem or secondary to hypertension caused by renal failure or administration of cyclosporine. The native kidneys, through effects on both local circulation and the renin–angiotensin system, can provide a chronic source of hypertension leading to heart failure. The relation of renal disease, hypertension, and heart disease in the cat has to be understood more fully before strong recommendations for treatment are made.

After maintenance of a functioning graft for 2 to 3 months, I recommend removal of the native kidneys if an indication arises. Native kidneys have been removed from feline transplant patients for the following reasons: recurrent UTI, polycystic kidney disease associated with polyuria and polydypsia, and slow enlargement of the kidneys associated with lower back pain (1).

Cyclosporine and prednisolone are used in combination for their synergistic effects. In addition to other mechanisms of action, together they produce an additive inhibitory effect on T-cell proliferation and interleukin-2 production (3). The dose level of cyclosporine can usually be reduced over the first several months of treatment without a reduction in the trough blood level, because the bioavailability of cyclosporine increases over time. However, if blood levels become too low, a rejection episode will occur.

Little correlation exists between the oral dose of cyclosporine and the trough whole blood level achieved in a particular patient. Because of interpatient and intrapatient variability in the absorption of oral cyclosporine and its metabolism during long-term therapy, cyclosporine blood levels should be regularly monitored to maintain therapeutic concentrations and to minimize toxic side effects. Fortunately, unlike in human patients, cyclosporine rarely produces nephrotoxicity or hepatotoxicity in the dog and cat (1, 2). A newer microemulsion form of cyclosporine (Neoral) has been approved for sale by the United States Food and Drug Administration. This form of cyclosporine has better absorption characteristics and may reduce the variability in the blood levels seen in the same and different animals following administration of cyclosporine.

Renal transplantation offers a unique opportunity to manage chronic renal failure successfully in the cat and, in some cases, the dog. Morbidity and mortality can be reduced by careful patient selection and proper preoperative and postoperative management of the patient. Despite thorough preparation with the best of candidates, renal transplantation is performed on critically ill animals, and graft failure and death occur in some patients. The transplant team and the client must understand this risk before the decision is made for surgery.

References

1. Gregory CR, Gourley IM, Kochin EJ, et al. Renal transplantation for the treatment of end-stage renal failure in cats. J Am Vet Med Assoc 1992;201:285–291.

2. Gregory CR, Gourley IM. Organ transplantation in clinical veterinary practice. In: Slatter DH, ed. Textbook of small animal surgery. Philadelphia: WB Saunders, 1993:95–101.

3. Gregory CR. Cyclosporine. In: Kirk RW, ed. Current veterinary therapy X. Small animal practice. Philadelphia: WB Saunders, 1989:513–515.

4. Gregory CR. Transplantation Immunology. In: Bonagura JD, Kirk RW, eds. Current veterinary therapy XII. Small animal practice. Philadelphia: WB Saunders, 1995:564–572.

5. Gregory CR, Gourley IM, Taylor NJ, et al. Preliminary results of clinical renal allograft transplantation in the dog and cat. J Vet Intern Med 1987;1:53–60.

6. Davies HffS, St. John Collier D, Thiru S, et al. Long-term survival of kidney allografts in dogs after withdrawal of immunosuppression with cyclosporine and azathioprine. Eur Surg Res 1989;21:65–75.

7. Lirtzman RA, Gregory CR, Levitski RE, et al. Combined immunosuppression with leflunomide and cyclosporine prevents MLR mismatched renal allograft rejection in a mongrel canine model. Transplant Proc (in press).

8. Lirtzman RA, Gregory CR. Long-term renal and hematologic effects of uninephrectomy in healthy feline kidney donors. J Am Vet Med Assoc 1995;207:1044–1047.

9. Cowgill LD. CVT update: use of recombinant human erythropoietin. In: Bonagura JD, Kirk RW, eds. Current veterinary therapy XII. Small animal practice. Philadelphia: WB Saunders, 1995:961–963.

10. Gregory CR, Lirtzman RA, Kochin EJ, et al. A mucosal apposition technique for ureteroneocystostomy after renal transplantation in cats. Vet Surg 1996;25:13–17.

26

URETER

Correction of Ectopic Ureter

Clarence A. Rawlings

Ectopic ureter is a congenital anomaly that can be operated on to redirect urine into the bladder, thereby producing continence. Preoperative signs of this anomaly include urinary incontinence and chronic vulvar dermatosis. The incontinence can be continual or intermittent. These incontinent animals frequently void normally in addition to dribbling between normal urination. Incontinence results when urine is not emptied from the ureter into the urinary bladder, but rather into either the distal portion of the urethra or the vagina. Because incontinence predisposes to urinary tract infections, another but less obvious sign of this anomaly is persistent urinary tract infection. Ectopic ureters may be intramural or extramural (Fig. 26.1). Both ureters are ectopic in more than one-third of the affected patients. Other ureteral abnormalities with similar signs are ureteral trough, branching ureter, and ureteroceles.

Ectopic ureters are diagnosed more often in female dogs than in males at a 25:1 ratio. Siberian huskies, West Highland white terriers, fox terriers, and poodles are overrepresented with ectopic ureters. The actual incidence of anatomic ectopic ureter in male dogs may be higher than its clinical frequency because urine exiting the ureter into the male urethra would more likely flow toward the bladder than toward the tip of the penis. In such a hypothetic location, urine could accumulate in the bladder rather than dribbling to the outside.

Diagnosis

In a young female dog with urinary incontinence and infection that has not responded to antibiotics, the top differential diagnostic choice is ectopic ureter. Confirmation of an ectopic ureter is by positive-contrast urinary radiography by either an intravenous urogram or a retrograde vaginogram. To diagnose an ectopic ureter with an intravenous urogram, the dog should be anesthetized, the bladder emptied and inflated with air, and then contrast media injected intravenously. The alternative contrast procedure is to inject contrast media in retrograde fashion as a vaginourethrogram. The diagnostic key is to identify the ureteral entrance into the lower urinary tract; some ectopic ureters also have an abnormally shaped ureterovesicular junction. The ectopic ureter may be seen to enter the urethra, the uterus, or the vagina. One-half of ectopic ureters are dilated, and many of these patients have hydronephrosis. This dilation of the ureter and renal pelvis develops in response to increased resistance of urine flow at the ureteral exit. My impression is that hydroureter most likely develops with intramural ectopic ureters. Approximately one-third of patients with ectopic ureters have bilateral ectopia. Because both ectopic ureters and upper urinary tract infections can produce dilatation of the ureter and renal pelvis, the abnormal ureteral entrance is essential to diagnose ectopia. Animals with dilated ureters, but not a well-defined ectopic ureter, may require an exploratory ventral cystotomy to determine whether an ectopic ureter is present.

Ultrasonography can be used to identify the ureteral "jet" injection of urine into the bladder. Administration of furosemide increases urine production and can

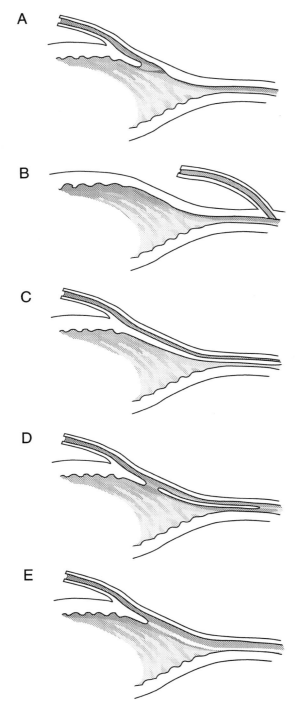

Fig. 26.1. Anatomic types of ureteral entrances into the lower urinary tract. **A.** Normal ureteral oblique intramural course of the ureter from the serosa to the mucosa with the entrance into the trigone. **B.** Intramural ectopic ureter with a normal entrance into the serosa, but a submucosal continuation from the trigone into the urethra to exit into the distal portion of the urethra or vagina. **C.** Extramural ectopic ureter in which the ureter bypasses the trigone and possibly the urethra. **D.** Trough ectopic ureter in which the ureter enters the trigone but continues distally as a trough. **E.** Branched ectopic ureter with double ectopic ureter openings, with one opening in the normal trigone location and the other opening distally. (Illustration by Dan Beisel.)

increase the probability of identifying the urine flow. Another alternative for identifying the ureteral orifice is endoscopy to examine the vagina and urethra.

Ectopic ureters may be intramural or extramural (see Fig. 26.1). Approximately two-thirds are intramural, in which the ectopic ureter enters the serosa and muscularis of the bladder in the usual fashion, and then the ureter continues submucosally through the bladder trigone to open distally in the urethra. The extramural ectopic ureter bypasses the bladder to open directly into the urethra or vagina. Other urinary abnormalities have been diagnosed with radiographic contrast studies in young incontinent dogs. Two bladder abnormalities have been described, a small bladder and an intrapelvic bladder. Incontinence has been attributed to an intrapelvic position of the bladder by some investigators, but this location is not considered abnormal by others. Investigators have also speculated that dogs with ectopic ureters have a small, unstretched, bladder. Many incontinent dogs have a short, wide urethra. An infrequent occurrence is a trough ectopic ureter, in which the ureter enters the trigone normally with a trough continuing from the ureteral orifice into the urethra. Rarely, double ureteral openings have been diagnosed in which the ureter branches with an opening in the usual trigone position and then a branched portion continuing distally within the urethral wall to exit into the distal urethra or vagina. Another unusual cause of incontinence is a ureterocele, a congenital abnormality with cystic dilation of the submucosal portion of the distal ureter. These ureteroceles are frequently associated with ectopic ureter, but the orthotopic (or simple) ureterocele also includes some located in the trigone of the bladder with the orifice at the normal intravesicular position.

Urinary tract infections occur in approximately two-thirds of the patients with ectopic ureters. These infections should be diagnosed by sediment examination and culture of urine, preferably obtained by cystocentesis. Antibiotic sensitivity should be determined, and treatment should be initiated before the surgical procedure. Renal function is usually normal, but it should be confirmed by blood urea nitrogen, serum creatinine, and urine specific gravity measurements.

Because surgical treatment produces continence in only approximately half the patients with ectopic ureter, the client appreciates an accurate prognosis for predicting incontinence after surgery. Postoperative incontinence is usually produced by decreased urethral sphincter competence. A urethral pressure profile, as used to assess urethral sphincters, has predicted postoperative incontinence. Dogs with ectopic ureters and low urethral pressures are more likely to leak urine after surgical correction. Dogs whose urethral pressures increase in response to phenylpropanolamine given preoperatively are more likely to become continent when treated with phenylpropanolamine for postoperative incontinence. A urethral pressure profile does not predict incontinence in dogs that also have decreased bladder capacity and compliance.

Surgical Techniques

Surgery is the definitive technique to diagnose ectopic ureters. A caudal midline celiotomy and a ventral cystotomy are performed to expose the ureters' entrance into the bladder (Fig. 26.2). If the ectopic ureter bypasses the bladder to enter caudal to the trigone (extramural), the ureter is transected and reimplanted into the bladder (also called extravesicular transplantation). If the ectopic ureter enters the bladder serosa in the normal position to run caudally within the bladder wall (intramural), the ureter is left in place and incised to produce a stoma opening directly from the ureter into the bladder (intravesicular diversion). Many sur-

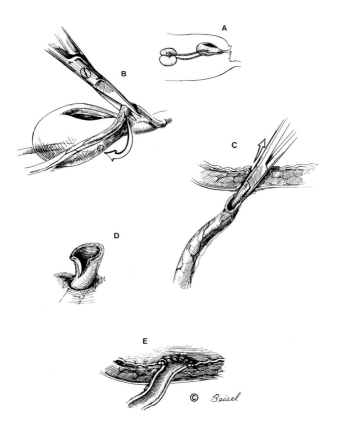

Fig. 26.2. Reimplantation of transected ureter to correct an extramural ectopic ureter. **A.** Caudal celiotomy and ventral cystotomy expose the ureters and trigone. **B.** The ureter that bypasses the bladder caudally is ligated and transected. The *dotted circle* indicates where the end will be passed through the dorsal cystic wall. **C.** A mosquito hemostat is passed from inside to outside the bladder wall and is used to draw the ureter into the bladder. **D.** The damaged portion of the ureter is excised, and the ureter is incised to provide a longer length for suturing. **E.** Simple interrupted sutures are placed between the ureteral wall and the cystic mucosa. (Copyright by the University of Georgia, Athens, GA.)

geons believe that the likelihood of postoperative strictures after reimplantation is high enough that reimplantation should be restricted to extramural ectopic ureters. A nephrectomy should be performed only when the opposite kidney appears to be capable of sustaining normal life and the affected kidney is nonfunctional or is large, hydronephrotic, and infected.

When the extramural ureter bypasses the trigone, it is doubly ligated, transected caudal to the trigone, and reimplanted into the bladder (see Fig. 26.2). Through a ventral cystotomy, a small circle of mucosa is excised from the dorsal cystic wall. A mosquito hemostat is plunged through the bladder wall at a slightly oblique angle starting at the area of excised mucosa. Although some surgeons have recommended long submucosal tunneling of the ureter to prevent vesicoureteral reflux, my experience is that a long tunnel increases resistance to urine flow, resulting in hydroureter and hydronephrosis. The shorter tunnel can be situated such that urine leakage is unlikely. The end of the excised ureter is drawn inside the bladder, is transected, and is incised 1 cm in the longitudinal direction. The ureter is sutured to the edges of the excised mucosa with an interrupted pattern of 4–0 or 5–0 synthetic absorbable suture. Twisting of the ureter must be avoided, and ureteral blood supply is preserved. If an upper urinary tract infection is suspected, a 3.5-French soft rubber catheter can be passed in a retrograde manner in the ureter to obtain a urine sample from the renal pelvis. The urinary bladder is closed in routine fashion, and omentum is placed over the cystotomy incision.

Most ectopic ureters enter the bladder's serosa dorsally in the normal position and then course within the cystic and urethral wall before entering the lumen of the genitourinary tract caudal to the bladder (intramural) (Fig. 26.3). These anatomic features are documented by ventral cystotomy and trigone exploration. These ureters can be dilated submucosally by simultaneous caudal obstruction of the ureter and diuresis with fluids and furosemide. The preferred correction is an intravesicular diversion, which has also been called neoureterostomy, intravesicular transplantation, and stomatization. To repair an intramural ectopic ureter, an incision is made to open the ureter into the trigone to permit urine to flow directly into the bladder. The ureteral wall and mucosa are then sutured to the cystic mucosa in an interrupted pattern with 4–0 or 5–0 synthetic absorbable suture. A catheter is passed caudally through the distal part of the ectopic ureter to identify its course. Several ligatures of nonabsorbable suture material (nylon or polypropylene) are placed to ligate the ectopic ureter distal to the trigone; these sutures should enter and exit through the serosa and should not include the mucosa. At least one ligature should be near the caudal end of the new entrance

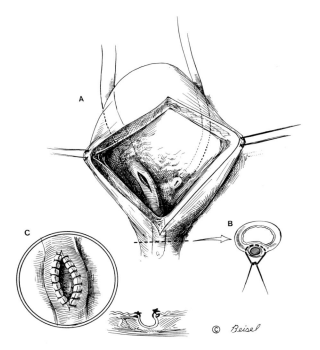

Fig. 26.3. Intravesicular diversion to correct an intramural ectopic ureter. **A.** The dilated ectopic ureter, which can be seen as a swelling under the mucosa, is incised to create an opening into the bladder. **B.** The ureter distal to this incision is ligated by placing several sutures from the outside to encircle the continuation of the ureter into the urethra; the cystic and urethral mucosa should be avoided. **C.** The edges of the incised ureter are sutured to the cystic mucosa in an interrupted pattern. (Copyright by the University of Georgia, Athens, GA.)

of the ureter into the bladder. The bladder is closed routinely, and omentum is secured over the cystotomy incision.

Repair of a trough ectopic ureter requires surgical confirmation that the ureteral orifice enters the trigone normally and that only a trough continues toward the urethra (Fig. 26.4). The trough should be closed with a simple continuous pattern using 4–0 or 5–0 synthetic absorbable suture material. When a branched ectopic ureter is suspected, the distal end should be probed with a small catheter in an attempt to identify the continuation into the urethra. If a ureteral tube continues into the urethra, the catheter is placed within it to serve as a reference for placing multiple enclosing ligatures about the ectopic ureter. When possible, ligature of the intramural ureters is done from the serosal surface to encircle the ureter with little or none of the suture exposed to mucosal surface. Ureters that have only an ureterocele without evidence of ectopic ureter should have the ureterocele incised to open a larger stoma into the lumen of the trigone. An alternative is to ligate the ureter, reduce any wall defect, transect the ureter, and reimplant it into the bladder. With any ureteral defect, nephrectomy should be considered if the affected kidney is nonfunctional and the contralateral kidney is healthy.

Postoperative Care and Complications

Medical care after repair of an ectopic ureter is the same as after any cystotomy. Postsurgical problems have included persistent urinary tract infections, strictures, and calculi formation near the orifice of the ureteroneocystostomy. Strict care must be taken to treat urinary tract infections. Dilated ureters and hydronephrosis typically decrease in size if surgical correction is done properly and no urinary tract infection is present. Dogs with persistent urinary tract infection that do not respond to appropriate antibiotic treatment and dogs with persistent incontinence should have their preoperative positive-contrast studies repeated. Abnormalities that permit pooling of urine may be associated with persistent infection and should be surgically corrected.

Approximately half the dogs with ectopic ureters become continent after proper surgical correction. Approximately half the others have no improvement, with the remainder having only modest improvement. Siberian huskies have an unusually high frequency of postoperative incontinence. Retrospective studies

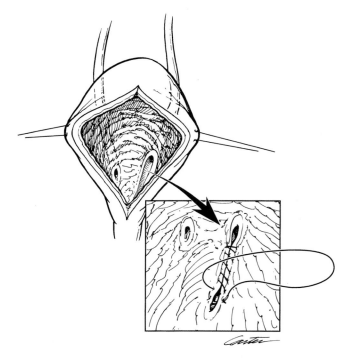

Fig. 26.4. Closure of an ectopic ureteral trough. The normal ureteral orifice with a trough continuing toward the urethra can be seen with a ventral cystotomy approach. *Inset,* The trough is closed with a simple continuous suture using synthetic absorbable suture material. (Illustration by Kip Carter.)

have found no difference in the frequency of postoperative incontinence between dogs with bilateral ectopic ureters and those with unilateral ectopic ureters. Dogs with persistent incontinence should be evaluated by urinalysis, intravenous urogram, and urodynamic tests. Even in dogs with abnormal urodynamic test results, multiple causes of the disorder always should be considered. If surgical correction appears to be satisfactory and no infection can be identified, trial therapy with phenylpropanolamine should be attempted. Urethral incompetence has been diagnosed by urethral pressure profile studies and has been successfully treated with phenylpropanolamine. Reduced bladder size and compliance in some dogs has been confirmed by cystometrography. Incontinent dogs may have both syndromes, a reason that phenylpropanolamine may fail to correct incontinence. Dogs with decreased bladder size may improve when treated with oxybutynin for its anticholinergic effect to reduce bladder spasms and sensitivity. Other suggested causes of urinary incontinence include hormonal imbalances, neurogenic abnormalities, and persistent urinary tract infection.

Suggested Readings

Dean PW, Bojrab MJ, Constantinescu GM. Canine ectopic ureter. Compend Contin Educ Small Anim Pract 1988;10:146.

Dingwall JS, Eger CE, Owen RR. Clinical experiences with the combined technique of ureterovesicular anastomosis for treatment of ectopic ureters. J Am Anim Hosp Assoc 1976;12:406.

Holt PE. Ectopic ureter in the bitch. Vet Rec 1976; 98:299.

Holt PE, Gibbs C, Pearson H. Canine ectopic ureter: a review of twenty-nine cases. J Small Anim Pract 1982;23:195.

Holt PE, Moore AH. Canine ureteral ectopia: an analysis of 175 cases and comparison of surgical treatments. Vet Rec 1995;136:345.

Lane IF, Lappin MR. Urinary incontinence and congenital urogenital anomalies in small animals. In: Kirk RW, ed. Current veterinary therapy XII. Philadelphia: WB Saunders, 1995:1022–1026.

Mason LK, Stone EA, Biery DN, et al. Surgery of ectopic ureters: pre- and postoperative radiographic morphology. J Am Anim Hosp Assoc 1990;26:73.

McLaughlin R, Miller CW. Urinary incontinence after surgical repair of ureteral ectopia in dogs. Vet Surg 1991;20:100.

McLoughlin MA, Hauptman JG, Spaulding K. Canine ureteroceles: a case report and literature review. J Am Anim Hosp Assoc 1989;25:699.

Osborne CA, Dieterich HF, Hanlon GF, et al. Urinary incontinence due to ectopic ureter in a male dog. J Am Vet Med Assoc 1975;166:911.

Owen RR. Canine ureteral ectopic: a review. 1. Embryology and aetiology. J Small Anim Pract 1973;14:407.

Owen RR. Canine ureteral ectopics: a review. 2. Incidence, diagnosis and treatment. J Small Anim Pract 1973;14:419.

Rawlings CA. Management of ectopic ureter. In: Bojrab MJ, ed. Current techniques in small animal surgery. 2nd ed. Philadelphia: Lea & Febiger, 1983:308.

Rigg DL, Zenoble RD, Riedesel EA. Neoureterostomy and phenylpropanolamine therapy for incontinence due to ectopic ureter in a dog. J Am Anim Hosp Assoc 1983;19:237.

Ross LA, Lamb CR. Reduction of hydronephrosis and hydroureter associated with ectopic ureters in two dogs after ureterovesical anastomoses. J Am Vet Med Assoc 1990;196:1497.

Stone EA, Mason LK: Surgery of ectopic ureters: types, method of correction, and postoperative results. J Am Anim Hosp Assoc 1990;26:81.

27

URINARY BLADDER

Cystotomy and Cystectomy

Andrew E. Kyles & Elizabeth Arnold Stone

Cystotomy is indicated to remove cystic and urethral calculi, to approach ectopic ureters, to examine the interior surface of the bladder for tumors, polyps, and ulcers, to remove blood clots, sloughed urothelium, or foreign bodies, and to repair some types of bladder rupture. Partial cystectomy is indicated to excise bladder neoplasms, polyps, ulcers, patent urachus, urachal diverticula, and infected urachal remnants. Total cystectomy has been used as a treatment for malignant tumors that are extensive or that involve the trigone and ureters. Various surgical techniques for urine diversion and for creation of a urine reservoir have been described, but all are associated with significant postoperative morbidity. Alternatives to total cystectomy include palliative treatment by placement of a permanent cystostomy catheter, chemotherapy, and radiation therapy.

Depending on the indication, preoperative assessment should include evaluation of renal function, urinalysis, and quantitative bacteriologic culture and diagnostic imaging of the bladder using plain radiography, contrast cystography, or ultrasonography.

Surgical Technique

Cystotomy

A caudal midline incision is made in female dogs and cats. In the male dog, a paraprepucial incision is used; the skin incision curves lateral to the prepuce, the prepuce is retracted laterally, and a midline abdominal incision is made through the linea alba.

A ventral cystotomy incision is recommended because it provides better access to the trigone, ureteral openings, and proximal urethra than a dorsal incision, and the risk of adhesions or leakage is similar (1). The bladder is isolated from the abdomen with moistened laparotomy sponges or towels. A retention suture is placed at the cranial end of the bladder, and a second suture is placed at the caudal end of the planned incision. The length of the incision is determined by the size of the calculi or by the extent of the planned exploration of the bladder interior. The bladder is emptied by cystocentesis using a 22-gauge needle and syringe (Fig. 27.1). A stab incision is made into the bladder with a scalpel. The incision is extended cranially and caudally with scissors (Fig. 27.2). Retention sutures can be placed lateral to the incision to help open the bladder and to allow inspection of the interior (Fig. 27.3).

Calculi are removed with a bladder spoon or forceps. Urethral calculi can often be dislodged by passing a urethral catheter and flushing the urethra from the bladder and from the urethral opening alternately. The bladder lining is inspected, and abnormal-appearing areas are sampled for biopsy. The ureteral openings

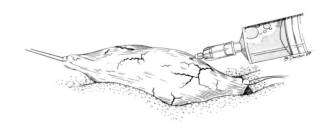

Fig. 27.1. Retention sutures are placed cranial and caudal to the ends of the proposed cystotomy incision. Urine is removed by cystocentesis.

451

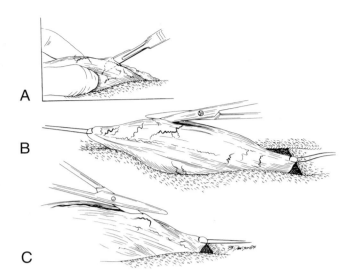

A

B

C

Fig. 27.2. **A.** A stab incision is made into the bladder. **B** and **C.** The incision is extended cranially and caudally with scissors.

can be identified in the trigone and catheterized if necessary. The bladder is flushed with warm saline before closure.

The bladder is closed in one layer with absorbable suture material. An inverting pattern (e.g., Cushing) is used in a bladder of normal thickness, and a simple interrupted pattern is used in a thickened bladder wall (Fig. 27.4). The suture material should not enter the lumen of the bladder, but should incorporate the submucosal layer. The bladder closure can be tested by injecting saline to distend the bladder and evaluating the incision for leakage. The abdomen is lavaged with warm saline and is closed routinely.

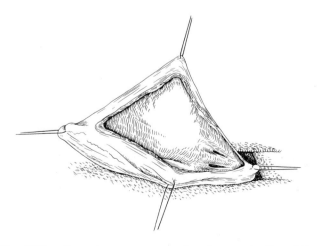

Fig. 27.3. Retention sutures are placed on each side of the incision and the interior of the bladder is inspected.

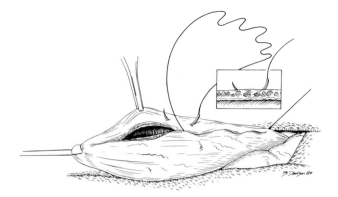

Fig. 27.4. The bladder is closed in a single-layer inverting pattern. In a thickened bladder wall, a simple interrupted appositional pattern is preferred.

Cystectomy

A cystotomy is performed to inspect the interior surface of the bladder. The bladder lesion is excised, taking care to preserve as much as possible of the blood supply to the bladder. It is preferable to preserve the trigone, although ureters can be reimplanted into the residual bladder. Closure of the bladder incision is similar to the cystotomy closure described previously. Up to 75% of the urinary bladder can be excised and the remaining tissue closed around a 5-mL Foley catheter bulb. A return to normal bladder volume and function within 3 months is anticipated.

If bladder neoplasia is suspected, the bladder wall is gently palpated and the bladder is incised 1 to 2 cm away from the bladder mass. The mass should not be manipulated during the procedure. The mass is excised with a 1- to 2-cm margin of grossly normal tissue. After tumor excision, gloves and drapes should be changed and new instruments used to close the bladder and abdomen, to prevent tumor seeding (2).

Postoperative Management

The patient should be allowed to urinate frequently. If this is not possible, the bladder should be kept empty for 2 to 3 days by intermittent catheterization or with an indwelling urethral catheter connected to a closed urine collection system. An indwelling urinary catheter should always be placed if more than 50% of the urinary bladder is excised. Any calculi are submitted for quantitative mineral analysis, and appropriate medical management is initiated to help prevent urolith recurrence. Excised tissue should be submitted for pathologic examination. With suspected bladder neoplasms, evaluation of the tissue margin is facilitated by pinning the specimen flat to a cork board and marking the edges of the excised tissue with India ink before fixing in formalin.

References

1. Desch JP II, Wagner SD. Urinary bladder incisions in dogs: comparison of ventral and dorsal. Vet Surg 1986;15:153.
2. Gilson SD, Stone EA. Surgically induced tumor seeding in eight dogs and two cats. J Am Vet Med Assoc 1990;11:1811.

Suggested Reading

Stone EA, Barsanti JA. Surgical therapy for urolithiasis. In: Stone EA, Barsanti JA, eds. Urologic surgery of the dog and cat. Philadelphia: Lea & Febiger, 1992:174.

Cystostomy Tube Placement

Julie D. Smith

Indications for cystostomy tube placement include temporary and permanent bypass of the urethra. Temporary bypass is indicated in patients with urethral obstruction due to urethral calculi, inflammation, or neoplasia. Temporary bypass may also be indicated in patients with bladder atonia while awaiting response to medication or for temporary urinary diversion after urethral surgery. Permanent cystostomy tubes can be used as palliative treatment for urethral neoplasia.

Preoperative Management

In a patient with suspected urethral obstruction, placement of a transurethral catheter should be attempted. If a transurethral catheter cannot be passed, urethral obstruction can be temporarily bypassed by placement of a cystostomy tube. The tube can be placed quickly and with minimal anesthetic compromise to the patient. This placement allows for drainage of urine while awaiting more definitive diagnostic procedures or for stabilization of a critically ill animal before instituting more definitive therapy.

If urethral or prostatic neoplasia is causing significant urethral obstruction, a cystostomy tube can be placed through a minilaparotomy or during a staging laparotomy. The cystostomy tube can be used as permanent palliative therapy, or it can be placed while awaiting response to more definitive therapy, such as chemotherapy or radiation.

Surgical Technique

A minilaparotomy (1- to 2-cm skin incision) is made in the caudal third of the abdomen. Usually, the bladder is easily palpable, and the incision is made over the bladder. The incision can be made on the midline through the linea alba, or it can be paramedian through the abdominal body wall. In male dogs, it is often easier to make a paramedian incision lateral to the prepuce, or alternatively, the prepuce can be retracted laterally to make a midline incision. The bladder is then exteriorized, and two retention sutures are placed to allow for retraction (Fig. 27.5**A**).

A pursestring suture is placed through the serosa and muscular layers of the bladder wall in the ventral portion of the exteriorized bladder. Synthetic absorbable suture is recommended. A stab incision is made into the bladder within the pursestring (Fig. 27.5**B**), and the cystostomy tube is introduced into the bladder (Fig. 27.5**C**). A Foley catheter is recommended (8- or 12-French) for temporary bypass, and the catheter is inflated with sterile saline. If the catheter is to remain in place for weeks to months, a mushroom-tip urinary catheter is recommended. The omentum can be incorporated around the catheter, or the retention sutures can be placed between the bladder and the body wall to help secure the pexy of the bladder (Fig. 27.5**D**). The incisions in the body wall and skin are closed around the catheter, and the catheter is secured to the skin. The catheter is connected to a closed drainage system, or alternatively, the bladder can be intermittently drained.

The catheter can be safely removed after 5 days, allowing for a strong adhesion to form between the bladder and the body wall. After tube removal, urine leaks from the stoma for 1 to 2 days.

Postoperative Management

After urine flow is restored by temporary bypass of the obstructed urethra, fluid therapy is instituted to correct dehydration, azotemia, and electrolyte and acid-base disturbances. Urine output is carefully monitored by continuous, closed-system drainage in the critically ill patient.

If the cystostomy tube was placed to remain for a longer period (i.e., urethral neoplasia, bladder atonia), the owners can be taught to drain the patient's bladder intermittently with a syringe. The cystostomy tube should be protected from self-mutilation by the patient with an Elizabethan collar or side brace if necessary.

Over time, the presence of the cystostomy tube will cause a urinary tract infection. Prophylactic antibiotics are not recommended, because of the potential devel-

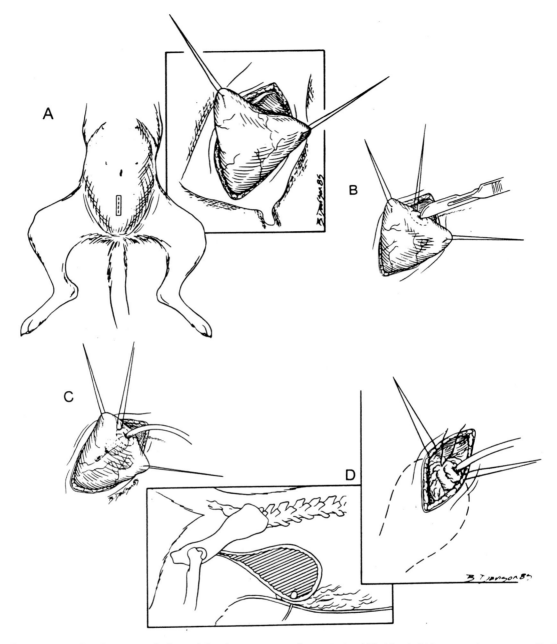

Fig. 27.5. Cystostomy tube placement. **A.** Site of the skin incision and exteriorized bladder held by retention sutures. **B.** Placement of the pursestring suture and stab incision into the bladder wall. **C.** Insertion of a Foley catheter into the bladder followed by inflation of the catheter. **D.** Securing the catheter to the body wall using the retention sutures. Sagittal section with catheter in place, with optional omentum wrapped around (*inset*). (From Stone EA. Contemporary issues in small animal practice; nephrology and urology. Breitschwerdt, EB, ed. WB Saunders, Philadelphia. 1986;4:86.)

opment of a resistant urinary tract infection. After removal of the tube, the urine should be cultured, and appropriate antibiotics should be administered. If the catheter is to remain permanently, the administration of antibiotics should be carefully considered only if the animal is showing systemic signs or discomfort from the infection.

Suggested Readings

Smith JD, Stone EA, Gilson SD. Placement of a permanent cystostomy catheter to relieve urine outflow obstruction in dogs with transitional cell carcinoma. J Am Vet Med Assoc 1995;206:496.

Stone EA, Barsanti JA. Surgical therapy for urethral obstruction in dogs. In: Stone EA, Barsanti JA, eds. Urologic surgery of the dog and cat. Philadelphia: Lea & Febiger, 1992.

Colposuspension for Urinary Incontinence

Peter E. Holt & Elizabeth Arnold Stone

Urethral sphincter mechanism incompetence is a common cause of urinary incontinence in the bitch. It can occur as a congenital or an acquired condition and has a multifactorial origin. Among factors contributing to the pathophysiology of the condition is a caudally located bladder neck ("pelvic bladder"), a common finding in bitches with urethral sphincter mechanism incompetence. The caudally located bladder neck may predispose to incontinence during increases in intra-abdominal pressure when this pressure acts on the (intra-abdominal) bladder but is transmitted less efficiently to the (extra-abdominal) intrapelvic urethra. A competent urethra maintains urinary continence under these conditions, but in a bitch with urethral sphincter mechanism incompetence, such disparity in pressure transmission can result in urinary incontinence. Thus, bitches with this disorder leak urine at times of abdominal pressure increases, mainly when they are recumbent.

Indication

Colposuspension treats urinary incontinence caused by urethral sphincter mechanism incompetence in bitches by moving the lower urogenital tract cranially, thereby moving the bladder neck and urethra to an intra-abdominal position. Thus, increased intra-abdominal pressure is transmitted simultaneously to the bladder and to the bladder neck and proximal urethra. In this way, increases in intravesical pressure resulting from raised intra-abdominal pressure may be counteracted by simultaneous increases in urethral resistance.

Because urethral sphincter mechanism incompetence is a multifactorial condition and colposuspension corrects only one of the factors, that is, the caudally positioned bladder neck, this treatment is not expected to cure all animals. However, in the long term, approximately 50% of bitches are completely cured, with the degree and frequency of incontinence significantly reduced in a further 40%. The severity of the incontinence remains unaltered in 10% of bitches.

Our approach is to perform surgery in affected younger bitches (less than 8 years of age) as the first form of treatment in the hope that long-term medical therapy with estrogens or α-adrenergic drugs and their potential side effects can be avoided. Colposuspension is delayed in juvenile bitches with congenital urethral sphincter mechanism incompetence until after the first estrus because more than half of such animals become continent after their first heat. Animals with severe congenital urethral hypoplasia may be unsuitable for colposuspension. In such animals, the bladder neck cannot be returned to an intra-abdominal position by colposuspension. Fortunately, such severe urethral hypoplasia is rare, and its treatment is described elsewhere (1). In older bitches, colposuspension is reserved for those animals which have failed to respond to medical therapy.

Surgical Technique

After general anesthesia is induced, the bitch is placed in dorsal recumbency with the hind limbs flexed. The ventral abdominal skin and vagina are prepared for aseptic surgery, the vagina by douching with dilute aqueous povidone–iodine solution (Betadine). An 8-French (smaller bitches—less than 35 kg) or a 10-French (larger bitches—more than 35 kg) Foley catheter is inserted through the urethra into the bladder, and the cuff is inflated. The catheter is then gently withdrawn until the cuff rests in the bladder neck. The presence of the catheter facilitates identification of the urethra and bladder neck during surgery.

A midline, caudal abdominal approach is made. The prepubic fat and fascia are separated by careful blunt and sharp dissection on both sides of the midline at the level of the pubic brim, and the prepubic tendons and external pudendal vessels are identified (Fig. 27.6**A**). These vessels must be avoided during subsequent placement of sutures around the prepubic tendon.

The midline incision is continued through the linea alba of the abdominal muscle wall and extends caudally to the pubic brim. Self-retaining (Gosset or Balfour) retractors are used to hold the rectus abdominis muscle edges apart, and the bladder is identified.

Cranial traction on the bladder allows the intrapelvic bladder neck to be pulled into the abdomen and identified by the presence of the inflated Foley catheter cuff. Visualization of the bladder neck and proximal urethra is often difficult because of the presence of local retroperitoneal fat.

The vagina is displaced cranially and is cleared of fat and fascia on both sides of the urethra. This is most easily accomplished by inserting a finger into the vagina (Fig. 27.6**B** and **C**). The urethra is palpated through the ventral vaginal wall and is displaced to the bitch's left. Using the finger in the vagina, the vaginal wall on the right side of the urethra is pushed cranially and ventrally toward the caudal end of the abdominal incision. The vaginal wall is exposed by using a dry swab to clean off the overlying fat and

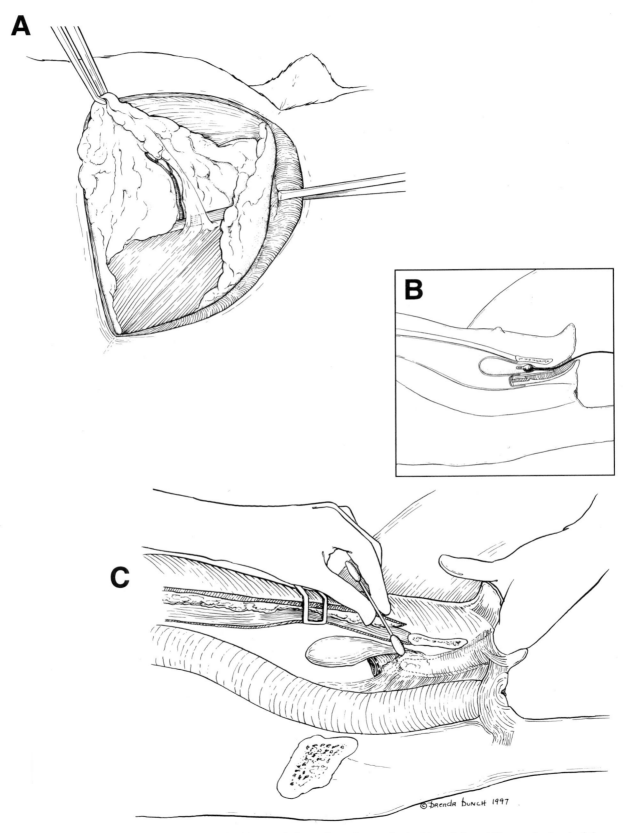

Fig. 27.6. A. Prepubic fat and fascia separated by blunt and sharp dissection on both sides of the midline at the level of the prepubic brim. **B.** A finger inserted into the vagina helps to clear out fat and fascia. **C.** The vaginal wall is exposed by using a dry swab to clean off the overlying fat and fascia in a caudolateral direction.

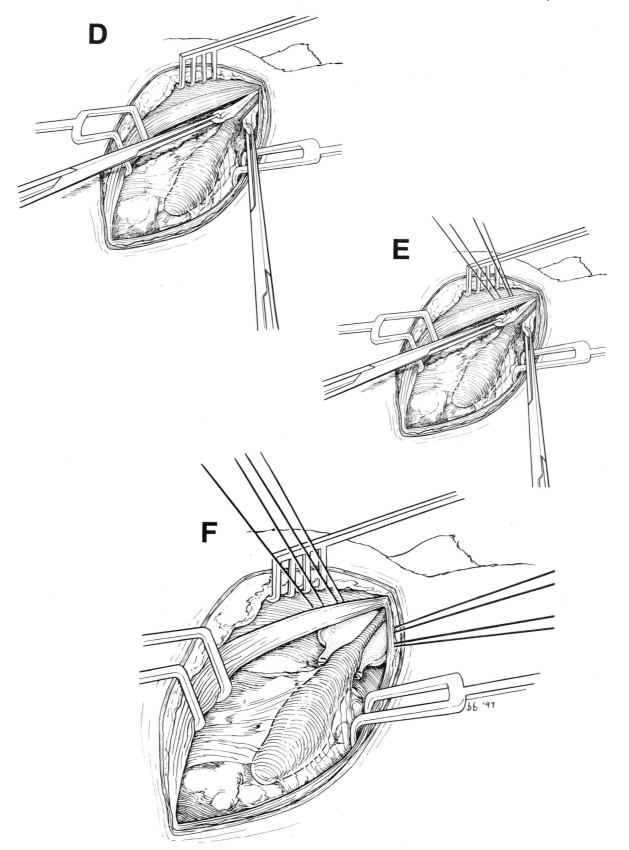

Fig. 27.6 (continued). **D.** Technique repeated on the other side of the vagina (see text). **E.** Sutures are passed through the abdominal wall caudal to the tendon, in and out of the vaginal wall, and back out of the abdominal wall cranial to the tendon. **F.** Sutures are placed around the prepubic tendon, depending on the size of the bitch and the position of the external pudendal vessels laterally. The optimal number of sutures in medium or large dogs is two.

fascia in a caudolateral direction (Fig. 27.6**C**). The bladder neck can be seen as a swelling because of the Foley catheter cuff in the bladder. The vaginal wall is grasped with Allis tissue forceps. The technique is repeated on the other side of the vagina (Fig. 27.6**D**). The surgeon then changes gloves, and the vulva is covered with a large sterile swab or surgical drape throughout the remainder of the procedure.

When the surgeon's finger and the patient's vagina are of incompatible sizes (very large or very small bitches or those with gross vaginal strictures or septa), the vagina has to be located by blunt and sharp dissection of the overlying fat and fascia on either side of the urethra, grasped with tissue forceps, and then pulled cranially. This is more difficult than the use of a finger in the vagina, and, fortunately, most bitches with urethral sphincter mechanism incompetence are of a size compatible with one's finger. It is sometimes helpful in extremely large or small bitches to identify the vagina by inserting a Poole suction tip or a closed Carmalt clamp.

The vagina must now be anchored cranially to maintain the bladder neck in an intra-abdominal position. The vagina is sutured to the prepubic tendon on each side of and approximately 1 to 1.5 cm away from the midline. The sutures (monofilament nylon) are passed through the abdominal wall caudal to the tendon, in and out of the vaginal wall (as far laterally as possible), and back out of the abdominal wall cranial to the tendon, avoiding any abnormal twisting of the vaginal wall (Fig. 27.6**E**). The sutures may enter the vaginal lumen during this procedure, hence the need to prepare the vagina for aseptic surgery.

One or two sutures are placed around the prepubic tendon, depending on the size of the bitch and the position of the external pudendal vessels laterally. Most affected bitches are medium to large breeds, and the optimum number of sutures is two around each tendon (Fig. 27.6**F**). Number 0 nylon is suitable for most bitches, but No. 1 nylon should be used in very large breeds. On the rare occasions when colposuspension is performed in small or toy breeds, it may only be possible to place one suture through each side of the vagina and around each prepubic tendon.

Before the sutures are tied, they are pulled tight to ensure that, after they are tied, the urethra will not be compressed against the pubis by an arch of vagina (see Fig. 27.6**F**). Compression on the urethra may result in postoperative dysuria. The surgeon should be able to insert the tip of a blunt instrument such as Mayo scissors or Carmalt forceps easily between the urethra and the vaginal arch and pubis. If the urethra is compressed, the sutures should be repositioned. This is rarely a problem when the sutures have been placed as laterally on the vagina as possible. After the sutures are properly placed, they are tied, the Foley catheter is removed, and the abdomen is closed routinely.

Postoperative Care

Preoperative, perioperative, and postoperative analgesics are used routinely. These are not usually required after the first 24 hours. Antibiotic therapy (e.g., amoxicillin) is used for 10 days postoperatively as a precaution to minimize the risk of peritonitis in case colposuspension sutures have entered the vaginal lumen. We have never encountered this complication. The use of a rectal thermometer to take the animal's temperature postoperatively is avoided because some bitches are sensitive in this area for a few days after surgery. In some bitches, local subcutaneous tissue swelling occurs, presumably because of the small dead spaces left after dissection to expose the prepubic tendons. Such swelling is not a problem and resolves spontaneously within 5 to 7 days. The animal is closely observed for signs of dysuria and to determine whether the incontinence has resolved. In most successful cases, the response is immediate, although some bitches remain incontinent for weeks before becoming continent. Conversely, animals that fail to respond to colposuspension in the long term all improve initially. Owners are warned, therefore, not to judge the success or failure of the operation until 3 months later. Skin sutures are removed routinely 7 to 10 days after the surgical procedure.

Possible Complications

Because the surgical procedure involves trauma to intrapelvic structures, some animals are stimulated to strain, usually immediately after recovery from general anesthesia. This can be controlled by the administration of appropriate analgesics. Rarely, some bitches find the first postoperative defecation uncomfortable if the feces are firm and bulky. This problem can be controlled with stool softeners.

Dysuria may occur immediately postoperatively. This complication is rare (approximately 5% of dogs in our experience) and may be caused by vaginal stimulation by the surgical procedure leading to suppression of the micturition reflex or reflex dyssynergia. Clinical observations and the response to diazepam suggest that reflex voluntary dyssynergia is the most likely cause of dysuria after colposuspension. It may be exacerbated by recent estrogen therapy, and so any estrogen therapy should cease at least 1 month before the operation. Voluntary dyssynergia usually responds to diazepam at a dose of 0.2 mg/kg by mouth two or three times daily. An indwelling urinary catheter can be used for a few days if necessary in the few animals that are unable to urinate at all. A further potential cause of dysuria is compression of the urethra against the pubis by the vagina. Care should be taken during surgery to avoid placement of vaginal sutures too close to the urethra.

Bitches that are allowed to be active after colposuspension may tear the sutures from the vagina. This is more likely to happen if these animals are allowed to run and jump, and owners should be advised of the necessity to restrict the exercise of their animals to leash walks only for 1 month postoperatively.

"Hymen" formation with accumulation of vaginal secretions causing dysuria or dyschezia is a rare, longer-term complication of colposuspension. This condition is caused by breakdown of a preexisting vestibulovaginal stricture during the operation and subsequent healing of apposing raw areas of vagina to form a barrier across the vaginal lumen. It can be treated by breaking down the "hymen."

Acknowledgment

We wish to thank Brenda Bunch, MA, of the College of Veterinary Medicine, North Carolina State University, for drawing the illustrations.

Reference

1. Holt PE. Surgical management of congenital urethral sphincter mechanism incompetence in eight female cats and a bitch. Vet Surg 1993;22:98–104.

Suggested Readings

Gregory SP. Review of developments in the understanding of the pathophysiology of urethral sphincter mechanism incompetence in the bitch. Br Vet J 1994;150:135–150.

Holt PE. Urinary incontinence in the bitch due to sphincter mechanism incompetence: surgical treatment. J Small Anim Pract 1985;26:237–246.

Holt PE. Long term evaluation of colposuspension in the treatment of urinary incontinence due to incompetence of the urethral sphincter mechanism in the bitch. Vet Rec 1990;127:537–542.

Holt PE. A color atlas and text of small animal urology. London: Mosby–Wolfe, 1994.

Stone EA, Barsanti JA, eds. Urologic surgery of the dog and cat. Philadelphia: Lea & Febiger, 1992.

—● 28 ●—

URETHRA

Surgical Management of Urethral Calculi in the Dog

Andrew E. Kyles & Elizabeth Arnold Stone

Urethral obstruction by uroliths occurs most frequently in male dogs, although it occurs occasionally in female dogs. Affected dogs try to urinate frequently and strain during urination, but they usually produce little urine. They may show anxiety, depression, and weakness, and the urinary bladder may be greatly distended. The dog's clinical condition can deteriorate rapidly.

Preoperative Management

An animal with complete urethral obstruction requires immediate treatment because this condition results in postrenal uremia and associated life-threatening water, electrolyte, and acid-base imbalances. Immediate treatment consists of intravenous fluid therapy and relief of the urethral obstruction. The aims of intravenous fluid therapy are to replace water, sodium, and chloride, to establish diuresis, and to correct the azotemia and hyperkalemia. Normal (0.9%) saline is the fluid of choice.

Urethral obstruction is relieved or bypassed with the least tranquilization or anesthesia possible. An attempt should be made to pass a small urethral catheter past the obstruction. The urinary catheter can further traumatize the urethra and should not be forced past the obstruction. If the patient cannot be catheterized, the bladder is decompressed by cystocentesis using a 22-gauge needle and syringe. Once the dog's condition is stabilized, definitive treatment can be initiated.

Patient assessment should include an evaluation of metabolic, fluid, and electrolyte abnormalities, urinalysis, and quantitative bacteriologic culture and radiographic imaging of urethral calculi with plain radiographs or positive-contrast urethrocystography. Urethral calculi can often be moved back into the bladder by retrograde hydropropulsion. This procedure involves injecting saline under pressure through a urethral catheter. The proximal urethra is palpated per rectum and is occluded with digital pressure to allow the saline to dilate the urethra. The occlusion of the urethra is removed, and the urethral calculi should be flushed back into the bladder. A cystotomy can be performed to recover the calculi from the bladder, or medical therapy can be instituted to dissolve the uroliths. Repeated episodes of urethral obstruction may occur during medical treatment.

A temporary cystostomy catheter can be placed to drain urine in a uremic patient with urethral calculi that cannot be removed by retrograde hydropropulsion or bypassed with a small urethral catheter. The catheter allows urine drainage while the patient's fluid, electrolyte, and metabolic imbalances are corrected. Use of a temporary cystostomy catheter is preferable to futile attempts to relieve obstruction that can further traumatize the urethra.

Surgical Techniques

Prescrotal Urethrotomy

A urethrotomy is used to remove urethral calculi in male dogs when hydropropulsion fails to flush the calculi into the bladder. Calculi most frequently lodge in the urethra just caudal to the os penis and can be retrieved through a prescrotal urethrotomy. More proximal urethral calculi can usually be flushed into the urinary bladder. A perineal urethrotomy should

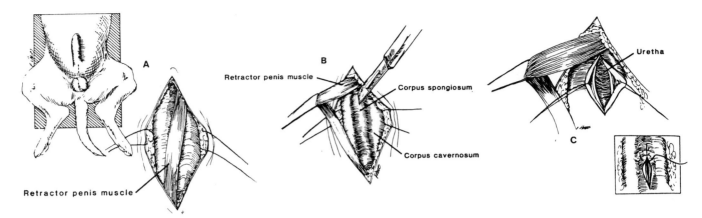

Fig. 28.1. Prescrotal urethrostomy. **A.** Site of skin incision and dissection of subcutaneous tissue to the retractor penile muscle. **B.** Longitudinal incision into the corpus spongiosum and urethra after lateral retraction of the retractor penis muscle. **C.** Retention sutures in the corpus cavernosum and exposure of the urethral interior. After removal of uroliths, the urethrotomy can be left open or closed in a simple interrupted pattern (*inset*). (From Stone EA. Urologic surgery: an update. In: Breitschwerdt, EB, ed. Contemporary issues in small animal practice. Vol. 4. Nephrology and urology. New York: Churchill Livingstone, 1986.)

be avoided if possible, because it causes greater hemorrhage and urine scalding than a prescrotal urethrotomy.

A skin incision is made from just caudal to the prepuce to just cranial to the scrotum (Fig. 28.1**A**). If the incision extends into the scrotum, the dog is more likely to excoriate the site, and the testicles may prolapse through the incision. Subcutaneous tissue is dissected to the level of the retractor penis muscle. The grayish corpus spongiosum surrounds the urethra with the paired white fibrous-covered corpora cavernosa lying on either side. The surgeon may need to rotate the animal's penis between thumb and forefinger to bring the retractor penis and corpus spongiosum to the midline.

The retractor penis muscle is retracted laterally, and a longitudinal incision is made in the corpus spongiosum and urethra (Fig. 28.1**B**). An exact midline incision avoids the highly vascular corpora cavernosa. The shiny, pinkish–white urethral mucosa lining contrasts with the surrounding corpus spongiosum. Retention sutures can be placed in the corpus spongiosum to aid in identifying and exposing the urethral mucosa (Fig. 28.1**C**). The uroliths are removed and saved for quantitative mineral analysis. A catheter is passed into the proximal urethra to identify additional uroliths or urethral obstruction. The catheter is also passed distally to dislodge calculi within the penile urethra and to assess patency.

The urethrotomy incision may be left open to heal by secondary intention and epithelialization. Primary closure of the urethrotomy site reduces postoperative hemorrhage (1, 2), but it increases operative time and requires gentle tissue handling and meticulous surgical technique to prevent postoperative stricture forma-

tion. Coagulopathies and anemia are indications for primary closure; the urethrotomy is closed with 4–0 synthetic absorbable suture in a simple interrupted pattern, with routine closure of the subcutaneous tissue and skin.

Postoperative Management

Urine output, hydration status, renal function, and electrolyte concentrations should be monitored for several days after relief of urethral obstruction. The kidneys may have an obligatory sodium and water diuresis for several days after urethral obstruction has been relieved. Lactated Ringer's solution supplemented with 20 mEq/L potassium chloride is the fluid of choice to avoid hypokalemia during the period of postobstruction diuresis.

If the urethrotomy incision is not sutured, the dog will urinate through both the urethrotomy site and the terminal urethra for up to 2 weeks. The urethrotomy incision heals completely in 2 to 4 weeks.

References

1. Waldron DR et al. The canine urethra. A comparison of first and second intention healing. Vet Surg 1985;14:213.
2. Weber WJ et al. Comparison of the healing of prescrotal urethrotomy incisions in the dog: sutured versus nonsutured. Am J Vet Res 1985;46:1309.

Suggested Reading

Stone EA, Barsanti JA. Surgical therapy for urethral obstruction in dogs. In: Stone EA, Barsanti JA eds. Urologic surgery of the dog and cat. Philadelphia: Lea & Febiger, 1992:149.

Nonsurgical Removal of Urocystoliths by Voiding Urohydropropulsion

Jody P. Lulich, Carl A. Osborne & David Polzin

Voiding urohydropropulsion is a nonsurgical technique for removal of small to moderately sized uroliths of any mineral composition from the urinary bladder of dogs or cats (1). This technique is effective because it takes advantage of gravity to reposition uroliths in the urinary bladder and of dilation of the urethral lumen during the voiding phase of micturition.

Technique

Voiding urohydropropulsion depends on first altering the patient's body position so gravitational force will reposition uroliths. The patient is positioned so the longitudinal axis of the spine is vertical. In this position, urocystoliths migrate into the neck of the urinary bladder, from which they can be easily voided.

Anesthesia is not necessary to perform voiding urohydropropulsion; however, sedation facilitates positioning of the patient and palpation of the urinary bladder, and it minimizes patient discomfort associated with urinary bladder compression. When anesthetics are used, the surgeon should consider agents that provide analgesia and muscle relaxation. We commonly use propofol (Diprivan) and a narcotic. Inhalation anesthetics also provide good analgesia and muscle relaxation.

Once the patient is anesthetized, we moderately distend the bladder with a sterilized physiologic solution (e.g., saline or Ringer's) injected through a transurethral catheter. As a general guideline, the normal empty urinary bladder can be moderately distended by injecting 6 to 9 mL of fluid per kilogram of body weight. To minimize overdistension of the bladder, its size should be assessed by abdominal palpation during infusion of fluid. If the urinary bladder is already moderately distended with urine, no additional fluid is needed.

After the bladder is distended, the surgeon removes the urinary catheter. If fluid is expelled prematurely, the urethra can be gently pinched closed using a thumb and finger. Next, the patient is positioned so the vertebral column is approximately vertical. The urinary bladder is then gently agitated by palpation to promote gravitational movement of all urocystoliths into the bladder neck. Steady digital pressure is applied to the urinary bladder to induce micturition. Once

voiding begins, the bladder is more vigorously compressed. The object is to sustain maximum urine flow through the urethral lumen to keep it dilated as long as possible. The urocystoliths are carried along with the voided urine (or infused saline) (Fig. 28.2).

If the number of uroliths voided is less than that previously detected by radiography, the procedure can be repeated. If uroliths detected by radiography are too numerous to count, we repeat voiding urohydropropulsion until uroliths are no longer detected in the voided fluid.

Visible hematuria is a common complication of voiding urohydropropulsion, and it is probably induced by manual compression of an inflamed urinary bladder. In our experience, hematuria and dysuria resolve in a few hours in dogs, but these complications can persist for up to 2 days in cats (1).

After voiding urohydropropulsion, we routinely perform abdominal radiography to determine whether all urocystoliths have been successfully removed. To remove urocystoliths that were not voided and are small enough to pass through the urethra, voiding urohydropropulsion should be repeated (2).

For patients with urocystoliths unassociated with bacterial urinary tract infection, antimicrobials are not needed, provided normal host defenses have not been disrupted by transurethral catheterization. However, in most of our patients, catheters are used either during voiding urohydropropulsion or for postprocedural radiography. To minimize catheter-induced urinary tract infection, one should consider administering therapeutic doses of antimicrobial drugs excreted in high concentrations in urine 4 to 8 hours before and for 2 to 5 days after catheterization (3). Urine collected by cystocentesis 5 to 7 days later can be cultured to verify that the urinary tract has not become infected.

If urocystoliths persist despite voiding urohydropropulsion, urethral obstruction with uroliths of appropriate size may occur, especially if the patient is dysuric. If urethral obstruction occurs, uroliths can be easily moved back into the urinary bladder by retrograde urohydropropulsion. Retrograde urohydropropulsion can also be used to flush uroliths back into the urinary bladder that become lodged in the urethra during voiding urohydropropulsion. Uroliths can then be dissolved with medical management or removed by cystotomy.

Limitations

Urolith removal by voiding urohydropropulsion depends on selecting patients with urocystoliths small enough to pass completely through the distended urethra (Table 28.1). The largest uroliths we have removed are a 7-mm diameter urolith from a 7.4-kg female dog, a 5-mm diameter urolith from a 4.6-kg

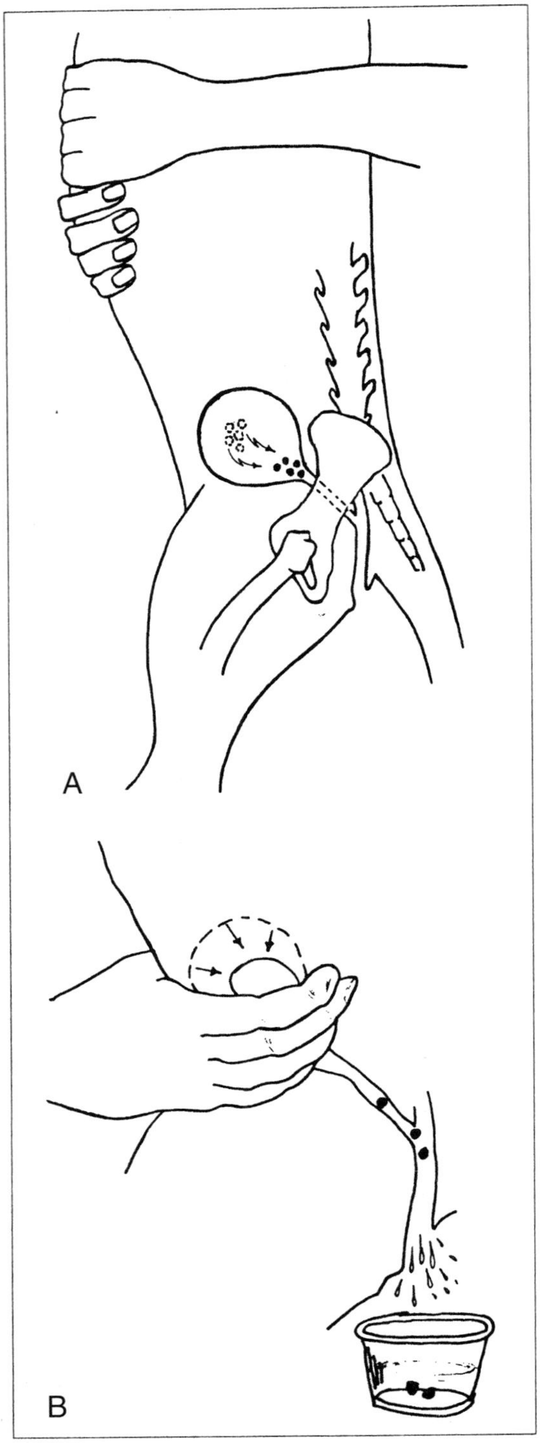

Fig. 28.2. Schematic illustration of voiding urohydropropulsion. **A.** To promote gravitational movement of urocystoliths into the neck of the urinary bladder, the animal is positioned so the vertebral column is approximately vertical. **B.** To induce voiding of urocystoliths, the urinary bladder is manually expressed, using steady digital pressure. Urine and uroliths are collected in a cup held beneath the external opening of the urogenital tract. (From Lulich JP, Osborne CA, Carlson M, et al. Nonsurgical removal of uroliths in dogs and cats by voiding urohydropropulsion. J Am Vet Med Assoc 1993;203:660.)

Table 28.1.
Limitations of Voiding Urohydropropulsion

Limitation	Resolution
Inexperience	Initially choose cases that have a high degree of success, for example, female dogs with small uroliths
Concomitant urinary tract infection (UTI)	Eradicate UTI first; to minimize hematuria and ascending UTI resulting from vesicoureteral reflux during bladder expression
Urethral obstruction	Uroliths are too large to pass through the urethra and therefore cannot be removed by voiding urohydropropulsion; consider medical dissolution of surgical removal

female cat, a 5-mm diameter urolith from a 9-kg male dog, and a 1-mm diameter urolith from a male cat (1). Larger urocystoliths can be removed from male dogs and cats with urethrostomies. Uroliths larger than the smallest diameter of any portion of the distended urethral lumen are unlikely to be voided. Therefore, voiding urohydropropulsion is usually ineffective in patients with uroliths lodged in the urethra at the time of diagnosis. However, uroliths amenable to dissolution that were initially too large to be voided may be easily removed once their size has been reduced by medical therapy (4).

Voiding urohydropropulsion should not be used if manual compression of the urinary bladder is likely to cause extravasation of urine into the peritoneal cavity. Consequently, this procedure should not be used during healing after urinary bladder surgery.

Manual compression of the urinary bladder to induce voiding is not without risk in patients with urinary tract infections. If excessive pressure is applied to the urinary bladder, vesicoureteral reflux of urine and bacteria can occur (5). Therefore, urinary tract infections should be controlled before voiding urohydropropulsion is performed. In addition, reduction of inflammation associated with control of infection lessens the severity of hematuria and dysuria induced by urinary bladder palpation.

References

1. Lulich JP, Osborne CA, Carlson M, et al. Nonsurgical removal of uroliths in dogs and cats by voiding urohydropropulsion. J Am Vet Med Assoc 1993;203:660.
2. Lulich JP, Osborne CA, Polzin DJ, et al. Incomplete removal of canine and feline urocystoliths by cystotomy. J Vet Intern Med 1993;7:124.
3. Osborne CA. Bacterial infections of the canine and feline urinary tract: cause, cure, and control. In: Bojrab MJ, ed. Disease mechanisms in small animal surgery. 2nd ed. Philadelphia: Lea & Febiger, 1993:458.
4. Osborne CA, Polzin DJ, Lulich JP, et al. Relationship of nutritional factors to the cause, dissolution, and prevention of canine uroliths. Vet Clin North Am Small Anim Pract 1989;19:583.

5. Feeney DA, Osborne CA, Johnston GR. Vesicoureteral reflux induced by manual compression of the urinary bladder. J Am Vet Med Assoc 1983;182:795.

Canine Scrotal Urethrostomy

Daniel D. Smeak & Jenifer D. Newton

Scrotal urethrostomy is the procedure of choice when creation of a new urethral orifice distal to the pelvic urethra is necessary. Scrotal urethrostomy has several advantages over prepubic or perineal urethrostomy. The membranous urethra in the region of the scrotum is larger and more distensible than the prepubic urethra. This reduces the risk of stricture formation and allows easier calculus passage after urethrostomy. The urethra in the scrotal area is more superficial and is surrounded by less cavernous tissue than in the perineal region (Fig. 28.3). Surgical exposure is easier, and the risk of hemorrhage or urine extravasation into periurethral tissues is reduced. Scrotal urethrostomy diverts urine directly downward and away from perineal skin. Skin surrounding the urethrostomy is kept dry, thereby reducing the risk of intractable dermatitis from urine scalding. Most urethral calculi are readily removed or flushed back to the bladder by scrotal urethrostomy. If castration is objectionable to the owner, however, other urethrostomy locations may be considered.

Indications

Scrotal urethrostomy is indicated for the following conditions: 1) recurrent urethral calculi that are not responsive to appropriate medical therapy; 2) acute calculi obstructions in dogs anticipated to have recurrent episodes (e.g., metabolic stone formers); 3) severe distal urethral wounds secondary to penile or os penis trauma; 4) urethral stricture distal to the scrotum from trauma or previous urethral surgery; and 5) diseases requiring amputation of the penis or prepuce and formation of a more proximal urethral stoma (e.g., extensive neoplasia, penile strangulation, certain congenital diseases such as severe hypospadias, and deficiency in penile or preputial length). Because a permanent stoma bypassing the normal opening of the urinary tract may increase the risk of ascending urocystitis, a urethrostomy should not be performed unless due consideration is given to the indications and complications of the procedure.

A modified urethrostomy technique is described here because the standard simple interrupted scrotal urethrostomy technique often results in unacceptable bleeding and bruising complications. In a retrospective study of dogs undergoing standard scrotal urethrostomy, active hemorrhage (requiring patient hospitalization) was noted an average of 4.2 days after surgery;

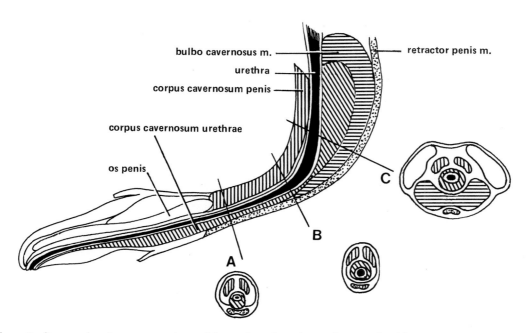

Fig. 28.3 Schematic diagram showing cross sections of the penis and urethra in the prepubic (*A*), scrotal (*B*), and perineal (*C*) locations. The urethra in the scrotal area is more superficial and is surrounded by less cavernous tissue than in the perineal area. The scrotal urethra is more distensible and larger than the prepubic urethra, allowing easier passage of calculi and reducing the risk of postoperative stricture formation.

in some patients, bleeding persisted for up to 10 days. The following modified scrotal urethrostomy technique uses a continuous suture pattern and a three-needle bite sequence for urethrostomy closure. In our hands, this modification has dramatically reduced active bleeding, bleeding after urination, and bruising postoperatively. Furthermore, no stricture or suture line breakdown has been observed to date in over 20 dogs. This closure is also faster to perform.

The rationale for the modified technique is several-fold. Simple continuous suture patterns produce a better seal by apposing tissues more completely. Continuous suture patterns require fewer knots, and irritation from ''prickly'' knot ears is reduced. Needle bites are placed closer together, and this also improves urethra-to-skin apposition. *Incorporation of a bite of tunica albuginea adds additional strength to the incision line and helps to seal incised cavernous edges* (see the section on surgical technique). When the needle is passed outward from the urethra to the skin, better apposition of cut surfaces results. All these advantages, we believe, help to reduce suture line breakdown and hemorrhage.

Surgical Technique

The surgeon must obtain the owner's consent for the animal's castration before attempting scrotal urethrostomy. Metabolic disturbances are stabilized in the obstructed patient preoperatively. While the patient is under general an-

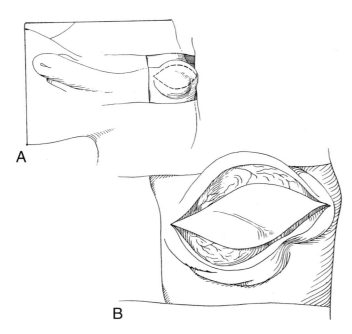

Fig. 28.4. **A** and **B.** An elliptic incision made around the scrotum. Enough lateral skin is retained to allow tension-free closure of the urethrostomy. Redundant skin can be resected later in the procedure.

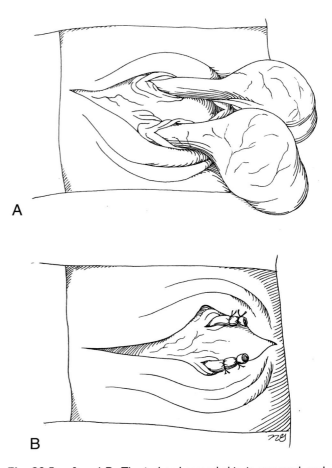

Fig. 28.5. **A** and **B.** The isolated scrotal skin is removed, and castration is performed.

esthesia, the surgeon places the patient in dorsal recumbency with the rear limbs gently abducted and secured caudally. The proposed surgery site, including the scrotum, is clipped and scrubbed routinely and is draped for aseptic surgery. An elliptic, full-thickness skin incision is made around the base of the scrotum. Hemostasis is maintained, and the isolated scrotal skin is discarded (Fig. 28.4). Enough skin should be left on the lateral aspect of the incision so no tension is placed on the urethrostomy during closure. Any redundant skin can be removed later in the procedure, if needed. If the dog is sexually intact, the testicles and spermatic cords are isolated, and the dog is neutered in a routine manner (Fig. 28.5). The underlying connective tissue is dissected to expose the paired retractor penis muscles, which appear as a brownish–tan band on the ventral surface of the penile shaft. The surgeon sharply dissects and mobilizes the retractor penis muscles and retracts them laterally to expose the bluish corpus spongiosum urethrae (Fig. 28.6). An appropriately sized urinary catheter is inserted retrograde from the normal penile opening, if possible, to outline and distend the urethra. The ventral midline of the urethra

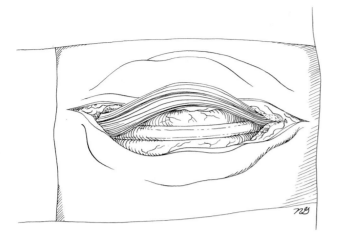

Fig. 28.6. A urinary catheter is placed retrograde from the penile orifice to help to identify the urethra. The retractor penis muscles are retracted laterally, and the ventral midline of the urethra is visualized.

is sharply incised over the catheter with a No. 15 Bard–Parker scalpel blade. If a catheter cannot be inserted, the incision must be made carefully, to avoid accidental laceration of the dorsal urethral surface. Blunt tenotomy scissors are used to enlarge the incision to 2.5 to 4 cm in length (approximately five to eight times the diameter of the urethra), to ensure sufficient urethral lumen size after healing is complete. The incision appears excessive at first, but after complete healing of

the urethrostomy, the opening is approximately one-third to one-half the original length. Stay directly on midline with your scissors to reduce intraoperative and postoperative hemorrhage from cavernous periurethral tissue. Intraoperative hemorrhage is controlled with direct digital pressure. The caudal limit of the incision is chosen to ensure that the new urethral stoma will allow urine to be diverted directly ventral from the ischial arch (Fig. 28.7). Monofilament, nonabsorbable suture material (size 4–0 or 5–0) is selected for the urethrostomy because this material incites little inflammatory response and has minimal tissue drag. A taper-cut swaged-on needle is preferred to reduce the size of the needle tract through the cavernous tissue. In addition, this needle can be inserted through the skin without difficulty and is much less apt to cut friable urethral mucosa.

Sutures should appose the skin and urethral mucosa accurately, to avoid possible stricture formation. When excess tension is present, the surgeon should try to adduct the patient's rear limbs before attempting closure. A deep suture line should be placed from the subdermal layer to the tunica albuginea if additional tension relief is necessary before closure of the skin and urethra.

The needle is inserted in an outward direction from the urethral lumen to the skin for best apposition. The first suture is placed from the corner of the caudal urethral incision to the corner of the caudal skin incision. Each suture pass comprises three tissue bites. The sequence begins with a 2-mm bite of urethral mucosa. Next, the needle is passed through a 2-mm bite of fibrous tunica albuginea and, finally a 2- to 3-mm split-thickness bite of skin (Fig. 28.8). A simple continuous suture line is used, with tissue bites 2 to 3 mm apart beginning caudally and working cranially (Fig. 28.9). The urethral mucosa and skin margins are grasped and manipulated to avoid excessive inflammation, which can lead to dehiscence and stricture. The urethral mucosa and skin are approximated without gapping. The suture line should not be tight, and each suture pass should have even tension. The sur-

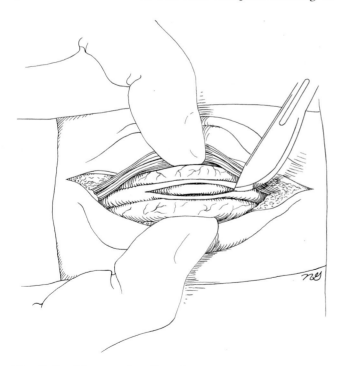

Fig. 28.7. The ventral midline of the urethra is incised for 2.5 to 4 cm. The incision extends far enough caudally to ensure that direct ventral urine drainage can occur from the level of the ischial arch.

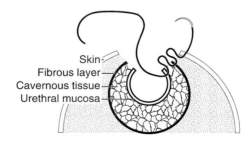

Fig. 28.8. Three-needle bite sequence. The needle is first inserted through the urethral mucosa, followed by the tunica albuginea, and split-thickness skin. The incised cavernous tissue is sealed between the urethral mucosa and the tunica albuginea.

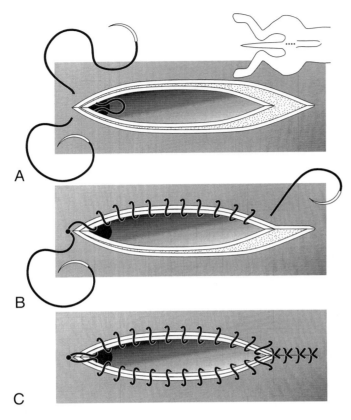

Fig. 28.9. The urethral mucosa is sutured to the skin, beginning at the caudal aspect of the wound and continuing cranially. **A.** The caudal suture is placed first. **B.** Subsequent sutures are placed to complete one side of the urethrostomy. **C.** Another continuous line on the opposite side of the incision completes the procedure. From Newton JD, Smeak DD. Simple continuous closure of canine scrotal urethrostomy: results in 20 dogs. J Am Anim Hosp Assoc 1996;32:531–534.

geon should excise any redundant skin in the cranial aspect of the incision to create a cosmetic closure. If the cranial aspect of the skin incision extends beyond the urethral incision, it is closed with simple interrupted sutures.

Postoperative Care and Complications

The urethrostomy is protected from self-mutilation by placing an Elizabethan collar or side body brace on the patient as soon as the surgical procedure is completed. Generous amounts of petroleum jelly are spread on the skin around the incision once or twice daily until postoperative swelling is reduced (generally 5 days) to decrease urine scald. Topical anesthetic agents (5% Xylocaine ointment, Astra Pharmaceutical Products, Inc., Westborough, MA) may reduce straining resulting from painful urination during the first 3 days after surgery. Exercise is strictly limited because any episodes of excitement could lead to excessive hemor-

rhage from the urethrostomy. Dogs should be hospitalized for the first 2 days because mild postoperative hemorrhage is common during this time. Owners should be warned at the time of patient release that scrotal urethrostomy reduces, but does not completely eliminate, calculi obstruction of the urethra. The animal's urine voiding habits should be monitored indefinitely to identify early signs of obstruction.

Sutures are removed 10 to 12 days after the surgical procedure. Removal of a continuous suture line is more difficult than removal of simple interrupted sutures placed in this area. Migrating epithelium often partially covers exposed suture, and sedation is necessary to remove sutures without causing pain and trauma.

Swollen, bruised, and painful areas of skin surrounding the urethrostomy may signal leakage of urine into the subcutaneous tissues. Placement of an indwelling urinary catheter is indicated in these dogs for 3 to 5 days, or until the edges of the urethrostomy are sealed. In general, catheters should be avoided because they increase the risk of bacterial contamination and may increase the risk of stricture. Because this urethrostomy is created some distance from the urethral "sphincter" area (pelvic urethra), incontinence is not a problem postoperatively. Urethrostomy dehiscence is allowed to heal by second intention unless the caudal area is involved. Dehiscence involving the caudal aspect of the urethrostomy should be repaired primarily, without tension, using the materials and technique described previously.

Suggested Readings

Brown SG, Greiner TP. Surgery of the urethra of the dog. In: Bojrab MJ, ed. Current techniques in small animal surgery. Philadelphia: Lea & Febiger, 1975:228–237.

Bilbrey S, Birchard SJ, Smeak DD. Scrotal urethrostomy: a retrospective review of 38 dogs (1973–1988). J Am Anim Hosp Assoc 1991;27:560–564.

Evans HE, Christenson GC. Miller's anatomy of the dog. 2nd ed. Philadelphia: WB Saunders, 1979.

Newton JD, Smeak DD. Simple continuous closure of canine scrotal urethrostomy: results in 20 dogs. J Am Anim Hosp Assoc 1996;32:531–534.

Perineal Urethrostomy in the Cat

M. Joseph Bojrab &
Gheorghe M. Constantinescu

Feline urologic syndrome (FUS), a synonym for lower urinary tract disease in the feline, can result from various single, multiple and interacting, or unrelated etiologic factors. Factors implicated in the development of FUS are infectious agents such as viruses and bacteria, diet, and urachal anomalies, especially bladder diverticula.

Crystalluria is a common clinical finding in cats and is characterized by microscopic precipitates in the urine. The most prevalent crystal type is struvite (magnesium ammonium phosphate). In normal cats, these crystals are passed in the urine during normal micturition. Urine from cats with FUS contains crystals that coalesce with a matrix of mucus and debris, to form a macroscopic semisolid mass, or concretion. Crystal formation is enhanced in an alkaline pH and is inhibited in a more acidic pH.

Urethral obstruction has been associated with concretions and urethral plugs. Other causes of urethral obstruction are strictures, lesions of the prostate gland, and extraluminal masses that compress the urethral lumen. Obstruction of the urethra by plugs occurs commonly in male cats but infrequently in females. The explanation for this difference resides in the anatomic differences in urethral structure between the sexes. The urethra in the male cat is long and narrow, whereas it is short and wide in the female.

Crystals composing a concretion have razor-sharp edges, which protrude from the concretion margins. In the male cat, at the root of the penis just proximal to the bulbourethral glands, the urethral lumen diameter narrows, creating a funnel effect. As a concretion passes down the urethra, it may become lodged at this point. Initially, the cat can usually force a concretion through the penile urethra by straining. This action, however, forces the sharp edges of the crystals into the urethral mucosa, resulting in multiple microlacerations. This trauma results in hemorrhage, urethral inflammation, edema, and swelling, which decrease the urethral diameter even further. Passage of another concretion through the urethra results in an obstruction that cannot be dislodged by the animal. This situation requires emergency treatment to unblock the urethral obstruction.

Diagnosis

The diagnosis of FUS is based on history, clinical signs, and palpation of a large, firm, tense bladder. The history may include urination in unusual locations along with increased frequency in attempts to urinate. This increased frequency may be mistaken for tenesmus by the client. Frequent licking at the genital area and occasional hematuria may also be present. With progression of the condition, the cat may become depressed, listless, or comatose. Prolonged obstruction results in hyperkalemia, which can lead to cardiac irregularities and subsequent death.

Medical Treatment

The first step in emergency treatment of urethral obstruction is to relieve obstruction. This can be done by catheterization of the urethra, which in the severely depressed or comatose patient can be accomplished without the use of anesthetics. If attempts to dislodge the obstruction are likely to result in additional urethral damage or to induce urinary tract infection, pharmacologic restraint should be considered. The anesthetic of choice is one of the ultrashort-acting barbiturates such as thiopental sodium. Anesthetics must be given cautiously, because effective doses in patients with postrenal azotemia tend to be lower than in animals with normal renal function.

To relieve the obstruction, concretions lodged in the distal penis are first milked out by gently rolling the penis between the thumb and forefinger. Additionally, massaging the urethra through the animal's rectum may help to dislodge abdominal or pelvic urethral concretions. Voiding is then induced by gentle urinary bladder palpation. If urethral massage and bladder expression fail to dislodge the obstruction, retrograde urethral flushing is attempted to dislodge the concretion into the bladder by hydropropulsion.

The penis is exposed, washed, and a 3.5-French open-ended tomcat catheter, lubricated with a sterile gel, is placed into the distal urethra. Once the catheter has been placed, the prepuce is grasped digitally and is retracted caudodorsally, so the urethra is parallel to the vertebral column. A 12-mL syringe containing sterile saline or lactated Ringer's solution is then connected to the catheter by an assistant. Subsequently, fluid is forced through the catheter while the catheter is gently advanced; the catheter should remain parallel to the spine during this maneuver. This technique should force the concretion into the bladder. The catheter is then advanced into the bladder, which is then repeatedly flushed and emptied to remove as much debris as possible. This catheter is then removed and is replaced with a 5-French catheter cut to a length of 6 cm. This catheter is positioned so the tip is just past the root of the penis. This reduces the possibility of ascending cystitis. The catheter is sutured in place and is removed in 5 days. If urethral patency cannot be restored by this method, one should suspect a mural or periurethral lesion with or without an associated urethral plug.

Antibiotics are given for 30 days; three different drugs are used for 10 days each. The cat's diet is changed to Prescription Diet Feline C/D (Hills Packing Company, Topeka, KS). This diet is low in magnesium and tends to acidify the urine, thus decreasing crystal formation. The food should be salted to increase fluid intake and to promote diuresis, to flush out urinary bacteria and precipitates. Instead of salting the food, the owner may administer a 1-g salt tablet orally once a day. If obstruction recurs, perineal urethrostomy is indicated.

Perineal Urethrostomy

Preoperative Considerations

Cats who have had urinary tract obstruction are poor anesthetic risks. Diuresis after unblocking is indicated. Induction of anesthesia with an ultrashort-acting barbiturate followed by maintenance with a gas anesthetic is recommended.

Surgical Technique

The animal is prepared for aseptic surgery. The hair is clipped from the entire perineal area including the base of the tail. A pursestring suture is placed in the anus, and a 3.5-French open-ended tomcat catheter is placed. The animal is positioned on the surgery table in ventral recumbency with the hind legs draped over the end of a titled table. The tail is taped up over the dorsal midline of the back, and the genital area is draped.

An elliptic incision starting halfway between the anus and scrotum is made around the scrotum and prepuce (Fig. 28.10). If the animal is sexually intact,

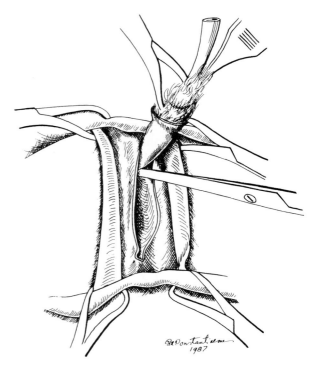

Fig. 28.11. The penis and prepuce are retracted dorsally, and ventral dissection is begun.

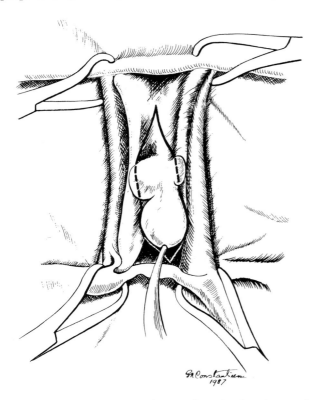

Fig. 28.10. After the perineal area is draped and a urinary catheter is placed, an elliptic incision is made around the scrotum and prepuce.

castration is performed. After the penis with accompanying prepuce and remaining scrotum are retracted dorsally, ventral dissection is begun with Metzenbaum scissors (Fig. 28.11). All preliminary dissection is done ventrally until the bilateral ischiocavernosus muscles are located and cut with scissors at their urethral attachments (Fig. 28.12). This technique frees the penis and allows the visualization of a ventral penile fibrous band from the pelvic diaphragm located on the midline between the penis and the ischial arch. This structure is then cut, further freeing the penis.

At this point, dorsal dissection is begun. All dorsal dissection is accomplished close to the urethra. Metzenbaum scissors are used to cut and bluntly dissect the attachments circumferentially, further freeing the urethra and allowing it to be retracted caudally. The dorsal white V-shaped uterus masculinus is now visible and is cut close to the urethra (Fig. 28.13). Care must be exercised during the entire dissection not to damage the rectum (dorsally) and the nerves that innervate the rectum and bladder neck. Such damage is avoided by keeping all dissection close to the urethra.

The dissected penis is grasped in the surgeon's left hand, with the index finger under the penile crus. A No. 10 scalpel is used to incise over the catheter on the dorsal midline of the urethra (Fig. 28.14). The incision is carried into the lumen. The incision is extended 1 cm cranial and 2 cm caudal to the crus of the penis. Extension of the pelvic urethral incision more than 1

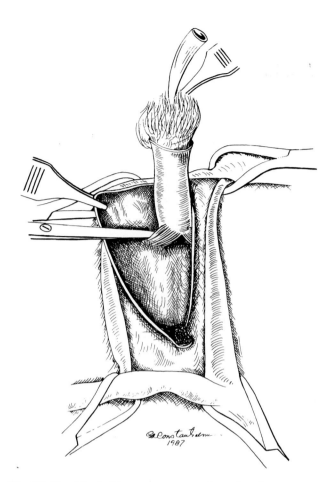

Fig. 28.12. The ischiocavernosus muscle is identified and is cut with scissors close to the penile attachment.

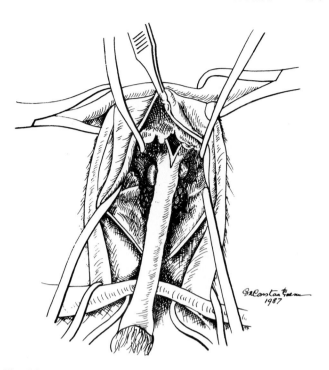

Fig. 28.13. Urethral dissection is completed by transecting the V-shaped uterus masculinus close to the urethra.

cm cranial to the crus leads to severe incisional invagination when the incision is sutured. A 1-cm incision in the pelvic urethra is adequate to provide the enlarged opening needed. The catheter is removed, and forceps are inserted into the pelvic urethra (Fig. 28.15). The incision is now ready for suturing.

We recommend using 4–0 Ethibond or Prolene (Ethicon, Inc., Somerville, NJ) with a swaged-on taper-cut needle for urethral suturing. The first suture is placed to approximate the most dorsal skin edges. The next suture, which begins the urethral suturing, picks up one skin edge and then passes through the dorsal roof of the urethra just cranial to the most cranial incision edge and then through the other skin edge (Fig. 28.16**A**). When this suture is tied, the roof of the urethra is pulled up to the skin edge, thus lifting the urethra to the surface. Suturing is continued down the skin incision on each side, including the cut edge of the urethral mucosa in each stitch (Fig. 28.16**B**). It is important also to include the edge of the corpus spongiosum (corpus cavernosum urethrae) within these urethral edge stitches to help control hemorrhage from the cut edge of the corpus spongiosum.

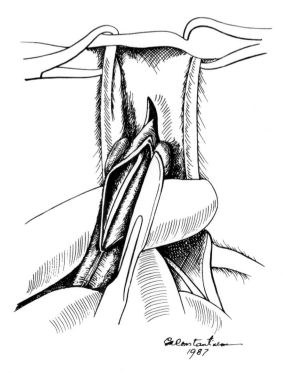

Fig. 28.14. The urethra is incised into the lumen with a No. 10 scalpel.

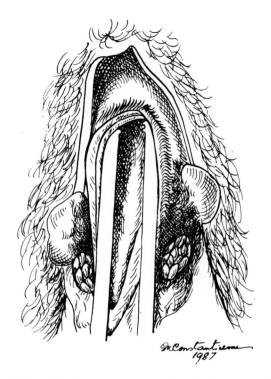

Fig. 28.15. After the incision is completed, the catheter is removed, and forceps are inserted into the pelvic urethra.

After both sides of the skin incision have been sutured, the penis is cut off with scissors (Fig. 28.17**A**) at the level of the caudal urethral incision. The cut end (Fig. 28.17**B**) is sutured as shown in Figure 28.18. This helps to seal the cut end of the corpus cavernosum penis and eliminates much of the excessive postoperative hemorrhage often encountered with this surgical procedure. The final sutures are placed approximating the caudal skin edges (Fig. 28.19). The wide end of the tomcat catheter is cut (approximately 2.5 cm), inserted into the new urethral opening, and sutured to the skin on each side (see Fig. 28.19).

Postoperative Care

The pursestring suture in the anus is removed. An Elizabethan collar is placed on the cat to prevent licking of the incision. The same medical therapy as outlined previously is begun. The collar is removed on the fifth postoperative day. The sutures and Elizabethan collar are removed on the tenth postoperative day.

The animal can be sent home during much of this postoperative period because urinary control is maintained even with the catheter, which is short and does not enter the bladder, in place. Owners must be in-

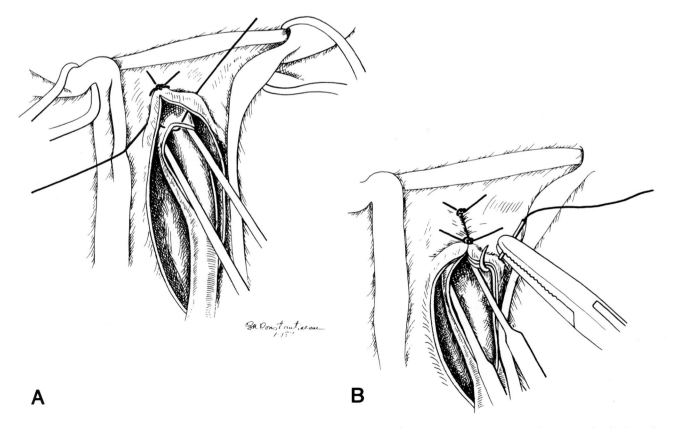

A **B**

Fig. 28.16. **A.** The first suture approximates the dorsal skin edges; then the first urethral suture is placed, engaging both skin edges and the pelvic urethral roof. **B.** Urethral suturing continues down the skin incision on each side.

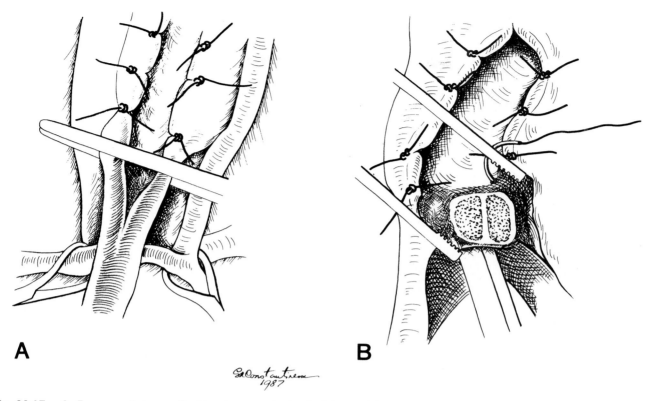

A

B

Fig. 28.17. **A.** Excess penis is cut off with scissors at the level of the caudal incision. **B.** The cut end of the penis is shown, revealing the corpus cavernosum penis.

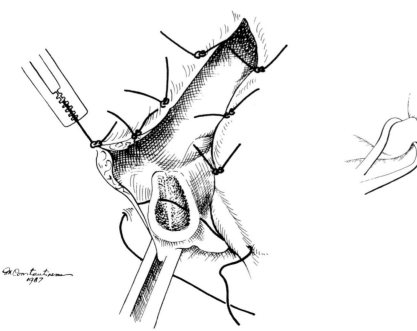

Fig. 28.18. The exposed cut surface of the corpus cavernosum penis is sutured.

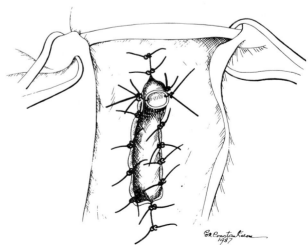

Fig. 28.19. After suturing of the incision is completed, a 2.5-cm segment of catheter is sutured into the urethrostomy opening.

structed not to allow the cat to go outside while the sutures are still in place and to place shredded papers in the cat's litter box, so litter will not stick to, contaminate, and irritate the incision.

Complications

The major complications of perineal urethrostomy are postoperative hemorrhage, subcutaneous urine leakage, infections, strictures, fecal and urinary incontinence, and rectal prolapse. Hemorrhage can be greatly reduced by taking care to include the cavernous tissue in the skin sutures. Infections can be decreased by eliminating postoperative contamination of the incision with litter and licking and by use of prophylactic antibiotics. Strictures can be prevented by adequate freeing of the urethra, to eliminate inpulling and suture line tension.

Urethroplasty for Stricture After Perineal Urethrostomy

Cats with urethrostomy stenosis present with stranguria producing only scanty urine and a palpably full bladder. If the stricture is due to improper dissection in the original surgical procedure (i.e., failure to transect ligaments and muscle attachments and free the urethra) or to failure to open the urethra properly, then the operation should be redone. If the original urethrostomy was done properly and a stricture subsequently occurred, a urethroplasty is performed.

The area around the stricture is clipped and prepared for surgery. The opening is located. The surgeon should use a 10× loupe to aid in visualization during surgery. A procedure similar to that for anal stricture (see Chap. 15) is used. Four cuts (dorsal, ventral, left lateral, and right lateral) are made with a No. 15 scalpel. Each cut incises the skin and underlying urethral mucosa. As each cut is made, the incisions open and form a diamond shape. The incisions are then sutured with 5–0 polydioxanone in the opposite direction in a manner similar to that shown in Figure 15.33. This technique alleviates the stricture.

Management of Urethral Trauma

Jamie R. Bellah

Blunt abdominal trauma and traumatic displacement of bone fragments, especially pubic fragments, can lacerate the membranous urethra (1). Urethral injuries from other sources are less common but include gunshots, bite wounds, and iatrogenic trauma. Absence of skeletal injury does not preclude urethral injury. Traumatic urethral injury usually occurs in male dogs because the postprostatic pelvic urethra is fixed at the greater ischiatic notch.

Diagnosis

Urethral injury is suspected when dysuria or anuria is observed. Hemorrhage from the urethral opening or hematuria, usually at the first portion of the urine stream, may be noted soon after injury. Urethral trauma is not excluded on the basis of an animal's ability to void urine, however. Animals with urethral rupture may be depressed and anorexic, and periurethral urine leakage may cause pyrexia and perineal or inguinal bruising and swelling. A distended urinary bladder may be palpable. Proximal urethral lacerations or rupture may result in uroperitoneum, and clinical signs mimic those of a ruptured urinary bladder. Urine leakage may be detected from open wounds in the region of the pelvic cavity.

Suspicion of urethral injury should be evaluated initially by positive-contrast urethrography using a water-soluble organic iodide preparation. Injection of air is avoided because it is difficult to delineate the site of urethral injury after air dissects periurethrally. Extravasation of contrast material occurs with both urethral laceration and urethral rupture, but in the latter instance, contrast material usually does not pass proximal to the complete tear. Animals with proximal urethral trauma should also be evaluated by intravenous pyelography because concomitant ureteral injury may present.

Surgical Techniques

Management of urethral injuries depends on the type of injury sustained and on the overall health of the animal. Uroperitoneum and its systemic metabolic effects must be resolved before lengthy surgical intervention. If uroperitoneum is present, its effects are resolved by urine diversion and intravenous fluid therapy to alleviate dehydration, acidemia, and hyperkalemia. Gentle catheterization of the urethra may be accomplished, depending on the site of the urethral laceration, but often the catheter tip finds the urethral defect and cannot be passed successfully. Urine can be diverted by percutaneous placement of a prepubic drainage catheter (Stamey catheter) or by insertion of a cystostomy tube (Foley catheter). Both techniques require sedation and (narcoleptic) local anesthesia unless the animal is moribund. Abdominal drains may be necessary if more proximal urinary tract injury does

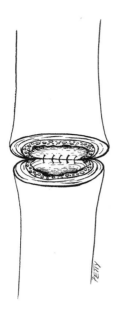

Fig. 28.20. Anastomosis of the urethra requires accurate apposition of the urethral mucosa. Failure to do so results in stricture and dysuria.

not allow urine diversion by the aforementioned techniques.

Definitive surgical treatment of urethral injuries requires careful preparation because often the site of injury is difficult to access (postprostatic rupture). Lacerations may be managed solely by urethral stenting if a catheter can be successfully manipulated into the urinary bladder, and it may need to remain in place for 7 to 10 days. Surgical correction of urethral rupture often requires pubic osteotomy to expose the severed urethra adequately. Sufficient exposure so debridement and precise anatomic anastomosis are feasible cannot be overly stressed. After debridement, simple interrupted sutures of absorbable material are used to perform the anastomosis over a urethral stent, with the knots outside the lumen of the urethra (Fig. 28.20). The urethral mucosa must be anatomically apposed or granulation tissue will be produced and contract the anastomosis, resulting in stricture despite the presence of a stent. Suture material appropriate for urethral anastomosis includes polydioxanone, polyglyconate (Maxon), and Monocryl. Monocryl maintains good tensile strength yet is absorbed more quickly. Nonabsorbable monofilament sutures such as nylon and polypropylene are also acceptable. Urine diversion is accomplished by cystostomy, and the urethral stent remains to support the anastomosis and to divert urine away from the urethral wound. The urethral stent should be large enough to maintain lumen size, but it should not be so large that it causes excessive pressure or tension on the anastomosis. If a large segment of urethra must be debrided, a permanent urine diversion procedure must be performed. Antepubic urethrostomy or extrapelvic urethral anastomosis may be done.

Postoperative Care

Postoperative management of patients with urethral trauma and obstruction is intensive. Management of pain is often required for 12 to 24 hours. Animals must be restrained from prematurely removing urethral stents and cystostomy tubes. This restraint may require Elizabethan collars, side braces, wire muzzles, and, in some instances, tranquilization. Prolonged catheterization (4 days or longer) often results in urinary tract infection, and periodic culture and sensitivity screening are important to avert a serious ascending infection. Proper use and care of closed urine drainage systems are mandatory. When urethral stents are removed, urine culture and sensitivity testing are done.

Urethral stents may be pulled when urothelium has bridged the urethral defect, as early as 5 days after repair. Careful injection of contrast material is done when contrast urethrograms are repeated, so the urethral wound is not disrupted. Difficult anastomoses when repair is tenuous (or unsutured defects) may require urethral stenting for as long as 14 to 21 days.

The most common complication of urethral trauma is stricture. Stricture may occur early, resulting from dehiscence of the anastomosis or a technically poor repair, caused by a fibrous scar that occludes the urethral lumen. Stricture may also occur months after surgery or conservative management if contraction of periurethral scar tissue results in stenosis of the urethral lumen. Correction of urethral stricture may require resection and anastomosis or a urinary diversion procedure. Distal strictures may be resolved by scrotal urethrostomy.

Reference

Bellah JR. Problems of the urethra. Probl Vet Med 1989:1;17.

Surgical Treatment of Urethral Prolapse in Male Dogs

Stephen J. Birchard

Prolapse of the urethral mucosa is a rare condition that occurs in male dogs. Young, intact, brachycephalic dogs, such as bulldogs or Boston terriers, are most commonly affected. The cause of the prolapse in most cases is unknown, but it may be related to excessive sexual excitement or underlying urogenital disorders such as urethritis or urethral calculi. Some authors believe that the relationship between brachycephalic breeds and urethral prolapse may be due to abnormal urethral development or increased abdominal pressure secondary to the upper airway obstruction typical of these breeds (1). Increased abdominal pressure could impair venous return and subsequently could cause chronic engorgement of the corpus spongiosum tissue surrounding the distal urethra (1). Further clinical studies are needed to elucidate the etiology of this disorder further.

Clinical signs of prolapsed urethra are bleeding from the prepuce, discomfort, and stranguria. Affected dogs may show excessive licking of the penis. Examination of the penis by extruding it from the prepuce reveals the protruding mucosa as a characteristic round, donut-shaped mass at the tip of the penis. The prolapsed mucosa is bright red to dark purple. A urethral catheter can be passed through the center of the tissue. The differential diagnosis includes other types of penile masses such as transmissible venereal tumors.

Preoperative Considerations

Dogs with urethral prolapse should be thoroughly examined and evaluated for underlying urogenital disease or other disorders. Urethral catheterization should be performed to evaluate for urethral lumen patency and other possible problems such as calculi. A rectal examination should be performed to ensure that the pelvic urethra feels normal. Urinalysis and urine culture should be performed to rule out bacterial infection of the urinary tract. Plain film abdominal radiographs should be obtained to evaluate the kidneys, urinary bladder, and prostate gland; positive-contrast studies can be done if indicated. Ultrasonography of any or all of the urogenital structures may also be helpful if indicated.

Because urethral prolapse occurs predominately in intact male dogs and may be related to sexual excitement, castration should be recommended to help prevent recurrence. Although medical approaches to treatment have been described (1), surgical resection of the prolapsed mucosal tissue is the best treatment in my experience. Simple reduction of the tissue is unlikely to result in long-term resolution of the problem.

Surgical Technique

The animal is anesthetized and placed in dorsal recumbency. The prepuce and surrounding area are clipped and aseptically prepared. The penis and interior of the

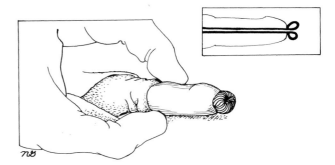

Fig. 28.21. Extrusion of the penis reveals the prolapsed mucosa.

prepuce are also gently scrubbed and irrigated with antiseptic solution. The surgical site is draped, and the penis is extruded either by using an assistant's fingers or by placing a Penrose drain around the caudal aspect of the penis to hold the prepuce caudally (Fig. 28.21).

A lubricated, sterile urinary catheter is passed into the urethra. A 180° incision is made at the base of the prolapsed mucosa, as close to the penile tunic as possible. The mucosa is not initially completely excised all the way around the urethral lumen because this will result in retraction of the mucosa and difficulty in suturing (Fig. 28.22). The incised mucosa is then sutured to the penile tunic with 4–0 or 5–0 polyglactin 910 (Vicryl) or polypropylene in a simple interrupted pattern. Sutures are placed about 2 to 3 mm apart.

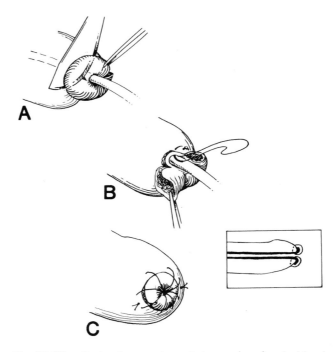

Fig. 28.22. **A.** A urinary catheter is inserted, and an incision is made at the base of the prolapsed mucosa. **B.** The prolapsed mucosa is partially resected, and the urethral mucosa is sutured to the penile mucosa in a simple continuous pattern. **C.** After resection and anastomosis are completed, the catheter is removed.

Care is taken to handle the healthy mucosa gently and to avoid excessive manipulation with thumb forceps. Fine-toothed thumb forceps, such as DeBakey forceps, are recommended. After the initial sutures are placed, the remainder of the prolapsed mucosa is resected and then sutured. The resected tissue is submitted for histopathologic examination if a disorder other than urethral prolapse is suspected.

Postoperative Care

The urinary catheter is removed after the procedure. An Elizabethan collar is placed on the dog to prevent licking of the surgical site. Intermittent bleeding from the penis may persist postoperatively for a few days. Tranquilization with acepromazine (0.2 mg/kg subcutaneously or intramuscularly, not exceeding a total dose of 4 mg) often is beneficial in reducing bleeding. Exercise is limited for 7 to 10 days to leash walking only. Treatment of underlying urinary problems, such as cystitis or prostatitis, should also be treated appropriately.

Prognosis for these animals is usually good. Urethral prolapse recurs in rare cases. Treatment is to repeat the resection as before. Penile amputation combined with scrotal urethrostomy may be necessary in the unusual patient that does not respond to repeated resection of the prolapsed tissue.

Suggested Readings

Hopson HP, Heller RA. Surgical correction of prolapse of the male urethra. Vet Med Small Anim Clin 1971;66:1177.

Osborne CA, Sanderson SL. Medical management of urethral prolapse in male dogs. In: Bonagura JD, Kirk RW, eds. Current veterinary therapy XII. Philadelphia: WB Saunders, 1995:1027–1029.

Sinibaldi KR, Green RW. Surgical correction of prolapse of the male urethra in three English bulldogs. J Am Anim Hosp Assoc 1973;9:450.

Smith CW. Surgical diseases of the urethra. In: Slatter DH, ed. Textbook of small animal surgery. 2nd ed. Philadelphia: WB Saunders, 1993;1462–1473.

29

PROSTATE GLAND

Surgery of the Prostate

Clarence A. Rawlings

Prostate disease includes hyperplasia, infection, cysts, abscesses, and cancer. Severe diseases of cysts, abscesses, and cancer are treated by excisional and partial prostatectomies. All prostatic disease, except cancer, can be prevented by castration during the first year of life. Castration, as a treatment of prostatic disease, reduces hyperplasia and the potential for persistent infections. Despite castration, prostatic abscesses can persist and present later as clinical problems. When prostatic disease develops, castration is recommended in all patients except those with prostatic cancer. The terminal prognosis for prostatic cancer mandates an attempt to early diagnosis.

Prostatic abscesses and cysts are difficult to treat. Surgery is required, and treatment is frequently complicated by disease recurrence, incontinence, infection, sepsis, and even death. Treatments initially attempted for abscesses and cysts included extra-abdominal drainage by Penrose drains or marsupialization. Early complications of these drainage procedures included sepsis in one-third of patients and death in one-fifth. The remainder of these dogs had transient improvement, but abscessation recurred in nearly one-fifth and incontinence in one-fourth of the dogs. To reduce the postoperative complications associated with prostatic tissue as a septic focus and mediator of infection, excisional prostatectomy was performed to remove all prostatic tissue. Although excisional prostatectomy reduced the incidence of early postoperative sepsis and eliminated recurrence, over 90% of dogs with excised diseased prostates also developed incontinence.

I prefer to treat most patients with abscesses and cysts by castration and partial prostatectomy using an ultrasonic aspirator. This technique eliminates nearly all the prostatic tissue while preserving the urethra and most nerves. Closed-suction drains have been successfully used to drain noninfected cysts, such as those with vascular and lymphatic drainage problems in perineal hernia. These dogs should be castrated. Many patients with abscesses and cysts appear to be adequately treated using peritoneal omentalization. All fluid-filled pockets must be explored and adequately drained. Before omentalization of paraprostatic cysts, the cysts should be excised as much as possible without damaging the urethra or the neurovascular supply.

Diagnosis

Diagnostic studies are designed to establish the anatomic distribution and histologic type of disease, to characterize the systemic response to the prostatic disease, to identify coexistent problems, to identify infections, and to characterize incontinence and outflow obstruction. The presenting complaints vary with the severity and type of disease. Tenesmus can be produced by any prostatic enlargement, that is, by hyperplasia, cyst, abscess, and neoplasia. Urethral obstruction is most typical of cancer, but it may occur in patients with cysts, abscesses, and hyperplasia. Incontinence is common in severe prostatic disease. Urethral discharge can be produced by nearly any prostatic disease with an opening into the prostatic urethra. Persistent urinary tract infections are frequently related to prostatic infections, particularly abscesses and infected cysts. Abdominal masses can be produced by cysts and abscesses. Many systemic responses develop in response to prostatic disease.

The size and character of the prostate should be determined by physical examination, including combined rectal and abdominal palpation, radiography, and ultrasonography. Contrast studies, especially retrograde urethrography, can be useful to identify the urethra, bladder, and prostate. Cystic structures as seen with an ultrasonogram have a more serious prognosis than hypertrophy, especially if a urinary tract infection is present. Cytologic and bacterial cultures can be obtained by sampling the urethral discharge, by semen ejaculation, by prostatic massage, by traumatic catheterization, or by direct sampling by needle aspiration or use of a larger biopsy needle. Placement of a needle into the prostate can be facilitated by ultrasonography or palpation. Care must be taken in placing a large-bore needle into a fluid-filled pocket of an infected prostate gland.

Most dogs with severe prostate disease do not urinate normally. Incontinence is common and frequently worsens after surgery. Even dogs that have undergone only a biopsy have dribbled urine after surgery, probably as a result of disease progression. Although obstruction in the absence of cancer is commonly thought to be infrequent, obstruction does occur and may be associated with calculi and strictures unrelated to cancer. Detrusor instability can develop in dogs with prostatic disease. A urethral pressure profile can identify decreased urethral pressures, which are common in dogs with prostatic disease, and a cystometrogram can identify an inability to develop a detrusor response or an irritable bladder. If incontinence persists after surgery, medical treatment can be attempted for each of these conditions.

Preoperative Care

Dogs with prostatic infections, especially those with abscesses, frequently become septic and develop toxic shock. Diagnosis is based on physical examination, urinalysis, complete blood and platelet counts, and serum chemistry profile, particularly liver enzymes, glucose, and albumin. Perioperative antibiotics must be given, preferably based on culture results. Although *Escherichia coli* is the most common organism isolated in bacterial prostatitis, some dogs have already been treated with long-term antibiotics and have developed resistant infections. Septic dogs, without culture results, are started on a combination of clindamycin and enrofloxacin. Measures to prevent and treat shock must be done and include fluid support, blockers of ischemia and reperfusion injury, and cardiotonic drugs (dopamine or dobutamine). Hypovolemia and hypotension must be treated by large volumes of intravenous fluids. If the albumin and total solids are low, plasma, hetastarch, or dextrans should be considered. Blockers commonly include dexamethasone (2 mg/kg intravenously), flunixin (1 mg/kg intravenously), and deferoxamine (20 to 40 mg/kg intramuscularly or slowly intravenously). Monitoring must include either indirect or direct arterial blood pressure. The anesthetic regimen should be based on the patient's disease status. Finally, surgery must be both expeditious and accurate to reduce the spread of sepsis.

Surgical Techniques

Excisional Prostatectomy

Excisional prostatectomy is used to treat cancer. This treatment is usually palliative, but it can be effective in extending the patient's normal life for several months because transitional cell carcinomas usually grow slowly. Another treatment option for proximal urethral cancer is excision of the lower urinary tract and implantation of the ureters into the colon. This produces ascending renal infections. Dogs with neoplastic urethral obstruction can be successfully managed for months by a cystostomy tube. Neither medical therapy nor radiation treatment provides significant benefits in patients with prostatic cancer. Urethral stents can provide temporary relief of urethral obstruction. Prostatectomy also can successfully cure prostatic abscesses and cysts, but the high rate of incontinence makes this procedure less desirable than partial prostatectomy or peritoneal omentalization.

Incisional biopsies are done by cutting deeply into the prostatic gland and then placing deep mattress sutures into the capsule to produce hemostasis (Fig. 29.1). The prostate is approached by a midline laparotomy (Fig. 29.2**A**). The periprostatic fat is incised on the ventral midline and is reflected laterally (Fig. 29.2**B**). An excisional prostatectomy requires dorsal dissection. Before prostatic surgery, a temporary tourniquet is placed about the distal aorta, just cranial to its bifurcation into the external iliac arteries. After placement of a urethral catheter, a retraction suture is placed around the urethra caudal to the prostate. Caudal dissection is facilitated by cranial incision of the ventral ligament of the penis. The prostate is rotated to ligate vessels close to the prostatic capsule and to ligate the vas deferens. The surgeon attempts to preserve the caudal vesical artery bilaterally and to preserve much of the urethra, both on the side of the neck and distally. Prostate tissue or fluid should be cultured. Multiple biopsy specimens are taken from the prostate and sublumbar lymph nodes. Neoplastic tissue must be excised, and this can require extensive urethral resection. Retraction sutures in the urethra caudal to the prostate can reduce traction problems. The urethra is transected cranial (Fig. 29.2**C**) and caudal to the prostate (Fig. 29.2**D**). The prostate is removed, and the urethral catheter is redirected into the bladder. The urethra is anastomosed with interrupted sutures using an absorbable monofilament synthetic

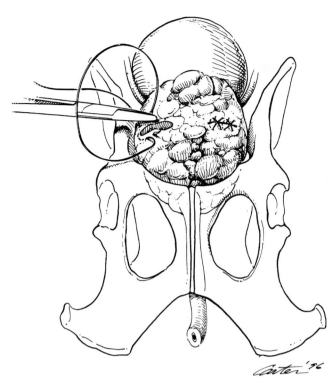

Fig. 29.1. Incisional biopsies are performed through a ventral midline laparotomy. Multiple biopsy specimens should be obtained, with each sample at least 1 cm wide and 2 cm deep. After each biopsy specimen is taken, interrupted cruciate sutures are placed at least 5 mm from the biopsy margins. Hemostasis is achieved as the sutures are tightened.

suture material, usually of 4–0 or 5–0 size (Fig. 29.2**E**). Some urethras are thick enough that a second layer of sutures can be placed in muscle tissue. A cystostomy catheter is placed in addition to the urethral catheter to ensure that urine is diverted and that little tension is placed on the anastomosis (Fig. 29.2**F**). Both catheters are left in place for 1 week, and urine is collected by a closed system. The balloon of the cystostomy catheter is deflated, and the catheter is withdrawn 1 week after the surgical procedure. The urethral catheter is left in place for half a day and then is withdrawn.

Partial Prostatectomy

Partial prostatectomy is my preferred procedure for treatment of patients with prostatic cysts and abscesses, but it is contraindicated for cancer. The use of the ultrasonic surgical aspirator permits removal of up to 85% of the prostatic glandular tissue in addition to all cysts and abscesses. Because the remaining prostatic tissue is dorsal and close to the urethra, most of the urethral innervation and muscles appear to be left intact. Incontinence is much less frequent and severe after partial prostatectomy of dogs with severe cavitary

disease than before the surgical procedure or after excisional prostatectomy. As with excisional prostatectomy, castration should be performed.

The prostate is approached in the same fashion as previously described, except dorsal and lateral dissections are avoided or at least limited. After obtaining biopsy specimens and after placing the aortic tourniquet and retraction suture about the urethra caudal to the prostate, the surgeon incises poles of the prostate ventrally with electrocautery (Fig. 29.3**A**). The Cavitron Ultrasonic Surgical Aspirator (CUSA System 200 Macro-Dissector, Valleylab, Inc., Pfizer Hospital Products Group, Boulder, CO) is used to fragment, irrigate, emulsify, and aspirate approximately 85% of the glandular tissue (Fig. 29.3**B** and **C**). A catheter is placed within the urethra to identify and avoid damaging it. Urethral fistulas are identified by inflating the urethra with fluid (Fig. 29.3**D**). After glandular resection and excision of the ventral hemisphere of the capsule, the dorsal prostatic capsule is sutured on the ventral midline to form a cuff around the prostatic urethra (Fig. 29.3**E**). A urethral catheter is secured in place for decompression of the urinary bladder during the initial 18 postoperative hours.

Postoperative Care and Complications

Early complications of prostatic surgery include shock potentially leading to death, infection (sepsis), pain, and renal shutdown. Fluid support should be continued at greater than maintenance rates based on monitoring results of, initially, arterial blood pressure and, later, volume of diuresis. If shock develops, treatment must be aggressive. Urinary output is recorded, and the bladder is evaluated frequently to ensure that it remains decompressed. Urinary catheters are usually removed during the first 2 days after partial prostatectomy. For excisional prostatectomy, catheters are left for 1 week and require protection with side braces or Elizabethan collars. Antibiotics are continued. Pain medications are normally given at least during the initial 8 hours after surgery. Intensive care monitoring is critical for several hours postoperatively. In addition to monitoring of urine output, temperature, pulse, and respiration, and attitude, complete blood counts with platelet counts, blood urea nitrogen, albumin, glucose, and urinalysis should be performed. Liver enzymes are also useful to detect signs of sepsis and septic shock. In dogs with signs of sepsis, decreasing albumin concentrations indicate a need for plasma. Nutritional status should be documented by measuring food intake and body weight daily. No deaths have been reported in dogs treated by partial prostatectomy.

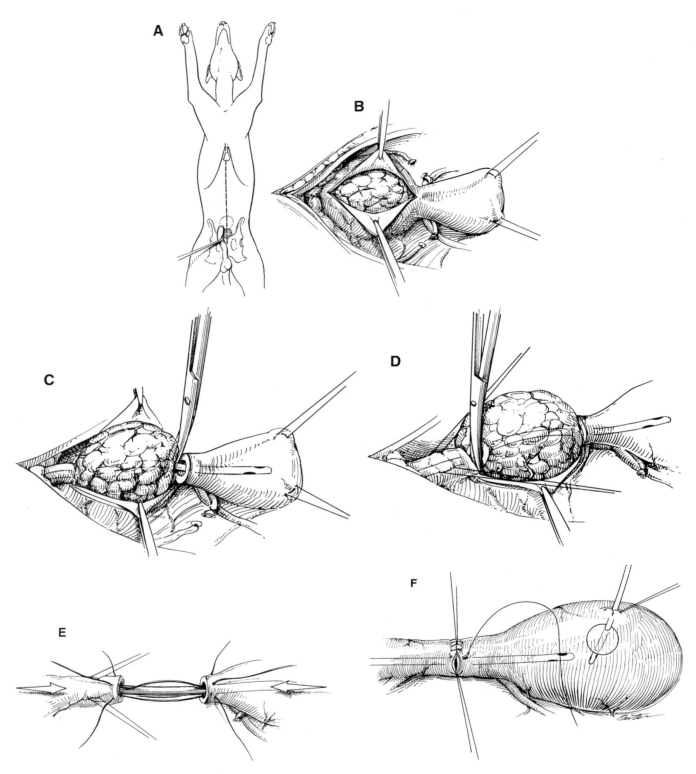

Fig. 29.2.   **A.** A ventral midline laparotomy is performed to approach the prostate for an excisional prostatectomy. Most prostate glands can be adequately exposed if the incision is extended caudally to the brim of the pubis. **B.** The periprostatic fat is incised on the midline and is reflected from the ventral and lateral surfaces. Hemostasis is improved if a tourniquet is placed about the aorta just cranial to its bifurcation. The vasa deferentia are ligated and divided, as are the prostatic vessels. Care must be taken to preserve the caudal vesical artery on both sides. Dissection should be close to the capsule, especially dorsal, cranial, and caudal to the prostate. A traction suture placed around the urethra, caudal to the prostate, and incision of the ventral ligament of the penis aid prostatic exposure. **C.** The urethra is transected cranial to the prostate. If excisional prostatectomy is done for cancer, the resection may need to be wider to ensure tumor-free margins. **D.** The urethra is transected caudal to the prostate. After the prostate is removed, the urethral catheter is replaced in the bladder. **E.** The urethral anastomosis is made with interrupted sutures of 4–0 or 5–0 absorbable synthetic monofilament material. The sutures are placed through all layers of the urethra, but additional sutures may be placed in a second pattern in some urethras. **F.** In addition to the urethral catheter, a cystostomy catheter is placed into the ventral region of the bladder. A double pursestring is used to secure the catheter.

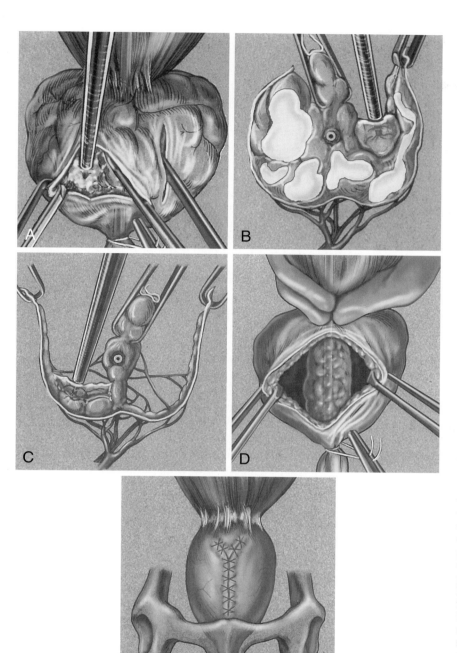

Fig. 29.3. **A.** Ventral view of a partial prostatectomy. After lymph node biopsy and placement of an aortic tourniquet, a 14- to 18-French urethral catheter is placed through a cystotomy, and a traction suture is placed about the urethral caudal to the prostate. Two parallel incisions are made into the ventral prostatic capsule using electrocautery. **B.** Transverse view. The ultrasonic aspirator is used to resect glandular tissue. All identifiable cystic pockets are entered. **C.** Transverse view. The surgeon attempts to remove 85% of the glandular tissue, including all abscess pockets. During ultrasonic aspiration, the urethral catheter and the dorsal capsule are frequently palpated and are avoided. **D.** Ventral view. The urethral catheter tip is withdrawn into the prostatic urethra, and the urethra is inflated by injecting saline. Urethral openings are identified and closed by suturing. **E.** Ventral view. Prostatic tissue between the paramedian incisions and ventral to the urethra and the excessive capsule are excised. The capsule is closed with interrupted sutures. An indwelling urethral catheter is left to decompress the bladder during the early postoperative period. From Vet Surg 1994;23:182–186.

Long-term complications of surgical treatment in dogs with severe prostatic disease include persistent infections and disease, as well as incontinence. Dogs usually urinate normally after partial prostatectomy, and fewer than 20% of dogs have even minor urinary control problems. After excisional prostatectomies, most dogs develop mild incontinence, and a few (approximately 10%) have continual dribbling of urine. Prostatectomy of normal dogs produces no decrease in urinary control function and only minor urodynamic changes, but the combination of prostatic disease and removal of the prostate increases incontinence. Some incontinent dogs with low urethral pressures have been successfully treated with phenylpropanolamine (1.5 mg/kg orally three times daily), and those with detrusor instability have been treated with oxybutynin (2.5 mg orally three times daily). Recurrent prostatic infections and disease should not occur when the prostate has been excised. Dogs with partial prostatectomy have not had recurrence during the first year after discharge from the hospital. Complications have been seen during hospitalization when a urethral to cyst fistula either persisted or recanalized. This fistula can been repaired during an additional surgery. Since a small amount of prostatic tissue is present and can be infected, at least two dogs have developed recurrent disease more than 1 year after surgery. The potential for urinary tract infection is high in any dog following surgery for major prostatic disease. These dogs must have regular urinalysis and cultures combined with aggressive antibiotic therapy. Intense surveillance and treatment should reduce problems with recurrent infections.

Acknowledgment

The illustrations by Dan Biesel and Kip Carter are appreciated.

Suggested Readings

Basinger RR, Rawlings CA. Surgical management of prostatic diseases. Compend Contin Educ Small Anim Pract 1987;9:993–1000.

Basinger RR, Rawlings CA, Barsanti JA, et al. Urodynamic alterations after prostatectomy in dogs without clinical disease. Vet Surg 1987;6:405–410.

Basinger RR, Rawlings CA, Barsanti JA, et al. Urodynamic alterations associated with clinical prostatic diseases and prostatic surgery in 23 dogs. J Am Anim Hosp Assoc 1989;25:385–392.

Cowan LA, Barsanti JA, Crowell W, et al. Effects of castration on chronic bacterial prostatitis in dogs. J Am Vet Med Assoc 1991;199:346–350.

Hardie EM, Barsanti JA, Rawlings CA. Complications of prostatic surgery. J Am Anim Hosp Assoc 1982;20:50–56.

Mullen HS, Mathieson DT, Scavelli TD. Results of surgery and postoperative complications in 92 dogs treated for prostatic abscessation by a multiple Penrose drain technique. J Am Anim Hosp Assoc 1990;26:369–379.

Rawlings CA, Crowell WA, Barsanti JA, et al. Intracapsular subtotal prostatectomy in normal dogs: use of an ultrasonic surgical aspirator. Vet Surg 1994;23:182–189.

Stone EA, Barsanti JA, eds. Urologic surgery of the dog and cat. Philadelphia: Lea & Febiger, 1992.

White RAS, Williams JM. Intracapsular prostatic omentalization: a new technique for managment of prostatic abscesses in dogs. Vet Surg 1995;24:390–395.

Use of Omentum in Prostatic Drainage

Richard A. S. White

Causes of Prostatic Abscesses and Cysts

Abscessation of the prostate gland in dogs is considered to result from an ascending bacterial infection that overcomes the normal urethral defense mechanisms and thereafter colonizes the prostatic parenchyma. A suppurative infection resulting in parenchymal microabscesses is thought to develop subsequently, but the precise mechanism by which these microabscesses coalesce into larger, loculated abscesses rather than remaining as diffuse prostatitis is unclear. The most commonly recovered organism is *Escherichia coli*, with *Staphylococcus* spp. and *Proteus* spp. occasionally encountered.

Discrete cysts involving the prostate gland are a well-defined but uncommon manifestation of prostatic disease. Two distinct categories of cyst are recognized, namely, *paraprostatic cysts* and *prostatic retention cysts*. Both types of cysts are capable of attaining considerable size and should be distinguished from the diffuse cystic changes that often occur in combination with benign prostatic hyperplasia. The cause of paraprostatic cysts has not been clearly established, and although investigators have suggested a congenital origin, the identity of the embryonic vestige from which they are suggested to arise has not been satisfactorily elucidated. Paraprostatic cysts have no structural communication with the prostate, urethra, or bladder. Prostatic retention cysts, however, are thought to develop as the result of obstruction of ducts within the parenchyma of the gland promoting the accumulation of prostatic secretions. Concurrent prostatic disease is always present, and this may include benign prostatic hyperplasia, squamous metaplasia, abscessation, or neoplasia.

Clinical Signs and Diagnosis

Dogs with *prostatic abscesses* are pyrexic and have signs of caudal abdominal pain on rectal and transabdominal palpation of the prostate gland. The prostate gland is invariably enlarged and may have a doughy feel when palpated. Many dogs have neutrophilia (white blood count higher than $17 \times 10^9/L$), but this is not a consistent feature of the disease. Alkaline phosphatase concentrations may be elevated in some patients. Radiography enables one to confirm the prostatic enlargement, but ultrasound imaging is necessary to demonstrate the characteristic loculation within the parenchyma that contains the slightly echodense purulent fluid. Fine-needle aspiration may be used to recover purulent material, but it should be performed with care to avoid the risk of peritonitis after this procedure.

Prostatic retention cysts are encountered mostly in large breed dogs, especially boxers. Signs of urinary dysfunction, including stranguria, dysuria, hematuria, and incontinence, are invariably seen. Palpation identifies a caudal abdominal mass. A presumptive diagnosis of prostatic cyst can be made by evaluation of survey abdominal radiographs and ultrasound examination of the prostate in all dogs. Mineralization of the cyst wall is evident in some dogs. Biopsy may be indicated because some retention cysts accompany prostatic neoplasia, but fine-needle aspiration should again be performed with care.

Conventional Drainage Strategies

Chronic parenchymal lesions of the prostate gland, most notably abscesses and discrete cysts, are difficult clinical entities to resolve consistently by means of medical or surgical therapy. Various surgical techniques have been described for the management of prostatic abscesses and cysts.

Abscesses

The use of antibiotic therapy, even in conjunction with castration, is notoriously ineffective in resolving prostatic abscessation because of its failure to achieve adequate therapeutic concentrations throughout the prostate. Previously described techniques for drainage or removal of abscesses include marsupialization of the abscess, local resection, subtotal prostatectomy, and excisional prostatectomy. Until recently, the most widely practiced technique was ventral drainage by means of dependent Penrose drains. All the foregoing techniques necessitate prolonged postoperative management, and long-term complications associated with these procedures include recurrent abscessation, chronic drainage after marsupialization, urinary incontinence, urinary tract infection, and the development of urethrocutaneous fistula.

Prostatic Retention Cysts

Marsupialization of prostatic cysts is a comparatively simple technique, but persistent discharge from the stoma, chronic urinary tract infection, and abscessation are recognized complications. Drainage and surgical resection of the cyst comprise a successful technique and should be regarded as the technique of choice for the management of paraprostatic cysts, for which the dissection is often uncomplicated. Many prostatic retention cysts, however, have extensive adhesions to the ureters, bladder neck, and prostate, and complete resection may increase the risk of postoperative incontinence or urinary retention resulting from neural or vascular compromise. Partial cyst resection may therefore be a preferable strategy to minimize the risk of incontinence, although this procedure may permit continued fluid secretion, redevelopment of the cyst, or formation of adhesions between the cyst remnant and other abdominal organs.

Omentum for Prostatic Drainage

The value of the omentum as an alternate source of vascularization and lymphatic supply in veterinary surgery is well established. Recognized applications include reconstruction of body wall deficits, filling of dead space, support for grafted tissue, reinforcement of gastrointestinal or urogenital repairs, and resolution of chronic wounds. The omentum is able to resolve bacterial contamination from perforated viscera and even can function in the presence of infection. The omentum can be used as a "physiologic drain" to resolve lesions of the prostatic parenchyma such as abscesses or to provide continued drainage of ongoing secretions from residual cystic tissue without merely walling them off from the abdominal cavity. Additionally, the omentum creates adhesions at the operative site, thereby minimizing the risk of visceral adhesion.

Intracapsular Prostatic Omentalization for Prostatic Abscesses

A caudal celiotomy extending from the umbilicus to the pubic brim is performed to permit adequate elevation of the prostate gland, which is then packed off from the remainder of the abdomen with moist laparotomy sponges. Stab incisions are made bilaterally in the lateral aspects of the prostate gland, and pus is removed by suction to minimize abdominal contamination. All abscess loculations within the parenchyma (Fig. 29.4) are explored and are broken down by digital exploration. The prostatic urethra is carefully preserved and can be identified by palpation of a previously placed urethral catheter. A Penrose drain may be temporarily placed around the prostatic urethra within the parenchyma to help elevate the gland and

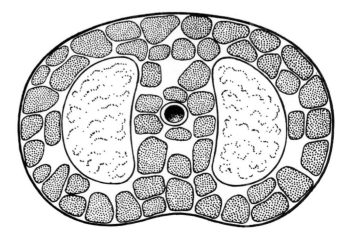

Fig. 29.4. Schematic representation of an abscessed prostate gland demonstrating abscess cavities before disruption and drainage. (The patient is in dorsal recumbency). From Vet Surg 1995;24:390–395.

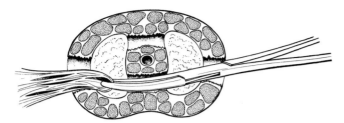

Fig. 29.5. Bilateral stab incisions are made into the abscess to permit drainage and digital disruption of the loculations within the cavities. The stab incisions are then enlarged by resection of the capsular tissue to permit the introduction of a leaf of omentum into the dorsal abscess cavity by means of forceps positioned through the contralateral capsulectomy wound. From Vet Surg 1995;24:390–395.

to facilitate irrigation of the abscess cavities with warm saline. The stab incisions are then enlarged by resection of the lateral capsular tissue. Artery or tissue forceps are introduced into one capsulectomy wound and are used to draw a leaf of omentum into the contralateral wound and through the dorsal abscess cavity (Fig. 29.5). The omentum is passed back through the ventral cavity, resulting in complete periurethral packing, to exit the prostate, and is then anchored to itself with absorbable mattress sutures outside the prostate gland (Fig. 29.6). The celiotomy wounds are closed routinely, and castration is performed. Dogs should receive broad-spectrum antibiotic therapy perioperatively, but this therapy does not need to be extended postoperatively unless complications occur, such as major contamination of the abdominal cavity before or during the surgical procedure.

Partial Resection and Omentalization for Prostatic Retention Cysts

A caudal celiotomy extending from the umbilicus to the pubic brim is performed. The cyst is identified (Fig.

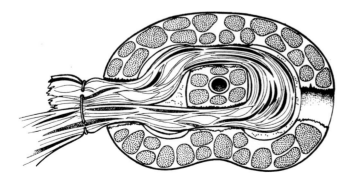

Fig. 29.6. The leaf of omentum is then returned through the ventral cavity of the abscess to complete the periurethral packing. The omentum is anchored to itself by means of horizontal mattress sutures using absorbable material. From Vet Surg 1995; 24:390–395.

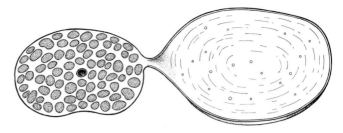

Fig. 29.7. Schematic illustration of a prostatic retention cyst in transverse section. The cyst wall develops as a dilatation of the prostatic parenchyma caused by the accumulation of secretions within the gland. From Vet Surg 1997;26:202–207.

29.7), and a single stab incision is made through the cyst wall. Complete drainage using suction to avoid contamination of the abdominal cavity is performed (Fig. 29.8), and the majority of the cyst wall is resected (Fig. 29.9). Extensive dissection of the cyst in the region of the bladder neck and prostate should be avoided, to minimize the risk of damaging nerves that control continence. Omentum is packed into the cyst remnant and is secured in place (Fig. 29.10) with mattress sutures of 2–0 absorbable suture material. The prostate gland should be carefully examined and palpated during the surgical procedure, and if neoplastic infiltration is suspected, an incisional biopsy should be performed. The celiotomy wounds are closed routinely, and castration is performed. Dogs should receive perioperative broad-spectrum antibiotics, which may need to be extended postoperatively if purulent debris is apparent in the cyst during the surgical procedure.

Postoperative Care and Complications

A significant advantage of omentalization drainage techniques for prostatic disease is that patients can normally be discharged from the hospital within 24 hours of the surgical procedure. As already indicated, prolonged antibiotic therapy is only necessary if complications are encountered.

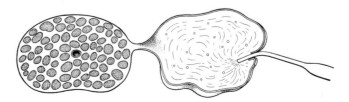

Fig. 29.8. The cyst is drained by a single stab incision into the lumen. Suction is used to minimize spillage of cyst contents into the abdominal cavity. From Vet Surg 1997;26:202–207.

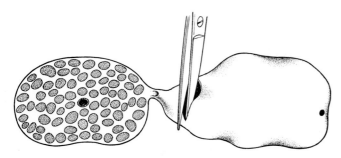

Fig. 29.9. After drainage, the cyst wall is partially resected. Extensive dissection about the bladder neck and prostate is avoided.

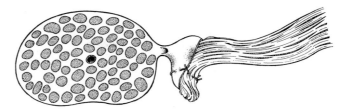

Fig. 29.10. After partial resection of the cyst wall, an omental pedicle is created to fill the residual prostatic cavity. The omentum is anchored in place with stay sutures. From Vet Surg 1997;26:202–207.

Abscesses may recur if insufficient omentum is packed into the abscess cavity. The surgeon should ensure that adequate lateral capsulectomy resections—normally sufficient to accommodate the easy entry of the forefinger into the abscess cavity—are performed to avoid this complication.

Urinary incontinence is a frequent presenting sign in patients with prostatic retention cysts, and this problem may persist even after successful omentalized drainage of the cyst. Therapy with phenylpropanolamine (1 mg/kg every 24 hours orally) to increase urethral sphincter tone may be appropriate in some of these patients. Urinary retention is less common, and the patient's urinary function should be monitored carefully during the first 24 hours after the surgical procedure.

Prognosis

Omentalized drainage has proved successful for the management of both prostatic abscesses and retention cysts. Compared with other drainage techniques, the level of surgical expertise required for successful omentalization is modest, hospitalization stays are brief, and postoperative complication rates are low.

Suggested Readings

Basinger RR, Rawlings CA, Barsanti JA, et al. Urodynamic alterations associated with clinical prostatic diseases and prostatic surgery in 23 dogs. J Am Anim Hosp Assoc 1989;25:385–392.

Gourley LG, Osborne CA. Marsupialization: a treatment for prostatic abscess in the dog. J Am Anim Hosp Assoc 1966;2:100–105.

Hardie EM, Barsanti JA, Rawlings CA. Complications of prostatic surgery. J Am Anim Hosp Assoc 1984;20:50–56.

Hardie EM, Stone EA, Spaudling KA, et al. Subtotal canine prostatectomy with neodymium yttrium–aluminium–garnet laser. Vet Surg 1990;19:348–355.

Hosgood G. The omentum—the forgotten organ: physiology and potential surgical applications in dogs and cats. Compend Contin Educ Pract Vet 1990;12:45–51.

Mullen HS, Matthiesen DT, Scavelli TD. Results of surgery and postoperative complications in 92 dogs treated for prostatic abscessation by a multiple Penrose drain technique. J Am Anim Hosp Assoc 1990;26:369–379.

Rawlings CA, Crowell WA, Barsanti JA, et al. Intracapsular subtotal prostatectomy in normal dogs: use of an ultrasonic surgical aspirator. Vet Surg 1994;23:182–189.

White RAS, Williams JM. Intra-capsular prostatic omentalization: a new technique for management of prostatic abscessation. Vet Surg 1995;24:390–395.

White RAS, Herrtage ME, Dennis R. The diagnosis and management of paraprostatic and prostatic retention cysts in the dog. J Small Anim Pract 1987;28:551–574.

30

UTERUS

Ovariohysterectomy

Roger B. Fingland

Indications

The most common indication for ovariohysterectomy is elective sterilization. Ovariohysterectomy is the treatment of choice for most uterine diseases including pyometra, uterine torsion, localized or diffuse cystic endometrial hyperplasia, uterine rupture, and uterine neoplasia (1). In a study of 1712 ovariohysterectomies in dogs, 82% were performed for elective sterilization, 18% for reproductive tract disease, and 7% as adjunctive therapy for mammary neoplasia (2). Ovariohysterectomy may be indicated for diabetic and epileptic animals to prevent hormonal changes that alter the effectiveness of medications.

Endogenous estrogen production plays a role in the etiology of spontaneous mammary tumors (3). Ovariohysterectomy before the first estrus provides a definitive protective factor, reducing the incidence of mammary neoplasia to 0.5% (1, 3). The risk factor is 8% when ovariohysterectomy is delayed until after one estrus, and after two or more estrus cycles, the risk rises to 26% (1, 3).

Ovariohysterectomy may be a justifiable adjuvant therapy for mammary neoplasia. Research on hormone receptors in canine mammary tumors is underway. Eventually, it may be possible to determine which dogs may respond to ovariohysterectomy at the time of mastectomy by analysis of specific tumor hormone receptors (3).

Surgical Anatomy

The ovaries, oviducts, and uterus are attached to the dorsolateral walls of the abdominal cavity and the lateral wall of the pelvic cavity by paired double folds of peritoneum called the right and left broad ligaments. Cranially, the broad ligament is attached by means of the suspensory ligament of the ovary (Fig. 30.1). The broad ligament is divided into three regions: the mesovarium, the mesosalpinx, and the mesometrium. The suspensory ligament runs from the ventral aspect of the ovary and mesosalpinx cranially and dorsally to the middle and ventral thirds of the last two ribs (3). The proper ligament is the caudal continuation of the suspensory ligament. The proper ligament attaches to the cranial end of the uterine horn. The round ligament of the uterus attaches to the cranial tip of the uterine horn and is a caudal continuation of the proper ligament. The round ligament extends caudally and ventrally in the broad ligament, and, in most bitches, it passes through the inguinal canal and terminates subcutaneously near the vulva (4).

The ovarian arteriovenous (AV) complex lies on the medial side of the broad ligament and extends from the aorta to the ovary. The distal two-thirds of the ovarian AV complex is convoluted, similar to the pampiniform plexus in males (2). The ovarian artery is less convoluted in cats (5). The ovarian artery supplies the ovary and the cranial portion of the uterine tube in the dog and cat. The arterial supply to the uterus in the nonpregnant dog and cat is relatively independent of the supply to the ovary. Small anastomoses in the broad ligament are present between branches of the ovarian artery and branches of the uterine artery (5).

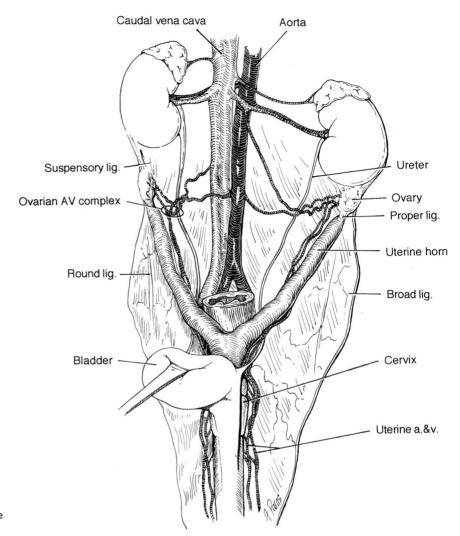

Fig. 30.1. The female canine reproductive tract.

Surgical Technique

The left ovarian vein drains into the left renal vein, and the right ovarian vein drains into the caudal vena cava. The uterine veins run in close association with the uterine arteries and terminate caudally into the internal iliac veins.

Surgical Technique

The urinary bladder should be manually expressed before ovariohysterectomy. A midline abdominal incision is made extending from the umbilicus to a point halfway between the umbilicus and the brim of the pubis in the dog. The incision begins approximately 1 cm caudal to the umbilicus in the cat and extends approximately 3 to 5 cm caudally. The abdominal incision must be carried further caudally in the cat to provide adequate exposure of the uterine body. A longer abdominal incision is required if the uterus is enlarged. The left uterine horn is located by using either an ovariohysterectomy (Snook) hook or the surgeon's index finger. A small hemostat may be placed on the proper ligament to aid in retraction of the ovary. The suspensory ligament is stretched or broken using the index finger (Fig. 30.2**A**). Tension must be directed caudally along the dorsal body wall rather than perpendicular to the incision to avoid tearing the ovarian AV complex. Separate ligation of the suspensory ligament is seldom necessary. The ovarian AV complex is located, and a "window" is made in the mesovarium immediately caudal to the complex (Fig. 30.2**B**). The ovarian AV complex is double clamped using Rochester–Carmalt hemostatic forceps (Fig. 30.3). The surgeon should maintain constant digital contact with the ovary when applying the first clamp to ensure that the entire ovary is removed. A third clamp is placed over the proper ligament between the ovary and uterine horn (Fig. 30.4). The pedicle is severed between the middle clamp and the ovary (Fig. 30.4). Alternately,

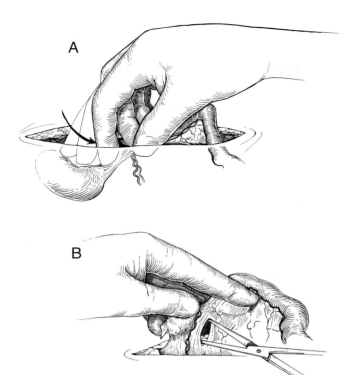

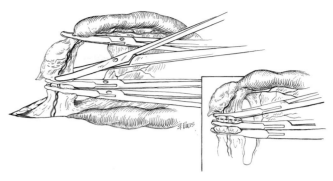

Fig. 30.4. The ovarian arteriovenous complex is transected between the ovary and the middle clamp. When all three clamps are placed proximal to the ovary (*inset*), the ovarian arteriovenous complex is transected between the middle clamp and the clamp closest to the ovary.

Fig. 30.2. Isolation of the left ovary. **A.** The ovary is grasped between the thumb and middle finger, and the suspensory ligament is stretched or broken with the index finger. Tension must be directed caudally along the dorsal body wall. **B.** A window is made in the mesovarium caudal to the ovarian arteriovenous complex.

the pedicle may be triple clamped (see Fig. 30.3, *inset*). When this technique is used, the pedicle is severed between the middle clamp and the clamp closest to the ovary (see Fig. 30.4, *inset*). Clamps should be placed on the ovarian pedicle as close to the ovary as possible to prevent accidental inclusion of the ureter.

Absorbable suture (e.g., chromic catgut) is preferred for all ligatures. A circumferential suture is loosely placed around the proximal clamp (Fig. 30.5). The clamp is removed while the circumferential suture is tightened so the circumferential suture lies in the groove of crushed tissue created by the clamp (Fig. 30.5, *inset*). A transfixation suture is placed between the circumferential suture and the cut end of the pedicle (Fig. 30.6). The pedicle is grasped (without grasping the ligature) with thumb forceps, the final clamp is released, and the pedicle is inspected for bleeding. If no bleeding occurs, the pedicle is replaced into the abdomen.

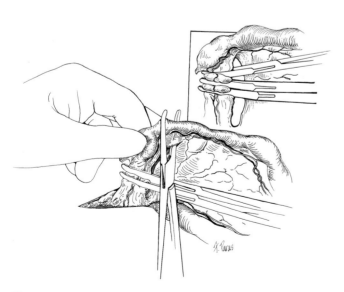

Fig. 30.3. Two clamps are placed on the ovarian arteriovenous complex proximal to the ovary, and a third clamp is placed over the proper ligament. Alternatively, all three clamps may be placed proximal to the ovary (*inset*).

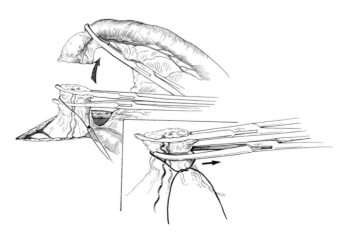

Fig. 30.5. A circumferential ligature is loosely placed around the most proximal clamp. The clamp is removed, and the ligature is tightened in the groove of crushed tissue created by the clamp (*inset*).

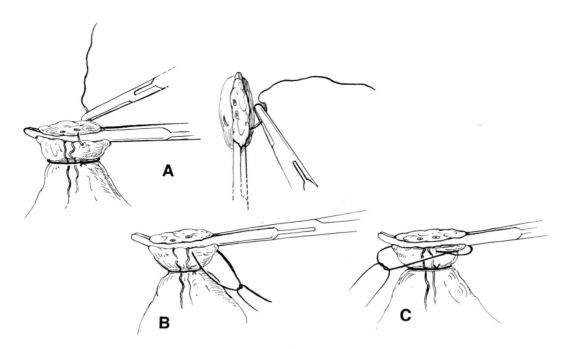

Fig. 30.6. A transfixation suture is placed between the circumferential suture and the cut edge of the ovarian arteriovenous complex. **A.** Approximately one-third of the width of the ovarian arteriovenous complex is included in the initial suture. **B.** The initial suture is tied. **C.** The ends of the suture are directed around the ovarian arteriovenous complex and are tied.

The right uterine horn is isolated by following the left uterine horn distally to the bifurcation. The ligation procedure is repeated on the right ovarian pedicle. A window is made in the broad ligament adjacent to the uterine artery and vein (Fig. 30.7A). The broad ligament is grasped and torn (Fig. 30.7**B** and **C**). Mass ligation of the broad and round ligament is seldom necessary; however, large vessels in the broad ligament should be ligated.

The uterine body is exteriorized, and the cervix is located. Various techniques may be used to ligate and divide the uterine body, depending on the size of the uterus and the surgeon's preference. The triple-clamp technique may be used when the uterine body is small, such as in cats and small dogs. Three clamps are placed immediately proximal to the cervix. Care must be taken when applying clamps to the uterine body because the clamps may cut rather than crush the tissue. The uterine body is severed between the middle clamp and the proximal clamp. The uterine arteries and veins are individually ligated between the distal clamp and the cervix. A circumferential suture is loosely placed around the distal clamp, the clamp is removed, and the suture is tightened in the groove of crushed tissue. A transfixation suture is placed between the circumferential suture and the remaining clamp. The remaining clamp is removed, and the uterine stump is evaluated for bleeding and replaced into the abdomen.

A second technique for ligation of the uterine body involves placement of bilateral transfixation sutures. The uterine body is exteriorized and retroflexed. Transfixation sutures that initially incorporate the uterine artery and vein and one-third the width of the uterine body are placed on either side of the uterine body (Fig. 30.8**A** and **B**). A clamp may be loosely placed proximal to the transfixation sutures to prevent backflow of blood after transection. The uterine body is severed between the clamp and the proximal transfixation suture (Fig. 30.8**C**). The uterine stump is evaluated for bleeding and is replaced into the abdomen. This technique is advantageous because clamps are not placed on the section of the uterine body that is ligated; therefore, the potential for cutting the tissue with the clamp is eliminated. I prefer the bilateral transfixation suture technique for routine elective ovariohysterectomy in dogs and cats.

A Parker–Kerr suture pattern may be used for ligation when the uterine body is greatly enlarged. The uterine arteries and veins should be ligated separately distal to the Parker–Kerr suture pattern.

The ovarian pedicles and uterine stump should be evaluated for bleeding before abdominal closure. The left ovarian pedicle is located by retracting the descending colon medially to expose the left paralumbar fossa. Retraction of the descending duodenum medially exposes the right paralumbar fossa and the right ovarian pedicle. The ovarian pedicles lie immediately caudal to the caudal pole of the kidneys. The uterine

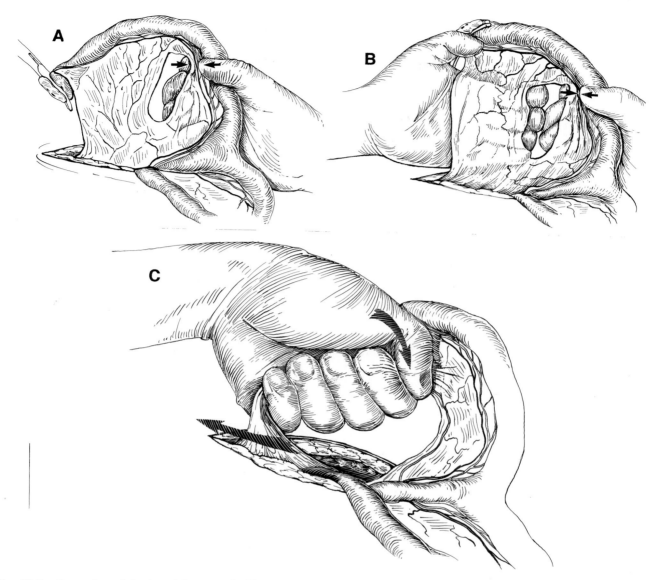

Fig. 30.7. Separation of the broad ligament. **A.** The uterine artery and vein are protected with the thumb and index finger, and a window is made in the broad ligament. **B.** The broad ligament is grasped. **C.** The broad ligament is torn. Large vessels should be individually ligated.

stump lies between the bladder and colon and is located by retroflexing the bladder. Sutures should not be grasped when evaluating the ovarian pedicles and uterine stump because excessive traction on the suture may cause it to loosen.

The abdominal incision is closed with either a simple interrupted suture pattern using absorbable suture or a simple continuous suture pattern using nonabsorbable (polypropylene or monofilament nylon) suture. Sutures should be placed in the external rectus sheath (6). It is not necessary to suture the internal rectus sheath or the peritoneum (6). The subcutaneous tissue and skin are closed routinely.

A flank approach for feline ovariohysterectomy has been suggested, but it is not recommended. Recovery of a dropped ovarian pedicle is problematic, and it may be difficult to expose the opposite ovary and the uterine bifurcation through this approach (7).

Complications and Sequelae

Hemorrhage

Intraoperative hemorrhage has been reported as the most common complication of ovariohysterectomy in dogs over 25 kg (8). Hemorrhage during ovariohyster-

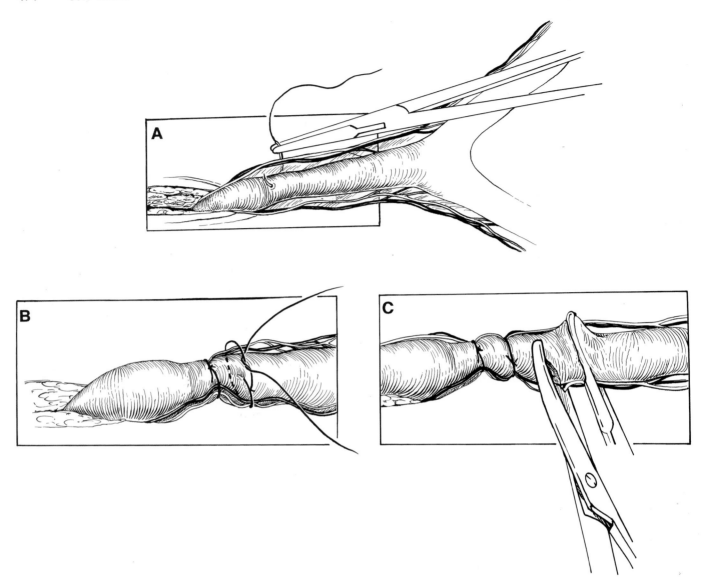

Fig. 30.8. Ligation of the uterine body. **A.** A transfixion suture is placed to include the left uterine artery and vein. **B.** A similar transfixion suture is placed to include the right uterine artery and vein. **C.** A clamp is placed across the uterine body proximal to the transfixion sutures, and the uterine body is transected.

ectomy may result from tearing of the ovarian AV complex while strumming the suspensory ligament. This complication may be avoided by carefully strumming the ligament as previously described. Intraoperative hemorrhage also may result from tearing of large vessels in the broad ligament, tearing of the uterine vessels by excessive traction on the uterine body, or accidental releasing of a clamp before placement of ligatures. Large vessels in the broad ligament should be individually ligated, and excessive traction on the uterine body should be avoided by lengthening the abdominal incision (1). Improperly placed sutures may result in intraoperative or postoperative hemorrhage. The ovarian pedicles and uterine stump should be dou-

ble ligated and evaluated for bleeding before abdominal closure.

Uterine Stump Pyometra

Uterine stump pyometra can occur if the entire uterine body or a portion of either uterine horn is not removed during ovariohysterectomy and the animal has elevated blood progesterone levels. The source of progesterone may be endogenous, from residual ovarian tissue, or exogenous, from progestational compounds used to treat dermatitis (1, 9). Uterine stump pyometra can be prevented by complete excision of the uterine horns and body.

Recurrent Estrus (Ovarian Remnant Syndrome)

Recurrent estrus usually results from functional residual ovarian tissue after incomplete ovariohysterectomy. Clinical signs associated with estrus and ovarian hormonal activity may be present (10). The hormonal effects may be delayed, depending on whether or not vascularity to the ovarian remnant has been maintained. Collateral circulation to the ovarian tissue may develop even though the ovarian AV complex has been ligated and transected (11). Treatment of recurrent estrus after ovariohysterectomy is surgical exploration and excision of residual ovarian tissue. Surgical exploration during estrus is preferable. Identification of an ovarian remnant on one side should not preclude inspection of the other ovarian site (10). Functional residual ovarian tissue is more commonly found on the right side (12). Residual ovarian tissue occasionally cannot be identified or palpated, and its presence is often made manifest by increased vascularity of the ovarian pedicle. All excised tissue should be submitted for histopathologic examination. A disproportionate number of cats that develop the ovarian remnant syndrome have been operated through a flank incision (10). Incomplete ovariectomy may be prevented by maintaining constant digital contact with the ovary during application of hemostatic clamps to the ovarian AV complex.

Ligation of Ureter

Accidental ligation of a ureter may occur during ligation of the uterine body or an ovarian AV complex (12). Ligation of a ureter results in hydronephrosis and may predispose to pyelonephritis. The ureter may be accidentally crushed or ligated if the ovarian AV complex is dropped and indiscriminate clamping of tissue occurs in the lumbar gutter. A ureter is more likely to be included in a uterine body ligature if the bladder is full because the trigone and vesicoureteral junction are cranially displaced, resulting in more slack on the ureters. Accidental ligation or crushing of a ureter may be prevented by ligating the ovarian AV complex as close to the ovary as possible, by evacuating the patient's urinary bladder preoperatively, and by isolating and ligating the uterine vessels carefully.

Urinary Incontinence

Urinary incontinence after ovariohysterectomy can be caused by a low systemic estrogen level, by adhesions or granulomas of the uterine stump that interfere with urinary bladder sphincter function, or by vaginoureteral fistulation from common ligation of the vagina and ureter (13). Estrogen-responsive urinary incontinence occurs in older bitches spayed at an early age and is an uncommon and poorly understood sequela of ovariohysterectomy (14). The onset of estrogen-responsive incontinence postoperatively is variable and may take several years (14). The mean reported age of onset is 8.3 years (14). The recommended therapy for estrogen-responsive urinary incontinence is oral administration of diethylstilbestrol at 0.1 to 1.0 mg per day for 3 to 5 days, followed by a maintenance dose of 1.0 mg per week (14).

Fistulous Tracts and Granulomas

The most common cause of sublumbar fistulous tracts in spayed bitches is adverse tissue reaction to implanted nonabsorbable multifilament suture material (e.g., polymerized caprolactam, Braunamid, B. Braun Melsurgen AG, Germany) used for ovarian or uterine ligature (12, 15–17). The high bacterial adherence and capillarity of multifilament suture may contribute to persistent and progressive infection when the suture is contaminated with bacterial organisms and is buried in tissue (18). No ovarian or uterine stump granulomas or fistulous tracts were reported in 377 bitches that had ovariohysterectomies using 2–0 chromic catgut suture (8).

The interval between ovariohysterectomy and appearance of fistulous tracts is often several months and may be several years (12). Fistulous tracts can occur anywhere on the trunk, although they most commonly occur in the flank when associated with ovarian pedicle ligatures and in the inguinal or thigh region when associated with a uterine ligature (18). Ovarian pedicle granulomas caused by adverse tissue reaction to suture material may involve the kidney or proximal ureter, resulting in hydronephrosis and pyelonephritis. Uterine stump granulomas may involve the urinary bladder, distal ureters, or colon, leading to cystitis, pollakiuria, urinary incontinence, or bowel obstruction (18). Exploratory laparotomy with excision of the offending ligature and of associated granulation tissue is the treatment of choice. All ovarian and uterine ligatures should be removed even though some appear uninvolved because they may subsequently provoke an adverse tissue response (12). Local exploration of fistulous tracts is seldom successful and is indicated only if exploratory laparotomy fails to identify the offending tissue (1). The use of absorbable suture material for ovarian and uterine ligatures during ovariohysterectomy reduces the incidence of this complication (18).

Body Weight Gain

Body weight gain was the most common long-term sequela reported in one study, occurring in 26.2% of bitches undergoing elective ovariohysterectomy (19).

The cause of excessive weight gain after ovariohysterectomy is poorly understood. One theory suggests that the fat deposits of the body possess receptors for specific steroid hormones so deposition is blocked or facilitated in a regional manner in response to testosterone, estradiol, progesterone, and cortisol. Estradiol inhibits lipoprotein lipase in adipocytes of fat deposits, so circulating fatty acids cannot be esterified and deposited (20). A low systemic estradiol level after ovariohysterectomy may lead to excessive fat deposition and weight gain.

Eunuchoid Syndromes

The eunuchoid syndrome is occasionally observed in working dogs after ovariohysterectomy. Affected dogs have decreases in aggression, interest in work, and stamina (20). Autotransplantation of an ovary to the subserosa of the stomach wall, which is drained exclusively by the portal vein, may prevent this complication (20). The graft produces estradiol and progesterone, which are partially metabolized by the liver. Circulating estradiol levels are inadequate to initiate estrus, but they are sufficient to prevent the eunuchoid syndrome (20).

Complications of Celiotomy

Accidental incision of the spleen or urinary bladder, failure to remove all gauze sponges from the abdominal cavity before closure, dehiscence, seroma formation, and self-mutilation may occur with any abdominal procedure. Self-inflicted trauma of the abdominal wound is the most commonly reported complication of ovariohysterectomy of dogs less than 25 kg (8). Most of these complications can be prevented by close attention to detail and by adhering to the basic principles of aseptic surgical technique.

Early Prepubertal Gonadectomy

Minimal scientific evidence exists to support the widely accepted practice of delaying elective sterilization until an animal is 5 to 8 months old. Veterinarians are comfortable with this practice because untoward effects occur infrequently. Early prepubertal gonadectomy (i.e., at 8 to 12 weeks of age) has been investigated because the efficacy of sterilization programs could be enhanced if all animals were neutered before adoption. Much has been learned about the effects of early prepubertal gonadectomy on skeletal growth, obesity, behavior, secondary sex characteristics, anesthetic risk, and immunology (21). The current body of knowledge does not summarily support or disprove the notion that early prepubertal gonadectomy is deleterious (21). Ongoing studies promise to bring more information to light in the near future.

References

1. Stone EA. Ovariohysterectomy. In: Slatter DH, ed. Textbook of small animal surgery. Philadelphia: WB Saunders, 1985:1667–1672.
2. Wilson GP, Hayes HM. Ovariohysterectomy in the dog and cat. In: Bojrab MJ, ed. Current techniques in small animal surgery. 2nd ed. Philadelphia: Lea & Febiger, 1983:334–338.
3. Farton JW, Withrow SJ. Canine mammary neoplasia: an overview. Calif Vet 1981;7:12.
4. Evans HE, Christensen GC. Miller's anatomy of the dog. 2nd ed. Philadelphia: WB Saunders, 1981.
5. DelCampo CH, Ginther OJ. Arteries and veins of uterus and ovaries in dogs and cats. Am J Vet Res 1974;35:409.
6. Rosin E. Single layer, simple continuous suture pattern for closure of abdominal incisions. J Am Anim Hosp Assoc 1985;21:751.
7. Krzaczynski J. The flank approach to feline ovariohysterectomy. Vet Med Small Anim Clin 1974;May :572.
8. Berzon JL. Complications of elective ovariohysterectomies in the dog and cat at a teaching institution: a clinical review of 853 cases. Vet Surg 1979;8:89.
9. Teale ML. Pyometritis in spayed cats (letter). Vet Rec 1972;90:129.
10. Stein BS. The genital system. In: Catcott EJ, ed. Feline medicine and surgery. 2nd ed. Santa Barbara, CA: American Veterinary, 1975.
11. Shenwell RE, Weed IC. Ovarian remnant syndrome. Obstet Gynecol 1970;36:299.
12. Pearson H. The complications of ovariohysterectomy in the bitch. J Small Anim Pract 1973;14:257.
13. Pearson H, Gibbs G. Urinary incontinence in the dog due to accidental vaginoureteral fistulation during hysterectomy. J Small Anim Pract 1980;21:287.
14. Rosin AH, Ross L. Diagnosis and pharmacological management of disorders of urinary continence in the dog. Compend Contin Educ Pract Vet 1981;3:601.
15. Osborne CA, Polzin DJ. Canine estrogen responsive incontinence: an enigma. DVM 1979;10:42.
16. Pearson H. Ovariohysterectomy in the bitch. Vet Rec 1970;87:257.
17. Borthwick R. Unilateral hydronephrosis in a spayed bitch. Vet Rec 1972;90:244.
18. Spackmann CJ, Caywood DD, Johnston GB, et al. Granulomas of the uterine and ovarian stumps: a case report. J Am Anim Hosp Assoc 1984;20:449.
19. Dorn AS, Swist RA. Complications of canine ovariohysterectomy. J Am Anim Hosp Assoc 1977;13:720.
20. LeRoux PH, Van Der Walt LA. Ovarian autograft as an alternative to ovariectomy in bitches. J S Afr Vet Med Assoc 1977;48:117.
21. Salmeri KR, Olson PN, Bloomberg MS. Elective gonadectomy in dogs: a review. J Am Vet Med Assoc 1991;198:1183.

Cesarean Section

Trevor N. Bebchuk & Curtis W. Probst

Cesarean section in the dog and cat usually is an emergency procedure because prolonged dystocia risks the life of the mother and neonate. Cesarean section can be planned and performed before the onset of active parturition when dystocia is predicted owing to preexisting injuries or abnormalities that compromise the birth canal. Cesarean section is indicated when dystocia results from primary uterine inertia, when secondary uterine inertia has occurred in protracted dystocia of over 24 hours' duration, when obstructive dystocia (e.g., grossly oversized fetus or abnormally narrow pelvic canal) is present, or when removal of the obstructed fetus is not likely to alter the ultimate outcome of the dystocia.

Surgical Anatomy

The gravid uterus lies on the abdominal floor during the last half of pregnancy. The heavily gravid uterine horns are parallel and in contact with each other, unlike the divergent uterine horns in the nonpregnant animal. As the horns enlarge, they also flex and bend the uterus cranially and ventrally on itself. When making the abdominal incision during cesarean section, the surgeon must be aware that the uterus is close to the thin, distended abdominal wall.

The uterus is composed of three layers: tunica serosa (perimetrium), tunica muscularis (myometrium), and tunica mucosa (endometrium). The tunica serosa is a layer of peritoneum that covers the entire uterus and is continuous with the mesometrium (broad ligaments). The muscular layer consists of a thin longitudinal outer layer and thick inner layer. The deeper myometrium contains blood vessels, nerves, and circular and oblique muscle fibers. The tunica muscularis is the layer of greatest tensile strength. The tunica mucosa is the thickest of the three layers.

The uterus is well supplied with arterial blood from the ovarian and uterine arteries (see Fig. 30.1). The uterine vessels greatly enlarge during gestation and potentially complicate an ovariohysterectomy performed in conjunction with a cesarean section. Lymphatic drainage of the uterus is through the internal iliac and lumbar lymph nodes. Autonomic nervous innervation is through the hypogastric and pelvic plexuses.

Preoperative Preparations

Animals considered for cesarean section are often in poor physiologic condition at the time of presentation and should be carefully examined. Abdominal radiographs are useful in documenting the presence and number of fetuses, thus helping the surgeon to avoid inadvertently leaving a fetus in the uterus or pelvic canal. Laboratory tests are often limited to measurement of the animal's hematocrit, total plasma protein, serum urea nitrogen, or urine specific gravity. These tests assist in evaluating the need for corrective fluid therapy or cross matching of potential blood donors. Most pregnant animals are mildly anemic because of an increase in plasma volume during gestation without a concomitant increase in red blood cells. The surgeon should consider this physiologic anemia when deciding whether the dam requires a whole-blood transfusion.

An intravenous fluid infusion should be established before any anesthesia is given. The preferred fluid is a balanced electrolyte solution such as lactated Ringer's solution. A solution of 2.5% dextrose and half-strength lactated Ringer's may be more appropriate if the animal has not eaten for some time and hypoglycemia is suspected. A baseline administration rate of 10 mL/kg per hour may be increased as indicated by physiologic parameters. All volume deficits should be corrected before the surgical procedure is begun, if possible. If the fetuses are known to be dead and decomposing or if uterine infection is established, intravenous antibiotic therapy (cephalothin sodium, 40 mg/kg IV, or cefazolin sodium 22 mg/kg IV) should be instituted at this time.

The surgeon and the client should discuss, before surgery, the nature of the surgical procedure, its potential complications, and the issue of simultaneous ovariohysterectomy. The length of the surgical procedure may be important, depending on the condition of the dam. The advisability of an additional operation for ovariohysterectomy should be carefully considered. Ovariohysterectomy may be better postponed until the litter is weaned and the uterine vasculature has returned to normal size.

Surgical Technique

The dam is clipped from the xiphoid to the pubis, and the ventral abdomen is initially prepared by surgical scrubbing before induction of anesthesia to reduce total anesthesia time. Anesthesia induction and intubation are performed on the operating table. Usually, the dam has not been fasted before anesthesia; therefore, the patient should be intubated rapidly to minimize the risk of aspiration should vomiting occur during induction of anesthesia.

Operative speed is important in cesarean sections because long "incision-to-delivery" time is associated with increased fetal asphyxia and depression. A 10 to 20° left or right lateral tilt from dorsal recumbency is frequently used in women to prevent supine hypotension syndrome, which is thought to result from compression of the gravid uterus on the posterior vena cava, thus reducing venous return. Supine hypotension syndrome does not occur in the term-pregnant bitch, and maternal posture has no effect on systemic blood pressure. Dorsal recumbency is therefore an acceptable position for cesarean sections in dogs and cats.

After induction of anesthesia, the patient's limbs are tied down, and the final surgical preparation of the ventral abdomen is rapidly completed. The ventral abdomen is four-quadrant toweled and is draped from the xiphoid to the pelvic brim, to allow room for extension of the abdominal incision if necessary.

A ventral midline incision is made commencing at the umbilicus. The length of the incision is determined by the estimated size of the uterus. The mammary glands often are hypertrophied, and the surgeon should not invade mammary tissue when making the skin incision. The surgeon should also remember that the uterus is enlarged and should not be lacerated when the abdominal cavity is entered. I prefer using thumb forceps and a scalpel to open the abdominal cavity; however, Mayo scissors also are acceptable.

Once an abdominal incision of adequate length is completed, the wound edges are protected with laparotomy pads moistened with sterile saline. The first uterine horn and then the second are exteriorized by careful lifting through the incision. The surrounding and underlying viscera are packed off with additional moistened laparotomy pads to prevent abdominal contamination with fetal fluids. A small incision with a scalpel is then made in a relatively avascular area on the dorsal or ventral aspect of the uterine body; one must be careful not to lacerate a fetus inadvertently with the scalpel. The uterine incision is then extended with scissors to a length sufficient for easy removal of the fetuses (Fig. 30.9).

In dystocia, the fetus present in the uterine body should be removed first. Each fetus is brought to the incision by gently "milking it down" the uterine horn. This is done by squeezing the uterine horn cranial to the enlargement. Once the fetus is near the incision, it may be grasped, and gentle traction may be applied to facilitate rapid removal from the uterus (Fig. 30.10). As each fetus is removed, the amniotic sac is broken to allow breathing to begin (Fig. 30.11). Fetal fluids should be removed from the operative field by suction to minimize contamination. The umbilical vessels are then clamped and are severed approximately 2 to 3 cm from the fetal abdominal wall (Fig. 30.12). The neonate is placed on a sterile towel, which is passed to an attendant. The associated placenta is then slowly removed from the endometrium by gentle traction to minimize hemorrhage. This procedure is repeated until all fetuses and placentas have been removed. If considerable difficulty is encountered in mobilizing the fetuses down the uterine horns, additional incisions can be made in the horns. Before closure, the uterus is palpated from the pelvic canal to each ovary to be

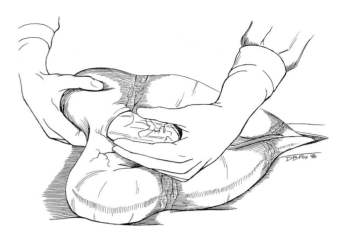

Fig. 30.10. Each fetus is brought to the incision by squeezing the uterine horn cranial to the enlargement; it may be grasped and gentle traction applied to remove it from the uterus.

certain that all fetuses and placentas have been removed.

Another method of delivery is to remove the neonate and placenta with the umbilical cord and fetal membranes still intact. The amniotic sac is broken, and the cord is clamped when the neonate has been handed to an attendant. More maternal hemorrhage may be noted with this method.

Once all fetuses have been removed, the uterus rapidly begins to contract; this contraction is important in arresting hemorrhage. If the uterus has not begun to contract at the time of closure, oxytocin (5 to 20 units intramuscularly can be administered.

I prefer absorbable suture material such as polydioxanone or polyglyconate with swaged-on noncutting needles for uterine closure. The edges of the uterine incision are carefully apposed with a double-layer, inverting, continuous Cushing pattern followed by a

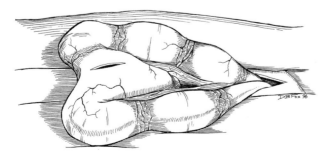

Fig. 30.9. The gravid uterus has been exteriorized and surrounded with moistened laparotomy pads. The *dashed line* indicates the proposed incision in the dorsal aspect of the uterine body.

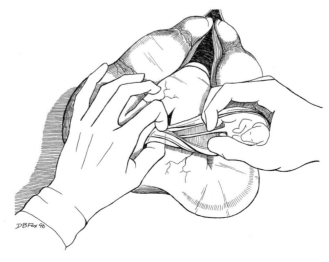

Fig. 30.11. As the fetus is removed from the uterus, the amniotic sac is broken to allow breathing to begin.

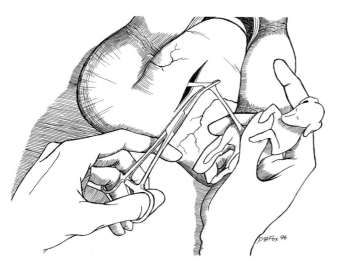

Fig. 30.12. The umbilical vessels are clamped and severed approximately 2 to 3 cm from the fetal abdominal wall.

continuous Lembert oversew (Fig. 30.13). Before the uterus is returned to the abdomen, the closure should be inspected, and the uterus should be cleansed with warmed sterile saline solution. If abdominal contamination has occurred during the surgical manipulations, the abdomen should be liberally lavaged with warmed sterile saline solution. The omentum is replaced over the uterus and other abdominal viscera before abdominal closure; the linea alba is closed with simple interrupted sutures of appropriate-sized absorbable suture material. Nonabsorbable suture material, such as polypropylene, nylon, or stainless steel wire, may also be used to close the linea alba. The subcutaneous tissue is closed with 3–0 or 2–0 absorbable suture, and the skin is closed with nonabsorbable suture.

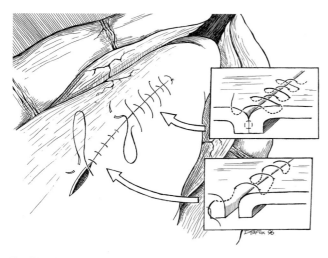

Fig. 30.13. Double-layer closure of the uterus. **A.** A continuous Cushing pattern is used for the first layer. **B.** The first-layer closure is oversewn with a continuous Lembert pattern.

Before the conclusion of the surgical procedure, all inhalation anesthetic agents are discontinued, and the dam is weaned from assisted ventilation by progressively decreasing the respiratory rate. The dam should then be given several maximal inspirations to reopen any atelectatic areas of lung before a return to breathing room air.

Extubation should not be too hasty because patients that undergo cesarean section may have full stomachs and may vomit during induction or recovery. Vomiting during recovery is a major problem in parturient women, but it is less important in the dog and cat.

Resuscitation of the Neonates

After the neonate has been handed to the assistant, its umbilical cord should be temporarily clamped, the fetal membranes should be removed (if this has not yet been done), and its viability should be ascertained. If a heartbeat can be palpated, the nasopharynx should be cleared of fluid and mucus by gentle suction or cotton swabs. If a suction apparatus is not available, a bulb syringe can be used for suction. A gentle, controlled, downward swing of the neonate may help to clear fluid from the upper airways by centrifugal force. The neonate is then vigorously dried because skin stimulation stimulates respiratory drive in a reflex manner.

The neonate should be breathing and crying by this stage. Other encouraging signs are pink mucous membranes and a strong pulse. More active resuscitative measures include narcotic antagonists such as naloxone (0.01 mg/kg IM or IV) and the respiratory stimulant doxapram (1 to 2 drops sublingual or 0.1 ml IV in the umbilical vein). In the event of cardiorespiratory collapse, an emergency endotracheal intubation may be attempted with a plastic intravenous catheter (18 to 20 gauge).

Postoperative Care of the Dam and Neonates

When the puppies or kittens have been resuscitated and dried, they should be kept in a warm environment to avoid chilling. The clamp is removed from the umbilical cord, which is checked for hemorrhage. If hemorrhage occurs, the cord should be ligated with 3–0 chromic gut.

While the mother is recovering from anesthesia, her mammary glands should be cleaned with warm water to remove any residual surgical preparation solutions, blood, or fetal fluids. The dam should be returned to her litter as soon as she has recovered. The dam should continue to be carefully watched by the veterinarian or the owner in the first hours after the operation because sudden lapses into shock can occur if uterine bleeding recommences.

Colostrum is important to the neonates. Although some transplacental acquisition of passive immunity occurs before birth, most antibodies are transferred through the colostrum after birth. Nursing also stimulates the release of oxytocin to mediate uterine contraction. Although drugs can be transferred to the neonate in the milk, this is not important unless drugs are administered to the mother on a continuing basis. Drugs that are weak bases and become ionized at a low pH usually accumulate in the milk at a higher concentration than in the dam's blood.

Before the litter is discharged, puppies or kittens should be inspected for obvious congenital abnormalities, such as deformed limbs, cleft palate, and imperforate anus. This check, together with advice to the owners on neonatal care, ensures good veterinarian–client relations. The dam and her litter can be discharged as soon as she is able to stand and appropriate behavior patterns toward the litter are confirmed. Owners should be instructed to monitor the dam carefully for the next 24 to 48 hours. They should look for evidence of continued uterine hemorrhage, anorexia, or signs of infection or dehiscence of the abdominal incision. The dam should be returned in 7 to 10 days for suture removal.

Postoperative Complications

Certain complications are associated with both emergency and elective cesarean section. Perioperative maternal mortality rates of over 4% have been reported, perhaps owing to the emergency nature of the operation and the patient's stressed condition at the time of surgery. Hypovolemia and hypotension are the most common complications and are treated with vigorous fluid therapy or blood replacement. Hemorrhage of uterine origin should be controlled with oxytocin (5 to 20 units IM or IV). In severe hemorrhage, the dosage may be repeated after 2 to 4 hours, and whole-blood transfusion may be started. Persistent hemorrhage may require an emergency ovariohysterectomy. If an infected uterus is encountered during the surgical procedure, ovariohysterectomy or packing of the uterus with antibiotic boluses and systemic antibiotics should be considered.

Postoperative peritonitis should not be a problem unless a break in surgical technique or abdominal contamination with septic uterine contents has occurred. Infection can be controlled with careful surgical technique, intraoperative abdominal lavage, and antibiotic therapy in most cases. Agalactia may occur in the queen or bitch after cesarean section, but normal milk flow usually occurs within 24 hours. Oxytocin (0.5 units/kg intramuscularly) may be administered to stimulate milk production if necessary. Excessive depression of either the mother or the offspring after

anesthesia indicates that one should critically review the anesthetic protocol for reduction in doses of analgesics or barbiturate depressants.

Suggested Readings

Abitbol MM. Inferior vena cava compression in the pregnant dog. Am J Obstet Gynecol 1978;130:194.

Probst CW, Webb AI. Postural influence on systemic blood pressure, gas exchange, and acid/base status in the term-pregnant bitch during general anesthesia. Am J Vet Res 1983;44:1963.

Probst CW, Broadstone RV, Evans AT. Postural influence on systemic blood pressure in large full-term pregnant bitches during general anesthesia. Vet Surg 1987;16(6):471.

Cesarean Section by Ovariohysterectomy

Holly S. Mullen

Traditional cesarean section (hysterotomy) has been the treatment of choice for canine and feline dystocia that is not responsive to medical management. Hysterotomy is a well-described and widely accepted technique. Most references advise against ovariohysterectomy at the time of hysterotomy, citing additional stress to the female, increased blood loss, longer anesthetic time, and problems with neonatal survival (1–3). Sometimes, no reason is specified (4). Many practicing veterinarians have performed ovariohysterectomy for dystocia in the dog and cat with excellent results. The technique of "en-bloc" cesarean section (ovariohysterectomy followed by rapid removal of neonates from the gravid uterus) has been shown to be safe and effective for both cats and dogs (5). Future reproduction is impossible after this technique, a fact that pleases most owners. The technique is easier, quicker, and has less chance for intraoperative contamination than traditional cesarean section.

Surgical Technique

Preoperative considerations and anesthetic techniques are identical to those for routine cesarean section. A caudal ventral midline incision is made through the skin, subcutis, and linea of the abdomen. The incision is packed off with sterile, saline-moistened laparotomy sponges. The gravid uterus is exteriorized, and the uterine horns are laid out laterally to the incision (Fig. 30.14). Next, the suspensory ligaments are cut or broken to allow mobilization of the ovaries by their vascular pedicles. No clamps are applied at this time. The broad ligament is broken down on both sides of the

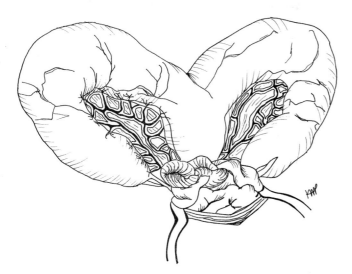

Fig. 30.14. The gravid uterus is exteriorized, and both horns are laid out laterally to the abdominal incision.

uterus from the ovarian pedicle to the cervix. This leaves the blood supply to the uterus and fetuses intact while freeing up all attachments except the ovarian pedicles and the uterine body (Fig. 30.15).

Ovariohysterectomy can now be performed rapidly and safely, with a maximum of no more than 45 to 60 seconds elapsed between clamping of the ovarian pedicles and uterine body and delivery of the neonates by assistants.

The surgeon palpates the patient's cervix and vagina to check for a fetus. If one is present, it is manipulated gently back into the uterine body. Two hemostatic

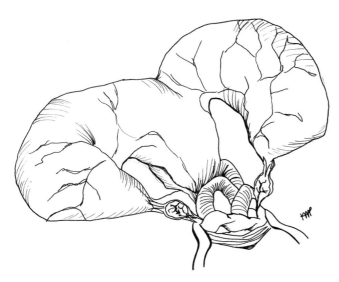

Fig. 30.15. The suspensory ligaments are broken down to exteriorize the ovaries, and the broad ligament is torn on both sides of the uterine horns. The ovarian pedicles and the uterine body provide blood supply to the uterus and are the only structures remaining that need to be transected and ligated to remove the gravid uterus.

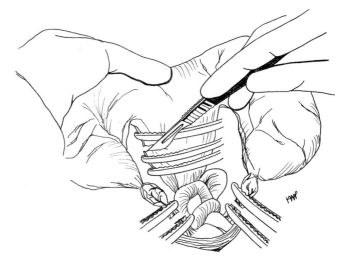

Fig. 30.16. The gravid uterus can be removed in 45 to 60 seconds by first placing two hemostats on each ovarian pedicle and then three clamps on the uterine body and transecting between them as shown.

clamps are placed across each ovarian pedicle, and three clamps are placed across the uterine body just distal to the cervix. The gravid uterus and ovaries are removed by dividing between the clamps (Fig. 30.16). The surgeon hands the gravid uterus to a team of assistants, who immediately open the uterus and resuscitate the neonates. The ovarian pedicles and uterine stump are ligated with chromic gut sized according to the surgeon's preference. The abdomen is closed routinely. Subcuticular sutures are preferred over skin sutures to prevent irritation of the suture line by the nursing pups. Appropriate postoperative pain relievers, such as butorphanol tartrate (0.1 to 0.4 mg/kg intravenously, intramuscularly, or subcutaneously), buprenorphine (5 to 10 μg/kg intravenously, intramuscularly, or subcutaneously), or oxymorphone (0.03 to 0.1 mg/kg intravenously, intramuscularly, or subcutaneously), are given just before the end of anesthesia.

Resuscitation of the Neonates

The gravid uterus is handed to an assistant after removal, who takes it from the sterile operating room to a location previously prepared for neonatal resuscitation. The uterus is opened with scissors or a scalpel blade (Fig. 30.17), taking care not to cut a fetus. The neonates are rapidly removed and resuscitated by the assistants. Ideally, one assistant should be available for each neonate, although one person can care for two or three neonates at a time if the neonates are healthy.

Hypoxia is thought to be one of the primary reasons for neonatal mortality (6). The mortality rate of puppies and kittens delivered by ovariohysterectomy is

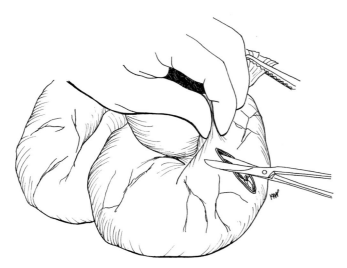

Fig. 30.17. An assistant opens the uterus with scissors or a scalpel blade and removes and resuscitates the neonates.

reportedly lower than the mortality rates by either traditional cesarean section or natural parturition (5). This finding suggests that ovariohysterectomy for the treatment of dystocia has no adverse effect on neonatal survival.

Contraindications for Ovariohysterectomy

No important complications or contraindications for this technique have been described (5). Some limitations include the need for multiple assistants for simultaneous neonatal resuscitation of a large litter and the loss of future reproductive capability (although this is usually considered an asset). Anemia is not a complication with this technique, because no significant decrease in packed cell volume was reported in either dogs or cats undergoing cesarean section by ovariohysterectomy (5). In a small, significantly anemic female with a markedly engorged uterus, however, hysterotomy followed by rapid involution of the uterus may allow return of some of the uterine blood to the peripheral circulation before removal of the nongravid uterus.

Advantages of Ovariohysterectomy

Ovariohysterectomy for dystocia is rapid and safe for both mother and babies. Use of this technique minimizes anesthetic time and reduces intraoperative peritoneal contamination by uterine contents, which may occur during hysterotomy. Both dogs and cats continue to lactate normally as long as the babies continue to nurse. There is scant to no postoperative lochial discharge, as is common for several days after birth, because the uterus has been removed. Ovariohysterectomy also provides an opportunity for future population control in pets that are unable to reproduce naturally or whose owners may not be able to afford a second operation for sterilization of the animal in the future. The health of the mother and of the neonates is not compromised when cesarean section by ovariohysterectomy is used as the surgical treatment for dystocia.

References

1. Herron MR, Herron MA. Surgery of the uterus. Vet Clin North Am 1975;5:471–476.
2. Probst CW, Webb AI. Cesarean section in the dog and cat: anesthetic and surgical techniques. In: Bojrab MJ, ed. Current techniques in small animal surgery. 2nd ed. Philadelphia: Lea & Febiger, 1983:346–351.
3. Gaudet DA, Kitchell BE. Canine dystocia. Compend Contin Educ Pract Vet 1985;7:406–418.
4. Probst CW. Uterus: cesarean section. In: Bojrab MJ, ed. Current techniques in small animal surgery. 3rd ed. Philadelphia: Lea & Febiger, 1990:404–408.
5. Robbins MA, Mullen, HS. En bloc ovariohysterectomy as a treatment of dystocia in dogs and cats. Vet Surg 1994;23:48–52.
6. Fox MW. Neonatal mortality in the dog. J Am Vet Med Assoc 1963;143:1219–1223.

— 31 —

VAGINA AND VULVA

Surgical Treatment of Vaginal and Vulvar Masses

Ghery D. Pettit

In the bitch, physiologic enlargement of the vulvar labia during proestrus and estrus is a normal estrogenic response. It may be mimicked or exaggerated by masses within the vestibule of the vulva or the vagina that cause the labia to protrude. Such masses include hyperplasia of the vaginal floor, vaginal prolapse, vestibular or vaginal tumors, and clitoral enlargement. Subtle perineal bulges may be detected, but the masses usually become apparent to an animal's owner when they protrude through the vulva, cause irritation and licking, or interfere with mating. They may cause dysuria. Prolonged estrogenic stimulation from follicular cysts or granulosa cell tumors can cause persistent hyperplasia of the labial and vaginal mucosa, making the labia larger, firm, pigmented, and hairless.

Inspection, digital vaginal or rectal palpation, and vaginoscopy provide preliminary identification of most vaginal lesions. In at least one instance, an intraluminal vaginal tumor was diagnosed by pneumovaginography. Surgical treatment of these lesions is facilitated by episiotomy. Excised neoplasms should be identified histologically.

Hyperplasia of the Vaginal Floor

During proestrus and estrus, the vestibular and vaginal mucosae normally become swollen, thickened, and turgid. Exaggeration of this estrogenic response occasionally leads to the development of a transverse mucosal fold on the floor of the vagina just cranial to the external urethral orifice. Although "hyperplasia" is the accepted term for this condition, histologically the swelling is mostly edema with some fibroplasia. If the redundant fold becomes large enough, it protrudes between the labia of the vulva as a red, fleshy mass (Fig. 31.1**A**). The disorder occurs most often during a bitch's first, second, or third estrus. Spontaneous regression occurs during metestrus, but recurrence is common at the next estrus. The condition has been reported in more than 20 breeds of dogs, with frequent mention of brachycephalic breeds, such as boxers and English bulldogs.

Because the protrusion is vulnerable to trauma, inflammation, and ulceration, tends to recur, and is aesthetically objectionable, amputation is frequently the treatment of choice. Recurrence after surgical excision is uncommon, and natural mating is possible at subsequent estrous periods. With or without surgical excision, ovariectomy provides permanent relief.

Alternatively, one can manage the condition conservatively until it regresses spontaneously by lubricating the mass with an antibiotic ointment and applying an Elizabethan collar to prevent self-abuse. If breeding during the same estrus is important, artificial insemination can be performed. Simultaneous excision of the mass and artificial insemination are technically possible but seldom indicated.

A third option is to try to shorten the duration of estrogenic stimulation of the vaginal tissue by inducing ovulation at the onset of clinical signs. A single dose of gonadotropin-releasing hormone or human chorionic gonadotropin has been used for this purpose. Regression of the prolapse occurs about 1 week after induction of ovulation.

Surgical Treatment

The animal is positioned in ventral recumbency with the hindquarters elevated, and the perineum is

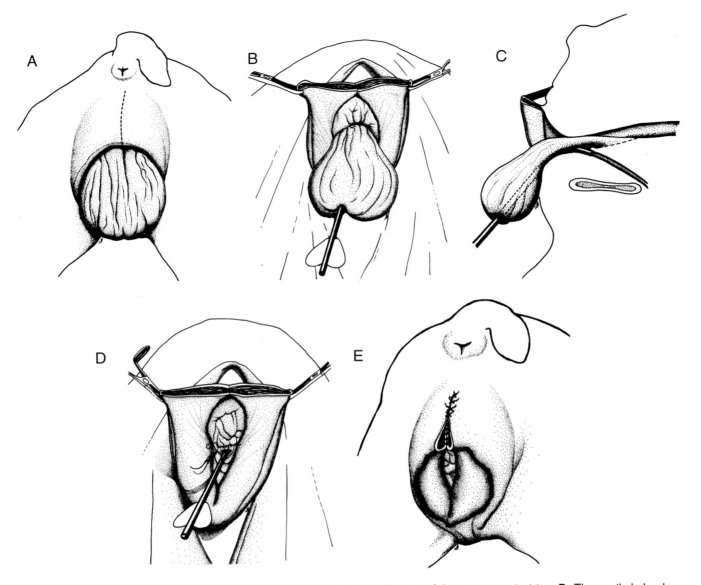

Fig. 31.1. Hyperplasia of the vaginal floor. **A.** The broken line indicates the site of the episiotomy incision. **B.** The vestibule has been opened by performing an episiotomy, and a urethral catheter has been inserted. **C.** Lateral view. Episiotomy and urethral catheterization have been performed. The broken line on the floor of the vagina indicates the incision site for amputation of the redundant mucosal mass. **D.** The mass has been amputated, and the mucosal incision is closed with a simple continuous suture. **E.** Postoperative view. The catheter has been removed, and the episiotomy incision is being closed.

prepared aseptically. The vestibule and vagina are cleansed with a mild antiseptic solution (1:10 povidone–iodine [Betadine] or 1:5000 benzalkonium chloride [Zephiran chloride] solution). A median episiotomy incision is begun with a scalpel or an electrosurgery unit and is completed with scissors. Doyen intestinal forceps can be positioned on each side of the incision to serve as a guide and to reduce bleeding. Hemorrhage is controlled with hemostatic forceps, ligation, or electrocoagulation. Retracting the margins of the episiotomy incision exposes the vaginal lumen. The mass must be elevated for catheterization of the urethra, to identify and protect that structure (Fig.

31.1**B** and **C**). The superfluous tissue is amputated by making connecting, curved, transverse incisions through its base. One incision is made on the dorsal surface of the mass (the cranial aspect of its base), and the other is made on its ventral surface (the caudal surface of the base of the mass). The incisions should be no deeper than necessary to excise the mass. The mucosal opening is closed with absorbable suture material in a transverse, simple continuous pattern (Fig. 31.1**D**). The catheter is removed, and the episiotomy incision is closed (Fig. 31.1**E**). The mucosa is apposed with simple interrupted absorbable sutures. In obese or heavily muscled animals, the musculature should be sutured separately with absorbable sutures. The skin incision is closed with simple interrupted nonabsorbable sutures. If bleeding persists, a vaginal tampon may be left in place for 12 hours.

Vaginal Prolapse

Cylindric prolapse of the vaginal wall is much rarer than hyperplasia of the vaginal floor. In this condition, which also occurs during estrus, a donut-shaped eversion of the entire vaginal circumference protrudes from the vulva (Fig. 31.2). Vaginal prolapse has been reported after forcible separation of the male and female during the genital tie. As in hyperplasia of the vaginal floor, the external urethral orifice is ventral to the entire mass, but access to the vaginal canal is through the center of the protrusion, rather than dorsal to it.

Complete vaginal prolapse also occurs during parturition or advanced pregnancy, as a prelude to prolapse of the cervix, uterine body, and one or both uterine horns. It results from excessive straining while the supportive tissues are relaxed. The everted organs are usually discolored from venous congestion, soiled, and traumatized.

Some authors prefer to classify hyperplasia of the vaginal floor as a type of vaginal prolapse. According to that interpretation, hyperplasia of the vaginal floor that does not protrude through the vulva is called type I prolapse, and hyperplasia that protrudes completely is called type II. A true cylindric prolapse is called type III.

A recent "type III" vaginal prolapse can be reduced, but recurrence is likely. Recurrence, hemorrhage, infection, and necrosis make amputation necessary. Shock and dehydration are common complications that must be treated appropriately.

Surgical Treatment

With the animal under general anesthesia, the protruding structures are washed gently with warm saline solution or a mild detergent. Additional trauma is avoided. The mass is compressed manually to reduce edema before reduction is attempted. Sprinkling the mucosal surface with table sugar may further reduce the swelling, and episiotomy makes reduction easier. Once accomplished, reduction is maintained by placing heavy nonabsorbable sutures across the vulvar labia.

Reduction of a vaginal prolapse can be facilitated by traction on the uterus through a ventral abdominal incision. When this technique is used, suturing the uterine body or horns to the abdominal wall (hysteropexy) provides protection against recurrence.

If reduction is impossible or inadvisable, the protruding tissue must be amputated. Paying careful attention to the distorted anatomy minimizes errors. With a catheter in place to identify and protect the urethra, a circumferential incision is made in stages through the vaginal wall. The outer, everted mucosa is incised first. The incision is deepened to penetrate all layers of prolapsed vaginal tissue until the inner, noneverted mucosa is reached. Hemostasis is maintained by ligation or electrocoagulation, and the proximal mucosal margins are united with horizontal mattress sutures. The incision is extended for another short distance, the exposed segment is sutured, and the process is repeated until the amputation is complete.

Tumors of the Vulva and Vagina

Vulvar and vaginal neoplasms, which usually occur in older bitches, account for no more than 3% of all canine tumors; 70 to 80% of them are benign. The most common tumors of the vulva and vagina are leiomyoma, fibroma, and lipoma. Leiomyosarcoma is the most common malignant vaginal tumor. Mast cell tumors, sebaceous adenomas, and epidermoid carcinomas have been reported.

Leiomyomas and fibromas are often grossly indistinguishable. They form smooth, firm, spheric masses that are often pedunculated and protrude into the vestibular or vaginal lumen. They may protrude from the vulva and resemble an early hyperplasia of the vaginal floor. Lipomas occur as a gradually enlarging mass un-

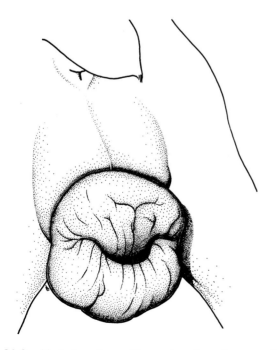

Fig. 31.2. Vaginal prolapse. The entire circumference of the vaginal wall has everted.

der the intact mucosa; they may protrude into the lumen, or they may become apparent under the perineal skin adjacent to the vulva. Surgical excision of benign vulvar and vaginal tumors combined with ovariohysterectomy is effective in preventing recurrence, but malignant tumors have been reported in spayed females.

The transmissible venereal tumor is an allogeneic cellular transplant that is transmitted by implantation of exfoliated cells into traumatized vaginal or penile epithelium. The condition is most prevalent and perhaps most severe when dogs are crowded and stressed. In females, the transmissible venereal tumor appears in the vagina as single or multiple projecting masses with roughened or reddened, ulcerated surfaces. Metastasis is rare. Spontaneous regression occurs after 2 to 6 months in about 60% of experimentally transplanted tumors, but reports of spontaneous regression in naturally occurring cases are inconsistent. Surgical excision is an appropriate initial treatment. If surgery is impossible or if recurrence or metastasis is noted, radiation therapy and chemotherapy are effective. Immunotherapy may be as effective as chemotherapy, but additional clinical trials are needed.

Surgical Treatment

Episiotomy is performed for better exposure. Pedunculated intraluminal tumors can be amputated, but encapsulated extraluminal tumors are removed by submucosal resection (Fig. 31.3). An incision is made through the mucosa, and the tumor is bluntly peeled away. The mucosal incision is closed with absorbable

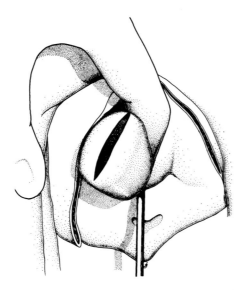

Fig. 31.3. Vestibular leiomyoma. Episiotomy has been performed, and a mucosal incision has been made to facilitate submucosal resection of the tumor.

sutures. Submucosal resection is especially useful for large or multiple tumors.

Clitoral Enlargement

Enlargement of the clitoris, sometimes with an os clitoridis, is an androgenic response. The condition has been caused by administration of exogenous androgens or anabolic steroids, and it has been reported in bitches with hyperadrenocorticism. Clitoral enlargement has occurred in puppies whose dams were treated with androgens during pregnancy. Friction between the protruding clitoris and the vulva may cause inflammation. Treatment includes topical antibiotic ointments, removal of the androgen source, or excision of the enlarged clitoris. If an os clitoridis is not present, the clitoris regresses to normal size when exogenous androgen is withdrawn.

Suggested Readings

Adams WM, Biery DN, Millar HC. Pneumovaginography in the dog: a case report. J Am Vet Radiol Soc 1978;19:80.

Alexander JE, Lennox WJ. Vaginal prolapse in a bitch. Can Vet J 1961;2:428.

Brodey RS, Roszel JF. Neoplasms of the canine uterus, vagina, and vulva: a clinicopathologic survey of 90 cases. J Am Vet Med Assoc 1967;151:1294.

Johnston SD. Vaginal prolapse. In: Kirk RW, ed. Current veterinary therapy X. Small animal practice. Philadelphia: WB Saunders, 1989:1302.

Krongthong M, Johnston SD. Clinical approach to vaginal/vestibular masses in the bitch. Vet Clin North Am Small Anim Pract 1991;21:509.

Madewell BR, Theilen GH. Tumors of the urinary tract. In: Theilen GH, Madewell BR, eds. Veterinary cancer medicine. 2nd ed. Philadelphia: Lea & Febiger, 1987:591.

Purswell BJ. Vaginal disorders. In: Ettinger SJ, Feldman EC, eds. Textbook of veterinary internal medicine. 4th ed. Philadelphia: WB Saunders, 1995:1642.

Richardson RC. Canine transmissible venereal tumors. Compend Contin Educ Pract Vet 1981;3:951.

Schutte AP. Vaginal prolapse in the bitch. J S Afr Vet Med Assoc 1967;38:197.

Soderberg SF. Vaginal disorders. Vet Clin North Am Small Anim Pract 1986;16:543.

Episioplasty

Sandra Manfra Marretta

Episioplasty is indicated in dogs with chronic perivulvar pyoderma resulting from redundant perivulvar skin and a recessed juvenile vulva. This condition is common in obese older female dogs that have infantile vulvae as a result of spaying at a young age. The vulva is recessed, resulting in retention of vaginal secretions and drops of urine in the folds of the perivulvar region stimulating bacterial growth and ulcerations. Episioplasty with dorsal fixation of the recessed vulva provides better ventilation of the area, thereby resolving perivulvar pyoderma.

Preoperative Care

Preoperatively, perivulvar pyoderma should be medically managed. Medical management of perivulvar pyoderma is similar to other skinfold pyodermas and includes gentle cleansing of the affected area with a benzoyl peroxide shampoo followed by rinsing and drying and application of a mild astringent such as Burow's solution. In patients with a severe inflammatory response, the first few days of treatment consist of twice-daily application of an antibiotic–steroid cream. Once the inflammatory reaction has subsided, an episioplasty can be performed.

After induction of anesthesia, the animal is placed in a perineal stand with adequate padding at the edge of the table. A pursestring suture is placed around the anus, and the hair is clipped from the perineal region, which is then surgically scrubbed in a routine manner. The surgical site is draped so the perivulvar area is exposed and the anus is covered.

Surgical Technique

Before initiation of the episioplasty, the surgeon must determine how much perivulvar skin needs to be removed by plicating the redundant skin between the thumb and index finger (Fig. 31.4). The goal is to re-

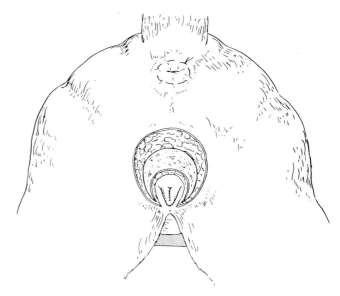

Fig. 31.5. Two crescent-shaped skin incisions are made around the vulva.

move redundant skin without creating excessive tension on the suture line postoperatively.

A No. 10 Bard–Parker scalpel blade is used to create a crescent-shaped skin incision around the vulva. The incision extends lateral to the ventral commissure of the vulva, curving laterally and dorsally to a point 1 cm dorsal to the dorsal commissure of the vulva and then curving ventrolaterally on the contralateral side. A second crescent-shaped incision begins and ends in the same area as the first incision, except the second incision swings in a wider arch around the vulva (Fig. 31.5). The second incision may be made in a relatively narrow arch initially and widened later if the surgeon is unsure about how much skin to remove. This approach prevents removal of too much perivulvar skin and unnecessary tension on the incision line.

The perivulvar skin lying between the two crescent-shaped incisions is excised with Metzenbaum scissors (Fig. 31.6). Excess subcutaneous fat dorsal to the vulva is removed. Hemorrhage is controlled with hemostats, ligation, and judicious use of electrocautery.

Before permanent closure, the skin edges are temporarily approximated with three skin sutures placed at the 9, 12, and 3 o'clock positions to determine the effectiveness of the plasty procedure (Fig. 31.7**A**). It the vulva remains recessed, then additional skin is removed by creating a slightly wider arch following the edge of the second perivulvar crescent-shaped incision and removing the additional narrow strip of perivulvar skin.

The subcutaneous tissues are closed using 3–0 absorbable suture in a simple interrupted pattern. The initial subcutaneous suture should be placed at the

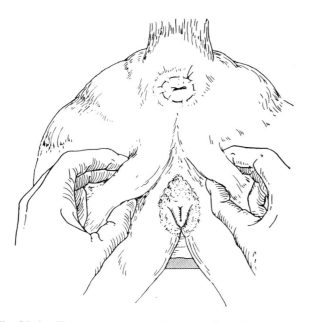

Fig. 31.4. The excess or redundant perivulvar skin is accessed by plicating the skin around the vulva with the thumb and index finger to determine how much perivulvar skin needs to be removed.

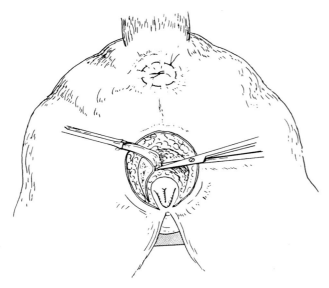

Fig. 31.6. The island of perivulvar skin lying between the two crescent-shaped incisions is excised with Metzenbaum scissors.

dorsal midpoint of the defect. Additional subcutaneous sutures are placed at the midpoints of the remaining defects until the edges of the skin are apposed. The skin is closed in a simple interrupted pattern using 3–0 monofilament nonabsorbable sutures (Fig. 31.7**B**). A cosmetic closure can be achieved by placing skin sutures initially at the 9, 12, and 3 o'clock positions. Additional sutures are then placed equidistantly between previously placed sutures until the incision is completely closed. The pursestring suture is removed postoperatively.

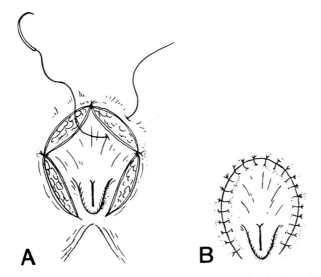

Fig. 31.7. **A.** Three skin sutures are placed at the 9, 12, and 3 o'clock positions to access the adequacy of the episioplasty. **B.** After closure of the subcutaneous tissues, the skin is closed with multiple simple interrupted sutures.

Postoperative Care

An Elizabethan collar should be used postoperatively to prevent self-mutilation. Systemic antibiotics should be used as needed to control any residual pyoderma. A weight-reducing diet is recommended in obese animals. Skin sutures are removed 10 to 14 days after the surgical procedure.

Complications

Surgical complications are minimal when an episioplasty is properly performed. Inadequate removal of perivulvar skin during the plasty procedure may result in persistence of perivulvar pyoderma. Removal of too much perivulvar skin may result in excessive surgical line tension and dehiscence. Careful evaluation of the surgical site during the episioplasty helps to prevent either of these complications.

Suggested Reading

Scott DW, Miller WH, Griffin CE. Environmental skin diseases. In: Scott DW, Miller WH, Griffin CE, eds. Small animal dermatology. 5th ed. Philadelphia: WB Saunders, 1995:859–889.

Episiotomy

Sandra Manfra Marretta

An episiotomy is a surgical procedure that temporarily enlarges the vulvar cleft. An episiotomy provides exposure of those structures of the female urogenital tract that cannot be approached by laparotomy, including the vestibule and the vagina. The main indications for an episiotomy in a dog are vaginal masses, lacerations, prolapsed tissue, strictures, congenital defects, and dystocia resulting from an inadequate vulvar cleft.

Preoperative Care

Episiotomies may be performed with the animal under local, epidural, or general anesthesia, depending on the patient's condition. The patient is positioned on the surgical table in a perineal stand with adequate padding at the edge of the table. The rectum and anal sacs are emptied, and several gauze sponges and a pursestring suture are placed in the rectum and anus before surgery to prevent intraoperative fecal contamination.

The hair from the perineal region is clipped, and the vestibule and vagina are liberally flushed with a diluted antiseptic solution such as a 1:10 povidone–

iodine (Betadine) solution. The perineal region is then scrubbed in a routine manner. A Foley catheter is aseptically placed through the urethral papilla into the urinary bladder so the exact location of the urethral papilla and urethra are apparent throughout the entire surgical procedure. Placement of an intraoperative urinary catheter helps to prevent inadvertent damage to the urethra or urethral papilla. The surgical site is draped so the vulvar cleft and the perineal skin dorsal to the vulvar cleft are exposed but the anus is covered.

Surgical Technique

Immediately before an episiotomy, a digital examination is performed to identify the caudodorsal aspect of the horizontal vaginal canal. To avoid incising the external anal sphincter, the episiotomy incision should not extend further dorsally than the caudodorsal aspect of the horizontal vaginal canal.

A median skin incision is made from the level of the caudodorsal aspect of the horizontal vaginal canal, extending to the dorsal commissure of the vulvar cleft using a No. 10 Bard–Parker scalpel (Fig. 31.8). The remaining layers of the episiotomy incision, including the thin musculature and mucosal layers, are cut with Mayo scissors, following the skin incision from ventral to dorsal (Fig. 31.9). Hemostats, ligation, and judicious use of electrocautery are used to control hemorrhage.

The procedure for which the episiotomy was per-

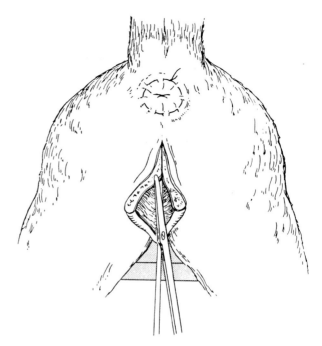

Fig. 31.9. The musculature and mucosal layers are cut with Mayo scissors following the skin incision.

formed can now be completed with adequate surgical exposure. The position of the urethral papilla and location of the urethra should be monitored throughout the surgical procedure with the aid of the preplaced

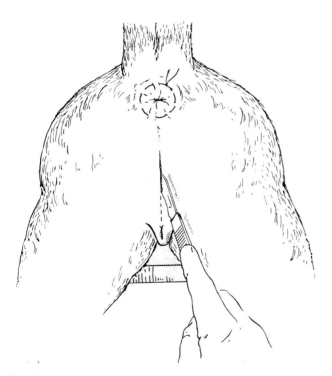

Fig. 31.8. A median skin incision is made from the caudodorsal aspect of the horizontal vaginal canal to the dorsal commissure of the vulvar cleft.

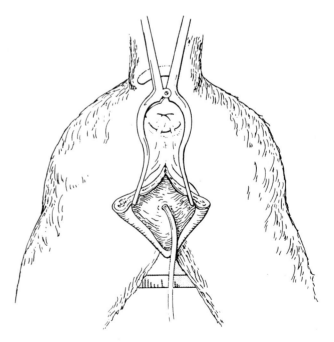

Fig. 31.10. The episiotomy has been completed. A Foley catheter is in place in the urinary bladder to aid in the localization of the urethral papilla and urethra during additional surgical procedures. A self-retaining retractor is in place to provide increased visibility of the vestibule and vagina.

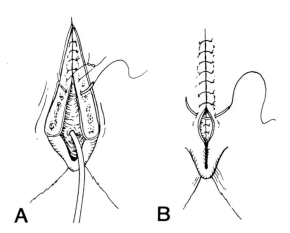

Fig. 31.11. A. The mucosal layer of the episiotomy is closed with simple interrupted sutures. **B.** The skin edges are apposed with simple interrupted monofilament nonabsorbable sutures.

Foley catheter to avoid surgical trauma to these structures (Fig. 31.10).

Closure of the episiotomy is completed in three layers: the mucosa, the muscular and subcutaneous tissues, and the skin. The mucosa is apposed with 3–0 absorbable suture material in a simple interrupted pattern (Fig. 31.11**A**). The musculature and subcutaneous tissues are closed in one layer using a simple interrupted pattern of 3–0 or 4–0 absorbable suture material. The skin edges are apposed with simple interrupted 3–0 nonabsorbable sutures (Fig. 31.11**B**). The urethral catheter is removed if no longer required, and the pursestring and gauze sponges are removed from the anus and rectum immediately after the surgical procedure.

Postoperative Care

An Elizabethan collar is recommended postoperatively to prevent the patient from disrupting the suture line. Any tissue samples obtained during surgery are submitted for histopathologic examination. The skin sutures are removed 10 to 14 days postoperatively.

Complications

Postoperative complications associated with the performance of episiotomy are rare and are often associated with poor surgical technique or inappropriate postoperative care. Poor surgical technique during closure of the incision, including inaccurate suture placement, tight sutures, or the use of through-and-through sutures, may result in unnecessary pain, self-mutilation of the incision site, and discomfort after an episiotomy. Appropriate suturing techniques minimize these problems.

Suggested Reading

van Sluijs FJ. Episiotomy. In: van Sluijs FJ, ed. Atlas of small animal surgery. New York: Churchill Livingstone, 1992:116–117.

32

TESTICLES

Prepubertal Gonadectomy

W. Preston Stubbs

Prepubertal gonadectomy (early-age neutering) refers to orchiectomy or ovariohysterectomy performed in a puppy or kitten before the onset of sexual maturity. Many animal shelter and animal control facilities currently use prepubertal gonadectomy as a means of ensuring that puppies and kittens are incapable of reproducing before adoption, thereby increasing the effectiveness of pet population management programs. Early neutering has also been used by dog and cat breeders to prevent selected animals from being irresponsibly bred. Although numerous concerns have been raised with respect to the safety of pediatric surgery and anesthesia and the potential side effects associated with prepubertal gonadectomy (1–3), increasing evidence suggests that these concerns are unfounded. Several studies have shown that anesthesia and early-age neutering can be performed with minimal complications and that the physical and behavioral development of puppies and kittens that have undergone prepubertal gonadectomy is similar to that of animals neutered at a more conventional age (4–9).

Surgical Anatomy

The relevant surgical anatomy of prepubertal puppies and kittens is similar to that of the adult, with a few exceptions. In male cats, the testes, although normally fully descended at birth, may move freely within the inguinal canal until puberty (10, 11). The testes are small but easily palpated in young (less than 8 weeks of age) tomcats and can be manipulated into the area of the immature scrotum without difficulty. The testes have descended into the scrotum in 50% of newborn pups (12) and may be palpated in the prescrotal or inguinal region in the remaining individuals. Testes palpated in the latter locations in pups can also usually be manipulated caudally into the scrotum (6).

Female kittens neutered between 6 and 14 weeks of age commonly have a persistent urachal remnant on the apex of the bladder (4), and substantial amounts of serous fluid may be present in the abdominal cavities of puppies and kittens as a normal incidental finding (4, 6).

Preoperative Considerations

Pups and kittens undergoing prepubertal gonadectomy should have a thorough physical examination, including assessment of hydration status, mucous membrane color and capillary refill time, thoracic auscultation, body temperature, overall body condition, and accurate body weight measurement. Preoperative laboratory studies consist of measurement of packed cell volume, serum total solids, and blood glucose. More extensive laboratory studies are usually not performed unless the physical examination reveals abnormalities that could require further diagnostic tests. Animals exhibiting signs of debilitation or infectious disease are not considered candidates for prepubertal gonadectomy.

Preoperatively, puppies and kittens should be handled minimally and housed in a warm, quiet environment, preferably with their dam and littermates. Because pediatric animals are more susceptible to hypoglycemia than adults, food should be withheld for no more than 3 to 4 hours in the youngest puppies and kittens (6 to 8 weeks of age). A preoperative fast of 8 hours is adequate in older patients. If necessary, corn syrup can be administered orally, or 50% dextrose can be given orally or intravenously before the surgical procedure. Female pups and kittens are usually administered dextrose-containing isotonic fluids intravenously at a rate of 4 mL/kg per hour during the ovariohysterectomy procedure. A pediatric infusion set (60 drops/mL) or an infusion pump is recommended to quantify fluid administration accurately and to prevent overhydration.

Puppies and kittens are also prone to hypothermia. Hypothermia can be minimized by placing patients on recirculating warm water blankets or water bottles or by placing them under infrared heat lamps. Extreme care should be taken with heat lamps and water bottles because they can cause thermal injury when placed too close to or against the skin. Hypothermia can also be prevented by administering warmed intravenous fluids, limiting hair removal adjacent to the operative site, and warming antiseptics used for skin preparation. Excessive wetting of the patient during skin disinfection should be avoided, and the use of alcohol-containing antiseptics is discouraged to decrease evaporative heat loss.

The use of prophylactic antibiotics is unnecessary because prepubertal gonadectomy is a clean, elective procedure of short duration.

Anesthetic Techniques

Pediatric dogs and cats differ from adults physiologically, and this difference has a profound influence on their successful anesthetic management. Pediatric patients have immature hepatorenal, respiratory, and cardiovascular system function, as well as differences in drug uptake, distribution, and action when compared with adults (13). Despite this, many techniques are available to anesthetize pups and kittens safely and effectively.

Ideally, agents chosen for preanesthetic medication and anesthetic induction and maintenance should provide adequate sedation for preoperative handling and sufficient analgesia during and after the surgical procedure, and they should allow rapid recovery of patients postoperatively. Anesthetic agents that predictably cause bradycardia and hypotension (e.g., xylazine and phenothiazines, respectively) should be avoided because cardiac output in pediatric animals depends on heart rate, and baroresponses are immature (13). Respiratory depression is also of concern because the high oxygen demand of young pups and kittens necessitates a greater respiratory rate than that of adults (13). Therefore, hypoventilation should be avoided, and assisted ventilation may be necessary to prevent hypoxemia in some patients. Anesthetics that rely heavily on hepatic biotransformation or redistribution (e.g., barbiturates) may have a prolonged duration of action in pediatric patients because of incompletely developed hepatic enzyme systems and low body fat levels

(13). Drug pharmacokinetics is further affected in pediatric patients by their increased volume of distribution, lower plasma albumin concentrations, and higher distribution of cardiac output to vessel-rich tissues as compared with adults (13).

The use of preanesthetic agents varies with the anesthetic technique used. I do not administer anticholinergics (atropine, 0.01 to 0.04 mg/kg, or glycopyrrolate, 0.01 to 0.02 mg/kg) routinely, but they may be beneficial in stabilizing heart rate and thus cardiac output in patients given anesthetics likely to cause bradycardia (e.g., opioids). Anticholinergics also decrease respiratory secretions and may prevent airway obstruction and aspiration (13).

Anesthesia can be easily induced and maintained with inhalant agents administered with or without premedication. Isoflurane or halothane and oxygen administered through a clear, tight-fitting mask produce a rapid, smooth anesthetic induction. Minimal restraint is required to induce anesthesia successfully in most pups and kittens. Alternatively, chamber induction can be performed, but it has the disadvantage of greater environmental pollution with anesthetic gases. Isoflurane is preferred to halothane in pediatric animals because of its rapid induction and recovery characteristics, inert (i.e., virtually unmetabolized) nature, and minimal cardiovascular depression (13). Pups and kittens undergoing orchiectomy are usually maintained on inhalant agents administered by mask because of the short duration of the procedure. Endotracheal intubation using an appropriately sized (2.0 to 3.5 mm in kittens) Cole or Magill endotracheal tube, is performed in pups and kittens undergoing ovariohysterectomy (4–6). Noncuffed tubes have the advantage of allowing the largest possible tube diameter to be used, decreasing airway resistance (14). A laryngoscope with a small Michael blade greatly facilitates gentle endotracheal tube placement, reducing the likelihood of laryngeal edema and obstruction of the small airway of pediatric patients. Endotracheal tubes should be of proper length to avoid endobronchial intubation and to minimize dead space. Ideally, the tube end should be level with the nasal planum (14). Tubes smaller than 3.0 mm diameter are prone to obstruction with respiratory secretions and should be aspirated every 30 minutes. A nonrebreathing anesthetic circuit (Ayre's T-piece, Norman elbow, Bain circuit) should be used in pediatric patients weighing less than 5 kg. A fresh gas flow rate between 200 and 500 mL/kg per minute is recommended.

Several injectable anesthetic combinations have been used for anesthetic premedication and for induction and maintenance of anesthesia in pups and kittens undergoing prepubertal gonadectomy. Induction of anesthesia in kittens is best performed using benzodiazepine–dissociative combinations. In male kittens, tiletamine–zolazepam (Telazol) administered at a dose of 11 mg/kg intramuscularly, produces a rapid anesthetic induction and good muscle relaxation, provides sufficient analgesia to perform orchiectomy, and has good recovery qualities (5). A combination of 0.22 mg/kg midazolam (Versed) and 11 mg/kg ketamine (Ketaset) given intramuscularly can also be used for anesthetic induction of kittens and is preferable to tiletamine–zolazepam in female kittens because it produces a shorter, smoother recovery and allows more accurate assessment of anesthetic depth (5). I have routinely induced anesthesia in male and female kittens using an intravenous combination of 0.2 mg/kg diazepam (Valium) and 10 mg/kg ketamine. In male kittens, supplemental inhalant anesthetic can be administered by mask if the level of analgesia achieved with the foregoing techniques is thought to be inadequate. Female kittens are always intubated and are maintained with inhalant anesthetic agents. Administration of inhalants by mask may initially be required in females if intubation cannot be accomplished with the benzodiazepine–dissociative combinations alone.

In pups, premedication with 0.04 mg/kg atropine and 0.11 to 0.22 mg/kg oxymorphone (Numorphan) given intramuscularly, followed by induction with 3 to 6.5 mg/kg propofol (Diprivan) intravenously, produces good preanesthetic sedation, a rapid, smooth induction and recovery, and analgesia sufficient to allow orchiectomy to be performed in male pups without the routine use of supplementary inhalant agents (6). This anesthetic combination may result in apnea and respiratory depression, however, so intubation and administration of oxygen are recommended in male pups (6). Females are intubated and are maintained with isoflurane or halothane and oxygen. Recovery may be hastened with the administration of an opioid antagonist or agonist–antagonist. Alternatively, mask induction can easily be performed in male and female pups after premedication with atropine and oxymorphone. Butorphanol (Torbugesic) at a dose of 0.2 to 0.4 mg/kg intramuscularly, with or without a benzodiazepine such as midazolam (0.44 mg/kg) intramuscularly, may be suitable for premedication, but it may not provide the sedation needed for patient restraint for administration of an intravenous induction agent (6). I have used benzodiazepine–dissociative combinations such as diazepam (0.2 mg/kg) and ketamine (10 mg/kg) given intravenously or tiletamine–zolazepam (13 mg/kg) intramuscularly for anesthetic induction of pups, and these agents are a reasonable alternative to the foregoing protocols because of their general safety and simplicity. In male pups, supplemental inhalant anesthetic should be provided by mask during orchiectomy because the muscle relax-

ation and analgesia provided by benzodiazepine–dissociative combinations are poor (6). In female puppies, administration of inhalant agents by mask may be necessary to facilitate endotracheal intubation.

Anesthetic monitoring is similar to that practiced in adult dogs and cats, with particular attention given to preventing bradycardia, hypotension, and hypoventilation. Heart rate can be monitored using an 18-gauge esophageal stethoscope or a Doppler ultrasound device (Ultrasonic Doppler Flow Detector Model 811-AL, Parks Medical Electronics), which, in combination with a sphygmomanometer and pediatric pressure cuff, can be used to determine blood pressure as well.

Surgical Techniques

The small blood volume of neonates relative to adult dogs and cats makes careful hemostasis of great importance when performing prepubertal gonadectomy. Pediatric tissues are also friable, so meticulous surgical technique is necessary to prevent excessive trauma and to avoid complications.

Orchiectomy

Scrotal and perineal hair is removed with a No. 40 clipper blade, and the skin is disinfected with warmed 4% chlorhexidine gluconate and sterile saline. The animal is positioned in either dorsal or lateral recumbency, depending on the preference of the surgeon. Placing the patient in dorsal recumbency at the end of the operating table with the hindquarters elevated on a sandbag, the hind limbs secured cranially, and the tail hanging affords ideal exposure of the small surgical field (Fig. 32.1). A small surgical drape should be placed to ensure sterility. A closed orchiectomy technique through a scrotal approach is used in both pups and kittens. The testes are palpated and maneuvered into the scrotum if they are in an inguinal or prescrotal location. With the testicle immobilized within the scrotum, a No. 15 scalpel blade is used to make an incision in the scrotal skin lateral to the median septum (Fig. 32.2**A**). In young cats, the scrotum is so immature that it may be difficult to identify because of its small size. In this case, the scrotal incisions are made just dorsal to the prepuce on either side of midline over the immobilized testes. The incision is continued through the tunica dartos and spermatic fascia, and the testicle is exteriorized by gently squeezing the base of the scrotum just proximal to the incision. Careful caudoventral traction on the testicle exposes the thin spermatic cord (Fig. 32.2**B**). Two Halsted mosquito hemostats are placed on the spermatic cord 1 cm from the scrotal incision, and a single ligature of 3–0 to 5–0 absorbable suture material is placed 0.5 cm proximal to the hemo-

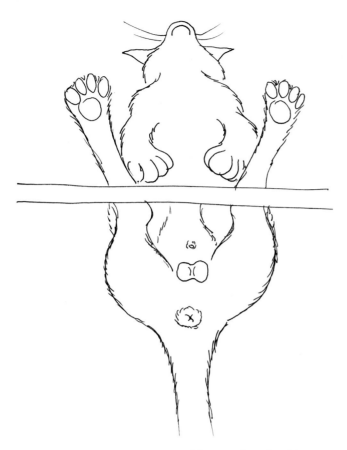

Fig. 32.1. Young kitten positioned for prepubertal orchiectomy. The kitten is in dorsal recumbency, its hindquarters secured cranially with 1-inch porous tape.

stats. Suture materials suitable for ligation of the spermatic cord include chromic gut, polyglycolic acid (Dexon, Davis & Geck, Wayne, NJ), polyglactin 910 (Vicryl, Ethicon, Somerville, NJ), polyglyconate (Maxon, Davis & Geck), and poliglecaprone 25 (Monocryl, Ethicon). Stainless steel hemostatic clips can also be used (4, 6). The spermatic cord is transected between the hemostats (Fig. 32.2**C**), and the testicle is set aside. The spermatic cord is grasped gently with Brown–Adson thumb forceps as the proximal hemostat is released, and the spermatic cord is checked for hemorrhage as it is delivered slowly into the scrotum. The procedure is repeated on the remaining testicle through a separate scrotal incision.

An alternate technique for orchiectomy can be used in kittens, although one author has discouraged its use because of the friable nature of the spermatic cord in such immature cats (4). The technique involves tying the spermatic cord on itself using a mosquito hemostat, thus eliminating the need for ligatures. I have performed prepubertal orchiectomy in this manner in a few young kittens without breakage of the spermatic cord or other complications.

The scrotal incisions are left to heal by second intention or, in pups, may be approximated using two or three simple interrupted subcuticular sutures of 3–0 to 4–0 polyglactin 910, polyglycolic acid, or poliglecaprone 25.

If the pup or kitten is a unilateral or bilateral cryptorchid, it is advisable to delay orchiectomy until the testicles can be palpated in the scrotum or until the animal is 5 to 8 months of age.

Ovariohysterectomy

Hair is removed from the ventral abdomen with a No. 40 clipper blade, and the skin is disinfected with warmed antiseptic solution. The patient is placed in dorsal recumbency, and an incision is made on the ventral abdominal midline using a No. 10 or 15 scalpel blade, starting at the umbilicus in puppies and 1 cm caudal to the umbilicus in kittens. The incision should extend 3 to 5 cm caudally (depending on patient size) and proceed through skin, subcutis, and linea alba in routine fashion. An ovariohysterectomy hook is introduced into the right side of the abdominal cavity and is advanced to the dorsal extent of the body wall, angled slightly toward the bladder. Because of the small size of the celiotomy incision, visualizing the uterine horn and exteriorizing it digitally may be difficult. The urinary bladder may be retracted caudally or momentarily exteriorized through the incision to aid in visualizing the uterine horns near the bladder trigone. The right uterine horn is exteriorized with the ovariohysterectomy hook, and the proper ligament is grasped with a Halsted mosquito hemostat (Fig. 32.3**A**), to facilitate exposure and manipulation of the ovary and vascular structures. Excessive traction should be avoided, particularly in dogs, because the proper ligament is friable (6). Rupture of the suspensory ligament is unnecessary in kittens, but pups may require gentle manual stretching of the ligament to gain sufficient exposure of the ovary. Another mosquito hemostat is used to make a window in the mesovarium adjacent to the ovarian arteriovenous complex. The small amount of adipose tissue in the area of the ovarian pedicle and bursa as compared with adult animals simplifies delineation of the ovary and vascular structures. Two mosquito hemostats are placed across the arteriovenous complex, just proximal to the ovary. A simple, circumferential ligature of fine (3–0 or 5–0) absorbable suture material is secured 0.5 cm proximal to the hemostats (Fig. 32.3**B**). The suture materials used for ligation are similar to those previously recommended for ligation of the spermatic cord. Alternatively, a stainless steel hemostatic clip can be used for pedicle ligation (4, 6). A single ligature is sufficient in the youngest (6- to 10-week old) pups and kittens, whereas a second simple ligature provides more secu-

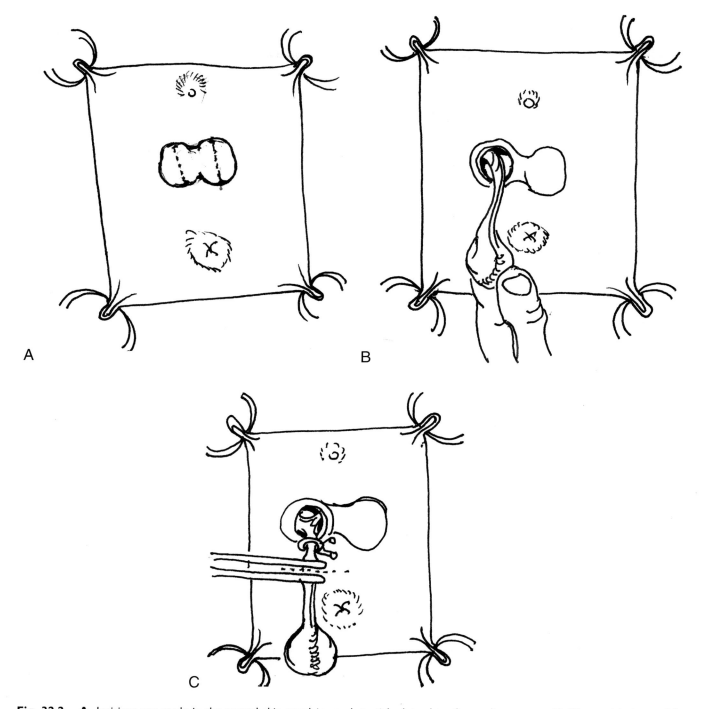

Fig. 32.2. **A.** Incisions are made in the scrotal skin overlying each testicle, lateral to the median septum. **B.** The testicle is carefully exposed using gentle caudoventral traction. **C.** A single ligature of fine suture material (or hemostatic clip) is placed 0.5 cm proximal to the hemostats. The *broken line* indicates transection of the spermatic cord between hemostats.

rity against hemorrhage in older or larger animals. Transfixation ligatures are not routinely used because of the small volume of tissue encompassed by the ligatures. The small amount of adipose tissue present poses little threat to ligature security, also obviating the need for transfixation of the pedicle. The pedicle is transected between the proximal hemostats (Fig. 32.3**C**), and the pedicle is delivered into the abdominal cavity after confirming that hemostasis has been achieved. The broad ligament can be broken down manually or sharply incised with fine scissors. Vessels in the broad ligament are small and need not be ligated. The left

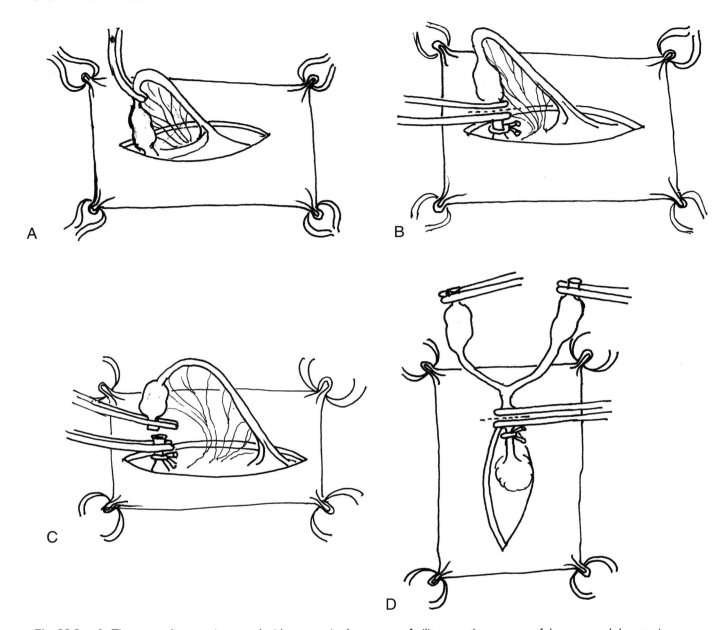

Fig. 32.3. **A.** The proper ligament is grasped with a mosquito hemostat to facilitate gentle exposure of the ovary and the arteriovenous complex. **B.** Hemostats are placed proximal to the ovary, and a single ligature of fine suture material (or hemostatic clip) is placed 0.5 cm proximal to the hemostats. The *broken line* indicates the proposed site of transection of the ovarian pedicle. **C.** The ovarian pedicle is transected between the hemostats, and the broad ligament is broken down. **D.** Two hemostats are placed on the uterine body. Two ligatures are placed proximal to the hemostats, and the uterine body is transected between the hemostats.

uterine horn is located by following the right uterine horn to the bifurcation, and the process described previously is repeated.

The uterine body is clamped with two mosquito hemostats distal to its bifurcation (Fig. 32.3**D**). The cervix is small and is difficult to use as a landmark for determining how much of the tract will be removed. Two simple ligatures of fine absorbable suture material are placed proximal to the hemostats. The second ligature may be a transfixation ligature in older or larger animals. The uterine body may also be ligated without

placing hemostats if it is extremely small or friable. The uterine body is transected between the hemostats, and the tract is removed (see Fig. 32.3**D**). The uterine stump is examined for hemorrhage and is returned slowly to the abdomen. The abdominal cavity is examined for hemorrhage from the ovarian pedicles, and the wound is closed. The linea alba is apposed with 3–0 or 4–0 absorbable or nonabsorbable monofilament suture material in a simple interrupted or simple continuous pattern.

Subcuticular closure is usually omitted in kittens

and is accomplished in pups using 3–0 or 4–0 absorbable suture material in a simple continuous pattern. Polydioxanone (PDS, Ethicon) should not be used for linea alba or subcuticular closure because of reports that it causes calcinosis circumscripta in young dogs (15). The skin is closed with 3–0 or 4–0 nonabsorbable monofilament (e.g., nylon, polypropylene) suture material. Some surgeons prefer to place only subcuticular sutures to decrease the risk that skin sutures will draw the animal's attention to the wound (4, 7).

Postoperative Care and Complications

Puppies and kittens should be placed in a quiet environment during recovery from anesthesia and surgery. The animals can be wrapped in warm towels or placed on warm recirculating water blankets to combat hypothermia. If recovery is prolonged, hypoglycemia should be suspected, and the animal's blood glucose concentration should be measured. Fifty percent dextrose can be given orally (1 to 3 mL) or intravenously (0.5 g/kg) empirically or administered based on results of the blood glucose determination (if lower than 80 mg/dL). Puppies and kittens should also be fed a small meal within 1 hour of standing. Animals are placed with their dam and littermates when ambulatory. Recovery is usually extremely rapid, with most animals returning to normal activities within a few hours of the operation.

Although animals that are neutered prepubertally are subject to the same postoperative complications as adults undergoing similar procedures, the actual reported complications of early neutering are few. Anesthetic deaths have not occurred in six studies evaluating various aspects of prepubertal gonadectomy (4–9). Female puppies and kittens may experience swelling and erythema at the incision that resolve with twice-daily application of warm compresses. Infection of the surgical wound is uncommon, and one author has experienced a wound infection rate of 0% in kittens neutered between 6 and 14 weeks of age (4). Premature removal of skin sutures has been mentioned as a common complication, and some surgeons recommend placing only subcuticular sutures to avoid this problem (4, 7).

The effect of prepubertal gonadectomy on physical and behavioral development continues to be debated; however, two studies (8, 9) demonstrated that pups and kittens neutered prepubertally (7 weeks of age) develop no differently from animals neutered at a more conventional age (7 months of age). Early neutering of puppies and kittens is a safe and effective method of pet population control. The risks and morbidity associated with pediatric anesthesia and surgery are minimal, and the advantages of a shorter operative time, better intraoperative visualization, decreased likelihood of hemorrhage, and more rapid recovery are significant.

References

1. Salmeri KR, Olson PN, Bloomberg MS. Elective gonadectomy in dogs: a review. J Am Vet Med Assoc 1991;198:1183–1192.
2. Stubbs WP, Bloomberg MS. Implications of early neutering in the dog and cat. Semin Vet Med Surg 1995;10:8–12.
3. Stubbs WP, Salmeri KR, Bloomberg MS. Early neutering of the dog and cat. In: Kirk RW, Bonagura JD eds. Current veterinary therapy XII. Philadelphia: WB Saunders, 1995:1037–1040.
4. Aronsohn MG, Faggella AM. Surgical techniques for neutering 6- to 14-week-old kittens. J Am Vet Med Assoc 1993;202:53–55.
5. Faggella AM, Aronsohn MG. Anesthetic techniques for neutering 6- to 14-week-old kittens. J Am Vet Med Assoc 1993;202:56–62.
6. Faggella AM, Aronsohn MG. Evaluation of anesthetic protocols for neutering 6- to 14-week-old pups. J Am Vet Med Assoc 1994;205:308–314.
7. Theran P. Early-age neutering of dogs and cats. J Am Vet Med Assoc 1993;202:914–917.
8. Salmeri KR, Bloomberg MS, Scruggs SL, et al. Gonadectomy in immature dogs: effects on skeletal, physical, and behavioral development. J Am Vet Med Assoc 1991;198:1193–1203.
9. Stubbs WP, Bloomberg MS, Scruggs SL, et al. Effects of prepubertal gonadectomy on physical and behavioral development in cats. J Am Vet Med Assoc 1996;11:1864–1871.
10. Scott MG, Scott PP. Post-natal development of the testis and epididymis in the cat. In: Proceedings of the Physiological Society. 1957:40–41.
11. Sojka NJ. The male reproductive system. In: Morrow DA, ed. Current therapy in theriogenology. Philadelphia: WB Saunders, 1980:844–845.
12. Mialot JP, Guerin C, Begon D. Growth, testicular development and sperm output in the dog from birth to post pubertal period. Andrologia 1985;17:450–460.
13. Grandy JL, Dunlop CI. Anesthesia of pups and kittens. J Am Vet Med Asoc 1991;198:1244–1249.
14. Robinson EP. Anesthesia of pediatric patients. Compend Contin Educ Pract Vet 1983;5:1004–1011.
15. Kirby BM, Knoll JS, Manley PA, et al. Calcinosis circumscripta associated with polydioxanone suture in two young dogs. Vet Surg 1989;18:216–220.

Orchiectomy of Descended and Retained Testes in the Dog and Cat

Stephen W. Crane

Castration (orchiectomy) is performed frequently, usually for reproductive neutering and for modifying or eliminating behavior patterns characteristic of intact males. Neoplasia, severe traumatic injury, and refractory orchitis or epididymitis are primary medical indications for orchiectomy. Castration also removes endocrine sources of androgenic hormones that may be mediators in benign prostatic hypertrophy, perianal adenoma, and perineal hernia. In addition, castration, coupled with scrotal ablation, is the initial surgical step in the perineal urethrostomy of the cat, a salvage procedure for the scar-damaged urethra. These procedures also initiate the permanent scrotal urethrostomy in the dog.

Surgical Anatomy

The spermatic cord, which requires transection in any castration procedure, originates at the vaginal ring as its individual components exit the abdominal cavity. In the center of the spermatic cord are the mesorchium, the testicular artery, the testicular vein and associated pampiniform plexus, the lymphatic vessels, the deferent duct with its associated vessels, and the testicular plexus of autonomic nerves. These structures are externally wrapped with the double tunicae of the vaginal process, which is covered by the spermatic fascia, an extension of the fascia of the abdominal wall. Between the visceral and parietal layers, the cavity of the vaginal process is continuous with the peritoneal cavity. Two thin connective tissue layers of spermatic fascia also invest the vaginal process. The cremaster muscle is a thin, flat extension of the internal abdominal oblique muscle that runs along the external surface of the parietal tunica of the vaginal process to insert on the spermatic fascia and parietal vaginal tunic. Surgically, the cremaster must be handled as though it were part of the spermatic cord.

Between the subcutaneous inguinal ring and the scrotum, the spermatic cords pass ventral to the adductor muscle groups of the pelvic limb in a subcutaneous position. Within the abdominal cavity, the deferent duct courses from the abdominal inguinal ring to its termination in the prostatic urethra. Each of the deferent ducts loops caudally and medially around the ipsilateral ureter at the level of the lateral ligaments of the bladder. The ureter is dorsal to the deferent duct, and the consistent relationships of these structures at this location can be used to help find an undescended gonad during exploratory celiotomy.

Surgical Techniques

Castration of the Dog

Orchiectomy in the dog is performed while the patient is under general anesthesia. The patency of the airway is always protected by an endotracheal tube. The dog is positioned in dorsal recumbency, with caudal restraint of the pelvic limbs to the operating table. The hair of the prescrotal area and medial thighs is clipped. These areas and the scrotum are scrubbed with water and mild soap. The prescrotal area is then prepared for aseptic surgery with skin-preparation soap and solution; the scrotum is not prepared with antiseptics

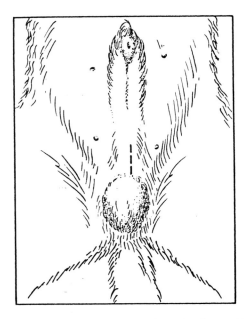

Fig. 32.4. Location of the prescrotal incision for orchiectomy.

because of the high incidence of contact dermatitis. Because the scrotum has not received aseptic preparation, the fully prepared prescrotal operative field is quadrant toweled to cover the scrotum. A fenestrated drape is positioned over the remainder of the dog. All further manipulations of the scrotum itself are performed through the sterile fabric of the towels and drape.

A skin and subcutaneous tissue incision is made on the ventral midline of the prepuce at the base of the scrotum (Fig. 32.4). The length of the incision allows for the outward expression of each testis (Fig. 32.5**A**). Next, one testis is manipulated craniad toward and into the incision by pressure on the scrotum through the drape and towel. The tissue that limits the outward extrusion of the testis at this point is the spermatic fascia, which must be incised to the parietal layer of the vaginal tunica. The latter structure is a distinct, white, glistening layer that surrounds the testis. Once the spermatic fascia has been divided, the tunica-covered testis can be delivered through the skin incision (Fig. 32.5**B**). Shortly after the testis appears, however, its outward progress is resisted by additional attachments of the spermatic fascia in the form of dense connective tissue between the tail of the epididymis and the scrotal wall, the ligament of the tail of the epididymis. It is isolated by blunt dissection, and hemostatic forceps are placed across the fascial condensation to crush small vessels. In the case of testicular neoplasia or orchitis, the ligament of the tail of the epididymis is ligated in addition to being clamped, to preclude the potential complication of postoperative scrotal hematoma. After clamping or ligation of the

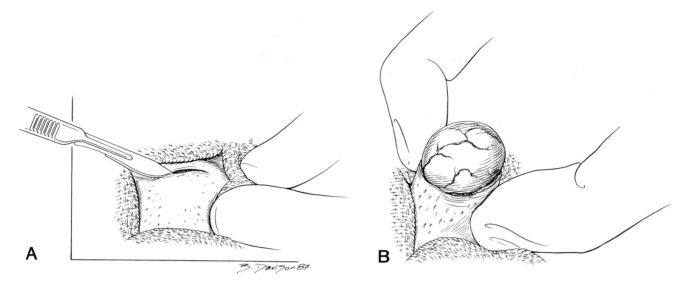

Fig. 32.5. **A.** The skin, subcutaneous tissue, and the spermatic fascia are incised. The body of the penis is visible deep to the incision. **B.** Once the spermatic fascia has been completely divided, the testis, covered by the vaginal process, can be manipulated cranially into the incision. The scrotum is handled only through the sterile fabric of the towel and drape.

ligament of the tail of the epididymis, the structure is divided to release the invagination of the scrotal skin and to allow further exteriorization of the testis (Fig. 32.6). The forceps can be left in place for the duration of the procedure.

Steady caudal and outward traction is next applied to the testis to break down connective tissue attachments between the spermatic cord and the spermatic fascia. As the cord emerges into the operative field, any fat around the cord is removed by proximal wiping with a moist sponge. At this stage, the testis and a considerable portion of the spermatic cord are exteriorized, and the cremaster muscle is clearly seen on the external surface of the vaginal tunicae. The technique for cord transection depends on the patient's size.

CLOSED CASTRATION

In patients under 20 kg, a "closed" castration technique is used. "Closed" means that the contents of the spermatic cord are triple clamped, ligated, and divided with the tunicae of the vaginal process intact around the cord (Fig. 32.7). Additionally, the vaginal process

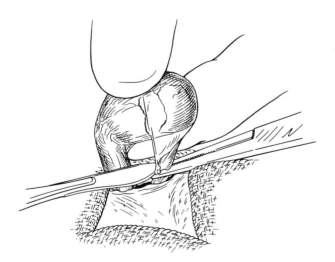

Fig. 32.6. The spermatic fascia is fenestrated to identify and isolate the ligament of the tail of the epididymis. This structure is clamped with hemostatic forceps before its sharp division. The clamp can be left in place until the incision is closed.

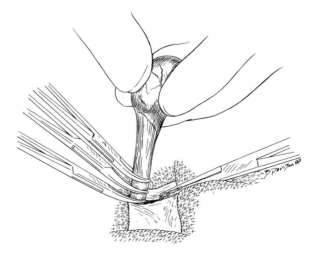

Fig. 32.7. After exteriorization of the testis and most of the spermatic cord, any fat around the cord is removed. The initial step in closed castration is the application of triple hemostatic forceps across the unopened vaginal process and the cremaster muscle.

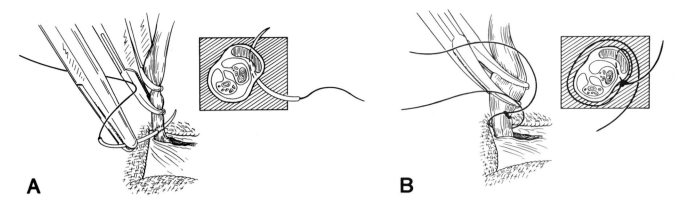

Fig. 32.8. **A.** A transfixing ligature is applied between the cremaster muscle and spermatic cord in the closed castration. The initial needle passage incorporates the parietal tunica of the vaginal process and the cremaster. **B.** After the ligature transfixing the vaginal process and cremaster is tied, the entire cord is encircled with ligature before forming the final knot.

is transfixed to the cremaster muscle for extra security in ligation. After triple hemostatic forceps are applied to the proximal portion of the exposed cord, the most proximal clamp is removed, and a slowly absorbable suture material, swaged on to a taper needle, is passed through the cremaster and tunica (Fig. 32.8A). In placing this transfixation ligature, the surgeon must take care to miss the vascular structures of the spermatic cord. The ligature is tied over the cremaster, and the ends of the suture are passed in opposite directions back around the spermatic cord to encircle it before forming a final knot and completing the ligation (Figs. 32.8B and 32.9). The transfixation method of securing the hemostatic ligature helps to prevent loosening or shifting of the ligature if the cremaster should contract.

Such loosening could cause a retraction of the testicular artery away from ligature control. The middle clamp is removed, and a second nontransfixing ligature is placed in the clamp's crush mark. The spermatic cord is severed along the proximal edge of the distal clamp to prevent backflow hemorrhage from the testis into the operative field (see Fig. 32.9).

OPEN CASTRATION

The "open" castration method is used for dogs over 20 kg. After each testis is exteriorized as described previously, the vaginal process is incised and opened longitudinally with scissors to expose the internal structures of the spermatic cord directly (Fig. 32.10).

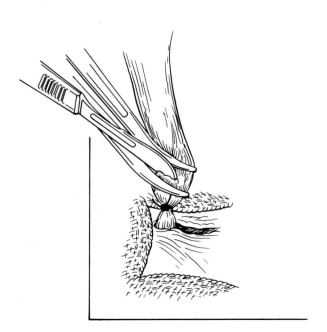

Fig. 32.9. The spermatic cord is severed between the two most distal clamps to prevent backflow hemorrhage from the testis into the operative field and to retain control of the cord.

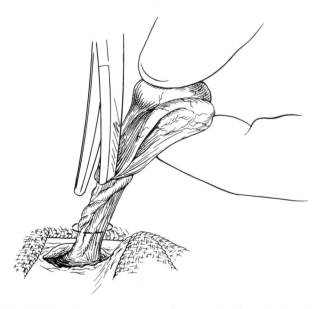

Fig. 32.10. Open castration involves opening the parietal tunica of the vaginal process with scissors to reveal the vascular structures of the spermatic cord directly. The vaginal process and cremaster muscle are amputated proximally (*dotted line*). Ligation of the vaginal process and cremaster is not usually performed, but it may be required if larger blood vessels are present.

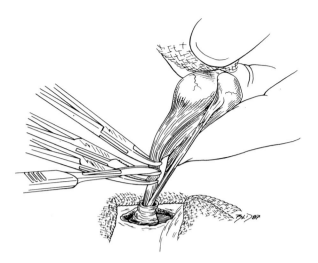

Fig. 32.11. The testicular artery and vein and then the deferent duct are triple clamped. They are ligated just distal to the most proximal clamp.

Proximally, most of the vaginal process and cremaster muscle are amputated; they are ligated only if large blood vessels are present. In returning to the spermatic cord itself, the testicular artery and vein and the deferent duct are ligated according to triple-clamp technique with slowly absorbable suture material and are divided (Figs. 32.11 and 32.12). The advantages of the open method are that the vascular ligations are direct and more secure. The disadvantages are the opening of an extension of the peritoneal cavity and a longer operative time.

After the spermatic cord is divided in either the open or closed castration technique, the remaining portion of the cord is released proximally into the subcutaneous tissue under direct control of thumb forceps (Fig. 32.13). Control during the release of the cord is important because the vessels shorten and dilate as

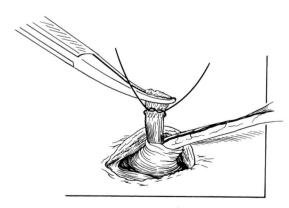

Fig. 32.12. After division of the vessels, single or double ligations are securely placed directly on the testicular artery and vein, using slowly absorbable suture material. In this drawing, the arteriovenous complex is receiving its first ligature, and the ductus is yet to be clamped and ligated.

tension on them is released, and any ligature slippage will probably occur at this time. If bleeding occurs, the vessels or cord can be immediately retrieved for further attention if held by thumb forceps.

The remaining testis is produced by incising the contralateral spermatic fascia, and the gonad is removed in the same manner to complete the castration. At no time is invasion of the scrotal wall or scrotal septum necessary, and doing so invites the complication of scrotal hematoma. After inspection for the complete arrest of bleeding, the deep and superficial subcutaneous layers and subdermal skin are closed with absorbable sutures in a simple interrupted pattern with the knots buried. Several of these sutures should pick up connective tissue surrounding the retractor penis muscle to ablate potential dead space. Finally, the skin edges are apposed with a fine nonabsorbable material in a simple interrupted pattern (Fig. 32.14). Skin sutures that are placed too tightly may attract the patient's attention. If self-mutilating tendencies develop postoperatively, restraint devices such as a head bucket or side bars, tranquilization, antilicking topical preparations, drainage, or removal and replacement of the sutures can be considered to facilitate wound healing.

MODIFIED TECHNIQUES

Some clients may prefer scrotal ablation with the orchiectomy. This orchiectomy is initiated by circumferential excision of the scrotum after full preoperative scrubbing and prepping. The incision is made slightly toward the scrotal side of the junction between skin and scrotum, because surgically induced spasms of the tunica dartos tend to reduce intraoperative hemorrhage. After orchiectomy, attention to dead space ablation during closure is important.

An alternative surgical approach for canine orchiectomy can be used for patients already positioned in sternal recumbency on an elevated platform for perineal surgery. Before the other perineal procedure is performed, a transverse incision is made dorsal to the scrotum at the junction with perineal skin. After the spermatic fascia is incised, the testes are delivered dorsocaudally into the operative field by upward pressure on the toweled scrotum. With outward traction applied, the ligament of the tail of the epididymis is identified, isolated, clamped, and divided; the spermatic cord is then delivered fully into the incision. The remainder of the operation is performed as previously described for a closed or open technique.

Castration of the Cat

Male cats are usually neutered at or before sexual maturity. The intact male cat is usually not tolerated as an exclusively indoor companion animal because of marking and spraying with an odoriferous urine. Nocturnal fighting and roaming are other behavior pat-

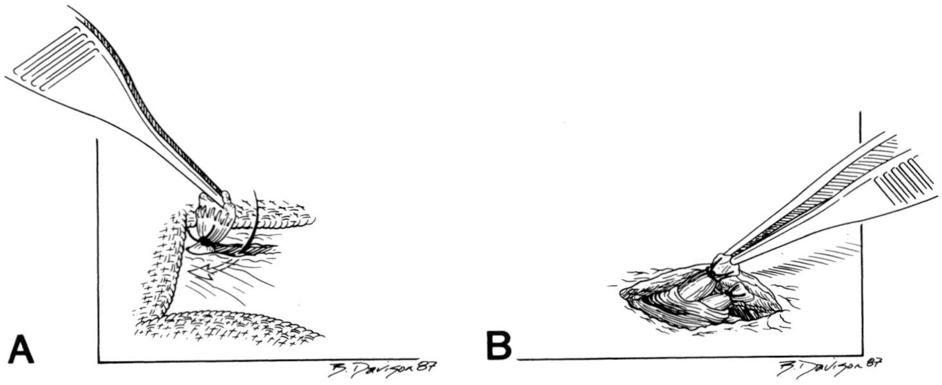

Figure 32.13. A and **B.** In either the closed or open technique, the remaining portion of the amputated spermatic cord is released into the subcutaneous tissue under direct thumb forceps control. This allows retrieval of the vessels or cord if hemorrhage should begin when the stretching in the vessels is relaxed.

terns of male cats that are often successfully controlled by orchiectomy.

The instruments needed for cat castration are two mosquito forceps, a pair of sharp–sharp scissors, a No. 10 scalpel blade, absorbable ligature material, and small, nonfenestrated paper drape. The cat, under ultrashort-acting general anesthesia, is placed in dorsal recumbency. The perineal area is conveniently exposed by bringing the cat's hindquarters to the edge of a table and allowing the tail to fall toward the floor. The patient's pelvic limbs are secured in an abducted position, and the hair covering the scrotum is either plucked with the fingers or clipped with a No. 40 clipper blade. The scrotal area is prepared with scrub soap and skin antiseptics and is draped. A handkerchief-sized drape is easily and economically made from paper drape material, which is sterilized with the other instruments. A fenestration about the size of a dime is cut in the center of the drape, and the prepared scrotum is expressed through the hole to create an acceptably draped surgical area with a minimum of exposed hair.

The skin, tunica dartos, and spermatic fascia over each testis are vertically incised with a finger-held No. 10 scalpel blade. The incision should extend amply from the dorsal to the ventral aspect of the scrotal compartments. An incision into the most ventral portion of the scrotum allows for any postoperative drain-

age. With a gentle pinching maneuver, the testis, still enclosed in the vaginal process, is "popped" out of the incision. The testis is pulled caudoventrally until considerable exposure of the spermatic cord is obtained and resistance to further traction is met. In a proximal position, the two Halsted mosquito forceps are placed across the spermatic cord. As the proximal forceps is removed, one ligature of absorbable suture material is tied tightly in the crush mark created by the forceps. The testis is then amputated proximal to the distal clamp, and the spermatic cord is released into the subcutaneous tissues under direct control of the remaining mosquito forceps. After the other testis is removed, both scrotal incisions are dilated by spreading the tips of mosquito forceps between the wound edges; dilatation is needed to preclude an early fibrin seal across the incision that may prevent drainage. Topical ointments or powders and systemic antibiotics are unnecessary. Proper ligature technique and avoidance of the scrotal septum prevent postoperative hemorrhage.

Cryptorchidism

Unilateral or bilateral cryptorchidism, especially in the dog, is encountered frequently. Canine cryptorchidism is transmitted as a hereditary disorder in a simple autosomal recessive manner. The condition occurs most

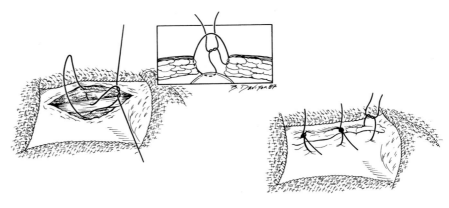

Fig. 32.14. Simple interrupted sutures, with the knots buried, are used to ablate dead space and to appose wound edges. In this drawing, each suture is just "catching" superficial portions of the retractor penis muscle. Ablation of dead space helps to prevent postoperative hematoma or seroma. Skin suture should loosely approximate wound edges.

frequently in small purebred dogs, with a right-to-left ratio of 2.3:1, and 14 breeds are identified as risk factors. Unilaterally cryptorchid males are typically fertile and possess normal libido. The trait is widely disseminated.

Testicular descent should be complete shortly after birth. Testes not located within the scrotum by 2 months of age should be considered permanently retained. Medical therapy using luteinizing hormone–releasing factor or human chorionic gonadotropin is useless, because no drug can stimulate testicular migration after the contractile mechanism of gubernaculum testis has regressed. Because orchiopexy or prosthetic testicular implantation is illegal and unethical for show purposes and can contribute to the perpetuation of cryptorchidism, and because testes retained in an inguinal or abdominal position are predisposed to malignant changes (seminoma and Sertoli cell tumor) in later life, the veterinarian should strongly recommend the castration of cryptorchid animals.

The palpable absence of one or both testes during several examinations confirms the diagnosis of cryptorchidism. Serial examination may be needed because a fear-induced spasm of the cremaster muscle can cause an artifactual elevation of descended testes in some young puppies. Once a diagnosis of cryptorchidism has been established, the surgeon must determine at what point along the normal path of descent testicular migration became arrested. This point can be anywhere from just cranial to the scrotum in the subcutaneous tissue of the groin region to the position in embryonic organogenesis, just caudal to the kidney. Careful palpation usually enables the examiner to detect most gonads if they are distal to the superficial inguinal ring in the subcutaneous tissue of the groin.

Many retained canine testes are located within the abdominal cavity, and exploratory celiotomy is required for their removal. With the patient under general anesthesia and the ventral abdominal wall prepared for aseptic surgery, a midline celiotomy is performed through the linea alba from the umbilicus to the prepuce.

Frequently, the testis is located in the midabdominal region as a highly movable organ smaller than the descended gonad. Arterial supply from the testicular artery, a direct branch of the aorta, and a small artery in the gubernacular remnant or the deferential fold of the peritoneum are typically visualized. The ductus deferens courses toward the caudal aspect of the abdomen and can be used as the primary landmark for finding the retained testicle.

If the testis cannot be located initially in the midabdominal area, the area of the inguinal ring is examined. When testicular descent is arrested at this location, the testis can usually be palpated by moving a finger along the abdominal wall toward the ring. If the testis still cannot be located, the celiotomy incision is extended caudally, and the ductus deferens is identified at the ureteral loop and then traced proximally to find the testis. After the cryptorchid testis is located, the testicular vessels and ductus are isolated, triple clamped, and doubly ligated either collectively or individually with slowly absorbable suture material. After division of vascular structures, the abdominal cavity is checked carefully for bleeding, and the celiotomy is closed. Agenesis of the testis and vas deferens is reported, but it is rare.

If the testis has descended through the inguinal canal and is located in the subcutaneous tissue of the groin, removal is by a standard prescrotal incision with manipulation of the testis into the incision by digital pressure.

Selected Readings

Baumans V, Dijkstra G, Hensing CJG. Testicular descent in the dog. Zentralbl Veterinaermed [A] 1981;10:97.

Evans HE. Miller's anatomy of the dog. 3rd ed. Philadelphia: WB Saunders, 1993.

Hates HM, Wilson GP, Pendergrass TW, et al. Canine cryptorchidism and subsequent testicular neoplasia: case control study with epidemiologic update. Teratology 1985;32:51.

Hudson LC, Hamilton WP. Atlas of feline anatomy for veterinarians. Philadelphia, WB Saunders, 1993.

Knecht CD. An alternative approach for castration of the dog. Vet Med Small Anim Clin 1976;71:469.

Reif JS, Moquire TG, Kenney RS. A cohort study of canine testicular neoplasia. J Am Vet Med Assoc 1979;175:719.

Caudal Castration in the Dog

F. A. Mann & Gheorghe M. Constantinescu

An alternative to standard prescrotal castration is desirable in dogs when castration is indicated in conjunction with perianal or perineal surgery. In the surgical treatment of perianal adenoma, excisional biopsy is indicated to confirm the diagnosis, and castration is performed to minimize recurrence (1). Although the role of castration in canine perineal hernia is debatable (2), many surgeons continue to perform castration in conjunction with perineal herniorrhaphy. In these two situations, or whenever a dog is undergoing castration at the same time as a procedure that requires perineal positioning, caudal castration can decrease operative time by eliminating the need for intraoperative repositioning (3).

Patient Preparation

For caudal castration, the dog must be surgically prepared such that the scrotum is in the aseptic surgical field once the surgical drapes are in place. Therefore,

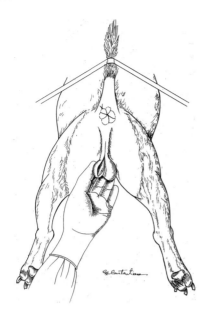

Fig. 32.15. Caudal castration skin incision. Surgical drapes are not shown to allow anatomic reference. Both testicles are removed through the same skin incision.

gentle clipping of scrotal hair with a cool clipper blade is performed before clipping of the remainder of the surgical field. After clipping and hair removal are complete, the dog is placed in the perineal position (Fig. 32.15; see also Chapter 16) for aseptic surgical preparation. We prefer to use chlorhexidine instead of povidone–iodine for scrotal disinfection, to minimize the chance of scrotal dermatitis. On completion of skin disinfection, surgical drapes are placed such that the scrotum is within the surgical field, and caudal castration is performed before the other scheduled surgical procedure (perianal adenoma excision, perineal herniorrhaphy). The anus and perianal region may be temporarily covered with drapes to minimize contamination of the castration procedure.

Surgical Technique

The skin incision begins on the median raphe and extends ventrally onto the scrotum over the left testicle (see Fig. 32.15). Open castration (as described in the previous section of this chapter) is then performed. The left testicle is pushed toward the skin incision to

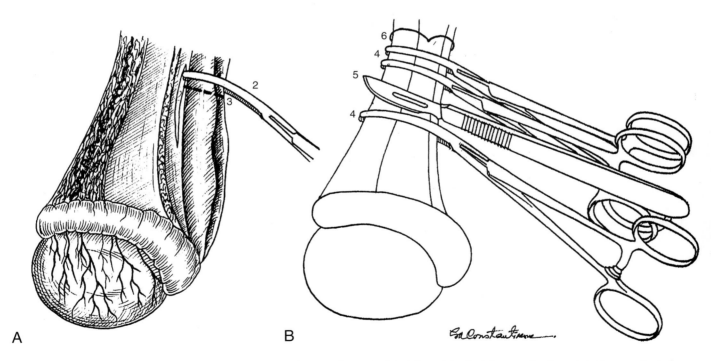

A   B

Fig. 32.16. Three-clamp technique for caudal castration (open technique) of the left testicle. **A.** A fenestration is made in the mesofuniculus to allow Carmalt forceps to be placed across the tunic containing the cremaster muscle. An incision (*dotted line*) is made distally to the Carmalt forceps. A transfixation ligature (not shown) is placed proximally to the Carmalt forceps and tied as the forceps are removed to control hemorrhage from the cremaster muscle. **B.** Three Carmalt forceps are placed across the mesorchium; the testicle is excised by cutting (scalpel) between the two most distal forceps, and a ligature is placed proximal to the most proximal Carmalt forceps and tightened as the most proximal forceps are removed. The numbers represent the steps of the procedure. (Alternately, the pampiniform plexus–testicular artery complex and the deferent artery and ductus deferens may be excised and ligated using two separate three-clamp procedures.)

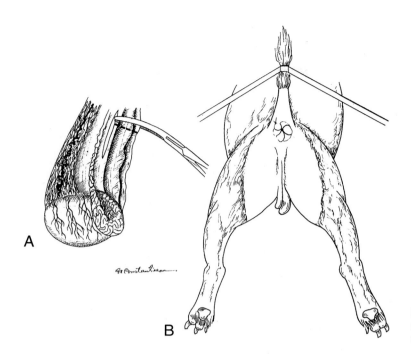

A

B

Fig. 32.17. **A.** Appearance of the right testicle for caudal castration (open technique). **B.** Perineal position and testicular bursae after castration is complete.

allow incision of the vaginal tunic exposing the testicle. The excess vaginal tunic is excised, and the testicle is removed using a three-clamp technique (Fig. 32.16). The right testicle (Fig. 32.17) is approached through the same skin incision through the interdartoic septum and is removed in a fashion similar to that of the left testicle. A few subcutaneous–subcuticular sutures of synthetic absorbable suture are used for closure. The perineal position (see Fig. 32.17) is maintained for the subsequent surgical procedure, and the scrotum may be draped out of the surgical field to minimize contamination of the castration incision.

References

1. Henderson RA, Brewer WG. Skin and subcutis. In: Slatter DH, ed. Textbook of small animal surgery. Philadelphia: WB Saunders, 1993:2075–2088.
2. Mann FA, Nonneman DJ, Pope ER, et al. Androgen receptors in the pelvic diaphragm muscles of dogs with and without perineal hernia. Am J Vet Res 1995;56:134–139.
3. Knecht CD. An alternate approach for castration of the dog. Vet Med Small Anim Clin 1976;71:469–473.

33

PENIS AND PREPUCE

Surgical Procedures of the Penis

H. Phil Hobson

Amputation Techniques

Partial or "complete" amputation of the penis may be indicated in certain congenital, traumatic, or neoplastic conditions. The most common neoplasm of this area, transmissible venereal tumor, is generally responsive to chemotherapy or radiotherapy. Thus, amputation of the penis should be considered rarely, if ever, as a corrective measure for this condition. Cryotherapy has also been used successfully for removal of benign tumors of the penis.

Partial Amputation

The exact location of the amputation is determined by the site of the lesion. In most cases, the penis can be extruded (Fig. 33.1**A**) and held in the extruded position by clamping the preputial orifice with a towel clamp just caudal to the bulbus glandis. The sheath can be opened full thickness on the ventral midline, when necessary, to expose the penis. The penis can be extruded through a ventral opening in the prepuce, or the entire length of the prepuce can be opened for better exposure. A Penrose drain tube works well as a tourniquet around the base of the penis.

Amputation of the tip of the penis may be necessary in patients with chronic or recurrent prolapse of the urethra (Fig. 33.1). Placing a catheter in the urethra helps to identify the limits of the lumen. The surgeon should make the incision partway across the tip, place a stay suture to unite the mucosa of the urethra with the mucosa of the penis, and then complete the exci-

sion of the tip of the penis (Fig. 33.1**B**). The triangulation technique (Fig. 33.1**C** and **D**) conserves a patent lumen to the tip of the urethra. Careful apposition of the cut mucosal edges to the penile tunica helps to avoid excessive scar tissue proliferation and stricture. A continuous suture pattern helps to control seepage from the cavernous erectile tissue. Synthetic absorbable suture is used for mucosal closure.

An Elizabethan collar or a side-bar restraint device should always be used to prevent the patient from licking the wound (see Chap. 5). Castration or careful hormone therapy may be indicated to help to prevent erection during healing.

Amputations of the main body of the penis require the severing of the os penis, as well as the salvaging of enough urethra distal to the severed os penis for a distance of 1 cm. The os penis and urethra are severed with bone-cutting forceps and a scalpel. The urethra is isolated subperiosteally from the groove of the os penis with a small dental chisel. The urethra is split, flared, trimmed, and sutured to the infolded tunica albuginea, as shown in Figure 33.2. Care should be taken to appose the mucosal surfaces. Although it is perhaps easier to achieve excellent apposition with fine, closely placed interrupted sutures, a continuous pattern is more likely to control bleeding. Some bleeding, especially at the end of urination, is common, even for several days after the operation. It is difficult to identify and to ligate individual vessels in this area. Releasing the tourniquet while the wound is open, in an effort to identify and to ligate the vessels within the corpus spongiosum penis, may prove unrewarding.

Preputial Amputation

When pooling of urine within the prepuce becomes a concern after partial amputation of the penis, shorten-

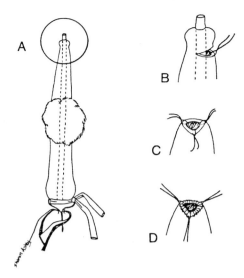

Fig. 33.1. **A.** Amputation of the tip of the penis. **B.** Securing the urethral mucosa to the penile mucosa. **C.** Triangulating the urethral orifice with stay sutures. **D.** Placement of a simple continuous pattern between the stay sutures with the orifice in maximal dilatation.

ing of the entire prepuce may be desirable. For the best cosmetic results, a full-thickness section of the prepuce can be removed (Fig. 33.3). The length of prepuce to be removed should be the same as the length of the penile resection. In patients with congen-

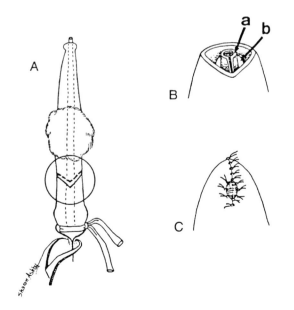

Fig. 33.2. **A.** Amputation of the penis proximal to a lesion. The corpus spongiosum penis is incised at a 45° angle. The os penis and urethra are incised 1 cm further distal than the corpus spongiosum penis. **B.** The urethra (*a*) is elevated subperiosteally from the groove in the os penis. The os penis (*b*) is trimmed away with a rongeur to the level of the corpus spongiosum penis. **C.** The urethra is sutured to the penile mucosa, and the remainder of the penile stump is closed.

ital micropenis, the tip of the prepuce should cover the tip of the penis by approximately 1 cm. The cranial transverse incision is made 2 cm caudal to the cranial junction of the prepuce and the body wall, to allow adequate circulation to the cranial end of the prepuce. The location of the caudal transverse incision is determined by the length of the penis. The two incisions are extended laterally in an elliptic fashion to facilitate a smooth closure of the skin.

Next, the dorsal aspect of the section of prepuce to be removed is dissected free from the body wall with scissors. With careful dissection, most of the preputial vessels, which lie immediately subcutaneously on both sides of the sheath, can be identified and preserved. To close the amputation, the preputial mucosa is apposed with 4–0 absorbable suture, using a submucosal pattern. If a continuous pattern is used around the circumference of the prepuce, care should be taken to avoid a pursestring effect, which limits the movement of the penis. The veterinarian may find it easier to close the dorsal mucosa if the penis is allowed to protrude through the incision site during this phase of closure.

Complete Amputation

The initial skin incision is made in an elliptic fashion around the entire external genitalia (Fig. 33.4**A**). The preputial vessels are ligated, as are any additional branches of the caudal superficial epigastric vessels that cross the incision line. The spermatic cords are isolated, ligated, and severed. Care must be taken to place the ligatures tightly enough to prevent retraction of the severed spermatic artery if the tunicae are incorporated in the ligature. When the penis and the prepuce have been stripped from the body wall in a caudal direction, the dorsal penile vessels are identified and ligated just caudal to the level of the desired penile amputation site. The retractor penis muscle is reflected from the urethra, and, with a catheter in place, a midline incision is made into the urethral lumen at the desire urethrostomy site. A 1–0 absorbable, ligature, which circumscribes the penis, is placed just caudal to the amputation site and just cranial to the urethrostomy site (Fig. 33.4**B**), to control seepage bleeding from the erectile tissue further, if necessary. The shaft of the penis is amputated in a wedge fashion, and the tunica albuginea is apposed over the amputation stump. The urethrostomy should be located in the scrotal area whenever possible. Careful apposition of penile urethra and skin edge, as the urethrostomy is completed, minimizes postoperative bleeding and scar tissue formation (Fig. 33.4**C**). Although suture patterns and materials are a matter of choice, a continuous pattern aids in controlling hemorrhage from any incised erectile tissue. The use of synthetic absorbable suture eliminates the need for suture removal.

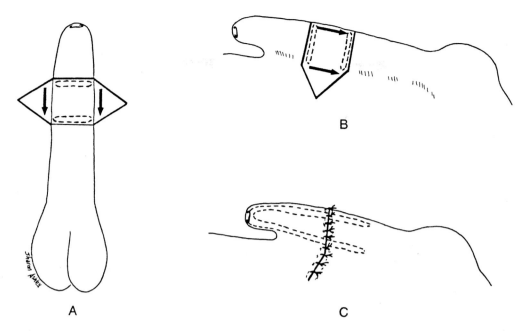

Fig. 33.3. Shortening of the prepuce in cases of pooling of the urine within its lumen. **A.** Removal of a section of the entire prepuce. **B** and **C.** Reapposition of the mucosa and skin.

Particular care should be taken to obliterate dead space, especially cranial to the stump of the amputated penis, when closing the subcutaneous tissue. The use of a restraint device to prevent licking of the surgery site by the patient is imperative.

Correction of Hypospadias

Hypospadias is a congenital anomaly of the external genitalia in which the penile urethra terminates caudal to its normal opening. The urethra can terminate at any level from the perineum to the tip of the penis (Fig. 33.5) because the urethral folds fail to fuse (see Fig. 33.9). In severe cases, the two halves of the scrotum can fail to fuse, the penis fails to develop normally, and the urethra fails to close in the perineal area (Fig. 33.6). Frequently, the analog of the urethra can be present as a fibrous cord that runs from the glans penis to the urethral opening and pulls the penis into a deforming ventral curvature (chordae) (see Fig. 33.6).

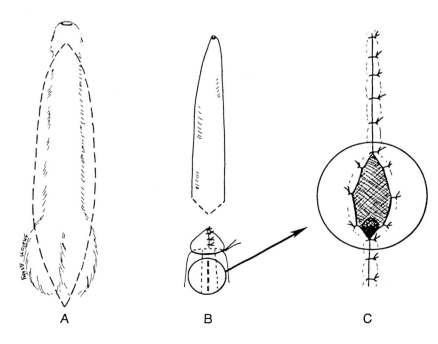

Fig. 33.4. Ablation of the external male genitalia. **A.** The skin incision extends from cranial to the prepuce to caudal to the scrotum. **B.** Amputation of the shaft of the penis in the area of the scrotum. The penis is ligated, incised, and sutured. **C.** The urethrostomy is established by careful apposition of the urethral mucosa to the edge of the skin.

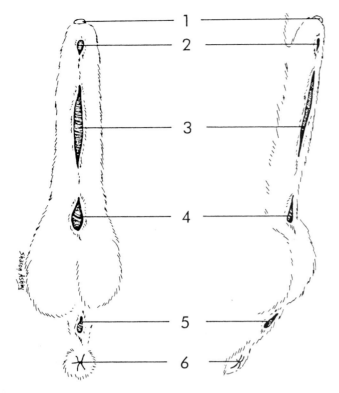

Fig. 33.5. Normal urethral meatus (*1*) and types of hypospadias: glandular (*2*); penile (*3*); scrotal (*4*); perineal (*5*); and anal (*6*).

Minimal defects usually require no urethral surgery. The constant extrusion of the tip of the glans penis can often be relieved by closing the prepuce to its normal extent (Figs. 33.7 and 33.8) on its caudoventral aspect. Should the resulting orifice be too small to allow extrusion of the penis, the opening can be increased to the desired diameter by enlarging the lumen of the craniodorsal aspect. Simply leaving the orifice larger by not closing the caudoventral defect to its fullest extent can cause the tip of the penis to continue to droop from the prepuce and may thus subject it to continual drying, licking, and trauma.

Caudoventral closure is accomplished by incising the mucocutaneous junction, separating the mucosa from the skin, and closing the two layers individually (Fig. 33.8**A**). Sutures of 4–0 to 6–0 absorbable synthetic material are preferred. Should the orifice need to be enlarged dorsally, one scissor jaw is inserted into the lumen of the prepuce, and the orifice is cut to the needed extent. With a minimum of undermining, the cut mucosal and skin edge can be apposed (Fig. 33.8**B**). Failure to appose the skin and mucosal edges adequately may result in closure by granulation, or, should the patient be allowed to lick out the sutures, stricture formation is likely to follow.

Small urethral defects can be closed successfully with a two-layer closure (Fig. 33.9). A catheter is in-

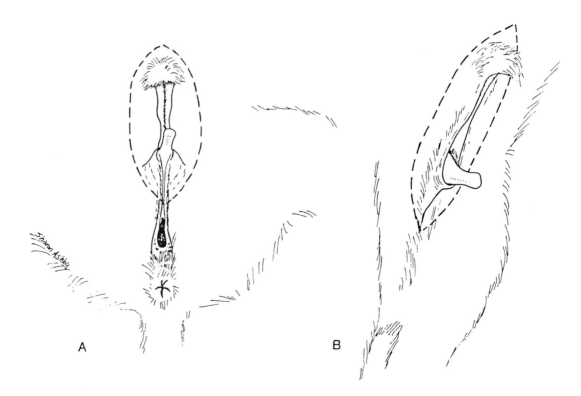

A   B

Fig. 33.6. **A** and **B.** Severe hypospadias with concurrent defects of penile and preputial development. Excision of the entire external genitalia is the approach of choice.

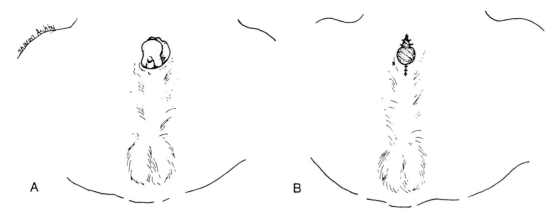

Fig. 33.7. **A.** Glandular hypospadias with a concurrent preputial defect. **B.** The defect is closed ventrocaudally. If the resulting orifice is too small, it is enlarged by incising the prepuce dorsocranially. The preputial mucosa is sutured to the skin edge.

serted past the defect, and an incision is made at the open mucocutaneous junction around the perimeter. The mucosa is undermined and is closed, as is the skin. Care must be taken not to create a stricture. Skin can be invaginated to close the urethral defect, provided the hair follicles have been destroyed previously.

Rectangular full-thickness bladder wall sections, rolled into a tube, have been used to replace surgically sacrificed sections of urethra (i.e., urethral neoplasms). Oral mucosa has been used as well. After suturing of the grafts into the urethral defect (over a catheter), the skin is undermined as in Figure 33.9**C** and is closed over the urethral graft. The catheter is left in place for 7 to 10 days. If open-ended catheters are used as stents, the catheter need not be introduced all the way to the bladder. Catheters remain in place much better if they are cut flush with the urethral orifice and are sutured in place by passing one or two sutures through the catheter and the tip of the penis. For major urethral defects, excision of the external genitalia and urine diversion by urethrostomy are the treatments of choice (see Fig. 33.4). An elliptic incision is made around the rudimentary penis, prepuce, and scrotum. Dissection from the body wall is carried out in a cranial-to-caudal direction; the surgeon should ligate preputial vessels as they are identified and isolated. Should penile tissue be present near the caudal end of the incision, it can be ligated in its entirety and excised. Ligation of the dorsal artery of penis is accomplished when necessary. The subcutaneous tissue and skin are closed in a routine fashion.

Correction of Phimosis

The inability to extrude the penis from the sheath (phimosis) is usually the result of too small a preputial orifice. Because surgical enlargement of the orifice with a ventrocaudal preputial incision can cause persistent extrusion of the glans, the orifice should be enlarged on the craniodorsal surface. A full-thickness incision is made to the desired length with heavy scissors. The severed preputial mucosa is then undermined sufficiently to allow apposition to the ipsilateral skin edge (see Fig. 33.8**B**). The use of a restraint device to prevent licking or chewing is imperative.

Correction of Paraphimosis

The inability to return the penis to the sheath can result in severe trauma or circulatory compromise. The

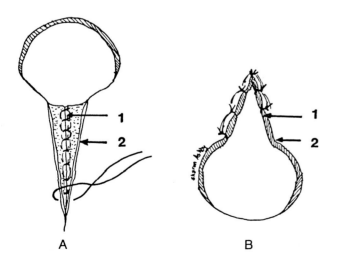

Fig. 33.8. **A.** Closure of a ventrocaudal preputial defect. The mucocutaneous junction is trimmed away, the skin is undermined, and the mucosa (*1*) and the skin edges (*2*) are closed as separate layers. **B.** Enlargement of the dorsocranial aspect of the preputial orifice. The prepuce is cut at full thickness. The mucosa (*1*) is sutured to the skin edge (*2*) along the margin of the incision.

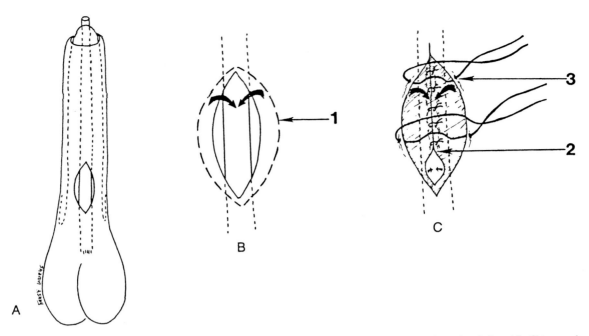

Fig. 33.9. **A.** Penile hypospadias with a catheter in the urethra. **B.** Incisions are made lateral to the defect (*1*). Skin can be used to reconstruct the ventral wall of the urethra if mucosa is insufficient. Hair follicles need to be destroyed if skin is invaginated. **C.** The tissue is undermined sufficiently to allow the ventral urethral wall to be reconstructed (*1*) and the skin to be closed (2) without undue tension.

animal can develop necrosis or injury sufficient to require penile amputation. Persistent exposure of the glans can also result in chapping and excessive licking.

Many patients with acute paraphimosis can be managed by noninvasive methods to return the penis to the lumen of the sheath. The extruded and visually edematous penis should be cleansed, and the sheath should be thoroughly irrigated with nonirritating soaps. A combination of massage and locally applied hypertonic and hygroscopic agents, such as sugar, can help to reduce swelling. Once swelling is reduced, the constricting preputial orifice can usually be pulled over the lubricated penile shaft. Preputial enlargement can be accomplished by incision and primary repair of the mucosal and skin layers, to reduce refractory paraphimosis.

On occasion, the tip of the penis can remain exposed when no obvious orifice defects are present. Once the mucosa has been exposed for some time and has become dry and cornified, the skin of the prepuce rolls inwardly as attempts are made to return the penis to its sheath. After adequate cleansing and lubrication, the penis can be returned to its sheath. If the tip of the penis is well covered by the prepuce (at least 1 cm), narrowing of the preputial orifice will probably prevent recurrence (see Fig. 33.8**A**). Should the prepuce not cover the tip of the penis well, cranial movement of the prepuce should be performed (Fig. 33.10). This translocation can be accomplished by removing a crescent-shaped piece of skin from the ventral body wall just cranial to its juncture with the prepuce. Care should be taken to preserve the preputial vessels. The preputial muscles, which lie superficial to the rectus abdominis muscles, can then be shortened by either an overlapping technique (Fig. 33.10**A**) or simple excision followed by reapposition (Fig. 33.10**B**). The closure of the subcutaneous tissue and skin is routine.

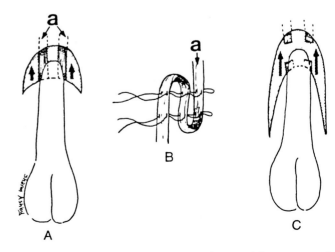

Fig. 33.10. **A** and **B.** A crescent-shaped piece of skin is removed with subsequent cranial movement of the cranial aspect of the prepuce by folding the preputial muscles (*a*). **C.** Excision of a segment of the preputial muscles.

Preputial Reconstruction

A hypoplastic prepuce can be lengthened in a two-step surgical procedure. The first step involves transplanting oral mucosa to a prepared graft site on the ventral body wall immediately cranial to the hypoplastic prepuce; in the second step, the lateral sides of the grafted mucosa are freed, are formed into a tube, and are anastomosed to the isolated mucosa of the cranial end of the prepuce. Single pedicle skin flaps are advanced to the ventral midline from both sides of the ventral body wall to cover the mucosal tube and to complete the cranial extension of the prepuce.

Preputial reconstruction is discussed in detail later in this chapter.

Correction of Ventral Deviation of the Penis

Wedge osteotomies reportedly have been successfully performed to correct ventral penile deviation. The os penis is approached on the dorsal midline over its greatest curvature. The os penis is fractured with a bone cutter, and a small pie-shaped wedge of bone is excised to allow for straightening of the os penis. After wound closure, an open-ended catheter is sutured in place within the urethra and is left for a minimum of 3 weeks. One disadvantage of this procedure is possible damage to the penile urethra at the time of surgery or during healing. Rigid fixation of the os penis should definitely be maintained to help alleviate the likelihood of nonunion or malunion. Animals with congenital anomalies should not be used for reproductive purposes.

Removal of Penile Urethral Calculi

Most urethral calculi causing impairment of urine flow are lodged just proximal to the os penis. On rare occasion, particularly when the groove within the os penis is narrowed, calculi lodge within the penile urethra. This narrowing can be the result of a congenital deformity or injury, with or without fracture of the os penis. Whenever possible, these calculi should be hydropulsed into the bladder. Extraordinary efforts should not be used to relocate these stones, however, because debridement of the urethral mucosa is likely to result in stricture formation.

The penile urethra is approached from a ventral midline incision, after exposure of the penis as in Figure 33.1**A** or by splitting the prepuce. A catheter is advanced from the urethral orifice caudally to determine the exact location of the obstruction. Ideally, the incision is made exactly on the ventral midline of the penis, to avoid the erectile tissue. The incision is extended caudally 1 to 2 cm, exposing the calculi. On rare occasion, the surgeon may need to rongeur away a part of the wall of the groove in the os penis after carefully elevating the soft tissue, including the urethra, from the bone.

The calculi are grasped with forceps and carefully are removed. The area is flushed with sterile saline, and the catheter is advanced to the bladder, while one checks for the presence of more calculi. A cystotomy is performed if indicated. The penile urethral incision is closed with fine absorbable suture over a catheter with a continuous suture pattern. The penile incision is then closed over the urethra in similar fashion.

Correction of Penile Urethral Strictures

Minimal stricturing of the penile urethra can often be managed by dilating the stricture and leaving an indwelling open-ended catheter in place for 7 to 10 days. More extensive strictures may be better managed with a prescrotal or scrotal urethrostomy, as discussed previously and in Chapter 28, because the urethra is immobile within the groove of the os penis and does not lend itself well to reconstruction.

Correction of Persistent Penile Frenulum

On rare occasions, the penile mucosa may fail to separate from the prepucial mucosa as the puppy matures, and it may serve as an irritant to the pup or may even impair breeding in the mature male. Rarely is this persistent attachment more than a narrow band of tissue that is easily severed.

Suggested Readings

Ader PL, Hobson HP. Hypospadias: a review of the veterinary literature and a report of three cases in the dog. J Am Anim Hosp Assoc 1978;14:721.

Bennett D, Baugham J, Murphy F. Wedge osteotomy of the os penis to correct penile deviation. J Small Anim Pract 1986;27:379.

Burger RA, Müller SC, et al. The buccal mucosal graft for urethral reconstruction: a preliminary report. J Urol 1992;147:662.

Chaffee VM, Knecht CD. Canine paraphimosis: sequel to inefficient preputial muscles. Vet Med Small Anim Clin 1975;70:1418.

Hayes AG, Pavletic MM, et al. A preputial splitting technique for surgery of the canine penis. J Am Anim Hosp Assoc 1994;30:291.

Leighton RL. A simple surgical correction for chronic penile protrusion (dog). J Am Anim Hosp Assoc 1976;12:667.

Pope ER, Swaim SF. Surgical reconstruction of hypoplastic prepuce. J Am Anim Hosp Assoc 1986;22:73.

Poppas DP, Mininberg LH, et al. Patch graft urethroplasty using dye enhanced laser tissue welding with a human protein solder: a preclinical canine model. J Urol 1993;150:648.

Proescholdt TA, DeYoung DW, Evans LE. Preputial reconstruction for phimosis and infantile penis. J Am Anim Hosp Assoc 1977; 13:725.

Smith MM, Gourley IM. Preputial reconstruction in a dog. J Am Vet Med Assoc 1990;196:1493.

Varshney AC, Sharma VK, et al. Surgical management of carcinomatous urethral obstruction in a dog. Indian Vet J 1985; 62:1073.

Preputial Reconstruction

J. David Fowler

Defects requiring preputial reconstruction may result from direct trauma or congenital anomalies. An understanding of preputial anatomy and function is necessary in determining appropriate methods of reconstruction.

Surgical Anatomy

The prepuce is a fold of skin that functions to cover the flaccid penis, thereby protecting the penis from desiccation and trauma. The prepuce consists of an outer, haired cutaneous layer (the external lamina) and an inner, nonhaired layer of stratified squamous epithelium (the internal lamina). The external and internal laminae are continuous with one another at the preputial ostium. The internal lamina is continuous with the skin of the glans at the level of the fornix. During erection, the internal lamina is everted from the preputial orifice and covers the bulbus glandis and body of the penis.

The blood supply to the prepuce is derived principally from the external pudendal artery and to a lesser extent from the preputial branch of the dorsal artery of the penis (1). The paired external pudendal arteries lie dorsolateral to the prepuce and interconnect by a network of fine vascular anastomoses along the ventral midline (Fig. 33.11). Blood supply from the preputial branch of the dorsal artery of the penis also communicates with this vascular plexus. Venous drainage occurs primarily through the external pudendal veins. Lymphatic drainage occurs through the superficial inguinal lymph nodes.

The paired preputial muscles are derived from the cutaneus trunci muscle. They originate from the area of the xiphoid cartilage and insert along the dorsal wall of the prepuce. The preputial muscles function to prevent an excessively pendulous prepuce and advance the prepuce over the nonerect penis.

Preputial Disorders

Congenital Deformities

Congenital deformities of the prepuce may include preputial aplasia, preputial hypoplasia, and defects of embryologic fusion (2). Such preputial defects are often accompanied by similar defects in penile development. An excessively pendulous prepuce may also be seen as a developmental disorder.

Clinical complaints associated with congenital preputial disorders most frequently are caused by expo-

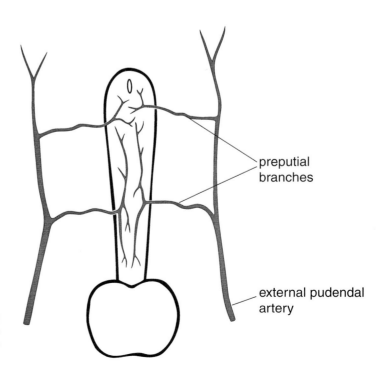

Fig. 33.11. The vascular supply to the prepuce is served primarily by the paired external pudendal arteries. The vasculature forms a fine anastomotic network along the ventral midline of the prepuce.

sure and trauma of the penis (3). Penile drying, inflammation, and self-mutilation are common. An abnormal urine stream and soiling of the hair with urine may be seen in dogs with an abnormally flaccid, or excessively taut, prepuce.

Traumatic and Neoplastic Conditions

Traumatic preputial injuries may result from animal altercations, thermal injury, or preputial foreign bodies. Lacerations may be full thickness, involving both the external and internal laminae, or they may be partial thickness, involving only the external lamina. Occasionally, large preputial defects occur secondary to significant tissue loss.

Neoplastic diseases that affect the skin can also present with preputial involvement. Owners may complain of a localized mass, or clinical signs may result from preputial stenosis or local ulceration and inflammation. Mast cell tumors are the most frequently reported tumors affecting the external genitalia. Transmissible venereal tumor, melanoma, squamous cell carcinoma, and perianal gland tumors are also reported. Diagnosis of preputial neoplasia should be based on cytologic or histopathologic examination of tumor tissue after biopsy. Treatment of preputial neoplasia is beyond the scope of this chapter, but it should be based on an accurate histopathologic diagnosis and a thorough knowledge of tumor behavior and response to therapy.

Congenital anomalies of the prepuce, preputial neoplasia, or healed preputial injuries may result in abnormalities of the preputial ostium. An abnormally constricted ostium prevents extrusion of the penis, a condition termed phimosis. Inversion and restriction of the preputial ostium after penile extrusion may prevent withdrawal of the penis into the prepuce, a disorder known as paraphimosis. Both phimosis and paraphimosis result in local inflammation and are common reasons for presentation for treatment, regardless of cause.

Preputial Reconstruction

Successful preputial reconstruction must provide protection of the flaccid penis, should allow extrusion and retraction of the penis from the prepuce, and should maintain normal anatomic alignment. To achieve these goals, anatomic alignment of tissue layers and prevention of scar contraction and infection are important. The vascular supply to the prepuce should be preserved in designing preputial reconstructive procedures.

In the event of full-thickness preputial lacerations, reconstruction of both internal and external laminae

are critical. Wounds should be thoroughly debrided and cleansed with a nonirritating antiseptic solution such as 0.05% chlorhexidine gluconate. If ongoing tissue necrosis is suspected, or if infection is established, wounds should be kept open until a clean-contaminated status has been achieved. The internal lamina should be sutured using a fine synthetic absorbable suture material. Knots should be buried to prevent irritation of the penis within the preputial cavity. The external lamina may be closed with externally placed skin sutures in a simple interrupted pattern. Accurate apposition of tissue layers limits postoperative scar contraction.

Management of Preputial Ostial Anomalies

Phimosis is caused by an abnormal narrowing of the preputial ostium and should be managed by surgical enlargement of the orifice. Preputial ostioplasty should be performed on the craniodorsal border of the prepuce because incision of the caudoventral border may allow exposure of the underlying penis. Enlargement of the preputial ostium is accomplished by sharp full-thickness incision of the craniodorsal aspect of the preputial orifice (Fig. 33.12). The incision is carried forward an adequate distance to ensure an unrestricted opening. The internal lamina of the prepuce is undermined and is sutured to the ipsilateral skin edges using a fine nonreactive suture material in a simple interrupted pattern.

The preputial ostium may be surgically narrowed in patients with excessive flaccidity of the prepuce (Fig. 33.13). The mucocutaneous junction of the prepuce is sharply incised along the ventrocaudal margin. The internal lamina of the prepuce is undermined circumferentially and is sutured in apposition using a fine absorbable suture material and buried knots. The external lamina of the prepuce is similarly closed in apposition using skin sutures. Care should be taken to avoid an excessively restrictive preputial orifice.

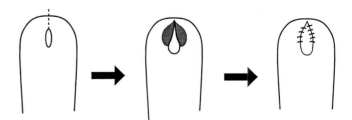

Fig. 33.12. Stenosis of the preputial ostium is addressed by surgical enlargement along the craniodorsal margin. A vertical full-thickness incision is extended from the ostium cranially. The incised edges of the internal preputial lamina are apposed to ipsilateral skin edges using simple interrupted sutures.

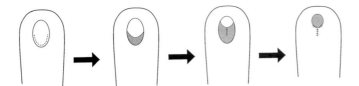

Fig. 33.13. The flaccid prepuce with an abnormally large preputial ostium may be corrected by surgical narrowing. A circumferential incision is made along the caudoventral margin of the ostium at the mucocutaneous junction. The internal and external laminae are separated by blunt dissection. The incised edge of the internal lamina is apposed using absorbable suture with buried knots. The incised external lamina is subsequently apposed using simple interrupted sutures.

Preputial Advancement

Chronic exposure of the tip of the penis is sometimes encountered in the absence of obvious preputial deficits. This condition is often cosmetically disconcerting to owners and may result in secondary penile trauma resulting from desiccation. Ability to reduce the penis to a normal location within the preputial cavity must be established. Lubricants and gentle cleansing of the penis and prepuce may be required in instances of chronic exposure. Once the ability to reduce the penis is established, preputial advancement may be performed (Fig. 33.14). This is accomplished by excising an elliptic or arrowhead-shaped portion of skin immediately cranial to the prepuce. The paired preputial vessels should be spared in performing this excision. The prepuce is then undermined. The paired protrac-

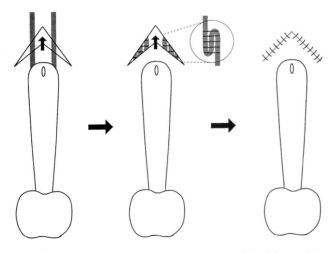

Fig. 33.14. Preputial advancement is accomplished by excision of an elliptic or "arrowhead" cutaneous flap immediately cranial to the prepuce. Incisions should be planned to avoid iatrogenic trauma to the preputial vasculature. Skin edges are undermined toward the prepuce, and the underlying paired preputial muscles are identified and elevated. The preputial muscles are then shortened by excision of a portion of the muscle or by using an overlap technique. Skin margins are subsequently sutured, thereby advancing the prepuce cranially.

tor preputii muscles are identified overlying the rectus abdominis muscles. These muscles are undermined and shortened, either by excision of a portion of the muscle and suture of muscle ends or by a simple overlap technique. The cutaneous deficit is then closed using simple interrupted skin sutures, thereby advancing the prepuce.

Correction of Preputial Hypoplasia

Reconstruction of the congenitally hypoplastic, or traumatically deficient, prepuce is difficult. When considering surgical techniques, both the mucosal internal lamina and the cutaneous external lamina must be reconstructed. Few reports detail reconstructive techniques. Reported techniques involve staged reconstruction of both internal and external preputial laminae using a combination of oral mucosal grafts and local skin flaps.

Pope and Swaim reported reconstruction of a congenital preputial hypoplasia in a 7-month-old Yorkshire terrier (4). Mucosal reconstruction was accomplished by grafting full-thickness oral mucosa onto the rectus abdominis muscle immediately cranial to the prepuce. Ten days after grafting, the edges of the mucosal graft were elevated and were sutured circumferentially around the exposed portion of the penis. External lamina reconstruction was accomplished by elevating bilateral advancement flaps from lateral to the prepuce. Functional recovery was good, although a third surgical procedure was required for repair of a fistula formed on the ventral midline of the reconstructed prepuce.

Smith and Gourley subsequently reported preputial reconstruction using a multiple-staged procedure in a 2-year-old Chesapeake Bay retriever (5). A bipedicle flap was elevated parallel to the traumatically hypoplastic prepuce. Two weeks after flap elevation, an oral mucosal graft was harvested and was transferred to the dermal aspect of the bipedicle skin flap. Multiple-delay procedures were subsequently used to raise the cranial and then the caudal pedicles of the skin flap gradually. The resulting flap of skin and oral mucosa was used to reconstruct the deficient prepuce functionally.

Both reports reveal the necessity, and difficulty, of replacing both the mucosal and cutaneous surfaces of the prepuce. In both instances, oral mucosal grafts were used for reconstruction of the internal lamina, but procedures differed with respect to the recipient site used. It is tempting to speculate that, with increasing use of microvascular technique in tissue transfer, single-stage reconstructive techniques may be possible using full-thickness cheek flaps, myoperitoneal flaps, or other novel donor sites. Based on current experience, recommendation of any one surgical reconstructive technique is difficult. Rather, the surgeon must use sound principles in guiding decisions regarding functional preputial reconstruction.

References

1. Hayes AG, Pavletic MM, Schwartz A, et al. A preputial splitting technique for surgery of the canine penis. Am Anim Hosp Assoc J 1994;30:291–295.

2. Hobson HP. Surgical procedures of the penis. In: Bojrab MJ, ed. Current techniques in small animal surgery. Philadelphia: Lea & Febiger, 1990:423–430.

3. Chaffee VM, Knecht CD. Canine paraphimosis: sequel to inefficient preputial muscles. Vet Med Small Anim Clin 1975;70:1418.

4. Pope ER, Swaim SF. Surgical reconstruction of a hypoplastic prepuce. Am Anim Hosp Assoc J 1986;22:73–77.

5. Smith MM, Gourley IM. Preputial reconstruction in a dog. J Am Vet Med Assoc 1990;196:1493–1496.

34

ENDOCRINE SYSTEM

Adrenalectomy

Thomas D. Scavelli

Adrenalectomy usually is performed in the dog to treat hyperadrenocorticism caused by an adrenocortical tumor. In addition, it can also be used to remove tumors of the adrenal medulla (pheochromocytoma) or to treat pituitary-dependent hyperadrenocorticism refractory to medical management. In the latter situation, bilateral adrenalectomies are performed to remove adrenal glands with adrenocortical hyperplasia secondary to pituitary microadenomas.

Surgical Anatomy

The normal anatomy of the adrenal glands as viewed from the ventral midline approach is depicted in Figure 34.1. The adrenal glands are craniomedial to the ipsilateral kidney and are retroperitoneal. The left adrenal gland is in a layer of loose connective tissue between the aorta and the left kidney. The right adrenal gland is in a layer of connective tissue between the caudal vena cava and the right kidney. The capsule of the right adrenal gland can be continuous with the tunica externa of the caudal vena cava (1). The phrenicoabdominal artery is present on the dorsal surface of the adrenal gland. The phrenicoabdominal vein courses over the ventral surface of the adrenal glands. Caudally, the adrenals are in close proximity to the ipsilateral renal artery and vein, which must be avoided during adrenalectomy.

Surgical Approach

Surgical examination and removal of the canine adrenal glands can be achieved using a ventral midline approach, with paracostal extension of the incision, if needed. Ventral midline celiotomy permits complete examination of the abdominal cavity, with inspection of both adrenal glands, and the identification of metastasis, if present. Disadvantages of this approach are the potential risk of dehiscence of the ventral abdominal incision and the potential for iatrogenic damage to the pancreas.

Another possible approach is the retroperitoneal (paracostal) approach (2–4). The retroperitoneal approach minimizes surgical dissection and provides adequate exposure of the adrenal gland, kidney, and retroperitoneal space on that side, while keeping anesthesia time to a minimum. This approach avoids a ventral weight-bearing incision and minimizes potential problems with wound healing. The disadvantages of the retroperitoneal approach are that one incision does not allow visualization of both adrenal glands, and complete abdominal exploration to identify metastatic adrenal neoplasms is not possible.

Anesthesia

Most dogs undergoing adrenalectomy are older animals with some degree of hyperadrenocorticism. In dogs with adrenocortical tumors, the contralateral adrenal gland is atrophied, and once the neoplastic adrenal gland is removed, a state of hypoadrenocorticism occurs rapidly. As a result, these dogs must be carefully monitored intraoperatively.

539

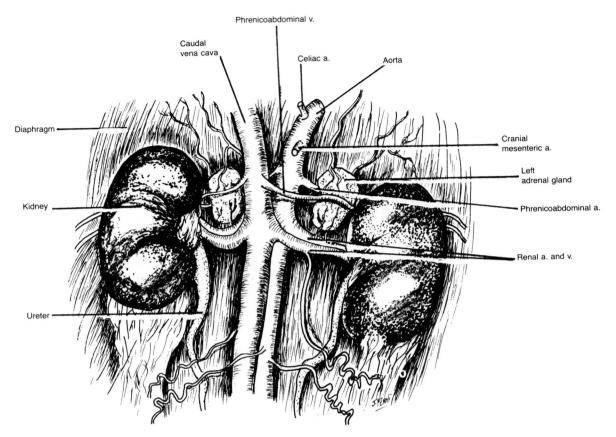

Fig. 34.1. Surgical anatomy for adrenalectomy by a ventral midline approach.

An intravenous catheter should be placed preoperatively for fluid and glucocorticoid administration. A broad-spectrum bactericidal antibiotic should be given as an intravenous bolus about 30 minutes before induction of anesthesia. Anesthetic induction can be successfully performed with thiamylal sodium (3 to 6 mg/kg intravenously) or oxymorphone (0.1 to 0.3 mg/kg intravenously). After the patient is intubated, anesthesia can be maintained with nitrous oxide, oxygen, and an inhalation anesthetic agent. Methoxyflurane, halothane, enflurane, or isoflurane can be used. Isoflurane is preferred because of its rapid onset of action and the patient's rapid recovery; in addition, isoflurane produces the least depression of the cardiovascular system. The use of isoflurane is especially recommended in a dog suspected of having a pheochromocytoma. This tumor produces high circulating levels of catecholamines that, in the presence of a drug such as halothane, can produce profound cardiac dysrhythmias. Because isoflurane does not sensitize the heart to catecholamines, it is the inhalation agent of choice in a dog with pheochromocytoma.

Throughout the surgical procedure, a balanced electrolyte solution (i.e., lactated Ringer's solution) should be administered at a dose of 10 mL/kg per hour.

When an adrenocortical tumor is suspected or when both adrenal glands are being removed for pituitary-dependent hyperadrenocorticism, corticosteroid supplementation in the form of dexamethasone (0.1 to 0.2 mg/kg intravenously) should be administered immediately before adrenalectomy. This glucocorticoid should be administered again at the completion of the operation.

Surgical Technique

The ventral midline approach is especially helpful when lateralization of the tumor cannot be determined preoperatively. The initial incision should be made on the midline of the ventral abdomen from the xiphoid to approximately 2 cm caudal to the umbilicus. The liver and regional lymph nodes should be carefully inspected for the presence of metastasis. The adjacent portions of the aorta, vena cava, and ipsilateral renal artery and vein should be carefully palpated for evidence of tumor thrombus. After exploration of the abdomen is complete, extension of the midline approach with a left or right paracostal incision increases exposure of the abnormal adrenal gland (Fig. 34.2). The paracostal incision is started at the most cranial

tery and vein should be ligated separately with the use of hemostatic clips. In some dogs, the adrenal gland also receives branches from the cranial abdominal, renal, celiac, and lumbar arteries (2). If present, these arterial branches should be ligated. Adrenal tumors are often extremely vascular, and hemostatic clips should be used as needed to ligate any vessels encountered during dissection and removal of the gland. The surgeon must avoid accidentally placing a hemostat or ligature on the adjacent renal artery or vein. After adrenalectomy is completed, the body wall should be apposed with nonabsorbable suture material (e.g., polypropylene).

The retroperitoneal approach has been described by Johnson (2). A 10-cm incision is made immediately caudal to the last rib, with its most dorsal aspect at the ventral aspect of the epaxial muscles (Fig. 34.3). A grid incision is made by incising the external abdominal oblique muscle, internal abdominal oblique muscle, and transversus abdominis muscle in the direction of their fibers. The peritoneum is entered, the kidney is palpated, and the adrenal is located within the perirenal connective tissue at the craniomedial aspect of the kidney (Fig. 34.4). Use of self-retaining retractors or an assistant with hand-held retractors facilitates dissection and removal of the adrenal gland, as described for the ventral midline approach.

Postoperative Complications and Management

Potential postoperative complications of adrenalectomy are cardiac arrest, fluid and electrolyte imbalances, pneumonia, pulmonary artery thromboembolism, pancreatitis, acute renal failure, and adrenal insufficiency (4). Mineralocorticoid and glucocorticoid

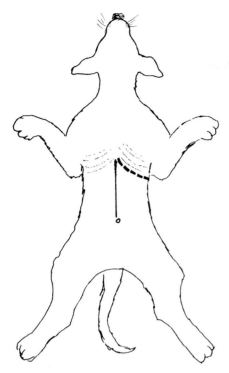

Fig. 34.2. Ventral midline approach. The *solid line* depicts the midline incision; the *broken line* portrays a paracostal extension that can be used to aid in visualization and dissection of adrenal gland.

aspect of the midline incision (near the xiphoid) and is continued parallel to the costal arch in a dorsocaudal direction (3).

The area adjacent to the adrenal gland is isolated with moistened laparotomy pads. The key to adrenalectomy is gentle dissection of the gland with special attention to hemostasis. The phrenicoabdominal ar-

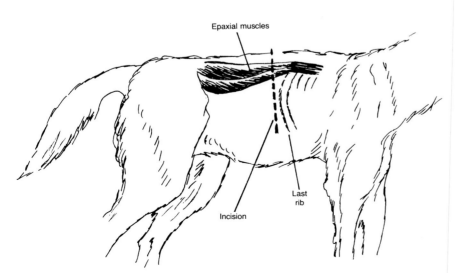

Epaxial muscles

Last rib

Incision

Fig. 34.3. Retroperitoneal approach for adrenalectomy is performed by making an initial incision in the skin and subcutaneous tissue immediately caudal to the last rib and ventral to the epaxial muscles. A grid incision through the abdominal wall muscles is made to enter the retroperitoneal space.

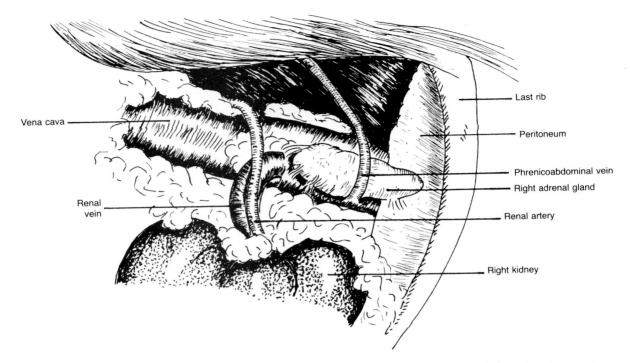

Fig. 34.4. Surgical anatomy of the retroperitoneal space in the area of the right kidney and adrenal gland. Careful attention must be directed to the location of the phrenicoabdominal vein and the adjacent renal vessels.

deficiencies occur after bilateral adrenalectomy and require permanent exogenous supplementation.

In patients that undergo unilateral adrenalectomy for an adrenocortical tumor, glucocorticoid deficiency develops unless large doses of glucocorticoids are given during and after the surgical procedure. To evaluate adrenal reserve, an adrenocorticotropic hormone (ACTH) stimulation test should be performed on the first postoperative day. In dogs with postoperative adrenal insufficiency, prednisone should be administered during the first 3 postoperative days at a dosage of 0.5 mg/kg orally twice a day; the dosage is gradually tapered over a 10- to 14-day period to an approximate oral daily maintenance dosage of 0.2 mg/kg. Glucocorticoid supplementation should be continued at this maintenance dosage until the remaining adrenal gland is functioning normally, as determined by ACTH stimulation testing. In most dogs, glucocorticoids can be discontinued within 2 months after unilateral adrenalectomy.

References

1. Evans HE, Christensen GC. Miller's anatomy of the dog. 2nd ed. Philadelphia: WB Saunders, 1979:618–625.
2. Johnson DE. Adrenalectomy in the dog. In: Bojrab MJ, ed. Current techniques in small animal surgery. 2nd ed. Philadelphia: Lea & Febiger, 1983:386–389.
3. Peterson ME, Birchard SJ, Mehlhaff CJ. Anesthetic and surgical management of endocrine disorders. Vet Clin North Am Small Anim Pract 1984;14:911–925.
4. Scavelli TD, Peterson ME, Matthiesen DT. Results of surgical treatment for hyperadrenocorticism caused by adrenocortical neoplasia in the dog: 25 cases (1980–1984). J Am Vet Med Assoc 1986;189:1360–1364.

Thyroidectomy in the Dog and Cat

Stephen J. Birchard

Thyroid neoplasia is the primary indication for thyroidectomy in dogs and cats. Thyroid tumors in dogs are usually malignant and nonfunctional, whereas in cats they are usually benign and functional. Thyroidectomy can range from a straightforward operation to a complex surgical procedure. However, a good working knowledge of the regional anatomy, the pathophysiology of thyroid and parathyroidectomy disorders, and the principles of preoperative and postoperative care is necessary for successful patient management. Animals with thyroid tumors tend to be geriatric. They fre-

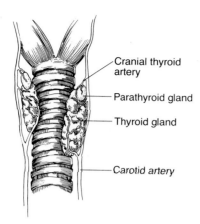

Fig. 34.5. Gross appearance of bilateral thyroid tumors in a cat. (From Graves TK, Peterson ME, Birchard SJ. Thyroid gland. In: Birchard SJ, Sherding, eds. Saunders manual of small animal practice. Philadelphia: WB Saunders, 1994:218–228.)

quently have disorders of other organ systems that should be recognized and treated appropriately.

The purpose of this discussion is to provide a brief overview of the pathophysiology of thyroid neoplasia, to review the anatomy of the thyroid and parathyroid glands, and to describe the surgical technique for thyroidectomy. Postoperative care and complications are also covered.

Surgical Anatomy

The thyroid gland in the dog and cat is divided into two lobes located adjacent to the trachea and just distal to the larynx. The left lobe is slightly caudal to the right (1). The normal gland is pale tan. The principal blood supply to each lobe is the cranial thyroid artery, a branch of the common carotid artery (1) (Fig. 34.5). The caudal thyroid artery in the dog arises from the brachycephalic artery. The caudal thyroid artery is absent in the cat (2). Venous drainage of the thyroid is through the cranial and caudal thyroid veins (1). The thyroid has a distinct capsule that can be bluntly separated from the gland. Small blood vessels may be located on the capsule surface and between the capsule and the parenchyma of the gland.

Two parathyroid glands are usually associated with each thyroid lobe. The external parathyroid gland usually lies in the loose fascia at the cranial pole of the thyroid lobe (2). The internal parathyroid gland is usually embedded in the thyroid parenchyma and is variable in location. The external parathyroid glands are much smaller than the thyroid lobe and can be distinguished from the thyroid tissue by their lighter color and spheric shape. The blood supply to the parathyroid glands also arises from the cranial thyroid artery (1).

Thyroid Tumors in Dogs

Pathophysiology

Thyroid tumors in dogs account for 1.2% of all canine tumors (3) (Fig. 34.6). Most of these tumors are malignant, and adenocarcinoma is the most common tissue type reported. Boxers, beagles, and golden retrievers appear to have a greater risk of developing thyroid carcinoma (4).

The most common presenting signs in dogs with thyroid tumors are the presence of a palpable neck mass and coughing (4). Signs of hyperthyroidism are usually not present because elevation of thyroid hormone levels is infrequent in dogs with thyroid neoplasia. However, I have seen two dogs with functional thyroid adenocarcinomas that had elevated triiodothyronine and thyroxine levels but did not have signs of hyperthyroidism.

Thyroid carcinomas in dogs most frequently metastasize to the lungs (4). Studies have indicated that over 50% of all thyroid carcinomas produce lung metastases (3, 5). The larger the primary tumor, the greater the chance for lung metastasis (5). The second most common site of metastasis is the cervical lymph nodes.

A key factor in the preoperative evaluation of a dog with suspected thyroid neoplasia is determining

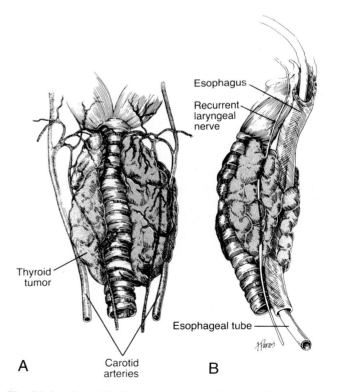

Fig. 34.6. **A** and **B.** Gross appearance of a thyroid carcinoma in a dog. (From Graves TK, Peterson ME, Birchard SJ. Thyroid gland. In: Birchard SJ, Sherding, eds. Saunders manual of small animal practice. Philadelphia: WB Saunders, 1994:218–228.)

whether or not the tumor is movable. Thyroid masses that are freely movable on palpation tend to be less invasive into surrounding tissues and are surgically resectable. One study found that, of 82 dogs with thyroid carcinoma, 20 had movable tumors. These tumors were resected, and median survival of the group was 20.5 months (3).

Diagnosis

Diagnosis of thyroid neoplasia in dogs is by physical examination (palpation of a neck mass) and biopsy of the tumor. Fine-needle aspiration of the mass should yield cells characteristic of a carcinoma. A Tru-cut needle biopsy of the tumor may be necessary if cytologic findings are inconclusive, but this procedure may cause hemorrhage because of the extensive neovascularization of the tumor. Thoracic radiographs are mandatory to rule out pulmonary metastases. Thyroid function should be evaluated with a thyroid-stimulating hormone stimulation test if the dog shows signs of hyperthyroidism or hypothyroidism. Routine preoperative tests, such as complete blood count, serum chemistry profile, and urinalysis, are also recommended.

Surgical Technique

Treatment of thyroid neoplasia involves both surgical and medical therapy. Small, freely movable tumors can be completely removed by thyroidectomy. The dog is placed in dorsal recumbency with the front legs tied caudally and the neck slightly hyperextended over a rolled towel or other cushion. The ventral cervical region from the caudal mandibles to the manubrium is prepared for aseptic surgery. A ventral midline cervical skin incision is made from the caudal aspect of the larynx to 2 to 3 cm cranial to the manubrium. The paired sternohyoideus and sternothyroideus muscles are separated on the midline and are retracted with self-retaining retractors (Gelpi or Weitlaner). The trachea is gently retracted, and both thyroid lobes are examined carefully. An attempt should be made to identify the parathyroid glands, although visualization may be impaired by larger neoplasms. The tumor is carefully dissected from surrounding tissues (Fig. 34.7). I usually start at the caudal aspect of the lobe and work cranially. Care is taken to avoid injury to the esophagus, carotid artery, jugular vein, vagosympathetic trunk, and recurrent laryngeal nerve. These tumors are extremely vascular, and strict hemostasis is important, to prevent serious blood loss. Even small vessels should be ligated or cauterized because surgery is hampered by a bloody operating field. Removal of large tumors results in dead space in the tissues; a Penrose drain should be placed in the area of resected tumor to prevent hematoma or seroma formation. The

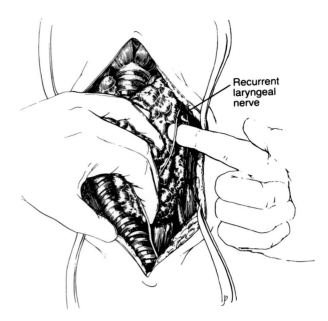

Fig. 34.7. Removal of a canine thyroid tumor with a combination of blunt and sharp dissection. The surgeon must identify and preserve the recurrent laryngeal nerve. (From Graves TK, Peterson ME, Birchard SJ. Thyroid gland. In: Birchard SJ, Sherding, eds. Saunders manual of small animal practice. Philadelphia: WB Saunders, 1994:218–228.)

sternohyoideus and sternothyroideus muscles are closed with absorbable suture (3–0 polyglactin 910 [Vicryl] or polydioxanone [PDS]) in a simple continuous pattern. The subcutaneous tissues are closed in the same fashion. Skin is closed with nonabsorbable suture (4–0 polyamide nylon [Ethilon]) in a simple interrupted pattern.

The thyroid tissue should always be submitted for histopathologic analysis. Results of histopathologic examination help to determine the need for adjunctive therapy, such as chemotherapy, and to evaluate the patient's long-term prognosis.

Postoperative Care

Postoperatively, the animal should be closely observed during recovery for bleeding at the surgical site. Serum calcium levels should be monitored daily for 2 to 4 days postoperatively if a bilateral tumor is resected. Hypocalcemia due to hypoparathyroidism is treated according to the protocol in Table 34.1.

The animal should be reevaluated at 2 weeks, 3 months, 6 months, and 1 year. Radiographs of the thorax should be obtained at these rechecks to monitor for metastasis. Prognosis obviously depends on tumor type and completeness of excision. As previously mentioned, even thyroid carcinoma can be associated with a good prognosis if the tumor is mobile and is completely excised.

Table 34.1.
Treatment of Postoperative Hypoparathyroidism in Dogs and Cats

Initial therapy
1. Calcium gluconate (10%) IV .... 1.0–1.5 mL/kg (administered slowly over 10 to 20 minutes; stop injection if bradycardia develops)
2. Calcium gluconate (10%) IV (after tetany stops) .... 2 mL/kg (slowly administered over 6 to 8 hours)
3. Oral calcium, calcium gluconate .... 500–750 mg/kg/d (divided into 3 or 4 doses)
   Discontinue IV calcium over 1 to 2 days
Long-term
1. Vitamin D dihydrotachysterol .... 0.03 mg/kg/d (2 days)
   0.02 mg/kg/d (2 days)
   0.01 mg/kg/d (long term)
2. Try to maintain serum calcium at 8 to 10 mg/dL (check weekly)
   Adjust vitamin D dose to maintain normal calcium
3. Usually can discontinue calcium therapy if animal is eating
4. Once animal is stable, recheck serum calcium every 3 to 4 months
5. Gradually "wean off" vitamin D therapy after a few months to see if parathyroid function returns

* Data from Peterson, M. E.: Treatment of canine and feline hypoparathyroidism. J Am Vet Med Assoc 1981;181:1434–1436.

Thyroid Tumors in Cats

Pathophysiology

Thyroid neoplasia in the cat is a much different disease than in dogs. The tumors are almost always benign and functional. These tumors produce excessive amounts of thyroxine, and cats develop the clinical syndrome of hyperthyroidism. Classic clinical signs of hyperthyroidism include tachycardia, hyperactivity, weight loss, polyphagia, and polyuria and polydipsia. Some cats have apathetic hyperthyroidism, a syndrome characterized by signs opposite to the classic presentation for hyperthyroidism, such as depression, lethargy, and anorexia.

Diagnosis

Diagnosis is based on the history and clinical signs, palpation of a neck mass, and elevated serum triiodothyronine and thyroxine concentrations. One or more thyroid nodules are palpable in approximately 85 to 90% of affected cats (6). These cats may also have leukocytosis, higher than normal packed cell volume, and high alkaline phosphatase (6). Hyperthyroid cats may also have hypertrophic cardiomyopathy with hypertrophy of the left ventricular free wall and ventricular septum (6).

Radionuclide scan of the thyroid gland in cats with hyperthyroidism reveals increased uptake and size of the affected lobes. Nuclear scanning can be a useful diagnostic tool in cats that do not have a palpable thyroid nodule or that have had relapse of hyperthyroidism after thyroidectomy. However, nuclear scans have limited practicality because of the specialized equipment and expertise needed to perform the studies.

Treatment options for hyperthyroidism in cats include use of methimazole (lowers thyroxine by blocking uptake of iodine by the thyroid), radioactive iodine treatment, or surgical removal of the gland.

Surgical Techniques

Thyroidectomy is a practical and usually curative procedure for hyperthyroidism that requires little in the way of special facilities or equipment (7). Preoperatively, I prefer to treat severely affected cats with methimazole to establish euthyroidism. This treatment makes the animal a much better candidate for anesthesia and surgery. Methimazole (Tapazole, 5 mg orally twice a day) is administered for 7 to 10 days before surgery. The patient's thyroxine levels are rechecked and, if normal or significantly reduced, surgery is scheduled. Cats that are only mildly affected by hyperthyroidism (i.e., only mildly elevated thyroxine, still normal weight, not severely tachycardic) are operated on without pretreatment.

The electrocardiogram is closely monitored during the surgical procedure because premature ventricular contractions are common. If these arrhythmias occur, the cat is given 0.1 mg of propranolol intravenously. Thyroidectomy in the cat is performed by the same approach as in the dog. Several techniques for thyroidectomy in cats have been described, some allowing for resection of the capsule (extracapsular dissection) and others preserving the capsule (intracapsular dissection). The choice of technique depends on personal preference. I typically use the extracapsular technique because of the reduced incidence of recurrence of hyperthyroidism from remnants of thyroid tissue left behind that can occur with intracapsular technique. However, when the parathyroid glands are not visible, I tend to rely on intracapsular dissection, to ensure preservation of at least one of the parathyroid glands. Both techniques are described here.

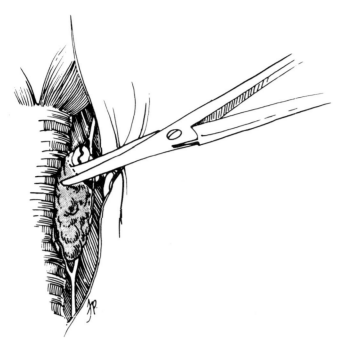

Fig. 34.8. Extracapsular dissection for removal of a thyroid lobe in a cat. (From Graves TK, Peterson ME, Birchard SJ. Thyroid gland. In: Birchard SJ, Sherding, eds. Saunders manual of small animal practice. Philadelphia: WB Saunders, 1994:218–228.)

EXTRACAPSULAR TECHNIQUE

The thyroid lobes are exposed through a ventral midline cervical approach, as described in dogs (Fig. 34.8). The affected thyroid lobe is dissected free from surrounding fascia, working caudally to cranially. The external parathyroid gland is identified at the cranial aspect of the thyroid gland. The thyroid gland capsule is incised adjacent to the parathyroid gland. Pinpoint electrocautery is used on any vessels encountered during this dissection, with care taken to avoid damage to the parathyroid gland or its blood supply. The parathyroid gland is then carefully separated from the thyroid using sterile cotton-tipped applicators. Once the parathyroid gland is completely separated from the thyroid, the thyroid gland is completely removed using blunt and sharp dissection and pinpoint cautery on all vessels.

INTRACAPSULAR TECHNIQUE

A small nick incision is made in an avascular area of the capsule (Fig. 34.9). This incision is extended with small scissors. The thyroid tissue then is separated gently from the capsule with sterile cotton-tipped applicators. Meticulous hemostasis is critical to maintain good visualization of the surgical field. Hemorrhage from small capsular vessels is controlled using pinpoint electrocautery. Extreme care is required during manipulation of the cranial pole of the thyroid to avoid injury to the blood supply of the extracapsular parathyroid gland. If the thyroid gland becomes fragmented during dissection, the surgical field is carefully examined for remnants of thyroid tissue that have not been removed. These remnants and the associated capsule to which they are attached are removed. The incision is closed as described in the dog. The resected tissue is submitted for histopathologic evaluation.

Preservation of the thyroid capsule ensures preservation of the extracapsular parathyroid gland, especially important during bilateral thyroidectomy. However, small pieces of thyroid tissue may remain

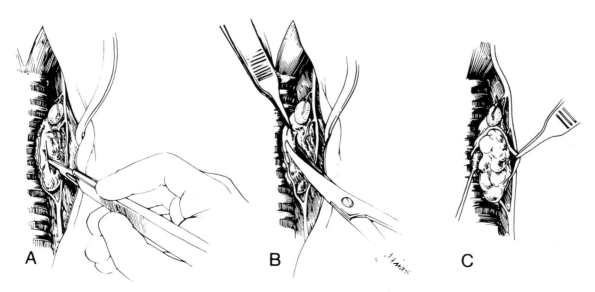

Fig. 34.9.   A–C. Intracapsular dissection for removal of a thyroid tumor in a cat. (From Graves TK, Peterson ME, Birchard SJ. Thyroid gland. In: Birchard SJ, Sherding, eds. Saunders manual of small animal practice. Philadelphia, WB Saunders, 1994:218–228.)

attached to the capsule. This remaining tissue can cause relapse of hyperthyroidism if it is not removed.

Postoperative Care

Postoperatively, the cat is closely monitored for evidence of hemorrhage from the surgical site. Serum calcium levels are monitored for at least 2 days postoperatively. If hypocalcemia develops because of removal or damage to the parathyroid glands, the cat is treated with calcium (parenteral or oral administration) and vitamin D (8). Early signs of hypocalcemia are muscle soreness or spasm, anorexia, and depression. Later signs are collapse and tetany. Thyroid replacement therapy (L-thyroxine, 0.1 mg orally once daily) is not given routinely, but it may be indicated for cats that have had bilateral thyroidectomy and show clinical signs of hypothyroidism.

I am careful to monitor renal function closely in cats after thyroidectomy, especially if they have evidence of chronic renal failure preoperatively. Renal function in some of these cats worsens after thyroidectomy, presumably because of decreased renal blood flow after lowering the thyroxine levels. Thyroid replacement therapy is indicated for these cats. The serum thyroxine level should be evaluated in these animals after 1 month of replacement therapy.

The prognosis for hyperthyroid cats after thyroidectomy is good. Histopathologic examination of the thyroid tissue usually reveals adenomatous hyperplasia. I have operated on a few cats with thyroid carcinoma. The tumors were much larger and more vascular than the more common benign neoplasms. Relapse of hyperthyroidism rarely occurs 1 to 2 years postoperatively because of regrowth of the adenoma. Postoperative hypocalcemia is more common after reoperation for thyroidectomy.

References

1. Evans HE, Christensen GC. The endocrine system. In: Evans HE, Christensen GC, eds. Miller's anatomy of the dog. Philadelphia: WB Saunders, 1979:611–618.
2. Nicholas JS, Swingle WW. An experimental and morphological study of the parathyroid glands of the cat. Am J Anat 1925; 34:469–508.
3. Brodey TS, Kelly DF. Thyroid neoplasms in the dog. Cancer 1968;22:406–416.
4. Birchard SJ, Roesel OF. Neoplasia of the thyroid gland in the dog: a retrospective study of 16 cases. J Am Anim Hosp Assoc 1981;17:369–372.
5. Leav I, Shiller AC, Rijnberk A, et al. Adenomas and carcinomas of the canine and feline thyroid. Am J Pathol 1976;83:61–93.
6. Peterson ME. Feline hyperthyroidism. Vet Clin North Am 1984;14:809–826.
7. Birchard SJ, Peterson ME, Jacobson A. Surgical treatment of feline hyperthyroidism: results of 85 cases. J Am Anim Hosp Assoc 1984;20:705–709.
8. Carothers M, Chew D, Van Gundy T. Disorders of the parathyroid gland and calcium metabolism In: Birchard SJ, Sherding, eds. Saunders manual of small animal practice. Philadelphia: WB Saunders, 1994:229–237.

— 35 —

HERNIAS

Incisional Hernia Repair

Daniel D. Smeak

Definition and Etiology

An incisional hernia results from disruption of an abdominal wall closure. Acute incisional hernias generally develop within the first 5 to 7 days after surgery, whereas chronic hernias are seen weeks to years postoperatively. Incisional hernia incidence is reported to be between 1 and 11% in human patients and up to 16% in large animals, depending on the surgical approach to the abdomen, certain predisposing factors, and the general status of the patient. Incisional herniation in small animals appears to be uncommon.

Predisposing causes of acute and chronic incisional hernia vary and are interrelated. Reported risk factors for acute incisional hernia include increased intra-abdominal pressure from pain, entrapped fat between hernia edges, inappropriate suture material use, infection, long-term steroid treatment, and poor postoperative care. *Technical error in surgery, however, is believed to be the most common cause of acute wound disruption.* Factors associated with chronic incisional hernia in human patients include obesity, hypoproteinemia, cardiopulmonary complications, abdominal distension, skin wound dehiscence, and deep fascial infection. *Local wound complications, especially deep infection, appear to be the most important predisposing cause of chronic incisional hernias.*

Incisional hernias result from either excessive forces acting on the abdominal incision or poor holding strength of the sutured wound. Forces acting to disrupt the abdominal incision are mainly derived from excessive intra-abdominal pressure or muscle tension. Increased intra-abdominal pressure is observed in such conditions as obesity, abdominal effusions, pregnancy, and organ distension from ileus or obstruction; all these problems significantly increase incisional hernia risk. Uncontrolled exercise after abdominal wall surgery, early in the postoperative period, increases the risk of wound breakdown.

The choice of suture material used for abdominal closure is rarely the sole cause of incisional hernia, provided the appropriate size is used. However, choice of suture type may be critical in patients that have prolonged wound healing or are severely catabolic, and when wound infection is present, particularly when an unpredictable, rapidly absorbable suture material such as chromic gut is used. Inappropriate knot tying technique or inappropriate number of knots in an abdominal wall closure increases the risk of herniation.

Whether suture is placed in an interrupted or a continuous pattern, or whether the abdomen is closed in a single or double layer, has little significance in incisional hernia formation, provided the strength-holding layer is incorporated. Interrupted suture patterns are more secure if wound edges have questionable viability or strength or if other predisposing incisional hernia risk factors are present.

The most common cause of incisional hernia in small animals is failure to place sutures in the strength-holding layer of the abdomen, with appropriately sized tissue bites. Successful lasting abdominal wall closures must include the external rectus fascia. Closure of the internal rectus fascia (including peritoneum) with the external fascia not only prolongs the procedure time and increases trauma from tissue manipulation, but also may

549

enhance adhesion formation. In addition, suture material penetrating the peritoneum is a known potent stimulus for adhesion formation. Thus, separate peritoneal closure is not required or recommended to ensure successful abdominal closure.

Clinical Signs and Diagnosis

Signs of acute incisional herniation usually develop within the first 3 to 5 days after surgery. Wound edema and inflammation are signals of altered wound healing, and these signs may be seen early in the sequence of events leading to herniation. Serosanguineous drainage from the incision and swelling are important and consistent signs of impending acute abdominal wound dehiscence across animal species. Swelling is usually soft and painless unless infection or organ compromise is present. Early diagnosis and treatment of incisional hernias are vital to reduce the possibility of dehiscence and evisceration (organ protrusion).

Any wound exhibiting signs of altered wound healing (edema, swelling, inflammation) should be examined carefully for incisional herniation. Seroma, hematoma, cellulitis, and excessive foreign body response to buried suture material are differential diagnoses for acute incisional hernias. The skin incision line should be manipulated laterally during deep palpation over the muscle wall closure to aid in definition of the abdominal suture line. Further diagnostic testing (radiography, ultrasound, and fine-needle aspiration) may be required for definitive diagnosis if displaced viscera or a hernial ring cannot be identified. Small amounts of omentum herniated through a small defect cause persistent wound swelling and are rarely detected without wound exploration.

Treatment

Acute Incisional Hernias

Most incisional hernias should be repaired without delay unless they are chronic and freely reducible. Prognosis dramatically worsens when evisceration occurs. Immediate hospitalization and support of the hernia with bandages should be performed as the patient is prepared for surgery. Early surgical intervention is recommended for those patients with eviscerated hernias and for those with overlying skin incision breakdown or devitalization.

The approach is made over the original incision unless organ damage is present; otherwise, a ventral midline approach may be used. When technical failure is suspected (knot, suture, or tissue failure) the *entire* wound is reopened and repaired. If one significant technical error is present in the obviously affected area, other areas are also affected to some degree. The surgeon should pay particular attention to identification of the strength-holding layer and to placement of appropriately sized tissue bites (at least 5 mm) in this layer. Acute incisional hernias are repaired with primary musculofascial reconstruction if adequate tissue is present to close the hernia without undue tension. The surgeon removes fat completely between edges to be approximated. Knots are carefully tied with the appropriate amount of snug square throws, and attention is paid to intrinsic suture tension to avoid crushing tissue. Debridement is contraindicated during repair of acute incisional hernias unless wound edges are nonviable or necrotizing infected fascial tissue is present. Removing healthy wound edges creates excessive and unnecessary tissue trauma and spreads contamination into sterile areas. Debridement of this actively healing tissue sets the wound back to the substrate phase and delays the onset of rapid wound strength gain.

Chronic Incisional Hernias

Chronic incisional hernias generally have enough strength in the overlying hernia sac and skin to prevent evisceration, so these hernias may be repaired on an elective basis or conservatively managed. Palpable adhesions to protruding organs are, however, indications for early surgical intervention because adhesions may cause obstruction, torsion, and vascular compromise of entrapped tissue.

Conservative management of asymptomatic patients with small hernias should be considered only if the patient's owners can be trusted with wound monitoring. Affected patients require daily hernia palpation. Pain, discoloration, incarceration, and rapid increase in hernia size are indications for immediate examination of the animal by the veterinarian. Chronic hernias usually do not cause significant patient discomfort; however, they may be of concern when the animal is used for breeding. Large hernias may prevent delivery because of uterine incarceration or lack of adequate abdominal contraction during labor.

Chronic incisional hernias are usually approached surgically over the original incision area. Muscle edges may retract some distance away from the defect, producing a *functional* loss of abdominal wall. This results in excessive tension during primary hernia repair and thus increases the risk of recurrence.

A major technical difficulty in repair of chronic incisional hernias is accurate identification of normal tissue. Surgical dissection and accurate identification of primary strength-holding tissue at hernia margins are critical for lasting repair. Simple imbrication of the hernial sac without extensive scar excision usually results in recurrence of the hernia because of attenuation of the scar tissue. In chronic hernias, muscle and subcutaneous tissues are scarred together in one layer. Conservative excision of surrounding scar tissue is recommended until identification of the strength-holding layer is possible.

A condition termed loss of domain occurs when the abdominal cavity has become accustomed to a small intra-abdominal volume. As a result, reduction of the hernia and primary closure of the (usually large) defect may be impossible. Closure of the abdominal wall by forcing herniated contents back into the abdomen results not only in excessive tension on the repair, but also in acute pulmonary compromise from restriction of diaphragmatic function. In most veterinary patients with large chronic defects or areas of abdominal tissue loss, surgical repair is performed with prosthetic materials such as polypropylene mesh.

Evisceration

Patients presenting with evisceration require early aggressive supportive therapy. Exposed organs are covered with sterile bandages to reduce contamination and tissue damage further until vital diagnostic tests are performed and stabilization is attempted. In addition, an Elizabethan collar is placed on the patient if constant monitoring is not possible. Exposed organs are quickly mutilated by animals, and the result is shock from fluid and blood loss. Sepsis may occur from severe wound contamination, particularly when intestines have been violated. Therefore, appropriate fluid and antibiotic therapy is critical to stabilize the patient's condition.

Wound preparation is performed in a clean area after the patient has undergone anesthetic induction. The surgeon should avoid contact between potentially irritating and toxic antiseptics and cleansing agents and the patient's exposed organs during skin preparation. Exposed tissue is covered with saline-soaked laparotomy sponges, and a larger area of the abdomen is clipped, if necessary. The skin surrounding the wound is prepared routinely. In an aseptic area, the original abdominal wound is extended, if necessary, to explore abdominal viscera fully. The surgeon copiously lavages exposed but viable organs before exploration. After isolating damaged areas from the rest of the viscera with laparotomy sponges, the surgeon resects nonviable and irreversibly damaged areas and repairs organs when necessary. Appropriate specimens are submitted for culture and susceptibility testing. The abdomen is copiously lavaged to help remove particulate foreign material and gross contamination.

The decision whether to close the abdominal wall and superficial tissues depends on the amount and location of tissue damage and wound contamination observed at surgery. Primary repair is appropriate for patients with acute herniation with little tissue damage or contamination. Patients with minimal intraperitoneal but significant superficial tissue damage or contamination should have routine abdominal wall closure, but superficial layers are left open for necessary drainage and tangential debridement. Deep, severely contaminated wounds are best managed by an open peritoneal drainage techniques.

Aftercare and Prognosis

Postoperative management of patients after repair of acute, closed incisional hernias is similar to postoperative care of patients that have undergone elective abdominal surgery. Exercise is strictly limited for at least 2 weeks. Careful observation of the wound is critical for detection of early signs of infection. If infection occurs, the skin and subcutaneous tissue sutures are removed, and the wound is left open for second-intention healing. A superficial infection is not necessarily fatal to the success of the repair, but the longer the infection is present before treatment, the more likely the wound is to disrupt.

When evisceration has occurred, the nature of the organ damage and repair and the patient's status dictate postoperative treatment and monitoring. Intense monitoring and treatment are needed if shock and septic peritonitis are present. Fluid deficits are replenished, and infection is treated with antibiotics and appropriate wound drainage. Nutritional management in these critically ill patients often is the major factor influencing prognosis.

Most patients with incisional hernias have a good prognosis after repair, provided initiating causal factors were eliminated and minimal damage occurred to deep structures. Consequently, because most incisional hernias are usually closed and are a result of technical failure, most patients have an excellent prognosis as long as appropriate repair was performed. Septic patients with severe peritoneal contamination and organ damage warrant a poor prognosis.

Suggested Readings

Alexander HC, Prudden JF. The causes of abdominal wound disruption. Surg Gynec Obstet 1966;122:1223–1229.

Smeak DD. Abdominal hernias. In: Slatter DH, ed. Textbook of small animal surgery. 2nd ed. Philadelphia: WB Saunders, 1993: 433–454.

Smeak DD. Management and prevention of surgical complications associated with small animal abdominal herniorrhaphy. Probl Vet Med 1989;1:254–267.

Inguinal Hernia Repair in the Dog

Paul W. Dean, M. Joseph Bojrab &
Gheorghe M. Constantinescu

A hernia is an abnormal protrusion of an organ or tissue through a normal body opening. True hernias have a hernial ring and a sac formed of peritoneum surrounding the hernia contents; false hernias lack the peritoneal sac. Hernias are either reducible or irreducible. Irreducible hernias can become strangulated if the circulation to the contents becomes interrupted.

Inguinal hernias are formed when an organ or tissue protrudes through the inguinal canal. Indirect inguinal hernias, the most common type, occur when tissue protrudes through the normal evagination of the vaginal process in females or the vaginal tunica in males. A direct inguinal hernia occurs when the peritoneal evagination occurs separate from and lies alongside the vaginal process or vaginal tunica as a separate outpouching of tissue.

Surgical Anatomy

The inguinal canal is a passage through the abdominal wall. During development, it is occupied by the gubernaculum of the testis, the vaginal tunica that will ensheathe the descended testis, the descending testis, and the spermatic cord, which consists of the vessels, nerves, and duct of the descended testis. In the bitch, the gubernaculum persists within the broad ligament of the uterus as the round ligament that traverses the inguinal canal (1). In veterinary anatomy, it is customary to consider the inguinal canal as the passage between the internal inguinal ring and the external inguinal ring (1). The cranial boundary of the internal inguinal ring is formed by the caudal edge of the insertion of the internal abdominal oblique muscle. It is bordered ventromedially by the rectus abdominis muscle and the prepubic tendon and caudally and laterally by the edge of the pelvis and the inguinal ligament. The external inguinal ring is formed as a slitlike orifice in the insertion of the external abdominal oblique muscle and overlies the internal inguinal ring. The anatomy of the inguinal canal varies among species, depending on the caudal extent of the attachment of the internal abdominal oblique muscle (1).

Etiopathogenesis

The exact etiopathogenesis of inguinal hernias is unknown. Congenital inguinal hernias have been noted in certain breeds. Inguinal hernias have been shown to be hereditary in the basenji, regressing spontaneously by 12 weeks of age (2). Other breeds exhibiting a greater risk of inguinal hernias include the basset hound, cairn terrier, Pekingese, and West Highland white terrier. The Pekingese also exhibits a greater incidence of concurrent umbilical hernia (3). The cause of congenital inguinal hernias is unknown, but the disorder has been attributed to normal anatomic variations, polygenic inheritance, and infectious diseases (3).

Acquired inguinal hernias are noted most often in the middle-aged intact bitch (4–6). Most cases of herniation occur in the estral or pregnant bitch, suggesting hormonal involvement. Inguinal hernia has not been reported in the neutered bitch (6). Other factors that may be involved include weakening of the abdominal wall, trauma, obesity, and the accumulation of fat in the vaginal process (1, 5).

Clinical Signs and Diagnosis

Most dogs with inguinal hernias have a soft, doughy mass in the inguinal region that is usually not painful on palpation. The mass can have been present for up to a year and may or may not be reducible on palpation. Elevation of the patient's hindquarters may aid the examiner in reducing the hernia and allows palpation of the defect in the abdominal wall. The hernia can contain a gravid or infected uterus that is unable to be reduced. Other tissues and organs that can be contained within the hernia include omentum, intestine, bladder, prostatic fat, and spleen. Diagnosis of inguinal herniation is aided by radiography demonstrating gas-filled loops of intestine or the appearance of the ossifying fetal skeleton after 43 to 45 days of gestation. The bladder can be identified by contrast radiography after catheterization and aspiration of bladder contents. Inguinal hernia must be differentiated from subcutaneous fatty tissue accumulation, abscess, hematoma formation, and mammary gland neoplasia. The hernia can appear as a swelling lateral to the vulva and must be differentiated from a perineal hernia (7).

Surgical Techniques

A ventral midline incision can be used for all inguinal hernias. This approach allows visualization of both inguinal rings and repair of bilateral herniation through a single incision. It also permits extension of the incision cranially, when necessary, without invasion of mammary tissue or its blood supply (5, 8).

The surgical incision extends from the cranial brim of the pelvis as far cranially as necessary to allow exposure of the hernial sac. This incision is continued through the subcutaneous tissue down to the ventral

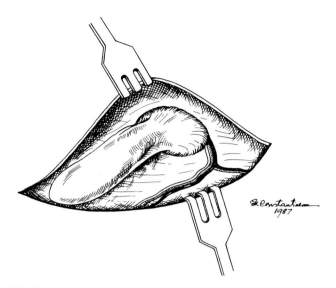

Fig. 35.1. Lateral retraction of the midline incision exposes the hernial sac and its contents.

rectus sheath. Dissection proceeds bluntly under the mammary tissue, and the mammary tissue is undermined and retracted laterally to expose the inguinal ring and hernial sac (Fig. 35.1). After the hernial sac is dissected from the subcutaneous tissue, the hernial sac is opened, and the contents are inspected (Fig. 35.2). Any adhesions between the sac and the viscera are broken down, and the contents are returned to the abdominal cavity.

In some cases, it may be necessary to enlarge the hernial ring cranially to facilitate reduction of the hernia. If the urinary bladder is included in the hernia,

aspiration of urine facilitates reduction. When one or both horns of the uterus are included and ovariohysterectomy is performed, extending the incision in a cranial and medial direction may be necessary to complete the procedure (4, 5). Should the hernia contain a gravid uterus, up to the seventh week of pregnancy the hernia can be replaced into the abdomen and the pregnancy can be allowed to continue to completion. After the seventh week of pregnancy, ovariohysterectomy is recommended, depending on the age and value of the bitch as a breeding animal (5).

After replacement of viscera into the abdomen, the redundant sac is trimmed at the margins of the inguinal ring. Twisting the redundant sac may help to maintain reduction of the contents within the abdomen (Fig. 35.3). The hernial ring is sutured with simple interrupted sutures of 2–0 nonabsorbable suture material (Fig. 35.4) (9). Care must be taken during closure to avoid the external pudendal vessels and genitofemoral nerve, which exit from the caudomedial aspect of the ring. In males, the inguinal ring must be closed without compromising the spermatic cord as it traverses the inguinal canal.

The inguinal ring on the other side is inspected, the vaginal process is removed, and the ring is sutured closed. The mammary tissue is then drawn back to the midline, and the subcutaneous tissues are closed using absorbable sutures, with care taken to eliminate potential dead space. If necessary, a Penrose drain can be placed before closure and made to exit from a separate stab incision ventrally if a large amount of dead space in which fluid could accumulate is present. The skin is closed routinely.

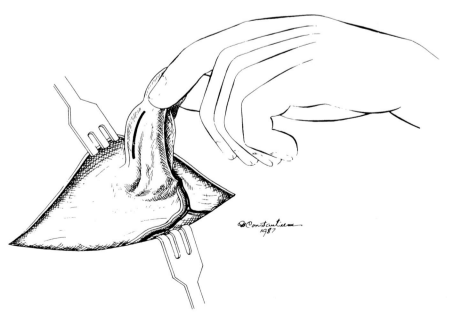

Fig. 35.2. The hernia sac is incised, and its contents are inspected and returned to the abdomen. (The *line* indicates the incision in the sac.)

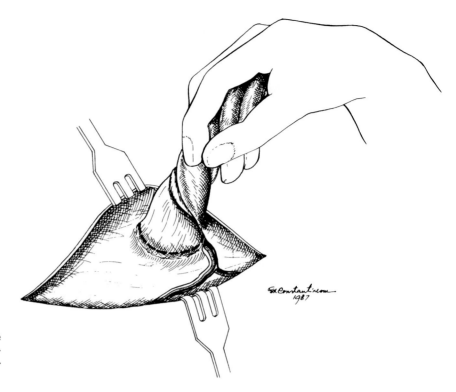

Fig. 35.3. The edges of redundant sac are excised. Twisting of the sac facilitates maintenance of the reduced contents within the abdomen.

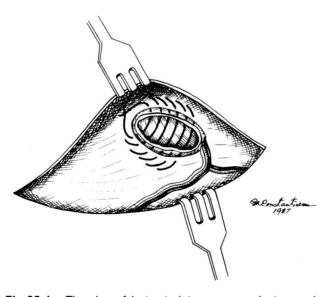

Fig. 35.4. The edges of the inguinal ring are apposed using nonabsorbable suture material in a simple interrupted pattern. Care must be taken not to compromise the external pudendal vessels and genitofemoral nerve as they exit the caudomedial border of the ring.

Postoperative Care

The caudal abdomen is bandaged immediately after the procedure. Bandaging helps to eliminate dead space and increases the comfort of the patient. If used, drains should be covered with an absorbent dressing and bandage and can be removed 3 to 5 days postsurgically, before the patient's discharge from the hospital. Broad-spectrum antibiotic treatment is used if a drain is in place and for 3 days after drain removal.

References

1. Ashdown RR. The anatomy of the inguinal canal in the domesticated mammals. Vet Rec 1983;75:1345–1351.
2. Fox MW. Inherited inguinal hernia and midline defects in the dog. J Am Vet Med Assoc 1963;143:602–604.
3. Hayes HM Jr. Congenital umbilical and inguinal hernias in cattle, horses, swine, dogs, and cats: risk by breed and sex among hospital patients. Am J Vet Res 1974;35:839–842.
4. Archibald J, Sumner-Smith G. Hernia. In: Archibald J, ed. Canine surgery. 2nd ed. Santa Barbara, CA: American Veterinary Publications, 1974.
5. North AF Jr. A new surgical approach to inguinal hernias in the dog. Cornell Vet 1959;49:379–383.
6. Smeak DD. Caudal abdominal hernias. In: Slatter DH, ed. Textbook of small animal surgery. 2nd ed. Vol. 1. Philadelphia: WB Saunders, 1985.
7. Blakely CL. Perineal hernia. In: Mayer K, LaCroix JV, Hoskins HP, eds. Canine surgery. 4th ed. Evanston, IL: American Veterinary Publishers, 1957.
8. Peddie JF. Inguinal hernia repair in the dog. Mod Vet Pract 1980;61:859–861.
9. Bojrab MJ. Inguinal hernias. In: Bojrab MJ, ed. Current techniques in small animal surgery. 2nd ed. Philadelphia: Lea & Febiger, 1983.

Perineal Hernia Repair in the Dog

Mark A. Anderson, Gheorghe M. Constantinescu & F. A. Mann

The perineum is the region that closes the pelvic outlet, surrounding the anal and urogenital canals (1). On the surface of the dog, the perineum is limited by the tail dorsally, the scrotum or beginning of the vulva ventrally, and the ischiadic tuberosity on both sides. Deeply, the perineum is bounded by the third caudal vertebra dorsally, the sacrotuberous ligaments on both sides, and the arch of the ischium ventrally. The pelvic diaphragm is the vertical closure of the pelvic canal through which the rectum passes (2).

Perineal hernia is the result of weakness and separation of the muscles and fascia that make up the pelvic diaphragm. The pelvic diaphragm is composed of the levator ani and coccygeus muscles and the internal and external fascia (1). The exact cause of the muscular weakness is unknown, but several factors have been proposed (3–11). As a result of the muscular weakness, caudal displacement of intra-abdominal organs or deviation or dilatation of the rectum into the perineum can occur (3, 4). Retroflexion of the bladder occurs in approximately 20% of patients (12, 13). Other intra-abdominal contents found within the hernial sac include jejunum, colon, and prostate (13). However, more commonly retroperitoneal fat and fluid fill the sac (14).

Perineal hernia has been reported in many different species, but it is most problematic in dogs. Some breeds of dogs are overrepresented in the occurrence of perineal herniation. Boston terriers, Pekingese, collies, boxers, Welsh corgis, kelpies, miniature poodles, German shepherds, bouviers de Flandres, old English sheepdogs, dachshunds, and mongrels all have an increased incidence of the condition (9, 12, 14). Perineal hernia occurs commonly in the male dog, particularly in sexually intact males, and rarely in females. Most dogs with perineal hernia are between 7 and 9 years of age (9, 15).

Perineal herniation may be unilateral or bilateral. Some investigators have reported an increased incidence of perineal herniation on the right side, but the criterion used to determine unilateral versus bilateral and left versus right is subjective. In fact, the occurrence of the hernia on one side as opposed to the other may be related to the rate and extent of tissue deterioration rather than to the preferential involvement of one side (14).

Clinical Signs

Tenesmus, constipation, and perineal swelling are the three most consistent clinical features of dogs presented with perineal hernia (3, 14). In as many as 80% of dogs presented for perineal hernia, straining to defecate is the primary compliant. Tenesmus is the result of the collection of excessive feces that a rectal dilatation or sacculation in the perineal hernia (4). Furthermore, the perineal swelling may be the combination of abdominal contents and a feces-filled rectum.

Retroflexion of the urinary bladder into the perineal hernia may result in urinary obstruction. The obstruction results from an abrupt change in direction of the urethra (13). Clinical signs of bladder retroflexion include stranguria, dysuria, and anuria (13). Although perineal hernia is not considered a surgical emergency, immediate repositioning of the bladder or urine evacuation is required. If the bladder cannot be reduced and urine evacuation cannot be achieved, surgical intervention on an emergency basis may be required. Other less commonly reported clinical signs are depression or lethargy, vomiting, anorexia, perineal pain, stringy stool, weight loss, and fecal incontinence (12).

Diagnosis

The diagnosis of a perineal hernia is based on the history, clinical signs, physical examination, and radiography. The diagnosis may be difficult during the early stages, when the hernia is forming (3). However, with progression of the clinical signs, the diagnosis generally becomes more obvious. Rectal palpation is the most important part of the physical examination when diagnosing perineal hernia. When performing a rectal examination, the veterinarian's index finger should be directed cranially into the middle of the herniated rectum, which lies lateral to the anus and medial to the wall of the pelvic canal (16). Generally, the rectum is filled with feces, making identification of the extent (unilateral versus bilateral) of the hernia difficult. Manual removal of the fecoliths from the rectum should be performed. This allows better assessment of the pelvic diaphragm muscles. When evaluating the rectum for abnormalities such as a deviation, sacculation, or diverticulum, a rectal barium enema (4) may be helpful, but it is usually not necessary. Differentiation between rectal sacculation (full-thickness outpouching of the rectal wall) and diverticulum (protrusion of mucosa or submucosa through a muscular defect) requires perioperative inspection of the rectal muscularis.

When a patient has clinical signs of urinary tract involvement with a perineal hernia, caudal abdominal radiography including the perineum should be performed. The contents of the perineal hernia and the location of the urinary bladder should be identified. If the urinary bladder cannot be visualized on routine radiography, retrograde urethrography or cystography should be done (3, 13). Ultrasonography is another noninvasive technique that can be used to identify the location of the urinary bladder (either within the hernia or the abdomen) and can be used to assist decompression by syringe and needle.

Conservative Therapy

Conservative management of perineal hernia includes the use of stool softeners, periodic enemas, and digital evacuation of the feces from the rectum as needed (3, 14). Dogs considered for conservative medical and dietary management include dogs that are poor surgical candidates and dogs with owners who refuse surgical treatment for the animal (3, 17). Dogs that present with straining during the initial examination are reported to have a poor long-term response to medical management (17).

Hormonal therapy by castration, low-dose estrogen therapy, or progestin administration can decrease the size of the prostate and can alleviate clinical signs associated with prostatic hyperplasia. However, no reported studies have evaluated the efficacy of hormonal therapy on controlling the long-term clinical signs associated with prostatomegaly and a concomitant perineal hernia (14). We recommend castration because of its beneficial effects on prostatic disease prophylaxis despite its questionable role in preventing the recurrence of perineal hernia. We caution against other forms of hormonal therapy for prostatic disease.

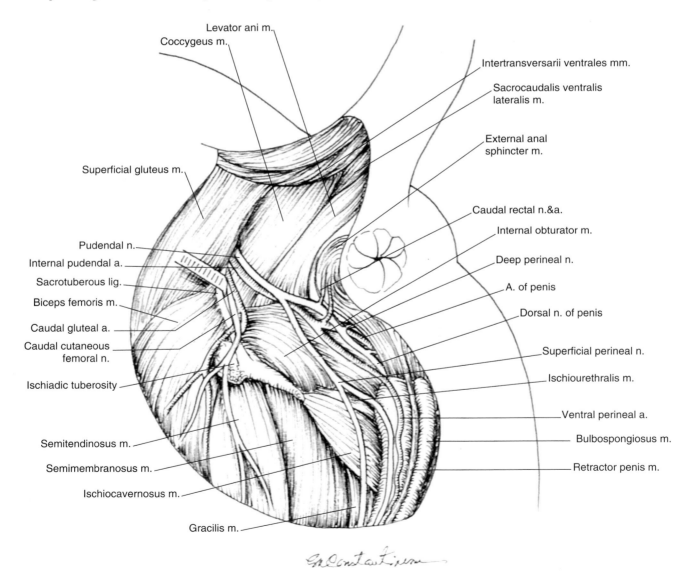

Fig. 35.5. Surgical anatomy of the left perineum, caudal aspect.

Surgical Anatomy

The structures involved in surgical repair of perineal hernia include the pelvic diaphragm, the perineal fascia, and the nerves and vessels in the proximity of these structures (Figs. 35.5 and 35.6) (18). Additionally, extraperineal muscle flaps can be transposed for perineal herniorrhaphy (i.e., the semitendinosus muscle flap) (19).

The levator ani and coccygeus muscles originate from the medial side of the ischial spine and the medial side of the body of the ilium–dorsal surface of the pubis cranial to the obturator foramen, respectively. The levator ani and coccygeus muscles insert on the second through fourth or fifth caudal vertebrae and on the fourth through the seventh caudal vertebrae, respectively. These two muscles form the lateral boundary of the rectum or the medial boundary of the pelvic diaphragm (2, 17).

The sacrotuberous ligament and the superficial gluteal muscle form the lateral aspect of the pelvic diaphragm. The sacrotuberous ligament originates from the tuber ischiadicum and inserts on the sacrum and first caudal vertebra. The superficial gluteal muscle originates on the lateral aspect of the sacrum, first caudal vertebra, and the cranial half of the sacrotuberous ligament. The superficial gluteal muscle forms a tendon lateral to the perineal region and runs over the dorsal aspect of the greater trochanter to insert on the third trochanter (2, 17).

The ventral aspect of the perineal region is bounded by the internal obturator muscle. The internal obturator muscle originates on the cranial and medial border of the obturator foramen and inserts as a flat tendon embedded in the muscle bellies of the gemelli muscles in the trochanteric fossa of the femur (2, 17).

The external anal sphincter muscle is a striated muscle that surrounds the anal canal. This muscle is divided into three parts: cutaneous, superficial, and deep. The cutaneous part lies directly under the skin in the subcutaneous fascia. The superficial part attaches to the third and fourth caudal vertebrae and passes around the lateral aspect of the anus and anal sacs to insert on the bulbocavernosus muscle (male) or the constrictor muscle of the vulva (female). The deep part surrounds the anal canal, passing medial to the anal sacs. The superficial and deep parts can interchange with each other (2, 14).

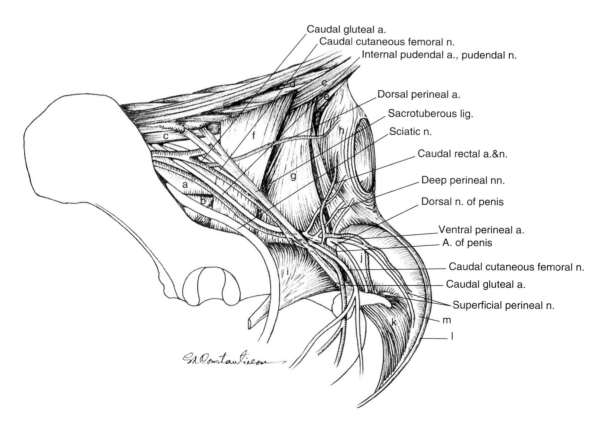

Fig. 35.6. Surgical anatomy of the left perineum, lateral aspect. *a*, rectum; *b*, urethralis muscle; *c*, sacrocaudalis ventralis lateralis muscle; *d*, intertransversarii ventrales muscles; *e*, rectococcygeus muscle; *f*, coccygeus muscle; *g*, levator ani muscle; *h*, external anal sphincter; *i*, internal obturator muscle; *j*, bulbus penis; *k*, ischiocavernosus muscle; *l*, retractor penis muscle; *m*, bulbospongiosus muscle.

The semitendinosus muscle is another striated muscle that originates from the tuber ischiadicum and inserts on the tibia and on the tuber calcanei (1), and it does not directly bound the perineal region. However, the semitendinosus muscle has been used to reconstruct perineal hernia defects (19).

The internal pudendal artery and vein and the pudendal nerve are bound together by loose connective tissue, and this neurovascular bundle passes ventrolaterally to the coccygeus muscle and continues caudomedially across the dorsal surface of the internal obturator muscle. At the caudal border of the ventral aspect of the external anal sphincter muscle, the pudendal nerve gives off the caudal rectal nerve. This branch of the pudendal nerve provides motor innervation to the external anal sphincter muscle (2).

The perineal fascia is the connective tissue covering of the perineal musculature and is divided into deep and superficial layers. The deep perineal fascia tightly covers the musculature. The superficial perineal fascia is the loose connective tissue that makes up the hernial sac. The superficial perineal fascia is not considered to be of adequate strength to suture as the primary layer for hernia repair.

Patient Preparation

A perineal hernia is not considered a surgical emergency unless the urinary bladder is retroflexed (13). If the urinary bladder is retroflexed into the perineal hernia, the urinary bladder should be manually reduced. If the urinary bladder cannot be reduced, a urinary catheter should be placed or paracentesis must be performed. Removal of urine from the urinary bladder should assist in reduction. Serum biochemistry studies (serum urea nitrogen and creatinine) should be evaluated. Dogs with azotemia should be treated appropriately, and the surgical procedure should be postponed until the patient's condition is stable (13).

If the perineal hernia does not contain the urinary bladder, the surgical repair is an elective procedure. Because most dogs with perineal hernias are geriatric, a minimum database including a complete blood count, serum biochemistry values, and a complete urinalysis should be obtained (3).

Some surgeons prepare the dog for surgery by having the animal's rectum cleaned of all feces with several enemas the day before surgery and by fasting the dog for 24 hours before the operation (3, 14, 16, 18). Enemas increase the risk of rectal trauma and make for fluid fecal material, which is difficult to contain during surgery; therefore, we prefer to avoid enemas. Instead, gentle digital extraction of feces is performed after the dog is anesthetized immediately before the surgical procedure.

After the dog is anesthetized, the perineal region is liberally clipped. The anal sacs are evacuated, a lubricated gauze tampon is inserted into the rectum, and a pursestring suture is placed in the anus. A preliminary scrub is performed to remove gross contamination from the perineum. The dog is positioned in sternal recumbency and is pulled to the end of the operating table (Fig. 35.7). The pelvic limbs are placed off the end of the table and are gently pulled forward. The table can either be tilted forward, or the dog can be placed in a perineal stand. If a perineal stand or tilt table is not available, sandbags or other padding can be used to elevate the dog's perineum. When pulling the animal's pelvic limbs over the end of the table, the surgeon should protect the front of the limb, to help prevent femoral and peroneal nerve injury (16). If a tilt table is used to help position the dog, excessive tilting of the table should be prevented because of concern for respiratory compromise. Because the perineal position causes the dog's head to be placed downward, the abdominal contents encroach on the diaphragm, and intermittent positive-pressure ventilation is required (18).

After the patient is positioned, the tail can be wrapped, and several pieces of adhesive tape can be placed several inches above the base of the tail and then directed toward the dog's head. This maneuver pulls the tail over the dog's back. After the tail has been positioned, a final scrub can be performed.

Perioperative antibiotics are used by some surgeons; however, the use of antibiotics should not preclude good aseptic surgical technique. If antibiotics are chosen, a broad-spectrum antibiotic with a spectrum of activity against gram-negative enteric organisms should be used (18).

Surgical Technique

The perineal region should be draped so none of the anus is exposed after the skin incision is made, but it remains accessible to visualization if necessary. For correction of bilateral perineal hernias, the dog should be redraped, the surgeon should reglove, and consideration should be given to changing instruments. Castration is performed on sexually intact male dogs before herniorrhaphy. Caudal castration (20) may be performed with the dog in the perineal position (see Chap. 32) to decrease the overall length of the surgical procedure by avoiding the repositioning associated with standard prescrotal castration.

The incision is made over the hernia from just lateral to the tail base to just below the hernial mass (see Fig. 35.7). The incision is curved slightly laterally in a dorsoventral direction. Care must be taken to not incise too deeply and injure the hernial contents.

Blunt dissection is used to enter the hernial sac (superficial perineal fascia) and expose the hernial con-

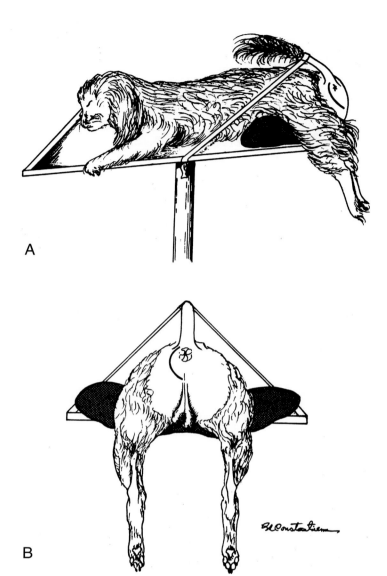

Fig. 35.7. Positioning for perineal herniorrhaphy. **A.** The sandbags provide padding. Tape secures the tail in a midline position over the back. Tape may also be used to secure the pelvic limbs in position, but care must be exercised to avoid excessive tension. **B.** The semicircular line to the left of the anus indicates the proposed incision. Surgical drapes are not pictured, to allow anatomic reference.

tents. Once the contents of the hernia are exposed, redundant fat can be excised and hernial fluid removed. If jejunum, prostate, colon, or urinary bladder is encountered, these structures can be reduced by digital manipulation in a cranial direction back to their pelvic or abdominal location and maintained with a gauze sponge. A suture can be tied to the gauze sponge to facilitate its removal before tying the herniorrhaphy sutures.

After reduction of the hernia, the muscular defect and landmarks for surgical closure are identified. The medial side of the defect is bounded by the rectum, ending with the anal sphincter muscle caudally. The coccygeus muscle and, if present, the levator ani muscle are dorsolateral. The sacrotuberous ligament can be palpated as the lateral landmark of the repair. This ligament is a broad fibrous cord that extends from the sacrum to the ischiadic tuberosity. The ventral boundary of the hernia is formed by the internal obturator muscle on the floor of the pelvis. Ventrolateral to the coccygeus and levator ani muscles and dorsal to the internal obturator muscle is the neurovascular bundle (internal pudendal artery and vein and pudendal nerve) of this region. Identification of the neurovascular bundle is important because the pudendal nerve supplies motor function to the external anal sphincter muscle. Bilateral pudendal nerve injury may result in permanent fecal incontinence (3). Unilateral pudendal nerve injury may lead to temporary incontinence until reinnervation or compensation from the opposite side occurs.

Before pelvic diaphragm repair, the presence or absence of rectal disease must be ascertained (4, 8). Rectal deviation occurs as a result of a potential space

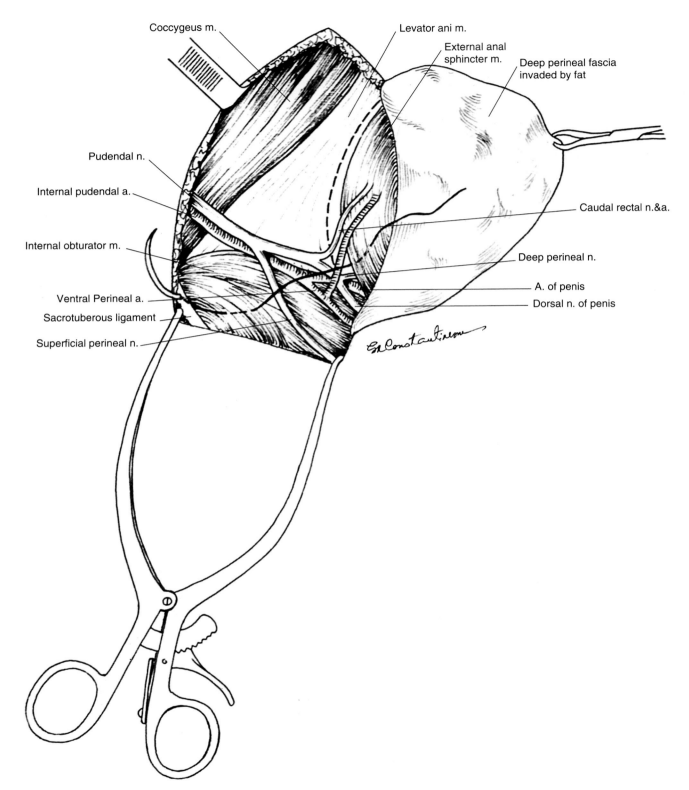

Coccygeus m.

Levator ani m.

External anal sphincter m.

Deep perineal fascia invaded by fat

Pudendal n.

Internal pudendal a.

Internal obturator m.

Ventral Perineal a.

Sacrotuberous ligament

Superficial perineal n.

Caudal rectal n.&a.

Deep perineal n.

A. of penis

Dorsal n. of penis

Fig. 35.8. Operative view of left perineal hernia with placement of the first suture using the standard herniorrhaphy technique. The first suture is placed in the most ventral position, from the internal obturator muscle to the external anal sphincter.

created by the hernia. Perineal herniorrhaphy should alleviate rectal deviation and small sacculation (18). Large rectal sacculation and rectal diverticulum may cause straining to expel feces. Therefore, surgical excision of rectal diverticulum or large sacculation, followed by a double-layer inverting suture pattern that does not enter the lumen of the rectum, should be performed to prevent perineal hernia recurrence resulting from straining caused by impacted feces (4).

All sutures should be preplaced before they are tied (Figs. 35.8 and 35.9). The selection of suture type has been controversial. We recommend synthetic nonabsorbable monofilament suture such as polypropylene for the primary closure of the hernial defect. Suture placement is begun from the most ventral aspect of the defect. The first suture is placed from the internal obturator muscle laterally to the external anal sphincter muscle medially, or vice versa, depending on the side of the hernia and the surgeon (right-handed versus left-handed). Care should be taken when passing sutures through the internal obturator muscle to not incorporate sutures into the neurovascular bundle in this region. Because the recurrence rate is high with the conventional suture technique, placement of an adequate number of sutures ventrally is important to success (3, 18). Several more sutures are placed dorsal to the internal obturator sutures, incorporating bites from the external anal sphincter into the sacrotuberous ligament, the coccygeus muscle, and, when present, the levator ani muscle (3, 18). When placing sutures through the sacrotuberous ligament, care must be taken to not include the caudal gluteal artery or vein or the sciatic nerve, which lie cranial to the ligament. Placing a finger medial and cranial to the sacrotuberous ligament may assist in determining the depth of suture placement by palpation of the caudal gluteal artery's pulse (3, 18). Furthermore, the suture should be placed through the fibers of the sacrotuberous ligament instead of encircling the entire structure. When placing sutures through the external anal sphincter muscle, multiple fibers are gathered onto the needle. Care should be taken to avoid penetration of the rec-

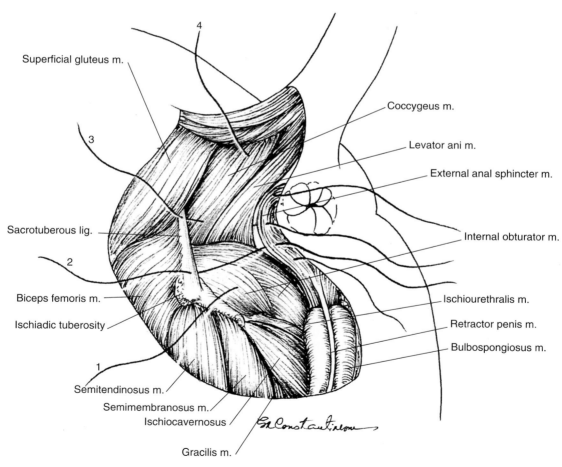

Fig. 35.9. Placement of sutures in the standard perineal herniorrhaphy technique. Suture placement is from ventral to dorsal: (*1* to *4*). All sutures are preplaced and then are tied. More than one suture may be placed in any of the four basic positions, depending on the size of the dog.

tum or anal sacs. Once all sutures are preplaced, they are tied from dorsal to ventral. As sutures are tied, the anus may be visualized to ensure that it has not been grossly distorted.

After closure of the hernial defect, the superficial perineal fascia is mobilized laterally from the skin. After mobilization, the perineal fascia can be used to reinforce the closure by suturing the fascia caudally to the external anal sphincter muscle using synthetic absorbable suture material. The subcutaneous tissue and skin are closed routinely. Strategic subcutaneous suture placement to minimize dead space eliminates the need for placement of drains. Drains are to be avoided in the perineal region because of postoperative contamination risks.

If bilateral hernia repair is considered, the hernias can be repaired at the same time; however, some surgeons wait 4 to 6 weeks between repairs to decrease the stress and distortion of the external anal sphincter muscle associated with standard herniorrhaphy technique (3, 18).

We believe that castration should be performed for its benefits relative to prostatic disease. Castration is unlikely to prevent perineal diaphragm muscle weakness (21–23).

After all procedures have been completed, the anal pursestring suture and rectal gauze tampon are removed. A thorough rectal examination should be performed to evaluate the integrity of the repair.

Postoperative Management

Efforts should be made to ensure a smooth recovery from anesthesia, to prevent undo stress on the repaired perineum. To this end, light sedation is occasionally necessary in conjunction with routine analgesics in the early postoperative period.

Prophylactic use of antibiotics to lower the incidence of infection with perineal hernia repair is not straightforward. In one report retrospectively evaluating 100 dogs, the investigators recommended the use of perioperative antibiotics rather than postoperative antibiotics unless an infection has been documented (12). We believe that good aseptic surgical technique is more important than antibiotics to prevent infection, and we select prophylactic antibiotics on a case-by-case basis.

A low-residue diet can be fed for the first few days to help prevent straining during defecation, which may lead to disruption of the perineal hernia repair. If straining to defecate does not resolve, digital palpation should be performed to rule out suture placement in the rectal mucosa. If a suture is not the cause for straining, the pain usually resolves, but analgesics may be necessary in the interim (18).

If the dog chews or licks excessively at the incision,

a side brace, Elizabethan collar, or plastic bucket can be used. Dogs should return in 10 to 14 days for suture removal.

Complications

Several potential postoperative complications are associated with repair of perineal hernia. These complications include sciatic nerve injury, fecal incontinence, infection around the incision site, rectal prolapse associated with excessive straining, misplacement of sutures into the anal sac or rectal lumen, urinary bladder necrosis, urinary incontinence, and recurrence of the perineal hernia (24). Recognition, prevention, and appropriate management of these postoperative complications are essential to a successful surgical outcome.

Sciatic nerve injury or entrapment can occur if the nerve becomes encircled or is penetrated by a suture passed either through or around the sacrotuberous ligament. Entrapment of the sciatic nerve is identified immediately after the animal recovers from the surgical procedure. The dog shows signs of extreme pain over the hip and perineal region. Furthermore, sciatic nerve palsy may be detected on a neurologic examination. The treatment of sciatic nerve entrapment is removal of the suture through a caudolateral approach to the hip (25). This surgical approach allows good visualization of the sciatic nerve and does not require disruption of the perineal hernia repair. Occasionally, epidural administration of medication is used for postoperative analgesia in patients that have undergone pelvic or perianal operations. Because this analgesic technique sometimes causes transient sciatic palsy, we recommend alternate means of controlling postoperative pain after perineal herniorrhaphy, to avoid confusion with the foregoing surgical complication. Observation of sciatic palsy subjects the dog to unnecessary sciatic nerve exploration if the neurologic deficit is due to the epidural analgesic technique.

Fecal incontinence may be only temporary, the result of postoperative pain and inflammation associated with the surgery. Unilateral damage to either the pudendal nerve or the caudal rectal nerve may be associated with temporary incontinence that resolves after the contralateral caudal rectal nerve reinnervates the damaged nerve's side (14, 24). Return of full fecal continence may take several weeks after unilateral caudal rectal nerve damage. Permanent fecal incontinence is likely if bilateral caudal rectal or pudendal nerve damage occurs or if damage to the external anal sphincter muscle or other pararectal tissue is excessive (24). Permanent fecal incontinence is best avoided because the reported prosthetic implants and muscle transpositions have been inconsistently successful in reestablishing fecal continence (19, 26).

Incisional complications have been reported frequently and are a function of the surgical location (12). Exposure of the incision to feces either during the surgical procedure or before a good fibrin seal has occurred can cause a wound infection. If an infection occurs, surgical drainage of the site and administration of antibiotics based on culture and susceptibility testing are ideal. If antibiotics need to be instituted before culture and susceptibility results are available, a broad-spectrum antibiotic with activity against *Escherichia coli* should be used (24).

Rectal prolapse is uncommon immediately after surgery. Rectal prolapse can occur as a result of excessive straining postoperatively because of placement of sutures in the rectal lumen or because of pain associated with bilateral hernia repair. Rectal disease and external anal sphincter nerve injury are two other predisposing factors to rectal prolapse. The rectal prolapse should be reduced, and a pursestring suture should be placed in the patient's anus. If straining is excessive and is unresponsive to narcotics, epidural medication can be administered. The pursestring suture should be maintained until the straining has resolved. Generally, this takes several days. If the rectal prolapse recurs after several attempts of reduction, colopexy should be performed (24).

Misplaced sutures into the rectal mucosa can occur because of difficulty in identifying perineal structures resulting from excessive tissue inflammation and swelling. Misplaced sutures can lead to excessive straining and, less commonly, to the development of a rectocutaneous fistula. Misplacement of sutures into the anal sac can also lead to draining tracts. The treatment of chronic fistulas associated with misplaced sutures is by fistulectomy and anal sacculectomy, depending on the anatomic structure involved (24).

Complications relative to retroflexion of the urinary bladder into the perineal hernia are seen infrequently. Retroflexion of the urinary bladder can stretch the nerves that supply the urinary bladder and urethral sphincter, stretch the detrusor muscle, or interfere with the blood supply to the bladder. Usually, clinical signs of this complication are temporary. Manual decompression of the urinary bladder or catheterization may be necessary to keep the urinary bladder empty until bladder tone recurs. Urinary bladder necrosis has been associated with long-standing cases secondary to urinary bladder obstruction and distension. The clinical signs of bladder necrosis are rupture and uroperitoneum. Exploratory celiotomy and resection of the necrotic portion of the urinary bladder may be required; however, in some cases, excessive urinary bladder necrosis may prohibit a successful resection (24).

Recurrence of perineal hernia after repair has ranged from 10 to 46% (8–10, 27). Although some surgical procedures offer better results and less chance of recurrence, the accurate identification of all ana-tomic structures is paramount to the success of any procedure. Furthermore, understanding the limitations of each particular technique is important in the surgical decision-making process and may help to prevent the failure of any technique.

The association between castration and the recurrence of a perineal hernia after surgical repair has been reported to be 2.7 times greater in dogs that were not castrated than in dogs that were castrated (9). In a more recent study, however, no correlation was found between castration and perineal hernia recurrence. Failure of perineal hernia repair was thought to be more closely related to lack of experience with the surgical technique than to any effect of castration (12).

References

1. Schaller O, Constantinescu GM, Habel RE, et al. Illustrated veterinary anatomical nomenclature. Stuttgart: Enke F, 1992:222.
2. Chibuzo GA. The digestive apparatus and abdomen. In: Evans HE, Christensen GC, eds. Miller's anatomy of the dog. Philadelphia: WB Saunders, 1979:491–492.
3. Bojrab MJ, Toomey A. Perineal herniorrhaphy. Compend Contin Educ Pract Vet 1981;8:8–15.
4. Krahwinkel DJ. Rectal diseases and their role in perineal hernia. Vet Surg 1983;12:160–165.
5. Spruell JSA, Frankland AL. Transplanting the superficial gluteal muscle in the treatment of perineal hernia and flexure of the rectum in dogs. J Small Anim Pract 1980;21:265–278.
6. Holmes JR. Perineal hernia in the dog. Vet Rec 1964;76:1250–1251.
7. Walker RG. Perineal hernia in the dog. Vet Rec 1965;77:93–94.
8. Pettit GD. Perineal hernia in the dog. Cornell Vet 1962;52:261–279.
9. Hayes HW, Wilson GP, Tarone RE. The epidemiologic features of perineal hernia in 771 dogs. J Am Anim Hosp Assoc 1978;14:703–707.
10. Burrows CF, Harvey CE. Perineal hernia in the dog. J Small Anim Pract 1973;14:315–332.
11. Sjollema BE, Venker-van Haagen, van Sluijs FJ, et al. Electromyography of the pelvic diaphragm and anal sphincter in dogs with perineal hernia. Am J Vet Res 1993;54:185–190.
12. Hosgood G, Hedlund CS, Pechman RD, et al. Perineal herniorrhaphy: perioperative data from 100 dogs. J Am Anim Hosp Assoc 1995;31:331–342.
13. White RAS, Herrtage ME. Bladder retroflexion in the dog. J Small Anim Pract 1986;27:735–746.
14. Bellenger CR, Canfield RB. Perineal hernia. In: Slatter DH, ed. Textbook of Small Animal Surgery. Philadelphia: WB Saunders, 1993:471–482.
15. Weaver AD, Omamegbe JO. Surgical treatment of perineal hernia in the dog. J Small Anim Pract 1981;22:749–758.
16. Dieterich HF. Perineal hernia repair in the canine. Vet Clin North Am 1975;5:383–399.
17. Harvey CE. Treatment of perineal hernia in the dog: reassessment. J Small Anim Pract 1977;18:505–511.
18. Dean PW, Bojrab MJ. Perineal hernia repair in the dog. In: Bojrab MJ, ed. Current techniques in small animal surgery. Philadelphia: WB Saunders, 1990:442–448.
19. Chambers JN, Rawlings CA. Applications of a semitendinosus flap in two dogs. J Am Vet Med Assoc 1991;199:84–86.
20. Knecht CD. An alternate approach for castration of the dog. Vet Med Small Anim Clin 1976;71:469–473.
21. Desai R. An anatomical study of the canine male and female pelvic diaphragm and effect of testosterone on the status of the levator ani of male dogs. J Am Anim Hosp Assoc 1982;18:195–202.
22. Mann FA, Boothe HW, Amoss MS, et al. Serum testosterone

and estradiol 17-beta concentration in 15 dogs with perineal hernia. J Am Vet Med Assoc 1989;194:1578–1580.

23. Mann FA, Nonneman DJ, Pope ER, et al. Androgen receptors in the pelvic diaphragm muscles of dogs with and without perineal hernia. Am J Vet Res 1995;56:134–139.

24. Matthiesen DT. Diagnosis and management of complications occurring after perineal herniorrhaphy in dogs. Compend Contin Educ Pract Vet 1989;11:797–823.

25. Piermattei DL, Greeley RG. Approach to the hip joint through a caudolateral incision. In: Piermattei DL, ed. Atlas of surgical approaches to the bones of the dog and cat. Philadelphia: WB Saunders, 1979:146–149.

26. Dean PW, O'Brien DP, Turk MA, et al. Silicone elastomer sling for fecal incontinence in dogs. Vet Surg 1988;17:304–310.

27. Orsher RJ. Clinical and surgical parameters in dogs with perineal hernia: analysis of results of internal obturator transposition. Vet Surg 1986;15:253–258.

Salvage Techniques for Failed Perineal Herniorrhaphy

F. A. Mann & Gheorghe M. Constantinescu

Recurrence of canine perineal herniation after traditional (standard) herniorrhaphy has been reported to be as high as 46% (1). Recurrent rates as low as 5% have been reported for the internal obturator muscle transposition herniorrhaphy technique (2). Nonetheless, until the cause of canine perineal hernia can be identified and controlled, a certain degree of recurrence can be expected regardless of refinements in surgical technique. This discussion describes techniques that can be used to salvage cases of failed perineal herniorrhaphy. When the traditional herniorrhaphy technique (discussed in an earlier section of this chapter) fails, the simplest and usually the most effective means of salvage is to perform an internal obturator muscle transposition (discussed in a later section of this chapter) to reconstruct the pelvic diaphragm. When the internal obturator muscle transposition fails or is deemed unlikely to succeed, we recommend choosing from one of the following two options: semitendinosus muscle transposition (3, 4) for perineal reconstruction or colopexy or cystopexy by deferent duct fixation (5) for preventing herniation of important structures.

Internal Obturator Muscle Transposition

With the dog ventrally recumbent in the perineal position, a semicircular skin incision similar to the one used for the traditional herniorrhaphy technique is made in the perineal skin from the tail base to the median raphe ventrally. After the hernial contents are isolated and reduced, the internal obturator muscle is

subperiosteally elevated from the ischiatic table and is lifted dorsally. The transposed internal obturator muscle is sutured medially to the external anal sphincter and laterally to the sacrotuberous ligament, the coccygeus muscle, and, if present, the levator ani muscle using polypropylene sutures (Figs. 35.10 and 35.11). Specific details of this technique are described in a later section of this chapter.

Failure of internal obturator muscle transposition most commonly occurs in the ventromedial aspect of the transposed muscle. To prevent failure, care should be exercised during subperiosteal elevation to prevent excessive trauma to the muscle, and the ventromedial sutures from the internal obturator muscle to the external anal sphincter should be secure.

Semitendinosus Muscle Transposition

The semitendinosus muscle transposition is particularly useful for reconstructions in which the ventral aspect of the perineum is severely affected, as is the case with some bilateral perineal hernias. For unilateral perineal herniation, the contralateral semitendinosus muscle is recommended for pelvic diaphragm reconstruction.

With the dog in the perineal position, a skin incision is made in the perineal skin from the tail base to the median raphe ventrally, just as for traditional and internal obturator muscle transposition repairs, and the incision is continued across the midline toward the ischiadic tuberosity, where it curves and progresses distally on the caudal aspect of the pelvic limb to end at the caudomedial aspect of the transition between the stifle and the crus (Fig. 35.12). The hernial contents are exposed and reduced, as in other herniorrhaphy techniques, before isolation of the semitendinosus muscle. The subcutaneous tissues over the semitendinosus muscle are incised to expose the muscle (Fig. 35.13). The semitendinosus muscle is bluntly isolated from surrounding structures, with care taken not to injure the proximal vascular pedicle (the caudal gluteal artery and vein). The semitendinosus muscle is transected as distally as possible near the stifle and is further isolated for mobilization to the perineal region. Incision of the lateral portion of the semitendinosus tendinous attachment to the ischium may be necessary for maximal mobilization, but care must be taken to avoid proximal vascular pedicle trauma or kinking that may occur with excessive mobilization. Using polypropylene or nylon suture, the transected portion of the semitendinosus muscle is sutured to the sacrotuberous ligament and the coccygeus muscle. The medial aspect of the semitendinosus muscle (now adjacent to the external anal sphincter muscle dorsally) is sutured to the external anal sphincter, and the lateral aspect of the semitendinosus muscle (now adjacent to the ven-

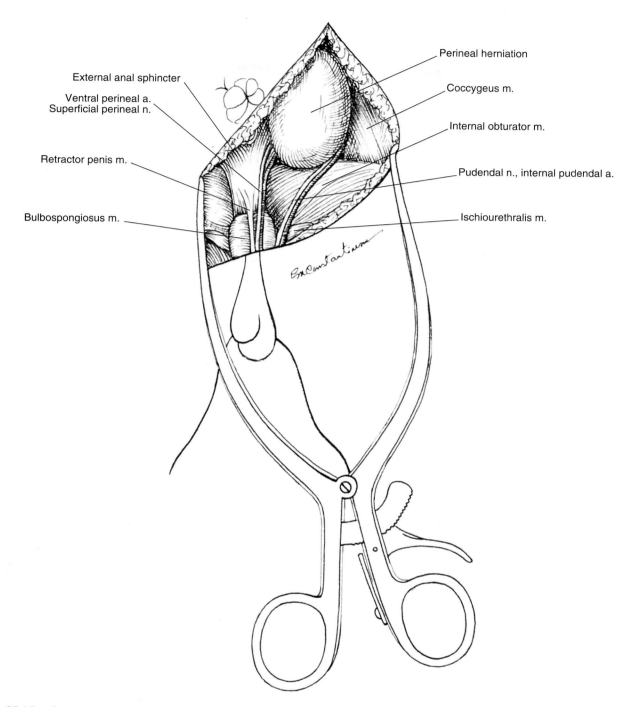

External anal sphincter

Ventral perineal a.
Superficial perineal n.

Retractor penis m.

Bulbospongiosus m.

Perineal herniation

Coccygeus m.

Internal obturator m.

Pudendal n., internal pudendal a.

Ischiourethralis m.

Fig. 35.10. Exposure of the right perineum for perineal herniorrhaphy using the internal obturator muscle transposition technique.

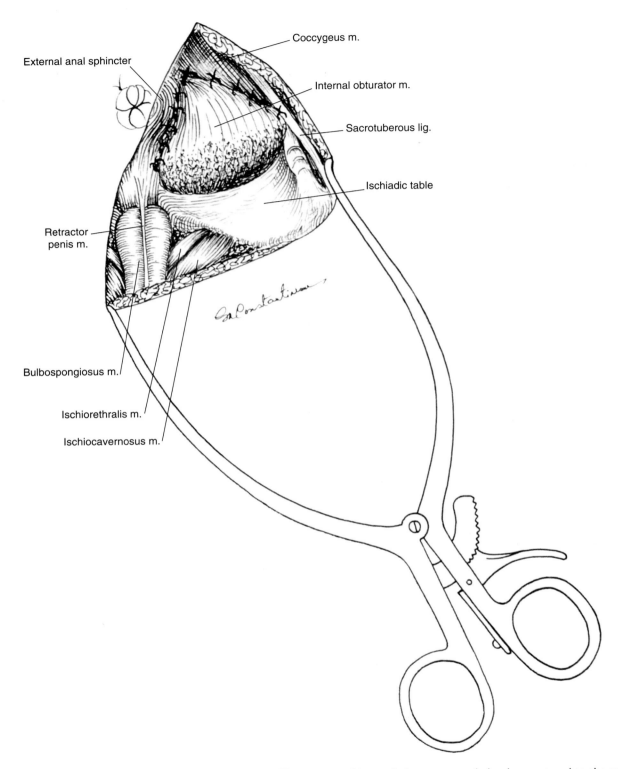

Fig. 35.11. Right internal obturator muscle transposition. The transposed internal obturator muscle has been sutured to the external anal sphincter medially and to the sacrotuberous ligament and coccygeus muscle laterally.

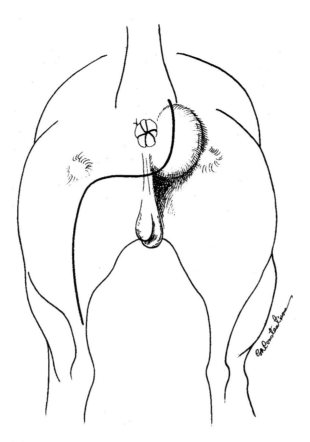

Fig. 35.12. Skin incision for left semitendinosus muscle transposition to repair a failed right perineal herniorrhaphy.

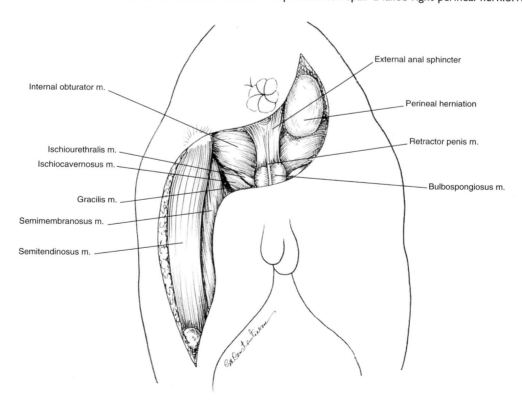

Internal obturator m.

Ischiourethralis m.

Ischiocavernosus m.

Gracilis m.

Semimembranosus m.

Semitendinosus m.

External anal sphincter

Perineal herniation

Retractor penis m.

Bulbospongiosus m.

Fig. 35.13. Left semitendinosus muscle exposed before isolation and mobilization to reconstruct a failed right perineal herniorrhaphy.

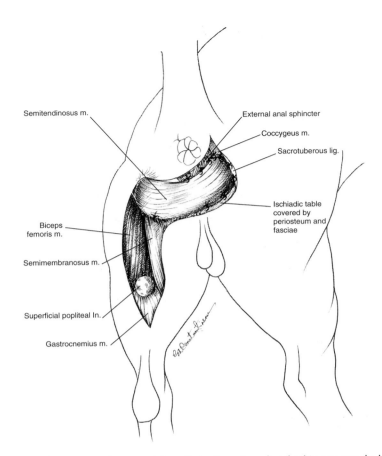

Semitendinosus m.

External anal sphincter

Coccygeus m.

Sacrotuberous lig.

Ischiadic table covered by periosteum and fasciae

Biceps femoris m.

Semimembranosus m.

Superficial popliteal ln.

Gastrocnemius m.

Fig. 35.14.   Transposed left semitendinosus muscle sutured dorsally to the external anal sphincter muscle, laterally to the right sacrotuberous ligament and coccygeus muscle, and ventrally to the internal obturator muscle fascia, the ischiourethralis muscle fascia, and the ischial periosteum.

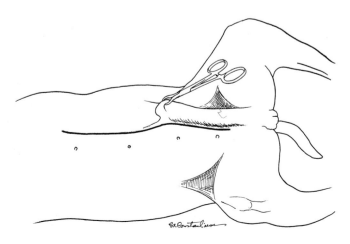

Fig. 35.15.   Skin incision for colopexy or cystopexy treatment of failed perineal herniorrhaphy.

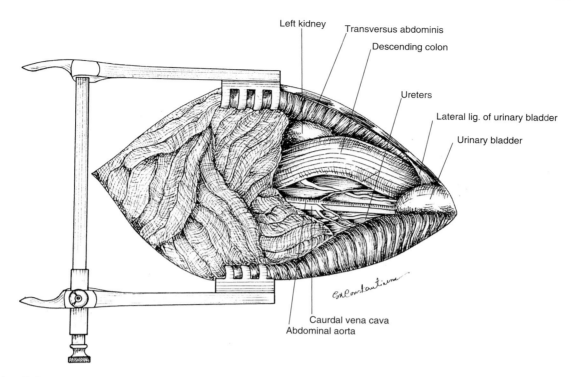

Fig. 35.16. Colopexy. Abdominal organs are packed cranially with moist laparotomy sponges. The colon has been pulled cranially and secured (sutures not shown) to the dorsolateral body wall.

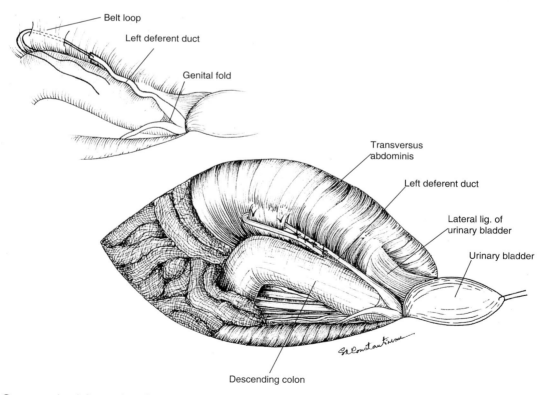

Fig. 35.17. Cystopexy by deferent duct fixation. The left deferent duct is passed through a belt loop created in the left transversus abdominis muscle with the aid of a stay suture (*inset*) and is folded onto itself and sutured to itself and to the belt loop.

tral aspect of the perineum) is sutured to the remnant of the internal obturator muscle, the ischiourethralis muscle, pelvic fascia, and the periosteum of the dorsal surface of the ischium (Fig. 35.14). Synthetic absorbable sutures are used to obliterate dead space and to close the subcutaneous tissues. Closed-suction wound drainage may be used at the surgeon's discretion. The skin is closed with the routine closure of the surgeon's choice.

Colopexy or Cystopexy for Failed Perineal Herniorrhaphy Salvage

Colopexy with cystopexy by deferent duct fixation is designed to prevent herniation of the most problematic organs (colon, prostate, urinary bladder) that may become entrapped in the perineal hernia space. This technique is typically reserved for when perineal reconstruction using muscle transpositions has failed or when the surgeon anticipates failure of muscle transposition.

The dog is positioned in dorsal recumbency for ventral midline celiotomy (Fig. 35.15). If the dog is not castrated, standard prescrotal castration is performed before celiotomy. Once the abdomen is open, the colon and urinary bladder are exposed by packing the other abdominal organs cranially with moist laparotomy sponges. Cranial traction is applied to the colon to reduce herniated rectum and to prevent the rectum from migrating into the perineal space. The colon is secured in this position to the dorsolateral body wall with multiple (six to eight) mattress sutures of polypropylene placed in full-thickness fashion through the colon (Fig. 35.16).

A stay suture is placed in the apex of the urinary bladder to aid in exteriorization and exposure of the deferent ducts. Both deferent ducts are gently pulled into the abdomen from the vaginal canals. A stay suture is placed at the severed end of the left deferent duct to assist manipulation. A 1- to 2-cm belt loop is created dorsolaterally in the left transversus abdominis muscle midway between the left kidney and the urinary bladder. The belt loop is created by making two stab incisions parallel to the transversus abdominis muscle fibers and bluntly dissecting beneath the muscle between the stab incisions with hemostatic forceps. The stay suture in the deferent duct is grasped with hemostatic forceps and is pulled from caudal to cranial through the belt loop to pull the deferent duct through the loop until it is taut. The deferent duct is then folded back (caudally) over the belt loop and is sutured to itself and to the belt loop with simple interrupted polypropylene sutures (Fig. 35.17). The manipulated end of the deferent duct with the stay suture is excised. The right deferent duct is secured to the right body wall

in the same fashion. After removal of the laparotomy sponges and urinary bladder stay suture, the celiotomy is closed routinely.

References

1. Burrows CF, Harvey CE. Perineal hernia in the dog. J Small Anim Pract 1973;14:315–332.
2. Sjollema BE, van Sluijs FJ. Perineal hernia repair in the dog by transposition of the internal obturator muscle. Part II. Complications and results in 100 patients. Vet Q 1989;11:18–23.
3. Chambers JN, Rawlings CA. Applications of a semitendinosus muscle flap in two dogs. J Am Vet Med Assoc 1991;199:84–86.
4. Philibert D, Fowler JD. Use of muscle flaps in reconstructive surgery. Compend Contin Educ Pract Vet 1996;18:395–405.
5. Bilbrey SA, Smeak DD, DeHoff W. Fixation of the deferent ducts for retrodisplacement of the urinary bladder and prostate in canine perineal hernia. Vet Surg 1990;19:24–27.

Perineal Hernia in the Cat

Julie M. Duval, Mark A. Anderson &
Gheorghe M. Constantinescu

The incidence of perineal hernias is lower in the cat than in the dog. The proposed hormonal influence on the occurrence of perineal hernias in dogs is probably not a factor in cats, because perineal hernias occur in both male and female cats, and most of the reported clinical cases have occurred in spayed or castrated animals (1–5). A breed predisposition has not been identified, and the median age at onset of clinical signs is 9 years. Unlike in dogs, most perineal hernias in cats are bilateral (1, 5).

Pathogenesis

In contrast to the proposed pathogenesis in the dog, hormonal influences are thought to be unimportant to the development of perineal hernia in the cat, because all but one reported case have been in spayed or castrated cats. Approximately half the cats with reported perineal hernia had no other disease processes associated with the perineum and were assumed to have idiopathic perineal hernias. The other cats had processes identified that were assumed to be associated with the incidence of the hernia. Many of these cats had previously had a perineal urethrostomy for feline lower urinary tract disease at a median of 3 years before diagnosis of the perineal hernia. Another predisposing factor identified was the presence of megacolon. Other causes of tenesmus, such as perineal masses or colitis, have also been implicated as predisposing factors for the development of perineal hernia (1). Most perineal hernias in cats are bilateral, with a tendency for the left side to be more severely affected than the right (1). Herniation of peritoneal contents is rare, although one cat was reported with retroflexion on the bladder into the hernia (1).

Diagnosis

Perineal hernia is usually diagnosed based on history, clinical signs, and rectal examination. Tenesmus and constipation are the most common historical findings in cats with perineal hernias (1, 6–8). Up to 50% of cats may have vomiting and anorexia associated with these episodes of constipation (1). On physical examination, large amounts of fecal material are usually present in the rectum and distal colon. Rectal examination frequently reveals rectal dilatation and sacculation with retention of feces and weakened pelvic musculature. Whereas visible bulging in the perineal area is a common finding in the dog (5), it is only occasionally seen in the cat with perineal hernia. Prolapse of the rectum is also occasionally seen because of persistent straining.

An effort should be made to identify predisposing factors such as megacolon, perineal masses, or colitis, because successful treatment may depend on management of these associated disorders. Abdominal radiography or colonoscopy may be useful in the diagnostic workup of patients with these diseases.

Nonsurgical Treatment

Medical treatment of perineal hernia in the cat consists primarily of relief of constipation by administration of laxatives, stool softeners, and enemas or manual removal of impacted stool. If a predisposing factor such as megacolon or colitis can be identified, response of that disorder to medical treatment may allow response of the hernia. In one study, 16% of cats treated medically had a complete response, and another 53% partially responded to medical treatment. The other 31% were unresponsive. Medical treatment seemed to have similar responses regardless of the cause of the hernia and seemed to be more effective when clinical signs were mild (1). Surgical treatment seems more consistently effective in the resolution of clinical signs and therefore is the treatment of choice.

Surgical Anatomy

The anatomic structures involved in the surgical repair of perineal hernia in the cat are similar to those in the dog, with some exceptions, and they have been described (Fig. 35.18) (6, 7). In general, the muscles of the perineum of the cat are smaller than in the dog (2). The sacrotuberous ligament is sometimes incorpo-

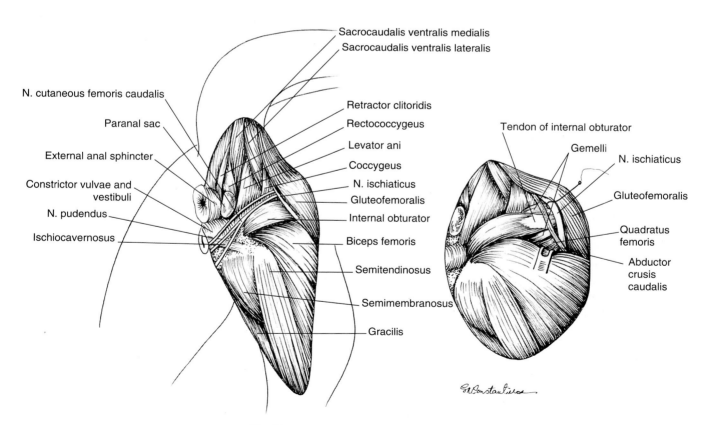

Fig. 35.18. Perineal anatomy of the cat.

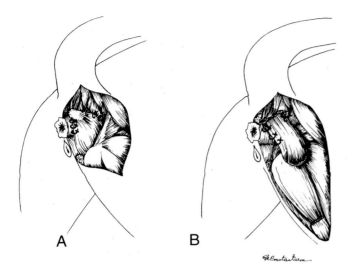

Fig. 35.19. Repair of perineal hernia by the use of an internal obturator muscle flap in the cat.

rated into surgical repairs in the dog, but it is absent in the cat (6–8).

Surgical Technique

If megacolon is diagnosed as the primary problem with a secondary perineal hernia, surgical treatment should be directed at resolution of the megacolon (1, 8). Subtotal colectomy (see Chap. 16) is the recommended treatment, and surgical correction of the perineal hernia is usually unnecessary. Surgical correction of the hernia without resolution of the megacolon, however, is unlikely to resolve the clinical signs. In addition, subtotal colectomy has not been successful in the treatment of idiopathic perineal hernia in the absence of megacolon (1). If a perineal mass seems to be the primary condition, an excisional biopsy should be the initial mode of surgical therapy. Colopexy has also been described as surgical treatment for those cats with rectal prolapse concurrent with perineal hernia (1).

Surgery is indicated for correction of idiopathic perineal hernias in cats as well as for correction of perineal hernias caused by conditions other than megacolon. Surgical techniques in cats are similar to those in dogs (see earlier sections of this chapter), except cats do not have a sacrotuberous ligament. Successful repairs have been described in the cat both with the conventional suture technique and with the use of an internal obturator muscle flap (Fig. 35.19) (1–4, 6).

Surgical Outcome and Complications

In one series of cases, the surgical success rate was 73% (11 of 15) for cats undergoing primary surgical repair of the hernia. An additional 20% (3 of 15) of cats had partial resolution of clinical signs for some time with recurrence later, and 7% (1 cat) was a surgical failure from the outset. No association was apparent in this study between surgical failure and type of surgical technique or suture material used or the experience of the surgeon. However, all three of the patients with recurrent hernias had visible perineal bulging preoperatively. Successful outcomes were also obtained when subtotal colectomy was performed on cats with megacolon and when excisional biopsies of perineal masses were performed (1).

Complications of surgical repair of perineal hernia in the cat seem to be less common than in the dog, but surgical wound infection and cellulitis have been described (1, 3). Appropriate aseptic technique, including draping out the area of the anus and using a pursestring suture, should be used to help avoid surgical contamination. Use of a broad-spectrum perioperative antibiotic effective against gram-negatives and anaerobes may also be considered.

References

1. Welches CD, Scavelli TD, Aronsohn MG, et al. Perineal hernia in the cat: a retrospective study of 40 cases. J Am Anim Hosp Assoc 1992;28:431–438.
2. Johnson MS, Gourley IM. Perineal hernia in a cat. Vet Med 1980;75:241–243.
3. Ashton DG. Perineal hernia in the cat: a description of two cases. J Small Anim Pract 1976;17:473–477.
4. Leighton RL. Perineal hernia in a cat. Feline Pract 1979;9:44.
5. Dean PW, Bojrab MJ. Perineal hernia repair in the dog. In: Bojrab MJ, ed. Current techniques in small animal surgery. 3rd ed. Philadelphia: Lea & Febiger, 1990:442–448.
6. Martin WD, Fletcher TF, Bradley WE. Perineal musculature in the cat. Anat Rec 1974;180:3–14.
7. Constantinescu GM, Amann JF, Anderson MA, et al. Topography and surgery in the regio perinealis of the cat. Wien Tierarztl Monatsschr 1993;80:208–211.
8. Bright RM, Bauer MS. Surgery of the digestive system. In: Sherding RG, ed. The cat: diseases and clinical management. New York: Churchill Livingstone, 1994:1384–1385.

Perineal Hernia Repair Using the Obturator Muscle Flap

Ronald J. Kolata

The traditional method of repairing a perineal hernia involves reconstructing the pelvic diaphragm by suturing the external anal sphincter to the internal obturator muscle ventrally and to the sacrotuberous ligament laterally and dorsally (1, 2). This repair has a reported recurrence rate of between 22 and 48% (1, 3). Many factors can contribute to recurrence of the hernia; one of these is the great amount of tension that must sometimes be applied to the sutures used to appose the

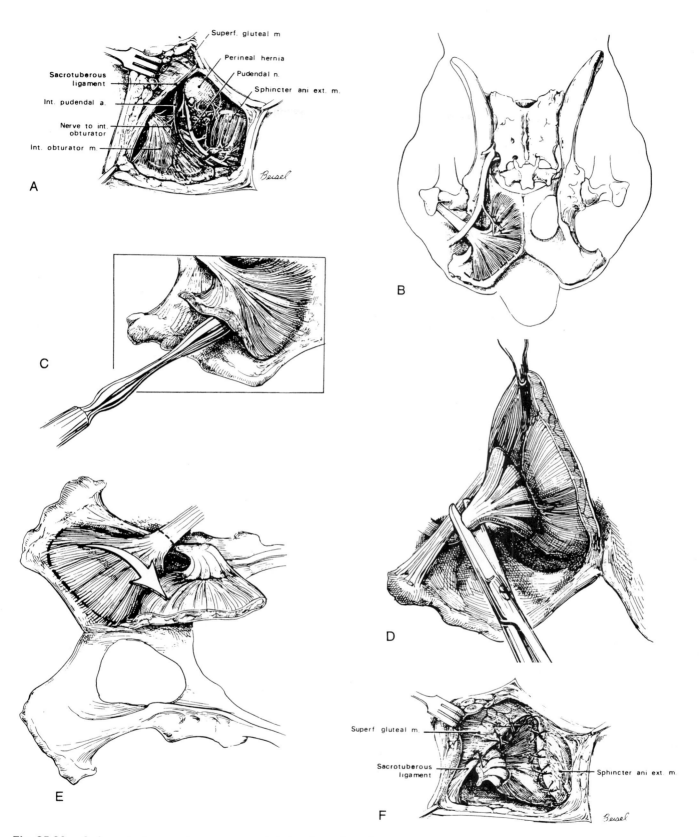

Fig. 35.20. **A.** Important anatomic structures and their relationships. **B.** The site of incision (*dashed line*) of the origin of the internal obturator muscle and the relation of the tendon to the ischiatic nerve. **C.** Elevation of the internal obturator muscle from the ischiatic table. **D.** Severance of the tendon of the internal obturator muscle. **E.** Orientation of the elevated internal obturator muscle for reconstruction of the pelvic diaphragm. **F.** The internal obturator muscle sutured in place and the pelvic diaphragm reconstructed. (Copyright by the University of Georgia. Reprinted by permission.)

573

components of the pelvic diaphragm. Our method for repairing perineal hernias reduces tension on the sutures approximating the reconstructed pelvic diaphragm and thereby decreases the likelihood of their cutting through tissues. This method brings into the area muscular tissue bulk and an additional blood supply that might also foster secure healing.

Surgical Techniques

The approach to the hernia is the same as in the traditional technique. Once exposed, the herniated structures are reduced into the abdomen, and redundant fat is excised. Care is taken to identify and to preserve the pudendal artery, vein, and nerve (Fig. 35.20).

Once the external anal sphincter, sacrotuberous ligament, and internal obturator muscle are identified, the caudal border of the origin of the internal obturator muscle is incised, and a periosteal elevator is used to elevate it from the ischiatic table (Fig. 35.20**B** and **C**). Elevation should not proceed beyond the caudal edge of the obturator foramen, to avoid injuring the obturator nerve and the artery supplying the internal obturator muscle. The tendon of the internal obturator muscle is severed at the point at which it condenses and begins to pass laterally over the body of the ischium (Fig. 35.20**D**). Care is taken to sever the tendon medial to the ischium where the ischiatic (sciatic) nerve crosses the tendon just lateral to the ischium (see Fig. 35.20**B**). Once the caudal portion of the internal obturator muscle is elevated and its tendon is severed, it is brought dorsally to fill the hernial defect (Fig. 35.20**E**). The attachment of the superficial gluteal to the sacrotuberous ligament is elevated, and the lateral margin of the internal obturator is sutured to the fascia of the superficial gluteal muscle. The lateral aspect of the external anal sphincter is freed of as much connective tissue as possible, to create a surface that will adhere to the internal obturator muscle. An initial suture is placed between the external anal sphincter and the sacrotuberous ligament and gluteal fascia as far dorsally as possible to create a point to which the apex of the internal obturator muscle is sutured. The caudolateral border of the internal obturator muscle is sutured to the caudomedial edge of the sacrotuberous ligament using four to six cruciate sutures of 1–0 nylon (Fig. 35.20**F**). *Care must be taken when placing these sutures to anchor them firmly in the sacrotuberous ligament, so the caudal gluteal artery and ischiatic nerve, which course just cranial to this ligament, are not injured.* As an alternative to using the ligament, the superficial gluteal muscle fascia can be dissected off the sacrotuberous ligament and sutured to the internal obturator muscle. A modification I prefer involves elevating the superficial gluteal fascia, sliding it medially (dorsal to the sacrotuberous ligament), and suturing the lateral margin of the internal obturator muscle to the gluteal fascia. This modification provides less tension on the suture margins and offers a more complete closure of the dorsal hernia.

The caudomedial border of the internal obturator muscle is similarly sutured to the external anal sphincter. Preplacement of all the sutures before knotting makes it easier to insert them accurately. Each suture should include a generous bite of the internal obturator muscle and should be drawn only as tightly as necessary to achieve apposition to the sacrotuberous ligament and the external anal sphincter. Closure is continued by apposing the subcutaneous tissues in one or two layers with chromic gut to obliterate dead space. If deemed necessary, a Penrose drain is placed in the depths of the wound and is made to exit ventral and lateral to the skin incision. The skin is closed routinely.

Postoperative Care

Postoperative care and potential complications are the same as for the traditional method of repair. We and our colleagues have used this method for perineal hernia repair in approximately 25 dogs during the last 2 years with no hernia recurrences or complications. Further evaluation is necessary before the merits of this method can be accurately assessed.

References

1. Burrows CF, Harvey CE. Perineal hernia in the dog. J Small Anim Pract 1973;14:315.
2. Petit GD. Perineal hernia in the dog. Cornell Vet 1962;52:261.
3. Hayes HM, Wilson GP, Tarone RE. The epidemiological features of the perineal hernia in 771 dogs. J Am Anim Hosp Assoc 1978;14:703.

Prepubic Hernia Repair

Daniel D. Smeak

Prepubic hernia or cranial pubic ligament (CPL) rupture is the most common abdominal hernia caused by blunt trauma in small animals. The flank region was once thought to be the most common site for traumatic hernias because of the lack of elasticity and support from the rectus abdominis muscle in this area. Perhaps these hernias should be considered one and the same because patients with prepubic hernias often have coexisting inguinal ligament rupture and extend into the femoral vascular lacuna area, causing ventral abdominal and flank swelling.

The CPL attaches to the cranial aspect of the pubis and extends from one iliopectineal eminence and pectineus muscle to the other. It serves as the attachment of the rectus abdominis muscle to the pelvis. Blunt trauma during which abdominal muscles are tight but little intra-abdominal pressure develops (glottis is open) causes traction or avulsion of the cranial pubic tendon from its attachment or, less commonly, a tear at the musculotendinous junction. In contrast, CPL rupture is spontaneous in large animals and most often occurs during the last 2 months of gestation, apparently because of increasing uterine weight.

Blunt trauma severe enough to cause rupture of the abdominal wall often also results in widespread crush, rupture, or avulsion damage to surrounding structures and intra-abdominal organs. As many as 75% of small animals with traumatic abdominal hernias have other significant injuries, mostly orthopedic (usually involving the pelvis). The second most common injuries are to soft tissues, including respiratory, gastrointestinal, and genitourinary systems. Therefore, a thorough physical examination and diagnostic workup are indicated for any patient with a traumatic hernia, to evaluate for more insidious, often life-threatening, injuries.

The diagnosis of prepubic hernia is often confirmed by palpating a defect in the caudal abdominal wall, by reduction of tissue back into the caudal abdomen, or by palpation of organs in the subcutaneous space near the pubic or thigh areas. Organs such as the intestine may not be confined to the local area and may migrate a considerable distance from the hernia, such as down the medial thigh or along the abdominal wall and thorax. Pain and swelling from trauma or hemorrhage may not allow detection of a hernial ring or herniated tissue. In these instances, radiographs or ultrasound examinations of the local area are indicated. Routine ventrodorsal and lateral plain radiographs aid in identifying the abdominal stripe, or lack thereof, the position of the abdominal contents, and the presence of fluid in the abdomen. When radiographs or ultrasound studies are not conclusive, a contrast peritoneogram may help to delineate the abdominal wall defect. Patients should be thoroughly evaluated for concurrent injuries such as urinary tract rupture, abdominal hemorrhage, fractures, and thoracic trauma. Survey thoracic and abdominal films (including the pelvic area) and blood workup are usually indicated for all severely traumatized patients. If electrocardiography is available, a rhythm strip should be evaluated; otherwise, detection of an irregular cardiac rhythm or dropped beats while checking the patient's pulse may indicate traumatic myocarditis.

Stabilization of the patient's condition takes precedence over hernia repair. Because these hernias are usually large, the risk of incarceration or strangulation is rare. Therefore, if the patient is stable, the hernia can be repaired several days later, after swelling and hemorrhage begin to subside and tissues reestablish their blood supply. If the patient does not stabilize with resuscitative measures, serious intra-abdominal injury should be suspected; further diagnostic tests or emergency exploratory laparotomy may be indicated.

Surgical Technique

Surgical correction is usually performed using a ventral midline approach. When an exploratory laparotomy is indicated, the entire abdomen should be prepared aseptically, and if the hernial sac extends to adjacent areas, these areas should be liberally prepared also. The way in which the patient is positioned on the operating table may be critical for successful closure of a prepubic hernia. Closure may be virtually impossible if the patient is placed in a routine dorsal recumbent position, with the limbs pulled caudally and abducted and the trunk in slight dorsal flexion (Fig. 35.21**A**). The rear limbs should be pulled cranially and the body

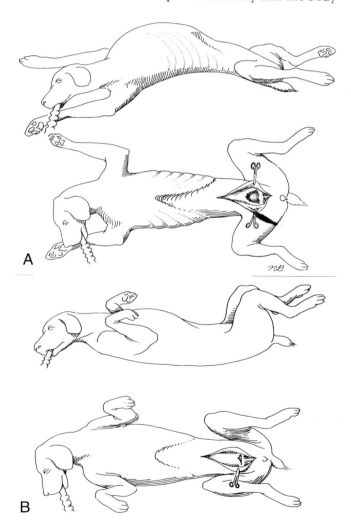

Fig. 35.21. **A.** Example of altering position to relieve tension on a hernia repair. Dorsal recumbency position for prepubic hernia repair; rear limbs are pulled caudally and are extended, causing undue tension. **B.** Modified dorsal recumbency position; rear limbs are flexed slightly and are pulled cranially. This creates truncal ventroflexion, reduces the defect size, and decreases tension during hernia repair.

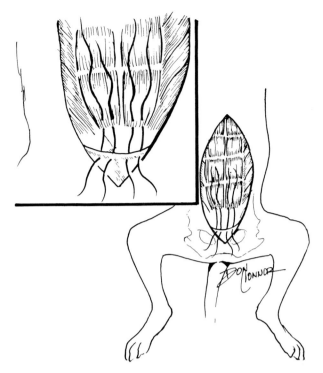

Fig. 35.22. A prepubic tendon is repaired by preplacing large gauge nonabsorbable sutures through holes in the cranial brim of the pubis and the avulsed tendon.

ventroflexed to relieve tension during hernia repair (Fig. 35.21**B**).

Besides hernia recurrence, wound infection and skin slough are the most common complications after repair. Therefore, traumatized skin and soft tissues are handled with utmost care because the vascular supply may be tenuous, and further insult could result in tissue loss. After abdominal exploration after attempts at necessary repair to vital organs, the abdominal cavity may be lavaged, and the linea alba is closed routinely.

The prepubic hernia is better defined by careful dissection and debridement of devitalized tissue. The surgeon carefully inspects the lateral margins to determine whether the hernia extends into the inguinal and femoral areas. Important vascular and neural structures are isolated and protected, particularly if the femoral area requires reconstruction. If femoral or inguinal areas are involved, the regional anatomy is studied carefully before undertaking herniorrhaphy. The prepubic hernia component is repaired first, to help align tissues correctly for anatomic reconstruction of the inguinal and femoral hernias, if present. The cranial pubic ligament is reattached with large 2–0 to 0 size monofilament (prolonged absorbable) suture or nonabsorbable suture. If enough healthy tendon is present, the surgeon anatomically repairs the hernia with preplaced interrupted sutures incorporating large bites of tissue. Alternately, holes may be drilled in the

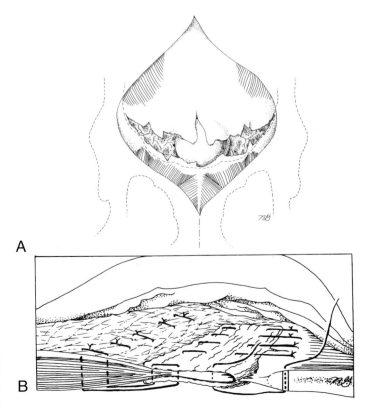

A

B

Fig. 35.23. Cuff mesh reinforcement of a prepubic hernia. **A.** Ventral view showing severe damage and loss of a portion of the prepubic tendon. **B.** Interrupted vertical mattress suture fixation of the mesh to the abdominal wall and interrupted sutures are placed between the reinforced prepubic tendon and pubic bone.

cranial brim of the pubis to anchor sutures (Fig. 35.22). When the hernia cannot be repaired without excess tension, a cuff mesh reinforcement of the prepubic tendon can be performed using Marlex mesh (Fig. 35.23). Concurrent femoral or inguinal hernias are repaired by isolating the hernia edges and anatomic reconstruction. Often, the inguinal ligament is ruptured, and sutures are placed between the abdominal oblique fascia and the musculature of the proximal medial thigh. Extreme care is required to avoid damaging or incorporating important vascular and neural structures.

Usually, a large amount of dead space is present in the subcutaneous tissues after herniorrhaphy. Gravity-dependent drains such as Penrose drains or closed-suction drain systems should be used in most cases. Avoid placing open-drain systems directly against buried mesh to reduce the risk of ascending infection.

Postoperative Care

Monitoring and postoperative care instructions are dictated by the nature and severity of the injury. The surgeon continues to monitor the patient's vital signs and remains aware of possible problems related to occult visceral damage. Patients should be given analgesic agents for at least 24 hours after the surgical procedure. Wounds and drains should be monitored for signs of infection or hernia recurrence. Drains should be bandaged, if possible, and removed when discharge has diminished. If infection occurs, wounds are opened, cultured, debrided, and secondarily closed. Strict exercise limitation is recommended for at least 4 to 6 weeks, particularly if a prosthetic mesh has been implanted. An Elizabethan collar is used to guard against premature drain removal or wound mutilation.

Prognosis

Based on a report of a series of patients undergoing prepubic herniorrhaphy, approximately 80% survive and have successful hernia repair. If a hernia recurs (about 15% do), the defect is usually evident by 1 month postoperatively. Repair of these recurrent hernias is usually successful, provided the repair is anatomic, is free of tension, and incorporates strong tissue. The remaining 20% have poor results because of the severity of accompanying injuries.

Suggested Readings

Mann FA, Tangner CH, Boothe HW, et al. Cranial pubic ligament rupture in dogs and cats. J Am Anim Hosp Assoc 1986;22: 519–523.

Smeak DD. Management and prevention of surgical complications associated with small animal abdominal herniorrhaphy. Probl Vet Med 1989;1:254–267.

Waldron DR. Abdominal hernias in dogs and cats: a review of 24 cases. J Am Anim Hosp Assoc 1986;22:817–823.

36

MAMMARY GLANDS

Mastectomy

H. Jay Harvey

Mastectomy, the removal of varying amounts of mammary tissue, is the primary method for treating breast tumors in dogs and cats. However, the amount of tissue to remove is a subject of some controversy. Cure rates for patients with malignant breast disease are still low even after massive amounts of tissue have been removed. The behavior of the tumor, not the extent of treatment, determines the eventual fate of the patient. Nonetheless, properly performed surgical treatment of mammary tumors can modify disease progression, prolong comfortable survival, and be curative in some instances.

Surgical Anatomy

Mammary glands in the dog and cat are modified sudoriferous skin glands with an apocrine compound lobuloalveolar structure. Mammary glands are arranged in two parallel paramedian rows from the axillary to the inguinal regions. The glands are surrounded by subcutaneous adipose tissue, which is scant in the thoracic region and abundant in the inguinal region.

Individual glands are discerned by the corresponding teat, although mammary tissue can be confluent between adjacent cranial and caudal glands. The midline separation between the mammary chains is distinct. Glands are signified by name (cranial and caudal thoracic, cranial and caudal abdominal, and inguinal) or by number (1 through 5 cranial to caudal). Dogs usually have five pairs of mammary glands, and cats have four, although the number can range from four to six in either species.

Thoracic glands adhere directly to the underlying pectoral muscles with little intervening fat or areolar connective tissue. Abdominal glands are loosely attached to fascia by filmy connective tissue and fat. Inguinal glands are suspended from the body wall by an extension of the cutaneus trunci muscle.

Blood is supplied to the thoracic glands by perforating branches of the internal thoracic artery, by cutaneous branches of intercostal arteries, and by the lateral thoracic artery. Cranial abdominal glands receive blood predominantly from the cranial superficial epigastric artery. Caudal abdominal and inguinal glands are supplied by the caudal superficial epigastric artery and by perivulvar branches of the external pudendal artery. Veins parallel arteries, except for numerous veins that traverse the midline during lactation.

Lymphatic drainage of the mammary glands is subject to individual variation and also is influenced by the stage of lactation and by the presence of space-occupying masses. Lymph generally flows from the cranial three pairs of mammary glands toward the axillary lymph nodes and from the caudal two pairs toward the inguinal lymph nodes. A lymphatic connection between the cranial and caudal abdominal glands is present in some bitches.

Mammary Gland Neoplasia: Incidence and Prognosis

Neoplasia is the major indication for mastectomy in dogs and cats. Mammary tumors are the most common type of neoplasia in dogs and the third most common type in cats. Mammary neoplasia affects middle-aged and older animals, with a median age of onset of 10 to 11 years.

Only about half of all canine mammary tumors are malignant, whereas nearly all (86%) feline mammary tumors are malignant. Prognosis for both dogs and cats with malignant tumors is guarded to poor. Although length of survival is inversely correlated with the growth rate of the tumor, the extent of regional infiltration, and the status of regional lymph nodes, the major statistically significant survival factor is tumor volume. Both dogs and cats with large mammary malignant tumors have significantly shorter survival times than those with small malignant tumors.

Treatment failure is represented by intractable local recurrence or, more commonly, by metastatic disease. Because metastatic mammary cancer is found most frequently in the lungs, thoracic radiography is a common screening test before mastectomy. Dogs with mammary cancer affecting the caudal mammary glands, especially when the inguinal lymph nodes are palpably enlarged, should also be radiographically or ultrasonographically checked for enlarged sublumbar lymph nodes, because metastasis through sublumbar lymphatics is often detectable before the radiographic appearance of lung metastases.

Mammary neoplasia can be prevented by ovariohysterectomy performed when the bitch is young (i.e., before the first estrus). However, although estrogen and other hormone receptors have been found in canine and feline breast tumors, no evidence suggests that ovariohysterectomy has any beneficial effect as a treatment for existing mammary neoplasia.

Selection of Surgical Procedure

The amount of mammary tissue to remove from a dog or cat with mammary neoplasia is influenced by several factors: the size, consistency, and location of the tumor; the size, age, and physiologic status of the patient; and the beliefs and prejudices of the surgeon. Unfortunately, subjective criteria still play a major role in the selection of a mastectomy procedure because the scientific bases for choice are inconclusive.

The extent of tissue removal with various mastectomy procedures is illustrated in Figure 36.1. For the purposes of this chapter, these procedures are defined as follows:

Lumpectomy (nodulectomy): Removal of the tumor only without any surrounding breast tissue. Generally, lumpectomy is used when a tumor is small, encapsulated, and noninvasive, thus requiring a minimum of surgical dissection for removal.
Partial mammectomy: Removal of the tumor and a surrounding margin of breast tissue. This procedure usually is indicated for tumors that are small to moderate in size (up to 2 cm in diameter) and occupy only a portion of an individual gland. The tumor may be suspected to be invasive and may or may not have readily palpable distinct margins.

Simple mastectomy: Removal of the entire mammary gland containing the tumor.
Regional mastectomy (modified radical mastectomy): Removal of groups of mammary glands depending on which glands contain tumor. The rationale for regional mastectomy depends on the presumed anatomy of mammary gland lymphatic drainage and the assumption that mammary cancer spreads from one gland to another along lymphatic pathways, which are not altered by space-occupying masses.
Complete unilateral mastectomy (radical mastectomy): Removal of all ipsilateral mammary glands, intervening tissues, and regional lymphatics.
Simultaneous complete bilateral mastectomy (bilateral radical mastectomy): Removal of both entire mammary chains, intervening tissues, and regional lymphatics.

Available data indicate that the extent of surgery has little influence on either the survival time or the rate of recurrence of breast cancer in dogs. In other words, no evidence indicates that complete unilateral mastectomy (radical mastectomy) is any more beneficial for treating a 2-cm tumor in the fourth mammary gland of a dog than is a simple mastectomy. Until more definitive information is available, selection of a procedure in dogs should be dictated by what is most efficient. Good oncologic surgical principles still apply, however: whatever procedure is used, invasive tumor should be widely resected with deep and centrifugal en bloc margins of normal tissue.

In cats, complete unilateral mastectomy is the traditional procedure of choice for all mammary tumors. This approach has been recommended by veterinary oncologists because most feline breast tumors are highly malignant. The 10 to 15% of cats with benign mammary nodules are overtreated by this philosophy.

Surgery is contraindicated for inflammatory carcinoma of the breast. Inflammatory carcinoma of the breast is a fulminant, aggressive malignant disease usually affecting the inguinal glands. Tissues are diffusely thickened, inflamed, painful, and frequently ulcerated. A space-occupying mammary mass may or may not be obvious. Commonly, the tissues are so diffusely thickened that discrete tumors are not apparent. The condition closely resembles severe mastitis and is frequently misdiagnosed as such. Surgery is unrewarding because it is virtually impossible to remove the affected tissues completely, and, more important, because most affected dogs also suffer from disseminated intravascular coagulation. Attempts at extensive surgical therapy often result in severe, intractable bleeding from the incision, deterioration of the patient over 12 to 24 hours, and death. Inflammatory breast carcinoma is invariably fatal, usually within a short time after clinical signs are obvious. Treatment is

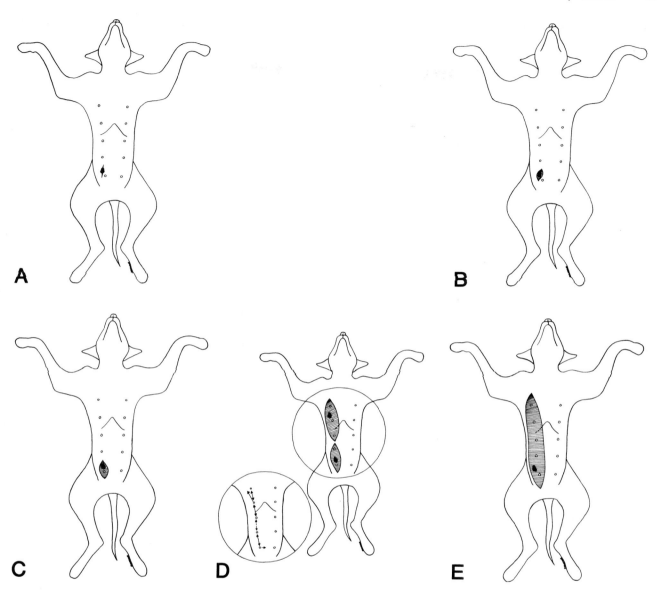

Fig. 36.1. Comparison of extent of tissue removal with different mastectomy procedures. **A.** Lumpectomy. Skin incision is made directly over the tumor. **B.** Partial mastectomy. An elliptic skin incision is made, encompassing the tumor and a portion of the surrounding mammary tissue. **C.** An elliptic skin incision is made to encompass the gland that contains the tumor completely. **D.** Regional mastectomy. An elliptic skin incision is made to encompass the glands to be removed, as determined by the location of tumor and the presumed pathways of lymphatic drainage (*inset*). Generally, the first three glands are removed en bloc when tumor exists in any one of them; likewise, the last two glands are removed en bloc when tumor exists in either of them. Some authors recommend that the third gland be removed whenever the fourth and fifth are excised because of the "inconstant" lymphatic drainage between the third and fourth glands. **E.** Complete unilateral mastectomy. The skin incision encompasses all ipsilateral mammary glands. See the text for details of the dissection.

strictly palliative and consists of anti-inflammatory drugs and antibiotics.

Surgical Techniques

Mastectomy procedures are performed similarly in cats and dogs, although the laxity of feline skin generally makes surgery easier in cats.

Lumpectomy

A lumpectomy is initiated by making a skin incision directly over the tumor. The breast tissue overlying the tumor is bluntly separated. The periphery of the tumor is grasped with forceps, and the natural tissue planes adjacent to the isolated tumor are defined by dissection with mosquito hemostats or by wiping the tissues away from the tumor with a sponge (sponge dissection). The tumor is removed, partially sectioned, and placed in 10% buffered formalin. After hemorrhage is controlled, the wound is closed by approximating breast tissue with fine (4–0) chromic catgut. Skin is closed with suture of the surgeon's choice.

Partial Mammectomy

A liberal incision is made over the tumor. If the tumor contacts or is adherent to the skin or subcutaneous tissue (i.e., if the tumor is "fixed" to skin), an elliptic incision is made that encompasses both the tumor and the affected skin. An artificial plane of dissection is developed in normal mammary tissue surrounding the tumor. A liberal amount of tissue, often approaching one-third to one-half of the breast, is removed. Closure of the defect in the breast tissue is done by direct apposition if possible. Subcutaneous apposition with 4–0 or 3–0 catgut is done to reduce tension on the skin closure. The skin is closed routinely.

Simple Mastectomy, Regional Mastectomy, and Complete Unilateral Mastectomy

The basic technique for simple mastectomy, regional mastectomy, and complete unilateral mastectomy is the same. All these procedures involve removal of the skin segment that encompasses the affected mammary gland or glands. Surgery is initiated by making an elliptic incision around the mammary gland or glands to be removed. The incision is extended sharply through the subcutaneous tissue to the body wall. In the thoracic region, the body wall is represented by the pectoral muscle and in the abdominal region by the cranial

rectus fascia. A plane of dissection that allows the skin segment and associated mammary tissues to be cleanly stripped from the body wall is then established. The proper plane of dissection is deep to the adipose tissue and directly on the muscle or fascia.

In the abdominal and inguinal regions, the glands are loosely adherent and can be stripped from the underlying fascia with a sponge (Fig. 36.2**A**). In the thoracic region, the glands adhere to the underlying muscle, and the plane of dissection must be developed by a combination of sharp and blunt dissection with scissors (Fig. 36.2**B**). The proper thoracic plane is represented by lacy but tough strands of fibrous connective tissue. Traction on the rostral portion of the skin segment facilitates dissection. Dissection proceeds from cranial to caudal without, in most cases, the need to damage underlying muscle. When removal of tissues is completed, intact muscle should be clearly visible in the thoracic region and rectus fascia should be seen in the abdominal region.

Invasion of underlying tissue by tumor, whether pectoral muscle in the thoracic region or rectus fascia in the abdominal region, requires en bloc resection of the affected body wall tissue along with the tumor. In extreme cases, full-thickness resection of the body wall must be done to remove all visible tumor, even though body wall invasion by tumor is a grave prognostic sign and even massive surgical resection is seldom curative.

Inguinal gland removal entails en bloc removal of the inguinal fat. Care must be taken to isolate and ligate the caudal superficial epigastric artery and vein, which emerge from the inguinal canal (Fig. 36.3). The vaginal process, the finger-shaped protrusion of fat extending through the inguinal canal, along with the artery, vein, and vaginal ligament, may be bluntly sep-

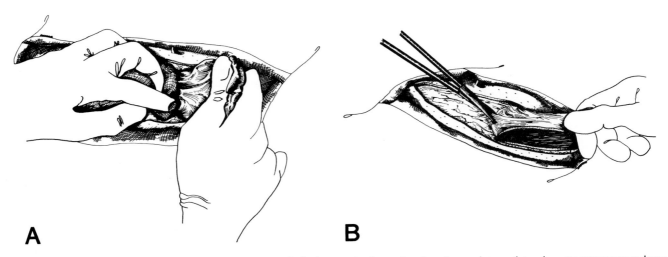

A   **B**

Fig. 36.2. Developing a proper plane of dissection greatly facilitates simple, regional, and complete unilateral mastectomy procedures. **A.** In the abdominal and inguinal regions, the loosely adherent mammary glands can be stripped from the underlying fascia with a sponge. **B.** In the thoracic region, the glands adhere to the underlying muscle, so dissection with scissors is required.

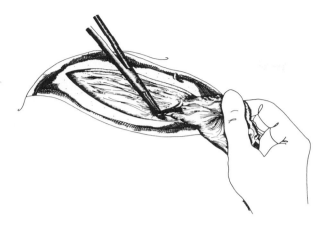

Fig. 36.3. The superficial epigastric artery and vein emerge from the inguinal canal deep to the fifth mammary gland. When this gland is excised, these vessels must be isolated, clamped, divided, and ligated.

arated from the inguinal fat and left behind or ligated and removed. Inguinal lymph nodes are removed along with the skin segment, mammae, and inguinal fat when the dissection is done correctly. Arteries and veins from the pudendal vessels enter the inguinal glands caudally from the tissues around the vulva and may require ligation or cauterization.

Closure of the tissue defect left after a simple, regional, or complete unilateral mastectomy must account for the considerable dead space created. In most instances, drains, stents, bandages, or exotic suturing techniques are not necessary. Even large defects can be closed by apposing skin edges with subcutaneous suture of chromic catgut. An interrupted pattern is

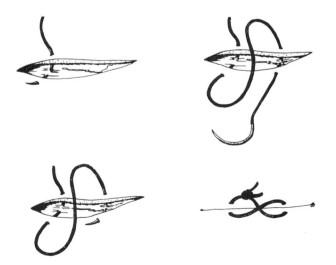

Fig. 36.4. An interrupted cruciate suture pattern is recommended for closure of skin incisions with simple, regional, or complete unilateral mastectomies.

preferred. The subcutaneous tissue may be tacked to the underlying body wall to reduce dead space. Skin is then closed according to the surgeon's preference. An interrupted cruciate suture pattern of 2–0 or 3–0 monofilament nylon can be placed quickly and distributes tension well (Fig. 36.4). This pattern has the advantage of being an interrupted pattern, but one that spans a longer segment of incision per suture than a simple interrupted pattern. Regardless of the suture pattern used for skin closure, the ultimate success of skin apposition depends on placement of a proper subcutaneous suture line.

Postoperative Care and Complications

Postoperative complications associated with mastectomy include seroma formation, wound dehiscence, and edema of one or both rear limbs. Seroma formation is most common in the groin region and may be treated by the use of warm, moist compresses. Drainage by aspiration helps temporarily but increases the risk of infection. Wound dehiscences, if not extensive, are best left to heal by second intention. Extensive dehiscences require debridement and closure.

Rear limb edema may occur because of the surgical procedure or because of the tumor. Removal of inguinal mammary tumors temporarily interrupts lymphatic drainage by also removing lymphatic vessels and nodes. Moderate exercise, warm compresses, diuretics, and time usually result in resolution. More ominous is the edema that results from tumor emboli in lymphatic vessels between the mammary glands and the sublumbar nodes and from tumor metastasis to sublumbar nodes. The latter situations are grave prognostic indications, and whereas edema may subside as potential lymphatic pathways become established, the chances for complete return to normal tissue fluid homeostasis are slim. Blockage of lymphatic vessels or nodes by tumor infiltration sometimes results in "retrograde metastasis." For example, inguinal tumor may extend distally in a string of nodules on the medial aspect of the hind leg.

Ovariohysterectomy, although not of proven benefit as a mammary cancer treatment, may be desired at the time of mastectomy for other reasons. Spaying can be done before or after the mastectomy. When circumstances permit, the approach for the procedure is made as usual. After the ovariohysterectomy and closure of the linea alba are completed, the skin incision forms part of the medial border of the mastectomy incision and is extended as needed to encompass the mammary gland or glands to be removed. Mammary tumors that extend across the midline should be removed before the ovariohysterectomy.

Suggested Readings

Anon. Breast cancer monograph. No. 17. New York: Memorial Hospital for Cancer and Allied Disease, 1973.

Bartels EK, et al. Simultaneous bilateral mastectomy in the dog. Vet Surg 1978;7:97.

Black MM. Human breast cancer: a model for cancer immunology. Isr J Med Sci 1973;9:284.

Bostock DE. The prognosis following the surgical excision of canine mammary neoplasms. Eur J. Cancer 1975;1:389.

Brodey RS. Canine and feline neoplasia. Adv Vet Sci 1969;23:309.

Brodey RS, Fidler IF, Beck-Nielsen S. Correction of in vitro immune response with clinical course of malignant neoplasia in dogs. Am J Vet Res 1975;36:74.

Brodey RS, Fidler IF, Howson AE. The relationship of estrous irregularity, pseudopregnancy, and pregnancy to the development of canine mammary neoplasma. J Am Vet Med Assoc 1966; 149:1047.

Cohen D, et al. Epidemiological analysis of the most prevalent sites and types of canine neoplasia observed in a veterinary hospital. Cancer Res 1974;34:2859.

Cotchin E. Neoplasia in the cat. Vet Rec 1957;69:425.

Cotchin E. Mammary neoplasms of the bitch. J Comp Pathol 1958; 68:1.

Dorn CR, et al. Surgery of animal neoplasms in Alameda and Contra Costa counties, California. I. Methodology and description of cases. J Natl Cancer Inst 1968;40:295.

Dorn CR, et al. Alameda and Contra Costa counties, California. II. Cancer morbidity in dogs and cats from Alameda County. J Natl Cancer Inst 1968;40:307.

Feller WF, Chopra HC. A small virus-like particle observed in human breast cancer by means of electron microscopy. J Natl Cancer Inst 1968;40:1359.

Fidler IJ, Abt DA, Brodey RS. The biological behavior of canine mammary neoplasms. J Am Vet Med Assoc 1967;151:1311.

Fowler EH, Wilson GP, Koestner A. Biologic behavior of canine mammary neoplasms based on a histogenic classification. Vet Pathol 1974;11:212.

Gross L, Feldman DG. Virus particles in guinea pig leukemia and cat mammary carcinoma. Proc Am Assoc Cancer Res 1969;10:33.

Hamilton JM. A review of recent advances in the study of the etiology of canine mammary tumors. Vet Annu 1975;15:276.

Hampe JF, Misdorp W. Tumors of dysplasia of the mammary gland. Bull WHO 1974;50:111.

Harvey HJ, Gilberston SR. Canine mammary gland tumors. Vet Clin North Am 1977;7:213.

Hayden DW, Nielson SW. Feline mammary tumors. J Small Anim Pract 1971;12:687.

Hayes AA. Feline mammary gland tumors. Vet Clin North Am 1977;7:205.

MacEwen EG. General concepts of immunotherapy of tumors. J Am Anim Hosp Assoc 1976;12:363.

MacEwen EG, et al. Evaluation of effects of levamisole and surgery on canine mammary cancer. J Biol Response Mod 1985;4:418.

Misdorp W, Hart AAM. Prognostic factors in canine mammary cancer. J Natl Cancer Inst 1976;56:779.

Misdorp W, Hart AAM. Canine mammary carcinoma. J Small Anim Pract 1979;20:385.

Misdorp W, et al. Canine malignant mammary tumors. II. Adenocarcinomas, solid carcinomas, and spindle call carcinoms. Vet Pathol 1972;9:447.

Mitchell L, et al. Mammary tumors in dogs: survey of clinical and pathological characteristics. Can Vet J 1974;15:131.

Moore DH, et al. Type B particles in human milk. Tex Rep Biol Med 1969;27:1027.

Moulton JE, et al. Canine mammary tumors. Pathol Vet 1970;7:289.

Nielson SW. The malignancy of mammary tumors in cats. North Am Vet 1952;245:252.

Nielson SW, et al. Canine mammary neoplasms and progestogens. JAMA 1972;219:1601.

Proud AJ. Measurement and treatment of mammary carcinoma in bitches. Vet Rec 1971;89:371.

Salnj PG, et al. Pituitary prolactin levels in canine mammary cancer. Eur J Cancer 1974;10:63.

Schmitt GH. Biology of lactation. San Francisco: WH Freeman, 1971.

Schneider R, et al. Factors influencing canine mammary cancer development and postsurgical survival. J Natl Cancer Inst 1969;43:1249.

Seman GB, et al. Présence de particules virales dans divers tumeurs transplantés de la souris. Rev Fr Etud Clin Biol 1968;12:1006.

Seman GB, et al. Studies on the relationship of viruses to the origin of human breast cancer. II. Virus-like particles isolated from human milk. Nature 1969;231:97.

Ulvand MJ. Cellular immunity to canine mammary tumor cells demonstrated by the leucocyte migration technique. Acta Vet Scand 1975;16:95.

Vallance DL, Capel-Edwards F. Chlormadinone and mammary nodules. Br Med J 1971;11:221.

Weider PL, et al. Immune reactivity in dogs with spontaneous malignancy. J Natl Cancer Inst, 53:1049, 1974.

Weijer K, et al. Feline malignant mammary tumors. II. Immunologic and electron microscopic investigations into a possible viral etiology. J Natl Cancer Inst 1974;52:673.

Wilkinson GT. The treatment of mammary tumors in the bitch and a comparison with the cat. Vet Rec 1971;29:13.

Withrow SJ. Surgical management of canine mammary tumors. Vet Clin North Am 1975;5:495.

— 37 —

SKIN GRAFTING AND RECONSTRUCTION TECHNIQUES

Skin Grafting Techniques

Michael M. Pavletic

Various skin flap and free grafting techniques can be used in the dog and cat to close wounds unamenable to simple apposition. Simple closure techniques, including undermining or simple tension-relieving procedures, should be considered to restore function to the area. The advanced techniques described in this discussion are suitable for more challenging wounds occasionally encountered in practice. Not every possible reconstructive surgical technique can be discussed here; only more commonly used techniques are reviewed. The reader is directed to the references listed for additional details on a given surgical procedure.

Wound contraction and epithelialization (second-intention healing) remain valuable options for wound closure if the advantages and disadvantages are kept in mind. Many of the techniques discussed here can be used to close wounds rapidly and economically, thus bypassing the inconvenience and costs associated with long-term management of an open wound.

Anatomic Considerations

The cutaneous vascular system of the hairy skin of the dog and cat is divided into three interconnected levels: 1) the deep, subdermal, or subcutaneous plexus; 2) the middle or cutaneous plexus; and 3) the superficial or subpapillary plexus (Fig. 37.1). These three plexus levels are interconnected and are supplied by direct cutaneous arteries, which travel parallel to the skin in the hypodermis (1, 2).

The deep or subdermal plexus is the major vascular network to the overlying skin and travels in the subcutaneous fatty and areolar tissue on the deep face of the dermis. Where there is a layer of cutaneous muscle, the subdermal plexus lies both superficial and deep to it. The major panniculus muscles in the dog include the cutaneous trunci, platysma, sphincter coli superficialis, and supramammarius muscles. Direct cutaneous arteries can be grossly visualized traveling in the hypodermis and associated panniculus muscle layer. In areas of loose skin in small animals, the direct cutaneous arteries are remarkably elastic and accommodate the stretching and shifting of the skin. Preservation of the blood supply is critical to the survival of skin.

General Surgical Considerations

The loose elastic skin over the neck and trunk of the dog and cat facilitates the closure of moderate-size skin defects by undermining alone or in combination with skin flap techniques. Based on the anatomy and circulation of the skin, the following general guidelines apply to undermining and elevation of skin (2–5):

1. Undermine skin below the panniculus muscle layer when present to preserve the subdermal plexus and associated direct cutaneous vessels.

2. Undermine skin without an underlying panniculus muscle layer (middle and distal portions of the extremities) in the loose areolar fascial beneath the dermis to preserve the subdermal plexus.

3. Preserve direct cutaneous arteries whenever possible during undermining.

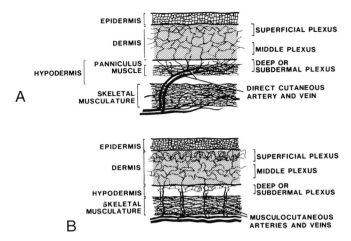

Fig. 37.1. A. Cutaneous circulation in the dog and cat. **B.** Human cutaneous circulation. The subdermal plexus is formed and supplied by terminal branches of direct cutaneous vessels at the level of the panniculus muscle in the dog and cat. Note the parallel relationship of the direct cutaneous vessels to the overlying skin in the dog and cat, in contrast to the perpendicular orientation of musculocutaneous vessels in the human. (From Pavletic MM. The integument. In: Slatter DH, ed. Textbook of small animal surgery. Philadelphia: WB Saunders, 1980.)

4. Elevate skin closely associated with an underlying muscle by including a portion of the outer muscle fascia with the dermis rather than undermining between these structures. This may help to minimize injury to the subdermal plexus.

5. Avoid direct injury to the subdermal plexus by using atraumatic surgical technique.

6. Avoid or minimize surgical manipulation of skin recently traumatized until circulation improves, as noted by the resolution of contusions, edema, and infection.

Atraumatic surgical technique is essential for consistent success in reconstructive surgery. Tissue trauma compromises vascular channels in the skin, damages and destroys cells, which may then serve as a bacterial growth medium and prolongs wound healing, further reducing the ability of the skin to resist infection. Sharp surgical blades should be used to cut skin; scissors crush skin and should be avoided. Skin hooks, Brown–Adson forceps, or stay sutures should be used to manipulate the flap. Allis tissue forceps and other crushing forceps should not be used.

Technique Selection

Selection of the most appropriate technique to close a wound includes the following considerations:
1. Wound size
2. Body region involved
3. Potential sources of donor skin
4. Condition of recipient bed
5. Functional results required
6. Cost

Cosmetic results generally are a secondary consideration in veterinary medicine, although the reconstructive surgeon tries to achieve optimal cosmetic results when these six general criteria are considered. Surgery solely for the sake of cosmetic improvement is to be discouraged (5).

Among the most difficult wounds to close are those of the lower third of the extremities because of the limited availability of loose skin in the dog and cat. Larger wounds approaching or beyond 180° of the limb's circumference are not ideal candidates for healing by second intention: closure with a skin graft or skin flap is required. In contrast, the trunk of the dog and cat has a comparatively ample amount of loose skin. This redundant skin can be used as a source of donor skin for closure of large trunk wounds, or it can be transferred to the extremities in the form of axial pattern flaps or free grafts. Larger wounds of the trunk, especially in immature dogs, can heal remarkably well by second intention. However, closure by contraction and epithelialization can be protracted. Excessive scarring, paucity of hair growth, or cessation in contraction or epithelialization can and does occur without surgical intervention. The costs associated with topical ointments, dressings, bandages, and hospital visits can approach or exceed the cost of several of the closure techniques discussed. Some wounds can be managed initially by contraction and epithelialization, with surgical intervention considered when a healing problem is recognized. In other cases, closure techniques may close the wound quickly and affordably, thus avoiding the inconveniences associated with prolonged open wound management (5).

In veterinary medicine, skin flaps frequently are the most practical means of closing wounds. Free grafts generally are reserved for lower extremity defects and for closure of larger surface area defects as a result of burns, massive bite wounds, and other forms of trauma capable of compromising large areas of skin. In time, experienced surgeons usually find that a half-dozen techniques work well for closure of most wounds. Other techniques are chosen for less common or more problematic regional defects (5).

Other techniques used more recently in human and small animal patients "stretch" skin before wound closure, thereby taking advantage of the natural elastic properties of the dermal collagen fibers. Tissue expanders and the use of externally applied elastic cable devices are described later in this discussion (5).

Skin Flaps (Pedicle Grafts)

Types and Uses

A pedicle graft, or skin flap, is a portion of skin and subcutaneous tissue with an intact vascular attachment that is transferred from one body area to another

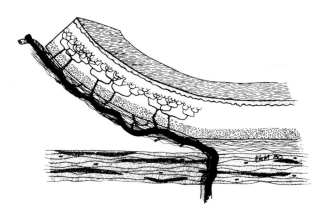

Fig. 37.2. Axial pattern flap (arterial pedicle graft) in the dog and cat. A flap created over the direct cutaneous vessels has an intact blood supply capable of supporting a flap of considerable size. An axial pattern flap in humans is similar, with the exception of their poorly developed panniculus muscle. (From Pavletic MM. Canine axial pattern flaps, using the omocervical, thoracodorsal, and deep circumflex iliac direct cutaneous arteries. Am J Vet Res 1981;42:391.)

(3, 5). Properly developed flaps survive because of their intact circulation. Flaps are versatile and have the following uses: covering defects with poor vascularity; improving regional circulation to an area; covering areas difficult to immobilize; covering holes overlying body cavities; providing a full-thickness skin surface over areas where padding and durability are essential; giving immediate protection to nerves, vessels, tendons, and other structures susceptible to exposure and injury; and providing a skin surface with hair growth comparable with that of the donor area (3, 5).

Pedicle grafts can be classified according to their circulation, location, or composition (3, 5). Pedicle grafts that incorporate a direct cutaneous artery and vein are termed *axial pattern flaps* (Fig. 37.2) (3, 5–7). Variations of the axial pattern flap include the island arterial flap (Fig. 37.3) and the secondary axial pattern flap (3, 5–7). Island arterial flaps have been transferred as free flaps by means of microvascular surgical techniques or pivoted up to 180° to close an adjacent defect (3, 5–7). Flaps elevated without the inclusion of direct cutaneous vessels primarily rely on circulation by the deep or subdermal plexus and are termed *subdermal plexus flaps* (Fig. 37.4). Axial pattern flaps have an excellent blood supply and enable the veterinary surgeon to create large flaps of considerable dimension in the cat and dog (3, 5–7).

Flaps also may be classified as *local flaps* and *distant flaps* according to their location and transfer to the recipient bed (3, 5–7). Local flaps are elevated adjacent to the defect and are advanced or rotated (pivoted) into place. Distant flaps, on the other hand, are almost always used for closure of defects involving the limbs (5).

Distant flaps generally are transferred as delayed tube flaps (indirect flaps) to the defect or by elevating the affected limb to a flap developed on the lower lateral thorax or abdomen (direct flap) (3, 5, 8, 9). Distant flaps have several disadvantages when they are used for extremity defects in small animals. Many cats do not tolerate their limbs bound to their trunk. In addition, the time and care required for distant flaps transfer preclude their use except in a few isolated instances. Because free grafts, axial pattern flaps, and

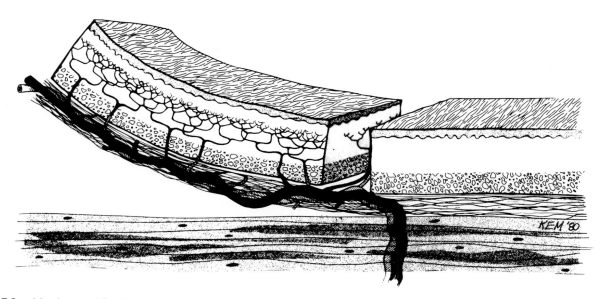

Fig. 37.3. Island arterial flap (island axial pattern flap) in the dog. The graft is nourished solely by the direct cutaneous artery and vein. Island flaps have greater mobility than axial pattern flaps. Vessels have the potential to be severed and reanastomosed with microvascular surgery at a distant recipient site. (From Pavletic MM. Canine axial pattern flaps, using the omocervical, thoracodorsal, and deep circumflex iliac direct cutaneous arteries. Am J Vet Res 1981;42:391.)

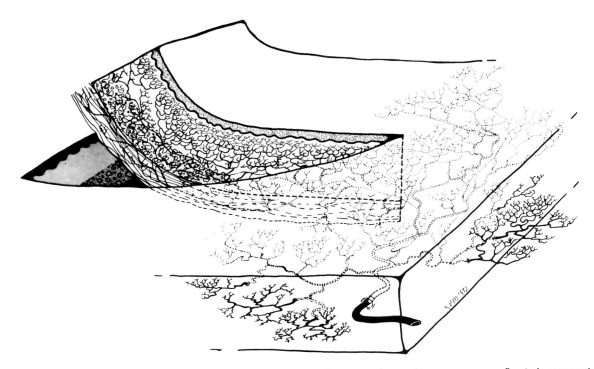

Fig. 37.4. The subdermal plexus flap in the dog and cat. This flap is analogous to the random or cutaneous flap in human patients. The flap is nourished by the subdermal plexus and attenuated branches of the direct cutaneous vessels some distance away. (From Pavletic MM. Canine axial pattern flaps, using the omocervical, thoracodorsal, and deep circumflex iliac direct cutaneous arteries. Am J Vet Res 1981;42:391.)

myocutaneous flaps are more effective and less costly to perform, the clinical need for distant flaps is rare (5).

Compound (composite) flaps are pedicle grafts that incorporate skin and other tissues including muscle, fat, bone, and cartilage (3, 5, 10). *Myocutaneous flaps,* one type of compound flap, are created by the submuscular elevation of a muscle segment with the overlying skin as a unit (Fig. 37.5). Myocutaneous flaps have been used effectively in human patients clinically and in dogs primarily on an experimental basis (3, 5, 10). Although these flaps have been used successfully in the cat and dog, the loose skin available in small animals enables the veterinarian to close wounds with simpler reconstructive techniques (5).

General Principles of Flap Development

The size, location, shape, and condition of a wound generally dictate the technique required to close the defect. The simplest method of satisfactory closing of a skin defect generally prevails in veterinary medicine because of cost considerations (3, 5).

The surgeon must consider all possible flap designs and combinations when choosing the method for closure. Skin tension and pliability are evaluated by manually lifting or pushing the adjacent skin toward the

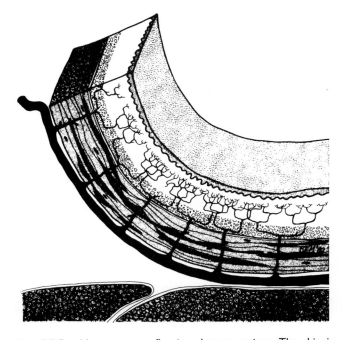

Fig. 37.5. Myocutaneous flap in a human patient. The skin is nourished by musculocutaneous vessels, which receive circulation from the intact skeletal muscle vasculature. (From Pavletic MM. Canine axial pattern flaps, using the omocervical, thoracodorsal, and deep circumflex iliac direct cutaneous arteries. Am J Vet Res 1981;42:391.)

center of the wound. Ideal donor areas have ample skin available to elevate a flap without creating a secondary defect in the donor bed unamenable to simple closure. The surgeon should avoid donor sites subject to excessive motion or tension, to minimize the potential of wound dehiscence or compromise of local mobility. However, it is occasionally preferable to close a wound to protect exposed structures despite the creation of a secondary defect that cannot be closed directly (3, 5). In this situation, the secondary defect can be closed by a second flap, by a free graft, or by healing by wound contraction and epithelialization (3).

Factors that maximize the circulation to a pedicle graft should be considered during flap planning. Increasing the width of a pedicle graft does *not* increase its total surviving length. Flaps created under the same conditions of blood supply survive to the same length regardless of flap width. The only effect of increasing the width of a pedicle graft is the chance of including direct cutaneous vessels in the flap (3, 5). Moreover, because the cutaneous circulation differs regionally, a set ratio of length to width is not applicable (3, 5). Narrowing of a pedicle can reduce the perfusion to the body of the flap and can increase the likelihood of necrosis; axial pattern flaps are an exception to this rule as long as the direct cutaneous artery and vein are preserved (3, 5). Creation of unduly long subdermal plexus flaps can also result in necrosis. As a result of these considerations, I generally design flaps with a base slightly wider than the width of the flap body, to avoid inadvertent narrowing of the pedicle and to limit flap length required to cover the recipient bed without excessive tension (3, 5).

Skin necrosis usually is attributed to insufficient vascular perfusion. Poor planning and traumatic surgical technique also contribute to flap failure. Thus, flaps should be planned with the blood supply as a primary consideration to restore the anatomic and functional continuity of the affected area. The direction of hair growth from the flap also is considered if other surgical factors are considered equal (5).

Preparation of the Wound (Recipient) Bed

The recipient bed should be free of debris, necrotic tissue, and infection. Flaps that are properly developed and transferred can survive on avascular beds. However, distant flaps require the establishment of circulation from the defect to divide the pedicles eventually for completion of flap transfer. Vascular tissue, such as healthy muscle, periosteum, and the paratenon, is capable of vascularizing an overlying skin flap or a free graft. Chronic granulation tissue usually is excised to reestablish a healthy granulation bed. A healthy flat granulation bed usually forms again within 3 to 5 days, when the surrounding tissues have sufficient circula-

tion. Epithelialized borders on the wound also are removed to cover the entire wound with the flap or graft skin (3, 5). With the increasing use of radiation therapy for the management of neoplasms, radiation ulcers may require surgical management. Chronic, infected radiation ulcers can be particularly difficult to close. Management of the avascular ulcers includes surgical debridement and closure with a skin flap, muscle flap, or myocutaneous flap (5). (Closure occasionally can be achieved with careful undermining and regional skin advancement over the prepared defect. This may be facilitated by using the skin stretching techniques discussed later in this chapter.)

Surgical Techniques

LOCAL FLAPS
Local flaps are a simple and practical method of closing wounds that cannot be adequately closed primarily. Their effective use generally requires loose elastic skin adjacent to the wound. Most local flaps are based on the subdermal plexus blood supply and do not achieve the potential size of axial pattern flaps. Despite this feature, local flaps can be extremely effective in closing many of the small to moderate-sized defects encountered in small animal practice. Local flaps also are more likely to maintain a similar color and hair growth pattern than skin transplanted from a distant location. Local flaps are subdivided into two general categories: advancement flaps and rotating flaps. The four local flap techniques considered most versatile are discussed (3, 5).

Single-Pedicle Advancement Flap
The single-pedicle advancement flap (sliding flap) is probably the most common local flap used in veterinary medicine because it has a simple design and does not create a secondary defect requiring closure (3, 5). Forward advancement of a pedicle graft is accomplished primarily by taking advantage of the elasticity or stretching of the skin (Fig. 37.6). Paired single-pedicle advancement flaps can be used to close square or rectangular defects, resulting in an H-closure design, (H-plasty) (Fig. 37.7). In fact, two shorter single-pedicle advancement flaps may be more effective than elevating one long advancement flap, which may have a greater likelihood of partial necrosis.

To create a single-pedicle advancement flap, two skin incisions equal to the width of the defect are made in incremental fashion. The distant edge of the flap borders the defect. I make the two incisions slightly divergent to ensure that creation of the pedicle (base) of the flap is not inadvertently too narrow, resulting in circulatory compromise. The flap is undermined and is advanced into the defect. Closure generally is with

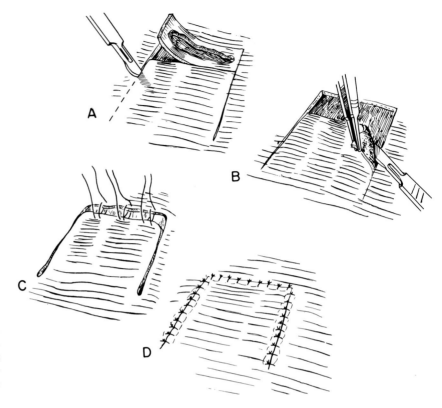

Fig. 37.6. Single-pedicle advancement flap. **A.** Removal of skin lesions and outline of intended flap incisions. **B.** The flap is lengthened and undermined enough to allow for closure without excessive flap tension. **C.** Preplacement of tension sutures may aid in flap alignment. **D.** Closure.

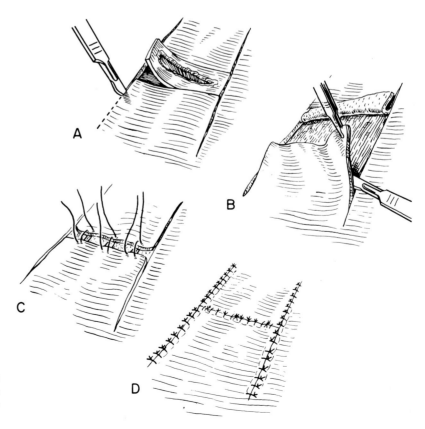

Fig. 37.7. Sliding H-plasty. **A.** Removal of lesion and outline of the flaps on both sides of the defect. **B.** Undermining of both flaps. **C.** Alignment. **D.** Closure.

monofilament nylon or polypropylene sutures (3–0) placed in a simple interrupted pattern.

A single-pedicle advancement flap should not be used in areas where skin tension must be avoided (e.g., wounds around the eyelids). Advancement flaps have a tendency to retract elastically, distorting structures under the influence of this force. A 90° transposition flap should be considered under the circumstances, because it donates loose skin into the defect, unlike the advancement flap, which primarily relies on stretching advancement to cover the wound.

Bipedicle Advancement Flap

Bipedicle advancement flaps are easily constructed by making an incision parallel to the long axis of a defect, the width of the flap generally being equal to the width of the adjacent defect (3, 5). Advancement may be facilitated if the relaxing incision is curved, with the concave side toward the defect. The flap is undermined and sutured into the defect (Fig. 37.8). The secondary defect usually is closed by undermining and suturing the adjacent skin edge. Two pedicles allow for longer flaps to be created. However, necrosis can occur at the vascular interface between the two pedicles. This does not necessarily correlate with the center of the flap unless the circulatory perfusion pressure from each pedicle is equal.

The release or relaxing incision, occasionally used to reduce tension to facilitate wound closure, is a bipedicle advancement flap in design. Release incisions can be effective for closure of wounds in difficult or high-priority areas. The secondary defect created may be strategically positioned in an adjacent area more amenable to healing by wound contraction and epithelialization. As a general rule, the release incision is no closer than 3 to 5 cm from a given incision.

Transposition Flap

A transposition flap is a rotating rectangular pedicle graft usually created with 90° of the long axis of the defect (3, 5). An edge of the defect comprises a portion of the flap border (Fig. 37.9). The width of the flap normally equals the width of the defect. The flap length, from the pivot point of the flap to its most

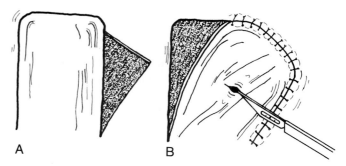

Fig. 37.9. **A** and **B.** When creating a transposition flap, adjustment should be made to allow for the length loss caused by rotation of the flap. A stab incision made over the line of greatest tension can be used to relieve any excessive tension developed on transfer. The secondary defect can be closed by undermining and direct suture closure. (Redrawn from Grabb WC, Myers MB. Skin flaps. Boston: Little, Brown, 1975.)

distant point, should be equal to the distance measured between the pivot point and most distant point of the defect (Fig. 37.10).

Although I have rotated transposition flaps beyond 90°, flap length decreases as the arc of rotation increases. The greater the flap rotation, the greater is the likelihood that a skin fold or "dog ear" will develop. Any secondary defect created is usually closed by direct apposition. A second local flap may be used to close this donor bed, if necessary. Mild tension along the line of greatest tension can be relieved with a small perpendicular stab incision. I have found the transposition flap to be the most useful local flap design for wound closure.

Z-Plasty

Z-plasty is used to lengthen a scar or contracture, alter or relieve tension on an incision, and make a scar less conspicuous and therefore more cosmetically acceptable (3, 5). In small animal surgery, this technique is most commonly used to lengthen restrictive scars

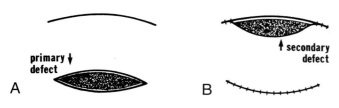

Fig. 37.8. Bipedicle advancement flap. **A.** The flap width generally equals the width of the defect. **B.** The secondary defect (donor bed) is closed by direct apposition. (Redrawn from Grabb WC, Myers MB. Skin flaps. Boston: Little, Brown, 1975.)

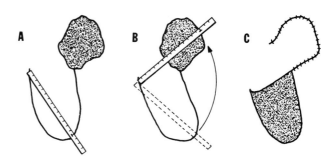

Fig. 37.10. Transposition flap. **A.** Removal of defect and outline of the intended flap incision. **B.** Rotation and alignment of flap. **C.** Closure. The ruler measurement from the pivot point to the tip of the flap must equal the distance between the pivot point and the most distant point of the defect (recipient bed). The secondary defect is sutured closed after local undermining.

involving flexion surfaces. Z-plasty, by placement of its central limb perpendicular to an incision site under excessive tension, also can be used to reduce this force in a fashion similar to the use of a release incision previously discussed. Z-plasty generally involves creating two equilateral triangular flaps adjacent to a resected linear scar and transposing them to their opposing donor bed. The rotation of each flap transplants adjacent loose skin into the previously restricted area (11–13). Although various Z-plasty designs have been used in human patients, the 60° Z-plasty is considered optimal in small animal surgery (Fig. 37.11). Single or multiple Z-plasties may be used (Fig. 37.12). Unfortunately, net gains in scar lengthening can be significantly less than the theoretic mathematic gains previously estimated. Transposition flaps and release incisions generally are simpler to execute than Z-plasty techniques.

AXIAL PATTERN FLAPS

Not every flap elevated on the patient can include a direct cutaneous artery and vein. However, axial pattern flaps can enable the surgeon to transfer large skin segments in a simple stage safely without the necessity of a delay procedure. To date, several axial pattern flaps are used to close various types of wounds (Table 37.1). They include the brachial, caudal superficial epigastric, cranial superficial epigastric, deep circumflex iliac (dorsal branch), deep circumflex iliac (ventral branch), genicular, omocervical, reverse saphenous, thoracodorsal, caudal auricular, and lateral caudal (tail) axial pattern flaps (Figs. 37.13 and 37.14) (3, 5, 11, 14–22).

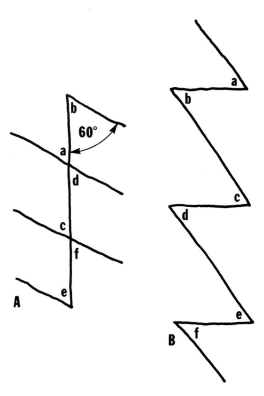

Fig. 37.12. Multiple Z-plasties have a cumulative lengthening effect and can be used effectively in areas in which a single Z-plasty procedure is impossible or unadvisable. **A.** Incision lines. **B.** After rotation of flaps.

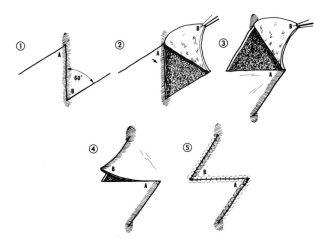

Fig. 37.11. Z-plasty technique to lengthen a restrictive scar (*shaded area*): (*1*) a central incision is made over the scar, and two additional incisions equal in length to the central incision are created at a 60° angle forming a Z; (*2*) triangular flaps A and B are elevated and (*3, 4*) are transposed to their opposing bed; (*5*) the equilateral triangular flaps are sutured into place, resulting in a lengthening of the previously restricted area by 75%.

Careful positioning of each patient is necessary before outlining the proposed flap onto the skin with a felt-tipped marking pen. Skin distortion in relation to the anatomic landmarks may result in failure to include the direct cutaneous vessels into the pedicle graft. Table 37.1 summarizes the outline of the listed axial pattern flaps in the dog.

Axial pattern flaps can be rotated into the adjacent defects or to distant sites of the lower trunk and extremities. A portion of the flap can be tubed to traverse the skin between the donor and recipient beds, or a bridge incision may be used to bypass tubing the flap. The flap body can be elevated as the standard (peninsular design) or the L (hockey stick) design, depending on the shape and size of the cutaneous defect (see Fig. 37.14).

Island arterial flaps depend on a single direct cutaneous artery and vein. They can be developed in each of the canine axial pattern flaps by dividing the cutaneous pedicle below the area where the direct cutaneous artery enters the outlined flap (3, 5, 18, 23). Island arterial flaps are more mobile than conventional axial pattern flaps, but they have more limited clinical use. However, island flaps are particularly useful for closure of large wounds that encroach on the base of a given axial pattern flap. As a result, the flap can pivot 180°

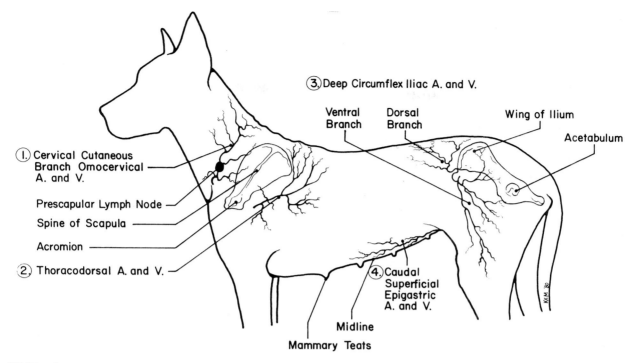

Fig. 37.13. Four major cutaneous arteries are illustrated in relation to their anatomic landmarks (*1* to *4*). (From Pavletic MM. Canine axial pattern flaps, using the omocervical, thoracodorsal, and deep circumflex iliac direct cutaneous arteries. Am J Vet Res 1981;42:391.)

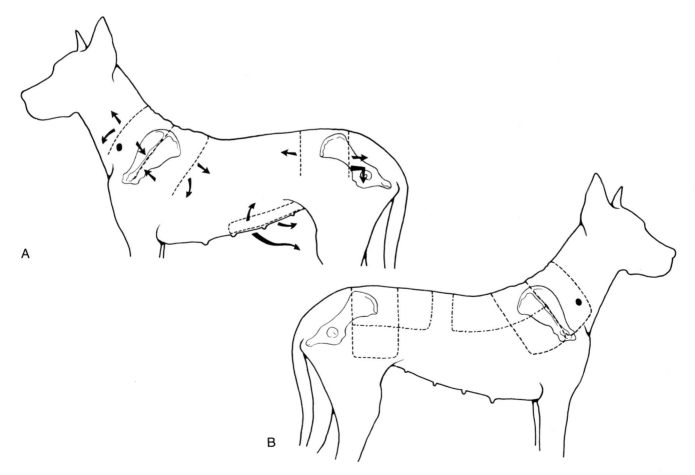

Fig. 37.14. Reference lines for the omocervical, thoracodorsal, deep circumflex iliac, and caudal superficial epigastric axial pattern flaps. **A.** Standard peninsula flaps (*dashed lines*). **B.** L or hockey-stick (*dashed and dotted lines*) configuration. (From Pavletic MM. Canine axial pattern flaps, using the omocervical, thoracodorsal, and deep circumflex iliac direct cutaneous arteries. Am J Vet Res 1981;42:391.)

Table 37.1.
Summary of Guidelines for Axial Pattern Flap Development

Artery	Anatomic Landmarks	Reference Incisions	Potential Uses[a]
Cervical cutaneous branch of the omocervical artery	Spine of the scapula Cranial edge of the scapula (cranial shoulder depression) Dogs in lateral recumbency, skin in natural position, thoracic limb placed in relaxed extension Vessel originates at location of the prescapular lymph node	*Caudal incision:* Spine of the scapula in a dorsal direction *Cranial incision:* Parallel to the caudal incision equal to the distance between the scapular spine and cranial scapular edge (cranial shoulder depression) *Flap length:* Variable; contralateral scapulohumeral joint	Facial defects Ear reconstruction Cervical defect Shoulder defect Axillary defects
Thoracodorsal artery	Spine of the scapula Caudal edge of the scapula (caudal shoulder depression) Dog in lateral recumbency, skin in natural position, thoracic limb in relaxed extension Vessel originates at caudal shoulder depression at a level parallel to the dorsal point of the acromion	*Cranial incision:* Spine of the scapula in a dorsal direction *Caudal incision:* Parallel to the cranial incision equal to the distance between the scapular spine and caudal scapular edge (caudal shoulder depression) *Flap length:* Variable; can survive ventral to contralateral scapulohumeral joint	Thoracic defects Shoulder defects Forelimb defects Axillary defects
Superficial brachial artery	Flexor surface of elbow Humeral shift Greater tubercle	*Incision lines:* Flap base includes flexor surface of elbow, anterior third; lateral and medial incisions parallel humeral shaft; flap progressively tapered approaching greater tubercle *Flap length:* Variable, flap ends at level of greater tubercle	Antebrachial defects Elbow defects
Caudal superficial epigastric artery	Midline of abdomen Mammary teats Base of prepuce	*Medial incision:* Abdominal midline; in the male dog, the base of the prepuce included in the midline incision to preserve adjacent epigastric vasculature *Lateral incision:* Parallel to medial incision at an equal distance from the mammary teats *Flap length:* Variable: may include last four glands and adjacent skin	Flank defects Inner thigh defects Stifle area Perineal area Preputial area
Cranial epigastric artery	Hypogastric region Abdominal midline Mammary teats Base of prepuce	*Base of flap:* Location in hypogastric region *Medial incision:* Abdominal midline *Lateral incision:* Parallel to midline incision at an equal distance from mammary teats *Flap length:* Glands 2, 3, 4; anterior to prepuce	Closure of wounds overlying sternal region
Deep circumflex iliac artery (dorsal branch)	Cranial edge of wing of ilium Great trochanter Dog in lateral recumbency, skin in natural position, pelvic limb in relaxed extension Vessel originates at a point cranioventral to wing of the ilium	*Caudal incision:* Midway between edge of wing of ilium and greater trochanter *Cranial incision:* Parallel to caudal incision equal to the distance between caudal incision and cranial edge of iliac wing *Flap length:* Dorsal to contralateral flank fold	Thoracic defects Lateral abdominal wall defects Flank defects Lateromedial thigh defects Defects over the greater trochanter
Deep circumflex iliac artery (ventral branch)	Anatomic landmarks of flap base same as dorsal branch of deep circumflex iliac artery Shaft of femur	*Caudal incision:* Extending distally, anterior to cranial border of femoral shaft *Cranial incision:* Parallel to caudal incision *Flap length:* Proximal to patella	Lateral abdominal wall defects Pelvic defects Sacral defects, as an island arterial flap
Genicular artery	Patella Tibial tuberosity Greater trochanter	*Base of the flap:* 1 cm proximal to patella and 1.5 cm distal to tibial tuberosity (laterally) *Flap borders:* Extending caudodorsally parallel to the femoral shaft; flap terminates at base of greater trochanter	Lateral or medial aspect of the lower limb, from the stifle to the tibiotarsal joint

Table 37.1 (continued).

Artery	Anatomic Landmarks	Reference Incisions	Potential Uses[a]
Lateral caudal arteries (left and right)	Proximal third of tail length Transverse processes of vertebrae	*Incision:* Dorsal or ventral midline skin incision, depending on intended flap usage; careful dissection along deep caudal fascia of the tail; vessels located lateral and slightly ventral to transverse processes, in proximal tail region; amputation of tail at third to fourth intervertebral space, preserving skin *Flap length:* Proximal third of tail length	Perineum, caudo-dorsal trunk
Caudal auricular artery	Wing of atlas Spine of the scapula	*Base of flap:* Palpable depression between lateral aspect of wing of atlas and vertical ear canal *Width of flap:* Central "third" of lateral cervical area over lateral aspect of wing of atlas *Flap length:* Up to spine of scapula (survival length variability)	Facial area Dorsum of head Ear
Reverse saphenous conduit flap[b]	Inner thigh Tibial shaft	*Proximal incision:* Central third of inner thigh at level of patella; ligate saphenous artery and vein at level of femoral artery and vein *Cranial and caudal incisions:* Skin incisions extended distally in converging fashion, 0.5–1.0 cm cranial and caudal to cranial and caudal saphenous artery and medial saphenous vein; flap undermined beneath saphenous vasculature; ligate and divide peroneal artery and vein *Flap length:* Variable, base of flap at level of anastomosis of cranial branches of medial and lateral saphenous veins	Defects of tarso-metatarsal regions Note: Use of flap requires intact collateral blood supply to lower extremity

[a] Major defects only.
[b] Axial pattern flap variation.

into the adjacent defect. The similar survival area of axial pattern flaps and island arterial flaps indicates that a backcut procedure at the pivot point of a skin flap can be performed to improve flap mobility safely in an axial pattern flap as long as the direct cutaneous artery and vein are preserved (18, 23). A variation of this procedure, neurovascular island flap, has been used to cover small trophic ulcers of the paw in dogs (24).

The thoracodorsal and caudal superficial epigastric axial pattern flaps are the most versatile in the dog and cat (5, 25). They can be used to close various defects at the cranial and caudal regions of each animal with their arc of rotation. They are particularly useful for closing defects of the upper to middle regions of the extremities (Figs. 37.14 to 37.16) (5, 19, 25). In cats and short-legged dogs, the flaps can extend down to the distal extremities. Readers are encouraged to review references to specific axial pattern flaps for additional details.

Compound and Composite Flaps

Musculocutaneous flaps based on the submuscular elevation of the gracilis muscle and a portion of the latissimus dorsi muscle with the overlying skin have been used for microvascular studies in dogs (12, 13, 26, 27). The latissimus dorsi myocutaneous flap and cutaneus trunci myocutaneous flaps have been developed for clinical use in the dog (Figs. 37.17 and 37.18) (5, 10). They can be rotated into various defects within their arc of rotation. The latissimus dorsi and cutaneous trunci myocutaneous flaps have special use for wounds of the thorax and upper forelimb, although the omocervical and thoracodorsal axial pattern flaps are better suited for larger wounds confined to the skin. The thicker latissimus dorsi myocutaneous flap is useful for closing wounds of the thoracic wall or areas where muscle bulk can have a cushion effect (e.g., elbow).

Secondary or revascularized musculocutaneous flaps also have been developed in dogs experimentally by suturing skin to portions of the adductor and sartorius muscles (28, 29). Vascularization subsequently occurs between the muscle–dermal interface, allowing the successful transfer of the muscle and attached island of skin to another region as a second procedure. As such, these flaps have limited clinical practicality in small animals.

Other examples of composite flaps in the dog in-

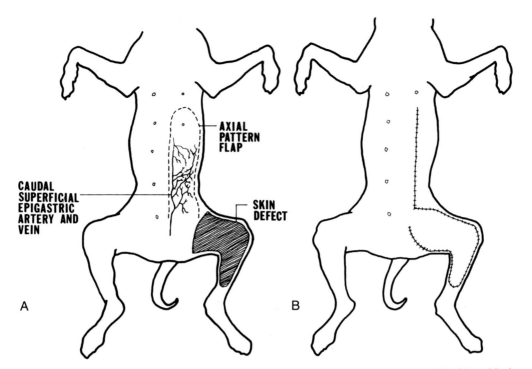

Fig. 37.15. Caudal superficial epigastric axial pattern flap. **A.** Vascular supply to the skin, outline of flap (*dotted line*), and defect to be covered. **B.** Suture line after rotation of flap and closure of initial defect and secondary defect. The flap can be rotated 180° as long as the direct cutaneous artery and vein are not twisted or kinked.

clude the labial advancement flap, buccal rotation flap and labial lift-up technique for full-thickness labial defects, and the composite mucocutaneous subdermal plexus flap for complete lower eyelid reconstruction (5, 30). By strict definition, skin flaps elevated in the dog and cat with subcutaneous fat and panniculus muscle can be considered composite flaps (3, 5).

The routine elevation of major skeletal muscles to transfer the overlying skin is fortunately unnecessary in the dog and cat. The ample amount of loose, elastic skin available and the comparable ease of elevating axial pattern flaps preclude the routine clinical use of this technique (3, 5, 7, 10).

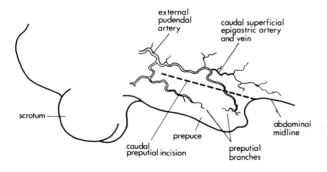

Fig. 37.16. During development of a caudal superficial epigastric axial pattern flap in the male, the prepuce should be included in the medial incision to avoid transection of the direct cutaneous artery and vein.

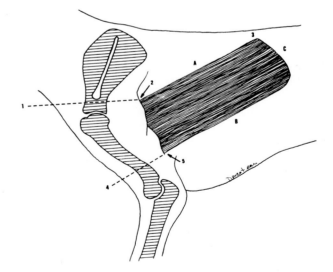

Fig. 37.17. Anatomic landmarks for the latissimus dorsi and cutaneus trunci myocutaneous flaps: (*1*) ventral border of the acromion and (*2*) adjacent caudal border of the triceps muscle; (*3*) head of the last rib; (*4*) distal third of the humerus, which corresponds to the (*5*) axillary skin fold. The flap is drawn onto the skin with a marking pen by connecting landmarks 2 and 3 to form the dorsal flap border (*A*). A second line is drawn from landmarks parallel to line *A* to the border of the last rib forming the lower flap border (*B*). A third line (*C*) is drawn along the caudal border of the last rib, connecting lines *A* and *B*. (From Pavletic M, Kostolich M, Koblik P, et al. A comparison of the cutaneus trunci myocutaneous flap and latissimus dorsi myocutaneous flap in the dog. Vet Surg 1987;16:283.)

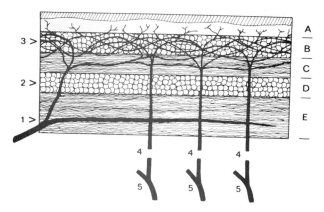

Fig. 37.18. Vascular levels of the latissimus dorsi myocutaneous flap: (*A*) skin, (*B*) subcutaneous flap, (*C*) cutaneous trunci muscle, (*D*) fat, and (*E*) latissimus dorsi muscle. The vessels involved include: (*1*) the main branch of the thoracodorsal artery traveling within the latissimus dorsi muscle; (*2*) short perforating branches of the thoracodorsal artery to the cutaneus trunci muscle and overlying skin; (*3*) the subdermal (deep) plexus to the skin associated with the cutaneous trunci muscle; (*4*) the proximal lateral intercostal arteries divided during elevation of the latissimus dorsi muscle demonstrating anastomotic connections with the thoracodorsal artery intramuscularly; and (*5*) the intercostal arteries. (From Pavletic M, Kostolich M, Koblik P, et al. A comparison of the cutaneous trunci myocutaneous flap and latissimus dorsi myocutaneous flap in the dog. Vet Surg 1987;16:283.)

Skin-Stretching Techniques

Human and animal skin is a nonhomogeneous viscoelastic tissue with the combined characteristics of a viscous fluid and an elastic solid. Skin extensibility depends on three factors occurring consecutively as a load, applied to the skin, is progressively increased: 1) progressive straightening of convolutions in dermal collagen; 2) parallel alignment of dermal collagen fibers in the direction of the applied load; and 3) extension of fully aligned collagen fibers only on application of great increases in tension. As skin progressively extends, it contracts in a plane at right angles to the applied load (31).

The *inherent extensibility* of the skin is subjectively assessed by gently grasping and lifting this skin between the thumb and index finger. *Mechanical creep* is the biomechanical property that enables skin to extend beyond the limits of its inherent extensibility. In mechanical creep, collagen fibers align, over time, with subsequent displacement of interstitial fluid surrounding the collagen fibers and fibrils that comprise individual collagen strands. *Stress relaxation* of the skin, the progressive reduction in force required to maintain the stretched skin's length, is a corollary of mechanical creep. Mechanical creep and stress relaxation can be achieved by application of a constant load to the skin or by intermittent stretching of the skin with periods

of relaxation (load cycling). Biologic creep has been recognized as the progressive increase in skin surface area that occurs when slowly expanding subcutaneous forces are applied to the overlying cutaneous tissues. Progressive enlargement of a gravid uterus, enlarging tumors, and obesity are examples of this natural phenomenon (31).

Surgical attempts at stretching skin to facilitate closure of wounds primarily rely on mobilization by taking advantage of the skin's inherent extensibility, mechanical creep, and stress relaxation. Tissue expanders and the presuturing technique take advantage of these biomechanical properties of skin. Each technique has advantages and limitations to clinical use. One common disadvantage of each of these methods, to a variable degree, is their proximity of placement to the surgical site. Recruitment of skin is limited to the immediate vicinity of their application. Additionally, each device requires insertion beneath or into the skin to exert their mechanical effect (31).

Skin Expanders

Skin expanders are inflatable devices composed of an expandable silicone elastomer bag, silicone connecting tube, and a self-sealing inflation reservoir that serves as an injection port (32, 33). Controlled inflation of this device creates a donor site for elevation of an advancement or transposition flap adjacent to a defect (traumatic or surgically induced) (Fig. 37.19) (32).

For skin expanders to be effective, they must be of sufficient size to exert their stretching effect on the overlying skin. The loose, elastic skin of the neck and trunk precludes the need for, and effective use of, skin expanders in most cases. The greatest clinical potential for skin expanders resides in repair of moderate-sized defects of the middle to lower extremities, as well as the head, where primary closure is not feasible, and alternate closure options are less satisfactory (32).

Skin expanders require a degree of skin laxity (inherent elasticity) to accommodate the mass of the collapsed unit. It is unrealistic to expect a skin expander to be effective for large defects of the extremities. These devices do not permit one-stage surgical reconstruction and are best used for secondary restorative procedures rather than for treatment of acute traumatic injuries (32).

The size of the implant is generally determined by the size of the defect. The base of the implant corresponds to the net gain expected. Not all body regions, however, can accommodate a skin expander of the size required achieve coverage. One can select two or more small expanders to accomplish this goal. Skin expanders can be hyperinflated beyond their designated volume capacity by 20 to 25%, for additional tissue gains. The 100-ml expander used in medium-

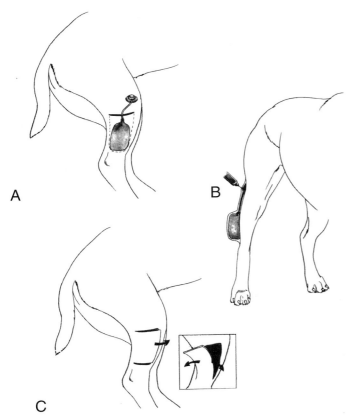

Fig. 36.19. A–C. Tissue expander. In this illustration, a 100-ml tissue expander has been inserted into a subcutaneous pocket created by careful undermining of the skin. The access incision is closed with an intradermal suture pattern and skin sutures; 15 mL of saline is injected into the inflation reservoir, using a 23- to 25-gauge hypodermic needle, on alternate days after implant insertion. In approximately 2 weeks, the implant is deflated and removed; the expanded skin can be advanced or transposed into an adjacent detect. (From Pavletic MM. Atlas of small animal reconstructive surgery. Philadelphia: JB Lippincott, 1992.)

sized dogs, when placed in the middle to lower tibial and radial region, has been effective experimentally. Two such expanders can be used in some situations in which additional skin is desirable (5, 32).

Variable rates of inflation have been used in human surgery. Although a slow rate of expansion may be preferable in elective reconstruction, in which time is not critical, other situations demand more rapid rates of expansion (32, 33). My research demonstrated that 100-ml expanders can be inflated with minimal complications within 2 weeks, using an alternate-day injection schedule. A more cautious (3-week) rate is indicated in delicate cutaneous tissues, especially tissues previously compromised by trauma. Use of expanders in previously irradiated tissues is best avoided (32).

Owners can be trained to inject the skin expander at home, or the patient can be handled on an outpa-

tient basis. Clinical guidelines for expansion rates in human patients include change in skin coloration (ischemia or cyanosis) and patient discomfort. In my study, no patient displayed discomfort during injection. Skin blanching or cyanosis was not noted. Unimpeded hair growth of the expanded skin, when compared with the regional skin, suggested that skin circulation and viability were not compromised throughout the procedure (32).

The expanded skin can be advanced or rotated into the recipient bed on completion of the injection schedule. The expander is drained of saline and removed through the original cutaneous access incision. The advancement flap design is simple to execute if the expander can be satisfactory positioned for this surgical technique. When used for advancement, at least one-third of the limb circumference must be preserved to provide an adequate base to support circulation to the flap. The transposition flap can be rotated into lower extremity defects, thus enabling the surgeon to develop a donor source proximal to the recipient area. The initial skin incision used for insertion of the implant should not be included into the base of a skin flap. I have noted circulatory compromise in flaps that incorporated a linear scar perpendicular to the length of the flap body (5, 32).

Complications noted with skin expanders include dehiscence, implant extrusion, seroma, infection, implant failure (leakage), and skin necrosis (32, 33). A thick, fibrous capsule forms around the implant and reduces the pliability of the flap created. Skin expansion takes time and requires two operations to complete flap transfer. In many situations, skin flaps and free grafts can close wounds effectively and more economically than skin expanders at their present cost. However, skin expanders do enable surgeons to create full-thickness donor skin of similar color, hair growth, and texture adjacent to a defect where no flap can be used otherwise. Moreover, the overall costs associated with tissue expanders may be similar to the total costs associated with mesh grafts. Skin expanders have clinical use in veterinary medicine, but their surgical niche is smaller than in human reconstructive surgery (32).

"Skin Stretchers"

This new method and kit for facilitating wound closure uses a system of externally applied Velcro hook pads, secured to the skin with an adhesive compound. Multiple hook pads can be applied in various locations around a wound or lesion before its elective surgical excision using cyanoacrylate glue. Elastic bands or cables have been designed with Velcro felt or "fuzzy" pads spaced along their surface. These pads engage the hook pads on opposing sides of the proposed surgical site. Bands are applied under tension and are adjusted periodically (three to four times daily) as the stretched skin relaxes and accommodates to a given tension. The skin stretchers are generally employed 3 to 4 days before the surgical closure of the defect created (31).

Although these devices are currently under further development, they show promise in stretching skin before an elective surgical procedure to close large cutaneous defects (e.g., scar revision, tumor removal), during open wound management, and postoperatively to reduce incisional skin tension. Disadvantages include the need to adjust the cables and the occasional necessity to reapply skin pads displaced during the stretching procedure. Skin pads can be peeled off the skin or allowed to separate spontaneously over the next 7 to 10 days. Glue solvent also may be used to facilitate their removal. Research is underway to define clinical guidelines for their application (31).

Free Skin Grafts

Free skin grafts lack a vascular attachment on transfer to the recipient graft bed. These grafts must survive the initial transfer by absorbing tissue fluid (plasmatic imbibition) from the recipient bed by capillary action during the initial 48 hours after transplantation. During this period, capillaries from the recipient bed unite with the exposed graft plexuses to reestablish vital circulation. New capillaries later grow into the graft, and the vascular channels remodel. In addition, fibrous connective tissue forms to hold the graft securely in place. Grafts assume a pink color in 48 hours if circulation is adequate. Grafts with venous obstruction have a cyanotic hue until circulation improves (5).

Any accumulation of material such as pus, serum, blood, hematoma, or foreign matter between the graft and the recipient bed delays or prevents graft revascularization. This delay often results in graft necrosis. Motion between the graft and the recipient bed has a similar effect. Fibrinolysis secondary to bacterial infection destroys the early fibrin glue between the graft and the bed, resulting in motion and graft necrosis. Improper contact between the graft and the recipient bed prevents proper surface-to-surface interdigitation and causes poor graft revascularization. This improper contact may occur if the graft is stretched over the bed like a drum skin or if an excessively large graft is applied to form graft folds that lack proper recipient bed contact (5).

Although free skin grafts require a vascularized recipient bed for survival, granulation tissue is not necessary before a graft is applied. Healthy pink granulation tissue, however, is an excellent recipient bed for skin grafts. Pale, collagen-laden chronic granulation tissue has a poor vascular supply and should be excised to promote formation of healthy granulation tissue. As noted, chronic radiation ulcers, which lack a satisfac-

tory blood supply, are poorly suited to support a free skin graft. Contamination and infection should be controlled, and the granulation surface must be free of any epithelial cover before graft application (5).

Types and Uses

Free grafts can be classified according to the source of the graft, the graft thickness, and the graft shape or

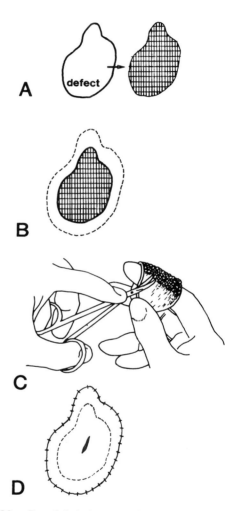

Fig. 37.20. Free full-thickness graft. The recipient is prepared for operation, and any epithelialized areas are excised to accept full graft coverage (cross-hatching). **A.** A sterile gauze or paper template is made of the recipient bed. **B.** After the template is transferred to the prepared donor site, a sterile ink applicator is used to outline the template on the donor site 1 cm outside its border. **C.** The graft is removed, and the donor bed is closed. The graft is "defatted" by trimming away all subcutaneous tissue. The resultant graft appears opaque when held to a light source and must be kept moist at all times. **D.** The graft is laid over the wound. Stab incisions may be used to prevent fluid accumulation beneath the graft. The graft overlaps the recipient bed and is sutured into place with a simple interrupted or continuous pattern. The overlapped border eventually sloughs, leaving complete graft coverage over the recipient bed. The graft is dressed and bandaged postsurgically.

design. Although autogenous grafts are used for permanent free graft coverage in the dog and cat, allografts (homografts) and xenografts (heterografts) can be used as a temporary biologic dressing until an autogenous graft can be successfully applied. Free grafts can be harvested as full-thickness or split-thickness skin grafts. Split-thickness grafts are harvested with razor blades, graft knives, or a dermatome. Graft thickness varies according to the amount of dermis included with the overlying epidermis. The donor bed of a split-thickness graft bed can be excised and closed, or it may be left to heal by adnexal reepithelialization (5, 34).

Thin split-thickness grafts "take" more readily than full-thickness grafts, but they lack durability and proper hair growth, and they are more susceptible to secondary graft contraction. Thin split-thickness grafts in conjunction with mesh graft expansion devices are reserved for coverage of large wounds, especially those secondary to burns (5, 34).

Full-thickness grafts are preferred by many veterinarians for their durability and better hair growth compared with thinner grafts. Free grafts can be applied as a sheet over the entire recipient bed, or they can be divided into various shapes or patterns (5, 34). Punch, strip, and stamp grafts are commonly used as partial-coverage grafts to increase the total recipient surface area that a small graft harvest can cover (5, 34). With these grafts, open spaces between the graft perimeters allow for drainage until the granulation tissue bed is covered by the advancing sheet of epithelial cells originating from the graft. For this reason, partial-coverage grafts are useful for recipient beds with low-grade infections. Small grafts also conform to irregular recipient beds, are simple to apply,

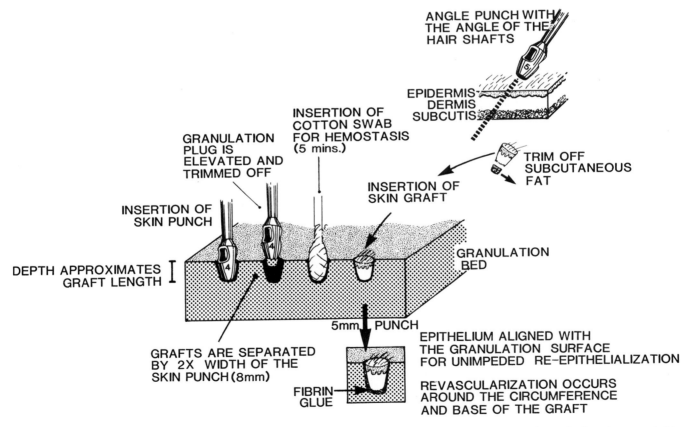

Fig. 37.21. Punch graft technique (pinch grafts). A sharp 5- or 6-mm biopsy punch is used to harvest the graft plugs from a suitable donor site. The donor area is clipped, leaving the hair shafts exposed. Subcutaneous fat is trimmed off the graft base. A single stitch is used to close the donor bed. The grafts are placed between two moistened saline pads until needed. A 4-mm biopsy punch is used to remove cores of granulation tissue in the recipient bed. Holes are spaced 8 mm apart (twice the width of the biopsy punch). Fine scissors are required to remove the granulation core. A sterile cotton swab is inserted into each hole for 5 minutes. The graft plugs are then inserted in the direction of natural hair growth. A firm dressing is applied postsurgically to maintain the position of the grafts. This procedure has the following advantages: 1) 4-mm granulation holes compensate for graft shrinkage and allow the grafts to fit more snugly; 2) the epithelial surface of the graft is level with the granulation bed, and re-epithelialization is unimpeded; 3) as many hair follicles as possible are included into each graft to promote hair growth; 4) re-epithelialization is possible despite partial graft necrosis from surviving hair follicles and skin adnexa deep in the graft; and 5) graft revascularization occurs around the circumferences as well as through the base of the graft plug, a comparatively large surface area.

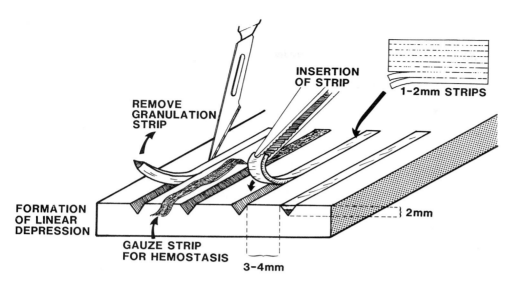

Fig. 37.22. Strip grafts. Application of strip grafts is similar to that of punch grafts. Linear strips of skin are laid in granulation troughs cut with a special blade. Granulation tissue between the strips is eventually reepithelialized from the graft.

and are economical to perform. Unfortunately, the resultant epithelialized surface lacks the durability and cosmetic results achievable with full-thickness graft coverage. Depending on the number and spatial arrangement of stamp, pinch, punch, and strip grafts, epithelialization may be prolonged. I prefer to use full-thickness hand mesh grafts to close wounds of the lower extremities and to use punch or strip grafts for smaller wounds that are not located over areas where skin durability is essential. Grafts using mesh graft expansion units are best suited for coverage of larger wound surface areas, especially when the donor source is limited (5).

Surgical Techniques

The techniques for developing full-thickness skin grafts, punch grafts, strip grafts, stamp grafts, and mesh grafts are illustrated and described in Figures 37.20 through 37.24.

Full-thickness skin grafts are the most useful of the grafting techniques to close small to moderate-sized wounds in areas where skin flaps are not feasible or impractical to use. This is especially true for defects involving the distal extremities. A template of the vascularized wound bed is obtained using sterile gauze or the paper liner from a pack of sterile surgical gloves. The moisture absorbed from the wound surfaces creates a general outline of the defect. This template is trimmed and placed on the prepared donor area. Although skin can be harvested from various body regions, most surgeons obtain their sample from the lateral thorax or abdomen because of its ease of accessibility and closure of the donor site. However, the surgeon can select another donor site that may match more closely the hair color and growth charac-

teristics of the skin lost to injury. The template is positioned on the proposed donor site to maintain the normal direction of hair growth. I prefer to harvest a rectangular segment of skin that encompasses the dimension of the template, including an additional 1-cm border of skin beyond the outer limits of the template border. Harvesting of a rectangular skin segment enables the surgeon to close the donor area more easily than attempting to harvest an irregularly shaped graft to conform exactly to the wound. Redundant skin can be trimmed and discarded to achieve optimal coverage (5).

All subcutaneous tissues must be removed from the graft to expose the dermal surface. When tissues are defatted properly, the surgeon sees the dermal collagen striations and speckled appearance of the compound hair follicles, giving the dermal surface a cobblestone appearance. Grafts are draped over the

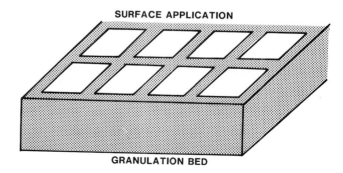

Fig. 37.23. Stamp grafts. Full-thickness or split-thickness grafts are harvested and are divided into squares. Size can vary up to the size of postage stamps. Grafts are laid over the recipient bed a few to several millimeters apart. Square depressions may be cut into a granulation bed if necessary to improve graft immobilization.

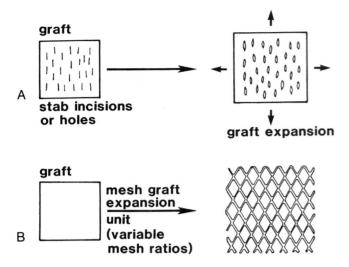

Fig. 37.24. Mesh grafts. Both full-thickness and split-thickness grafts may be used. **A.** Multiple stab incisions or holes are cut into the graft to allow the graft to expand and to provide adequate drainage. The graft is sutured at the periphery. **B.** Mesh-graft expansion units have been developed to expand the graft into a uniform mesh. A graft can be expanded 1.5 to 9 times its original surface area to cover extensive skin defects.

vascular wound bed, with the borders overlying the borders of the defect. Skin staples are useful to secure the graft border to the underlying skin rapidly. Skin tension is adjusted by stapling one side and slightly stretching the graft before stapling the opposing side of the graft. The process is repeated in the opposite plane. The graft is applied with sufficient tension to allow the graft to flatten and conform to all surface areas; graft holes are stretched to allow a gap of a few millimeters to form to facilitate drainage. As a general rule, grafts are not sutured to the wound bed, to avoid hemorrhage and injury to this recipient surface. A fibrin glue forms within hours to help secure the graft. Redundant skin is trimmed with scissors and is discarded when no further grafting is necessary. Staples and the necrotic, overlapped border of skin are easily removed 7 to 10 days postoperatively (5).

Pad Grafting

More recent articles have discussed the clinical feasibility of grafting foot pads to areas denuded of this highly specialized cutaneous surface (5, 35, 36). Readers should closely review these articles to assess their potential use in similar clinical situations.

Postoperative Care

Proper protection is essential for survival of a skin graft. The animal should be confined to a cage, and sedatives should be administered if the patient is excitable. The type of bandage, the dressing, and the sequence of bandage changes may vary. I prefer to cover grafts postoperatively with a nonadherent pad (Adaptic [Johnson & Johnson, New Brunswick, NJ] or Telfa [Kendall Company Hospital Products, Boston, MA]) and a bland antimicrobial ointment, followed by an even layer of gauze pads. Alternate layers of adherent gauze and cotton are applied. A layer of elastic tape is applied to complete the bandage. Such bandages are bulky and restrict motion to the graft. Additional external support (e.g., splints, casts, slings, and reinforcement rods) is used if necessary. Schroeder–Thomas splints are ideal for immobilizing grafts overlying the elbow, carpus, knee, or tibiotarsal joints. Spica splints are used for grafting the upper extremity, especially in cats, whose reputation for extricating themselves from bandages is legendary (5).

The bandage is changed 3 to 5 days postsurgically with the patient under light anesthesia or sedation and restraint. Earlier bandage changes risk graft motion during the critical 48-hour period of graft revascularization. The veterinarian must resist the tremendous temptation to check the graft in the early stages. To remove the bandage, the outer layers are cut away, and the dressing is removed carefully. However, any bandage materials sticking to the graft should be removed carefully to avoid lifting or damaging the graft. "Nonadherent" dressings frequently stick to the areas of exposed granulation tissue from dried blood or granulation tissue extension into the interstices of the dressing. Warm saline, however, can be applied to soften the dressing to facilitate its removal. If visible, the graft is inspected for signs of infection, necrosis, or elevation from the graft bed. Cultures are taken if infection is a concern. However, this is seldom necessary. Early signs of graft necrosis are discouraging, but not always catastrophic, because hair follicles and cutaneous adnexa in the deep portion of the graft may survive and may serve as a source for wound epithelialization. Subsequent bandage changes are repeated in similar fashion every 2 to 4 days, depending on the condition of the graft. This routine is continued for approximately 2 weeks, followed by application of a lighter bandage for an additional 10 to 14 days if necessary. An Elizabethan collar is advisable to prevent self-mutilation of the graft site. Eventually, the owner can remove the collar temporarily with the pet under close observation. If the animal does not rub or lick the area, the collar can be eliminated completely, approximately 1 month after surgery (5).

Bandages have potential adverse effects. Excessive pressure or application of wrinkled bandage material over the graft can result in graft necrosis. In addition, bandage materials can act as an abrasive on the graft if immobilization of the affected area is inadequate (5).

References

1. Pavletic MM. The vascular supply to the skin of the dog: a review. Vet Surg 1980;9:77.
2. Pavletic MM. The integument. In: Slatter DH, ed. Textbook of small animal surgery. Philadelphia: WB Saunders, 1994.
3. Pavletic MM. Pedicle grafts. In: Slatter DH, ed. Textbook of small animal surgery. Philadelphia: WB Saunders, 1994.
4. Pavletic MM. Undermining the skin in the dog and cat. Mod Vet Pract 1986;67:16.
5. Pavletic MM. Atlas of small animal reconstructive surgery, Philadelphia: JB Lippincott, 1992.
6. Pavletic MM. Caudal superficial epigastric arterial pedicle grafts in the dog. Vet Surg 1980;9:103.
7. Pavletic MM. Canine axial pattern flaps, using the omocervical, thoracodorsal, and deep circumflex iliac direct cutaneous arteries. Am J Vet Res 1981;42:391.
8. Alexander JW, Hoffer RE, MacDonald JM. The use of tubular flap grafts in the treatment of traumatic wounds on the extremity of the cat. Feline Pract 1976;6:29.
9. Yturraspe DJ, Creed JE, Schwach RP. Thoracic pedicle skin flap for repair of lower limb wounds in dogs and cats. J Am Anim Hosp Assoc 1976;12:581.
10. Pavletic MM, Kostolich M, Koblik P, et al. Comparison of the cutaneous trunci myocutaneous flap and latissimus dorsi myocutaneous flap in the dog. Vet Surg 1987;16:283.
11. Smith MM, Carrig CB, Waldron DR, et al. Direct cutaneous arterial supply to the tail in dogs. Am J Vet Res 1992;53:145.
12. Krizek TJ, Tani T, Desprez JD, et al. Experimental transplantation of composite grafts by microsurgical vascular anastomoses. Plast Reconstr Surg 1965;36:538.
13. Tsai TJ, et al. The effect of hypothermia and tissue perfusion on extended myocutaneous flap viability. Plast Reconstr Surg 1982;70:444.
14. Kostolich M, Pavletic MM. Axial pattern flap based on the genicular branch of the saphenous artery in the dog. Vet Surg 1987;16:217.
15. Pavletic MM, Macintire D. Phycomycosis of the axilla and inner brachium in a dog: surgical excision and reconstruction with a thoracodorsal axial pattern flap. J Am Vet Med Assoc 1982;180:1197.
16. Pavletic MM. Combined closure techniques for a large skin defect in a cat. Feline Pract 1982;12:16.
17. Henney LHS, Pavletic MM. Axial pattern flap based on the superficial brachial artery in the dog. Vet Surg 17:311, 1988.
18. Sardinas JC, Pavletic MM, Ross JT, et al. Comparative viability of peninsular and island axial pattern flaps incorporating the cranial superficial epigastric artery in dogs. J Am Vet Med Assoc 1995;207:452.
19. Remedios AM, Bauer MS, Bowen CV. Thoracodorsal and caudal superficial epigastric axial pattern skin flaps in cats. Am J Vet Res 1992;53:145.
20. Smith MM, Payne JT, Moon ML, et al. Axial pattern flap based on the caudal auricular artery in dogs. Am J Vet Res 1991; 52:922.
21. Pavletic MM, Watters J, Henry RW, et al. Reverse saphenous conduit flap in the dog. J Am Vet Med Assoc 1982;182:380.
22. Cornell K, Salisbury K, Jakovljevic S, et al. Reverse saphenous conduit flap in cats: an anatomic study. Vet Surg 1995;24:202.
23. Milton SH. Experimental studies of island flaps. I. The surviving length. Plast Reconstr Surg 1971;48:574.
24. Gourley IM. Neurovascular island flap for treatment of trophic metacarpal pad ulcer in the dog. J Am Anim Hosp Assoc 1978;14:119.
25. Pavletic MM. Surgery of the skin and management of wounds. In: Sherding R, ed. Diseases of the cat: diagnosis and management. New York: Churchill Livingstone, 1994.
26. Harii K, Ohmori K, Sekiguchi J. The free musculocutaneous flap. Plast Reconstr Surg 1976;57:294.
27. Schlenker JD. Discussion: the effect of hypothermia and tissue perfusion on extended myocutaneous flap viability. Plast Reconstr Surg 1982;70:453.
28. Erol OO, Spira M. Secondary musculocutaneous flap: an experimental study. Plast Reconstr Surg 1980;65:277.
29. Schechter GL, Biller HF, Ogura JH. Revascularized skin flaps: a new concept in transfer of skin flaps. Laryngoscope 1969; 79:1647.
30. Pavletic MM, Nafe LA, Confer AW. Mucocutaneous subdermal plexus flap from the lip for lower eyelid restoration in the dog. J Am Vet Med Assoc 1982;180:921.
31. Pavletic MM, Hoffman A. Skin stretchers: an externally applied device to facilitate wound closure utilizing the inherent viscoelastic properties of skin. A preliminary report. Vet Surg 1994;23:413.
32. Spodnick G, Pavletic MM, Schelling S, et al. Controlled tissue expansion in the distal extremities of dogs. Vet Surg 1993; 22:436.
33. Keller WG, Anon DN, Rarich PM, et al. Rapid tissue expansion for the development of rotational skin flaps in the distal portion of the hind limb of dogs: an experimental study. Vet Surg 1994;23:31.
34. Swaim SF. Principles of plastic and reconstructive surgery. In: Slatter DH, ed. Textbook of small animal surgery. Philadelphia: WB Saunders, 1994.
35. Bradley DM, Swaim SF, Alexander CM, et al. Autogenous pad grafts for reconstruction of a weight-bearing surface: a case report. J Am Anim Hosp Assoc 1994;30:533.
36. Pavletic MM. Foot salvage by delayed reimplantation of several metatarsal and digital pads using a bipedicle direct flap technique. J Am Anim Hosp Assoc 1994;30:539.

Mesh Skin Grafting

Eric R. Pope

Skin defects in dogs and cats are routinely reconstructed by skin grafting. The most common use of grafts is for reconstructing degloving injuries on the extremities, although these grafts also are used for treating burn wounds. Both full-thickness and split-thickness grafts are used. Full-thickness grafts consist of the epidermis and entire dermis, whereas split-thickness grafts consist of the epidermis and variable portions of the dermis (Fig. 37.25). Of the various types of skin grafts described in the literature, the mesh skin graft offers many advantages for the veterinary surgeon. A mesh graft is a full-thickness or split-thickness skin graft in which parallel rows of staggered slits have been cut either manually with a No. 11 scalpel blade or mechanically with a commercial mesh dermatome (Mesh-Skin Graft Expander No. P-160, Padgett Instruments, Kansas City, MO). Mesh grafts have the following advantages: 1) they can be expanded to cover large defects if donor sites are limited (e.g., burns); 2) they conform well to irregular surfaces; 3) the numerous slits allow drainage from underneath the graft; and 4) they can be placed over areas that are difficult to immobilize. The primary disadvantage of mesh grafts is that when they are expanded, the interstices heal by epithelialization, resulting in islands of nonhaired epithelium throughout the graft. For this reason, a nonexpanded or minimally expanded graft is preferred.

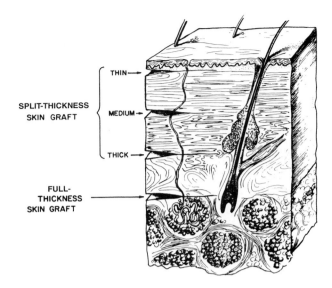

THIN

SPLIT-THICKNESS
SKIN GRAFT

MEDIUM

THICK

FULL-
THICKNESS
SKIN GRAFT

Fig. 37.25. Full-thickness skin grafts consist of the epidermis and entire dermis. Split-thickness grafts consist of the epidermis and variable portions of the dermis. (Courtesy of Swaim SF, DVM, Auburn University, Auburn, AL.)

Preoperative Considerations

Recipient Bed

Skin grafts can be successfully placed on freshly created surgical wounds or on healthy granulation beds. A freshly created wound can be grafted immediately if the surface of the wound has a blood supply sufficient enough to produce granulation tissue if left ungrafted. Muscle and fascia generally support grafts well. Bone, cartilage, and tendon covered by their supporting structures also support grafts. Grafts placed over avascular areas less than 1 cm in width (0.5 cm from each margin) generally survive because of the extensive interconnection of blood vessels within the dermis; this is referred to as the bridging phenomenon.

If any doubt exists about the condition of a wound, I prefer to allow a healthy granulation bed to form before grafting. A granulation bed should be sufficiently formed within 5 to 7 days. A healthy granulation bed is smooth and pink; the migration of epithelium from the wound margin also is a good indicator that the granulation tissue is healthy. Chronic granulation tissue is rough and dark red and may be infected. Chronic granulation tissue should be excised to its base and a fresh granulation bed allowed to form before any skin-grafting procedure is performed. Culture and sensitivity testing should be considered if infection is suspected.

In most instances, traumatic wounds are best managed conservatively initially, followed by grafting after a healthy granulation bed has formed. Obviously, devitalized tissue should be debrided from the wound, and the surface should be covered with wet-to-dry dressings (e.g., wet saline dressings [Kendall Company Hospital Products, Boston, MA]) until a granulation bed forms. Once a granulation bed forms, the wound surface should be protected with nonadherent dressings (e.g., Telfa pads [Kendall Company Hospital Products]) until grafting is performed.

Donor Sites

Important criteria in selecting a donor site are the color and length of hair with respect to that surrounding the recipient site and also the ability to close the donor site after harvesting the graft. Because abundant skin generally is present on the thorax and neck, large grafts can be harvested from these areas, and primary closure of the donor site is possible.

Split-Thickness Versus Full-Thickness Graft

Split-thickness grafts can be classified as thin (less than 0.008-inch thick), intermediate (0.010- to 0.015-inch thick), or thick (0.015- to 0.025-inch thick), depending on the amount of dermis included. Thin and intermediate-thickness grafts generally do not grow hair well and may have a scaly appearance because of the lack of glandular structures. Thick split-thickness grafts approach full-thickness grafts in depth and therefore grow hair better and result in a more normal appearance. If thick grafts are harvested, the donor site should be excised and closed primarily, if possible, because healing is usually prolonged, and hair growth may be poor.

Full-thickness grafts have several advantages over split-thickness grafts. Because full-thickness grafts contain all the adnexal components, they are more likely to resemble normal skin than split-thickness grafts. They also generally grow hair well and are able to withstand trauma as well as the surrounding normal skin. In contrast to split-thickness grafts, no specialized equipment is required to harvest full-thickness grafts. Finally, the success rate with full-thickness grafts is at least as good as that obtained with split-thickness grafts. For these various reasons, I recommend using full-thickness grafts unless donor skin is limited (e.g., large burn wounds or multiple degloving injuries). Therefore, the rest of this discussion is limited to a practical full-thickness mesh grafting technique that I have used almost exclusively.

Surgical Technique

The mesh grafting procedure involves four basic steps: 1) preparing the donor and recipient sites; 2) harvesting the graft from the donor site; 3) meshing the graft; and 4) applying the graft on the recipient bed.

Preparing Donor and Recipient Site

The patient is anesthetized following a standard protocol, and the donor and recipient site are prepared for aseptic surgery. The donor site should be widely clipped in case a plasty procedure is required for closure. The recipient bed is prepared first, so hemorrhage can be controlled before the graft is applied. Strong antiseptic solution should be avoided, but a dilute solution of chlorhexidine (0.05%) does not affect graft "take" and is used routinely.

On fresh granulation beds, the surface is lightly scraped with a scalpel blade to remove any surface debris and to expose capillary ends. On more established granulation beds, a thin layer (0.5 to 2 mm) may be shaved off with a scalpel blade or grafting knife. All epithelium migrating from the wound edge should be removed. At this point, a blood imprint of the recipient site is made if a full-thickness graft is to be used (see later). Finally, saline-moistened sponges are applied to the surface of the recipient bed, and digital pressure is used to control hemorrhage. Excessive use of cautery or ligatures should be avoided.

Donor sites for full-thickness grafts usually are abundant. Large grafts can be harvested by the technique described here, and the donor site can be closed primarily. The first step is to make a pattern of the defect if a nonexpanded technique is to be used. A pattern can be made by obtaining a blood imprint of the recipient site after it is prepared as described previously. After the pattern is made, it is placed on the donor site, with care taken not to reverse the pattern (i.e., turning the pattern over so the dermal side is up and a mirror image of the needed graft is harvested). The pattern should also be placed so the direction of hair growth of the graft matches that of the skin surrounding the wound. A skin scribe, sterile new methylene blue, or a scalpel blade can be used to transfer the pattern to the skin before cutting the graft. This is done so the borders of the pattern can still be followed if the skin is distorted while the graft is being cut.

If the wound edges are fairly regular (e.g., rectangular) or if the graft will be expanded, an exact pattern is not necessary. For nonexpanded grafts, the length and width of the defect are measured at their widest point, and a segment of skin of those dimensions is harvested. Excess skin is trimmed from the edge after the graft is placed on the recipient site. When expanded grafts are needed, the graft should be cut longer in the direction parallel with the mesh incisions to account for the loss of length that occurs as the graft is expanded.

The graft can be harvested from the donor site by one of two techniques. In the first technique, the dermis of the graft is dissected from the underlying subcutaneous tissue as the graft is being harvested. I find this

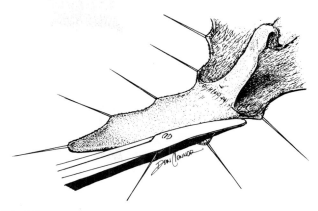

Fig. 37.26. The graft is sutured, subcutaneous side up, to a piece of sterile cardboard, and the subcutaneous tissue is removed with sharp scissors. The base of the hair follicles should be visible in a properly prepared graft.

technique tedious, and frequently some subcutaneous tissue is left on the graft and must be removed. In the second technique, the graft is harvested at the level of the superficial subcutaneous tissue; after the graft is dissected free from the donor site, the subcutaneous tissue is removed. Removal of the subcutaneous tissue is enhanced by suturing the graft, dermal side up, to a piece of sterile cardboard with silk sutures (Fig. 37.26). Sharp scissors are then used to cut the subcutaneous tissue from the graft. The base of the hair follicles is visible when the subcutaneous tissue is removed, giving the graft a cobblestone appearance. Because the hair follicles extend into the subcutaneous tissue in part of the hair growth cycle, the hair follicles may be damaged and hair growth reduced. Failure to remove all the subcutaneous tissue impairs revascularization of the graft and is an important cause of graft loss.

Meshing the Graft

Meshing can be accomplished with a No. 11 scalpel blade or a mesh dermatome. If a scalpel is used, the graft is left attached to the sterile cardboard, and staggered rows of parallel slits (approximately 0.5 to 1 cm in length) are cut in the graft (Fig. 37.27). The length of the slits determines the degree of expansion. If a mesh dermatome is used, the graft is placed dermal side down on the mesher, and a Teflon roller is used to cut the slits (Fig. 37.28). The mesher most commonly used in veterinary surgery produces a 3:1 maximum expansion ratio.

Application of the Graft

After the skin graft is harvested and prepared as previously described, it is placed on the recipient bed. To

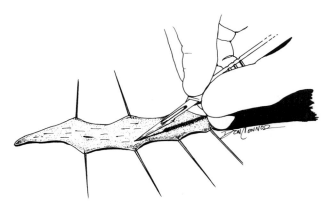

Fig. 37.27. Meshing graft with a No. 11 scalpel blade. The rows of slits are placed, especially if graft will be expanded.

avoid disrupting the fibrin seal that begins to form soon after the graft is placed on the recipient bed, the graft should be manipulated as little as possible. The edge of the graft is sutured to the edge of the recipient bed using either nonabsorbable monofilament suture material or surgical staples. Tacking sutures may be placed between the graft and graft bed on large grafts to help immobilize the graft.

Postoperative Care

Proper postoperative management is essential to successful skin grafting. Complete immobilization of a

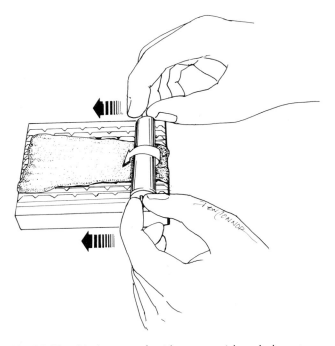

Fig. 37.28. Meshing a graft with commercial mesh dermatome.

graft is necessary until a fibrous union occurs between graft and bed. Immediately after the surgical procedure, the graft is covered with a nonadherent pad (a broad-spectrum antibiotic ointment may be applied on the pad first). A layer of absorbent material (e.g., Telfa WetPruf pads [Kendall Company Hospital Products] or cast padding) is applied next and is covered with elastic gauze. The entire bandage is covered with porous adhesive tape. The bandage should provide moderate pressure. If the graft crosses a joint, the leg should be immobilized with a splint. The dressing usually is changed in 48 hours. Care must be taken not to disturb the graft. Fractious animals should be sedated if necessary.

Because a moderate amount of drainage from the graft bed is common, waiting longer than 48 hours to change the bandage is not recommended. If a large amount of drainage is expected, the bandage can be changed as early as 24 hours after surgery, but the risk of disrupting the fibrin seal between the graft and the recipient bed is increased. Bandages usually are changed every other day for the first 10 days and then as needed for 2 more weeks. Splinting usually can be discontinued after 10 days if the graft has healed normally. Healing grafts normally pass through a series of color changes during the healing process. Initially, a graft appears pale because of the lack of blood supply. After 2 to 3 days, a graft normally develops a dark red or bruised appearance as the blood supply is reestablished. The graft may also appear edematous because of venous congestion. Graft areas that remain white or turn black will probably slough. Unless the entire graft is obviously nonviable, questionable areas are left until healing is complete. Attempts to remove small areas of nonviable graft may disrupt healing of surrounding areas.

Postoperative infection can have devastating results. Infection between the graft and the recipient bed may result in dissolution of the fibrin seal, or the graft may be physically elevated from the graft bed by the exudate produced. Care must be taken not to contaminate the graft when bandages are changed. Full-thickness skin grafts may develop a superficial infection, especially if revascularization is delayed. This generally is the result of the overgrowth of normal skin flora on abnormal skin and does not affect graft take. Infection usually is controlled by swabbing the graft lightly with an antiseptic solution when the bandages are changed and applying a topical antibiotic ointment. Sutures are removed 10 days postoperatively. The patient's owner should be cautioned to watch for developing paresthesia, as evidenced by constant licking and chewing at the graft. This problem is not common, but it is distressing if the patient chews off a successful graft.

Suggested Readings

Converse JM, McCarthy JG, Braue RO, et al. Transplantation of skin: grafts and flaps. In: Converse JM, ed. Reconstructive plastic surgery: principles and procedures in correction, reconstruction and transplantation. Philadelphia: WB Saunders, 1977.

Crabb WC, Smith JW. Basic techniques of plastic surgery. In: Grabb WC, Smith JW, eds. Plastic surgery: a concise guide to clinical practice. 2nd ed. Boston: Little, Brown, 1973.

McGregor IA. Fundamental techniques of plastic surgery. 7th ed. New York: Churchill Livingstone, 1980.

Pope ER, Swaim SF. Wound drainage from under full-thickness skin grafts in dogs. II. Effect on cosmetic appearance. Vet Surg 1986;15:72.

Probst CW, Peyton LC. Split-thickness skin grafting. In: Bojrab MJ, ed. Current techniques in small animal surgery. 2nd ed. Philadelphia: Lea & Febiger, 1983.

Swaim SF. Surgery of the traumatized skin. In: Swain SF, ed. Surgery of traumatized skin: management and reconstruction in the dog and cat. Philadelphia: WB Saunders, 1980.

Reconstructive Microsurgical Applications

J. David Fowler

Reconstructive microsurgery refers to the use of the operating microscope and microvascular technique in facilitating reconstruction of difficult or complex wounds. The premise of reconstructive microsurgery involves harvesting autogenous tissue from a body part distant to the wound, transferring that tissue into the wound bed for reconstruction, and reestablishing the transferred tissue's blood supply by microvascular anastomosis of vessels feeding the flap to vessels adjacent to the wound bed. Tissues transferred in this manner are most commonly termed "free flaps." Microvascular tissue transfer, free tissue transfer, and vascularized grafts are terms also used to refer to microsurgically transplanted tissue.

Free flaps are further described according to the tissue or tissues comprising the flap. Cutaneous free flaps refer to flaps incorporating skin and subcutaneous tissue. Free muscle flaps, omental flaps, jejunal flaps, and autogenous vascularized bone grafts are other examples of tissue transfers incorporating a single tissue type. Compound flaps incorporate more than one tissue type and are described accordingly. Myocutaneous flaps incorporate both muscle and skin; myo-osseous flaps incorporate muscle and bone; osteomusculocutaneous flaps incorporate bone, muscle, and skin.

Successful application of microvascular tissue transfer was first reported in human patients in the early 1960s. The development of instrumentation, suture, and needles appropriate to the repair of small vessels

was a prerequisite. Throughout the 1970s and 1980s, a plethora of manuscripts detailing microvascular flaps and techniques in human patients appeared in the literature. Free tissue transfer is now strongly integrated into orthopedic and reconstructive surgery.

Veterinary reconstructive microsurgery is comparatively in its infancy. However, several microvascular flaps have been described experimentally and have been applied clinically to reconstructive problems in dogs. The purpose of this discussion is to detail the latest developments in veterinary reconstructive microsurgery and to provide the reader with some insight into future potential applications.

Recipient Site Requirements

Tissues used in free flaps vary according to the requirements of the recipient wound. A detailed assessment of the wound bed should be performed to obtain an optimal outcome after reconstruction. One of the greatest advantages of microvascular tissue transfer is the ability to select from various tissues and donor sites to best suit the patient's specific reconstructive requirements. Timing of reconstruction may also vary according to the status of the wound or exposure of vital structures.

Vascular supply is paramount to successful wound healing. Complex and high-velocity impact wounds are often associated with extensive vascular disruption. Loss of blood supply delays wound healing and increases the incidence of complications, especially in instances of orthopedic injury with associated soft tissue disruption (1). Adequate debridement of devitalized tissue, followed by vascular enhancement through early reconstruction, is beneficial in these patients. Muscle is most efficacious in the revascularization of ischemic wound beds (2–6). Free microvascular transfer of muscle into the wound bed assists in neovascularization of the wound and provides a source of systemic factors reducing the incidence of wound sepsis.

Structural requirements of the recipient site must also be considered in selecting appropriate tissues for microvascular transfer. In the simplest of cases, the wound may simply require a volume of tissue to replace a tissue deficit. This may be accomplished using various tissues and flaps. The specific selection of donor site depends, in these instances, on ease of access and volume of tissue required. More complex wounds, such as segmental bone loss, may have specific structural requirements that are the major determining factors in selection of donor tissue.

Functional requirements of the recipient site frequently play a role in determining the optimal donor tissue. For example, little benefit results from reconstructing a wound with loss of a vital functional muscle group unless that function is restored. Functional muscle transfer has not been reported clinically in the dog, but is used in human patients for facial reanimation and restoration of flexor function after forearm trauma (7, 8). The functional requirements of weight-bearing surfaces are particularly problematic after extensive injury to the footpads. Reconstruction using "like tissue" is ideal in such circumstances. Sensory reinnervation, although not of certain necessity, may also be accomplished through the use of a neurovascular free flap that incorporates a sensory nerve as well as a vascular pedicle. Sensory nerve repair of the donor nerve to an appropriate recipient nerve may assist in the ultimate protection of the transferred tissue against ongoing weight-bearing stresses.

Donor Site Selection

Selection of an appropriate donor tissue depends on the requirements of the recipient site. Factors to consider in the specific selection of a donor site include ease of surgical dissection, morbidity associated with loss of the donor tissue, matching of donor tissue to recipient requirements, and the ability to access both donor and recipient sites simultaneously. Free tissue transfer has been described as the art of "robbing Peter to pay Paul." The surgeon must ensure that Peter does, in fact, have what Paul needs and that, by stealing it, Peter will not suffer undue consequences.

Technical Considerations

Successful free tissue transfer depends on detailed advance planning. Familiarity of the surgical team with the procedure, patient positioning, stability of the patient under anesthesia, and selection and preparation of recipient vessels all may affect outcome.

Angiosomes

An angiosome is defined as a region of tissue or tissues perfused by a single-source artery and vein (Fig. 37.29) (9). Adjacent angiosomes are interconnected by vessels termed choke anastomoses. These communications are of obvious biologic advantage. After vascular injury, an angiosome normally dependent on the injured vessel generally receives adequate vascular supply from adjacent angiosomes. However, anatomic continuity of angiosomes does not necessarily ensure physiologic continuity of vascular supply in the event of vascular injury.

The concept of the angiosome is central to the development of free tissue flaps. Tissue incorporated in a free flap should lie, ideally, entirely within the primary angiosome of the source artery and vein, to ensure

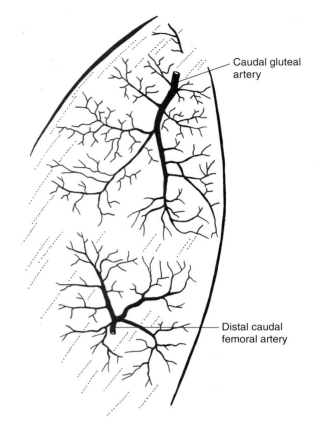

Fig. 37.29. The biceps femoris muscle contains two distinct angiosomes. The proximal half of the muscle is vascularized by the caudal gluteal artery and vein, whereas the distal half of the muscle is vascularized by the distal caudal femoral artery and vein.

survival after revascularization. Demonstration of tissue survival beyond the primary angiosome has been demonstrated with cutaneous axial pattern pedicle flaps and with some pedicled muscle flaps (10–12). As a general rule, a single, smaller angiosome adjacent to the primary angiosome survives when incorporated into the flap design. Dissection beyond the level of a single secondary angiosome should be considered tenuous and likely to lead to partial flap failure.

Anatomic descriptions of many cutaneous and muscle angiosomes have been provided for the dog, with few specific descriptions for the cat (13–22). Based on this information, as well as on experimental data, several regional angiosomes and free flaps have been described. The importance of understanding the anatomy, consistency, and variability of regional vascular patterns cannot be overstated when undertaking microvascular tissue transfer.

Flap Dissection

The particular approach to flap dissection depends on the tissue harvested. Several guidelines and recommendations are common to dissecting all flaps for microvascular transfer. The tissue to be harvested must be isolated to the level of its source artery and vein. All supporting microvasculature must be preserved during this process. All underlying subcutaneous tissue should be incorporated with cutaneous flap dissections; underlying superficial cutaneous musculature should be incorporated in regions where such musculature exists. For example, the cutaneus trunci muscle should be incorporated with elevation of the thoracodorsal cutaneous flap. Muscle is readily dissected because of surrounding fascial sheaths. A soft tissue envelope is incorporated with dissection of vascularized bone grafts to preserve myoperiosteal vasculature. The reader should consult references pertaining to specific flaps, as well as the first section of this chapter, for details of surgical harvest.

Tissue is generally elevated beginning at a site distant to the vascular pedicle. Flap dissection is then continued until the source artery and vein are identified. Bleeding vessels encountered during this process should be meticulously controlled with bipolar electrocoagulation, suture ligation, or vascular clips. Once the vascular pedicle is identified, the artery and vein are skeletonized. Small branches encountered during vascular dissection may be electrocoagulated or clipped with vascular clips, depending on size. The surgeon must avoid damage to the intima of the parent vessel by excessive traction on small vascular branches or aggressive electrocautery. As much surrounding adventitia as possible should be removed during initial dissection of the vascular pedicle. Surgical loupes providing a magnification of 3× to 4× facilitate identification of fine anatomic detail and atraumatic dissection of the vascular pedicle.

The length of vascular pedicle depends primarily on the anatomy of the donor flap. As a general rule, as much length as possible should be included with the initial vascular dissection. Excess length may be trimmed after transfer to the recipient site. A minimum vascular pedicle length of 1 cm is preferred, to allow manipulation of vessels during microanastomosis.

To minimize flap ischemia time, the vascular pedicle should not be ligated and divided before preparation of the recipient site. At that time, the artery and vein are independently ligated with vascular clips and are transected using fine vascular scissors.

Recipient Site Preparation

The recipient site should be free of devitalized tissue or active infection. Judicious debridement and lavage should be used to minimize contamination and necrotic tissue in open wounds. Early reconstruction of open wounds using vascularized tissues minimizes the risk of wound complications. In my experience, most open wounds can be converted to a state suitable for microvascular reconstruction within 48 hours of injury. Minimal debridement should be required at the time of microsurgical reconstruction. The wound bed may be lavaged preoperatively with an antibacterial solution, such as 0.05% chlorhexidine gluconate, to decrease bacterial contamination.

Recipient vessels, appropriate for anastomosis to the artery and vein of the flap to be transferred, must be identified and dissected. A knowledge of regional vascular anatomy is obviously a prerequisite. In patients with severe trauma, or a past history of trauma or surgery involving the affected area, preoperative angiography should be considered to identify variations in vascular anatomy. Recipient vessels should approximate the diameter of donor vessels, assuming end-to-end anastomosis. End-to-side technique is often used for arterial anastomosis, to preserve arterial supply distal to the wound. In this event, the recipient artery should be of larger diameter than the donor artery. Recipient vessels should be dissected beyond the wound's zone of trauma. The surgical approach used for vascular dissection should involve elevation of a skin flap such that the incision will not directly overlie the vascular anastomosis after skin closure.

The free flap is secured at the recipient site before initiating microvascular anastomosis. In the case of soft tissue flaps, this is accomplished using a few strategically placed simple interrupted sutures. Cutaneous flaps are sutured under minimal tension. Muscle flaps are sutured under sufficient tension to approximate their initial resting length at the donor site. Vascularized bone grafts are stabilized using suitable orthopedic fixation. Microvascular anastomosis of the donor and recipient artery and vein is then completed using an operating microscope and standard microvascular technique. Approximating clamps are not released until the completion of both artery and vein repair.

Pedicle length must be planned to avoid excessive length and redundancy of the pedicle or insufficient length resulting in tension or kinking. The vascular pedicle must be carefully positioned to avoid compression of the anastomosed vessels during closure. The venous pedicle is particularly sensitive to these effects. The vascular pedicle is assessed for patency, and remaining sutures are placed between the flap and the recipient wound bed. Patency should be reassessed before final skin closure. Total operative time is minimized by using two surgical teams. One team harvests the donor tissue while the second simultaneously prepares the recipient site.

Flap Perfusion and Anticoagulation

Uncomplicated free tissue transfer generally requires approximately 4 hours of general anesthesia. More complicated procedures, such as those requiring orthopedic fixation, may necessitate 6 to 10 hours of general anesthesia. Adequate flap perfusion depends on maintaining the cardiovascular stability of the patient during the operative and postoperative periods. Intravenous fluid support during and after surgery is an absolute requirement.

Hypothermia must be controlled to avoid peripheral vasoconstriction and deleterious effects on flap perfusion. Patients are maintained on circulating water blankets, and temperature is monitored both during and after the surgical procedure. A heat lamp may be placed over the flap during the immediate postoperative period, before the patient's recovery from anesthesia. Bandaging of flaps using a lightly applied, heavily padded bandage protects the flap from trauma and assists in trapping body heat.

No consistent recommendation exists on the use of antithrombotic agents before, during, or after microvascular tissue transfer. The most critical factor in preventing thrombosis of the microvascular anastomosis is appropriate surgical technique, and no amount of antithrombotic therapy can salvage a poorly performed anastomosis. Heparin and saline (10 units heparin per 1 mL saline) are used topically at the anastomotic site to clear the lumen of vessels before anastomosis. Other antithrombotic therapy is determined by the preference of the surgeon and identified patient risk factors.

Aspirin may be used at a dose of 5 to 10 mg/kg body weight preoperatively, to inhibit platelet aggregation (23). I routinely administer dextran 40 at a dose of 10 mL/kg body weight intraoperatively. Dextran administration expands the vascular space, thereby improving flap perfusion, and it may have an inhibitory effect on platelet function (24). Anticoagulation using systemic heparin is rarely indicated.

Tolerated flap ischemia times vary according to the tissue transferred (25–27). Skin is considered resistant to the detrimental effects of ischemia and reperfusion. Cutaneous free flaps tolerate 6 to 8 hours of warm (room temperature) ischemia before the onset of significant injury. Muscle is sensitive to ischemia and reperfusion and may demonstrate detrimental effects after 2 to 4 hours of warm ischemia. Total ischemia times in clinical free tissue transfer rarely exceed these time frames. In my experience, flap ischemia times have varied from 60 to 180 minutes.

Occasionally, a flap fails to perfuse after an apparently successful microvascular anastomosis. This is termed a "no-reflow" phenomenon and may be attributed to many causes. In this event, the vascular pedicle extending from the anastomotic site to the flap should be inspected under the operating microscope. Active bleeding through any previously unidentified branches from the pedicle is controlled with vascular clips. Specific attention is paid to areas of potential vascular injury and vasospasm. If a region of vasospasm is identified, 2% lidocaine is placed topically on the vessel. If focal vasospasm persists, then damage to the vessel may be assumed, and microvascular anastomosis should be repeated distal to this site. No reflow may occasionally be caused by inappropriate or traumatic dissection of the flap, with subsequent injury to the supportive microvasculature. This problem is easily avoided through meticulous attention to flap dissection. Little can be done to rectify the situation after its occurrence. Extended ischemia time may lead to reperfusion injury and subsequent occlusion of venous microvasculature by neutrophil adhesion. Therapy aimed at alleviating ischemia–reperfusion injury is indicated, but it is of questionable benefit after the period of reperfusion.

Postoperative Monitoring

Free flaps entirely depend on the integrity of the microvascular anastomsoses. Free flap failure may be caused by venous or arterial thrombosis, either of which must be recognized early and investigated aggressively if the flap is to be salvaged. Venous failure of cutaneous flaps is most easily recognized by the onset of congestion in the flap (Fig. 37.30). A purplish–blue discoloration is noted. Bandaged flaps may be assessed by creating a window in the bandage to allow visualization of a portion of the flap. Flaps tolerate venous outflow occlusion poorly. At the earliest indication of this problem, the patient should be returned to the operating room, and the vascular pedicle should be dissected using the operating microscope. Careful attention is paid during the approach to look for evidence of vessel compression or kinking caused by positioning of the vascular pedicle or restrictive skin closure. If this is the case, the anastomosis may actually be patent, and the problem is addressed by simple repositioning of the pedicle or release of the overlying skin incision. In the event of a thrombosed anastomosis, the region of thrombosis is excised, and venous effluent from the flap is documented. Once flow through the flap is established, venous anastomosis is repeated. Sluggish venous outflow may also be treated by application of medicinal leeches. Leeches reduce flap congestion by direct ingestion of blood and by promoting continued hemorrhage from bite wounds resulting from local infusion of hirudin (28).

Arterial failure can be more difficult to diagnose because it is not associated initially with overt color change of the flap. Flap temperature can be monitored; a drop in temperature indicates arterial insufficiency. This method is unreliable in bandaged flaps, because

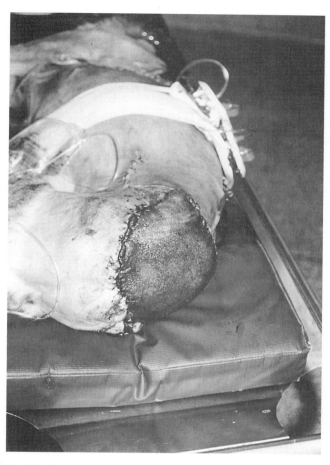

Fig. 37.30. A latissimus dorsi myocutaneous flap has been used to reconstruct a large deficit over the rear quarters in this dog. Venous compromise of the flap is visually apparent because of the onset of congestion and purplish discoloration of the flap. Reexploration of the venous pedicle and, possibly, medicinal leech therapy are indicated.

the bandage traps body heat and artificially elevates flap temperature. Doppler flow probes may be used to monitor arterial patency more reliably in the postoperative period. A window is created in the bandage overlying the arterial pedicle distal to the anastomosis. A pencil Doppler probe is then easily inserted through the window to monitor arterial patency. Bleeding may be a useful indicator of flap perfusion. Cutaneous flaps are punctured with a 20- or 22-gauge hypodermic needle and are monitored for active bleeding from the site. More specialized monitoring techniques such as laser Doppler flowmetry or fluorescein clearance have been described, but they are usually beyond the realm of clinical necessity.

Monitoring of flaps that do not incorporate a cutaneous component is more difficult. Doppler techniques are useful for monitoring arterial adequacy in such flaps. Venous monitoring is difficult or impossi-

ble. Vascularized bone grafts should be assessed using [^{99m}]technetium scintigraphy within 5 days of operation.

Free Flaps in the Dog and Cat

Several free flaps have been described experimentally, clinically, or both in the dog and cat. Other flaps have been described as pedicled flaps, maintaining a vascular attachment to the donor site. These flaps may be used reliably for free transfer as well, assuming adequate dimensions of the vascular pedicle. Vessel diameters for most described flaps in the dog approximate 1 to 2 mm. Vessel diameters of less than 0.5 mm are associated with increased rates of anastomotic thrombosis.

Cutaneous Flaps

Cutaneous angiosomes have been described extensively, and anatomic landmarks for dissection of pedicled cutaneous axial pattern flaps are well documented. Axial pattern skin flaps may be used for free transfer as well.

The superficial cervical axial pattern flap, based on the direct cutaneous pedicle of the prescapular branch of the superficial cervical artery and vein, has been documented as a free flap in a series of cases (Fig. 37.31) (29, 30). The vascular pedicle perforates the septum formed by the omotransversarius, cleidocervicalis, and trapezius muscles. The cutaneous angiosome extends dorsally from the point of origin to the midline and roughly incorporates the caudal two-thirds of the cervical skin in a craniocaudal direction. The amount of skin harvested for transfer is determined, first, by the requirements of the recipient site and, second, by the ability to close the donor site primarily.

I have also used the caudal superficial epigastric axial pattern flap sporadically for microvascular transfer. The primary advantage of selecting an axial pattern skin flap for microvascular transfer is ease of dissection. Disadvantages include excessive bulk from inclusion of associated subcutaneous tissue and poor cosmetic result caused by differential hair growth characteristics between donor and recipient sites.

The saphenous fasciocutaneous free flap has been documented in experimental and clinical cases (28, 31). The flap is based on the medial saphenous artery and vein and includes the skin overlying the medial aspect of the thigh (Fig. 37.32). Flap dissection includes the superficial fascia of the medial gastrocnemius muscle, giving the flap its designation as fasciocutaneous. Numerous small direct cutaneous vessels arise from the saphenous vessels as they course through the flap. The saphenous fasciocutaneous flap

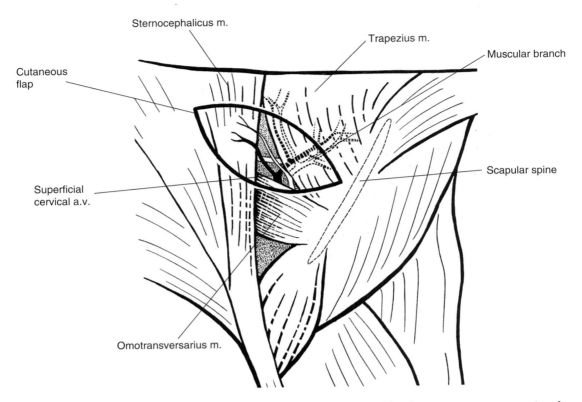

Fig. 37.31. The anatomy of the superficial cervical cutaneous free flap is indicated. The direct cutaneous artery arises from a septum formed by the trapezius, omotransversarius, and sternocephalicus muscles. The muscular branch to the cervical portion of the trapezius muscle also arises from the superficial cervical artery.

has the advantage of less bulk and improved cosmetic results compared with other free axial pattern skin flaps. The width of the flap is limited by the ability to close the donor site primarily.

Muscle Flaps

Muscle probably has the greatest utility of any tissue used for microsurgical reconstruction. Muscle flaps are, for the most part, easily dissected. Most muscles may be harvested with minimal donor site morbidity because of the function of synergic muscle groups. Neovascularization of compromised wound beds is facilitated to a greater degree by muscle than by other tissues. Finally, donor muscles may be selected that closely match the dimensional and functional requirements of nearly any wound reconstruction.

The angiosomes of muscles may be classified into one of five types (Fig. 37.33). Type I muscles have a single dominant vascular pedicle. Type II muscles have a single dominant pedicle and one or more minor pedicles. Type III muscles contain two dominant vascular pedicles, each of which has an approximately equal contribution to the muscle's blood supply. Type IV muscles have a segmental blood supply formed by numerous small pedicles of approximately equal contribution. Type V muscles have a single dominant vascu-

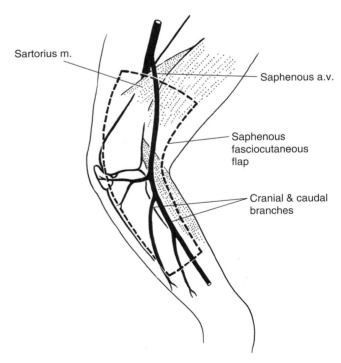

Fig. 37.32. The saphenous fasciocutaneous flap is composed of skin and underlying fascia overlying the medial aspect of the thigh and tibia. The flap is based on the medial saphenous artery and vein. Inclusion of the caudal sartorius muscle is possible, by preservation of muscular branches from the saphenous vessels.

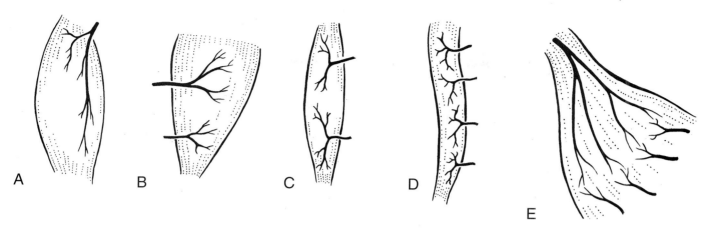

Fig. 37.33. Diagrammatic representation of the five basic vascular patterns to skeletal muscles. **A.** Type I muscles have a single vascular supply. **B.** Type II muscles have one dominant pedicle and one or more minor pedicles. **C.** Type III muscles contain two equally dominant pedicles. **D.** Type IV muscles have a segmental blood supply derived from numerous small pedicles. **E.** Type V muscles have a single dominant pedicle near their insertion and a second segmental system near their origin. Type IV muscles are the least suitable for microvascular application.

lar pedicle near their insertion and a segmental system near the origin of the muscle. Based on assumptions of physiologic blood supply through angiosomes, one can surmise that any type I muscle will survive entirely after free transfer based on the single dominant pedicle. Most type II muscles willl survive based on the dominant pedicle, depending on the number and relative contribution of the minor pedicles. Type III muscles are expected to survive after free transfer based on either dominant pedicle system. Type V muscles generally will survive based only on the single dominant pedicle. Type IV muscles are generally poor candidates for microvascular transfer because of the large number and small contribution of each pedicle system to the muscle's blood supply. Detailed descriptions of the vascular supply to muscles of the dog have been published (21, 22). The foregoing assumptions given serve as guidelines only. The ultimate reliability of any muscle in reconstructive microsurgery is proved only through experimental or clinical trials that establish its utility. If at all possible, muscle transfers should be limited to single angiosomes or previously documented free flaps.

TRAPEZIUS MUSCLE FLAP

The vascular supply of the cervical portion of the trapezius muscle has been thoroughly described, as has the entire angiosome of the prescapular branch of the superficial cervical artery and vein (Fig. 37.34) (32). The cervical portion of the trapezius muscle has a type II vascular supply, with the prescapular branch of the superficial cervical artery forming the dominant pedicle. Experimentally and clinically, survival of the entire cervical portion of the muscle has been consis-

tently documented based solely on this dominant pedicle.

Dissection of the trapezius muscle flap is through a curvilinear incision beginning approximately 2 to 3 cm cranial to the point of the shoulder, extending dorsally parallel to the scapular spine and curving cranially below the dorsal midline (33). Skin and subcutaneous tissue are dissected from the superficial fascia of the muscle, with care taken to identify and ligate the direct cutaneous branch as it exits the septum formed by the trapezius, omotransversarius, and cleidocervicalis muscles. The cervical portion of the trapezius muscle is sharply incised from its attachment to the scapular spine. Fascial attachments dorsally are incised, and the muscle is elevated carefully. Several muscle branches extending into deep musculature of the neck are identified and are ligated with vascular clips. At this point, the vascular pedicle should be located. The location of the pedicle is variable as it courses deep to the trapezius muscle. It is most commonly located immediately beneath the cranial border of the muscle coursing from ventral to dorsal. In a few instances, the vascular pedicle lies immediately cranial to the cranial border of the trapezius muscle and gives off several smaller muscular branches to the muscle as it extends dorsally. Dissection in these patients must be performed with caution, to preserve the integrity of the vascular pedicle. After identification of the prescapular branch of the superficial cervical artery and vein, remaining muscle attachments are dissected. One or two small muscular branches to the omotransversarius muscle are identified and clipped, and the artery and vein are skeletonized and dissected for a length of at least 2 to 3 cm. The prescapular lymph node is intimately associated

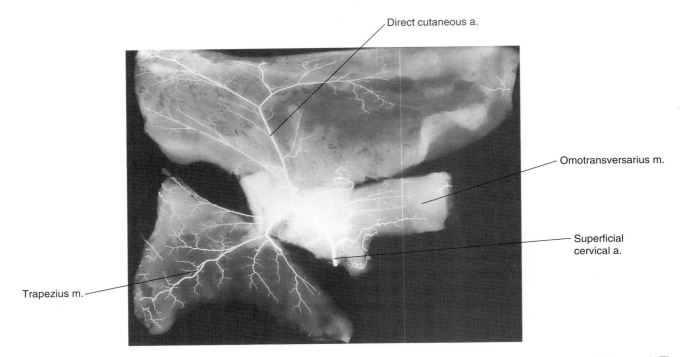

Direct cutaneous a.

Omotransversarius m.

Superficial
cervical a.

Trapezius m.

Fig. 37.34. Barium has been infused into the superficial cervical artery to demonstrate the regional angiosome of this vessel. The superficial cervical artery gives rise to the dominant pedicle of the cervical portion of the trapezius muscle, the superficial cervical direct cutaneous artery, and a minor pedicle to the omotransversarius muscle. Any or all of these tissues may be included in a microvascular flap based on this vascular pedicle.

with the vascular pedicle and may either be included with the pedicle or carefully excised.

I used the trapezius muscle free flap for distal extremity reconstruction in a series of 20 cases. The trapezius muscle is broad and flat, lending itself well to conformation to many wound beds. Bulk of the flap is minimal and decreases dramatically over the course of several weeks because of denervation atrophy. Despite denervation atrophy, transferred muscle maintains a constant vascular density beneficial to the wound bed. The trapezius muscle is resurfaced using a full-thickness skin graft harvested from a donor site with hair growth characteristics similar to those of the recipient site. This technique has resulted in improved cosmetic results, compared with cutaneous or musculocutaneous free flaps (Fig. 37.35). Seroma formation at the donor site is common and should be managed with drain placement for 5 to 7 days.

LATISSIMUS DORSI MUSCLE FLAP
The latissimus dorsi muscle has, historically, been the workhorse for microsurgical reconstruction of complex distal extremity wounds in human patients. Pedicled latissimus dorsi muscle flaps have been used for chest wall reconstruction and experimental cardiomyoplasty in the dog and have been described experimentally for microsurgical transfer in the cat (34). The latissimus dorsi muscle reliably survives in its entirety

based solely on the dominant thoracodorsal artery and vein, which enter the deep surface of the muscle near its insertion (Fig. 37.36). The muscle is approached through a curvilinear skin incision beginning at the axilla and extending dorsally and caudally to the level of the muscle's origin. Skin and subcutaneous tissues are dissected from the superficial muscle fascia, with care taken to identify and ligate the direct cutaneous branch of the vascular pedicle, located near the caudal shoulder depression. The origin of the latissimus muscle is identified and is sharply incised. Muscle elevation reveals numerous small muscular branches extending from the intercostal arteries. Segmental pedicles are cauterized or ligated and are transected as they are encountered. Dissection continues toward the muscle's insertion, and the dominant thoracodorsal artery and vein are identified on the deep surface of the muscle. After identification of the vascular pedicle, the muscle's tendon of insertion is transected, and the thoracodorsal artery and vein are skeletonized for a length of at least 2 to 3 cm. The cat occasionally has a minor pedicle originating from the lateral thoracic artery and vein, which enter the deep surface of the muscle ventrally near its tendon of insertion. This pedicle must be identified and ligated. The thoracodorsal pedicle in the cat has a diameter of approximately 0.4 mm, making microvascular anastomosis difficult. Dissection in the cat is therefore continued to the level

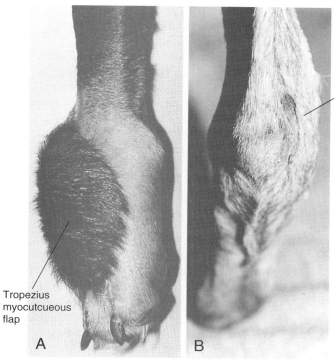

Trapezius muscle
flap & skin graft

Tropezius
myocutcueous
flap

A   B

Fig. 37.35. **A.** Cosmetic results are less than optimal after reconstruction using the trapezius myocutaneous flap because of the excessive subcutaneous bulk and poor match of hair characteristics. **B.** Contour and hair characteristics are much more closely matched by using the trapezius muscle flap and resurfacing with a full-thickness skin graft.

of the origin of the subscapular artery and vein from the axillary vessels to facilitate subsequent anastomosis.

The dimensions of the latissimus dorsi muscle exceed the requirements of most wound beds in the dog. Its clinical use therefore has been sporadic. The latissimus dorsi muscle is useful as a free flap in patients with massive soft tissue loss secondary to trauma or ablative cancer surgery. I have used the latissimus dorsi free flap for cranial reconstruction after partial craniectomy and orbitectomy for a sebaceous adeno-

carcinoma in a dog and for reconstruction of a massive rear limb degloving injury with associated orthopedic trauma. Clinical experience with this flap, however, is limited.

Vascularized Bone Grafts

The veterinary literature has no clinical reports, and few experimental descriptions, of autogenous vascularized bone grafts. Numerous reports of vascularized canine bone grafts appear as experimental models in the human literature. The indications, contraindications, and clinical utility of nonvascularized cortical bone grafts are well established. Nonvascularized cortical bone grafts provide immediate structural support in orthopedic reconstruction. Ultimate success depends on revascularization of the cortical graft from the wound bed, followed by gradual resorption and new bone deposition. This process requires years to complete and depends on a favorable wound environment. Osteomyelitis, structural weakening of the graft, and delayed healing of graft–bone interfaces are common complications.

Autogenous vascularized bone grafts are advantageous in that they maintain a vascular supply and, therefore, viability of cellular elements within the graft. Graft bone actively contributes to bone healing and remodeling. Vascularized grafts are more resistant to infection than nonvascularized grafts, lending themselves to the reconstruction of large segmental

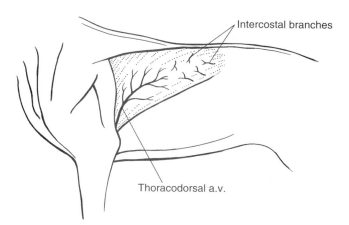

Intercostal branches

Thoracodorsal a.v.

Fig. 37.36. The latissimus dorsi flap is based on the dominant thoracodorsal vascular pedicle. The entire muscle survives based on this dominant pedicle.

defects or vascularly compromised wound beds. Vascularized bone grafts described in the dog include rib, fibula, proximal ulna, and distal ulna (35).

VASCULARIZED FIBULA GRAFT

The canine fibula graft has been used as an experimental model for the study of vascularized bone graft biology (Fig. 37.37) (36). The popliteal artery branches into a larger cranial tibial and a smaller caudal tibial artery. The caudal tibial artery enters the interosseous space between the fibula and tibia and is intimately associated with the flexor hallucis longus muscle. The nutrient artery of the fibula arises from the caudal tibial artery and enters the fibula medially in its central third. Dissection of the fibula is performed to maintain a surrounding muscle cuff. Particular care is taken to preserve the flexor hallucis longus muscle with the graft. Subperiosteal dissection of the tibia is required to preserve vasculature within the interosseous space. The fibula may be transferred based either on the cau-

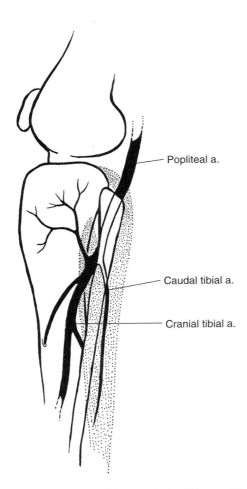

Fig. 37.37. The anatomy of the vascularized fibula graft is demonstrated. The fibula may be harvested based on the caudal tibial artery. Dissection to the level of the popliteal artery gives rise to a more manageable pedicle for microvascular anastomosis, but it necessitates ligation of the cranial tibial artery.

dal tibial artery or on the popliteal artery. Dissection to the level of the popliteal artery necessitates ligation and transection of the cranial tibial artery. Use of the caudal tibial artery as a pedicle may be limited by the diameter of these vessels. Iatrogenic damage to the peroneal nerve must be avoided during proximal dissection of the graft and vascular pedicle. The vascularized fibula graft has not been used clinically in the dog and likely has limited utility for segmental long bone reconstruction because of its poor structural integrity.

VASCULARIZED RIB GRAFT

Microsurgical transfer of the rib has been used in the dog as an experimental model for bone transfer (37). Either the dorsal or the ventral part of the intercostal vascular system may be used as a vascular pedicle for rib transfer. Inclusion of the nutrient artery with the transfer mandates dorsal dissection. Ventrally dissected grafts survive based on an intact musculoperiosteal vascular supply. The dorsal intercostal arteries arise from the thoracic aorta. Immediately before entering the intercostal space, a dorsal branch supplying the spinal cord and epaxial muscles is given off. The nutrient artery branches from the dorsal intercostal artery just distal to the tubercle of the rib and extends dorsally to enter the nutrient foramen. The dorsal intercostal artery continues distally in the costal groove on the caudal aspect of the rib, giving off numerous periosteal branches. A lateral cutaneous branch is formed from the dorsal intercostal artery before its anastomosis with the ventral intercostal artery. Intercostal veins parallel the arterial supply, with eventual drainage into the azygous vein. Clinical utility of the rib graft likely will be limited by its curvature and weak structural characteristics. Vascularized rib grafts may prove to have some usefulness in mandibular reconstruction, although this remains to be documented.

VASCULARIZED PROXIMAL ULNA GRAFT

The canine ulna may be harvested with little resulting functional impairment to limb use. This fact, along with the obvious structural integrity of the ulna, makes it a logical choice for segmental long bone reconstruction. The proximal ulna bone graft is harvested based on the common interosseous vascular pedicle (38). The common interosseous artery arises from the median artery at the level of the proximal radius, immediately enters the interosseous space from the medial side, and bifurcates into caudal and cranial interosseous branches. The caudal interosseous artery continues distally in the interosseous space, where it gives rise to the nutrient arteries of the radius and ulna, as well as to multiple periosteal branches. The nutrient artery of the ulna enters near the junction of the proximal and central thirds of the bone. The cranial interosseous artery emerges from the interosseous space laterally, where it gives rise to muscular branches to the extensor carpi ulnaris and the lateral and common digital extensor muscles.

Dissection of the proximal ulna graft is performed through a curvilinear caudolateral skin incision. Fasciotomy of the flexor and extensor muscle groups facilitates muscle dissection and identification of vascular structures. Separation between the extensor carpi ulnaris and the lateral digital extensor muscles proximally reveals vascular branches to these muscles. These muscular branches serve as a consistent landmark indicating the level of the vascular pedicle of the flap (Fig. 37.38). The lateral radial periosteum is incised along the cranial surface of the abductor pollicis longus muscle, and subperiosteal dissection of the radius is continued into the interosseous space. The medial radial periosteum is similarly incised and elevated. Distal osteotomy of the ulna is then performed using an oscillating bone saw. The caudal interosseous artery and vein are identified within the interosseous space, ligated, and divided. Proximal osteotomy of the ulna is performed proximal to the level of the vascular pedicle. Circumferential subperiosteal dissection of the ulna is performed at this level, and the ulna is osteotomized. Muscular branches to the extensor muscles

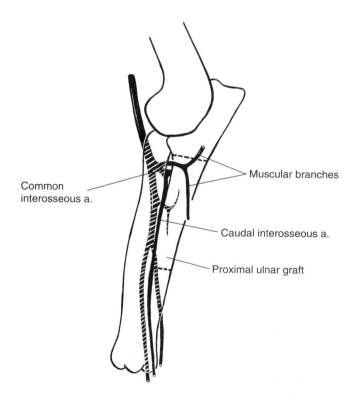

Fig. 37.38. The proximal ulna vascularized bone graft is based on the common interosseous pedicle and preserves both the periosteal and nutrient vascular systems. Muscular branches to extensor muscles indicate the approximate level of the common interosseous pedicle.

Common interosseous a.

Muscular branches

Caudal interosseous a.

Proximal ulnar graft

are ligated and divided. Cautious elevation of the osteotomized ulna reveals the common interosseous pedicle on the medial aspect of the graft. The common interosseous artery and vein are dissected to their point of origin from the median artery and vein.

Advantages of the proximal ulna graft include structural integrity and provision of a nutrient blood supply. Primary disadvantages include the necessity of proximal osteotomy adjacent to the elbow joint, difficult dissection of the vascular pedicle because of its medial location, and limited length of the vascular pedicle. The proximal ulna graft has been documented experimentally, but it has not yet been used clinically in the dog.

VASCULARIZED DISTAL ULNA GRAFT
The distal ulna graft has great potential for clinical use in the dog (39). The approach to initial dissection of the graft is identical to that described for the proximal ulna graft. After fasciotomy of the flexor and extensor muscle groups, the caudal interosseous artery and vein are identified as they exit the interosseous space caudomedially at the level of the distal ulna. These vessels are ligated and transected. The ulna is circumferentially dissected immediately distal to this level and is osteotomized using an oscillating bone saw. Dissection of the medial and lateral radial periosteum is performed as described for the proximal ulna transfer and is continued proximally. Subperiosteal dissection of the radius must be performed with great caution to avoid damage to the caudal interosseous vessels as they course through the interosseous space. The length of graft required for recipient site reconstruction is calculated. Proximal osteotomy is performed after circumferential subperiosteal dissection of the ulna. The proximal osteotomy should be performed such that the resulting length of bone graft is 2 to 3 cm longer than that required for the reconstructive procedure (Fig. 37.39). The caudal interosseous artery and vein are located within the interosseous space, ligated with vascular clips, and transected. Once harvested, the interosseous artery and vein are dissected for a length of approximately 3 cm. The bone graft is then shortened to its required length by osteotomizing that portion of proximal ulna from which the vascular pedicle has been dissected.

The distal ulna graft depends entirely on an intact musculoperiosteal circulation for survival. An intact musculoperiosteal cuff must be included with the dissection, to include the ulnar head of the deep digital flexor, the pronator quadratus, and the abductor pollicis longus muscles. External skeletal fixation is recommended to minimize implant-associated embarrassment of the periosteal vasculature.

The utility of the vascularized distal ulna graft has been demonstrated experimentally (40). I have used

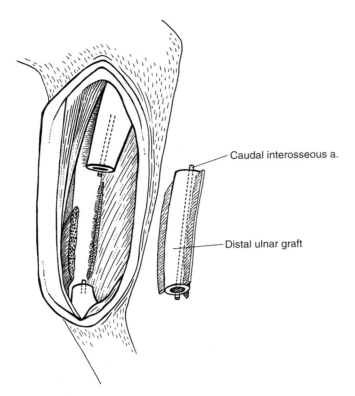

Caudal interosseous a.

Distal ulnar graft

Fig. 37.39. The distal ulna vascularized bone graft is based on the caudal interosseous artery and vein. Dissection preserves only the periosteal vascular supply. Inclusion of a surrounding muscle cuff is required to preserve this blood supply.

the distal ulna graft for reconstruction of the distal radius after limb-sparing surgery for osteosarcoma and for reconstruction of a mandibular nonunion and segmental defect caused by a gunshot injury.

Compound Flaps

Compound free flaps incorporate tissues of more than one type. They may be useful for the reconstruction of complex trauma involving loss of multiple tissue types. A detailed knowledge of vascular anatomy allows the surgeon the flexibility of designing many compound flaps.

Musculocutaneous flaps combine both muscle and skin in the transfer. The superficial cervical axial pattern skin flap may easily be included with the cervical portion of the trapezius muscle by maintaining the direct cutaneous branch rather than by ligating it during dissection. The vascular supply to both muscle and skin is based on the prescapular branch of the superficial cervical artery and vein. Similarly, the thoracodorsal axial pattern skin flap may be incorporated with the latissimus dorsi muscle flap. Dissection of musculocutaneous free flaps must be carefully planned to include appropriate dimensions of the cutaneous com-

ponent. With inclusion of an axial pattern skin flap, the cutaneous component may be used to overlie the transferred muscle directly and to reconstruct an associated cutaneous defect. The axial pattern skin flap may also be dissected free of the muscle flap, with care taken to maintain the direct cutaneous artery and vein. This allows use of both the muscle and cutaneous components for reconstruction of adjacent portions of large wound beds (Fig. 37.40).

Myo-osseous flaps incorporate both muscle and bone. By strict definition, all vascularized bone grafts may be considered myo-osseous because of the preservation of an intact musculoperiosteal cuff. However, the term is recognized to designate the inclusion of a significant muscle component used in the reconstruction. The successful inclusion of the scapular spine with the cervical trapezius muscle flap has been demonstrated experimentally (Fig. 37.41) (41). Survival of the scapular spine depends on its periosteal vascular supply. Unfortunately, the scapular spine lies outside the primary angiosome of the prescapular branch of the superficial cervical artery, and this causes some concern relative to the reliability of its vascular integrity after transfer. I have used the cervical trapezius myo-osseous flap for reconstruction of metatarsal segmental defects and overlying soft tissue loss caused by a gunshot injury in a Chesapeake Bay retriever. Survival of the muscle flap and its overlying free skin graft was evident. However, postoperative [99m]technetium scintigraphy of the bone graft was negative. This bone graft proceeded to rapid incorporation and healing, a finding suggesting either an intact vascular supply or rapid revascularization. Based on the negative scintigraphy results in this dog and the tenuous vascular integrity of the flap design, the cervical trapezius myo-osseous flap should be used with caution.

The vascularized rib graft may be harvested as an osteocutaneous flap by preserving the cutaneous branch of the dorsal intercostal artery and its associated skin paddle. Maintenance of the skin paddle facilitates postoperative monitoring of vascular integrity of the flap. This flap may also be of benefit in mandibular reconstruction with associated skin loss.

Reconstruction of Weight-Bearing Surfaces

Reconstruction of weight-bearing surfaces poses a particular problem because of the stresses placed on the repair. Tissue used for such reconstruction must be durable and resilient. Local footpad transposition techniques and free pad grafts have been described for footpad reconstruction (42–45). Marginal recipient beds may compromise the success of free grafts, and extensive trauma may preclude local transposition techniques. Free vascularized transfer of footpads may be used for reconstruction in such cases.

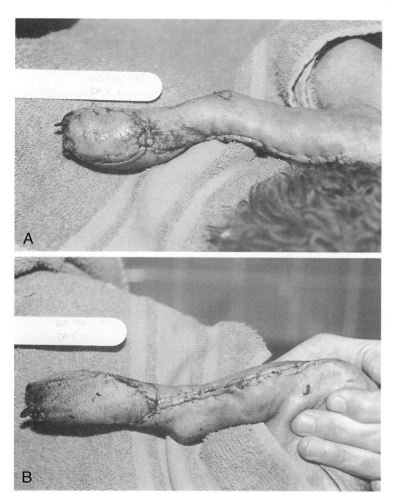

Fig. 37.40. The cutaneous portion of myocutaneous flaps incorporating a direct cutaneous artery may be dissected independent of the underlying muscle. In this dog, the trapezius muscle was used to reconstruct the lateral aspect of a large degloving injury (**A**) while the cutaneous portion of the flap was rotated to cover the defect medially (**B**). The muscle was subsequently resurfaced with a full-thickness skin graft. Both components of the flap are based on the superficial cervical artery and vein.

A microvascular transfer of the fifth digital footpad was described previously (Fig. 37.42) (46). This procedure involves a digital fillet of the fifth rear digit. All phalangeal bones are dissected extraperiosteally and are excised through a dorsal skin incision. The digital pad and surrounding skin are then harvested, based on the deep plantar metatarsal artery IV and the superficial dorsal metatarsal vein IV. Sensory innervation is provided by the deep plantar metatarsal nerve IV and parallels the arterial supply to the footpad. Transfer may be accomplished as a microvascular free flap or as a neuromicrovascular free flap with repair of the donor nerve to a sensory nerve branch at the recipient site. The absolute necessity of sensory reinnervation in such flaps is not established.

The carpal pad may also be transferred as a microvascular free flap. This flap is advantageous in that a larger area of surrounding skin may be included with the flap, and harvest does not necessitate digital amputation. The smaller size and conical shape of the carpal pad make initial resurfacing of the weight-bearing sur-

face more difficult compared with the digital pad flap. The carpal pad flap is dissected based on the caudal interosseous artery as it courses through the carpal tunnel. Two to three small venous branches from the medial aspect of the flap drain into the cephalic vein, which serves as the venous pedicle.

Both the digital pad flap and the carpal pad flap have been used for reconstruction of severely traumatized feet in dogs. The transferred pads have proved resilient to weight-bearing stresses and have undergone hypertrophic change in response to continued weight bearing. Precise positioning of the pad is essential to avoid trauma to surrounding hirsute skin. The most common complication of microvascular footpad transfer has been chronic incisional breakdown at the junction of donor and recipient skin caused by repeated tensile stresses placed on the wound. Functional reconstruction of weight-bearing surfaces is difficult. Further research and experience are needed before firm recommendations can be made regarding optimal techniques.

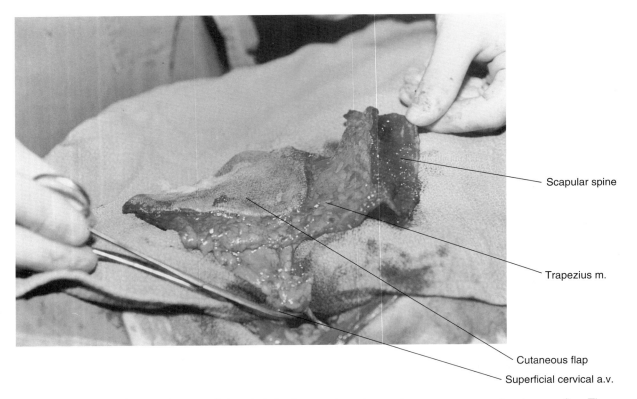

Fig. 37.41. The trapezius flap may be extended to include the scapular spine, to form an osteomusculocutaneous flap. The scapular spine lies outside the primary angiosome of the flap, but experimentally it has been shown to survive based on perfusion through "choke" anastomoses from the trapezius muscle. Elevation of the flap based on the superficial cervical vessels is demonstrated.

Complications of Free Flaps

Complications associated with microvascular tissue transfer may be divided into recipient site and donor site problems. Donor site complications are site specific, depending on the tissue harvested. Difficulties arising from loss of the donor tissue should not be seen if appropriate consideration has been given to selection of a donor site. Seroma formation is common after harvest of soft tissue flaps, particularly muscle flaps. The large amount of dead space and inherent movement between tissue planes in these instances makes prevention of seromas difficult. Tacking or walking sutures are not recommended for dead space management after dissection of muscle flaps because they restrict movement and increase postoperative discomfort. Dead space is managed by provision of surgical drainage; drainage for 5 to 7 days is adequate in most instances.

Cross-contamination from the recipient site to the donor site may result in donor site infection. Care should be taken to use separate instrumentation in

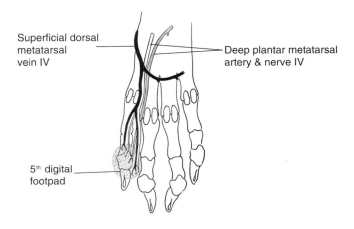

Fig. 37.42. The fifth digital footpad may be harvested as a microvascular free flap for reconstruction of weight-bearing surfaces. Elevation of the flap involves a fillet of the digit through a dorsal incision. The vascular pedicle consists of the deep plantar metatarsal artery IV and the superficial dorsal metatarsal vein IV. Sensory innervation may be provided by including the deep plantar metatarsal nerve IV with subsequent repair of the nerve to an appropriate sensory recipient nerve.

each surgical field. The surgical team responsible for dissection of the donor site should avoid contact with the recipient site, and vice versa.

Recipient site complications may be caused by inappropriate preparation of the recipient wound bed or by flap-related complications. Microsurgically transferred flaps are excellent sources of vascularized tissue for reconstruction, but they should not be viewed as a panacea for a poorly prepared wound bed. Necrotic tissue and debris must be surgically removed from the wound before transfer. In the case of osteomyelitis, infected bone must be thoroughly debrided. Free flaps should not be placed onto heavily contaminated or overtly infected wound beds. Such wounds should be aggressively converted to a clean contaminated state and subsequently reconstructed.

Flap-related complications may be specific to the tissue transferred, such as loss of orthopedic fixation in vascularized bone grafts or incisional dehiscence of transferred footpads. Complications common to all flaps relate to the integrity of the microvascular anastomosis. Meticulous attention to anastomotic technique, astute postoperative monitoring and early surgical re-exploration of compromised flaps are mandatory.

The relative advantages and disadvantages of microsurgical reconstruction are well documented in the human literature. Our understanding of the potential of these techniques in veterinary surgery is expanding. Successful use of microsurgical tissue transfer requires appropriate instrumentation and a familiarity with microvascular technique, both of which are increasingly available at larger veterinary referral centers. Further experience with, and definition of, these techniques will inevitably lead to increased veterinary clinical application.

References

1. Gustilo RB, Merkow RL, Templeman D. Current concepts review: the management of open fractures. J Bone Joint Surg Am 1990;72:299–304.
2. Asaadi M, Murray KA, Russell RC, et al. Experimental evaluation of free tissue transfer to promote healing of infected wounds in dogs. Ann Plast Surg 1986;17:6–12.
3. Richards RR, Schemitsch EH. Effect of muscle flap coverage on bone blood flow following devascularization of a segment of tibia: an experimental investigation in the dog. J Orthop Res 1989;7:550–558.
4. Richards RR, McKee MD, Paitich B, et al. A comparison of the effects of skin coverage and muscle flap coverage on the early strength of union at the site of osteotomy after devascularization of a segment of canine tibia. J Bone Joint Surg Am 1991; 73:1323–1330.
5. Anthony JP, Mathes SJ, Alpert BS. The muscle flap in the treatment of chronic lower extremity osteomyelitis: results in patients over 5 years after treatment. Plast Reconst Surg 1991; 88:311–318.
6. Jaeger K, Stark GB. Clinical and experimental evidence for the improvement of perfusion from free myocutaneous flaps. In: Stuttgart DR, ed. Microsurgical tissue transplantation. Chicago: Quintessence, 1989:217–222.
7. McKee NH, Kuzon WM. Functioning free muscle transplantation: making it work? What is known? Ann Plast Surg 1989; 23:249–254.
8. Manktelow RT, Zuker RN. The principles of functioning muscle transplantation: applications to the upper arm. Ann Plast Surg 1989;22:275–281.
9. Taylor GI, Minabe T. The angiosomes of the mammals and other vertebrates. Plast Reconst Surg 1992;89:181–215.
10. Gregory CR, Gourley IM, Koblik PD, et al. Experimental definition of latissimus dorsi, gracilis, and rectus abdominis musculocutaneous flaps in the dog. Am J Vet Res 1988;49:878–884.
11. Weinstein MJ, Pavletic MM, Boudrieau RJ. Caudal sartorius muscle flap in the dog. Vet Surg 1988;17:203–210.
12. Solano M, Purinton PT, Chambers JN, et al. Effects of vascular pedicle ligation on blood flow in canine semitendinosus muscle. Am J Vet Res 1995;56:731–735.
13. Pavletic MM. Canine axial pattern flaps, using the omocervical, thoracodorsal, and deep circumflex iliac direct cutaneous arteries. Am J Vet Res 1981;42:391–406.
14. Pavletic MM. Caudal superficial epigastric arterial pedicle grafts in the dog. Vet Surg 1980;9:103–107.
15. Henney LHS, Pavletic MM. Axial pattern flap based on the superficial brachial artery in the dog. Vet Surg 1988;17:311–317.
16. Smith MM, Shults S, Waldron DR, et al. Platysma myocutaneous flap for head and neck reconstruction in cats. Head Neck 1993;15:433–439.
17. Smith MM, Payne JT, Moon ML, et al. Axial pattern flap based on the caudal auricular artery in dogs. Am J Vet Res 1991; 52:922–925.
18. Remedios AM, Bauer MS, Bowen CV. Thoracodorsal and caudal superficial epigastric axial pattern skin flaps in cats. Vet Surg 1989;18:380–385.
19. Weinstein MJ, Pavletic MM, Boudrieau RJ, et al. Cranial sartorius muscle flap in the dog. Vet Surg 1989;18:286–291.
20. Degner DA, Bauer MS, Steyn PF, et al. The cranial rectus abdominis muscle pedicle flap in the dog. Vet Comparative Orthop Traumatol 1994;7:21–24.
21. Purinton PT, Chambers JN, Moore JL. Identification and categorization of the vascular patterns to muscles of the thoracic limb, thorax, and neck of dogs. Am J Vet Res 1992;53:1435–1445.
22. Chambers JN, Purinton PT, Allen SW, et al. Identification and anatomic categorization of the vascular patterns to the pelvic limb muscles of dogs. Am J Vet Res 1990;51:305–313.
23. Jackson M. Platelet physiology and platelet function: inhibition by aspirin. Compend Contin Educ Pract Vet 1987;9:627–638.
24. Concannon KT, Haskins SC, Feldman BF. Hemostatic defects associated with two infusion rates of dextran 70 in dogs. Am J Vet Res 1992;53:1369–1372.
25. Zelt RG, Olding M, Kerrigan CL, et al. Primary and secondary critical ischemia times of myocutaneous flaps. Plast Reconstr Surg 1986;78:500–503.
26. Picard-Ami LA, Thomson JG, Kerrigan CL. Critical ischemia times and survival patterns of experimental pig flaps. Plast Reconstr Surg 1990;86:739–743.
27. Kerrigan CL, Zelt RG, Daniel RK. Secondary critical ischemia time of experimental skin flaps. Plast Reconstr Surg 1984; 74:522–526.
28. Degner DA, Walshaw R. Medial saphenous fasciocutaneous and myocutaneous free flap transfer in eight dogs. Vet Surg 1997; 26:20–25.
29. Fowler JD, Miller CW, Bowen V, et al. Transfer of free vascular cutaneous flaps by microvascular anastomosis: results in six dogs. Vet Surg 1987;16:446–450.
30. Miller CW, Fowler JD, Bowen CVA, et al. Experimental and clinical free cutaneous transfers in the dog. Microsurgery 1991;12:113–118.
31. Degner DA, Walshaw R, Lanz O, et al. The medial saphenous fasciocutaneous free flap in dogs. Vet Surg 1996;25:105–113.
32. Philibert D, Fowler JD, Clapson JB. The anatomic basis for a trapezius muscle flaps in dogs. Vet Surg 1992;21:429–434.
33. Philibert D, Fowler JD, Clapson JB. Free microvascular transfer of the trapezius musculocutaneous flap in dog. Vet Surg 1992;21:435–440.

34. Nicoll SA, Fowler JD, Remedios AR, et al. Development of a free latissimus dorsi muscle flap in cats. Vet Surg 1996;22:40–48.

35. Fowler JD, Levitt L, Bowen CVA. Microsurgical free bone transfer in the dog. Microsurgery 1991;12:145–150.

36. Brown K, Marie P, Lyszakowski T, et al. Epiphysial growth after free fibular transfer with and without microvascular anastomosis. J Bone Joint Surg Br 1983;65:493–501.

37. Ostrup LT, Fredrickson JM. Distant transfer of a free, living bone graft by microvascular anastomoses. Plast Reconstr Surg 1974;54:274–285.

38. Levitt L, Fowler JD, Longley M, et al. A developmental model for free vascularized bone transfers in the dog. Vet Surg 1988;17:194–202.

39. Szentimrey DG, Fowler JD. The anatomic basis of a free vascularized bone graft based on the distal canine ulna. Vet Surg 1994;23:529–533.

40. Szentimrey DG, Fowler JD, Johnston C, et al. Transplantation of the canine distal ulna as a free vascularized bone graft. Vet Surg 1995;24:215–225.

41. Philibert D, Fowler JD. The trapezius osteomusculocutaneous flaps in dogs. Vet Surg 1993;22:444–450.

42. Swaim SF, Bradley DM, Steiss JE, et al. Free segmental paw pad grafts in dogs. Am J Vet Res 1993;54:2161–2170.

43. Swaim SF, Riddell KP, Powers RD. Healing of segmental grafts of digital pad skin in dogs. Am J Vet Res 1992;53:406–410.

44. Gourley IM. Neurovascular island flap for treatment of trophic metacarpal pad ulcer in the dog. J Am Anim Hosp Assoc 1978;14:119–125.

45. Basher A. Foot injuries in dogs and cats. Compend Contin Ed Pract Vet 1994;16:1159–1176.

46. Basher AWP, Fowler JD, Bowen CV, et al. Microneurovascular free digital pad transfer in the dog. Vet Surg 1990;19:226–231.

Surgical Treatment of Hygroma of the Elbow

Eric R. Pope

Hygromas usually are seen in dogs of large or giant breeds between 6 and 18 months of age. Although hygromas can occur over any bony prominence (e.g., greater trochanter, tuber ischiadicum), the most common site is over the olecranon. Hygromas develop as the result of repeated trauma to the soft tissues overlying the olecranon. In most instances, this trauma results in the formation of a protective callus, but when this does not occur, a hygroma may develop.

A hygroma is a well-delineated sac composed of fibrous connective tissue and lined by granulation tissue (1). A hygroma begins as a pressure sore, which progresses in severity as the trauma continues. Initially, the pressure compromises the circulation to the soft tissues over the bone. If the pressure continues, local ischemia develops, resulting in cellular death and edema (2). Because the surrounding tissues also are involved, the fluid is not reabsorbed. As the inflammation increases, a fibrous capsule is formed to wall off the area.

Awareness of the tendency of larger breeds of dog to develop hygromas and appropriate client education are especially important in the prevention of hygromas. Owners should be instructed to provide soft bedding and to avoid kenneling the dog on a hard surface until a protective callus has formed over the bony prominences. If developing hygromas are suspected because of the presence of inflammation and edema over the elbow but a fluid-filled cavity is not detectable, the animal's legs should be protected from further trauma by the application of a soft padded bandage for 2 to 3 weeks. A donut made from a foam pad can be incorporated into the bandage to relieve all pressure over the area of the developing hygroma.

Once a cavity has formed, conservative therapy usually is ineffective. Aspiration of the fluid followed by bandaging can be attempted, but recurrence and infection are common sequelae. If aspiration is performed, strict aseptic technique must be used to decrease the possibility of infection.

Indications

The indications for surgical management of hygromas include hygromas that fail to respond to conservative management, long-standing hygromas with a thick, well-developed capsule, infected hygromas after repeated aspiration, and ulcerated neglected hygromas. The objective is to remove the fluid and allow the granulating surfaces that line the cavity to heal together. Because the lining of the cavity is not secretory, complete excision of the hygroma is not necessary. Moreover, complete removal typically necessitates excision of the overlying skin, which is best avoided because the skin is responsible for callus formation and because of a risk of complications exists.

Surgical Techniques

Drainage of Cavitary Lesions

After aseptic preparation of the forelimb, stab incisions are made in the skin proximal and distal to the hygroma. Dissection is continued into the hygroma from both directions. A finger can be inserted into the holes to break down any loculi and to remove the fibrin masses that are commonly present. Traditionally, drainage is maintained by placing a quarter-inch Penrose drain through the stab incisions and secured at each end with sutures (Fig. 37.43). Postoperatively, Telfa WetPruf pads (Kendall Company Hospital Products, Boston, MA) are placed over the ends of the drain, and a Robert Jones bandage is applied. The bandages are changed at 4- to 5-day intervals unless the bandage becomes wet. The drain usually is removed in 2 to 3 weeks (3). By that time, the surfaces of the hygroma should be healed together. Bandaging is continued for 2 to 3 more weeks after the drain is re-

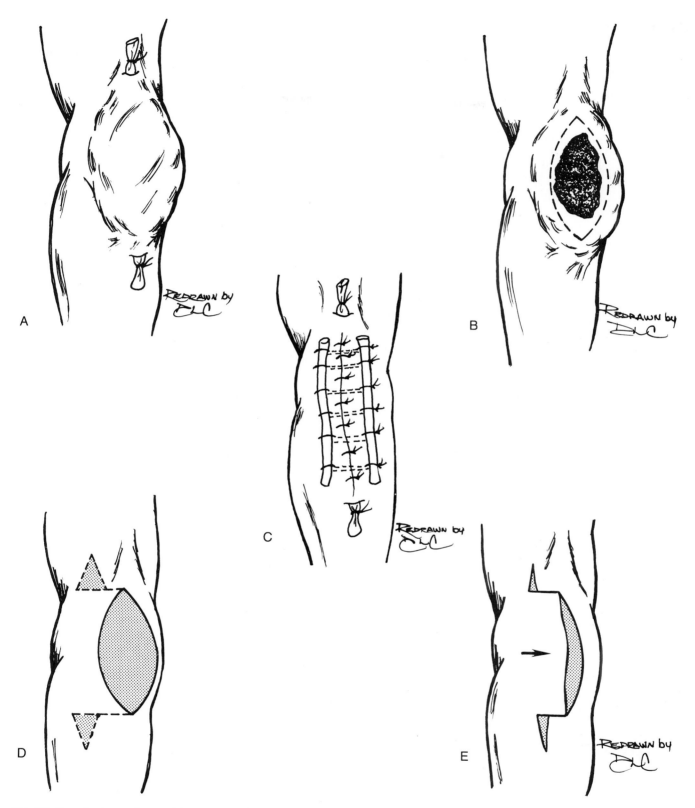

Fig. 37.43. **A.** A nonulcerated hygroma can be treated by placement of a Penrose drain. **B.** The edges of an ulcerated lesion are debrided, and the skin is undermined. **C.** Quill sutures are placed to relieve tension, and the skin edges are apposed with simple interrupted sutures. **D.** A single-pedicle advancement flap can be created on the lateral surface of the elbow (Burow's triangles removed to distribute tension). **E.** Advancement flap sutured in place. The suture line is off the caudal surface of the elbow. (From Toomey AA, Bojrab MJ. In: Bojrab MJ, ed. Current techniques in small animal surgery. 2nd ed. Philadelphia: Lea & Febiger, 1983; **C** and **E** redrawn from Krahwinkel DJ. Elbow hygroma. In: Swaim SF, ed. Surgery of traumatized skin: management and reconstruction in the dog and cat. Philadelphia: WB Saunders, 1980.)

moved. An alternative is to place a closed-suction drain through a single stab incision. The drain can be exteriorized through the bandage to allow access for changing the reservoir. Because minimal wound fluid contacts the skin, complications, such as maceration of the surrounding skin and ascending infection typically associated with passive drains, are likely to be decreased. The excess skin that remains after drainage of a hygroma decreases with time and should not be removed. Removing this skin may also remove any protective callus that is beginning to form (4).

Infected hygromas that have not ulcerated can be managed with the same technique. Infection most commonly results from repeated aspiration, although hematogenous spread of organisms is possible (3). Culture and sensitivity testing should be performed on the fluid, and appropriate antimicrobial therapy should be instituted. The frequency of bandage changes is increased until the infection is controlled. In advanced infections, the skin over the hygroma may ulcerate.

Reconstructive Procedures for Ulcerated Lesions

Ineffective conservative management, infection, and wound dehiscence after surgical removal may result in chronic ulceration of the skin over the elbow. These wounds may be difficult to manage because of the limited mobility of the skin surrounding the ulcer and the tension on the suture line when the elbow is flexed. Generally, the simplest technique that provides secure closure should be chosen. If the ulceration is chronic, samples should be collected for bacterial culture and antibiotic sensitivity testing before surgery. Deep cultures are warranted in chronic cases, and radiographs of the elbow can be used to assess involvement of the underlying bone or elbow joint. Antimicrobial therapy should be instituted before surgical intervention. Removal of a portion of the caudal aspect of the olecranon may also be advantageous, to decrease pressure on the overlying skin when the dog lies down. Care must be taken to avoid disruption of the insertion of the triceps tendon.

SMALL LESIONS
Small ulcers can be closed by undermining the surrounding skin and advancing it over the defect. The ulcerated tissue and thin epithelium surrounding the ulcer are removed before closure. If possible, the skin should be undermined from only one side, so the suture line will not lie directly over the caudal surface of the elbow (see Fig. 37.43**C**). If necessary, a single-pedicle advancement flap can be created to increase the mobility of the skin along the margin of the ulcer (see Fig. 37.43**D** and **E**) (5). Quilled sutures (vertical

mattress sutures incorporating tubing or gauze in the external loops) decrease the tension on the primary suture line. A quarter-inch Penrose drain may be placed if extensive undermining has created dead space.

LARGE LESIONS
If a large ulcer is present or if dehiscence occurs after the previously described procedure, reconstruction using a skin flap may be necessary. The superficial brachial artery axial pattern flap, the single-pedicle direct flap transferred from the lateral thorax, and the thoracodorsal artery axial pattern flap can be used to resurface the elbow. The superficial brachial artery and thoracodorsal artery axial pattern flap techniques are discussed in an earlier section of this chapter. When these flaps are used, the ulcer tissue and the thin contracted skin surrounding the ulcer are completely excised. The elbow is then resurfaced with fully haired skin. The superficial brachial artery axial pattern flap has the advantage of not requiring immobilization of the limb, but the size of the flap may not allow reconstruction of large lesions. The single-pedicle direct flap and, sometimes, the thoracodorsal artery axial pattern flap require immobilization of the limb for at least 2 weeks while the flap becomes vascularized from the recipient bed. Although prolonged immobilization may result in restricted range of motion in the joints of immature animals, the duration of the immobilization with these procedures is not long enough to result in this problem (1).

The thoracodorsal artery axial pattern flap allows the development of a large and long flap because it incorporates a direct cutaneous artery (6). In some instances, the flap can be made long enough that immobilization postoperatively is not necessary. In this case, a bridging incision can be made between donor and recipient sites so the entire procedure can be completed during one operation. The edges of the flap are sutured to the edges of the bridging incision. This may result in redundant skin in that area, but it avoids multiple surgical procedures. Even if immobilization is necessary to avoid excessive tension, the limb is generally still free enough that physical therapy and range-of-motion exercises can be performed when the bandages are changed (7). If a bridging incision is not used, the portion of the flap between donor and recipient sites is sutured into a tube. The flap should be allowed to develop a vascular supply from the recipient bed for at least 2 weeks before the tube is severed.

The single-pedicle direct flap is an easy procedure to perform, but disadvantages include the necessity for multiple operations and for immobilization of the limb. After induction of anesthesia, the forelimb is clipped from the shoulder to the carpus, and the foot is wrapped to cover any exposed hair. The lateral thorax is clipped from the scapula to the flank. The skin of the leg and thorax is routinely prepared, and drapes are applied. The leg is positioned against the thorax in what appears to be a comfortable position, so the length and width of flap necessary to cover the defect can be determined. A dorsally based single-pedicle flap is created by incising three sides of the flap (Fig. 37.44). The flap should include the cutaneus trunci muscle to prevent damage to the subdermal plexus, which is the major blood supply to the skin. The donor site is closed as much as possible before the leg is repositioned against the side. The edges of the flap and elbow defect are approximated with simple interrupted sutures of nonabsorbable monofilament suture material. The edges should be sutured as completely as possible to ensure good contact between the flap and the elbow.

Postoperatively a sling is placed around the foot and attached to the body to reduce the tension on the flap. The sling also helps to hold the leg against the thorax when the bandages are changed. Telfa WetPruf pads are placed between the leg and body wall and over the elbow, and then a soft padded bandage is applied over the entire limb and thorax. The frequency of bandage changes is determined by the amount of discharge from the donor site. The skin should be kept as dry as possible to prevent irritation and maceration.

Two weeks after the initial surgical procedure, the flap is cut free, and the donor site and remaining edge of the flap are sutured as previously described. A padded bandage should be applied to the elbow for 2 to 3 more weeks to allow the flap to adapt completely to its new environment. Sutures are removed in 10 to 14 days.

No matter what technique is used to manage hygromas, the patient's owner should be instructed to provide soft bedding at least until a protective callus forms or preferably for the rest of the animal's life, to decrease the possibility of recurrence.

References

1. Newton CD, Wilson GP, Allen HL, et al. Surgical closure of elbow hygromas in the dog. J Am Vet Med Assoc 1974;164:147.
2. Shea JD. Pressure sores: classification and management. Clin Orthop 1975;112:89.
3. Johnston DE. Hygroma of the elbow in dogs. J Am Vet Med Assoc 1975;167:213.
4. Johnston DE. Hygroma of the elbow in dogs. Compend Contin Educ Pract Vet 1979;1:157.
5. Krahwinkel DJ. Elbow hygroma. In: Swaim SF, ed. Surgery of traumatized skin: management and reconstruction in the dog and cat. Philadelphia: WB Saunders, 1980.
6. Pope ER, Swaim SF. Chronic elbow ulceration repair utilizing an axial pattern flap based on the thoracodorsal artery. J Am Anim Hosp Assoc 1986;22:89.
7. Shires PK, Braund KC, Milton JL, et al. Effect of localized trauma and temporary splinting on immature skeletal muscle and mobility of the femorotibial joint in the dog. Am J Vet Res 1982;43:454.

Paw and Distal Limb Salvage and Reconstructive Techniques

Steven F. Swaim & M. Stacie Scardino

Indications

The paws of a dog and cat play a significant roll in their ambulatory abilities. Thus, when an animal has paw skin defects, some form of reconstruction or salvage surgery is necessary to maintain these abilities. Paw defects may be small and simple, requiring a simple reconstructive surgical technique, such as suture of a pad laceration. Conversely, defects may be large, requiring a more involved reconstruction or salvage surgical technique as with a skin graft to reconstruct a massive skin defect. With severe paw trauma, limb amputation is often performed, whereas if paw salvage techniques were available, limb amputation possibly could be avoided. In other instances of severe paw

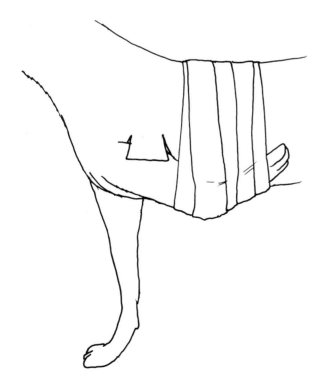

Fig. 37.44. The leg is placed in a comfortable position along the thorax, and a dorsally based single-pedicle flap is created and undermined. The donor site is closed as much as possible before the flap is sutured in place. The flap is sutured around as much of the defect as possible.

trauma, limb amputation is not an option, and reconstruction or salvage is necessary, such as loss of both forepaws of a cat because of avascular necrosis from tight bandages after onychectomy. In the working dog and canine athlete, in which limb and paw function are essential for the animal to perform its working or athletic endeavor, strong functional reconstructions and salvage procedures are important.

Defects of the paws can involve the dorsal surface, palmar or plantar surface (pads), interdigital surfaces, or interpad surfaces. Some of the larger wounds on the dorsum of the paw and distal limb can be managed by techniques such as skin grafts and flaps, which are described in earlier sections of this chapter. This discussion describes some of the techniques that have particular application for reconstruction and salvage of the unique injuries of the specialized structures of the paws.

Dorsal Paw Wounds

Dorsal paw wounds may be such that the wound edges can be easily apposed after wound debridement and lavage. In other instances, tension in wound closure may need to be overcome by using some type of tension suture pattern, such as vertical mattress sutures, horizontal mattress sutures, or far-near-near-far sutures. Other sutures can be used to relieve tension by gradually stretching skin around a wound so it can be apposed or nearly apposed. Examples of these latter sutures are presutures and adjustable horizontal mattress sutures.

When wound tension is too great to be overcome by undermining, tension sutures, or skin stretching sutures, relaxing incisions can be considered when wound size permits. These are used in lieu of skin grafts or flaps. A simple relaxing incision made adjacent to the wound can be used; however, such incisions commonly result in wounds about as large as the one that is closed as a result of their use. Multiple punctate relaxing incisions provide cosmetic and quickly healing small wounds while giving skin relaxation.

Although other familiar tension suture patterns and simple relaxing incisions can be used to aid in closure of dorsal paw wounds, this section describes presutures, adjustable horizontal mattress sutures, and multiple punctate relaxing incisions. These techniques have been found unique and useful in closure of distal limb and dorsal paw wounds.

Presutures

Presutures are particularly useful in the distal limb and paws, in which "walking" sutures can encroach on vessels, nerves, and tendons. Presutures are thus

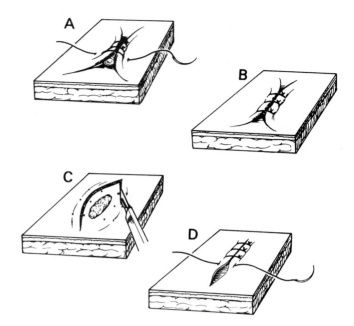

Fig. 37.45. Presutures. **A** and **B.** The day before definitive surgical treatment, skin adjacent to the lesion is sutured over the lesion using a Lembert suture pattern. **C.** The next day, the presutures are removed, and the lesion is excised. **D.** The resulting defect or wound is closed using the stretched skin made available by the presutures.

termed because they are placed before excision or debridement of a lesion. They stretch surrounding skin so it can be used to close a distal limb or paw defect after definitive surgery. Presutures are placed in a Lembert suture pattern with 2–0 or 3–0 polypropylene or nylon sutures, with bites taken in skin on either side of the defect (Fig. 37.45**A** and **B**). They are placed with some tension in tying several hours before excision or debridement. Presutures are placed while the animal is under the effects of a tranquilizer or neuroleptanalgesia and local analgesic agent in the skin to be sutured. The area is placed under a bandage between presuturing and lesion excision or debridement.

At the time of definitive surgery, the presutures are removed. The lesion is removed or debrided, and the skin, which has been stretched gradually by stress relaxation, is used to close the defect (Fig. 37.45**C** and **D**).

Presutures have the advantage that they can be used in conjunction with other tension-relieving techniques to provide wound closure. Between the time they are placed and the time they are removed, the surgeon can note any swelling of the limb distal to the sutures. This swelling indicates the possibility of a biologic tourniquet developing at the time of definitive surgery, and another form of reconstruction may be considered.

Adjustable Horizontal Mattress Sutures

A continuous adjustable horizontal mattress suture may be used to aid wound contraction by applying continuous tension to the skin edges of a wound that cannot be closed initially because of tension. The suture may be placed early in wound management or after granulation tissue has formed.

Synthetic 2–0 monofilament suture (nylon or polypropylene) on a cutting needle is used to place a half-buried horizontal mattress suture at one end of the defect. The suture is continued as an intradermal horizontal mattress suture along the length of the wound. Each suture bite is advanced slightly, so the suture passes at an angle across the wound. Thus, as the suture is tightened, it slides through the tissues more easily. Care is taken not to disturb the attachment of skin to any granulation tissue present in the wound. At the opposite end of the wound, the needle is passed through the entire skin thickness and through a hole in a sterile button. Traction on the suture moves the wound edges toward each other. The skin edge advancement is maintained by a small fishing weight (split shot) placed on the suture adjacent to the button. To prevent slippage, a second weight is placed against the first (Fig. 37.46). Excess suture is cut off about 2 inches beyond the weights, and a bandage is applied over the wound.

On succeeding days, suture beyond the weights is grasped with forceps, and gentle traction is applied while the limb is steadied. The wound edges move closer together, and the fishing weights are pulled away from the button. Two additional weights are placed against the button to maintain suture advancement. Because of inherent skin elasticity, skin advancement is greatest in the first 2 to 3 days. When the wound edges are apposed or when they have advanced to their limit and further tension does not result in wound edge advancement or movement of the suture, the suture is removed.

Modified placement can be performed by placing the fishing weight-button apparatus at both ends of the suture to allow tightening from both ends. With longer wounds, this maneuver is helpful because, the further the button is from the point of traction, the less suture slippage through the tissues occurs. Therefore, pulling at each end of the wound distributes tension more evenly along the wound. During the use of an adjustable horizontal mattress suture, wounds can be treated with a topical antimicrobial or wound-healing stimulant in combination with a protective bandage.

Multiple Punctate Relaxing Incisions

Multiple punctate relaxing incisions are small, parallel staggered skin incisions made adjacent to a wound

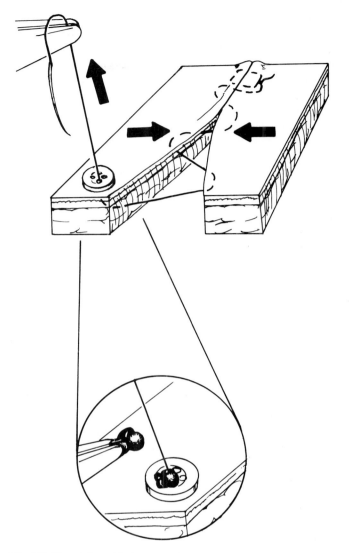

Fig. 37.46. Adjustable horizontal mattress suture placement: A half-buried horizontal mattress suture starts the suture at one end. The suture is advanced as an intradermal horizontal mattress suture with each bite advanced slightly. On the final bite, the needle is passed through the entire skin thickness and through a hole in a sterile button. Tension on the suture (*vertical arrow*) results in wound edge advancement toward the wound center (*horizontal arrows*). After wound edge advancement as far as possible, two split shots are used to hold the suture tight (*inset*). The suture is similarly tightened daily.

to release tension and to allow wound closure. The surgeon may want to use presutures or an adjustable horizontal mattress suture before making these relaxing incisions.

A continuous intradermal suture of 3–0 synthetic absorbable suture material, such as polydioxanone or polyglactin 910, is begun at one end of the wound. If the skin edges do not appose or appose with tension while placing and tightening this suture, punctate relaxing incisions are made in the skin adjacent to the wound edges on both sides of the wound. These incisions are usually 1 cm from the wound edge, 1 cm long, and 0.5 cm apart. They are made in parallel staggered rows (Fig. 37.47**A**). After the skin edges are apposed, simple interrupted 2–0 or 3–0 polypropylene or nylon sutures are then placed in the wound edges (Fig. 37.47**B**).

An alternate method for performing the procedure entails placing the continuous intradermal absorbable suture along the length of the wound, but not tightening or tying it at one end. Tension is applied to the free end of the suture, and hemostats are placed under a loop of suture near its origin. If the skin edges do not appose when the hemostats are elevated, bilateral punctate incisions are made in the area of tension (Fig. 37.48**A** and **B**). The procedure is repeated along the suture line to bring the wound edges into apposition (Fig. 37.48**C** and **D**). Final closure is with simple interrupted 2–0 or 3–0 polypropylene or nylon sutures (Fig. 37.48**E**).

The more punctate incisions that are made and the larger they are, the greater the tension relief. However, the chance of damaging the skin vasculature is increased, thus resulting in necrosis. Therefore, no more punctate incisions should be made than are necessary to provide wound closure without tension.

The sutured wound is routinely bandaged, with daily changes in the early postoperative period to remove drainage from the wound site that occurs through the punctate incisions. As healing occurs and drainage decreases, bandages are changed less frequently.

Multiple punctate relaxing incisions break up the relaxing incision in numerous small incisions that are more cosmetic, heal rapidly, and are more acceptable to the animal's owner. However, the amount of ten-

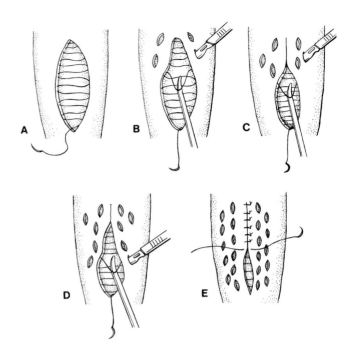

Fig. 37.48. Alternate technique for multiple punctate relaxing incisions. **A.** A continuous intradermal suture is placed. **B.** If tightening a section of suture results in tension, multiple punctate relaxing incisions are made. **C** and **D.** The suture is progressively tightened, and incisions are made. **E.** Final closure is done with simple interrupted sutures. (From Swaim SF, Henderson RA. Small animal wound management. Philadelphia: Lea & Febiger, 1990:105.)

sion relief may not be as great as that attained by one large relaxing incision.

Palmar or Plantar Pad Wounds

Wounds on the palmar or plantar surface of the paw often involve the digital or metacarpal or metatarsal pads. These wounds may be as simple as a laceration or as serious as loss of an entire pad. Because of their specialized function of providing a shock-absorbing tissue and a tough tissue to withstand frictional wear, surgical techniques and aftercare require some special features for adequate healing.

Suturing Pad Lacerations

Suturing of pad lacerations is indicated when the edges of the traumatized pad can be apposed. Pad lacerations require special attention before closure, first to assess the depth of the laceration and second to determine the degree of contamination of the wound. Wound depth may be assessed by placing a pair of hemostats in the wound and separating the blades. Some wounds may be partial thickness; however, some may be full thickness. In the latter case, as the hemostats separate the wound edges, digital flexion tendons may be ob-

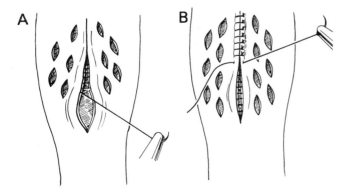

Fig. 37.47. Multiple punctate relaxing incisions. **A.** As a continuous intradermal suture is placed, if wound edges do not appose, multiple punctate relaxing incisions are made bilaterally in parallel staggered rows. **B.** Once apposed, the skin edges are routinely sutured. (After Swaim SF, Henderson RA. Small animal wound management. Philadelphia: Lea & Febiger, 1990:105.)

served through the pad separation. This applies mainly to the metacarpal and metatarsal pads.

Because of the location and function of pads, they are subject to considerable contamination because the animal may place the paw on the ground after injury. This forces contaminants into the tissues. Before suturing the pad, dirt and other contaminants should be thoroughly debrided and lavaged from the tissues. If the laceration has extended through the entire metacarpal or metatarsal pad, thorough lavage is indicated, as well as placement of a small, soft, latex Penrose drain under, *not through*, the pad.

Although the deep pad tissue may appear to be apposed, placement of some deep 3–0 simple interrupted sutures of polydioxanone gives support to the tissues (Fig. 37.49**A**). The superficial pad tissues are sutured with 3–0 far-near-near-far sutures of nylon or polypropylene (Fig. 37.49**B**).

A *small* amount of powder and a small amount of cotton are placed between the digits and in the space between the digits and the metacarpal or metatarsal pad to help keep these areas dry. A nonadherent bandage pad is placed over the incision line. The success of pad sutures in helping to provide early strong healing depends on proper bandaging to help prevent spreading of the pad when weight is borne on it. To help prevent pad spreading, a bulky secondary bandage wrap is placed on the paw. In addition, the cup portion of a metal splint is incorporated into the bandage under the pads. A tertiary bandage layer of adhesive tape is placed. The bandage is changed every 2 to 3 days unless a drain has been placed under the metacarpal or metatarsal pad. In this case, more frequent bandage changes are indicated to remove drainage fluid. Sutures are usually left in place for 10 to 14 days. These times are subject to change, depending on the severity of injury and the size of the animal; for example, a severe laceration on a large dog needs sutures and bandages longer than a minor laceration on a cat's paw.

Phalangeal Fillet

The phalangeal fillet technique is the removal of the proximal, middle, and distal phalanges from a digit to free the pad so it can be used to replace or fill defects in a metacarpal or metatarsal pad. The technique is indicated when conservative therapy has not resulted in effective healing of the pad or when the entire pad is missing.

In patients with chronic nonhealing of metacarpal or metatarsal pad wounds that have not resulted from trauma, a thorough examination should be performed preoperatively. This should include cytologic examination, fungal and bacterial culture, and sensitivity testing, as well as histopathologic examination. Appropriate medical and surgical therapy should be done if cultures reveal fungal or neoplastic tissue. Surgical therapy may range from limb amputation to pad amputation and replacement (phalangeal fillet), depending on test results. If histologic examination reveals chronic nonhealing tissue, the wound should be thoroughly debrided and lavaged because the granulation tissue may have embedded dirt and sand embedded.

Phalangeal fillet may be performed from the palmar or plantar surface of the paw. The digit nearest the metacarpal or metatarsal pad defect is selected for filleting. This is usually the second or fifth digit. A rectangular skin segment is removed from the palmar or plantar skin between the digital pad and the edge of the metacarpal or metatarsal pad defect (Fig. 37.50**A**). The proximal, middle, and distal phalanges of the digit are removed by incising the joint capsules and ligamentous attachments to the bones (Fig. 37.50**B**). The phalanges and nail are removed using blunt dissection as close to the bone as possible, thus leaving the blood and nerve supply intact in this digital flap. The edge and surface of the metacarpal or metatarsal pad defect are debrided, and the pad of the filleted digit is folded back on its neurovascular pedicle of skin to fill the metacarpal or metatarsal pad defect (Fig. 37.50**C**). The edges of the digital pad are sutured to the edges of the pad defect using 3–0 polypropylene or nylon suture material with simple interrupted or far-near-near-far sutures (Fig. 37.50**D**). The paw is bandaged as described for pad laceration repair.

A second technique for phalangeal fillet entails phalangeal removal through a single longitudinal incision on the dorsal surface of the digit (Fig. 37.51**A** and **B**). The skin is then closed with simple interrupted sutures of 3–0 polypropylene or nylon suture material (Fig. 37.51**C**). The area where the nail was removed is left

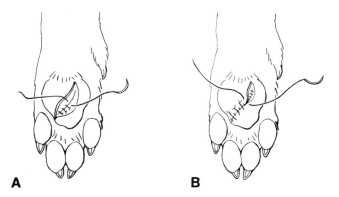

Fig. 37.49. Suturing pad lacerations. **A.** Simple interrupted sutures are placed in deep pad tissue. **B.** Far-near-near-far sutures are placed in superficial pad tissue. (From Swaim SF, Henderson RA. Small animal wound management. Philadelphia: Lea & Febiger, 1990:208.)

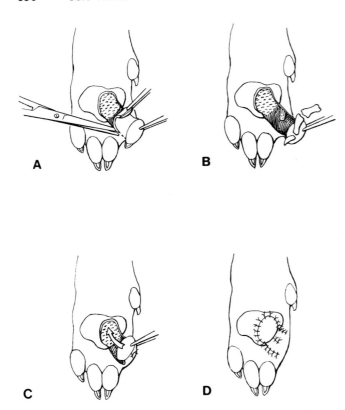

Fig. 37.50. Palmar and plantar phalangeal fillet technique for pad replacement. **A.** A rectangle of skin is removed between the metacarpal and second digital pads. **B.** The proximal, middle, and distal phalanges and nail are removed. **C.** The second digital pad is folded back into the metacarpal pad defect (*arrow*). **D.** The second digital pad is sutured in place. (From Swaim SF, Henderson RA. Small animal wound management. Philadelphia: Lea & Febiger, 1990:212.)

open for drainage. The paw is bandaged with periodic bandage changes, and it is allowed to heal for 14 days. At this time, the rectangle of palmar or plantar skin is removed, and the digital pad is folded back and is sutured into the defect as previously described (Fig. 37.51**D–F**). Bandaging is as previously described.

Palmar or plantar filleting has the advantage of being a one-step procedure; however, it is more difficult, and the potential for damage to the blood supply of the digital pad is greater. Dorsal filleting is easier, but the technique takes longer because it is a two-step procedure, with digital pad transposition performed 14 days after the phalanges have been removed.

In some instances, if a metacarpal or metatarsal pad wound has resulted from abnormal paw position because of tendon malfunction, bone misalignment, or nerve damage, digital pad transposition may not be successful. Unless the underlying cause of abnormal pad wear is corrected, the new pad may wear through just as did the original pad.

Pad Grafts

Paw pad grafts are small full-thickness segments of pad tissue that are placed in a granulation tissue bed around the edges of a wound where weight-bearing tissue is missing. They are indicated in patients with loss of the metacarpal or metatarsal pad as well as loss of some or all the digital pads, thus precluding phalangeal fillet.

After a paw wound has been managed to the point that it has a healthy bed of granulation tissue, rectan-

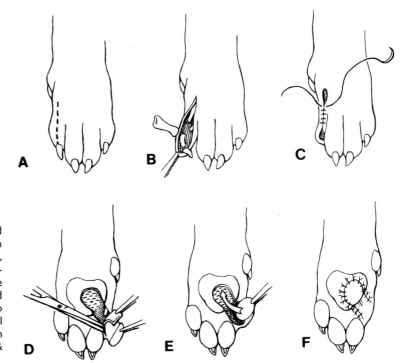

Fig. 37.51. Dorsal phalangeal fillet technique for pad replacement. **A.** A longitudinal incision line is made on the dorsum of the second digit. **B.** The proximal, middle, and distal phalanges and nail are removed. **C.** The longitudinal incision is closed. **D.** Fourteen days later, a rectangle of skin is removed between the metacarpal and second digital pads. **E.** The second digital pad is folded back into the metacarpal pad defect (*arrow*). **F.** The second digital pad is sutured in place. (From Swaim SF, Henderson RA. Small animal wound management. Philadelphia: Lea & Febiger, 1990:213.)

gular tissue segments measuring 6 × 8 mm are traced around the periphery of the wound using a template of x-ray film with a hole in its center and a splintered applicator stick dipped in methylene blue (Fig. 37.52**A**). The rectangles of tissue are incised with a No. 11 scalpel blade, and the tissue is excised using iris scissors and thumb forceps, leaving a series of rectangular depressions about 2 mm deep around the wound (Fig. 37.52**B** and **C**).

In the center of other digital pads on the same animal, possibly the same paw, the template, splintered applicator stick, and methylene blue are used to trace the same number and size of rectangles (Fig. 37.52**C**). Again, a No. 11 scalpel blade is used to incise the grafts, and iris scissors and thumb forceps are used to remove the grafts (Fig. 37.52**D**). All subcutaneous tissue is removed from the grafts with iris scissors.

A graft is placed in each of the rectangular depressions and is sutured in place. Two simple interrupted sutures of 5–0 polypropylene can be used, with one suture on each side of the graft on the long sides of the graft (Fig. 37.53**A**). An alternative suture pattern is a simple interrupted suture placed at each corner of the graft (Fig. 37.53**B**).

A nonadherent bandage pad with a *small* amount of 0.1% gentamicin sulfate ointment is placed over the grafted site. The remainder of the bandage is as described for pad lacerations. The graft donor sites are allowed to heal by second intention and are bandaged in a similar manner. If remaining digital pad tissue is pliable enough to allow suture closure of the donor sites, these sites may be closed with 3–0 polypropylene or nylon, far-near-near-far sutures, followed by bandaging. The initial bandage is usually left in place for 3 days, followed by bandage changes every other day until 21 days postoperatively. A bootie may be indicated for a transitional period between bandage and no bandage. Sutures in the grafts are removed between 10 and 14 days postoperatively.

When sutures are removed from the grafts, the hard and dark stratum corneum usually lifts off of the graft to reveal underlying viable graft tissue that will form

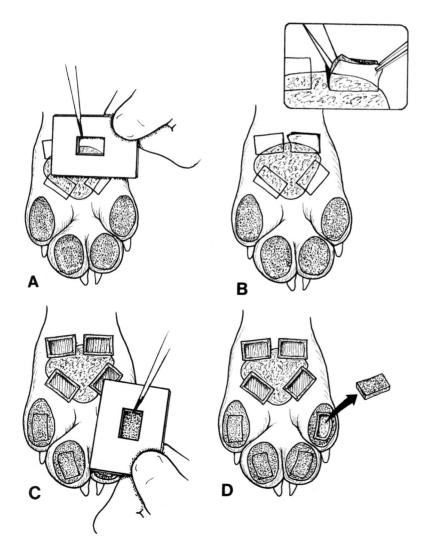

A   **B**

C   **D**

Fig. 37.52. Pad grafts. **A.** A piece of x-ray film with a 6 × 8-mm hole in its center is used with a splintered applicator stick dipped in methylene blue to trace graft recipient sites around the wound. **B.** After incision, thumb forceps and iris scissors are used to remove rectangles of tissue from recipient sites. **C.** With recipient sites prepared, the x-ray film applicator stick and methylene blue are used to trace segmental grafts on digital pads. **D.** A segmental pad graft has been removed from a digit. (From Swaim SF, Bradley DM, Steiss, JE, et al. Free segmental paw pad grafts in dogs. Am J Vet Res 1993;54:2161–2170.)

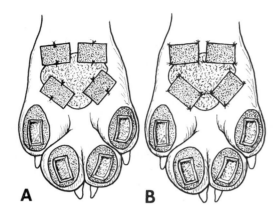

Fig. 37.53. Pad graft sutures. **A.** Two simple interrupted sutures are used to suture each long side of the grafts into the recipient site. **B.** Simple interrupted sutures are used at each corner of the grafts to suture them into recipient sites. (From Swaim SF, Bradley DM, Steiss, JE, et al. Free segmental paw pad grafts in dogs. Am J Vet Res 1993;54:2161–2170.)

a new stratum corneum. As the grafts heal, two phenomena occur that provide a tough tissue on which the animal can ambulate. First, with wound contraction, the grafts coalesce toward the wound's center. Second, the epithelial tissue that grows from the grafts to cover the remainder of the wound is tough keratinized epithelium that withstands the stress placed on pad tissue. If paw trauma has been severe enough so bone is present directly under the healed pad grafts, weight bearing may cause pad trauma.

Carpal Pad Flaps

Carpal pad flaps are flaps of skin on the distal forelimb that incorporate the carpal pad. They are used to provide a structure on which an animal can ambulate after amputation at the carpometacarpal articulation. These flaps may be single-pedicle or bipedicle advancement flaps. They have been described as successful when used bilaterally on a small dog (single-pedicle flap) and unilaterally on a cat (bipedicle flap).

SINGLE-PEDICLE CARPAL PAD FLAPS

For a single-pedicle advancement flap, a transverse skin incision is made over the cranial aspect of the limb at the carpometacarpal level. A dorsally based single-pedicle advancement flap is created on the palmar aspect of the limb such that it includes the carpal pad. The skin flap distal to the pad should extend to the midmetacarpal level, to allow sufficient length for suturing the flap to the skin on the dorsum of the limb after advancement into position (Fig. 37.54**A**).

After blunt dissection of the skin flap from underlying structures, the flexor carpi ulnaris tendon is transected, and the prominence of the accessory carpal

bone is removed. The distal limb is then amputated at the carpometacarpal joint. The flap is advanced distally until the carpal pad is located at the caudodistal end of the amputation stump. The pad is anchored in position with 3–0 chromic gut subcutaneous simple interrupted sutures, and the skin is sutured with simple interrupted sutures of 2–0 polypropylene (Fig. 37.54**B**).

The limb is immobilized in a padded metal splint. Sutures are removed and splinting is discontinued 2 weeks postoperatively.

BIPEDICLE CARPAL PAD FLAPS

With a bipedicle advancement flap, parallel horizontal skin incisions, one proximal to and one distal to the carpal pad, are made on the palmar aspect of the limb. The proximal incision is curved 2 to 3 mm proximally at each end to facilitate flap transposition (Fig. 37.55**A**). After advancement of the flap under the end of the amputation stump, the flap is sutured in place with simple interrupted 3–0 nonabsorbable sutures. The palmar donor site is allowed to heal as an open wound (Fig. 37.55**B**).

A padded splint is applied to the limb. A supplemental bar may be added to allow ambulation without disturbing the flap. Periodic bandage or splint changes are performed until healing has occurred.

With both carpal pad flap procedures, if they are successful, use by the animal results in thickening and

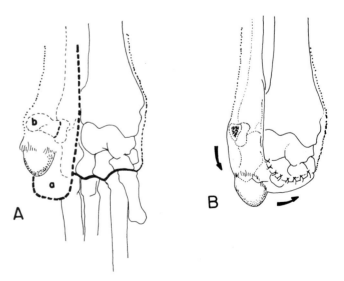

Fig. 37.54. Single-pedicle carpal pad flap. **A.** A dorsally based single pedicle advancement flap is designed to incorporate the carpal pad (*a*). The prominence of the accessory carpal bone (*b*) will be removed. **B.** After amputation at the carpometacarpal joint, the pad is advanced on the flap (*arrows*) and is sutured in position at the caudodistal end of the amputation stump. (From Barclay CG, Fowler JD, Basher AW. Use of the carpal pad to salvage the forelimb in a dog and cat: An alternative to total limb amputation. J Am Anim Hosp Assoc 1987;23:527–532.)

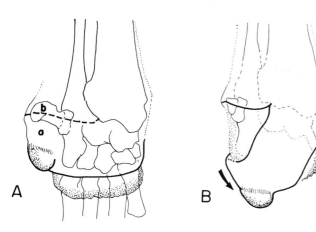

Fig. 37.55. Bipedicle carpal pad flap. **A.** A bipedicle advancement flap is designed to incorporate the carpal pad and is undermined (*a*). The prominence of the accessory carpal bone (*b*) will be removed. **B.** After amputation at the proximal metacarpal area, the pad is advanced on the flap (*arrow*) and is sutured in position under the end of the amputation stump. (From Barclay CG, Fowler JD, Basher AW. Use of the carpal pad to salvage the forelimb in a dog and cat: an alternative to total limb amputation. J Am Anim Hosp Assoc 1987;23:521–532.)

enlargement of the pad. This provides functional weight-bearing tissue.

Before performing carpometacarpal amputation and carpal pad flap repositioning, the animal's activity, its use, and the owner's expectations after surgery should be considered. The technique has potential for use on larger dogs; however, accurate placement of the pad may be more critical when considering the greater weight to be placed on it. Moreover, when the procedure is performed unilaterally, that limb is significantly shorter than the other limb, and the animal may tend to carry the limb or only use it intermittently.

Digital, Interdigital, and Interpad Wounds

Paw lesions may involve the interdigital skin or the interpad skin on the palmar or plantar surface of the paw. The lesions are usually traumatic or infectious. The phalangeal fillet technique and a fusion podoplasty technique may be used to reconstruct or to salvage paws thus involved.

Phalangeal Fillet for Digital and Dorsal Paw Resurfacing

The phalangeal fillet technique can be used as a salvage technique when patients have sustained considerable digital trauma to osseous structures of a digit with skin deficits of adjacent digits or the dorsum of the paw. If

the digital and interdigital skin of the digit with osseous damage is viable, phalanges may be removed from the digit and its skin, and adjacent interdigital skin may be used to replace the skin deficit of the adjacent digits or dorsum of the paw.

The digits with severe osseous damage are carefully debrided, and the remaining proximal, middle, and distal phalanges and tendon fragments are removed (Figs. 37.56**A** and 37.57**A**). The skin of this digit and any available interdigital skin are cut and trimmed such that they can be used as a flap to resurface adjacent digits with large skin deficits or the dorsum of the paw (Figs. 37.56**B** and **C** and 37.57**B** and **C**). The digital and interdigital skin should be cut and trimmed with care, to ensure that sufficient skin and subcutaneous tissue remain at the base of the flap to provide blood supply. The flap is sutured to the remaining skin of the adjacent digits or dorsum of the paw with simple interrupted sutures of 2–0 or 3–0 polypropylene (Figs. 37.56**D** and 37.57**D**).

Small amounts of cotton and powder are placed between remaining digits and in the space between remaining digits and the metacarpal or metatarsal pad

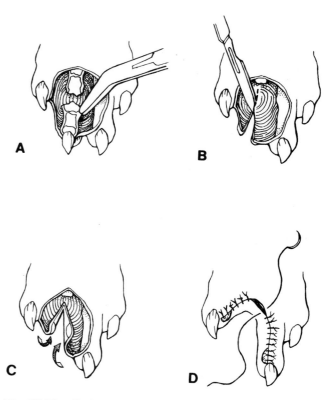

Fig. 37.56. Phalangeal fillet for digital resurfacing: two flaps. **A.** The wound area is debrided, and bone and tendon fragments are removed. **B.** Digital and interdigital skin were used to create flaps. **C.** Flaps will be rotated to resurface adjacent digits (*arrows*). **D.** The flaps are sutured in place. (From Swaim SF, Henderson RA. Small animal wound management. Philadelphia: Lea & Febiger, 1990:217.)

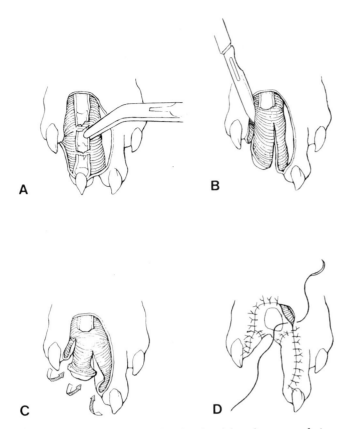

Fig. 37.57. Phalangeal fillet for digital and dorsal paw resurfacing: three flaps. **A.** The wound area is debrided, and bone and tendon fragments are removed. **B.** Digital and interdigital skin are used to create flaps. **C.** Flaps will be rotated to resurface the dorsum of the paw and adjacent digits (*arrows*). **D.** Flaps are sutured in place. (From Swaim SF, Henderson RA. Small animal wound management. Philadelphia: Lea & Febiger, 1990:218.)

for dryness. A strip of nonadherent bandage pad is placed over suture lines. Absorbent secondary bandage and adhesive tape tertiary bandage are then applied. The cup of a metal splint may also be incorporated in the bandage. Bandages are changed periodically for 7 to 10 days. The length of time sutures should remain in place, the frequency of bandage changes, and the length of time bandages are needed are variable factors dependent on wound tension, wound healing rate, and amount of drainage.

The disadvantages of the procedure are that filleting of digit 3 or 4 leaves a cosmetic defect in the center of the paw, and a defect in this area can cause lameness. If digits 3 and 4 have been filleted to resurface digits 2 and 5 or the dorsum of the paw, the second and fifth digits protrude and may be subject to snagging on carpets or vegetation. If the pads of the filleted digits are needed for resurfacing procedures, they should be used. However, pad tissue in an abnormal location on the digits or the dorsum of the paw may be uncosmetic.

Fusion Podoplasty

Fusion podoplasty is a paw salvage technique whereby all interdigital and interpad skin is removed from a paw, and the remaining strips of skin on the dorsum of the digits are sutured together, as are the digital and metacarpal or metatarsal pads. The technique is indicated for treating chronic fibrosing interdigital pyoderma in dogs when other forms of medical therapy or conservative surgical approaches have been unsuccessful. The procedure is usually performed on two paws at a time when all four paws are involved. The most severely involved paws (usually the forepaws) are operated on first, followed 1 month later by the hind paws. The technique has also been described for use in treating abnormalities associated with severed digital flexion tendons to fuse the digits back against the metacarpal or metatarsal pad to provide a functional paw.

When this technique is used to treat chronic fibrosing interdigital pyoderma, the dog is given systemic antibiotics based on the results of culture and sensitivity tests before the surgical procedure. At the time of surgery, a sterile marking pen is used to outline the interdigital skin to be removed. On the dorsum of the paw, lines are drawn on the digits at the junction of normal and affected skin. Lines are drawn near the nails, so 2 to 3 mm of skin are adjacent to the nail on

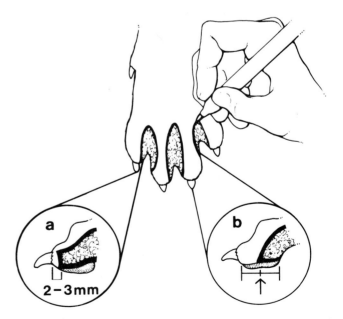

Fig. 37.58. Fusion podoplasty. Interdigital skin to be removed from the dorsum of the paw is marked (*bold lines*). Inset: (*a*) 2 or 3 mm of skin is left near the nails on the axial surface of digits; (*b*) excision lines on the abaxial surfaces of digits 3 and 4 bisect the length of the pad (*arrow*). (After Swaim SF, Lee AH, MacDonald JM, et al. Fusion podoplasty for the treatment of chronic fibrosing interdigital pyoderma in the dog. J Am Anim Hosp Assoc 1991;27:264–274.)

the axial surfaces of the digits. Because the third and fourth digits extend beyond the second and fifth, respectively, lines on the abaxial surfaces of the third and fourth digits are drawn so they intersect the digital pad midway between their cranial and caudal ends. This technique provides skin excisions on the abaxial surfaces of the third and fourth digits that match the axial surface excisions on digits 2 and 5, respectively (Fig. 37.58). This method usually incorporates all affected skin between the fourth and fifth as well as the second and third digits.

On the palmar or plantar paw surfaces, lines are drawn to enclose all interpad skin and the cranial portion of the metacarpal or metatarsal pad. Lines are drawn around the caudal aspects of the pads at the junction of pad and interpad skin. No lines are drawn around the cranial edge of the pads under the claws or around the abaxial surface of pads 2 and 5. From the caudoabaxial aspect of the second and fifth digital pads, lines are drawn along the skin fold that extends from this point to the base of the metacarpal or metatarsal pad. The line is continued across the cranial surface of the metacarpal or metatarsal pad. This line is 3 to 5 mm cranial to the level at which the caudal

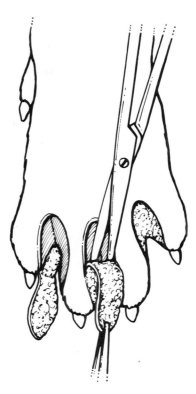

Fig. 37.60. Fusion podoplasty. The dorsal interdigital skin is dissected from the interdigital spaces progressing from the digital cleft to the fold of the web. (After Swaim SF, Lee AH, MacDonald JM, et al. Fusion podoplasty for the treatment of chronic fibrosing interdigital pyoderma in the dog. J Am Anim Hosp Assoc 1991;27:264–274.)

edges of the digital pads contact the metacarpal or metatarsal pad when the digits are flexed back against this pad (Fig. 37.59).

A half-inch Penrose drain is stretched around the limb just distal to the carpus or tarsus and is fixed, with large hemostatic forceps, as a tourniquet. This tourniquet is released twice for 1 minute each during the excisional procedure after all skin incisions and after excision of all interdigital skin. A scalpel blade is used to incise along all previously drawn lines.

Starting at one dorsal interdigital cleft, interdigital skin is dissected from the cleft toward the cranial fold of this skin. Dissection is performed as close to the dermis as possible to avoid damage to the axial and abaxial dorsal and palmar or plantar proper digital vessels and nerves. When dissection becomes difficult near the fold of the web, dissection is discontinued and an adjacent interdigital space is dissected (Fig. 37.60). After all interdigital spaces have been dissected, blunt and sharp dissection is done around the caudal aspects of the pads and along the palmar or plantar surface of each digit, again dissecting as close to the dermis as possible. At the base of the metacarpal or metatarsal pad, dissection of the dermis and epidermis is carried

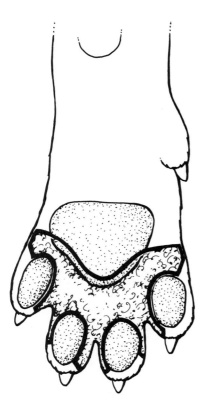

Fig. 37.59. Fusion podoplasty. Interpad skin to be removed from the palmar or plantar surface of the paw is outlined (*bold line*) to include some skin from the cranial surface of the metacarpal or metatarsal pad. (After Swaim SF, Lee AH, MacDonald JM, et al. Fusion podoplasty for the treatment of chronic fibrosing interdigital pyoderma in the dog. J Am Anim Hosp Assoc 1991;27:264–274.)

across the cranial surface of the pad from the lateral to the medial aspects of the pad. Underlying pad tissue is undisturbed (Fig. 37.61). Deep connective tissue pockets containing exudate are carefully removed. After removal of the tourniquet, fine-point electrocoagulation is used for hemostasis. The paw is soaked in a 0.05% chlorhexidine diacetate solution for 1 to 2 minutes. The paw is wrapped in a snug pressure bandage, and the same procedures are performed on the opposite paw.

After pressure wrapping the second paw, the pressure wrap is removed from the first paw. Adjacent digital pads are united with three simple interrupted 3–0 polypropylene sutures (Fig. 37.62). The four united digital pads are flexed back against the cranial surface of the metacarpal or metatarsal pad from which skin has been removed. Simple interrupted 3–0 polypropylene sutures are placed alternately on either side of a central suture to affix the united digital pads to the metacarpal or metatarsal pad (Fig. 37.63). The primary purpose of these sutures is to hold the digital pads in position against the metacarpal or metatarsal pad while the healing process begins in the deeper tissues.

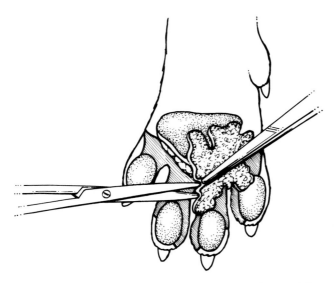

Fig. 37.61. Fusion podoplasty. Interpad skin is dissected from the palmar or plantar surface of the paw. Dissection is done first along the palmar or plantar surface of the digits, then across the cranial surface of the metacarpal or metatarsal pad. (After Swaim SF, Lee AH, MacDonald JM, et al. Fusion podoplasty for the treatment of chronic fibrosing interdigital pyoderma in the dog. J Am Anim Hosp Assoc 1991;27:264–274.)

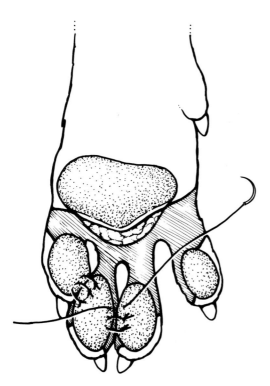

Fig. 37.62. Fusion podoplasty. The digital pads are united with three simple interrupted sutures. (After Swaim SF, Lee AH, MacDonald JM, et al. Fusion podoplasty for the treatment of chronic fibrosing interdigital pyoderma in the dog. J Am Anim Hosp Assoc 1991;27:264–274.)

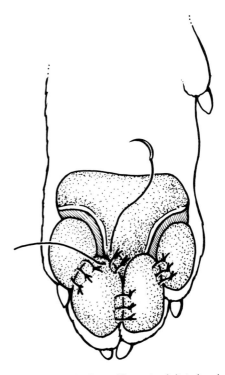

Fig. 37.63. Fusion podoplasty. The united digital pads are flexed back against the metacarpal or metatarsal pad. Suturing progresses alternately to each side from a central suture using simple interrupted sutures. (After Swaim SF, Lee AH, MacDonald JM, et al. Fusion podoplasty for the treatment of chronic fibrosing interdigital pyoderma in the dog. J Am Anim Hosp Assoc 1991;27:264–274.)

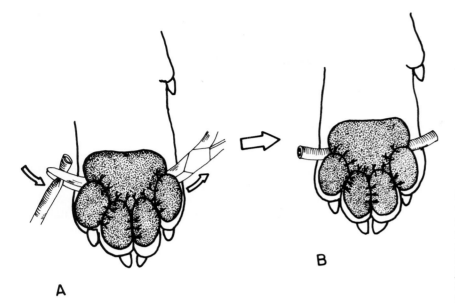

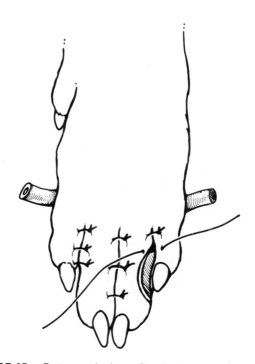

Fig. 37.64. Fusion podoplasty. **A.** Curved Carmalt forceps are passed across the cranial surface of the metacarpal or metatarsal pad deep to the sutures to grasp a quarter-inch Penrose drain to be pulled through the area. **B.** The drain is in place. (After Swaim SF, Lee AH, MacDonald JM, et al. Fusion podoplasty for the treatment of chronic fibrosing interdigital pyoderma in the dog. J Am Anim Hosp Assoc 1991;27:264–274.)

Before placing the final two sutures on either side of the paw, the blades of a pair of Carmalt forceps are passed deep to the digital metacarpal or metatarsal pad sutures across the cranial surface of the metacarpal or metatarsal pad. A quarter-inch diameter Penrose drain is grasped and pulled through the wound. It is cut with half an inch protruding on each side of the paw. The drain is anchored in place by passing the final suture on each side through the skin and drain (Fig. 37.64).

The skin strips on the dorsum of each digit are sutured together with three to four simple interrupted sutures of 3–0 polypropylene (Fig. 37.65). Areas at the ends of the digits are not sutured, to allow for drainage. After suturing the first paw, the pressure wrap is removed from the second paw, and it is sutured in like manner.

Gauze sponges are placed on the dorsal and palmar or plantar surfaces of the paws. A thick absorbent secondary wrap is placed over the sponges. On the forelimbs the wrap goes over the elbow, and on the hind limb the wrap goes just above the hock. Plastic spoon-like splints have been found to provide the best support when they are placed and taped in place over the bandages. These splints go as high as the elbow on the forelimbs and as high as the hocks on the hind limbs. Bandages are changed daily as long as drainage is significant, usually 10 to 14 days. With decreased drainage, bandages are changed every second or third day until 21 days. A small amount of gentamicin sulfate ointment may be placed over the suture lines and at points allowed for drainage. If at bandage change, the area has a characteristic odor of *Pseudomonas*, the paw may be soaked in 0.5% chlorhexidine solution before rebandage.

Drain tubes are removed at 10 days. Sutures are removed from the dorsal paw skin and from between digital pads at 10 to 14 days. Sutures between the digital pads and the metacarpal or metatarsal pad are removed at variable times, depending on when the

Fig. 37.65. Fusion podoplasty. Simple interrupted sutures are used to suture the skin strips on the dorsum of each digit. (After Swaim SF, Lee AH, MacDonald JM, et al. Fusion podoplasty for the treatment of chronic fibrosing interdigital pyoderma in the dog. J Am Anim Hosp Assoc 1991;27:264–274.)

tissues appear healed or whether the sutures are still apposing tissues in patients with some tissue separation in this area. Generally, all sutures and splints are removed by 21 days. A light bandage or a protective bootie may be used for a period as a transition between full bandaging and no bandage.

The most common complication of the procedure is separation of the suture line between the digital pads and the metacarpal or metatarsal pad. The spoonlike splint helps to prevent this complication; however, separation may occur and can expose an area of granulation tissue. If it appears that individual sutures are not functioning to hold the digital pads against the metacarpal or metatarsal pad, these sutures are removed, and the area is allowed to heal as an open wound. A nonadherent bandage pad is used with the remainder of the bandage until the area has epithelialized, usually by 21 days.

Massive Digital Wounds

Pandigital Amputation

Pandigital amputation is a salvage operation in which all digits are amputated at the metacarpophalangeal or metatarsophalangeal level, and the metacarpal or metatarsal pad is positioned under the ends of the metacarpal or metatarsal bones to provide a weight-bearing tissue on which the animal can ambulate. The procedure is indicated in cases of severe damage to all digits as the result of pressure necrosis, phlebitis, trap injury, or other sources of trauma.

A transverse incision is made in the dorsal paw skin over the metacarpophalangeal or metatarsophalangeal articulation (Fig. 37.66A). On the palmar or plantar surface of the paw, the incision is made at the junction of the metacarpal or metatarsal pad with the interpad skin (Fig. 37.66B). If a line of demarcation is present

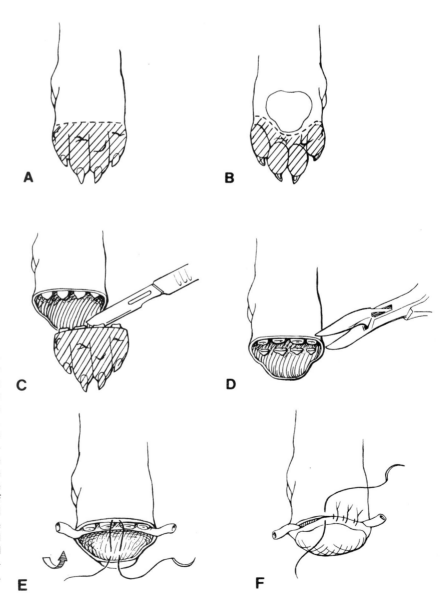

Fig. 37.66. Pandigital amputation. **A.** A transverse incision is made on the dorsum of the paw proximal to the line of demarcation between viable and nonviable skin. **B.** A similar incision is made on the palmar or plantar surface of the paw cranial to the metacarpal or metatarsal pad. **C.** After severance of deep structures, the digits are removed. **D.** The distal heads of the metacarpal or metatarsal bones are removed, and the bones are trimmed to allow proper fit of the pad under their ends. **E.** A quarter-inch Penrose drain is placed between the pad and the ends of the bones, and series of interrupted horizontal mattress subcuticular sutures are used to suture the pad under the metacarpal or metatarsal bones. **F.** Far-near-near-far skin sutures are used to complete the closure. (From Swaim SF, Henderson RA. Small animal wound management. Philadelphia: Lea & Febiger, 1990:221.

between viable and nonviable skin on either surface of the paw, the incision should be made approximately 3 mm proximal to the line in viable tissue.

Working from the dorsum of the paw, the skin is reflected, and dorsal axial and abaxial common or proper digital vessels are ligated with 3–0 polydioxanone ligatures and are severed distal to the ligatures. Associated nerves, extensor tendons, collateral ligaments and metacarpophalangeal or metatarsophalangeal joint capsules are severed. The sesamoid ligaments are cut, and the sesamoid bones are removed on the palmar or plantar surface of the limb. The palmar or plantar common or proper digital vessels are ligated and are severed along with associated nerves and flexion tendons. The digits are removed (Fig. 37.66**C**).

Bone rongeurs are used to remove the heads of the metacarpal or metatarsal bones if no infection is present. Metacarpal or metatarsal bones, especially the third and fourth bones, are trimmed back until the metacarpal or metatarsal pad can be folded cranially and positioned such that the thickest part of the pad is directly beneath the ends of the metacarpal or metatarsal bones (Fig. 37.66**D**). If infection is present, the heads are not removed from these bones in an effort to avoid the possibility of ascending infection in the marrow cavities of the bones. After infection is controlled, the area may undergo reoperation to remove the heads and trim the bones.

After the metacarpal or metatarsal pad has been folded cranially into position, a quarter-inch diameter Penrose drain is placed between the pad and the ends of the bones. The pad is rotated under the ends of the bones. Interrupted horizontal mattress sutures of 2–0 or 3–0 polydioxanone are used to suture the subcutaneous tissue on the cranial edge of the metacarpal or metatarsal pad to the subcutaneous tissue overlying the cranial aspect of the metacarpal or metatarsal bones after the pad is rotated into position (Fig. 37.66**E**). Far-near-near-far sutures of 2–0 or 3–0 polypropylene or nylon are used to complete the closure of the metacarpal or metatarsal pad to the skin on the cranial surface of the metacarpal or metatarsal bones. Simple interrupted tacking sutures are placed at each end of the drain to hold it in place (Fig. 37.66**F**).

Bandaging the area is as described for pad lacerations, with abundant secondary bandage layer for padding and a metal cup in the bandage. The drain is removed in 4 to 5 days. Sutures are removed at 10 to 14 days, and bandage support is used for 21 days. These times are subject to variation, depending on healing and the size of the animal.

Occasionally, because of a combination of the way an animal bears weight and the lack of secure connective tissue fixation of the metacarpal or metatarsal pad to underlying structures, the pad may not remain in the desired position under the metacarpal or metatar-sal bones, and ulceration may develop in an area adjacent to the pad. Repositioning of the pad and placement of fixation sutures under the pad may help to secure it in place. Placement of pad grafts in the area of wear may also be considered.

Suggested Readings

Barclay CG, Fowler JD, Basher AW. Use of the carpal pad to salvage the forelimb in a dog and cat: An alternative to total limb amputation. J Am Anim Hosp Assoc 1987;23,527–532.

Basher AW. Foot injuries in dogs and cats. Compend Contin Educ Pract Vet 1994;16:1159–1178.

Bradley DM, Shealy PM, Swaim SF. Meshed skin graft and phalangeal fillet for paw salvage: a case report. J Am Anim Hosp Assoc 1993;29:427–433.

Bradley DM, Swaim SF, Alexander CN, et al. Autogenous pad grafts for reconstruction of a weight-bearing surface: a case report. J Am Anim Hosp Assoc 1994;30:533–538.

Newman ME, Lee AH, Swaim SF, et al. Wound healing of sutured and nonsutured canine metatarsal foot pad incisions. J Am Anim Hosp Assoc 1986;22:757–761.

Pavletic MM. Atlas of small animal reconstructive surgery. Philadelphia: JB Lippincott, 1993:292.

Pavletic MM. Foot salvage by delayed reimplantation of severed metatarsal and digital pads by using a bipedicle direct flap technique. J Am Anim Hosp Assoc 1994;30:539–547.

Swaim SF. Management and bandaging of soft tissue injuries of dog and cat feet. J Am Anim Hosp Assoc 1985;21:329–340.

Swaim SF. Wound management of distal limbs and paws: reconstruction and salvage. Vet Med Rep 1990;2:128–139.

Swaim SF, Garrett PD. Foot salvage techniques in dogs and cats: options, "do's and don'ts." J Am Anim Hosp Assoc 1985;21:511–519.

Swaim SF, Henderson RA. Small animal wound management. Philadelphia: Lea & Febiger, 1990:181.

Swaim SF, Milton JL. Fusion podoplasty to treat abnormalities associated with severed digital flexion tendons. J Am Anim Hosp Assoc 1994;30:137–144.

Swaim SF, Riddell KP, Powers RD. Healing of segmental grafts of digital pad skin in dogs. Am J Vet Res 1992;53:406–410.

Swaim SF, Bradley DM, Steiss JE, et al. Free segmental paw pad grafts in dogs. Am J Vet Res 1993;54:2161–2170.

Swaim SF, Lee AH, MacDonald JM, et al. Fusion podoplasty for the treatment of chronic fibrosing interdigital pyoderma in the dog. J Am Anim Hosp Assoc 1991;27:264–274.

Vig MM. Management of integumentary wounds of extremities in dogs: An experimental study. J Am Anim Hosp Assoc 1985;21:187–192.

Antidrool Cheiloplasty

Daniel D. Smeak

Antidrool cheiloplasty (ADC) is a surgical procedure in which the everted mucocutaneous border of the lower lip is affixed in a dorsally suspended position to the buccal surface of the upper lip. The purpose of this procedure is to reduce the loss of food and saliva from the lateral vestibules of the oral cavity. Indications for ADC include congenital overabundance and eversion of the lower lip, as frequently seen in large breed dogs such as the St. Bernard, and acquired loss of lower lip motor function from trauma or nerve damage.

Surgical Technique

Food is withheld from patients for 12 hours before the surgical procedure, and no prophylactic antibiotics are required. Inhalant anesthesia is recommended. The cuff of the endotracheal tube must is properly inflated to prevent aspiration of blood during the procedure. Food and saliva are irrigated from the oral cavity with water before aseptic preparation of the lip. The dog is placed in lateral recumbency, and the oral cavity and lip skin are prepared with three to five povidone-iodine soap scrub cycles and sprayed with povidone-iodine solution. Chlorhexidine scrub should not be used on the face because accidental contact with the eye causes severe chemosis. The animal's head is stabilized and draped without altering lip position or the surgeon's ability to open the patient's mouth fully.

The lower lip is grasped about 2 to 3 cm rostral to

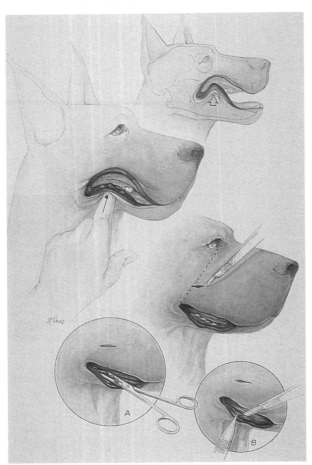

Fig. 37.67. The lower lip, 2 to 3 cm rostral to the commissure, is digitally elevated until the lip is taut when the mouth is fully opened to mark the dorsal extent of the horizontal cheek incision.
Fig. 37.68. Completed full-thickness horizontal cheek incision. The caudal aspect of the incision intersects a line drawn from the medial canthus to the commissure (*dotted line*).
Fig. 37.69. **A.** A 2.5-cm long mucocutaneous border is excised from the lower lip. **B.** The incised edge of the lower lip is split in half to form a cutaneous and a mucosal flap.

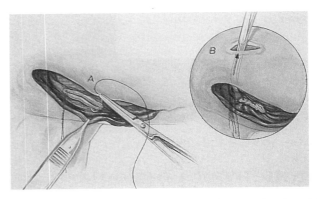

Fig. 37.70. **A.** Stay sutures are placed in the rostral and caudal aspects of the lower lip incision. **B.** The lower lip flaps are pulled through the cheek incision with the stay sutures. From Smeak DD. Antidrooling cheiloplasty clinical results in 6 dogs. J Am Animal Hosp. Assoc. 1989;25:181–185.

the commissure and the lip is elevated dorsally until it is taut when the dog's mouth is fully opened (Fig. 37.67). This spot is lightly marked on the upper lip skin (cheek) with a scalpel blade. In most patients, this mark roughly corresponds to the level of the caudal root of the upper fourth premolar. The surgeon starts a horizontal full-thickness lip incision, 2.5 to 3 cm long, from a point that intersects the marked lip area and an imaginary line drawn from the medial canthus of the eye to the commissure of the lip (Fig. 37.68). If possible, one should avoid the dorsal labial vein that lies just rostrodorsal to this incision. Bleeding vessels are electrocoagulated or ligated with 4–0 chromic gut suture material. A 2-mm mucocutaneous margin of the lower lip is resected with Mayo scissors beginning 2 cm rostral to the commissure, and the cut is continued rostrally for 2.5 cm (Fig. 37.69**A**). The cut edge of the lip is split with a scalpel blade to a depth of 0.5 to 0.75 cm; this incision creates a mucosal and a cutaneous flap (Fig. 37.69**B**). The flaps are everted and are pulled through the cheek incision with stay sutures (Figs. 37.70**A** and **B**). The key to creating a permanent lip adhesion in this procedure is to appose as much raw tissue as possible between the upper and lower lip incisions. The incised edges of the lip and cheek are apposed with horizontal mattress sutures using 0 monofilament nonabsorbable suture material. Each mattress suture is formed by two series of five needle bites. For bite 1, a large cutting needle is passed through the cheek (split-thickness) 1 to 1.5 cm from the incision. Bite 2 is taken through the raw edge side of the mucosal flap of the lower lip. Bite 3 is taken through the base of the lower lip, and then bite 4 is passed through the opposite cutaneous side of the lower lip flap. Finally, bite 5 is taken through the cheek, again split-thickness (Fig. 37.71). About 1 to 1.5 cm away from the needle exit site, the direction of the needle is reversed, and the entire procedure

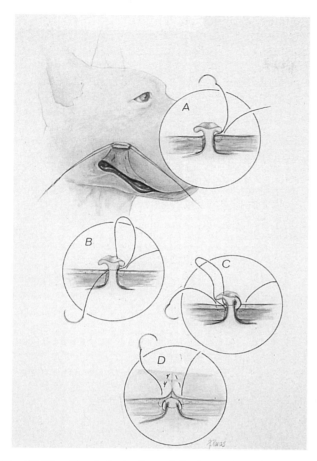

Fig. 37.71. The incised edges of the lower lip and cheek are apposed with horizontal mattress sutures. The needle is passed split thickness through the cheek into the incision (**A**) then through the mucosal flap, through the base of the lower lip (**B**), up through the cutaneous flap, and finally through the opposite side of the cheek (**C**). The needle is reversed and is passed through in an opposite direction to complete the pattern. **D.** Two or three mattress sutures appose the lip flaps to the cheek. From Smeak DD. Antidrooling cheiloplasty clinical results in 6 dogs. J Am Animal Hosp. Assoc. 1989;25:181–185.

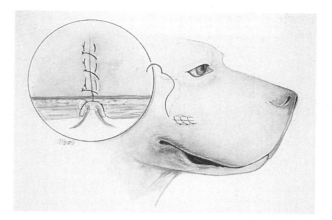

Fig. 37.72. Cheek skin is closed with simple interrupted sutures to complete the antidrool cheiloplasty. From Smeak DD. Antidrooling cheiloplasty clinical results in 6 dogs. J Am Animal Hosp. Assoc. 1989;25:181–185.

is repeated in an opposite direction to complete the mattress suture. The surgeon preplaces two or three mattress sutures and tightens each suture just enough to appose the incised edges of the lip and cheek, while avoiding the tendency to tighten these sutures excessively. Moderate swelling occurs after the procedure, and this may cause excess intrinsic suture tension. Cheek skin is closed routinely with simple interrupted 3–0 or 4–0 monofilament nonabsorbable suture material (Fig. 37.72). If bilateral ADCs are planned, the surgeon undrapes the dog, turns it over, and repeats the procedure on the other side. Bilateral ADCs take approximately 45 minutes to complete.

Patients are usually released from the hospital 1 to 2 days postoperatively. The oral vestibules are irrigated after meals with water-filled syringes to remove food debris. The animal's owners are instructed to remove all items available for their dog to chew for 2 months

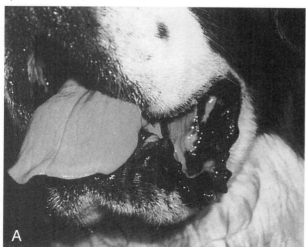

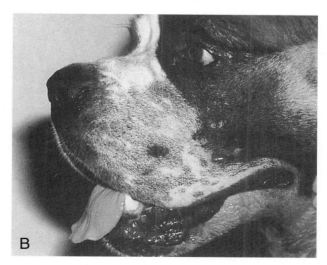

Fig. 37.73. Gross appearance of a patient before and after antidrool cheiloplasty (ADC). **A.** Preoperative appearance. **B.** Appearance after suture removal 24 days after bilateral ADC was performed. Notice the draining wounds around the upper lip incision.

after surgery. A short Elizabethan collar is worn by the patient until suture removal to prevent self-mutilation. Sutures are removed 2.5 to 3 weeks after surgery (Fig. 37.73).

This procedure is successful in *reducing* drooling associated with congenital lower lip eversion and lip paralysis. It does not totally eliminate drooling. Owners should be advised that drooling is reduced to a level similar to that seen in dogs with minimal lip redundancy and normal lip conformation. ADC does not appear to cause excessive discomfort after surgery. Dogs are not reluctant to open their mouths the day after the operation, and they eat without difficulty. Slight puckering occurs in the area of the mattress sutures for 1 to 2 months. Over time, only a small indentation or a fine incision scar is evident. Excessive tension on the mattress sutures causes suture cutout and sometimes abscessation. If this occurs, sutures should be removed as soon as possible after the mucosal incisions have healed. The wound should be treated open and left to heal by second-intention closure.

References

Harvey CE. Diseases of the oral cavity and pharynx. In: Slatter DH, ed. Textbook of small animal surgery. Philadelphia: WB Saunders, 1985:629–643.

Smeak DD. Anti-drool cheiloplasty: clinical results in six dogs. J Am Anim Hosp Assoc 1989;25:181–185.

Stoll SG. Cheiloplasty. In: Bojrab MJ, ed. Current techniques in small animal surgery. Philadelphia: Lea & Febiger, 1983:446–451.

—•38•—

HEART AND GREAT VESSELS

Principles of Vascular Surgery

Kyle K. Kerstetter & Jill E. Sackman

Many veterinary surgeons believe that vascular surgery is beyond the scope of general surgical practice; however, this is not true. Any surgeon who has performed a splenectomy, limb amputation, ovariohysterectomy, or castration has performed basic vascular surgery. Many of the same principles used for these operations are employed in much more complex vascular procedures. Vascular surgical principles are useful tools for veterinary surgeons and have many applications in both clinical and research settings.

Vascular reconstruction has gained popularity in human surgery only during the last 50 years, although the first description of a successful repair was in 1762. Reports of success were sporadic over the next two centuries, and the modern era of vascular surgery did not arrive until technologic advances in surgical technique, blood cross-matching, suture and needle design, and the availability of heparin had occurred. These advances have given the vascular surgeon of today many high-quality materials as well as an excellent understanding of vascular and hemostatic physiology, all of which are necessary for success.

Instruments and Suture Material

A good general surgery pack contains most instruments needed for basic vascular surgery, with the exception of vascular forceps, fine vascular needle holders, right-angle forceps, and fine scissors. Assorted atraumatic vascular clamps are also required in more complex vascular procedures; however, heavy suture material, umbilical tape, or Silastic tubing can be used

to gain vascular and hemostatic control in simple procedures such as cardiac catheterization.

The goal of vascular forcep and clamp design is to grasp the vessel wall without slipping or traumatizing it. This is best accomplished with a gripping surface consisting of several interdigitating rows of teeth, exemplified by the DeBakey atraumatic tissue forceps, Satinsky tangential clamp, Cooley clamp, or the handleless DeBakey bulldog clamp (Fig. 38.1). All these instruments have the same atraumatic gripping surface, and the bulldog clamp is useful in procedures requiring a limited exposure or in repair of smaller vessels in which handled clamps may clutter the surgical field. Clamps such as Kelly or Halsted forceps grip tissue by crushing it and are considered too traumatic to be used on vascular tissue.

Silastic tubing, moistened umbilical tape, heavy silk suture material, or sterile rubber bands can offer an inexpensive and atraumatic method of vessel control. Doubly looped around a vessel then clamped to a surgical towel out of the operative field, these materials offer an excellent method of controlling and manipulating vessels without the addition of vascular clamps into the surgical field. Vascular clamps are recommended in more complex anastomoses because of the ease of vessel manipulation they allow.

Right-angle forceps (Fig. 38.2) are invaluable when dissecting, freeing, and encircling vessels. The tips of these forceps must be fine but not sharp, to lessen the risk of inadvertent perforation of the vessel wall. Small Metzenbaum scissors (Fig. 38.3**A**) with a blunt–blunt tip are especially suited for dissection on or around the vessel because they are less likely to injure the vessel wall. Incision into the vessel wall requires scissors with delicately pointed tips such as angled or straight Pott scissors (Fig. 38.3**B**).

Several different types of suture material are acceptable for vascular anastomosis, and the selection ulti-

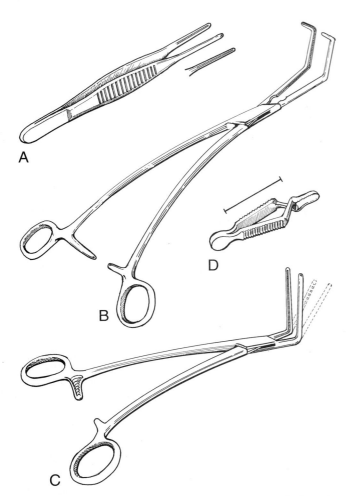

Fig. 38.1. A. DeBakey atraumatic tissue forceps. B. Satinsky tangential vascular clamp. C. Cooley vascular clamp. D. DeBakey bulldog clamp.

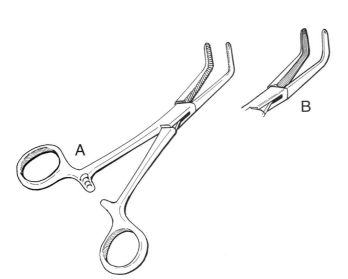

Fig. 38.2. Mixter right-angle forceps with horizontal striations (A) and longitudinal striations (B).

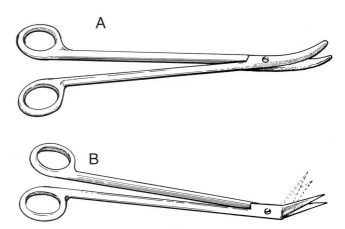

Fig. 38.3. A. Blunt-blunt tip Metzenbaum scissors. B. Angled and straight Pott–Smith scissors.

mately is the surgeon's preference. Fine braided silk is acceptable for venous anastomosis; however, lubrication with sterile mineral oil or bone wax is recommended to decrease tissue drag. Monofilament polypropylene or nylon is popular for both venous and arterial reconstruction because of its strength and low tissue reactivity. Polytetrafluoroethylene suture mate-

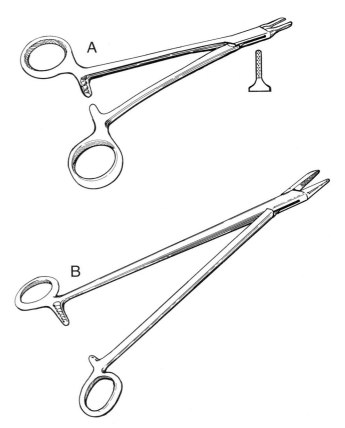

Fig. 38.4. A. Ryder needle holder. B. Crile–Wood needle holder.

rial has excellent strength, durability, and handling characteristics, but its cost makes routine use impractical. All vascular suture should be swaged onto a fine one-half to three-eighths round needle with a taper point, making the use of fine vascular needle holders necessary to avoid destroying the needle (Fig. 38.4). The lack of atherosclerotic plaques in veterinary patients makes the use of cutting point needles and flattened needle bodies unnecessary. Double swaged-on needles allow more flexibility and are recommended for more complex anastomosis procedures.

Vascular Exposure and Control

When systemic heparinization is going to be used, such as during vascular division and anastomosis, it should be withheld until exposure of the vessel is completed. An understanding of the anatomic relation of the vascular segment to surrounding structures is important, to avoid unnecessary dissection and to place the initial incision properly. In most instances, the incision is made over the longitudinal course of the vessel and should extend 1 to 2 cm beyond the anticipated vascular exposure. Under emergency conditions, when venous pressure is low and vascular access is required for patient resuscitation, an incision perpendicular to the long axis of the vessel allows for more error in incision placement and is recommended. After the initial incision, subcutaneous fat and muscle bellies should be retracted for vascular exposure. A self-retaining retractor such as a Gelpi perineal or Weitlaner retractor is helpful. A sheath of fatty tissue often surrounds delicate structures such as blood vessels and nerves. In healthy vessels, a pulse may be palpated through this sheath and aids in vascular dissection When the artery is visualized, the surgeon should stay as close to the vessel wall as possible for the entire length of the exposure. Many inexperienced surgeons make the mistake of attempting to "stay a safe distance" from the vessel when, in reality, the safest area is in direct contact with the vessel. The use of traction and countertraction on the vessel is helpful in identifying the proper adventitial plane of dissection, marked by a white line in the adventitia called the adventitial white line. Traction and countertraction also help one to identify collateral branches and crossing veins while pulling the vessel away from surrounding structures (accompanying vessel or nerve) to avoid inadvertent damage. By following the white line, the surgeon may safely dissect an adequate vascular segment using Metzenbaum scissors. Moreover, the majority of dissection should be sharp, especially when exposing the aorta, to avoid tearing collateral vessels. Periadventitial vessels exposed during the dissection should be temporarily controlled with a suture or ligated and divided.

To complete the dissection of a vascular segment, right-angle forceps are carefully passed deep to the vessel. A moistened umbilical tape is placed into the forcep jaws, and the forceps are withdrawn (Fig. 38.5). Traction on this tape eases identification of collateral branches and makes further vascular exposure much easier. Greater hemostatic control can be achieved in simple arteriotomies or venotomies by doubly looping the tape to form a "Pott loop" or by forming a Rumel tourniquet (Fig. 38.6). Cannulas or other intravascular instruments can be easily passed into the vessel by simply loosening the loop. Further control of the vascular segment can be accomplished by placing a second moistened umbilical tape or Silastic tubing (vessel loop) around the vessel so the proposed arteriotomy site is between the two tapes or vessel loops. This tech-

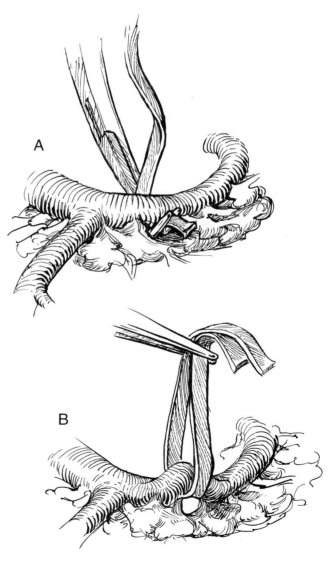

Fig. 38.5. A. Proper dissection plane for isolation of a vessel. **B.** Placement of an umbilical tape as a traction aid for vascular dissection and temporary vascular control.

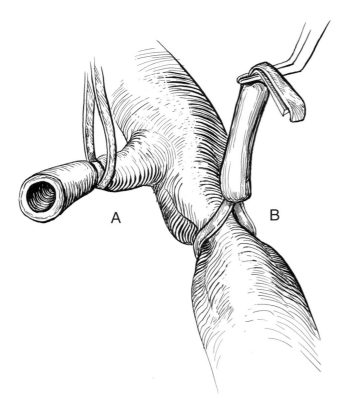

Fig. 38-6. Greater hemostatic control is achieved with a Pott loop (*A*) or a Rumel tourniquet (*B*).

nique is useful for simple procedures because it maintains an uncluttered surgical field and avoids potential injury to the vessel wall from a vascular clamp. Excessive tension on the vessel wall by the tape or Silastic tubing can also cause damage; therefore, the tension should be periodically reassessed during the procedure. For more involved procedures (i.e., vascular division and anastomosis), vascular clamps or a proximal clamp and distal vessel loop are recommended.

When a vascular segment is being prepared for an incision, the immediate area of the incision should be cleared of any periadventitial tissue. The vessel should not be completely stripped, however, because this could disrupt the vasa vasorum, potentially leading to vascular disruption. Incorporation of adventitia into the suture line should be avoided because of its propensity to act as a thrombus focus.

Anticoagulation

Hemostasis and anticoagulation are important aspects of vascular surgery. Only brief procedures requiring interruption of the flow of blood can be undertaken without the use of an anticoagulant. The success of many vascular surgeries lies in anticoagulation The most commonly used anticoagulant is heparin, given at 100 μ/kg intravenously at 1.5-hour intervals. Hepa-

rinization should not be done until vascular dissection is completed and preclotting of any vascular prosthesis has been accomplished. Heparin reversal can be accomplished with an equal volume of protamine zinc; however, this agent is rarely indicated because of the short half-life of heparin and the risk of hypotension associated with rapid protamine zinc administration.

Vascular Interruption

The most basic vascular surgical procedure is vascular interruption. Several methods may be safely used to interrupt vascular continuity permanently. Small vessels may simply be divided between two hemostats before ligation. If vessel exposure is adequate, the surgeon should doubly ligate the vessel before division. This is accomplished by placing two ligatures beneath a vessel using curved or right-angle forceps. The ligatures are then tied, leaving ample space between them so the vessel will not retract beyond the ligature when the vessel is divided. This technique is acceptable when ligating even large veins, although three ligatures should be placed, leaving two on the patient side after vascular division. Pulsations in the blind end of a ligated artery have the potential to force the ligature off the artery, causing uncontrolled hemorrhage. For this reason, the proximal arterial segment should be doubly ligated. The second ligature should be placed distal to the first and should transfix the vessel, especially large artery segments. To accomplish a transfixation suture, the surgeon places two circumferential ligatures as stated previously with 10 to 12 mm between them. The transfixation suture is placed at least 3 mm from the proximal ligature by penetrating the middle of the vascular lumen with the suture needle. This ligature is then tied on both sides of the vessel. A vascular clip is an acceptable alternative to a transfixation suture. The vessel is divided 3 mm distal to the transfixation suture.

When interruption of blood flow is all that is desired without division of the vessel, such as with a patent ductus arteriosus, the foregoing ligation techniques can still be used, with the exception of the distances between ligatures, which only need to be 1 mm apart. Optimally, ligation in continuity should be performed using two heavy sutures with a transfixation suture between them to destroy intimal continuity and to promote thrombotic occlusion. This procedure is not always possible in short vascular segments such as a patent ductus arteriosus, and the potential risk of vascular disruption must be considered.

Vessel Catheterization

Vessel catheterization is commonly performed through the common carotid artery or jugular vein for the purpose of pressure recordings, blood gas collection, cardiac output determinations, and angiographic studies. Both vessels can be easily approached through one incision, and the surgeon should use vessels on the right side because of the difficulty and confusion that may result in animals with a persistent left vena cava. To accomplish this end, the right lateral aspect of the animals cervical region is prepared for aseptic surgery. The jugular vein is temporarily occluded by the surgeon's finger to act as a landmark. The incision is made ventral to the jugular vein and caudal to the larynx. After incision of the platysma muscle, the subcutaneous fat and fascia are dissected to the level of the sternothyroideus and sternocephalicus muscles. The jugular vein lies just deep to the platysma muscle and can be easily identified at this point. To identify the carotid artery, the fascial plane between the sternothyroideus and sternocephalicus muscle bellies is identified and is bluntly dissected. The pulse of the carotid artery may be palpable. When the pulse is located or the vascular sheath is identified, the carotid artery can be lifted from the incision using right-angle forceps as a "hook." The accompanying vagosympathetic trunk and recurrent laryngeal nerve may also be incorporated in the sheath and should be carefully dissected free and replaced into the incision. Pott loops may be placed around the vessels at this point and the vessels prepared for cannulation.

Vascular Incision and Closure

An arteriotomy or venotomy is a simple and highly useful procedure. This maneuver is used clinically to introduce cannulas or pressure transducers into vessels, to remove vascular thrombi, and to repair specific vascular anomalies. Although, in many instances, these vessels simply can be ligated after cannulation, it is often desirable to maintain vascular integrity for future cannulation, blood sampling, and drug delivery. Before any vascular incision, vascular and hemostatic control must be adequate. The direction of incision and the type of closure is often based on individual preference and vessel size. A longitudinal incision provides excellent exposure and can easily be extended if the need arises; however, it is much more prone to stenosis than a transverse incision. Vascular stenosis secondary to vessel closure can cause turbulence and intravascular thrombosis, especially in vessels smaller than 4 mm; therefore, a transverse incision is recommended for smaller vessels.

A longitudinal vascular incision commences with a stab incision in the vessel wall using a No. 11 scalpel blade. Care must be taken not to penetrate the back wall of the vessel. This incision is completed with Pott scissors to a sufficient length. The incision should be closed using two continuous patterns initiated at either end of the incision and tied in the middle (Fig. 38.7). In small vessels, smaller than 4 mm, the incision should be closed using preplaced interrupted sutures to avoid vascular stenosis. If double-armed suture material is not used, a helpful technique is to leave the free end long and uncut until closure is completed to aid in vessel manipulation.

A transverse arteriotomy is made perpendicular to the vessel. The incision may be initiated with a No. 11 blade as described earlier and continued with Pott scissors, or, in small vessels, it may be completed with one smooth motion of the blade (Fig.38.8**A**). The incision should extend laterally up to one-half of the circumference of the vessel. Closure should commence at either end of the incision using either double-armed or single-armed suture material, with the free ends left long for manipulation of the vessel (Fig. 38.8**B**). The suture knot should be placed in the middle of the incision site. In vessels smaller than 4 mm, interrupted sutures may result in less stenosis (Fig. 38.8**C**).

Suture material should be of the smallest diameter possible to decrease the amount of suture material exposed to the blood and to minimize hemorrhage through suture holes in the wall of the vessel or graft. To minimize suture contact with blood further, suture knots are placed outside the lumen of the vessel, and continuous suture lines are started in a horizontal mattress pattern. In addition, the vessel wall should be slightly everted with forceps while suturing. These techniques should provide a smooth intimal lining at the suture line.

The most common suture sizes used are 5–0 and 6–0, and a good starting point for suture placement is 1 mm from the edge the incision and 1 mm apart. Strict attention to surgical technique also minimizes

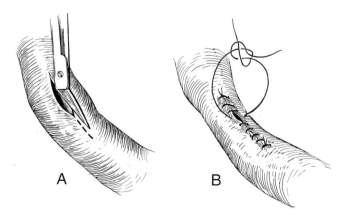

Fig. 38.7. **A.** Longitudinal vascular incisions are initiated with a No. 11 scalpel blade and completed with Pott's scissors. **B.** Closure of the vascular incision should begin at the proximal and distal end of the incision, progressing toward the midpoint, where it is tied. Note the stenosis, which may occur during closure of a longitudinal vascular incision.

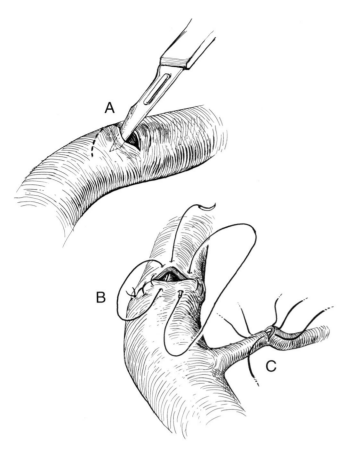

Fig. 38.8. **A.** Initiation of a transverse vascular incision. **B.** Continuous closure of the incision should begin at either end and is completed by tying at the midpoint of the incision. **C.** Preplaced interrupted sutures may prevent stricture in vessels smaller than 4 mm.

the suture hole size. The vessel or graft wall should always be penetrated at a 90° angle, the wrist supinated through 180° between needle insertion and withdrawal, following the curve of the needle precisely to eliminate iatrogenic vessel tears. All layers of the vessel wall should be penetrated by the suture material to provide adequate suture line strength. Before tightening the suture line and tying the knot, vascular clamps or tapes should be loosened to allow flow across the vessel, pushing thrombi and air out of the vessel lumen.

A simplified method of cannulation (Seldinger technique) that can often be used minimizes suture time and is technically easier than a vascular incision. A large-bore needle (14 to 16 gauge) is introduced into the vessel. A guidewire is placed through the needle, the needle is removed, and a vessel dilator or cannula is placed over the wire, into the vessel, and the wire is removed. When the cannula is introduced into the vessel lumen and is placed at the desired position, the vessel dilator is removed, completing the cannulation

process. When the cannula is removed from the vessel, the hemostatic tapes or vascular clamps are loosened to allow escape of intravascular air or thrombi, and a simple cruciate mattress suture is placed through the needle defect, with care taken not to incorporate the back wall. If a leak is present, another suture is carefully placed to complete vessel closure.

Vascular Anastomosis

The techniques used for vascular anastomosis apply to both vessel-to-vessel anastomosis and vessel-to-prosthesis anastomosis. The simplest method is end-to-end anastomosis. A double-armed suture is placed at the 12 o'clock and 6 o'clock positions (Fig. 38.9**A**). The 6 o'clock suture line is run in a continuous pattern half of the width of the vessel on the anterior and posterior aspects (Fig. 38.9**B**). The 12 o'clock suture is then run in a continuous pattern to meet the 6 o'clock suture, with the knots tied in the 3 o'clock and 9 o'clock positions. Before tying the last knot, flow should be restored to remove thrombi and air from the vessel lu-

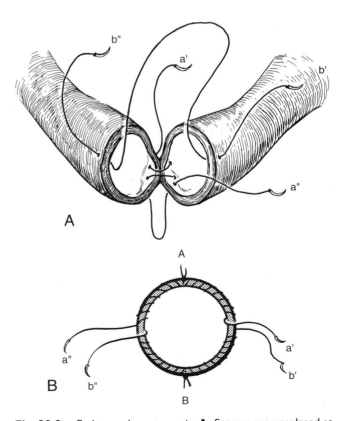

Fig. 38.9. End-to-end anastomosis. **A.** Sutures are preplaced at the 12 o'clock and 6 o'clock positions and are tied. **B.** *a'* is placed in a continuous manner from 12 o'clock to the 3 o'clock position; *b'* is placed in like fashion from the 6 o'clock position to the 3 o'clock position and is tied to *a'*. This is repeated from 12 o'clock to 9 o'clock for *a"* and at 6 o'clock to 9 o'clock for *b"*, completing the anastomosis.

men and to allow the vessel to "stretch," to avoid stricture at the anastomotic site. The use of polypropylene suture is recommended to allow the suture to slip during this maneuver. Although placement of interrupted suture lines is more time-consuming, these suture lines minimize stenosis at the anastomotic site.

Small vessels that are mobile can be anastomosed using a triangulation technique. This is accomplished by placing sutures at the 12 o'clock, 4 o'clock, and 8 o'clock positions (Fig 38.10). The sutures can be used to rotate the vessel to facilitate easier closure, by running each suture to its nearest neighboring suture in a continuous manner.

Stenosis associated with perpendicular end-to-end anastomosis, particularly in small vessels (less than

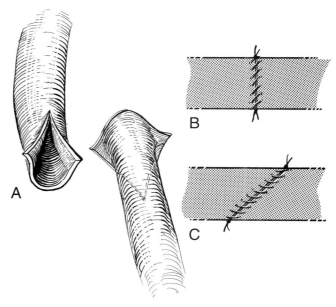

Fig. 38.11. Beveled end-to-end anastomosis. **A.** Incision for the formation of a bevel for vascular anastomosis. Comparison of perpendicular (**B**) and beveled (**C**) end-to-end anastomosis.

4 mm), can be avoided by using an oblique or beveled end-to-end technique. The vessels are incised longitudinally at the 12 o'clock and 6 o'clock positions (Fig. 38.11**A**). The angled corners can be removed before initiating the anastomosis, or they can be grasped with forceps to aid in positioning of the vessel and removed at the end of the procedure. The sutures should be placed at the 12 o'clock ("toe") and 6 o'clock ("heel") positions. The 6 o'clock suture is run in a continuous fashion to the midpoint of the anastomosis; this should be repeated using the 12 o'clock suture, so the sutures meet at the midpoint and are tied.

The end-to-side anastomosis is the most useful anastomosis technique available and is used in both research and clinical settings. One of the main advantages of this technique is that, if thrombosis of the anastomotic site occurs, flow distal to the anastomosis is usually maintained. After routine mobilization and hemostatic control, the wall of the recipient vessel is prepared by making an elliptic or longitudinal incision. The shape of this incision depends on the size of the donor vessel lumen. The donor vessel lumen should be incised at a 45° angle to create an ellipse. The elliptic shape of the donor vessel lumen may be created by direct incision at the desired angle, or the vessel may be incised along one side in a manner similar to that for a beveled end-to-end anastomosis. The angle of the anastomosis varies, but it should be 30 to 45° or less for an arterial anastomosis, to minimize turbulence.

The anastomosis should begin at the lower (underneath) corner, the "heel," of the elliptic donor lumen (Fig. 38.12**A**). A horizontal mattress suture, with the

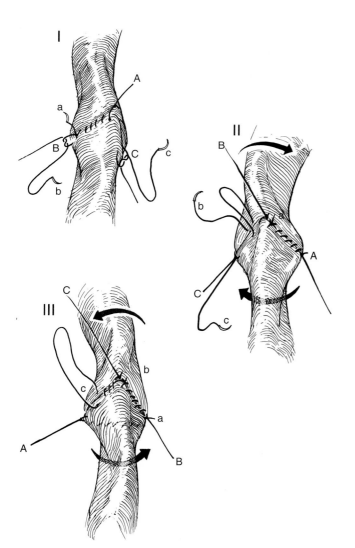

Fig. 38.10. Triangulation technique. **I–III.** Sutures are placed at 12 o'clock (*A*), 8 o'clock (*B*), and 4 o'clock (*C*). One suture arm is used to rotate the vessel while the other arm is run in a continuous manner to its nearest neighbor where it is tied, that is, *a′* to *B*, *b′* to *C*, and *c′* to *A*.

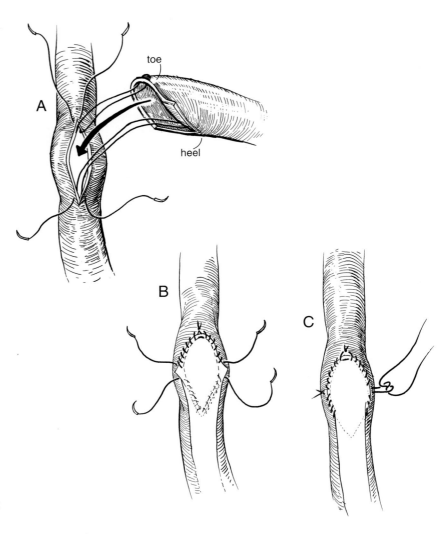

Fig. 38.12. A. Careful placement of a horizontal mattress suture in the "heel" and "toe" is crucial to success. **B.** Continuous sutures are placed between the "heel" and the "toe," joining at the midpoint (**C**), where they are tied.

knot outside the lumen, is placed using a double-armed suture (Fig. 38.12**A**). The same technique should be repeated for the upper (superior) corner of the donor vessel, the "toe" (Fig. 38.12**A**). Occasionally, the "heel" and "toe" must be reinforced with polytetrafluoroethylene (Teflon) pledgets. Suturing commences at the "heel" and continues along each side to the midpoint of the anastomosis (Fig. 38.12**B**). The "toe" is then sutured toward the "heel," with the knot placed at the midpoint. The surgeon must start at the "heel" because it is the more difficult segment of the vascular closure. The last few bites from each suture line are placed blindly across the vessel wall. Beginning the suture line with a mattress pattern and slightly everting the vessel walls will aid in the placement of these sutures.

Suggested Readings

Breznock EM, et al. Surgical manipulation of intrahepatic portocaval shunts in dogs. J Am Vet Med Assoc 1983;182:798–805.

Buchanan JW, et al. Aortic embolism in cats: prevalence, surgical treatment and electrocardiography. Vet Rec 1966;79:496.

Gregory CR, et al. Renal transplantation for the treatment of end-stage renal failure in cats. J Am Vet Med Assoc 1992;201:285–291.

Kempczinski RF, Rutherford RB. Fundamental techniques in vascular surgery. In: Rutherford RB, ed. Vascular surgery. 3rd ed. Philadelphia: WB Saunders 1989.

Rutherford RB. In: Rutherford RB, ed. Vascular surgery. 3rd ed. Philadelphia: WB Saunders 1989.

Conventional Ligation of Patent Ductus Arteriosus in Dogs and Cats

Eric Monnet

Patent ductus arteriosus is the most common congenital heart defect diagnosed in dogs. Physical findings include a continuous murmur auscultated at the left heart base and a hyperkinetic pulse. Chest radiographs show dilation of the descending aorta, the left atrium, and the pulmonary artery. Pulmonary overcirculation is also present. Surgical correction of the defect should be performed as soon as possible after diagnosis. Most animals with patent ductus arteriosus die within 1 year from congestive heart failure. Pulmonary hypertension may cause reversal of flow through the ductus arteriosus in few cases. Dogs presenting with pulmonary edema should be treated with furosemide preoperatively.

Surgical Technique

Ligation of a patent ductus arteriosus is accomplished through a fourth intercostal thoracotomy in dogs or through a fourth or fifth intercostal thoracotomy in cats. The left cranial lung lobe is reflected caudally and is packed with a laparotomy sponge. The vagus nerve courses over the ductus arteriosus and can be used as a landmark to locate the ductus arteriosus. The vagus nerve is elevated from the mediastinum by sharp dissection. The laryngeal recurrent nerve should be identified as it passes caudal to the ductus. The vagus nerve is retracted gently with a suture. Dissection of the patent ductus arteriosus should be performed outside the

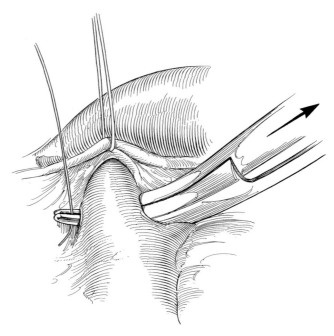

Fig. 38.14. Patent ductus arteriosus ligation. Two sutures are passed from cranial to caudal around the ductus with right-angle forceps after complete dissection of the ductus arteriosus. (From Orton EC. Congenital heart defect. In: Orton EC, ed. Small animal thoracic surgery. Baltimore: Williams & Wilkins, 1995:206.)

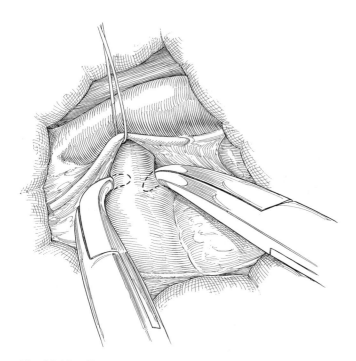

Fig. 38.13. Patent ductus arteriosus ligation. The patent ductus arteriosus is isolated by blunt dissection without opening the pericardial sac. Right-angle forceps are parallel to the transverse plane for the caudal dissection of the ductus. Right-angle forceps are angled caudally 45° for the cranial dissection of the ductus. (From Orton EC. Congenital heart defect. In: Orton EC, ed. Small animal thoracic surgery. Baltimore: Williams & Wilkins, 1995:205.)

pericardial sac with right-angle forceps. Dissection of the patent ductus arteriosus starts on its caudal aspect (Fig. 38.13). The forceps should be kept parallel to the transverse plane during this part of the dissection. Dissection of the cranial portion of the ductus is performed at an angle of approximately 45° to the transverse plane in a triangle delimited by the aortic arch, the pulmonary artery, and the patent ductus arteriosus (Fig. 38.13). Careful sharp dissection with scissors is sometimes necessary to reflect the attachment of the pericardium ventrally from the aorta to expose this triangle. The medial aspect of the patent ductus arteriosus is dissected by passing the right-angle forceps caudally to cranially (Fig. 38.14). Dissection should be as gentle as possible, with small movements of the right-angle forceps to avoid tearing the medial wall of the ductus. When the tip of the right-angle forceps is clear of tissue, a 1 silk suture is grasped by the forceps and is passed around the ductus. A second suture is passed around the ductus in the same manner. The ligature closest to the aorta is slowly tightened and is tied first (Fig. 38.15). The second ligature is then tightened and tied. The palpable thrill in the pulmonary artery present before ligation should be completely eliminated after ligation. If the medial wall of the ductus is ruptured during dissection, light pressure should be applied to control the bleeding. If the tear is not too large, the bleeding will stop. However, continuing the

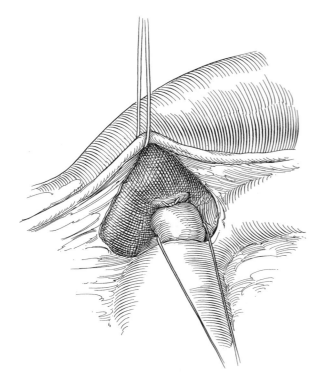

Fig. 38.15. Patent ductus arteriosus ligation. The suture closest to the aorta is ligated slowly first. (From Orton EC. Congenital heart defect. In: Orton EC, ed. Small animal thoracic surgery. Baltimore: Williams & Wilkins, 1995:206.)

dissection may worsen the tear and may lead to uncontrollable hemorrhage. At this point, the options depend on the experience of the surgeon and on the availability of vascular instruments. One option is to divide the ductus between two vascular forceps and to close both ends with 4–0 polypropylene suture using a continuous mattress pattern. Alternatively, the operation may have to be aborted and the animal referred to a surgeon experienced in cardiovascular surgery for later closure. At the end of the surgical procedure, the cranial lung lobe is unpacked, replaced in its normal position, and reinflated. A thoracostomy tube is placed, and the thoracotomy is closed in a routine fashion.

Suggested Readings

Birchard SJ, Bonagura JD, Fingland RB. Results of ligation of patent ductus arteriosus in 201 cases (1969–1988). J Am Vet Med Assoc 1990;196:2011.

Eyster GE. Basic cardiac surgical procedures. In: Slatter DH, ed. Textbook of small animal surgery. Philadelphia: WB Saunders, 1993:893–918.

Eyster GE, Probst MR. Basic cardiovascular surgery and procedures. In: Fox PR. Canine and feline cardiology. New York: Churchill Livingstone, 1988:605–624.

Orton EC. Congenital heart defect. In: Orton EC, ed. Small animal thoracic surgery. Baltimore: Williams & Wilkins, 1995:203–227.

Modified Double Ligation and Division of Patent Ductus Arteriosus

Ralph A. Henderson & William F. Jackson

Normal Cardiopulmonary Development

Postnatal patency of the ductus arteriosus (PDA) is the most common pathologic cardiac or vascular condition requiring surgical intervention in the dog. In the fetus, the right and left ventricles have similar wall thickness and pump equal quantities of blood at a pressure of about 60/0 mm Hg. Because the nonaerated pulmonary tissue resists flow, the majority of the right ventricle output bypasses the lung to the fetal aorta through the fetal ductus arteriosus, where it mixes with the left ventricular output.

After normal birth and neonatal development, the lungs inflate, pulmonary vascular resistance drops, and specialized smooth muscle fibers in the wall of the ductus contract and close the channel. Simultaneous with a decreased pulmonary resistance is a requirement for the left ventricle to supply the systemic vasculature alone. Thus, lessened pulmonary resistance, closure of the ductus, and high pressure demands of the systemic circulation cause the well-known differences in wall thickness and pressures that distinguish the right and left ventricles.

Abnormal Cardiopulmonary Development with Patent Ductus Arteriosus

Pathologic shunting results when the ductus fails to close. The direction of shunted blood flow depends on pulmonary development, inflation, and duration of the shunting. If the lungs do not develop normally, or if the lungs fail to inflate, the ductus remains patent, and a congenital right-to-left shunt persists. Congenital right-to-left shunting is rare in our experience. Surgical closure of this type shunt is disastrous, as described later. Usually, right-to-left shunting is a late acquired change and results from pulmonary hypertension, left heart dilatation, and right heart compensatory hypertrophy.

Most PDAs result in a left-to-right shunt if pulmonary development is normal. When the ductus fails to close, the autonomy of the pulmonary and systemic circuits is not established. The shunt direction is from left to right because the circulatory resistance of the inflated lung is less than that of the systemic circulation. The left-to-right shunting initiates a vicious cycle in which a portion of the systemic (left ventricular) cardiac output shunts into the pulmonary circulation with each cardiac contraction. Gradually, the pulmonary system becomes overcirculated (Fig. 38.16). At first, the lung accommodates to the increased volume by vascular expansion, but eventually the vessels fill to capacity. During the early phases, the right ventricle empties with little pulmonary resistance, but increased pulmonary venous return immediately begins overloading the left ventricle (Fig. 38.17). The left ventricle accommodates for volume overloading initially by hypertrophy; however, later it undergoes decompensating dilatation.

When untreated, a left-to-right shunt may progress to a right-to-left shunt. This progression is explained by the increasing inability of the pulmonary vasculature to accommodate the shunting blood fraction. The lung is the Achilles' heel of the pathologic blood shunting. Concomitant with increasing pulmonary volume are increased intrapulmonary vascular pressures and increased tension in the vascular walls. Eventually, the lungs become hypertensive. The pulmonary arteries undergo muscular hypertrophy as a countermeasure to arterial stretching. With continued pulmonary hypertension as a stimulus, the hypertrophy progresses to fibrosis, and fibrotic contracture leads to vascular narrowing and decreased pulmonary volume. The rapidity of progression of this process depends on the volume of flow across the PDA.

Once pulmonary vascular fibrosis begins, many changes become irreversible. Advanced compensatory changes in the right side of the heart caused the increased resistance of fibrotic stenosis of the pulmonary vasculature, and the decompensating left side of the heart can cause the left-to-right shunting to reverse. When right-to-left shunting is present, the pulmonary circulation becomes minimally competent, and the cyanotic patient becomes partially dependent on the shunt for systemic perfusion from the right ventricle.

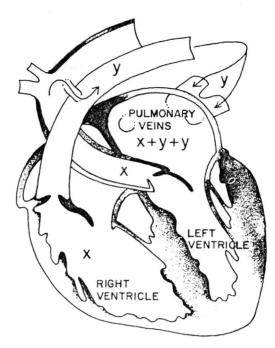

Fig. 38.17. Left ventricular volume overloading results from the increased pulmonary venous return ($x + y + y$) (see Fig. 38.16). The left ventricle accommodates for the increased volume poorly, but even this poor accommodation is defeated because, during each contraction, blood escapes into the pulmonary circulation (y) through the patent ductus arteriosus.

Death is likely after surgical intervention in right-to-left shunts because of acute right heart pressure overload, which precipitates ventricular failure.

Most dogs affected by PDA develop cardiopulmonary failure within a few years, but a few dogs remain clinically normal for a decade or longer. Surgical correction should be performed before significant cardiopulmonary changes have developed. Early changes such as left atrioventricular enlargement, ductus dilatation, poststenotic aortic dilatation, and pulmonary hypertension are reversible with early surgical correction. Late changes such as biventricular enlargement, pulmonary fibrosis, heart failure, and right-to-left shunting are usually not reversible. Other congenital heart or physical anomalies may coexist, and adult dogs with untreated PDA are also reported to be predisposed to infectious endocarditis. Diagnostic tests should be planned and interpreted based on the pathophysiologic features.

Diagnostic Protocol and Patient Selection

PDA is usually suspected first because of the characteristic continuous or machinery murmur. Flow across the PDA results in turbulence. More turbulence is usually associated with more murmur. Accordingly, the

PULMONARY CIRCULATION

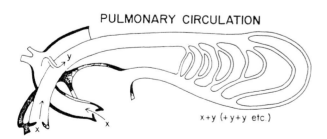

$x+y$ ($+y+y$ etc.)

Fig. 38.16. Mechanism of hyperperfusion of lungs with patent ductus arteriosus. Normally, the cardiac outputs (x) of the right and left ventricle are equal. In the presence of a patent ductus, however, with each cardiac cycle, a portion of aortic blood (left ventricular output) (y) shunts into the pulmonary circulation. Because this is repetitive, the lungs become hyperperfused with additional volume ($x + y + y + y$, etc.).

intensity of the murmur does not necessarily correlate with the size of the PDA. The murmur is continuous but usually is auscultated to have two phases, an initial loud phase and a secondary softer phase. It is usually a mistaken interpretation that the two phases result from bidirectional flow through the shunt. In fact, flow is unidirectional: the first, loud phase of murmur is due to the higher pressure associated with ventricular contraction, and the second, softer phase is associated with the secondary aortic elasticity that completes the dicrotic notch pulse wave. The murmur may become difficult to hear or may disappear completely when a large PDA is present and when, in long-standing PDA, the pressures in the pulmonary and systemic circuits are nearly equal.

A second characteristic physical feature of PDA is the "BB shot" or "water-hammer" pulse. This pulse is characterized by an intense initial vascular expansion, followed by near-complete vessel collapse. This pulse phenomenon occurs because systolic pressures are likely to be normal or even high, but blood is rapidly drained from the systemic circuit into the pulmonary circuit in the earlier stages of PDA, with resulting low diastolic pressure and vascular collapse.

Clinically, results of hematology and biochemistry tests are usually normal. Predominance of early left heart hypertrophy creates electrocardiographic changes characterized by increased rate widened P wave and an R wave that usually exceeds 3.5 mV. Turbulent blood flow results in enlargement of the PDA and adjacent aorta and pulmonary vein. Increased pulmonary venous return results in an enlarged left atrium. The aorta, ductus "bump" and enlarged left atrial appendage form a pathognomonic triad which together with vascular congestion of the lung form the typical ventrodorsal radiographic image. Echocardiographic evaluation reveals characteristic ventricular wall and valve changes, atrial dilatation and the PDA.

In the young dog with no other apparent abnormalities, the minimum database acquired for PDA should include the medical history and examinations including physical, endoparasites, complete blood count, total protein, blood urea nitrogen, urinalysis, electrocardiogram, thoracic radiographs, and echocardiogram. If the dog has a history of exercise intolerance, weight loss, general or differential (caudal versus cranial membranes) cyanosis, ascites, or paraparesis, multiple anomalies or right-to-left shunting may exist. For these dogs and for dogs older than 2 years, additional examinations are warranted, including additional biochemistry values, electrolytes, blood gases and acid-base status, and flow Doppler echocardiography or cardiac catheterization.

The ideal time for surgical correction is between 3 and 6 months of age or as soon as practical after diagnosis. Patients with long-standing PDAs have greater vessel fragility and are more likely to have surgical complications. The contraindications to closure of a PDA include right-to-left shunting and the presence of tetralogy of Fallot, or the association of the PDA with an inoperable cardiovascular anomaly. If PDA coexists with pulmonic stenosis, both lesions may be operated on simultaneously or at staged operations. The patient's size is of little consequence, except fluid and anesthetic administration, ventilation, and control of body temperature are more critical in smaller patients.

Anesthesia and Analgesia

Our technique for anesthesia is to administer buprenorphine (P/M Oxymorphone HCl, 0.015 mg/kg intramuscularly), acetylpromazine (Promace, 0.05 mg/kg IM) and glycopyrrolate (Robinul, 0.01 mg/kg subcutaneously). Puppies are given 1 to 2 tablespoons of corn syrup or honey the morning of the surgical procedure and are provided a 0.25% sodium chloride and 5% dextrose drip (11 to 22 mL/kg per hour) during anesthesia and recovery through a cephalic catheter. General anesthesia is induced with thiopental (about 5 mg/kg intravenously) or by mask inhalation of isoflurane, the maintenance anesthetic. Hyperventilation during surgery ensures that the patient is well oxygenated and, because of hypocarbia, that spontaneous respiration (diaphragmatic movement) ceases, thereby reducing movement during dissection.

Although puppies seem remarkably resilient to surgery and anesthesia, some puppies hypoventilate without sufficient analgesia, and adult and larger dogs always require postoperative analgesia. We routinely continue analgesics for a minimum of 24 hours. Initial excellent analgesia can be provided with local anesthesia. After the ductus is ligated, and before the thora is closed, bupivacaine (Marcaine, 0.25 to 0.5 mL) is infiltrated near each costovertebral junction (emergence of the intercostal nerve), including the incised intercostal space and one or two spaces on either side. Systemic analgesics are readministered at the time of endotracheal intubation. Buprenorphine (Buprenex) .005–.01 mg/kg may be repeated at 6- to 8-hour intervals as needed. Oxymorphone (0.1 mg/kg), a schedule II agent, is a superior analgesic, but it must be given at 4- to 6-hour intervals. Butorphanol (0.2–0.4 mg/kg) is a weak analgesic that can be substituted in this protocol, but it must be readministered at 2- to 4-hour intervals.

Surgical Anatomy

Most surgical procedures for closure of PDA patency require that the medial aspect of the ductus be exposed

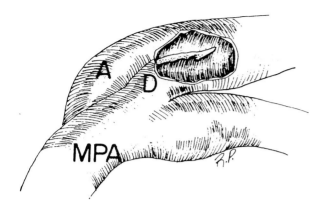

Fig. 38.18. Anatomy of patent ductus arteriosus. The patent ductus (D) blends with the aorta (A), but its actual opening is caudal to its apparent union because of an intra-aortic shelf (seen with left lateral aortic wall removed). The fetal blood flow from main pulmonary artery (MPA) into the aorta is not obstructed by this shelf, but the flow is turbulent when the flow is from left (aorta) to right (pulmonary arteries). This turbulence is responsible for vascular dilatation of the aorta, patent ductus, and pulmonary arteries.

or otherwise dissected to allow passage of ligatures, clips, or vascular forceps. The main pulmonary artery bifurcates at the same level as the opening of the ductus arteriosus (Fig. 38.18). The origin and course of the right pulmonary artery are invisible to the veterinary surgeon, but the conjoining of the ductus and the right pulmonary artery forms an abrupt right angle that is thin and fragile when aneurysmic dilatation has occurred (Fig. 38.19).

Surgical Techniques

Nonsurgical transvascular occlusion of PDA with radiographically imaged assistance has been performed in dogs, but the treatments most commonly used for PDA are surgical occlusion and division.

The decision between occlusion and division is made at the time of surgery. In our experience, occlusion is always possible, and we prefer double ligation to single ligation or the application of clips, because we believe the incidence of recanalization or inadvertent tearing is reduced. The discovery of an aorticopulmonary fusion or "window" would require division. Division and oversewing are also required when the ductus is accidentally lacerated or avulsed.

The suture material used for ligature of a PDA is the prerogative of the surgeon, but some general observations assist in avoiding mistakes. Size 0 to 2 suture is used, depending on the size of the dog. Braided synthetic nonabsorbable suture is soft, supple, and permanent; however, if contaminated during placement, it can harbor microorganisms. Natural fiber silk may weaken over time and may permit recanalization.

Monofilament synthetic nonabsorbable suture passes with little resistance, but it is more difficult to knot securely, and if it is cut too short, the constant movement of the beating heart may cause the sharp suture ends to erode through the major vessels. Therefore, monofilament suture ends should be cut at a *minimum* of 2 cm.

Overview of the Conventional Approach

The conventional approach to dissection of the medial aspect of the PDA requires separation of the mediastinal pleura, retraction of the phrenic and vagus nerves, and protection of the left recurrent laryngeal nerve. After the pleura has been removed from the lateral aspects of the aorta, pulmonary artery, and PDA, right-angled forceps are used to dissect caudally to cranially between the left pulmonary artery and the aorta. During dissection medial to the PDA, the medial aspect of the ductus may stretch and tear at the right pulmonary arterial junction. Additionally, the natural tendency is to try to dissect as superficially and conservatively as possible. In fact, deeper, more dorsal dissection placed toward the medial side of the aorta puts less stress on the PDA. Additional hazards in conventional dissection include variations in toughness of the ductus and differences in pleural reflections. These dissection

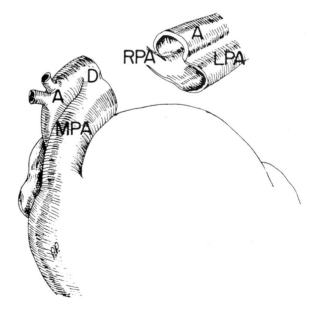

Fig. 38.19. Anatomy of the patent ductus arteriosus with transverse section through main pulmonary artery (MPA), patent ductus (D), and aorta (A). The intra-aortic shelf of the ductus (see Fig. 38.18) has been omitted. The right pulmonary artery (RPA) arborizes from the main pulmonary artery at the level and immediately ventromedial to the patent ductus. The angle of the right pulmonary artery–patent ductus junction is the most common location of tearing during dissection. LPA, left pulmonary artery.

techniques are mentioned in the previous section of this chapter.

Modified Double-Ligation Occlusion of the Ductus

The patient's left shoulder, brachium, and hemithorax are routinely prepared for left lateral thoracotomy.

After thoracotomy, the mediastinal pleura dorsal to the aorta, but ventral to the thoracic duct, is incised with scissors from the left subclavian artery to the first aortic intercostal artery, which branches at the fifth rib. This wound is deepened by digital dissection to the medial (right) side of the aorta, and the aortic arch is freed (Fig. 38.20A). The ventral incised border of the mediastinal pleura is elevated with forceps, and

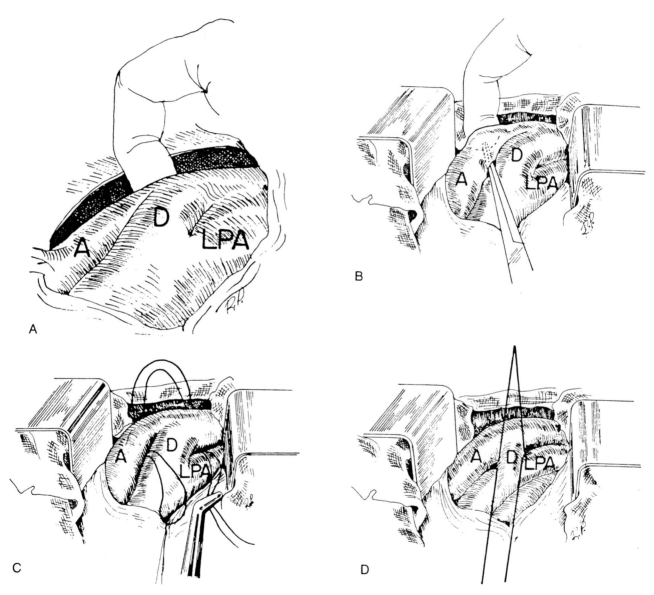

Fig. 38.20. Double-ligation occlusion of patent ductus arteriosus. **A.** After incision of the mediastinum dorsal to the aorta, the dissection of the medial aspect of the aorta (A) is performed digitally. Between the left subclavian and first intercostal vessels (at the fifth space) there are no vessels, nor are there fragile structures medial to the aorta in the mediastinum. The aorta is thoroughly mobilized on its medial aspect. **B.** Ligature placement. A pair of blunt, smooth hemostats are passed ventral to the aortic arch (A), aided by the index finger. The tips of the instrument should be kept close to the aorta. The instrument should be thin enough to ensure that stretching of the patent ductus (D) and of the pulmonary artery is minimal. Once passed, the instrument grasps the midpoint of a suture, which is drawn to the lateral aortic aspect. **C.** The maneuver used in **B** is repeated caudal to the ductus (D) around the descending aorta (A), and the two free ends of the looped ligature are pulled laterally. Care is taken to prevent the ligatures from becoming entwined. **D.** The suture is placed under tension, and the medial aortic lengths are gently placed by traction medial to the ductus (D). The looped cranial suture is cut in two, forming two separate ligatures encircling the ductus that are carefully and slowly tied. A, aorta; LPA, left pulmonary artery.

dissection is continued to expose the lateral aspect of the descending aorta and the PDA to the main and left pulmonary arteries. The mediastinal pleura is retracted ventrally; this maneuver retracts and protects the vagus and phrenic nerves. The left recurrent laryngeal nerve can be tagged if desired. The pericardium is avoided entirely.

When the ductus arteriosus is plainly visualized, a pair of ligatures is readily placed by passing a fine, blunt, curved hemostat or Mixter forceps from ventral to dorsal around the medial aspect of the aorta cranial to the ductus. Elevation of the aortic arch with an index finger while keeping the hemostat close to the aorta aids the initial passage. The instrument picks up the midpoint of the ligature on the dorsomedial aspect of the aortic arch (Fig. 38.20**B**). The ligature is drawn to the lateral aspect of the aortic arch. Forceps should not be opened too widely to receive the looped end, or a tear could result. The jaws of the forceps should be sufficiently long that the instrument does not engage tissue in the vascular triangle as they are closed.

Forceps are introduced a second time, medial to the descending aorta and caudal to the ductus. The instrument grasps and withdraws the free ends of the ligature (Fig. 38.20**C**). The ductus arteriosus has now been loosely encircled, and preparation is made to slide the ligatures into position medial to the ductus. The ends of the suture should not be intertwined; if they are, the ligature will not be separated on the medial aspect of the ductus and will not allow proper double ligation.

The looped cranial and free caudal ends of the ligature are next placed under traction to advance the ligature from the dorsomedial aspect of the aorta to the aorta and right pulmonary artery. The ligature thus dissects the loose stroma between the vessels and incorporates a small amount of cushioning areolar tissue on the medial aspect of the ductus arteriosus (Fig. 38.20**D**).

The looped end is divided to form two complete ligatures. The occlusion procedure is completed by tying the ligatures slowly to allow time for compensation of the vascular dynamics. The aortic side is closed first. While the ligatures are being tied, the heart rate and rhythm are observed for bradycardia. Before the left cranial lung lobes are replaced, the heart and major vessels are palpated to be certain that no fremitus resulting from an incompletely closed ductus or an unsuspected pulmonic stenosis remains.

Ductus Division

If a ductus arteriosus is too short to ligate with a double or single ligature, or if iatrogenic trauma has caused hemorrhage, the ductus must be divided and sutured. Technical skill in dissection and suturing and adequate instrumentation should be available in the event the PDA tears. Dissection for division and over-sewing can be conducted rapidly by passing a ligature as with the modified double-ligation technique, but ligature must be removed before placing the vascular clamps. An identical pair of patent ductus or coarctation forceps (pediatric cardiovascular forceps, American V. Mueller, Chicago, IL) specifically designed for this application are applied with the tips directed cranially. By being identical, they can be placed in close approximation. Alternatively, a Pott–Smith aortic clamp (American V. Mueller) may be used on the aortic side (Fig. 38.21).

The occluding forceps are placed to allow at least 2 to 3 mm of vessel to lie between the forceps. The ductus arteriosus is divided, and the forceps are rolled

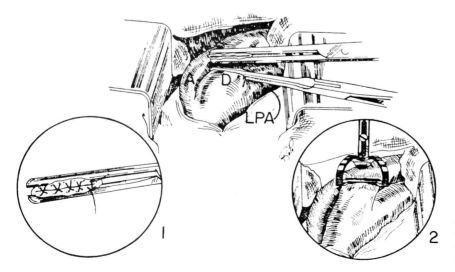

Fig. 38.21. Ductus division and control of hemorrhage. Patent ductus or coarctation forceps are applied with the tips directed cranially. Modern instruments have fine teeth that are atraumatic and prevent slippage. A, aorta; D, ductus; LPA, left pulmonary artery. *Inset 1,* The ductus may be sutured with a simple continuous overlap (baseball or shoelace pattern), as shown, or with a fine simple continuous pattern. Small leaks are best managed with cruciate (X) mattress sutures. *Inset 2,* An alternative instrument, especially for short "windows," is Pott's aortic clamp. This instrument includes a section of aortic wall, which is especially useful if the ductus has torn. Various sizes are made, and one size is not satisfactory for all dogs.

laterally to expose the cut ductus edge for suturing. Size 5–0 sutures swaged onto a cardiovascular needle and a closely approximated simple continuous suture pattern or the over-and-over pattern are adequate (Fig. 38.21, *inset 2*). The needle is passed in an arc following its natural curve with an arced wrist motion to prevent vascular tearing. The clamps are removed slowly to check for bleeding. Slight seepage is common, but it stops with digital pressure. Pulsatile hemorrhage is inhibited by cruciate or simple interrupted sutures. A small piece of oxidized cellulose sponge is interposed between the suture lines before closure to minimize suture abrasion.

Thoracotomy Closure

The ribs are approximated with heavy absorbable suture material, and the muscle, fascias, subcutis, and skin are closed in layers. Before rib closure, an intercostal nerve block is applied as previously described. A thoracic catheter is optional, but is rarely indicated. Air is removed from the pleural space by inflation of the lungs as soon as the layers of muscle sutured can provide a seal. However, if persistent pneumothorax is anticipated, a thoracic catheter should be placed before rib closure, even if it is only to be left in place for a few hours to assist in postoperative management.

Complications

Intraoperative complications include tearing of the major vessels, air embolization, central nervous or myocardial hypoxia, hypothermia, and hypercapnea or hypocapnea and attendant respiratory acidosis or alkalosis, respectively. In the event of severe hemorrhage, digital pressure should be immediately applied to retard bleeding, and suction should be used to clear the operative field. If possible, the tear is sutured by briefly releasing the digital occlusion, placing a needle pass, and reapplying digital occlusion. This sequence is continued until the tear is closed. If digital pressure cannot occlude flow, the aortic arch, left pulmonary artery–ductus junction, and descending aorta can be cross-clamped to attenuate hemorrhage during the repair. Continued suction is important to facilitate visualization. The duration of cross-clamping should be minimized. Spinal cord ischemia for longer than 20 minutes increases the probability of permanent injury. With patience, finesse, and good technique, most iatrogenic tears can be repaired.

Postoperative complications include recanalization, congestive heart failure, lung torsion, infection, thromboembolism, pneumothorax, cardiac tamponade, and adhesions. Careful technique and attention to detail limit these sequelae.

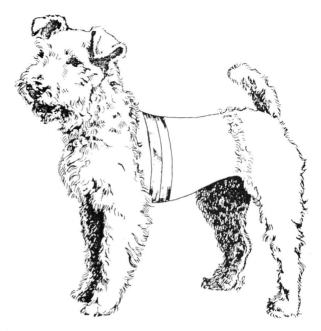

Fig. 38.22. Chest bandage after a routine surgical procedure for patent ductus arteriosus. The functions of a bandage are to protect the wound, apply pressure to prevent hematoma, and mechanically stabilize to minimize pain and assist sutures. These functions can be performed by a snug bandage over only the surgical site. Tape is applied directly to the hair of the right side to prevent slippage. A narrow bandage improves respiration and allows aseptic preparation for thoracentesis without removing a full chest wrap.

Postoperative Care

Injectable analgesics are administered as described earlier. As a routine, pneumothorax must be considered as a possible complication. Immediately after skin closure, thoracentesis is performed, bilaterally, and the volume is recorded. In the postoperative period, any deterioration in ventilation should cause clinical reevaluation for pneumothorax. The routine evaluations of temperature, pulse rate and quality, and respiratory rate and quality are continued at 15-minute intervals until the dog's condition is stable. If a thoracic catheter was placed, it is removed as soon as practical. In the postoperative period, fluid administration is usually not required. Weak pulse and pallor are corrected by the administration crystalloids, but total fluid administration in the routine correction of PDA usually should not exceed 20 to 40 mL/kg.

Mechanical stabilization of the thoracic wound further decreases the discomfort of surgical wounding. Sterile dressings are applied over the wound, and one or two strips of 2-inch tape should compress the sterile dressing tightly over the wound and should circumferentially encompass the torso from the third through the fifth rib spaces (Fig. 38.22). Tape is applied directly to the skin and hair to prevent slippage. Full thoracic bandages are contraindicated because they compromise ventilation and make thoracentesis difficult.

Suggested Readings

Eyster GD. Patent ductus arteriosus in the dog: characteristics of recurrence and results of 100 consecutive cases. J Am Vet Med Assoc 1976;168:435.

Goodwin JK, Lombard CW. Patent ductus arteriosus in adult dogs: clinical features of 14 cases. J Am Anim Hosp Assoc 1992; 28:349–354.

Grifka RG, Miller MW, Frischmeyer KJ, et al. Transcatheter occlusion of a patent ductus arteriosus in a Newfoundland puppy using the Gianturco–Grifka vascular occlusion device. J Vet Intern Med 1996;10:42–44.

Snaps FR, McEntee K, Saunders JH, et al. Treatment of patent ductus arteriosus by placement of intravascular coils in a pup. J Am Vet Med Assoc 1995;207:724–725.

Weirich WE, Blevins WE, Rebar AH. Late consequences of patent ductus arteriosus in the dog: a report of six cases. J Am Anim Hosp Assoc 1978;14:40.

Surgical Correction of Persistent Right Aortic Arch

Gary W. Ellison

Incidence

Persistent right aortic arch (PRAA) accounts for approximately 95% of all reported vascular ring anomalies in the dog. It is the fourth most common cardiovascular malformation in dogs; only patent ductus arteriosus, pulmonic stenosis, and aortic stenosis have a higher incidence. Other vascular ring anomalies that are occasionally seen include double aortic arch, aberrant left and right subclavian arteries, and persistent right ligamentum arteriosum (1).

Purebred dogs are more susceptible than mongrels to PRAA. The condition is likely heritable with German shepherds, and Irish setters appear to have a higher incidence than the general canine population. Increased numbers of offspring with PRAA have been observed in certain family lines. Because single or multiple recessive genes appear to be responsible for the trait, breeding of affected animals is discouraged (2, 3).

In cats, the exact incidence of PRAA is unknown, but the anomaly appears to be less common than in dogs. About half the feline cases occur in Siamese and Persian cats, although the absolute numbers are insufficient to make conclusions on breed predisposition (4).

Persistent left cranial vena cava occurs in conjunction with PRAA about 40% of the time. The left cranial vena cava is not clinically significant, because it empties into the right atrium and does not act as a constricting vascular ring. However, its presence may make surgical dissection more difficult because it passes over the pulmonary artery and partially obliterates visualization of the ligamentum arteriosum. PRAA is rarely associated with concurrent patent ductus arteriosus. When patent ductus arteriosus is present, diagnosis is usually made at the time of surgery. Minimal blood flow occurs through the ductus, and insufficient turbulence is produced to create a murmur.

Animals with PRAA usually are diagnosed early in life, usually before 6 months of age. Exceptions sometimes occur, however, and diagnosis in dogs as old as 10 years have been reported. Whereas in humans, PRAA often is asymptomatic, virtually all cases in the dog and cat involve some degree of esophageal constriction and resultant regurgitation.

Embryologic Development

PRAA occurs when the right fourth arch, instead of the left, enlarges and becomes the functional adult aorta. The right ductus arteriosus degenerates, and the left ductus arteriosus remains. This configuration forms a strap that constricts the esophagus between the left pulmonary artery and the anomalous right aorta. The vascular ring is thus formed by the aorta on the right, the ligamentum arteriosum on the left dorsolaterally, the pulmonary trunk on the left, and the base of the heart ventrally (1, 2).

Diagnosis

Dogs and cats affected with PRAA usually are asymptomatic when nursing, but postprandial regurgitation of solid food may occur as early as 4 to 8 weeks of age. A ravenous appetite is typically reported, but the animal usually lags behind littermates in size and body weight. Regurgitation often occurs shortly after eating, although it may be delayed for several hours. The regurgitated food usually is undigested, covered by mucus, and has a neutral pH. With long-term retention, fermentation may occur, giving the regurgitated food a characteristic foul odor. A cough may be reported, indicating the presence of aspiration pneumonia.

Auscultation of the heart is usually normal; even in animals with PRAA with patent ductus arteriosus, no murmur is present. Lung sounds can be normal, or rales can be heard if aspiration pneumonia is present. Food retained in the dilated esophagus may produce a gurgling sound on auscultation. If dilation extends up into the central esophagus, a characteristic postprandial bulge may be seen or palpated at the thoracic inlet. Simultaneous closing of the mouth and external nares while gently squeezing the abdomen may produce bulging of the cervical esophagus (1–3).

Radiographic signs that may be observed on plain thoracic films include ventral tracheal displacement, mediastinal widening, and occasionally a right-sided descending aortic shadow. Ventral tracheal displacement is caused by the dilated esophagus. If only the cranial thoracic esophagus is dilated, the trachea returns to a normal position at the tracheal bifurcation over the heart base, and the trachea and heart are displaced ventrally. Mediastinal widening is caused by the dilated esophagus and usually is confined to the cranial mediastinum. With both a prestenotic and poststenotic esophageal dilation, the mediastinum is wide throughout the entire thorax.

An esophagogram should be performed to confirm the diagnosis. Esophagographic findings may consist of cranial thoracic esophageal dilation alone or cranial and caudal thoracic esophageal dilation associated with abrupt esophageal narrowing over the heart base at the fourth rib. On the ventrodorsal view, the esophagus may be displaced to the left just proximal to the stricture, with an indentation into the right side of the esophagus. If available, fluoroscopic evaluation determines the quality of esophageal peristalsis in the dilated esophagus both preoperatively and postoperatively. Endoscopy can also be a useful tool in evaluating the magnitude of esophageal dilation and in demonstrating constriction of the intrathoracic esophagus over the base of the heart.

Presurgical Considerations

Definitive treatment for PRAA involves surgical ligation and division of the ligamentum arteriosum. Dietary management alone is usually unrewarding because, without relieving the esophageal constriction, the prestenotic dilation often enlarges with age. Animals with PRAA often present in a debilitated, cachectic, and dehydrated state that requires special presurgical considerations. Any fluid or electrolyte imbalances should be corrected preoperatively. Aspiration pneumonia, if present, compromises the patient's ability to ventilate the lungs effectively. Placement of gastric feeding tubes for an esophageal bypass in combination with broad-spectrum antibiotics may be indicated to pretreat patients with severe aspiration pneumonia.

We use propofol for rapid intravenous induction of anesthesia and tracheal intubation. Immediately after induction, the patient should be assisted in its ventilatory effort. A grossly enlarged cranial esophagus may inhibit the inflatability of cranial and middle lung lobes during anesthesia. Anesthesia is maintained with inhalants such as isoflurane or halothane.

Surgical Technique

Surgical ligation of the ligamentum arteriosum is best accomplished through a left fourth thoracotomy (see Chap. 23). The cranial and middle lung lobes are packed caudally with moistened surgical sponges. The esophagus, aorta, main pulmonary artery, and left vagus nerve are identified. The mediastinal pleura is transected longitudinally, and the vagus nerve is reflected dorsally with 2–0 silk. The ligamentum arteriosum usually is longer than normal and often is difficult to visualize within the fibrous ring. It is most easily located cranial to the recurrent laryngeal nerve. If a persistent left cranial vena cava is present, it may have a hemizygous branch that obscures the ligamentum arteriosum. This stricture can be ligated and reflected ventrally. If an aberrant left or right subclavian artery is also compressing the esophagus, it must be elevated and divided between ligatures. Adequate collateral circulation is provided by the vertebral arteries.

Blunt dissection of the ligamentum arteriosum is performed in a caudal to cranial direction with right-angle forceps (Fig. 38.23**A**). The ligament is elevated off the esophagus from its left lateral aspect. Care must be taken during dissection near the pulmonary artery, because this vessel is easily torn. When the ligament is successfully freed, two ligatures of 1–0 surgical silk are placed as close to the aorta and pulmonary artery, respectively, as possible (Fig. 38.23**B**). The ligamentum arteriosum is then divided between the ligatures. Traction then is placed on the ligatures, and the esophagus is dissected free of any residual fibrous bands between the aorta and the pulmonary artery (Fig. 38.23**C**). Extreme care is necessary during this dissection because the esophagus is thin and easily perforated. A 22-French Foley catheter is then introduced through the mouth into the esophagus and is passed down to the constriction. Inflation of the cuff at the constriction helps to visualize any residual fibrous constricting bands and facilitates their removal. Passage of the inflated cuff back and forth at the stricture site indicates when sufficient esophageal lumen size has been obtained (Fig. 38.23**D**).

Resection of the dilated cranial esophagus is usually not attempted because of its thin walls and inherent tendency for leakage. With moderate esophageal dilation, passage of food improves once the constriction is relieved. If severe chronic dilation is present, plication of a redundant esophagus with Lembert-type gathering sutures of 4–0 nylon or polypropylene can be attempted. Care must be taken not to penetrate the mucosa of the esophagus, because leakage around the sutures may occur and postoperative pleuritis or pyothorax may result. For intractable regurgitation, resection of a dilated esophagus with thoracoabdominal

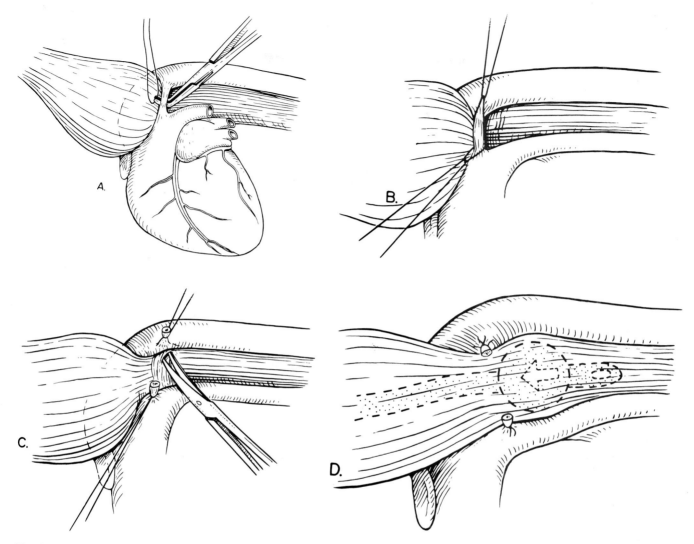

Fig. 38.23. Surgical ligation and division of ligamentum arteriosum. **A.** Blunt dissection and ligamentum arteriosum and right-angle forceps and insertion of ligature. **B.** Location of silk sutures around the ligamentum arteriosum. **C.** Blunt dissection of remaining fibrous bands after division of the ligamentum arteriosum. **D.** Use of Foley catheter to ensure that constriction has been relieved. See text for details.

(TA-55) autostapling equipment has been attempted but with only fair results. Plication or resection of a dilated esophagus only reduces redundant tissue and does not restore normal esophageal peristalsis.

After ligation and division is completed, a thoracostomy tube is placed, and routine thoracic closure is performed. Postoperative antibiotics are continued if aspiration pneumonia is present. Parenteral analgesics or infusion of local anesthetics into the pleural cavity can be used to manage postsurgical pain.

Postoperative Care

Postoperative management of animals with PRAA involves reestablishment of an adequate plane of nu-

trition and efforts to prevent further regurgitation. Elevated feedings of small amounts of canned or moistened kibbled food are started the day after the surgical procedure. The animal is fed from a stool or platform that requires the forelimbs to be elevated off the ground. Feeding small quantities of food provided three or more times daily is generally more successful than single large feedings. Small portions of the solid food usually do not pocket in the cervical esophagus and do not reflux into the trachea as easily as liquid diets if regurgitated. If solid food does not pass into the stomach, gruel is used. Holding the patient upright while rocking it slowly back and forth may also facilitate passage of the food. Elevated feedings are continued for at least 8 weeks before normal feedings are attempted. Some animals resume regurgitation with horizontal feedings and require vertical feedings as a lifelong procedure.

Prognosis

Morbidity and mortality associated with PRAA are usually seen in the perioperative period and are usually due to aspiration pneumonia. Animals surviving the postoperative period and leaving the hospital stand a good chance to improve clinically. A contrast esophagogram performed 24 to 72 hours after surgery serves as a baseline and documents release of the constriction. Contrast studies performed 3 to 4 months postoperatively are then helpful in evaluating the esophagus for decreasing dilation. Esophageal dilation usually decreases with time, but it is not reversible. Likewise, esophageal peristalsis also usually improves with time, but it does not return to normal. Although these radiographic changes remain, many animals regurgitate much less regularly after surgical treatment (5, 6). In one study of 45 dogs, good to excellent results with either no regurgitation or only sporadic regurgitation occurred in about 90% of animals that survived beyond 6 months. Fewer than 10% of the animals failed to respond to surgery and required euthanasia. In general, dogs or cats with esophageal dilation caudal to the heart are poor surgical candidates. The exact cause of postcardial esophageal dilation associated with PRAA is unknown, but interference of the vagus nerves at the constriction may play a factor.

At the present time, early surgical ligation and division of the ligamentum arteriosum offer patients with PRAA a reasonable long-term prognosis. Reversal of clinical signs is less likely as the age of the animal increases. In addition to surgical management, medical dietary therapy is required. Esophageal dilation usually remains, but it may be decreased enough that the animal is free of symptoms.

References

1. Helphrey ML. Vascular ring anomalies in the dog. Vet Clin North Am 1979;9:207.
2. Ellison GW. Vascular ring anomalies in the dog and cat. Compend Contin Educ Pract Vet 1980;2:693.
3. Van Gundy T. Vascular ring anomalies. Compend Contin Educ Pract Vet 1989;11:36.
4. Wheaton LG. Persistent right aortic arch associated with other vascular anomalies in two cats. J Am Vet Med Assoc 1984; 184:848.
5. Shires PK. Persistent right aortic arch in dogs: a long-term follow-up after surgical correction. J Am Anim Hosp Assoc 1981;17:773.
6. Muldoon MM, Birchard SJ, Ellison GW. Long-term results of surgical correction of persistent right aortic arch in dogs: a retrospective study. In: Abstracts of the 31st Annual ACVS Scientific Meeting. American College of Veterinary Surgeons, San Francisco 1996:16.

Surgical Correction of Pulmonic Stenosis

D. J. Krahwinkel, Jr. & Jill E. Sackman

Pulmonic stenosis is reported to be the third most common congenital heart disease in the dog, with patent ductus arteriosus and aortic stenosis being first and second, respectively (1). The English bulldog is the most common breed represented; however, other dogs at risk include the beagle, samoyed, chihuahua, schnauzer, Boykin spaniel, mastiff, and various terrier breeds (2). The disease occurs equally between males and females, except in the bulldog, in which the incidence in males predominates. The disease is rare in cats. Pulmonic stenosis has a genetic basis in dogs, although this basis is uncertain in the cat (3).

The lesion may occur as supravalvular, valvular, or subvalvular stenosis. With any of the three, infundibular stenosis may occur in which the hypertrophied musculature obstructs the right ventricular outflow tract. The valvular site is by far the most common and is manifested by thickening, fibrosis, and hypoplasia of the valve leading to outflow obstruction.

Diagnosis

Many animals with pulmonic stenosis are asymptomatic early in life; some remain asymptomatic indefinitely. Animals with more severe cases display exertional fatigue, dyspnea, and syncope. Signs of right heart failure, including ascites, hepatomegaly, and arrhythmia, may be present in advanced cases (4). Physical examination reveals a systolic ejection murmur heard over the pulmonic valve that often radiates along the sternum to both sides of the thorax. A holosystolic murmur of tricuspid insufficiency may sometimes be auscultated over the right hemithorax.

The electrocardiogram (ECG) usually indicates right ventricular hypertrophy, including right axial deviation and S waves in leads I, II, III, and aVF. Thoracic radiographs reveal varying degrees of cardiomegaly. The right side of the heart predominates in the enlargement. A poststenotic dilatation of the main pulmonary artery is seen on the dorsoventral view. The pulmonary vessels appear normal or underperfused. Cardiac catheterization helps to locate the specific site of the stenosis and to measure pressure gradients for prognosis. Measuring gradients under anesthesia gives pressure readings that are usually much lower than actually exist. Angiographic features of pulmonic stenosis include thickened and dysplastic valve leaflets, narrowing of the outflow tract and valve orifice, post-stenotic dilatation of the pulmonary artery, and right ventricular hypertrophy. In English bulldogs, an anomalous left coronary artery may be seen crossing the ventricle at the level of the stenosis.

In many cases, echocardiography and Doppler examination provide sufficient data making cardiac catheterization unnecessary. Typical findings are hypertrophy of the right ventricle, muscular narrowing of the right ventricular outflow tract, deformity and narrowing of the pulmonic valve, and poststenotic dilatation of the pulmonary artery. Pressure gradients measured by Doppler are more likely than catheterization to give an accurate assessment of the severity of disease because the examination does not require general anesthesia. Echocardiography or cardiac catheterization can usually demonstrate the severity of the disease and can locate the stenosis at the supravalvular, valvular, subvalvular, or infundibular site. This information is crucial in determining surgical candidates, selecting the correct surgical procedure, and giving a prognosis. In some patients, it is difficult to delineate between a pure valvular stenosis and one that is both valvular and subvalvular. This ambiguity makes selection of the proper surgical technique more difficult.

Surgical Guidelines

Nonanesthetized pressure gradients that are less than 50 mm Hg are generally considered mild, and such patients do not require surgical intervention. Severe gradients exceeding 80 mm Hg place the patient at risk of heart failure and death. These animals should have surgical intervention (3, 4). Dogs with moderate disease (gradients of 50 to 80 mm Hg) may or may not require surgical correction, depending on the progression of the disease. One author has recommended surgery when: 1) the right ventricular pressure exceeds 120 mm Hg or a gradient exceeds 100 mm Hg in a mature dog, or 2) the right ventricular pressure is 90 to 120 or a gradient of 70 to 100 in an immature dog (5). Others recommend surgery any time the gradient exceeds 50 mm Hg and right ventricular hypertrophy is significant (6).

Any animal not undergoing surgery should be reevaluated at 3-month intervals to determine whether the disease is progressing. Symptomatic animals should have surgical intervention regardless of their pressure gradients. One problem with waiting to see whether a patient's disease is progressive based on pressure measurements or disease signs is that these animals may become poorer surgical candidates with time. These animals may develop secondary infundibular muscular stenosis, worsening hypertrophy and fibrosis of the right ventricle and right heart failure. If possible, surgery should be delayed until the animal is mature, so the procedure is done on a fully developed heart that will not outgrow the correction.

Even though various authors have stated guidelines for surgical intervention, most of these are based on personal observations. No clinical trials have been conducted in dogs with long-term follow-up to validate criteria for surgical intervention or to determine which corrective procedure gives the best results.

Anesthesia

Nearly all anesthetic agents depress cardiopulmonary function directly or alter reflex regulatory mechanisms (7). Patients with cardiac disease may have little to no reserve for compensation; therefore, anesthetic agents must be administered carefully and in reduced dosages. Preanesthetic agents should be administered to relieve anxiety and to reduce the amount of depressant general anesthetic required. A combination of a benzodiazepine (diazepam or midazolam) and an opioid (morphine or oxymorphone) is used for sedation. Opioid-induced respiratory depression may occur; therefore, oxygen by mask should be provided during the induction process. Anticholinergics, especially atropine, are not used unless bradycardia occurs, because of their propensity to induce tachycardia.

Anesthetic induction is completed by administering low-concentration isoflurane in oxygen until tracheal intubation can be accomplished. Anesthetic maintenance is by continued low concentration of isoflurane supplemented with intermittent doses of opioid (morphine, oxymorphone, or fentanyl). Intermittent positive-pressure ventilation is provided either manually or mechanically. Profound muscle relaxation can be produced by intravenous administration of atracurium, a nondepolarizing muscle relaxant.

Patients with pulmonic stenosis must be closely monitored for cardiopulmonary function. Monitoring parameters should include heart rate, ECG, pulse quality, direct or indirect blood pressure, pulse oximetry, and central venous pressure. Assessment of blood volume and hemodilution is by serial determinations of packed cell volume and total plasma proteins. Renal function is assessed by measuring urine production. Blood pressure is maintained by a maintenance flow of intravenous crystalloids supplemented with colloids (dextran or hetastarch). Cross-matched whole blood must be available should major hemorrhage occur.

Surgical Procedures

Various surgical procedures have been described for correction of pulmonic stenosis (8). These include balloon dilatation, open valvulotomy or valvulectomy, closed valvulotomy or dilatation, patch grafting, bypass conduit, and open heart repair with cardiopulmonary bypass. The specific procedure depends on the location of the stenosis, the size of the patient, the severity of the disease, the expertise of the surgeon, and the equipment available. Many of the procedures have been adapted from techniques used to correct pulmonic stenosis in children, although direct application to animals may be erroneous. For example, valvular stenosis in children is commonly a fusion of the valve leaflets, whereas in dogs it is usually a fibrotic, thickened, dysplastic valve. Direct comparison of the techniques or the expected results between children and dogs should not be made.

Balloon Valvuloplasty

The technique of percutaneous balloon valvuloplasty has been used extensively for the treatment of valvular pulmonic stenosis in children (9). The technique has been applied to the dog as a noninvasive way to dilate the stenotic valve mechanically in high-risk patients without infundibular hypertrophy (10–14). Balloon valvuloplasty is performed in patients after angiocardiographic studies are used to evaluate the location and extent of the stenotic lesion. Selective coronary angiography to evaluate for possible single right coronary artery is recommended in bulldogs and boxers before balloon valvuloplasty because balloon dilation in these patients has been associated with sudden death (15).

Cardiac catheterization provides important information regarding pressure gradients across the stenotic valve, cardiac output, and oxygen tension. Potential complications include vascular damage during catheter placement, emboli, and dysrhythmias. In anticipation of potential catheter-induced dysrhythmias, antidysrhythmic drugs and a defibrillator should be readily available. Catheterization is performed with the patient under general anesthesia. The right external jugular vein is surgically isolated, and pressures in the right ventricle and pulmonary artery are measured after placement of an appropriately sized end-hole catheter suitable for pressure recording. The normal gradient recorded from the right ventricle to the pulmonary artery should be less than 5 mm Hg. Pulmonic stenosis produces a pressure gradient from the right ventricle to the pulmonary artery that varies based on the degree of the lesion.

Valvuloplasty is performed after a pullback pressure recording across the pulmonic valve. The cardiac catheter is repositioned in the pulmonary artery, and an angioplasty guidewire is passed through the catheter. The cardiac catheter is removed, and a balloon dilation catheter (i.e., Owens balloon dilation catheter, Mansfield Scientific) with an inflatable balloon (approxi-

mately 10% greater than the angiographically determined diameter of the valve annulus) is advanced over the guidewire (Fig. 38.24). The balloon is centered across the stenotic valve and, using a syringe and pressure gauge, is rapidly inflated by hand with a 1:1 mixture of saline and contrast medium (Fig. 38.25). The balloon should be inflated and deflated several times. Inflation time should be maintained for 6 to 8 seconds. After deflation, an indentation in the stenotic valve caused by the balloon may be visualized. Ventricular premature beats and transient (1- to 3-minute) right bundle branch block have been observed during the procedure (10, 11). The balloon catheter should then be replaced by an end-hole catheter, and pressures again should be recorded across the valvular lesion. Reported peak systolic pressure gradient reductions after balloon dilation have been from 46 to 80% (11, 14).

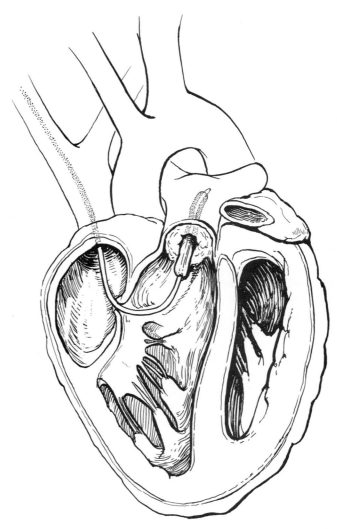

Fig. 38.24. Placement of the balloon catheter. (Copyright 1996, University of Tennessee College of Veterinary Medicine, Knoxville, TN.)

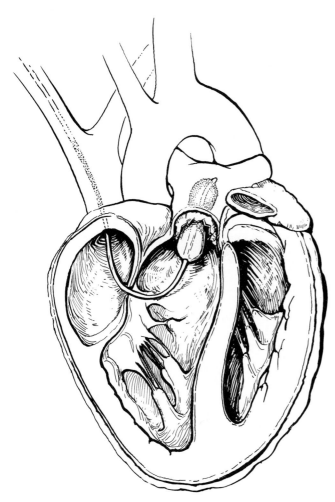

Fig. 38.25. Inflation of the balloon catheter. (Copyright 1996, University of Tennessee College of Veterinary Medicine, Knoxville, TN.)

Although pulmonary valvuloplasty is a well-established technique in pediatric cardiology, its use in the dog is recent, and long-term efficacy is unknown. Recatheterization of patients 3 months after valvuloplasty showed sustained hemodynamic improvement and pressure gradient reductions (11). Balloon valvuloplasty has been most successful in children whose pulmonic valve leaflets are fused but relatively thin (16). In patients with thick, dysplastic valves and a hypoplastic annulus, the technique is significantly less effective (16). The lesion in the dog frequently involves thickened fibrotic valves and a hypoplastic annulus, indicating that long-term results of balloon valvuloplasty in this species may be less than successful. Many patients undergoing balloon procedures will probably need additional intervention at a later time. The procedure may provide a "bridge" to allow small patients to reach adequate size for definitive correction.

Open Valvulotomy or Valvulectomy

This procedure is a modification of the technique developed by Swan (17) using transient venous inflow occlusion and a pulmonary arteriotomy. The technique is used in patients with a valvular stenosis and minimal to no subvalvular component. The thorax is opened by a thoracotomy at the left fourth intercostal space. The cranial vena cava is isolated by dissecting between the thymus and the cranial aspect of the pericardial sac. The cranial vena cava is located on the right side of the thorax and ventral to the brachycephalic artery. A Rumel tourniquet of umbilical tape is placed on the vessel. The caudal vena cava is approached by incising the caudal mediastinum immediately behind the pericardial sac and ventral to the phrenic nerve. The vessel can be visualized deep in the mediastinal space to the right side of the thorax. Right-angle forceps are used to place a Rumel tourniquet similar to that used in the cranial vena cava. Dissection of the caudal vena cava may be impossible from the fourth intercostal space in dogs with severe cardiac enlargement. In these instances, the caudal edge of the incised skin is retracted, and a small thoracotomy incision is made at the sixth intercostal space. The caudal vena cava is easily isolated from this position.

The pericardial sac is incised parallel and ventral to the phrenic nerve. Four to six stay sutures are placed in the pericardial sac and are secured to the surgical drapes to "cradle" the heart (Fig. 38.26). Lidocaine applied topically to the heart and an intravenous lidocaine drip help to minimize surgically induced arrhythmias. Stay sutures of 5–0 polypropylene are placed in the dilated pulmonary artery immediately distal to the pulmonary valve. Venous inflow occlusion is accomplished by tightening the caval tourniquets. After waiting a few seconds for the heart to empty partially, a 1- to 2-cm incision is made between the two stay sutures (Fig. 38.27). A small retractor at the ventral end of the incision and the two stay sutures retract the arteriotomy site (Fig. 38.28). Suction is used to empty the right ventricle and to visualize the pulmonic valve. The dysplastic leaflets are grasped with forceps, with scissors or a scalpel used to excise the valve (Fig. 38.29). After all three leaflets have been excised or incised, forceps are used to dilate the valve annulus. A "pop" can be felt as the annulus stretches. One finger is inserted into the outflow tract to ensure that the stenosis is relieved. The cranial Rumel tourniquet is released, and the heart and pulmonary artery are permitted to fill to remove all intravascular air. The stay sutures are used to elevate the edges of the artery, and a Satinsky clamp is placed on the arteriotomy site (Fig. 38.30). The secondary Rumel tourniquet is released. Cardiovascular resuscitation is accom-

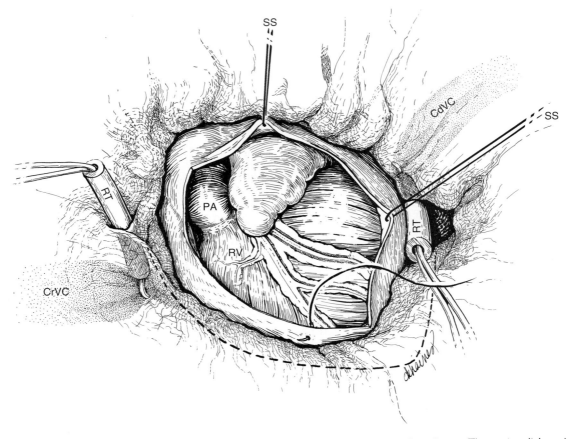

Fig. 38.26. Surgical approach to the right ventricular outflow tract and pulmonary artery (*PA*) is shown. The pericardial sac is opened and is retracted with stay sutures. Rumel tourniquets (*RT*) are placed around the cranial vena cava (*CrVC*) and caudal vena cava (*CdVC*). The pulmonary artery and right ventricle (*RV*) are exposed. (Copyright 1996, University of Tennessee College of Veterinary Medicine, Knoxville, TN.)

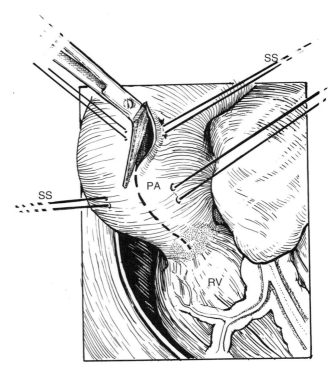

Fig. 38.27. Stay sutures (*SS*) are placed in the dilated pulmonary artery. The pulmonary artery (*PA*) is opened to just above the level of the pulmonic valve (*PV*).(Copyright 1996, University of Tennessee College of Veterinary Medicine, Knoxville, TN.)

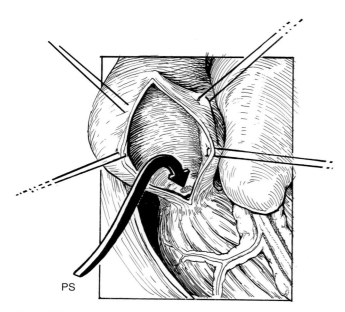

Fig. 38.28. The pulmonic stenosis (*PS*) is observed near the ventral end of the arteriotomy. (Copyright 1996, University of Tennessee College of Veterinary Medicine, Knoxville, TN.)

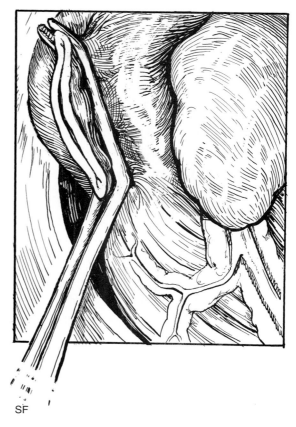

Fig. 38.30. Satinsky forceps (*SF*) are used to occlude the arteriotomy site. (Copyright 1996, University of Tennessee College of Veterinary Medicine, Knoxville, TN.)

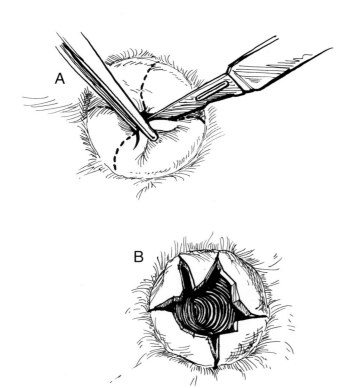

Fig. 38.29. **A.** The dysplastic leaflets are excised using a No. 11 scalpel or scissors. **B.** The appearance of the valve after the leaflets have been partially excised and dilated. (Copyright 1996, University of Tennessee College of Veterinary Medicine, Knoxville, TN.)

plished by digitally occluding the thoracic aorta to increase coronary and cerebral blood flow. Cardiac massage and an intravenous infusion of dopamine may be required to reestablish normal cardiac function. Total inflow occlusion of a diseased heart should not exceed 2 minutes. If this is not sufficient time to complete the procedure, then inflow is terminated, and 10 to 15 minutes of normal cardiac function should be established. A brief second inflow occlusion can be used to complete the procedure. Normal hearts can tolerate 4 minutes or more of inflow occlusion; however, diseased hearts often fibrillate and are difficult to defibrillate.

The arteriotomy is closed with a double row of continuous 5–0 polypropylene suture, and the stay sutures are removed (Fig. 38.31). The pericardial sac is loosely closed with 3–0 absorbable suture. Closing the sac tightly could result in tamponade if the arteriotomy site should leak. The tourniquets are removed, and the thorax is lavaged with warm saline to remove all blood. The intercostal nerves are blocked with local anesthetic for analgesia, a thoracic tube is placed, and the thorax is closed in a routine manner.

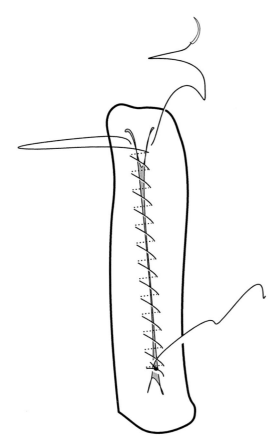

Fig. 38.31. The arteriotomy is closed with a double row of continuous monofilament sutures. (Copyright 1996, University of Tennessee College of Veterinary Medicine, Knoxville, TN.)

Closed Valvulotomy or Dilatation

This procedure is used in patients who likely cannot tolerate even brief inflow occlusion. The surgical approach is as described previously, but without inflow occlusion. A pursestring suture is placed in the right ventricular outflow tract just below the pulmonic valve or in the dilated pulmonary artery above the valve. The suture ends are placed through a piece of tubing similar to the Rumel tourniquet. A stab incision is made through the pursestring and into the lumen of either the right ventricle or the pulmonary artery. A blunt-tipped tent bistoury or valvulotome is passed through the valve, and several blind cuts are made through the stenotic valve by cutting against backpressure applied by the surgeon's finger (Fig. 38.32). A forcep jaw is then placed through the pursestring, and the valve annulus is dilatated to break down the stenotic ring completely. In dogs with severe muscular hypertrophy and a narrow outflow tract, this procedure is more easily accomplished through a pursestring in the dilated pulmonary artery. Simple dilatation without first cutting the stenotic valve may only pro-

vide temporary relief because the torn and stretched tissue may heal with scar tissue, resulting in a new stenosis.

Open Patch Grafting

The use of patch grafting for repair of pulmonic stenosis in the dog was first reported in 1976 (18). The graft extends from the pulmonary artery to the right ventricle and as a result is effective in correcting valvular and subvalvular stenosis as well as alleviating infundibular lesions. Patch grafting may be performed by either a closed or open technique. The closed patch graft technique (18, 19) relies on the placement of a cutting wire across the stenotic lesion under the applied patch. Unfortunately, the technique does not allow excision of the dysplastic valve and relies on the surgeon's ability to place a cutting wire blindly across the defect.

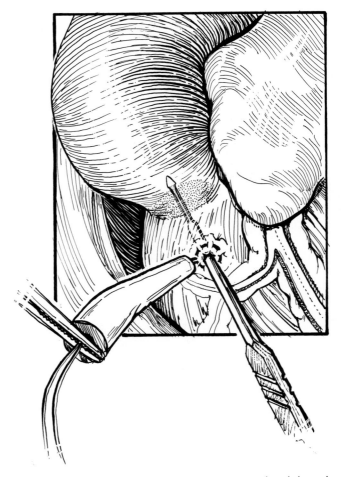

Fig. 38.32. A closed valvulotome or bistoury is placed through a pursestring in the right ventricle, and the dysplastic valve leaflets are incised. (Copyright 1996, University of Tennessee College of Veterinary Medicine, Knoxville, TN.)

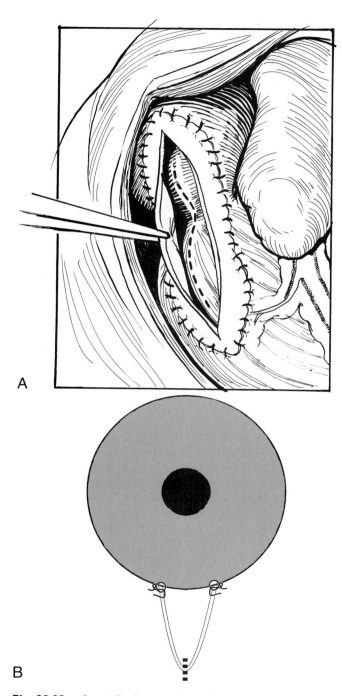

Fig. 38.33. **A** and **B.** Open patch grafting technique. See text. (Copyright 1996, University of Tennessee College of Veterinary Medicine, Knoxville, TN.)

An open technique for patch grafting has been described (20, 21). We prefer a modification of this technique that is performed through a left lateral thoracotomy at the fourth intercostal space. The lungs are retracted dorsally to expose the caudal mediastinum. Umbilical tape is placed around the cranial and caudal vena cava, and a Rumel tourniquet is formed as for

open valvulotomy or valvulectomy. The pericardium is incised parallel and ventral to the phrenic nerve, with an extension ventral and perpendicular. Pericardial basket sutures are placed. An elliptic polytetrafluoroethylene (Gortex, W.L. Gore and Assoc. Elkton, MD) patch is cut so the graft will extend both proximal and distal to the stenotic lesion. The patch is sutured to the outflow tract using 4–0 polypropylene and a double-armed taper-point needle. Suturing is started at the ventral tip of the patch, which is placed on the ventricle with an interrupted suture. The margins are sutured in a continuous fashion up onto the pulmonary artery. The patch must be sutured so at least 1 cm can be "tented" up over the outflow tract. This extra graft allows for expansion of the stenotic area. Once the patch has been applied, it is cut longitudinally at an equal distance between the cranial and caudal margins (Fig. 38.33). The caval tourniquets are tightened to accomplish venous inflow occlusion. A stab incision with a No. 11 scalpel blade is made into the pulmonary artery and is extended to the dorsal and ventral margins of the patch with Metzenbaum scissors. The valve is inspected, and the leaflets are excised (Fig. 38.34). A forcep jaw may be used to dilate the valve and annulus further. A finger is inserted into the annulus to ensure that the stenosis has been

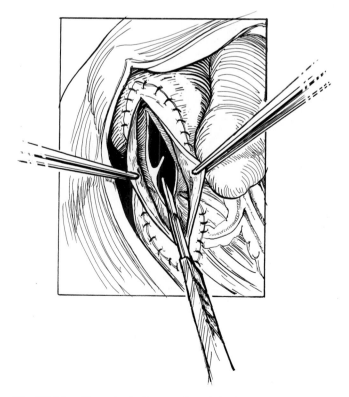

Fig. 38.34. The valve is inspected, and the leaflets are excised. See text. (Copyright 1996, University of Tennessee College of Veterinary Medicine, Knoxville, TN.)

relieved. Air is evacuated from the heart by releasing the cranial Rumel tourniquet. The incised patch graft is clamped using Satinsky tangential vascular occlusion clamps, and the patch graft is sutured with 4–0 polypropylene in a continuous pattern (Fig. 38.35). The caudal Rumel tourniquet is then released. Total inflow occlusion time should not exceed 2 minutes. The pericardium is closed loosely with interrupted sutures. A thoracostomy tube is placed, and the thoracotomy incision is closed in routine fashion.

Open patch grafting is effective in young animals with severe valvular, subvalvular, and infundibular stenosis. Care must be taken in identifying an aberrant

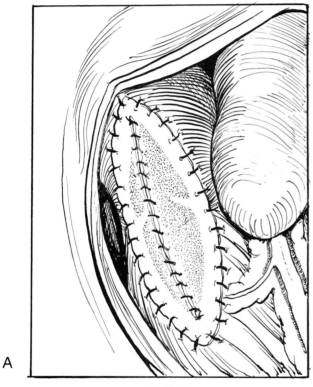

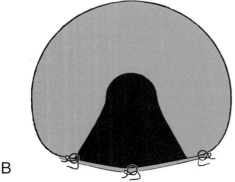

Fig. 38.35. **A** and **B.** Suturing of the patch graft. See text. (Copyright 1996, University of Tennessee College of Veterinary Medicine, Knoxville, TN.)

coronary artery, which crosses the right ventricular outflow tract occasionally in boxers and bulldogs and negates the use of this procedure.

Conduits

Vascular grafts or conduits have been used to repair supravalvular pulmonic stenosis in the dog (22). Conduits from the pulmonary artery to the right ventricle may be used to bypass the stenotic pulmonary valve in animals with an aberrant coronary artery. The technique is performed through a left lateral thoracotomy at the fifth intercostal space. The pericardium is opened and sutured as previously described. The stenotic region is observed, and an appropriately sized Dacron or polytetrafluoroethylene conduit is chosen. A Satinsky partially occluding vascular clamp is applied to the pulmonary artery above the site of the lesion. An arteriotomy is made with a No. 11 scalpel blade and is extended with Pott's scissors. The conduit is cut at an oblique angle and is sutured from end to side to the pulmonary artery with continuous 5–0 to 6–0 polypropylene suture on a double-armed taperpoint needle. The conduit is anastomosed to the ventricular wall in end-to-side fashion after coring a hole in the ventricular wall. Closure of the pericardium and thoracotomy incisions is routine.

Conduits, with the exception of those used in supravalvular stenosis (pulmonary artery to pulmonary artery), have had limited success in veterinary medicine. The procedure may be best applied during cardiopulmonary bypass operations.

Cardiopulmonary Bypass

Pulmonic stenosis can be repaired effectively using cardiopulmonary bypass (see the discussion in a later section of this chapter). This technique permits direct visualization and repair of the lesion without the time constraints of inflow occlusion. Valvuloplasties, patches, and conduits can all be performed during cardiopulmonary bypass, which permits the surgeon to do precise surgical repairs (23).

References

1. Buchanan JW. Causes and prevalence of cardiovascular disease. In: Kirk RW, Bonagura JD, eds. Current veterinary therapy XI. Philadelphia: WB Saunders, 1992:647–655.
2. Buchanan JW. Changing breed predispositions in canine heart disease. In: Proceedings of the tenth ACVIM forum. American College of Veterinary Internal Medicine, San Diego, CA 1992:213–215.
3. Bonagura JD, Darke PG. Congenital heart disease. In: Ettinger SJ, Feldman EE, eds. Textbook of veterinary internal medicine. Philadelphia: WB Saunders, 1995:892–943.
4. Thomas WP. Therapy in congenital pulmonic stenosis. In: Kirk RW, Bonagura JD, eds. Current veterinary therapy XII. Philadelphia: WB Saunders, 1995:817–821.

5. Eyster GE. Basic cardiac surgical procedure. In: Slatter DH, ed. Textbook of small animal surgery. Philadelphia: WB Saunders, 1993:462–469.
6. Orton EC. Pulmonic stenosis and subvalvular aortic stenosis: surgical options. Semin Vet Med Surg 1994;9:221–226.
7. Hellyer PW. Anesthesia in patients with cardiovascular disease. In: Kirk RW, Bonagura JD, eds. Current veterinary therapy XI. Philadelphia: WB Saunders, 1992:655–660.
8. Breznock EM. Surgical relief of pulmonic stenosis. In: Bojrab MJ, ed. Current techniques in small animal surgery. 3rd ed. Philadelphia: Lea & Febiger, 1990:513–522.
9. Kveselis DA, Rocchini AP, Snider AR, et al. Results of balloon valvuloplasty in the treatment of congenital valvular pulmonary stenosis in children. Am J Cardiol 1985;56: 527–532.
10. Bright JM, Jennings J, Toal R, et al. Percutaneous balloon valvuloplasty for treatment of pulmonic stenosis in a dog. J Am Vet Med Assoc 1987;191:995–996.
11. Sisson DD, MacCoy DM. Treatment of congenital pulmonic stenosis in two dogs by balloon valvuloplasty. J Vet Intern Med 1988;2:92–99.
12. DeMadron E, Bussadori C. Five cases of valvuloplasty with a balloon catheter for stenotic pulmonary valves in dogs. Prat Med Chir Anim Comp 1994;29:383–391.
13. Brownlie SE, Cobb MA, Chambers J, et al. Percutaneous balloon valvuloplasty in four dogs with pulmonic stenosis. J Small Anim Pract 1991;32:165–169.
14. Martin MWS, Godman M, Fuentes VL, et al. Assessment of balloon pulmonary valvuloplasty in six dogs. J Small Anim Pract 1992;33:443–440.
15. Buchanan JW. Pulmonic stenosis caused by single coronary artery in dogs: four cases (1965–1984). J Am Vet Med Assoc 1990;196:115–119.
16. Sullivan ID, Robinson PJ, Macartney FJ, et al. Percutaneous balloon valvuloplasty for pulmonic stenosis in infants and children. Br Heart J 1985;54:435–441.
17. Swan H. Surgery by direct vision in the open heart during hypothermia. JAMA 1953;153:1081–1086.
18. Breznock EM, Wood GL. A patch-graft technique for correction of pulmonic stenosis in dogs. J Am Vet Med Assoc 1976; 169:1090–1097.
19. Shores A, Weirick WE. A modified pericardial patch graft technique for correction of pulmonic stenosis in the dog. J Am Anim Hosp Assoc 1985;21:809–812.
20. Orton EC, Bruecker KA, McCracken TO. An open patch graft technique for correction of pulmonic stenosis in the dog. Vet Surg 1990;19:148–154.
21. Hunt GB, Pearson MRB, Bellenger CR, et al. Use of a modified open patch-graft technique and valvulectomy for correction of severe pulmonic stenosis in dogs: eight consecutive cases. Aust Vet J 1993;70:244–248.
22. Ford RB, Spaulding GL, Eyster GE. Use of a extracardiac conduit in the repair of supravalvular pulmonic stenosis in a dog. J Am Vet Med Assoc 1978;172:922–925.
23. Orton EC. Cardiopulmonary bypass for small animals. Semin Vet Med Surg 1994;9:210–216.

Surgical Treatment of Pericardial Diseases and Cardiac Neoplasms

R. John Berg

Diseases affecting the canine pericardium can result in either pericardial effusion or pericardial constriction, both of which can be managed surgically. Antemortem diagnosis of feline pericardial disease is rare.

Anatomy and Physiology of the Pericardium

The pericardium is a fibrous sac composed of an outer fibrous layer and an inner serous layer. The serous layer is divided into the visceral pericardium (epicardium), which adheres firmly to the surface of the heart, and the parietal pericardium, which lines the interior surface of the fibrous pericardium. The pericardial cavity lies between the serous layers and normally contains a small quantity of clear fluid.

The fibrous pericardium forms a tough, thick sac that blends with the adventitia of the great vessels at the base of the heart. It is attached to the diaphragm in the xiphoid region by the thin sternopericardiac ligament ventrally and by pleural reflections caudally. The phrenic nerves course across the dorsal third of the pericardium on both left and right sides.

The functions of the pericardium are not completely understood, and its physiologic significance has been debated in the literature. The following functions have been attributed to the pericardium: prevention of overdilatation of the heart, protection of the heart from infection and from formation of adhesions to surrounding tissues, maintenance of the heart in a relatively fixed position within the chest, regulation of the interrelation between the stroke volumes of the two ventricles, and prevention of right ventricular regurgitation when ventricular diastolic pressure is increased.

Suggestions that the pericardium serves no vital functions have arisen from observations that humans and animals can live normally after pericardiectomy. Studies in animals suggest that the heart probably undergoes some minor dilatation after pericardiectomy, although significant impairment of cardiac function has not been demonstrated (1).

Pericardial Effusion

Pathophysiology

Pericardial effusion is an abnormal accumulation of fluid within the pericardial sac. Severe pericardial effusion may result in *cardiac tamponade*, a potentially life-threatening compression of the heart in which intrapericardial pressure rises sufficiently to affect cardiac function. Cardiac tamponade occurs when enough pericardial fluid accumulates to exhaust the limits of pericardial elasticity. Once the pericardium can no longer stretch to accommodate additional fluid, the addition of small amounts of fluid begins to produce rapid increases in intrapericardial pressure.

Cardiac tamponade primarily affects cardiac function during diastole and has little effect on systolic function. Because intrapericardial pressure is transmitted directly through the ventricular wall, diastolic filling pressures rise until the diastolic pressures within each ventricle are equal to one another and to intrapericardial pressure. As predicted by the Frank–Starling law, the decreased diastolic filling results in decreased myocardial stretching, force of contraction, and cardiac output.

The cardiovascular system attempts to compensate for falling cardiac output through peripheral arterial and venous vasoconstriction and increased heart rate. However, these compensatory mechanisms may themselves stress the heart. The catecholamines responsible for vasoconstriction increase myocardial oxygen consumption, and tachycardia decreases coronary blood flow by decreasing the proportion of the cardiac cycle spent in diastole, when coronary flow occurs. Coronary flow is further compromised by low cardiac output and pressure on the coronary vessels produced by the pericardial fluid. These factors produce myocardial ischemia and can eventually lead to cardiac decompensation.

Causes

The most common causes of pericardial effusion in the dog are neoplasia and idiopathic hemorrhagic pericardial effusion. Most neoplastic effusions are hemorrhagic and probably result from acute or chronic hemorrhage from the tumor surface. Intrapericardial cysts (2), infectious pericardial effusion (3), and other uncommon causes of pericardial effusion have also been reported (4).

The most common neoplastic cause of pericardial effusion is right atrial hemangiosarcoma. This tumor generally involves the right auricular appendage, although the right atrial wall may be involved. German shepherd dogs and other large breeds are predisposed to this tumor. The tumor is highly metastatic and almost always spreads to other organs such as the liver or lungs before it is discovered in the heart.

Chemodectomas arise from the aortic bodies located around the aorta at the heart base. The aortic bodies are composed of chemoreceptor tissue sensitive to blood pH, carbon dioxide content, and oxygen tension, and they are involved in the regulation of ventilation. Chemodectomas vary in their location around the aorta and in their degree of local invasiveness. The metastatic rate of this tumor is unknown. Although chemodectomas may occur in any breed, most of these tumors are reported to occur in brachycephalic breeds, a finding suggesting that chronic hypoxia may be an underlying cause (5). Anecdotally, the apparently high incidence of chemodectoma among dogs in Colorado further implicates chronic hypoxia in the pathogenesis of the tumor.

Other neoplastic causes of pericardial effusion are much less common. Malignant diseases that may metastasize to the heart or pericardium include hemangiosarcoma, lymphosarcoma, melanoma, and mammary adenocarcinoma. Mesothelioma rarely causes pericardial effusion, either alone or in combination with pleural or peritoneal effusion.

Idiopathic hemorrhagic pericardial effusion, a poorly understood syndrome, is probably the second most common form of pericardial effusion in the dog. It occurs predominantly in large and giant breeds, has a distinct male predilection, and affects dogs of all ages (6). Patients have signs of acute or chronic cardiac tamponade, which may respond to either conservative treatment or surgical management. Although the cause of this syndrome is unknown, a similar syndrome in humans is suspected to be either viral or immune-mediated. Histologically, blood vessels of the canine parietal (and possibly visceral) pericardium appear to be the targets of the disease process and are the source of pericardial hemorrhage (6).

Intrapericardial cysts are large, benign mass lesions that occasionally cause effusion and cardiac tamponade in young dogs (2). The cysts arise from the apex of the pericardial sac and resemble acquired cystic hematomas grossly and histologically. Although the cause of intrapericardial cysts is unknown, they may possibly develop from herniated omental or falciform fat in dogs born with small peritoneopericardial diaphragmatic hernias. Intrapericardial cysts usually are diagnosed in dogs between 6 months and 3 years of age, although these cysts occasionally are identified later in life.

Infectious pericardial effusion is reported to be caused most commonly by migrating grass awns (3). Many different bacteria have been cultured from the pericardial fluid of affected dogs.

Other potential causes of pericardial effusion include congenital and acquired peritoneopericardial hernias, left atrial rupture, blunt or penetrating trauma, congestive heart failure, and uremia. Pericardial effusion in the latter two conditions is usually inconsequential and tends to be a postmortem finding only.

History and Clinical Signs

Dogs with cardiac tamponade usually present with acute or chronic histories of nonspecific signs suggestive of right-sided heart failure (4). These signs include lethargy, dyspnea, cough, abdominal distension, anorexia, weight loss, and exercise intolerance. Acute collapse with no prior history of suggestive signs is seen occasionally. In general, the history is not helpful in differentiating neoplastic from idiopathic hemorrhagic pericardial effusion; signs may be acute or chronic in either condition.

Several physical findings may suggest cardiac tamponade as the cause of right-sided heart failure. These include muffled heart sounds, pronounced jugular pulses and jugular distension, and weak arterial pulses. Pulsus paradoxus and pericardial friction rubs are commonly seen in human patients, but they are rarely detected in dogs.

Diagnostic Evaluation

The diagnostic evaluation of dogs with signs compatible with cardiac tamponade should be aimed at demonstrating pericardial effusion and determining its underlying cause. Pericardial effusion can be demonstrated in most cases using a combination of electrocardiography, thoracic radiography, and M-mode echocardiography. Diminished QRS voltages and electrical alternans are seen in a significant proportion of electrocardiograms. Diminished QRS amplitudes usually are explained by decreased conduction of electrical impulses through fluid media, although decreased ventricular filling also may be involved (7). Pleural effusion as well as pericardial effusion can produce decreased QRS voltages. Electrical alternans is a beat-to-beat variation in QRS amplitude produced by a swinging motion of the heart within the pericardial sac.

Thoracic radiography demonstrates pericardial effusion if the volume of effusion is substantial. Generalized heart enlargement is seen, and the heart may have a characteristic globoid appearance, which is demonstrated best on dorsoventral views. Pleural effusion may also be present.

M-mode echocardiography is the most sensitive test available for detecting pericardial effusion (4). Effusions are demonstrated in approximately 90% of cases, and volumes as small as 75 mL can be detected (8).

Because pericardial effusions caused by neoplasia have a distinctly poorer prognosis than idiopathic hemorrhagic and other effusions, the detection of cardiac masses, particularly right atrial hemangiosarcomas, is an important part of the diagnostic evaluation. Cytologic examination of fluid obtained by pericardiocentesis (discussed later) generally does not differentiate neoplastic from idiopathic hemorrhagic effusions (4, 9). In both cases, the fluid is hemorrhagic and non-clotting, and it contains predominantly red blood cells, macrophages, and reactive mesothelial cells. Demonstration of neoplastic cells is extremely rare, and care must be exercised in cytologic interpretation because reactive mesothelial cells can have neoplastic characteristics.

Two-dimensional echocardiography is the most sensitive test available for detecting cardiac masses and for determining preoperatively whether a mass is likely to be surgically resectable. Because right atrial hemangiosarcomas are often small (1 to 2 cm in diam-

eter), they occasionally escape detection. Examination from both sides of the thorax allows more accurate localization (10). Involvement of the right atrial wall, which increases the difficulty of surgical excision, often can be detected echocardiographically. Chemodectomas often can be visualized in association with the ascending aorta. Small, discrete chemodectomas confined to the aortic area may prove resectable, whereas larger, more invasive masses are less likely to be resectable. Chemodectomas may be situated on either the right side or the left side of the aorta, and ultrasonography can assist in the selection of a surgical approach. Mesotheliomas have a diffuse growth pattern and usually are not detected with ultrasonography. Intrapericardial cysts are large lesions that are detected easily by echocardiography.

Unfortunately, it may be difficult to make a definitive diagnosis, and particularly to differentiate right atrial hemangiosarcoma from idiopathic hemorrhagic pericardial effusion, without exploratory thoracotomy.

Treatment

PERICARDIOCENTESIS
Indications
Pericardiocentesis is performed for both diagnostic and therapeutic purposes. The removal of small volumes of pericardial fluid in patients with cardiac tamponade can result in tremendous decreases in intrapericardial pressure and is often a lifesaving measure. Idiopathic hemorrhagic pericardial effusion occasionally can be treated definitively by periodic pericardiocentesis, performed when necessary to relieve cardiac tamponade. Multiple pericardiocenteses, days to weeks apart, may be necessary to produce a resolution, and recurrence of pericardial effusion is reported to occur as late as 4 years after pericardiocentesis (6). Owners of dogs treated by pericardiocentesis alone should be made aware of the potential for sudden recurrence of cardiac tamponade. The advantages of pericardiectomy over pericardiocentesis are discussed later.

Technique
Pericardiocentesis is performed at the right third, fourth, or fifth intercostal space near the costochondral junction. An excellent description of this procedure is available (11).

PERICARDIECTOMY
Indications
Pericardiectomy is used most often to treat pericardial effusions caused by neoplasia, idiopathic hemorrhage, intrapericardial cysts, infection, and penetrating foreign bodies. Effusions caused by congestive heart fail-

ure or uremia usually are treated medically. The specific goals of pericardiectomy depend on the primary disease treated.

In pericardial effusion caused by neoplasia, the pericardium is often excised to allow surgical exploration of the heart, but pericardiectomy alone is of little value. Excision of right atrial hemangiosarcomas, chemodectomas, and intrapericardial cysts is discussed later.

Idiopathic hemorrhagic pericardial effusion can be treated successfully by total or subtotal pericardiectomy, which allows any persistent effusion to be removed by the large absorptive area of the pleural space. Although the condition often is manageable by periodic pericardiocentesis, early pericardiectomy has some advantages (6). Treatment by pericardiocentesis alone risks a sudden recurrence of life-threatening cardiac tamponade. Pericardiectomy does not entail long-term risks for the patient and, unlike pericardiocentesis, removes most of the diseased organ responsible for the effusion. Some evidence suggests that idiopathic pericardial effusion may progress to pericardial constriction, although this appears to be uncommon (12, 13). Surgery is technically simpler, and is associated with a better prognosis, for pericardial effusion than for pericardial constriction. Finally, early surgical exploration may allow detection of small tumors, particularly right atrial hemangiosarcomas, and may offer the best chance for their removal.

Technique
When the cause of pericardial effusion is unknown, either a right fifth intercostal thoracotomy or a median sternotomy may be performed. Excision of right atrial tumors may be accomplished with similar ease through either approach. Subtotal pericardiectomy is easier to perform through a median sternotomy because a right intercostal approach does not allow good visualization of the left side of the thorax. In addition, if an intercostal approach is used, the heart must be elevated as the left side of the pericardial sac is excised, a maneuver that impairs venous return temporarily. Chemodectomas are approached through either a right or a left fourth intercostal thoracotomy, depending on the location of the tumor as determined by ultrasonography. Intrapericardial cysts are best approached through a median sternotomy, which facilitates subtotal pericardiectomy and allows inspection of the diaphragm for a peritoneopericardial hernia (2).

Once the thoracotomy is completed, the phrenic and vagus nerves are identified. The phrenic nerve may be isolated and gently retracted with a Penrose drain, although retraction of the nerve usually is unnecessary. The vagus nerve is located more dorsally and is unlikely to be damaged during pericardiectomy.

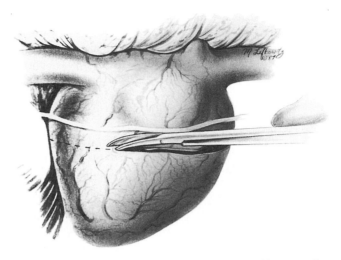

Fig. 38.36. Subtotal pericardiectomy is performed by circumferentially excising the pericardial sac below the level of the phrenic nerves.

A stab incision is made in the pericardium ventral to the phrenic nerve, and pericardial fluid is removed by suction. The incision is then continued cranially and caudally until it is complete circumferentially (Fig. 38.36). If an intercostal approach has been used, completion of the pericardiectomy on the left side requires elevation of the heart. An assistant should cradle the patient's heart in one hand and gently rotate the apex of the heart laterally and dorsally to permit incision of the pericardium below the level of the left phrenic nerve. Because elevation of the heart impairs venous return, this maneuver should be performed as quickly as possible. Diseased pericardia are often extremely vascular, and care must be taken to limit hemorrhage with electrocautery. A thoracostomy tube is placed before closure, and postoperative management generally is uncomplicated. The thoracostomy tube may be removed after 12 hours if it is unproductive.

For dogs with infectious pericardial effusion, long-term antibiotics, selected on the basis of culture and sensitivity testing, should be administered postoperatively (3). The prognosis for these dogs is extremely good (3).

EXCISION OF RIGHT ATRIAL HEMANGIOSARCOMAS
Indications
Excision of right atrial hemangiosarcomas should be considered purely palliative. The goal of surgery is to prevent a recurrence of cardiac tamponade, because most of these tumors have metastasized before surgical treatment. Mean survival time after surgery is reported to be approximately 4 months (4, 14).

Technique

After right thoracotomy, an incision is made in the pericardial sac approximately 1 cm below and parallel to the phrenic nerve. The incision is extended cranially and caudally as far as necessary to expose the auricular appendage fully. Exposure may be improved by using stay sutures or Babcock forceps to retract the incised edges of the pericardial sac.

Either conventional suturing or surgical stapling equipment may be used to remove right atrial masses. If conventional suturing is elected, a tangential vascular clamp is placed across the base of the auricular appendage. The appendage is transected immediately distal to the clamp, leaving a cuff of auricular tissue (Fig. 38.37). The margin of the excised tumor should be inspected to ensure that excision was complete; if possible, at least 1 cm of normal auricular tissue should be removed with the tumor. The auricle is then oversewn with two rows of simple continuous sutures, with the rows oriented perpendicularly to each other (Fig. 38.38). Either 3–0 or 4–0 nylon or polypropylene suture may be used.

Surgical stapling is faster and less technically demanding than hand suturing. A 55-mm thoracoabdominal stapler is used, with 4.8-mm staples (United States Surgical Corp, Norwalk, CT). The stapler should be positioned to provide a 1-cm resection margin. If there is room, a tangential vascular or other noncrushing clamp should be placed across the base of the auricle before releasing the stapler; the clamp should be slowly released as the staple line is inspected for bleeding. If necessary, the staple line may be oversewn with

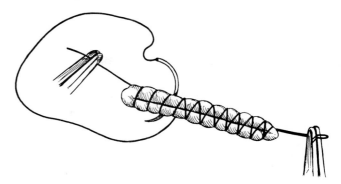

Fig. 38.38. After excision of the mass, the auricle is oversewn with two rows of simple continuous sutures. (From Orton EC, ed. Small animal thoracic surgery. Baltimore, Williams & Wilkins, 1995.)

a layer of simple continuous sutures. After tumor excision, a subtotal pericardiectomy should be performed.

Prognosis

Because right atrial hemangiosarcoma is a highly metastatic tumor, surgical excision is purely palliative. Euthanasia is performed in most affected dogs because of distant metastases, usually to the lungs, within a few months of surgery. Unfortunately, no compelling evidence indicates that survival times in dogs with either splenic or right atrial hemangiosarcoma can be significantly prolonged with adjuvant chemotherapy, and controlled clinical trials are needed.

EXCISION OF CHEMODECTOMAS

Technique

Chemodectomas are extremely vascular tumors, and control of hemorrhage is the major difficulty encountered during excision. Because of their location, chemodectomas must be marginally excised at the gross limits of the tumor; wide margins are impossible to provide. Excision is best accomplished by slow, meticulous, sharp dissection with the help of electrocoagulation. Care must be taken to avoid perforating the aorta or pulmonary artery; cotton-tipped swabs are useful for slowly dissecting the tumor away from these structures. Before closure, the tumor bed should be closely inspected, and residual points of hemorrhage should be controlled with electrocoagulation.

Prognosis

Chemodectomas seem to be slow-growing tumors, and limited experience suggests that dogs undergoing excision of small chemodectomas can have prolonged survival postoperatively (10). No evidence indicates that adjuvant chemotherapy improves the prognosis for dogs with this tumor.

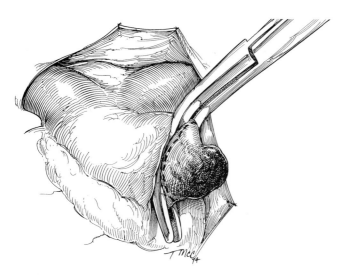

Fig. 38.37. A tangential vascular clamp is placed across the base of the right auricular appendage before excision of a right atrial mass. (From Orton EC, ed. Small animal thoracic surgery. Baltimore: Williams & Wilkins, 1995.)

EXCISION OF INTRAPERICARDIAL CYSTS

Intrapericardial cysts are usually located at the apex of the pericardial sac and can be excised readily by routine subtotal pericardiectomy. If the patient has an associated peritoneopericardial hernia, the edges of the hernia are incised, and the defect is closed with a row of simple continuous sutures.

Pericardial Constriction

Pathophysiology and Causes

As in cardiac tamponade resulting from pericardial effusion, pericardial constriction restricts diastolic volume. Diastolic filling is limited by the fibrotic pericardium, which acts as a noncompliant shell around the heart (12).

Pericardial constriction in dogs usually is idiopathic. Like idiopathic hemorrhagic pericardial effusion, the condition occurs predominantly in medium-size and large breeds, although no evidence of male sex predilection exists. Some evidence based on isolated cases indicates that idiopathic hemorrhagic pericardial effusion can progress to pericardial constriction, although this situation is uncommon (12, 13). Whether idiopathic pericardial constriction and idiopathic hemorrhagic pericardial effusion are different manifestations of the same syndrome or are separate disease entities altogether is unknown. Pericardial constriction is also reported as a sequela of fungal bacterial pericarditis (12) (*Coccidioides immitis* and *Actinomyces* spp.), gunshot trauma (12, 13), and pericardial fenestration (13).

History, Clinical Signs, and Diagnosis

Dogs with constrictive pericardial disease usually present with signs of chronic right-sided heart failure. Abdominal distension, dyspnea, weakness or syncope, exercise intolerance, and weight loss are common signs. Typical physical examination findings are ascites, jugular distension, and weak arterial pulses. Poorly auscultable heart sounds are also common.

Definitive diagnosis of pericardial constriction may require surgical exploration, although a presumptive diagnosis can often be made preoperatively based on a combination of physical, electrocardiographic, radiographic, and hemodynamic findings. One or more abnormalities may be present on electrocardiographic examination. Decreased QRS amplitudes and increased P-wave duration are most common. Radiographs may reveal free pleural fluid and mild to moderate cardiomegaly. Echocardiographic findings that support the diagnosis include decreased end-diastolic diameter, decreased fractional shortening, flattening of left ventricular free-wall motion during late diastole,

and rapid premature diastolic closure of the mitral valve. Right-sided heart manometry, if performed, shows prominent x and y descents on the atrial pressure tracing and prominent early diastolic dips and midsystolic plateaus on the ventricular pressure tracing. In general, a diagnosis of pericardial constriction should be considered in dogs with signs of right-sided heart failure that cannot be explained by pericardial effusion, congenital or acquired heart disease, or pulmonary hypertension. Surgical exploration should be performed if the condition is suspected.

Treatment: Subtotal Pericardiectomy

Because significant epicardial fibrosis rarely is present in dogs, most dogs can be treated successfully by subtotal pericardiectomy, as previously described. Median sternotomy is the preferred approach because it allows visualization and division of any epicardial adhesions that may be present. In dogs with significant epicardial fibrosis, epicardial decortication may be necessary. This difficult procedure may require partial removal of myocardial tissue. Caution is necessary to avoid inadvertent damage to coronary vessels. Epicardial decortication is associated with significant perioperative morbidity and mortality.

References

1. Holt JP. The normal pericardium. Am J Cardiol 1970;26:455.
2. Sisson D, Thomas WP, Reed J, et al. Intrapericardial cysts in the dog. J Vet Intern Med 1993;7:364–369.
3. Aronson LR, Gregory CR. Infectious pericardial effusion in five dogs. J Vet Surg 1995;24:402–407.
4. Berg RJ, Wingfield WE. Pericardial effusion in the dog: a review of 42 cases. J Am Anim Hosp Assoc 1984;20:721–730.
5. Patraik AK, Liu SK, Hurvitz AI, et al. Canine chemodectoma (extra-adrenal paragangliomas): a comparative study. J Small Anim Pract 1975;16:785–801.
6. Berg RJ, Wingfield WE, Hoopes PJ. Idiopathic hemorrhagic pericardial effusion in eight dogs. J Am Vet Med Assoc 1984;185:988–992.
7. Manoach M. The relation between the conductivity of the blood and the body tissue and the amplitude of the QRS during heart filling and pericardial compression in the cat. Am Heart J 1972;84:72.
8. Christensen EE, Bonte FJ. The relative accuracy of echocardiography, intravenous CO_2 studies, and blood pool scanning in detecting pericardial effusions in dogs. Radiology 1968;91:265.
9. Sisson D, Thomas WP, Ruehl WW, et al. Diagnostic value of pericardial fluid analysis in the dog. J Am Vet Med Assoc 1984;184:51–55.
10. Thomas WP, Sisson D. Bauer TG, et al. Detection of cardiac masses in dogs by two-dimensional echocardiography. Vet Radiol 1984;25:65–72.
11. Lombard CW. Pericardial disease. Vet Clin North Am 1983; 13:337.
12. Thomas WP, Reed JR, Bauer TG, et al. Constrictive pericardial disease in the dog. J Am Vet Med Assoc 1984;184:546–553.
13. Schwartz A. Constrictive pericarditis in two dogs. J Am Vet Med Assoc 1971;159:763.
14. Aronsohn M. Cardiac hemangiosarcoma in the dog: a review of 38 cases. J Am Vet Med Assoc 1985;187:922.

Transdiaphragmatic Pacemaker Implantation

Eric Monnet

Pacemaker therapy is indicated in veterinary medicine for symptomatic bradyarrhythmias including high-grade second-degree atrioventricular (AV) block, third-degree AV block, sick sinus syndrome, and persistent atrial standstill with a slow ventricular escape rate. Pacemaker implantation is indicated when clinical signs such as exercise intolerance, syncope, or congestive heart failure are related to the bradycardia. Pacemaker therapy improves cardiac output and prevents sudden death associated with bradyarrhythmias by maintaining the heart rate above a predetermined rate.

Several types of pacemaker generators and pacing modalities are available. Pacemaker function is identified by a three-letter code. The first letter indicates which cardiac chamber is paced, the second letter indicates which cardiac chamber is sensed, and the third indicates the electronic response to sensing. The most common pacemaker function used in veterinary patients is VVI in which the ventricle is the site of both pacing and sensing, and the pacing impulse is inhibited when a naturally occurring heartbeat is sensed. Electrodes may be unipolar or bipolar. With unipolar electrodes, the electric current goes from the tip of the electrode (cathode) to the metallic box of the generator (anode). With bipolar electrodes, the anode and cathode are at the tip of the electrode. Transvenous electrodes are usually bipolar, whereas epicardial electrodes are usually unipolar. Transvenous electrodes can be used for either temporary or permanent pacemaker therapy.

The natural escape rhythm associated with a third-degree AV block is a slow ventricular rate (30 to 50 beats per minute). Administration of lidocaine to an animal with this rhythm is contraindicated. Before implantation of the permanent pacemaker, the animal's heart rate must be increased either with a temporary external pacemaker or pharmacologically. If a temporary external pacemaker is available, a flow-directed balloon-tip bipolar electrode is introduced into the jugular vein and is wedged in the trabeculae of the right ventricle with the patient under local anesthesia and light sedation. The transvenous electrode is introduced into the jugular vein either through a venous introducer or a cutdown of the jugular vein. Transvenous electrode placement can be performed either by monitoring the electrocardiogram (ECG) or under fluoros-copy. Before introduction, the transvenous electrode is connected to an external pacer set up at 5 V and a rate of 100 beats per minute. The transvenous electrode is advanced into the right atrium, where the balloon at the tip is inflated. The electrode is carried by the blood flow into the right ventricle. The ECG documents capture of the ventricle when the electrode is properly wedged in a trabecula. Fluoroscopy can be used to assist with placement of the electrode and to confirm its position. For sick sinus syndrome, the right atrium can be paced instead of the right ventricle. If a temporary external pacemaker is not available, constant intravenous infusion of a β agonist (isoproterenol, 0.01 μg/kg per minute) can be used during anesthesia to increase the rate of the escape rhythm, but this method is less reliable.

Surgical Technique

Intraoperative antibiotic therapy is recommended during pacemaker implantation to reduce the risk of im-

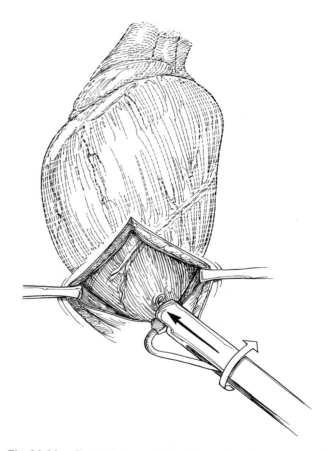

Fig. 38.39. Electrode implantation. The pericardial sac is opened and is retracted with tissue forceps. An epicardial screw-in electrode is implanted into the apex of the left ventricle. (From Orton EC. Congenital heart defect. In: Orton EC, ed. Small animal thoracic surgery. Baltimore: Williams & Wilkins, 1995:243.)

plant infection. Permanent transdiaphragmatic pacemaker implantation is accomplished through a ventral midline celiotomy. Balfour retractors are placed, the liver is gently retracted caudally, and the phrenicohepatic ligament is incised. A midline incision is made in the diaphragm to expose the heart. Stay sutures are placed on the edge of the diaphragm for retraction. The pericardium is opened and retracted with tissue forceps to expose the apex of the left ventricle. A screw-in unipolar epicardial electrode is implanted in the myocardium at the apex of the left ventricle, with care taken to avoid coronary arteries (Fig. 38.39). The screw-in electrode is turned clockwise into the myocardium; the number of turns is specified by the manufacturer. Ideally, electrical impedance of the electrode should be measured to confirm appropriate implantation of the electrode. Lead impedance at implantation should be between 250 and 1000 ohms. A broken lead has an impedance over 1000 ohms, whereas a lead leaking because of damage to the insulation has an impedance below 250 ohms. The capture voltage (i.e., the lowest voltage at which the heart is paced) also can be determined. The other end of the unipolar electrode is connected and is tightly secured with the pacemaker. For the pacemaker generator, a pouch is made between the transverse abdominal muscle and the internal oblique muscle (Fig. 38.40). As soon as the pacemaker is placed in the muscular pouch, the temporary pacemaker is stopped and the permanent pacemaker paces the heart. A subcostal thoracostomy tube is implanted. The diaphragmatic incision, the muscular pouch and the celiotomy are closed in a routine fashion. Care should be taken not to damage the electrode during suturing.

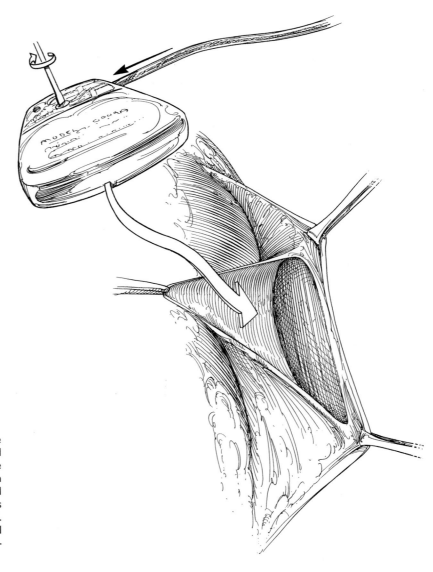

Fig. 38.40. Pulse generator implantation. The lead wire is brought through the diaphragm and is connected to the pulse generator. The pulse generator is placed in a pouch created between the transverse abdominal and internal abdominal oblique muscles. As soon as the pacemaker touches the muscle, the heart is paced. (From Orton EC. Congenital heart defect. In: Orton EC, ed. Small animal thoracic surgery. Baltimore: Williams & Wilkins, 1995:244.)

Postoperative Care

After surgery, animals should undergo continuous ECG monitoring for 24 hours to confirm proper function of the pacemaker. The heart rate should not drop below the preset rate of the pacemaker. Pacemakers are usually set at an impulse rate between 80 and 100 beats per minute, according to the size of the dog and its activity level. Ventricular premature contractions often are seen after surgery because of the myocardial trauma from the lead implantation. Lidocaine can be used to suppress ventricular premature contractions, but usually this is not necessary. The temporary transvenous lead is left in place for 24 hours as a backup in case the permanent pacemaker shows problems. The voltage output of the pacemaker is set at twice the measured capture voltage if known, or at 5 V and 0.5 milliseconds. Lower voltages spare the pacemaker battery. Current pacemaker batteries last approximately 5 to 6 years, but this depends on generator use or shelf life before implantation.

Pacing complications are due to failure to capture, failure to sense, failure to capture and sense, or battery failure. Failure to capture is characterized on an ECG by pacemaker spikes not followed by a QRS-T complex. Increased lead impedance from fibrous tissue deposition around the lead is the most common cause of this problem. It takes approximately 4 to 6 weeks for sufficient fibrous tissue to develop and to increase impedance. The problem is treated by increasing the output voltage. Other causes are a lead fracture, a lead insulation failure, or a lead dislodgment. Failure to sense a nonpaced heartbeat results from lead fracture, lead insulation failure, lead dislodgment, or increased impedance at the lead–myocardium interface. Failure to sense is recognized on an ECG by the presence of a nonpaced heartbeat between two normally timed paced beats. Sometimes, sensitivity threshold can be adjusted to correct the problem. Failure to sense places the animal at risk for competitive tachycardia and ventricular fibrillation. Battery failure is characterized by erratic behavior of the pacemaker (i.e., inconsistent failure to capture, or to sense, or both). Confirmation of a battery failure is usually made after elimination of the other problems. The battery level of newer generation of pacemaker can be measured. A failing pacemaker generator must be surgically replaced.

Suggested Readings

Orton EC. Pacemaker therapy. In: Orton EC, ed. Small animal thoracic surgery. Baltimore: Williams & Wilkins, 1995:239–247.

Tilley LP. Special methods for treating arrhythmias: cardiopulmonary arrest and resuscitation, pacemaker therapy. In: Tilley LP, ed. Essentials of canine and feline electrocardiography. Philadelphia: Lea & Febiger, 1992:365–382.

Cardiopulmonary Bypass

E. Christopher Orton

Cardiopulmonary bypass is a procedure whereby an extracorporeal system diverts blood away from the heart and lungs and provides flow of oxygenated blood to the rest of the body during open cardiac repair. Cardiopulmonary bypass can be performed in dogs with low morbidity and mortality to treat congenital or acquired cardiac defects. Several advances make cardiopulmonary bypass feasible in dogs, including the development of membrane oxygenators, improved methods of myocardial protection, increased availability of monitoring technologies, and advances in veterinary critical care and anesthesia. The physiologic principles and methods for cardiopulmonary bypass are reviewed elsewhere (1–4). In this discussion, the surgical techniques of cannulation for cardiopulmonary bypass applicable to the dog are reviewed.

Surgical Technique

Cannulation for cardiopulmonary bypass may be accomplished from a right or left thoracotomy or a median sternotomy, depending on the cardiac procedure to be performed. Intercostal thoracotomy, especially on the right side, is preferred for most cardiac procedures in dogs. Arterial cannulation in the femoral artery is preferred over aortic cannulation in dogs. If a thoracotomy approach is chosen, the dog is placed in lateral recumbency with the upper hind limb abducted and extended to expose the contralateral femoral artery for cannulation (Fig. 38.41). After bypass, the femoral artery either may be repaired with 6–0 suture or ligated.

Venous cannulation can be accomplished by one of two methods. Bicaval venous cannulation is the most efficient method of venous drainage for cardiopulmonary bypass (Fig. 38.42). It is required for procedures that involve isolation of the right atrium, such as septal defect repairs and tricuspid valve surgery. Bicaval venous cannulation can be accomplished in dogs through a right thoracotomy or a median sternotomy. Cannulation of the right atrium with a single cannula is simpler than bicaval cannulation and can be accomplished from any thoracic approach (Fig. 38.43).

A left ventricular vent keeps the ventricle dry during left-sided procedures and protects the ventricle from distension during bypass. Ventricular venting can be accomplished by one of two methods. From a lateral thoracotomy, a left ventricular vent cannula is introduced through a pulmonary vein and is passed

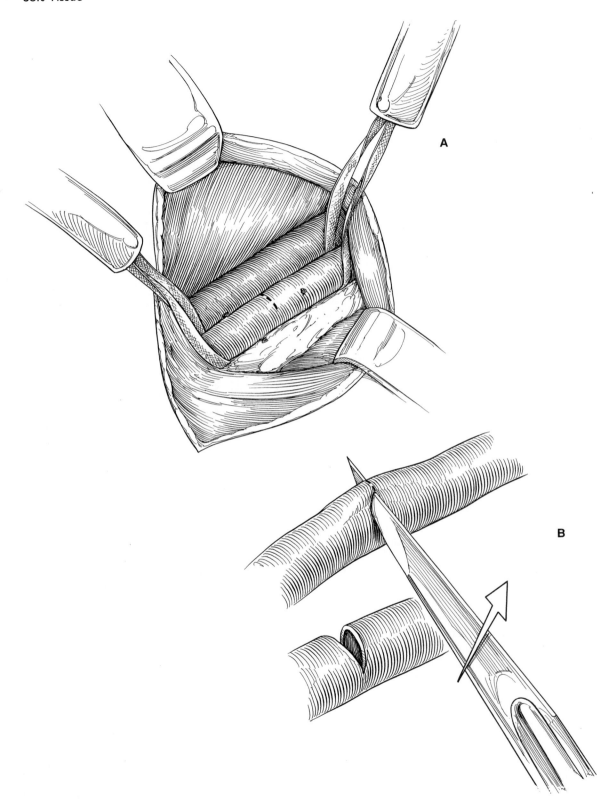

Fig. 38.41. Femoral arterial cannulation. **A.** The femoral artery is surgically exposed high in the femoral triangle close to the inguinal region, small collateral branches are ligated and divided, and two tourniquets are placed around the artery. **B.** The artery is incised transversely with a No. 11 scalpel blade.

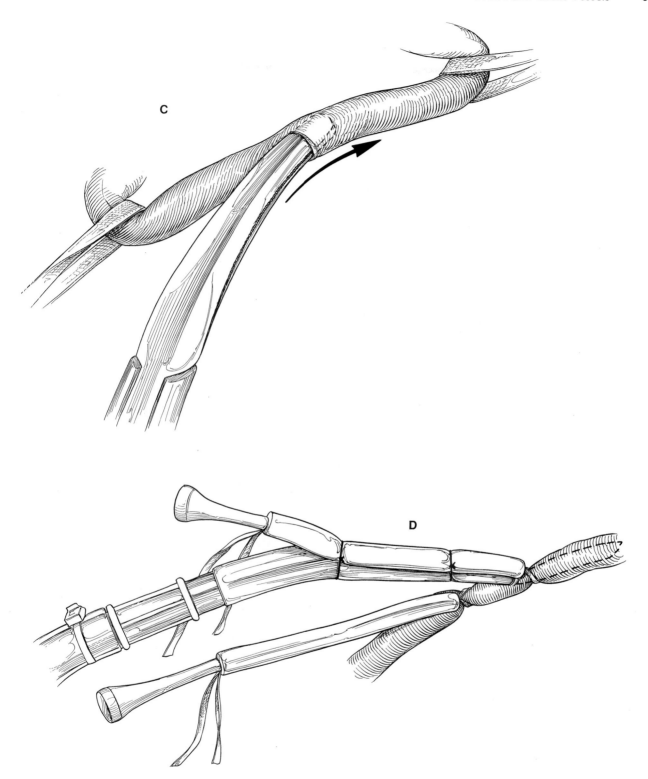

Fig. 38.41. (continued). **C.** The artery then is dilated with a blunt instrument. An arterial cannula is passed into the artery to the level of the external iliac artery. **D.** The proximal tourniquet is tightened around the cannula and then is tied to the cannula to secure it. Golf tees or hemostatic clamps can be used to secure the tapes in the tourniquets. (From Orton EC, ed. Small animal thoracic surgery. Baltimore: Williams & Wilkins, 1995.)

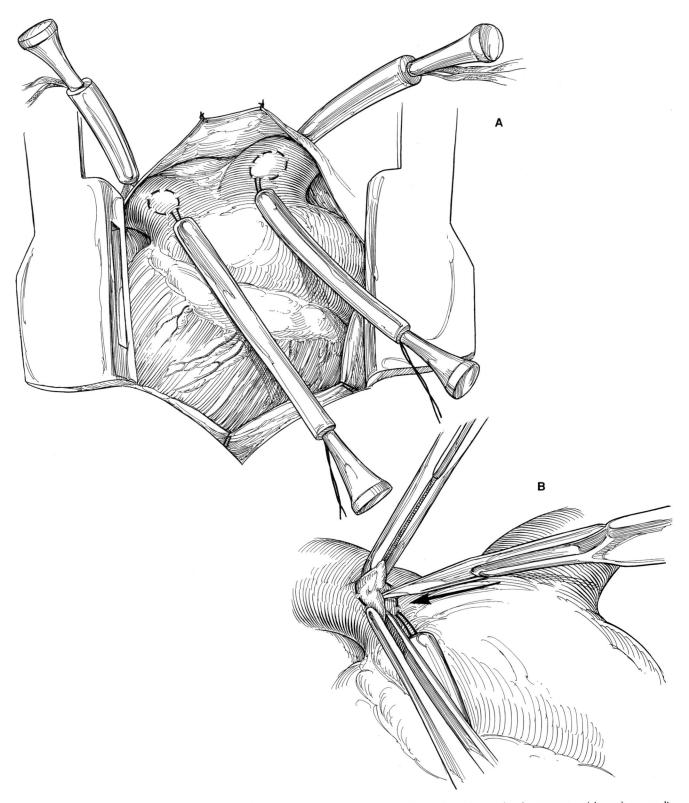

Fig. 38.42. Bicaval venous cannulation. Bicaval venous cannulation is accomplished through a right thoracotomy (shown) or median sternotomy to achieve isolation to the right atrium. Tape tourniquets may be passed around the cranial and caudal vena cava and azygous vein and are eventually tightened around the venous cannula to ensure complete diversion of venous blood from the right atrium. The pericardium is opened. **A.** Pursestring sutures are placed at each caval–atrial junction and are passed through tourniquets. **B.** The cannulation site is grasped with two forceps and is incised with a No. 11 blade. Hemorrhage is controlled during cannula insertion by holding the forceps together.

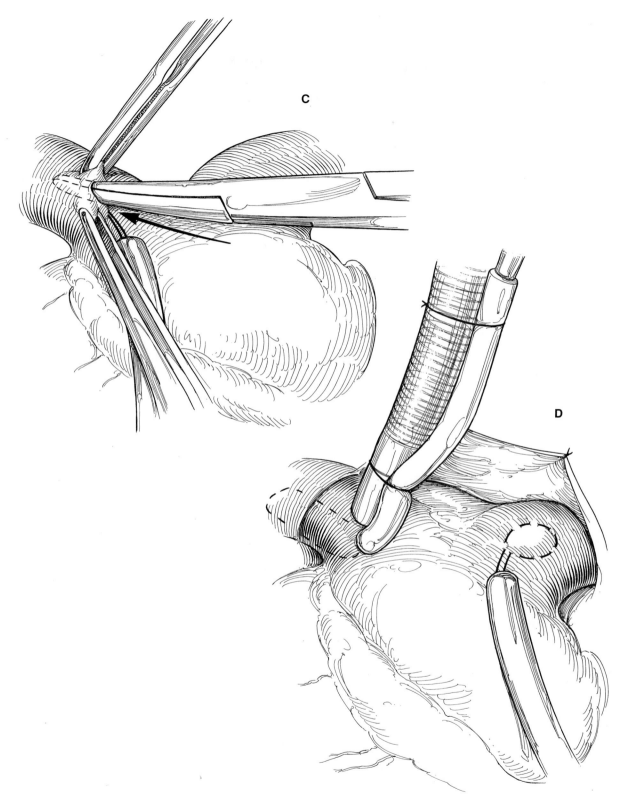

Fig. 38.42. (continued). **C.** The cannulation site is dilated with a blunt instrument. **D.** An angled venous cannula is placed into the caudal vena cava, the pursestring is tightened to control hemorrhage, and the tourniquet is tied to the cannula.

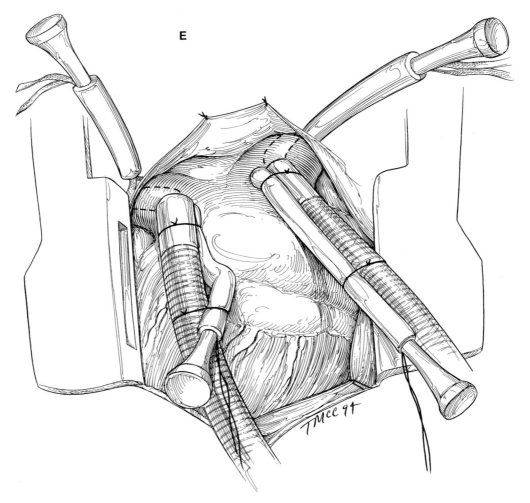

Fig. 38.42. (continued). E. The process is repeated to place the cranial cannula. Total bypass and atrial exclusion are accomplished by tightening the extrapericardial tourniquets around the venous cannulas. The pursestring sutures are tied to close the cannulation incisions after cannula removal. (From Orton EC, ed. Small animal thoracic surgery. Baltimore: Williams & Wilkins, 1995.)

through the mitral valve into the ventricle (Fig. 38.44). If a median sternotomy approach is used, the vent may be introduced through a buttressed mattress suture placed in the left ventricular apex.

Complete isolation of the heart for open heart surgery is accomplished by cross-clamping the ascending aorta (Fig. 38.45). Because coronary blood flow is arrested when the aorta is cross-clamped, the myocardium must be protected from ischemic injury during this period. Myocardial protection is accomplished by immediate cessation of electromechanical activity and by rapid and even cooling of the myocardium. This is accomplished by infusion of the heart with a cardioplegic solution (5). Cardioplegic solutions may be administered by several methods. The most common is in an antegrade fashion by a cannula placed in the ascending aorta proximal to the aortic cross-clamp (Fig. 38.46). Alternatively, cardioplegic solution may be administered in a retrograde fashion by a cannula

placed in the coronary sinus for procedures such as aortic valve surgery involving the aortic root or when substantial aortic insufficiency is present (Fig. 38.47). Last, if the aortic root is open, the coronary ostia may be directly catheterized with small cannulas to administer cardioplegic solution.

Postoperative Care

The first 12 hours after cardiopulmonary bypass are most critical. Thrombocytopenia and mild coagulopathy commonly are present after surgery. Administration of 1 or 2 units of fresh whole blood is indicated to correct thrombocytopenia and to replace clotting factors. Although some bleeding into the thoracic cavity is expected postoperatively, major bleeding into the thoracic cavity after bypass is a concern. Autotransfusion of blood collected from the pleural space may be necessary after surgery. The packed cell volume should

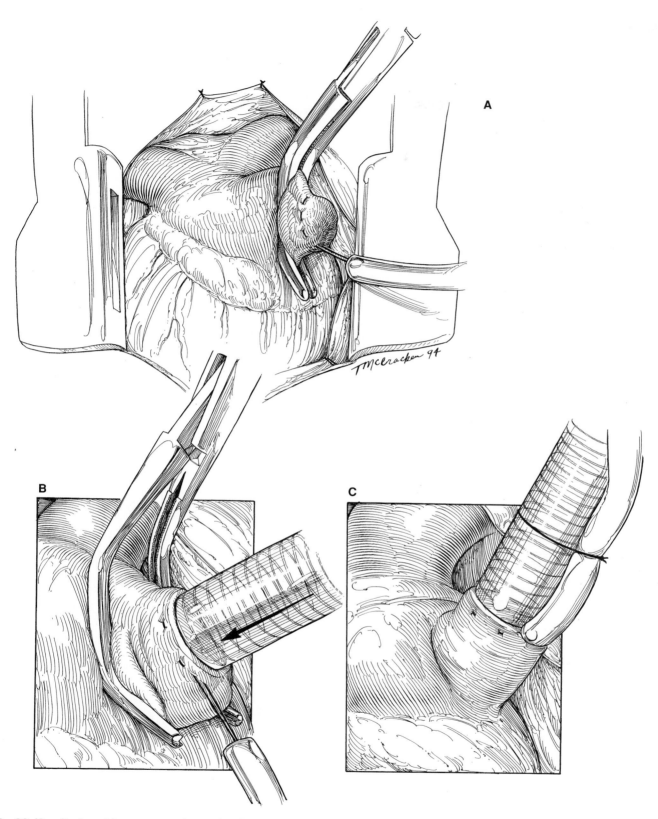

Fig. 38.43. Single atrial venous cannulation. Atrial venous cannulation is accomplished by placing a single cannula through the right atrial appendage. **A.** A pursestring suture is placed around the circumference of the atrial appendage and is passed through a tourniquet. A vascular clamp is placed at the base of atrial appendage, and the end of the atrial appendage is excised. **B.** A straight venous cannula is passed through the atriotomy as the vascular clamp is released. **C.** The pursestring tourniquet is tightened and is secured to the cannula. The pursestring suture is tied after removal of the cannula, and a second ligature is tied around the appendage. (From Orton EC, ed. Small animal thoracic surgery. Baltimore: Williams & Wilkins, 1995.)

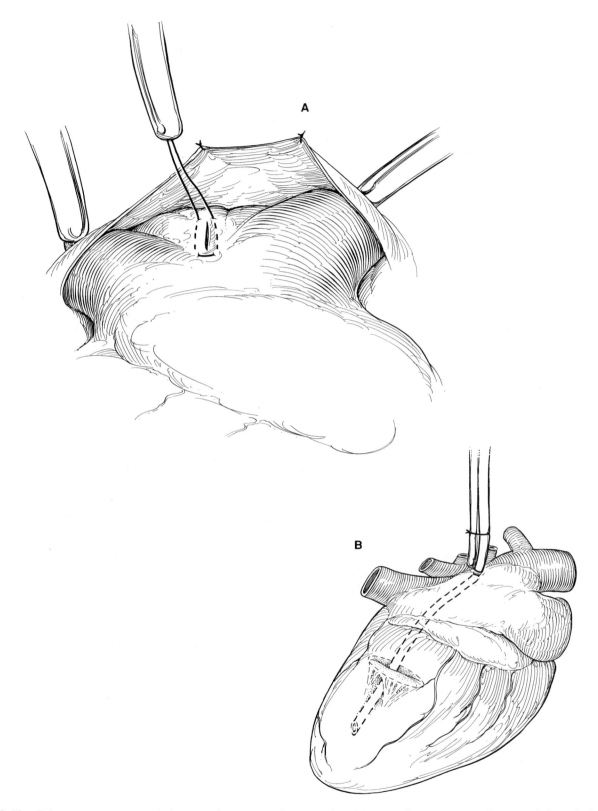

Fig. 38.44. Pulmonary venous ventricular vent. A vent cannula is introduced into a pulmonary vein and is passed through the mitral valve to decompress the left ventricle during bypass. **A.** A mattress suture is placed at the base of a pulmonary vein inside the pericardium and is passed through a tourniquet. The pulmonary vein is incised with a No. 11 blade and is dilated with a blunt instrument. **B.** The vent is passed into the left atrium and through the mitral valve. The vent cannula is tied to the tourniquet to secure it. The mattress suture is tied to close the site after cannula removal. (From Orton EC, ed. Small animal thoracic surgery. Baltimore: Williams & Wilkins, 1995.)

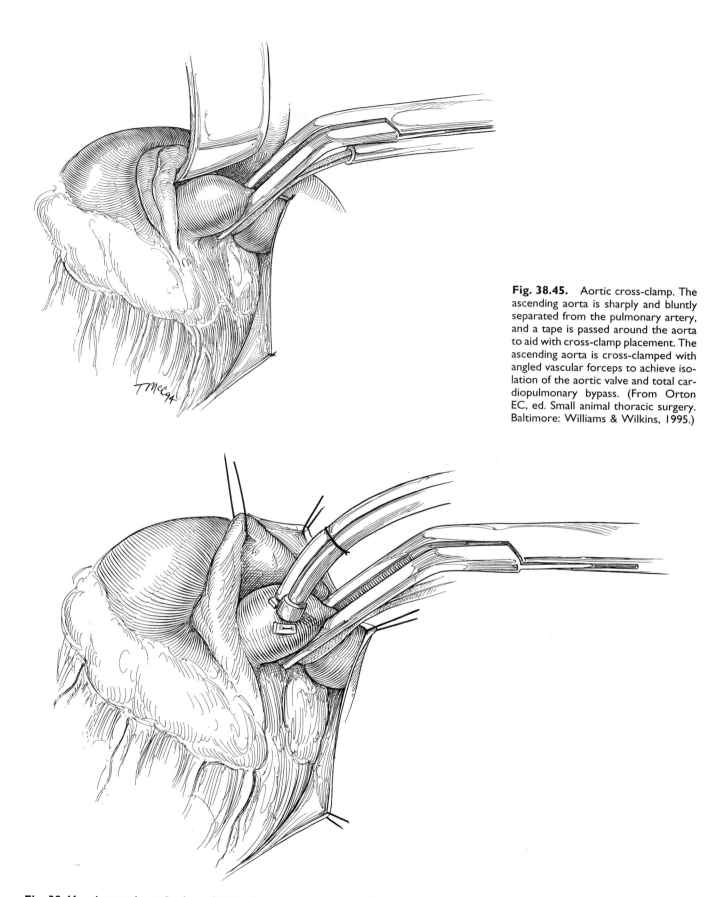

Fig. 38.45. Aortic cross-clamp. The ascending aorta is sharply and bluntly separated from the pulmonary artery, and a tape is passed around the aorta to aid with cross-clamp placement. The ascending aorta is cross-clamped with angled vascular forceps to achieve isolation of the aortic valve and total cardiopulmonary bypass. (From Orton EC, ed. Small animal thoracic surgery. Baltimore: Williams & Wilkins, 1995.)

Fig. 38.46. Antegrade cardioplegia. Antegrade administration of cardioplegic solution is accomplished by a cannula placed in the aortic root. The cannula is introduced through a double-buttressed mattress suture tourniquet. The mattress suture is tied after removal of the cannula. (From Orton EC, ed. Small animal thoracic surgery. Baltimore: Williams & Wilkins, 1995.)

687

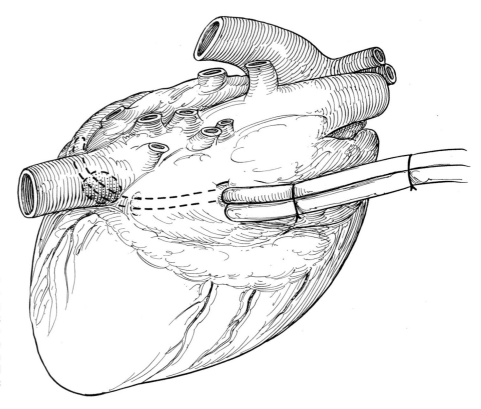

Fig. 38.47. Retrograde cardioplegia. Cardioplegia can be administered in a retrograde fashion through a balloon cannula placed in the coronary sinus. The cannula is introduced through a right atrial pursestring tourniquet. Administration of cardioplegic solution by this route should not exceed a pressure of 50 mm Hg. (From Orton EC, ed. Small animal thoracic surgery. Baltimore: Williams & Wilkins, 1995.)

be kept above 30% and the total protein above 3.5 g/dL in the postoperative period. Arterial blood gases should be monitored for evidence of metabolic acidosis, hypoventilation, or impaired gas exchange. Although some pulmonary injury is invariably present after cardiopulmonary bypass, continued tracheal intubation and ventilatory support rarely are necessary after surgery. Supplemental oxygen should be administered by intranasal cannula for 12 to 24 hours postoperatively, to correct moderate gas exchange impairment. Hypokalemia and hypocalcemia are frequently encountered postoperatively and should be corrected by judicious intravenous administration of potassium chloride and calcium chloride. Systemic arterial and central venous pressures should be monitored after surgery. Inotropic drugs such as dobutamine may be administered as necessary to keep mean systemic arterial pressure above 65 mm Hg and venous oxygen saturation above 65%. Patients should be kept relatively volume loaded postoperatively by keeping the central venous pressure between 5 and 10 cm H_2O. Ventricular arrhythmias may be encountered in the postoperative period and should be managed with intravenous lidocaine therapy.

References

1. Gravlee GP, Davis RE, Utley JR, eds. Cardiopulmonary bypass: principles and practice. Baltimore: Williams & Wilkins, 1993.

2. Klement P, del Nido P, Mickleborough L, et al. Technique and postoperative management for successful cardiopulmonary bypass and open-heart surgery in dogs. J Am Vet Med Assoc 1987;190:869–874.
3. Monnet E, Orton EC, Gaynor J, et al. Open resection of subvalvular aortic stenosis in dogs. J Am Vet Med Assoc 1996;209:1255–1261.
4. Orton EC. Inflow occlusion and cardiopulmonary bypass. In: Orton EC, ed. Small animal thoracic surgery. Baltimore: Williams & Wilkins, 1995:185–201.
5. Chitwood WR. Retrograde cardioplegia: current methods. Ann Thorac Surg 1992;53:352–355.

Open Resection for Subvalvular Aortic Stenosis

E. Christopher Orton

Congenital subvalvular aortic stenosis is the second most common congenital heart defect diagnosed in dogs. Newfoundlands, German shepherd dogs, boxers, golden retrievers, and rottweilers are predisposed. The condition is considered heritable in all these breeds. The typical lesion is a discrete subvalvular fibrous ring or membrane just below the aortic valve cusps that traverses the ventricular septum and reflects onto the septal leaflet of the mitral valve. This lesion often is complicated by varying degrees of muscular septal hy-

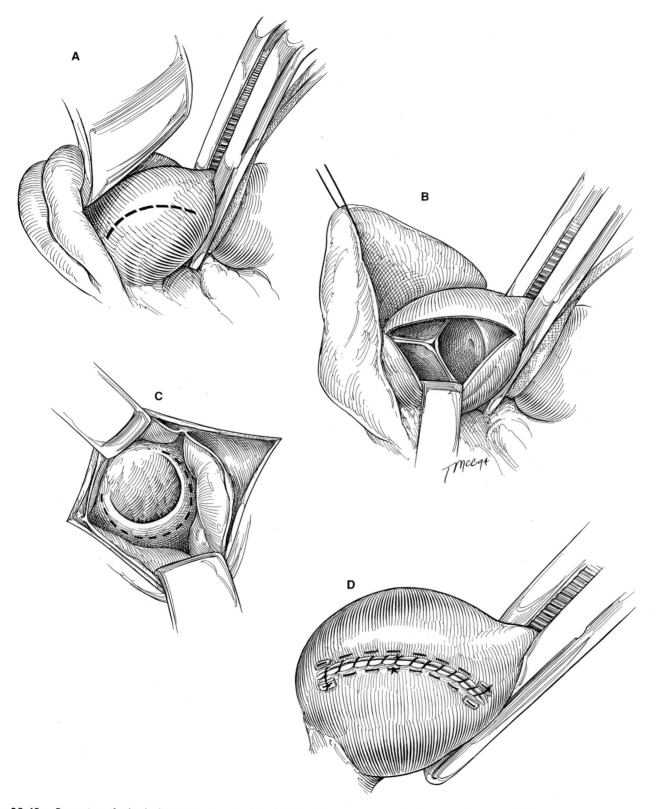

Fig. 38.48. Resection of subvalvular aortic stenosis. **A** and **B.** Curvilinear aortotomy in the ascending aorta. **C.** Excision of the subvalvular membrane from the ventricular septum and mitral valve. **D.** Closure of the aortotomy. (From Orton EC, ed. Small animal thoracic surgery. Baltimore: Williams & Wilkins, 1995.)

pertrophy and fibrosis of the outflow tract. The most severe lesions are associated with an immobile septal mitral leaflet that effectively results in a "tunnel-like" stenosis. Left ventricular hypertrophy, coronary artery disease, and myocardial ischemia result from the ventricular pressure overload imposed by the stenosis. Prognosis for subvalvular aortic stenosis depends on its severity. Dogs with Doppler-measured peak systolic aortic pressure gradients of 80 mm of Hg or greater have a substantial risk of sudden death early in life.

Open resection of subvalvular aortic stenosis during cardiopulmonary bypass is currently the most promising treatment for dogs with severe aortic stenosis. Excision of the discrete fibrous membrane (i.e., membranectomy) is the primary goal of surgery. Septal myectomy is performed in most cases to relieve obstruction resulting from septal hypertrophy. This procedure can be performed with low operative mortality in dogs and results in a 70 to 80% reduction of the systolic pressure gradient. Dogs with isolated discrete membranes are most likely to benefit from this operation, whereas dogs with complicated obstructions or tunnel-like lesions benefit less.

Surgical Technique

The surgical procedure is performed through a right fourth intercostal thoracotomy. Arterial cannulation for cardiopulmonary bypass is in the left femoral artery, and venous cannulation is bicaval (see the previous section of this chapter on cardiopulmonary bypass). A vent cannula is introduced through a pulmonary vein and is passed into the left ventricle. The ascending aorta is cross-clamped. The first dose of cardioplegic solution is administered in an antegrade fashion into the aortic root. After the aorta is opened, subsequent doses of cardioplegic solution may be administered in a retrograde manner into the coronary sinus or by direct cannulation of the coronary ostia.

The cardiac approach is through an incision in the aorta (Fig. 38.48). The aortic valve leaflets are gently retracted, and the subvalvular fibrous membrane is sharply excised with a No. 11 scalpel. The membrane usually reflects onto the septal leaflet of mitral valve, which tethers the leaflet to the outflow tract. This portion of the membrane must be excised to achieve good results; however, great care must be taken to avoid injury to the mitral valve. Injury to the mitral valve can be a fatal complication. After resection of the subvalvular membrane, the outflow tract is evaluated for the need to perform a septal myectomy. A large sponge is placed under the left ventricle to cause the septum to bulge into the left ventricular outflow tract. Most dogs with subvalvular aortic stenosis benefit from a septal myectomy. Septal myectomy is accomplished by making two partial-thickness parallel incisions in the

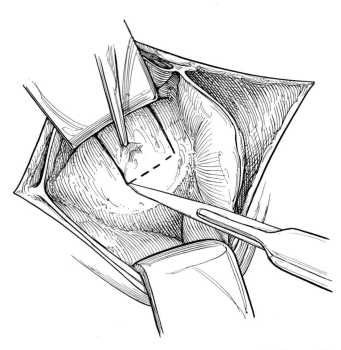

Fig. 38.49. Septal myectomy. (From Monnet E, Orton EC, Gaynor J, et al. Open resection of subvalvular aortic stenosis in dogs. J Am Vet Med Assoc 1996;209:1255–1261.)

ventricular septum (Fig. 38.49). The two incisions are connected by a transverse incision, and a portion of the muscular septum is excised. The conduction system is situated at the junction of the noncoronary and right coronary cusps, so the myectomy is performed to the left of this area.

The aortotomy is closed with a Teflon pledget-buttressed continuous horizontal mattress pattern oversewn with a simple continuous pattern (see Fig. 38.48). The left heart is de-aired just before final closure of the aortotomy. The aortic cross-clamp is removed, and the dog is weaned from cardiopulmonary bypass.

Suggested Readings

Kienle RD, Thomas WP, Pion PD. The natural clinical history of canine congenital subaortic stenosis. J Vet Intern Med 1994; 8:423–431.

Komtebedde J, Ilkiw JE, Follette DM, et al. Resection of subvalvular aortic stenosis: surgical and perioperative management in seven dogs. Vet Surg 1993;22:419–430.

Lupinetti FM, Pridjan AK, Callow LB, et al. Optimum treatment of discrete subaortic stenosis. Ann Thorac Surg 1992;54:467–471.

Monnet E, Orton EC, Gaynor J, et al. Open resection of subvalvular aortic stenosis in dogs. J Am Vet Med Assoc 1996;209:1255–1261.

O'Grady MR, Holmberg DL, Miller CW, et al. Canine congenital aortic stenosis: a review of the literature and commentary. Can Vet J 1989;30:811–815.

Pyle RL, Patterson DF, Chacko S. The genetics and pathology of discrete subaortic stenosis in the Newfoundland dog. Am Heart J 1976;92:324–334.

Cardiac Septal Defect Repair

E. Christopher Orton

Three general types of cardiac septal defect occur in small animals: atrial septal defect (ASD), atrioventricular (AV) septal defect, and ventricular septal defect (VSD). Three types of ASD are recognized: *patent foramen ovale, sinus venous type,* and *fossa ovalis type.* All three of these defects occur in the septum secundum. Defects of the septum secundum are located dorsally and are bordered ventrally by a septal rim that rises from the

AV valves. Patent foramen ovale results from enlargement of the foramen ovale relative to its valve and occurs secondary to pressure or volume overload conditions involving the right heart. Sinus venous defects occur cranial in the atrial septum and frequently are associated with anomalous pulmonary venous drainage, whereas fossa ovalis defects occur in the caudal septum and result from a true deficiency in the development of the septum secundum.

AV septal defects represent a spectrum of malformations that involve the septum primum, the inlet portion of ventricular septum, and the AV valves. Ostium primum ASD is currently considered to be a *partial AV septal defect* that consists of the ostium primum defect

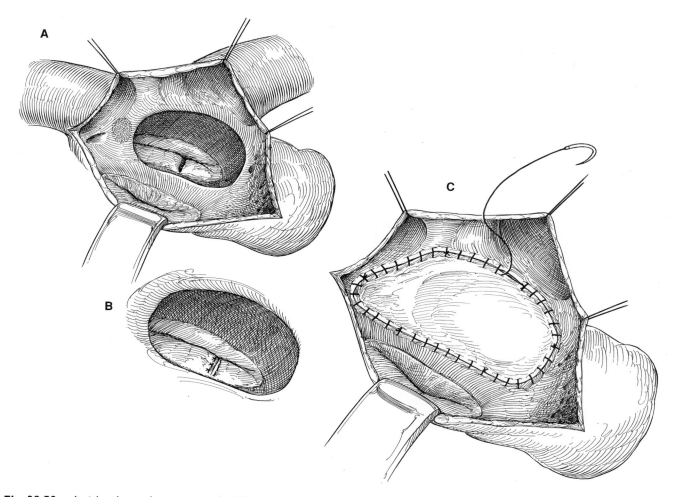

Fig. 38.50. Atrial and partial atrioventricular (AV) septal defect repair. **A.** Repair of an atrial or partial AV septal defect is accomplished through a right atriotomy approach during cardiopulmonary bypass. Bicaval venous cannulation is necessary to isolate the right atrium during bypass. **B.** Partial AV septal defects are associated with a cleft of the septal leaflet of the mitral valve that is repaired with mattress sutures before closure of the septal defect. **C.** The septal defect is closed with an autogenous pericardial patch using a continuous suture pattern. In partial AV septal defects, the AV node is located between the coronary sinus and the septal (ostium primum) defect and is susceptible to injury during patch closure. The patch can be extended beyond the margin of the defect to the caudal aspect of the coronary sinus to reduce risk of AV node injury. If anomalous pulmonary venous drainage is present, the patch is extended in a similar manner around the ostia of the abnormal veins to redirect anomalous flow to the left side. After repair of the septal defect, the atriotomy incision is closed with a continuous mattress suture pattern oversewn with a simple continuous pattern. (From Orton EC, ed. Small animal thoracic surgery. Baltimore: Williams & Wilkins, 1995.)

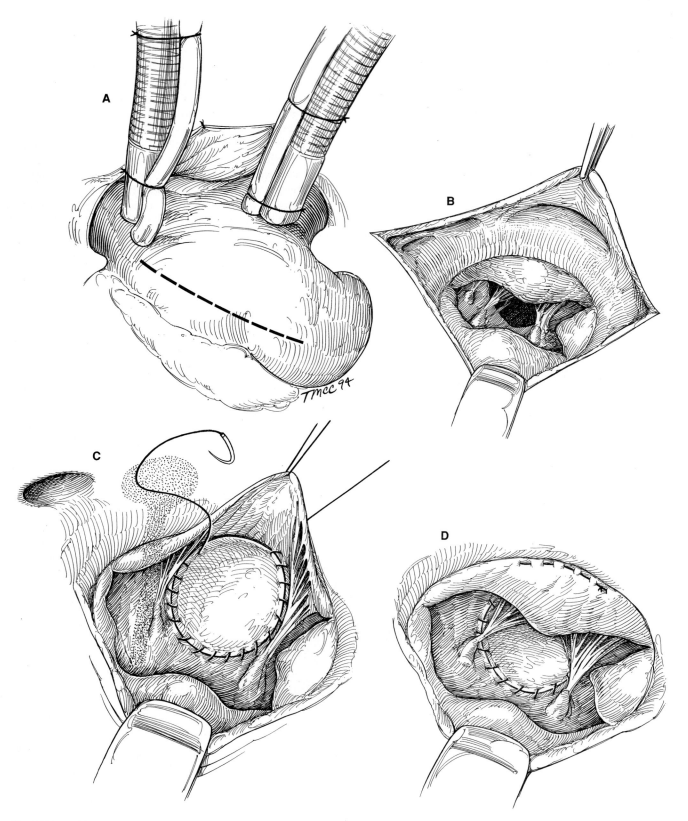

Fig. 38.51. Ventricular septal defect repair. **A.** Patch repair of a perimembranous ventricular septal defect is accomplished through a right atriotomy approach during cardiopulmonary bypass. Bicaval venous cannulation is necessary to isolate the right atrium during bypass. **B.** Perimembranous ventricular septal defects are located adjacent to the membranous ventricular septum medial to the septal leaflet of the tricuspid valve. **C.** The tricuspid valve is retracted gently, and a synthetic patch graft is sutured into the defect using a buttressed mattress or continuous suture pattern. Conduction bundles usually are located close to the caudal margin of the defect and are susceptible to injury during suture placement. Sutures in this portion of the defect should not be placed through the margin of the defect, but rather they should be placed superficially on the right ventricular side of the defect. **D.** The patch closure is completed at the base of the tricuspid valve by passing the sutures through the tricuspid valve annulus. After the repair is completed, the atriotomy incision is closed with a continuous mattress suture pattern oversewn with a simple continuous pattern. (From Orton EC, ed. Small animal thoracic surgery. Baltimore: Williams & Wilkins, 1995.)

and a malformation of the mitral valve. The mitral valve defect is characterized by a cleft in the septal leaflet that changes the valve into a trileaflet structure. This malformation usually causes hemodynamically significant mitral insufficiency. A *complete AV septal defect* consists of an ostium primum defect above, a ventricular septal defect below, and a single AV valve that is common to the right and left ventricle. The complete form of AV septal defect is formally termed an *endocardial cushion defect.*

VSDs occur anywhere in the muscular or membranous ventricular septum. *Perimembranous* defects are bordered by the fibrous tissue of the AV valve leaflets, the central fibrous body, and the inlet, trabecular, or infundibular (outlet) portion of the muscular septum. These defects are medial to the septal tricuspid leaflet and are closely associated with the conduction tissues of the heart. *Muscular* defects are bordered entirely by muscle and occur in the inlet, trabecular, or infundibular muscular septums.

Indications for Surgery

Patent foramen ovale is usually an acquired defect and generally is not an indication for surgery. Closure of other cardiac septal defects is indicated when they are hemodynamically unrestrictive. Such defects place the animal at risk for development of progressive heart failure, pulmonary hypertension, or both. Findings that support a hemodynamically significant defect include cardiac chamber dilation, radiographic evidence of pulmonary vessel enlargement, Doppler-measured peak pulmonary systolic velocity greater than 3.5 m/s, pulmonary-to-systemic flow (Q_p/Q_s) ratio greater than 1.5, or evidence of increased pulmonary vascular resistance. Associated valvular insufficiencies that are likely to be progressive such as mitral insufficiency with partial AV septal defects or aortic insufficiency with VSD should also be considered in the decision to operate. Repair of cardiac septal defects generally is considered curative.

Surgical Technique

Cardiac septal defect repair can be accomplished with cardiopulmonary bypass in dogs weighing 10 kg or more (see the earlier section of this chapter on cardiopulmonary bypass). Repairs in smaller animals can be attempted using special bypass techniques and equipment or whole-body hypothermia; however, the risk of operative mortality is increased. Repair of most septal defects is accomplished through a right fifth intercostal thoracotomy and a right atriotomy. Bicaval venous cannulation is required to isolate the right atrium for this approach. Ostium secundum ASD, partial AV septal defects, and perimembranous and inlet muscular VSD are reparable through the right atrium. Trabecular and infundibular muscular defects are sometimes reparable through the right atrium. If not, these defects are closed through a right ventriculotomy.

Fossa ovalis–type, sinus venosus–type, and partial AV septal defects are closed with autogenous pericardium using a continuous suture pattern (Fig. 38.50). Secundum-type ASD should be carefully evaluated for the concurrent presence of partial anomalous pulmonary venous return. If this condition is present, flow from pulmonary veins emptying into the right atrium can be redirected to the left side by extending the pericardial patch around the ostia of the abnormal veins. With partial AV septal defects, the mitral valve cleft is repaired through the septal defect before patch closure.

Small or medium VSDs may be closed directly with buttressed mattress sutures. Large VSDs are closed with a synthetic patch using either a continuous or an interrupted technique with buttressed mattress sutures (Fig. 38.51). Sutures should not be placed in the margin of the defect, especially over its caudal aspect, to avoid injury to conduction tissues.

Suggested Readings

Backer CL, Idriss FS, Zales VR, et al. Surgical management of the conal (supracristal) ventricular septal defect. J Thorac Cardiovasc Surg 1991;102:288–296.

Eyster GE, Anderson LK, Krehbeil JD, et al. Surgical repair of atrial septal defect in a dog. J Am Vet Med Assoc 1976;169:1081–1084.

Jeraj K, Ogburn PN, Johnston GR, et al. Atrial septal defect (sinus venosus type) in a dog. J Am Vet Med Assoc 1980;177:342–346.

Stark J, de Level M, eds. Surgery for congenital heart defects. New York: Grune & Stratton, 1983.

Weirich WE, Blevins WE. Ventricular septal defect repair. Vet Surg 1977;1:2–7.

39

LYMPHATICS AND LYMPH NODES

Surgical Management of Chylothorax

Theresa W. Fossum

Etiology

Chyle is the term used to denote lymphatic fluid arising from the intestine and therefore containing a high quantity of fat; *chylothorax* is a collection of chyle in the pleural space. The thoracic duct (TD) is the cranial continuation of the cisterna chyli and is generally said to begin between the crura of the diaphragm. In cats, the TD lies between the aorta and azygous vein on the left side of the mediastinum, whereas in dogs it lies on the right side of the mediastinum until it reaches the fifth or sixth vertebra, where it crosses to the left side. The TD terminates in the venous system of the neck (left external jugular vein or jugulosubclavian angle).

In most animals, abnormal flows or pressures within the TD are thought to lead to exudation of chyle from intact, but dilated, thoracic lymphatic vessels (known as thoracic lymphangiectasia). These dilated lymphatic vessels may form in response to increased lymphatic flows (resulting from increased hepatic lymph formation), decreased lymphatic drainage into the venous system because of high venous pressures, or both factors acting simultaneously to increase lymph flows and decrease drainage. Any disease or process that increases systemic venous pressures (i.e., right-sided heart failure, mediastinal neoplasia, cranial vena cava thrombi, granulomas) may cause chylothorax (Table 39.1). Trauma is an uncommonly recognized cause of chylothorax in dogs and cats be-

cause the TD heals rapidly after injury, and within 1 to 2 weeks the effusion resolves without treatment.

Possible causes of chylothorax include anterior mediastinal masses (i.e., mediastinal lymphosarcoma, thymoma), heart disease (e.g., cardiomyopathy, pericardial effusion, heartworm infection, foreign objects, tetralogy of Fallot, tricuspid dysplasia, cor triatriatum dexter), fungal granulomas, venous thrombi, and congenital abnormalities of the TD. Chylothorax may occur in association with diffuse lymphatic abnormalities including intestinal lymphangiectasia and generalized lymphangiectasia with subcutaneous chyle leakage. In most animals, despite extensive diagnostic workups, the underlying cause is undetermined (idiopathic chylothorax). Because the treatment of this disease varies depending on the underlying origin, clinicians must identify concurrent disease processes before instituting definitive therapy. A flow chart for managing an animal identified as having a chylous effusion is presented in Figure 39.1.

Diagnosis

Signalment and History

Any breed dog or cat may be affected; however, a breed predisposition has been suspected in the Afghan hound for years. More recently, investigators have suggested that the shiba inu breed may also be predisposed to this disease. Among cats, Asian breeds (i.e., Siamese and Himalayan) appear to have an increased prevalence. Chylothorax may affect animals of any age; however, in one study older cats were more likely to develop chylothorax than were young cats. This finding was believed to indicate an association between chylothorax and neoplasia. Whereas Afghan

Table 39.1.
Abnormalities Associated with Chylothorax in Dogs and Cats

Cardiomyopathy
Mediastinal lymphosarcoma or thymoma
Cranial vena cava thrombi
Heartworm disease
Fungal granulomas
Pericardial effusion or heart base tumors
Foreign objects
Tetralogy of Fallot
Tricuspid dysplasia
Cor triatriatum dexter
Congenital thoracic duct abnormalities
Lymphangioleiomyomatosis

hounds appear to develop this disease when middle aged, affected shiba inus have been less than 1 year of age. A sex predisposition has not been identified.

Coughing is often the first (and occasionally the only) abnormality noted by owners until the animal becomes dyspneic. Many owners report that they first noticed coughing months before presenting the animal for veterinary care; therefore, animals that cough and do not respond to standard treatment of nonspecific respiratory problems should be evaluated for chylothorax. Coughing may be a result of irritation caused by the effusion, or it may be related to the underlying disease process (i.e., cardiomyopathy, thoracic neoplasia).

Physical Examination Findings

The most common physical examination finding in animals with pleural effusion is dyspnea. The dyspnea may be marked by a forceful inspiration with delayed expiration, making the animal appear to be holding its breath. This respiratory pattern is particularly noticeable in cats. Increased bronchovesicular sounds may be heard dorsally, and lung sounds may be absent ventrally (usually bilaterally, but occasionally unilaterally). Most animals with chylothorax present with a normal body temperature, unless they are extremely excited or severely depressed. Additional findings in patients with chylothorax may include muffled heart sounds, depression, anorexia, weight loss, pale mucous membranes, arrhythmias, heart murmurs, and pericardial effusion.

Radiography and Ultrasonography

If the animal is not overtly dyspneic, thoracic radiographs should be taken to confirm the diagnosis of pleural fluid. Taking dorsoventral (rather than ventrodorsal views) and "standing lateral" radiographic views, minimizing handling, and supplementing oxygen by face mask during the radiographic procedures may help to prevent further compromise of respiration. If the animal is not dyspneic and only small amounts of fluid are suspected, ventrodorsal and expiratory views may help to delineate the effusion. Radiographic signs associated with pleural effusion include blurring of the cardiac silhouette, interlobar fissure lines, rounding of lung margins at the costophrenic angles, widening of the mediastinum, separation of the lung borders from the thoracic wall, and scalloping of the lung margins at the sternal border. The last may be the earliest radiographic sign of pleural effusion.

Ultrasonography should be performed before fluid removal because the fluid acts as an "acoustic window" enhancing visualization of thoracic structures. Ultrasonography is used to evaluate cardiac function, valvular lesions and function, congenital cardiac abnormalities, the presence of pericardial effusion, and mediastinal masses. The presence of pleural fluid often prevents satisfactory radiographic evaluation of the structures of the thoracic cavity. Because adequate visualization of the entire thorax is necessary to rule out anterior mediastinal masses such as lymphosarcoma or thymoma, radiographs should be repeated after removal of most of the pleural fluid.

Animals with collapsed lung lobes that do not appear to reexpand after removal of pleural fluid should be suspected of having underlying pulmonary parenchymal or pleural disease, such as fibrosing pleuritis. Although the cause of this fibrosis is unknown, it apparently can occur subsequent to any prolonged exudative or blood-stained effusion. Diagnosis of fibrosing pleuritis is difficult. The atelectatic lobes may be confused with metastatic or primary pulmonary neoplasia, lung lobe torsion, or hilar lymphadenopathy. Radiographic evidence of pulmonary parenchyma that fails to reexpand after removal of pleural fluid should be considered possible evidence of atelectasis with associated fibrosis. Fibrosing pleuritis should also be considered in animals with persistent dyspnea but minimal pleural fluid.

Laboratory Findings

Fluid recovered by thoracentesis should be placed in an ethylenediaminetetraacetic acid (EDTA) tube for cytologic examination. Placing the fluid in an EDTA tube rather than a "clot-tube" allows cell counts to be performed. Although chylous effusions are routinely classified as exudates, the physical characteristics of the fluid may be consistent with a modified transudate (Table 39.2). The color varies, depending on fat content of the diet and the presence of concurrent hemorrhage. The protein content is variable and often inaccurate because of interference of the refractive index

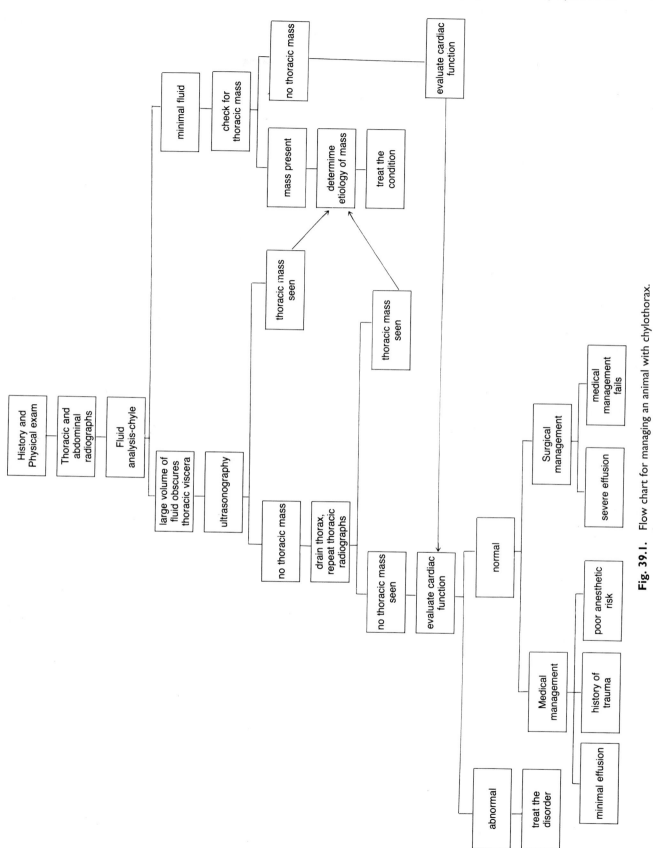

Fig. 39.1. Flow chart for managing an animal with chylothorax.

Table 39.2.
Characteristics of Chylous Effusions

	Cats	Dogs
Color	white or pink (occasionally red)	same
Clarity	opaque remains opaque when centrifuged	same
Specific gravity	1.019–1.050	1.022–1.037
Total protein (g/dL)	2.6–10.3	2.5–6.2
Total white cells/μL	~8,000	~6,000
Triglyceride content > serum		
Cholesterol content ≤ serum		
Chylomicrons are present		
Predominant cell type may be lymphocyte or neutrophil		
Sudanophilic fat globules present		
Clearance with ether		

by the high lipid content of the fluid. The total nucleated cell count is usually less than 10,000/μL and consists primarily of small lymphocytes or neutrophils, with lesser numbers of lipid-laden macrophages.

Chronic chylous effusions may contain low numbers of small lymphocytes because of the body's inability to compensate for continued lymphocyte loss. Nondegenerative neutrophils may predominate with prolonged loss of lymphocytes or when multiple therapeutic thoracocenteses have induced inflammation. Degenerative neutrophils and sepsis are uncommon findings because of the bacteriostatic effect of fatty acids, but these findings can occur iatrogenically as a result of repeated aspirations. To help determine whether a pleural effusion is truly chylous, several tests can be performed, including comparison of fluid and serum triglyceride levels, Sudan III stain for lipid droplets, and ether clearance test. The most diagnostic test is comparison of serum and fluid triglyceride levels. *If the effusion is truly chylous, it will contain a higher concentration of triglycerides than simultaneously collected serum.*

Differential Diagnosis

Any cause of respiratory distress or coughing should be considered in the differential diagnosis. Once pleural effusion has been identified, differential diagnoses include diseases causing exudative pleural effusion, such as pyothorax. Although chylous effusions have a characteristic appearance, the physical characteristics of chylous effusions and other exudative effusions may be similar. Additionally, the appearance and cell populations of chylous effusions can be altered by diet and chronicity.

"Pseudochylous effusion" is a term that has been *misused* in the veterinary literature to describe effusions that look like chyle, but in which a ruptured TD is not found. Given the known causes of chylothorax in dogs and cats, this term should be reserved for effusions in which the pleural fluid cholesterol is greater than the serum cholesterol concentration and the pleural fluid triglyceride is less than or equal to the serum triglyceride. Pseudochylous effusions are rare in veterinary patients, but they may be associated with tuberculosis.

Medical Management

If an underlying disease is diagnosed, it should be treated and the chylous effusion managed by intermittent thoracocentesis. If the underlying disease is effectively treated, the effusion often resolves; however, complete resolution may take several months. Surgical intervention should be considered only in animals with idiopathic chylothorax or in those that do not respond to medical management. Chest tubes should only be placed in those animals with suspected chylothorax secondary to trauma (extremely rare), with rapid fluid accumulation, or after surgical procedures. Electrolytes should be monitored because hyponatremia and hyperkalemia have also been documented in dogs with chylothorax undergoing multiple thoracentesis. A low-fat diet may decrease the amount of fat in the effusion, which may improve the animal's ability to resorb fluid from the thoracic cavity.

Commercial low-fat diets are preferable to homemade diets; however, if commercial diets are refused, homemade diets are a reasonable alternative. Medium-chain triglycerides (once thought to be absorbed directly into the portal system, bypassing the TD) are transported through the TD of dogs. Thus, they may be less useful than previously believed. Dietary therapy is unlikely to "cure" this disease, but it may help in the management of animals with chronic chylothorax. Clients should be informed that, with the idiopathic form of this disease, no effective treatment is available to stop the effusion in all animals. However, the condition may spontaneously resolve in some animals after several weeks or months.

Benzopyrone drugs have been used for the treatment of lymphedema in human patients for years. Whether these drugs may be effective in decreasing pleural effusion in animals with chylothorax is not known; however, preliminary findings suggest that more than 25% of animals treated with benzopyrones (e.g., Rutin) had complete resolution of their effusion at 2 months after initiation of therapy. Determination of whether the effusion resolved spontaneously in these animals or was associated with the drug therapy requires further study. Because the efficacy and potential side effects of these drugs have not been determined in a large clinical study, they should be used with caution.

Surgical Treatment

Surgical intervention may be warranted in animals that do not have underlying disease and in which medical management becomes impractical or is ineffective. Surgical options in animals that do not have severe fibrosing pleuritis include mesenteric lymphangiography and TD ligation, passive pleuroperitoneal shunting, active pleuroperitoneal or pleurovenous shunting, and pleurodesis. Only TD ligation and active pleuroperitoneal shunting are described here. The mechanism by which TD ligation is purported to work is that, after TD ligation, abdominal lymphaticovenous anastomoses form for the transport of chyle to the venous system. Therefore, chyle bypasses the TD, and the effusion resolves. Unfortunately, TD ligation results in complete resolution of pleural effusion in only about 50% of animals that undergo operation. The advantage of TD ligation is that, if it is successful, the result is complete resolution of pleural fluid (as compared with palliative procedures such as passive or active pleuroperitoneal shunting). Disadvantages include a long operating time (problematic in debilitated animals), a high incidence of continued or recurrent chylous or nonchylous (from pulmonary lymphatics) effusion, and difficulty in performing mesenteric lymphangiography (particularly in cats). Without mesenteric lymphangiography, complete ligation of the TD cannot be ensured; however, this technique may not be uniformly successful in verifying complete ligation of the TD. Some small branches of the TD system may be present and yet not fill with dye during lymphangiography.

Food is withheld 12 hours preoperatively. Cream or oil may be fed 3 to 4 hours before the surgical procedure, to help visualize lymphatics, or alternately, methylene blue may be injected into a lymph node at surgery. If a thoracic approach to the TD is used (see later), the left side (cats) or right side (dogs) of the thorax and abdomen are prepared for aseptic surgery. If a transdiaphragmatic approach is used, the cranial abdomen and caudal chest are prepared.

Surgical Techniques

MESENTERIC LYMPHANGIOGRAPHY

For a thoracic approach, the surgeon makes a left paracostal incision (or, for a transdiaphragmatic approach, a cranial midline abdominal incision), exteriorizes the cecum, and locates an adjacent lymph node (Fig. 39.2). If necessary, a small volume (0.5 to 1 mL) of methylene blue is injected into the lymph node to increase lymphatic visualization. Repeated doses of methylene blue are avoided because of the risk of inducing Heinz body anemia or renal failure. The surgeon finds a lym-

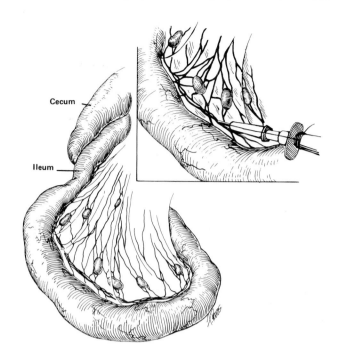

Fig. 39.2. Arrangement of lymphatics near the cecum and insertion of a catheter into a major lymphatic channel (*inset*).

phatic vessel near the node to catheterize by gently dissecting the mesentery (Fig. 39.2, *inset*). The lymphatic vessel is cannulated with a 20- or 22-gauge over-the-needle catheter, and a three-way catheter and extension tubing (filled with heparinized saline) are attached to the catheter with a suture (3–0 silk). An additional suture is placed around the extension tubing and through a segment of intestine to prevent dislodgment of the catheter. After diluting 1 mL/kg of a water-soluble contrast agent (i.e., Renovist) with 0.5 mL/kg of sterile saline, the surgeon injects this mixture into the catheter and takes a lateral thoracic radiograph while the last milliliter is being flushed into the catheter. This lymphangiogram helps to identify the number and location of branches of the TD that need to be ligated. The lymphangiogram is repeated after TD ligation (see later) to identify branches that were not occluded. Embolization of the TD with cyanoacrylate injected through a mesenteric lymphatic catheter has been reported in dogs. Advantages of TD embolization are that direct visualization of the TD is not required, thereby negating the need for a thoracotomy or diaphragmatic incision. Disadvantages of this procedure are the same as those for mesenteric lymphangiography and TD ligation (i.e., not all TD branches may fill with the cyanoacrylate mixture, and collateralization may occur past the obstruction).

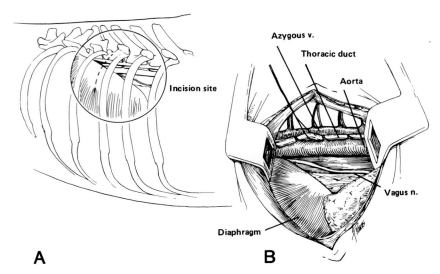

Fig. 39.3. Thoracic duct ligation. **A.** Incision through the right tenth intercostal space. **B.** Ligature around the thoracic duct.

A

B

THORACIC DUCT LIGATION

An intercostal thoracotomy (right side for dogs, left side for cats) is performed at the eighth, ninth, or tenth intercostal space, or an incision is made in the diaphragm. The surgeon locates the TD (Fig. 39.3) and uses hemostatic clips or silk (2–0 or 3–0) suture to ligate it. Visualization of the TD can be aided by injecting methylene blue into the lymphatic catheter.

ACTIVE PLEUROPERITONEAL OR PLEUROVENOUS SHUNTING

Commercially made shunt catheters are available and can be used to pump pleural fluid into the abdomen or into a vein (i.e., jugular, azygous, caudal vena cava). Two types of shunts are available: a pleuroperitoneal shunt (Fig. 39.4); and an ascites (peritoneovenous) shunt. The latter is meant to pump fluid from the abdomen into a vein and does not require manual pumping (i.e., it acts in an active fashion). This shunt can be placed from the pleural space into a vein (pleurovenous); when used in this manner, manual pumping is required (the shunt does not act in an active fashion). A potential complication of pleurovenous shunt placement is formation of a right atrial or ventricular thrombi. This complication may be life-threatening; therefore, pleuroperitoneal shunting is preferred if the surgeon has no reason to believe that the animal may not reabsorb the fluid from its abdominal cavity (e.g., presence of diffuse lymphatic disease or cardiac disease). Close observation of these patients for several weeks after pleurovenous shunt placement is necessary, and preoperative heparinization and maintenance on heparin, aspirin, or other anticoagulants may be warranted. Pleuroperitoneal shunts go from the pleural space to the abdomen. They are generally safer than pleurovenous shunts. Both types of catheters are placed while the animal is under general anesthesia.

The pump chamber and tubing are placed in a bowl of sterilized, heparinized saline. The pump is primed by compressing the valve repeatedly until the system is filled with fluid and flow is established. Any remaining air bubbles are expelled from the tubing or valve. A vertical incision is made over the middle of the sixth, seventh, or eighth rib. The surgeon bluntly inserts the pleural end of the shunt catheter into the thoracic cavity. For a pleuroperitoneal shunt, a tunnel is created under the external abdominal oblique muscle using blunt dissection, and the pump chamber is pulled through the tunnel. The surgeon places the efferent (peritoneal) end of the catheter into the abdominal cavity just caudal to the costal arch through a small skin incision and a preplaced pursestring suture in the abdominal musculature. For a pleurovenous shunt, the efferent (venous) end of the catheter is tunneled over the shoulder to the ventral cervical region.

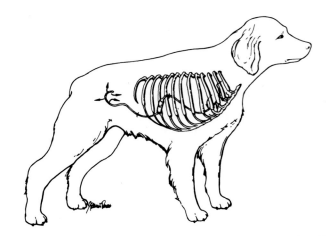

Fig. 39.4. Placement of a pleuroperitoneal shunt. (From Smeak DD, et al. Management of intractable pleural effusions in a dog with pleuroperitoneal shunt. Vet Surg 1987;16:212.)

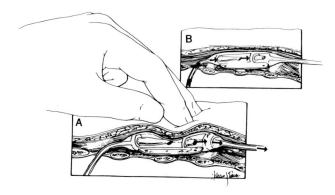

Fig. 39.5. Operation of a pleuroperitoneal shunt. **A.** Emptying of the pump chamber by percutaneous digital pressure. **B.** Filling cycle. (From Smeak DD, et al. Management of intractable pleural effusion in a dog with pleuroperitoneal shunt. Vet Surg 1987;16:212.)

A small incision is made over the jugular vein, and the venous end of the catheter is inserted into the vein. Using fluoroscopy, the surgeon places the distal end of the catheter at the caudal aspect of the cranial vena cava, just proximal to the right atrium (the venous end of the catheter may be shortened if necessary). Alternately, the venous end of the catheter may be placed in the azygous or caudal vena cava through an abdominal incision. The pump chamber must overlie a rib so the chamber can be effectively compressed (Fig. 39.5).

Postoperative Care

If chylothorax resolves spontaneously or after surgery, periodic reevaluations for several years are warranted to detect recurrence. Fibrosing pleuritis is the most common, serious complication of chronic chylothorax. Immunosuppression may occur in patients undergoing repeated and frequent thoracentesis because of lymphocyte depletion. This condition may resolve spontaneously or after surgical treatment. Untreated or chronic chylothorax may result in severe fibrosing pleuritis and persistent dyspnea. Euthanasia is frequently performed in animals that do not respond to surgical or medical management.

Suggested Readings

Birchard SJ, Smeak DD, Fossum TW. Results of thoracic duct ligation in dogs with chylothorax. J Am Vet Med Assoc 1988;193:68.

Fossum TW, Birchard SJ. Lymphangiographic evaluation of experimentally induced chylothorax after ligation of the cranial vena cava in dogs. Am J Vet Res 1986;47:967.

Fossum TW, Birchard SJ, Jacobs RM. Chylothorax in 34 dogs. J Am Vet Med Assoc 1986;188:1315.

Fossum TW, Jacobs RM, Birchard SJ. Evaluation of cholesterol and triglyceride concentrations in differentiating chylous and nonchylous pleural effusions in dogs and cats. J Am Vet Med Assoc 1986;188:49.

Fossum TW, Evering WN, Miller MW, et al. Severe bilateral fibrosing pleuritis associated with chronic chylothorax in 5 cats and 2 dogs. J Am Vet Med Assoc 1992;201:317.

Fossum TW, Forrester SD, Swenson CL, et al. Chylothorax in cats: 37 cases (1969–1989). J Am Vet Med Assoc 1991;198:672.

Fossum TW, Miller MW, Rogers KS, et al. Chylothorax associated with right-sided heart failure in 5 cats. J Am Vet Med Assoc 1994;204:84.

Kerpsack SJ, McLoughlin MA, Birchard SJ, et al. Evaluation of mesenteric lymphangiography and thoracic duct ligation in cats with chylothorax: 19 cases (1987–1992). J Am Vet Med Assoc 1994;205:711.

Martin RA, Leighton D, Richards S, et al. Transdiaphragmatic approach to thoracic duct ligation in the cat. Vet Surg 1988;17:22.

Meadows RL, MacWilliams PS. Chylous effusions revisited. Vet Clin Pathol 1994;23:54.

Willard MD, Fossum TW, Torrance A, et al. Hyponatremia and hyperkalemia associated with idiopathic or experimentally induced chylothorax in four dogs. J Am Vet Med Assoc 1991;199:353.

Transdiaphragmatic Approach to Thoracic Duct Ligation in Cats

Robert A. Martin

This technique is one of several surgical procedures used in an attempt to disrupt the flow of abdominal lymph drainage through the thoracic duct system in cats; it is specifically aimed at resolving chylothorax when no identified underlying cause can be found. Occlusion of the thoracic duct system results in the formation of alternate abdominal lymphaticovenous communications to return chyle to the circulation (1). After a ventral midline celiotomy, a left transdiaphragmatic thoracotomy exposes the thoracic duct system for occlusion with hemostatic clips (1). The procedure allows vital staining and immediate ligation of the thoracic duct system through a single body wall incision. The technical description of the procedure follows.

Surgical Technique

The cat is placed in dorsal recumbency, and the abdomen is prepared for aseptic surgery. A ventral midline incision is made from the xiphoid cartilage caudal to the umbilicus. The jejunum, ileum, and ascending colon are identified and are exteriorized to locate the mesenteric lymph nodes. A more caudal lymph node is selected, usually the right colic, for injection of 1% Evans blue solution (Sigma Chemical Co., St. Louis, MO). Direct puncture with a 25-gauge needle on a 1-mL syringe is used to deliver 0.1 to 0.2 mL of dye into the selected node. A dry surgical sponge is used to contain any leakage of dye on removal of the needle, thus minimizing abdominal contamination. Lymphatic drainage of the injected dye is immediate. By retracting the descending duodenum ventrally and to the left, the stained intestinal lymphatic trunk is easily visualized as it courses through the duodenal mesentery dorsally toward the cisterna chyli. The transparent wall of the intestinal trunk is covered by visceral peritoneum, which can be delicately dissected away to improve the ease of cannulation of the intestinal trunk with a 22-gauge, over-the-needle catheter (Jelco intravenous catheter × 1 inch, Johnson & Johnson, Inc., Arlington, TX). After stylet removal, spillage of dye from the catheter should be contained by capping the catheter either with an injection cap (PRN Adapter, Becton Dickinson Vascular Access, Sandy, UT) or by attaching the 1-mL syringe containing the Evans blue solution. The catheter is fixed to the mesoduodenum with circumferential ligatures of small-diameter suture material (4–0 or 5–0), and the viscera are returned to the abdomen. Gentle manipulation of viscera minimizes disruption of the catheter.

The left side of the diaphragm is identified by retracting the stomach and left liver lobes caudomedially. A left transdiaphragmatic thoracotomy is performed by incising the diaphragm from a point 2 cm dorsolateral to the xiphoid cartilage dorsally toward the left diaphragmatic crus until adequate exposure of the caudal thoracic aorta is achieved. By curving the diaphragmatic incision to parallel the costal arch, the medial portion of the incised diaphragm can more readily be used as a retractor to contain and displace the abdominal viscera caudomedially. Several stay sutures in the medial margin of the diaphragmatic incision are used for retraction.

The left caudal lung lobe is displaced cranially with a moistened sponge to expose the caudal thoracic aorta. The thoracic duct system should be identified in the areolar tissues surrounding the aorta by its staining from the previously injected Evans blue solution. An additional injection through the catheter in the intestinal trunk may be necessary to improve visualization of the thoracic duct branches. The thoracic aorta is dissected from the thoracic duct system just cranial to the aortic hiatus of the diaphragm. The least number of branches of the thoracic duct system is present for ligation at this location (2). The aortic dissection is performed by beginning directly along its ventral adventitia to minimize disruption of any of the thoracic duct branches, which are incorporated in areolar tissue dorsally and laterally. A moistened umbilical tape is passed around the aorta, which is then retracted ven-

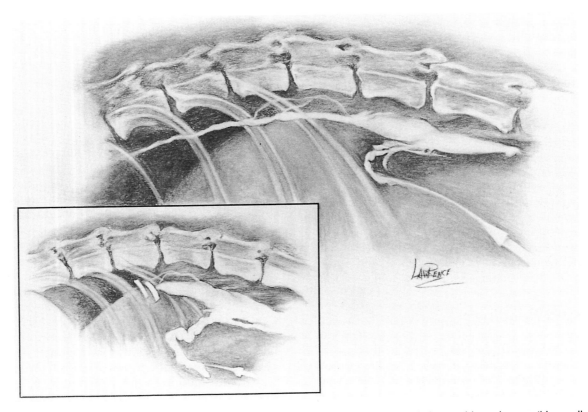

Fig. 39.6. A lymphangiogram of the cisterna chyli and thoracic duct system in the caudal thorax. Note the possible small collateral branches coursing through the diaphragm dorsal to the major duct. *Inset:* the correct location of hemostatic clip mass ligation at a point immediately below thoracic vertebra 13.

trally to expose the stained thoracic duct system completely within the mediastinal tissues. Contraction of aorta occurs during dissection and retraction. Without immobilization of the thoracic aorta by complete circumferential dissection and isolation, complete exposure to the thoracic duct system cannot be achieved consistently.

Multiple hemostatic clips (Hemoclip [medium], Edward Weck, Inc., Research Triangle Park, NC) are used to mass ligate any visible thoracic duct branches, without an attempt to isolate individual ducts before ligation. Usually, a single duct arising from the cranial pole of the cisterna chyli abdominally passes through the diaphragm and gives rise to one or two main thoracic branches, which can be identified at this site along with occasional minor collateral branches (2). A major thoracic duct branch courses on the left dorsolateral aspect of the thoracic aorta. Looping collateral branches or a major or minor thoracic duct may be identified along the right dorsolateral aspect of the thoracic aorta, and multiple cross-communications between longitudinal ducts usually exist more cranially. The number of cross-communications increases cranial to the preferred site of ligation (Fig. 39.6), which is just cranial to the aortic hiatus of the diaphragm (ventral to T13). The paired sympathetic trunks that lie lateral to the thoracic duct system should not be included in the ligation.

After thoracic duct system ligation, a second injection of dye into the intestinal trunk catheter is performed to highlight any collateral branches at the site of ligation that may have been unidentified but require ligation. The moistened sponge on the left caudal lung lobe is removed, and the lobe is reinflated. The thorax is lavaged with warm balanced electrolyte solution, and all fluid is removed from the thorax with suction. The diaphragm is closed in a simple continuous suture pattern dorsally to ventrally with 3–0 monofilament absorbable suture material. Thoracentesis may be performed through diaphragmatic puncture or through a previously placed thoracostomy tube until negative intrathoracic pressure is established. The abdominal lymphatic catheter is removed, and two-layer or three-layer abdominal closure is performed.

Postoperative Care

Postoperatively, a thoracostomy tube is maintained for 24 hours or until thoracic effusion becomes minimal. The success of the procedure is determined by resolution of the chylothorax without recurrence. Perioperative antibiotics are indicated and should be continued until after the thoracostomy tube is removed. Frequent short-term follow-up evaluations are indicated to monitor the cat for recurrent thoracic effusion.

References

1. Martin RA, Richards DLS, Barber DL, et al. Sufit E. Transdiaphragmatic approach to thoracic duct ligation in the cat. Vet Surg 1988;17:22–26.
2. Martin RA, Barber DL, Richards DLS, et al. A technique for direct lymphangiography of the thoracic duct system in the cat. Vet Radiol 1988;29:116–121.

Lymph Node Biopsy

Theresa W. Fossum

Indications and Contraindications

Lymph node biopsy is a valuable tool for differentiating neoplastic from nonneoplastic lymph node enlargement, for determining whether a neoplastic disease has metastasized, for histologically classifying diseases such as lymphosarcoma, and for evaluating immune-mediated disease. If a preoperative biopsy indicates that a neoplasm has metastasized to the local lymph nodes, ancillary chemotherapeutic or radiation modalities may be warranted and, in some cases, may be commenced before the definitive surgical procedure. A lymph node biopsy is easy to perform, is relatively inexpensive, and can provide valuable information. For these reasons, lymph node biopsy should be performed routinely when indicated as a diagnostic aid.

When proper clinical judgment is used, no absolute contraindications exist to lymph node biopsy. In animals with hemostatic disorders, the disorder should be corrected preoperatively if possible, and care should be taken to ensure that blood vessels are properly ligated. Removal of a single lymph node does not usually result in lymphedema. When it does occur, it is usually temporary (1) and seldom requires specific therapy.

A common objection to lymph node biopsy is that it may increase the likelihood of metastasis either by spreading neoplastic cells in the tissues peripheral to the node or by encouraging seeding of the hemic and lymphatic systems with these cells. However, only 1% or less of the millions of tumor cells that escape from primary tumors into the circulation survive to become a viable metastasis (2). The death of most of these cells has been attributed to several factors: mechanical shear forces, loss of attachment of substrate and shedding, oxygen toxicity, and destruction by host-derived circulating natural killer cells (2). Although manipulation of a tumor during biopsy procedures probably transiently increases the number of neoplastic cells present in the lymphatic and vascular systems, and isolated reports of local tumor spread in human patients after punch biopsy do exist in the literature, metastasis after biopsy has seldom been substantiated. Berg and Robbins in 1962 demonstrated the safety of aspiration biopsy by comparing women treated by radical mastectomy for breast cancer whose cancer had been diagnosed by aspiration biopsy with a comparable group who had not undergone biopsy. They concluded that "by no method of comparison that they could devise was there a short or long term increase in cancer mortality associated with aspiration biopsy" (3). The benefits of an accurate, early, easily obtained diagnosis by biopsy outweigh the theoretic and unsubstantiated

disadvantage of increased metastasis as the result of this procedure.

Choice of Biopsy Site

The selection of a lymph node for biopsy should be based on clinical findings. In patients with generalized lymphadenopathy, the popliteal, inguinal, and prescapular lymph nodes are preferred sites for biopsy. At least two nodes should undergo biopsy in such patients. In generalized lymphadenopathy, the mandibular lymph node and lymph nodes draining the gastro-

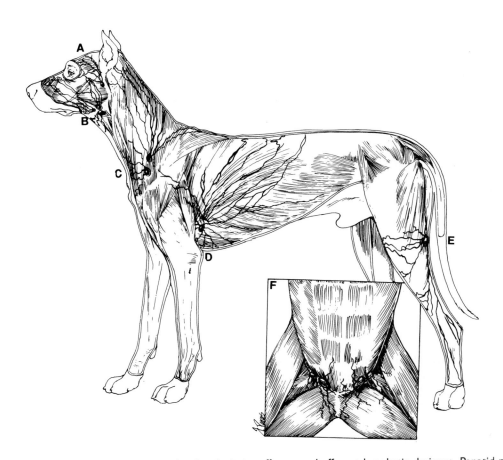

Fig. 39.7. Diagram of superficial lymph nodes in the dog depicting afferent and efferent lymphatic drainage. Parotid nodes (A): afferent lymphatics drain the cutaneous area of the posterior half of the dorsum of the muzzle and side of the cranium, including the eyelids and associated glands, external ear, temporomandibular joint, and parotid gland. Efferent lymphatics go to the retropharyngeal lymph nodes. Mandibular nodes (B): afferent lymphatics drain all parts of the head not drained by the parotid lymph node; the areas of drainage overlap so the eyelids and their glands, the skin of the dorsum of the cranium, and the temporomandibular joint drain into both mandibular and parotid lymph nodes. Efferent lymphatics go to the medial retropharyngeal lymph nodes. Superficial cervical nodes (C): afferent lymphatics drain the skin of the posterior part of the head (including the pharyngeal region and part of the pinna), the lateral surface of neck, the entire thoracic limb (except for the variable region on the medial side of brachium and antebrachium), the shoulder, and the cranial part of the thoracic wall. Efferent lymphatics on the right side go to the right lymphatic duct and on the left side go to the thoracic duct; either side may empty into the external jugular vein directly. Axillary nodes (D): afferent lymphatics drain the thoracic wall and deep structures of thoracic limb and the thoracic and cranial abdominal mammary glands of each side. Efferent lymphatics empty into the thoracic duct (right lymphatic duct on the right side), tracheal duct, external jugular vein, or all of these. Popliteal nodes (E): afferent lymphatics drain all parts of the pelvic limb distal to the location of the popliteal lymph node. Efferent lymphatics go to the superficial inguinal and external iliac lymph nodes. Superficial inguinal nodes (F): afferent lymphatics drain the ventral half of the abdominal wall including the caudal abdominal and inguinal mammary glands, the penis, the skin of prepuce and scrotum, ventral parts of pelvis, the tail, the medial side of thigh, the stifle joint, the crus, and the efferents from the popliteal node. Efferent lymphatics go to the external iliac lymph node.

intestinal tract should not be chosen for biopsy because their morphologic appearance is often distorted by reactive hyperplasia caused by constant exposure to lesions and exogenous antigens (1, 4).

Knowledge of the peripheral lymph nodes and of the areas they drain is essential in selecting a biopsy site. Figure 39.7 depicts lymph nodes commonly sampled for biopsy in the dog and delineates areas drained by these nodes.

Surgical Techniques

Among the techniques available to the clinician for obtaining biopsy samples of lymph nodes are fine-needle aspiration, incisional (wedge) biopsy, and excisional biopsy.

Fine-Needle Aspiration

Fine-needle aspirations can be performed on any lymph node, provided the lymph node can be adequately stabilized during palpation. Once the lymph node has been localized, the skin over the lymph node may be prepared as for surgery; however, lymph nodes have been routinely aspirated at Texas A & M University without skin preparation, and no complications have been noted. Because minimal discomfort is felt by the patient, superficial lymph nodes usually can be aspirated without the use of local anesthetics.

The lymph node is immobilized with one hand while the other hand guides a 20- to 25-gauge needle attached to a 12- to 20-mL syringe into the node. A commercial aspiration gun (Aspir-gun, Everest Co., Inc., Linden, NJ) may also be used (Fig. 39.8). Negative pressure is created in the syringe by pulling the syringe plunger outward to the 3- to 5-mL mark while the needle is alternatively advanced through two or three different planes into the parenchyma of the lymph node. Perforating the capsule of the node may lead to contamination of the sample with fat and blood. The

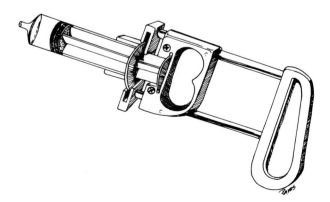

Fig. 39.8. The syringe plunger of a commercial aspiration gun can be manipulated easily with one hand.

central portion of the lymph node should be avoided when possible because this area is predisposed to degenerative changes and may not yield a representative sample.

Before the needle is removed from the lymph node, the plunger should be gently returned to the starting position. If negative pressure is not released before removal of the needle from the lymph node, the biopsy sample may be inadvertently sucked into the syringe barrel and lost, or the biopsy sample may be contaminated with tissue located between the skin and the lymph node (1).

Two or three drops of material should be located within the hub of the needle (only rarely is material present within the barrel of the syringe). This material should be rapidly expelled from the syringe onto glass microscopic slides. Removing the needle and putting 3 to 5 mL of air into the syringe barrel before reattaching the needle may help to expel the obtained sample onto the slides. A film is then made by using a second slide to spread the sample (as for making a blood smear), or squash preparations are made by placing two slides at right angles and sliding them in opposite directions. A single layer of intact cells is obtained if the smears are properly made. The slides should then be air dried and appropriately stained.

Incisional Biopsy

Incisional (wedge) biopsy of lymph nodes is indicated primarily in areas where excisional biopsy may be difficult to perform because of a node's size or location. For example, nodes located close to major vascular or nervous structures would be difficult to spare if excisional biopsy were performed. I commonly use incisional biopsy techniques to obtain samples from mesenteric and sublumbar lymph nodes.

To obtain an incisional biopsy, a No. 15 scalpel blade is used to remove a wedge-shaped section of the parenchyma of the node. The sample is placed in a buffered formalin solution. To provide hemostasis, a horizontal mattress suture of absorbable suture material such as 3–0 chromic catgut may be placed to close the incision site (Fig. 39.9). If bleeding continues, light pressure on the node usually can stop it.

The sample is submitted for histopathologic examination. Alternatively, before placing the sample in formalin solution, an impression smear can be made by lightly touching the cut surface to a glass slide. Bacterial and fungal cultures also can be obtained before placing the sample in formalin.

Excisional Biopsy

Excision of superficial lymph nodes, such as the popliteal lymph nodes, can be performed with the area un-

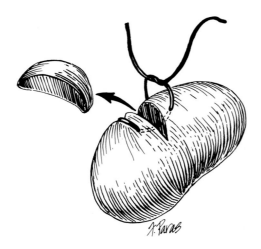

Fig. 39.9. Incisional lymph node biopsy. A wedge-shaped section of the parenchyma of the node is removed, and a horizontal mattress suture (absorbable suture material) is placed to provide hemostasis.

der local anesthesia if the patient's condition permits; however, short-duration general anesthesia facilitates extirpation of lymph nodes in most patients.

The skin overlying the lymph node should be prepared for aseptic surgery. The lymph node is firmly immobilized with one hand, and an incision is made in the skin overlying the node. The node is bluntly dissected from surrounding tissue. Generally, a vessel near the hilus of the lymph node requires ligation to prevent postoperative hemorrhage. The node must be handled gently to prevent damage and distortion of the lymph node tissue. At this point, the lymph node can be sectioned to provide samples for aerobic and anaerobic cultures, fungal cultures, histopathologic examination, and cytologic study. Impression smears can be made by lightly blotting the cut edge of the node with absorbent paper and then touching the sample lightly to a glass slide before placing the sample in formalin solution.

Diagnostic Accuracy of Aspiration Biopsy

The accuracy of aspiration biopsy for diagnosis of neoplastic disease is high when the procedure is performed properly. For example, in a retrospective study of 996 aspiration biopsies from human patients that were performed at a single institution over a 2-year period, 84% of the 682 patients with cancer were accurately identified on aspiration smear (5). In the patients with neoplastic disease that were not identified, the samples were judged to be poor, and neoplastic cells either were not present on the smears or were too sparse for a positive diagnosis. This study shows the importance of using proper technique in collecting the samples and in making the smears. It also emphasizes the need for sound clinical judgment in deciding whether fine-needle aspiration should be followed by incisional or excisional biopsy.

The techniques for lymph node biopsy, when properly performed, are easy, accurate, and valuable, both for diagnosis and for assessing the prognosis of animals with neoplastic disease.

References

1. Perman V, et al. Lymph node biopsy. Vet Clin North Am 1974; 4:281.
2. Schumacher V. Cancer metastasis. Adv Cancer Res 1985;43:1.
3. Berg JW, Robbins GF. A late look at the safety of aspiration biopsy. Cancer 1962;15:826.
4. Thrall MA. Cytology of lymphoid tissue. Compend Contin Educ Pract Vet 1987;9:104.
5. Hajda SI, Melamed MR. The diagnostic value of aspiration smears. Am J Clin Pathol 1973;59:350.

Suggested Reading

Evans HE, Christensen GC. Regional anatomy of the lymphatic system. In: Evans HE, Christensen GC, eds. Miller's anatomy of the dog. Philadelphia: WB Saunders, 1979.

40

SPLEEN

Surgery of the Spleen

Dale E. Bjorling

The spleen is suspended in a portion of the greater omentum (the gastrosplenic ligament) that extends from the diaphragm, fundus, and greater curvature of the stomach to the spleen (1). The splenic artery arises from the celiac artery and supplies branches to the left lobe of the pancreas as it courses to the splenic hilus (Fig. 40.1). The splenic artery divides into a dorsal and a ventral branch several centimeters from the spleen. The dorsal branch continues to the dorsal portion of the spleen, where it gives off the short gastric arteries. The left gastroepiploic artery arises from the ventral branch of the splenic artery before it contacts the spleen. Venous drainage from the spleen is through the portal vein.

The spleen contains smooth muscle and is innervated by both sympathetic (from the celiac plexus) and parasympathetic (from the vagus) nerve fibers. The spleen also has a considerable population of α-adrenergic receptors that control contraction and relaxation (2).

Multiple spleens are uncommon in dogs, but trauma may result in the widespread dissemination of splenic tissue throughout the abdomen. Such fragments of splenic tissue become revascularized, and the resultant condition (splenosis) may be confused with neoplasia. Intentional splenic reimplantation during surgery has been recommended as a means of salvaging splenic function (3), but the mere presence of tissue of splenic origin does not ensure that normal splenic function will be maintained (4, 5).

The spleen may have white fibrin deposits or siderotic plaque on its surface. Siderotic plaque consists of iron and calcium deposits and is brown or rust colored. This appearance should not be considered abnormal. Similarly, splenic nodules (areas of benign hyperplasia) may be confused with neoplasia. Distinguishing splenic nodular hyperplasia from neoplasia may be difficult without a biopsy. The size of the spleen is variable, and the spleen may appear abnormally large during barbiturate anesthesia or when it is relaxed during minimal cholinergic stimulation. Anemia, blood loss, and stress all cause the spleen to contract.

The spleen has several functions: blood storage; blood filtration and phagocytosis of particles, parasites, bacteria, and damaged or aged red blood cells, contributions to the body's immune defenses; hematopoiesis; and iron metabolism. The spleen may retain as much as 10% of the total red blood cell mass (6, 7), which can be discharged into the general circulation in response to cholinergic stimulation during stress or blood loss. The structure of the spleen places red blood cells in close contact with macrophages; therefore, red cells that are damaged, contain parasites, or have immunoglobulins attached to the surface are removed from circulation in the spleen. The spleen also appears to remove blood-borne bacteria efficiently (8). It also produces immunoglobulins (particularly IgM) and opsonins (9). Although not reported in animals, overwhelming sepsis after splenectomy has occurred in human patients (10). Hematopoiesis is not a significant function of the spleen in adult animals unless it is necessitated by decreased function of the bone marrow. Iron is extracted from hemoglobin as red blood cells are broken down and is stored in the spleen for future transport to the bone marrow for production of more hemoglobin.

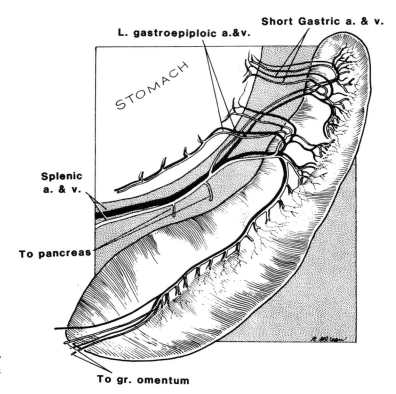

L. gastroepiploic a.&v.

Short Gastric a. & v.

STOMACH

Splenic a. & v.

To pancreas

To gr. omentum

Fig. 40.1. Vasculature of the spleen. The splenic artery and its branches give off vessels that supply the pancreas and the greater curvature of the stomach.

Indications

Indications for removal of the spleen include neoplasia, torsion of the splenic pedicle (isolated or in conjunction with gastric dilatation–volvulus), and severe traumatic injuries. Splenectomy has been recommended as adjunctive treatment for immune-mediated thrombocytopenia and hemolytic anemia unresponsive to medical therapy (11). The spleen is often removed in dogs used as blood donors to prevent undetected infection with *Haemobartonella canis* or *Babesia canis*. Because the spleen has several functions, partial splenectomy should be considered (when feasible) to retain functional splenic tissue.

Hemangiosarcoma is the most common primary tumor of the spleen. Other tumors of the spleen include hemangioma, leiomyosarcoma, fibrosarcoma, lymphosarcoma, plasma cell sarcoma, mast cell sarcoma, and reticular cell sarcoma. Euthanasia of an animal should not be recommended to an owner solely because of the presence of a splenic tumor. Splenectomy prevents intra-abdominal bleeding subsequent to rupture of the tumor, and mean survival times of at least 4 to 6 months in the dog (12, 13) and longer in the cat (14) may be expected after splenectomy for hemangiosarcoma. Removal of the spleen for treatment of splenic leiomyosarcoma in dogs resulted in a median

survival of 10 months (15). The spleen may also be enlarged because of infiltration with mast cells in association with feline systemic mastocytosis. Splenectomy appears to improve the duration of survival in affected cats (16).

Determining exactly when irreversible splenic injury has occurred after torsion of the splenic pedicle is difficult. The onset of clinical signs may be insidious or peracute, necessitating emergency surgery (17). Occlusion of the splenic vein causes vascular stasis, and the vessels ultimately become thrombosed. If the spleen is engorged and blue black, or if thrombi are observed within the vasculature, the spleen should probably be removed. Untwisting the splenic pedicle to restore circulation may release toxic byproducts of anaerobic metabolism.

Preoperative Considerations

Intravenous fluid administration should begin before, and should continue during and after, splenectomy. The rate of administration and total volume given depend on the animal's condition. If the hematocrit is low (less than 18 to 20%), a transfusion of whole blood before surgery should be considered. Although a certain percentage of the red cell mass is removed with the spleen, this volume of cells does not contribute to the peripheral hematocrit at the time of the surgical procedure. Removal of the spleen, however, has a negative effect on the body's ability to compensate for subsequent blood loss. Primary splenic tumors are rare in dogs and cats, and the patient should be thoroughly evaluated in an effort to detect primary tumors or other sites of metastasis that would seriously diminish the animal's ability to tolerate anesthesia and surgery or would decrease its life span after surgery.

Surgical Techniques

Splenorrhaphy

Superficial lacerations of the capsule of the spleen may be closed with sutures. If hemorrhage from the splenic wound is brisk, the injured tissue can be devascularized by ligation of the arteries supplying the wounded area near their junction with the spleen (Fig. 40.2**A** and **B**). This tissue does not remain ischemic, and collateral circulation develops within 3 weeks (18). Large, isolated arteries within the splenic parenchyma that

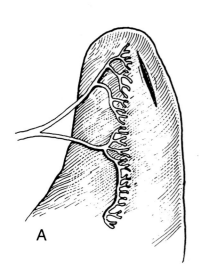

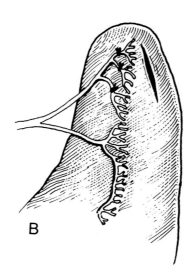

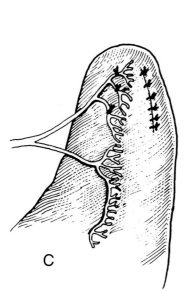

Fig. 40.2. Splenorrhaphy. **A.** Laceration of the spleen. **B.** The vessels supplying the injured area of the spleen are ligated to control hemorrhage. **C.** The laceration in the capsule of the spleen is closed with absorbable sutures in a simple interrupted or continuous pattern.

have been injured can be individually ligated. The splenic capsule is closed with 3–0 or 4–0 absorbable suture swaged onto an atraumatic needle in a continuous pattern (Fig. 40.2**C**). Pressure may be applied to the surface of the spleen to control continued hemorrhage. The omentum may also be wrapped around the spleen. If complete hemostasis cannot be achieved, a partial or total splenectomy should be performed.

Partial Splenectomy

A portion of the spleen can be removed for biopsy purposes or to treat localized splenic trauma or abscessation. A partial splenectomy can be performed with sutures or a mechanical stapling device. The vascular supply of the area to be removed is isolated, ligated, and divided. The tissue to be removed soon assumes an ischemic appearance. The parenchyma is compressed between the fingers along the proposed line of excision. Two pairs of forceps are applied to the spleen, so 1 to 2 cm is between them (Fig. 40.3**A**). A pair of atraumatic forceps (large, straight vascular forceps or Doyen intestinal forceps) should be applied to the splenic remnant to be retained; crushing forceps may be applied to the portion to be excised. The spleen is completely incised between the two forceps approximately 3 to 5 mm from the atraumatic forceps. The capsule is closed with 3–0 or 4–0 absorbable suture in a simple continuous pattern, and the forceps are removed (Fig. 40.3**B**). A second suture line is placed proximal to the first suture line using the same suture material in a continuous horizontal mattress pattern to ensure hemostasis. Partial splenectomy can be performed easily with stapling devices. Staples of a length sufficient to incorporate all tissue when applied must be used. In most animals, staples at least 3.5 mm in

length are adequate; if splenic tissue cannot be compressed to a width less than 2 mm, staples 4.8 mm in length should be used (19). If hemorrhage is observed after application of staples and excision of a portion of the spleen, individual vessels can be ligated.

Splenectomy

Splenectomy usually is performed from a midline celiotomy. The incision should be of sufficient length to allow the spleen to be easily delivered from the abdomen. If an essentially normal spleen is being removed (e.g., to prevent hidden parasitemia or to treat an autoimmune disorder), 1 to 2 mL of 1:100,000 epinephrine can be applied to the surface to cause the spleen to contract. Use of larger volumes or higher concentrations may predispose the animal to cardiac arrhythmias, especially if anesthesia is maintained with halothane.

Vessels should be ligated as close to the hilus of the spleen as possible, to minimize the potential for damage to the left gastroepiploic and short gastric vessels, which supply the greater curvature of the stomach, or the vessels passing to the left lobe of the pancreas. Ligation of vessels during splenectomy can be achieved with suture, metal clips, or a mechanical stapling device. Although absorbable suture may be used for ligation of vessels, I prefer 2–0 or 3–0 silk. The vasculature of the spleen usually is isolated, ligated, and then divided. Alternatively, two rows of hemostatic forceps may be applied to the vasculature. The vasculature is divided, and ligatures are placed after the spleen has been removed. This technique often results in placement of ligatures some distance from the spleen, thereby increasing the potential for incidental ligation of vessels supplying the stomach and

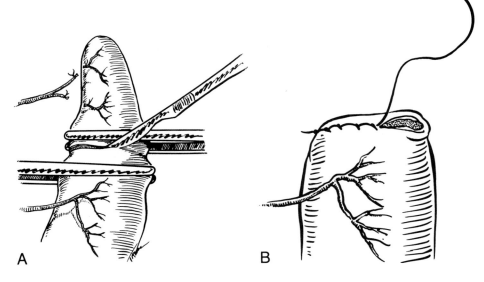

Fig. 40.3. Partial splenectomy. **A.** After the vessels supplying the portion to be removed are ligated and divided, crushing forceps are applied to the tissues to be removed and atraumatic forceps to the splenic remnant. The spleen is then divided between these forceps a few millimeters from the atraumatic pair. **B.** The capsule of the spleen is closed with absorbable suture in a simple continuous pattern. A second suture line is placed proximal to the first to control hemorrhage.

pancreas. As previously mentioned, when splenectomy is performed for treatment of splenic torsion, the splenic pedicle should not be untwisted. The vessels are usually adequately accessible to allow individual ligation near the spleen. If this is not possible, forceps can be applied, and the vessels then can be ligated individually after the spleen has been removed.

The abdomen should be explored thoroughly after removal of the spleen. When the spleen has been removed because of neoplastic disease, particular attention should be paid to the liver and lymph nodes, and biopsy specimens should be obtained if these structures appear abnormal. The pancreas and stomach should be examined to be sure that these structures and their vasculature have been damaged during surgery.

The splenic bed should be examined for hemorrhage before closure of the abdomen. Lavaging the abdomen with sterile saline or another balanced salt solution helps to remove blood clots and improves the surgeon's view of the splenic pedicle.

Postoperative Complications

Hemorrhage as a result of displacement of a ligature is the most common complication of splenectomy. Intraabdominal hemorrhage causes a progressive decline in the packed cell volume and plasma protein concentration when these values are repeatedly measured. Abdominal paracentesis and peritoneal lavage also are useful for detecting hemorrhage after splenectomy. If diagnostic tests support a diagnosis of intra-abdominal hemorrhage after splenectomy, the abdominal incision should be reopened, and the splenic bed should be directly examined. A transfusion of whole blood may be required to compensate for blood loss. If a donor is not available, blood may be retrieved from the patient's abdomen, mixed with an appropriate volume of anticoagulant, and given back to the patient (autotransfusion). This blood should be filtered as it is administered to remove microemboli and other debris. Blood should be removed from the abdomen by some means (suction or sponges), and clots should be removed from the splenic bed to allow direct observation of the splenic vessels.

Damage to the vasculature of the stomach or pancreas can cause ischemic necrosis of these organs. Pancreatitis may result from traumatic handling of the pancreas during surgery. These complications occur infrequently.

As previously mentioned, overwhelming septicemia (occasionally observed in humans after splenectomy) has not been reported after splenectomy in dogs and cats. Splenectomy may render animals more susceptible to infection by blood-borne organisms (*Haemobartonella, Babesia*), however. Other, as yet undetected, immunologic abnormalities possibly may result from splenectomy in dogs and cats.

Anemia after splenectomy is of limited duration if the bone marrow is functioning satisfactorily. Splenectomy does impair the capacity of the animal to maintain the circulating red blood cell volume during hemorrhage. Removal of the spleen 2 to 3 weeks before experimentation impaired the ability of anesthetized dogs to respond to hypoxemia (20). Although this phenomenon may be transient, it does suggest that animals that have undergone splenectomy may be less able to maintain cardiovascular homeostasis during surgery, anesthesia, or other stressful situations.

References

1. Evans HE. Miller's anatomy of the dog. 3rd ed. Philadelphia: WB Saunders, 1993.
2. Opdyke DF, Ward CJ. Spleen as an experimental model for the study of vascular capacitance. Am J Physiol 1973;225:1416.
3. Millikan JS, et al. Alternatives to splenectomy in adults after trauma: repair, partial resection, and reimplantation of splenic tissue. Am J Surg 1982;144:711.
4. Cooney DR, Swanson SE, Dearth JC. Heterotopic splenic autotransplantation in prevention of overwhelming postsplenectomy infection. J Pediatr Surg 1979;14:337.
5. Cooney DR, et al. Relative merits of partial splenectomy splenic reimplantation, and immunization in preventing postsplenectomy infection. Surgery 1979;86:561.
6. Prankerd TAJ. The spleen and anemia. Br J Med 1963;2:517.
7. Song SH, Groom AC. Storage of blood cells in the spleen of the cat. Am J Physiol 1971;220:779.
8. Sullivan JL, et al. Immune response after splenectomy. Lancet 1978;1:178.
9. Andersen V, et al. Immunological studies in children before and after splenectomy. Acta Paediatr Scand 1976;65:409.
10. Krivit W. Overwhelming postsplenectomy infection. Am J Hematol 1977;2:193.
11. Feldman BF, Handagama P, Lubberink AAME. Splenectomy as adjunctive therapy for immune-mediated thrombocytopenia and hemolytic anemia in the dog. J Am Vet Med Assoc 1985;187:617.
12. Fees DL, Withrow SJ. Canine hemangiosarcoma. Compend Contin Educ Pract Vet 1981;3:1047.
13. Frey AJ, Betts CW. A retrospective study of splenectomy in the dog. J Am Anim Hosp Assoc 1977;13:730.
14. Scavelli TD, et al. Hemangiosarcoma in the cat: retrospective evaluation of 31 surgical cases. J Am Vet Med Assoc 1985;187:817.
15. Kapatkin AS, Mullen HS, Matthiesen DT, et al. Leiomyosarcoma in dogs: 44 cases (1983–1988). J Am Vet Med Assoc 1992;201:1077–1079.
16. Liska WD, et al. Feline systemic mastocystosis: a review and results of splenectomy in seven cases. J Am Anim Hosp Assoc 1979;15:589.
17. Montgomery RD, Henderson RA, Horne RD, et al. Primary splenic torsion in dogs: literature review and report of five cases. Canine Pract 1990;15:17–21.
18. Keramidas DC. Ligation of the splenic artery in the treatment of traumatic rupture of the spleen. Surgery 1979;85:530.
19. Bellah JR. Surgical stapling of the spleen, pancreas, liver, and urogenital tract. Vet Clin North Am Small Anim Pract 1994;24:375–394.
20. Ffoulkes-Crabbe DJO, et al. The effect of splenectomy on circulatory adjustments to hypoxaemia in the anaesthetized dog. Br J Anaesth 1976;48:639.

—• *41* •—

MICROSURGERY

Microvascular Instrumentation

Otto Lanz & R. Avery Bennett

The genesis of microvascular instrumentation occurred in the 1930s and progressed further in 1952 with the creation of the Microsurgical Instrumentation Research Association (1). The early improvements to microinstrumentation included spring handles, ratchets, stops, short handles, body skeletonization, and the use of new metal alloys (1, 2). To reduce the amount of shaking and vessel damage, early instrumentation was created that was powered pneumatically, hydraulically, electrically, and manually (1). These powered instruments soon became obsolete because of high maintenance, decreased precision, and lack of improvement in the ability to perform vascular anastomoses (3).

Plastic surgeons began modifying ophthalmic and neurosurgical equipment for their own specific use. The early instruments consisted of jeweler's forceps, needle holders that did not have ratchets, dissecting microscopes, and modified bipolar cautery. Atraumatic microvascular clamps that could approximate severed vessels for microvascular anastomosis were developed. Thanks to the work of Acland, Buncke, Tamai, and others, many different instruments have been designed specifically for every need (1). Surgeons now have a wide range of microvascular instruments, some sophisticated and some basic.

Most of the maneuvers performed in microvascular surgery are delicate, refined motions. Under magnification, even slight aberrant movements are exaggerated. Efforts are directed at preventing hand tremors, which result in tremor at the instrument tips that inhibits accurate manipulations. Substances and activities that predispose to trembling, such as alcohol, coffee, and heavy exercise, are avoided before performing microsurgery. Microsurgery is performed with the surgeon in a sitting position to minimize fatigue, which results in muscle tremors. The surgeon's antebrachium rests on the table, with the heels of the hands resting comfortably on the table as well. The instruments are held as one holds a pen or pencil, with most movements carried out by the fingers while the wrists remain motionless on the table.

Microsurgical instruments have fine tips like ophthalmic instruments, but they differ in that they are a more standard length, whereas ophthalmic instruments are generally short. The length of the instruments varies with the type of surgery performed. With plastic and reconstructive surgery, the operative field is superficial, and the average length of the instruments is 14 to 16 cm (2). In contrast, in brain and thoracic surgery, the average length of instruments is 20 to 24 cm, because structures are located more deeply (2).

In microvascular surgery, most of the instruments are spring loaded to reduce cramping of the hand muscles during long procedures that can lead to shaking and tremors. The handles are generally rounded to facilitate maneuvering the instruments in the fingers and allowing them to be rolled in the fingers, as necessary for suture placement and tissue manipulation. Many microsurgical instruments are grooved near the head to make them conform to the notch created between the surgeon's thumb and index finger. This groove allows the instrument to rest in the notch without being actively held, to minimize muscle fatigue from grasping the instrument, which can result in tremors. Additionally, many instruments are counter-

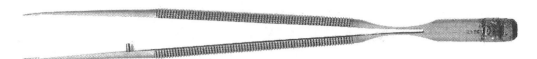

Fig. 41.1. These microsurgical tying forceps are of standard length with miniaturized tips, rounded shanks; this instrument is contoured to fit in the notch between the base of the thumb and the index finger and is counterbalanced.

balanced with a weight at the head of the instrument to minimize the amount the fingers must grip the instruments, thereby preventing fatigue (Fig. 41.1).

The instruments are generally made of stainless steel with tips containing chromium to increase their strength. Some surgeons advocate the use of titanium instruments, which are lighter and stronger and have antimagnetic properties that prevent the fine microneedles from sticking to instruments (1, 2). Unfortunately, titanium instruments are more costly than stainless steel.

This discussion focuses on the instruments and suture material that are essential and are most commonly used for various types of microsurgery.

Jeweler's Forceps

Jeweler's forceps consist of two flat, narrow legs connected at the head that narrow to form the jaws of the instrument (1–3). The contact surface at the tips is referred to as the bit. The distance between the jaws is 8 mm. Jeweler's forceps are numbered according to the width of the bit and legs and their overall shape (1). Five basic jeweler's forceps are used in microvascular surgery: Nos. 2, 3, 4, 5, and 7 (Fig. 41.2). The No. 2 forceps have the largest contact surface and have been advocated for use as needle holders. The No. 3 forceps can be used for testing vessel patency. Nos. 4 and 5 forceps are useful for delicate tissue handling; the No. 4 forceps have a slightly larger bit (1, 2). The

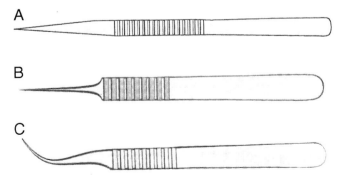

Fig. 41.2. Jeweler's forceps are available in different sizes and configurations. **A.** No. 3 jeweler's forceps are used to test the patency of small vessels by occluding the flow with the forceps and allowing the vessel to refill after the forceps are removed. **B.** No. 5 jeweler's forceps have fine, delicate tips for microsurgical applications. **C.** No. 7 jeweler's forceps have a curve enabling the surgeon to gain access to remote areas of the surgical field.

No. 7 forceps have the unique feature of having curved tips, which are useful to access obstructed areas or to prepare small vessels (Fig. 41.2**C**).

Special care must be taken to avoid bending the tips of the jeweler's forceps. The tips should be examined under a microscope before the beginning of each surgical procedure to assess the alignment of the tips. Bent tips catch on adventitia, tear vessel walls, and inhibit proper handling of the microneedle. The tips of some jeweler forceps are pointed or rough, leading to tissue or vessel damage and inadvertent cutting of the suture material. For these reasons, microsurgeons frequently recommend filing the tips of jeweler's forceps with an emery board or Arkansas stone before their first use (1).

The jeweler's forceps are inexpensive ($30 to $100) and have a wide range of styles and usefulness during microvascular surgery; however, they do not have round handles, are not counterbalanced, and are of short length. Microsurgical forceps are available in a variety of styles and designs but are considerably more expensive ($300 to $600). Microvascular DeBakey forceps, micro ring-tipped forceps, and a variety of curved or straight microforceps are available. These forceps are an appropriate length, have round handles and are usually counterbalanced.

Needle Holders

Reconstructive surgeons have spent much time and effort creating a needle holder that can hold microneedles and can tie microsuture. Some surgeons use No. 2 jeweler's forceps for needle holders for simplicity, ease of knot tying, lack of worry about entrapment of the suture in the lock mechanism, and low cost. The major disadvantage of jeweler's forceps is that the needle is not held securely and may slip at an inopportune moment. Additionally, these forceps do not have round shanks, lack a grooved head, and are not counterbalanced. Rounded shanks are particularly important in needle holders because passage of the microneedle through the vessel wall requires that the instrument be rolled in the fingers (Fig. 41.3).

The three basic parts of the needle holder are the jaws, the lock, and the shank. The jaws are usually flat and not grooved. Castroviejo developed the modern spring-handle needle holders, which have fine-pointed round jaws, round-handled pencil shape, and

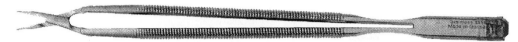

Fig. 41.3. A microneedle holder has all the characteristics desirable in a microsurgical instrument. Care must be taken to avoid catching the fine suture in the hinge mechanism.

a mechanism that disengages for cleaning (4). Castroviejo needle holders are usually short and contain a ratchet mechanism; however, this mechanism can be removed.

Although jeweler's forceps and Castroviejo needle holders are inexpensive and useful, some available microneedle holders are counterbalanced and contoured, with rounded shanks ($30 to $600). Generally, curved needle holders are used because they have less of a tendency to obstruct the surgeon's view of the operating field. Ratchetless needle holders are used almost exclusively in microsurgery because of the delicate nature of the microneedles (Fig. 41.4). Additionally, the locking and unlocking of the ratchet causes motion at the tips that can damage the vessel.

Scissors

Microvascular scissors are among the more expensive instruments in the microvascular surgical pack ($300 to $600). They should have rounded shanks, be spring loaded, and have fine, delicate tips. They are used for delicate dissection, for cutting suture, and for trimming adventitia during vessel preparation.

Scissors are composed of blades, lock, and shanks. The blade tips are pointed or slightly rounded, and the blades are only sharp along their inner surface. The blades may be straight, curved, or angled at 45° (Fig. 41.5). The shanks are spring loaded so the blades are open at rest, and when the shanks are compressed, they come together with a cutting action. These instruments are used for blunt tissue dissection by closing the blades, inserting them into a fascial plane, and allowing the spring action to open the blades within the tissue plane. Scissors must be thoroughly cleaned, well protected, and always sharp. Ophthalmic tenotomy scissors can be used in microvascular surgery for dissecting or cutting larger tissues.

Vessel Dilators

Vessel dilators are modified jeweler's forceps with a narrower, smoother, nontapering tip (Fig. 41.6) (3). The tips of this instrument are inserted into the vessel lumen and are opened slightly to dilate the vessel gently as part of vessel preparation. They may also be used as a counterpressor when suturing vessels. They should be inspected under high magnification to ensure alignment of the tips. The tips must be smooth and unbent to prevent injury to the vascular intima when they are inserted into the vessel lumen.

Microvascular Clamps

Microvascular clamps are used to occlude the vessel, to prevent intraoperative hemorrhage. These clamps must be atraumatic yet have adequate closing pressure to prevent hemorrhage from the vessel. The blades should be flat to disperse the pressure evenly across the vessel, and they should have a rough surface to hold the vessel securely (1–3). Clamps should be easy to apply with finger pressure or applicator forceps (Fig. 41.7). Most clamps are small enough to fit in the operating field but large enough to be easily manipulated. Clamps are available in various sizes with varying closing pressure to accommodate variation in vessel size. The closing pressure of the clamps should be less than 30 g/mm to avoid endothelial damage (1, 2). The surfaces of the clamps are usually dull, to minimize light reflection.

The approximating clamp facilitates retraction and reapproximation of vessels for suturing. The purpose of the approximator clamps is to decrease the amount of tension between two vessels being anastomosed, thereby allowing for atraumatic vascular anastomosis. In the simplest form, an approximating clamp is composed of two microvascular clamps joined by a con-

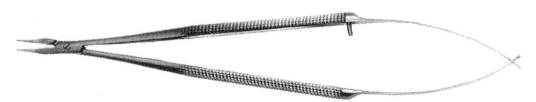

Fig. 41.4. Another microneedle holder design with rounded shanks that is not counterbalanced. This microneedle holder is spring loaded. Neither needle holder contains a ratchet mechanism.

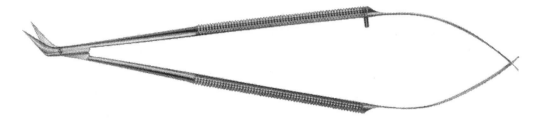

Fig. 41.5. These Potts microvascular scissors are spring loaded, have round shanks, and have blades angled at 45°.

necting bar. The clamps may be movable along the connecting bar to allow for the distance between vessels to be adjusted (Fig. 41.8) or fixed in position to the connecting bar, a position requiring that the clamps be placed at the appropriate distance along the vessels because the interclamp distance cannot be adjusted. The entire apparatus should fit in the operating field, yet be large enough to be easily maneuvered and turned over for suturing both sides of the vessels. The Acland framed nonmovable approximator clamps have two cleats on the frame that facilitate vessel anastomosis, especially when a surgical assistant is not available (Fig. 41.9). Because they are the most expensive microvascular instruments, extreme care should be taken when cleaning and storing microvascular clamps and approximator clamps to prevent damaging them.

Coagulators

Hemostasis is essential for creating a clear field for microvascular surgery. Because of the magnification required to perform microsurgery, even the smallest amount of blood can obscure the operating field and can thereby make surgery virtually impossible. Because of the small vessel size, bleeding cannot be stopped by ligation, so a microcoagulator is essential. Unipolar coagulators damage surrounding tissue because the current passes from the cautery tip, through surrounding tissues, into the patient, and out to the ground plate (Fig. 41.10). This dissipation of current and associated heat generation can damage the parent vessel of interest. Bipolar cautery has the advantage that current and heat are only produced in the small space between the tips of the coagulating forceps. This restricts the amount of tissue damage, yet it provides for accurate hemostasis. A thin layer of sterile petrolatum applied to the tips of bipolar cautery forceps helps to prevent charred tissue from adhering to the tips of the forceps (2).

If bipolar coagulation is not available, jeweler's forceps can serve as cautery forceps. Although this appli-

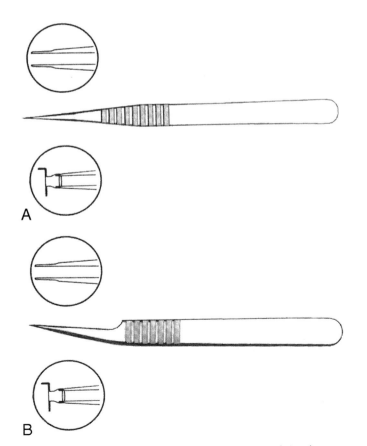

Fig. 41.6. Vessel dilators have smooth, nontapered tips that are inserted into the vessel lumen and are opened gently to dilate the vessel. **A.** No. 3 jeweler's forceps modified for use as a vessel dilator. **B.** Another vessel dilator with angled legs.

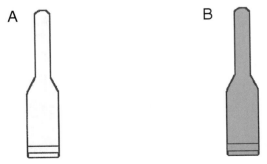

Fig. 41.7. **A** and **B.** Vessel clamps are precisely manufactured to provide adequate pressure to occlude blood flow without damaging the vessel.

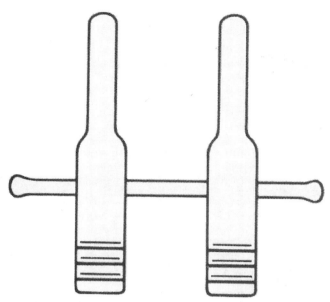

Fig. 41.8. This vessel approximator clamp consists of two vessel clamps that are movable along the bar. Vessels to be anastomosed are placed one in each clamp; then the distance between the vessel ends can be adjusted.

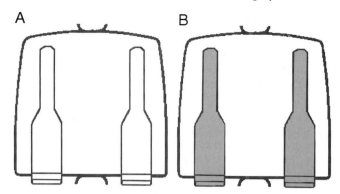

Fig. 41.9. **A** and **B.** Another vessel approximator clamp in which the clamps do not move along the bar. With this type of clamp, the vessels must be positioned precisely to allow the ends of the vessels to be sutured because the distance between them cannot be adjusted.

cation is monopolar, it is more precise and minimizes the amount of lateral heat and damage to adjacent tissues compared with the standard cautery pencil. Using this technique, a small vessel is grasped with the jeweler's forceps, and the tip of the cautery pencil is touched to the forceps such that the current passes along the legs of the forceps, coagulates the vessel held in the tips of the jeweler's forceps, and passes through the patient to the ground.

The amount of cautery used in microsurgery should be kept to a minimum, to avoid damage to vessels or other important structures that may be in the vicinity of the operating field. For vessels larger than 1.5 mm in diameter, hemostatic clips are effective in achieving hemostasis without damaging adjacent structures. Clips are used judiciously because too many hemostatic clips can interfere with the microvascular procedure (1, 2).

Suction

Vacuum suction is an optional tool in microvascular surgery. If mechanical suction is used, care must be taken to avoid contact with vessels or nerves. Endothelial damage from suction can lead to complete thrombosis of the vessel and surgical failure. Standard suction tips are generally too large for microsurgical application. A 20-gauge catheter may be connected to appropriately sized Silastic tubing, then connected to the suction unit to create a fine-tipped suction device. A small fenestration created in the Silastic tubing allows the surgeon some control over the strength of the vacuum. The surgeon's finger is placed over the hole to occlude the fenestration partially or completely, thereby adjusting the amount of suction at the catheter tip. This control over the strength of suction aids in minimizing vascular injury.

Buncke recommends "siphon suction," in which the corner of a sponge is placed in the most dependent part of the wound and the rest is of the sponge is draped over the wound margin (1). Fluid in the surgical field is drawn away along the sponge by capillary action, rather than by mechanical suction. Sterile applicators can also be used for fluid absorption, but care must be taken to avoid damaging vessels or nerves.

Irrigators

Irrigation of the wound is essential in microvascular surgery to decrease the amount of desiccation caused by the intense light source of the operating microscope. Irrigation is also used to remove clots and

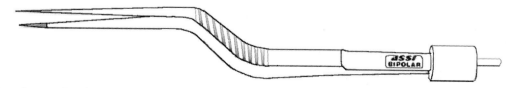

Fig. 41.10. These bayonet bipolar electrocautery forceps have insulated shanks so only tissue held within the tips is affected by the current.

to float the vessel edges apart. Standard irrigation syringes are too bulky and flood the microsurgical field. A simple irrigator can be made for microsurgery using a 10-mL syringe attached to a 20-gauge needle or catheter using either saline or heparinized saline. Irrigation is applied in a gentle stream. The catheter tip is not inserted into the vessel, to avoid damaging the vascular endothelium.

The Bishop–Harmon anterior chamber irrigator is used extensively in ophthalmic surgery and is applicable to microvascular surgery. It consists of a small bulb that contains fluid, an adapter to connect the bulb to a needle, and the cannula. Many cannulas are available. The advantage of this system is that it is easier to operate and to control the flow of the fluid with the small bulb than with a syringe.

Background Material

When performing microvascular surgery, a background is used to set the vessels out from surrounding structures. Background material is placed behind the structures of interest to improve their visualization through the operating microscope. Various colors have been advocated to maximize visualization of these structures. Use of dark colors, such as green or blue, enhances visualization of both the artery and vein, as well as the suture material. Background materials are commercially available, but a rectangular section of a balloon can be sterilized and used as an inexpensive background.

Counterpressor

Counterpressors are used to avoid suturing the opposite wall of a vessel during creation of an anastomosis. When the surgeon passes the needle through the vessel wall, counterpressure must be applied, or the wall is pushed away. The counterpressor provides resistance for passing the microneedle. The instrument must be sturdy, small enough to fit in the vessel, and easily maneuverable. The counterpressor has either a circular or a double-pronged tip, so the microneedle can be passed through the circle or between the tips. A counterpressor can be constructed by twisting 34-gauge wire onto itself, creating a tiny loop at the end. The free end is connected to a disposable tuberculin syringe or a metal bar to serve as a handle (1).

Maintenance of Instruments

Microvascular instruments are delicate and easily damaged. Extreme care is exercised when cleaning and storing instruments. After use, instruments are soaked in warm water containing a commercially available enzymatic cleaner, rinsed in distilled water, and air dried. Ultrasonic instrument cleaners offer the best way of cleaning microinstruments. Care should be taken when instruments are dried with a cloth, because the delicate tips of the microinstruments bend easily. After all the instruments have been thoroughly cleaned and dried, tipped instruments should be covered with rubber tubing to protect them from bending. Because of the amount of electrical instrumentation in the operating room, microinstruments become magnetized, causing the microneedle to become attracted to clamps and other instruments during surgery. This problem can be solved by running the instruments through a demagnetizer coil before backing and autoclaving them.

Storage boxes should contain specially shaped, troughlike receptacles made of foam to prevent damage to instruments. Instruments must not be stored in such a fashion that they are in direct contact with metal or other instruments. Microinstruments can be steam autoclaved without damage or dulling.

Microvascular Suture

The creation of microsuture enabled surgeons to anastomose vessels with a diameter of 1.0 to 2.0 mm. The microvascular needle consists of a point, blade, body, and swage. The needle may be straight or curved, and the curve may be one-half, three-eighths, or one-fourth (Fig. 41.11). A 3- to 4-mm length needle is used most commonly. The diameter of the needle is important because it is directly related to the amount of trauma the needle inflicts on the vessel. Most microneedles contain a tapered point, which is the least traumatic to tissue. Currently, flat needles are used almost exclusively because a flat needle is more secure in the needle holder than a round needle, which can roll between the microneedle holder jaws. Because of the extreme difficulty in threading needles, all microsutures are swaged sutures. Swaged sutures also cause little trauma when passed through tissue. The needle may be made from carbon steel, stainless steel, or other

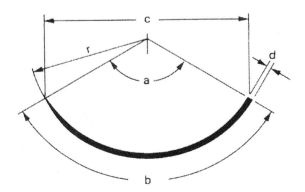

Fig. 41.11. Microneedles are fine, with a taper point and swaged-on suture. They are available straight or with a one-half, three-eighths, or one-quarter curve. *a*, angle; *b*, arch length; *c*, chord length; *d*, diameter; *r*, radius.

metal alloys, with carbon steel the strongest and least malleable.

Nylon is the most commonly used suture material in microvascular surgery (1, 2). It is smooth, allowing it to glide easily through tissue, and it has a high tensile strength while causing minimal tissue reaction. The major disadvantage of nylon is that additional throws may be needed to ensure knot security. In 1966, Ethicon was able to make 10–0 nylon suture on a BV2 needle (1). The most commonly used suture in microvascular surgery is 10–0 nylon.

Acknowledgment

We would like to thank Accurate Surgical & Scientific Instruments Corporation and Debby Sunstrom for technical assistance with the illustrations.

References

1. Daniel RK, Terzis JK, eds. Reconstructive microsurgery. Boston: Little, Brown and Company, 1977.
2. Zhong-wei C, Dong-yue Y, De-sheng C, eds. Microsurgery. New York: Shanghai Scientific and Technical Publishers, 1982.
3. Acland RD. Practice manual for microvascular surgery. 2nd ed. St. Louis: CV Mosby, 1989.
4. Blake HJ. Microsurgery: Transplantation-Replantation: an atlas-text, Philadelphia, Lea & Febiger, 1991.

Applications of Microvascular Techniques

Daniel A. Degner & Richard Walshaw

In veterinary medicine, microvascular surgical techniques are essential to free tissue transfer, renal transplantation in the cat, and reimplantation of appendages (1–11). Using well-established techniques, the success rate of microvascular anastomosis in human patients has ranged from 91 to 97% (11). In our clinical and experimental experience, the long-term patency rate of microsurgically anastomosed vessels in the dog is approximately 95% (1–4). Therefore, because microvascular surgery is becoming more accepted for clinical use in veterinary medicine, the veterinary surgeon should become familiar with these techniques. Performing microsurgical anastomosis of an artery or vein has three steps: 1) vessel preparation; 2) vessel anastomosis; and 3) evaluation of vessel patency.

Vessel Preparation

Vessel preparation is one of the most critical steps in performing a microvascular anastomosis. Failure to pay detailed attention to this part of the microsurgical

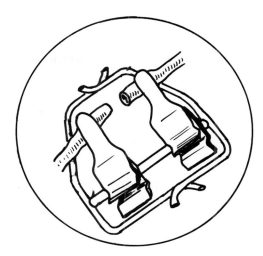

Fig. 41.12. Vessel ends placed in an approximator clamp.

procedure increases the risk of failure. Vessel preparation includes vessel irrigation, trimming of the adventitia away from the vessel ends, and vessel dilation. The ends of the vessels to be anastomosed are placed in an approximator clamp, with care taken not to twist the vessels axially (Fig. 41.12). First, the ends of the vessels are irrigated with heparinized saline to remove all intraluminal blood (Fig. 41.13). This procedure prevents blood located at the ends of the vessels from developing into a thrombus. Flushing out the entire vascular bed of a free tissue flap is not necessary because blood does not clot in untraumatized blood vessels (13–15). Second, the adventitia from the end of the vessel is removed. Adventitia that drapes over the vessel edge and becomes intraluminal at the anastomotic site potentiates the formation of a blood clot because of its thrombogenic properties. Frequently, the adventitia drapes over the cut edge of the vessel in the form of

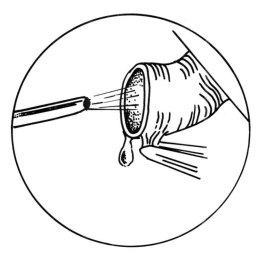

Fig. 41.13. Irrigation of vessel ends to remove intraluminal blood.

an adventitial skirt. This tissue is grasped with the tips of a pair of forceps and is retracted until slight tension on the adventitia is felt. A small hole is made in the adventitia at the end of the vessel wall with adventitia scissors, and one blade of the scissors is placed in this hole (Fig. 41.14). The scissor blade is moved adjacent to the attachment of the adventitia on the vessel, and the adventitia is excised around the circumference of the vessel wall. If the adventitia does not drape completely over the end of the vessel, the portions of redundant adventitia are grasped and are carefully excised at the attachment to the vessel wall (tunica media).

Vessel dilation results in temporary mechanical paralysis of the smooth muscle wall, thereby preventing vasospasm at the level of the anastomotic site. Moreover, it opens the lumen of the vessel and thus helps to define the front and back walls of the vessel. Vessel dilation also is useful to accommodate the disparity in vessel diameters. A vessel that is significantly smaller

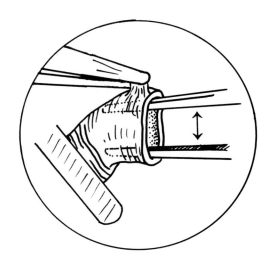

Fig. 41.15. Vessel dilation is performed to prevent vasospasm and to improve definition of the vessel lumen.

may be dilated to the size of a larger vessel (14). A vessel dilator is introduced into the lumen of the vessel and is opened and closed gently several times to dilate the vessel (Fig. 41.15). Only specialized microvascular dilators with blunt tips should be used for this purpose because they do not damage the endothelium.

Preparation of veins for anastomosis is more difficult than preparation of arteries, because venous walls are much thinner. Peripheral veins have a thicker wall than veins located more deeply in the body. For example, in the dog, the vein of the omocervical free skin flap is much thinner walled and more difficult to work with than the vein of the medial saphenous fasciocutaneous free flap (2). Special care must be taken while trimming the adventitia from the end of a vein because the wall of the vessel is thin, and inadvertent damage to the tunica media can result, thus weakening the vessel. Irrigation of the end of the vein, using a syringe and a 20-gauge intravenous catheter, can aid in locating the lumen of the vessel and may assist in identifying the layers of the vessel. Thin-walled veins also may be prepared while submerged in a pool of saline, to improve visibility of the vessel lumen (13).

End-to-End Anastomosis

The end-to-end anastomosis is usually performed by using a full-thickness simple interrupted pattern. For free tissue transfer in the dog, 10–0 nylon on a 100-μm flat-bodied needle is used. The ends of the vessels, held by an approximator clamp, are moved together to create a gap of about 1 to 2 mm between the vessels.

For the right-handed surgeon, when possible, the axis of the proposed anastomosis is aligned so it is oriented from the upper left to the lower right of the microsurgical field (Fig. 41.16). This alignment pro-

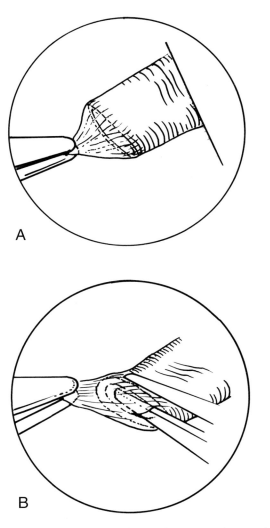

Fig. 41.14 A. The adventitial skirt is drawn over the vessel end with a pair of forceps. **B.** The adventitia is then excised.

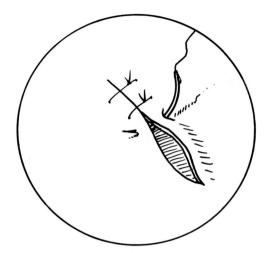

Fig. 41.16. This axis of the proposed anastomosis, oriented from the upper left to the lower right of the field, provides the right-handed surgeon with the most comfortable hand position.

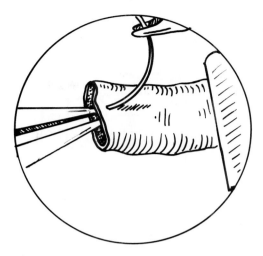

Fig. 41.17. Atraumatic manipulation of the vessel wall is performed by inserting the tips of a pair of forceps slightly into the vessel lumen.

vides the right-handed surgeon with the most comfortable hand position for suturing. For the left-handed surgeon, the axis of the anastomosis should be rotated 90°. The surgeon should, however, become adept at suturing vessels positioned in different orientations.

The needle is held just behind its midpoint with the needle holder. The suture bites are placed about three to four needle widths from the edge of the vessel and penetrate the vessel wall perpendicular to the surface of the vessel. This technique usually necessitates everting the edge of the vessel wall slightly. The vessel wall should not be grasped directly with forceps because this maneuver traumatizes the tissues and may contribute to thrombus formation and thus failure of the anastomosis. To manipulate the vessel wall atraumatically, the tips of a pair of forceps may be inserted into the lumen of the vessel and elevated slightly (Fig. 41.17). Residual adventitia on the vessel wall or the tags of an adjacent suture may also be grasped with a pair of forceps to manipulate the vessel. When passing the needle through the wall of the other vessel, counterpressure may be applied adjacent to the site of exit of the needle to facilitate passing the needle through the tissues (Fig. 41.18). Care must be taken while placing the sutures not to incorporate the back wall of the vessel.

The delicate vessel wall of veins can be torn simply by pulling the suture through the wall. This occurs when the suture is pulled at an angle to the entry and exit points of the bite. Thus, the surgeon should use the back side of the jaw of a curved needle holder as a pulley to redirect the suture so it travels along the same axis as the entry and exit points of the suture. The needle should be placed within the microscopic field before the suture is tied, so it can be located easily.

Microscopic suture tying is similar to macroscopic instrument ties; however, the nondominant hand holds the long end of the suture with a pair of jeweler's forceps instead of the fingers. If the vessel ends do not approximate easily while tying the first suture, the approximating clamps should be moved together slightly to eliminate excessive tension on the anastomosis, because this may damage the vessel wall. Three throws should be placed to complete the knot.

The first two sutures are placed at the 10 o'clock and 2 o'clock positions. A tag is left on each of these two stay sutures so the assistant surgeon can hold these with forceps to manipulate the vessel during the anastomosis. If the approximator clamp has a suture-holding frame, each of these sutures is wrapped once

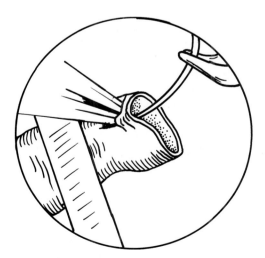

Fig. 41.18. Counterpressure is applied adjacent to the site of exit of the needle to facilitate passage of the needle through the vessel wall.

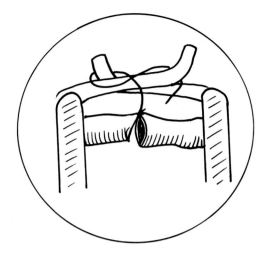

Fig. 41.19. The stay sutures are wrapped around the suture cleats of the approximator clamp in a figure-of-eight pattern.

around the corresponding suture cleat in a figure-of-eight pattern (Fig. 41.19). Placement of these two stay sutures around the suture cleats of the approximator causes the back wall of the vessel to separate from the front wall (Fig. 41.20). The remaining sutures are placed evenly between the two stay sutures. The approximator clamp is turned over to expose the back wall. To ensure that the back wall of the vessel has not been incorporated with the front wall, the luminal aspect of the suture line is inspected. The remaining unsutured vessel circumference is divided in half, and the third stay suture is placed and tied (Fig. 41.21**A**). One of the first two stay sutures is released from the suture cleat, and the third stay suture is placed around the cleat. The remaining sutures of the second third of the vessel circumference are then placed. The last third of the vessel circumference is placed in position for suturing by releasing the appropriate stay suture and fastening the other around the cleat. As the anastomosis nears completion, visualization of the lumen becomes more difficult, thus increasing the chance of incorporating the back wall with the front wall of the vessel in the suture. To increase the visibility of the lumen, the last two sutures are preplaced and then

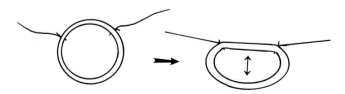

Fig. 41.20. Two stay sutures are first placed in the vessel one-third of the circumference apart. Tension placed on these two sutures, which are wrapped around the cleats on the approximator clamp, results in separation of the back wall of the vessel from the front wall.

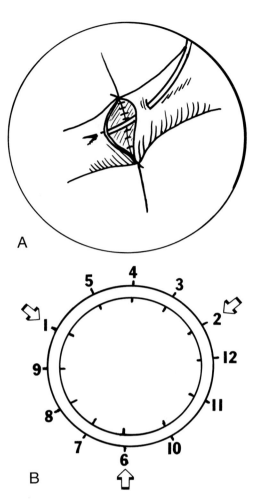

Fig. 41.21. **A.** The approximator clamp is flipped over to suture the remaining circumference of the vessel. **B.** Sequence of placement of sutures to perform the microvascular anastomosis; *arrows* denote stay sutures.

tied. For a typical arterial anastomosis, about 12 simple interrupted sutures are needed (Fig. 41.21**B**).

For a vascular pedicle consisting of an artery and a vein, the clamps occluding the venous blood supply are removed first, followed by those occluding the arterial supply. The clamp distal to the anastomosis is always removed before the proximal clamp (Fig. 41.22). This sequence of clamp removal is important because the systemic blood pressures may potentiate leakage of blood at the arterial anastomotic site if the clamps are removed in the incorrect order.

End-to-Side Anastomosis

Traumatic injuries sometimes result in significant vascular damage to the distal extremity; thus, the use of an end-to-end technique, which sacrifices one of the arteries to the distal aspect of the extremity, may "embarrass" the blood supply to that part of the limb.

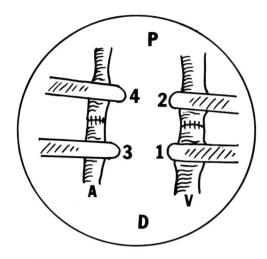

Fig. 41.22. Clamps are removed in a distal (*D*) to proximal (*P*) direction. The clamps are removed first from the vein (*V*) and then from the artery (*A*).

In this situation, the use of an end-to-side technique is recommended. Another use of the end-to-side anastomosis is for the accommodation of significant disparity of vessel diameters (13).

The end-to-side anastomosis involves preparing the vessels, creating an arteriotomy in the "side" vessel, performing the anastomosis, and evaluating the anastomosis for patency. An approximator clamp is placed on the isolated "side" vessel, and a single clamp is placed on the "end" vessel. The adventitia is removed completely from the proposed arteriotomy site (Fig. 41.23**A**). This area should be twice as long and twice as wide as the arteriotomy. A stay suture of 10–0 nylon is placed in the center of the proposed arteriotomy site. The stay suture is elevated as two scissor cuts are made from opposite directions at an angle of 45° to the surface of the vessel (Fig. 41.23**B**). The diameter of the arteriotomy should approximate the diameter of the "end" vessel (Fig. 41.23**C**). Intraluminal blood is flushed with heparinized saline from the segment of the clamped vessel through the arteriotomy site. The first two sutures are placed at the most proximal and distal aspects of the arteriotomy site to situate the "end" vessel in position (Fig. 41.23**D**). The remaining sutures are placed on the front and back walls of the vessels to complete the anastomosis (Fig. 41.23**E**).

Interpositional Grafts

Sometimes, a recipient artery or vein is not available adjacent to a wound that is to be reconstructed with a free tissue flap, or the vascular leash of a flap is of an inadequate length to reach to the recipient vessels. In these situations, a segment of a peripheral vein from the medial saphenous or cephalic vein is harvested and is anastomosed to the flap vessels in an end-to-end fashion, and it is anastomosed to the recipient vessels adjacent to the wound in an end-to-end or end-to-side fashion. The interpositional graft should be oriented in the appropriate direction so the valves of the vein graft remain open when blood flows through the vessel segment. Interpositional vein grafts used for arteries undergo hypertrophy of the tunica media (arterialization) with time. Clinical use of interpositional grafts in human patients has a failure rate five times that of simple end-to-end anastomosis. Therefore, if possible, this technique should be reserved for when a simpler technique is not possible.

Evaluation of Patency

After the anastomosis has been completed, patency of the vessel is evaluated. The trained eye can evaluate arterial patency without manipulation of the vessel by observing the pulse character. Expansile pulsation of the vessel distal to the anastomotic site is the increase and decrease in the diameter of the vessel with each pulse beat. A second sign of patency is "wriggling" or the change of curvature of the vessel branches distal to the anastomosis with each pulse. On the other hand, the occluded anastomotic site may have a longitudinal pulse character. This form of pulsation emanates distally in the recipient vessel, proximal to the anastomosis, and is concentrated at the anastomotic site. The phrase "hammering against the anastomosis" has been used to describe the longitudinal pulse (12). In free tissue transfer, examination of the arterial bed of the transplanted tissue flap for pulsation and evaluation of the cut edges of the flap for capillary bleeding can document arterial patency.

If patency of the artery is evident by evaluation for the signs described, additional testing should not be performed because such maneuvers may be traumatic to the vessels. Several tests of patency have been described. One such test involves lifting the vessel just distal to the anastomosis with a curved instrument under gentle pressure until the lumen almost becomes occluded. The patent artery demonstrates a visible filling and collapsing of the vessel with blood over the instrument with each pulse beat (Fig. 41.24). Finally, the most traumatic test involves occluding the vessel just distal to the anastomosis with a pair of forceps, stripping the blood from this point distally with another pair of forceps, and observing a refill of that segment of vessel with blood as the first pair of forceps is released (Fig. 41.25).

Patency of the venous anastomosis also is made at the time of removal of the microvascular clamps. Because venous walls are translucent, a column of blood that rapidly moves across the anastomotic site when the first clamp is removed can be visualized if the anas-

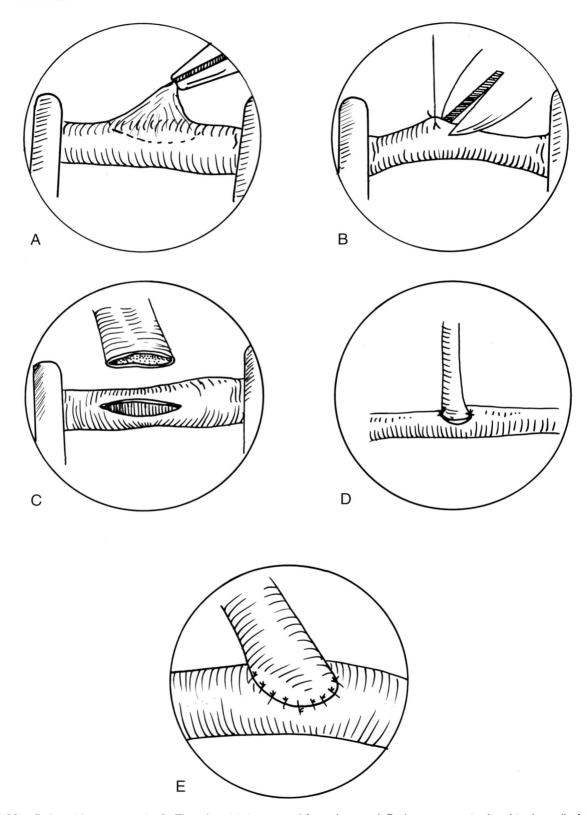

Fig. 41.23. End-to-side anastomosis. **A.** The adventitia is removed from the vessel. **B.** A stay suture is placed in the wall of the vessel, and the arteriotomy is performed. **C.** The diameter of the arteriotomy site should approximate the diameter of the "end" vessel. **D.** The first two sutures are placed 180° apart to position the vessels for the anastomosis. **E.** The sutures are placed perpendicular to the anastomotic line in a radiating fashion.

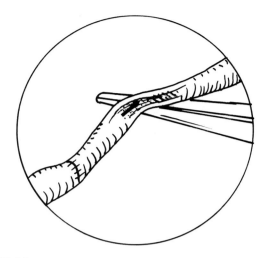

Fig. 41.24. A test of arterial patency involves lifting the vessel with an instrument to observe the visible filling and collapsing of the vessel over the elevated instrument with each pulse beat.

tomosis is patent. An occluded vein, however, becomes dilated distal to the anastomosis and contains dark blood.

Tests can also be used to evaluate the patency of veins. In a less traumatic test, a pair of curved forceps is placed beneath the vein proximal to the anastomosis and is elevated to occlude the column of blood within the vessel. The instrument is then drawn proximally along the vessel. If the column of blood briskly follows the movement of the uplifted instrument, the vessel is patent. A more traumatic form of this test involves stripping a segment of the vein proximal to the anastomosis with a pair of forceps (as previously described for the arterial anastomosis) and observing refill of the vessel segment with blood (13, 14).

Anastomotic Devices

Anastomotic coupling devices (3M Precise Microvascular Anastomotic Device, Medical and Surgical Products, 3M Health Care, St. Paul, MN) may be used in place of hand suturing for microvascular anastomosis, because they provide a high patency rate and dramatically decrease the time required to perform the anastomosis. Because of the increased risk of technical error associated with performing a microvascular venous anastomosis, we routinely use a microvascular anastomotic device for this purpose. This device consists of a pair of polyethylene rings with six small pins on one side of each ring. The anastomosis is performed by drawing the end of the vessel through the ring and impaling the wall of the vessel over the six pins (Fig. 41.26**A–C**). The other end of the vessel likewise is impaled on the pins of the other ring, and the two rings are precisely mated together with an anastomotic

instrument (Fig. 41.26**D** and **E**). This device ensures accurate intima-to-intima contact, hence preventing adventitia from entering the lumen of the vessel at the anastomotic site. Surgeons with some specific training can perform an anastomosis in as little time as 3 minutes using this device (15). Furthermore, extensive training to perform this technique is not needed, as it is for traditional hand suturing of vessels. Experimental studies in the dog and clinical studies in human patients have demonstrated high patency rates associated with the use of this device (17, 18).

Disadvantages of this coupling device are few. The cost of using the device to perform the anastomosis is approximately four times that of using suture material. We have found that the use of the device on thick-walled arteries may cause tearing of the vessel wall as it is being impaled on the pins of the anastomotic device. Anastomosis of vessels, in areas of limited exposure, precludes the use of this device because of the size of the anastomotic instrument. Finally, the use of this device on vessels 1.0 mm or smaller in diameter is associated with an increased clinical failure rate (17).

Causes of Microvascular Anastomosis Failure

Failure of microvascular anastomosis is frequently due to technical errors made at the time of the surgical procedure. Incomplete excision of adventitia prevents accurate placement of the sutures. Moreover, adventitia that drapes over the vessel edge and becomes intraluminal at the anastomotic site potentiates the formation of a blood clot because of its thrombogenic properties. One of the commonest technical errors made by novices is "through-stitching," or incorporation of the back wall of the vessel with the front wall in the suture. This error results in obstruction to blood flow with subsequent thrombosis of the vessel. Traumatic handling of the tissues by grasping the entire thickness of the vessel wall may damage the vessel, with resultant vessel thrombosis. Venous anastomoses are more difficult to perform than arterial anastomoses because venous walls are thin. As a result, venous anastomoses become thrombosed more often than arterial anastomoses because of technical errors. Inversion of the wall of the vein can result from improper placement of sutures. This exposes thrombogenic material to the lumen of the vessel (13). Vessel redundancy increases the tendency for kinking and occlusion of the vessels at the site of the anastomosis. This is more of a problem with veins than arteries because veins are low-pressure vessels. Excessive tension on the microvascular anastomosis has also been reported to cause thrombosis (19).

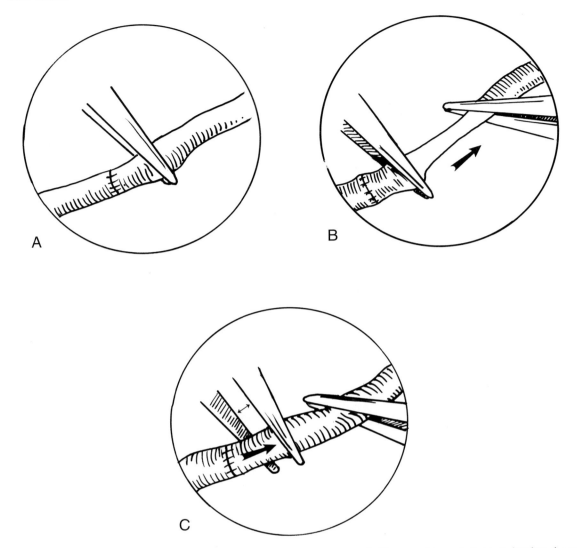

Fig. 41.25. Test used to evaluate the patency of arterial or venous anastomoses. **A.** The vessel is occluded just distal to the anastomosis. **B.** Blood is stripped from a segment of the vessel in a distal direction. **C.** The proximal clamp is released, and refill of the stripped vessel segment is observed.

The vascular surgeon's adage, "vessel vasospasm is spelled 'CLOT' and means vascular damage," should be strongly heeded (19). Vasospasm of the vessels at the anastomotic site decreases the flow of blood at the level of the anastomosis, thus increasing the likelihood of thrombus formation. Another cause of vasospasm is poor hemostasis. Exposure of the vessels to free blood while the anastomosis is performed causes vasospasm because of the presence of vasoconstricting substances. Prolonged anesthesia time results in hypothermia of the patient, a condition known to induce vasospasm. Lidocaine 1% should be used after the anastomosis has been completed, to paralyze the smooth muscle of anastomosed vessels (13).

Normal blood pressure and thus perfusion must be maintained through the anastomosed vessels both during and after surgery. Medications that can induce hypotension should be used judiciously to ensure that adequate perfusion pressures are maintained. The use of aggressive fluid therapy both intraoperatively and postoperatively may decrease the chance of hypotension and subsequent microvascular thrombosis (19).

The use of anticoagulants is controversial. Preoperative administration of heparin has not been recommended for dogs undergoing free tissue transfer (1–8, 10). However, we routinely administer aspirin, 2 mg/kg every 12 hours orally 1 day before the operation, and we continue the medication for 3 days postoperatively, to decrease platelet adhesion (2–4).

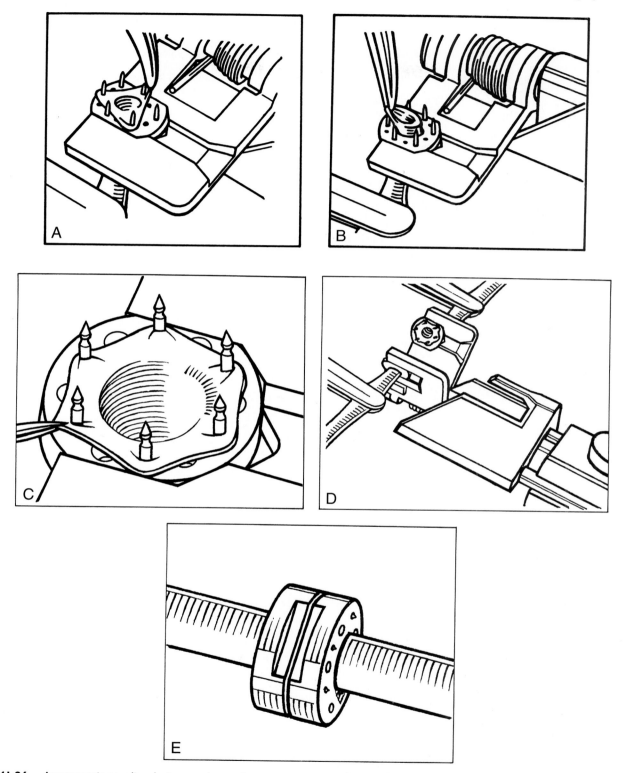

Fig. 41.26. Anastomotic coupling devices can be used to anastomose vessels instead of hand suturing. **A–C.** The vessel is drawn through the lumen of the anastomotic ring device, and the vessel wall is impaled on alternate pins of the ring. **D** and **E.** The ends of the vessels are approximated by precisely mating the anastomotic rings together with the anastomotic instrument.

References

1. Degner DA, Walshaw R, Kerstetter KK. Vascular anomaly of the prescapular branch of the superficial cervical artery and vein of an omocervical free skin flap in a dog. Vet Comp Orthop Traumatol 1995;8:102–106.

2. Degner DA, Walshaw R, Lanz OI, et al. The medial saphenous fasciocutaneous free flap in the dog. Vet Surg 1995; 24:424 (abstract).

3. Degner DA, Walshaw R. Medial saphenous fasciocutaneous and myocutaneous free flap transfer in eight dogs. Vet Surg 1997; 26:20–25.

4. Degner DA, Lanz OI, Walshaw R, et al. Myoperitoneal microvascular free flaps in dogs: an anatomical study and a clinical case report. Vet Surg 1996;25:463–70.

5. Miller CW, Chang P, Bowen V. Identification and transfer of free cutaneous flaps by microvascular anastomosis in the dog. Vet Surg 1986;2:199–204.

6. Miller CW, Fowler JD, Bowen V, et al. Experimental and clinical free cutaneous transfers in the dog. Microsurgery 1991; 12:113–117.

7. Miller CW, Bowen V, Chang P. Microvascular distant transfer of a cervical axial–pattern skin flap in a dog. J Am Vet Med Assoc 1987;190:203–204.

8. Fowler JD, Miller CW, Bowen V, et al. Transfer of free cutaneous flaps by microvascular anastomosis: results in six dogs. Vet Surg 1987;16:446–450.

9. Philibert D, Fowler JD, Clapson JB. The anatomic basis for a trapezius muscle flap in dogs. Vet Surg 1992;21:429–434.

10. Philibert D, Fowler JD, Clapson JB. Free microvascular transplantation of the trapezius musculocutaneous flap in dogs. Vet Surg 1992;21:435–440.

11. Gregory CR. Renal transplantation in cats. Compend Contin Educ Pract Vet 15:1325–1338, 1993.

12. Khouri RK, Shaw WW. Reconstruction of the lower extremity with microvascular free flaps: a 10-year experience with 304 consecutive cases. J Trauma 1989;54:1337–1354.

13. Acland RD. Practice manual for microvascular surgery. 2nd ed. St. Louis: CV Mosby, 1989:1–126.

14. Berezniak R. Creating, developing, and mastering a superior microsurgical technique. Sharpoint, LR. Reading, PA, 1991:1–89.

15. Harii H. Microvascular tissue transfer fundamental techniques and clinical applications. New York: Igaku–Shoin, 1983:3–8.

16. Ostrup LT, Berggren A. The Unilink instrument system for fast and safe microvascular anastomosis. Ann Plast Surg 1986; 17:521–525.

17. Steichen JB, Clandruccio JH, McClinton MA, et al. Clinical results of vessel repair by the 3M mechanical anastomotic coupling device. Presented at the 46th annual meeting of the American Society for Surgery of the Hand, October 2–4, 1991 Orlando, FL.

18. Falconer DP, Lewis TW, Lamprecht EG, et al. Evaluation of a Unilink microvascular anastomotic device in the dog. J Reconstr Microsurg 1990;6:215–222.

19. Khouri RK. Avoiding free flap failure. Clin Plast Surg 1992; 19:773–781.

42

ENDOSURGERY

Endosurgery

James E. Bailey, Lynetta J. Freeman &
Robert J. Hardie

Minimally invasive surgery is a collection of techniques designed to minimize the extent of the anatomic approach while still maintaining precision and efficiency. Endoscopic surgery (endosurgery) involves performing a minimally invasive surgical procedure with visualization provided by an endoscope. Endosurgery is only one specialty within the domain of minimally invasive surgery. Laparoscopic surgery and thoracoscopic surgery entail endoscopic approaches to abdominal and thoracic surgery, respectively. The purpose of this chapter is to introduce the fundamentals of endosurgery to surgeons untrained in these techniques and to entice the adept to do more.

History

The historical development of endoscopic surgical techniques in animals has been reviewed (1), and only an abbreviated history is presented here. Endoscopy was first described in the early 1800s by Bozzini (2), but the discipline made no great advances until the late 1800s, when optical lenses were incorporated into viewing devices and incandescent bulbs were invented. Although von Ott (3) first described viewing the abdominal cavity with a lighted speculum through what amounted to be a modified laparotomy in 1901, Kelling is most often credited as pioneering laparoscopy by inserting a cystoscope into the abdomen of a living dog at the seventy-third Congress of German Naturalists and Physicians and then publishing the technique in 1902 (4). The next step was to develop a clinical operative endoscopic technique. Jacobaeus first used the terms "laparoskopie" and "thorakoskopie" (5); however, historians still debate whether Kelling or Jacobaeus first developed a clinical endoscopic surgical technique. Certainly, the gynecologists and theriogenologists of the world have driven much of the development of laparoscopic surgery through the 1980s. Nevertheless, in 1987 Mouret (6) performed the first laparoscopic cholecystectomy, and what followed was an explosion of simultaneous work developing endless endoscopic surgical techniques and equipment under the philosophy, *if it can be done open, it can be done with endosurgery.* Bozzini's endosurgical vision of 1806, in which "Surgery will not only develop new and previously impossible procedures, but all uncertain operations which depended on luck and approximation will become safe under the influence of direct vision, since the surgeon's hand will now be guided by his eyes" (7), has come to light.

Advantages and Disadvantages

Some endosurgical procedures may appear to the anesthesiologist as mere surgical dawdling or purposeless attempts at academic self-promotion. However, emerging clinical evidence provides justification for these new methods. Innovation is no stranger to the veterinary surgeon, but economic constraints often dictate one's indulgence in modernization. The veterinary surgeon must examine the risks and benefits of innovative procedures carefully, forcing change at whatever cost when it is truly justified.

Every veterinary surgeon is charged to restore biologic form and function. Of equal importance is the veterinary surgeon's management of pain associated with the condition or the restorative procedure. Advantages of endosurgical techniques include reduced incision size, closing time, and scar formation, as well as improved visualization of the surgical site. Evidence of rapid return to work and better cosmetic appearance in human patients does not necessarily apply to veterinary medicine. On the other hand, the improved visualization is dramatic in many cases and is an invaluable teaching tool. Although moderate savings have been demonstrated when endosurgery is chosen in human medicine, the same issues do not apply to veterinary medicine. In fact, the initial investment to begin veterinary endosurgery is considerable. Disadvantages of endosurgery include the equipment cost and the technique learning curve, with its associated mishaps. So why should veterinary surgeons consider endosurgical methods as an alternative, let alone a principal choice? The veterinary surgeon's innate hunger for precision and technical skill may be enough to answer this question. Minimally invasive surgery is a state of mind—a creed. Furthermore, as the pioneer endosurgeon Nadeau pointed out in 1925, "How often is not the surgeon or the diagnostician confronted with a case in which the difficulties of reaching a decision urge the desire to get a glimpse of the body interior!" (8) Still more important is the issue of pain management. The surgical entry wound with endosurgery is smaller. A surgical entry wound often causes greater associated morbidity and pain than the operation itself. The simple reduction in entry wound size of endosurgery has led to reduced postoperative pain, reduced requirement for narcotic analgesics, fewer respiratory difficulties, reduced adhesion formation, earlier ambulation and return to feeding, and rapid return to self-sufficiency (9–18). The veterinary surgeon must investigate all means of pain management (see also Chap. 1).

Indications

As new endosurgical procedures were developing at an exponential rate in human medicine, veterinarians were still describing the primary indication for laparoscopy and thoracoscopy as diagnostic (19, 20). This is no longer true. Endosurgery is simply an alternative approach to a surgical problem. If reduction in adhesion formation, postoperative pain, and recovery time, as well as improved visualization or micromanipulation, are desired, then endosurgery is indicated. The indication for a specific surgical procedure is no different from the open approach. Financial issues have delayed the veterinary response. The economics of human endosurgery led to reduced costs and enhanced surgeons' incomes, thus promoting endosurgery. Human patients further persuaded surgeons to convert by specifically requesting the endosurgical approach. Conversely, the cost for startup and for necessary expendable items is high for veterinarians, hospital stays are already minimal, and the benefit to the patient may not be clear. For example, an endosurgical ovariohysterectomy in a healthy young cat may take longer, cost more, and not provide less incisional pain than the typical minilaparotomy open technique. On the other hand, thoracoscopic partial lobectomy for bulla rupture in a young dog reduces postoperative pain, the requirement for narcotic analgesics, respiratory depression, and adhesion formation. When applied to the appropriate patient, endosurgery can become a practice builder, especially as educated clients increasingly request its use.

Safety and Efficacy (Complications and Contraindications)

The veterinary surgeon must have a thorough understanding of each specific surgical therapeutic technique, including associated complications and contraindications. Those same classic complications and contraindications also apply to the endosurgical approach. Because the number of possible endosurgical procedures is almost endless, no purpose exists in listing all associated complications here. However, a few complications are specific to endosurgical approaches. Although the incidence of these complications is extremely low, some may be lethal (life-threatening complication rate lower than 0.5% [21]), and discussion is mandatory.

Several complications are associated with patient positioning and the use of insufflation gases. The use of Trendelenburg positioning (head-down tilt) and pneumoperitoneum (abdominal gas insufflation) in laparoscopy increases the risk of gastrointestinal reflux and acid aspiration. Proper fasting, endotracheal intubation with a cuffed tube, and prompt attention to reflux are necessary. Pneumoperitoneum may also lead to the development of subcutaneous emphysema. If ignored, this condition can become life-threatening. Simply reducing the insufflation pressure and securing the peritoneum resolve the problem. Excessive subcutaneous emphysema necessitates conversion to an open technique. If a defect is present in the diaphragm, pneumothorax or pneumomediastinum may develop when pneumoperitoneum is used. The anesthesiologist must be alert to any pulmonary function changes during anesthesia.

Surgeons must be attentive to the position of their surgical instruments at all times. One should never cut what one cannot see clearly. Even so, most injuries to viscera (stomach, bowel, ureters, and lung) are due to blind placement of Verres-type insufflation needles and trocars. Large-vessel injury can occur as well, causing severe retroperitoneal bleeding, or worse, venous air embolism through entrainment of insufflation gases. Diagnosis and treatment require cooperation between the surgeon and the anesthesiologist. Monitoring of end-tidal carbon dioxide (CO_2) can be invaluable in these cases (precipitous drop). The patient should always be surgically prepared for conversion to an open technique.

Contraindications are everchanging as these complications are investigated. Many previously absolute contraindications, such as adhesions and diaphragmatic hernia, have become relative. In fact, in the hands of skilled surgeons and anesthesiologists, these patients may fare better with endosurgery. Known adhesions may be broken down endosurgically, with a reduced likelihood of recurrence. Diaphragmatic hernia repair may be performed with the patient in the Fowler position (head-up tilt) while the surgeon uses a suspension technique to lift the abdominal wall rather than the pneumoperitoneum.

Anesthesia

The anesthesiologist should be prepared for the unique aspects of anesthesia in the endosurgical patient. The distension produced by gas insufflation used in laparoscopy and occasionally in thoracoscopy can trigger vasovagal reflexes, decrease venous return and cardiac output leading to hypotension, and compress the diaphragm leading to ventilation–perfusion mismatch, as well as decreased vital capacity, functional residual capacity, and compliance. Positioning (head-up or head-down tilt) contributes to this cardiopulmonary insult. Ventilatory support is mandatory in most cases. An intimate knowledge of one-lung ventilation techniques is also necessary for thoracoscopic techniques. The differential diagnosis of cardiopulmonary collapse in these cases includes hemorrhage, pneumothorax, or pneumomediastinum, aspiration, diaphragmatic rupture, excess cavity pressure (tension pneumothorax or pneumoperitoneum), vasovagal reflex, pulmonary thromboembolism, and gas embolus. Anesthetic considerations for endosurgery are reviewed in the literature (22).

Light, Optics, Video, and Television

Veterinarians are generally directly responsible for hospital instrument purchases, and review of recommended equipment is obligatory. The standard endosurgical optical system has a light source, fiberoptic light cable, rigid operating endoscope, video camera, video monitor, and often a video recorder. Adequate illumination of the endosurgical field is essential to completion of the procedure. Although a 150-watt tungsten *light source* is less expensive, it may not be adequate in some situations. Greater illumination can be produced by a 300-watt xenon source, but many of today's more sensitive cameras do not require excessive lighting. Although these modern external light sources may operate at scorching temperatures, little of this heat ever reaches the patient. However, if a xenon light source is used, cloth surgical drapes are recommended to prevent burns and fires induced by excessive heat production at the interface between the fiberoptic light cable and the rigid operating endoscope. For this same reason, the light source should not be left turned on when the fiberoptic cable is detached from the rigid operating endoscope.

The development of fiberoptics in the 1960s made it possible to present this intense light to the endosurgical field without burning the patient. An incoherent bundle of glass fibers, 10 to 25 μm in diameter, connects the light source to the rigid surgical endoscope. Fiberoptic bundles fan around the inner core lens system of the endoscope, carrying light to the surgical field. Because of the air-to-glass interfaces at connecting points and fiber mismatching, only approximately one-quarter of the original light is transmitted.

Light transmitted from the tip of the endoscope must reflect and be picked up by the lens system of the endoscope. Light emitted into the body cavity reduces in intensity by the square of the distance traveled. Changing focal points changes light intensity. Such changes demand an adjustable light source output control; however, low-quality automatic illumination control devices can be visually bothersome. The term *dynamic range* is used to describe the capability of the system to reproduce high-quality images under many different illumination conditions. Adequate dynamic range depends not only on the automatic illumination control, but also on the image-processing circuitry and camera chip sensitivity. Reflected light, incident with the operating endoscope, is captured by the lens system. The diameter of the standard lens system ranges from 1 to 5.5 mm. Endoscopes lacking an instrument channel allow larger lenses and the optimum number of light-emitting fibers, and they provide the best visualization. Finally, superior light transmission is accomplished with the now commonplace *Hopkins rod-lens system*.

Light captured by the rigid operating endoscope can be viewed directly or with greater ease and resolution using a miniature, photosensitive silicone chip, video camera (also called a charge-coupled-device or CCD). The light sensitivity of the camera is vital to the quality of the image. Cameras having a lower *lux* (lumen per square meter) illumination requirement are more sensitive to any incident light. Cameras having a lux greater than 5 may strain to provide an acceptable image. Cameras with a lux of 1 or 2 are superior (beware: measurements are not yet standardized). Camera *resolution* is also important. Resolution is compromised in cameras with less than 400 vertical rows of image-sensing picture elements or *pixels* (common matrix size 768 × 494 pixels). The *signal-to-noise ratio* of the chip can affect the final image quality as well and should be 50 dB or more. Additionally, in single-chip cameras, each pixel of the chip is filtered to detect red, blue, or green (or green, yellow, cyan, and magenta) and then sends a signal to the video monitor's amplifier. Three-chip cameras may provide better color resolution, with each chip detecting one of the foundation colors. Still, light sensitivity is more important than color separation. A high-quality single-chip camera can outperform some three-chip systems.

The method of communicating the image affects resolution. The standard *NTSC*, one-wire, composite video signal is simple and familiar, but component video signals (two-wire *Super-VHS* and three-wire *RBG*) reproduce more monochrome and color image detail. The monitor resolution should reflect the resolution of the camera or image quality may be lost. Most surgical monitors have 550 to 700 vertical lines of resolution, at least a 13-inch diagonal screen, and are medical grade, to limit chassis electrical current leakage. The monitor must also be compatible with the method of communicating the image from the camera (NTSC, Super-VHS, or RBG). The video system component with the lowest resolution capabilities defines the resolution for the system. Finally, as hospitals purchase extravagant video systems to avoid equipment obsolescence and to enhance image quality, such as three-chip cameras and three-dimensional imaging technology, veterinarians will find opportunities to purchase good-quality used equipment at reasonable prices.

Gas Insufflation

The purpose of gas insufflation of a potential space (e.g., peritoneal, pleural, retroperitoneal) during endosurgery is to produce dissection, to create a viewing cavity, or to lift the body wall, thereby producing a protective distance between the viscera and sharp instruments. The ideal insufflation gas would be transparent, colorless, nonexplosive, physiologically inert, and either nonabsorbed or eliminated by the pulmonary system. Automatic insufflators are used to regulate the gas pressure. Typical pressures range from 8 to 15 mm Hg, and pressures exceeding 20 to 25 mm Hg cause significant cardiopulmonary embarrassment. CO_2, nitrous oxide, medical-grade air, oxygen, argon, and helium have all been used as insufflation gases. CO_2 is most commonly used because it is cheap, it is most soluble (perhaps reducing the likelihood of developing gas embolus), it is rapidly resorbed and eliminated by the lungs, and it does not support combustion when electrocautery is used. However, CO_2 may cause irritation to the body cavity through formation of carbonic acid on visceral surfaces and is ab-

sorbed into the blood, possibly leading to hypercarbia, stimulation of the sympathetic nervous system, vasodilation, hypertension, and tachycardia and other arrhythmias. The second favored choice, nitrous oxide, is less irritating, but it supports combustion, leads to distension of hollow viscera, may cause diffusion hypoxia on recovery, and may affect operating personnel if it escapes the body cavity. As for the remainder, air may be more likely to cause gas emboli while also supporting combustion, oxygen supports combustion, and argon has not proved to be physiologically inert. Nitrogen has been applied experimentally; however, nitrogen has low diffusibility and high lipid solubility, increasing the risk of embolism formation. Helium, however, is chemically inert, colorless, and nontoxic, and it does not support combustion. Helium is less soluble than CO_2, but it is more highly diffusible (perhaps enhancing dissolution), making it a suitable alternative to CO_2 insufflation when hypercarbia cannot be controlled by ventilation. Automatic insufflators are used to regulate the gas pressure strictly.

Endosurgical Instrumentation

Basic veterinary endosurgical instrumentation has not changed dramatically since it was reviewed in 1980 (23), and it has been reviewed again recently (22). Major advancements in endosurgical instrumentation have come in the form of endoscopic clip appliers, staples, stapling-cutting devices, and automated suturing instruments. One of the most promising devices, the endoscopic harmonic scalpel, provides a bloodless operation with reduced lateral thermal spread and burn. To review this instrumentation is beyond the scope of this chapter.

Endosurgical Methods of Hemostasis

Several methods of hemostasis are available for veterinary endosurgery, including electrocoagulation, endoscopic hemostatic clips, endoscopic stapling devices, endoscopic loops, sutures and knots, and laser coagulation. The surgeon's ability to perform more than one technique ensures the fastest, safest endoscopic surgery.

Electrosurgical techniques are discussed in Chapter 4. Both monopolar and bipolar electrocautery are available for endosurgery. A long, insulated instrument passing through a trocar–cannula placed in the body wall is used to apply endoscopic electrosurgery. Many endoscopic surgical instruments have monopolar cautery attachments. Electrical current reaching the tissues behaves as it would in conventional surgery. However, some unique issues arise with the use of endoscopic electrosurgery.

If the shaft of the instrument for application electrocautery is not well insulated or the insulation is defective, burns may occur where the shaft contacts tissues. Bowel burns are of particular concern because the compromised bowel may leak postoperatively. Another issue is *capacitance coupling*. When the high-frequency electrosurgical current travels down the shaft of the application instrument and passes through a metal trocar–cannula or a metal operative endoscope channel, some electrical charge "couples" to the surrounding metal, even if the instrument is well insulated. The electrical charge is stored in the metal cannula or channel (the capacitor) until it makes contact with body tissues, possibly causing a burn. Nonconductive threaded mounts insulate the cannula from the abdominal wall, allow excessive charge to build in the metallic cannula, and increase the possibility of distal cannula coupled energy discharge with associated visceral injury. The use of nonconductive materials in trocar–cannulas has helped to minimize this concern. Care should be taken when using reusable, metallic trocar–cannulas.

Endoscopic clips have greatly facilitated endosurgical procedures and have proved secure. Multiple clip appliers allow rapid and repeated placement of clips. These clips are used to occlude blood vessels and other small, hollow structures. They are useful in controlling acute bleeding episodes; however, secure ligature is only accomplished with complete skeletonization of the vessel (see Figs. 42.4**D** and 42.5**C**).

Endosurgical staple-and-cut devices place multiple rows of staples, providing hemostasis, and cut between the rows. Staple leg length varies according to purpose, from bowel transection to great vessel occlusion. Staples may be arranged linearly or in a circle. Linear staple-and-cut devices are used to transect (see Fig. 42.8**B** and **D**), and circular staple-and-cut instruments create anastomoses, hemostatically.

Laser coagulation techniques are covered in Chapter 4. Concerns specific to the endosurgeon relate to plume formation. High-density laser energy bursts cells, sending cellular debris into the body cavity and obscuring the view. The plume must be evacuated, necessitating use of a high-flow abdominal insufflator. Additionally, the combination of this cloud of particulate matter with a gas supporting combustion could result in explosion. For this reason, nitrous oxide should not be used as the insufflation gas for laser endosurgery.

Endosurgical Loops, Sutures, and Knot Tying

The cost of materials for endoscopic suturing is far less than for endoscopic clips and staplers, but manual suturing is more time-consuming. A description of all aspects of laparoscopic suturing techniques is beyond the scope of this chapter. Discussion is limited to endoscopic loop ligatures and sutures, with extracorporeal and intracorporeal knot tying.

Extracorporeal Knot Tying

This technique is defined as throws created outside of the body under direct vision transferred to the body cavity by a device called a knot pusher.

ENDOSCOPIC KNOT (ENDOKNOT) TYING
Equipment

Pretied endoknot or long suture (endosuture) (at least 48 cm)
Knot pusher
Two endoscopic needle drivers or graspers
Endoscopic scissors

Technique
The structure to be ligated is identified and isolated. The free end of the ligature is grasped with a needle driver and is passed into the body cavity through a cannula. The ligature is passed around the structure to be ligated with the assistance of a second needle driver entering from another cannula. The ligature is pulled through the first cannula using the original needle driver. The remainder of the ligature is fed into the cannula while the surgeon simultaneously pulls the free end of the ligature from the body cavity. Additionally, the second needle driver is used to prevent pulling and sawing to the tissue being ligated. The free ends of ligature are tied in a Roeder knot (Fig. 42.1). The knot is transferred to the body cavity with a knot pusher.

ENDOSCOPIC LOOP (ENDOLOOP) LIGATURES
Equipment

Pretied endoloop or long ligature (48 cm or greater)
Knot pusher
Endoscopic grasper or needle driver
Endoscopic scissors

Technique
Pretied endoloops most often use a modified Westin knot. The endoloop is passed through the contralateral working cannula, and the endoscopic grasper is passed through the ipsilateral cannula. The grasper is passed through the endoloop ligature to grasp the tissue pedicle to be ligated. The knot is placed at the level of intended ligation, and the loop is slowly closed with a knot pusher (Fig. 42.2). Endoscopic scissors are used to cut the suture tail.

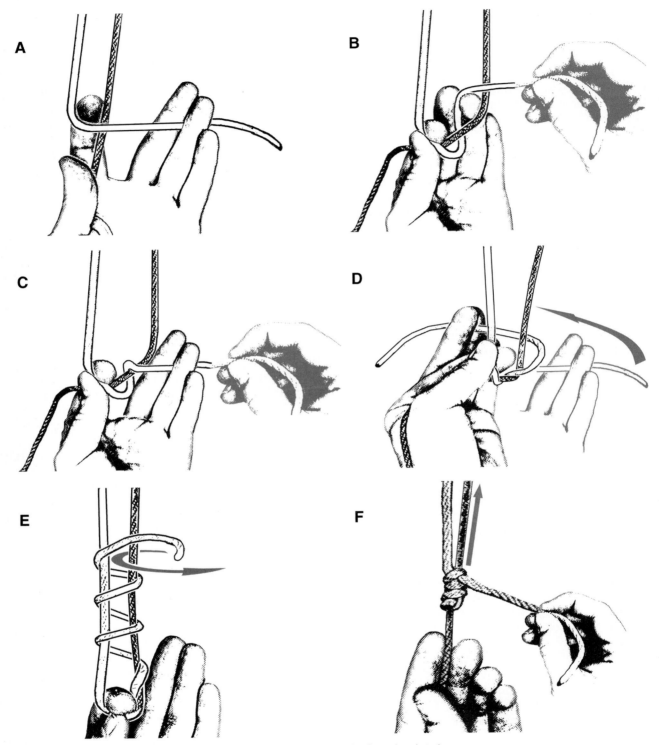

Fig. 42.1. **A–F.** Roeder knot hand tied.

Intracorporeal Instrument Knot Tying

ENDOSCOPIC SUTURING

Equipment

Short ligature (10 to 15 cm) with a curved needle
Two endoscopic graspers or needle drivers
Endoscopic scissors

Technique

Proper suture placement requires proper trocar–cannula placement. Intracorporeal knot tying requires placement of two working cannulas and one cannula for the laparoscope. Ideally, the insertion point of the laparoscope and the two cannulas form an isosceles triangle, with the line of suturing equidistant from either of the working cannulas and nearly parallel to the shaft of the active needle holder. One simple intra-corporeal suture technique is diagramed in Figure 42.3.

CLOSURE OF ENTRY WOUNDS

Closure of trocar–cannula entry wounds is performed in two layers. Buttonhook suture devices are available to ease closure. Some surgeons have proposed that closure of 5-mm puncture sites is unnecessary with the exception of bandaging. However, omental herniation has been reported, and wound closure is recommended (22).

OPEN VERSUS CLOSED APPROACH

The closed approach uses a Verres-type insufflation needle and blind placement of the primary trocar–cannula. The body wall is grasped and lifted while the

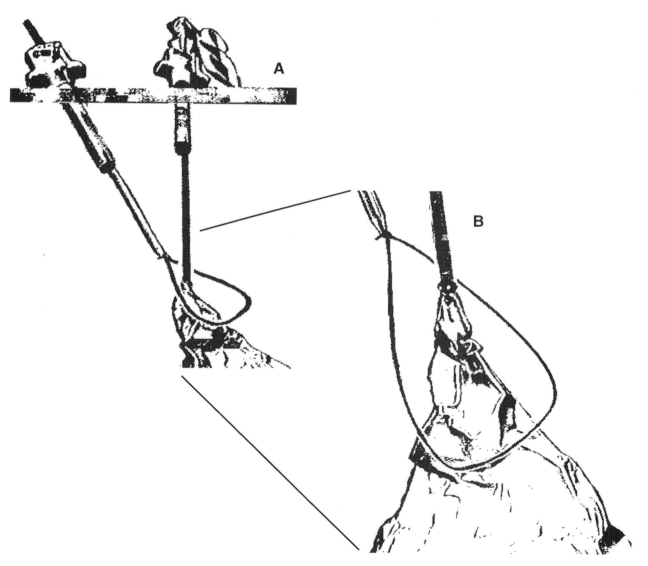

Fig. 42.2. **A** and **B.** Pretied, modified Westin knot, endoloop. See text for description.

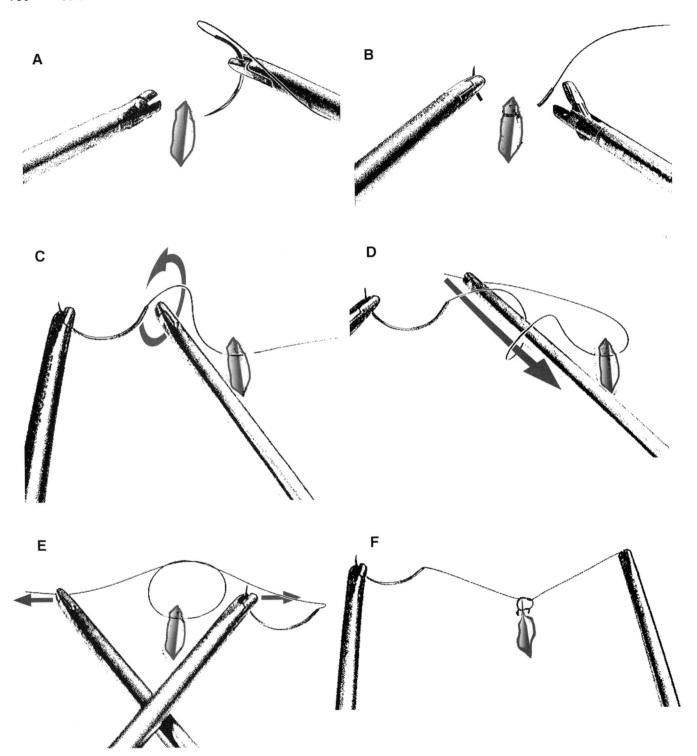

Fig. 42.3. A–F. Interrupted intracorporeal suture technique. Steps **A** through **E** yield the first throw of a square knot. Repeating steps **C** through **E** on the opposite side leads to step **F** and the completed square knot.

Verres needle is passed in the direction predicted to be devoid of viscera (depending on tilt). Proper needle placement is confirmed by aspiration and hanging-drop techniques. The body cavity is insufflated with gas, and the needle is removed. After placing a 1-cm skin incision, the primary sharp trocar–cannula is then blindly placed in a similar fashion to the needle. The open approach uses a small abdominal incision to advance the blunt primary cannula and surgical endoscope into the body cavity under continuous visual control. Many endoscopic surgeons prefer this approach to avoid visceral injury resulting from blind placement of insufflation needles and sharp trocar–cannulas. The open method should be used by the amateur endosurgeon. Advanced trocar–cannulas, such as the Optiview (Ethicon Endosurgery, Cincinnati, OH), allow continuous visualization while providing simple penetration, but they are not for the amateur endosurgeon.

Laparoscopic Endosurgical Procedures

Patient Positioning

The patient may be placed in several different positions, depending on the goal of the procedure. Various procedures can be accomplished with the patient in dorsal recumbency and either a Trendelenburg (head-down tilt) or a reverse Trendelenburg (head-up or Fowler tilt) position.

Insufflation

Generally, insufflation of the abdominal cavity with gas is performed with CO_2 to provide a viewing cavity in which to work. Intra-abdominal gas pressures of 8 to 15 mm Hg are usually adequate for viewing. A pressure of 10 mm Hg provides adequate visualization with minimal effect on diaphragmatic excursions and cardiac output in normal patients. Pressure should not exceed 20 to 25 mm Hg.

Cryptorchid Castration

INDICATIONS
This therapeutic procedure is indicated for animals that have intra-abdominal retained testicles, which are susceptible to torsion and neoplasia.

INSTRUMENTATION

Blunt-tip 12-mm obturator–cannula
Sharp 12-mm trocar–cannula
Sharp 5-mm trocar–cannula
Laparoscopic multiple clip applier medium to large, or

polyglactin 910 endoscopic knot (endoknot) suture (×6)
5-mm Maryland dissecting forceps
5-mm Metzenbaum scissors
10-mm Babcock grasping forceps

PATIENT PREPARATION
The patient should be fasted for 12 hours to prevent food from remaining in the stomach, to minimize bowel contents, and to allow easier identification of the retained testicle. The urinary bladder should be expressed before the surgical procedure.

PATIENT POSITIONING
The patient is placed in the Trendelenburg position (head-down tilt), with all four limbs secured to the table.

GAS INSUFFLATION
After open approach, the abdomen is insufflated with CO_2. Intra-abdominal gas pressures of 8 to 15 mm Hg are usually adequate for viewing. Pressure should not exceed 20 to 25 mm Hg.

TROCAR–CANNULA PLACEMENT

Camera port: One 12-mm obturator–cannula placed on the ventral midline just cranial to the umbilicus
Contralateral operative port: One 5-mm trocar–cannula placed paramedian, 5 to 10 cm cranial to the inguinal region
Ipsilateral port: One 12-mm trocar–cannula placed paramedian, 5 to 10 cm cranial to the inguinal region

SURGICAL TECHNIQUE
The camera port is placed using a blunt obturator-cannula and the open technique. A 10-mm, 0° viewing laparoscope is placed through the port and is used to transilluminate the abdominal wall to identify epigastric vessels as well as visually to guide the placement of the other two cannula. Skin incisions of 1 and 0.5 cm are necessary for introduction of the second 12-mm sharp trocar–cannula and the 5-mm sharp trocar–cannula, respectively (Fig. 42.4**A**). The abdomen is explored, and the intra-abdominally retained testicle is identified. The testicle is held with Babcock grasping forceps from the ipsilateral port, and a window is made through the visceral vaginal tunic with a dissecting instrument or scissors from the contralateral port (Fig. 42.4**B**). Hemostasis can be maintained using monopolar electrocautery attached to the laparoscopic instruments. The cremaster muscle is skeletonized and is ligated with endosurgical clips (or endoknot sutures): two on the patient side; one on the testicle side (Fig. 42.4**C** and **D**). Metzenbaum scissors are used to cut between the clips. The remaining spermatic cord is

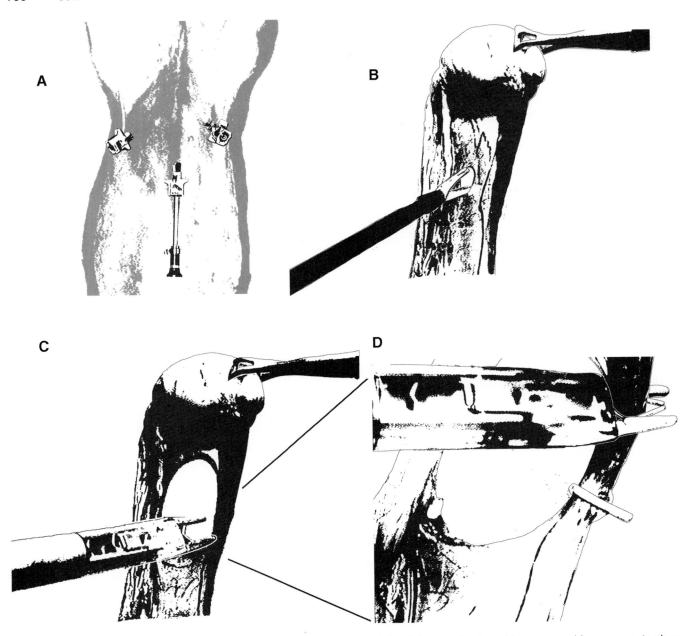

Fig. 42.4. A–D. Laparoscopic cryptorchid castration. **A.** Ventral view of the abdomen of a dog with trocars and laparoscope in place. The top is the caudal end of the dog. See text for additional description.

ligated and is transected in a similar fashion. The clips are inspected for security and hemostasis. After completing the procedure, the abdomen is explored a final time before removing the cannulas and deflating the abdomen. The testicle is pulled into the 12-mm cannula, and the cannula is removed. Alternatively, an 18- or 33-mm trocar–cannula replaces the 12-mm trocar–cannula, or a minilaparotomy is used to remove larger testicles. Any subcutaneous emphysema can be manually expressed through the skin incisions. The abdominal incisions are closed routinely in two layers.

POSTOPERATIVE CARE
Standard care is maintained after the surgical procedure, and food is resumed within 12 to 24 hours. Skin sutures can be removed in 7 to 10 days.

Ovariohysterectomy

INDICATIONS
This therapeutic procedure is indicated for animals that require elective sterilization or treatment of ovarian and uterine disease.

INSTRUMENTATION

Blunt-tip 12-mm obturator–cannula
Sharp 12-mm trocar–cannula
Sharp 5-mm trocar–cannula (×2)
Laparoscopic multiple clip applier medium to large, or polyglactin 910 endoknot suture (×6)
5-mm Maryland dissecting forceps
5-mm Metzenbaum scissors
10-mm Babcock grasping forceps
±35-mm linear staple-and-cut device
±Hernia stapler

PATIENT PREPARATION

The patient should be fasted for 12 hours to prevent food from remaining in the stomach, to minimize bowel contents, and to allow easier identification of the uterus and ovaries. An enema may be necessary preoperatively. The urinary bladder should be catheterized to minimize bladder size.

PATIENT POSITIONING

The patient is placed in the Trendelenburg position (head-down tilt), with all four limbs secured to the table.

GAS INSUFFLATION

After an open approach, the abdomen is insufflated with CO_2. Intra-abdominal gas pressures of 8 to 15 mm Hg are usually adequate for viewing. Pressure should not exceed 20 to 25 mm Hg.

TROCAR–CANNULA PLACEMENT

Camera port: One 12-mm obturator–cannula placed on the ventral midline at the umbilicus
Lateral operative ports: One 5-mm trocar–cannula placed paramedian, 5 to 10 cm cranial to the inguinal region on both the right and left sides
Midline operative port: One 12-mm trocar–cannula placed on the ventral midline, 5 to 10 cm cranial to the pubis

SURGICAL TECHNIQUE

The camera port is placed using a blunt obturator–cannula and the open technique. A 10-mm, 0° viewing laparoscope is placed through the port and is used to transilluminate the abdominal wall to identify epigastric vessels as well as visually to guide the placement of the other three cannula. Skin incisions of 1 and 0.5 cm are necessary for introduction of the 12-mm sharp trocar–cannula and the 5 mm sharp trocar–cannula, respectively (Fig. 42.5**A**).

The abdomen is explored, and the uterus and ovaries are identified. The intercornual ligament of the uterus is held with Babcock grasping forceps from the midline operative port, and the ureters are identified

traversing the dorsal broad ligament. An ovary is grasped from the ipsilateral port. The suspensory ligament of the ovary is cut using Metzenbaum scissors from the contralateral port, and hemostasis is maintained with monopolar cautery attached (Fig. 42.5**B**). The incision is carried to the level of the ovarian artery. A window is made through the broad ligament with a dissecting instrument or scissors from the contralateral port. The ovarian artery is skeletonized and is ligated with endosurgical clips (or endoknot sutures): two on the patient side; one on the ovary side (Fig. 42.5**C**). Metzenbaum scissors are used to cut between the clips. The clips are inspected for security and hemostasis.

The incision is carried through the broad ligament to the level of the uterine artery. The uterine artery is skeletonized and is ligated with endosurgical clips (or endoknot sutures): two on the patient side; one on the ovary side. The clips are inspected for security and hemostasis. The incision is then carried through the broad ligament to the level of the uterine body and cervix. This process is duplicated for the second ovary.

The cervix is identified by visualization and instrument palpation. Two endoloop ligatures are placed around the uterine body proximal to the cervix and are tightened (Fig. 42.5**D**). Care must be taken to avoid ligation of the ureters. Alternatively, a 35-mm staple-and-cut device is placed proximal to the cervix and is discharged. Care should be taken to view both sides of the cutter before discharge, to ensure that no structures are cut unintentionally. Transfixing endoknot sutures may be placed from each side as a third option. Metzenbaum scissors with a monopolar cautery attachment are used to transect the uterine body. After completing the procedure, the abdomen is explored before removing the cannulas and deflating the abdomen. A small uterus may be pulled partially into the 12-mm cannula, and the cannula is removed. Alternatively, the surgeon may change camera ports, bring the uterus to the midline port, and extend the port incision as necessary to remove a larger uterus. Endoscopic bags are available to collect tissues for controlled removal, particularly if the uterus is infectious or cancerous. Any subcutaneous emphysema can be manually expressed through the skin incisions. The abdominal incisions are closed routinely in two layers.

POSTOPERATIVE CARE

Standard care is maintained after the surgical procedure, and food is resumed within 12 to 24 hours. Skin sutures can be removed in 7 to 10 days.

Laparoscopic Stapled Gastropexy

INDICATIONS

This prophylactic procedure is indicated for dogs that have previously experienced gastric dilatation and are

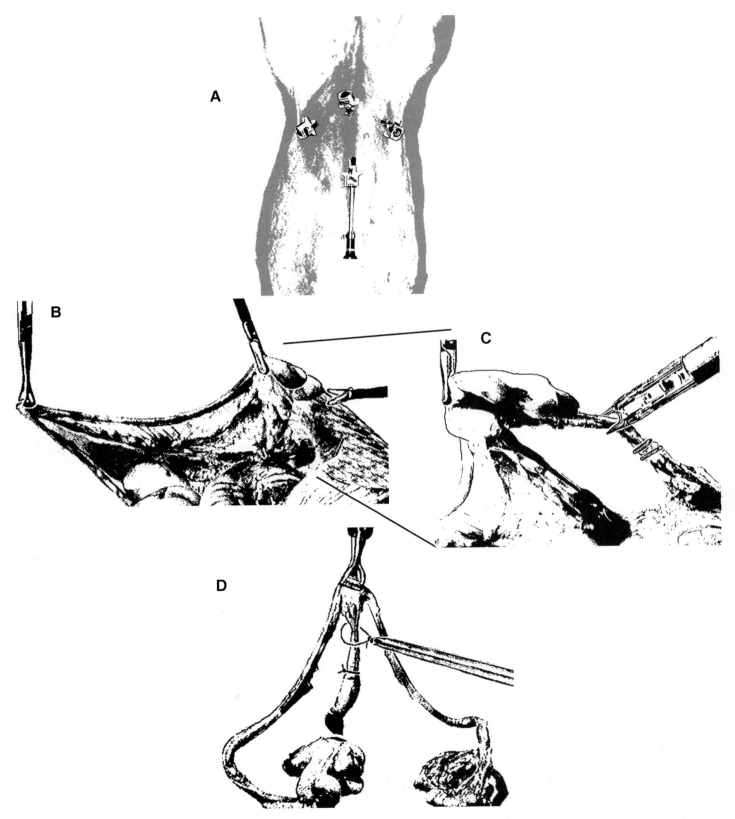

Fig. 42.5. A–D. Laparoscopic ovariohysterectomy. **A.** Ventral view of the abdomen of a dog with trocars and laparoscope in place. The top is the caudal end of the dog. See text for additional description.

at risk for developing gastric dilatation–volvulus in the future.

INSTRUMENTATION

Blunt-tip 12-mm obturator-cannula
Sharp 12-mm trocar-cannula (×3)
35-mm linear staple-and-cut device
10-mm Kelly forceps
10-mm Metzenbaum scissors
10-mm grasping forceps
10-mm Babcock forceps (×2)
Modified Kitner dissector ("peanut sponges")
Hernia stapler

PATIENT PREPARATION

The dog should be fasted for 12 hours to prevent food from remaining in the stomach and to allow easier manipulation of the stomach.

PATIENT POSITIONING

The dog should be placed in dorsal recumbency, with all four limbs secured to the table. Tilting the table is not necessary for this procedure.

GAS INSUFFLATION

Pneumoperitoneum is created with a Verres needle placed in the cranial aspect of the right side of the abdomen. Insufflation pressure of 8 to 15 mm Hg is maintained.

TROCAR–CANNULA PLACEMENT

Three 12-mm trocar–cannulas are placed in the caudal aspect of the right side of the abdomen in a triangle formation. The cannulas can be placed through small skin incisions using the sharp trocar or with the "open technique" using a blunt obturator–cannula. A 10-mm, 0° laparoscope is then placed through the first cannula and is used visually to guide the placement of the other two cannulas (Fig. 42.6**A**).

SURGICAL TECHNIQUE

The abdomen is explored, and the gastric antrum and the proposed gastropexy site on the adjacent right lateral abdominal wall are identified. The gastric antrum is held with grasping forceps, and a 2 × 5 cm submucosal tunnel is made in a caudal-to-cranial direction. The tunnel is made with laparoscopic Metzenbaum scissors and Kelly forceps using both sharp and blunt dissection; the surgeon must be careful not to penetrate the gastric mucosa (Fig. 42.6**B**). Hemostasis can be maintained using monopolar electrocautery attached to the laparoscopic instruments. Peanut sponges can be used to dry the surgical field and to help identify the proper tissue plane for dissection. A tunnel of similar size is made between the transverse and internal abdominal

oblique muscles on the right lateral abdominal wall caudal to the last rib (Fig. 42.6**C**). The 35-mm laparoscopic stapler is then inserted into the dissected tunnels, and the stomach is stapled to the right abdominal wall (Fig. 42.6**D**). The stapler is removed, and the gastropexy is inspected for defects in the staple lines or for perforations of the gastric mucosa. If a perforation is suspected, it may be necessary to pass a stomach tube and to distend the stomach with air and observe the mucosa for leaks. Any defects or perforations can be repaired with individual staples. The opening of the tunnel is closed by apposing the tissue edges with a grasping instrument and by stapling them together using the hernia stapler (Fig. 42.**E**). The completed gastropexy is firmly manipulated to make sure that it is securely attached to the abdominal wall. After completing the procedure, the abdomen is explored a final time before removing the cannulas and deflating the abdomen. Residual subcutaneous emphysema can be manually expressed through the skin incisions. The abdominal incisions are closed routinely in two layers.

POSTOPERATIVE CARE

Standard care is maintained postoperatively, and food is resumed within 12 to 24 hours. Skin sutures can be removed in 7 to 10 days.

Thorascopic Endosurgical Procedures

The American Association for Thoracic Surgery has changed the name of thoracoscopy to video-assisted thoracic surgery (VATS).

Patient Positioning

The patient may be placed in several different positions, depending on the goal of the procedure. Various procedures can be accomplished with the patient in right lateral recumbency with the forelimbs extended forward.

Insufflation

Generally, insufflation of the thoracic cavity with gas is not necessary because of the rigid cavity structure. Initial puncture of the thoracic cavity disrupts the coherence of the lung with the pleura, and the lung collapses. If bronchial outflow is obstructed by a poorly placed endobronchial tube or a bronchial blocker, the lung may not collapse completely, and the operative field of view may be obscured. In a similar fashion, continuous positive airway pressure of the collapsed lung may improve ventilation, but it may obscure the operative field of view. Additionally, lung disease or adhesions may prevent complete collapse.

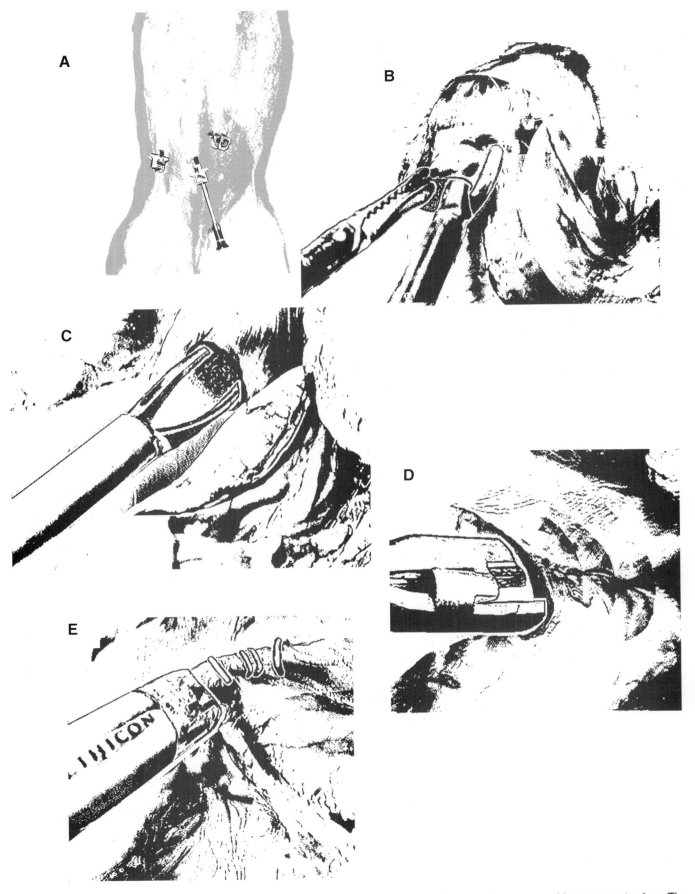

Fig. 42.6.   A–E. Laparoscopic stapled gastropexy. **A.** Ventral view of the abdomen of a dog with trocars and laparoscope in place. The top is the cranial end of the dog. See text for additional description.

Trocar–Cannula Placement

Because insufflation is not often necessary in thoracoscopy, valved trocars are not required. However, rigid or flexible cannulas do protect soft tissues from excessive damage and reduce postoperative pain.

Pericardial Window Pericardiectomy

INDICATIONS

This therapeutic procedure is indicated to relieve pericardial effusion or to obtain a pericardial biopsy.

INSTRUMENTATION

Blunt-tip 12-mm thoracic obturator–cannula (×3)
5-mm grasping forceps
5-mm Metzenbaum scissors

PATIENT PREPARATION

The patient should be fasted for 12 hours. After the patient is anesthetized and positioned for surgery, one-lung ventilation is initiated. One lung ventilation may be produced using a double-lumen endotracheal tube, endobronchial intubation, or bronchial blocker.

PATIENT POSITIONING

The patient is positioned in right lateral recumbency, with the forelimbs extended forward.

INSUFFLATION

None is indicated.

TROCAR–CANNULA PLACEMENT

Camera port: One 12-mm flexible thoracic trocar–cannula placed on the midaxillary line in the fifth or sixth intercostal space

Dorsal operative port: One 12-mm flexible thoracic trocar–cannula placed in the dorsal third of the fourth or fifth intercostal space

Ventral operative port: One 12-mm flexible thoracic trocar–cannula placed in the ventral third of the fourth or fifth intercostal space

SURGICAL TECHNIQUE

A 1-cm skin incision is made, and standard curved Kelly forceps are used to penetrate the thoracic cavity bluntly. The camera port is placed first using this blunt technique. A 10-mm, 30° viewing laparoscope is placed through the port and is used visually to guide the placement of the other two cannulas (Fig. 42.7).

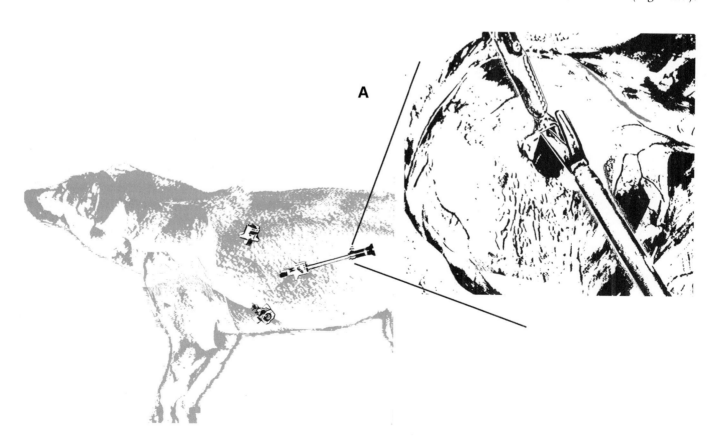

A

Fig. 42.7. Thoracoscopic pericardial window pericardiectomy. See text for additional description.

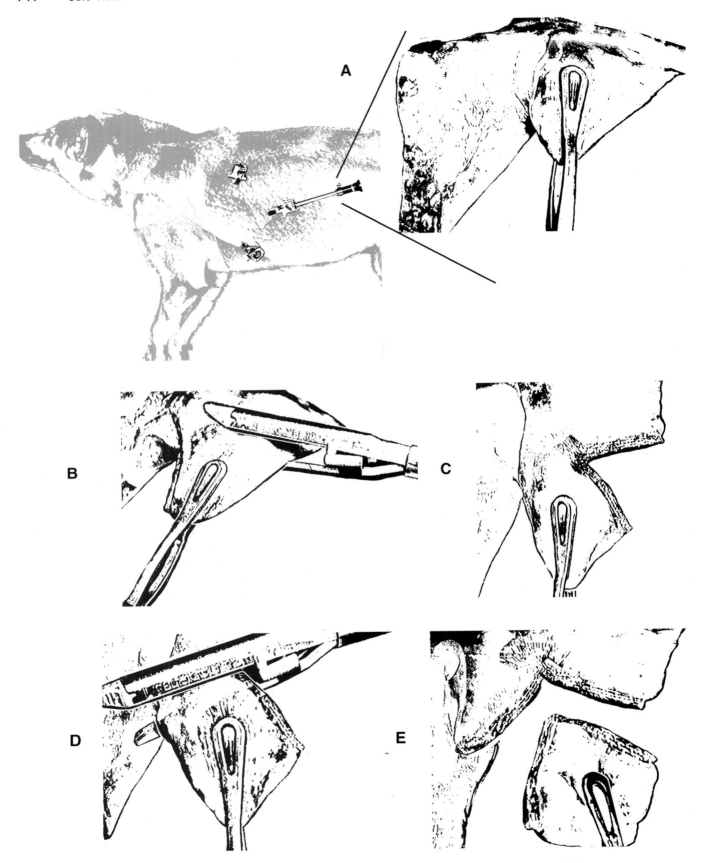

Fig. 42.8. **A–E.** Thoracoscopic lobar apical biopsy or wedge resection. See text for additional description.

The thorax is explored, and the pericardium is identified. The pericardium is held with the grasping forceps from the ventral port, and a small window is cut from the pericardium with Metzenbaum scissors from the dorsal port (Fig. 42.7). Care should be taken to avoid the phrenic nerve as it traverses the pericardium. Hemostasis can be maintained using monopolar electrocautery attached to the laparoscopic instruments (not in proximity to the heart). The operative incisions are closed routinely in two layers.

POSTOPERATIVE CARE
Standard care is maintained postoperatively, and food is resumed within 12 to 24 hours. Skin sutures can be removed in 7 to 10 days.

Lobar Apical Biopsy or Wedge Resection

INDICATIONS
This therapeutic procedure is indicated to remove a peripheral mass, bulla, or bleb or to obtain a lung biopsy.

INSTRUMENTATION

Blunt-tip 12-mm thoracic obturator–cannula (×3)
10-mm lung forceps
5-mm Metzenbaum scissors
35-mm linear staple-and-cut device with multiple cartridges
Endoscopic loop ligatures

PATIENT PREPARATION
The patient should be fasted for 12 hours. After the patient is anesthetized and positioned for surgery, one-lung ventilation is initiated. One-lung ventilation may be produced using a double-lumen endotracheal tube, endobronchial intubation, or bronchial blocker.

PATIENT POSITIONING
The patient is positioned in right or left lateral recumbency, with the forelimbs extended forward.

INSUFFLATION
None is indicated.

TROCAR–CANNULA PLACEMENT

Camera port: One 12-mm flexible thoracic trocar–cannula placed on the midaxillary line in the fifth to seventh intercostal spaces
Dorsal operative port: One 12-mm flexible thoracic trocar–cannula placed in the dorsal third of the third to fifth intercostal spaces
Ventral operative port: One 12-mm flexible thoracic trocar–cannula placed in the ventral third of the fourth or fifth intercostal space

SURGICAL TECHNIQUE
A 1-cm skin incision is made, and standard curved Kelly forceps are used to penetrate the thoracic cavity bluntly. The camera port is placed first using this blunt technique. A 10-mm, 30° viewing laparoscope is placed through the port and is used visually to guide the placement of the other two cannulas (Fig. 42.8A). The thorax is explored, and the affected lung lobe is identified. The site is held with the lung forceps from the ventral port (Fig. 42.8A, *inset*). Small peripheral lesions (smaller than 2 cm) may be ligated proximally with endoscopic loop ligatures, cut free, and removed. Large peripheral lesions require stapling. The 35-mm linear staple-and-cut device is passed through the dorsal port and is used to make a wedge cut to remove the affected region (Fig. 42.8B–E). Some overlap of staple lines is necessary to prevent leaks. Care should be taken to view both sides of the cutter before discharge, to ensure that no structures are cut unintentionally. Larger lesions may require multiple staple lines. Added hemostasis can be maintained using monopolar electrocautery attached to the laparoscopic instruments (not in proximity to the heart). The tissue is removed though the ventral trocar if size permits. An endoscopic bag can be used to assist removal and to contain infectious or cancerous tissues. The operative incisions are closed routinely in two layers.

POSTOPERATIVE CARE
Standard care is maintained after the surgical procedure, and food is resumed within 12 to 24 hours. Skin sutures can be removed in 7 to 10 days.

Acknowledgment

All line diagrams were created from actual instruments and procedures digitally captured using a 510 × 492 pixel, high-resolution, 2.5-lux, color, charge-coupled device-type camera with a 5-mm lens.

References

1. Harrison R. Historical development of laparoscopy in animals. In: Harrison R, Wildt D, eds. Animal laparoscopy. Baltimore: Williams & Wilkins, 1980:1–14.
2. Bozzini P. Lichtleiter, eine erfindung zur anschauung innerer Theile und Krankheiten nebst der Abbildung. J Pract Arzneykunde Wundarzneykunst 1806;24:107–124.
3. von Ott D. Illumination of the abdomen (ventroscopia). J Akush Zhensk Boliez 1901;15:1045–1049.
4. Kelling G. Ueber oesophagoskopie, gastroskopie und kölioskopie. Munch Med Wochenschr 1902;49:21–24.
5. Jacobaeus H. Ueber die Möglichkeit die Zystoskopie bei Untersuchung seröser höhlungen Anzuwenden. Munch Med Wochenschr 1910;57:2090–2092.
6. Cushieri A, Dubois F, Mouiel J. The European experience with laparoscopic cholecystectomy. Am J Surg 1991;161:385–387.
7. Bush R, Leonahardt H, Bush I, et al. Dr. Bozzini's lichtleiter: a translation of his original article (1806). Urology 1974;3:119–123.

8. Nadeau O, Kampmeier O. Endoscopy of the abdomen; abdominoscopy: a preliminary study, including a summary of the literature and a description of the technique. Surg Gynecol Obstet 1925;41:259–271.

9. Schirmer B, Edge S, Dix J, et al. Laparoscopic cholecystectomy: treatment of choice for symptomatic cholelithiasis. Ann Surg 1991;213:665–677.

10. Cigarini I, Joris J, Jacquet N, et al. Pain and pulmonary dysfunction after cholecystectomy under laparoscopy and laparotomy. Anesthesiology 1991;75:A122.

11. McAnena O, Austin O, Hederman W, et al. Laparoscopic versus open appendectomy. Lancet 1991;338:693.

12. Messina, MJ, Garavaglia M, Walsh R, et al. Laparoscopy-assisted vaginal hysterectomy: cost analysis and review of initial experience in a community hospital. J Am Osteopath Assoc 1995;95:31–36.

13. Group OLS. Postoperative adhesion development after operative laparoscopy: evaluation at early second-look procedures. Fertil Steril 1991;55:700–704.

14. Nezhat C, Nezhat F, Metzger D, et al. Adhesion reformation after reproductive surgery by videolaseroscopy. Fertil Steril 1990;53:1008–1011.

15. Erice F, Fox G, Salib Y, et al. Diaphragmatic function before and after laparoscopic cholecystectomy. Anesthesiology 1993;79:966–975.

16. Frazee R, Roberts J, Okeson G, et al. Open versus laparoscopic cholecystectomy: a comparison of postoperative pulmonary function. Ann Surg 1991;213:651–653.

17. Lewis R, Caccavale R, Sisler G, et al. One hundred consecutive patients undergoing video-assisted thoracic operations. Ann Thorac Surg 1992;54:421–426.

18. Joris J, Cigarini I, Legrand M, et al. Metabolic and respiratory changes after cholecystectomy performed via laparotomy or laparoscopy. Br J Anaesth 1992;69:341–345.

19. Jones B. Laparoscopy. Vet Clin North Am Small Anim Pract 1990;20:1243–1263.

20. McCarthy T, McDermaid S. Thoracoscopy. Vet Clin North Am Small Anim Pract 1990;20:1341–1352.

21. Hulka J, Reich H. Textbook of laparoscopy. 2nd ed. Philadelphia: WB Saunders, 1994.

22. Freeman L. Veterinary endo-surgery. St. Louis: Mosby–Year Book (in press).

23. Harrison R, Wildt D. Laparoscopic instrumentation. In: Harrison R, Wildt D, eds. Animal laparoscopy. Baltimore: Williams & Wilkins, 1980:199–229.

43

EXOTIC SPECIES

Avian Soft Tissue Surgery

James K. Morrisey & R. Avery Bennett

Avian surgery has made many advances in recent years, and procedures that were once considered beyond the scope of general surgeons are now performed routinely. Because of the small size and delicate nature of the tissues of avian patients, special instrumentation and techniques similar to microsurgery are used (see Chap. 41). In many situations, magnification is essential. Bipolar electrosurgery and hemostatic clips are vital for performing surgery in the recesses of the avian coelomic cavity. For surgical preparation of avian patients, the feathers are plucked rather than cut. A cut feather does not regrow until the next molt, whereas a plucked feather begins to regrow immediately. Feathers should be pulled individually in the direction of growth. Standard surgical preparation solutions are used in avian surgery; however, alcohol is avoided because of its cooling properties. Avian patients are susceptible to hypothermia, and using alcohol for surgical preparation can potentiate this complication.

Ingluviotomy

The primary function of the crop, or ingluvies, is for the storage of food. The crop allows the bird to eat a large amount of food quickly but maintain a more continuous presentation of food to the digestive portion of the gastrointestinal tract (1). Ingluviotomy is indicated for foreign body removal, for full-thickness biopsies (for the diagnosis of potential myenteric ganglioneuritis or proventricular dilatation disease), for placement of an enteric feeding tube, and as an approach for endoscopy of the proventriculus (2–4).

Neonates are especially prone to ingesting foreign bodies such as bedding material, toys, feeding tubes, and unhulled seeds. The foreign bodies can cause ingluvieitis, which can lead to crop stasis, regurgitation, or obstruction. Some foreign bodies can be removed manually by digital manipulation of the objects into the oropharynx, where they can be grasped with fingers or hemostats. Extending the bird's head makes manipulation easier. Alternatively, especially in smaller birds, a hemostat may be passed directly into the crop, and the object may be grasped and removed. The esophagus and crop are lubricated with a water-based lubricant to minimize the risk of iatrogenic injury to the esophageal or crop wall (3).

Crop burns are a result of feeding (especially tube or gavage feeding) overheated materials. The result can be necrosis of the crop and, in many cases, fistula formation. Repair of crop burns and fistulae involves debridement of necrotic tissue or the fistula margin and closure as for an ingluviotomy (3).

Surgical Procedure

An ingluviotomy may be necessary for the removal of any foreign body, particularly large or multiple foreign bodies. The patient is anesthetized, intubated, and placed in dorsal recumbency on a restraint board with the head and shoulders slightly elevated. Moist gauze is placed in the pharynx to prevent fluids from entering the oral cavity and being aspirated during manipulation of the ingluvies. An area over the crop and to the left of the midline should be plucked and prepared for aseptic surgery. The size of the prepared area depends on the size of the foreign body to be removed or the size of the instruments to be placed into the crop for endoscopy (2). The skin incision is made using an electrosurgical unit (Surgitron, Ellman International, Inc., Hewlett, NJ). Care must be taken with the fine-wire electrode to avoid penetrating the ingluvies while making the skin incision. After incision, the skin is gently dissected from the wall of the ingluvies in the area of the proposed ingluviotomy. The incision into the crop is made with a blade or electrosurgical fine-wire electrode over the left portion of the crop (Fig. 43.1). In cases of crop burn, when significant amounts of the wall are lost and the ability to close is a concern, electrosurgery is avoided because the associated lateral necrosis may compromise incisional healing. The incision is made in the left area of the crop to avoid large vessels and because it is less subject to stress as the crop fills or as a feeding tube is placed in the crop (4). Bipolar electrocautery is then used for hemostasis of specific vessels. The length of the incision should be approximately half the length necessary because it will enlarge as a result of the elasticity of the crop. The incision can be lengthened as needed for adequate exposure. The retrieval of large objects through a small incision should not be attempted. Stay sutures can be placed on all four sides to facilitate visualization of the lumen. Full-thickness biopsies for the potential diagnosis of proventricular dilatation disease should be taken from a moderately vascularized portion of the crop wall for the best diagnostic capability (5).

The incision is closed with a synthetic monofilament absorbable material, swaged onto an atraumatic needle (3, 4). Several patterns have been described (2, 4); however, a simple continuous appositional pattern oversewn with an inverting pattern provides mucosal apposition and serosa-to-serosa healing. When only a small incision is made, as for endoscopy, an inverting mattress suture is sufficient. The crop can be distended with air or saline to evaluate for the presence of leaks in the incision. The skin is closed with a simple continuous, Ford interlocking, or simple interrupted pattern using monofilament material.

Postoperative Management

Postoperative complications are usually minimal. Birds being hand fed are given smaller, more frequent meals for 3 to 5 days postoperatively, to avoid overstretching the crop wall. The amount fed may then be gradually increased to the presurgical amount over the next 10 to 14 days. Birds generally do not eat enough voluntarily to place unnecessary tension on the crop wall; however, offering multiple small meals may be of benefit, especially when resection of a large portion of the crop wall has been necessary, as in some patients with crop burns.

Proventriculotomy

The avian stomach has two compartments: the proventriculus and the ventriculus. The proventriculus is the more orad, glandular portion, and the ventriculus is the aborad, grinding portion. The proventriculus and ventriculus are connected by a narrowing called the isthmus. The isthmus is more highly developed in psittacines and less so in carnivorous birds. A proventriculotomy is indicated to remove impacted material, toxic material, or foreign bodies that cannot be removed endoscopically and to obtain biopsy samples for the potential diagnosis of proventriculus dilatation disease (2–7). The proventriculotomy incision can also be used to remove debris from the ventriculus. The muscular walls of the ventriculus make adequate closure of this organ difficult; however, some surgeons prefer to approach it directly (2).

Surgical Procedure

A left lateral celiotomy approach is used to access the proventriculus (Fig. 43.2). The bird is placed in right lateral recumbency with the left leg pulled caudally and externally rotated. The feathers are plucked in the left flank 1 cm cranial to the last two ribs extending to the right of the ventral midline and caudally past the pubis to include the vent. The area is prepared for aseptic surgery. A skin incision is made from the pubis to the level of the uncinate process between the sixth and seventh ribs (most psittacines have eight ribs) using a fine-wire electrode and an electrosurgical unit. The incision is best initiated at the knee web (a web of skin extending from the stifle to the sternum), extending it craniodorsally into the area cranial to the thigh where the ribs are palpable and caudally paramedian to the level of the pubic bone. Once the skin

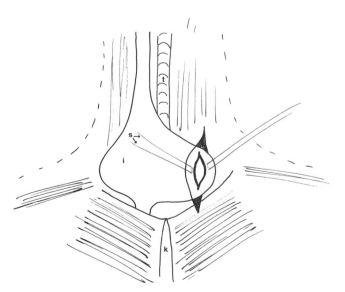

Fig. 43.1. An ingluviotomy incision is made in an avascular area over the left lateral portion of the crop. Stay sutures (s) are used to allow manipulation and improve visualization of the crop. *I,* ingluvies; *t,* trachea, *k,* keel.

joint. These vessels are ligated and coagulated, or hemostatic clips are applied to control hemorrhage.

The abdominal musculature is incised carefully with a fine-wire electrode on the electrosurgical unit to avoid damaging underlying structures. The last two (seventh and eighth) ribs are transected 2 to 4 mm dorsal to the junction between the sternal and vertebral portions and are spread to provide adequate exposure for a proventriculotomy. If the ribs are transected too far dorsally, the incision will damage lung parenchyma, and if transection is too far ventral, the exposure will not be adequate. Some authors recommend removing these ribs for better visualization and access to the proventriculus (2, 3, 8). Removing these ribs makes closure difficult and is not usually necessary. The intercostal artery and vein are located along the cranial border of the corresponding rib and are coagulated using radiosurgery before transection of the ribs. The ribs of most species are thin and can easily be cut with scissors. Retractors such as Heiss, Alm, or mini-Balfour are used to retract the ribs, thereby providing exposure through the cranial aspect of the incision, as is necessary for a proventriculotomy.

Once the approach is made, the caudal thoracic air sac has been entered and abdominal air sac is visible. The caudal extent of the lung is visualized at the cranial extent of the incision and can be gently manipulated with a cotton-tipped applicator if necessary. The air sacs and suspensory ligaments of the proventriculus are bluntly dissected to allow the ventriculus to be manipulated out of the celiotomy. The caudal portion of the left liver lobe lies over the isthmus and is readily visualized. Stay sutures should not be placed in the proventriculus because its thin, glandular wall tears when traction is applied. The thick muscular walls of the ventriculus are more suited for the placement of stay sutures. Stay sutures are placed in the white tendinous portion of the ventriculus, not in the muscle itself. These sutures are then used to elevate the isthmus and aborad portion of the proventriculus to the body wall. Care is taken in manipulating the proventriculus because it is fragile and can be easily torn. The areas surrounding the proventriculus and isthmus are packed off with moist gauze sponges to avoid leakage of proventricular contents into the coelom. The caudal portion of the left liver lobe is gently elevated and is retracted medially with a moist cotton-tipped applicator exposing the isthmus. Many small vessels are present between this portion of the liver and the proventriculus. If excessive traction is applied, severe hemorrhage will result.

The incision should be made at the isthmus with a scalpel and should be extended orad using scissors, while avoiding the superficial vessels of the proventriculus (Fig. 43.3). Bipolar coagulation is used to control hemorrhage, but it should not be used to make the incision because lateral necrosis can have a negative

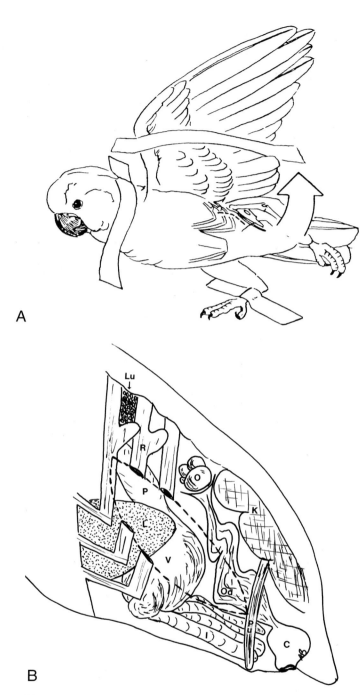

A

B

Fig. 43.2. **A.** Positioning of the patient for left lateral celiotomy. (Reprinted with permission from Bennett RA, Harrison GJ. Soft tissue surgery. In: Ritchie BW, Harrison GJ, Harrison LR, eds. Avian medicine and surgery: principles and applications. Lake Worth, FL: Wingers, 1996:1096–1136.) **B.** The left lateral celiotomy provides access to the proventriculis (*P*), ventriculis (*V*), and oviduct (*Od*). *R*, seventh rib; *Lu*, lung; *O*, ovary; *K*, kidney; *C*, cloaca; *I*, intestines; *L*, liver; *Pu*, pubis.

is incised, the leg is extended more caudally and is rotated externally for better exposure of the abdominal musculature. The superficial branches of the medial femoral artery and vein course perpendicular to the midline emerging from the area of the coxofemoral

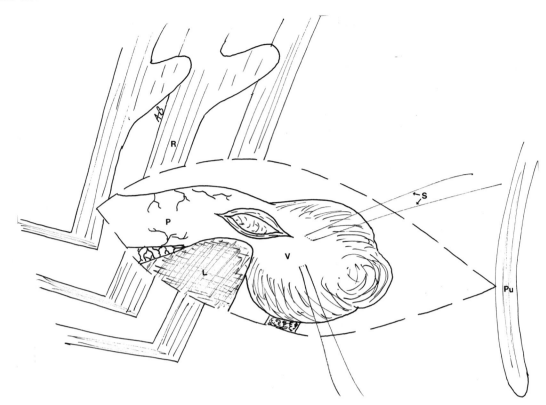

Fig. 43.3. The proventriculotomy incision is initiated at the isthmus. Stay sutures (*S*) are placed in the ventriculus (*V*). The left lobe of the liver (*L*) may be gently retracted using a cotton-tipped applicator to provide access to the isthmus. This portion of the liver is used to provide a serosal patch at closure. *R*, seventh rib; *P*, proventriculus; *Pu*, pubis.

effect on incisional healing. Sharp-toothed forceps are avoided because they can cause severe damage including perforation of the proventricular wall. Suction is used immediately to remove any liquid contents and thus to minimize the risk of coelomic contamination. Small bladder spoons, ear curettes, bone curettes, suction, or forceps can be used to remove foreign materials. A combination of irrigation and suction is useful to remove all material from the proventriculus and the ventriculus (3, 4).

The proventriculus is closed using a 4–0 to 8–0 synthetic monofilament material with a fine, small, swaged-on atraumatic needle. A two-layer closure is recommended, although a single-layer continuous Cushing pattern has also been described (4). The two-layer closure consists of an initial simple continuous layer oversewn with a second inverting layer, such as a Lembert or Cushing pattern, which overextends the initial closure (2, 3). The two-layer closure is recommended because postoperative incisional leakage occurs more frequently than in mammals (6). The incision is checked for leakage using air or saline infused through a feeding tube passed through the patient's mouth and into the proventriculus. The rib retractor is removed, and no effort is made to stabilize the tran-

sected ribs. The intercostal and abdominal muscles are closed with a monofilament absorbable suture in a simple continuous or simple interrupted pattern. The skin is closed using a monofilament suture in a simple interrupted, simple continuous, or Ford interlocking pattern.

Postoperative Management

Leakage from the proventriculotomy incision is of concern even with the most careful closure. That birds do not have an omentum to aid in sealing serosal incisions has been cited as a cause of the increased incidence of leakage after proventriculotomy (6). Birds should not be fasted postoperatively for longer than 12 hours because the incision is stronger immediately postoperatively than it is during the debridement phase of wound healing, which occurs approximately 3 to 5 days postoperatively (3). Dehiscence and leakage are most likely to occur during the debridement phase. However, the patient should be fed smaller meals more frequently, to decrease expansion of the proventriculus. If the proventricular wall appears especially thin or fragile, or if one is concerned about the security of the closure, a serosal patch with the liver or adjacent intestine, or placement of a duodenal feeding tube to bypass the proventriculus, may be warranted.

Cloacopexy

Cloacopexy is indicated in cases of chronic cloacal prolapse. The etiology of this syndrome is uncertain, although chronic gram-negative enteritis has been cited as an initiating factor (9). Other suspected causes include hormonal influence causing sphincter muscle weakness and chronic masturbation behavior. Old World species, especially cockatoos and African gray parrots, are more commonly affected. Prolapse can cause damage to the cloacal attachments and loss of muscle tone to the cloacal wall and vent sphincter. Prolapsed cloacal tissue may also obstruct the ureters, colon, or oviduct, which open into the cloaca.

Surgical Procedure

Minor prolapses may be temporarily or permanently repaired by placing two simple interrupted or mattress sutures transversely across the vent. These sutures must be close enough together to prevent the cloaca from prolapsing but far enough apart to allow passage of fecal material. The placement of an appropriately sized red rubber feeding tube or moist cotton-tipped applicator is used to ensure that adequate space is left for feces to pass. These sutures may be left in for several days to weeks, depending on the clinical situation (3). A pursestring suture is not recommended because it causes more damage to the vent sphincter muscle or its nerve supply.

A percutaneous cloacopexy can be performed on patients with minor disorders to alleviate a cloacal prolapse temporarily. The surgeon reduces the prolapse by using a lubricated gloved finger or a cotton-tipped applicator. The applicator is placed in a dorsolateral corner of the cloaca, and one or two sutures are blindly placed through the skin, body wall, and cloacal wall. The process is then repeated on the opposite side. The sutures should be removed in 2 to 4 weeks, to allow for adhesions to form around the sutures. Possible risks associated with this procedure are entrapment of bowel or ureters within the sutures.

Severe, chronic, recurrent cloacal prolapse requires more invasive techniques. The simplest of these procedures is an incisional cloacopexy (Fig. 43.4). A midline or transverse abdominal incision is made, and an assistant's finger or cotton-tipped applicator is placed into the cloaca to reduce the prolapse fully and to identify the limits of the cloaca clearly. Generally, an accumulation of fat along the ventral aspect of the cloaca prevents adhesion formation. This fat is excised, and the body wall incision is closed incorporating the cloacal wall into the body wall closure (3, 10). The sutures

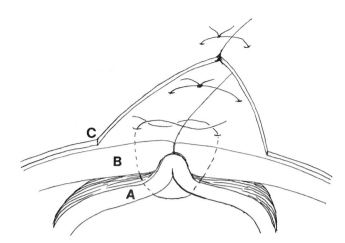

Fig. 43.4. An incisional cloacopexy incorporates the cloaca (A) into a ventral midline or transverse abdominal incision. The simple interrupted sutures pass full-thickness through the cloaca. The skin (C) is closed routinely. B, body wall.

penetrate the body wall on one side, the full thickness of the cloaca, then the body wall on the other side. A monofilament, absorbable, or nonabsorbable suture is used in a simple interrupted pattern. A transverse approach may provide more even distribution of tension than a midline approach (9).

Another method for cloacopexy involves making a 2- to 5-mm incision into the ventral serosal surface of the cloaca parallel to its length and 5 to 10 mm from the midline. A similar incision is made on the peritoneal surface of the body wall. This incision is placed so the two incisions are apposed when the cloaca is reduced and traction causes the vent to be slightly inverted. Three or four sutures are placed on each side of the two corresponding incisions between the serosal layers of the peritoneum and the cloaca, to appose the subserosal tissues. The procedure is repeated on the opposite paramedian side. This procedure forms stronger adhesions between the cloaca and the body wall and should last longer than the methods previously described (4). The abdominal wall and skin are closed routinely. This procedure can only be accomplished in large avian patients with a thick cloacal wall.

A rib cloacopexy is an alternative for severe cases of prolapse (Fig. 43.5). A ventral midline approach to the cloaca is made. The cranial extent of the incision should be at the level of or slightly cranial to the last rib (most psittacine birds have eight ribs). To provide better exposure of the last rib, the ventral midline incision is extended laterally along the sternal border, thus creating a T-shaped or Y-shaped celiotomy. The last rib is pushed caudally and medially with a finger while the body wall is retracted to expose the serosal surface covering the last rib. Two sutures are preplaced around

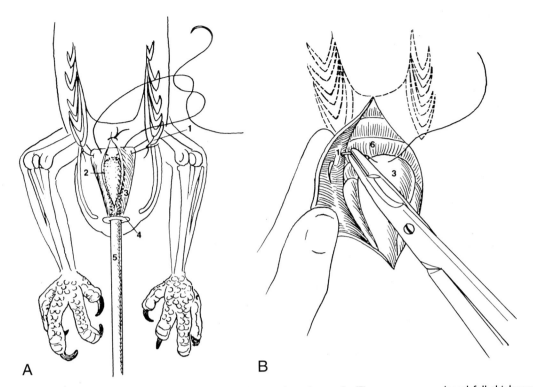

Fig. 43.5. A rib cloacopexy is performed on chronic cases of cloacal prolapse. **A.** The sutures are placed full thickness through each craniolateral aspect of the cloaca and are secured to the last rib on each side. **B.** Placing pressure on the eighth rib while simultaneously retracting the skin helps to visualize the rib for suture placement. 1) eighth rib, 2) skin incision, 3) cloaca, 4) rents, 5) swab, 6) intestines (Reprinted with permission from Bennett RA, Harrison GJ: Soft tissue surgery. In: Ritchie BW, Harrison GJ, Harrison LR, eds. Avian medicine and surgery: principles and applications. Lake Worth, FL: Wingers, 1996:1096–1136.)

the last rib and through the craniolateral extent of the cloaca on each side. The sutures should incorporate large sections of the cloaca and should pass full-thickness into the lumen. A monofilament nonabsorbable suture is used, and the suture is tied with enough tension to invert the cloaca slightly. Alternatively, the cranioventral border of the cloaca may be sutured to the caudal border of the sternum if the rib sutures place excessive tension on the cloaca (3). Finally, the ventral cloacal wall is also incorporated into the closure of the body wall as previously described for incisional cloacopexy. If the cloacal wall is thin or friable, the rib cloacopexy can damage the cloaca.

When atony of the vent sphincter is present in conjunction with cloacal prolapse, the size of the vent opening can be reduced using a ventplasty to prevent cloacal prolapse. A 2- to 3-mm strip of tissue is removed along the mucocutaneous junction of the vent at each lateral aspect (Fig. 43.6). One-quarter to one-third of the vent skin may be excised from each side. This maneuver exposes the sphincter muscle. A horizontal mattress suture of absorbable material on an atraumatic needle is placed in the sphincter muscle between the cranial and caudal aspects on each side. The skin is closed with a nonabsorbable material in a simple interrupted pattern. Sutures are removed in 10 to 14 days.

Postoperative Management

Postoperative care is aimed at the treatment of any underlying conditions that may cause or contribute to the cloacal prolapse. Because most of the techniques discussed involve sutures entering the cloacal lumen,

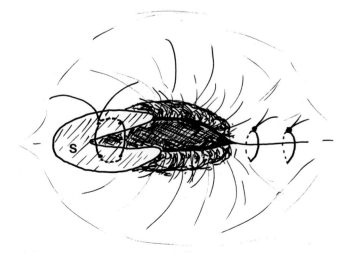

Fig. 43.6. A ventplasty can be performed when tone is lost in the cloacal sphincter muscle. The mucocutaneous junction is excised at each commissure, and a horizontal mattress suture is placed through the vent sphincter muscle (S). The skin is closed with simple interrupted sutures.

a broad-spectrum antibiotic is indicated. The duration and selection of antibiotic therapy varies, depending on culture results. Stool softeners may prevent excessive straining associated with defecation and may diminish stress on the surgical area. Stool softeners are continued for at least 2 weeks to minimize straining during the weakest phases of wound healing. Owners should be warned that recurrence is possible, especially in birds with behavioral causes of prolapse. Clients should also be advised that if severe damage to the nervous supply to the cloaca has occurred, flatulence and abnormal defecation may result (10). Other complications include vent stricture, cloacitis, and peritonitis.

Salpingohysterectomy

Salpingohysterectomy or removal of the oviduct and uterus (shell gland) is indicated to treat egg binding, persistent egg laying, abnormal egg production, ruptured or infected oviduct, and recurrent oviductal prolapse (2–4, 11, 12). The ovary is not removed because it is not possible to ligate the ovarian artery and veins,

which enter the broad dorsal surface in the ovarian hilus (13). Cockatiels and budgerigars are most often affected with chronic or pathologic egg laying; however, salpingohysterectomy carries risks and is not generally recommended as a preventive measure (3).

Surgical Procedure

Salpingohysterectomy has been described using a transverse or a left lateral celiotomy (2, 3, 11, 12). A left lateral approach is preferred because it gives better access to the entire length of the reproductive tract. The transverse approach provides access to the right and left coelom. Because most pet avian species have only a left-sided reproductive tract, this factor is less important.

The left lateral celiotomy is described in the previous discussion on proventriculotomy. Some surgeons do not transect the ribs for this procedure (Fig. 43.7). Once the coelom is entered, the proventriculus is retracted medially and ventrally to expose the ovary. The oviduct extends caudally from the ovary along

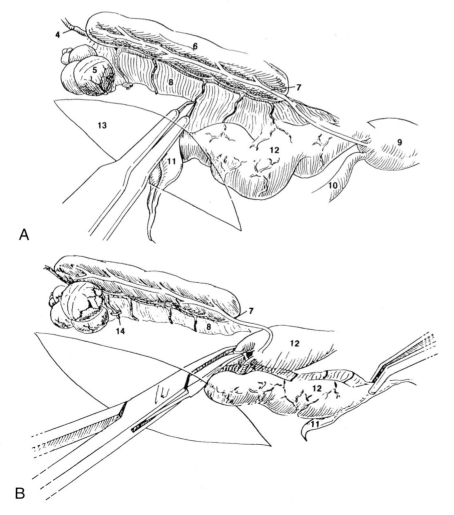

Fig. 43.7. The salpingohysterectomy is performed through the left lateral celiotomy, as shown in Figure 43.2. **A.** A hemostatic clip is placed on the cranial oviductal artery, and bipolar cautery is used to dissect the dorsal oviductal ligament. **B.** Hemostatic clips are applied to the uterus (shell gland) at its junction with the vagina before transection and removal: *4*, aorta; *5*, ovary; *6*, kidney; *7*, ureter; *8*, suspensory ligament of oviduct; *9*, cloaca; *10*, rectum; *11*, infundibulum; *12*, oviduct; *13*, celiotomy incision; *14*, surgical clip (Hemoclip).

the dorsal body wall. The size of the oviduct varies, depending on the reproductive status of the bird and on any underlying pathologic process. The oviduct is carefully elevated from the caudal vena cava to expose the ventral ligament. This ligament causes the convolutions of the uterus and oviduct and courses caudally to form a muscular cord at the vagina. This ligament has no major vessels, and it is transected to allow the oviduct and uterus to be stretched into a linear configuration.

The oviduct is followed cranially and the infundibulum is identified and elevated to expose the dorsal suspensory ligament of the oviduct. This ligament contains a branch of the ovarian artery (the cranial oviductal artery) that is identified and ligated with a hemostatic clip, ligature, or bipolar cautery. If this artery is not ligated or coagulated before transection, it will retract under the ovary and become virtually irretrievable (2, 3). The remainder of the dorsal ligament can be dissected caudally using bipolar electrocautery to coagulate vessels. Many small branches of the ovarian artery can be seen in the ligament, and each is coagulated. As the dorsal ligament is dissected, the oviduct and uterus are elevated to expose the junction with the vagina dorsolateral to the colon. The uterus is ligated at this site using two hemostatic clips or ligatures. If the vaginal wall is damaged or infected, the ligatures or clips are placed at the junction of the vagina with the cloaca. Care is taken to avoid entrapping the ureter. The surgeon must ensure that the entire width of the uterus is within the ligature to prevent the reflux of cloacal contents into the coelom.

Postoperative Management

Postoperative complications are more common when uterine disease, such as salpingitis or rupture, is present. Should rupture or leakage occur, gentle cleansing of the coelom with moist cotton-tipped applicators helps to prevent inflammation. Irrigation of the avian coelom is not recommended because of the anatomy of the respiratory system.

Egg yolk peritonitis caused by continued yolk release after salpingohysterectomy has been reported in a domestic duck and a California quail (14). A study of cockatiels that underwent salpingohysterectomy showed continuation of breeding behavior without evidence of peritonitis caused by egg yolk deposition into the coelom (15). Endoscopic examinations performed several months postoperatively confirmed ovarian activity without visible signs of egg release after salpingohysterectomy. Another study of six birds followed for 1 year after surgery did not show reproductive behaviors or signs of egg yolk peritonitis (13). A hormonal feedback mechanism between the uterus or oviduct and the ovary is believed to be necessary for follicular development and release of ova (12, 14). Investigators have speculated that yolk release occurs if the entire uterus is not removed.

References

1. Duke GE. Alimentary canal: anatomy, regulation of feeding and motility. In: Sturkie PD, ed. Avian physiology. 4th ed. New York: Springer-Verlag, 1986:239–288.
2. Altman RB. Soft tissue surgical procedures. In: Altman RB, Clubb SB, Dorrestein GM, et al, eds. Avian medicine and surgery. Philadelphia: WB Saunders, 1996:704–732.
3. Bennett RA, Harrison GJ: Soft tissue surgery. In: Ritchie BW, Harrison GJ, Harrison LR, eds. Avian medicine and surgery: principles and applications. Lake Worth, FL: Wingers, 1996:1096–1136.
4. Jenkins JR. Avian soft tissue surgery. Part 2. In: Proceedings of the American College of Veterinary Surgeons Annual Conference.: American College of Veterinary Surgeons, 1992:634–636.
5. Ritchie BW. Proventricular dilatation disease and chlamydiosis. In: Proceedings of the North American Veterinary Conference. Orlando, FL. 1997:700–701.
6. McCluggage D. Proventriculotomy: a study of selected cases. In: Proceedings of the Association of Avian Veterinarians Annual Conference.: New Orleans, LA. Association of Avian Veterinarians, 1992:195–198.
7. Rosskopf WJ, et al: Pet avian emergency care. In: Proceedings of the Association of Avian Veterinarians Annual Conference.: Chicago, IL. Association of Avian Veterinarians, 1991:349.
8. Harrison GJ. Selected surgical procedures. In: Harrison GJ, Harrison LR, eds. Clinical avian medicine and surgery. Philadelphia: WB Saunders, 1986:577–595.
9. Avgeris S, Rigg D. Cloacopexy in a sulphur-crested cockatoo. J Am Anim Hosp Assoc 1988;24:407–410.
10. Rosskopf WJ, Woerpel RW. Cloacal conditions in pet birds with a cloacopexy update. In: Proceedings of the Association of Avian Veterinarians Annual Conference.: Seattle, WA. Association of Avian Veterinarians, 1989:156–163.
11. Wissman MA. Unusual C-section and hysterectomy in an Isle of Pines Amazon. In: Proceedings of the Association of Avian Veterinarians Annual Conference.: Chicago, IL. Association of Avian Veterinarians, 1991:265–266.
12. Smith RE. Hysterectomy to relieve reproductive disorders in birds. Avian Exotic Pract 1985;2:40–43.
13. King AS, McLelland J. Birds: their structure and function. 2nd ed. Philadelphia: Bailliere Tindall, 1984:147.
14. Rosskopf WJ, Woerpel RW. Pet avian obstetrics. In: Proceedings of the 1st International Conference on Zoological and Avian Medicine. 1987:213–231.
15. McCluggage D. Hysterectomy: a review of selected cases. In: Proceedings of the Association of Avian Veterinarians Annual Conference.: New Orleans, LA. Association of Avian Veterinarians, 1992:201–206.

Avian Laparoscopy

Darryl J. Heard

Indications

Gender Determination

The earliest use of avian laparoscopy was for sex identification (1–3), a technique that revolutionized captive breeding of monomorphic birds, most notably parrots (4). Laparoscopic sex determination has been partially superseded by testing systems based on karyo-typing (5) and DNA fingerprinting (6). The advantages of these tests are that they can be used in neonatal birds and they avoid many of the complications of laparoscopy (see later). However, they have the disad-vantages of slow turnaround, high cost, and validation in only a limited number of avian families (although this number is increasing) (6). Furthermore, by allowing direct visualization, laparoscopy enables one to assess gonadal maturity, reproductive status, and the presence or absence of disease.

Disease Diagnosis

Laparoscopy provides direct visualization of many coe-lomic cavity organs. With appropriate equipment (see later), one can obtain swabs or biopsy samples of sus-pected pathologic lesions for cytologic study, bacterial and fungal culture, and histopathologic examination. Biopsies are valuable in disease diagnosis because di-rect visualization of an organ surface is often insuffi-cient to identify a pathologic process.

Surgery

Laparoscopic surgery offers the advantages of a small surgical wound, minimal trauma, and faster recovery. Some veterinarians use laparoscopy for male steriliza-tion by electrocauterizing the vas deferens. The future development of suitable instruments should allow more complex surgical procedures to be performed (e.g., removal of air sac granulomas).

Contraindications

Ascites

Avian ascites is usually due either to congestive heart failure or to end-stage liver disease, both diseases that increase anesthetic risk (7, 8). Ascitic fluid accumula-tion in the peritoneal cavities not only compresses air sacs, but also it may enter the lungs and drown a recumbent bird if the peritoneal cavities are ruptured. When laparoscopy is considered necessary, the fluid should be drained. However, rapid removal of a large volume of protein-containing fluid may result in car-diovascular collapse.

Crop and Proventricular Distension

Although this condition is not an absolute contraindi-cation, laparoscopy should not be performed in birds with a distended proventriculus or crop because of the possibility of perforation of the former and regurgita-tion from the latter. The crop and proventriculus are likely to be distended in unweaned parrots, nonfasted and recently tube-fed birds, and parrots afflicted with proventricular dilatation syndrome (8).

Impaired Hemostasis

Abnormal hemostasis predisposes birds to severe hem-orrhage, even with the minor trauma associated with laparoscopy. Unfortunately, other than determina-tions of thrombocyte count and bleeding time and pre-operative examination for bruising, few diagnostic tools are available for evaluation of avian hemostasis. The coagulation tests used in mammals are not valid in birds. Bleeding disorders are frequently associated with hepatic disease.

Inexperience

The most common cause of complication is inexperi-ence of the clinician. The practitioner who wishes to perform laparoscopy should participate in a formal training course or should practice on cadavers and in-expensive birds. The inexperienced laparoscopist is more likely to perforate an organ, produce hemor-rhage, and prolong the duration of the procedure.

Obesity

Obese birds have increased coelomic fat that decreases air sac and peritoneal cavity volumes. Decreased air sac volume impairs ventilation and impedes visualiza-tion, an effect compounded by fat covering organ sur-faces. I have also observed that portions of fatty tissue readily obstruct and smear the lens and sheath.

Ovulation

In some avian species, gonadal size varies dramatically between breeding and nonbreeding seasons. These en-larged gonads are predisposed to laparoscopic injury (e.g., a ruptured follicle and associated egg yolk perito-nitis). Additionally, large gonads are difficult to visual-ize because of the small field of view of the endoscope relative to the size of the organ.

Physiologic Instability

As with other invasive procedures requiring anesthe-sia, laparoscopy ideally should be performed in birds that are physiologically stable. An exception would be those birds in which the need for a diagnosis out-weighs the risks of performing the procedure.

Equipment

Laparoscopic examination minimally requires a light source, a fiberoptic cable, a trocar and sheath, and the endoscope.

Light Source

Several companies produce powerful light sources adequate for avian laparoscopy (see the appendix at the end of this discussion). An important feature is portability, particularly for surgical sexing, for which the practitioner may need to travel to the breeding facility.

Fiberoptic Cable

Light transmission along the cable through fiberoptic glass bundles is based on total internal light reflection within the glass fibers (9). Although the cable should be of sufficient length to allow a comfortable distance between the light source and the working space, long cables are more likely to be damaged. Care must be taken to prevent the cable from being twisted or chewed by the patient, both of which result in broken fibers and loss of light transmission. For the same reason, the cable is gently coiled and protected during storage and sterilization.

Trocar and Sheath

The trocar and sheath combination is used to penetrate the abdominal wall and occasionally the walls of the coelomic cavities. The sheath also protects the delicate laparoscope. However, in small birds (smaller than 500 g) the sheath, by increasing the outside laparoscope diameter, makes it cumbersome and more hazardous. An alternative is to dissect the approach to the coelomic cavity bluntly and to introduce the laparoscope directly. A sheath that allows the introduction of flexible biopsy forceps alongside a 2.7-mm diameter endoscope has been developed for avian laparoscopy (Karl Storz Veterinary Endoscopy—America, Ovledo, FL).

Endoscope

The earliest avian surgical sexing technique involved direct visualization through a large paralumbar incision (10, 11). Later, visualization was improved and incision size was decreased by using an otoscope (2, 3). Although the latter technique is adequate for gender determination, the otoscope is inappropriate for routine laparoscopy. Rather, laparoscopy should be performed using a rigid fiberoptic endoscope (1, 9, 12, 13). These instruments are expensive, but if appropriately cared for, they have a long working life. If a practitioner does not wish to purchase this equipment, then referral to a qualified laparoscopist is advised.

The commercially available avian laparoscopes are actually human arthroscopes. They range in outside diameter from 1.7 to 5.0 mm (14). The most frequently recommended avian laparoscope for use in small to medium-sized birds is 2.7 mm in outer diameter because it provides good illumination and is rugged (14). In addition to their small diameter, the most useful avian endoscopes are 170 to 180 mm long and have a viewing angle 10 to 30° from the axis (9, 14). This angle improves visualization in confined spaces and, by rotation, around visceral edges (14). Further, the beveled end is less traumatic and facilitates easy penetration of air sac walls (14). The 1.7- and 1.9-mm arthroscopes are useful in extremely small patients (e.g., smaller than 100 g) and for visualization in small anatomic sites (9, 14). However, smaller laparoscopes provide less illumination because they contain fewer light-carrying fibers. Small laparoscopes also have the disadvantages of visual obstruction and frequent fogging.

Instrument Care

The rigid endoscope and associated equipment are expensive and unfortunately are easily damaged. The equipment should be handled carefully during manipulation, cleaning, sterilization, and storage. This also includes training all personnel in the appropriate care of the equipment.

The endoscope is picked up by its eyepiece and not by the distal tip (15). Additionally, it must not be bent or dropped, and both ends should be supported during handling and storage (16). Flexing the barrel either fractures the fiberoptic bundles, leading to black dots in the field of view, or dislodges the lens (16). When possible, the endoscope is stored in a protective sheath, and during sterilization and storage, all equipment is protected in a rigid padded container. At the end of each procedure, the endoscope, trocar, and sheath are gently rinsed with clean water to remove all organic material. The lens is then wiped with lens paper or a cotton swab dampened in alcohol (16). One should always follow the manufacturer's directions for cleaning, handling, and storage.

Sterilization

Sterilization of equipment is important because of the potential for disease transmission among birds. The two recommended techniques for the endoscope and light cable are gas and cold sterilization, the latter being recommended for use between multiple patients.

Although gas sterilization using ethylene oxide gas is effective, it requires a prolonged aeration period (8 to 12 hours) and expensive equipment, and it is a human health hazard. Hence, the most practical and safest technique is immersion in a 2% glutaraldehyde solution of a type approved by the equipment manufacturer (15). The activated life span of these products is short, and they should be changed frequently. For effective sterilization, the instruments should be free of all organic material, they should not touch each other, and they should remain immersed for 15 to 20 minutes (15). Prolonged immersion is avoided, to prevent instrument damage. After soaking, the equipment is immersed in sterile water and is rinsed thoroughly to remove the irritant glutaraldehyde. When the endoscope is to be used immediately, one should use a warm water rinse and dry the scope with a sterile towel to prevent fogging (16).

Anesthesia

Although laparoscopy in awake birds has been performed by some practitioners (1), I consider it to be both inhumane and unnecessary. Some large birds (e.g., cranes), which are able to be manually restrained, can undergo laparoscopy after local anesthetic infiltration of the surgical site. However, general anesthesia using isoflurane anesthesia offers the advantages of good muscle relaxation, decreased likelihood of visceral lacerations from struggling, and an ability to regulate anesthetic duration. When gas anesthesia is not available, I have found that, during surgical sexing of large numbers of parrots, ketamine hydrochloride (10 to 15 mg/kg intravenously in the metatarsal vein) gives a short anesthetic period with a brief recovery. However, it is necessary either to recover the birds in a darkened container or to wrap them in a towel to prevent struggling.

Fasting overnight is indicated in most birds to decrease the likelihood of proventricular distension. This protocol not only lowers the risk of proventricular perforation, but also it improves ventilation.

Positioning

Correct positioning is essential for accurate endoscope placement and identification of visceral landmarks. For lateral recumbency, the bird's wings are stretched above the back and pulled forward while simultaneously the legs are stretched either caudally or cranially and downward, depending on the approach. The wings and legs are either held in place by an assistant or are taped or Velcroed in place on a board. For dorsal recumbency, the birds are taped flat with the wings slightly extended and the legs abducted slightly and pulled backward, and a piece of tape is placed across the neck.

Preparation

Laparoscopy is a surgical procedure and therefore is performed as aseptically as possible. The entry site is cleared of feathers by either plucking or wetting down with antiseptic or a sterile water-soluble lubricant. The site is disinfected with either an alcohol and povidone–iodine or chlorhexidine scrub. Care is taken to prevent excessive wetting, which may promote hypothermia. A clear, sterile adhesive drape is placed over the entry site when prolonged procedures or complex cases are anticipated.

In each approach described in this discussion, the surgeon must make a small skin incision with a scalpel blade to allow penetration of either the trocar and sheath or the endoscope. The underlying muscle and subcutaneous tissues are either bluntly dissected with a sterile hemostat or penetrated with the blunt trocar and sheath.

Surgical Technique

The surgeon must be comfortable when performing laparoscopy; the support table should be at an appropriate height to prevent prolonged bending. To reduce trauma to the patient, movement of the trocar and sheath and the endoscope is controlled and deliberate at all times. To achieve this goal, the trocar and sheath and the endoscope are held at their respective bases. The surgeon then uses the free hand, which rests on the table, to steady each instrument at the entry site. In medium-sized to large birds, the trocar and sheath are gently drilled through the underlying tissues with alternating clockwise and counterclockwise twisting wrist motions. Frequently, a decrease in resistance or ''pop'' is felt as the endoscope enters the coelomic cavity. The entry angle varies with the approach and the laparoscopist; some authors recommend an acute approach angle (less than 45°) to reduce the likelihood of organ perforation, whereas others appear satisfied with a perpendicular angle. In small birds (smaller than 500 g), the coelomic cavity can be entered by blunt dissection with a hemostat and either the endoscope alone or the endoscope in combination with the sheath placed through this opening. Regardless of the type of entry, the surgeon should check for hemorrhage either by direct visualization or by wiping the trocar over the back of the glove. If severe hemorrhage is noted, the procedure should be discontinued, and the surgeon should follow the recommendations described later in this discussion. When penetration of an air sac or peritoneal space is necessary, the surgeon should place either the sheath and reinserted trocar or the endoscope against the membrane at a site free of blood vessels and underlying structures, then gently push forward with the same controlled twisting motion used to enter the coelomic cavity. Once again, one usually feels the membrane tear and the resistance change on entry into the next cavity.

Surgical Anatomy

Birds are well suited to laparoscopy because of their unique respiratory system, which includes large air sacs that ramify throughout the viscera. This anatomic configuration allows excellent visualization without the need for artificial insufflation. Although birds lack a diaphragm, the term "diaphragm" is occasionally but erroneously applied to the horizontal and oblique septa (17). The avian embryo has six pairs of air sacs. In most birds, two of these pairs have fused at or soon after hatching to form the midline clavicular sac (17). In chickens and many other avian species, an additional pair of sacs fuses to form the cervical sac. The three pairs of air sacs most important to avian laparoscopy, the cranial thoracic, caudal thoracic, and abdominal, do not fuse (17). The symmetric cranial thoracic air sacs lie dorsolaterally within the thoracic cage (17), and in parrots they are the smallest of the three pairs (17). The caudal thoracic air sacs also lie in a dorsolateral position but caudal to the cranial air sacs (17). In chickens, they are small and are covered medially by the cranial thoracic and abdominal air sacs, which compress them against the body wall (17). In parrots, the caudal thoracic air sacs do not extend as far caudally as in pigeons (15). In most birds, the largest air sacs are the abdominal sacs (15), which spread caudally from the lungs between the intestinal loops, except where they are attached to the dorsal abdominal wall (17). Paired diverticula spread dorsally between the kidneys and the pelvis and synsacrum (17).

In addition to the air sacs, the avian coelomic cavity contains eight other distinct and separate cavities (17). Five of these (left and right ventral hepatic, left and right dorsal hepatic, and intestinal) are peritoneal cavities formed by peritoneal partitions not present in mammals (Figs. 43.8 and 43.9) (17). The intestinal peritoneal cavity is a single elongated space extending in the midline from the liver to the vent between the left and right hepatic cavities. It touches the body wall in the caudal region, where it can be entered directly through the abdominal wall (17). The intestines and the gonads and their ducts are suspended by mesenteries within the intestinal peritoneal cavity (see Fig. 43.9) (17).

Approaches

All of the following approaches require the bird to be in lateral recumbency, except the midline approach. They can be performed from either the left or right side.

Paralumbar Fossa Entry Site

The legs are pulled caudally and downward (Fig. 43.10). Entry is made immediately in front of the cranial iliotibialis muscle approximately one-third down the length of the femur. In small birds, this site is behind the last rib, whereas in large birds it is between the last two ribs (9, 18).

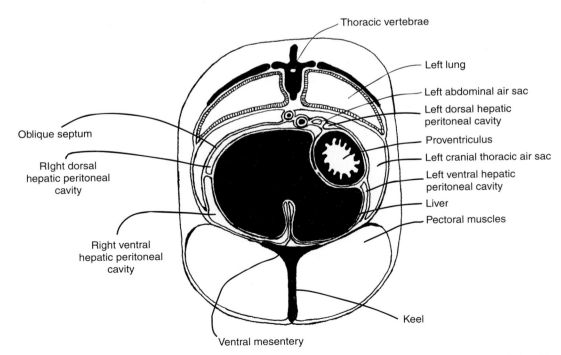

Fig. 43.8. Schematic diagram of a transverse section through the midthoracic area of a pigeon showing the relationship among some of the peritoneal and air sac cavities. (Modified, in part, from King AS, McLelland J. Birds: their structure and function. 2nd ed. Philadelphia: Bailliere Tindall, 1984.)

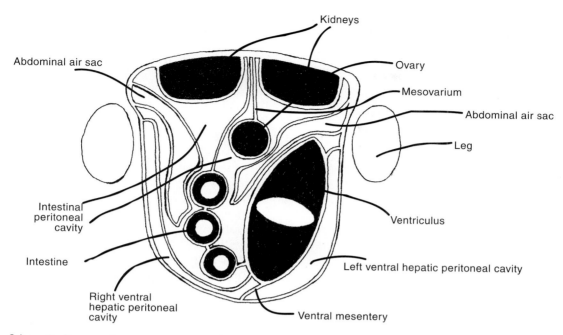

Fig. 43.9. Schematic diagram of a transverse section through the midcoelomic cavity of a pigeon showing the relationship among some of the peritoneal and air sac cavities. Note the location of the gonad in the intestinal peritoneal cavity and the position of the abdominal air sac. (Modified, in part, from King AS, McLelland J. Birds: their structure and function. 2nd ed. Philadelphia: Bailliere Tindall, 1984.)

VISIBLE ANATOMY

The abdominal air sac, occasionally the caudal thoracic, is entered using this approach (15). Although this approach is usually used for sex determination, it allows visualization of the cranial pole of the kidney (dorsocranial), the adrenal glands (dorsocranial), the abdominal air sac and its ostium (cranial), the caudal lung (cranial), the intestinal peritoneal cavity, the pro-ventriculus (cranioventral) and ventriculus (cranioventral), the intestines (ventral), the spleen (ventral), and portions of the liver (cranioventral). The paired, triple-lobed kidneys are deep red, are cranially rounded, and lie in the dorsal midline immediately ventral to the synsacrum. The adrenal glands are paired, white to yellow to orange triangular structures lying on each side of the midline at the cranial ends

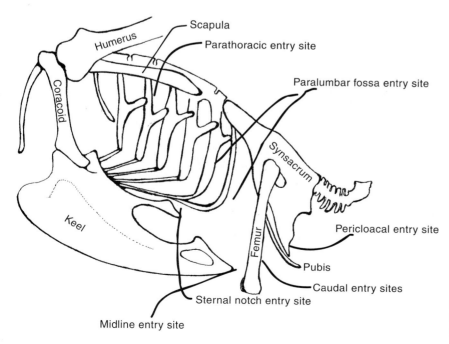

Fig. 43.10. Schematic partial diagram of the skeleton of a pigeon showing described entry sites for avian laparoscopy.

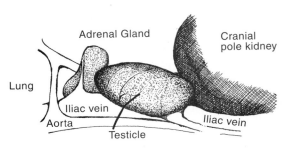

Fig. 43.11. Diagram of the left testicle of a cockatoo showing the geographic relationship of the lung, adrenal gland, gonad, and cranial pole of the kidney as viewed from a paralumbar laparoscopic approach.

of the kidneys and craniodorsal to the gonads (Fig. 43.11). During breeding season, these structures may be obscured by the enlarged gonadal tissue. From either air sac can be observed cranially a large ostium leading into the pink lung tissue.

REPRODUCTIVE ANATOMY

The left approach is used for sex determination because, in most avian species, the female oviduct and ovary develop only on this side. The right ovary is normally quiescent and may resemble a small testis located near the right adrenal gland. The avian gonads are located in the intestinal peritoneal cavity. It is therefore necessary when using a lateral approach either to penetrate the air sac–peritoneal interface or to push the membrane against the gonad for visualization. The gonads are located caudal to the lungs and adrenal gland and ventromedial to the cranial pole of the kidney (see Fig. 43.11).

In most birds (except several hawk species), the left testis in the immature bird tends to be larger than the right, although both are much smaller than those of the adult (17). The immature testes are tubular to ellipsoid and are distinctly rounded at both ends (15). In the immature bird, visualization of the right testis through the dorsal mesentery indicates a male. In immature macaws, the ductus deferens is a thin, white, tubular structure, usually about one-third of the diameter of the ureter (19).

The mature testicle is ellipsoid to bean shaped and in most species is creamy white (see Fig. 43.11). However, in several groups of birds (e.g., quail, cockatoos, mynahs, and toucans), testicles may be pigmented, varying from green to gray to black. The amount of color depends on testicular size; larger testicles appear whiter with increased spermatogenesis. Testicular size varies seasonally in many avian species. Some testicles become so large that gonadal identification is made difficult because of the small field of view of the endoscope. Accompanying this size increase is an increased surface vascularization, enlargement of the epididy-

mis, and an increase in the convolutions of the ductus deferens (15).

The juvenile ovary is comma shaped and dorsoventrally flattened. It is closely applied to and partially covering the adrenal gland and cranial pole of the kidney (19). In extremely young macaws (younger than 10 weeks), the ovary has a faintly granular surface with fine sulci. As the bird ages, the sulci deepen, giving the ovary a furrowed appearance resembling that of the cerebral cortex. With maturation, the primary oocytes enlarge, the sulci disappear, and the ovary becomes distinctly granular. The oviduct is pale white with a thicker, more substantial appearance than the vas deferens. In immature macaws, the oviduct was generally two to four times the thickness of the ureter (19). Close inspection of the oviduct often shows spiral bands, which are hypothesized to be spiral folds of the mature oviductal mucosa. A useful anatomic feature for sex determination in the female macaw is the presence of the supporting ligament of the infundibulum (Fig. 43.12). This structure is clearly visible crossing the cranial division of the kidney. In the mature female, the ovary has the appearance of tapioca pudding, with many small follicles visible during the nonbreeding season. Under hormonal influence, these follicles enlarge to give the appearance of a bunch of grapes. A large ovum is occasionally mistaken for a testis.

Caudal Entry Site

Two similar entry sites have been described (12, 15), and both require the uppermost leg to be cranially extended (see Fig. 43.10). The first entry site is delineated by a triangle formed by the proximal femur, the last rib, and the cranial edge of the pubis (12). After making a small skin incision, the trocar and sheath are gently pushed through the underlying muscle at right angles to the abdominal wall (12). Once into the cav-

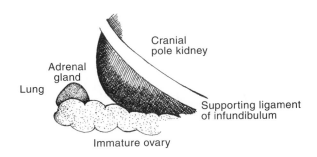

Fig. 43.12. Diagram of an immature parrot ovary showing the geographic relationship of the lung, adrenal gland, gonad, and cranial pole of the kidney as viewed from a paralumbar laparoscopic approach. Note the position of the supporting ligament of the infundibulum, an important aid for sex determination in juvenile parrots. (From Taylor M. A morphologic approach to the endoscopic determination of sex in juvenile macaws. J Assoc Avian Vet 1989;3:199–201.)

ity, the endoscope and sheath are craniodorsally directed for visualization of the organs. In penguins, large fat deposits surround the main viscera and are attached to the walls of the air sacs, making this an impossible approach (12). In one report using this approach, some birds belonging to the orders Ciconiiformes, Falconiformes, Strigiformes, and Psittaciformes were difficult or impossible to sex owing to large visceral fat deposits, peritoneal fluid, or air sac opacity (12).

The second entry site is where the semimembranosus muscle crosses the last rib (15). The ventral fascia is separated from the body wall, the muscle is dorsally reflected, and a blunt entry is made just caudal to the last rib. Placement of the leg forward allows the lateral body wall to be approached more easily without the interference of the femoral musculature.

VISIBLE ANATOMY

The caudal thoracic air sac is entered at or near its caudal border (15), and within it can be visualized the caudal lung and ostium (craniodorsal), the proventriculus (cranioventral), and the liver (cranioventral). The membranes between the caudal thoracic and abdominal (caudodorsal), and the caudal and cranial thoracic air sacs (craniodorsal), can also be observed (15).

Pericloacal Entry Site

A trocar–cannula or blunt entry is made ventral to the ischium and just caudal to the pubis (14) (see Fig. 43.10).

VISIBLE ANATOMY

The endoscope enters the caudal portion of the intestinal peritoneal cavity and is directed cranially to view the gonads and kidney. This approach avoids penetration of air sac walls and is used for biopsy of the caudal kidney.

Sternal Notch Entry Site

The uppermost leg is placed either caudally or cranially depending on the species (20) (see Fig. 43.10). The entry site is at the sternal notch, a V shape formed where the last sternal rib joins the sternum, or slightly dorsal to this site and caudal to the last rib (20). The notch can be palpated as an indentation. During entry, the plane of the trocar–cannula is parallel to the thoracolumbosacral vertebrae with the point of the trocar directed cranially (20). The trocar–cannula is used in birds weighing more than 500 g, whereas in smaller birds or when hepatomegaly is suspected, the laparoscope alone is inserted through the abdominal wall (20).

VISIBLE ANATOMY

The laparoscope first enters the cranial thoracic air sac, from which one can observe the liver (craniodorsal), heart (craniodorsal), lungs (dorsal), and posterior wall of the air sac (caudodorsal) (20). The kidneys and gonads may either be observed directly through the air sac membrane or after its penetration when fat or air sacculitis renders it opaque. Penetration into the intestinal peritoneal cavity also allows visualization of the adrenals (dorsal), ventriculus (dorsal) and proventriculus (craniodorsal), spleen (caudodorsal), and intestines (caudodorsal).

Midline Entry Site

The entry site is in the midline just behind the sternum (see Fig. 43.10).

VISIBLE ANATOMY

Although this approach is used primarily for liver biopsy, it allows good visualization of the heart and pericardium, the caudal borders of both lungs, and the cranial aspects of the abdominal air sacs (21). The avian liver is composed of two main lobes that join cranially in the midline (17). The left and right liver lobes protrude into the left and right ventral hepatic cavities, respectively (17). The left and right ventral hepatic peritoneal cavities are large, elongated cavities extending along the lateroventral body wall from the liver to the caudal body wall (17). To access the liver, one or both of the ventral cavities must be entered either directly or laterally from the caudal thoracic air sac.

Parathoracic Entry Site

This approach is used to access the dorsolateral aspect of the lung (22) (see Fig. 43.10). This is done through the third intercostal space, located by counting cranially from the last (seventh in pigeons) rib (22). The intercostal space is palpated just ventral to the scapula, a small skin incision is made, and the intercostal muscles are bluntly separated to the level of the pleura.

VISIBLE ANATOMY

The laparoscope and sheath are inserted into the incision and are maneuvered between the ribs for visualization of the lung surface. If indicated, a biopsy sample can then be obtained (22).

Biopsy
Equipment

The experienced and confident laparoscopist can, with the appropriate equipment, progress to biopsy collection for culture and histologic examination (23). The

Storz company has developed an endoscope sheath that allows the parallel insertion of flexible biopsy forceps. Forcep biopsy cups come in two forms; the elliptical cup penetrates tissue more readily than the round. For birds larger than 200 g, the 3.0-mm elliptic cup is recommended.

Technique

Organs sampled for biopsy include the lung, air sacs, kidneys, ventriculus, liver, and spleen (9, 22, 23). The technique is the same as described in mammals.

Complications

Hemorrhage

Whenever significant hemorrhage is observed, the procedure is immediately discontinued. A common source of hemorrhage is the cutaneous and subcutaneous tissue including muscle. Good hemostasis before to insertion of the endoscope reduces this seepage and improves visualization. If major hemorrhage occurs, the bird should be placed in an upright position to allow blood to accumulate in the dependent portions of the air sacs. Intravenous or intraosseous administration of fluids or whole blood is indicated when large volumes of blood are lost.

Organ Trauma

An organ can be pierced by either the trocar or the endoscope. This complication is best prevented by controlled and deliberate movement of the endoscope. If the proventriculus is perforated, I recommend removal of the endoscope and administration of a combination of broad-spectrum antibiotics (e.g., amikacin and ampicillin). If a large tear is present, surgical correction will be necessary.

Subcutaneous Emphysema

Subcutaneous emphysema is an uncommon postoperative problem, and it is usually associated with large wounds that allow air to escape from the air sacs. Most openings into the coelomic cavity rapidly seal over once the leg is returned to the normal position. When the emphysema is not severe, no treatment is necessary for the first 24 hours. If the problem persists or appears to be worsening, a pressure bandage, depending on the site, may be adequate to resolve the problem. If this is not successful, sutures will be required to close the body wall and overlying muscles.

Air Sac and Peritoneal Bacterial Infections

Air sac and peritoneal granulomas or abscesses are uncommon and usually result from contamination during laparoscopy. Granulomas, coelomitis, or air sacculitis should be suspected in the weeks after a procedure if a bird becomes anorectic, loses weight, or has persistent to increasing heterophilia with increased radioopaque densities in the coelomic cavity. Granulomas may develop coincidentally. Fungal and mycobacterial granulomas usually stimulate marked heterophilia (more than 30,000 cells/μL). However, this is also observed in chlamydiosis. Chronic bacterial infections rarely initiate heterophilias of more than 20,000 cells/μL. Suspicion of a granuloma is an indication for surgical biopsy. Treatment is then based on culture and histologic examination of the biopsy sample. Until aerobic and anaerobic microbial culture results are obtained, the bird should be treated with a broad-spectrum bactericidal antibiotic and itraconazole.

Appendix: Companies Selling Endoscopic Equipment

Olympus Corp.
4 Nevada Dr.
Lake Success, NY 114042–1179

Karl Storz Veterinary Endoscopy—America, Inc.
2220 Edgar Ct.
Ovledo, FL 32765
(800–955–7832)

Richard Wolf Medical Instruments Corp.
7046 Lyndon Ave.
Rosemont, IL 60018

References

1. Harrison GJ. Endoscopic examination of avian gonadal tissues. Vet Med Small Anim Clin 1978;73:479–484.
2. Ingram KA. Laparotomy technique for sex determination of psittacine birds. J Am Vet Med Assoc 1978;173:1244–1246.
3. Ingram KA. Otoscopic technique for sexing birds. In: Kirk RW, ed. Current veterinary therapy VII. Philadelphia: WB Saunders, 1980:656–658.
4. Low R. Parrots: their care and breeding. 3rd ed. London: Blandford Press, 1992.
5. Clubb SL. Sex determination techniques. In: Harrison GJ, Harrison LR, eds. Clinical avian medicine and surgery. Philadelphia: WB Saunders, 1986:613–619.
6. Halverson J. What do I tell my clients about DNA fingerprinting? In: Proceedings of the Association of Avian Veterinarians Annual Conference. Nashville, TN. Association of Avian Veterinarians, 1993:27–29.
7. Julian RJ. Ascites in poultry. Avian Pathol 1993;22:419–454.
8. Lumeij JT. Gastroenterology. In: Ritchie BW, Harrison GJ, Harrison LR, eds. Avian medicine: principles and application. Lake Worth, FL: Wingers, 1994:482–521.
9. Kollias GV. Avian endoscopy. In: Jacobson ER, Kollias GV, eds. Exotic animals. New York: Churchill Livingstone, 1988:75–106.
10. Bailey RE. Surgery for sexing and observing gonad condition in birds. Auk 1953:497–499.
11. Risser AC. A technique for performing laparotomy on small birds. Condor 1971:376–379.

12. Jones DM, Samour JH, Knight JA, et al. Sex determination of monomorphic birds by fibreoptic endoscopy. Vet Rec 1984; 115:596–598.

13. Bush M, Wildt DE, Kennedy S, et al. Laparoscopy in zoological medicine. 1978;173:1081–1087.

14. Taylor M. Endoscopy: practical lab. In: Proceedings of the Association of Avian Veterinarians Annual Conference. Phoenix, AZ. Association of Avian Veterinarians, 1990:319–324.

15. Taylor M. Endoscopic examination and biopsy techniques. In: Ritchie BW, Harrison GJ, Harrison LR, eds. Avian medicine: principles and application. Lake Worth, FL: Wingers, 1994: 327–354.

16. Harrison GJ. Endoscopy. In: Harrison GJ, Harrison LR, eds. Clinical avian medicine and surgery. Philadelphia: WB Saunders, 1986:234–244.

17. King AS, McLelland J. Birds: their structure and function. 2nd ed. Philadelphia: Bailliere Tindall, 1984.

18. McDonald SE. Endoscopic examination. In: Burr EW, ed. Companion bird medicine. Ames, IA: Iowa State University Press, 1987:166–174.

19. Taylor M. A morphologic approach to the endoscopic determination of sex in juvenile macaws. J Assoc Avian Vet 1989; 3:199–201.

20. Bush M. Laparoscopy in birds and reptiles. In: Harrison RM, Wildt DE, eds. Animal laparoscopy. Baltimore: Williams & Wilkins, 1980:183–197.

21. Kollias GV. Liver biopsy techniques in avian clinical practice. Vet Clin North Am Small Anim Pract 1984;14:287–298.

22. Hunter DB, Taylor M. Lung biopsy as a diagnostic technique in avian medicine. In: Proceedings of the Association of Avian Veterinarians Annual Conference. New Orleans, LA. Association of Avian Veterinarians, 1992:207–211.

23. Taylor M. Biopsy techniques in avian medicine. In: Proceedings of the Association of Avian Veterinarians Annual Conference. Philadelphia, PA. Association of Avian Veterinarians, 1995:275–280.

Suggested Readings

King AS, McLelland J. Birds: their structure and function. 2nd ed. Philadelphia: Bailliere Tindall, 1984.

Kollias GV. Avian endoscopy. In: Jacobson ER, Kollias GV, eds. Exotic animals. New York: Churchill Livingstone, 1988:75–106.

Taylor M. Endoscopic examination and biopsy techniques. In: Ritchie BW, Harrison GJ, Harrison LR, eds. Avian medicine: principles and application. Lake Worth, FL: Wingers, 1994: 327–354.

Surgery of Pet Ferrets

Neal L. Beeber

In recent years, the domestic ferret has had a dramatic increase in popularity. In 1990, the number of pet ferrets in the United States was estimated to be more than 7 million (1). As these animals have increased in popularity, they have become more common in veterinary practices. This discussion deals with some of the more common surgical procedures in ferrets.

Preparation and Fasting

Healthy ferrets make excellent surgical candidates. They are hardy, and with attention to certain parameters, they do not present any unusual anesthetic risks.

The intestinal tract is short, resulting in a gastrointestinal transit time of 3 to 4 hours (2). For this reason, patients are only fasted for 4 to 5 hours before surgery, except in the case of insulinoma resection, for which the fast is 3 hours.

Sedation and Anesthesia

Isoflurane is the anesthetic of choice; however, halothane can also be used, except in critically ill patients. A nonrebreathing system is used with a flow rate of 0.6 to 1.0 L per minute. No premedication is required. In many cases, ferrets can be masked until they are sufficiently anesthetized to allow endotracheal intubation. This can usually be accomplished with a flow rate of 2 L and a 4 to 5% isoflurane concentration. The animal relaxes in 2 to 5 minutes. Because struggling or excitement is minimal, chamber induction is not usually necessary. Maintenance level of isoflurane is 1.75 to 2.5%. It is often necessary to use a small amount of lidocaine (0.1 mL) to paralyze the larynx to accomplish intubation, as in the feline species. All ferrets are intubated except for the most minor procedures. Use of 1.5- to 4.5-French endotracheal tubes is sufficient for most ferrets. If the tubes are allowed to become cold in a refrigerator, they will become stiff and more easily introduced into the trachea. Because ferrets vary in body size, several tube sizes should be available. Some breeding establishments have been importing European ferrets, which are generally larger than the American breeds and commonly weigh up to 5 to 6 lb. These ferrets need slightly larger endotracheal tubes. Whenever possible, a cuffed tube is recommended.

Ketamine and diazepam–ketamine combinations can be used as a preanesthetic, for intubation, or for short procedures intramuscularly at a dose of 10 to 20 mg/kg for ketamine and 1 to 2 mg/kg for diazepam. In my opinion, acepromazine should not be used in ferrets because of this agent's vasodilatative properties and the possibility of heat loss. Ferrets should be placed on a warm water recirculating system to prevent heat loss, and any intravenous fluids to be administered should be warmed to 85 to 90°F. The patient's rectal temperature should be monitored during the surgical procedure. A simple and inexpensive way to accomplish this is to use a digital outdoor thermometer available commercially for under $15 (indoor–outdoor thermometer, Radio Shack catalog No. 63–854). The probe can be inserted directly into the rectum or attached to a red rubber catheter as a stylet.

Except for a routine spay, neuter, or other minor procedure, a 24-gauge intravenous catheter (Baxter Quickcath 24-gauge 1.6 cm) should be placed for all surgical procedures. The cephalic vein is the most common site for placement, but lateral saphenous, jugular, and intraosseous catheters can also be used. When a jugular catheter is necessary, a 24-gauge cephalic catheter can be placed in the jugular vein. The types of fluids administered depend on the type of surgical procedure performed and are discussed under the appropriate section. Ferrets are monitored with a pulse oximeter, which works well in this species. Recovery time depends on the animal's condition and length of anesthesia; however, when isoflurane is used alone, recovery is remarkably fast and smooth.

General Surgical Considerations

Ferret skin is tougher than dog or cat skin, so slightly more pressure may need to be exerted. One often sees a thick subcutaneous fat layer, which should be dissected bluntly. The lineal alba is readily apparent. A stab incision should be made into the abdominal cavity and extended. Care should be taken to avoid the spleen because it is often large in this species. Most common types of sutures can be used depending on the operation performed. I prefer to close the abdomen with 4–0 polydioxanone (PDS), polypropylene (Prolene), or nylon. Most nonabsorbable suture material with a cutting needle can be used for skin sutures. Ferrets rarely chew external sutures.

Ovariohysterectomy

Most ferrets sold as pets in the United States are neutered before 6 or 7 weeks of age, so ovariohysterectomy is not a common procedure, as in dogs and cats. Ferrets should be spayed by 6 months of age, however, if they are not to be used for breeding. Ferrets are induced ovulators. If they are allowed to remain in estrus, potentially fatal bone marrow suppression may result from estrogen toxicity. Medical treatments to terminate estrus are available (3); however, spaying is recommended.

The surgical procedure is similar to that for cats. The ferret is placed in dorsal recumbency, and the abdomen is shaved and prepared. A 3- to 4-cm midline incision is made 1 cm posterior to the umbilicus. Blunt dissection is used to dissect through the fat layer and subcutaneous tissue to expose the linea alba. An incision is made through the linea and is extended. Usually, a layer of fat is encountered. The uterus of ferrets is bicornate, as in cats. The uterus can be elevated by using a spay hook, or sometimes it can be seen lying just under the incision by bluntly moving the fat. The uterus of the ferret is not nearly as friable as that of the rabbit. Ferrets have a high degree of body fat, and the ovarian tissue and vessels may be obscured. The surgeon must be certain to ligate the ovarian vessels completely using 2–0 or 3–0 gut. The uterus is easily exteriorized and the suspensory ligament is readily torn. The uterus is ligated with gut and is removed. The abdomen can be closed with any of several suture types in a simple interrupted pattern using 4–0 monofilament absorbable or nonabsorbable material. The same suture or gut can be used for the subcutaneous or subcuticular layer. The skin can be closed with 3–0 or 4–0 nylon. Chewing of sutures has not been a problem. If the surgical procedure is performed in the morning, the ferret is released the same day. Postoperative antibiotics are not necessary. Skin sutures are removed in 7 to 10 days.

Orchiectomy

Like ovariohysterectomy, orchiectomy (castration) is usually done in young ferrets before they are sold to pet stores. For this reason, the average practitioner is not called on to perform this operation routinely. If an intact male ferret is presented, the owners should be encouraged to have the ferret castrated. In some cases, intact male ferrets are more aggressive, especially if intact females are nearby. The main objection to intact males is the heavy musky odor they produce. Many times, castration alone is enough to control odor, making descenting unnecessary. Testicular tumors have been reported, but a true incidence is difficult to estimate because most domestic ferrets are neutered (4, 5).

Castration in the ferret is similar to castration in the dog. The ferret is placed in dorsal recumbency, and the prescrotal area is shaved. One prescrotal incision is made through which both testicles may be exteriorized. An open or closed method can be used. The spermatic cord and vessels are ligated with 4–0 gut, are incised, and are allowed to retract into the incision. The subcutaneous tissue is closed with gut, and the skin is closed with 4–0 nonabsorbable suture, which is removed in 7 to 10 days. Chewing the sutures has not been a problem. Alternatively, two incisions can be made in the scrotum, and the vessels can be clamped and ligated with 4–0 chromic gut. With this method, the scrotal incisions are not closed, similar to the procedure in cats. The ferrets are released the same day.

Adrenalectomy

Adrenal tumors are among the most common neoplasms of ferrets. In our practice, adrenalectomy is the single most common surgical procedure performed in these animals, followed by insulinoma resection. In a retrospective study performed at our hospital and the Animal Medical Center from 1987 to 1991, the following types and frequency of biopsy results were recorded: adrenocortical adenoma, 64%; nodular adrenocortical hyperplasia, 26%; and adrenocortical carcinoma, 10%. In the patients with adrenocortical carcinoma, no gross or microscopic evidence of metastasis was seen. In addition, 70% of the cases occurred in females (6). Since this study, I have had the opportunity to operate on many more cases and have found that the biopsy percentage has shifted to adrenocortical adenoma, hyperplasia now accounts for 95% of the cases, and the ratio of males to females has equalized. In addition, the earlier study found that 64% of ferrets had disease of the left adrenal gland, 20% had disease of the right gland, and 16% had bilateral disease. In the years after the study, my colleagues and I have seen left-sided disease in 75% of patients, right-sided disease in 15%, and bilateral disease in 10%.

Clinical signs, in order of decreasing frequency, are vulvar swelling, alopecia, pruritus, polydipsia, and polyuria. The diagnosis is based on clinical signs and abdominal ultrasonography. The accuracy of the ultrasound diagnosis depends on the experience of the ultrasonagrapher. Recently, a study indicated that the concentrations of certain plasma steroid hormones can be used as a marker for the disease (7). Even though the clinical signs may indicate the presence of an adrenal tumor, the clinician should obtain a presurgical ultrasound study whenever possible. This examination helps to rule out other causes of the clinical signs and indicates which adrenal gland is diseased. This distinction becomes important because removal of the right gland is technically more difficult, owing to its location under the caudate liver lobe and its proximity to the vena cava. The differential diagnosis of adrenal gland disease includes ovarian remnants, an intact female reproductive tract, pheochromocytoma, seasonal hair loss of ferrets, nutritional deficiencies (8, 9), mycosis fungoides (10), and infestation by external parasites. I have also seen a ferret with cutaneous *Malassezia pachydermatis* infection that caused generalized hair loss. Adrenal disease in ferrets is not the same as Cushing's disease because the clinical signs and pathologic changes are not caused by an increase in plasma cortisol concentration.

Preparation

After the diagnosis is made, a complete blood screen and chemistry panel should be evaluated for each patient. Any abnormalities should be investigated and treated preoperatively. One of the most common abnormalities is hypoglycemia because many ferrets concurrently have insulin-secreting tumors of the pancreas. Because these islet cell tumors are generally malignant, the prognosis should be discussed with the owners before proceeding. In addition, an in-hospital blood glucose determination should be made immediately before anesthesia is induced, to make certain the blood sugar is still normal after the presurgical fasting period. Another important presurgical consideration is the possibility of underlying cardiac disease. Both hypertrophic and dilated forms of cardiomyopathy are seen in ferrets (11). At this time, clients are advised that a presurgical echocardiogram should be performed if possible. If this is not feasible, chest radiographs and careful cardiac auscultation should be performed. Every patient undergoing adrenalectomy receives an intravenous catheter. Various fluid types may be used; however, if one has any question about the presence of an insulinoma, 5% dextrose is the fluid of choice. Each patient receives a presurgical injection of antibiotics.

Left Adrenalectomy

The ferret is placed in dorsal recumbency, and the abdomen is shaved from the area of the xiphoid cartilage to the inguinal area. An incision is made starting 1 to 2 cm from the xiphoid and extending 4 to 5 cm caudally. After dissecting through the fat and subcutaneous tissue, a stab incision is made in the linea alba and is extended with scissors. A self-retaining Gelpi retractor should be used for good exposure. As in other species, a complete abdominal exploratory operation should be performed. It is especially important to check the pancreas for the possibility of insulinoma nodules (see later). In addition, all male ferrets should be examined for the presence of paraurethral cysts (discussed later). The surgeon generally must retract the spleen and intestines toward the right side of the ferret's body. A laparotomy pad soaked in warm saline can be used to hold structures away from the surgical site. Alternately, the spleen and small intestines can be exteriorized through the incision and placed to the right. This maneuver pulls the mesentery away from the area of the adrenal gland and affords excellent exposure. Any exteriorized tissues should be covered with a warm moist lap pad to prevent tissue drying. The left adrenal gland is located just medial and proximal to the left kidney. This gland is located within a fat pad, and if diseased, it is usually irregular in shape and readily seen. In some cases, one sees a brownish–yellow discoloration. Digital palpation reveals the presence or borders of the mass. The dissection is begun on the medial side of the gland through the fat layer using Mayo scissors and is continued bluntly with mosquito forceps and sterile cotton-tipped applicators. The gland is gently elevated as the dissection is continued. The small blood vessels in the fat generally do not have to be ligated. The adrenolumbar vein runs laterally and caudally from the ventral surface of the adrenal gland. It can be seen as the gland is elevated. This vessel is ligated using 4–0 chromic gut or a surgical clip (Hemoclip). The gland is continually elevated and dissected until a suture can be placed below it.

The tissue is then incised, and the gland is removed. Closure is the same as for an ovariohysterectomy. Because this is a major abdominal procedure, patients are hospitalized for 1 to 2 days postoperatively. Amoxicillin oral suspension at a dose of 10 mg/lb is dispensed for 7 days.

Right Adrenalectomy

As mentioned previously, removal of the right adrenal gland is a technically more difficult procedure. After entry into the abdominal cavity, and a general exploratory operation, the spleen and intestines are moved to the left or are exteriorized. The right adrenal gland is located under the caudate liver lobe. The hepatorenal ligament must be incised to elevate the tip of the liver lobe. The lobe is then reflected cranially. The adrenal gland is usually directly adhered to the vena cava (Fig. 43.13). One must be careful to avoid lacerating this major vessel. The surgeon begins shelling out the gland by sharp dissection of the surface furthest from the vena cava and continues around the gland using iris scissors, mosquito forceps, and sterile cotton swabs. When the gland is mostly peeled away, a Hemoclip or a ligature using 5–0 absorbable suture is placed between the gland and the vena cava. Any remaining glandular tissue is trimmed using the iris scissors. One should have available 5–0 and 7–0 suture as well as sterile sponges (Gelfoam) in the event that the vena cava is lacerated. When one is certain that all hemorrhage has been controlled, closure is as described earlier.

Bilateral Adrenal Disease

When both adrenal glands are abnormal, the surgeon removes the left entirely and debulks the right. If incised, the adrenal gland bleeds profusely. One begins

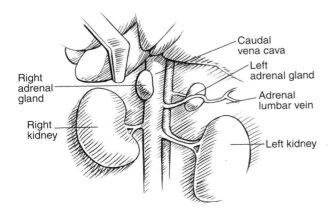

Fig. 43.13. Appearance of the adrenal glands. The caudate lobe of the liver has been reflected cranially. The right adrenal gland usually adheres to the vena cava.

dissecting the gland and places a crushing suture around the part that has been freed, using 4–0 or 5–0 monofilament absorbable or nonabsorbable material. Iris scissors can then be used to cut above the suture. The surgeon removes 50 to 75% of the right adrenal tissue.

Complications

The most common complication of adrenalectomy is prolonged or difficult recovery resulting from hypoglycemia secondary to an undiagnosed insulin-secreting tumor of the pancreas. In fact, when ferrets are referred to my practice for postsurgical problems, low blood glucose concentrations are frequently found. For this reason, a blood glucose determination is performed before the surgical procedure and 1 to 2 hours postoperatively. Many times, fluids containing dextrose are used as a precaution. Ferrets are encouraged to eat after they are fully awake, and Deliver (Deliver 2.0, Mead Johnson Nutritionals, Evansville, IN) is often administered orally within 3 to 4 hours postoperatively. Vomiting has not been a problem.

Another problem commonly encountered is hypothermia. Intravenous fluids should be warmed before administration. We use a warm water heating pad and heat lamp during and after surgery. Ferrets are generally hardy and are good surgical candidates. Postoperative infections appear to be rare.

Even with the removal of the left adrenal gland and part of the right, most patients do not appear to require hormonal supplementation. Vital signs in these ferrets should be monitored closely in the immediate postoperative period. If recovery is prolonged or if the patient is doing poorly, a blood glucose determination should be made. If the blood glucose level is normal, corticosteroids can be administered, and blood can be saved for a resting cortisol level to ascertain the need for continued cortisone supplementation.

Paraurethral Cysts

One problem encountered with male ferrets with adrenal disease is the presence of paraurethral cysts. Animals with this condition present with dysuria or total blockage along with other signs of adrenal disease. The cysts are thought to arise from prostatic tissue that has been stimulated by the hormones released from the adrenal gland. These cysts are present just caudal to the bladder and can usually be felt by external abdominal palpation (Fig. 43.14). If the urinary tract is totally obstructed, the blockage must be relieved. This procedure can be challenging because the penis is difficult to catheterize as a result of the os penis. I have been most successful using a tomcat catheter or 3-French red rubber catheter. At the present time, the best treat-

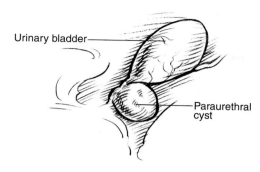

Fig. 43.14. A paraurethral cyst around the neck of the urinary bladder.

ment appears to be adrenalectomy. In addition, one should attempt to aspirate material from the cyst during the surgical procedure using a 22-gauge needle and a 3-mL syringe. The material in the cysts appears flocculent. Because the cysts are usually multiloculated, a few attempts should be made into different areas. Leakage from the cysts after this procedure has not been a problem. The cysts regress after the adrenal tumor has been removed. The ferret is kept on postoperative antibiotics for 14 days. In a few cases, cysts that have not regressed and that cause reobstruction need to be marsupialized. In severe cases, prescrotal or perineal urethrostomies can be performed. In these patients, the cysts should regress after 3 to 4 weeks of antibiotic therapy.

Prognosis

The prognosis for patients undergoing adrenalectomy is excellent. It is the treatment of choice for this condition. In females, the swollen vulva may begin to shrink within 1 to 2 days. Hair loss takes longer to resolve. My impression is that the longer the interval between the onset of clinical signs and surgery (and usually the more extensive the alopecia), the longer the hair takes to regrow. Clinical signs return in some patients, and a second surgical procedure will be needed to remove the other gland, which has since become diseased.

Insulinoma

As previously mentioned, insulinoma surgery is the second most common procedure performed in my practice. Signs are due to hypoglycemia and range from ferrets who begin to sleep more and seem lethargic, act nauseated, and paw at their mouths, to episodes of "vacant expressions" and staring into space, to hind limb weakness and collapse, to seizures and coma. Signs can be intermittent and can resolve quickly. Because this disease is commonly seen in ferrets over 3 years of age, early signs may be interpreted

as normal aging. Diagnosis is based on the demonstration of low blood glucose concentrations and hyperinsulinemia. After a 3-hour fast, normal blood glucose should be above 80 mg/dL. Levels below 65 mg/dL suggest the diagnosis. Prolonged anorexia or starvation can produce a blood glucose level this low, but the presence of an insulinoma is much more common. Many times, the blood glucose level is below 50 mg/dL. Blood glucose levels between 65 and 80 mg/dL are suggestive of this diagnosis, and the fast should be continued for another 1 to 2 hours and an insulin level checked. An abnormally high insulin level along with low blood glucose is diagnostic.

Often, treatment begins with medical intervention. It is effective in the early course of the disease and has been used for 3 months to 2 years. Therapy is begun with prednisone at a dose of 0.5 to 2 mg/kg. The dose can be increased over time to keep clinical signs under control. Diazoxide (Proglycem), at a dose of 5 to 10 mg/kg, can be added to the prednisone regimen. It inhibits insulin release and stimulates hepatic gluconeogenesis (12). Sometimes, the dose of prednisone can be lowered when diazoxide is added. Side effects in other species include vomiting and anorexia, but these effects are rare in ferrets. The easiest form to administer is the suspension, which is expensive.

Owners are instructed to feed ferrets with insulinomas frequently. Owners are also instructed to avoid high sugar or carbohydrate-containing supplements unless treating a hypoglycemic episode. These foods or treats can stimulate insulin secretion and can cause rebound hypoglycemia. These ferrets should be fed a high-quality ferret or cat food containing an animal protein source. Brewer's yeast should be added to the diet at a rate of one-quarter teaspoon twice daily because it is a good source of chromium, which helps to stabilize blood glucose and insulin levels in humans (13). Deliver makes an excellent supplement because of its high fat content and acceptance by almost every ferret. Medical treatment is indicated in ferrets that are poor surgical candidates or whose owners decline surgery for their pet. Clients should be informed that the β cell tumors are almost always malignant, and surgical treatment appears to slow the progression of the disease. Many ferrets become normoglycemic at least for a time after surgery. Clinical impression is that ferrets seem to do better for longer with a combination of surgical and medical treatment. In dogs with insulinomas, surgical treatment prolongs life span over medical management alone (14).

Surgery is generally recommended in ferrets younger than 5 or 6 years of age. All ferrets should be carefully screened for other diseases, especially cardiac disease. As mentioned in the discussion of adrenal surgery, a cardiac ultrasound study is recommended as a presurgical screen. Often, surgery is performed concurrently for adrenal disease and insulinoma. Presurgical fasting is usually limited to 3 to 4 hours. An intravenous catheter is placed in all cases, and warmed 5% dextrose is administered during the surgical procedure.

As with adrenal surgery, a midline incision is made, and a standard exploratory operation is performed. I have seen metastasis of β cell carcinoma to the spleen and liver. In patients with splenic metastasis, splenectomy was performed. Most commonly multiple, and infrequently solitary, nodules are present. The entire pancreas should be inspected visually and also palpated. The nodules usually appear as raised areas that may be lighter in color. Sometimes, the nodules are not evident visually, yet they are firmer than the surrounding tissue, so careful digital palpation is imperative. In most cases, blunt dissection enables the surgeon to shell out the affected areas. Some minimal bleeding occurs, but it usually stops with pressure or Gelfoam application. In some cases, 5–0 or 6–0 polyglycolic acid (Dexon), polyglactin 910 (Vicryl), or polydioxanone (PDS) can be used to ligate larger vessels. If numerous nodules are present, a partial pancreatectomy can be performed. The previously listed absorbable suture can be used to ligate the pancreatic tissue in a crushing manner. If the area is small enough, one circumferential ligature can be placed around the area to be removed, or the suture can be placed in the center of the area and transfixed in both directions (Fig. 43.15). In this manner, less tissue is included in each tie. Pancreatitis does not seem to be a problem after surgery.

Blood glucose should be measured postoperatively and at reasonable intervals during recovery. Some ferrets become normoglycemic 1 to 2 days postoperatively. In many cases, I observe only a slight increase in measured blood glucose, although the ferrets appear to improve clinically. Often, medical management must be continued. Some patients have postoperative hyperglycemia, which is usually transient and resolves with 3 to 5 days.

The surgeon must inform clients that this is a malignant neoplasm (15), and a cure should not be expected. One should also be sure that clients understand that medical intervention may need to be continued or resumed as the disease progresses. Even with all these caveats, I believe, based on many cases, that a combination of surgical and medical management yields the best results for the longest period.

Foreign Body Surgery

Foreign body ingestion by ferrets is common, especially in young animals. The most common materials are pieces of a ferret's plastic or rubber toys. For this reason, I recommend that owners do not provide ferrets with the soft squeaky toys commonly sold for use by ferrets or with toys made of any other material soft enough to be chewed apart. Hard nylon (Nylabone-type) toys are acceptable. Other foreign bodies seen include trichobezoar, pieces of foam rubber, cork, the hard ends of shoe laces, and almost anything one could imagine.

Clinical signs include anorexia, vomiting, diarrhea, and weakness. In general, ferrets do not exhibit vomiting as often as dogs and cats, but they appear nauseated by stretching the neck and retching, salivating, and pawing at the mouth.

Diagnosis is made by history, abdominal palpation, and plain and contrast radiography. Ferrets often exhibit pain on abdominal palpation. In my experience, ferrets with trichobezoars exhibit less severe clinical signs. The most common location for foreign bodies is the small intestine, but they may also be located in the stomach or esophagus (16, 17).

In some cases, endoscopy may be helpful to remove esophageal and gastric foreign bodies. I use a pediatric bronchoscope. The diameter is too large to be useful for the small intestine.

Surgical Procedure

In many cases, ferrets with foreign body ingestion exhibit anorexia and are dehydrated. Therefore, adequate rehydration is important. Surgery should be considered an emergency and performed as soon as possible. A standard midline approach is used, and a complete examination of the intestinal tract is performed to check for multiple foreign bodies. In patients with esophageal or proximal duodenal obstruction, the surgeon should retropulse the material into the stomach and perform a simple gastrotomy. Gastric surgery

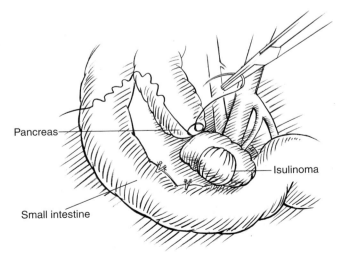

Fig. 43.15. Transfixation and removal of a portion of the pancreas containing a nodule of moderate size.

Pancreas

Small intestine

Isulinoma

is similar to that in the dog or cat. Closure is accomplished with a double-layer simple interrupted pattern using 4–0 absorbable material.

Because of the small diameter and fragility of the intestines, gentle tissue handling is important, to minimize stricture of the surgical site. The incision is made on the antimesenteric border and is closed with 4–0 or 5–0 monofilament nonreactive suture in a simple interrupted pattern. Because of its handling characteristics, I prefer 5–0 polydioxanone (PDS). If the section of intestine appears devitalized, an intestinal resection and anastomosis should be performed. The procedure is the same as in dogs and cats. The surgical site and abdomen should be flushed completely with warmed saline solution. The omentum should be placed over the area to aid healing. Closure is routine, and as in all gastrointestinal surgery, care must be taken to avoid contamination.

Ferrets are offered water and Deliver about 12 hours postoperatively, and they are encouraged to eat solid food within 24 hours. Intravenous fluids should be continued until the patient is eating well.

References

1. Rupprecht CE, Gilbert J, Pitts R, et al. Evaluation of an inactivated rabies virus vaccine in domestic ferrets. J Am Vet Med Assoc 1990;193:1614–1616.
2. An NQ, Evans HE. Anatomy of the ferret. In: Fox JG, ed. Biology and diseases of the ferret. Philadelphia: Lea & Febiger, 1988:100–134.
3. Bernard, SL, Leathers, CW, Brobst, DF, et al. Estrogen induced bone marrow depression in ferrets. Am J Vet Res 1983;44:657.
4. Meschter CL. Interstitial cell adenoma in a ferret. Lab Anim Sci 1989;39:353–354.
5. Goad MEP, Fox JG. Neoplasia in ferrets. In: Fox JG, ed. Biology and diseases of the ferret. Philadelphia: Lea & Febiger, 1988:278–280.
6. Rosenthal KL, Peterson ME, Quesenberry KE, et al. Hyperadrenocorticism associated with adrenocortical tumor or nodular hyperplasia of the adrenal gland in ferrets: 50 cases (1987–1991). J Am Vet Med Assoc 1993;203:271–275.
7. Rosenthal KL, Peterson ME. Evaluation of plasma androgen and estrogen concentrations in ferrets with hyperadrenocorticism. J Am Vet Med Assoc 1996;209:1097–1102.
8. Ryland LM, Bernard SL. A clinical guide to the pet ferret. Compend Contin Educ Pract Vet 1983;5:25–32.
9. Ryland LM, Gorham JR. The ferret and its diseases. J Am Vet Med Assoc 1978;173:1154–1158.
10. Rosenbaum MR, Affolter VK, Usborne AL, et al. Cutaneous epitheliotropic lymphoma in a ferret. J Am Vet Med Assoc 1996;209:1441–1444.
11. Stamoulis ME, Miller MS. Cardiovascular diseases. In: Hillyer EV, Quisenberry KE, eds. Ferrets, rabbits, and rodents: clinical medicine and surgery. Philadelphia: WB Saunders, 1997:67–68.
12. Feldman EC, Nelson RW. Canine and feline endocrinology and reproduction. Philadelphia: WB Saunders, 1987:259, 304–327.
13. Balch JF, Balch PA. Prescription for nutritional healing. Garden Park City: Avery, NY. 1990:18–19, 211–213.
14. Leifer CE, Peterson ME, Matus RE. Insulin secreting tumor: diagnosis and medical and surgical management in 55 dogs. J Am Vet Med Assoc 1986;188:60–64.
15. Caplan ER, Peterson ME, Mullen HS, et al. Surgical treatment of insulin secreting pancreatic islet cell tumors in 49 ferrets: ACVS abstract. Vet Surg 1995;24:422.
16. Caligiuri R, Bellah JR, Collins BR, et al. Medical and surgical management of esophageal foreign body in a ferret. J Am Vet Med Assoc 1989;195:969–971.
17. Mullen HS, Scavelli TD, Quesenberry KE, et al. Gastrointestinal foreign body in ferrets: 25 cases (1986–1990). J Am Anim Hosp Assoc 1992;28:13–19.

Anal Sac Resection in the Ferret

James E. Creed

The ferret is a popular house pet; however, odor emitted from the anal sacs of both sexes is often objectionable. Like nearly all carnivores (1) and all mustelids (2), the ferret has an anal sac on each side of the anus. The ducts open at 4 o'clock and 8 o'clock positions on the inner cutaneous zone of the anus, adjacent to the mucocutaneous junction. The sacs are interposed between the internal and external anal sphincter muscles. Material stored within the sac is secreted by a glandular complex surrounding the neck of the sac and 3 to 4 mm of the duct. This complex is evident without magnification, but a binocular loupe enhances visualization. The sebaceous gland component surrounding the distal part of the duct is covered asymmetrically by an apocrine gland component (3). Surgical removal of the anal sacs and their ducts eliminates the odor of anal sac secretions, but some odor from sebaceous and apocrine tubular glands in the perianal region typically persists.

Indications

Client request is the principal indication for performing this procedure. However, veterinarians should recommend this operation for all ferrets at 6 to 8 months of age to make them more acceptable pets. Neutering should be recommended at this age in ferrets of both sexes to reduce odor further. Neutering also prevents development of aplastic anemia in nonbreeding females, which can develop from hyperestrinism associated with prolonged estrus (3, 4). The client must be made aware that anal sac resection and neutering do not eliminate all "musky" odor, because of sebaceous and apocrine glands in the ferret's perianal skin.

Preoperative Considerations

In addition to a complete physical examination, the patient's packed cell volume of blood and total serum protein level should be determined. One study of 11 healthy male ferrets reported an average packed cell volume of 52.4% and average total serum protein of 6.0 g/dL (3). Food should be withheld for 12 hours. Anesthesia is induced with oxygen and an appropriate gaseous agent in an anesthesia chamber; it can be maintained with a mask or an endotracheal tube 2.5 mm in inner diameter (12-French outer diameter, Cole, Intermountain Veterinary Supply, N. Kansas City, MO). An alternate method is intramuscular injection of ketamine hydrochloride (26 mg/kg) and acepromazine (0.2 to 0.3 mg/kg) (5).

The ferret may be positioned for anal gland resection in dorsal or ventral recumbency. Because neutering is frequently performed and is best accomplished in dorsal recumbency, all ferrets should be positioned in this way, to provide consistent orientation of anatomic structures. The ferret is placed at the end of a table on a sandbag or similar pad to prevent loss of body heat, with its pelvic limbs pulled craniad and its tail dropped. The scrotal or ventral abdomen and perianal regions are prepared and draped for the surgical procedure. Aseptic neutering is accomplished, and then the surgical drape is shifted to expose the anal region.

Surgical Technique

A binocular loupe should be used to locate the minute opening of each anal sac duct and to aid visualization throughout the procedure. The opening of each duct and the surrounding 2 mm of skin and mucous membrane are grasped with mosquito forceps. A circumferential incision is made with a No. 15 Bard–Parker scalpel blade immediately distal to the forceps tip; one must be careful not to incise too deeply. Using a gentle scraping action with the blade, skin and mucosa are reflected from the duct (Fig. 43.16). The glandular complex surrounding the terminal 3 to 4 mm of the duct makes dissection difficult (Fig. 43.16, C). This complex has a nodular surface, with skeletal muscle fibers inserting into the glandular tissue. One should not attempt to find a fascial plane at this level, and dissection should be superficial with respect to overlying tissue. Shifting the mosquito forceps to clamp them across skin, mucous membrane, and terminal duct should prevent tearing the duct as caudal traction is applied with the forceps (Fig. 43.16, E). Applying another forceps parallel to the first provides even more support.

A fascial plane is encountered as dissection is carried beyond the glandular complex (Fig. 43.16, B). The anal sac can be removed readily by reflecting sphincter muscles off the sac wall with a scraping action of the scalpel blade. Staying on the proper fascial plane not only enhances sac removal, but also minimizes hemorrhage and damage to internal and external anal sphincters. If the fascial plane is followed, little muscle

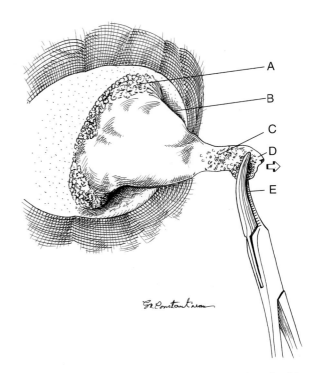

Fig. 43.16. Resection of the anal sac. External anal sphincter muscle (*A*). Wall of the anal sac (*B*). Nodular glandular complex surrounding the duct (*C*). End of the anal sac duct (*D*). Tip of mosquito forceps grasping skin, mucous membrane, and terminal duct (*E*).

will be left on the sac wall. The wall appears yellowish white; it is thin, and glandular secretions are yellow. It is easy to rupture the duct and sac, particularly if the veterinary surgeon is inexperienced. Trying to establish a fascial plane before dissecting beyond the nodular glandular complex is futile and particularly hazardous, because it is easy to cut into the duct lumen. If the duct or sac is incised, surgical extirpation can still be accomplished, but the absence of a distended sac makes the operation more tedious. Odor from an incised or ruptured sac is obnoxious, but not overwhelming.

Intraoperative hemorrhage is negligible, although sterile cotton-tipped applicator sticks work well to clear oozing blood from the surgical field. Placement of sutures and administration of local or systemic antibiotics are not required.

Postoperative Care

The patient is normally discharged when recovery from anesthesia is complete. Although no serious postoperative sequelae have been observed, complications can occur. Persistent minor hemorrhage may develop postoperatively, but this ceases spontaneously. Potential complications include prolapsed rectum and fecal incontinence if trauma to the anal sphincter muscles is excessive. Staying on the proper fascial plane minimizes trauma and the possibility of these serious sequelae.

References

1. Ewer RF. The carnivores. Ithaca, NY: Cornell University Press, 1973:95.
2. Ryland LM, Gorham JR. The ferret and its diseases. J Am Vet Med Assoc 1978;173:1154.
3. Creed JE, Kainer RA. Surgical extirpation and related anatomy of anal sacs of the ferret. J Am Vet Med Assoc 1981;179:575.
4. Kociba GJ, Caputo CA. Aplastic anemia associated with estrus in pet ferrets. J Am Vet Med Assoc 1981;178:1293.
5. Muir WW III, Hubbell JAE. Handbook of veterinary anesthesia. 2nd ed. Philadelphia: Mosby, 1995:368.

Soft Tissue Surgery In Reptiles

R. Avery Bennett

Reptiles have become increasingly popular as pets. Veterinarians are called on to perform various medical and surgical procedures on these animals (1, 2). The anatomy and physiology of reptiles differ from those of the more familiar mammalian patients, and the surgeon must be familiar with these differences. Skin incisions are generally made in the thin, softer tissue between the scales. Healing in this skin is assumed to be more rapid than when an incision is made through the tough scales. A No. 11 scalpel blade is particularly useful for skin incision because its fine tip allows the surgeon to incise with more precision in the zigzag pattern required to cut between scales. In a retrospective report, no difference in healing was seen when the incision for celiotomy in snakes was made through the scutes (large ventral scales) on the midline compared with a lateral incision between scales (5).

The incised skin of most reptiles has a tendency to invert. Because of this, an everting skin closure pattern, such as an interrupted horizontal mattress pattern, is commonly used. Alternatively, skin staples are designed to evert the skin edges slightly when applied and serve nicely for skin closure in reptiles. Reptiles have little subcutaneous tissue, and most incisions are closed with sutures in the deep tissues and skin only. The skin of reptiles is tough and is considered the holding layer for wound security. For example, when closing a celiotomy in an iguana, the body wall muscle is thin and does not hold suture well. No distinct fascia is identified, and the muscle does not easily separate from the skin. A two-layer closure is used with a simple continuous pattern in the body wall and an everting

pattern in the skin, in recognizing that the skin is the holding layer. Sutures are tightened to appose the skin edges gently. Sutures tightened excessively cause necrosis of the skin within the suture and dehiscence of the incision. Reptiles do not traumatize their skin incisions or remove sutures.

The absorption time and tissue reaction associated with various suture materials has not been studied in reptiles; however, chromic catgut has induced granuloma formation and was not absorbed 12 weeks postoperatively (3). For this reason, this suture material is not recommended in reptiles. Synthetic absorbable materials are preferred, but absorption appears to be prolonged compared with mammals. If these absorbable materials are placed in the skin, the surgeon should anticipate that they will require removal. Polyglactin 910 placed in the skin of a common boa constrictor (*Constrictor constrictor*) was intact 4 weeks after placement. Skin suture removal is generally not attempted for at least 4 weeks postoperatively. At that time, incisional healing is assessed by teasing the incision edges gently to determine wound security. Often, only every other suture is removed at 4 weeks, and the remaining sutures are removed 2 to 3 weeks later. Ecdysis (skin shedding) is considered to speed wound healing because during this time the epidermis is metabolically active. Therefore, many surgeons prefer to wait for suture removal until after the subsequent ecdysis. Environmental temperature has an effect on wound healing in reptiles (4). The patient is maintained at the upper end of its preferred optimum temperature range during the recovery period to promote healing. After suture removal, the skin frequently sticks to the incisional scar for several sheds, but this condition eventually resolves.

Anatomy

Before undertaking a surgical procedure in a reptile patient, the surgeon must become familiar with the unique anatomy of the particular family of reptiles to which the patient belongs (1, 2, 5). Anatomic features vary among families of reptiles; for example, crocodilians are considered to have a four-chambered heart, whereas squamates (lizards and snakes) and chelonians (turtles and tortoises) have a three-chambered heart. Variation also exists within a family of reptiles. In green iguanas, the kidneys are normally located within the pelvic canal, whereas in monitor lizards they are within the coelomic cavity.

Some features are consistent across species of reptiles. In general, reptiles do not have a muscular diaphragm and, as such, have a coelomic cavity rather than thoracic and abdominal cavities; however, crocodilians do have a well-developed septum between the thoracic viscera and the abdominal viscera. Reptiles do not have lymph nodes. They do not store fat in the subcutaneous tissue, but they have discrete fat bodies within the coelom. In some species, the spleen and pancreas are intimately associated with each other and form a splenopancreas.

The urinary system of reptiles is substantially different from that of mammals. Reptiles have a renal portal system such that, when the portal vein is open, blood from the caudal half of the body passes through the kidney before reaching the systemic circulation. Urine leaves the kidneys through the ureters, which empty into the cloaca, not the urinary bladder. Urine then travels from the cloaca into the bladder of those species with a urinary bladder (chelonians and some lizards) or into the colon in those species without a bladder (snakes, crocodilians, and some lizards), where absorption and ion exchange occur. Urine does not flow through the reproductive system, and the short urethra only connects the bladder to the cloaca.

The cloaca receives excretions from the ureters, from the colon and urinary bladder in those species with a bladder, and from the reproductive system. Chelonians and crocodilians have a single copulatory organ (penis), whereas squamates have paired copulatory organs called hemipenes (hemipenis, singular). The copulatory organs do not contain tubular structures such as a urethra. Semen travels along a groove in the hemipenis into the cloaca of the female. The female reproductive tract is bilateral in reptiles, with each oviduct having a separate opening into the cloaca.

Celiotomy

The approach for celiotomy in reptiles varies with the family of reptiles. Because reptiles lack a diaphragm, celiotomy can allow access to both thoracic and abdominal viscera.

Lizards and crocodilians have a body structure more similar to that of mammals than do chelonians and snakes. A paramedian incision is recommended in these species because of the ventral abdominal vein. This vein receives blood from the caudal abdominal wall and courses along the ventral midline 2 to 3 mm inside the body wall. It is located between the umbilical scar and the pubic bones and is suspended by a short mesovasorum. Some surgeons prefer a midline approach using meticulous dissection to avoid damaging this large vein (5). Making a paramedian incision 2 to 4 mm lateral to the midline minimizes the risk of lacerating this vessel. This vein may be ligated without consequence (2, 5).

Closure is accomplished using a simple continuous pattern with a synthetic absorbable material on a fine, atraumatic swaged-on needle. Because the muscle of the body wall is thin and tightly adheres to the skin,

care must be taken with suture placement and tension on the suture or tearing through the muscle will occur. Suturing the body wall pulls the skin edges into apposition. Skin staples or an everting pattern of a nonabsorbable material maintain skin apposition.

In laterally compressed lizards, such as chameleons, a flank incision is more appropriate. The incision is initiated 2 to 4 mm caudal to the last rib on one side of the body, through the skin and then through the body wall. Closure is as described previously.

Snakes have organs arranged in a linear configuration. In most cases, the specific organ approached must be identified preoperatively because celiotomy does not allow access to all the viscera (Fig. 43.17). The surgeon must know the location of the specific organ approached and whether ligation or clipping can be performed without consequence to gain the necessary surgical exposure.

The coelomic membrane may be closed at a separate layer or incorporated in the body wall closure. The body wall is a thin, pale muscle that is tightly adhered to the skin. The coelomic membrane is not attached to the skin. The muscle of the body wall is closed with a simple continuous pattern using a synthetic absorbable material on a fine atraumatic needle that also approximates the skin edges. The skin is closed with either skin staples or an everting suture pattern such as a horizontal mattress pattern.

Chelonians present a unique challenge for celiotomy because of their shell. For most procedures, a plastron osteotomy is required. In species with a small plastron, such as snapping turtles and sea turtles, many procedures can be accomplished through a flank incision. Some procedures, such as cystotomy, can be accomplished through this approach in other chelonians (5).

The pelvic bones are avoided during plastron osteotomy to avoid injury to the appendicular skeleton. Radiographs are helpful in assessing the location and extent of the pelvic bones. In most species, osteotomy

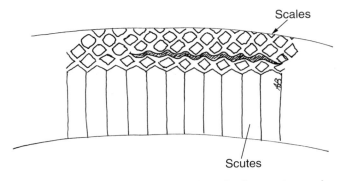

Fig. 43.17. The skin incision for a lateral celiotomy in a snake is made between the first two rows of scales dorsal to the large ventral scales (scutes). The incision is made in the soft skin between the scales.

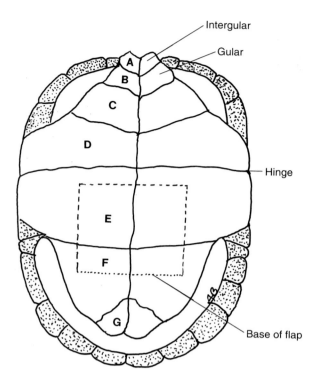

Fig. 43.18. The plastron osteotomy for celiotomy in chelonians is generally made in the femoral (F) and abdominal (E) epidermal shields. If the osteotomy is made too cranially, the heart can be injured, and if too caudally, the pelvic bones can be damaged. *A,* intergular; *B,* gular; *C,* humeral; *D,* pectoral; *G,* anal.

through the femoral and abdominal epidermal shields (Fig. 43.18) allows access to coelomic viscera while avoiding injury to the appendicular skeleton and heart. The osteotomy must be large enough to allow the procedure to be accomplished and located in a position to allow access to the target organ.

Plastron osteotomy is performed using a power or pneumatic bone saw or a sterile motorized woodworking tool with a fine circular saw blade. Standard bur bits are not recommended because they cut an excessively wide osteotomy that will delay bone healing. Standard surgical preparation is performed, and the surface of the plastron must be completely free of keratin debris and soil. This cleansing requires a surgical scrub brush. Alcohol, ether, or acetone is used to remove grease from the surface of the plastron, to allow a better bond to form between the epithelium and the epoxy resin that will be used to stabilize the plastron osteotomy postoperatively.

The plastron is dermal bone, and efforts are made to improve the environment for bone healing. The osteotomy cut is beveled slightly, and the blade should be as thin as possible so when the segment of plastron is replaced, bone-to-bone contact will be achieved (Fig. 43.19). The blade is irrigated during the osteotomy to dissipate heat and to control bone dust. The surgeon

should make a three-sided osteotomy in species with a hinge (e.g., box turtles). An osteotomy is made on both sides as well as on the caudal margin of the proposed flap. The segment of plastron is then reflected craniad based on the intact hinge that will provide blood supply to the segment of bone. For those species without a hinge (most tortoises), the segment is cut along the cranial border and the two sides. The fourth (caudal) side is partially cut with the saw, and then, as the section of bone is elevated, it is cracked along the caudal border to preserve some blood supply as well as some stability. The flap is based caudally because the attachments of the pelvic musculature insert on the plastron in the caudal area of the flap, providing a blood supply to the segment of bone.

After the bone has been osteotomized, a periosteal elevator is used to dissect the body wall off the plastron, thereby preserving the attachments of the pelvic musculature caudally. Bending the segment beyond 90° may be difficult, and one may need an assistant to hold the segment up and out of the surgeon's field during the procedure. A large venous sinus is found within the coelomic membrane located paramedian on each side between the midline and the bridge (junction of the plastron with the carapace). These sinuses are generally obvious during the initial approach but, once manipulated, they undergo vasospasm and become imperceptible. Care is taken not to damage these vessels so fatal hemorrhage does not occur when they dilate after closure. Some investigators have reported that these vessels can be ligated without consequences (2, 5). The incision into the coelom is made along the ventral midline. The membrane is thin and transparent in the central region, where no muscle is present.

Closure is accomplished using a synthetic absorbable material in the coelomic membrane and body wall. The bone flap is replaced and secured using epoxy resin and fiberglass cloth. Epoxy is mixed and applied 2 to 3 cm around the periphery of the plastron

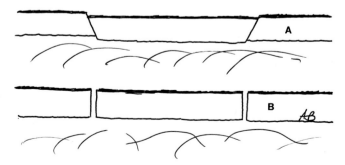

Fig. 43.19. A bevel cut is recommended for plastron osteotomy to achieve postoperative bone-to-bone contact for more rapid bone healing. When the flap is replaced after a bevel cut, the bone contacts bone (*A*). With a vertical cut, a gap is created (*B*).

osteotomy and over the entire bone segment, leaving a 3- to 4-mm border around the osteotomy on both sides to prevent the resin from flowing into the osteotomy, which would delay healing. A sterile autoclaved piece of fiberglass cloth is placed over the plastron flap with a 2- to 3-cm border extending over the osteotomy onto the plastron. The epoxy already in the plastron is worked gently into the cloth, with care taken not to allow the resin to seep into the osteotomy. The epoxy is allowed to cure, and a second layer is applied over the entire patch. This layer should be thin enough that the resin does not soak through the cloth and into the osteotomy. Enough layers of epoxy are applied to create a completely smooth surface with no texture from the cloth remaining. During the final curing process, a piece of plastic sheeting or wax paper is applied to the patch to prevent paper or soil from adhering to the resin. This does not stick to the epoxy and is removed the next day. Within 24 hours, the resin is completely cured, and the turtle can resume normal activity, including swimming. Some surgeons prefer to apply a thin layer of antibiotic cream along the osteotomy site to prevent resin from entering and to provide some antibacterial activity.

Healing of a plastron osteotomy requires 1 to 2 years (7). Patches have remained intact for over 5 years and are generally not removed. Often, the patch falls off on its own; however, if the borders become elevated from the plastron, the patch can be pried off. In young growing chelonians, the patch is cut at the growth rings after bone healing is complete to allow for shell growth. Because the epoxy is potentially carcinogenic, the cuts are best made while the surgeon is under a hood or, at least, in a well-ventilated area and using a respirator mask. Copious irrigation helps to prevent aerosolization of the toxic dust.

Flank celiotomy is used in chelonians with a small plastron or in tortoises with small cystic calculi or a small intestinal foreign body (5). With the animal in dorsal recumbency, the left hind limb is pulled caudally to expose the inguinal depression. The skin is incised in either a longitudinal or a transverse manner, and the muscles are bluntly separated until the coelomic membrane is identified. The membrane is grasped with tissue forceps and is incised to allow access to the coelomic cavity. Through this approach, the left lobe of the bladder can be accessed, and with digital exploration, small intestinal foreign bodies can be exteriorized. This approach is not adequate for access to the entire female reproductive tract for ovariohysterectomy; however, focal oviductal lesions may be approached through the flank. Two-layer or three-layer closure is performed, with the coelomic membrane and muscle sutured either as separate layers or together.

Surgery of the Female Reproductive Tract

Female reptiles have a bilateral reproductive tract, but their reproductive physiology varies considerably. Some reptiles lay eggs (crocodilians, chelonians, and some squamates), whereas others deliver live babies (some lizards and some snakes). Dystocia and prevention of reproduction are the major indications for surgery of the female reproductive tract. Surgical management of dystocia is indicated when husbandry changes and medical management have failed to relieve the dystocia or when evidence (e.g., radiography) indicates that the eggs are unable to pass because they are too large or are abnormally shaped. Ovariosalpingectomy is performed to treat dystocia or to prevent future problems related to the reproductive tract such as yolk peritonitis, dystocia, and salpingitis.

Preovulatory egg stasis is characterized by the development of yolks on the ovary that are not subsequently released. Postovulatory stasis occurs when the eggs or fetuses are within the oviduct but do not pass normally. In either case, the ovaries as well as the oviducts should be removed (5). Apparently, if the oviduct is removed without removing the ovary, yolks will be released into the coelom and potentially can induce yolk peritonitis. If the ovaries are removed and the oviducts are left, the oviducts simply atrophy and are unlikely to cause problems. Removal of one side of the reproductive tract (unilateral ovariosalpingectomy) for treatment of reproductive disease allows the patient to remain reproductively viable, which may be important for herpetoculturists.

The female reproductive tract is mobile within the coelom. In lizards and chelonians, this tract is readily accessible through a standard celiotomy approach. In snakes, the tract is long, and if the entire oviduct contains eggs or fetuses that must be removed, one must often make several celiotomy approaches. Generally, three to six eggs can be manipulated from a single salpingotomy incision.

When the patient is active reproductively, the blood vessels supplying the ovary and oviduct become engorged and hypertrophied, making surgical removal more challenging. For this reason, in pet reptile species with a high incidence of dystocia, prepubertal elective ovariosalpingectomy should be considered. The procedure is much easier when the vessels, ovary, and oviduct are small and the patient is in good metabolic condition.

The oviduct wall is thin and transparent. In patients with salpingitis, the wall becomes thicker but more friable, making it a challenge to suture closed. Cultures and biopsy specimens should be obtained from the oviduct for diagnostic purposes to guide postoperative management and to determine the prognosis for future reproductive capability. Once the oviduct is identified, an incision is made over an egg or fetus approximately the length of the egg or fetus. If the salpingotomy incision is too small, the oviduct will tear while the eggs or fetuses are manipulated through the incision. The first egg or fetus is generally removed without much effort. Eggs or fetuses that have been in place a long time adhere to the oviduct wall. A 20-gauge catheter on a 20-mL syringe filled with saline is inserted between the egg or fetus and the oviduct wall, and saline is injected to separate the wall from the egg or fetus. This procedure not only frees the egg or fetus from its adhesions to the oviduct, but also provides some lubrication. After the first egg or fetus is removed, adjacent eggs or fetuses are massaged toward the salpingotomy using saline injection, finger dilation, and digital manipulation to separate adhesions between the egg or fetus and the oviduct and to extrude the egg or fetus from the salpingotomy. Once all the eggs or fetuses have been removed, the salpingotomy is closed using a fine (6–0 to 8–0) monofilament, synthetic absorbable material on a fine atraumatic needle in a two-layer inverting pattern or a simple continuous pattern oversewn with an inverting pattern. After a properly performed salpingotomy, the prognosis for reproductive viability is good.

When damage to the reproductive tract is irreparable, or when the owner desires to prevent future episodes of dystocia, ovariosalpingectomy is performed. The following discussion applies primarily to green iguanas. Other lizards and chelonians have some variation in anatomy, but the procedure is similar. In snakes, with their longitudinal configuration, the ovary is cranial to the oviduct and must be approached through a separate incision or by extending the celiotomy craniad until the ovary is identified.

In iguanas, the right ovary is close to the right external iliac vein, whereas the left ovary is more loosely attached, with the left adrenal gland interposed between the left renal vein and the ovary (Fig. 43.20). When the ovary is active, as with preovulatory egg stasis, the ligament is stretched out, and it is easy to apply hemostatic clips to the vessels supplying the ovary. Two clips are applied to each vessel, and the vessel is transected between the clips. The process is continued until all vessels are clipped and the ovary with its multitude of yolk follicles is removed.

When the ovary is not active, removal is more challenging. Removal of the right ovary is accomplished by gently elevating the ovary, applying one or two clips between the right ovary and the right renal vein, and then transecting the tissue distal to the clip to allow removal of the ovary. The left ovary is removed in a similar manner, with the clips applied between

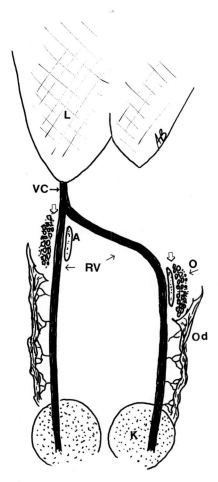

Fig. 43.20. Anatomy of the female reproductive tract of a green iguana. Hemostatic clips are applied between the right ovary and the right external iliac vein and between the left ovary and the left adrenal gland (*open arrows*). The tissue distal to the clip is incised, allowing the ovaries to be removed. *L*, liver; *VC*, vena cava; *RV*, renal vein; *O*, ovary; *Od*, oviduct; *K*, kidney; *A*, adrenal gland.

the ovary and the left adrenal gland. The tissue distal to the clips is transected, allowing removal of the ovary without damaging the adjacent adrenal gland.

After removal of the ovaries, the oviducts are removed. Dissection is initiated at the infundibulum and is continued to the cloaca. With preovulatory egg binding, the oviduct is empty, and vessels are easily controlled either with hemostatic clips or bipolar cautery. One or two clips are applied to the base of each oviduct at the cloaca before their transection and removal.

In patients with postovulatory egg binding in which the oviducts are full of eggs, the ovaries are small and inactive because they have already released their yolks. The oviducts full of eggs obscure visualization of the ovaries and are removed before ovariectomy. The vessels to the oviducts are generally engorged and are numerous. Each vessel is identified, two hemostatic clips are applied, and the vessel is transected between them. Dissection is initiated at the ovaries and is continued caudad until the oviducts can be ligated or clipped at the cloaca before transection. After the oviducts are removed, the ovaries are visualized as described previously. Closure is routine.

Postoperative care is supportive. Most patients are anorectic for 2 to 4 weeks before the surgical intervention. Fluid therapy is administered through an intravenous or an intraosseous catheter. Antibiotics are indicated in the management of bacterial salpingitis. Again, the patient should be maintained at the upper end of its preferred temperature range for proper function of the immune and digestive systems.

Orchidectomy

Castration is primarily performed in male green iguanas that have become aggressive toward their owners (5). Castration decreases testosterone levels and sexually aggressive behaviors in other lizard species (8–10). Most commonly, orchidectomy is performed in iguanas after the aggressive behavior has developed; it may be more appropriate to perform the procedure in prepubertal iguanas before the inappropriate behaviors develop. When the procedure is performed in an aggressive animal, the aggression does not appear to be ameliorated until the following breeding season. The prognosis for attenuation of the behavior has been reported anecdotally to be around 50% after orchidectomy (5).

Orchidectomy is performed through a standard celiotomy. As with the ovaries, the right testicle is more closely attached to the right renal vein by its short, vascular mesorchium. The right adrenal gland is located on the other side of the renal vein. The left testicle is more loosely attached to the left renal vein, and the left adrenal gland is located between the left testicle and the renal vein (Fig. 43.21). The adrenals are elongated, granular, pink glands easily distinguished from the smooth, white testicles. The testicles are covered by a capsule that can be ruptured during aggressive manipulations. Rupture of the capsule does not result in hemorrhage, but the contents flow out, making it difficult to continue with the dissection.

The testicles are removed in a manner similar to that described for removal of inactive ovaries. The right testicle is gently elevated, and one or two hemostatic clips are applied between the testicle and the renal vein. The tissue distal to the clips is transected, allowing removal of the testicle. The left testicle is removed after application of hemostatic clips between the left adrenal gland and the testicle. If hemorrhage from the external iliac vein occurs, one or two hemo-

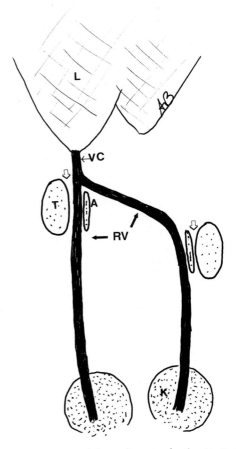

Fig. 43.21. Anatomy of the male reproductive tract of a green iguana. The testicles are removed as described for ovariectomy in Figure 43.20. *Open arrows* demonstrate the location where clips are applied. *L,* liver; *VC,* vena cava; *RV,* renal vein; *T,* testis; *K,* kidney; *A,* adrenal gland.

static clips are applied longitudinally along the damaged side of the vessel (Fig. 43.22). Partial occlusion of the external iliac vein has not been associated with clinical disease; however, if over half the diameter of the external iliac vein is attenuated, signs of vascular obstruction should be anticipated.

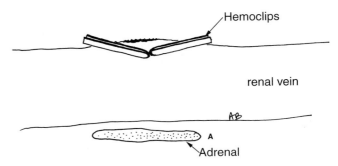

Fig. 43.22. Hemostatic clips are applied to the renal if there is damage to the vein. Partial occlusion does not generally cause clinical problems. *A,* adrenal gland.

Cystotomy

Urinary calculi can develop in any species of reptiles with a urinary bladder, but they but seem to occur most frequently in desert tortoises (*Gopherus agassizi*) and green iguanas. Improper nutrition and inadequate access to water or dehydration have been suggested as initiating causes (5). Clinical signs of cystic calculi include anorexia, depression, constipation from occlusion of the colon, dystocia from occlusion of the oviduct, cloacal prolapse from tenesmus, and paraparesis secondary to compressive injury to the pelvic nerves (5). A definitive diagnosis is made based on radiographs or palpation. Calcium urate calculi are radioopaque, whereas ammonium urate calculi can be difficult to visualize radiographically.

In chelonians, cystic calculi are palpated in the left inguinal fossa. The urinary bladder of chelonians is bilobed, and the right liver lobe lies over the right lobe of the urinary bladder. Because the right portion of the bladder is compressed by the right liver lobe, most cystic calculi are present in the left lobe of the bladder. The examiner's finger is inserted into the fossa with the chelonian in a sternal recumbency. With the finger left in place, the tortoise is tipped vertically (90°), and the stone is felt hitting the finger as it falls to the dependent portion of the bladder. In lizards, cystic calculi are easily identified by abdominal palpation.

Cystotomy is performed through a standard celiotomy approach. The bladder is large and easily identified when a calculus is present. The bladder wall is thin and transparent, but it becomes thicker because of the cystitis usually associated with a calculus. The bladder is isolated with moist gauze sponges or laparotomy pads before making the cystotomy to minimize coelomic contamination. The urine of reptiles contains mucus and urates that give it a thick, cloudy appearance, and it may not be aspirated easily through small suction tips. After removal of the calculus, the bladder is irrigated to remove residual debris. Closure is accomplished using a fine (5–0 to 7–0) monofilament, absorbable material on a small, swaged-on, atraumatic needle in a simple continuous appositional pattern oversewn with an inverting pattern. Celiotomy closure is routine.

Because dehydration may cause desiccation of urates within the bladder, thereby initiating calculus formation, attention must be paid to maintaining adequate hydration. Antibiotics are indicated if bacterial cystitis is present. Husbandry changes (nutrition, temperature, access to water) are made when appropriate.

Other Procedures

Various surgical procedures, such as enterotomy for removal of foreign bodies, may be performed in rep-

tiles once the surgeon is familiar with the unique anatomy of and surgical approaches used in these patients. Once the approach to the celomic cavity is made, most procedures are analogous to those performed in domestic animals.

References

1. Bennett RA. Reptilian surgery. Part I. Basic principles. Compend Contin Educ Pract Vet 1989;11:10–20.
2. Bennett RA. Reptilian surgery. Part II. Management of surgical diseases. Compend Contin Educ Pract Vet 1989;11:122–133.
3. Millichamp NJ, Lawrence K, Jacobson ER, et al. Egg retention in snakes. J Am Vet Med Assoc 1983;183:1213–1218.
4. Smith DA, Barker IK. Preliminary observations on the effects of ambient temperature on cutaneous wound healing in snakes. In: Proceedings of the American Association of Zoo Veterinarians.: Tampa, FL. American Association of Zoo Veterinarians, 1983:210–211.
5. Bennett RA. Soft tissue surgery. In: Mader DR. Reptile medicine and surgery. Philadelphia: WB Saunders, 1996:287–298.
6. Russo EA. Diagnosis and treatment of lumps and bumps in snakes. Compend Contin Educ Pract Vet 1987;9:795–807.
7. Barten SL. Shell damage. In: Mader DR. Reptile medicine and surgery. Philadelphia: WB Saunders, 1996:413–416.
8. Moore MC. Castration affects territorial and sexual behavior of free-living male lizards, *Sceloporus jarrovi*. Anim Behav 1987;35:1193–1199.
9. Cooper WE, Mendonca MT, Vitt LJ. Induction of orange head coloration and activation of courtship and aggression by testosterone in the male broad-headed skink (*Eumeces laticeps*). J Herpetol 1987;21:96–101.
10. Mason P, Adkins EK. Hormones and social behavior in the lizard, *Anolis carolinesis*. Horm Behav 1976;7:75–86.

Abdominal Surgery of Pet Rabbits

Robert F. Hoyt Jr.

Because of their relative ease of care and their docile dispositions, rabbits are becoming more and more popular as pets in today's transient society. They are now estimated to be found in more than 1% of households in the United States, and represent some 4 million animals. As such, requests to small animal practitioners to provide rabbits with both medical and surgical care are increasing. In many areas, practitioners are responding to the increase in popularity of this animal species, with resulting supplemental income to many practices. In some cases, rabbits comprise a significant percentage of the total number of patients, and the result is that some practices are devoted exclusively to exotic animals. Unfortunately, some clinicians are failing to take advantage of this emerging "pocket pet" clientele and to incorporate these patients into their practices. Practitioners' reluctance to provide such veterinary care, especially surgery on rabbits, may, in part, be due to a lack of formal training in the species at their veterinary colleges. It may also be due to a lack of confidence based on clinical experience with the species; no mentor may have been available for guidance.

The intent of this discussion is to provide veterinary practitioners with basic information to perform common abdominal surgical procedures in rabbits. Included are a general overview of anatomy, indications for each type of surgical procedure, and detailed descriptions of commonly performed procedures: gastrotomy, cystotomy, ovariohysterectomy, orchiectomy (castration), and vasectomy. Because each procedure occurs within the abdominal cavity, several areas are common to all and warrant discussion beforehand: a review of unique properties of rabbit skin, preoperative considerations, guidelines for preparation of the surgical area, general surgical principles particular to the rabbit, and useful suture patterns for closure.

Anatomy of the Skin

Except for some of the heavy-skinned rabbit breeds whose pelts are used in the fur trade, a rabbit's skin is thin relative to body size (1). The full thickness of the skin, including the hypodermis and panniculus carnosus, is generally only 1.0 to 2.0 mm thick. Except for the tip of the nose and the inguinal region (in both sexes) and a small area on the scrotum in bucks, a rabbit's skin is covered with fine-textured hair, and both underfur and guard hairs are present. Rabbits generally molt their hair coats annually, with hair loss starting on the shoulders and moving caudally. Frequently, patterns and rates of hair growth and regrowth (where the hair has been clipped for a surgical procedure) do not appear uniform; this is often a concern of clients. After the rabbit's hair has been clipped, it may not begin to grow back uniformly and may look patchy, with some areas of hair longer and appearing to grow faster than others. This unusual, seemingly abnormal skin coat can be more pronounced in young, white animals when the hair on the animal's flank has been removed. It does, however, represent normal skin responses to variations in rabbit hair growth cycles. The raised, blotchy areas are areas of active hair growth. Beginning with the second coat of hair, waves of hair growth periodically move caudally and ventrally from the neck region. These "growth waves" occur in areas of the skin where all the hair follicles are simultaneously in an active growth cycle.

The hair growth cycle has been divided into three main phases: anagen, catagen, and telogen. The anagen, or growing, phase is the time when the germ cells undergo a burst of mitotic activity, leading to the formation of the sheathed hair bulb and papillary cavity and emergence from the skin surface. The catagen,

or transition, phase is a brief period in which mitotic activity slows and the follicle shortens. The hair then passes into the telogen phase, which is a resting period. Changes in the vascularity of the skin and skin thickness are associated with these phases of the hair growth cycle. The skin thickness is approximately 1.0 mm during the telogen phase and may become 2.0 mm thick during the anagen period. As rabbits become older, the waves become less frequent and more patchy in their distribution.

Preoperative Considerations

Normal rabbit behavior and activity are typically sedentary and stoic when compared with dogs and cats. As such, they may have preexisting health problems that may not manifest themselves clinically to their owners and easily could be overlooked preoperatively in today's busy veterinary practices. Therefore, each animal must have a complete presurgical workup including physical examination, history, and, if possible, complete blood count and urinalysis. Diet, eating habits, and volume or consistency of fecal production are important items to be addressed. Clinical or subclinical problems, such as dehydration or emerging septicemia, should be corrected before any surgical procedure, to maximize the potential for a successful outcome. Because rabbits cannot vomit, withholding of food and water before the surgical procedure is not necessary.

As in other species, prophylactic antibiotics may be used in rabbits undergoing surgical procedures. The surgeon must know which antibiotics to use and which to avoid. Because of the predominance of gram-positive bacterial flora in the rabbit gastrointestinal tract, especially the cecum, any antibiotic that affects those populations, such as aminoglycosides, should be avoided. Antibiotics, such as trimethoprim–sulfa combinations, or fluorinated quinolone such as enrofloxacin, given either individually or together, can be used effectively with minimal side effects. These drugs are generally started the day before surgery, or they are administered at induction of anesthesia and are maintained for 3 days to ensure adequate blood levels should unexpected contamination occur during the surgical procedure.

Preparation of the Surgical Site

For all procedures described in this discussion, the rabbits are placed in dorsal recumbency on heated water blankets with all four limbs fully extended. The animals are preanesthetized with a combination of ketamine hydrochloride (35 mg/kg intramuscularly), xylazine (5 mg/kg intramuscularly), and glycopyrrolate (0.1 mg/kg subcutaneously); they are intubated and placed on inhalational isoflurane for general anesthesia during the procedure. Intravenous access is established with a 22-gauge catheter (Angiocath) placed in the marginal ear vein and maintained by the slow administration of an isotonic crystalloid. The reader is referred to the literature for additional information on anesthetic protocols used in rabbits (2, 3).

Preparing the rabbit skin for surgery can be a challenge to a practitioner inexperienced with the species. Removing hair at and around the incision site without damaging the skin can be frustrating. Although many clinicians use traditional clinic clippers with a No. 40 clipper blade to remove hair, variable high-speed clippers (e.g., Double K Industries, Inc., Model 401) specifically designed for animals with fine hair, such as cats, rabbits, and rodents, are recommended. These clippers make hair removal easier and reduce the incidence of accidental cutting or burning of the skin. If possible, hair should be removed at least 5 to 10 cm in every direction from the incision site.

Rabbit skin can be sensitive to alcohol. Care should be taken to avoid excessive scrubbing when preparing the skin for surgery. After clipping the hair, the surgical site is vacuumed to remove any remaining hair and is wiped with a saline-soaked gauze. The skin is then surgically prepared using alternating applications of povidone–iodine soap and either alcohol or sterile saline for a total of three applications each. Each application begins at the center of the surgical site and works outward in larger and larger circles. Povidone–iodine solution should next be sprayed over the entire surgical site and allowed to dry.

General Surgical Principles

Because of their increased susceptibility to develop abdominal adhesions when compared with other species, rabbits are used as animal models of adhesion formation in biomedical research (4). Such adhesions can develop from any uncorrected abdominal hemorrhage, from contamination with foreign materials, and from the inappropriate apposition of the peritoneum during closure (5). Using electrosurgical instruments for skin incisions helps to minimize any bleeding. These versatile instruments can be used alone for cutting the skin and at the same time inducing vessel coagulation (in a blended current mode), or they can be used as an adjunct to a scalpel blade to provide coagulation only. They can be especially useful in obese animals or in pregnant or postpartum does, in which bleeding can become a major problem. Whenever these instruments are used on rabbits, the dialed settings should be reduced to facilitate control over the depth of the skin incision made in such thin-skinned patients. Metzenbaum scissors should be used to enter the abdomen through the linea alba. At this layer, the tissue is thin and often lies directly over the cecum or

other viscus organ, which may or may not be evident. Once inside the abdomen, the surgeon must handle the tissues delicately, and only when necessary. From experience, rabbit tissues appear to be more friable than tissues of species of comparable size, such as cats and small dogs, and they often have many microhemorrhages. This is especially true with manipulation of the uterus and intestines. Moving the organs around by handling adjacent adipose tissue rather than the organ directly helps to reduce these microhemorrhages, which later may lead to adhesion formation.

Taking steps to minimize inclusion of foreign materials such as gauze lint, surgical glove powder, and talc also decreases the opportunity for adhesion formation. After donning a surgical gown and gloves and before beginning the procedure, the surgeon needs to take the time to wash the powder and talc off the surgical gloves with sterile saline–soaked gauze. In addition, any gauze sponges with frayed ends should be removed from the surgical tray because these may fall into the rabbit's abdomen and become a nidus for adhesion formation (5).

Another important practice for avoiding adhesion formation is applied during closure of the abdomen. The two cut peritoneal surfaces from the incision must be brought into apposition when closing the muscle–fascia layer. This maneuver reestablishes continuity of the nonadherent peritoneal surface, which directly contacts the underlying organs. Failure to restore the peritoneal barrier often results in adhesions involving the muscle–fascia layer with one or more abdominal organs, often with adverse outcomes.

Wound Closure

Various suture materials can be used to close wounds, including absorbable and nonabsorbable materials. I believe that two suture materials meet most surgical indications: 1) a long-acting synthetic absorbable suture material that is broken down by enzymatic hydrolysis, such as 3–0 polyglactin 910 or polydioxanone suture, and 2) nonabsorbable stainless steel. Rabbits tolerate these materials readily and have minimal adverse tissue reactions.

Closure of the abdomen in most rabbits is difficult in more than two layers. The muscle–fascia layer (with underlying peritoneum) is the primary weight-supporting layer of the abdomen. As such, this layer should be closed using a tapered swaged-on needle and a simple interrupted suture pattern. These sutures should be placed close together. Elevating the muscle–fascia layer with towel clamps placed at each end of the incision during the closure is useful and reduces suturing time. The added visualization helps to avoid accidental suturing of an underlying organs and at the same time ensures approximation of the two edges of "glistening" peritoneum with each stitch. When completed, the suture line should be evaluated for potential herniation using Brown–Adson thumb forceps. The tips of the forceps are held together, and the surgeon gently probes between each suture. If the forceps can easily enter the abdomen, a potential for abdominal organ herniation exists, and additional sutures should be placed. This process is continued until sufficient sutures are placed to prevent forcep entry.

The skin may be closed using various different suture patterns and materials. I prefer to close the skin using either absorbable suture material, as mentioned earlier, on a swaged-on, reverse-cutting needle in a subcuticular pattern or surgical staples. Surgical staples are usually reserved for linear skin incisions on flat surfaces. The site and nature of the skin lesion generally dictate which method to use.

Adjustable Cervical Collars ("Scratch Guards")

Rabbits have an almost compulsive desire to keep themselves well groomed. This behavior is often exaggerated by surgery to a level to which, unless they are inhibited, the animals literally lick and bite themselves down to muscle and bone, removing skin, sutures, and anything else in an attempt to eliminate the incision site pain. Unfortunately, rabbits usually do not tolerate the traditional Elizabethan collar well postoperatively. Although this device does keep them from removing the sutures or traumatizing the incision, the animals seem frightened and frequently do not eat, drink, or even move around. Often, they just stay in one location with their heads down. One soft, adjustable type of cervical collar overcomes many of the problems associated with Elizabethan collars (6). It can be easily constructed using available clinic materials and is reusable. Preparation begins with an initial circular ring made from roll gauze or flexible anesthetic gas tubing approximately 14 inches in circumference. Four by four gauze sponges are next wrapped around the ring to provide both padding to the animal's neck and external diameter enlargement to the collar. The gauze is secured in place by wrapping over it with both surgical adhesive tape and Vetwrap (3M, Minneapolis, MN) applied sequentially. This not only reinforces the gauze ring, but provides for a consistent collar diameter and water resistance. The finished collar is simply placed over the animal's head, and the slack in the ring is compressed until it's snug. The collar can then be secured by adhesive tape so it resembles a yoke (Fig. 43.23). It was coined "scratch guard" by staff members because the animals did not scratch the surgical site. When this collar is used, the affected animals seem distracted from surgical site discomfort and even ap-

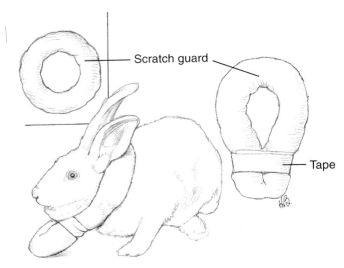

Fig. 43.23. Adjustable cervical collar ("scratch guard").

pear entertained. They quickly return to near-normal movement, begin eating and drinking, and may even appear content to "groom" the scratch guard. In a report of more than 1500 abdominal surgical procedures, only about 2.5% resulted in self-mutilation episodes, and those episodes occurred primarily because of the rabbit's ability to remove the scratch guard (6).

Postoperative Considerations

Postoperative care plays an important part in successful surgery in rabbits. Postoperative care can be broken down into two time periods: the first 24 hours after the surgical procedure and the next 13 days. After surgery, the animal is allowed to recover in a warmed, intensive care cage where the endotracheal tube is removed (on return of the animal's gag reflex). Once the rabbit is fully conscious, a scratch guard cervical collar is fitted, and food and water are offered. Close monitoring of the animal is important during the first 24 hours postoperatively, and, therefore, the animal should remain where it can be observed frequently by staff members. During this period, the animals should have complete health checks a minimum of twice a day. This examination includes rectal temperature, pulse count, chest auscultation, monitoring of fluid and water intake, monitoring of urination (volume) and defecation (amount and consistency), and monitoring of the incision line and the animal's behavior (activity and body language). In addition, the animals are continually evaluated for signs of pain, which may be obvious, such as vocalizations, to subtle, including reluctance to move, abnormal (hunched) posture, anorexia, grinding of teeth, elevated body temperature, increased respiratory rate, and unexpected aggression. If pain is present, pain relief can be provided (buprenorphine, 0.05 mg/kg subcutaneously twice daily) as needed. Minimal to no fecal production suggests potential trichobezoar (hairball) formation. A "cow paddy" stool may indicate bacterial enteritis. The animals must resume eating and drinking as soon as possible. Rabbits normally have a small amount of ileus in the postoperative period, and the return to voluntary food and water consumption helps to prevent this normal occurrence from developing into something deleterious. Offering the animals hay, either alfalfa or, preferably, timothy, or even shredded wheat usually stimulates reluctant animals to eat immediately.

If the animal returns to near-normal behavior, especially regarding food and water consumption, urination, and defecation, within 24 hours of the surgical procedure, the surgeon can send it home. To help facilitate a successful outcome, the owner should perform as many health-monitoring techniques as possible, especially monitoring body temperature, incision site, food and water intake, urination and defecation (volume and consistency), movement, and overall attitude. Owners appreciate participating in the rabbit's postoperative care and in becoming more aware of their pet's health.

Common Surgical Procedures

The common surgical procedures performed in the peritoneal cavity are discussed in this section. The techniques presented focus on procedures that I believe are easily learned and successful. No attempt is made to discuss all available techniques. In addition, the description of each technique begins as if the surgeon had already opened the abdomen as discussed previously.

Gastrotomy

Rabbits are hindgut fermenters and have a simple, glandular stomach. The stomach serves as a reservoir for most of the ingested food, and it is never empty in a healthy animal. The stomach acids in the rabbit are among the most acidic of those of any species, with a pH of 1.2 to 1.5. This high acidity enables rabbits to use plant proteins more efficiently than most mammals and normally minimizes problems with ingested hair.

Unlike other species with incessant grooming behaviors, such as cats, rabbits physiologically cannot vomit. Consequently, ingested foreign materials, especially hair, which would normally induce a protective emetic reflex in other species, have the potential to form life-threatening obstructions. Because constant grooming is a lifelong normal behavior for rabbits with minimal adverse side effects, the mechanism that triggers the routine digestive process suddenly to decrease

and cause the development of an obstructive trichobezoar is unclear. Whatever the predisposing cause—boredom, inadequate dietary roughage, anorexia because of off-flavor or off-odor feed, inability to smell from rhinitis, pain from sore hocks, malocclusion, lack of fresh water, or other stressors—the animals stop eating and drinking, and critical metabolic problems can result if this problem is not corrected (4, 7–13).

Common presenting complaints include anorexia, lethargy, weight loss, oligodipsia, diarrhea, or conversely, small or scant, dry feces. Other frequent clinical signs are dehydration, depression, hunched posture, tense abdomen, hypothermia, and bloating.

Although definitive diagnosis of trichobezoar cannot be made without surgical exploration, a tentative diagnosis can be made based on history, clinical signs, palpation of an abdominal mass in the vicinity of the stomach, and contrast radiography, especially with fluoroscopy. Care should be taken when palpating the upper abdomen because the liver in these animals is often friable.

Rabbits with trichobezoars are frequently dehydrated and cachectic and should be treated as medical emergencies. Initial efforts should be directed at reestablishing normal homeostasis, including aggressive parenteral fluid administration before definitive therapy is pursued. Initial medical therapy involves the administration of oral fluids, including fresh pineapple juice or crushed papain tablets in water. These fluids should be given in small amounts (10 to 20 mL) four to six times a day for up to 3 to 4 days. Often, this oral fluid administration both "refloats" the hair mass in the stomach and aids in quickly rehydrating the animal. Refloating allows the proteolytic enzymes to penetrate the trichobezoar and to begin digesting the hair. A valuable tool in assessing the efficacy of medical treatment is the production of fecal pellets in increased quantities.

Other medical treatment strategies for treating trichobezoars, formerly a strictly surgical condition, have been successful in recent years, including the use of metoclopramide (4, 8–10). These newer regimens have reduced the number of animals that ultimately undergo surgical procedures. As a general rule, if no improvement is seen with medical therapy for trichobezoars after 3 days, these animals become surgical candidates for an exploratory gastrotomy. Animals presented for gastric foreign bodies other than trichobezoar are surgical candidates for gastrotomy (Fig. 43.24).

All animals having a gastrotomy are given prophylactic antibiotics, as previously mentioned, which are maintained generally for 5 days. Postoperatively, these animals resume food and water consumption as soon as possible. I recommend maintaining these animals in the hospital for several days until the rabbits return

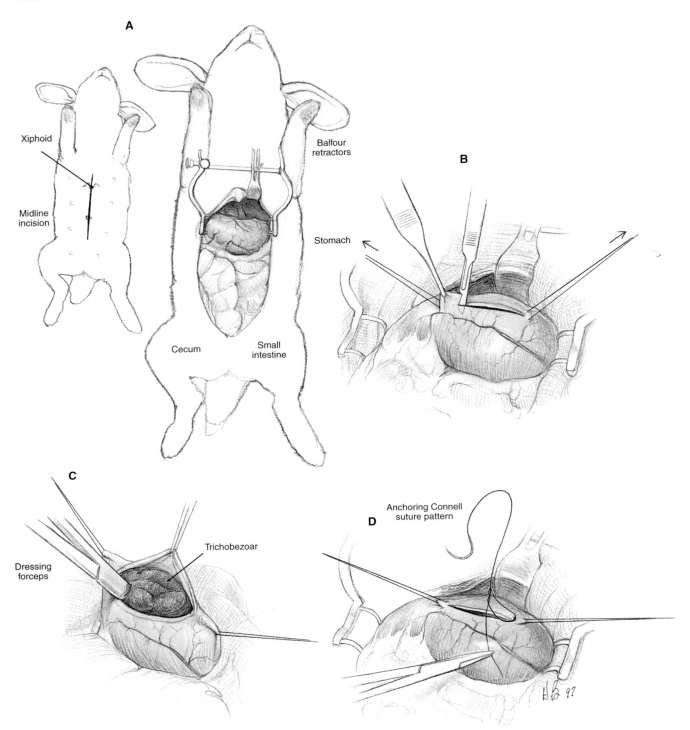

Fig. 43.24. Gastrotomy. **A.** The animal is placed in dorsal recumbency, and the surgical site draped from 4 cm anterior to the xiphoid cartilage to 5 cm caudal to the umbilicus. A midline skin incision is made extending from 2 cm cranial to the xiphoid cartilage to 3 cm caudal to the umbilicus. Using thumb forceps and Metzenbaum scissors, incision is continued through the linea alba down through the muscle–fascia layer into abdomen. The surgeon must identify and avoid cutting the xiphoid cartilage when cutting the muscle cranially. When reaching the caudal edge of the xiphoid, the surgeon redirects the scissors and continues cutting the muscle along the edge of the cartilage for the remaining 2 cm. Both sides of the abdominal incision are lined with moistened laparotomy sponges. Exposure is maximized by placing pediatric self-retracting Balfour abdominal retractors just caudal to the xiphoid. The two fenestrated retractor blades are spread laterally, and the xiphoid cartilage is elevated gently with the center Balfour blade to visualize the stomach, the cecum, and portions of the small intestine. **B.** Two stay sutures are placed 5 to 6 cm apart midway between the greater and lesser curvature of the stomach in a visibly avascular area. The sutures are lifted in opposite directions to elevate the stomach out of the abdomen and to provide a taut area for entering the stomach. The surgeon packs off the elevated portion of the stomach from the rest of the abdomen with moistened laparotomy sponges. Waterproof drapes are placed over the laparotomy sponges to prevent abdominal contamination from gastric contents

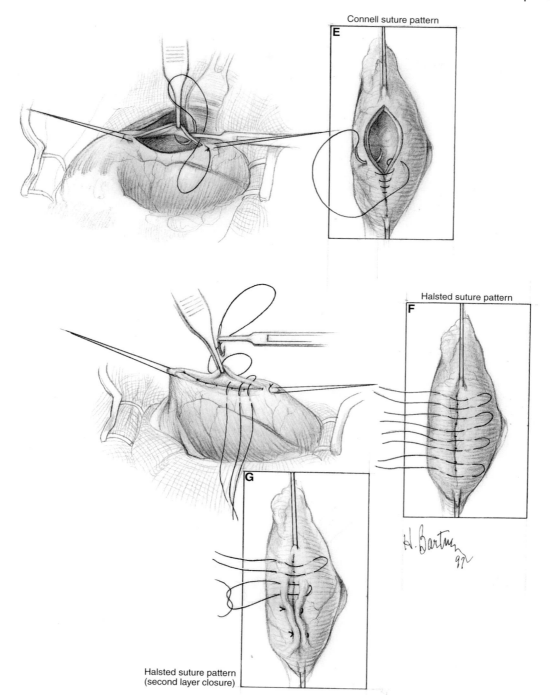

Connell suture pattern

E

Halsted suture pattern

F

G

Halsted suture pattern
(second layer closure)

H. Bartman
97

Fig. 43.24 (continued). when the stomach is opened. In addition, separate instruments should be available for entering and closing the stomach. A stab incision is made with a scalpel into the stomach. Suction is used to prevent accidental spillage of gastric juices onto the stomach serosal surface. This incision is extended as needed with a scalpel or with Metzenbaum scissors until a desired opening is achieved. **C.** The stomach contents are examined. If a trichobezoar is present, the hair mass is broken up and is removed with a pair of dressing forceps. The stomach is lavaged with warm saline solution and is suctioned. All instruments involved with entering the stomach are discarded. The surgeon should reglove, change or discard drapes, and begin closing the stomach with clean instruments. **D and E.** Closure of the stomach is accomplished with two inverting suture patterns using 3–0 polyglactin 910 or polydioxanone on a tapered needle. The first layer is a Connell pattern followed by a Halsted oversew. When performing the Connell pattern, full-thickness bites should be placed from the edges of the incision, and the anchoring knots should be placed 2 to 3 mm from the incision at both ends. **F and G.** The second layer is closed using a Halsted suture pattern, which further inverts the incision and helps to ensure a complete seal. Each suture should be preplaced before being tied, to provide for even tissue inversion and tension distribution. Once the second layer is completed, the closure is checked for any leakage. The abdominal cavity should be lavaged with warmed saline and suctioned if one sees evidence of gastric spillage. The stomach is returned to its normal anatomic position, and the abdomen is closed routinely.

to normal food and water intake and begin to make fecal pellets.

Orchiectomy (Castration)

Orchiectomy (castration) is one of the most common surgical procedures performed in rabbits. The usual indications for removing testicles are for birth control or to modify or eliminate certain offensive behaviors intact male rabbits (bucks) often develop when they reach sexual maturity: urine spraying, territory marking with both urine and feces, and aggression toward their owners or other rabbits. Although not a total panacea, castrating bucks generally makes them more docile, reduces fighting, and diminishes urine spraying. Other indications for castration are related to scrotal injury, including trauma from fighting or severe urine scalding (4).

Male rabbits have two separate scrotal sacs, rather than one, as found in other placental mammals. These hairless structures, which lie slightly cranial to the penis, more closely resemble the genitalia of male marsupials (T Donnelly, unpublished data). The testes are found in the abdomen at birth and descend into the scrotal sacs at approximately 3 months of age. Bucks reach sexual maturity between 4 and 5 months of age, and the animals should be at least that age before castration is performed. In addition to their peculiar scrotal anatomy, rabbits have open inguinal canals that allow the testicles to move easily between the scrotal sacs and the abdomen (8). In intact bucks, epididymal fat, which lies cranial and medial to the inguinal canal on each side, normally is inhibited from entering the scrotal sac by each testicle. Because this fat lies on the abdominal side of the inguinal ring, it, in turn, inhibits intestinal herniation through the canal. Castration techniques involving incision of the scrotal sac and removal of the testicle could potentially lead initially to epididymal fat herniation and, subsequently, herniation of the intestine into the scrotum.

Most of the techniques described for castrating male rabbits are adaptations of techniques used in dogs and cats: scrotal approach—open castration with incised tunica albuginea and preservation of the epididymal fat; scrotal approach—closed castration without incising the tunica albuginea; and prescrotal approach—over the inguinal rings with inguinal ring closure (4, 6, 10, 12). From experience, each technique is easily learned and has minimal complications. However, the scrotal–perineal area is traumatized or irritated either by the surgical procedure or by surgical preparation using any of these techniques. This trauma or irritation potentiates iatrogenic injury and the opportunity for subsequent bowel herniation or infection. I describe another castration technique, the abdominal castration technique, which is easily learned, quick to perform, and avoids traumatizing the scrotal or perineal areas (Fig. 43.25). Another advantage is that, with an abdominal incision, scratch guard cervical collars can be used with greater success to overcome a talented rabbit's ability to injure itself.

When the animal is discharged from the clinic, the owners must be advised that the desired effects of castration are not instantaneous. Although the animal's testicles have been surgically removed, male hormone levels have not been eliminated. Urine spraying, territory marking, and aggression continue for a few weeks. In addition, libido and probably viable sperm (remaining in the vas deferens) are present for a month, and with that is a real potential for impregnating intact does.

Cystotomy

Urinary calculi (urolithiasis) are commonly encountered in clinical practice in pet rabbits. A healthy adult rabbit produces an average of 130 mL/kg of urine each day; this urine is usually turbid and varies from yellow to brown to orange to bright red (8–11, 14–16). The turbidity of the urine is due primarily to mineral precipitates. Because urine is the primary route for calcium and magnesium excretion in rabbits, various crystals, including ammonium magnesium phosphate, calcium carbonate monohydrate, and anhydrous calcium carbonate precipitates, are normally found on urinalysis (8). The wide spectrum of colors and intensity is related to the dietary pigments and the animal's hydration status; higher alkalinity and dehydration are associated with brighter, more intense colors (8). The etiology of urolithiasis is still not clear, but several predisposing factors have been proposed, including urine stasis, genetic predisposition, dietary imbalances (especially elevated calcium levels), chronic urinary tract infections, and inadequate water intake (8, 9, 14). Normal urine pH in rabbits is around 8.2, but at 8.5, calcium carbonate and phosphate crystals precipitate.

The most common presenting complaint in rabbits with urolithiasis is hematuria. As mentioned previously, rabbit urine may be any of several colors, depending on urine pH and diet. Diets high in calcium, such as alfalfa, can cause the urine to become bright red orange to red. Hematuria should, therefore, be confirmed by urinalysis or urine dipstick. This condition is often diagnosed after the animal has been presented for other problems. Hematuria was reported as the chief complaint in only one of seven rabbits with urinary calculi (10). Other signalments may include polyuria, perineal irritation from urine scalding, stranguria, lethargy, anorexia, hunched posture, abdominal distension, and chronic or intermittent cystitis (4, 9–11). Diagnosis can be confirmed through physical examination, palpation, and radiography.

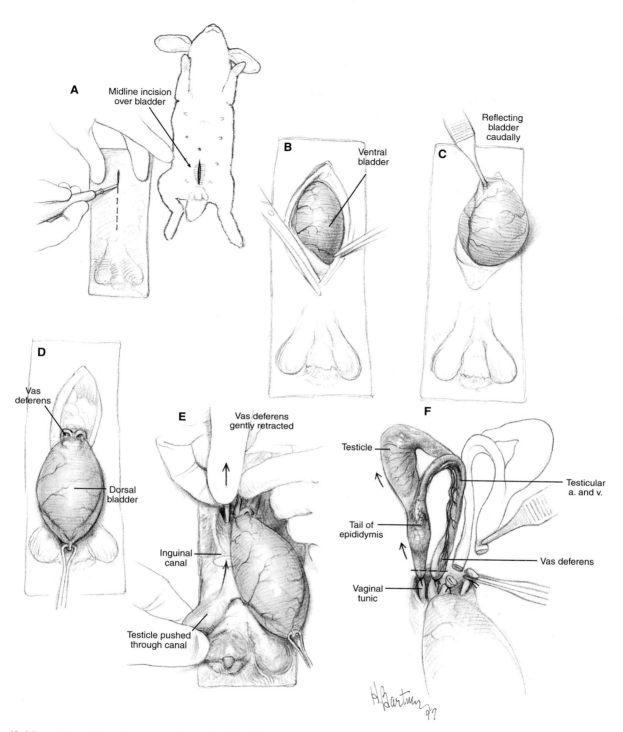

Fig. 43.25. Abdominal orchiectomy (castration). **A.** The animal is placed in dorsal recumbency, and the surgical site is draped off to include the scrotum and penis. A midline skin incision is made extending from 5 cm caudal to the umbilicus to the level of the pelvis or 2.5 cm anterior to the genitalia or to the level of the last set of nipples. **B.** Using a pair of thumb forceps and Metzenbaum scissors, incision is continued through the linea alba down through the muscle–fascia layer into the abdomen, exposing the ventral surface of the bladder. **C.** The apex of the bladder is next grasped with a pair of Babcock (or other atraumatic) forceps and is reflected caudally, exposing the dorsal side of the bladder. **D.** Further gentle caudal retraction of bladder with Babcock forceps exposes the two vasa deferentia emerging near the base of the bladder. **E.** Removing the testicle involves performing the two procedures almost simultaneously: each vas deferens is gently retracted cranially (either with a spay hook or manually) while one gently pushes the testicle (often located within the scrotal sac) through the inguinal canal into the abdomen. **F.** This retraction continues until the entire testicle and blood supply are removed from the scrotal sac. These procedures are repeated for the other testicle. A ligature is placed around both vasa deferentia and their associated blood supply near the base of bladder. A second ligature is then placed between the head of the epididymis and its scrotal attachment (at vaginal tunic). The testicle can now be removed by cutting above both ligatures. After removal of both testicles, each side of the invaginated scrotal sac and its associated epididymal fat is pushed back to its normal position. The bladder is returned to its anatomic position, and the abdomen is closed routinely.

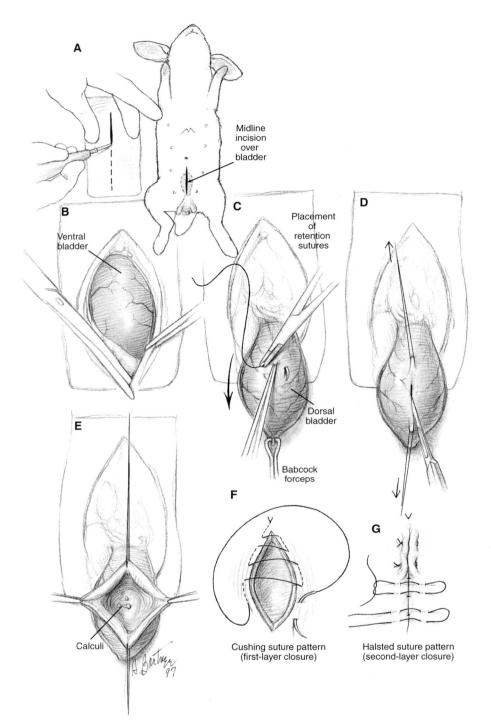

Fig. 43.26. Cystotomy. **A.** With the animal placed in dorsal recumbency, a midline skin incision is made extending from a point 5 cm caudal to the umbilicus to the level of the pelvic brim. **B.** Using Metzenbaum scissors and forceps, the incision is continued through the thin linea alba down through the muscle–fascia layer into the abdomen, exposing the ventral surface of the bladder. **C.** The apex of the bladder is next grasped with a pair of Babcock (or other atraumatic) forceps and is reflected caudally, exposing the dorsal side of the bladder. The bladder is then isolated from the abdomen with moistened laparotomy pads. Then, using 3–0 polyglactin 910 or polydioxanone suture on a taper needle, two retention sutures are placed 3 cm apart in an avascular location of the bladder. The bladder is then emptied by cystocentesis using a 25-gauge needle on a 20-mL syringe in a visibly avascular area of the fundus of the bladder. **D.** Lifting both retention sutures in opposite directions further elevates the bladder out of the abdomen and provides a taut area between them for entering the bladder. A stab incision is then made into this taut area with a scalpel. This incision is then extended cranially and caudally with Metzenbaum scissors. **E.** The bladder incision is then spread to allow inspection of the bladder contents. Any urinary calculi are removed with forceps or irrigation and suction. A specimen of bladder mucosa may be obtained for culture. **F.** The bladder is then closed in two layers using 3–0 polyglactin 910 or polydioxanone suture on a taper needle. The first layer is a Cushing suture pattern, which inverts the suture line when completed. The suture should not penetrate the lumen of the bladder. **G.** The second layer is closed using a Halsted suture pattern, which further inverts the incision and helps to ensure a complete seal. Each suture should be preplaced before being tied, to provide for even tissue inversion and tension distribution. Once the second layer is completed, the closure is checked for any leakage. The bladder is returned to its normal anatomic position, and the abdomen is closed routinely.

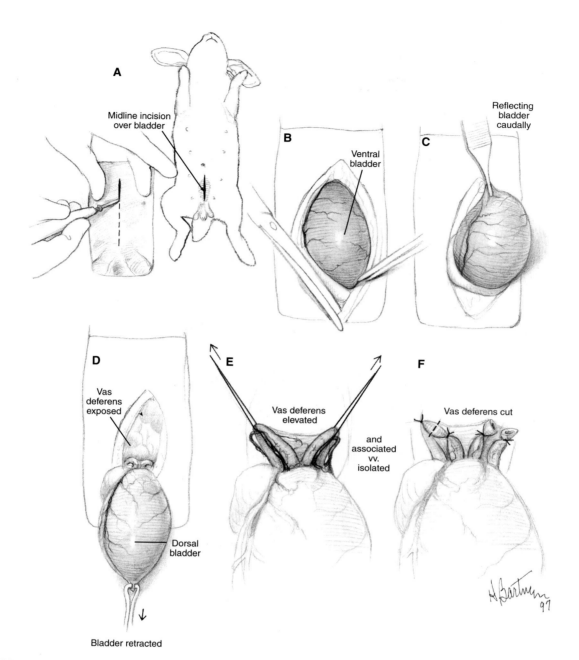

Labels in figure:

A — Midline incision over bladder

B — Ventral bladder

C — Reflecting bladder caudally

D — Vas deferens exposed; Dorsal bladder; Bladder retracted

E — Vas deferens elevated; and associated vv. isolated

F — Vas deferens cut

H Bartmann 97

Fig. 43.27. Vasectomy. **A.** With the animal placed in dorsal recumbency, a midline skin incision is made extending from 5 cm caudal to the umbilicus to the level of the pelvis or 2.5 cm anterior to the genitalia or to the level of the last set of nipples. **B.** Using a pair of Metzenbaum scissors and forceps, the incision is continued on the linea alba down through the muscle–fascia layer into the abdomen, exposing the ventral surface of the bladder. **C.** The apex of the bladder is next grasped with a pair of Babcock (or other atraumatic) forceps and is reflected caudally, exposing the dorsal side of the bladder. **D.** Further gentle caudal retraction of the bladder with the Babcock forceps exposes the two vasa deferentia emerging near the base of the bladder. **E.** A ligature is placed around each vas deferens, with care taken not to include the adjacent associated blood vessels. Each ligature is retracted to allow more exposure of each vas deferens for placement of second ligatures approximately 3 mm from the first. **F.** Each vas deferens is divided between the two ligatures with Metzenbaum scissors to complete the vasectomy. The bladder is returned to its normal anatomic position, and the abdomen is closed routinely.

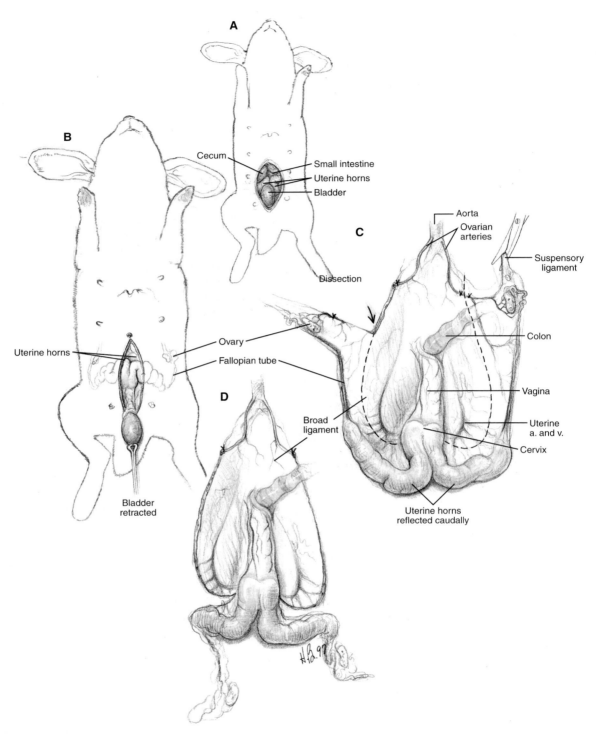

Fig. 43.28. Ovariohysterectomy. **A.** With the animal placed in dorsal recumbency, a midline skin incision is made extending from the umbilicus to the level 2 cm caudal to the last pair of nipples. Using Metzenbaum scissors and forceps, the incision is continued through the linea alba down through the muscle–fascia layer into the abdomen, exposing small portions of cecum, small intestines, uterine horns, and the bladder (if distended). Gentle retraction of the cecum laterally exposes the uterus. **B.** The bladder is retracted caudally with Babcock forceps to aid in visualizing the cervix and vagina. Using either Balfour or malleable retractors, the surgeon spreads the abdominal incision to aid in exposing the complete reproductive tract. **C** and **D.** Retracting the uterus caudally helps to expose the complete reproductive tract: vagina, cervix, two uterine horns, both fallopian tubes and ovaries, and the major blood supplies. With moistened cotton-tipped applicators, the fat is dissected gently to expose the abdominal aorta and the two ovarian arteries. Each ovarian artery is followed to the point where it branches to the ovary and the rest of the uterus. The surgeon places two ligatures around the vessel 3 mm apart above the branching and transects between them. The ovary is elevated, and the suspensory ligament identified and cut. The long fallopian tube and uterine horn are bluntly dissected from the broad ligament to the level 5 mm above the cervix, with care taken to control any hemorrhage from the many small vessels within the broad ligament supplying the uterine horn. This process is repeated on the other side.

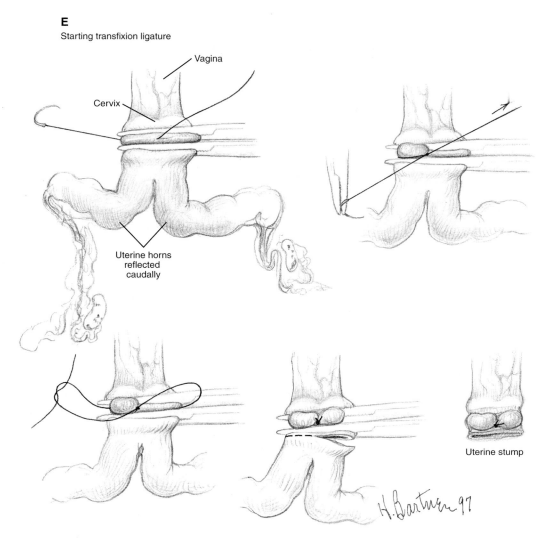

E
Starting transfixion ligature

Vagina

Cervix

Uterine horns
reflected
caudally

Uterine stump

H.Bartner 97

Fig. 43.28 (continued). **E.** Continuing (with the uterus reflected caudally), the cervix is identified and is palpated to identify its anatomy. Two Kelly forceps are placed 4 mm apart on the uterus just below the cervix. Using 3–0 absorbable suture on a taper needle, a transfixion ligature is started midway between the clamps. The transfixion ligature is completed, and the uterus is transected below the most distal clamp from the cervix with a scalpel. The uterine stump is examined for hemorrhage and is allowed to retract into the abdomen. The bladder is returned to its normal position, and the abdomen is closed routinely.

The treatment of choice for urinary calculi is cystotomy (Fig. 43.26). A urine culture should be taken by cystocentesis during the surgical procedure, before entering the bladder, and submitted for culture and sensitivity testing. Any calculi removed also should be analyzed for possible dietary adjustment as part of the treatment.

The animals should undergo diuresis for 2 to 3 days postoperatively with either intravenous or subcutaneous fluids, and appropriate antibiotic therapy should be instituted, if indicated. Once the calculi have been analyzed, adjustments in the diet can be made. In my experience, attempts at correcting other underlying problems, such as acidifying the urine, are futile. Affected animals should be monitored radiographically for recurrence (10).

Vasectomy

Vasectomy is generally performed on male rabbits for birth control purposes only (12). However, unlike castration, all the adverse side effects of an intact buck remain, including libido, urine spraying, aggressiveness, and hormonal urge to mark territory with urine and feces. The technique involves the resection of a portion of each vas deferens just cranial to the bladder after a midline laparotomy (Fig. 43.27). This surgical technique is currently gaining more use in biomedical research because of interest in producing transgenic animals. Bucks that have undergone vasectomy are used to induce ovulation in embryo-recipient does at the same time as the embryo-donor female is mated to an intact male (17). As previously suggested in the discussion of orchiectomy, bucks that have undergone vasectomy should be separated from intact does for at least 30 days postoperatively, to prevent possible pregnancy resulting from viable sperm remaining in the vas deferens.

Ovariohysterectomy

Ovariohysterectomy (OVH) is a commonly performed procedure in small animal practice and involves the surgical removal of the ovaries, fallopian tubes and the uterus. Performing an OVH on female rabbits (does) is similar to the procedure performed on dogs and cats and only requires a knowledge of the anatomic differences of rabbits for the procedure to be adapted. One major difference is that rather than having two uterine horns, a uterine body and one cervix (uterus bicornis bicollis) as in dogs and cats, rabbits have two uteri, each opening into the vagina through a separate cervix (duplex uterus) and no uterine body. These anatomic peculiarities, at first glance, appear to complicate the traditional OVH surgery techniques taught for cats and dogs where excision of the uterus is completed at the level of the uterine body. Carefully placing a transfixion ligature just anterior to the cervix (analogous to placement in the uterine body of a dog or cat), however, enables the complete removal of the doe's reproductive tract (see Figure 43.28).

Like cats, rabbits are induced ovulators with ovulation occurring 10–13 hours following copulation or after orgasm induced by another doe (8, 10). The gestation period is from 30–32 days. Female rabbits normally reach sexual maturity at 4–5 months, but it is best to wait until they reach at least 6 months of age before performing an OVH.

Indications for performing OVH in rabbits are: (1) to prevent or treat uterine adenocarcinoma (a very common neoplasia found in 50–80% of does over the age of 3); (2) to correct repeated false pregnancies; (3) to prevent pregnancy; (4) to treat pyometra or uterine hyperplasia; (5) to modify aggressive behavior and biting; and (6) to decrease urine spraying (4, 8, 10–12).

Figure 43.28 details the procedure for ovariohysterectomy in rabbits.

References

1. Marcella KL, Wright EM, Foresman PA, et al. What's your diagnosis: raised skin patches? Lab Anim 1986;15:13–15.
2. Flecknell P. Anesthesia and analgesia for rodents and rabbits. In: Laber–Laird K, Swindle MM, Flecknell P, eds. Handbook of rodent and rabbit medicine. Tarrytown, NY: Elsevier Science, 1996:219–237.
3. Wixson SK. Anesthesia and analgesia. In: Manning PJ, Ringler DH, Newcomer CE, eds. Biology of the laboratory rabbit. 2nd ed. San Diego: Academic Press, 1994:87–109.
4. Jenkins JR. Soft tissue surgery and dental procedures. In: Hillyear EV, Quesenberry KE, eds. Ferrets, rabbits and rodents: clinical medicine and surgery. Philadelphia: WB Saunders, 1997:227–239.
5. Crowe DT Jr, Bjorling DE. Peritoneum and peritoneal cavity. In: Slater D, ed. Textbook of small animal surgery. 2nd ed. Philadelphia: WB Saunders, 1993:413–415.
6. Hoyt RF Jr, DeLeonardis J, Clements S, et al. Post-operative use of adjustable cervical collars in rabbits. Contemp Top Lab Anim Sci 1994;33:822.
7. Gillett NA Brooks DL, Tillman PC. Medical and surgical management of gastric obstruction from a hairball in the rabbit. J Am Vet Med Assoc 1983;183:1176–1178.
8. Harkness JE. Rabbit husbandry and medicine. Vet Clin North Am Small Anim Pract 1987;17:1019–1044.
9. Harkness JE, Wagner JE. The biology and medicine of rabbits and rodents. 3rd ed. Philadelphia: Lea & Febiger, 1989:86–90.
10. Hillyer EV. Pet rabbits. Vet Clin North Am Small Anim Pract 1994;24:25–65.
11. Stein S, Walshaw S. Rabbits. In: Laber-Laird K, Swindle MM, Flecknell P, eds. Handbook of rodent and rabbit medicine. Tarrytown, NY: Elsevier Science, 1996:219–237.
12. Swindle MM, Shealy PM. Common surgical procedures in rodents and rabbits. In: Laber-Laird K, Swindle MM, Flecknell P, eds. Handbook of rodent and rabbit medicine. Tarrytown, NY: Elsevier Science, 1996:239–254.
13. Wagner JL, Hackel DB, Samsel AG. Spontaneous deaths in rabbits resulting from gastric trichobezoars. Lab Anim Sci 1974;24:826.
14. Garibaldi BA, Fox JG, Otto G, et al. Hematuria in rabbits. Lab Anim Sci 1987;37:769.
15. Kozma C, Macklin W, Cummins LM, et al. Anatomy, physiology, and biochemistry of the rabbit. In: Weisbroth SH, Flatt RE, Kraus AL, eds. The biology of the laboratory rabbit. New York: Academic Press, 1974:62–63.
16. Kraus AL, Weisbroth SH, Flatt RE, et al. Biology and diseases of rabbits. In: Fox JG, Cohen BJ, Loew FM, eds. Laboratory animal medicine. San Diego: Academic Press, 1984:207.
17. Robl JM, Heideman JK: Production of transgenic rats and rabbits. In: Pinkert CA, ed. Transgenic animal technology. New York: Academic Press, 1994:265–277.

Suggested Readings

Jenkins JR, Brown SA. A practitioner's guide to rabbits and ferrets. Denver, CO: American Animal Hospital Association, 1993.

Kaplan HM, Timmons EH. The rabbit: a model for the principles of mammalian physiology and surgery. New York: Academic Press, 1979:137–142.

Sebesteny A. Acute obstruction of the duodenum of a rabbit following the apparently successful treatment of a hairball. Lab Anim 1977;11:135.

Sedgewick CJ. Spaying the rabbit. Mod Vet Pract 1982;63:401.

Part II

Bones and Joints

44

NEUROLOGIC DIAGNOSIS

Algorithm for Diagnosis of Surgical Diseases of the Nervous System

James F. Biggart, III

Figures 44.1 to 44.9 are algorithms for the diagnosis of surgical diseases of the nervous system.

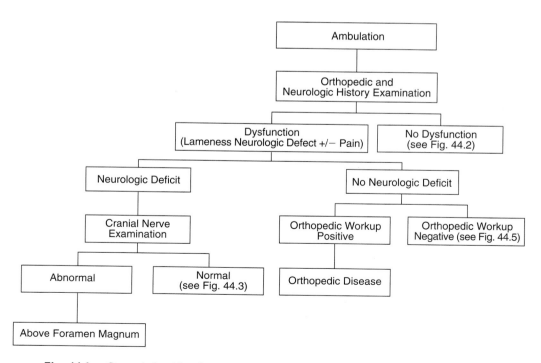

Fig. 44.1. General algorithm for the diagnosis of surgical diseases of the nervous system.

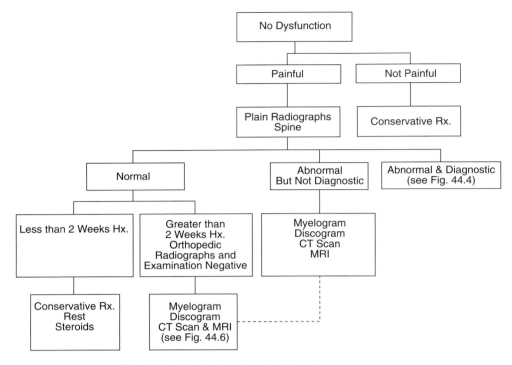

Fig. 44.2. No dysfunction: algorithm for management.

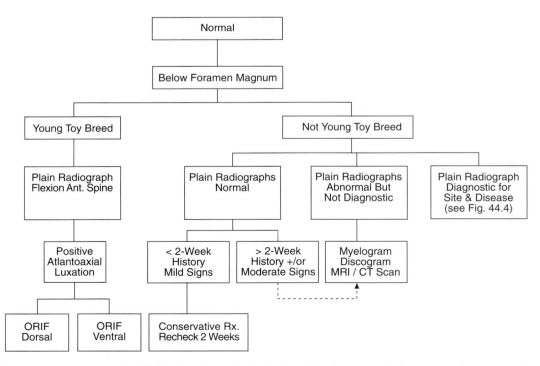

Fig. 44.3. Cervical vertebral instability (CVI) often has multiple levels and both static and dynamic cord pressures. A myelogram is helpful to add information not visible on plain films. Even if only one level is involved, a myelogram rules out other lesions at other levels. The variables in CVI are many, and a myelogram is usually indicated. *ORIF,* open reduction with internal fixation.

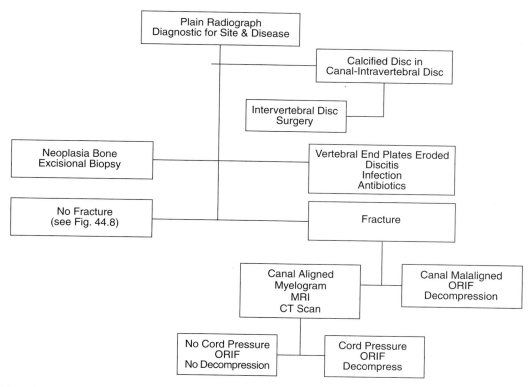

Fig. 44.4. Plain radiographs diagnostic for site and disease. Radiographs show a lesion so one can establish the disease possibilities and the location in the spine to one level. If a lesion cannot be located to one level, then a myelogram is needed. *ORIF*, open reduction with internal fixation.

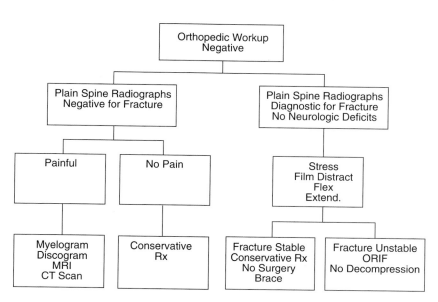

Fig. 44.5. Ambulation. The musculoskeletal and nervous systems contribute to ambulation. Eliminating orthopedic disease or verifying neurologic disease early allows the surgeon to concentrate on the spinal cord and nervous system. Few significant neurologic diseases of the spine occur without affecting ambulation. Pain limits generalized spine mobility, and this affects ambulation. Pain can be intermittent and is often absent when a patient is presented to the clinician. Clinicians often hesitate to evaluate patients that do not exhibit any other ambulation abnormalities when these animals have no history of pain (constant or intermittent) for several weeks. Subtle ambulation defects should be noted early. *ORIF*, open reduction with internal fixation.

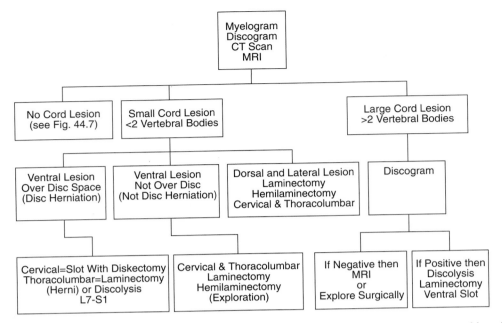

Fig. 44.6. Neurologic examination. Finding neurologic deficits pinpoints the abnormality to the nervous system. Musculoskeletal systems may also be involved, but the clinician can concentrate on the spine (or skull). Asymmetry in neurologic reflexes helps to confirm neurologic disease. Some orthopedic diseases can mimic neurologic diseases. Dementia and cranial nerve deficits place a lesion above the foramen magnum.

Generally, clinicians should localize neurologic lesions to one anatomic region of the spine and should make the differential diagnosis based on potential disorders in that region. Single lesions are more common than multifocal diseases and are more amenable to surgical treatment. More time should be spent on identifying treatable diseases than on differentiating nontreatable diseases. Treatable diseases should be ruled out first. Because surgery can treat spinal disease and can aid in making a prognosis, localization to one surgical level is helpful. Often, exploration of spinal disease at one level may be more cost-effective than the use of multiple diagnostic tests that do not also provide a treatment. Most owners cannot or will not take care of patients with painful spine disease or those that cannot walk or control their bladder and bowel function for long, and usually euthanasia is performed on these pets. Therefore, the veterinarian must diagnose and treat these patients quickly. The "do no harm" rule in medicine may need to be modified in these cases because prolonged diagnostic steps may lead to frustration. The worst risk to these patients is for clinicians to be too conservative and do too little.

Usually, the more severe the neurologic deficit, the more rapid is the need for diagnosis and treatment. That is not to say that a delay before treatment should preclude any type of therapy, but only that the prognosis may be worse with delay. The severity of the neurologic deficit influences the decision process less than is described in the literature because all neurologic lesions are serious, and until a diagnosis is made, all patients have the same chance of deterioration as of recovery. Most patients with neurologic disease benefit from medical or surgical intervention, yet clients' finances or their lack of understanding the potential for improvement with care and the severity of the consequences without it often influence our ability to treat their pets.

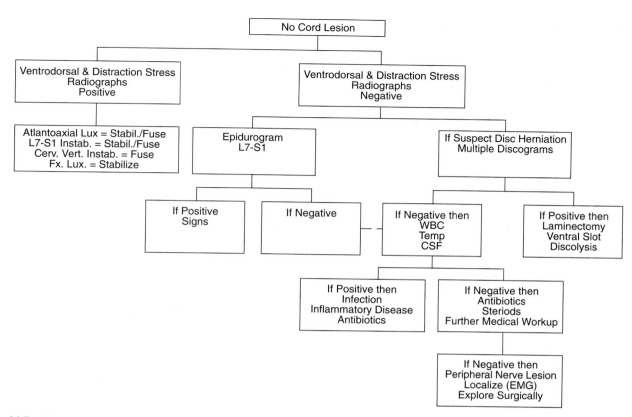

Fig. 44.7. History. The time of onset (acute versus chronic), a history of pain, previous trauma, progression of signs, and the patient's age aid in decision making. Patients deteriorating or remaining static while receiving adequate medical treatment need more aggressive care, such as surgery. Patients improving rapidly require less aggressive measures. I have not included euthanasia in the medical decision-making process because this is a socioeconomic decision made by the owner, not the veterinarian.

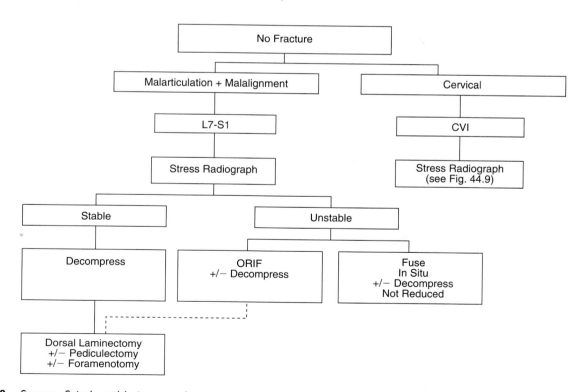

Fig. 44.8. Surgery. Spinal cord lesions are due to injury, inflammation, degeneration, neoplasia, or malformation. The types of spinal cord lesion amenable to surgery are subarachnoid cysts, external injury, such as fractures and gunshot wounds, internal injury, such as neoplasia, intervertebral disc disease, multicartilaginous exostosis, vertebral malformation, and discospondylitis, suppurative meningitis, and intramedullary neoplasia.

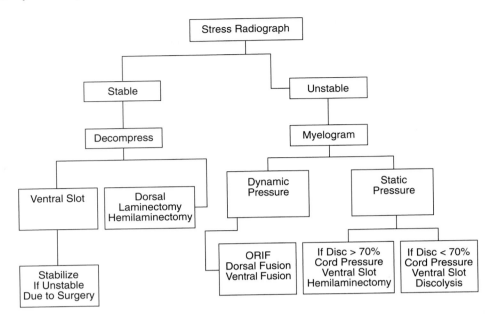

Fig. 44.9. The myelogram is the single most useful test to determine the need and type of surgery to perform in the spinal canal. Most spinal cord lesions amenable to surgery involve pressures on the spinal cord or nerve roots. Myelography demonstrates spinal cord pressures well with few false-negative results and usually allows visualization of the entire spine. Negative myelograms preclude surgery because the level of injury must be known in order to operate. Myelography is inexpensive compared with MRI, or CT, and is readily performed without elaborate instrumentation. Surgery can be performed during the same anesthesia. MRI, CT scans, and discography require some localization of the region to be studied because of the impracticality and cost of using these modalities as scanning devices of the entire spine. *ORIF,* open reduction with internal fixation.

Determination and Localization of Spinal Cord and Peripheral Nerve Lesions

Linda Blythe

Animals with an acute onset of deficits of the spinal cord or peripheral nerves present with clinical signs relative to pain, sensory ataxia (loss of proprioception), or weakness of voluntary movement. Pain and reluctance to move resulting from musculoskeletal lesions or from generalized motor weakness induced by metabolic disorders must be differentiated from the same signs caused by neurologic dysfunction. Often, assessments of the presence or absence of reflexes and proprioceptive (knowing where one's body is relative to the environment) deficits are the best differentiating tests. A complete history including signalment, onset, and progression of clinical signs, vaccinations, and exposure risks to infectious diseases needs to be collected, and both physical and neurologic examinations are required. Although this discussion focuses on determination and localization of spinal cord and peripheral nerve disorders, the veterinarian must be sure that the patient has no cranial nerve deficits, no changes in behavior or mentation, and no past seizure activity

that would indicate a lesion localized in the head or diffusely throughout the central nervous system.

The use of the concept of upper motor neuron (UMN) versus lower motor neuron (LMN) lesion is valuable in localizing the lesion to specific areas of the spinal cord or peripheral nerves. UMN have their cell bodies (neurons) in the brain with axons that course distally through the spinal cord to synapse on and direct the LMNs to excite a skeletal muscle (Fig. 44.10). LMN are those neurons with cell bodies scattered throughout the ventral horn of the gray matter of the spinal cord and with axons distributed in peripheral

Table 44.1.
Comparison of Clinical Signs Present with Lower Motor Neuron (LMN) and Upper Motor Neuron (UMN) Disease

	LMN Signs	UMN Signs
Voluntary movement	←——Paresis to Paralysis——→	
Sensory perception	←——Loss of Proprioception——→	
	←——Hypalgesia——→	
	←——Analgesia——→	
Reflexes	Hyporeflexia → Areflexia	Normal → Hyperreflexia
Muscles	Hypotonic Neurogenic atrophy EMG abnormalities (after 5 days)	Hypertonic Mild disuse atrophy No EMG changes

nerves to innervate skeletal muscles directly. Table 44.1 compares the similarities and differences in clinical signs seen in UMN and LMN disease. The presence or absence of reflexes and the finding of denervation (LMN) muscle atrophy (in lesions present for more than 2 weeks) are the keys to localization of a lesion within the spinal cord or peripheral nerves. Figure 44.11 is a schematic illustration dividing the spinal cord into functional segments that can be tested for localization of a lesion within that segment, and Table 44.2 lists the defects that may be present in each area.

The initial examination should evaluate the animal's gait (if ambulatory) and the presence of muscle atrophy. With the latter, careful comparison of the muscle mass of the right and left sides may assist in determination if an asymmetric LMN spinal cord lesion or a peripheral nerve dysfunction is more chronic (duration longer than 2 weeks). Gait should be evaluated for normal functioning of each of the major joints of the limbs, for example, the ability to flex the elbow, extend the hock, and support the body in the weight-bearing phase of the gait. Presence of ataxia (lack of coordination) and motor weakness in either the thoracic or the pelvic limbs should be noted. Testing of reflexes, evaluation of the presence or absence of conscious proprioception, and assessments of touch and pain response follow. If the results of these tests are abnormal (see later), neurologic dysfunction is suggested and can be localized to the specific functional spinal cord segment or peripheral nerves. Peripheral nerve injury most commonly affects only one limb, but a diffuse acute onset of LMN peripheral nerve diseases, such as botulism, tick paralysis, and polyradiculoneuritis ("coonhound paralysis"), is not uncommon. In addition, chronic dieback peripheral neuropathies occur in various metabolic diseases, such as hypothyroidism. Figure 44.12 illustrates a stepwise approach that may assist in the localization of a spinal cord lesion.

Clinically, the most useful reflexes to test are the pain-induced limb withdrawal reflex, the patellar tendon tap (phasic stretch reflex), the perineal or anal

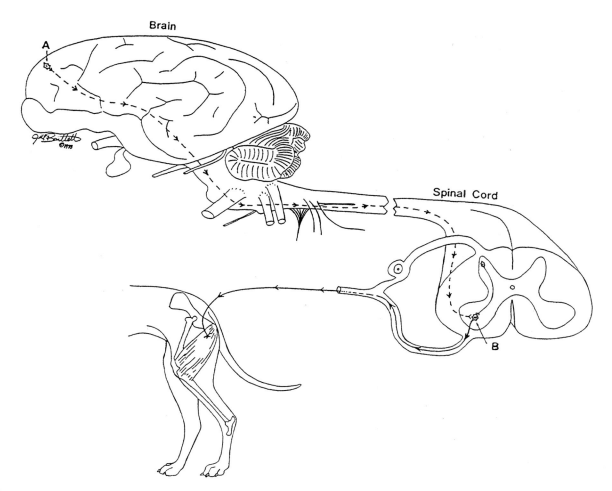

Fig. 44.10. Schematic illustration of the location of upper motor neurons (**A**) in the brain and their effect on lower motor neurons (**B**) found in the ventral horn of the spinal cord of a dog.

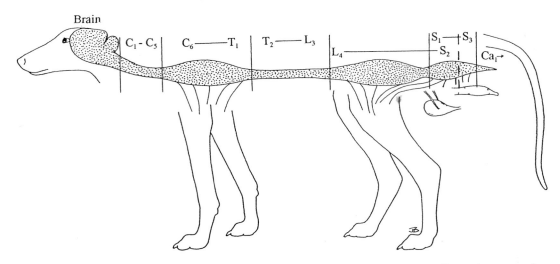

Fig. 44.11. Schematic illustration of the functional spinal cord segments of the dog. Neurologically, each segment has a grouping of clinical signs that are unique to it and are detailed in Table 44.2.

Table 44.2.
Summary of Clinical Signs Seen With Spinal Cord Lesions at Various Levels[a]

Focal Lesion	Clinical Signs
Upper cervical (C1–5)	Ataxia and paresis of all four limbs to quadriplegia (may be more obvious in pelvic limbs)
	Normal or exaggerated reflexes and muscle tone in all four limbs (UMN)
	Normal to hyper tail and anal tone and reflexes (UMN)
	± Hypoesthesia caudal to lesion
	± Urinary incontinence with automatic bladder (UMN) depending on severity of lesion
	± Horner's syndrome
	± Respiratory death in acute trauma cases from loss of input to the phrenic nerve
Brachial enlargement (C6–T1)	Ataxia and paresis of all four limbs to quadriplegia
	Depressed or absent thoracic limb reflexes and muscle hypotonia with atrophy (LMN)
	Normal or hyperreflexia in pelvic limb with muscle hypertonicity (UMN)
	Normal to hyper tail and anal tone and reflexes (UMN)
	Hypoesthesia or analgesia caudal to lesion
	± Urinary incontinence with automatic bladder (UMN) depending on severity of lesion
	± Horner's syndrome (T1–3)
Thoracolumbar area (T2–L3)	Thoracic limbs normal (Schiff–Sherrington syndrome[b] is the only exception in acute severe cord trauma)
	Pelvic limb ataxia and paresis to paraplegia
	Normal to hyper tail and anal tone and reflexes
	Normal to exaggerated pelvic limb reflexes with normal to hypertonicity of muscles (UMN)
	Hypoesthesia of muscles (UMN)
	Hypoesthesia or analgesia caudal to lesion
	Urinary incontinence with automatic bladder (UMN)
Pelvic enlargement (L4 through caudal segments)	Thoracic limbs normal
	Ataxia and paresis to paraplegia in the pelvic limbs
	Decreased or absent pelvic limb reflexes
	Muscle hypotonia and atrophy
	Hypoesthesia or analgesia caudal to lesion
	Urinary incontinence and constipation:
	Automatic bladder if above S2
	Overflow flaccid bladder if below S2
	Decreased or absent tail tone and anal reflexes if below S2

[a] With spinal cord trauma, *pain perception* is the best prognostic indicator. If it is gone after 48 hours, prognosis is guarded but *not always hopeless.* Withdrawal flexor reflex should not be confused with pain perception.
[b] Schiff–Sherrington syndrome is an extension of the thoracic limbs when the dog is at rest in lateral recumbency. However, when the dog stands, walks, or is neurologically tested, the thoracic limbs test normal. This is the only instance in which a clinical sign is evident in front of a spinal cord lesion.

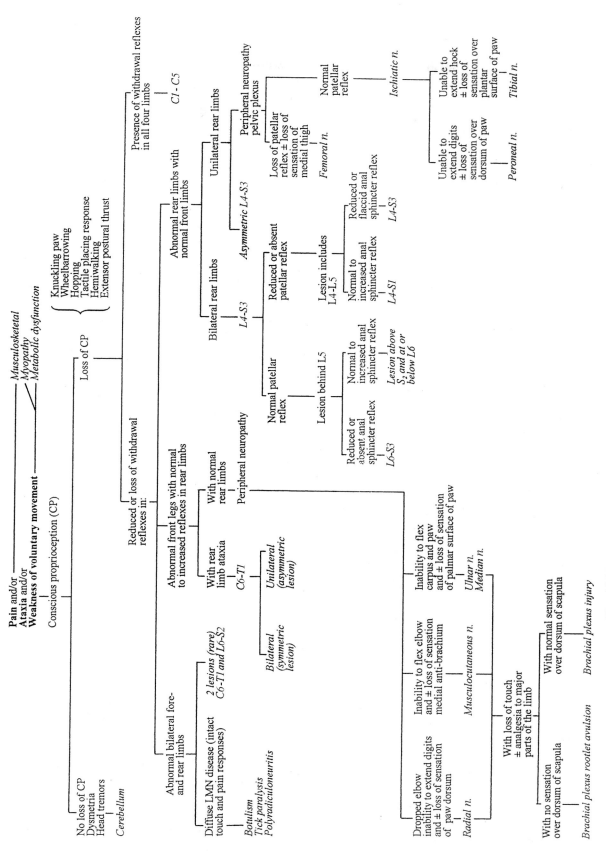

Fig. 44.12. Algorithm for localization of lesions in the spinal cord of a dog.

sphincter reflex, the panniculus or cutaneus trunci reflex, and muscle tone (tonic stretch reflex). In addition to watching the animal's ability to ambulate and testing reflex arcs, the veterinarian can test the sensory components of each segment for the perception of touch and pain and intact proprioception. The cutaneous maps for the dog's autonomous (single nerve supply) and overlap (more than a single nerve supply) zones have been published by Bailey, Kitchell, and Johnson (1, 2). Figure 44.13 illustrates the autonomous zones (skin areas with a single nerve supply) of the peripheral nerves of the forelimb that are commonly affected by trauma (3). These cutaneous maps are especially useful in localizing unilateral peripheral nerve deficits. Brachial plexus injuries often involve multiple nerves with large areas of skin analgesic to perception of both touch and pain. Loss of pain indicates a more severe lesion with possible disruption of the nerve fibers. When the autonomous zone of the

dorsal cutaneous branch of cervical nerve VI is analgesic, irreversible brachial plexus rootlet avulsion must be suspected (2).

Presence of proprioception is best tested by knuckling the animal's paw to rest on the dorsum of the foot, while the veterinarian supports the animal's body, and seeing whether the animal does not immediately correct it. This maneuver should be done sequentially with all four paws. Other tests of conscious proprioception are hopping, wheelbarrowing, hemiwalking, and extensor postural thrust (picking an animal up and slowly lowering it to the ground while observing the correct positioning of the limbs under the body to support weight or the failure to do so). The last test can be done both in thoracic and pelvic limbs. Visual and tactile (without visual input) placing responses are also useful tests in detecting lack of proprioception and in differentiating between spinal cord and cerebellar lesions. With a cerebellar lesion, dysmetria of the placing responses is evident, as opposed to failure to respond to this sensory stimulus when spinal cord compression or disease is present. Presence of proprioceptive deficits is a hallmark of neurologic dysfunction and often the earliest evident neurologic deficit.

Ancillary radiologic tests including myelography, scintigraphy, magnetic resonance imaging, and computed tomography are all useful in localizing a morphologic lesion of the spinal cord. Cerebrospinal fluid analysis is optimal in detecting inflammatory or infectious diffuse spinal cord disease. The most readily available neurodiagnostic tests are electromyography (EMG) and nerve conduction velocity measurements. Somatosensory-evoked potentials recorded from the spinal cord or the head are commonly available only in veterinary colleges, as reviewed by Holliday (4).

EMG is a diagnostic technique that evaluates muscle for the presence or absence of spontaneous abnormal electrical activity and for the presence and character of evoked motor unit potentials. Essentially a sophisticated voltmeter with an oscilloscope and audiomonitor, the electromyograph detects and displays differences in membrane potentials between an active and a reference electrode placed within a muscle (often using a concentric needle that contains both electrodes within the same needle). Amplification of sounds characteristic of certain spontaneous electrical discharges assists the electromyographer in detecting abnormalities in the muscle fibers.

The most common veterinary use of EMG is in animals either with muscle wasting or suspected traumatic injuries to the nervous system. The presence of spontaneous electrical activity in resting muscle indicates that either the muscle or the nerve supplying that muscle has been affected. Fibrillation potentials have a wave form that is low in amplitude (20 to 250

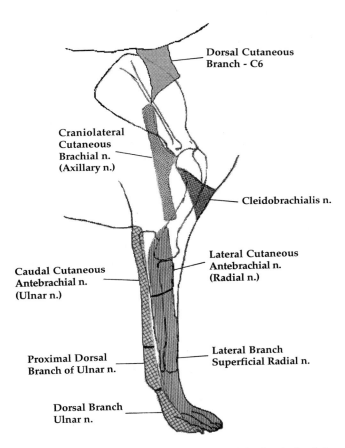

Fig. 44.13. Autonomous sensory areas of the forelimb of the dogs. Each nerve with a shaded area provides the sole cutaneous innervation for that section of the body. (From Engel HN. Multimedia guide to the study of the anatomy of the dog. Corvallis, OR: Oregon State University Press, 1996.)

Labels on figure:
Dorsal Cutaneous Branch - C6
Craniolateral Cutaneous Brachial n. (Axillary n.)
Cleidobrachialis n.
Caudal Cutaneous Antebrachial n. (Ulnar n.)
Lateral Cutaneous Antebrachial n. (Radial n.)
Proximal Dorsal Branch of Ulnar n.
Lateral Branch Superficial Radial n.
Dorsal Branch Ulnar n.

μV) and short in duration (1 to 5 milliseconds), with a characteristic "frying eggs" or "rain on a tin roof" sound. Positive sharp waves have an amplitude of 10 to 1000 μV and a longer duration of 10 to 100 milliseconds, with the characteristic sound of an idling motor boat. Although both these spontaneous potentials can be present in myopathies, they are most commonly associated with muscles that have lost part or all of their nerve supply. In injuries causing peripheral nerve or lower motor neuron damage in the spinal cord, it takes 5 days for the affected muscles to develop detectable abnormal electrical potentials.

Nerve conduction velocity measurements are the optimal way to test the integrity of peripheral nerves, both motor and sensory. With motor nerves, one uses two stimulation sites over the nerve and records the evoked motor unit action potential of the innervated muscle. Both the latency (the time for the stimulus to cause a response) and the distance between the cathode-stimulating electrode and the recording electrodes are measured for each stimulation site. The differences in distance between the two sites divided by the differences in latency between the two sites gives the nerve conduction velocity of the proximal segment of the nerve. With sensory nerve conduction velocity measurements, one records the evoked action potential direct off the sensory nerve with one stimulation site, but a signal averager and multiple stimuli are needed to visualize the evoked potential. Nerve conduction velocities vary among nerves within an animal and among animal species; for example, the cat has faster nerve conduction velocities than the dog. Generally, nerve conduction velocities slower than 50 m/second when measured at normal room temperatures are considered abnormal and reflect demyelination (i.e., from compression) of the peripheral nerve (5). Electrical stimulation of a nerve and observation of the contraction of the respective innervated muscles are also useful tools in evaluating acute injuries such as humeral, femoral, or pelvic fractures, to ensure the integrity of adjacent nerves to the limbs.

References

1. Bailey C, Kitchell R. Cutaneous sensory testing in the dog. J Vet Intern Med 1987;1:128–135.
2. Bailey C, Kitchell R, Johnson R. Spinal nerve root origins of the cutaneous nerves arising from the canine brachial plexus. Am J Vet Res 1982;43:820–825.
3. Engel HN. Multimedia guide to the study of the anatomy of the dog. Corvallis, OR: Oregon State University Press, 1996.
4. Holliday T. Electrodiagnostic examination: somatosensory evoked potentials and electromyography. Vet Clin North Am Small Anim Pract 1992;22:833–857.
5. Chrisman C. Special ancillary investigations. In: Problems in small animal neurology. 2nd ed. Philadelphia: Lea & Febiger, 1991:81–118.

Myelography of Disc Disease

Barclay Slocum,
Theresa Devine Slocum &
James F. Biggart, III

Myelography is a contrast imaging technique of the spine that is ideally suited for the practicing veterinarian. Iohexol contrast material is injected in the intrathecal space, which contains the cerebrospinal fluid (CSF). Standard radiography is used to image the spinal area. The procedure can be performed in a hospital setting at a reasonable cost. The primary prerequisite is precision, attention to detail, and patience.

The primary purpose of a myelogram is to locate the site of a lesion before surgical intervention for decompression of a herniated intervertebral disc or tumor. The diagnosis of the disease process may be based on clinical signs, progression of the disease process, and signalment. If the client rejects the surgical option and elects a medical course of treatment, then a myelogram will have no benefit to the outcome of the case and may add some additional insult to an already compromised spinal cord. If the client accepts the surgical option for treatment of a suspected herniated intervertebral disc, then a myelogram is mandatory to locate the site of spinal cord compression.

The second purpose of a myelogram is to define the extent of spinal cord compromise and thereby to assist in rendering a more accurate prognosis. This is especially useful when spastic paresis has given way to flaccid, areflexic hind limbs, because the owner needs to know whether the disease process involves widespread spinal cord swelling and a grave prognosis.

Although myelography allows visualization of spinal cord lesions, the myelographic contrast material is irritating to the central nervous system and can precipitate seizures. An improperly performed myelogram at the cisterna magna can pith the patient or cause respiratory paralysis by damaging the brainstem. If the brainstem is abnormal, a properly performed myelogram at the cisterna magna may cause respiratory compromise. In patients with little neurologic reserve, a transient reduction in neurologic function is often observed for 1 day to 2 weeks. Patients with mild neurologic signs seldom experience a reduction in neurologic function after a myelogram.

In short, a myelogram has some inherent risks that should be conveyed to the client before the procedure, and the procedure itself should be performed when the potential knowledge gained will benefit the patient or client, change the course of treatment, and clarify the diagnosis or prognosis.

Cisternal Injection

Lateral and ventrodorsal radiographs of the spine are taken before contrast injection to survey for lesions and to ensure proper exposure and positioning. Separate films are necessary in large-chested dogs to obtain properly exposed C1–4 vertebrae and C5 through the thoracic vertebrae. Visualization of the thoracic region is often obscured by overlying ribs on the lateral radiograph. By placing a foam wedge beneath the animal's chest, the spine rotates around its long axis, and the oblique projection then allows a clear view of the thoracic region.

The equipment necessary for a cisternal injection is a 20-gauge spinal needle, 2.5 inches in length, iohexol 180 mg Iodine/mL, an extension set with a "T," an appropriately sized syringe, and a sterile collection tube for the CSF. Preparation of contrast media for injection is done before insertion of the spinal needle, so no delay occurs during the procedure. The sterile extension set with the "T" is placed on the end of the syringe and is filled with the iohexol media; all bubbles are eliminated. The spinal epaxial muscles may not support the spinal needle with the "T" extension in place. Increased support of the needle eliminates movement of the needle tip in the subarachnoid space.

The dosage of iohexol for myelography depends on the severity and location of the lesion; it is 0.2 mL/kg for cervical filling and 0.4 mL/kg for lumbar filling. If the patient is ambulatory, in pain, and only mildly affected neurologically, then the subarachnoid space will be incompletely compressed; the contrast material usually flows past the lesion. For most patients, 0.4 mL/kg is necessary to permit the dye to occupy the area cranial and caudal to the lesion to demonstrate the lesion.

If the patient is nonambulatory because of a herniated intervertebral disc, then the occlusion of the subarachnoid space will inhibit the flow of contrast material past the lesion. A dosage of 0.2 mL/kg should be considered because the dye will occupy the space cranial to the lesion, and that is the region outlined by contrast material. Excessive volume forces the contrast media to occupy the ventricles within the brain, predisposing the patient to seizures.

In preparation for cervical myelography, the dorsal midline cranial to the occiput and caudal to the axis, 7.5 cm wide, is clipped and prepared for sterile surgery. The animal's ears are taped ventrally to prevent contamination of the injection site. The anesthetized and intubated patient is positioned in lateral recumbency, with the head flexed at 90° to the cervical spine at the occipitoatlantal articulation. The technician who holds the patient in this position must be stable and comfortable, with body weight resting on the table.

The injection site is the cisterna cerebellomedullaris.

The anatomic landmarks for tapping the cisterna magna are the occiput and the cranial margin of the dorsal spinous process of the axis. A 20-gauge, 2.5-inch spinal needle is introduced through the skin in the dorsal midline, halfway between the occiput and the axis. The needle is slowly and carefully advanced in the ventral direction. The needle tends to be unstable in the soft tissues until the dura mater is pierced by the tip of the needle. As soon as the resistance of piercing the dura matter is overcome, the tip of the needle should be in the cisterna magna. The stylet of the spinal needle is withdrawn, and spinal fluid is allowed to flow freely. After the first 0.5 mL of CSF has passed the needle hub, the next 5.0 mL of CSF is collected in a sterile test tube for laboratory analysis.

Tilting the table slightly is helpful, so the patient's head is lower than the lumbar spine to drain the CSF from the spinal cord. This maneuver allows the subarachnoid space of the spinal cord to be filled more easily with contrast medium. The table is leveled, and the filled extension set is placed between the spinal needle and the syringe to prevent unwanted movement at the needle during injection of the contrast material. Injection of the contrast media is extremely slow, to allow the dye to flow into the subarachnoid space without excessive pressure. The syringe should have no back pressure during injection. Back pressure indicates too rapid an injection or incorrect placement of the needle tip in the cisternal magna. The patient's respiration should be monitored continuously. Diminished respiration is a reason for decreasing the injection rate to lessen pressure. Immediately after injection of the contrast material, the spinal needle is withdrawn. Slight negative pressure on the syringe during withdrawal minimizes leakage of contrast media from the needle through the puncture site or contamination of the epidural space. Tilting the table so the patient's head is slightly higher than the spinal cord facilitates filling of the subarachnoid space of the caudal cord. Lateral and ventrodorsal radiographs of the spine are taken after injection in the same sequence as the flow of dye, cranially to caudally.

Lumbar Injection

Survey radiographs are taken of the spine. The equipment is the same for both injection sites, except a longer spinal needle is often required in large dogs or obese animals. We find that 3.5 inches in length is most frequently used. The contrast medium is prepared in the syringe and extension set before lumbar injection. Dosage in most cases is 0.4 mL/kg for a complete spinal series.

In preparation for lumbar myelography, an area from L2 to the sacrum, 10 cm wide, is clipped and prepared for sterile surgery. The anesthetized and intubated patient is positioned in lateral recumbency with the lumbar spine flexed by a technician holding the animal's hocks to the rib cage. The technician holding the patient in this position must be stable and comfortable, with body weight resting on the table. The dorsal acetabular rim (radiographic position), with the dog in sternal position and the hind legs pulled forward, is an alternative position for a lumbar myelograph. The preferred injection site is between the L6 and L7 vertebrae because the sacral segments of the spinal cord end at the body of L5. Performing a myelogram at this level reduces the possibility of trauma to the spinal cord by the needle. The dorsal spinous process of L7 is the landmark for injection at L6–7. This process is shorter than the dorsal spinous process of L6, and it may be difficult to palpate if the patient is obese. The L5–6 vertebral space is also used for lumbar injection in patients with severe spinal facet arthritis or a collapsed space. The L6 dorsal spinous process is the landmark for injection at L5–6.

A 3.5-inch 20-gauge spinal needle is introduced through the skin in the dorsal midline at the caudal margin of the dorsal spinous of L7. The needle is carefully advanced in the cranioventral direction parallel to the dorsal spinous process. The ligamentum flavum is penetrated at the dorsal intervertebral space.

If the patient has spinal facet arthritis, this space may be so small that the spinal needle is pinched by the lamina cranially and caudally as it passes through the space. If the spine is arthritic and a lumbar myelogram is mandatory, then the surgeon must be prepared to make a surgical exposure of the dorsal lamina of L6. The dorsal lamina is penetrated by a small, 1-mm bur, and the spinal needle is passed through the bur hole in the lamina to complete the myelogram in a routine manner.

The needle is advanced through the spinal cord to come rest on the floor of the spinal canal. The viable cord reacts to this penetration by the spinal needle, and muscular "twitch" of the rump or tail region is noted. If the needle is believed to be on the floor of the spinal canal and no "twitch" is noted, then the spinal cord is nonresponsive because of the lesion or the depth of anesthesia or because the needle is not positioned correctly. Without moving the patient, the position of the needle can be confirmed by a lateral radiograph.

The tip of the spinal needle is withdrawn 2 to 3 mm to lie in the subarachnoid space. The stylet of the spinal needle is withdrawn, and spinal fluid is allowed to flow freely. After the first 0.5 mL of CSF has passed the needle hub, the next 5.0 mL of CSF is collected for laboratory analysis. A small patient such as a dachshund may only produce 1 mL of CSF. If no CSF flows from the needle, then the needle is improperly located, or the spinal cord lesion is compressing the subarach-

noid space. Occlusion of the jugular may increase CSF flow.

The filled extension set is attached between the spinal needle and the syringe to prevent unwanted movement at the needle during injection of the contrast material. Care must be taken to prevent any air bubbles from entering the needle before injection. Injection of the contrast is slow to allow the dye to flow into the subarachnoid space without excessive pressure. The syringe should have no back pressure during injection. If one has any question about the position of the needle or the dye, a lateral radiograph is taken without moving the patient. Immediately after injection of the contrast material, the spinal needle is withdrawn. Negative pressure on the syringe during the withdrawal minimizes the leakage of the dye through the puncture site.

Tilting the table so patient's head is lower than the lumbar spine may be helpful, so the subarachnoid space of the cervical spinal cord can be filled more easily with contrast media. Because the volume of contrast provides the pressure for movement of contrast material, tilting the table is usually necessary only if the lesion is in the cervical region.

Radiographs follow the direction of dye flow from lumbar to the cervical region. As described previously, the thoracic region is rotated to prevent the ribs from obscuring the spinal column on the lateral radiograph of this region.

Radiography

Before contrast injection, whether the site is cisternal or lumbar, lateral and ventrodorsal radiographs of the spine are taken to survey for lesions and to ensure correct exposure and positioning. Properly exposed films of all areas are critical for diagnosis. Large-chested dogs require separate films for adjoining areas in the cervical region. The thoracic area should be rotated with a radiolucent foam wedge for the lateral radiograph so the ribs do not obscure the spinal area. After injection of contrast material, radiographs should be taken sequentially to follow the dye flow. In large-chested dogs, the head and hip should be raised to obtain adequate dye flow in the thoracic region.

Myelographic dynamics of the cervical region can be demonstrated by specific radiographic views. Traction on the cervical spine during contrast radiography often differentiates between a herniated disc within the cervical spinal canal and a redundant dorsal anulus that compresses the ventral dye column. In patients with cervical vertebral instability, flexion and extension radiographs of the cervical spine demonstrate that the cranial portion of the body of the caudal vertebra pathologically projects into the cervical spinal canal, greatly compressing the spinal cord and dye columns.

Stenosis of the cervical spinal canal can cause a neurologic deficit and sometimes accompanies the cervical vertebral instability.

The lumbosacral region is frequently subjected to contrast radiography to demonstrate compression of the L7–S1 cauda equina by a redundant dorsal anulus fibrosis or herniated intervertebral disc. Because the dural sac normally extends to the midsacrum, a cervical injection allows the dye to flow unobstructed to the midsacrum and to end in a point. The ventrodorsal radiograph demonstrates the dural sac in the midline. Neither lateral nor ventrodorsal radiographs of the myelogram show the nerve roots as they exit the L7–S1 foramina. In some patients, the normal dural sac may end in a point as far cranially as the midbody of L6. An epidurogram may be used in these patients to demonstrate L7–S1 dorsal annular redundancy or disc herniation.

Lateral radiographs of the lumbosacral region, first in a neutral position, second in flexion, and third in extension, can demonstrate the dynamic redundancy of the dorsal anulus of the L7–S1 disc causing compression of the cauda equina. In mild cases of cauda equina compression, the dye column is not compressed in flexion, but it is compressed on the extended lateral radiograph. This provides graphic evidence of the mechanism of trauma that causes the patient to be sore after activity.

If a relaxed lateral radiograph of the lumbosacral region demonstrates compression of the cauda equina, then redundancy of the dorsal anulus of the L7–S1 disc can be distinguished from a herniated disc or spondylosis deformans within the spinal canal by a flexion radiograph. If the dye column is restored by flexion of the L7–S1 region, then the cause is redundancy of the dorsal anulus, which is responsive to the L7–S1 fixation fusion procedure. If the dye column is not restored or is increased in the flexion radiograph, then exploration and decompression of L7–S1 are indicated to visualize and correct the cause.

If clinical signs are associated with the L7–S1 junction and are lateralized to one limb with fixed lateral deviation of the caudal dural sac, then a herniated disc impinging the L7–S1 nerve root in the foramen is the probable cause.

Interpretation

The myelogram is used to provide a positive contrast image of the space in which the CSF resides. On the ventrodorsal radiograph of the spine, one sees right and left columns of contrast material. The ventrodorsal radiograph often shows a loss of dye column with a herniated intervertebral disc. The dye is centered over the space where the herniation occurs. Most often, the

dye loss is bilaterally symmetric. If a small amount of disc herniation is centrally located in the spinal canal, the dye column may deviate and may have diminished contrast axially. If the dye loss is greater on one side, this indicates lateralization of the herniation. The side of greatest dye loss is usually the side of greatest neurologic deficit. Sometimes, the only deviation of the dye column is to the side opposite the herniation.

On the lateral radiograph of the spine using contrast, one sees dorsal and ventral columns of contrast material. A widened portion of the spinal canal in the region of the nerve roots to the limbs is visible. The caudal cervical intumescence, C4–T1, is the widened region of the spinal cord supplying the forelimb nerve roots. The lumbar intumescence, L3–5, is the widened region of the spinal cord supplying the hind limb nerve roots. Nerve rootlets can be seen as parallel striations on the myelogram running caudoventrally in the region of the lumbar intumescence. The myelogram does not demonstrate compression of nerve roots as they pass through the intervertebral foramen because no subarachnoid space is present around the nerve roots, and the contrast material does not flow laterally. Pain and ventral column compression infer intervertebral disc herniation against the nerve roots as they pass through the foramen. Diminished spinal cord function, in the absence of pain and ventral column compression, infers a centrally located intervertebral disc herniation.

A myelogram of a patient with a herniated intervertebral disc usually shows compression of the dye column centered over a disc space. The disc space may or may not appear collapsed. The disc space may or may not have calcified disc material (Fig. 44.14). Calcified disc material in the spinal canal often makes the intervertebral foramen at the site of herniation appear lighter than the adjacent foramina. Calcified disc material may or may not be seen in the spinal canal.

If the patient is ambulatory, then the occlusion of the subarachnoid space is usually incomplete, and the contrast material usually flows past the lesion. The

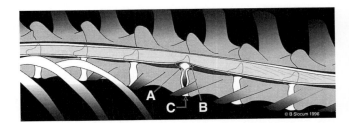

Fig. 44.14. The mild herniation of an intervertebral disc at L2 (A) has only a mild compression of the ventral dye column (B) without narrowing of the disc space (C). The prognosis is good.

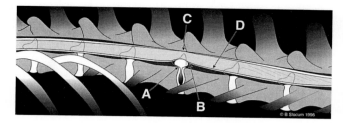

Fig. 44.15. Herniation of the intervertebral disc at L2 (*A*) has caused loss of the ventral dye column (*B*), dorsal dye column (*C*), and dorsal deviation of the cord (*D*). The prognosis is good.

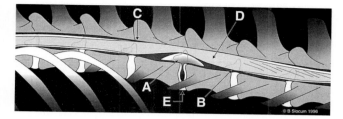

Fig. 44.17. Herniation of the intervertebral disc at L2 (*A*) has caused loss of the ventral dye column over the length of the vertebra (*B*), dorsal column over the length of the vertebra (*C*), swelling of the spinal cord without definition adjacent to the herniated disc (*D*), and a collapsed disc space (*E*). The prognosis is poor.

volume provides contrast media to the regions cranial and caudal to the lesion that demonstrate the pathologic features (Fig. 44.15). With a lumbar injection, the dural sac is a closed space, and hydraulic pressure forces the contrast material past the lesion. As the resistance to injection increases with increasing compromise of the cord and subarachnoid space, the incidence of epidural spillage of the contrast is increased. With a cisternal injection, when the contrast material is less concentrated caudal to the lesion, the pressure of the spinal cord on the subarachnoid space is considerable. This condition is reason to recommend decompression of the spinal cord. The prognosis for this type of patient is good with surgical intervention.

Patients with spastic paresis usually have a viable spinal cord caudal to the lesion (Fig. 44.16). If deep pain is present even in the absence of conscious proprioception, the prognosis is still good. Loss of contrast material of one-half the vertebral body length cranial and caudal to the herniated disc approaches the limit of the ischemic insult that the spinal cord can withstand without permanent long-term neurologic deficit. One usually sees a slightly diminished "twitch" reaction at the time of lumbar tap. A limited amount of CSF is available because the cord swelling is marked. The prognosis is good for return of function, which may take 3 to 6 months. Full urinary and fecal control usually returns.

If loss of contrast material of one vertebral body length cranial and caudal to the herniated disc occurs, the ischemic insult to the spinal cord usually results in a permanent long-term neurologic deficit (Fig. 44.17). The patient often has spastic paresis, but less severely than earlier in the disease process. That the patient feels less pain is a sign of deterioration misinterpreted by owners as an improvement. The patient usually has a barely noticeable "twitch" reaction at the time of lumbar tap. CSF is limited to the hub of the needle because the cord swelling is severe. The prognosis is fair for return of function, which may take 6 months. Full urinary and fecal control does not usually return.

A swollen spinal cord with the loss of contrast material over several vertebrae is usually recognized clinically as flaccid paralysis with no proprioception, no deep pain, and no urinary or bowel control (Fig. 44.18). Some of these patients have no "twitch" when the spinal needle is placed with the lumbar tap. Usually, no CSF is obtained because of the massive swelling. Some patients have a "star gazing" behavior with mental detachment that usually accompanies myelomalacia of the spinal cord secondary to cord ischemia. The prognosis is grave for these patients.

Patients often have additional lesions, such as calcified nucleus pulposus, narrowed disc space, spon-

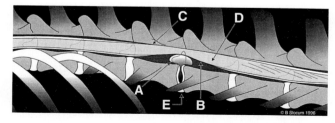

Fig. 44.16. Herniation of the intervertebral disc at L2 (*A*) has caused loss of the ventral dye column over half the vertebra (*B*), dorsal column over half the vertebra (*C*), dorsal deviation of the spinal cord without definition adjacent to the herniated disc (*D*), and a collapsed disc space (*E*). The prognosis is fair.

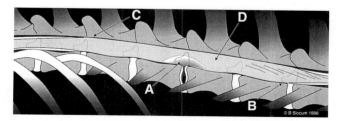

Fig. 44.18. Herniation of the intervertebral disc at L2 (*A*) has caused loss of the ventral dye column over the length of four vertebrae (*B*), dorsal column over the length of four vertebrae (*C*), and swelling of the spinal cord without definition (*D*). The lumbar tap rarely produces cerebrospinal fluid or a "twitch" response. The prognosis is grave.

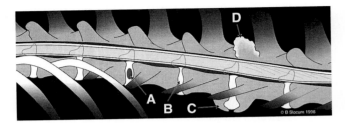

Fig. 44.19. The calcified disc at L1 (*A*), the narrow disc space at L2 (*B*), the spondylosis deformans at L3 (*C*), and the spinal facet arthritis (*D*) are all abnormal. Although these lesions do not necessarily cause neurologic signs or pain, they may accompany other lesions that do.

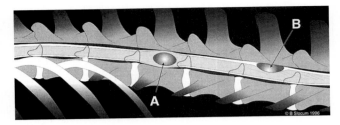

Fig. 44.21. An intramedullary tumor (*A*) lies within the substance of the spinal cord and flares the dye column. A solitary subdural mass is partially outlined by the dye column (*B*).

dylosis deformans, and facet arthritis, that can be diagnosed without the aid of contrast material and usually do not affect the dye columns (Fig. 44.19). These lesions seldom contribute a neurologic deficit directly, but they do represent weakened structures that may secondarily lead to nerve or spinal cord compression.

Discospondylitis, infection of the nucleus pulposus, initially causes intense pain without much distortion of the surrounding tissues (Fig. 44.20). Later, as the process progresses, the disc space collapses, and the infected nucleus pulposus causes resorption at the end plates of the adjacent vertebral bodies. Reactive tissue is often found in the spinal canal and displaces the ventral column dorsally. The infection and pain remain until the avascular end plates are resorbed and the infection is overcome. The final results of this process are usually fusion of the two vertebrae adjacent to the infected disc and loss of pain.

Intradural tumors are usually found within the substance of the spinal cord, or they may be a solitary mass that lies between the spinal cord and the dura mater (Fig. 44.21). The tumors within the substance of the cord flare the dorsal and ventral dye column both cranial and caudal to the lesion. In patients with

a solitary tumor, the contrast usually starts to surround the lesion.

Extradural tumors compress the spinal cord from outside the dura mater (Fig. 44.22). The lesions may come from origins as diverse as a primary or secondary tumor in the adjacent bone, hematoma from trauma or von Willebrand's disease, or migrating parasites. Neurofibromas are usually painful and cause an irregular, undulating appearance around the nerve rootlets and nerve roots.

Ischemic insults to the spinal cord can occur at any level. These lesions are usually from fibrocartilaginous emboli or thrombosis. If they are small and localized, they may not be detectable by myelography. This type of lesion usually has a transitory neurologic effect. Larger regions of ischemia may cause extensive spinal cord swelling and paralysis, and these patients have a grave prognosis. These lesions have no specific relation to the intervertebral foramen.

In summary, myelography is a visual representation of the internal pathologic features of the spinal cord. It gives important diagnostic information and is essential in locating a lesion preoperatively. The appearance of the myelogram yields information that confirms the prognosis generated by neurologic examination. Through flexion, extension, and traction views, one can gain information critical to understanding the underlying pathologic process.

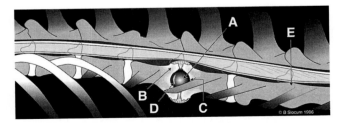

Fig. 44.20. Discospondylitis (*A*) is an infection of the nucleus pulposus with an inflammatory reaction shown by bone proliferation (*B*). This painful process causes cavitation of the end plates (*C*). Often, an avascular fragment of the end plate (*D*) persists as long as the infection and pain. Resolution results in fusion of the vertebral bodies, as in *E*. The inflammatory reaction can impinge on the spinal cord, but it seldom causes paralysis.

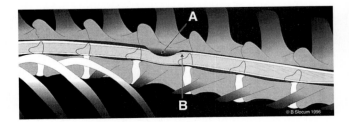

Fig. 44.22. An extradural mass (*A*) forms without regard to the intervertebral foramen. The cord is compressed, and the dye column shows the compression at the margin of the lesion (*B*).

Discography for Diagnosis of Neurologic Disease

James F. Biggart, III

Discography, the radiographic study of the percutaneous injection of contrast material into the nucleus pulposus of the intervertebral disc, aids in the diagnosis of degenerated or herniated discs. In human medicine, spinal pain can be recreated in the awake patient by injecting contrast material into the disc. The general anesthesia required in animal patients generally precludes this diagnostic test.

The advantages of discography include minimal toxicity of the contrast agents to the injected discs, diagnosis of herniated discs after false-negative myelograms, and the diagnosis of far lateral disc herniations. The technique is minimally invasive.

The disadvantages include requirements for general anesthesia, for fluoroscopy to aid in needle placement, and for some localization of the area of the spine affected because of the impracticality of injecting more than four or five discs. Usually, physical examination, history, and plain radiographic evaluation help to localize spinal disorders to cervical, thoracolumbar, or lower lumbar regions. Discography does not determine

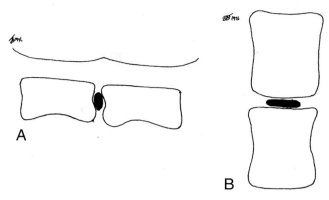

Fig. 44.24. Discogram of a normal disc. **A.** Lateral view. **B.** Ventrodorsal view.

when herniations occur. Many old asymptomatic discs show degeneration or herniation on a discogram (1).

Discographic Patterns

The patterns of discograms comprise the following four categories:

1. A normal nucleus without disc degeneration (Figs. 44.23 and 44.24)
2. A degenerated asymptomatic disc (Fig. 44.25)
3. Annular disruption, tears, or bulges without dye penetration of the outer anulus or dorsal longitudinal ligament (the most common pattern in humans), known as a protruded disc (Fig. 44.26)

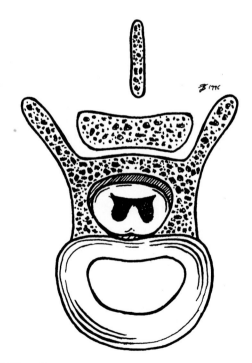

Fig. 44.23. Cross section of a normal nucleus without disc degeneration.

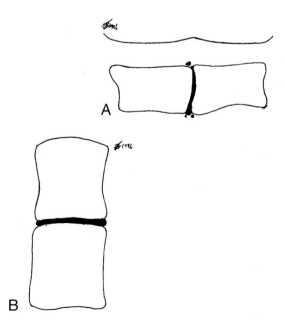

Fig. 44.25. Discogram of a degenerated asymptomatic disc. **A.** Lateral view. **B.** Ventrodorsal view.

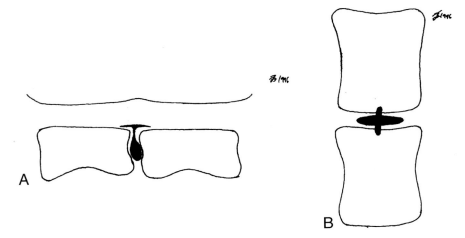

Fig. 44.26. Discogram of a protruded disc. **A.** Lateral view. **B.** Ventrodorsal view.

4. Leakage of dye outside the anulus into surrounding tissue or into the spinal canal or adjacent foramen, with three variations of this pattern of extruded discs:

a. Dye that leaks laterally or ventrally and thus does not involve the spinal cord (false-negative myelogram)

b. Dye that enters the spinal canal but stays mixed with and remains adjacent to the disc space (Figs. 44.27 and 44.28)

c. Discs that herniate such that the dye flows up and down or dorsally in the spinal canal without concentration over the disc space; this so-called sequestered disc or extruded discogram pattern is the most common pattern in dogs; sequestered disc material is not adjacent to the disc space and may be separate from the site of herniation (Figs. 44.29 to 44.31)

Anatomy

Exiting nerve roots through the foramen and blood vessels are the structures potentially encountered in discography (2). In the cervical region, the vertebral artery poses a hazard (3). Keeping the needle below the upper dorsal third of the disc space usually avoids this structure. This artery was only damaged in 2 of more than 700 cervical discograms. In both instances, a large hematoma developed but was managed with pressure. No sequelae occurred, and both patients remained unaffected. The nerve roots especially at C5–6 and C6–7 were the only roots encountered. In all 11 instances, the 18-gauge needle caused twitching of the upper left foreleg and shoulder. Repositioning the needle allowed successful discography.

In the lumbar region, no major blood vessels have been encountered. Several caudal nerve roots have

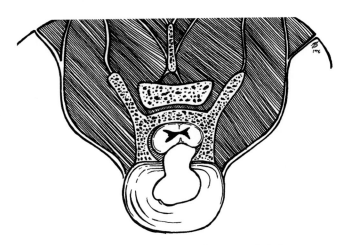

Fig. 44.27. Cross section of a protruded disc.

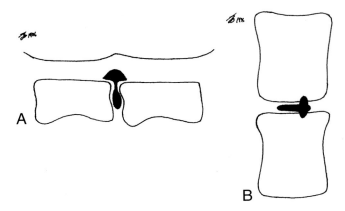

Fig. 44.28. Discogram of an extruded disc. **A.** Lateral view. **B.** Ventrodorsal view.

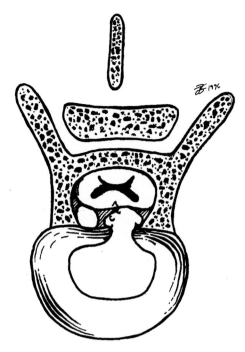

Fig. 44.29. Cross section of a sequestered disc.

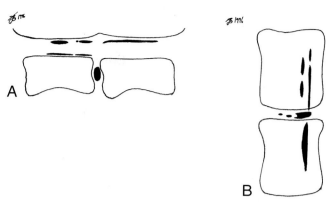

Fig. 44.31. Discogram of a sequestered disc. **A.** Lateral view. **B.** Ventrodorsal view.

been stimulated, but repositioning the needle proves successful in avoiding root damage. The aorta is just beneath the spine and always poses a risk, but keeping the needle perpendicular to the spine and directly lateral to the nucleus avoids this hazard.

In the thoracic region, the needle penetrates the pleural space, especially in barrel-chested dogs with arching rib heads. Lung penetration is possible, but no radiographs have demonstrated pneumothorax or pulmonary hemorrhage. No clinical respiratory signs have been seen postoperatively. The aorta is nearby, but it poses no more hazard than in the lumbar region. Intercostal vessels may be damaged, but keeping the

needle dorsal to the ribs and rib heads is helpful in avoiding these structures. Generally, when discography is performed more cranial to T13, the needles should be kept dorsal to the dorsal rib, and one should avoid the pleural cavity altogether.

Indications

Discography is useful in diagnosing degenerated or herniated discs in patients with normal myelograms. Patients likely to have disc herniations can be diagnosed with multiple discograms. Once a level of spine involvement is narrowed to three or four discs, discography can demonstrate a disc hernia. If a myelogram shows a swollen spinal cord over several disc spaces with not enough subarachnoid dye filling to be diagnostic, a discogram can verify disc herniation. If a myelogram is normal or equivocal, or if it shows a rare pattern, a discogram can rule out a disc hernia. Because disc hernias are common and treatable, and because statistical prognoses are possible, veterinarians would like not to miss these lesions.

Contraindications

Discography has few contraindications, except known allergy to contrast media or those contraindications peculiar to general anesthesia. Because tissue invasion is minimal, animals with known bleeding disorders can safely undergo discography.

Technique

The anesthetized patient is placed in right lateral recumbency on a movable plastic radiolucent form on top of the x-ray table such that biplane radiographs can be taken of the patient's spine without rotating the patient. The left lumbar skin over the disc or discs

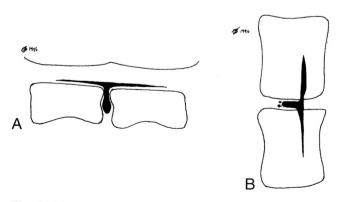

Fig. 44.30. Discogram of a sequestered disc. **A.** Lateral view. **B.** Ventrodorsal view.

to be injected (usually determined by myelography) is prepared for sterile surgery. The patient is draped, and a metal location marker is placed on the drape and is viewed through the fluoroscope. A stab incision in the skin is made over the disc, and a 3-inch, 18-gauge needle is placed through the lateral lumbar muscle into the outer edge of the anulus a distance of a few millimeters. A 3.25-inch, 22-gauge needle replaces the 18-gauge stylet and penetrates the nucleus (Fig. 44.32) Biplane radiographs document proper needle placement. The patient should not be rotated because the needles are easily dislodged. Biplane radiography or fluoroscopy is essential to measure proper needle depth.

For cervical discography, the patient's uppermost left foreleg is tied to both back legs, and a radiolucent sponge is placed beneath the neck between C1 and the shoulder to arch the neck upward, thereby widening the left lateral disc space and allowing easy needle penetration. The dog is placed on a movable form on top of the x-ray table. Taping the left foreleg to the rear legs instead of to the table allows one to slide the form (and the dog) across the table to allow biplane radiographs without rotating the dog. A floating four-way moving x-ray table accomplishes the same end without using the plastic form. Pulling the upper leg caudally moves the scapula caudally, allowing the needle direct lateral access to C5–6. To access C6–7 and C7–T1, the needle must be started in the skin more cranially, to avoid the cranial scapula, and must be placed in the lateral anulus in a cranial to caudal direction. Once the 18-gauge outer needle is lodged in the outer anulus of C6–7 or C7–T1, the hub of the needle is levered caudally and is maintained until the 22-gauge inner needle is placed in the nucleus. The caudal hub pressure is released; the scapula pushes the needle anteriorly, leaving the 22-gauge needle shaft bent at the outer anulus but centered in the nucleus.

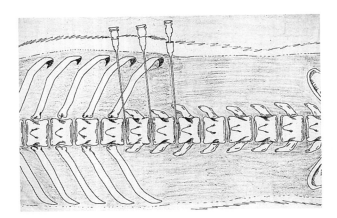

Fig. 44.32. Lateral approach of double needles into the nucleus of T13–L1 through L2–3.

Because the foramen allows access to the spinal canal and cord inside, it is avoided in needle placement. Starting the needle entrance slightly caudal and dorsal to the center of the nucleus allows accidental needle slippage off the outer anulus in a ventral anterior direction without cord damage. Some collapsed arthritic disc spaces require force to enter the nucleus, and slippage is common. It is better to slip ventrally than dorsally. Right-handed surgeons using a right lateral recumbency positioning for their patients find it easier to angle the needle slightly caudally to cranially than cranially to caudally.

For thoracolumbar discography, a direct lateral needle path perpendicular to the long axis of the spine is preferred. A radiolucent sponge is placed beneath the lumbar spine between the last rib and the wing of the ilium, thereby widening the lateral disc space. The patient's forelegs are stretched cranially and the rear legs caudally. A sponge is placed beneath the sternum to elevate it, giving a direct lateral view of the spine as viewed through the fluoroscope. The rib heads hinder penetration of the outer anulus in the thoracic spine and become more centered over the disc space as you go forward from T13. Twisting force on the needle is required to penetrate the rib head joint, to allow access to the nucleus. The 18-gauge needle can be embedded in this joint, and the sharper 22-gauge needle finishes the penetration into the nucleus.

The L6–7 disc injection requires a more cranial to caudal needle path starting cranial to the wings of the ilium and angling caudal to the outer anulus. Contrary to the movable scapula, the ilium is immovable, and the center of the L6–7 nucleus is reached by annular penetration at the caudal end plate of L6.

The L7–S1 disc space cannot be approached by lateral needle penetration percutaneously. A dorsolateral or dorsal approach is needed (4). This is the only disc space in the dog not approachable laterally. A dorsal approach exposes the terminal cord and nerve roots to needle damage, but the nucleus can be reached easily. Although root sleeve or dural penetration of the terminal cord by the needle and the introduction of modern myelographic contrast material do not harm the nervous tissue, the entrance of nucleolytic enzymes (chymopapain, collagenase, and ABC chondroitinase) is harmful. Contrast material and enzymes are often introduced during the same needle placement procedure. Discography combined with epidurography is effective in demonstrating degenerated or herniated discs at L7–S1 (5). Once needle placement is satisfactory, iohexol (Omnipaque), 0.2 mL, is injected into the disc and is flushed with 0.2 mL saline or sterile water. Half the dose is still in the needle, so flushing the needle is needed to insert all the contrast material into the nucleus. A normal disc with an intact anulus in a 40-lb dog accommodates only 0.1 mL. Giant dogs take 0.2 mL, and smaller dogs take 0.05 mL. High-pressure "pumping" of the syringe plunger is necessary to administer the full dose of the dye to a normal nucleus. Annular tears allow dye to escape into adjacent tissue and allow larger amounts of dye to be injected. The presence of high intradiscal pressure indicates an intact anulus or annular injection. Low intradiscal pressure and easy injection indicate a torn anulus, dye leakage into extradiscal tissue, or needle hub leakage (loose syringe). Radiographs taken immediately after or during injection document the discographic appearance of the nucleus (6). Usually, the needles are removed from the disc, and routine radiographs are taken. If questions arise regarding proper needle placement or if the diagnosis is ambiguous, then biplane radiographs can be taken without rotating the patient before needle removal.

Materials

Needle Sets

1. Hemostats hold hubs steady while attaching syringes.
2. Luer-Lok gastight 1 cc syringes are indicated.
3. An 18-gauge Luer-Lok 3-inch spinal needle should have the tips filed blunt enough not to penetrate intact skin; blunt needles do not damage nerves and blood vessels as easily and tend to push them out of the way rather than skewer them, and they can be forced between collapsed arthritic end plates more easily than sharp needles.
4. Sharp 22-gauge Luer-Lok 3.5-inch spinal needles are placed inside the 18-gauge needle penetrating the anulus, stopping in the nucleus.
5. Three needle sets are packaged to allow for differences in disc size:

  a. Small discs in animals smaller than 15 lb: the 22-gauge needle is 2 to 4 mm longer than the 18-gauge needle when inserted fully.

  b. Medium discs in animals 15 to 60 lb: the 22-gauge needle is 4 to 8 mm longer than the 18-gauge needle.

  c. Dogs weighing more than 60 lb: the 22-gauge needle is 6 to 12 mm longer than the 18-gauge needle.

Contrast Material

1. Iohexol in a concentrated form (240 mg Iodine/mL) is satisfactory in medium to large dogs, but the volume of small dogs' discs may fail to allow enough dye in the nucleus to allow visualization.
2. Double-strength (1:1) metrizamide is easier to see in small volumes and is biochemically compatible with chymopapain and collagenase enzymes; both iohexol and metrizamide are safe to use in and around the spinal cord.

Fluoroscopy

1. Percutaneous placement of a contrast dye intradiscally requires fluoroscopic guidance.
2. Although needles can be placed and dye introduced by open surgical techniques, this practice negates the less traumatic and much faster advantage of fluoroscopic needle placement.

References

1. Biggart JF. What's new: intradiscal therapy. In: Proceedings of the American Animal Hospital Association, Denver, CO. 1984.
2. Norby EJ, Brown MD, Dawson EC, et al. Glossary of spinal terminology. Am Acad Orthop Surg 85;32.
3. Wrigley RH, Peuter R. Canine cervical discography. Vet Radiol 1984;25:274–279.
4. Sisson AF, LeCouter RA, Ingram JT, et al. Diagnosis of cauda equina abnormalities by using electromyography, discography, and epidurography in dogs. J Vet Intern Med 1992;6:253–263.
5. Barthez PY, Morgan JP, Lipsitz D. Discography and epidurography for evaluation of the lumbosacral junction in dogs with cauda equina syndrome. Vet Radiol Ultrasound 1994;35:152–157.
6. Kahanovitz N, Arnoczky SP, Sisson HA, et al. The effects of discography on the canine intervertebral disc. Spine 1986;11:329–340.

Magnetic Resonance Imaging

Barbara Watrous

The purpose of magnetic resonance imaging (MRI) is to create an anatomic two- or three-dimensional computer-generated image of an area of interest. This imaging modality detects changes in the magnetic properties of atomic nuclei of cells within tissues. This is accomplished in MRI by using the inherent magnetism of tissue to create a representative image proportional to the concentration of hydrogen protons. Because water is prevalent in tissues, the hydrogen proton usually represents distribution of water.

MRI takes advantage of the fact that a hydrogen nucleus has a magnetic moment. The *frequency* at which the nucleus precesses in an applied magnetic field is specific to the nucleus and the magnetic field strength. When an equivalent energy radiofrequency (RF) pulse is applied, usually at 90 or 180° to the axis of the magnetic field, the energy is absorbed by the proton, and its alignment relative to the surrounding magnetic field is changed. After the RF pulse ceases, the proton flips back to align with the externally applied magnetic field and emits the absorbed energy as an induced current, which is recorded. This relaxation results in return of the longitudinal component of the magnetism (parallel to the applied magnetic field) and is referred to as T_1 relaxation. T_1 is a measure of the

Table 44.3.
Contrast Characteristics in Head and Brain Imaging

Entity Imaged	Image Contrast	
	T_1	T_2
Cerebrospinal fluid	dark (black)	bright
Gray matter	gray (intermediate)	light gray
White matter	light gray	gray or dark
Fat	bright	gray
Cortical bone	dark	dark
Calcifications	gray or dark	dark
Air	dark	dark
Blood (fast flow)	dark	dark
Edema	gray or dark	bright
Protein	bright	bright

time in which the longitudinal component has increased to a given percentage of its original value. Relaxation time of the transverse component resulting in decaying back to its initial zero state is referred to as T_2 relaxation.

The pulse of RF applied to the magnetically aligned tissue deflects the nuclear field. The most often used sequence causes a 90° deflection, and after a specified time a second pulse produces an 180° deflection. This process is repeated after a delay during which the emitted RF waves are sampled by the coil. The time interval between the 90° pulse and detection of the RF waves by the coil is termed the echo time or TE. The time between each pulse sequence is termed the repetition time or TR.

The ability to manipulate scan parameters to acquire images with differing T_1 (spin–lattice relaxation) and T_2 (spin–spin relaxation) "weighting" provides both anatomic and pathologic information. This method is ideally suited to image joints, muscles, brain and spinal cord, and noncontrasted vascular structures. Soft tissue differentiation is with gray-scale image production allowing differentiation of synovial fluid, cartilage, synovium, fibrous connective tissue and fascia, muscle and bone, hemorrhage and edema of spinal cord, disc herniation, ligamentous and osseous disruption, and epidural fluid.

MRI allows division of the patient into three basic planes: axial (or transverse orientation splitting the body into cranial and caudal or proximal and distal portions), sagittal (or right and left halves), and coronal (or front and back or dorsal and ventral halves) planes. Any oblique variations are also possible.

MRI contrast-enhancing media alter the relaxation times T_1 or T_2. They are often used to alter different tissues with similar signal intensities. Positive enhancement occurs when the tissue of interest produces a signal that is brighter than normal. Negative contrast enhancement results when the target tissue appears darker on enhancement. Contrast agents include paramagnetic, superparamagnetic, and ferromagnetic sub-

stances. Formulations include metal chelate complexes, salts, acyclic complexes, cyclic complexes, and particulates.

Tissues with a high proportion of bound water, such as white matter or fat, have a shorter T_1, meaning they relax to equilibrium more quickly than tissue with more free water such as fluids that have a longer T_1. T_1-weighted images are generated using a short TR (repetition time or time between successive pulse sequences) and short TE (echo time or time from the original RF pulse to the peak of the echo). The result of T_1 weighting produces bright signals for fat, dark or low signal intensity for cerebrospinal fluid (CSF), cortical bone, and ligament, and intermediate pathologic brain signal when edema is present.

Tissues with a short transverse relaxation time, such as muscle and liver, produce an intermediate signal. Tissues with an extremely short T_2 such as cortical bone produce a dark signal. The long T_2 of CSF and of pathologic tissue that commonly contains pathologic fluid produces bright signals.

Head and brain imaging routinely uses both T_1 and T_2 relaxation times. Tissue characteristics are summarized in Table 44.3.

The spinal cord and other neural tissues are imaged without the need for an intrathecal contrast medium, thus eliminating loss of image information from obstructed flow of contrast. Large fields of view are not affected by image distortion often encountered with the diverging angle of an x-ray beam in routine diagnostic radiology or artifacts from beam-hardening from CT imaging. Heavily weighted T_2 images produce the so-called myelographic effect. Sagittal images produce excellent information on disc protrusion, cord compression, intradural lesions, and extradural lesions. Vertebral bodies with lesions alter the normal homogeneous signal, most often by causing a decreased signal in T_1-weighted images. Discospondylitis disrupts the vertebral end plates (Table 44.4).

Musculoskeletal MRI produces superior soft tissue contrast and is the modality of choice for disorders of bone marrow and soft tissues. Inherent contrast comes from high signal intensity of fat highlighted against

Table 44.4.
Contrast Characteristics in Imaging of the Spinal Cord and Vertebrae

Entity Imaged	Image Contrast	
	T_1	T_2
Cerebrospinal fluid	dark or black	bright
Spinal cord	intermediate gray	gray or dark
Vertebral body	intermediate or bright	intermediate gray
Disc (young patient)	intermediate gray	bright
Disc degeneration	gray or dark	gray
Anulus	dark gray	dark gray

Table 44.5.
Contrast Characteristics in Musculoskeletal Imaging

Entity Imaged	Image Contrast	
	T_1	T_2
Cortical bone	dark or black	dark or black
Bone marrow	intermediate or bright	intermediate or gray
Articular cartilage	bright	gray
Ligament	dark	dark
Meniscus	dark or black	dark or black
Muscle	intermediate	dark or gray
Edema	dark	bright

lower signal intensities generated by bone and muscle. T_1-weighted images produce excellent contrast, and T_2-weighted images show conspicuous normal and pathologic fluid collections. In patients with avascular necrosis of the femoral head (Legg–Calvé–Perthes disease), the bone marrow has a low signal in T_1 and a bright signal on T_2-weighted images (Table 44.5).

Applied variations in TE, TR, pulse sequence, flip angle, spin-echo sequence, or gradient-echo sequence, multiechoes, and techniques such as inversion recovery sequence, fast spin echo, and time-of-flight MR angiography are beyond the scope of this discussion.

Suggested Readings

Newhouse JH, Wiener JI. Understanding MRI. Boston: Little, Brown, 1991.
Shores A. Magnetic resonance imaging. Vet Clin North Am Small Anim Pract 1993;23:437–459.
Woodward P, Freimarck RD. MRI for technologists. San Francisco: McGraw-Hill Health Professions Division, 1995.

Computed Tomography

Barbara Watrous

The purpose of the diagnostic imaging modality computed tomography (CT) is to produce two- or three-dimensional images of an area of interest. This process uses a computer to reconstruct tomograms or slices of images and records them as digital information. The principle of CT relies on an x-ray tube and a series of radiation detectors that rotate around a patient within a circular aperture or gantry. The transmitted pencil-like or fan-shaped x-ray beam is gathered at each degree of arc during rotation as data by a scintillation crystal detector or xenon gas–filled detector, and these data are converted mathematically to a cross-sectional image. A CT study may be recorded at 1.0-mm to no more than 5-mm slice thicknesses through the region of interest to avoid "losing" small lesions because of partial volume artifact. Slice intervals or spacing

should be similar in thickness to avoid omitting slices of tissue. Three-dimensional reconstruction may further be accomplished depending on the sophistication of the computer. Helical (spiral) CT combines continuous movement of the patient with concurrent scanning by a rotating gantry and detector system with a 360° arc over a 1-second interval. Breath holding is required, and therefore positive-pressure ventilation would be necessary in an anesthetized patient. Helical CT allows detection of small lesions that may be missed or duplicated by conventional CT because of motion artifact of respiration. This modality readily facilitates three-dimensional imaging.

Contrast enhancement is frequently used to augment the conventional CT image. Small boluses of intravascular organic iodide contrast medium depict arteries and veins in thoracic and abdominal studies. Orally administered barium is frequently used to highlight the gastrointestinal tract in abdominal examinations. A process called segmentation removes the bony structures and adjacent soft tissues to isolate the desired vessels in three-dimensional reconstruction.

Peak kilovoltage settings are constant for a given study, but they range from 77 to 140 kVp, depending on the machine and the given study. Milliamperage range is usually 120 to 1200. Milliamperage setting is determined by the size and tissue composition of the body part, the slice thickness, and the number of slices.

Density and contrast of the images are viewer-specific. Vast numbers of density gradations are generated from the numeric raw data that are converted to Hounsfield units (HU), which assign a relative numeric measure to tissue physical density. Water is assigned a value of 0 HU. Tissues of greater density are assigned positive HU. Tissues of lower physical density are assigned negative HU. HU scales are often −1000 to +2000 HU up to +4000 HU. From this scale, the viewer determines the center or level and the range or window of gray-scale densities to be displayed. The level setting determines the center of the gray scale. Increasing the level tends to make all tissues appear darker. The window width establishes the extent of the gray scale. Commonly used specifications are for either "bone" or "soft tissue" modes. A bone or wide window results in an image with more shades of gray, tending to improve both spatial and contrast resolution in musculoskeletal tissues, which have high inherent contrast. A soft tissue window is a low-level and narrow window resulting in a lighter, more strongly black-and-white image. Thus, contrast resolution is improved in tissues with low inherent contrast.

The digital format of the image results in precise measurement and location of objects in the image. This provides exact information for surgical planning, localization for transcutaneous biopsy, and monitoring of response to chemotherapy or radiation therapy.

Density measurements provide information on mineral content of bone. Computer manipulation enables one to display images in any plane from axial to longitudinal, frontal, or oblique.

CT has many possible applications. Abdominal, thoracic, central nervous system, and orthopedic disorders are studied. CT is ideally suited to osseous imaging. Cross-sectional slices of the skull provide anatomic images of the bones, teeth, sinuses, oral and nasal cavities, hyoid apparatus, and temporomandibular joints. Cranial trauma, nasal and sinus neoplasia and inflammation, and upper airway malformations are readily evaluated. CT is considered the procedure of choice for orbital trauma. The overlap of structures such as complex joints of the limbs (especially the carpus and tarsus) that occurs with conventional radiography is avoided with CT. The sensitive density discrimination of CT provides clear differentiation of soft tissue structures. Fluid can be discerned from synovium and from fibrous connective tissue in joint regions. The CNS is imaged both without and with intravenous contrast media to visualize space-occupying lesions if they are associated with altered tissue density or if they displace the cerebral ventricles. Contrast enhancement may highlight a vascular mass or may diffuse into a region in which the blood–brain barrier is disrupted, such as in inflammation, hemorrhage, or neoplasia. The cross-sectional images of the spinal cord, accompanied by myelography, display anatomic information that far exceeds that of conventional radiographic imaging.

Suggested Readings

Curry TS III, Dowdey JE, Murry RC. Christensen's physics of diagnostic radiology. 4th ed. Philadelphia: Lea & Febiger, 1990: 289–322.

Dalley RW. Intraorbital wood foreign bodies on CT: use of wide bone window settings to distinguish wood from air. AJR Am J Roentgenol 1995;164:434–435.

Hathcock JT, Stickle RL. Principles and concepts of computed tomography. Vet Clin North Am Small Anim Pract 1993;23:399–415.

Jones JC, Wilson ME, Bartels JE. A review of high resolution computed tomography and a proposed technique for regional examination of the canine lumbosacral spine. Vet Radiol Ultrasound 1994;35:339–346.

Touliopoulos P, Costello P. Helical (spiral) CT of the thorax. Radiol Clin North Am 1995;33:843–861.

45

CERVICAL SPINE

Atlantoaxial Instability Algorithm

Kurt Schulz & Peter K. Shires

Figure 45.1 is an algorithm for the management of atlantoaxial instability.

Tests for Diagnosis of Atlantoaxial Instability

Kurt Schulz & Peter K. Shires

History and Signalment

The initial test for diagnosis of atlantoaxial instability should be confirmation of an appropriate signalment and history. The disease almost exclusively affects small breed dogs in the first few years of life. Cervical pain is the most common clinical complaint, although neurologic deficits in the absence of pain do not rule out atlantoaxial instability. Demonstration of pain with or without neurologic deficits by physical and neurologic examination further supports the presumptive diagnosis.

Initial Radiologic Examination

Patients with appropriate signalment demonstrating severe cervical pain should undergo plain lateral cervical radiologic examination for confirmation of disease before further manipulation that could worsen the neurologic status. Positive radiographic findings include an increased space between the dorsal arch of C1 and the dorsal spinous process of C2 (Fig. 45.2). In severe cases, the obvious malarticulation may be evident. Observation of the dens is usually more difficult on lateral views than on dorsoventral views; however, in some cases, the absence of the dens may be evident on these initial survey studies. If needed, further radiographic studies are performed with the patient under general anesthesia in most cases.

Neurologic Examination

If neurologic deficits are present, they will be reflected as an anatomic diagnosis of the cranial cervical spinal cord. These signs may include quadriparesis, normal or increased reflexes of all limbs, and postural reaction deficits of all limbs. In rare cases of severe cervical myelopathy in association with atlantoaxial instability, signs may include respiratory difficulty, urinary incontinence, and Horner's syndrome.

Further Radiologic Studies

Radiographs performed while the animal is under anesthesia begin with a lateral study as described previously. Supportive findings on ventrodorsal radiographs include absence of the dens and obvious malarticulation. If all these studies are normal but atlantoaxial instability is still suspected, flexed lateral views or myelography may be pursued. Flexion and extension studies must be done with great care to avoid worsening neurologic deficits. Fluoroscopy can aid in visualization of instability during flexion and extension, and myelography may delineate spinal cord compression if present at the area of the C1–2 joint.

817

Atlantoaxial Instability

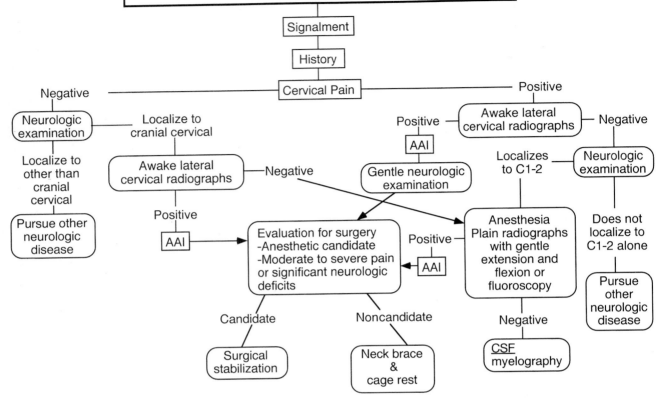

Fig. 45.1. Algorithm for the management of atlantoaxial instability (*AAI*).

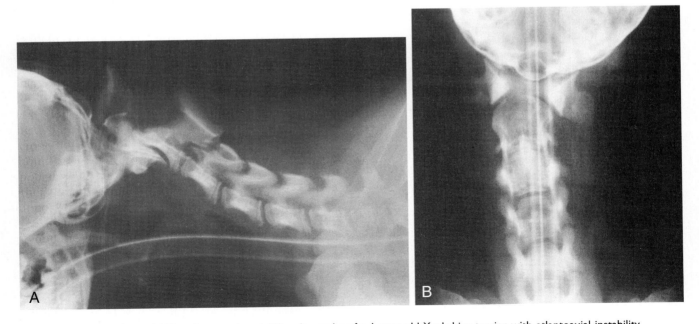

A

B

Fig. 45.2. Lateral (**A**) and ventrodorsal (**B**) radiographs of a 1-year-old Yorkshire terrier with atlantoaxial instability.

Surgical Treatment of Atlantoaxial Instability

Kurt Schulz & Peter K. Shires

Two categories of surgical techniques have been described. Both dorsal and ventral approaches aim to stabilize the atlantoaxial joint in the normal position; however, only ventral approaches allow for complete fusion of the involved cervical vertebrae and permit excision of the dens if necessary.

Ventral Approach

Atlantoaxial instability can be resolved permanently by fusing the two vertebrae in anatomic alignment, a procedure that is easier from a ventral approach. This approach also allows access to the dens if removal is indicated because of fracture or severe dorsal displacement. With the dog in dorsal recumbency, the head and neck should be extended and supported by padding under the cervical area (Fig. 45.3**A**). The surgical approach is made through a ventral midline incision extending from the larynx to the manubrium, followed by separation of the paired sternothyroid muscles. The trachea, esophagus, and carotid sheath are bluntly dissected to allow lateralization. The paired hypaxial muscles ventral to the atlas and axis then are separated carefully on the midline and are lateralized with self-retaining retractors.

The joint capsule of the atlantoaxial articulation should be identified and opened with a No. 11 Bard–Parker blade (Fig. 45.3**B**). In chronic cases, the joint capsule may be thickened and may contain increased

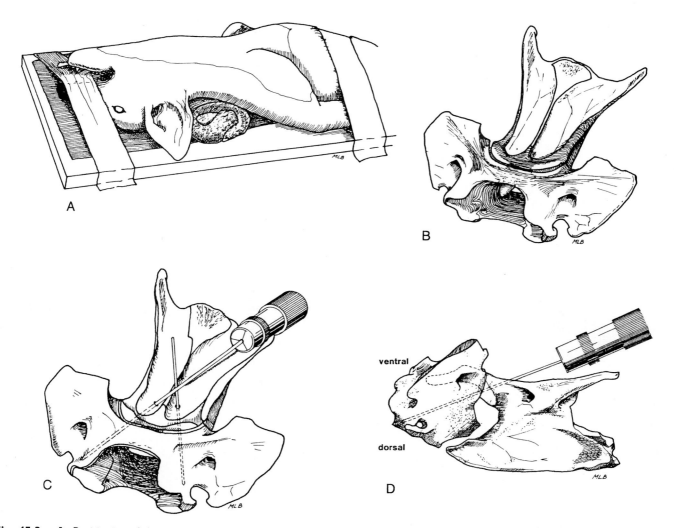

Fig. 45.3. **A.** Positioning of the patient for a ventral approach to the atlantoaxial joint. **B.** The ventral aspect of the atlantoaxial joint seen from a craniolateral view. **C.** Pin placement through the atlantoaxial joints from the ventral body of the axis. Accurate seating of the pins into the medial side of the alar notch is essential. **D.** A lateral view of the stabilization pin placement from the ventral body of the axis, through the atlantoaxial joint, and into the heavy bone surrounding the neural canal.

volumes of joint fluid. The joint may be reduced to normal position by retraction with small, pointed reduction forceps on the caudal body of the axis. If the dens is fractured or ununited, it should be removed through an incision through the membrane between the two articulations. The ligaments attached to the apex of the odontoid process are exposed through a ventral opening in the fascia covering the foramen magnum. The dens may be removed after careful severance of these apical and alar ligaments. Removal of the dens should not be necessary if it is united to the body of C2 and if accurate, stable realignment can be accomplished.

Arthrodesis of C1 and C2 is optimized by removal of the articular cartilage from the joint spaces and placement of a cancellous bone graft obtained from the proximal humerus. Access to the joints may be increased by gentle caudal retraction of C2 with reduction forceps, and the cartilage may be removed with rongeurs or an air drill. Because of the architecture and location of the joints, it is unrealistic to expect removal of all the articular cartilage; removal of the ventral 75% from all four articular surfaces is probably adequate. The bone graft is packed into the joint spaces after adequate removal of cartilage and lavage of the surgical site.

Ventral stabilization of the atlantoaxial joint may be achieved using pins alone, pins and polymethylmethacrylate, lag screws, or bone plates. A power drill is necessary for accurate placement of pins and screws. If pins alone are to be used, two small Steinmann pins or large Kirschner wires are driven from the center of the axis across the atlantoaxial joint and are seated in the atlas just medial to the alar notch (Fig. 45.3**C** and **D**) (1). The point of each pin must be kept as ventral as possible to avoid penetrating the dorsal surface of the thin wings of the atlas. The length of the pins is premeasured from the point of entry into the axis to the palpable medial aspect of the alar notches on the atlas. When both pins are seated, they are cut off close to the body of the axis. The protruding ends are crimped and bent to prevent cranial migration of the pins into the occipital condyles.

The addition of polymethylmethacrylate to the stabilization technique may increase the odds of successful arthrodesis by enhancing stability and may reduce the risk of pin migration (KS Schultz, Waldron DR, unpublished data). Pins are first placed into the atlas (Fig. 45.4**A**). This placement is facilitated by gentle dorsiflexion of the atlantoaxial joint that allows visualization of the spinal canal. Kirschner wires or small threaded pins are directed perpendicular to the long axis of the spine from ventral to dorsal into each of the pedicles of the atlas. The atlantoaxial joint is then reduced, and pins are placed across the joints as described for pin stabilization alone. One or two pins are then placed into the caudal body of the axis (Fig. 45.4**B**). All pins are cut short and are bent, leaving enough pin length to engage a small mass of polymethylmethacrylate (Fig. 45.5). Antibiotic powder should be added to the cement, and cool saline flush should be applied during polymerization of the cement to dissipate heat.

The surgical approach and preparation of the atlantoaxial joints are identical for stabilization with lag screws (2). In small dogs, 1.5-mm cortical screws are placed across each of the joints in a lag fashion. This technique may be facilitated by use of a cannulated drill and screw system. In either case, placement of the screws is in a direction similar to that of the trans-

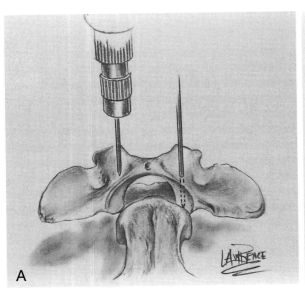
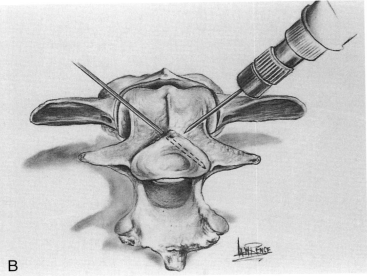

Fig. 45.4. **A.** Pin placement into the lateral masses of C1. **B.** Pin placement into the caudal body of C2.

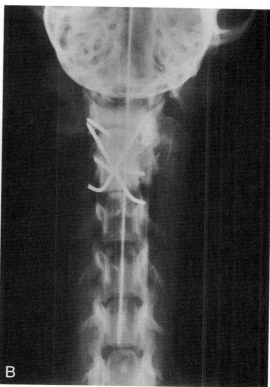

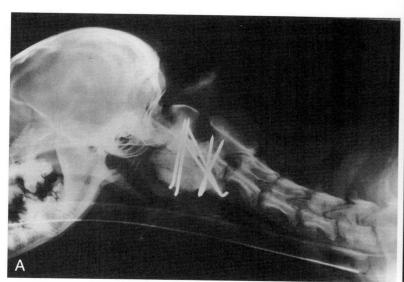

Fig. 45.5. Lateral and ventrodorsal radiographs showing stabilization of the atlantoaxial joint with ventral pins and polymethylmethacrylate.

articular pins. Ventral application of bone plates has also been described; however, the size of most patients may limit the practical application of this technique (3).

Postoperative radiographs should be obtained after stabilization with any of the ventral techniques to demonstrate reduction of the atlantoaxial joint and accurate placement of implants. Neck braces should be maintained if possible for several weeks, and initial cage rest is strictly enforced. Radiographs may be obtained 8 weeks postoperatively to evaluate maintenance of reduction and progression of arthrodesis.

Complications of ventral stabilization techniques include implant migration and loosening (4). The result may be subsequent instability and recurrence of neurologic signs. Placement of pins or screws within the vertebral canal may also worsen the neurologic signs. Tracheal necrosis has been reported with the ventral approach; therefore, gentle dissection and attention to preservation of the delicate blood supply of the region are indicated. As with any surgical implantation of polymethylmethacrylate, concern exists for thermal injury and infection.

Dorsal Approach

The dorsal arch of the atlas is secured to the dorsal spine of the axis with heavy suture material, orthope-

dic wire, or grafts of the nuchal ligament. Descriptions of these techniques are available in the third edition of this text. Although ventral techniques are more difficult, we recommend them because of their lower failure rate (4). Complications of dorsal techniques include instability resulting from breakage of the suture, wire, or graft and fracture of the axis or atlas. Wire stabilization may fail because of cycling, and the addition of polymethylmethacrylate to the wire technique has been recommended to alleviate this complication. Fracture of the axis may be due either to inappropriate placement of the holes or to the remaining motion of the joint, which places excessive forces on the stabilization technique.

Medical management including cervical splinting has been successful in selective cases; however, surgical therapy is recommended for patients demonstrating significant neurologic signs that have no other contraindications for anesthesia or surgery (5). Ventral techniques are technically challenging, but because of the higher failure rates of dorsal techniques, the routine use of dorsal procedures should be avoided (4).

References

1. Sorjonen DC, Shires PK. Atlantoaxial instability: a ventral surgical technique for decompression, fixation, and fusion. Vet Surg 1981;10:22–29.

2. Denny HR, Gibbs C, Waterman A. Atlanto-axial subluxation in the dog: a review of thirty cases and an evaluation of treatment by lag screw fixation. J Small Anim Pract 1988;29:37–47.
3. Thomas WB, Sorjonen DC, Simpson ST. Surgical management of atlantoaxial subluxation in 23 dogs. Vet Surg 1991;20:409–412.
4. McCarthy RJ, Lewis DD, Hosgood G. Atlantoaxial subluxation in dogs. Compend Contin Educ Pract Vet 1995;17:215–226.
5. Gilmore DR. Nonsurgical management of four cases of atlanto-axial subluxation in the dog. J Am Anim Hosp Assoc 1984; 20:93–96.

Cervical Disc Fenestration

*M. Joseph Bojrab &
Gheorghe M. Constantinescu*

Indications

Ventral fenestration for cervical disc disease is advocated in animals demonstrating pain, stiffness of the neck, or foreleg paresis. This technique is effective when degenerating discs protrude and cause nerve fiber and rootlet disorders, which account for most cervical disc problems. This procedure accomplishes intervertebral disc decompression by opening the ventral annular fibers for removal of the nucleus pulposus.

Cervical fenestration is not effective if foreleg paralysis or tetraplegia results from the presence of disc material within the spinal canal. These circumstances indicate a decompressive procedure.

Surgical Technique

The animal is placed in dorsal recumbency with a sandbag under the neck to produce dorsal flexion of the cervical spine, facilitating exposure. A ventral midline skin incision is made from the larynx to the thoracic inlet. The paired bellies of the sternohyoid muscle are separated (Fig. 45.6), and the trachea is displaced laterally and is held with a self-retaining retractor. Blunt dissection of the deep fascia reveals the V-shaped longus colli muscles of the neck (Fig. 45.7), which lie on the midline. Locating these muscles is essential to ensure midline identification. The ventral prominence of the first and second cervical vertebrae is located at the level of the wings of the atlas (Fig. 45.8**A**) for orientation. Because a disc is not present at this interspace, it is not fenestrated. The remaining ventral prominences are midline projections that are directed caudally from the caudal ventral aspect of the vertebrae and provide the insertion site for the longus colli muscles (Fig. 45.8**B**). The ventral entrance to the intervertebral space is covered by these projections and their associated muscle attachment. The muscle attachment is snipped with scissors, exposing the ventral longitudinal ligament. A No. 10 scalpel blade is used to cut the longitudinal ligament and ventral annular fibers (Fig. 45.9**A**). A tartar scraper (SCLB Miltex Tartar Scraper, Victor Medical, Irvine, CA) (Fig. 45.10) is used to fenestrate the disc (see Fig. 45.9**B**). All readily accessible cervical discs (C2–3, C3–4, C4–5, C5–6) are fenestrated.

The self-retaining retractor is removed, and the sternohyoid muscle bellies are sutured with a 3–0 polydi-

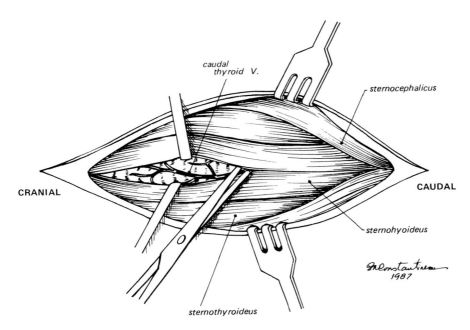

caudal
thyroid V.

sternocephalicus

CRANIAL

CAUDAL

sternohyoideus

sternothyroideus

GMConstantinescu
1987

Fig. 45.6. Ventral cervical incision from the larynx to the thoracic inlet exposing the trachea by separating between the sternohyoid muscles.

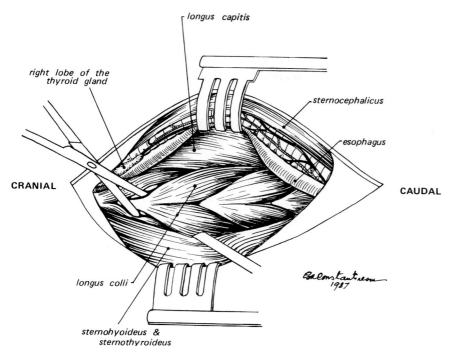

Fig. 45.7. Trachea and esophagus are retracted to the left, and the longus colli muscle insertions are identified and cut with scissors.

oxanone (PDS, Ethicon, Somerville, NJ). The skin is then closed.

Postoperative Care

Antibiotics are given for 5 to 10 days postoperatively. Corticosteroids (dexamethasone, 1 mg/lb body weight) are administered intramuscularly once or possibly twice each week. Buffered aspirin is given for 7

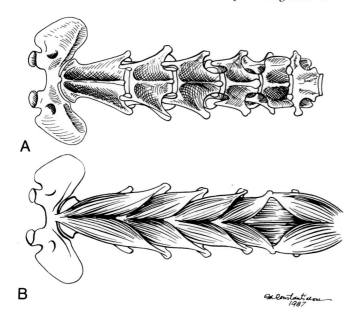

Fig. 45.8. **A.** Ventral aspect of the cervical vertebral column. **B.** Longus colli muscle identification and placement.

to 10 days if pain persists. After 10 to 14 days, complete remission of signs is expected.

Ventral Slot Decompression of the Herniated Cervical Disc

Kenneth A. Bruecker

The ventral approach to the cervical spine allows for direct access to the vertebral bodies and intervertebral discs.

Patient Positioning

The patient is placed in dorsal recumbency with the forelimbs secured caudally. The cervical spine should be supported by placing a vacuum positioner or rolled towel beneath the neck. Excessive dorsiflexion (hyperextension) should be avoided. The head can be secured by tying a rope around the upper canine teeth to the front of the table and placing tape across the hard palate. Gentle traction can thus be applied to the cervical spine resulting in distraction of the intervertebral disc spaces and enhanced access to the spinal canal (Fig. 45.11).

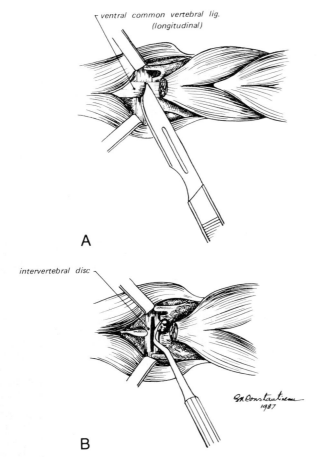

Fig. 45.9. A. After the longus colli muscle attachment is cut, a No. 10 scalpel is used to incise the ventral longitudinal ligament and annular fibers. **B.** A tartar scraper is used to fenestrate the disc.

Approach to the Cervical Vertebrae and Intervertebral Discs

A cutaneous incision is made from the larynx to the manubrium (1). The paired muscle bellies of the sternocephalicus muscles are sharply separated. The paired sternohyoideus muscles are sharply separated on the midline, exposing the trachea. The thyroid ima, a single unpaired blood vessel, lies between the left and right sternohyoideus muscles. If the branches of the thyroid ima are ligated and transected on the right, then this vessel can be reflected with the left sternohyoideus muscle.

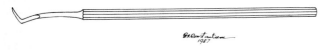

Fig. 45.10. A schematic drawing of the Miltex Scaler B tartar scraper.

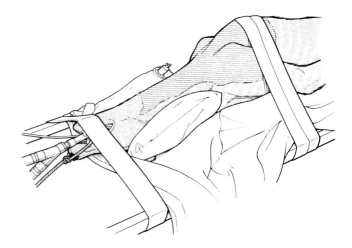

Fig. 45.11. Proper position of the patient with the head and neck stretched for ventral decompression. (From Bruecker KA, et al. Clinical evaluation of three surgical methods for treatment of caudal cervical spondylomyelopathy of dogs. Vet Surg 1989;18:197.)

Blunt dissection along the right side of the trachea allows retraction of the trachea to the left lateral area and retraction of the right carotid sheath to the right lateral area. Care should be taken to identify and protect the right recurrent laryngeal nerve. The endotracheal tube must be of sufficient length to avoid collapse of the trachea during retraction. The esophagus should also be retracted to the left, exposing the longus colli muscle. An esophageal stethoscope or soft rubber tube placed in the esophagus enhances palpation of the esophagus during retraction. Care should be used when retracting these tissues.

The tendon of the longus colli muscle is transected from its origin on the caudoventral midline aspect of the cervical vertebral body, thus exposing the underlying intervertebral disc. This maneuver can be done at each disc space intended for surgery. The location of the intended intervertebral disc can be determined by palpating the large, prominent transverse processes of C6. The C5–6 intervertebral disc lies on the midline at the cranial aspect of the C6 transverse processes. Palpating along the midline, the large ventral prominence of the caudal aspect of each vertebral body and the origin of the tendon of the longus colli muscle can be palpated. The transverse processes of C1 can also be used as a point of reference.

Surgical Technique

Further elevation of the longus colli muscle with a periosteal elevator should be performed in preparation for the ventral slot (2, 3). The retractors can be repositioned between the muscle bellies of the longus colli muscles. The prominence of the point of origin of the longus colli muscle on the caudoventral midline aspect of the cervical vertebral body can be removed with rongeurs, and the intervertebral disc can be fenestrated.

Using a No. 11 blade to fenestrate, a defect is made in the ventral anulus fibrosus. Starting on the midline of the cranial aspect of the vertebral body caudal to the disc, with the cutting edge of the blade directed toward the surgeon, the blade is gently advanced until the disc is reached. Alternatively, a hypodermic needle can be used to localize the intervertebral disc space. With the blade directed in a slightly cranial direction, the blade is inserted to the level of the dorsal anulus fibrosus, against and parallel to the vertebral end plate. This distance can be estimated from the lateral radiographic view of the cervical spine. The blade is advanced to no more than one-half the width of the intervertebral disc. The cutting edge of the blade is then directed cranially and is advanced up to the caudal end plate of the cranial vertebra. The blade is then directed to the left lateral area and is advanced to no further than one-half the width of the disc space. Again, the blade is angled cranially such that it is against and parallel to the caudal end plate of the cranial vertebral body. The blade is directed caudally and is advanced up until the cranial end plate of the caudal vertebral body is reached. The blade is then directed and advanced toward the midline to complete the rectangular excision (window) (Fig. 45.12). This portion of excised ventral anulus fibrosus can then be removed with rongeurs, and the nucleus pulposus gently can be removed with curettes or dental scraper (Fig. 45.13). Care must be taken such that additional disc material is not forced dorsally into the spinal canal.

After fenestration, a high-speed bur is used to create a slot in the vertebral bodies cranial and caudal to

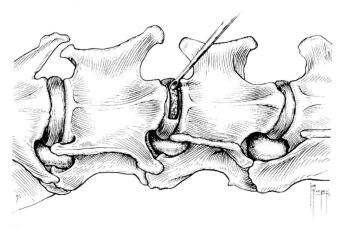

Fig. 45.13. Removal of the nucleus pulposus to complete the fenestration in preparation for a ventral slot procedure. (From Wheeler SJ, Sharp NJH. Small animal spinal disorders: diagnosis and surgery. St. Louis: CV Mosby, 1994:76.)

the intervertebral disc. Overheating of the bur can be prevented with saline lavage. I prefer a long, narrow slot for removal of herniated disc material. The slot should be no wider than one-third the vertebral body width and no longer than one-third the vertebral body length (Fig. 45.14). Because the disc space angles craniodorsally, the caudal aspect of the slot can begin at the end plate of the caudal vertebral body (Fig. 45.15). The slot can be deepened to the level of the cortical bone of the ventral spinal canal. The depth of the defect can be determined by identifying the difference in bone density of the cortical and cancellous bone. Once the bur has penetrated the inner cortical layer, a small bone curette can be used to enlarge the slot. The remaining dorsal anulus fibrosis and dorsal longitudinal ligament can be removed with rongeurs, forceps, curettes or hemostats. Small instruments such as ophthalmic spatulas, loop curettes, fine curved forceps, and suction can be used to retrieve herniated disc ma-

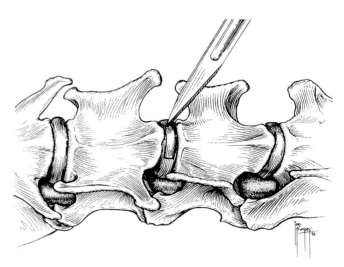

Fig. 45.12. Creation of fenestration window in the ventral aspect of the cervical disc. (From Wheeler SJ, Sharp NJH. Small animal spinal disorders: diagnosis and surgery. St. Louis: CV Mosby, 1994:76.)

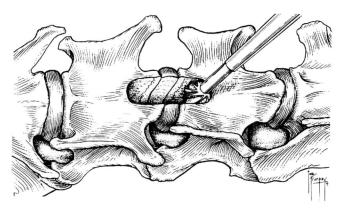

Fig. 45.14. Long, narrow slot created with a high-speed bur. (From Wheeler SJ, Sharp NJH. Small animal spinal disorders: diagnosis and surgery. St. Louis: CV Mosby, 1994:79.)

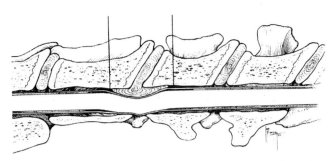

Fig. 45.15. Sagittal section of cervical spine indicating the orientation of the slot with respect to the disc space and spinal canal. (From Wheeler SJ, Sharp NJH. Small animal spinal disorders: diagnosis and surgery. St. Louis: CV Mosby, 1994:78.)

terial from the canal (Fig. 45.16). Disc material on the midline should be removed first, and then laterally extruded disc material can be removed to avoid damage to the venous sinus.

Damage to the venous sinus results in excessive hemorrhage and obstruction of visualization of the spinal cord. This can be controlled with suction and hemostatics, such as surgical sponge (Gelfoam, Upjohn Co., Kalamazoo, MI) or Surgicel (Johnson & Johnson, Arlington, TX). Suction can be used to evacuate the blood. A small piece of precut Gelfoam, presoaked in saline, can be placed at the site of the hemorrhage. Cottonoid (Codman and Scurtleff, Randolph, MA) or sponge is placed over the Gelfoam to prevent inadvertent aspiration of the hemostatic. Suction of the overlying sponge or Cottonoid is performed until hemorrhage has stopped. The sponge or Cottonoid can then be removed. The hemostatic agent can be removed after 5 minutes, and disc material retrieval can be resumed.

Monofilament absorbable suture material is used to close the sternohyoideus and sternocephalicus mus-

cles. Closure of subcutaneous tissues and skin is routine.

Postoperative Management

Analgesics may be necessary for 24 to 48 hours postoperatively. Anti-inflammatory drugs are not generally indicated in the postoperative period. A cervical bandage of rolled cotton and stretch gauze can be placed postoperatively to prevent excessive head and neck movements. This bandage can remain in place for 3 weeks. A thoracic harness should be used instead of a neck collar.

Postoperative management of patients that have undergone cervical decompressive slot procedures is generally divided into ambulatory and nonambulatory convalescence. Patients with an ambulatory status postoperatively are generally managed in the following manner: cage confinement, brief exercise two to three times a day for 2 to 3 weeks, serial neurologic examinations, and home on restricted exercise or passive range-of-motion exercises. Nonambulatory patients are managed in the following manner: elevated padded cage rack or waterbed, turning every 2 to 4 hours, bladder expressions four to five times a day, passive range-of-motion exercises, serial neurologic evaluations, and frequent hydrotherapy until their return to ambulatory status. Crate or pen confinement is recommended for 3 weeks, with a gradual return to normal activity to follow.

Neurologic recovery is generally rapid. Neck pain usually subsides within 24 to 48 hours. Tetraparetic patients may begin to show improvement within days, as well.

References

1. Piermattei DL. An atlas of surgical approaches to the bones and joints of the dog and cat. 3rd ed. Philadelphia: WB Saunders, 1993:54–59.
2. Swaim SF. Ventral decompression of the cervical spinal cord in the dog. J Am Vet Med Assoc 1974;164:491–495.
3. Seim HB, Prata RG. Ventral decompression for the treatment of cervical disc disease in the dog: a review of 54 cases. J Am Anim Hosp Assoc 1982;18:233–240.

Slanted Slot for Cervical Decompression

Barclay Slocum & Theresa Devine Slocum

The purpose of the slanted slot procedure is to allow access to the dorsal anulus fibrosis, vertebral end plate, and ventral spinal canal for decompression of the spi-

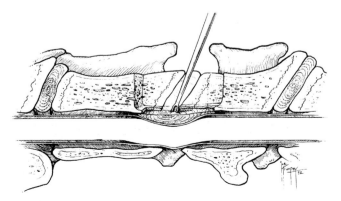

Fig. 45.16. Sagittal section depicting removal of disc material from the spinal canal through the slot. (From Wheeler SJ, Sharp NJH. Small animal spinal disorders: diagnosis and surgery. St. Louis: CV Mosby, 1994:81.)

nal cord from a herniated intervertebral disc, while maintaining the integrity of the ventral anulus fibrosis. The diagnosis of herniated intervertebral disc is made by neurologic, physical, radiographic, and myelographic examination. A headlight, high-speed bur, and neurosurgical instrumentation are necessary for this operation.

Surgical Procedure

The patient is prepared for aseptic surgery of the ventral cervical region and is placed in dorsal recumbency with a small pad under the dorsal neck. The right-handed surgeon can most easily perform the operation from the left side of the patient. The left-handed surgeon can most easily perform the procedure from the right side of the patient.

A ventral approach is made to the cervical spine. The intervertebral disc space, which has undergone dorsal herniation, is identified. The longus colli muscle is elevated from the ventral body of the vertebra cranial to the offending disc. Retraction of the muscles is maintained with deep Gelpi retractors.

A high-speed 4-mm bur is used to perforate the ventral cortex of the vertebral body 5 mm cranial to the disc space of dorsal herniation. A tunnel is made with the bur dorsally and slightly caudally until the caudal end plate of the cranial vertebra is penetrated. The deep portion of the tunnel is expanded and deepened until the cavity for the nucleus, the dorsal anulus, the dorsal limit of the cranial end plate, and the dorsal limit of the caudal end plate are identified (Fig. 45.17). If hemorrhage from the body of the vertebra is encountered, bone dust or bone wax can be used for hemostasis.

If the herniation is recent and clinical signs are limited to spinal cord compression, the dorsal portion of the caudal end plate of the cranial vertebra and the dorsal anulus fibrosis are removed. The herniated disc material can be removed with a right-angle manipulator.

If the herniation is of long standing and the disc is fibrosed to the cord, the dorsal portion of the caudal end plate of both the cranial and caudal vertebrae and the dorsal anulus fibrosis are removed. As much material as possible is removed from the spinal canal without undue manipulation of the cord. The enlarged cavity created by removing the cranial end plate of the caudal vertebra allows redundant disc material and fibrosis to fill the cavity created by this approach. Thus, the spinal cord is decompressed.

If the herniation is recent and clinical signs involve spinal cord compression and nerve root pain, the dorsal portion of the caudal end plate of the cranial vertebra and the dorsal anulus fibrosis are removed. In addition, the dorsolateral third of the end plate is removed to gain access to the laterally herniated disc material

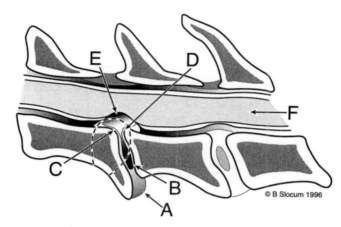

Fig. 45.17. The ventral cortex is perforated 5 mm cranial to the disc (A). The cavity is expanded (*dotted line*) until the nucleus pulposus (B), caudal end plate of the cranial vertebra (C), and the cranial end plate of the caudal vertebra (D) are identified. Extension of the cavity caudodorsally allows access to the spinal canal for retrieval of the disc material (E) and decompression of the spinal cord (F).

and redundant anulus. The herniated disc material can be removed with a right-angle manipulator. The redundant anulus is drawn into the cavity and is trimmed. If fusion between the two vertebra is desired, the cranial end plate of the caudal vertebra is perforated, leaving the ventral anulus intact, and bone graft is added.

The advantage of the slanted slot technique for cervical decompression is that the integrity of the ventral anulus fibrosis is maintained, while permitting access to herniated disc material and decompressing the spinal cord.

In a normal disc, the anulus provides containment for the nucleus pulposus. This enables the disc to undergo elastic deformation and the capability to withstand tremendous compressive, shear, and rotatory forces. The anulus also guides the movement between two vertebral bodies, much like a ligament. It controls dorsal and ventral translation, medial and lateral translation, distraction and compression, and rotation between the adjacent vertebrae. The ventral anulus fibrosis is the thickest portion of the anulus and offers the most resistance to motion between the vertebral bodies. In addition, the three junctions between two vertebrae, the two facets and anulus, offer stability to the spine as a whole, if the ventral portion of the vertebral bodies remain connected. The stabilizing effect of spondylosis deformans is manifested by a large ventral proliferation and sometimes a ventral osseous bridge.

When the nucleus pulposus herniates, besides the damage done to the spinal cord and nerve roots, the disc itself loses much of its ability to absorb compressive loads. Nonetheless, much of the ligamentous function of the anulus fibrosis remains after disc herniation. To maintain as much function as possible, the integrity of the remaining anulus must be respected.

Although the ventral slot technique has been the standard in the past for gaining access to the ventral cervical spinal cord, access to herniated disc material is limited without widening the slot. This maneuver weakens the bone, predisposes the vertebrae to fracture, and creates instability by loss of the anulus fibrosis, especially the ventral anulus.

The inverted cone technique improves on the ventral slot technique by making a small opening in the ventral anulus and ventral midline of the adjacent vertebral bodies. This respects the bone ventrally while creating greater access to the spinal canal and the herniated disc material. However, the stability of the ventral anulus fibrosis is lost. The slanted slot procedure is designed to respect the integrity of the bone of the vertebra, as does the inverted cone procedure, but additionally to maintain the stability of the ventral anulus.

The unique shape of the canine cervical vertebrae allows access to the dorsal anulus while maintaining an intact ventral anulus fibrosis. As viewed from the lateral perspective, the cervical vertebral body is roughly shaped like a parallelogram with the ventral portion of the body shifted caudally with respect to the dorsal portion of the vertebral body. By creating an opening cranial to the caudal end plate of the vertebral body, direct access to the dorsal anulus and vertebral end plates can be achieved by burring through the caudal end plate of the cranial vertebra and into the nucleus pulposus. The slanted slot procedure allows treatment of the herniated disc while minimizing the negative aspects of the surgical approach to the area. By preserving the ventral anulus fibrosis, the function of the patients is improved.

As with the other surgical procedures, care must be taken to prevent fracture of the caudoventral portion of the cranial vertebra from the rest of the vertebral body. Creating a small ventral vertebral body perforation and limiting bone removal to the dorsal portion of the vertebral end plate minimize this risk.

Caudal Cervical Spondylomyelopathy in Large Breed Dogs

Kenneth A. Bruecker

Surgeons have two separate philosophic approaches to the operative treatment of caudal cervical spondylomyelopathy (CCSM) in large breed dogs: direct decom-

pression and decompression by distraction and stabilization. In general, patients with malformation or malarticulation or static compressive lesions benefit from direct decompressive surgical techniques, whereas patients with dynamic compressive lesions such as cervical vertebral instability (CVI) require distraction and stabilization.

Treatment by Direct Decompression Using an Inverted Cone Modified Ventral Slot

The inverted cone modified ventral slot is a direct decompressive technique for the removal of hypertrophied dorsal anulus fibrosus associated with CVI (1). This technique is most useful in patients with a static lesion, unchanged by distraction. The hypertrophied dorsal anulus fibrosus can be difficult to remove from the canal using the classic ventral decompressive slot technique (1–4). This technique or a combination of this technique with the classic approach may have merit in allowing better retrieval of the anulus from the canal. The slot resembles an inverted cone wherein the base of the cone is at the ventral spinal canal (1) (Fig. 45.18).

The approach to the affected intervertebral disc space is the same as described in an earlier section of this chapter for the ventral cervical slot procedure. Using a high-speed bur, the slot is created from the caudal aspect of the intervertebral disc to involve the caudal one-quarter of the cranial vertebral body. The width of the slot is limited to one-fifth the width of the vertebral body. The slot is enlarged as it is deepened by moving the bur in a sweeping motion laterally, creating an elliptic slot. The slot is carried to the level of the inner cortical layer while preserving the dorsal anulus fibrosus. The dorsal anulus fibrosus can then be retracted back into the slot and excised (Figs. 45.19 and 45.20). The inner cortical bone layer is removed with the high-speed bur, and additional anulus and dorsal longitudinal ligament can be excised (Fig. 45.21). Closure is routine.

Treatment by Distraction and Stabilization Using Pins and Polymethylmethacrylate

Distraction and stabilization using Steinmann pins and polymethylmethacrylate comprise the technique I prefer for the treatment of a single dynamic compressive lesion associated with CVI (5, 6). Advantages of this technique include adequate spinal cord decompression without entering the spinal canal, reduced risk of iatrogenic cord trauma, and improvement in the percentage, rate, and duration of recovery as compared with

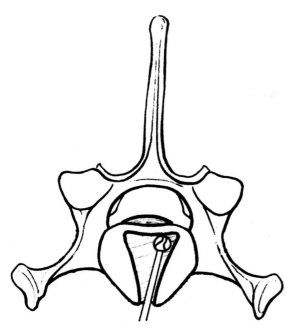

Fig. 45.18. Diagrammatic cross-sectional representation of the inverted cone decompressive slot at the level of the intervertebral disc space. (From Goring RL, Beale BS, Faulkner RF. The inverted cone decompression technique: a surgical treatment for cervical vertebral instability "wobbler syndrome" in Doberman pinschers. Part 1. J Am Anim Hosp Assoc 1991;27:405.)

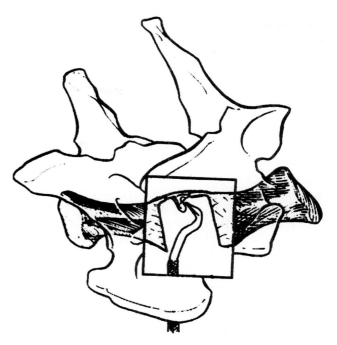

Fig. 45.20. Retrieval of additional compressive material into the slot. Note retention of dorsal cortical bone shelf and progressive spinal cord decompression. (From Goring RL, Beale BS, Faulkner RF. The inverted cone decompression technique: a surgical treatment for cervical vertebral instability "wobbler syndrome" in Doberman pinschers. Part 1. J Am Anim Hosp Assoc 1991;27:406.)

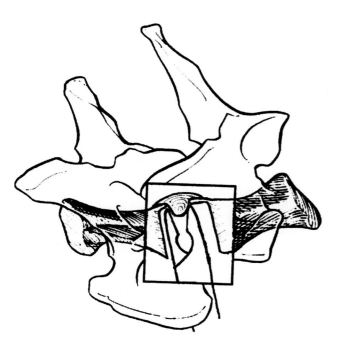

Fig. 45.19. The dorsal anulus fibrosus (*DAF*) is retrieved into the slot by applying traction before removal with a rongeur. (From Goring RL, Beale BS, Faulkner RF. The inverted cone decompression technique: a surgical treatment for cervical vertebral instability "wobbler syndrome" in Doberman pinschers. Part 1. J Am Anim Hosp Assoc 1991;27:405.)

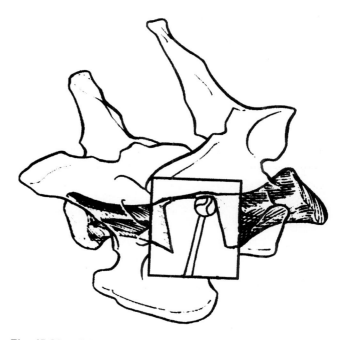

Fig. 45.21. A high-speed bur is used to remove the dorsal cortical bone shelf, thereby providing surgical access to the spinal canal. (From Goring RL, Beale BS, Faulkner RF. The inverted cone decompression technique: a surgical treatment for cervical vertebral instability "wobbler syndrome" in Doberman pinschers. Part 1. J Am Anim Hosp Assoc 1991;27:406.)

other techniques. In addition, a neck brace is not required.

A ventral approach, as described for the ventral decompressive slot technique, is performed to expose the vertebral bodies and intervertebral spaces cranial and caudal to the affected intervertebral space (5). The patient is positioned in dorsal recumbency with the cervical spine distracted, as described for the ventral slot technique. The affected intervertebral space is then pulled into additional linear traction by one of two techniques. A Gelpi retractor, modified by blunting the tips, is inserted into the fenestrated disc spaces cranial and caudal to the affected disc space to act as a vertebral spreader. The retractor is engaged, and the affected intervertebral space is spread an additional 2 to 3 mm. Alternately, a defect is created in the vertebral bodies cranial and caudal to the affected vertebral bodies with a high-speed surgical bur. The defects are created just large enough to accept the tips of the modified Gelpi retractor. The retractor is engaged, and the affected intervertebral space is spread an additional 2 to 3 mm (Fig. 45.22). This technique of vertebral spreading may have merit over insertion of the tips of the Gelpi retractor into fenestrated disc spaces. Fenestration of the intervertebral discs may predispose them to degenerative changes and collapse (7). Distraction results in decompression of the spinal cord (8, 9).

A ventral slot technique is performed at the affected intervertebral space; however, the slot is wider and shorter than a classic ventral decompressive slot. The depth is carried only to the level of the inner cortical bone layer. The spinal canal is not entered. The width of the slot should be no more than one-half the width of the vertebral body. The length of the slot is determined by the thickness of the vertebral end plates. Once the cortical end plate on each vertebral body has been removed, burring should cease. Autogenous cancellous bone is harvested from the heads of the humeri and is placed into the distracted slot. Two $\frac{7}{64}$- or $\frac{1}{8}$-inch Steinmann pins are inserted into the ventral surface of the vertebral body cranial to the affected intervertebral space. Two pins of similar pins are inserted into the vertebral body caudal to the affected intervertebral space. The pins are inserted on the ventral midline of the vertebral body and are directed 30 to 35° dorsolaterally to avoid entering the spinal canal. Two cortices must be engaged by each pin. The pins are cut, leaving approximately 1.5 to 2 cm exposed. The exposed portion of each pin is notched with pin cutters, allowing the bone cement to grip and prevent pin migration. Sterile polymethylmethacrylate powder is mixed with liquid monomer until it reaches a doughy consistency and can be handled without sticking to the surgeon's gloves. The cement then is molded meticulously around each pin (Fig. 45.23). Irrigation with sterile saline solution for 5 to 10 minutes dissipates the heat of polymerization. The vertebral spreaders are removed once the cement has hardened. Closure of the longus colli muscle is performed cranial and caudal to the cement mass. The remainder of the closure is routine. Postoperative care includes strict confinement for 4 to 6 weeks.

Treatment by Distraction and Stabilization Using a Harrington Rod

The Harrington rod distracts the cervical spine and stabilizes it during healing (10). This technique is most useful in patients with dynamic compression resulting from hypertrophied dorsal anulus fibrosus associated with CVI involving two adjacent lesions (generally C5–6 and C6–7). Advantages of this technique include adequate spinal cord decompression of two adjacent intervertebral disc spaces without entering the spinal canal, reduced risk of iatrogenic spinal cord trauma, and improvement in the recovery rate of patients with two lesions over that seen with the pins and polymethylmethacrylate technique. Two disadvantages are that distraction and stabilization of only one intervertebral disc space is not possible and the incidence of implant failure may be higher in patients that do not tolerate a neck brace.

With the patient in dorsal recumbency, the ventral cervical area is approached as with other ventral stabilization techniques. In patients with CVI, Harrington spinal distraction rods provide distraction and stabilization without the need for a vertebral spreader. The Harrington spinal distraction rod consists of a threaded

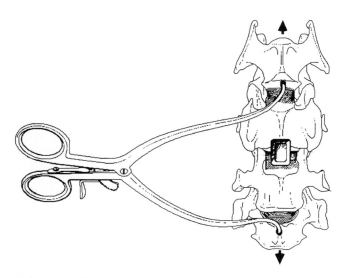

Fig. 45.22. Gelpi retractors, modified by blunting the tips, are inserted into the slots created in the vertebral bodies adjacent to the affected disc spaces. (From Bruecker KA, Seim HB. Caudal cervical spondylomyelopathy. In: Slatter DH, ed. Textbook of small animal surgery. Philadelphia: WB Saunders, 1993:1064.)

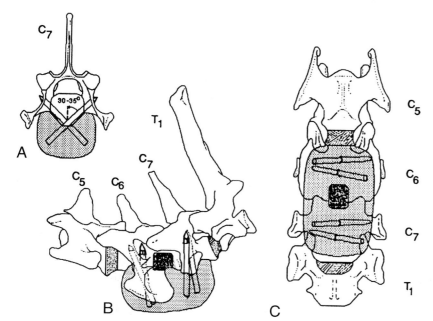

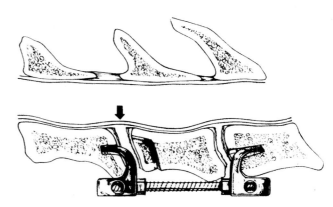

Fig. 45.23. **A–C.** Placement of cancellous bone, pins, and bone cement to treat cervical vertebral instability. (From Bruecker KA, Seim HB. Caudocervical spondylomyelopathy in large breed dogs. In: Bojrab MJ, ed. Current techniques in small animal surgery. 3rd ed. Philadelphia: Lea & Febiger, 1989:583.)

58-mm bolt, two nuts, and two distraction hooks (Harrington No. 1256 hooks and No. 1257 rods and nuts, Zimmer, Warsaw, IN). The threaded distraction bolt is cut twice the length of C6, and two nuts are threaded onto the center of the bolt. The distraction hooks slide over the threaded rod such that the tips of the hooks point away from each other.

The intervertebral disc spaces of C5–6 and C6–7 are fenestrated. Defects are created in the caudal end plate of C5 and the cranial end plate of C7 with a high-speed bur to accept the tips of the distraction hooks precisely (Fig. 45.24). An angled attachment allows better access to the caudal C5 end plate. Conservation

of as much cortical bone at the end plates as possible is necessary to prevent collapse and subsequent implant failure. The hooks are placed within the defects, and the rod is inserted with the nuts placed centrally. The centrally placed nuts are then turned such that one nut moves toward each end to contact the hooks. Distraction of both hooks and intervertebral disc spaces occurs with further tightening of the nuts (Fig. 45.25). Loosening of the nuts may be prevented by crimping the bolt or securing cerclage wire to the bolt adjacent to each nut. In large patients, two additional nuts may be placed between the hooks to act as lock nuts. Each lock nut is tightened against each of the nuts distracting the hooks. Cancellous bone is placed into the slotted defects to promote interbody fusion. The paired

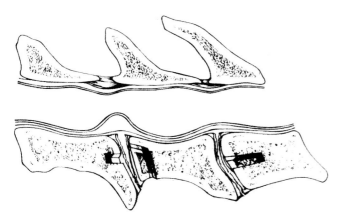

Fig. 45.24. A limited slot is made into the end plate of the primary site of compression. Defects are created in the caudal end plate of C5 and the cranial end plate of C7 to allow Harrington hook placement. (From Walker TL. Use of Harrington rods in caudal cervical spondylomyelopathy. In: Bojrab MJ, ed. Current techniques in small animal surgery. 3rd ed. Philadelphia: Lea & Febiger, 1989:585.)

Fig. 45.25. The nuts are turned to contact and distract the hooks. Distraction results in decompression of the cervical vertebral instability lesion. (From Walker TL. Use of Harrington rods in caudal cervical spondylomyelopathy. In: Bojrab MJ, ed. Current techniques in small animal surgery. 3rd ed. Philadelphia: Lea & Febiger, 1989:586.)

bellies of the longus colli muscle are approximated, and the remaining closure is routine. Because rotational stability is not immediately achieved with this technique, a neck brace may be required for 4 to 6 weeks postoperatively.

Treatment by Distraction and Stabilization Using a Polymethylmethacrylate Plug

Recently, another technique using an intervertebral plug of polymethylmethacrylate to accomplish distraction and stabilization has been described (11). As of this writing, I have had only limited experience with this distraction and stabilization technique. However, I believe the polymethylmethacrylate plug (PMP) technique may have merit over other techniques for the treatment of CVI. It has no apparent advantage in rates of recovery and overall success over distraction and stabilization using pins and polymethylmethacrylate; however, the risk of implant failure or iatrogenic spinal cord trauma from improperly placed pins is less with this technique. In addition, this technique can be performed at multiple disc spaces if necessary (11).

A ventral approach, as described for ventral decompression, is performed to expose the vertebral bodies and intervertebral spaces cranial and caudal to the affected intervertebral space. The affected intervertebral space is then pulled into additional linear traction, as previously described for the pins and polymethylmethacrylate technique. The original authors of the PMP technique have successfully used other vertebral spreaders, as well.

The affected disc material is removed to the level of the dorsal anulus fibrosus. To anchor the PMP, troughs are cut into the end plates using a high-speed drill and a 2- to 4-mm bur. These anchor troughs should be made approximately 5 to 10 mm in lateral width and 4 mm in depth and 4 mm in dorsoventral height (Fig. 45.26). An angled attachment allows better access to the caudal vertebral end plate. One gram of sterile cefazolin powder can be mixed with the sterile polymethylmethacrylate. The polymethylmethacrylate powder is mixed with liquid monomer until it reaches a liquid consistency and can be infused into the intervertebral disc space to the level of the ventral aspect of the vertebral bodies and gently packed digitally. Irrigation with sterile saline solution for 5 to 10 minutes dissipates the heat of polymerization. The vertebral spreaders are removed once the cement has hardened. Autogenous cancellous bone is harvested from the heads of the humeri and is placed ventral to the vertebral bodies and PMP to stimulate osseous fusion (Fig 45.27). Closure of the longus colli muscle is performed

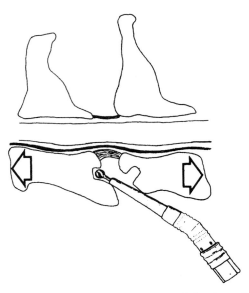

Fig. 45.26. Partial discectomy is performed, leaving only a thin layer of dorsal anulus fibrosus (*DAF*). Creation of anchor holes is accomplished with a high-speed bur and angle attachment. (From Dixon BC, Tomlinson JL, Kraus KH. Modified distraction–stabilization technique using an interbody polymethylmethacrylate plug in dogs with caudal cervical spondylomyelopathy. J Am Vet Med Assoc 1996;208:63.)

over the cancellous bone graft. The remainder of the closure is routine. A neck brace may be used postoperatively to limit excessive movement, but it may not be required (11).

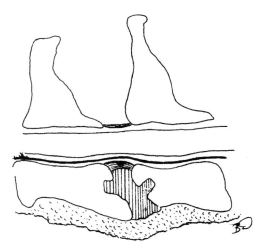

Fig. 45.27. The polymethylmethacrylate plug (*PMP*) is placed into the prepared disc space while traction is maintained. After the PMP hardens, the traction device is removed and cancellous bone graft (*CG*) is liberally packed along the ventral aspect of the vertebral bodies. The remaining thin layer of dorsal anulus fibrosus protects the spinal cord from the PMP. (From Dixon BC, Tomlinson JL, Kraus KH. Modified distraction–stabilization technique using an interbody polymethylmethacrylate plug in dogs with caudal cervical spondylomyelopathy. J Am Vet Med Assoc 1996;208:63.)

Treatment by Direct Decompression Using a Continuous Dorsal Laminectomy

Continuous dorsal laminectomy is a decompressive technique. This technique is most useful in patients with multiple lesions and those with dorsal lesions (12). Although this technique does not address the underlying pathophysiologic features associated with CCSM, relief of spinal cord compression is achieved.

With the patient in sternal recumbency, the front feet are secured cranially and the head and neck are elevated from the surgical table (13). Tape is placed over the muzzle and thorax to help secure the neck. A midline incision is made in the skin over the dorsal processes of the cervical spine from the poll of the cranium to T3. After the subcutaneous fascia and aponeurosis of the platysma muscle are incised, an incision is made through the median fibrous raphe. The origins of the splenius and serratus dorsalis muscles can be incised from the raphe and reflected to expose the nuchal ligament, the dorsal spinous processes of the thoracic vertebrae, and the long spinal muscles. These muscles are separated from the midline and are reflected from the dorsal spinous processes to expose the dorsal laminae.

After exposure of the cervical vertebrae, the dorsal spinous processes of the affected vertebrae are removed with rongeurs (12). The dorsal lamina is removed carefully using a high-speed surgical bur. The length of the laminectomy may be from three-quarters the length of each vertebrae up to a continuous laminectomy extending from C4 to C7. The width of the laminectomy is limited by the medial aspect of the articular facets of the cranial vertebrae. The initial depth of the laminectomy defect is to the periosteum of the inner cortical layer of the laminae. After penetration into the spinal canal, the remaining laminae and ligamenta flava are gently excised and are removed en bloc (Fig. 45.28). If needed, resection of the lateral aspects of the vertebral arches can be continued to the level of the ventral vertebral veins using rongeurs. The surgeon must preserve the articular facets. Hypertrophied joint capsule and ligamentum flavum are resected to achieve decompression of the spinal cord.

Transarticular hemicerclage wires or lag screws may need to be placed through the facets for additional stability. If stabilization is required, an appropriately sized hole is drilled through the articular facet. Removal of the articular cartilage is achieved using a high-speed surgical bur. An 18-gauge stainless steel wire is placed through the hole and is twist tightened, or alternatively, the hole is tapped and a lag screw is

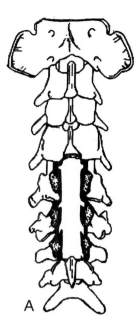

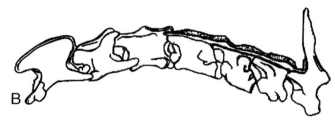

Fig. 45.28. A and **B.** The dorsal laminae have been removed from C4 through C7 to provide direct decompression of the caudal cervical spinal cord. (From Bruecker KA, Seim HB. Caudal cervical spondylomyelopathy. In: Slatter DH, ed. Textbook of small animal surgery. Philadelphia: WB Saunders, 1993:1067.)

placed. Cancellous bone is placed around the joint to promote arthrodesis (14–17).

An autogenous fat graft placed over the laminectomy site prevents the formation of a fibrous laminectomy membrane with subsequent stricture and spinal cord compression. Paraspinal muscles and fascia are approximated, and the remaining closure is routine. A cervical bandage or brace is generally required.

Postoperative Management

Analgesics may be necessary for 24 to 48 hours postoperatively. Anti-inflammatory drugs are not generally indicated in the postoperative period. A cervical bandage of rolled cotton and stretch gauze can be placed postoperatively to prevent excessive head and neck movements. This bandage can remain in place for 3 weeks. If warranted and tolerated, a neck brace constructed of fiberglass cast material or a heat-moldable splint material, incorporating the cervical and cranial aspect of the thoracic spine, may limit movement, thereby promoting fusion. Handles built into the brace may allow for better assistance when the animal is rising and walking. A thoracic harness should be used instead of a neck collar.

Postoperative management of patients with CCSM is generally divided into ambulatory or nonambulatory convalescence. Patients with an ambulatory status postoperatively are generally managed in the following manner: cage confinement, brief exercise two to three times a day for 2 to 3 weeks, serial neurologic examinations, and home on restricted exercise or passive range-of-motion exercises. Nonambulatory patients are managed in the following manner: elevated padded cage rack or waterbed, passive range-of-motion exercises and turning every 2 to 4 hours, bladder expressions four to five times a day, serial neurologic evaluations, and frequent hydrotherapy (swimming with support) until their return to ambulatory status. Crate or pen confinement is recommended for 3 weeks, with a gradual return to normal activity to follow.

Neurologic recovery is generally rapid. Neck pain usually subsides within 24 to 48 hours. Tetraparetic patients begin to show improvement within days, as well. Any neurologic improvement within 3 weeks of surgery is encouraging. The neurologic status 6 weeks postoperatively is a good indication of ultimate neurologic recovery; however, patients may show improvement in function up to 6 months postoperatively (4, 5).

Iatrogenic spinal cord trauma, irreversible demyelination, and myelomalacia or agenesis of the affected spinal cord limit the success of surgical techniques used to treat CCSM.

References

1. Goring RL, Beale BS, Faulkner RF. The inverted cone decompression technique: a surgical treatment for cervical vertebral instability "wobbler syndrome" in Doberman pinschers. Part 1. J Am Anim Hosp Assoc 1991;27:403–409.
2. Chambers JN, Betts CW. Caudal cervical spondylopathy in the dog: a review of 20 clinical cases and the literature. J Am Anim Hosp Assoc 1977;13:571–576.
3. Chambers JN, Oliver JE, Bjorling DE. Update on ventral decompression for caudal cervical disc herniation in Doberman pinschers. J Am Anim Hosp Assoc 1986;22:775–778.
4. Bruecker KA, Seim HB, Withrow SJ. Clinical evaluation of three surgical methods for treatment of caudal cervical spondylomyelopathy of dogs. Vet Surg 1989;18:197–203.
5. Bruecker KA, Seim HB, Blass CE. Caudal cervical spondylomyelopathy: decompression by linear traction and stabilization with Steinmann pins and polymethylmethacrylate. J Am Anim Hosp Assoc 1989;25:677–683.
6. Ellison, GW, Seim HB, Clemmons RM. Distracted cervical spinal fusion for management of caudal cervical spondylomyelopathy in large breed-dogs. J Am Vet Med Assoc 1988;193:447–453.
7. Lincoln JD, Pettit GD. Evaluation of fenestration for treatment of degenerative disc disease in the caudal cervical region of large dogs. Vet Surg 1985;14:240–246.
8. Seim HB, Withrow SJ. Pathophysiology and diagnosis of caudal cervical spondylomyelopathy with emphasis on the Doberman pinscher. J Am Anim Hosp Assoc 1982;18:241–251.
9. Seim HB, Bruecker KA. Caudal cervical spondylomyelopathy (wobbler syndrome). In: Bojrab MJ, ed. Disease mechanisms in small animal surgery. 2nd ed. Philadelphia: Lea & Febiger, 1993:979–983.
10. Walker TL. Use of Harrington rods in caudal cervical spondylomyelopathy. In: Bojrab MJ, ed. Current techniques in small animal surgery. 3rd ed. Philadelphia: Lea & Febiger, 1989: 584–586.
11. Dixon BC, Tomlinson JL, Kraus KH. Modified distraction–stabilization technique using an interbody polymethylmethacrylate plug in dogs with caudal cervical spondylomyelopathy. J Am Vet Med Assoc 1996;208:61–68.
12. Lyman, R. Continuous dorsal laminectomy for the treatment of Doberman pinschers with caudal cervical vertebral instability and malformation. In: Abstracts of the 5th Annual Meeting of the American Animal Hospital Association. Denver, CO: American Animal Hospital Association, 1987:303–308.
13. Piermattei DL. An atlas of surgical approaches to the bones and joints of the dog and cat. 3rd ed. Philadelphia: WB Saunders, 1993:60–69.
14. Walker TL, Tomlinson JL, Sorjonen DC, et al. Diseases of the spinal column. In: Slatter DH, ed. Textbook of small animal surgery. Philadelphia: WB Saunders, 1985:1367–1391.
15. Trotter EJ, deLahunta A, Geary JC, et al. Caudal cervical vertebral malformation–malarticulation in great Danes and Doberman pinschers. J Am Vet Med Assoc 1976;10:917–930.
16. Dueland R, Furneaux RW, Kaye MM. Spinal fusion and dorsal laminectomy for midcervical spondylolisthesis in a dog. J Am Vet Med Assoc 1973;162:366–369.
17. Hurov LI. Treatment of cervical vertebral instability in the dog. J Am Vet Med Assoc 1979;175:278–285.

46

THORACOLUMBAR SPINE

Intervertebral Disc Fenestration

James E. Creed & Daniel J. Yturraspe

Indications

Fenestration of thoracolumbar intervertebral discs is appropriate for dogs of breeds predisposed to disc herniation (such as the dachshund and Pekingese), with clinical signs ranging from lumbar pain to paresis, that are otherwise in good health and are less than 8 years of age. One study indicated that only 5% of dogs with thoracolumbar disc herniations are more than 8 years of age (1). Whether older dogs are less likely to have recurrent problems is unknown, but in such dogs a conservative approach seems advisable initially.

Fenestration should be considered when signs of disc herniation are first evident; the operation is definitely recommended if signs progress in severity or on the first recurrence. Dogs presented with caudal motor paralysis should undergo spinal cord decompression, because disc fenestration alone is not appropriate treatment for paralysis. If the dog still perceives pain in the rear toes, fenestration should also be accomplished. Fenestration can be performed within a variable period after disc herniation; we prefer to operate within the first 2 to 3 days. The patient can then recuperate from surgery while hospitalized to treat signs produced by that herniation.

Preoperative Preparations

Corticosteroids and antibiotics are administered preoperatively, and anesthesia is induced with a short-acting barbiturate and maintained by endotracheal administration of an acceptable volatile agent. Intravenous fluids are administered during surgery and postoperatively. An area of the back extending from the vertebral border of each scapula to the crest of each ilium is clipped and prepared for surgery. The dog is positioned in ventral recumbency on an insulating pad to conserve body heat. It is most convenient for surgeons to operate from the side of the patient opposite that of their dominant hand. Radiographs and a skeleton should be available for reference.

Surgical Technique

A dorsolateral approach (2) is used to gain access to eight intervertebral discs between T10 and L5. Discs between T9–10 and L5–6 can also be fenestrated if they are calcified or partially herniated. These discs are not routinely fenestrated because of their low incidence of herniation. They are also technically more difficult to fenestrate because of anatomic differences. Not only is the L5–6 disc more difficult to fenestrate, but also considerable risk of creating a femoral nerve deficit exists if the adjacent ventral nerve branch is damaged.

A skin incision is made from a point one to two spinous processes rostral to the anticlinal vertebra (T11) to a point one vertebra rostral to the ilium. This incision may be made directly on the dorsal midline or 1 to 2 cm lateral to the midline on the side from which the discs are to be fenestrated. The cutaneous trunci muscle, subcutaneous fat, and superficial fascia are incised in the same plane and are reflected sufficiently to expose the lumbodorsal fascia 1 to 2 cm lateral to the dorsal midline (Fig. 46.1**A**). The lumbodorsal fascia and aponeurosis of the longissimus thoracis et lumborum muscle are incised along an imagi-

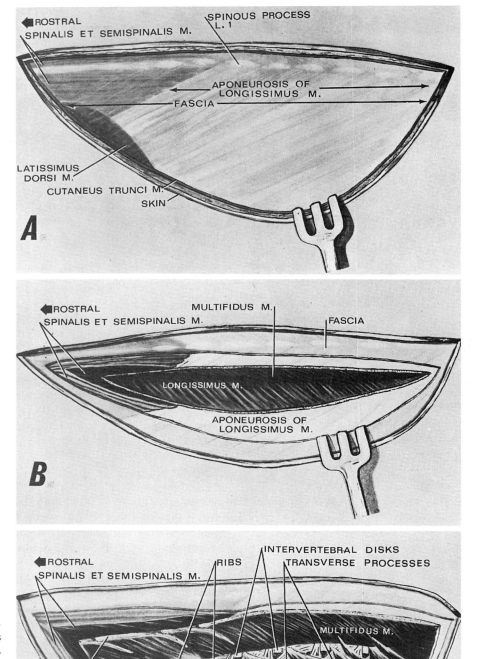

Fig. 46.1. Surgical anatomy of the dorsolateral approach to the thoracolumbar discs of the dog. **A.** The skin, subcutaneous fascia, fat, and cutaneous trunci muscle have been incised and reflected laterally on the left side of the dog. **B.** The deep external fascia of the trunk, the aponeurosis of the longissimus thoracis muscle, and the caudal edge of the spinalis et semispinalis muscles have been incised to expose the underlying multifidus and longissimus muscles. **C.** The multifidus muscle is separated from the longissimus thoracis muscle by blunt dissection to expose the thoracolumbar spine for intervertebral disc fenestration.

nary line drawn from a point 5 mm lateral to the spinous process of T9 to a point 1 to 2 cm lateral to the comparable process of L6 (Fig. 46.1**B**). In the rostral portion of the surgical field, the caudal border of the spinalis and semispinalis thoracis muscles, interposed between the lumbodorsal fascia and the aponeurosis of the longissimus thoracis muscle, is also incised (Figs. 46.1**B** and 46.2).

Access to intervertebral discs is gained by opening the intermuscular septum between the multifidus lumborum and thoracis muscles medially and the longissimus dorsi and sacrococcygeus dorsalis lateralis muscles laterally (Figs. 46.1**C**, 46.2, and 46.3). This septum is the first one lateral to the dorsal spinous processes; it is easiest to locate in the midlumbar region, where fat is interposed superficially between the muscles. Muscles are easily divided by blunt dissection in the lumbar region; however, the septum is less distinct over the ribs. All blunt dissection is done with an Adson semisharp, or comparable, periosteal elevator in each hand. As the tubercles of the last four ribs are exposed, care should be taken not to disturb the small nerves and vessels coursing craniolaterally immediately dorsolateral to each tubercle. Separation of musculature is carried to the base of the lumbar transverse processes.

The novice should completely separate muscles to this level and should be careful to avoid dorsal branches of the spinal nerves (see Fig. 46.1**C**). This maneuver provides good visualization of the intervertebral discs and adjacent structures. The experienced surgeon can "tunnel" down to each lumbar transverse

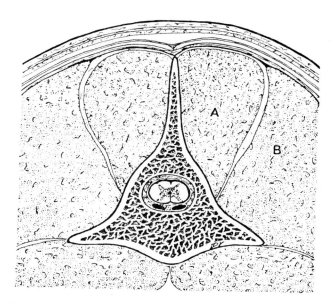

Fig. 46.3. Cross section through L4. **A.** Multifidus lumborum muscle. **B.** Longissimus lumborum muscle.

process, thereby avoiding considerable tedious dissection and trauma. The short transverse process of L1 lies adjacent to the last rib, assuming the thirteenth rib is present, and is used as an anatomic reference point. All other lumbar transverse processes can be "tunneled" down to by referring to the lateral radiograph and estimating the distance between each process. If judgment is correct, the veterinary surgeon will never see the dorsal branch of each rostral spinal nerve or its allied vessels. As the operation proceeds caudally from T13 to L1, succeeding transverse processes are progressively deeper.

As the surgeon exposes the lumbar transverse processes (L1–5), the lumbar discs are exposed. The lateral anulus of the intervertebral discs lies immediately rostral to the base of each transverse process (Fig. 46.4). In the caudal thoracic area, the disc lies rostromedial to the head of each rib. The T10–11 disc is difficult to expose because it is situated 1 to 2 cm ventromedially and is partially covered by the rib tubercle. Each disc can be visualized by elevating tissue off the lateral anulus with a periosteal elevator. The use of a small self-retaining retractor (Gelpi or Weitlaner) or hand-held retractors enhances visualization. Care should be taken not to invade the intervertebral foramen, which lies immediately dorsal to each disc and contains a spinal nerve and allied vessels. The inexperienced surgeon may overcompensate in avoiding the intervertebral foramina and work too far ventrally, where one risks injuring the ventral branches of the spinal nerves. Ventral branches of spinal nerves pass adjacent to the ventrolateral aspect of each disc (see Fig. 47.4).

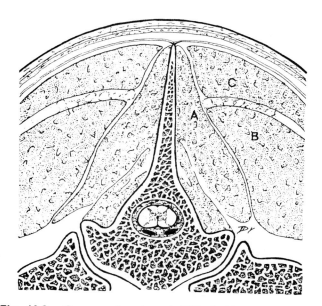

Fig. 46.2. Cross section through T12. **A.** Multifidus thoracis muscle. **B.** Longissimus thoracis muscle. **C.** Spinalis et semispinalis muscles.

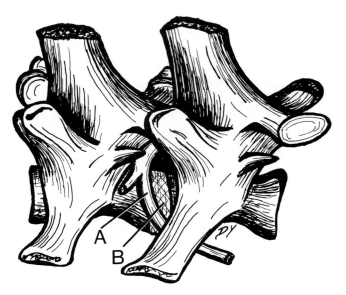

Fig. 46.4. L3–4 showing the relation of the spinal nerve to the intervertebral disc. **A.** Ventral branch of L3 spinal nerve. **B.** Intervertebral disc.

In the lumbar area, ventral branches of spinal nerves are located under the intertransverse fascia and are not visible in the surgical field unless an attempt is made to expose them. To ensure that a ventral branch is not traumatized, the tip of a curved mosquito hemostat can be introduced into the intertransverse fascia adjacent to the ventrolateral border of the anulus and the jaws can be spread gently. This maneuver exposes the ventral nerve branch occasionally, and the tissue defect also creates a landmark for the surgeon to avoid. If the L5–6 disc is fenestrated, the ventral branch of the fifth lumbar nerve should be identified and avoided to ensure that it is not damaged.

A disc's lateral anulus is visualized best for fenestration if adjacent muscle is retracted rostrodorsally with a curved periosteal elevator. This instrument also protects the dorsal branch of the spinal nerve and associated vessels. A pointed scalpel blade is used either to incise or to remove an elliptic section of the anulus fibrosus. The anulus should not be cut where it cannot be visualized. Fenestration is accomplished with a modified dental-claw tartar scraper or the eye portion of a large suture needle held in a needle holder. The nucleus pulposus is removed using a circular motion. The tip of the hook or needle eye is directed upward, with care taken not to break through the dorsal anulus. A partially herniated disc must be fenestrated cautiously, to avoid forcing additional nucleus pulposus into the spinal canal (Fig. 46.5). The surgeon must remove as much disc material as possible.

Fenestrating the T10–11 disc requires special care to avoid creating pneumothorax; the pleura, directly ventral to this disc, rises and falls with respiratory movement. If the existence of pneumothorax is in question, irritation of the area with saline solution and expansion of the lungs by compressing the ventilation bag should provide an answer; air bubbles will appear in the surgical field if significant pneumothorax exists.

Minimal hemorrhage associated with exposure and fenestration of thoracolumbar discs can be controlled usually by topical pressure on bleeding tissue with a periosteal elevator. Rarely, hemostatic forceps or electrocautery techniques are required to control bleeding.

Every disc fenestrated should be identified to ensure that no discs are missed between T10 and L5. If clinical signs merit decompression of the spinal cord, spinal cord decompression should be performed first, followed by disc fenestration. Fenestration is more compatible with hemilaminectomy than it is with dorsal decompression. Hemilaminectomy and fenestration can be performed from the same side; although the multifidus muscle is badly traumatized, no adverse clinical signs have been observed. Lateralization of signs often dictates performing a decompressive surgical procedure and fenestration on opposite sides of the spinal column.

Debridement of tissue is not necessary when the "tunnel" technique is used to expose the lumbar discs. Performing a hemilaminectomy on the same side, or division of the multifidus and longissimus dorsi muscles down to the level of transverse processes for improved exposure, may necessitate some debridement. The aponeurosis of the longissimus muscle and the spinalis et semispinalis muscle in the caudal thoracic area and the overlying thoracolumbar fascia are approximated with one suture line of absorbable suture

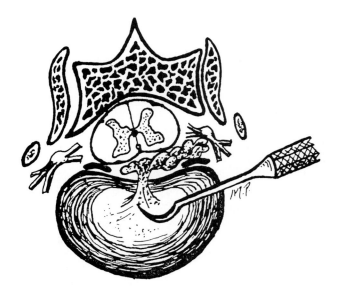

Fig. 46.5. The correct position of a modified dental claw tartar scraper to fenestrate a disc, in this case a partially herniated disc.

material. Subcutaneous tissues are apposed with similar material, catching the underlying fascia occasionally to obliterate dead space. The skin incision is closed with any dermal suture. A light-pressure bandage may be applied around the trunk of the dog and is left in place for 4 to 7 days.

Postoperative Care and Prognosis

Corticosteroid and analgesic agents should be administered for 1 to 3 days postoperatively because most dogs experience some discomfort. Thereafter, treatment depends on clinical signs. Because corticosteroids are used in association with this operation, skin sutures should not be removed for at least 3 weeks to avoid incisional dehiscence. Dogs routinely go home 48 to 72 hours after the surgical procedure, or as soon as voluntary urination is evident. In addition to preventing subsequent attacks of disc prolapse, fenestration eliminates the need for prolonged confinement of dogs with functional ambulatory ability. Physical therapy can be initiated within a day or so of surgery in patients with caudal paralysis.

The degree of paresis, if present, remains unchanged in most animals immediately postoperatively. Because clinical signs occasionally are more severe immediately after the procedure, the client must be forewarned of this possibility. Deterioration in neurologic status can be associated with the operation. If pathologic changes in the spinal cord, which may or may not be known, are progressive at the time of surgery, disc fenestration itself will not be responsible for a worsened neurologic state. Such a condition may result from spontaneous herniation of additional nucleus pulposus while the dog is anesthetized for radiographs or surgery. Overzealous fenestration of a partially herniated disc may also force additional material into the spinal canal. Trauma to the spinal cord from the fenestration hook is an unlikely cause of increase in neurologic deficit. The client should be advised that some dogs suddenly deteriorate neurologically without radiographs or operation.

The most likely potential surgical complications are 1) failure to fenestrate a disc, 2) creation of a pneumothorax, 3) injury to spinal nerves, 4) damage to the spinal cord, and 5) cutting of spinal arteries.

In most dogs, evidence of some degree of spinal nerve injury exists for a least a few days postoperatively. Dogs may have slight scoliosis, with deviation to the operated side, and sag (paralysis) of abdominal muscles ipsilateral to the operated side may be noticeable. If the ventral branch of the fifth lumbar (L5–6) has been damaged, the dog will have at least a temporary femoral nerve deficit. Severity of these signs is directly correlated with the expertise of the veterinary surgeon (3).

We are aggressive in promoting thoracolumbar disc fenestration because it is impossible to predict the severity of a recurrent disc attack. Herniation of a cervical disc has not been observed to cause permanent caudal paralysis or death from diffuse myelomalacia; in the thoracolumbar region, however, such a sequela is not unusual. Fenestration, properly performed, should minimize the chance of a subsequent disc episode, and the dog's locomotion should not be compromised.

The dorsolateral approach is preferred for fenestration of thoracolumbar discs because it 1) permits decompression by hemilaminectomy when this procedure is also indicated, 2) results in minimal trauma, and 3) provides easy access to nine discs. Thoracolumbar intervertebral disc fenestration is more difficult than cervical disc fenestration, and the potential for severe and possibly permanent neurologic injury cannot be overemphasized. Success with this procedure requires a thorough understanding of anatomy and basic surgical principles. Consequently, the novice should perform this surgical procedure on a cadaver before attempting it on a clinical patient.

References

1. Gage ED. Incidence of clinical disc disease in the dog. J Am Anim Hosp Assoc 1975;11:135.
2. Yturraspe JD, Lumb WV. A dorsolateral muscle separating approach for thoracolumbar intervertebral disc fenestration in the dog. J Am Vet Med Assoc 1973;162:1037–1040.
3. Bartels KE, Creed JE, Yturraspe DJ. Complications associated with the dorsolateral muscle-separating approach for thoracolumbar disc fenestration in the dog. J Am Vet Med Assoc 1983;183:1081–1083.

Prophylactic Thoracolumbar Disc Fenestration

M. Joseph Bojrab &
Gheorghe M. Constantinescu

Surgical fenestration of the intervertebral space provides a means of prophylaxis in disc disease. If protrusion exists, surgical removal of the nucleus remaining in the intervertebral area will eliminate the pressure causing the protrusion. When all other discs that are potential problems (T9–10 to L5–6) are fenestrated at the same time, complete prophylaxis against future disc protrusions is achieved. The material already extruded into the canal cannot be removed by disc fenestration alone; however, fenestration of other degenerated discs is recommended, so vigorous physical therapy, such as hydrotherapy and cart walking, can

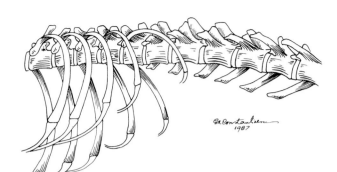

Fig. 46.6. Diagrammatic representation of the ventral vertebral column from the left lateral view. Note the relation of the lateral vertebral processes and the rib heads to the various disc spaces.

be prescribed without fear of causing another protrusion or even extrusion.

The ventral fenestration technique described here facilitates access to all potentially offending discs with a minimum of surgical trauma. Ten discs are fenestrated (T9–10 to L5–6). The thoracic discs are exposed through a left tenth intercostal thoracic approach, and the lumbar discs are exposed through a paracostal abdominal incision (Fig. 46.6).

Surgical Technique

The patient is medicated preoperatively with corticosteroids (dexamethasone 1 mg/lb) and antibiotics. The patient is placed in right lateral recumbency, and the left lateral side is clipped and prepared aseptically. The skin incision is made over the thirteenth rib from the dorsal to the ventral midline. The subcutaneous tissue is dissected, the incision is slid caudally, and a paracostal incision is made into the abdomen. The left kidney is located and is reflected ventrally with the peritoneum. Frazier laminectomy retractors are positioned (Fig. 46.7), and the abdominal viscera are packed off with a laparotomy pad. This retroperitoneal abdominal exposure affords access to the L1–2 through L5–6 intervertebral spaces. The iliopsoas (psoas minor) muscle is hooked with a muscle retractor and is retracted away from the ventral midline (Fig. 46.8). The ventral intervertebral prominences can be palpated.

The lateral transverse processes are identified and are numbered for orientation. Medial to the first transverse process is the T13–L1 intervertebral space. This space is not easily exposed from the abdominal approach and thus is fenestrated from the thorax. The remaining intervertebral spaces (L1–2 to L5–6) are fenestrated by first cutting the ventral longitudinal ligament and ventral annular fibers with a scalpel. The nucleus pulposus is removed with a Miltex scaler B tartar scraper. An inward, upward, and outward motion is used to clear the intervertebral space of as much nucleus as possible. Once this maneuver has been completed, the retractors are removed, and the muscle layers are individually sutured with 2–0 synthetic absorbable suture material.

The skin incision is slid in the cranial direction, and an incision is made into the thorax between the tenth and eleventh ribs. Frazier laminectomy retractors are placed (Fig. 46.9), and ventilation is instituted. The

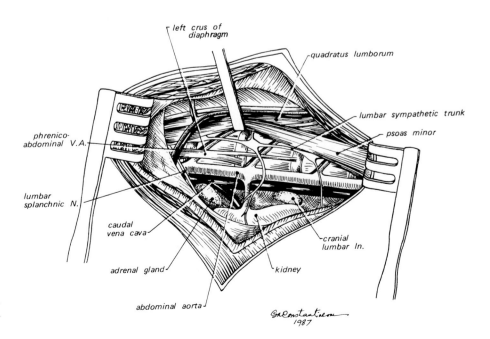

Fig. 46.7. Paracostal incision by retroperineal exposure for lumbar disc fenestration.

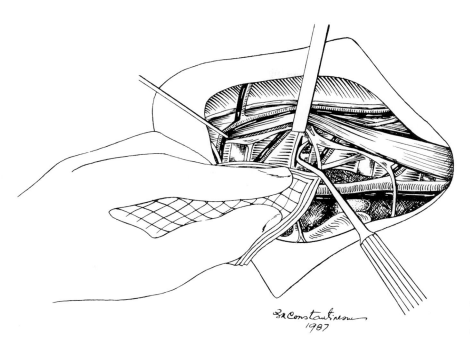

Fig. 46.8. The sublumbar muscles and sympathetic trunk have been elevated, and the crus of the diaphragm and the aorta have been depressed during a lumbar disc procedure.

T9–10 through T13–L1 intervertebral spaces are located and are dissected free of pleura; the sympathetic trunk and intercostal vessels are carefully avoided. When the dissection is complete, the discs are fenestrated in the same manner as already described (Fig. 46.10). The thorax, latissimus dorsi muscle, and skin are closed in a routine manner.

Postoperative Care

The animal is monitored closely during the anesthetic recovery period. Antibiotics are given, the bladder is

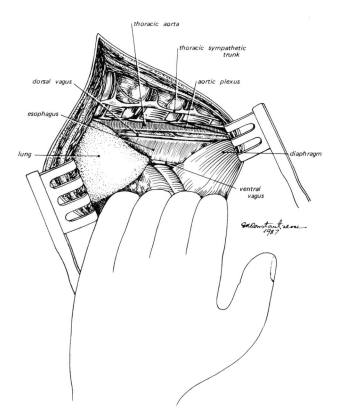

thoracic aorta

thoracic sympathetic trunk

dorsal vagus

aortic plexus

esophagus

lung

diaphragm

ventral vagus

Fig. 46.9. Exposure for thoracic disc fenestration.

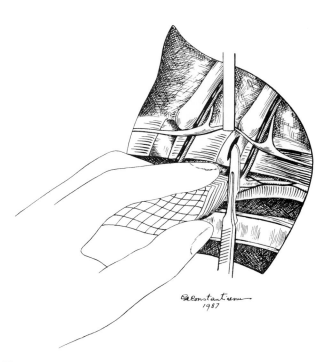

Fig. 46.10. The aorta is protected and depressed with a gauze sponge, and the thoracic disc is incised with a scalpel.

kept evacuated, and intensive physical therapy is instituted. Physical therapy includes hydrotherapy and cart walking.

Hemilaminectomy of the Cranial Thoracic Region

James F. Biggart, III

Indications

The most common indication for surgery of the thoracic spinal cord is the removal of extradural masses usually diagnosed by myelography. Disc herniations in the thoracic spine are rare, and many surgeons ignore the few disc lesions seen there. The intercapital ligaments occupying the floor of the canal between T2–10 help to protect the spinal cord from disc herniation. Neoplasia in the thoracic spine is more common than in other areas of the spine because of the lack of thoracic disc herniation. Therefore, exploration of the thoracic cord is likely to yield a tumor more often than in other areas of the spine.

Thoracic spinal fractures are rare because of the stabilizing influence of the ribs and long dorsal spines that help to prevent rotational deformities as well as flexion extension injuries. The mobile spine anterior and posterior to the thorax suffers more traumatic lesions.

The degenerative changes seen in the cervical and lumbar spine are not so common in the thoracic spine. Disc degeneration occurs as frequently as elsewhere in the spine, but disc herniations into the canal are rare. Redundancy of the ligamentum flavum is rare. Acquired bony stenosis is not often seen. Facet degenerative changes, synovitis, and synovial proliferation seldom cause cord stenosis or cord pressure. Bony stenosis, such as seen in the cervical region of caudal cervical spondylopathies of large dog breeds, has not been reported. Because many of these degenerative changes occur in more mobile segments of the spine, the more rigid thoracic spine is believed to be spared these changes.

Positioning of the Patient

The patient is placed in ventral recumbency. Elevation of the sternum (but not the elbows) by pillows, sandbags, or padding raises the spine in relation to the scapula. Pulling the forelegs forward usually loosens the adduction of the scapula to the spine, thereby allowing lateralization of the scapula. However, positioning the forelimbs posterior or crossing them under the sternum may aid in spinal visualization, so experimentation with foreleg positioning may be helpful.

Surgical Approach and Anatomy

A midline incision is made through the skin, subcutaneous fat, and fascia to the midline over the dorsal thoracic spinous processes. Just off the midline, the approach continues ventral alongside the dorsal spines to the dorsal lamina, which forms the base of the dorsal spines. The cutaneous trunci, trapezium, and cleidocephalicus are the first muscles encountered and are incised along their attachment to the dorsal spine processes on the midline. The latissimus dorsi and rhomboideus muscles are likewise incised, allowing lateralization of the scapula by self-retaining rib, Gelpi, or Weitlaner retractors. The cranial serratus dorsalis insertions are incised, as are the insertions of the thoracic spinalis and semispinalis muscles on the dorsal spines. The spinalis thoracis muscles are elevated by periosteal elevators to expose the lateral dorsal spines. The longissimus muscles are lateralized with retraction and do not require incision. The thoracic multifidus muscles are elevated with periosteal elevators or are incised at their origins. The supraspinatus ligament and interspinales muscles are left intact. The longi and breves rotatores muscles are incised at their origins exposing the dorsal lamina (Fig. 46.11). The levator costae muscle can be spared unless rib head exposure is needed.

Once the lamina is exposed, a high-speed drill is needed to remove the dorsal lateral lamina. For right-handed surgeons, a left-sided hemilaminectomy is preferred (Fig. 46.12). The dorsal spine can be undercut to the off side of the spinal canal. The ventral 1 to 2 cm of the dorsal spine can be removed, allowing wide lateral exposure to the off side (Fig. 46.13). The resultant floating dorsal spine, suspended by interspinous

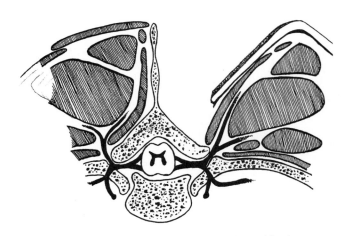

Fig. 46.11. Exposure of the dorsolateral lamina.

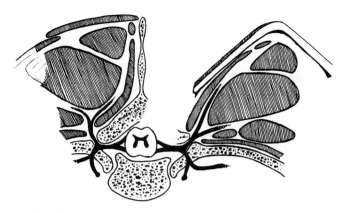

Fig. 46.12. Hemilaminectomy exposing the spinal cord.

muscles and supraspinous ligament, produces no noticeable effect. Likewise, the rib head, neck, and tubercle can be removed as needed for lateral cord exposure on the near side. The resultant floating rib seldom causes problems because it is supported by adjacent ribs through the intercostal muscles. As the surgeon moves forward in the thoracic spine, the ribs articulate higher in the interdiscal space and may necessitate rib head, neck, and tubercle resection. Resection of the proximal rib head, neck, and tubercle allows adequate spinal cord visualization. Care must be taken to avoid dissection below the rib that could allow penetration into the chest cavity, thereby creating a pneumothorax.

The length of the dorsal spines in some breeds may create a deep surgical field. Proper instrumentation and lighting allow careful cord evaluation. The arteries encountered are the dorsal branches of the intercostal arteries. The spinal branches supply the spinal cord through the foramen just above the rib neck. These vessels can be avoided by staying close to the midline along the dorsal spines. The veins encountered parallel the arteries and join the azygos posterior to the heart and the costocervical–vertebral trunk anterior to the heart.

Wound closure is similar to that of lumbar or cervical hemilaminectomy. A free fat graft harvested from the subcutaneous tissue is placed into the hemilaminectomy defect. Careful cord hemostasis lessens the hemorrhage under the fat graft that increases scar invasion of the graft. The more graft that undergoes revascularization, the less restrictive scar forms above the cord (1–3). The trapezius, rhomboideus, serratus dorsalis, and cranialis muscles should be reattached to preserve scapular function. The rest of the epaxial muscles reattach to the spine without direct suturing.

Postoperative care is similar to that after other spine approaches. Lameness is common for a few days until the scapular sling muscles lose their tenderness.

Benefits

Inclusion of this approach to the thoracic spine with well-known approaches to the neck and lumbar spine allows the surgeon to explore any lesion in the spinal canal from the foramen magnum to the coccygeal vertebrae. Most extradural lesions can be removed from the spinal canal, especially if undercutting the dorsal lamina or removal of the base of the dorsal spine is used to gain access to the far side of the spinal cord.

Limitations

Long, wide laminectomies over many disc spaces entail removal of the bases of many dorsal spines. The need for stabilization of these spines to prevent their ventral collapse into the laminectomy site adds additional hardware, expertise, and complexity to an already challenging approach. In addition, visualization, especially under the spinal cord, is sometimes poor.

The scapula prevents a lateral view of the cord in the cranial thoracic spine. Instruments have to be placed from a dorsal aspect. This necessitates using right-angled instruments that are not used in cervical and lumbar spine operations. Removal of the rib head and neck, especially over many disc spaces, adds complexity.

A surgical headlamp and 2× loop magnification are helpful in visualizing the spine especially in deep surgical fields. Bipolar cautery and fine tip suction are essential in providing hemostasis. The added visual acuity gained by hemostasis is more beneficial than the more obvious benefit of preventing blood loss and shock.

Because of the stabilizing influence of the adjacent dorsal spines and ribs, the destabilizing effects of wide deep laminectomy over the thoracic spine are less than those of the cervical or lumbar spine. Wider exposure

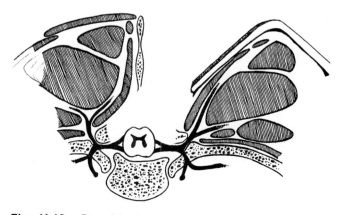

Fig. 46.13. Dorsal laminectomy necessitating removal of the dorsal spine.

of the spinal cord is possible, allowing a greater amount of adjacent tissue excision for biopsy or tumor removal. However, the close proximity to the aorta, azygos vein, and chest cavity makes exposure ventral to the cord or rib head hazardous. Damage to the nerve roots exiting the foramen cause some loss of forelimb function as well as loss of intercostal function affecting respiration.

Variations: First and Second Thoracic Cord Exposure

The first and second thoracic vertebral cord can be approached as a posterior extension of a seventh cervical dorsal laminectomy (4, 5). The thoracic dorsal spines can be exposed anteriorly without disturbing the ligamentum nuchae or supraspinous muscles, which are retracted laterally. The drill is angled from anterior to posterior, with the right-handed surgeon positioned on the right side of the patient that has been placed in sternal recumbency. Removal of the lamina between the base of the dorsal spine and first rib head exposes the spinal cord and canal over one side. Care must be used to leave enough of the base of the first dorsal spine to maintain the strength necessary to support the head and neck through its attachment of the nuchal ligament. This limits the exposure of the first thoracic spinal cord. If complete removal of the base of the first dorsal thoracic spine is needed, then enough of the base of the spine should be removed to prevent downward pressure of the spine stump on the exposed cord. Support of the head by the nuchal ligament, which attaches to the first three dorsal spines, pushes the remaining spine ventrally when its lower base is removed.

Approaching the anterior thoracic cord in this way avoids the disruption of the musculature along the dorsal spine and attachments to the scapula. The scapula influences the approach to the thoracic spine only anterior to T6 or T7. Posterior to these areas, the approach is similar to that of the lumbar spine.

References

1. Biggart JF III. Laminectomy membrane: etiology and prevention. In: Proceedings of the American College of Veterinary Surgeons Annual Meeting. Denver, CO: American College of Veterinary Surgeons, 1981.
2. Biggart JF III. Prevention of laminectomy membrane by free fat grafts after laminectomy in dogs with disc herniations. Vet Surg 1988;17:29.
3. Gill GG, Sakovich L, Thompson E. Pedicle fat grafts for the prevention of scar formation after laminectomy. Spine 1979;4:176.
4. Piermatei DL, Greeley RG. An atlas of surgical approaches to the bones of the dog and cat. 2nd ed. Philadelphia: WB Saunders, 1979:46–49.
5. Parker AL. Surgical approach to the cervico-thoracic junction. J Am Anim Hosp Assoc 1979;9:374–377.

Hemilaminectomy of the Caudal Thoracic and Lumbar Spine

Stephen T. Simpson

Hemilaminectomy provides rapid and safe exposure to one side of the spinal cord and the floor of the vertebral canal. Although less common, a bilateral approach can provide access to both sides and the floor of the vertebral canal (1). A unilateral exposure usually is adequate for the removal of herniated disc material that has not become fibrosed to the spinal cord and also provides easy access for fenestration. Disc fenestration and hemilaminectomy are more easily accomplished from the patient's left side by right-handed surgeons and from the right side by left-handed surgeons. A herniated disc can be removed from either side.

Hemilaminectomy can be combined with various fixation techniques to provide decompression and adequate stability of spinal fractures and luxations. Hemilaminectomy has been combined with spinous process plating (2, 3), vertebral body plating (4), spinal instrumentation procedures (5), and various pinning techniques (6–8). Although hemilaminectomy can be performed anywhere on the spinal column, modifications are necessary in the cervical and lumbosacral regions. The procedure is most commonly used for the surgical treatment of thoracolumbar intervertebral disc herniation.

Surgical Techniques

The patient can be anesthetized with any standard inhalant anesthetic. Standard monitoring and safety procedures should be established and used. Normally, the patient is anesthetized, radiographed, and treated surgically. Once the decision to operate is made, the patient is placed in sternal recumbency, and an area ap-

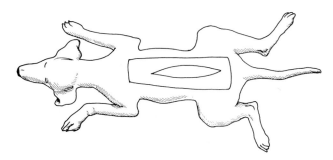

Fig. 46.14. A skin incision is made on the dorsal midline from the ninth thoracic vertebra to the sixth lumbar vertebra.

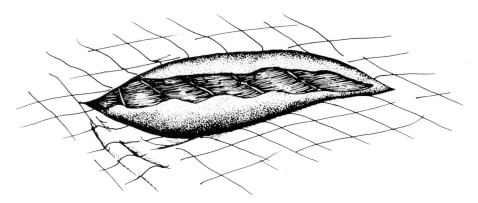

Fig. 46.15. The thoracolumbar fascia is cut at the midline, scalloping around the spinous processes, from T10 or T11 to L4.

proximately 10 cm wide centered on the midline and extending from the level of the scapula to the tuber coxae is prepared for surgery.

The skin is incised on the midline from T9 to L6 and is toweled in (Fig. 46.14). The subcutaneous fat is incised on the midline from the cranial to the caudal extent of the skin incision. Excessive retraction of the subcutaneous fat layer promotes seroma formation and should be avoided. The dense thoracolumbar fascia is incised on the midline, allowing the incision to scallop laterally to the spinous processes (Fig. 46.15).

Muscle Dissection

Dissection of muscles is a three-step procedure, one step for each of the major muscle attachments to the vertebrae. In stable injuries, periosteal elevation of muscle is preferred. Sharp dissection is required when spinal segments are unstable as a result of fracture or luxation. Each muscle layer is removed separately. Many surgeons prefer to work from caudal to cranial, but I find it easier to start in the middle of the incision and work toward the ends of the incision. Because the incised fascia has less tension in the middle than at either end of the incision, a less traumatic exposure is possible by working from the middle toward the ends of the incision. A periosteal elevator or the back end of a scalpel handle is inserted between the multifidus muscle and the spinous process. The instrument is pushed ventrally while firm contact is maintained with bone. The elevator is then levered laterally to produce a larger defect between the multifidus muscle and the spinous process. Moving cranially and caudally, similar elevation and levering are performed until the T10 through L4 processes are exposed. The multifidus muscle is loosely attached to the spinous processes laterally, but it is attached by strong tendons to their caudal edge. The tendons should be cut close to the caudal edge of each spinous process, and the muscles further retracted.

In the second step, muscle attachments are separated from the articular processes. The muscle elevation previously performed is continued by placing the elevator against the lamina at the medial base of the articular pedicle and elevating loosely attached muscle up to the pedicle and retracting it laterally. During this lateral retraction, the articular process is exposed by cutting the tendons attached to the cranial edge of the articular process (Fig. 46.16). The surgeon should use a shaving or fraying motion, rather than a slicing motion, to cut the tendons. A small bleeding vessel frequently is cut during this part of the procedure, but bleeding usually stops when the vessel is packed with gauze. The remaining muscular attachments are cut on the lateral side and the caudal edge of the articular process. The periosteal elevator is then pressed firmly on the lateral side of the articular process, and the muscle is elevated from the lateral, cranial, and caudal sides of the articular process. On the lateral side, elevation is stopped at the accessory process, which guards the dorsal entrance to the intervertebral foramen. The same procedure is performed at each articular process,

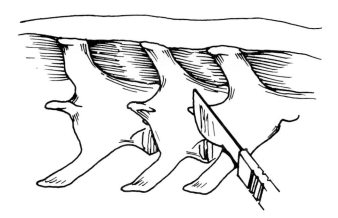

Fig. 46.16. The tendinous attachments are severed at the cranial, lateral, and caudal edges of the articular processes.

working cranially and caudally from the middle. For optimal visualization, the articular processes from T11–12 through L3–4 should be exposed.

Detachment of muscle from the accessory process is the third step in muscle dissection. It is an optional step and may be delayed until positive identification of the surgical site has been made. A longissimus tendon lies between the accessory process and ventral to the articular process. This tendon should be incised carefully about 0.5 cm from the bone. The spinal nerve and artery are ventral and close to this tendon; care must be exercised to avoid them. No further dissection beyond incision of this tendon is required.

Two Gelpi retractors are inserted near each end of the muscle dissection. The medial tine is inserted between spinous processes, and the lateral tine is inserted as deeply into the lateral muscle tissue as possible. After maximum retraction is obtained, any tags of tissue that have remained attached to bone are removed.

Access to the Spinal Cord

Identification of the lesion site is crucial to successful surgery. The surgeon must ascertain the location of the lesion from radiographs; if an unpaired last rib is present, the side must be defined. A transverse process emerges ventrally and cranially from each lumbar vertebral body. A rib proceeds laterally and curves caudally and ventrally from each thoracic vertebral body. The junction of the most cranial transverse process and most caudal rib identifies the articular process at the thoracolumbar junction (Fig. 46.17). Adjacent articular processes are counted to the appropriate site.

The articular processes are removed with rongeurs, and the pedicle is smoothed to the lamina. Several techniques have been described for gaining entrance to the vertebral canal. Use of a power drill and bur is the fastest method to produce a large laminar defect, but the equipment is expensive and may not always

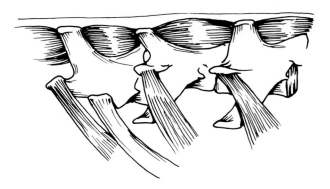

Fig. 46.17. The most cranial transverse process and the most caudal rib should be identified to localize the thoracolumbar junction from which the correct vertebra can be determined.

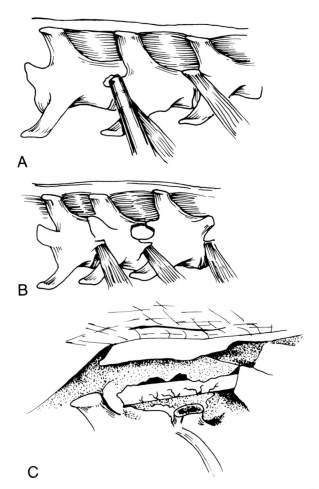

Fig. 46.18. Trephine method for exposing vertebral canal. **A.** A trephine is placed on the lamina directly over the location of the previously removed articular processes and pedicles. **B.** A laminar defect created by a trephine. **C.** The hemilaminectomy defect is extended with rongeurs as far as necessary cranially and caudally until normal epidural fat is seen and the cord is not compromised. See text for details.

be available. A procedure in which only rongeurs are used to gain access is used frequently; it requires some patient manipulation but the least instrumentation. The use of a Michele trephine—an old procedure—is still favored by many surgeons. Although this procedure involves blind penetration, which has some inherent risks, when properly used, it provides rapid access to the spinal canal. The laminar defect created with the trephine is enlarged with rongeurs.

TREPHINE METHOD

After the articular processes have been removed by rongeurs or bone cutters, the trephine is placed on the lamina at the articulation. It is maintained at approximately a 45° angle from vertical and 90° to the long axis of the vertebral column (Fig. 46.18A). An assistant provides manual support for the vertebral column. The trephine is turned alternately clockwise and counterclockwise on its own axis. The trephine can be tilted a few degrees in any direction for selective cutting. This allows the operator to know whether all quadrants of the hole are still being cut. The trephine can be removed frequently and the plug tested for looseness; before the trephine cuts through completely, the plug becomes loose. Early withdrawal of the superficial portion of the bone plug with rongeurs may produce a deep shelf of bone in the trephine hole that may prove difficult to remove. Proper use of the trephine allows adequate bone removal with no additional damage to the spinal cord (Fig. 46.18**B**). Often, the joint capsule and ligamentum flavum remain in the bottom of the trephine hole. This ligament should be left in place until the trephine hole is enlarged with rongeurs, and then the ligament can be cut away.

Lempert rongeurs are inserted into the laminar defect created by the trephine, and the edge of the hole is enlarged in all directions. The hemilaminectomy should be extended cranially and caudally until normal epidural fat is encountered or normal spinal cord is seen. The opening should be extended dorsally to the base of the spinous process and ventrally to the junction of the lamina and vertebral body (Fig. 46.18**C**). Care should be exercised when removing the accessory process because the spinal nerve emerges from the canal ventral and caudal to its junction with the lamina.

RONGEUR METHOD

The rongeur method for gaining access to the spinal column requires upward traction on the vertebral column (9). This is accomplished by applying towel forceps to the interspinous ligament of the vertebra that is cranial to the lesion and pulling upward. This maneuver opens the interarcuate space and allows insertion of a Lempert rongeur jaw under the caudal lip of the dorsolateral lamina of the vertebra (Fig. 46.19).

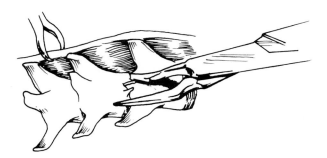

Fig. 46.19. The hemilaminectomy can be created with the use of rongeurs by opening the interarcuate space with dorsal traction and inserting a rongeur jaw into the interspinous ligaments and removing a bite of bone from the dorsolateral lamina. The opening is then enlarged by using the rongeur as in the trephine method.

The defect is begun by removing a bite of bone from the dorsolateral lamina with the rongeur. Traction is then removed, and the original defect is extended as described in the trephine method.

POWER DRILL METHOD

Use of a pneumatic drill (10) or electric drill (11) provides safe and rapid bone removal. A pineapple (6 to 8 mm) bur is used to outline the expected limits of the hemilaminectomy site; bone is then brushed away within these limits until a thin layer of cortical bone remains. The bur must be sharp, and the bone is flushed with saline. The thin layer of bone that remains can be removed with a tartar scraper and rongeur. Enlargement of the laminar defect, if needed, should be accomplished with rongeurs.

Removal of Extruded Disc Material and Disc Fenestration

Adequate removal of extruded disc material is accomplished with a narrow, dulled tartar scraper or thin ear curette. These thin instruments can be passed beneath the spinal cord to the other side of the canal if they are inserted horizontally. Disc material lying ventral to or lateral (same side) to the spinal cord can be removed completely by manipulating the material with these instruments. Disc material lying laterally on the opposite side from the laminar defect is more difficult to remove. Usually, it can be "snagged" by the tartar scraper and manipulated underneath the cord and out the laminar defect. Other options are to leave some material on the far side while relying on the laminar defect to provide decompression or to perform a hemilaminectomy on the other side.

After removing extruded disc material from the spinal canal, the surgeon should remove the rest of the affected disc and adjacent discs. The herniated disc can be fenestrated by inserting the point of the tartar scraper into the anulus from the dorsolateral corner of the disc at the level of the spinal canal and pushing the point into the disc in a ventromedial direction, thus encircling a portion of the nucleus pulposus. The handle of the scraper then is lifted upward and is pulled laterally, tearing a hole in the lateral side of the anulus. Incision of the anulus usually is not necessary.

Prophylactic fenestration of adjacent discs is slightly more difficult. Lumbar discs are located by identifying the junction of the transverse process with the vertebral body; the disc is immediately cranial to it. After the tendons of the longissimus muscle that were attached to the accessory process are carefully retracted cranially, the disc can be identified by observation or by sounding with a 22-gauge hypodermic needle. The needle does not penetrate bone, and if it enters soft tissue ventral to the vertebral body, it will not be firm. If the needle is placed in the disc space, it can be inserted and will remain firm. Once identified, the lateral anulus is incised with a No. 11 or 15 blade, and a tartar scraper is inserted into the incision. The curvature of the tartar scraper should always be down; it should be inserted with an encircling motion and withdrawn laterally. Other directions of insertion increase the risk of forcing disc material or the tartar scraper into the spinal canal. An auger device (Sismey fenestration auger, Arnolds Veterinary Products, Reading, Berkshire, UK) has been developed that both sounds the disc and incises the anulus (Fig. 46.20). Because removal of sufficient disc material often is not possible with this device, a tartar scraper or similar instrument generally must also be used to remove additional material. The surgeon must remove as much disc material as possible (12).

The major landmark used for locating thoracic discs is the site of rib articulation with the vertebral body. The ribs articulate caudally, so the disc resides 1 to 3 mm farther forward from the rib than from the transverse process. The thoracic vertebrae also are more superficial and have a smaller diameter than lumbar vertebrae. There is a tendency to fenestrate ventral to thoracic discs. The discs can be identified by observation or sounding and fenestrated similarly to lumbar discs. Discs from T11–12 through L3–4 should be fenestrated.

A potential complication of fenestration is acciden-

tal entry into the thoracic cavity. This is possible when fenestrating as far caudally as L1–2. This problem usually is not serious unless it occurs without the surgeon's knowledge. When entry does occur, pneumothorax results, and assisted ventilation is necessary. Complete lung distension during closure is usually definitive treatment.

Ancillary Procedures

A durotomy may be performed during a hemilaminectomy. Usually, this procedure is reserved for the patient that has a poor prognosis, is early in the course of the disease, and has a pale or blue spinal cord area that appears distended before the durotomy. A durotomy is not performed routinely.

Spinal cord perfusion is beneficial in patients with experimentally traumatized spinal cords, but it is of questionable value in patients that have been severely traumatized as little as several hours earlier. Normothermic perfusion is as effective as hypothermic perfusion. Like durotomy, perfusion should be reserved for the acutely ill patient with a poor prognosis. It is not a routine procedure.

A three-layer closure is used routinely with a hemilaminectomy. The thoracolumbar muscle fascia is sutured to the dorsal midline with one or two absorbable sutures placed between each spinous process. Because dorsal incisions generally have poor drainage, closure of the second layer—the subcutaneous tissue—is most important in preventing seroma formation. This layer should be closed with an absorbable suture in a continuous pattern; the knot is buried. The first bite of suture is subcuticular near the skin edge; the second bite is deep into the blind pocket created by the skin and the subcutaneous fat layer (Fig. 46.21). The third and fourth bites may be combined and should be near the midline in the fascia. The bites are repeated on the other side of the incision. The skin can be closed in a continuous or interrupted pattern with nonabsorbable suture material. Sutures should not be removed for 2 weeks because of the strain on the dorsal incision.

Postoperative Care

Postoperative care includes physical therapy and management of the incision. Generally, the incision is dry and closed by the third day after the surgical procedure. Physical therapy should be delayed until the incision is closed. If the patient is nonambulatory, the closed incision is coated with collodion and the patient is placed in a whirlpool tub for 10- to 15-minute exercise periods two or three times a day. If the patient is ambulatory, physical therapy consists of walking, and the collodion is not necessary. Additional physical therapy should include selective passive muscle exer-

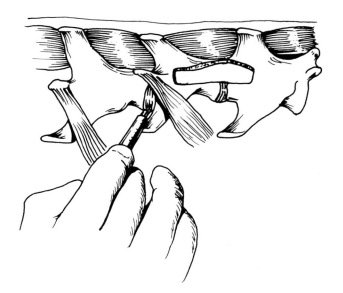

Fig. 46.20. Fenestration of a lumbar disc can be accomplished with a fenestration auger, which sounds the disc and then cuts a hole in its side. Additional removal of the nucleus pulposus is accomplished with a tartar scraper or a large bone needle. See text for details.

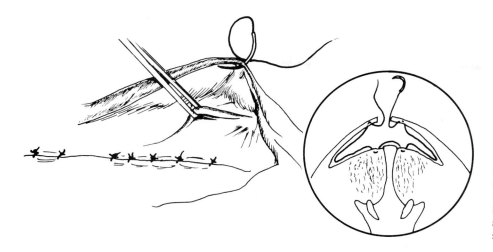

Fig. 46.21. Closure of the subcutaneous layer in a six-bite pattern incorporates the subcutaneous fat from the blind pouch created by the skin layer and deep muscle layer. *Inset,* cross-sectional view.

cises. Spastic muscles, which usually occur in extensor muscle groups, should not be exercised. A reasonable regimen is to use the whirlpool to relax spastic muscle groups, followed by isometric exercises of the flexor groups. This can be accomplished by encouraging a flexor reflex in the pelvic limbs. The stimulus should be enough to elicit a reflex but not enough to hurt the patient. The patient eventually will dislike the exercises, but they should be continued until the patient is ambulatory. Isometric exercises for 10 minutes twice a day is enough.

Most patients with spinal cord trauma have urinary incontinence and a spinal bladder. Appropriate care for these conditions includes meticulous attention to asepsis, frequent bladder evacuation either by expression or catheterization, and antibiotic therapy based on culture and sensitivity results.

References

1. Swaim SF, Vandevelde M. Clinical and histologic evaluation of bilateral hemilaminectomy and deep dorsal laminectomy for extensive spinal cord decompression in the dog. J Am Vet Med Assoc 1977;170:407.
2. Hoerlein BF. Canine neurology. 3rd ed. Philadelphia: WB Saunders, 1978.
3. Yturraspe DJ, Lumb WV. The use of plastic spinal plates for internal fixation of the canine spine. J Am Vet Med Assoc 1972;161:1651.
4. Swaim SF. Vertebral body plating for spinal immobilization. J Am Vet Med Assoc 1971;158:1683.
5. McAnulty JF, Lenehan TM, Maletz LM. Modified segmental spinal instrumentation in repair of spinal fractures and luxations in dogs. Vet Surg 1986;15:143.
6. Gage ED. A new method of spinal fixation in the dog (a preliminary report). Vet Med Small Anim Clin 1969;64:295.
7. Gage ED. Surgical repairs of spinal fractures in small breed dogs. Vet Med Small Anim Clin 1971;66:1095.
8. Gage ED. Modifications in dorsolateral hemilaminectomy and disc fenestration in the dog. J Am Anim Hosp Assoc 1975;11:407.
9. Swaim SF. A rongeuring technique for performing thoracolumbar hemilaminectomies. Vet Med Small Anim Clin 1976;71:172.
10. Swaim SF. Use of pneumatic surgical instruments in neurosurgery. Part 1. Spinal surgery. Vet Med Small Anim Clin 1973;68:1275.
11. Walker TL, Roberts RE, Kincaid SA, et al. The use of electric drills as an alternative to pneumatic equipment in spinal surgery. J Am Anim Hosp Assoc 1981;17:695.
12. Shores A, et al. Structural changes in thoracolumbar discs following lateral fenestration. Vet Surg 1985;14:117.

Modified Dorsal Laminectomy for Thoracolumbar Disc Disease

Eric J. Trotter

Various surgical procedures have been described for decompression of the spinal cord and removal of extruded or protruded intervertebral disc material from the vertebral canal in the thoracolumbar region of dogs. The procedures differ in the amount of bone removed and, thus, are referred to as hemilaminectomy, dorsal laminectomy, and modifications of these techniques, including laminotomies and laminoplasties. Each technique has its own inherent advantages and disadvantages, and most, if performed properly, satisfy the two basic tenets of spinal cord surgery for thoracolumbar disc disease: spinal cord decompression and mass removal. Objective comparison of the techniques has been precluded by the many variables associated with spontaneous extrusion or protrusion of intervertebral discs. Personal preference and the individual surgeon's training heretofore most frequently determined the type of decompressive procedure used. Previously, severely limited imaging modalities, that is, flat films and myelography, also made selection of the most appropriate technique for the individual patient difficult. With the increasing availability of computed tomography (CT) and magnetic resonance imaging (MRI), selection of the most appropriate decompressive technique based on the location of the extradural mass has become far more objective. In some instances, laminectomy is the procedure of choice.

After confirmation of the neuroanatomic lesion by myelography, CT, or MRI, the patient is placed in sternal recumbency and is prepared for aseptic surgery of the thoracolumbar spine. Prophylactic antibiotics (cefazolin) and corticosteroids (methylprednisolone sodium succinate) are administered intravenously at the time of surgical intervention. Only antibiotic therapy is continued in the postoperative period.

The skin incision, centered over the area of involvement, is made slightly lateral to the dorsal midline. Moistened laparotomy tapes are clipped to the reflected subcutaneous tissue or superficial fascia on each side of the incision to cover any exposed skin. The thoracolumbar fascia is incised bilaterally immediately lateral to the spinous processes. Periosteal elevators are used to lever or reflect the epaxial muscles bilaterally to a level just ventral to that of the accessory processes (Fig. 46.22). Use of self-retaining (Gelpi) retractors allows for atraumatic dissection under tension. Small branches of the paired lumbar or intercostal arteries are cauterized by means of bipolar cautery as they are exposed both cranially and caudally to the cranial articular processes of each adjacent vertebra. Care must be exercised during both periosteal elevation and the cauterization of small bleeding vessels around the articular processes to avoid exacerbation of spinal cord ischemia by interruption of the, at best, tenuous spinal cord blood supply through the varying

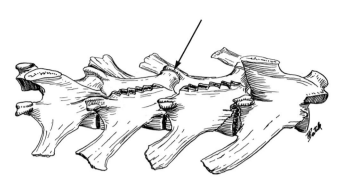

Fig. 46.23. The arrow indicates the joint space between the cranial and caudal articular processes, which is used as a guideline for the lateral extent of the laminectomy.

intervertebral foramina (dorsal and ventral radicular branches) (1–3).

The thirteenth rib and first lumbar transverse process are readily identifiable landmarks to confirm the appropriate site for laminectomy. The thirteenth rib arcs dorsocaudally and is located far more superficially than the cranioventrally directed first lumbar transverse process. The spinous processes of the vertebrae cranial and caudal to the involved disc space are removed by means of bone rongeurs (Fig. 46.23). This is preferable to the use of a bone cutter, which can apply excessive torque to the vertebral column of small breed dogs.

By means of a high-speed air drill with a new 4-mm egg-shaped bur with notched flutes, the rest of the dorsal spines are removed. Irrigation with either sterile saline or lactated Ringer's solution and fluid removal by suction maintain a clear field, remove the bone dust produced by the air drill, and dissipate the minimal amount of heat produced by a new bur. Old, dull burs should not be used for this laminectomy technique because they generate significant heat by sanding rather than cutting away the bone. In most instances, the laminectomy defect is centered over the area of involvement and extends cranially and caudally to the adjacent interarcuate ligaments. The width of the defect is determined by the joint spaces between the cranial and caudal articular processes at the involved interspace (see Fig. 46.23, *arrow*). The bone structure and color are reliable indexes of the depth of drilling: 1) outer cortical bone is dense and white; 2) middle cancellous bone is spongy and red; 3) inner cortical bone is dense, white, and thin. Once the limits of the laminectomy defect have been defined, drilling continues, to remove completely the outer layer of cortical bone and then the middle layer of spongy red cancellous bone (Fig. 46.24). The surgeon is removing the top of a cylinder while maintaining bone at the pedicles dorsal to the dorsal tangent of the spinal cord. The inner layers of the pedicles are excavated bilaterally to

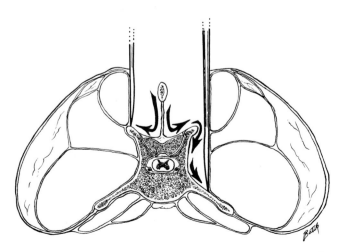

Fig. 46.22. Periosteal elevation of the epaxial musculature for dorsal laminectomy. Arrows indicate the direction of force applied to the elevator for atraumatic periosteal elevation.

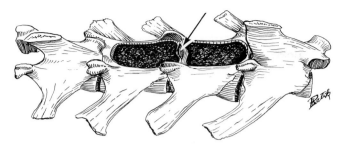

Fig. 46.24. The outer cortical bone and most of the middle layer of cancellous bone, including that of the caudal articular processes, have been removed. The *arrow* indicates the dense cortical bone at the intervertebral space and the interarcuate ligament.

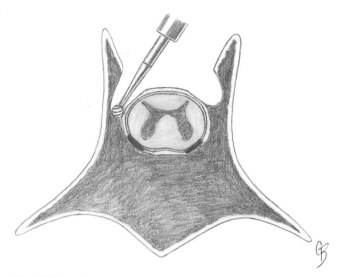

Fig. 46.26. Further excavation of the middle layer of cancellous bone of the lateral laminae is performed with one of the small round burs.

provide complete exposure of the epidural space (Fig. 46.25). When the thin layer of inner cortical bone begins to sag under the pressure of the drill, a 2.3- or 1.6-mm round carbide-tip bur is substituted for the large bur (Fig. 46.26). A thin plate of inner cortical bone remains to protect the spinal cord during most of the drilling. This thin plate of inner cortical bone is isolated by drilling around the periphery of the laminectomy defect with a small drill with approximately a 45° angle away from the spinal cord (Figs. 46.27 and 46.28). The angled approach avoids drilling directly over the spinal cord and results in smooth, deeply undercut edges of the laminectomy with excellent exposure of the full width of the vertebral canal. Some additional undercutting is necessary to remove the remainder of the cranial articular processes of the caudal of the two vertebrae located in the frontal plane, deep to the caudal articular processes of the cranial of the

two vertebrae. Complete excision of the caudal articular processes and undercutting in this region allow more than sufficient access to the vertebral canal for the removal of extruded or protruded intervertebral disc material from either side or from the ventral aspect of the canal. Excavation of the pedicles, that is, removal of the inner cortical and middle layer of cancellous bone of the pedicle, while preserving the outer layer of cortical bone of the pedicle, increases exposure without predisposing the patient to constrictive fibrosis (see Fig. 46.26) (4–7). The bone of the pedicles on both sides of the defect must be maintained at a level dorsal to the dorsal tangent of the spinal cord to prevent secondary spinal cord flattening during healing of the laminectomy defect. When the thin remaining layer of inner cortical bone has been completely isolated (Fig. 46.29), it is grasped with a hemostat and is removed as a complete bony shelf. In most instances, laminectomy over two vertebrae is sufficient to decompress the entire edematous section of spinal cord.

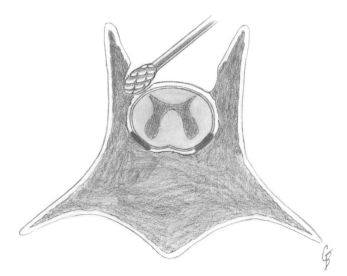

Fig. 46.25. After excision of the middle layer of cancellous bone, excavation of the pedicles is begun with a 4-mm-diameter bur.

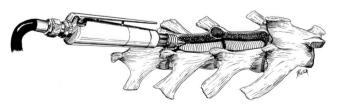

Fig. 46.27. Angled drilling into the cancellous bone around the periphery of the thin plate of inner cortical bone avoids drilling directly over the spinal cord and results in smooth, deeply undercut edges. This technique increases both exposure and decompression and facilitates removal of extruded disc material.

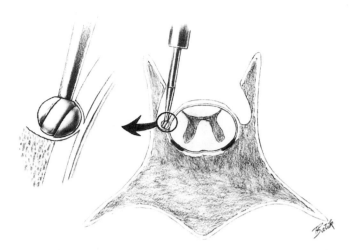

Fig. 46.28. The inner cortical bone shelf is cut around the periphery with the smallest bur.

In other cases, extension of the defect both cranially and caudally may be necessary until normal amounts of epidural fat are visualized in the epidural space. Because a higher incidence of laminectomy scar formation and secondary spinal cord compression is related to increased laminectomy length, the length of the defect should be only that necessary to decompress the involved segments of spinal cord (5).

Because of the undercutting procedure, removal of extruded disc material is uncomplicated, even with the minimal epidural space of the most frequently affected chondrodystrophic dogs with relative vertebral canal stenosis. Minimal spinal cord manipulation is necessary. When such manipulation is necessary, the spinal cord may be retracted gently by means of a small suture placed in the dura mater in a relatively avascular area. Fine-tipped suction and various ophthalmic and dental instruments have proved useful in the removal of the compressive mass of disc material from the vertebral canal. Bleeding from the internal vertebral venous plexus, when present, is easily controlled by means of absorbable gelatin sponge.

Durotomy is now only performed in paraplegic, analgesic patients to confirm or deny the presence of segmental, focal spinal cord necrosis. Durotomy is performed with either Potts–Smith 60° angled cardiovascular scissors or a bent disposable 20- to 22-gauge needle. The dura mater is incised on the dorsal midline for the full length of the laminectomy defect. Incision of the inelastic dural sheath and frequently the underlying pia mater may result in greater intramedullary decompression of the spinal cord and spinal cord vasculature. In most instances, however, durotomy is used more for the formulation of an accurate prognosis

because it permits the direct observation of superficial or deep focal malacia, thrombosis, and spinal cord blanching. In chronic cases, loss of spinal cord substance and glial scarring may be evident. Myelotomy, either superficial or deep, is only performed in paraplegic, analgesic patients in which the prognosis is in question. Continued leakage of cerebrospinal fluid has not been a problem with durotomy. A mild, transient neurologic deficit may be evident postoperatively. The dura appears to heal rapidly by neomembrane formation (5).

Torn or devitalized epaxial musculature is excised before closure. This maneuver also appears to limit infolding of the epaxial musculature into the laminectomy defect. A piece of absorbable gelatin sponge, creased on the midline and shaped to conform to the laminectomy defect, is carefully placed in direct apposition to the remaining pedicles (marginal fitting). With this particular technique in the thoracolumbar region of dogs, the healing pattern after implantation of absorbable gelatin sponge is predictable and innocuous (5). Other implants such as absorbable gelatin film, muscle, and free or pedicle fat grafts have met with variable and often unsatisfactory results in this laminectomy technique (5–7 and EJ Trotter, unpublished data). Although satisfactory in other locations, fat grafts in this location with this technique actually increase spinal cord compression postoperatively (7, 8). Cosmetically unacceptable scars or structural defects have not been a problem with this technique.

Corticosteroid therapy is no longer continued in the postoperative period because of the possibility of catastrophic gastrointestinal complications and the limited

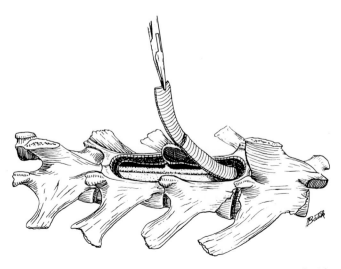

Fig. 46.29. The thin shelf of inner cortical bone is grasped with a hemostat and is removed as a unit.

benefits of these drugs, as confirmed by experimental studies. Postoperative therapy includes manual expression of the urinary bladder, whirlpool hydrotherapy, and general supportive care. Patients are discharged from the hospital as soon as conscious control of micturition is regained. Early return to familiar surroundings seems to promote enthusiasm on the part of the patient and owner and an early return to function.

References

1. Caulkins SE, Purinton PT, Oliver JE. Arterial supply to the spinal cord of dogs and cats. Am J Vet Res 1989;50:425–430.
2. Parker AJ. Distribution of spinal branches of the thoracolumbar segmental arteries in dogs. Am J Vet Res 1973;34:1351–1353.
3. Parker AJ, Park RD, Stowater JL. Traumatic occlusion of lumbar segmental arteries. J Trauma 1974;14:330–333.
4. Funkquist B, Schantz B. Influence of extensive laminectomy on the shape of the spinal canal. Acta Orthop Scand Suppl 1962; 56:1–50.
5. Trotter EJ, Crissman J, Robson D, et al. Influence of nonbiologic implants on laminectomy membrane formation in dogs. Am J Vet Res 1988;49:634–643.
6. Trotter EJ. Dorsal laminectomy for treatment of thoracolumbar disc disease. In: Bojrab MJ, ed. Current techniques in small animal surgery. 3rd ed. Philadelphia: Lea & Febiger, 1990:608–621.
7. Trevor PB, Martin RA, Saunders GK, et al. Vet Surg 1991; 20:282–290.

Pediculotomy in the Thoracolumbar Vertebra

Barclay Slocum & Theresa Devine Slocum

A pediculotomy is a surgical procedure that allows access to the spinal canal for removal of discrete herniated disc material. The offending disc must first be located precisely by means of a myelogram. This procedure has little surgical morbidity because the exposure stretches tissues but does not disrupt the osseous support of the spine. Access to the lateral and ventral aspects of the spinal cord is provided by openings in both right and left pedicles, both cranial and caudal to the foramen. In addition, chronic herniated intervertebral discs or spondylosis invading the spinal canal and adherent to the ventral cord can be removed without damage to the cord with this technique.

Surgical Procedure

The patient is placed in ventral recumbency and is prepared and draped for surgery. A dorsal skin incision with a lateral muscle-splitting approach is used. A 5- to 10-cm dorsal midline skin incision is centered over the offending disc. The superficial thoracolumbar fas-

cia is incised 5 mm lateral to the dorsal midline on the side of the lesion, as indicated by the myelogram and neurologic examination. On the vertebra immediately caudal to the herniated intervertebral disc, Kelly forceps are used to separate between the spinalis et semispinalis and the longissimus muscles. Two Gelpi retractors are used to spread the muscle groups apart, to expose the transverse process and the pedicle of the vertebra.

Using a 4-mm spheric bur, the surgeon makes a small hole in the cranial pedicle of the vertebra just caudal to the intervertebral foramen and ventral to the articular facets. A Lempert rongeur is used to enlarge the pediculotomy, opening cranially to join the intervertebral foramen. The spinal canal is examined. Herniated disc material can be removed by a small curette or iris spatula.

If the spinal cord is pressed against the wall of the spinal canal on the side of the surgeon, fat will be absent. This finding indicates that the disc herniation is most likely on the opposite side. The pediculotomy is then performed on the opposite side (Fig. 46.30). When the spinal cord is tented upward, the mass of disc material is probably cranial to the intervertebral foramen or centrally located in the spinal canal. A right-angle blunt probe is used to explore the foramen for disc material.

When the spinal canal examination indicates that the disc material is located cranially to the intervertebral foramen or the disc material is found, a pediculotomy is made in the caudal pedicle of the cranial vertebra, just cranial to the foramen. A Lempert ron-

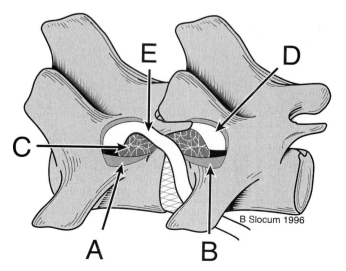

Fig. 46.30. A pediculotomy can be performed cranially (*A*) or caudally (*B*) to retrieve herniated disc material (*C*) and to decompress the spinal cord (*D*) and nerve root (*E*).

geur is used to enlarge the pediculotomy opening caudally to join the intervertebral foramen. Particular attention is warranted when opening the pediculotomy because the spinal nerve lies just medial and caudal to this portion of the pedicle. Careful elevation of all muscles and fibrous tissue optimizes visual control of the extension of the pediculotomy to the foramen. Disc material is removed from both cranial and caudal pediculotomy openings until the cord lies flat on the dorsal longitudinal ligament within the spinal canal. The intervertebral disc is fenestrated to prevent any further herniation of disc material.

The pediculotomy procedure can also be used for relieving spinal cord compression by a spondylotic lesion that has expanded dorsally into the spinal canal (Fig. 46.31). Chronic herniated intervertebral discs or spondylosis invading the ventral spinal canal adherent to the ventral cord can be removed without damage to the cord.

First, a routine pediculotomy is made caudal to the intervertebral disc, and the lesion is explored to confirm the diagnosis and pathologic features. A 3- to 4-mm bur is used to enlarge the pediculotomy into the body of the vertebra just caudal to the cranial end plate. The floor of the spinal canal is perforated from the ventral direction. If bleeding from the basivertebral veins within the body of the vertebra is excessive, bone wax is used to stop the hemorrhage. The dorsal portion of the cranial end plate of the vertebra, caudal to the disc space of concern, is removed by the high-speed bur. The dorsal portion of the caudal end plate of the vertebra, cranial to the disc space of concern, is also removed. The high-speed bur is used to remove the adherent disc or spondylosis dorsal to the cavity just

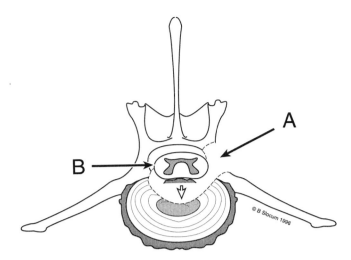

Fig. 46.32. The cavity (*dotted line*) formed by an extension of the pediculotomy (A) allows decompression of the spinal cord with the adherent disc (B). Notice the shift of the cord (*open arrow*).

created. No attempt is made to pull or manipulate the mass that is adherent to the cord; rather, most of the mass can be removed by burring, with the remainder falling into the cavity created by burring (Fig. 46.32). Direct closure of the superficial thoracolumbar fascia, subcutaneous fascia, and skin is performed.

A pediculotomy can be made cranial and caudal to an intervertebral foramen on both right and left sides without compromise to the bony support or the soft tissues. The pedicle can be removed on one side of the vertebra, but not on both sides of the same vertebra, because osseous support between the lamina and body of the vertebra would be lost. The pedicle can be thought of as having cranial and caudal halves. This means that any one vertebra has two right pedicle halves and two left pedicle halves, a total of four halves. Each vertebra maintains sufficient strength if no more than two pedicle halves in any combination are sacrificed to gain exposure.

This procedure provides no direct access to the dorsal spinal cord. Hemilaminectomy is the procedure of choice, when treating severe herniation with spinal cord swelling requiring durotomy, because of the limited access with a pediculotomy. However, if a hemilaminectomy is performed and disc material is found to be on the opposite side of the spinal cord, pediculotomies can be done cranial and caudal to the foramen on the opposite side of the vertebral canal, to remove the herniated disc material. Care must be taken to minimize bone removal of the opposite pedicle for the sake of stability. By using a pediculotomy, potential trauma caused by the surgeon to reach, manipulate, and remove disc material from the opposite side of the spinal cord is avoided.

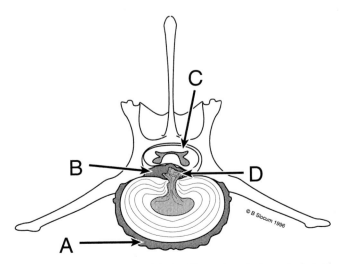

Fig. 46.31. Chronic spondylosis (A) may invade the spinal canal (B) and may become adherent to the spinal cord (C). The disc (D) may rupture, adding further spinal cord compression.

Discolysis

James F. Biggart, III

Discolysis (chemonucleolysis, disc injection) is the chemical dissolution of the nucleus pulposus of the intervertebral disc. The technique involves fluoroscopically controlled percutaneous placement of double needles into the nucleus and the deposition of nucleolytic enzymes. These enzymes follow the path of disc herniation, mixing with the herniated nucleus in the spinal canal with subsequent dissolution of the nucleus and lessening the mechanical pressure on the spinal cord or nerve roots (Fig. 46.33).

Indications

The indications are the same as for surgical treatment (laminectomy or hemilaminectomy in the thoracolumbar spine and ventral decompression in the cervical spine). Any patient that needs surgery for a herniated disc can be just as effectively treated with discolysis. Patients that have pain as the sole sign of disc herniation and have been unsuccessfully treated with rest and anti-inflammatory drugs for more than 2 weeks are candidates for this treatment. Patients that improve while rested but return to a painful state on cessation of drugs and rest are candidates. Any patient with neurologic deficits, especially if severe, should have treatment sooner rather than later. Patients without deep pain and voluntary motor function should have surgical treatment, but the results are the same as with discolysis. Both cervical and lumbar herniated discs can be treated. In fact, all canine and feline discs can be treated effectively with discolysis.

Contraindications

The contraindications are those associated with enzyme-produced anaphylactic reactions (not reported in the dog or cat) and those associated with general anesthesia and myelography. Lack of dural integrity adjacent to enzyme deposition sites is a relative contraindication. Durotomies, traumatic dural tears secondary to fractures, disc hernias, and dural punctures done during myelography are potential sources of dural tears. Enzyme leakage into the spinal canal adjacent to these tears may allow subdural access.

Advantages

Discolysis allows treatment of intervertebral disc disease with minimal blood loss, and it is especially useful in treating patients with disc disease and bleeding disorders. Von Willebrand–positive Doberman pinschers with herniated discs can be successfully treated with no unusual precautions. The routine testing of patients for von Willebrand's disease is not necessary. Patients with a high anesthetic risk can be treated quickly by discolysis. The total anesthesia time for a myelogram and discolysis often is less than an hour. The depth of anesthesia can be kept lighter because percutaneous needle placement is less painful than surgical intervention.

More than one herniated disc can be treated at a time, even if these discs are widely separated anatomically. Cervical lesions and thoracolumbar disc lesions can be treated at the same time. Prophylactic discolysis can be performed in conjunction with a specific hernia and can involve widely separated discs. Patients with painful discs that are difficult to localize anatomically or patients with negative myelograms can have many discs injected. This procedure is less traumatic than multiple surgical explorations. Far lateral disc hernias or those that involve nerve roots lateral to the foramen can be successfully treated. Patients with disc disorders and myelograms showing large areas of cord swelling can have multiple discs injected, preventing long laminectomies used to find and decompress the hernia site.

Disadvantages

Enzyme dissolution of the disc and relief of clinical signs may take several days despite the immediate chemical reaction. Verification of disc dissolution is difficult to obtain without repeat myelography or magnetic resonance imaging. Postinjection pain can be increased for several days, especially with the use of collagenase. Usually, this pain can be managed with steroids and analgesics, but it is more problematic than

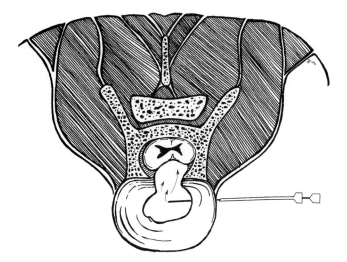

Fig. 46.33. Extruded disc with needle penetration of the anulus in preparation for enzyme deposition.

postsurgical pain in 10 to 15% of patients, especially patients with pain as the only clinical sign of disease. The reportedly high rate of failure of discolysis in treating sequestered discs in human patients has not been seen in dogs in which many discs are sequestered. The successful recovery with disc injections is the same as with surgical treatment in these patients with sequestered disc (1). The treatment of type II discs has not been as successful in dogs as in human patients. The associated ligamentous changes and osteophytes that often contribute to cord pressure are unaffected by nucleolytic enzymes. In type II discs without these changes, having only a bulging anulus, discolysis works well.

Technique

The enzymes are introduced into the nucleus with needles using a dorsal or dorsolateral approach (see Chap. 44) and follow the path of herniation, mixing with the disc material in the canal as well as the normally located nucleus pulposus. Half the dosage is in the needle, which is flushed with contrast media so all the enzyme reaches the nucleus. The dye marks the path of the enzyme. Not all the enzyme needs to mix with the herniated disc. If the herniated disc is contained, then all the enzyme is contained and is available for reaction. If the herniated disc is sequestered, the enzyme may mix entirely with the disc, only coat the disc if it is consolidated and hard, or go up and down the canal and not mix with the herniated material at all. In fact, in some cases the dye is seen many vertebrae away from the hernia site. Despite this lack of full dose contact of the disc and enzyme, clinical results are good. I have not been able to see a difference in results between sequestered discs and contained discs.

Choice of Enzymes

Chymopapain

Chymopapain is the most widely used enzyme in the human and veterinary field. It works well in dogs even with calcified discs. Postinjection pain and muscle spasm are minimal. Chemically, it works by destruction of the hygroscopic ground matrix of the nucleus, thereby releasing water and decreasing the intradiscal pressure. The protein disaccharide polymer is responsible for the water-binding property of the ground substance and is depolymerized by chymopapain.

The disc space collapses within days after injection, with the nucleus turning green. Some annular involvement occurs with chymopapain, but changes in the end plate are few (2). Approximately 20% of the discs rehydrate and rewiden several months after injection. Reherniation has been seen, but less often than reherniation of noninjected herniated disc spaces. Most discs stay narrowed, without progressive end plate changes or progressive degeneration. Calcified discs are decalcified about 50% of the time. Decalcification is not necessary for good results because the discs narrow but remain calcified. Disc material herniated into the canal frequently decalcifies, but this may take weeks (1). Clinical improvement occurs long before complete decalcification and removal of the disc in the canal, a finding that emphasizes the importance of the biochemical pathologic features, as well as the more mechanical pathologic features of cord compression most frequently associated with disc hernia. The dose is 400 to 800 units per disc, depending on the size of the patient and the amount of disc in the canal. As many as six discs can be injected at one time. Low doses give satisfactory disc dissolution without the side effects of muscle spasm and associated pain.

Collagenase

Collagenase is the second most widely used enzyme. It is noted for consistently decalcifying calcified discs even in the canal. Postinjection pain and spasm are more common than with chymopapain and are more intense, lasting many days. These sequelae usually are controlled successfully with steroids and muscle relaxants or analgesics. Chemically, collagenase works by specifically degrading collagen-sparing cell membranes and noncollagenous protein. Type I and type II collagen are broken down by collagenase as well as the protein polysaccharides of the matrix. Contact by serum inactivates collagenase. The disc space collapses within days after injection and remains collapsed 90% of the time. Rewidening seldom occurs, and reherniation is rare. The nucleus is completely dissolved, with little ground matrix left for rehydration. Less of the anulus is involved than with chymopapain, and a void is present where the nucleus pulposus was. The end plate has minimal changes (2). Progressive changes to the disc space occur, especially end plate sclerosis and spondylosis. Clinical signs have not been associated with these postinjection changes. Decalcification occurs 92% of the time without rewidening, whether the disc hernia is the sequestered type or not. The dose is 400 to 600 units per disc. As many as six discs can be injected at a time, depending on the volume of the nucleus and the amount of nuclear material in the canal. Low doses minimize postinjection pain and muscle spasm (1).

Chondroitinase ABC

Chondroitinase ABC is a disaccharidase with an affinity for chondroitin sulfate. Vascular toxicity and neurotoxicity are minimal. Normal injected discs show disc space collapse within 5 days. Treatment of spontaneous disc herniations in dogs has not undergone significant clinical trials to state efficacy. The low neurotoxicity makes the enzyme useful in dogs, but only if sequestered discs can be removed. More clinical studies are needed to establish the safety and efficacy of this agent (3).

Toxicity

None of the enzymes commonly used are especially toxic to tissue, except with dural penetration. The intact dura acts as a barrier to enzyme-produced toxic cord changes. The epidural space accommodates enzymes well, as do the anulus, end plates, and nerve roots. Dural penetration into the subarachnoid space by enzyme is catastrophic. Subarachnoid and parenchymal hemorrhage occurs. Capillary wall integrity is lost, producing diapedesis of blood into surrounding tissue. Transverse myelopathy is the typical result and appears to be permanent. Fortunately, the dura is seldom torn in canine disc herniation, so enzymes are relatively benign in the extradural spaces (1, 4).

Initial techniques whereby physicians introduced enzymes into the nucleus with transdurally placed needles allowed enzyme access to the subdural space, and several transverse myelopathies occurred. These accidents produced bad publicity for discolysis. Once the technique was changed to avoid dural penetration, results with discolysis improved (5). The introduction of skin tests for papain allergy avoided the last major complication of discolysis. Anaphylaxis has not been reported in dogs. Chymopapain is a protein, and so eventually this reaction may occur. Dogs are not commonly exposed to papain drugs to the extent humans are (e.g., meat tenderizers, contact lens cleaners) and thus have few anaphylactic reactions to similar drugs. Collagenase is a common enzyme found throughout mammalian tissue and has not been associated with anaphylaxis.

Postinjection Tissue Changes

Collapse of the disc space occurs rapidly after disc injection (discolysis), causing the now redundant dorsal longitudinal ligament to push outward, along with the outward bulging of the anulus. The disc space is more unstable for 6 to 8 weeks until collapse and stabilization occur by scar formation. Rest for 6 to 8 weeks after the procedure is needed to prevent pain from disc space instability.

Once several months elapse, the facets, disc space, and anulus stabilize in their new locations. The once redundant bulging dorsal longitudinal ligament flattens out along the ventral canal without compression of the cord. The adjacent vertebral bodies "fuse" with a fibrous fusion that produces less pain than immediately after injection. These changes are all produced by disc collapse of any origin and are not peculiar to enzyme-induced collapse.

Diskitis is a rare complication of injection. In my experience of injecting 1500 discs, I have seen this complication in 12 discs in a total of 7 patients. Most of these patients had no pain or other symptoms. One patient developed discospondylitis 1 year after chymodiactin injection and was successfully treated with cephalosporin antibiotics. The remaining patients resolved their radiographically dissolved discs with no treatment. All previously eroded end plates fused or became quiet again. The enzymes may damage the end plate, leading to erosion.

Chemical Fenestration

The nearly 100% rate of disc space collapse, even of calcified discs, makes collagenase an excellent choice for prophylactic "chemical" fenestration. Disc rewidening is less than with chymopapain, but both enzymes effectively lower the odds that a given disc will herniate in the future. Using collagenase, more than 200 discs have been injected prophylactically in the past 10 years, with fewer than 10 discs rewidening and only 1 disc herniating. The atraumatic percutaneous method of nucleolysis using fluoroscopically placed needles makes surgical fenestration less appealing. Discolysis can be used under direct vision to fenestrate discs chemically in conjunction with laminectomy.

Combination With Laminectomy

In patients with large discs that are difficult to remove during a laminectomy, nucleolytic enzymes can be injected into the herniated disc material in the canal to soften it, allowing easier piecemeal extraction. Some discs can be made liquid to allow suction removal. In patients with cervical spondylopathy or cauda equina syndrome, dorsal laminectomy can remove dorsal and lateral stenosis, whereas direct vision disc injection can lessen the ventral cord compression caused by the protruding disc. Dorsal and ventral compression can be relieved in this manner (6).

References

1. Biggart JF III. Collagenase vs. chymopapain. In: Proceedings of the International Intradiscal Therapy Society. Denver, CO: International Intradiscal Therapy Society, 1994:34.
2. Biggart JF III. Surgery of thoracolumbar disc disease. In: Proceedings of the 51st annual meeting of the American Animal Hospital Association. Denver CO: American Animal Hospital Association, 1984:365–369.

3. Fry TR, et al. Evaluation of chondroitinase abc for chemonucleo-lysis of canine lumbar intervertebral discs. Vet Surg 1990;19:65.
4. Biggart JF III. Collagenase: toxicity and efficacy. Proc Abbott Soc 1985;16:56–65.
5. Bailey CS. Chymopapain chemonucleolysis. In: Kirk RW, Bonagura JD, eds. Current veterinary therapy XI. Small animal practice. Philadelphia: WB Saunders, 1992:1018.
6. Biggart JF III. Results of discolysis in the treatment of 125 patients with herniated discs. Vet Surg 1988;17:29.

Suggested Readings

Brown MD. Intradiscal therapy: chymopapain or collagenase. Chicago: Year Book, 1983:43.
Biggart JF III. Discolysis: an introduction. Calif Vet 1984;38:10.
Javid MJ, Nordby EJ. Current status of chymopapain for herniated nucleus pulposus. Neurosurg Q 1994;4:92–101.
Nordby EJ, Wright PH. Efficacy of chymopapain in chemonucleolysis: a review. Spine 1994;19:2578–2583.

— 47 —

LUMBOSACRAL SPINE

Surgical Treatment of Cauda Equina Compression Syndrome by Laminectomy

Timothy M. Lenehan & Guy B. Tarvin

A definitive preoperative diagnosis of cauda equina syndrome can be difficult to make. Not all practitioners have access to magnetic resonance imaging. Access to computed tomography (CT) is equally limited, and often myelography or epidurography is required in concert with the CT scan to demonstrate soft tissue lesions such as nerve root entrapment. Epidurography is difficult both to perform and to interpret if it is performed only on occasion. Electrodiagnostic testing and electromyography require special equipment and expertise to perform and to evaluate, and not all dogs with cauda equina syndrome have electrophysiologically demonstrable signs of lower motor neuron disease.

Furthermore, most pathologic processes involving the nerve roots of the cauda equina are not readily demonstrable with myelography in the lumbosacral area of the dog. Stressed radiographs (hyperextension–flexion) of the spine demonstrate hypermobility, but they are not necessarily diagnostic of neurologic involvement. In fact, many animals affected by cauda equina syndrome have normal spinal radiographs. Hence, the veterinarian must use clinical acumen along with one or more of these diagnostic modalities to build a case for a diagnosis of cauda equina syndrome before recommending surgical intervention. An accurate diagnosis many times can be achieved only through an exploratory laminectomy. In such instances, laminectomy can prove both diagnostic for and curative of the disease process. The purpose of the surgery is to decompress the conus medullaris or those nerve roots of the cauda equina that are causing clinical symptoms. The surgeon should be vigilant to remove only as much bone as needed to accomplish this task, especially when dealing with cauda equina syndrome secondary to lumbosacral instability.

Surgical Procedure

The animal is placed in ventral recumbency with the stifles and hips flexed and the hocks extended. If extensive foraminal exploration is anticipated, then placement of the patient's hind legs in the forward extended position combined with padding placed under the belly in the lumbosacral region will accentuate lumbosacral kyphosis to open the foramina widely at the lumbosacral junction.

A dorsal midline approach to the lumbosacral spine is performed. Several large Gelpi or hinged Weitlaner retractors facilitate muscle retraction (Fig. 47.1). Suction is essential for good visualization, and most typically a No. 10 or 12 Frazier suction tip is adequate. Electrocautery, surgical sponge (Gelfoam), and bone wax are essential for adequate hemostasis in large breed dogs.

A modified dorsal laminectomy is performed over the affected interspaces (generally L7 to S1–2–3), initially leaving the caudal pedicles of L7 intact. If the compression is due to either midline disc bulging or hypertrophy of the interarcuate ligament, then this surgical approach alone should result in decompression. If the surgeon is unsure of complete decompression, then extradural fat and fibrous connective tissue are retrieved from the spinal canal as needed to facilitate visualization of the various nerve roots and ganglia of the cauda equina. A nerve hook helps to isolate and trace the individual nerves as they enter their

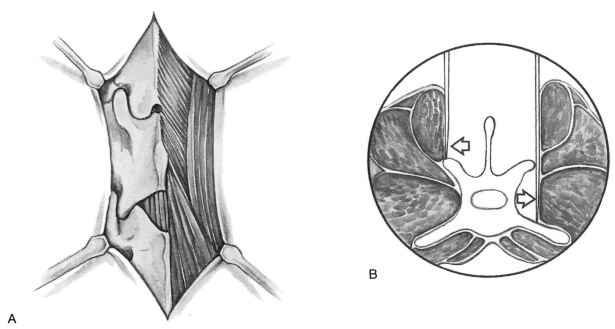

Fig. 47.1. Muscle elevation for dorsal laminectomy.

respective foramina to exit the spinal canal. Unilateral or bilateral pediculectomy is performed as needed to gain further exposure and decompression of the affected nerves. Tethered nerve roots are freed of any fibrous connective tissue constraints. In the case of a Hansen type I disc rupture, the ruptured nuclear material is removed (generally by suction). If a Hansen type II disc rupture is present, the location of the bulging anulus in relation to midline determines the surgical procedure. Any bulging disc material that is entrapping a nerve root is either cut away or, alternatively, is left alone and the nerve is decompressed by facetectomy, pediculectomy, or foraminotomy, depending on the location of compression.

Once decompression has been achieved and hemostasis is complete, an autologous free fat graft is harvested from the subcutaneous region and is placed over the laminectomy site to minimize cicatrix formation. Muscle, fascia, and subcutaneous layers are closed, respectively, with synthetic absorbable suture material. Inaccurate closure of the muscle fascia results in a palpable midline divot, whereas inattention to subcutaneous closure results in seroma formation. The application of a compression bandage is optimal, yet it is difficult to perform and maintain, given the location of the operative site, especially in male dogs.

Postoperative Care

Postoperative recommendations include strict confinement to house and leash activity only for 8 weeks' time, before a return to full function. This confinement allows time for the musculature to adhere to the lamina and for the spine to adjust to the added instability imposed by the surgical procedure.

In most cases, a modified dorsal laminectomy is sufficient to gain good visualization of the problem and to effect decompression. Whereas removal of the dorsal spinous processes and the caudal facets of L7 increases the mechanical instability of the spine, the instances of clinically significant sequelae seem to be few. Lumbosacral subluxation (acute or chronic) and cicatrix formation remain possible sequelae of the procedure, especially if the animal resumes heavy exercise. These complications are rare, however. Most animals experience relief of nerve root symptoms and only occasionally have mild to moderate osteoarthritic symptoms, (i.e., morning and exercise-induced stiffness with occasional episodes of low back pain lasting several days).

Decompressive laminectomy in a hypermobile lumbosacral segment should be undertaken with caution, particularly if discospondylitis is suspected. In such instances, laminectomy only destabilizes an already unstable situation further and may have orthopedic and neurologic sequelae, if the infection is not rapidly brought under control.

Bony or soft tissue disease at any of the L5–6–7 to S1–2–3 vertebral interspaces potentially can result in clinical signs of cauda equina syndrome (sciatic or sacral nerve root involvement) (Fig. 47.2). The clinician must attempt to localize the lesion to a specific area of the spinal cord or nerve roots preoperatively, or else a "routine" dorsal laminectomy at the L7–S1 interspace

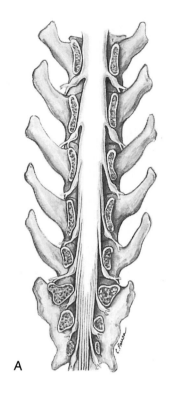

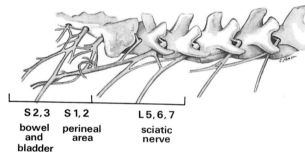

S 2,3	S 1,2	L 5,6,7
bowel and bladder	perineal area	sciatic nerve

Fig. 47.2. A. Dorsoventral view of the cauda equina. **B.** Nerve distribution of the cauda equina.

may miss the underlying disorder entirely, if the signs of the cauda equina syndrome are, for example, due to a nerve root tumor affecting the L6 segment of the spinal cord.

L7–S1 Fixation–Fusion Technique for Cauda Equina Syndrome

Barclay Slocum & Theresa Devine Slocum

Cauda equina syndrome is the intermittent or constant compression of the nerve roots that are confined within the terminal dural sac. This definition must be

expanded to include the spinal nerves arising from the L6 vertebra caudally, because of the practical difficulty in determining the exact source of nerve root compression. Nerve root compression occurs within the spinal canal and at the intervertebral foramen from mechanical factors such as dorsal protrusion of an intervertebral disc, herniation of the nucleus pulposus, spondylosis, spinal canal stenosis, or abnormal motion between vertebrae at this location.

Compression of the L7–S1 cauda equina has a high incidence in active medium and large breed dogs. Patients with cauda equina syndrome are presented with two basic histories. First, the intermittent pinching of the cauda equina by compression during extension can be determined by a history of pain after activity that resolves with rest. The animal has a diminished desire to jump, a positive stand test, pain on digital palpation of L7–S1, and pain on the lordosis test at L7–S1. Confirmation of L7–S1 compression is seen by myelogram or epidurogram in spinal extension, but not in flexion.

The second history is of disc herniation causing constant compression of the cauda equina at L7–S1. This is characterized by constant and severe unilateral or bilateral pain, loss of the desire to do any activity, a positive stand test, pain on digital palpation of L7–S1, and pain on the lordosis test at L7–S1. Confirmation of L7–S1 compression is seen by myelogram or epidurogram in spinal flexion or extension. Electromyelography is helpful in demonstrating a neurologic lesion in the presence of spondylosis at L7–S1 but without overt pain or proprioceptive deficits. Magnetic resonance imaging and computed tomography may be helpful to demonstrate compression at the intervertebral foramen.

Because the pain and dysfunction from cauda equina syndrome wax and wane depending on the amount of activity with increasing intensity over time, the optimal time to treat this disease surgically is after 2 to 3 months of fruitless conservative treatment, before constant nerve root compression. Once the diagnosis is clearly established, and the owners realize that the condition will not improve without intervention, then consent for surgery is usually forthcoming.

Surgical Techniques

The surgical treatment by L7–S1 fixation–fusion alone is limited to intermittent cauda equina compression at L7–S1 because constant compression requires an adjunct surgical decompression. Any history of proprioceptive deficits or urinary or fecal incontinence requires a laminectomy in addition to L7–S1 fixation–fusion to restore function.

The patient is positioned in ventral recumbency with the hips flexed and the hocks pulled forward along the side of the thorax (DAR position). This position opens the articular facets and stretches the liga-

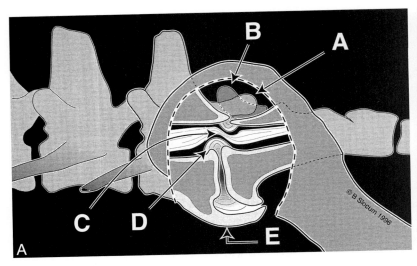

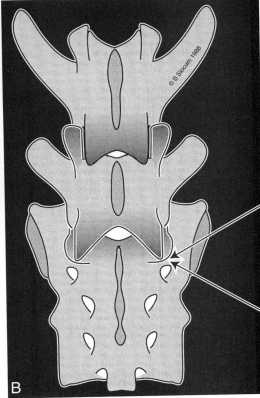

Fig. 47.3. **A.** Collapse of the L7–S1 disc space causes the L7 caudal articular process (A) to overlap the S1 cranial articular facet (B). The cauda equina (C) is compressed by the disc protrusion (D). Ventral spondylosis of the L7–S1 (E) is indicative of degeneration, but causes no direct cauda equina compression. **B.** Notice the collapse of the L7–S1 dorsal articular facets indicated by the *arrows*.

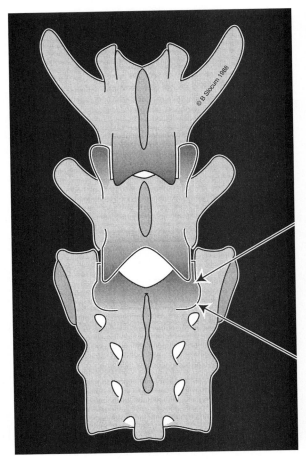

Fig. 47.4. The facts are repositioned so the articular surfaces of L7 and S1 match, as indicated by the *arrows*.

Table 47.1.
Levels of L7–S1 Exploration and Treatment (L7–S1 Fixation–Fusion Used at All Levels of Intervention)

Level	Exploration or Treatment
1	Ligamentum flavum left intact + L7–S1 fixation–fusion
2	Removal of ligamentum flavum to observe cauda equina + L7–S1 fixation–fusion
3	Level 2+: Movement of cauda equina to observe dorsal anulus fibrosis of L7–S1 disc
4	Level 3+: Dorsal sacral laminectomy
5	Level 4+: Caudal seventh lumbar laminectomy
6	Level 5+: Removal of dorsal anulus + fenestration of L7–S1 nucleus pulposus
7	Level 6+: Removal of caudal L7 articular process; freeing of L7 nerve root; stabilization with a plate using the pedicle for area of L7 fixation and S1 sacral segment lateral to the S1 nerve root for caudal fixation

mentum flavum and dorsal anulus of L7–S1. After surgical preparation and draping, the skin is incised in the dorsal midline from L7 to S3. The sacrocaudalis dorsalis medialis muscles are separated to provide access. Use of several Gelpi retractors is helpful for deep retraction. The dorsal spinal musculature is elevated off the lateral aspect of the dorsal spinous process and dorsal lamina, laterally to the mammillary process on both the L7 vertebra and sacrum. The articular facets are checked to ensure matching of articular surfaces (Fig. 47.3). A vertebral spreader may be helpful to position the facets (Fig. 47.4), although this is often unnecessary with the DAR positioning of the patient on the surgical table. Care must be taken to avoid overrotation. Overdistraction minimizes bone purchase of internal fixation and stability between the fusing elements. Removal of the fat over the dorsal S1 lamina completes the surgical exposure of the dorsal L7–S1 area.

The options for exploration and treatment of the cauda equina depend on the severity of the neurologic compromise and are listed in order of increasing intensity of clinical signs. The L7–S1 fixation–fusion technique is performed with all levels of exploration, to stop motion and the resulting trauma (Table 47.1). Levels 1 to 4 are for the purpose of assessment, including information from the preoperative evaluation. Levels 5 to 6 also include treatment of the bulging L7–S1 disc. Level 7 includes removal of the herniated L7–S1 disc from around the nerve root in and lateral to the L7–S1 foramen.

Fixation

The L7 articular process and the S1 articular facet are matched caudally (see Fig. 47.4). The fixation of the articular process of L7 to the S1 sacral articular facet

is accomplished by predrilling a hole at a location one-half the distance from medial to lateral across the L7 articular process and an equal distance just cranial to the caudal margin of the articular process. The pre-drilled hole is made with a $\frac{1}{16}$-inch pin in a small dog or a $\frac{3}{32}$-inch pin in a large dog, angled at 30 to 45° from the caudal margin of the apex of the L7 dorsal spinous process. A $\frac{3}{32}$-inch threaded pin (for a small dog) or a $\frac{1}{8}$-inch threaded pin (for a large dog) is inserted into the predrilled hole to prevent the L7 articular process from fracturing. The pin is advanced to the ventral sacrum and then is cut level with the dorsal spinous process (Fig. 47.5). Ellis pins are preferred. Pins placed in the described manner provide stability of L7–S1 without any compromise to the sacroiliac joint, sacral nerve roots, or L7–S1 foramen. Screws can be used in lieu of the pins, but the pins are much easier to retrieve if the need should arise.

Fusion

A free fat graft is placed over any laminectomy, if this is performed. The graft bed on the L7 and sacrum is

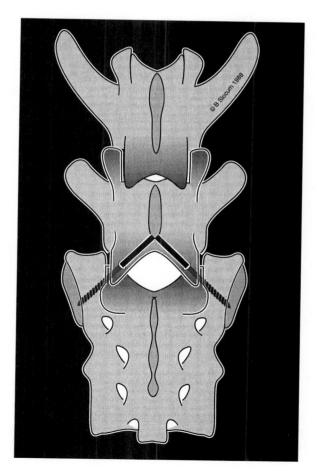

Fig. 47.5. The dorsal articular facets are held in position by threaded pins.

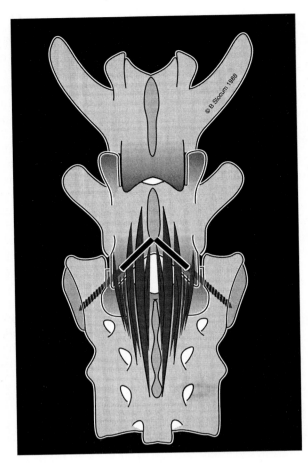

Fig. 47.6. A bone graft is placed over the dorsal aspect of the L7–S1 lamina to assist in the fusion process.

prepared by scarification. Bone graft assists in the fusion process (Fig. 47.6). The ilial cancellous and corticocancellous strip graft provides a good lattice for early fusion. Bone from a commercial bone bank reduces

surgical time dramatically. The lumbosacral fascia is sutured over the bone graft to hold it in place. The subcutaneous tissue and skin are closed routinely.

The history of the patient is important in the treatment of cauda equina syndrome to determine whether the L7–S1 fixation–fusion technique alone is sufficient to accomplish surgical objectives or whether laminectomy and surgical decompression are needed as part of the surgery. If the patient is presented with intermittent pain, then only L7–S1 fixation–fusion is necessary. If, however, the patient is presented for constant pain with times of relief with rest, then L7–S1 fixation–fusion and a small dorsal laminectomy are the preferred techniques. When the patient has constant pain without times of relief, L7–S1 fixation–fusion and a wide dorsal laminectomy for decompression are necessary. Constant pain and intense lateralizing neurologic signs are indications for an L7–S1 plate or pin fixation–fusion with one facet removed and a wide dorsal laminectomy for decompression and removal of the herniated disc material. When the articular facet is removed, a bur is used to prepare a surface for a plate, which is oriented on the dorsum of the pedicle. Two long screws are placed vertically in the pedicle. The remaining screws are placed in the S1 segment of the sacrum. The plate bridges the L7–S1 foramen, avoiding the L7 nerve.

Expansion of the L7–S1 disc space causes the L7 caudal articular process to align with the S1 cranial articular facet. The cauda equina is decompressed, and the disc is flattened. Ventral spondylosis of the L7–S1 assists in the stability between the vertebrae (Fig. 47.7).

The L7–S1 fixation–fusion technique for cauda equina syndrome is effective with proper case selection. This procedure is easy on the patient, the owner, and the surgeon.

Fig. 47.7. Expansion of the L7–S1 disc space causes the L7 caudal articular process (A) to align with the S1 cranial articular facet (B). The cauda equina (C) is decompressed, and the disc (D) is flattened. Ventral spondylosis of the L7–S1 (E) assists in the stability between the vertebrae.

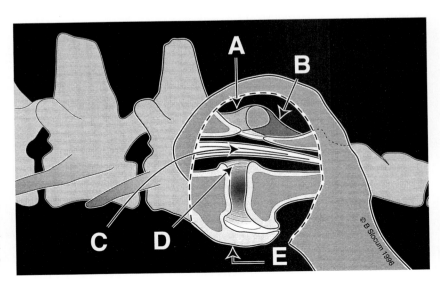

48

GENERAL PRINCIPLES

Algorithm for Bone Healing and Clinical Time Line for Fractures

Charles D. Newton

Bone healing is an inflammatory process that progresses in a logical fashion to bone union, if local and systemic factors are ideal (Table 48.1). This process, even with some motion at the fracture site, proceeds through a continuum of cellular and vascular changes that result in the production of collagen and mineral. In most instances, the process is described as classic fracture healing (inflammatory phase, reparative phase, remodeling phase) (1–3). In instances of extremely rigid fixation, primary fracture healing can occur (4, 5). Given ideal conditions of adequate rigid immobilization, bones heal on an age-related time line; immature animals heal in less time than mature animals, and mature animals require less time than aged animals (Table 48.2 and Fig. 48.1). All fractures, regardless of an animal's age, take longer to heal if

unfavorable conditions, either locally at the fracture site or systemically, prevail during the time of bone union (Table 48.3) (6).

Idealized representations of bone union are demonstrated radiographically as follows: union in an immature dog in external fixation (Fig. 48.2); union in an immature dog with an intramedullary pin fixation (Fig. 48.3); union in a mature dog with plate and screw fixation (Fig. 48.4); union in the face of contamination (Fig. 48.5); and union in an aged dog (Fig. 48.6).

Table 48.1.
Favorable Conditions Influencing the Rate of Bone Union

Rigid immobilization, whether using external fixation or internal fixation

Fractures at the ends of bones in areas of cancellous bone and an adequate blood supply

Minimal surrounding soft tissue damage

Fracture site free of infection

Age: young animals heal faster than older animals

Table 48.2.
Time to Bone Union Given Favorable Conditions

Immature animals: union rapid, 3–6 weeks
Mature animals: union less rapid, 5–8 weeks
Aged animals: union slow, 7–12 weeks

Table 48.3.
Unfavorable Conditions Influencing the Rate of Bone Union

Local factors
  Insufficient immobilization of fracture
  Inadequate blood supply to fracture
  Gaps between fracture ends
  Malposition of fracture fragments
  Severe comminution
  Infection
  Severe soft tissue damage with dispersal of the fracture hematoma
Systemic factors
  Poor nutrition or starvation
  Steroids
  Nonsteroidal anti-inflammatory drugs
  Some antibiotics
  Age: aged animals heal more slowly than young animals

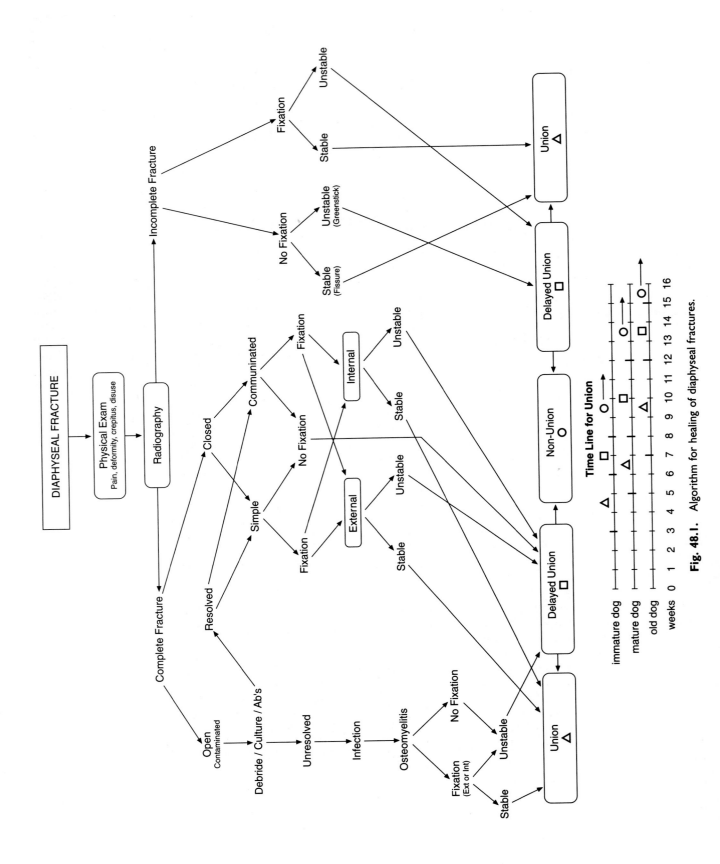

Fig. 48.1. Algorithm for healing of diaphyseal fractures.

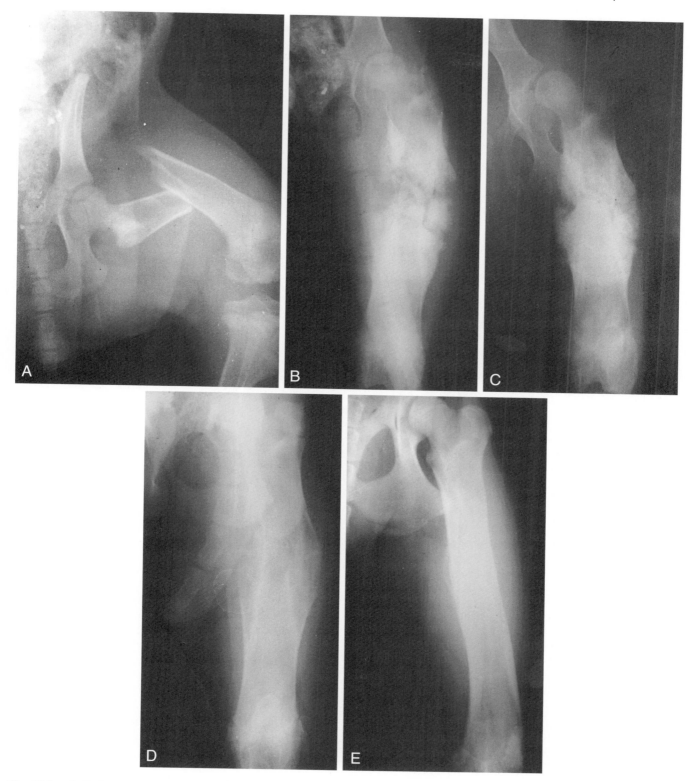

Fig. 48.2. **A.** Radiograph of a comminuted diaphyseal femoral fracture in a 4-month-old mixed breed dog. The fracture was subsequently reduced and immobilized in a Schroeder–Thomas splint. **B.** Three weeks after fixation. **C.** Five weeks after fixation; union has occurred. **D.** Seven weeks after fixation. **E.** Twenty weeks after fixation.

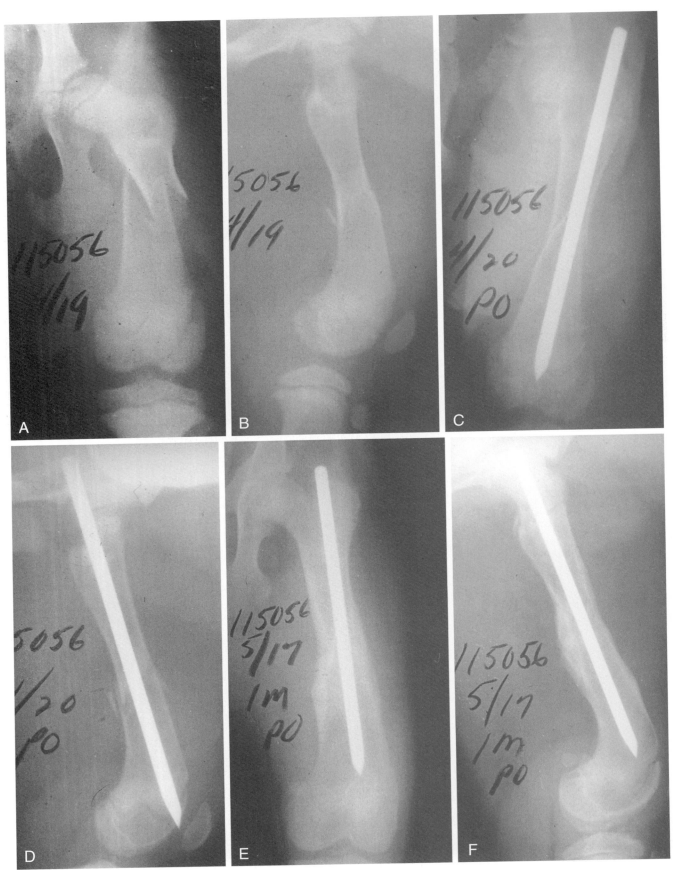

Fig. 48.3. Craniocaudal (**A**) and lateral (**B**) radiographs of a midshaft femoral fracture in a 5-month-old mixed-breed dog. **C** and **D.** Postoperative radiographs after placement of a single intramedullary pin. **E** and **F.** Radiographs taken 4 weeks postoperatively, documenting bone union.

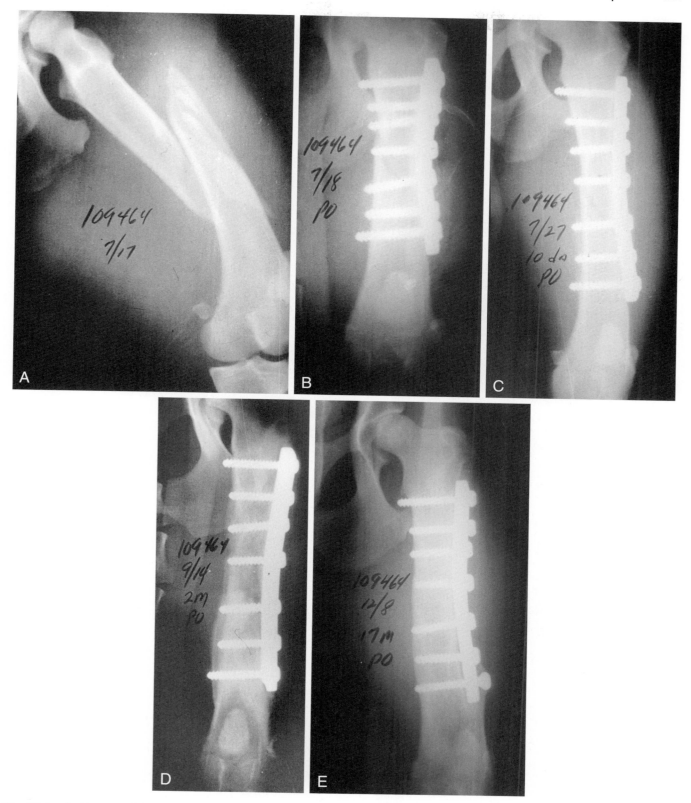

Fig. 48.4. **A.** Craniocaudal radiograph of a comminuted femoral fracture in a 4-year-old mixed breed dog. **B.** Postoperative radiograph demonstrating bone reduction and fixation using a bone plate. **C.** Ten days after fixation. **D.** Eight weeks after fixation; union has occurred. **E.** Seventeen months after fixation.

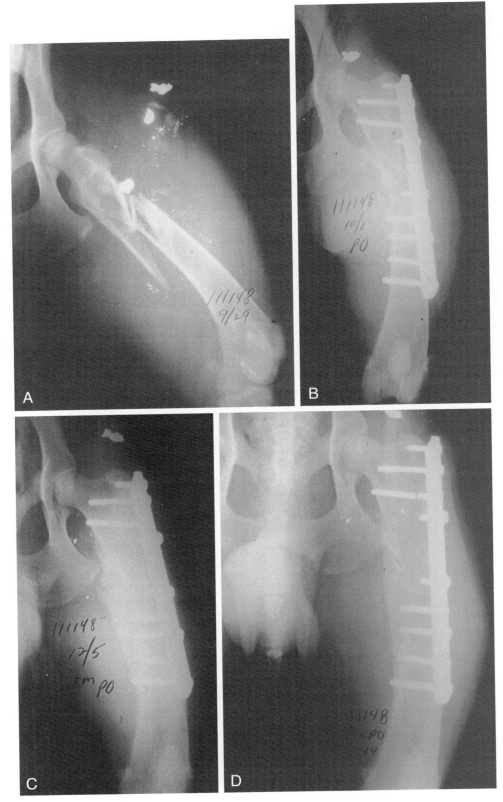

Fig. 48.5. **A.** Craniocaudal radiograph demonstrating a comminuted, open fracture of the femur in a 5-year-old dog caused by gunshot. **B.** Postoperative radiograph demonstrating bone reduction and fixation using a bone plate. **C.** Eight weeks after fixation; union has occurred. **D.** Seven months after fixation. Note callus remodeling.

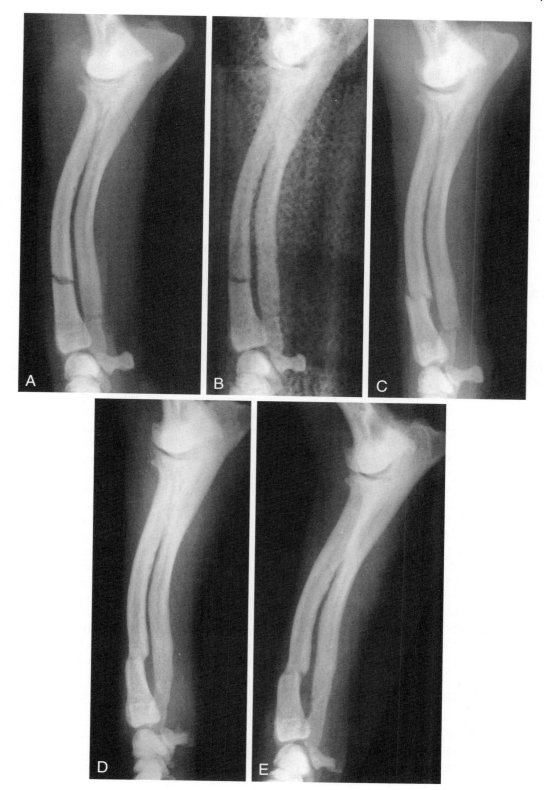

Fig. 48.6. A. Lateral radiograph demonstrating a fracture of the radius and ulna in a 13-year-old Yorkshire terrier. **B.** Postoperative radiograph after external fixation. **C.** Six weeks after fixation; union is incomplete. **D.** Fifteen weeks after fixation; union is complete. **E.** Eighteen weeks after fixation.

References

1. Cruess RL, Dumont J. In: Rockwood CA, Green DP, eds. Healing of bone, tendon and ligament. Philadelphia: JB Lippincott, 1975:988.
2. Cruess RL, Dumont J. Basic fracture healing. In: Newton CD, Nunamaker DM, eds. Textbook of small animal orthopaedics. Philadelphia: JB Lippincott, 1985:35–61.
3. Newton CD. Orthopedic basic sciences. In: Harvey, CE, Newton, CD, Schwartz, A, eds. Small animal surgery. Philadelphia: JB Lippincott, 1990:533–559.
4. Rahn BA, Gallinaro, P, Perren SM. Primary bone healing. J Bone Joint Surg Am 1971;53:783.
5. Schenk RF. Histology of fracture repair and non-union. A-O Bull Bern 1978:1–14.
6. Newton CD. Fracture repair. In: Lipowitz AJ, Caywood DD, Newton CD, et al. Complication in small animal surgery. Baltimore: Williams & Wilkins, 1996:563–595.

Stages of Bone Healing

Dennis N. Aron

When mechanical instability from a fracture is present, the body undergoes a healing process producing external callus that functions as a mechanical supporting structure. This external callus healing is the natural indirect process induced by injury and mechanical instability and is modulated by mechanical stability, vascular supply, local cell donor population, and local and systemic factors. Direct bone healing occurs in stable injuries or rigidly fixed fractures and does not need external callus formation, because no mechanical instability is present. This occurs in anatomically reduced, fixed stable fractures without comminution. It is mediated by a microscopic unit composed of osteoclasts, osteoblasts, and capillary cells, referred to as an osteonal unit that crosses the fracture site and bridges the fracture segments.

Arbitrarily, indirect fracture healing tends to be divided into stages or phases. Each phase extends into the next phase. These phases are well documented and are described in numerous reviews.

Inflammatory Stage

This phase begins with the development of the fracture and involves damage to the bone and soft tissue. The fracture trauma creates injury to blood vessels depriving cells of physiologic functions and causing death of bone and soft tissue extending back to regions of viable vascularity. The intensity and duration of this inflammatory phase is proportional to the amount of necrotic tissue produced. Involved with this phase are vasodilatation and plasma exudation resulting in acute edema and migration of polymorphonuclear leukocytes and macrophages to the inflammatory region. This phase must succeed in "cleaning up" the necrotic debris adequately before bone formation can advance. The stimulus for bone formation has been postulated to be from chemical mediators, pH changes, and electronegativity in the region of the healing fracture.

Reparative Stage

Cells of mesenchymal origin are pluripotential and can form collagen, cartilage, or bone. Small variations in the microenvironment and mechanical stresses probably determine the tissue type formed. This phase is completely linked with arrival of capillary buds into the healing region. Cells come from periosteum, endosteum, and elsewhere, but most cells enter the healing region with granulation tissue capillary buds. Origin of the capillary buds with indirect callus healing, early on, is from the surrounding soft tissue extraosseous blood supply of healing bone, whereas later it is from the medullary blood supply of the bone. The cells invade the fracture hematoma and make callus composed of fibrous tissue, cartilage, or bone, depending on the regional microenvironment. The callus envelops the bone ends and gradually increases stability of the fracture. Bone and fibrous tissue formation requires a microenvironment of high oxygen tension, whereas cartilage is produced in an environment of low oxygen tension, a situation reflective of decreased vascularity. Early on, fibrous tissue and cartilage predominate (substage of soft callus), but later mineralization occurs (substage of hard callus). The cartilage formed is absorbed through a process similar to endochondral ossification. Moreover, necrotic bone must be reabsorbed, and this is accomplished by osteoclasts derived from circulating monocytes, which are not recruited locally and depend on ingrowth of blood vessels to provide the osteoclasts. Collagen fibers have their own organization that produces hole zones in which bone mineral initially appears. The result is a series of organized collagen fibrils within and around which are clustered crystals of calcium hydroxyapatite. As this mineralization takes place, bone segments become more rigidly stable as they are enveloped in this mass of bone tissue.

Remodeling

During this stage, osteoclastic resorption of mechanically disadvantageous bone occurs, and new bone is laid down parallel to tension lines of force. The control mechanism is believed to be electrical, with electronegativity stimulating osteoblastic activity and electropositivity stimulating osteoclastic activity. Electropositive potentials are noted on the convex side of bone, and electronegative potentials occur on the concave side. The osteonal unit performs the remodeling process. The end result is a bone that is returned to its original form or to a form allowing it best to perform the intended biomechanical function.

From the previous discussion, it is obvious that bone healing is intimately linked to both bone stability and vascularity of bone and surrounding soft tissues. For healing to proceed unabated, balance between these parameters is necessary. When stability and vascularity are not in appropriate balance, healing is prolonged, or does not occur at all, and patient morbidity is high. This situation challenges the clinician with regard to fracture management. Attempts to provide stability by providing rigid internal fixation compromise soft tissues and ultimately the development of capillary buds, whereas not providing rigid internal fixation risks inadequate stability and compromises the developing capillary buds. The clinician must understand the mechanisms of fracture healing and the different stabilization methods available, to provide the best possible balance for treatment of a particular fracture.

References

Aron DN, Palmer RH, Johnson AL. Biologic strategies and a balanced concept for repair of highly comminuted long bone fractures. Compend Contin Educ Pract Vet 1995;17:35–49.

Russell TA. General principles of fracture treatment. In: Crenshaw AH, ed. Campbell's operative orthopaedics. 8th ed. St Louis: Mosby–Year Book, 1992:725.

Cruess RL. Healing of bone, tendon, and ligament. In: Rockwood CA Jr, Green DP, eds. Fractures: In adults. 2nd ed. Philadelphia: JB Lippincott, 1984:147.

Algorithms for Fracture Management

Jack Brinker & Wade Brinker

Figures 48.7 through 48.23 are algorithms for the management of fractures in small animal practice.

Table of Implant Biomechanics

Randy J. Boudrieau

Table 48.4 describes biomechanics related to implant selection for repair of long bone fractures.

Plate Selection by Bone and Body Weight

Barclay Slocum & Theresa Devine Slocum

Plate selection is based on the experience of the surgeon and the common properties of 316L stainless steel. Because stainless steel plates are similar in composition, their tensile strength varies by how the metal is work-hardened. This variable among different brands is minimal compared with the cross-sectional area (CSA) of the plate.

The CSA is given in the technical description of the implant. The CSA can be calculated by multiplying the width of the plate times the thickness. For example, if a plate is 10 mm wide and 3.5 mm thick, its cross-sectional area is 35 mm. In general, a plate with a CSA of 30 mm^2 is more capable of maintaining fixation of a tibia on a 25-kg dog than a plate with a CSA of 21 mm^2. Figures 48.24 to 48.32, representing the CSA as a function of bone and patient weight, also permit a general comparison among similar-size plates by different manufacturers.

The comparison is a guideline for the practicing veterinary orthopedist who wishes to purchase plates from different companies that have size selections unfamiliar to the surgeon. Because holes are present in plates, the implants are weaker than strictly a function of cross-sectional area. The different configurations of plate shape also affect plate strength. Figures 48.24 to 48.32 allow the surgeon to make proper size selection of plates for the different bones.

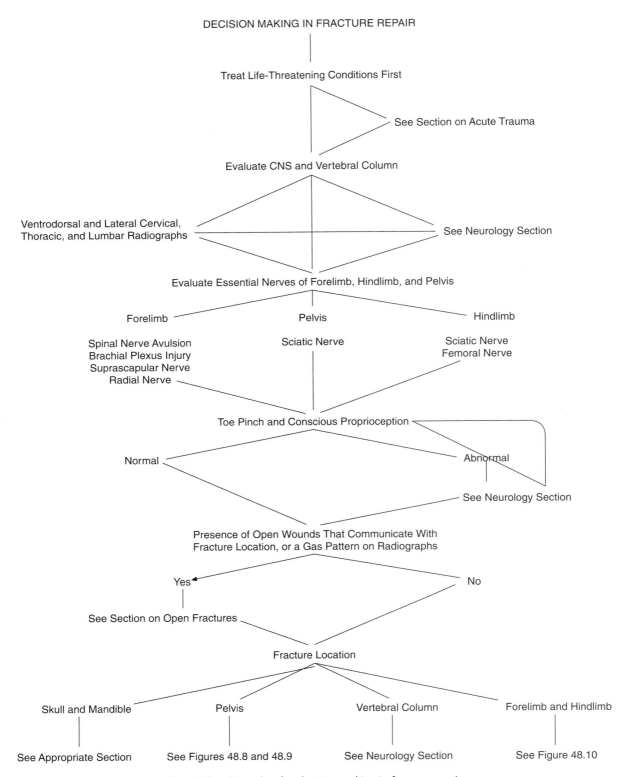

DECISION MAKING IN FRACTURE REPAIR

Treat Life-Threatening Conditions First

See Section on Acute Trauma

Evaluate CNS and Vertebral Column

Ventrodorsal and Lateral Cervical, Thoracic, and Lumbar Radiographs

See Neurology Section

Evaluate Essential Nerves of Forelimb, Hindlimb, and Pelvis

Forelimb   Pelvis   Hindlimb

Spinal Nerve Avulsion   Sciatic Nerve   Sciatic Nerve
Brachial Plexus Injury   Femoral Nerve
Suprascapular Nerve
Radial Nerve

Toe Pinch and Conscious Proprioception

Normal   Abnormal

See Neurology Section

Presence of Open Wounds That Communicate With Fracture Location, or a Gas Pattern on Radiographs

Yes   No

See Section on Open Fractures

Fracture Location

Skull and Mandible   Pelvis   Vertebral Column   Forelimb and Hindlimb

See Appropriate Section   See Figures 48.8 and 48.9   See Neurology Section   See Figure 48.10

Fig. 48.7. Algorithm for decision making in fracture repair.

Table 48.4.
Biomechanics and Implant Selection: Decision Making for Repair of Long Bone Fractures

Implant	Forces Neutralized
Intramedullary pin[a]	
Smooth Steinmann pin	Bending
Stack pin[b]	Bending (rotation)[c]
Interlocking nail	Bending
	Rotation
	Compression
Wire[d]	
Full-cerclage	Shear (compression,[e] rotation[e])
Hemicerclage	Shear
Skewer-pin techniques	
Full-cerclage	Shear (compression,[e,f] rotation[e,f])
Figure-of-eight	Shear
Tension-band	Tension[g]
Plate[h]	Bending
Neutralization	Rotation
Compression	Compression
Buttress	Shear
External skeletal fixator	
Primary fixation[i]	Bending
Type I	Rotation
Type II	Compression
Type III	Shear
Secondary (ancillary) fixation[j]	
Two-pin (or three-pin) type I	Rotation[k]
	Compression (bending)[l]
Four-pin type I	Rotation
	Compression
	Shear (bending)[l]

[a] An intramedullary (IM) pin is effective with neutralization of bending forces; however, if the IM pin fills the entire medullary cavity, shear forces will be neutralized in some fracture configurations. The latter is not a desirable situation, however, as the medullary blood supply becomes compromised. An interlocking nail, on the other hand, additionally allows compressive and rotational forces to be neutralized by virtue of allowing a screw (usually two screws on each side of the fracture) to be placed transversely into the bone and through the IM pin. Because these screws do not attain a direct purchase into the IM pin (they simply pass through a predrilled hole in the pin), shear forces are not neutralized.

[b] Stack pins most often are composed of multiple, smaller-diameter, IM pins placed into the bone; technically, this also refers to more than one IM pin placed into the bone, regardless of their size.

[c] Multiple IM pins improve rotational stability; however, as the only method used to neutralize rotational forces, this technique usually is inadequate.

[d] Wire primarily is used to rebuild the fracture fragments into their anatomic position and, as such, is most useful in neutralizing shear forces. Wire is used to supplement another form of "primary" fixation, such as an IM pin, plate, or external skeletal fixator (ESF). In certain circumstances, with some fracture configurations in simple fractures, wire may neutralize rotational and compressive forces (see [c]).

[e] Successful neutralization of these forces requires a fracture configuration such that multiple (more than two) full-cerclage wires can be placed across the fracture; therefore, a long oblique fracture configuration is required, most often defined as the length of the fracture line obliquity that is equal to or greater than twice the bone diameter.

[f] The skewer pin anchors the wire onto the tip of the pin. To neutralize these forces effectively, a criterion identical to that in [e] must exist for the fracture configuration; however, in this instance, the pin is used to secure the cerclage wire in areas of changing bone diameter, such as the flaring of the metaphysis.

[g] Tension forces primarily are observed in areas where the bone fragments at the fracture site will become distracted when subjected to a muscular contraction; for example, in an olecranon fracture, the triceps muscle creates the tension force to pull these fragments apart, and in a malleolar fracture, a varus or valgus stress to the joint causes the ligament attachments to the bone fragments to distract the fragments apart. The tension-band technique essentially uses a wire in a figure-of-eight pattern to bridge the fracture and prevent the distraction, a mechanism identical to the cables spanning the truss of a crane.

[h] All forces are effectively neutralized using a plate regardless of the method of application: neutralization, compression, or buttress. The differing applications depend on the ability to rebuild the fracture. The applied forces are shared by both the implant and the bone with either neutralization or compression plate fixation; however, if compression plate fixation can be applied (by providing tension to the implant, which, in turn compresses the bone fragments together) greater stability is obtained because of the generation of high frictional forces at the fracture site. The latter generally requires a simple fracture configuration. With buttress plate fixation, the applied forces must be borne totally by the implant.

[i] All forces are effectively neutralized using an ESF as the primary means of fracture fixation regardless of the methods of application, most commonly as a neutralization or buttress device. The primary limitation of the ESF is with upper extremity fractures in the larger patients; a type II or III ESF cannot be placed because of interference with the trunk of the animal. Additionally, a much greater amount of soft tissue impingement by the fixation pins results in more potential soft tissue complications.

[j] An ESF also may be used as an ancillary device to supplement the primary fixation, usually supplementing IM pin and wire fixation, in which not all the distracting forces have been sufficiently neutralized; most often, this involves rotational instability in transverse–short oblique or comminuted fractures. In comminuted fractures, the ESF as an ancillary device also is effective in neutralizing compressive forces to prevent fracture collapse.

[k] As an ancillary device, a type I, two-pin ESF adequately neutralizes rotational forces, provided shear forces already have been addressed, such as using wire fixation. If shear forces are not neutralized, the two-pin fixator continues to allow motion around the axis of the fixation pins. The addition of one additional pin on each side of the fracture, a four-pin, type I ESF, eliminates this motion and therefore also neutralizes shear forces in the absence of direct fixation (wire) at the fracture site.

[l] As an ancillary device, a type I ESF supplements the neutralization of bending forces. This property may be useful in the event that an inadequately sized IM pin is present in the bone (fills less than two-thirds of the medullary canal diameter).

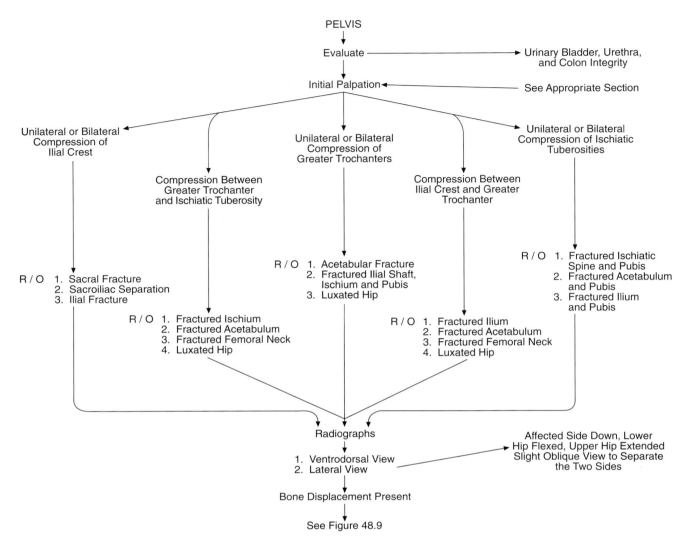

Fig. 48.8. Algorithm for evaluation of pelvic fractures. *R/O,* rule out.

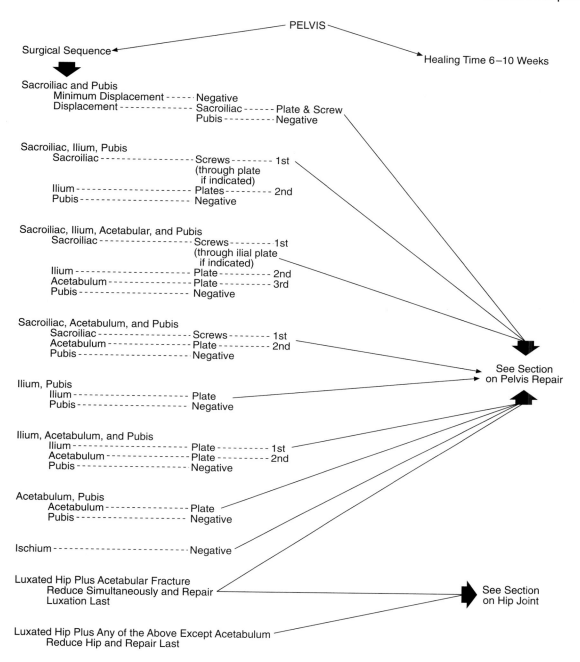

Fig. 48.9. Algorithm for surgical treatment of pelvic fractures. *Negative,* no repair needed.

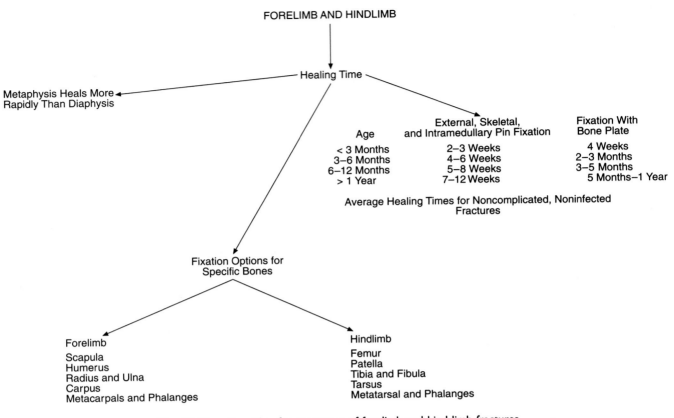

Fig. 48.10. Algorithm for treatment of forelimb and hind limb fractures.

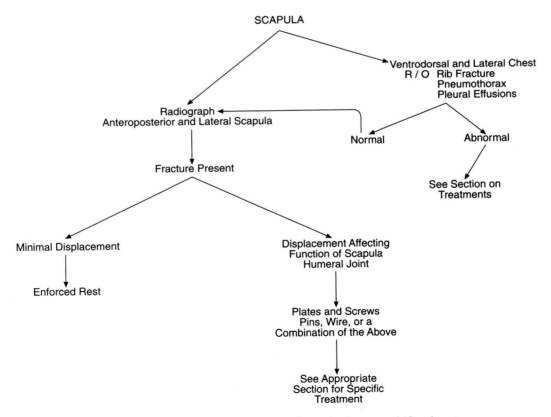

Fig. 48.11. Algorithm for evaluation of scapular fractures. *R/O*, rule out.

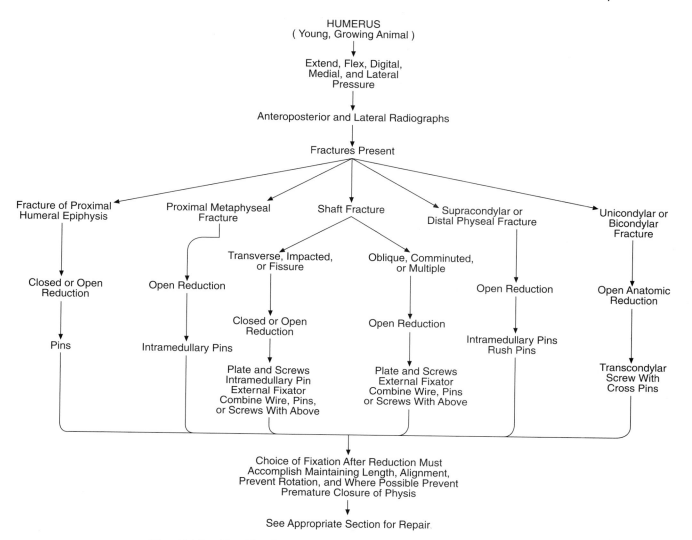

Fig. 48.12. Algorithm for evaluation of humeral fractures in young animals.

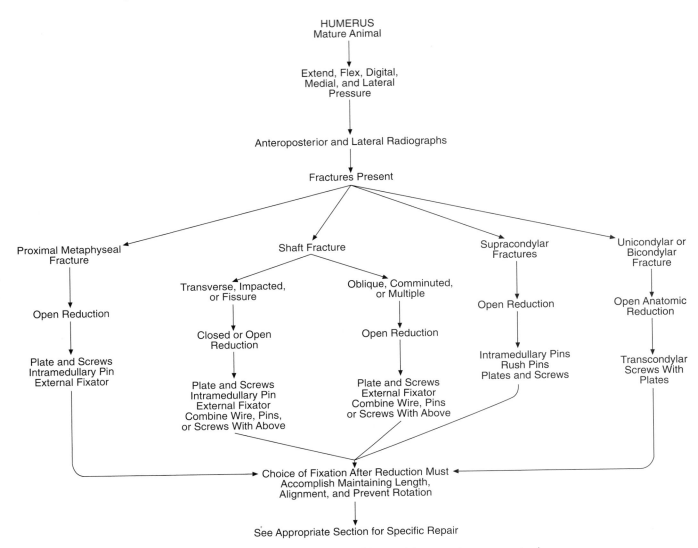

Fig. 48.13. Algorithm for evaluation of humeral fractures in mature animals.

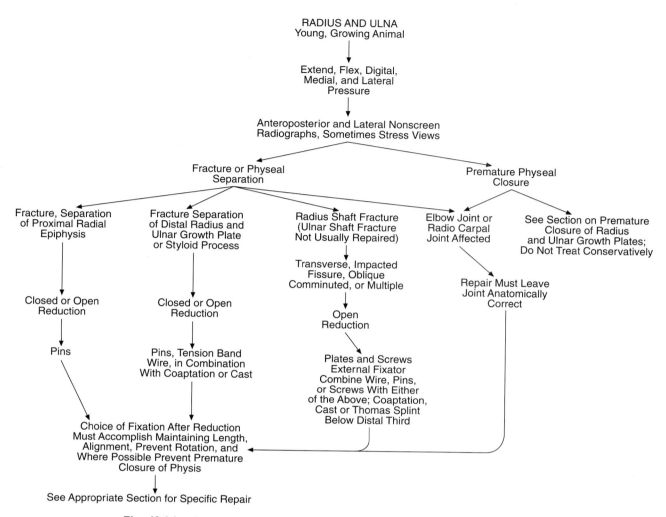

Fig. 48.14. Algorithm for evaluation of radial and ulnar fractures in young animals.

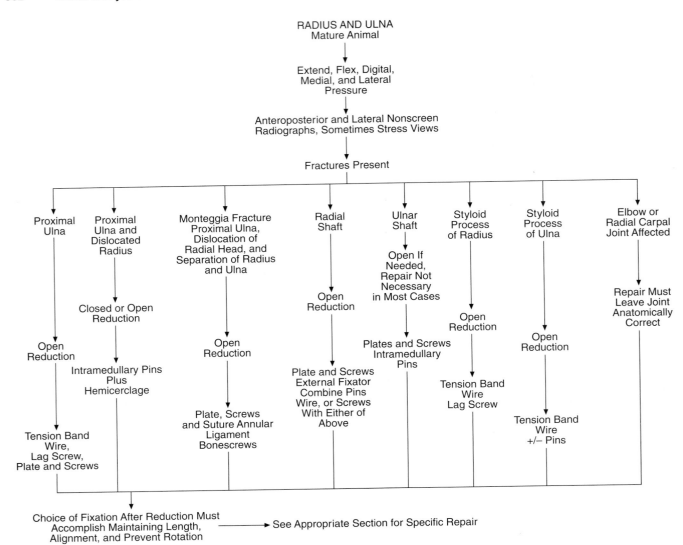

Fig. 48.15. Algorithm for evaluation of radial and ulnar fractures in mature animals.

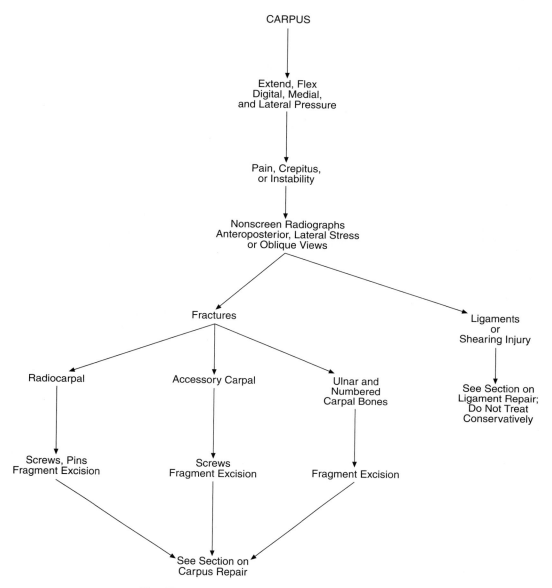

Fig. 48.16. Algorithm for evaluation of carpal injury.

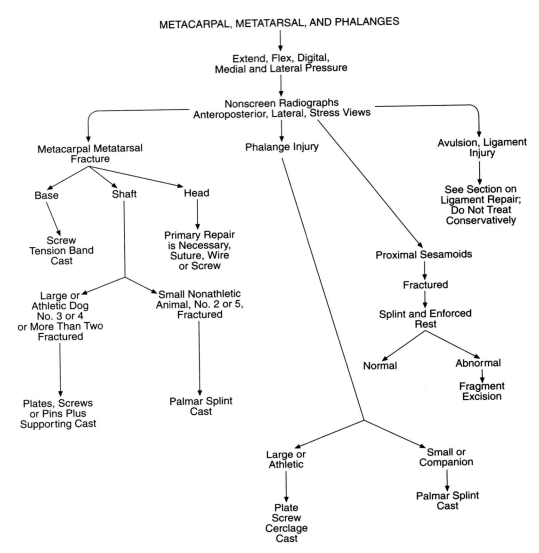

Fig. 48.17. Algorithm for evaluation of metacarpal, metatarsal, and phalangeal injury.

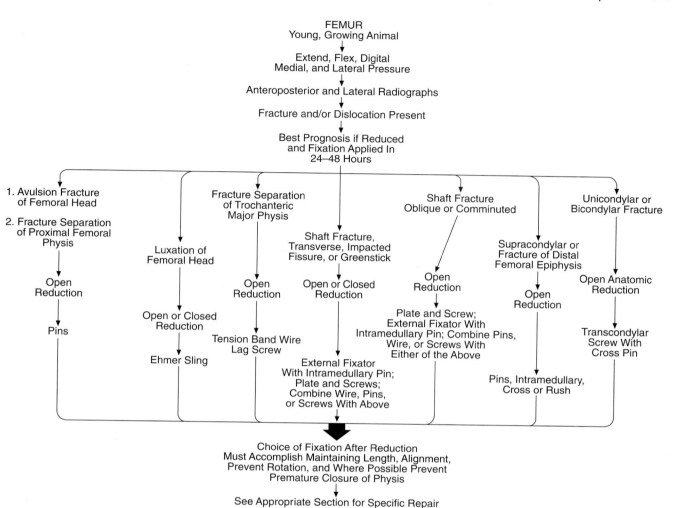

Fig. 48.18. Algorithm for evaluation of femoral injury in young animals.

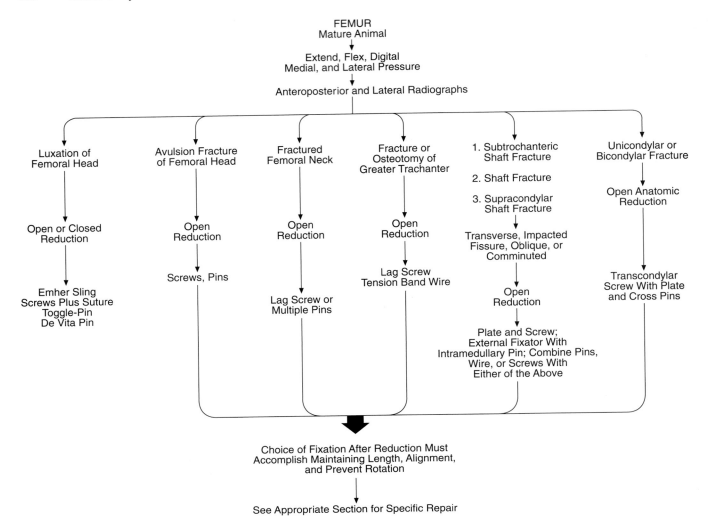

Fig. 48.19. Algorithm for evaluation of femoral injury in mature animals.

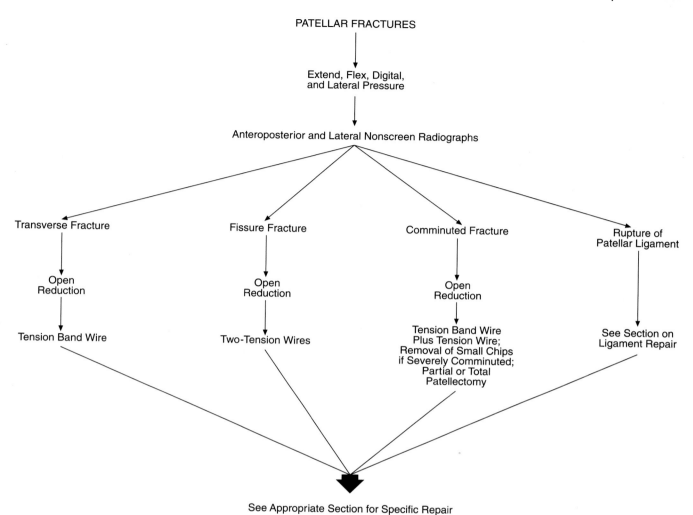

Fig. 48.20. Algorithm for evaluation of patellar fractures.

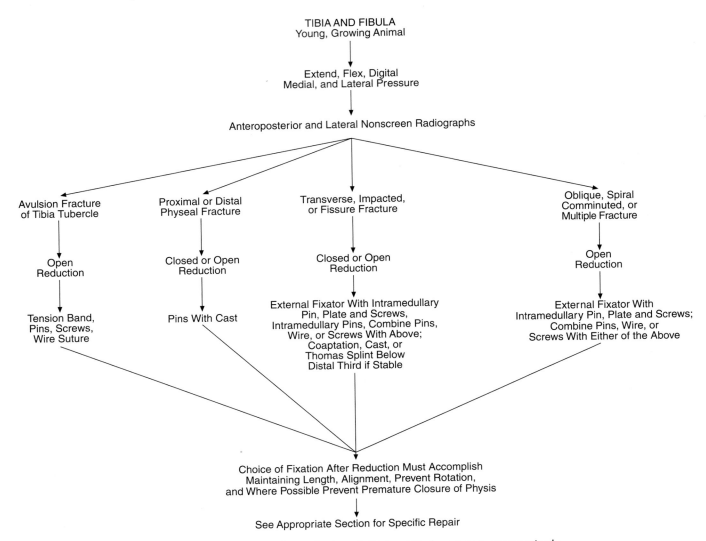

Fig. 48.21. Algorithm for evaluation of tibial and fibular injury in young animals.

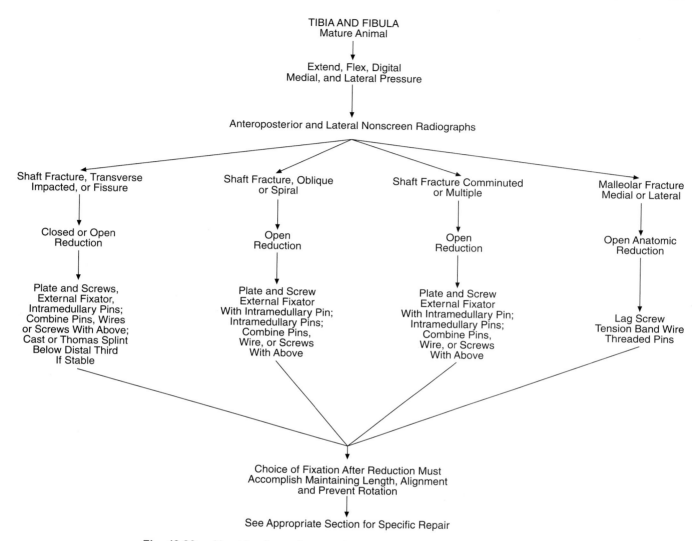

Fig. 48.22. Algorithm for evaluation of tibial and fibular injury in mature animals.

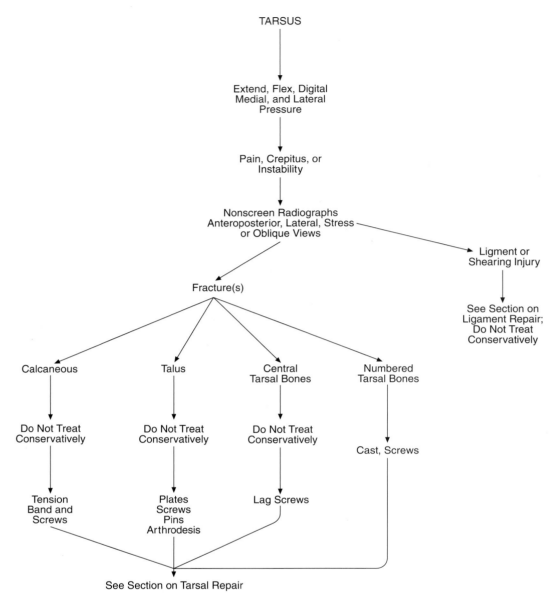

Fig. 48.23. Algorithm for evaluation of tarsal injury.

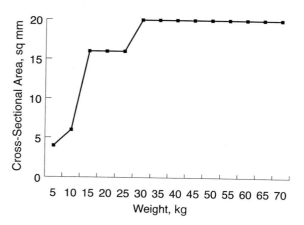

Fig. 48.24. Plate size for the mandible.

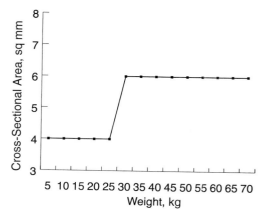

Fig. 48.27. Plate size for the metacarpals.

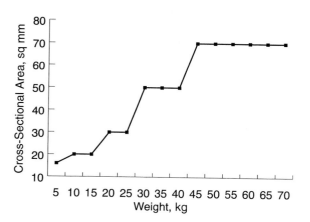

Fig. 48.25. Plate size for the humerus.

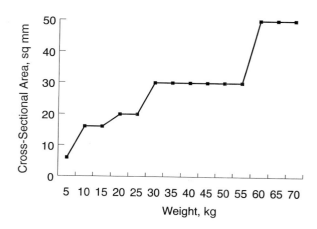

Fig. 48.28. Plate size for the ilium.

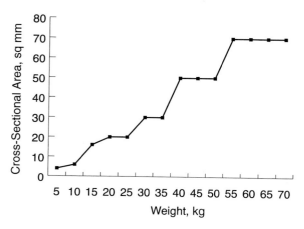

Fig. 48.26. Plate size for the radius.

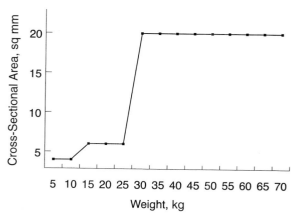

Fig. 48.29. Plate size for the acetabulum.

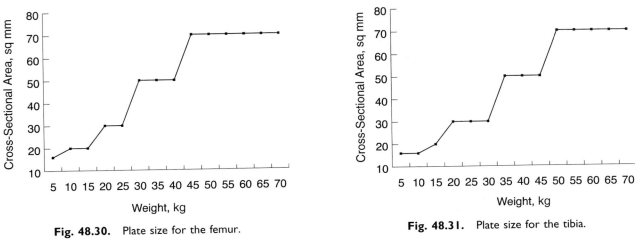

Fig. 48.30. Plate size for the femur.

Fig. 48.31. Plate size for the tibia.

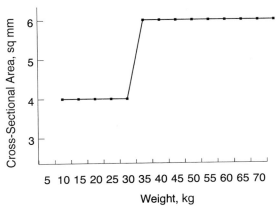

Fig. 48.32. Plate size for the metatarsals.

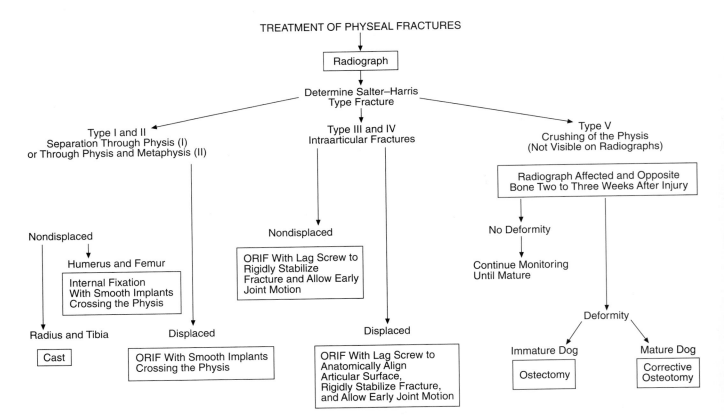

Fig. 48.33. Algorithm for the treatment of physeal fractures. *ORIF*, open reduction with internal fixation.

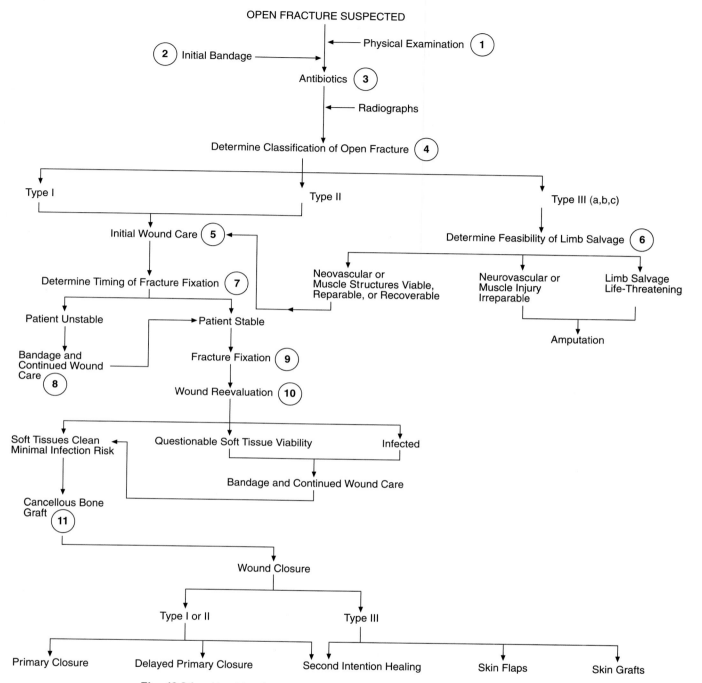

Fig. 48.34. Algorithm for treatment of open fractures. See text for explanation.

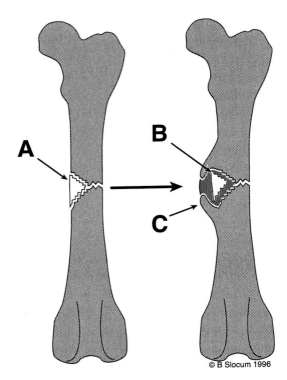

Fig. 48.35. An avascular bone fragment (A) can become an infected avascular sequestra (B), which lies within a concavity of reactive bone called an involucrum (C).

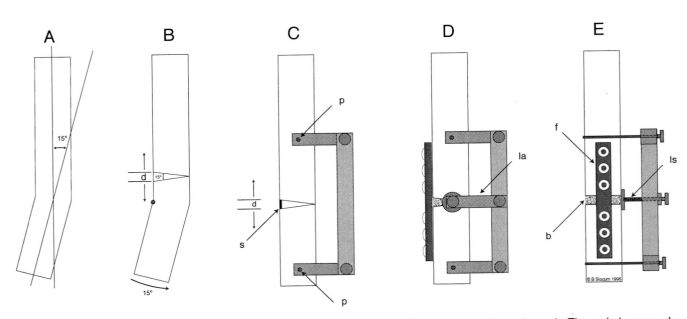

Fig. 48.36. Opening wedge osteotomy. **A.** Angular deformity is measured on the anteroposterior radiograph. The angle between the two lines is the angular correction necessary. **B.** The wedge needed for angular correction is drawn on the radiograph of the limb. The distance (d) measured from the radiograph is used as the amount of wedge opening in surgery. **C.** The tibial plateau leveling osteotomy jig is placed on the bone in the frontal plane. An eighth-inch threaded pin is placed through the jig holes and into the bone (p). The osteotomy cut is made through the bone, and a temporary spacer (s) is placed to maintain the opening distance for plate application. **D.** A leveling arm (la) is placed over the osteotomy to help stabilize the frontal cortices for plate application. **E.** In the sagittal plane view, the leveling screw (ls) is tightened to align the frontal cortices of the osteotomy site. Bone graft (b) is applied to assist with healing. A plate (f) is applied to maintain the angular correction.

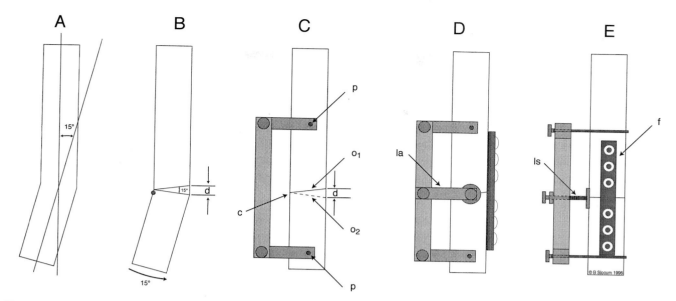

Fig. 48.37. Closing wedge osteotomy. **A.** Angular deformity is measured on the anteroposterior radiograph. The angle between the two lines is the angular correction necessary. **B.** The amount of the closing wedge osteotomy (*d*) is drawn on the radiograph. **C.** The jig is positioned on the bone in the frontal plane by two partially threaded eighth-inch pins (*p*). The first osteotomy (*O₁*) is made in the front cortex but is not completed through the bone. The second cut (*O₂*) is also partially completed through the bone to check for correct plane alignment and distance (*d*). **D.** The leveling arm of the jig (*la*) is positioned over the osteotomy site to assist in correct alignment of the cortices. **E.** As viewed from the sagittal plane, the leveling screw (*ls*) is tightened, and a plate (*f*) is applied.

Algorithm for Treatment of Physeal Fractures

Ann L. Johnson

Figure 48.33 is an algorithm for the repair of physeal fractures.

Algorithm for Treatment of Open Fractures

Richard P. Suess, Jr.

Figure 48.34 is an algorithm for the treatment of open fractures, as follows:

1. Most open fractures in dogs and cats are caused by vehicular trauma. Many other nonskeletal injuries occur with this type of trauma, so the surgeon must detect and address life-threatening problems first. The recognition of other significant injuries may influence treatment of the open fracture. Open fractures are emergencies. Prompt appropriate treatment is crucial to reduce potential complications.

2. A fracture should be treated as open if any full-thickness skin wound is present near the fracture site. To prevent contamination by hospital bacteria, the wound should be covered with a sterile bandage while the initial patient assessment is performed. Probing of the wound or reduction of the bone ends back underneath the skin should be avoided until initial wound care is provided.

3. All open fractures are contaminated and, if left untreated for 8 hours or more, are considered infected. Administration of intravenous bactericidal antibiotics is always indicated. Knowledge of commonly isolated bacteria from dogs with osteomyelitis is useful in the initial selection of an antibiotic. These bacteria include *Streptococcus* spp., *Staphylococcus* spp., and gram-negative enteric organisms. A first-generation cephalosporin is a good choice. If heavy soil or feces contamination is present or if the fracture is a result of a bite wound, administration of antibiotics effective against a broader spectrum of gram-negative and anaerobic bacteria should be considered. The appropriate length of time for antibiotic therapy is still debatable. Guidelines for treatment of humans with open fractures suggest antibiotics for the first 3 days. Antibiotics are then discontinued unless obvious clinical signs of infection are present or postdebridement cultures (see item 5 in

this list) are positive. At the time of wound closure, another culture is taken, and antibiotic therapy is reinstituted. If this second culture is negative and no overt signs of infection are present, the antibiotics are discontinued. The advantage of discontinuing the antibiotics after the first 3 days is that the drug is not present when the second culture is taken. If wound infection occurs or if culture results are positive, antibiotics may be necessary for 3 to 6 weeks.

4. Type I open fractures are caused by low-energy forces and have a wound less than 1 cm long. Most often, the wound is caused by piercing of the skin by the bone, rather than by a penetrating object. Muscle damage is minimal. The fracture is usually simple. Fractures of this type that occur in highly contaminated environments such as farmyards are classified as type III. Type II open fractures have moderate soft tissue damage caused by high-energy forces. The wounds are generally larger than 1 cm, no soft tissue flaps or avulsions are present, and a crushing component is minimal to moderate. The fracture is usually simple. Type III open fractures are the result of high-energy trauma. The soft tissue injuries are extensive and severe, and the wound is usually larger than 10 cm long. The fractures are often highly comminuted. Type III open fractures have been further subdivided to reflect the various degrees of soft tissue and vascular injuries seen in this group. Although extensive soft tissue trauma is present in type IIIa, major plastic reconstructive procedures such as skin flaps or grafts are not necessary to cover bone and close the wound. In type IIIb open fractures, soft tissue and skin are insufficient for primary closure, so reconstructive procedures are indicated. Type IIIc open fractures have a major vascular (arterial) injury that requires repair.

5. Initial wound care includes debridement, lavage, and bacterial culture and sensitivity testing. Debridement in the most important step in the treatment of open fractures. The goal is to convert a contaminated wound into a clean one. Sterile technique must be used when debriding and flushing the wound. Surgical preparation and draping of the limb should be performed. Sterile water-soluble lubrication jelly can be placed on the wound to prevent hair from entering it when the limb is clipped. All nonviable tissues are removed by sharp dissection. Removal of devitalized skin should be conservative but complete. Determination of muscle viability is based on established criteria of consistency, contractility, ability to bleed, and color. Bullets do not need to be sought unless they are intra-articular or interfering with vessels or nerves. Any bullets found should be saved because of the potential for lawsuits involving gunshot injuries. Small unattached bone pieces can be removed. However, larger pieces of bone should be retained even if they are devitalized because they are often important to fracture recon-

struction and stabilization. All bone with soft tissue attachments should remain in the fracture site. Copious lavage is the next step in initial wound management. A minimum of 2 L of sterile isotonic solution such as 0.9% sodium chloride is recommended. Greater volumes are necessary for severely contaminated and infected fractures. Physicians prefer commercial jet lavage systems for wound flushing. If one is not available, an effective system can be made with a 1-L bag of sterile isotonic saline, 10 drip/mL intravenous administration set, three-way stopcock, 18-gauge needle, and 60-mL syringe. The benefits of saline solutions containing certain antibiotics (neomycin–polymyxin) or antiseptics (0.05% chlorhexidine) are reported. However, use of large volumes of saline rather than inclusion of additives probably is more important in effective wound lavage. This described aseptic wound care is often necessary on a daily basis for type III fractures. Bacterial aerobic and anaerobic cultures and sensitivity tests are best taken immediately after debridement and lavage. Cultures obtained at this time, rather than before initial wound care, more accurately reflect the bacteria responsible for any resulting infection.

6. Early in the management of type III fractures, the surgeon should consider the long-term prognosis for limb usage. Recognition of appropriate amputation situation saves the patient, owner, and surgeon from an unrewarding limb-salvage attempt. If irreparable neurovascular or muscle damage has occurred, amputation is preferable to a nonfunctional limb. Amputation is also indicated when limb salvage would be life-threatening, such as in a patient with sepsis from an infected open wound.

7. In the stable patient, fracture fixation should immediately follow initial wound care. If the patient is unstable, a sterile bandage needs to be placed over the wound. If further debridement is anticipated, a wet–dry bandage is a good choice. Fractures below the elbow and stifle also benefit from a support bandage for temporary fracture stabilization. Fractures of the humerus and femur cannot easily be immobilized without placement of a cumbersome spica-type splint. Analgesics, gentle limb handling, and a stent bandage to cover the wound are often a better alternative for open fractures above the elbow and stifle.

8. Continued wound care includes daily debridement and lavage as described for initial wound care. In patients with extensive soft tissue injury, debridement and lavage are often necessary for 1 to 3 days.

9. The goals of fracture fixation, such as rigid stability, anatomic reduction, gentle tissue handling, and early return to function, must be maximized. Although an intramedullary pin and wires can be used in certain cases, bone plates or crews and external fixators generally are preferable. The more rigid fixa-

tion provided by the latter two devices encourages and enhances revascularization of the fracture. Revascularization, in turn, promotes bone healing and resistance to infection.

10. After fracture fixation, timing of cancellous bone grafting and wound closure needs to be considered. Both should be done once the wound is judged to be clean and the risk of infection is minimal.

11. Delayed union and nonunion are common complications of open fractures. For this reason, cancellous bone grafting is indicated, particularly in comminuted fractures and those with cortical defects.

Suggested Readings

Chapman MW. Open fractures. In: Chapman, MW, ed. Operative orthopedics. Philadelphia: JB Lippincott, 1993;365–372.

Dirschl DR, Wilson FC. Topical antibiotic irrigation in the prophylaxis of operative wound infections in orthopedic surgery. Orthop Clin North Am 1991:22:419–426.

Fischer MD, Gustillo RB, Varecka TF. The timing of flap coverage, bone grafting, and intramedullary nailing in patients who have a fracture of the tibial shaft with extensive soft tissue injury. J Bone Joint Surg Am 1991;73:1316–1322.

Georgiades GM, Behrens FF, Joyce MJ, et al. Open tibial fractures with severe soft tissue loss: limb salvage compared with below-the-knee amputation. J Bone Joint Surg Am 1993:75:1431–1441.

Gustilo RB. Management of open fractures and their complications. Philadelphia: WB Saunders, 1982.

Gustillo RB, Mendoza RM, Williams DN. Problems in the management of type III (severe) open fractures: a new classification of type III open fractures. J Trauma 1984;24:742–746.

Johnson KA. Osteomyelitis in dogs and cats. J Am Vet Med Assoc 1994;205:1882–1887.

Lincoln JD. Treatment of open, delayed union, and nonunion fractures with external skeletal fixation. Vet Clin North Am Small Anim Pract 1992;22:195–207.

Merrit K. Factors increasing the risk of infection in patients with open fractures. J Trauma 1988;28:823–827.

Tillson DM. Open fracture management. Vet Clin North Am Small Anim Pract 1995;25:1093–1110.

Wilkins J, Patzakis M. Choice and duration of antibiotics in open fractures. Orthop Clin North Am 1991:22:433–437.

Treatment of Sequestra

Mary Lynn Stanton

Once a sequestrum has been identified, the surgeon must use all principles of therapy to maximize chances for a successful outcome. Debridement, rigid internal fixation, antimicrobial therapy, patient medical status, and owner compliance all must be addressed.

Because sequestra are avascular segments of bone, they generally need to be removed. Otherwise, they serve as a constant source of infection and prevent callus formation in fractures, with resulting wound drainage and lameness. The surrounding bone may undergo curettage. The surgeon need not excise all

fistulous tracts because they should resolve with sequestra removal (Fig. 48.35).

Soft tissues should be generously lavaged with sterile isotonic saline at surgery. They may be left open, closed with a drainage system, or closed primarily. The choice depends on the degree of infection and the amount of drainage. Open wound management with sterile dressings of 1:20 chlorhexidine is effective in severely infected cases, but it requires at least one additional surgical procedure to stabilize and graft the fracture. Strict asepsis in bandaging techniques is required with either drains or open techniques, because secondary contamination of the fracture site with gram-negative opportunistic organisms can occur.

If sequestered bone is in continuity with vascularized cortical bone, it may become incorporated, if rigid fixation and appropriate antimicrobial therapy are used. However, if these segments are large or involve the full diameter of bone, they will lead to chronic osteomyelitis. Large sequestered segments may make amputation necessary.

Rigid internal fixation is required for fracture repair to progress after the sequestrum is removed. Maintenance of stability is best accomplished with an external fixator. These devices allow for the least amount of soft tissue and vascular disruption at the fracture site. Intramedullary pins are contraindicated because of their disruption of the medullary blood supply. Plate fixation is useful if the surgeon believes that it is the best method for rigid stability. Any implants from prior surgery that do not contribute to stability should be removed.

Along with fixation, autogenous cancellous grafting of the defect left by the sequestrum is indicated. Grafting should be done when open wound management or use of drainage systems is complete. As the progress of fracture healing is monitored radiographically, it may be necessary to regraft if healing is slow.

Cultures should be taken from the sequestrum site during the surgical procedure, rather than from draining tracts preoperatively. These tracts often have contaminants and do not give a true result of a deeper bone infection. Antimicrobial therapy should be discontinued 48 to 72 hours preoperatively. After samples are obtained, intraoperative intravenous antibiotics are given. *Staphylococcus* is a common finding, making cefazolin or clindamycin a good first treatment choice until culture and sensitivity results are known.

An important consideration is the patient's own ability to overcome infection and to be capable of normal bone healing. Patients with preexisting medical conditions such as diabetes or hyperadrenocorticism are at a disadvantage to handle what is a difficult clinical problem even under ideal conditions.

Client compliance plays a critical role in the outcome of these cases. Proper patient confinement, maintenance of the follow-up schedule, diligence in administering medications, and maintenance of bandages are all considerations when pursuing treatments. These patients can be costly to manage, and all these factors must be understood by the owner to maximize a successful outcome.

References

Bardet JF, Hohn RB, Basinger R. Open drainage and delayed autogenous cancellous bone grafting for treatment of chronic osteomyelitis in dogs and cats. J Am Vet Med Assoc 1983;183:312–317.
Lenehan T, Smith G. Management of infected tibial nonunions with sequestration in the dog. Vet Surg 1984;13:115–121.
Smith M. Orthopedic infections. In Slatter DH, ed. Textbook of small animal surgery. Philadelphia: WB Saunders, 1994.

Wedge Osteotomy Technique

Barclay Slocum & Theresa Devine Slocum

Varus or valgus deviation of the femur, tibia, humerus, or radius and ulna has a dramatic impact on the health of the joints within the limb. The greatest disorder occurs on the portion of the joint of the lesser curvature of the deviation because this is the articular surface under compression. The compression caused by limb deviation causes fibrillation of the cartilage, which leads to erosion of the cartilage and the onset of chronic pain. The problem with freehand methods of surgical repair is the imprecision of the osteotomy produced, as well as the inadvertent creation of devastating torsional deformities from the surgical procedure. Use of the tibial plateau leveling osteotomy jig (Slocum Enterprises, Eugene, OR) provides a simple, straightforward method of performing both an opening wedge osteotomy and a closing wedge osteotomy precisely.

Method of Opening Wedge Osteotomy

Cuneiform osteotomy in the frontal plane using the tibial plateau osteotomy jig prevents the introduction of torsional deformities into the surgical procedure. Preoperatively, the angle of varus or valgus deformity is measured from the anteroposterior radiograph (Fig. 48.36A). A wedge necessary for correcting the angular deviation is drawn on the radiograph, and the distance between where the lines cross the cortex is measured (Fig. 48.36B, d). This distance is the amount to be used for the opening wedge at the operating table.

An eighth-inch threaded pin is placed perpendicular to the frontal plane through the jig pin holes (Fig. 48.36C, p) and into the bone both proximal and distal to the osteotomy site. The osteotomy, consisting of one cut, is made in the bone. A spacer (Fig. 48.36C, s) is placed to maintain the predetermined amount of the opening wedge. The leveling arm of the jig (Fig. 48.36D, la) is positioned over the osteotomy, and the leveling screw (Fig. 48.36E, ls) is used to match the cortices in the frontal plane. A plate (Fig. 48.36E, f) is applied to the bone in the sagittal plane with the osteotomy in the separated position. The spacer is removed, and a cancellous bone graft is placed in the open wedge (Fig. 48.36E, b).

Method of Closing Wedge Osteotomy

The preoperative measurement from the anteroposterior radiograph is performed as described for the opening wedge osteotomy. Preoperatively, the angle of varus or valgus deformity is determined from the radiograph (Fig. 48.37A). A wedge of the angle necessary to correct the deviation is drawn on the radiograph. The distance of the wedge on the cortex is measured (Fig. 48.37B, d). This is the amount of the wedge to be removed at the operating table.

An eighth-inch threaded pin is placed through the jig pin holes (Fig. 48.37C, p) and into the bone perpendicular to the frontal plane both proximal and distal to the osteotomy site. The closing wedge osteotomy technique consists of two cuts to form a wedge in the bone, which is removed to correct the angular deviation. The first osteotomy cut is started in the bone (Fig. 48.37C, O₁), perpendicular to the frontal plane, but it is not completed through the back cortex. A stainless steel ruler is placed in the kerf. A second osteotomy is made in the bone perpendicular to the frontal plane (Fig. 48.37C, O₂), but again, it is only three-quarters completed. A second ruler placed in the kerf confirms the accuracy of the plane of the cut and the distance of the wedge (Fig. 48.37C, d). The saw blade replaces the ruler in the first osteotomy kerf, and the cut is completed through the back cortex. The second osteotomy is similarly completed. The wedge is removed. The leveling arm of the jig (Fig. 48.37D, la) is positioned over the osteotomy site, and the leveling screw (Fig. 48.37E, ls) is used to match the cortices in the frontal plane. A plate (Fig. 48.37E, f) is applied to the bone in the sagittal plane with the osteotomy in the compressed closed position. Cancellous bone graft is optionally applied to the osteotomy site.

The opening wedge osteotomy and closing wedge osteotomy are effective methods of correcting varus and valgus deviations of the long bones. The use of the tibial plateau leveling osteotomy jig allows for ease in maintaining alignment of the bone segments in the frontal plane. Because large muscle groups such as the quadriceps must be retracted to attain the necessary surgical exposure, distortion at the osteotomy in the sagittal plane (recurvatum) is controlled by the leveling screw. Thus, the problem of the creation of iatrogenic torsion at the operating table is eliminated. By simplifying the osteotomy procedure, the surgeon's focus can be directed to accurate plate application with the confidence of a precise correction of the deformity.

49

BONE GRAFTING PRINCIPLES AND TECHNIQUES

Bone Grafting Principles

Kenneth R. Sinibaldi

Bone grafting has become commonplace in most small animal fracture repairs. The use of these techniques can give the surgeon an advantage, especially in highly comminuted fractures or those fractures with large amounts of bone loss, and it is often the determining factor in success (healing) or failure (nonunion) of the repair. The most common grafts are cancellous, cortical, and corticocancellous bone.

Autogenous cancellous bone is the most common bone graft used in fracture repair. It is readily available and is easily harvested, but it lacks mechanical strength. Cortical allograft is not as commonly used, but it has specific indications, especially when mechanical strength is needed.

The purpose of this section is to discuss the clinical aspects of bone grafting principles, so the veterinary surgeon can use and understand these techniques for application in everyday practice. The principles, physiology, types, indications, and contraindications are discussed, as well as the theory of their use.

Types of Bone Grafts

Bone grafts are described based on their origin. An *autograft* is bone transferred from a donor site to a recipient site in the same individual. This type of graft is the most desirable because it is most compatible with the host immune system. An *allograft* is bone transferred from one individual to another individual of the same species. This type of graft elicits a greater immune response because of foreign cellular antigens of the allograft and the reaction of the host immune system. Allografts can also be considered *alloimplants* because they are a nonviable material (dead bone), and, by definition, the term *implant* refers to any nonviable material placed in the body (1). A *xenograft* is bone of one species transferred to an individual of a different species and is not commonly used in veterinary medicine.

Bone grafts are also described based on their composition. Cancellous bone, which is mostly cellular trabecular bone, cortical bone, and corticocancellous bone, which is a combination of the two, are the most commonly used. An allograft or alloimplant used with fresh cancellous bone is termed a *composite* graft (1). A graft made up of bone and articular cartilage is termed an *osteochondral* graft. *Vascularized autografts* and *allografts* are bone grafts harvested with their blood supply intact and require vascular anastomosis at the time of implantation.

Bone grafts can be harvested fresh and used immediately, or they can be preserved by freezing, freeze-drying, chemical preservation, irradiation, or autoclaving. Because cell death occurs with these preservation techniques, sterility in handling the graft material is important.

Function of Bone Grafts

Bone grafts function as a source for osteogenesis, osteoinduction, osteoconduction, and mechanical support. These functions vary with the different types of grafts.

Osteogenesis, or the formation of bone, can be derived from cells that survive a transfer, as in a fresh autogenous cancellous graft (2, 3), or from pluripotential cells of the host (4). Cancellous bone has a much greater surface area because of its "spongy" structure, which allows for a much greater source of cells for bone formation. Cortical allografts or alloimplants have undergone preservation and have no potential for viable surface cells to stimulate osteogenesis. Osteoinduction is the process by which host mesenchymal cells differentiate and regional cells dedifferentiate to form bone. This process is controlled by certain bioactive factors such as bone morphogenic protein (5), cytokines (6), interleukin-1 (6, 7), prostaglandin-E (PGE) (8), transforming growth factor-β (9, 10), platelet-derived growth factor (11), and PGE$_2$ (12). These factors stimulate osteoblasts, osteoclasts, endothelial cells, fibroblasts, and other cells to perform various tasks in the production of new bone (8, 13–15). Bone grafts are osteoconductive in that they provide a template or scaffolds for ingrowth of new host bone (16). This process is characterized by ingrowth of capillaries, perivascular tissue, and osteoprogenator cells from the recipient bed that leads to bone formation.

Bone Healing

All these functions of the graft and host lead to bone healing. Distinct phases of bone healing are associated with bone grafts. Healing of both autogenous cancellous and cortical allografts is essentially the same, but some differences exist.

Healing of autogenous cancellous bone involves hematoma formation and an inflammatory response resulting from the surgical procedure and some cell death. Vascular buds invade the graft, along with plasma cells, lymphocytes, and monocytes (17, 18). As vascularization continues, trabecular bone is lined by osteogenic cells derived from mesenchymal cell differentiation. Osteoblasts deposit osteoid along trabecular cores of dead bone and eventually become mineralized to form bone. Osteoclast activity begins as cores of necrotic bone are resorbed (17). At the same time, hematopoietic bone marrow elements accumulate within the remodeled graft. Once the graft is completely resorbed, the new host bone is remodeled into cortical bone in response to mechanical forces placed on the graft (17, 18). This osteoconductive phase can last up to several months. The final phase involves the mechanical strengthening of the graft. In the healing of autogenous cancellous bone, in which resorption and replacement are rapid, the final phase usually does not occur (17). Nonviable and nonabsorbed graft materials, along with natural stress from weightbearing, add to the mechanical strength of the graft.

Cortical allograft healing responds and stimulates the host in a fashion similar to that of autogenous cancellous bone. The entire process takes much longer because of the dense structure of cortical bone (17).

The host immune system can be sensitized to donor antigens, which may stimulate a humeral cellular response that slows incorporation (1). Cortical allograft incorporation also differs from autogenous cancellous bone in that initial repair is due to osteoclasts rather than to osteoblasts (19). Resorption is greater at 2 weeks after transplantation than resorption of normal bone. This increases up to the sixth week and gradually declines to normal levels within a year (19). Resorption of the graft and replacement by host bone begin at the host–graft interface and move toward the center of the graft, with marked proliferation of periosteal and endosteal bone covering the graft surfaces (20). This process can take years, depending on the length of the graft. Biopsy specimens taken at the center of long allografts at 45.5 months after implantation showed graft bone still present (20). As this process continues, mechanical strength is added to the graft.

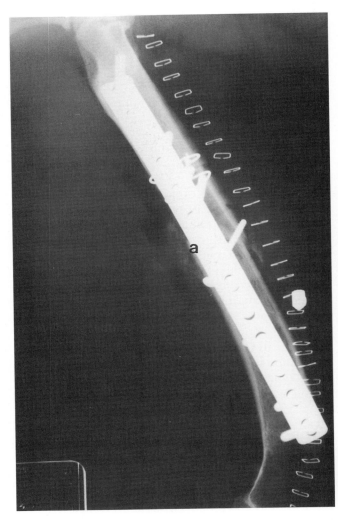

Fig. 49.1. Postoperative radiograph of a fractured femur repaired with a plate and autogenous cancellous bone (*a*) placed over fracture lines.

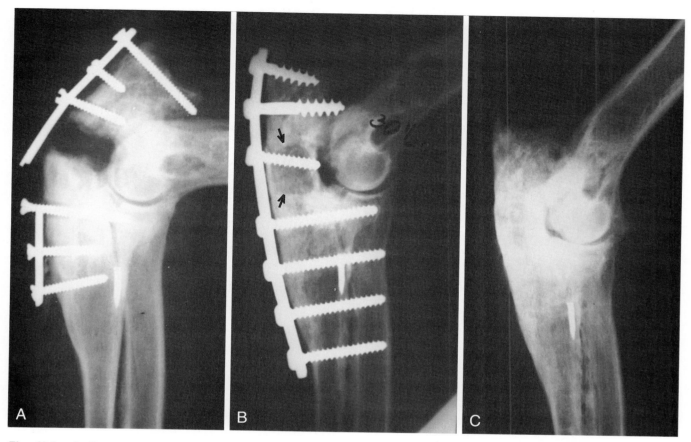

Fig. 49.2. **A.** Delayed union of the ulna. **B.** Fracture repaired with an allograft showing progressive healing with remodeling and incorporation of the allograft (*arrows*). **C.** Healed fracture 5 years postoperatively with establishment of cortices and a medullary canal.

The presence of dead bone matrix from the graft interspersed with interstitial lamellar and host osteons affords strength to the bone (19).

Clinical monitoring of bone healing can be evaluated radiographically. With autogenous cancellous grafts, the postoperative radiographs show the area grafted as cancellous bone (Fig. 49.1). Radiographs obtained 2 to 3 weeks postoperatively may show a slightly increased density or less density, depending on the host response, with deposition of new bone or resorption of necrotic bone. The graft eventually is resorbed with host cortical bone. This process can occur within 3 to 4 weeks in young patients and in 8 to 12 weeks in older patients. Usually, autogenous cancellous grafts reach their maximal clinical effect at 4 to 6 weeks. Radiographically, the increased bone density can be seen at the new host cortical bone with remodeling and reestablishment of a medullary canal.

With cortical allografts, initially the allograft can be seen easily on postoperative radiographs (Fig. 49.2). Healing begins at the host–graft interfaces. Between 4 and 8 weeks, the host–graft interface starts to demonstrate remodeling, with loss of density mostly on the

host side. The gradual incorporation of the graft varies and can take from 9 to 57 weeks, with a mean of 25 weeks (20). As this progresses, the density of the allograft decreases initially, and one sees a gradual transition of host cortical bone and allograft, with the cortex eventually regaining its density. The radiographic appearance of healing should not be mistaken for complete incorporation of the graft, which can take years to be completed. With such a long healing time, these grafts must be stabilized with rigid internal fixation to achieve success.

Autogenous Cancellous Bone

Autogenous cancellous bone grafting is indicated when early production of bone and rapid healing is desired. Any fracture repair benefits from cancellous bone grafting, whether applied to the fracture line or to fill any defects or areas of bone loss. Highly comminuted fractures (Fig. 49.3) and fractures with avascular segments and bone loss are the most common indications. Bone defects treated by curettage, such as bone cysts and benign tumors, can be filled with autogenous

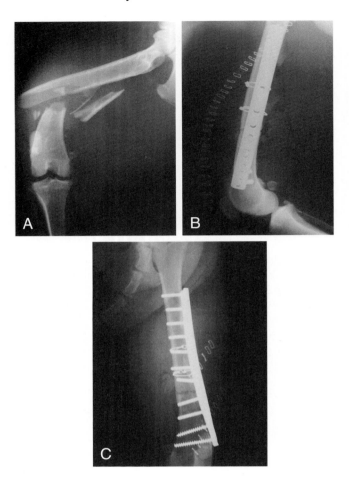

Fig. 49.3. **A.** Comminuted fracture of a femur. **B** and **C.** Fracture repaired with a plate and autogenous cancellous bone graft.

cancellous bone. Healing of nonunions, especially avascular nonunions, can be enhanced with autogenous cancellous bone. Autogenous cancellous bone has been used successfully in the treatment of osteomyelitis (21). Autogenous cancellous bone is indicated in arthrodesis of any joint and is useful in the healing of screw holes left empty by plate removal (22).

Cortical Allografts

Cortical allografts or alloimplants are used whenever mechanical strength is needed during the healing of a fracture. Highly comminuted fractures with many small fragments that cannot be reconstructed are the most common indications (see Fig. 49.3). Limb-sparing procedures in which large amounts of cortical bone involved with tumor must be removed are also indications. Bone lengthening and correction of malunions (Fig. 49.4), delayed unions, and nonunions have been reported (20). Osteomyelitis with sequestra formation can be treated with cortical allografts successfully, but this treatment requires absolutely rigid

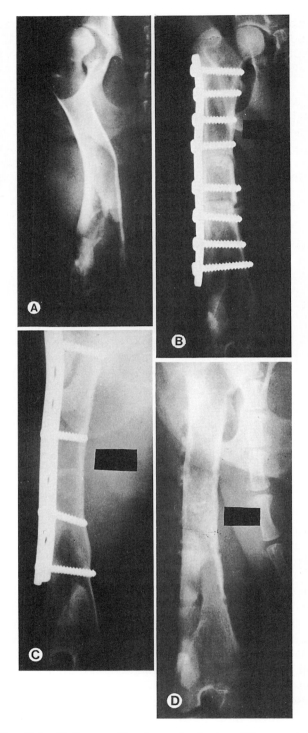

Fig. 49.4. **A.** Fractured left femur that healed with a malunion, diaphyseal valgus, some shortening, and subluxation of the femoral head. A cortical allograft was cut to lengthen the limb, and the host bone was cut to correct the valgus deformity. **B.** Notice the return to a normal joint in the hip on the postsurgical radiographs. The plate was gradually removed by first taking all but four screws (**C**) at 26 months, followed by complete removal 5 months later (**D**). (From Sinibaldi KR. Evaluation of full cortical allografts in 25 dogs. J Am Vet Med Assoc 1989;194:1570–1577.)

stabilization, meticulous flushing of the surgical site, and culture-confirmed antibiotic therapy (20). This grafting is considered a salvage procedure in lieu of amputation.

Autogenous cancellous bone can be harvested from any area in the body that has an adequate amount of trabecular bone. The proximal humerus and wing of the ilium are used most commonly. They are easy to approach and yield the greatest quantity of cancellous bone. Equipment needs are minimal. The harvesting and clinical use of autogenous cancellous bone and cortical allografts are discussed in later sections of this chapter.

References

1. Stevenson S. Bone grafting. In: Slatter DH, ed. Textbook of small animal surgery. Vol 2. Philadelphia: WB Saunders, 1993:1694–1703.
2. Bassett CAL. Clinical implications of cell function in bone grafting. Clin Orthop Rel Res 1972;87:49–59.
3. Gray JC, Elves MW. Osteogenesis in bone grafts after short term storage and topical antibiotic treatment. J. Bone Joint Surg Br 1981;63:441–445.
4. Olds RB, Sinibaldi KR, DeAngelis M, et al. Autogenous cancellous bone grafting in small animals. J Am Anim Hosp Assoc 1973;9:454–457.
5. Lindholm TS, Urist MR. A quantitative analysis of new bone formation by induction in composite grafts of bone marrow and bone matrix. Clin Orthop Rel Res 1980;150:288–300.
6. Gowen M, Murdy GR. Action of recombinant interleukin 1, interleukin 2, and interferon on bone resorption in vitro. J Immunol 1986;136:2478–2482.
7. Thompson BM, et al. Osteoblasts mediate IL-1 stimulation of bone resorption by rat osteoblasts. J Exp Med 1986;164:104–112.
8. Harvey W, Bennett A. Prostaglandins in bone resorption. Boca Raton, FL: CRC Press, 1988.
9. Centrella M, et al. Transforming growth factor β is a bifunctional regulator of replication and collagen synthesis in osteoblast-enriched cell cultures from fetal rat bone. J Biol Chem 1987;262:2869–2874.
10. Triffitt JT. Initiation and enhancement of bone formation: a review. Acta Orthop Scand 1987;58:673–684.
11. Nemeth GG, et al. Growth factors and their role in wound and fracture healing. In: Barbul A, et al. eds. Growth factors and other aspects of wound healing: biological and clinical implications. New York: Alan R. Liss, 1988:1–17.
12. Tashjian AH, et al. PDGF stimulates bone resorption via PG-mediated mechanism. Endocrinology 1982;111:118–124.
13. Dewhurst FE, et al. Purification and partial sequence of human osteoblast activating factor: identity with interleukin 1β 1985;135:2562–2568.
14. Gowen M, et al. Stimulation of the proliferation of human bone cells in vitro by human monocyte products with IL-1 activity. J Clin Invest 1985;75:1223–1229.
15. Rifas L, et al. Macrophage-derived growth factor for osteoblast-like cells and chondrocytes. Proc Natl Acad Sci USA 1984;81:4558–4562.
16. Burwell RG. The fate of bone grafts. In: Apley AG, ed. Recent advances in orthopedics. Baltimore: Williams & Williams, 1969:115–207.
17. Burchardt H, Enneking WF. Transplantation of bone. Surg Clin North Am 1978;58:403–427.
18. Heiple KG, Goldberg VM, Powell AE, et al. Biology of cancellous bone grafts. Orthop Clin North Am 1987;18:179–185.
19. Enneking WF, et al. Physical and biological aspects of repair in dog cortical bone transplants. J Bone Joint Surg Am 1975;57:237–252.
20. Sinibaldi KR. Evaluation of full cortical allografts in 25 dogs. J Am Vet Med Assoc 1989;194:1570–1577.
21. Olds RB, Sinibaldi KR, DeAngelis M, et al. Autogenous cancellous bone grafting in problem orthopedic cases. J Am Anim Hosp Assoc 1973;9:430–435.
22. Lesser AS. Cancellous bone grafting at plate removal to counteract stress protection. J Am Vet Med Assoc 1986;189:696–699.

Cortical Allograft: Harvest and Application

Kenneth R. Sinibaldi

The procurement of cortical allografts begins with proper donor selection. Donors should be mature, healthy animals, preferably between 1.5 and 8 years of age, with no preexisting neoplastic, metabolic, bacterial, or viral diseases. Immature donors have bones that may be brittle and less developed than older donors, and this factor may cause problems during implantation with stability (screw purchase).

Although allografts can be harvested from dead donors and then sterilized with ethylene oxide (1), live harvesting and preservation are more practical and are preferred. Preserved allografts are preferred over fresh allografts because fresh allografts have unaltered cellular antigens, whereas freezing alters cellular antigenicity (2). Absolute aseptic surgical technique is required. All donors should be prepared as for any standard surgical orthopedic procedure, with proper aseptic scrubbing and draping.

Donors are placed under general anesthesia, and standard approaches to the long bones are used. The bone should be exposed from metaphysis to metaphysis by removing as much of the soft tissues (muscle and periosteum) as possible. An oscillating bone saw is used to cut the bone. This saw should be cooled with liquid during cutting. After the bone is removed, it is placed in a solution of lactated Ringer's or saline with gentamicin sulfate added. This is temporary before final preparation of the graft. Once all donor graft has been harvested, euthanasia is performed on the donor.

The grafts are then stripped of all remaining soft tissue attachments, and the medullary contents are removed. A sharp periosteal elevator or scalpel blade works best for stripping, whereas a bone curette works best for removal of medullary contents. The medullary cavity should be flushed out with lactated Ringer's or saline solution. Once the graft is clean, it can be cut into proximal, middle, and distal thirds, halved or maintained in its full length. The graft's medullary cavity is cultured for aerobic and anaerobic organisms. The graft is then placed in a suitable glass jar that has been autoclaved previously and covered. Each jar with the graft should be marked, indicating left or right, with the name of the bone, segment of bone, date of harvesting, and donor identification. The jar and graft are then immediately placed in a household freezer at a temperature of −20°C. Any temperature warmer than this leads to improper freezing and possible autolysis. These grafts can be held safely for 1 year. Ethylene oxide and freeze-drying are other methods of preparation (1, 3–6). Although these methods are satisfactory, they are more involved technically and are not practical for the general practitioner.

The most common indication for use of cortical allograft is replacement of bone in patients with highly comminuted fractures (Fig. 49.5). Other indications are correction of nonunions, delayed unions, and mal-

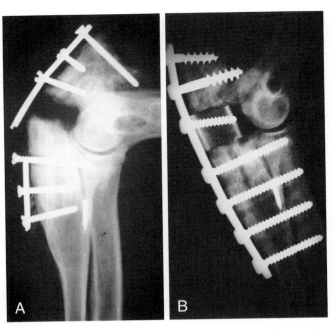

Fig. 49.6. **A.** Fractured ulna with a broken plate and nonunion of 2 years' duration. **B.** Fracture repaired with an allograft (femur) and plated.

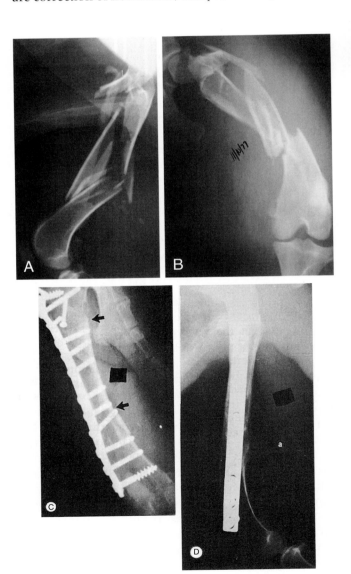

Fig. 49.5. **A** and **B.** Highly comminuted fracture of the femur. **C** and **D.** Comminuted fragments were replaced with a 9.7-cm allograft (*arrows*) and plated. (**C** and **D** from Sinibaldl KR. Evaluation of full cortical allografts in 25 dogs. J Am Vet Med Assoc 1989;194:1572.)

unions with or without bone loss, limb-sparing procedures for bone tumors, and, in selected cases, osteomyelitis with bone loss due to sequestrum formation (KR Sinibaldi, unpublished data). This last case should be considered a salvage procedure if amputation is not an option.

In preparation for surgical implantation of an allograft, radiographs of the opposite limb should be made, and bone length should be measured. An estimate of the graft length needed can be made by comparing the intact cortical segments on the lateral projection of the affected limb and subtracting this from the total length of the normal bone. A graft is then selected based on this estimate as well as by visually comparing the width of the host and graft bone. Usually, the femur is used to replace a segment of femur, but the use of other long bones should not be discouraged because the width of other bones may be adequate if a perfect match cannot be made with similar bones (Fig. 49.6).

Surgical Technique

Prophylactic antibiotics are administered at the time of induction of anesthesia and during the operation. An appropriate cancellous bone graft site is prepared. Before the surgical procedure, the cortical allograft is allowed to thaw in a bowl of lactated Ringer's or normal saline solution with gentamicin sulfate added. Strict aseptic surgical technique is required. If large segments of bone are to be removed, the surgeon must have a point of reference proximally and distally to maintain proper alignment for rotation, varus or valgus. This is best done with small Kirschner wires placed parallel to each other, one in the proximal fracture segment and one in the distal fracture segment. The fracture is exposed, and the comminuted fragments are removed. The fractured bone ends proximally and distally are cut with a bone saw perpendicular to the long axis of the bone in preparation for the cortical allograft. The allograft is cut to the correct size; the surgeon must ensure that it is perpendicular to the long axis. This cut should allow 360° of cortical contact at the host–graft interface. A dynamic compression plate is selected to allow for a minimum of five cortices (three screws) above and below the graft. Standard ASIF plating technique is used. The plate is contoured to both the host and the allograft. An alternate technique is to contour the plate preoperatively from the radiograph of the normal intact bone and to make adjustments at the time of surgery. The plate is first applied to the allograft with a minimum of two screws (four cortices) in a neutral position. The allograft is aligned to the host bone to ensure 360° cortical contact. This is not always possible, but the closer to 360°, the better the stability. Care should be taken to align the bone and to correct for any rotation, valgus or varus. The preplaced Kirschner wires and temporary cerclage wires or bone clamps aid in proper positioning. If any correction is needed for valgus or varus, the plate can be removed from the allograft, and the allograft can be recut for correction. If the correction will cause the total bone length to be shorter, a new allograft should be used. Depending on the bone, most patients can tolerate shortening of 2 to 3 cm in the limb without an impact on function. The screw holes above and below the allograft are placed in the loaded position. This maneuver results in compression at the host–graft interfaces. The remaining screws are placed in a neutral position. The entire surgical site is flushed with lactated Ringer's solution before placing a cancellous bone graft around the host–graft interfaces. Commercially prepared cancellous bone chips or powder can also be used (Veterinary Transplant Services, Seattle, WA). The surgical site is cultured for aerobic and anaerobic organisms before routine wound closure.

Postoperative care consists of an appropriate coaptation with a modified Robert Jones dressing or a padded bandage, depending on the long bone repaired, for 2 to 3 weeks. Activity should be restricted to leash activity only, and the patient should be confined to a cage or playpen turned upside down or similar confinement during this period. Antibiotics are continued for 7 to 10 days postoperatively and are adjusted or discontinued as soon as culture results are known. Radiographs are taken at 3- to 4-week intervals, to follow healing and implant stability.

Decreased surgical time, stability of the fracture repair, and rapid return to function are definite benefits of this procedure. Harvesting of bone, adherence to aseptic technique, and bone plating principles may be a limitation, depending on training and surgical experience. The added cost of proper surgical equipment and the time spent to set up the bone bank are also possible limitations. As a general rule, infected or open fractures and metaphyseal fractures that do not allow for proper screw purchase are not indications for cortical allografts.

References

1. Johnson AL, Roe SC, Harari J. Ethylene oxide sterilization of cortical bone for bone banking: Technique and results in three dogs and one cat. Vet Surg 1986;15:49–54.
2. Friedlaender GE, Strong DM, Sell KW. Studies on the antigenicity of bone. Part I. Freeze-dried and deep-frozen bone allografts in rabbits. J Bone Joint Surg Am 1976;58:854–858.
3. Johnson AL. Principle and practical applications of cortical bone grafting techniques. Compend Contin Educ Pract Vet 1988; 10:906–913.
4. Johnson AL, Moutray M, Hoffmann WE. Effects of ethylene oxide sterilization and storage conditions on canine cortical bone harvested for banking. Vet Surg 1987;16:418–422.
5. Johnson AL, Stein LE. Morphologic comparison of healing patterns in ethylene oxide-sterilized cortical allografts and untreated control autografts in the dog. Am J Vet Res 1988;49:101–105.
6. Stevenson S. Bone grafting In: Bojrab MJ, ed. Current techniques in small animal surgery. 3rd ed. Philadelphia: Lea & Febiger, 1990.

Bone Graft Harvest From the Proximal Tibia, Proximal Humerus, and Rib

Robert G. Roy

Selecting a donor site for harvesting autogenous bone for grafting depends on factors particular to the recipient site and the patient's status and concurrent medical problems. Consideration must be given to the type and quantity of bone graft needed for a specific application, as well as to patient morbidity associated with autogenous bone harvest. Multiple musculoskeletal injuries may influence the choice of sites for autogenous bone harvest. In addition, the potential problems of bone harvest in compromised patients must be considered.

A patient's position on the operating table during repair of an orthopedic injury is also considered when choosing a bone harvest site. In most dogs and cats, quantities of cancellous bone sufficient for most applications can be harvested from the humerus and tibia. Cancellous bone collection from these sites is technically simple and usually is associated with only mild to moderate postoperative morbidity. Corticocancellous bone for strut or onlay grafting can be harvested from the rib and ilial crest. However, donor site morbidity may be significantly greater than with harvest sites from the appendicular skeleton. The following describes the method of bone graft harvest from the tibia, humerus, and rib.

The largest reservoir of tibial cancellous bone is located within the proximal metaphysis. However, the triangular shape, in the coronal plane, of the proximal metaphysis necessitates placing the skin incision over the caudal half of the bone. Additionally, the medial approach is preferred because of the lateral location of the extensor muscles of the hock and digits. Therefore, a medial skin incision is made approximately two-thirds of the metaphyseal width caudal to the tibial crest and is centered just distal to the level of the tibial tuberosity. The approach requires cutting through the crural fascia, which is the confluence of the combined tendons of the gracilis, semimembranosus, and caudal belly of the sartorius muscles. The edges of the fascia are retracted, and the periosteum is elevated. An appropriately placed incision avoids damage to the distal insertion of the medial collateral ligament of the stifle. Cortical penetration can be performed using a drill bit or Steinmann pin, and a hole large enough to accommodate an appropriately sized curette should be made. The curette is then used to harvest the cancellous bone, which is appropriately stored (e.g., in a bloody sponge or sterile bowl) until used. Overzealous use of a curette during bone harvest may compromise the subchondral bone or the lateral tibial cortex, particularly cranially within the thin tibial crest. Once the bone has been harvested, routine closure of the soft tissues may be performed.

A greater amount of cancellous bone can be harvested from the humerus compared with the tibia. The mostly tubular shape of the proximal humeral metaphysis contains a large amount of cancellous bone. Although this structure is covered by many heavy muscles of the shoulder, proper incision placement allows easy access to the humeral cortex. A craniolateral skin incision is centered approximately one-third to one-half the distance from the greater tubercle to the deltoid tuberosity, and just cranial to the tricipital line. During the approach, the cranial edge of the acromial head of the deltoideus muscle and the caudal edge of the cleidobrachialis muscle are retracted caudally and cranially, respectively. As in harvesting bone from the tibia, the humeral cortex may be drilled with a standard drill bit or Steinmann pin, and cancellous bone can be harvested with a curette. Similar to harvesting cancellous bone from the tibia, overzealous use of the curette may compromise the subchondral bone or the medial humeral cortex. Soft tissue closure is routine.

The rib may be used when corticocancellous bone is needed for grafting. Rib bone is versatile and may be used as a single piece, split along its length or shaped to fit a particular site. Although virtually any rib seg-

ment may be used, the easiest access and greatest yield are available from the distal one-third of the sixth through tenth ribs, proximal to the costal cartilage. In addition, harvesting an entire rib supplies a large quantity of bone and results in little or no long-term consequences. Short segments of bone from adjacent ribs may be harvested; however, collecting more than three consecutive rib segments increases patient morbidity.

Morbidity may be high with rib harvest, and precautions must be taken in anticipation of complications associated with penetration of the pleural space. In addition, pain associated with the bone harvest site is frequently greater than that seen with bone harvest from the appendicular skeleton. To harvest the bone, an appropriate rib is selected, and the soft tissues are incised over it. Depending on the rib selected, several different muscles may be encountered including the latissimus dorsi, external abdominal oblique, scalenus medius, and serratus ventralis muscles. These may be either reflected or elevated from the rib. In most situations, the latissimus dorsi muscle can be reflected dorsally. If more exposure is needed, then it too may be incised; however, this incision usually increases postoperative pain. An incision is made in the rib periosteum, which is elevated from all sides of the desired segment. The bone is then excised at the costochondral junction and proximally for the needed length. An oscillating saw, bone scissors, or Gigli wire may be used to cut the rib. Rib periosteum is then apposed, and overlying soft tissues are routinely closed. The pleural space is commonly violated, and positive-pressure ventilation must be initiated during bone harvest. After rib collection, a thoracic catheter is placed, and careful closure of the overlying soft tissues is performed to avoid continued air leakage into the thoracic cavity. Postoperatively, a chest wrap may be applied to help seal tissue planes and to ease discomfort. Postoperative management including the use of analgesics and oxygen therapy should be consistent with the principles applicable to thoracotomy patients.

Bone Graft Harvest: Wing of the Ilium

Barclay Slocum & Theresa Devine Slocum

Bone graft from the wing of the ilium is plentiful in volume (12-mL syringe case loose pack per 50-lb dog) and has both corticocancellous and cancellous properties. The corticocancellous strips are pliable and can be molded to conform to the shape of the recipient graft site.

Procedure

The patient is placed in lateral recumbency. An area 3 cm cranial to the wing of the ilium to the greater trochanter and 3 cm dorsal to the wing of the ilium distally to the third trochanter is prepared for surgery. A headlight is useful to the surgeon to help visualize the harvest of the graft.

A 4-cm incision is made from the cranial border of the wing of the ilium, equidistant from the dorsal and ventral borders of the wing, in a caudal direction toward the greater trochanter. The fat and fibrous covering of the middle gluteal muscle are incised with sharp dissection. A Langenbeck periosteal elevator is used to penetrate the middle gluteal muscle at the cranial limit of the ilium and to elevate subperiosteally and undermine the middle gluteal muscle from the ilium for 8 cm toward the greater trochanter. With the tip of the elevator maintaining contact with the ilium, the handle of the elevator is raised to a position perpendicular to the ilium that causes the fibers of the middle gluteal muscles to separate, parallel to the incision. This gives access to the ilium while preventing damage to the cranial gluteal nerve. A Gelpi retractor is used to maintain an opening in the access window in the middle gluteal muscle. The middle and deep gluteal muscles are elevated from the wing and cranial body of the ilium without disrupting the marginal attachments of gluteal muscle mass (Fig. 49.7).

A sharp, curved $\frac{3}{8}$-inch gouge is used to penetrate the lateral cortex at the cranial wing of the ilium and to cut a 5-mm wide corticocancellous strip graft 8 cm in length, parallel to the original skin incision. The harvest is done without the aid of a mallet, which may cause deep penetration of the ilium, rather than the 3-mm thick corticocancellous graft obtained by the gouge. The remaining strip grafts are taken with ease from the lateral cortex. The osteonal pattern of the strips is parallel to the long axis of the strip graft, to provide graft pliability. The ventral portion of the ilial wing is thin and has only corticocancellous bone, whereas the dorsal wing has abundant cancellous bone beneath the lateral cortex. Closure of the fibrous covering of the middle gluteal muscle, subcutaneous fascia, and skin is direct.

Harvesting bone graft from the adolescent patient is done with great ease and speed, but additional effort is required in older patients because the hardness and brittleness of the lateral cortex increases with age. Use of a mallet to harvest graft is discouraged because of the high potential for damage to the ilium during the procedure. In over 100 clinical cases, only 1 nondisplaced fracture of the ilium was created postoperatively, and it healed without incident. The wing of the ilium for corticocancellous bone graft is highly recommended for ease of harvest and high quantity of bone.

Bone Graft Harvest: Distal Femoral Condyles

Barclay Slocum & Theresa Devine Slocum

The distal femur is an excellent source of cancellous bone for a bone graft. The approach can be made from either the medial or the lateral side. More than adequate graft can be obtained for most purposes in the dog, with minimal time and low tissue morbidity. The cat has little bone graft available at this site.

Surgical Procedure

The description of this procedure applies to either the medial or lateral aspect of the stifle. The distal femur is shaved, prepared, and draped for surgery. A 1.5-cm incision is made halfway between the fabella and the proximal patella, parallel to the margin of the patella. The incision is made from the skin to bone on the medial or lateral aspect of the femoral condyle. A Gelpi retractor is used to open the incision and to maintain exposure.

The exposure reveals the stifle at the caudal margin of the reflection of the joint capsule. The cortex is perforated with an appropriately sized trocar-tip Steinmann pin. A curette is used to scoop cancellous bone from the opening in the cortex. Approximately 5 to 7 mL of cancellous bone may be recovered from this site (Fig. 49.8).

Closure is simple and direct. A single mattress suture is placed in the synovium to cover the cortical

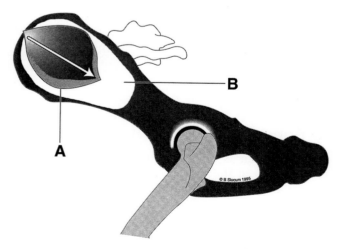

Fig. 49.7. Bone graft from the wing of the ilium is taken through an incision (A) by separating the middle gluteal muscle fibers in line with the *white arrow* and harvesting the corticocancellous bone from the ilial wing (B).

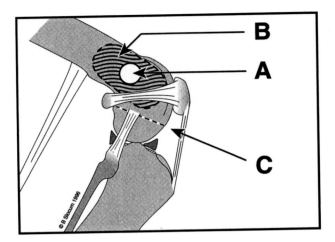

Fig. 49.8. A Steinmann pin is used to perforate the lateral cortex of the distal femur at the level of the proximal trochlea (*A*). A curette is used to remove cancellous bone (*B*). The surgeon must avoid perforating the cortex, subchondral bone, or intercondylar shelf (*C*).

perforation, to arrest hemorrhage. Three or four simple interrupted sutures are used to close the parapatellar fibrocartilage. The skin is closed with subcuticular sutures.

High-quality cancellous bone may be obtained from this location in adequate quantities in most dogs. Approximately 1 cm can be obtained per 10 lb body weight. However, the cat has little bone graft available at this site. In over 500 consecutive cancellous bone graft harvests from this site, the minor complications of small seroma formation or partial skin dehiscence were occasionally encountered. The harvesting of bone graft from the distal femur should not be coincident with surgical procedures such as a trochlear recession, which conflict with the area of graft harvest.

Banked Allogeneic Bone Grafts: An Overview of Current Theory and Uses

Helen Newman-Gage

Historical Perspective on the Development of Tissue Banking

The earliest recorded use of bone in transplantation describes the repair of a cranial defect in a soldier with canine calvarial bone. As the history is reported, religious elders subsequently threatened the surgeon with excommunication unless the canine bone was removed. When the surgeon attempted to retrieve the bone graft, it could not be removed because it had fused into place (1). The earliest published record of the transplant of human frozen allograft was presented by MacEwen in 1881, who reported the successful transplantation of a humeral shaft in a child with osteomyelitis. This history documents the early development of the concept of replacing damaged or defective bone with transplantation, and it presaged the development of the ideas that would culminate in orthopedic transplantation and tissue banking today.

In the last half-century, human bone banking has developed substantially to support the growing need for bone graft material and to foster development of new surgical options for patients. These new directions include limb-salvage procedures for tumor or trauma, prosthetic joint revisions, periodontic augmentation, and plastic surgery, among others. By 1992, the United States had more than 300 human allograft bone banks, providing bone grafts for more than 280,000 surgical procedures per year (2). Nearly 25 years ago, the American Association of Tissue Banks emerged as a forum for development of tissue bank activities, and its efforts have promulgated research, legislation, a tissue bank accreditation program, and the establishment of standards for tissue banking. The standards are intended to provide a framework for safety and consistency in basic requirements for donor screening, tissue processing, preservation, distribution, and tracing (3). Although most accredited tissue banks provide musculoskeletal tissues, many also provide allograft skin and corneas, and some also provide reproductive tissues, allograft heart valves, and research tissues.

With development of our basic understanding of the biology of bone repair and the advent of tissue banks capable of providing safe and needed allografts, surgeons have widely adapted bone grafting procedures to the many needs of patients and surgeons. Tissue banks and surgeons, in concert, have fueled the broadening of the spectrum of options available for surgical patients.

Fundamental Biology of Bone Transplantation

Autograft bone is considered ideal for orthopedic repair because of the rapidity of incorporation and the lack of concern regarding histocompatibility and disease transmission; however, allograft is often desirable for numerous reasons. The limited volume, size, or type of autologous bone and the potential additional morbidity of autologous sites, including infection, fracture, increased anesthesia time, disruption of normal structures, bleeding, and additional pain, can offset the drawbacks of bone allografts. Furthermore, for many surgical procedures, no appropriate autologous bone graft material is available, or what is available is less suitable than allograft. In addition to the obvious lack of a good substitute for massive allografts (e.g., distal femur or radius), a veterinary example may be illustrative: the cancellous bone commonly available from the canine proximal humerus is much less dense than the cancellous bone available from the canine distal femur or proximal tibia, and for some applications, the structural integrity of the cancellous allograft may be important. Ultimately, for many cases, allograft material provides suitable, biologically and mechanically functional graft material.

Substantial research efforts have begun to elucidate mechanisms of bone healing, the effect of the immune response, the role of exogenous growth factors, and other factors intrinsic to the use of bone material as a substitute for autografts (4). Three distinct mechanisms of bone healing have been described. These are osteogenesis, osteoconduction, and osteoinduction.

Osteogenesis

With the transfer of viable osteocytes, osteoblasts, and other cells in autografts, osteogenesis can occur rapidly. This mechanism for bone repair pertains primarily to cancellous autografts because they can revascularize more rapidly than cortical autografts and their repair appears to be rapidly effected by the transferred intrinsic osteoclasts and osteoblasts. Both autologous and allogeneic cancellous bone grafts are normally completely incorporated within 1 year. With cortical autografts, although one sees some evidence of osteogenesis, much of the viable autograft becomes necrotic, ostensibly as a result of interruption of the vasculature, and it is subjected to healing by "creeping substitution" or osteoconduction (5).

Osteoconduction

Osteoconduction refers to the process whereby implanted material (e.g., autograft, allograft, synthetic) provides a scaffolding for inward migration of osteoclasts, osteoblasts, and ingrowth of vasculature. With allograft or autograft bone and some synthetic implants as the osteoconductive implant material, this scaffolding is biodegradable. For cortical bone grafts, in contrast to cancellous grafts, evidence suggests that the osteoconductive process continually proceeds over the course of many years (6). Large cortical grafts of either allogeneic or autogenous bone may never be replaced completely with new host bone. This resorption of old bone and redistribution of new bone is the normal metabolic process for maintenance of bone, and Wolff's law describes the remodeling of intact bone based on the compressive load borne by the bone. This underscores the importance of good compressive fixation for cortical allografts. To stimulate the continual remodeling of a cortical bone graft, it follows that, in addition to having adequate vascular access and ingress of viable cells, bone must bear some compressive load.

Osteoinduction

Mineralized bone grafts (autologous or allogeneic) are remodeled at first by recruitment of osteoclasts and stimulation of bone-resorptive activity. Mesenchymal cells, potentially derived from the bone marrow, are stimulated by the subsequently exposed growth factors within the matrix to proliferate and differentiate into chondroblasts, and by day 10 osteoblasts can be found (6). These cells actively produce matrix that subsequently becomes mineralized. This *induction* of chondroblastic proliferation and matrix production with mineralization of the matrix is osteoinduction (endochondral ossification).

Investigators have suggested that a potential drawback for some allogeneic bone grafts is the lack of transferred viable osteocytes and the subsequent lack of immediate osteogenesis. Several studies, however, indicate that mesenchymal cells for osteogenesis are derived from marrow and that addition of autologous marrow to allograft preparations provides a source of osteogenic progenitor cells (7–10). As a result, many surgeons mix autologous marrow with allogeneic grafts for this purpose.

The interactive cellular cascade of inward migration and activation of osteoclast activity and then, ultimately, generation of new bone by osteoblast activity in transplanted mineralized bone autografts or allografts is analogous to that found with simple fracture wound healing. Investigators have postulated that exposure of the mineral-containing bone matrix, normally covered with a lining layer of osteoblasts, stimulates ingress and activation of the osteoclastic resorptive cells (11).

Unlike mineralized bone, when demineralized bone is implanted, the process of osteoinduction occurs directly, without recruitment of osteoclasts and without stimulation of the process of resorption (12, 13). When bone is demineralized by exposure to acid, not only mineral but acid-soluble constituents are lost from the matrix. Osteocalcin, an acid-soluble matrix component, has a significant role in recruitment and stimulation of osteoclast activity (14). With the diminished availability of osteocalcin, resorption is not stimulated by demineralized bone grafts. Furthermore, numerous acid-resistant growth factors are present in bone matrix (bone morphogenic proteins, and others); these factors are exposed in the demineralized bone matrix and activate the endochondral osteoinductive process (15, 16). The activity and effectiveness of these endogenous matrix bone morphogenic proteins do not require viable cells of donor origin.

Immunogenicity and Bone Processing

Bone contains some cell types that are capable of stimulating an immune response (17). Transplantation of fresh, untreated allogeneic bone stimulates a significant immune response that often results in excessive resorption and interferes with the ability of the bone to engraft. Consequently, most bone grafts are processed to reduce their antigenicity. Purging and freezing are commonly used to remove and destroy viable cells. These techniques reduce the immune-stimulatory features of bone allografts. These practices are based on the early studies by Chase and Herndon and their colleagues in the 1950s that demonstrated attenuation of the immune response to allograft bone that had been frozen (18, 19). Substantial numbers of clinical studies followed, validating this early work. Further studies have shown little effect on the compressive, torsional, or bending strength of bone that has been frozen compared with fresh bone (20, 21).

Freeze-drying (lyophilization), irradiation, and chemical treatments have also been used to decrease immunogenicity and contamination and to facilitate storage of grafts. Irradiation and postprocessing sterilization with ethylene oxide are typically used to reduce contaminating microorganisms, if the grafts are not processed aseptically. Each of these treatments has some degree of degratory effect on the bone graft. The large body of work evaluating the impacts of such treatments on the mechanical integrity and clinical outcome is beyond the scope of this chapter. Ultimately, the choice of graft type should balance the needs of the surgeon and patient with the available types of materials.

Current Clinical Uses of Allograft Bone

Because allografts are osteoconductive and osteoinductive, they have been used widely and successfully in human surgical procedures requiring arthrodesis, arthroplasty, bone replacement, augmentation, and segmental repair (4). Soft musculoskeletal (tendon and fascia) allografts are also frequently used to treat avulsion and rupture injuries. A commonly reported success rate combining all types of use of allograft bone is 85% (22). Typical features of failures include fracture, recurrence of tumor, nonunion, and infection. Success rates for simple allografts (e.g., intercalary grafts, cancellous bone chips, and blocks) are higher, whereas those for large segmental osteochondral allografts are lower.

Frozen and freeze-dried bone grafts are made available from tissue banks in many different shapes and sizes. Grafts typically available for human surgical procedures include whole bone grafts (e.g., femur, tibia, hemipelvis, rib), partial or segmental grafts (e.g., proximal femur or tibia, femur shaft segments of varying lengths, condyles), and morselized grafts (i.e., cancellous chips, corticocancellous chips, bone powder), as well as demineralized grafts and specifically shaped bone grafts (e.g., cancellous blocks, tricortical blocks, dowels, matchsticks, struts). During processing, grafts are cleaned of nonusable tissues and attachments, including the periosteum. The grafts can be cut and fashioned to specific requirements. The following sections describe the types of allografts typically used for several common indications in human surgery.

Spinal Fusions

Tissue banks routinely provide blocks and dowels for use in spinal fusions. A common procedure for cervical spinal fusion involves cutting hemicircular spaces in two adjacent cervical vertebrae using a Cloward dowel drill bit. The tissue bank prepares dense cancellous dowels from femoral condyles or the tibial plateau that fit tightly into the drilled circular space between the vertebrae. If needed, at the time of surgery, autologous dowels can also be procured from the ilium. A slightly different procedure is often used in lumbar spinal fusions. Rectangular blocks are cut from the wing of the ilium. The cancellous interior has two or three surfaces covered with a thin cortical layer (bicortical or tricortical blocks). These are placed between adjacent vertebral bodies that have had their cancellous interior exposed. The cortex lends some structural support for weightbearing, whereas the cancellous interior provides a good osteoconductive environment to promote fusion. Two or more of these grafts are packed side by side, depending on the width of the vertebral bodies, often with additional spaces filled with cancellous chips or demineralized powder. Struts or "matchsticks" are made from cortical bone and can be used as onlay grafts to bridge between vertebrae. Cortical "rings" made from femoral segmental cross sections provide a strong cortical support for spinal fusions with a medullary canal that can be packed with autogenous cancellous graft or an allogeneic dowel or cancellous chips and patient marrow. Allograft bone is frequently used across many vertebrae to correct severe congenital scoliosis or kyphosis.

Fracture Repair

Segmental shafts can be used to replace bone in severely comminuted fractures or cases of nonunion or malunion. Rigid fixation is critical for successful union when allografts are used. Hemishafts or cortical struts can be cerclaged in place as onlay support for fracture sites. These eventually fuse to the underlying cortical bone. Cancellous bone chips and demineralized powder can be used to augment osteoinduction at fracture sites, as commonly used for cases of nonunion or malunion. Struts can be used to buttress pelvic fractures. Ribs or segments of mandibular rami are used to replace severely fractured mandibles.

Replacement for Bone Loss

Allografts are commonly used to replace bone lost for many reasons (e.g., infection, trauma, tumor). Demineralized powder is used routinely in periodontics to augment alveolar ridge defects. Tumors that would ordinarily require limb amputation can be excised, and the bone segment can be replaced with allograft of matched size. Bone with malignant tumors involving the growth plate or close to the joint surface has been replaced with fresh or cryopreserved cartilage-bearing osteochondral allografts. Voids created by benign tumors and cysts can be filled with cancellous bone or demineralized bone or both. Pelvic bone lost to tumor, infection, or degenerative disease and inadequate pelvic structures secondary to congenital abnormalities have been replaced or rebuilt with allografts of many sorts, including partial-pelvis or hemipelvis allografts. Loss of bone as a result of wearing from prosthetic joint implants results in loosening of the prosthesis. Bone stock in these cases can be augmented with banked allograft. Cancellous allograft is commonly packed around prosthetic implants at wear sites, especially after total hip arthroplasty. In cases of acetabular protrusion, cortical struts and cancellous bone can be used to rebuild the deficit deep to the cup. With massive acetabular bone loss, the entire acetabulum has been replaced with allograft inset with a prosthetic implant. Proximal femurs are used regularly to repair complications related to prosthetic implants, including full proximal femoral segment replacement. Cortical strut allografts have been used to cover cortical defects or to bridge allograft–host junctions of large segmental grafts.

Musculoskeletal Soft Tissues

These tissues typically include fascia, dura, menisci, ligaments, and tendons. Cryopreserved allograft menisci with tibial bone blocks have been used to replace damaged menisci. These grafts have had limited success. Dura has been banked for transplantation in patients with dural defects. Fascia has been commonly used for hernia, pericardial, and dura repair procedures. It has also been used rolled as a ligament replacement, primarily for the anterior cruciate ligament (ACL). Although the bone–tendon–bone block from the ACL itself has been used as an allograft in the autologous site, preservation methods appear to diminish the ability of tendons to withstand strain. As a result, many orthopedic surgeons have turned to using a bone–tendon–bone graft obtained from the patella and patellar ligament with tibial bone block. This tendon is thicker and stronger than the ACL and, in human patients, performs well in its stead. Achilles' tendons with a calcaneal bone block are also used for ACL repair as well as for repair of ruptured or avulsed tendons. Smaller tendons with or without bone blocks have been used for other ruptures or avulsions (e.g., hand operations).

Miscellaneous Uses

Demineralized segments of bone (ribs, shafts) have been used in craniofacial cosmetic or restorative surgery (e.g., to sculpt the nasal bridge or zygoma). Costal cartilage has also been used for these purposes. These grafts are useful for such applications because they can be easily shaped and carved. Although tissue banks commonly provide packaged morselized bone grafts such as cancellous bone chips or demineralized powder, they also provide whole femoral heads, whole condyles or hemicondyles, and tibial plateaus, because these are often used as a source of cancellous bone stock to be milled or rongeured as needed at the time of surgery. To extend available graft material, allogeneic cancellous chips are often mixed with autologous cancellous bone to provide a fully adequate supply of graft.

Allografts encompass a wide spectrum of applications, only briefly touched on here. Applications are limited only by the inherent biology of the materials and the skill and imagination of the surgeons who apply their knowledge and technical abilities for the benefit of their patients.

Allograft tissue transplantation and tissue banking have undergone considerable development. As a result, allogeneic bone grafts have provided practitioners of human orthopedic surgery with a broad range of surgical options for their patients. Because many of these procedures were developed with the use of animal models, it seems evident that these developments in allograft transplantation could provide the same advantages for patients of veterinary general orthopedic surgeons, orthopedic oncologists, plastic surgeons, and periodontal specialists.

References

1. Haeseker B. VanMeekerin and his account of the transplantation of bone from a dog into the skull of a soldier (letter). Plast Reconstr Surg 1991;88:173–174.
2. Mowe J. Annual questionnaire of accredited tissue banks:-1992. McLean, VA: American Association of Tissue Banks, 1993.

3. Linden JV, et al., eds. American Association of Tissue Banks: standards for tissue banking. McLean, VA: American Association of Tissue Banks, 1996.

4. Friedlaender GE, Goldberg VM, eds. Bone and cartilage allografts: biology and clinical applications. American Academy of Orthopaedic Surgeons, 1991.

5. Burchardt H. The biology of bone graft repair. Clin Orthop 1983;174:28–42.

6. Goldberg VM, Stevenson S, Shaffer JW. Biology of autografts and allografts. In: Friedlaender GE, Goldberg VM, eds. Bone and cartilage allografts: biology and clinical applications. American Academy of Orthopaedic Surgeons, 1991.

7. Nade S. Osteogenesis after bone and bone marrow transplantation. Part II. The initial cellular events following transplantation of decalcified allografts of cancellous bone. Acta Orthop Scand 1977;48:572–579.

8. Ashton BA, Allen TD, Howlett CR, et al. Formation of bone and cartilage by marrow stromal cells in diffusion chambers in vivo. Clin Orthop 1980;151:294–307.

9. Wittbjer J, Palmer B, Rohlin M, et al. Osteogenetic activity in composite grafts of demineralized compact bone and marrow. Clin Orthop 1983;173:229–238.

10. Burwell RG. The function of bone marrow in the incorporation of a bone graft. Clin Orthop 1985;200:125–141.

11. Glowacki J, Lian JB. Impaired recruitment and differentiation of osteoclast progenitors by osteocalcin-depleted bone implants. Cell Growth Differ 1987;21:247–254.

12. Glowacki J, Altobelli D, Mulliken JB. Fate of mineralized and demineralized osseous implants in cranial defects. Calcif Tissue Int 1981;33:71–76.

13. Glowacki J. Cellular responses to bone-derived materials. In: Friedlaender GE, Goldberg VM, eds. Bone and cartilage allografts: biology and clinical applications. American Academy of Orthopaedic Surgeons, 1991.

14. DeFranco D, Glowacki J, Lian J. The recruitment and differentiation of bone-resorbing cells by normal and osteocalcin-deficient bone particles (letter). Calcif Tissue Int 1988;42(Suppl):A29.

15. Urist MR, Iwata H, Ceccotti PL, et al. Bone morphogenesis in implants of insoluble bone gelatin. Proc Natl Acad Sci USA 1973;70:3511–3515.

16. Reddi AH. Regulation of local differentiation of cartilage and bone by extracellular matrix: a cascade type mechanism. Prog Clin Biol Res 1982;110:261–268.

17. Horowitz M, Friedlaender GE. Immunologic aspects of bone transplantation. Orthop Clin North Am 1987;18:227–233.

18. Chase SW, Herndon CH. The fate of autogenous and homogenous bone grafts: a historical review. J Bone Joint Surg Am 1955;37:809–841.

19. Curtiss PH Jr, Powell AE, Herndon CH. Immunological factors in homogenous-bone transplantation. Part III. The inability of homogenous rabbit bone to induce circulating antibodies in rabbits. J Bone Joint Surg Am 1959;41:1482–1488.

20. Pelker RR, Friedlaender GE, Markham TC. Biomechanical properties of bone allografts. Clin Orthop 1983;174:54–57.

21. Sedlin ED. A rheologic model for cortical bone: a study of the physical properties of human femoral samples. Acta Orthop Scand Suppl 1965;36:1–77.

22. Mankin HJ, Doppelt SH, Tomford WW. Clinical experience with allograft implantation: the first ten years. Clin Orthop 1983;174:69–86.

— • 50 • —

TECHNIQUES OF FRACTURE FIXATION

Algorithms for Implant Selection for Fracture Fixation

Terry D. Braden

Figures 50.1 through 50.10 are algorithms for implant selection and treatment of fractures.

Cerclage Wiring

Randy Willer

The use of cerclage wires in fracture repair management has achieved widespread acceptance in veterinary orthopedics because of continued successful results, increased versatility, ease of application, and economic feasibility. Understanding the principles behind cerclage wiring is important to ensure successful outcomes. Many principles of cerclage wire use have remained unchanged over the past 15 years (1). When used properly, cerclage wires do not interfere with bone healing (2, 3), nor do they have detrimental effects on the bones of young growing animals (4). Fixation failure is most often caused by disobeying proper principles of cerclage wire application and failing to understand the limitations of its use with fracture management (1).

Materials and Instrumentation

Orthopedic cerclage wires should be made of 316L stainless steel and can be purchased on wire spools or as preformed loop cerclage wires. Different sizes are available, most commonly 22-, 20-, 18-, and 16-gauge diameters, or 0.64-, 0.8-, 1.0-, and 1.25-mm diameters, respectively. On rare occasions, for large giant breed dogs, larger diameter cerclage wires (1.5 mm) may be used. Sizes smaller than 0.64 mm are often too weak to counteract the forces on the fracture. Clinical judgment is required to determine the wire size necessary because the decision is based on the bone fragment size, the size of the animal, the anatomic location of its intended use, and the desired clinical goal. For example, the choice of wire size used in reconstruction of an oblique femoral fracture may differ from that chosen for an oblique metatarsal fracture in a 40-kg animal, and it also depends on whether the fracture will be additionally supported with an intramedullary pin, bone plate, external skeletal fixation, or other methods of stabilization.

Many wire tighteners are available, and the instrument chosen depends on whether a twist knot (twist cerclage) or loop knot (loop cerclage) wire is used (Fig. 50.11). I predominantly use, with good success, the Richards loop wire tightener and the similar ASIF (Association for the Study of Internal Fixation) loop wire tightener for applying loop cerclage wire and wire twisting forceps or pliers for twist cerclage wire application. Use of strain gauges on the wire tighteners is probably unnecessary because acceptable wire tension is not difficult to achieve without these devices (5, 6). Experience allows for consistent and reproducible wire tightness, but practice is mandatory.

Commercially available wire passers can be used to pass wire properly around the bone. The wire may also be pushed around the bone in a fashion similar to passing a suture needle, or it may be pulled around the bone after placing a hemostat. Applying interfragmentary wires requires a pin and hand chuck or power drill to create holes in the bone for wire placement. After loop cerclage is placed around the bone, it is

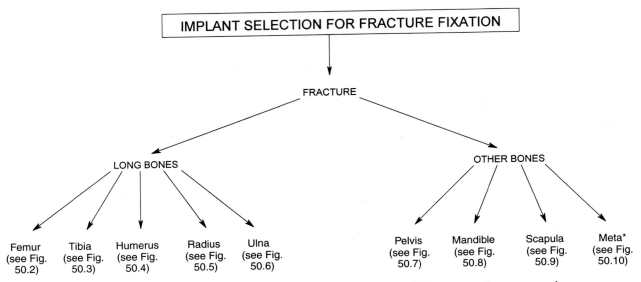

Fig. 50.1. Algorithm for implant selection for fracture fixation. *META*, metacarpal or metatarsal.

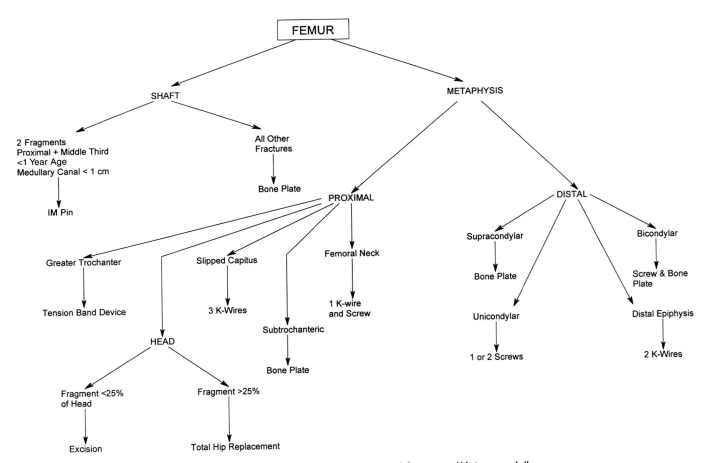

Fig. 50.2. Algorithm for treatment of femoral fractures. *IM*, intramedullary.

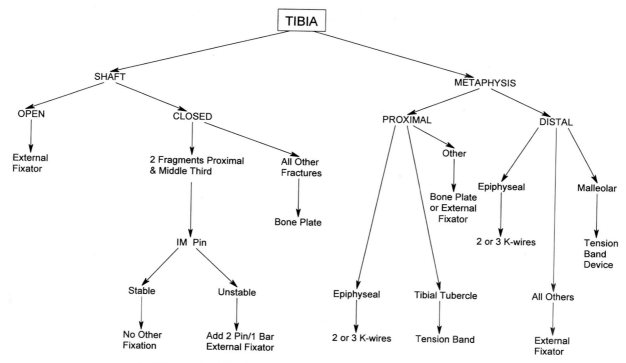

Fig. 50.3. Algorithm for treatment of tibial fractures. *IM,* intramedullary.

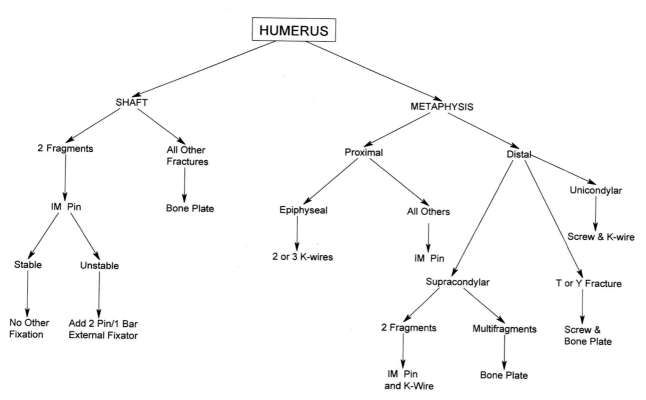

Fig. 50.4. Algorithm for treatment of humeral fractures. *IM,* intramedullary.

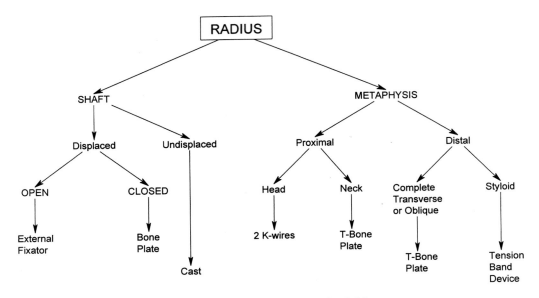

Fig. 50.5. Algorithm for treatment of radial fractures.

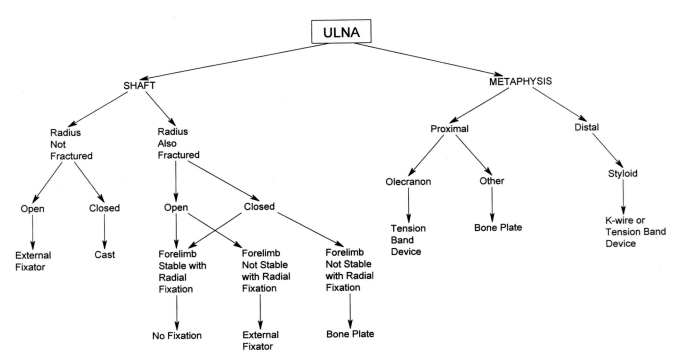

Fig. 50.6. Algorithm for treatment of ulnar fractures.

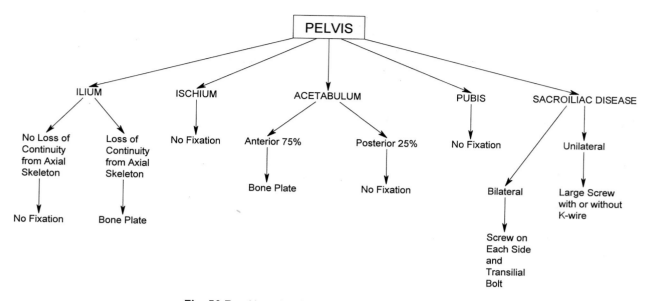

Fig. 50.7. Algorithm for treatment of pelvic fractures.

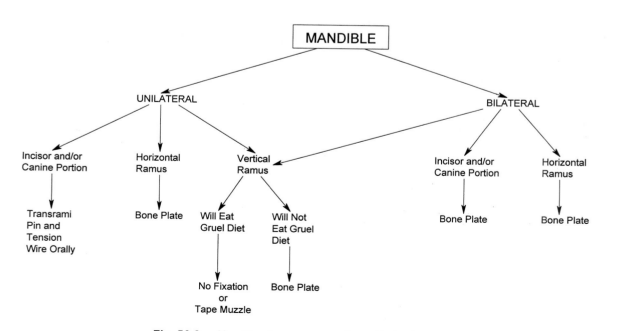

Fig. 50.8. Algorithm for treatment of mandibular fractures.

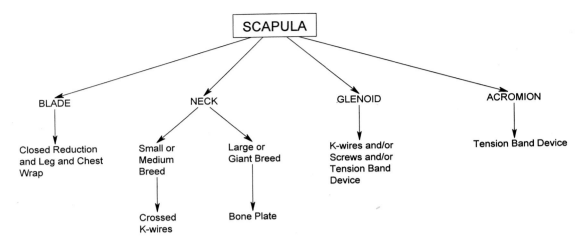

Fig. 50.9. Algorithm for treatment of scapular fractures.

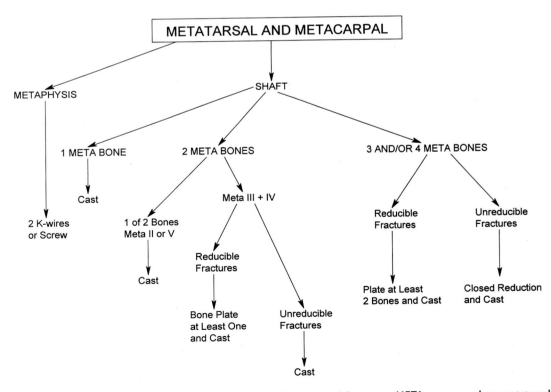

Fig. 50.10. Algorithm for treatment of metacarpal and metatarsal fractures. *META*, metacarpal or metatarsal.

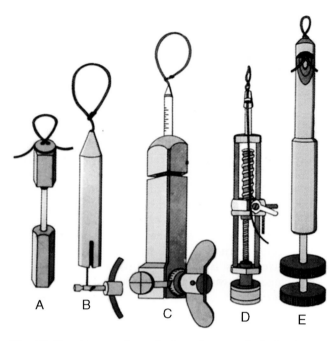

Fig. 50.11. Commonly used wire tighteners. **A.** Richards standard wire twister. **B.** Richards loop wire tightener. **C.** Osteo Systems through Richards wire tightener. **D.** Rhinelander wire tightener-twister. **E.** Bowen wire twister-cutter. **A** and **B** use loops; **C** and **D** feature strain gauges. **E** is designed to both twist and cut the wire in the same motion. Standard hardware pliers are not shown because they do not produce consistent results. (From Straw RC, Withrow SJ. Cerclage wiring. In: Bojrab MJ, ed. Current techniques in small animal surgery. 3rd ed. Philadelphia: Lea & Febiger, 1990.)

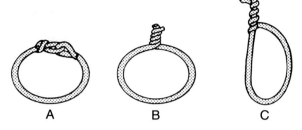

Fig. 50.12. Methods of securing a cerclage wire. **A.** A loop-knotted wire is secured by turning the wire back on itself. **B.** Twist-knotted wires should have each arm equally twisted. **C.** Slip knots should be avoided because they loosen easily and also put excessive stress on the twisted arm. (From Straw RC, Withrow SJ. Cerclage wiring. In: Bojrab MJ, ed. Current techniques in small animal surgery. 3rd ed. Philadelphia: Lea & Febiger, 1990.)

placed through the eye of the loop. The loop wire tightener is passed over the free end of the wire, and the free end of the wire is placed through the hand-held tightening device. The instrument tightens and secures the loop cerclage wire in two steps. The wire is tightened to an acceptable tension, and while tension is maintained, the wire is bent over on itself 180°. The tension on the tightening device is released and backed off, and the wire is cut. When a twist-type knot is applied, the instrument creates twisting and tension at the same time (7). The two strands of the wire should be twisted evenly to avoid creating a slip knot, which loosens easily (Fig. 50.12). When testing the knots experimentally, the loop knot develops a greater final static tension than the twist knot (5), a feature that translates into greater interfragmentary compression, but twist knot wires are more resistant to knot slippage under greater tensile loads (6). The loop knots fail by unbending and the twist knots by untwisting. The combined procedure of cutting the twisted portion and bending it over may create as much as 70% loss of tension on the wire (6). If twist knot wires are used, cutting the wire approximately at the level of the third

twist and leaving it unbent or bending it over perpendicular to the wire while applying the last twist may help to maintain tension on the wire (7). To maintain optimal tension, the twist knot can be applied by placing the twisting device approximately 1 cm from the bone, twisting the wire with equal tension on both strands after the slack is removed, and twisting until the wire breaks in the middle of the twist (between the second and third twist) (6). With this method, neither cutting the wire nor bending it is necessary. The disadvantage of this technique is that the twisted knot is left perpendicular to the bone and may irritate overlying soft tissues. The loop cerclage wire is cut after it has been bent and secured; therefore, cutting the wire does not decrease tension on the wire (7). Clinically, both methods can be used successfully. I prefer using the loop cerclage wire for ease and speed of application and greater interfragmentary compression.

General Indications and Application Principles

The use of cerclage wires has many indications. Fractured bones are subjected to forces that may displace the fracture segments. Cerclage wires may be used to stabilize and prevent nondisplaced fissures from propagating into larger displaced fragments during surgery and the healing period. Long oblique fractures or spiral fractures are optimal for full-cerclage wiring. A rule of thumb is that the length of the obliquity of the fracture should be at least twice the diameter of the diaphysis of the bone to apply full-cerclage wires (3). This rule also allows for a minimum of at least two cerclage wires to be placed and ensures adequate interfragmentary compression, whereas shear forces are amplified in short oblique fractures stabilized with a single full-

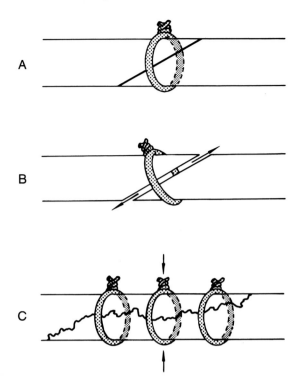

Fig. 50.13. When a short oblique fracture is encircled by a wire (**A**), compression of the wire potentiates gliding and distraction of the bone (**B**). Wiring of fractures with a longer obliquity, however, produces direct compression perpendicular (*arrows*) to the fracture line (**C**). (From Straw RC, Withrow SJ. Cerclage wiring. In: Bojrab MJ, ed. Current techniques in small animal surgery. 3rd ed. Philadelphia: Lea & Febiger, 1990.)

cerclage wire (Fig. 50.13). Short oblique or transverse fractures are best stabilized with a form of interfragmentary or hemicerclage wiring. Anatomic reconstruction of comminuted fractures can be achieved with cerclage wires. If the fragments cannot be reconstructed anatomically, cerclage wires should not be used to gather up fragments in a bundle at the fracture site (8). Cerclage wires should only be used to secure anatomically reconstructed segments rigidly. Unstable fragments bundled together with wire disrupt blood supply at the fracture site, and delayed or nonunion fracture healing may occur. If possible, placement of the full-cerclage wire should be planned such that the knot is located away from any potential interference with soft tissues or other implants to be applied such as a bone plate.

Application Techniques

Full-Cerclage Wires

Full-cerclage wires are wires placed around the entire circumference of the bone. Care must be taken to minimize the disruption of soft tissue attachments re-

sulting in transient loss of blood supply to the bone during application. Whichever instrumentation method is used for wire placement, the wire should be passed through the soft tissues and placed as close to the bone as possible (Fig. 50.14). Entrapping muscle or soft tissue between the wire and bone results in an apparently tight wire, but eventually it loosens when the tissues undergo ischemic necrosis after the surgical procedure. Elevating the periosteum to place the wire directly on the bone is not necessary (4) (Fig. 50.15).

Whichever type of full-cerclage wire (twist or loop cerclage wire) and method of application are chosen by the surgeon, the wire must be secured tightly to provide any benefit. Loose wire allows movement of the fracture segments, and their presence may impede early callus formation and revascularization of the outer cortex by soft tissue attachments.

Cerclage wire should be placed perpendicular to the long axis of the bone for maximal long-term stability. If the wire is placed obliquely to the long axis of the bone, it will often shift, resulting in a loose wire (3) (Fig. 50.16). A rule of thumb when placing full-

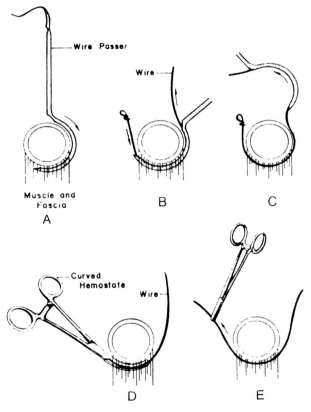

Fig. 50.14. Techniques for passing wire close to bone. A wire passer is inserted adjacent to and around the bone (**A**), the wire is then pushed through the passer (**B**), and finally the passer is removed (**C**). Alternatively, hemostats can be used to pull wire around the bone (**D** and **E**). (From Straw RC, Withrow SJ. Cerclage wiring. In: Bojrab MJ, ed. Current techniques in small animal surgery. 3rd ed. Philadelphia: Lea & Febiger, 1990.)

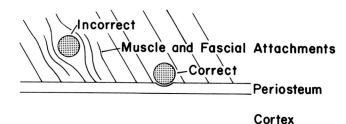

Fig. 50.15. Wire should lie directly on the bone, over the periosteum, rather than away from the bone and in soft tissues. (From Straw RC, Withrow SJ. Cerclage wiring. In: Bojrab MJ, ed. Current techniques in small animal surgery. 3rd ed. Philadelphia: Lea & Febiger, 1990.)

cerclage wires is to place them approximately 1 cm apart and a minimum of 5 mm from the ends of the fracture (3). They should never be placed within a fracture line or within a cortical defect because this can result in delayed union or nonunion. If a minimum of two cerclage wires cannot be placed, one should question the placement of any full-cerclage wires at this location, but instead interfragmentary wire placement should be considered. Near the distal and proximal ends of the bone, the changing diameter of the bone creates a taper where the wires may tend to slip. Placing a transcortical Kirschner wire to prevent the full-cerclage wire from slippage may be considered. Other methods to prevent the wire from slipping are notching and scoring the outer cortex to seat the wire

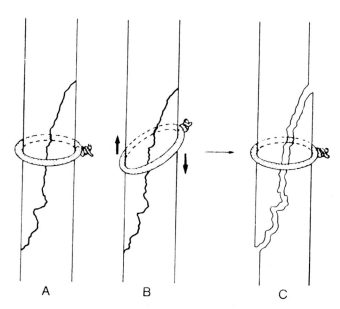

Fig. 50.16. **A.** Cerclage wire should be placed perpendicular to the diaphysis. If a wire is placed obliquely to the diaphysis, it will often shift position (**B**), resulting in fracture instability (**C**). (From Straw RC, Withrow SJ. Cerclage wiring. In: Bojrab MJ, ed. Current techniques in small animal surgery. 3rd ed. Philadelphia: Lea & Febiger, 1990.)

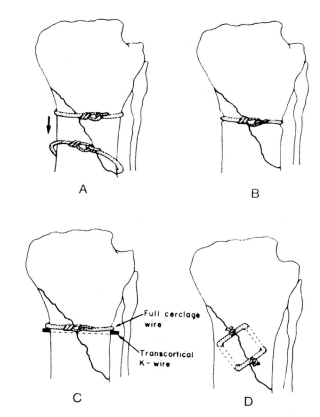

Fig. 50.17. **A.** Cerclage wire placed on a conical bone often slips to a narrower area. Slippage can be prevented by notching the bone slightly (**B**), by passing a Kirschner wire below the cerclage wire (**C**), or by placing interfragmentary wires (**D**). (From Straw RC, Withrow SJ. Cerclage wiring. In: Bojrab MJ, ed. Current techniques in small animal surgery. 3rd ed. Philadelphia: Lea & Febiger, 1990.)

(Fig. 50.17). Care must be taken with this approach because even small notches can decrease the strength of the bone significantly (9). Alternatively, interfragmentary wires may be applied to prevent slippage. Cerclage wires should not be used as the sole fixation method, but they should be applied in conjunction with other stable fixation methods. Stabilization with bone plates, intramedullary pins, external skeletal fixation, rigid splints, or a combination of these is required to help neutralize the forces. Full-cerclage wires are placed before seating the intramedullary pins. When full-cerclage wires are used with bone plates, the cylinder of the bone is reconstructed with the use of cerclage wires and the bone plate can be placed over the wires without compromising the stability of bone plate fixation and healing potential (10). Full-cerclage wires may also be placed around the plate and bone in certain tenuous situations in which additional stabilization is required, such as when a fissure line develops during screw tightening of a bone plate, to prevent further propagation, or when added stabilization of the plate is necessary in a comminuted fracture repaired with a bone plate (7). After the wires are placed, they should be tested for tightness by taking an instrument and firmly pushing against them. If they move, they should be replaced. On occasion, they may appear tight after application, and as the fixation repair progresses, they loosen from minor shifting of the bone segments. Therefore, the wires should be rechecked for tightness periodically throughout the repair process. Removal of cerclage wires after healing is not necessary unless complications develop from their presence.

Interfragmentary (Hemicerclage) Wires

Cerclage wires placed through holes in the cortex of the bone not passing around the entire circumference and crossing the fracture line are termed interfragmentary wires. Interfragmentary wires are indicated in short oblique or transverse fractures for which full-cerclage wires are not indicated and when rotational forces are a concern or slippage of the wire is a problem. These wires are used most commonly with intramedullary pinning. Types of interfragmentary wire configurations include cruciate, horizontal mattress, and simple interrupted patterns (Fig. 50.18). Cruciate wires, also called figure-of-eight wires, produce the greatest resistance to rotation and provide increased interfragmentary compression (11). When cruciate or horizontal mattress wires are placed, holes are drilled transversely across the cortex approximately 1 cm from the fracture ends perpendicular to the long axis of the bone. Both the holes on the same side should be drilled with the same drill or Kirschner wire to facilitate passage of the wire and to maintain the alignment of the fracture when the wires are tightened (Fig. 50.19). Two separate strands of wire are replaced in the holes, the fracture is reduced, the intramedullary

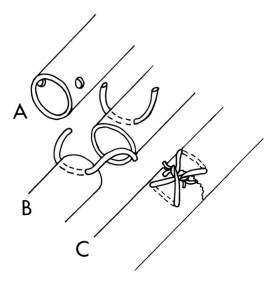

Fig. 50.19. Placement of cruciate interfragmentary wire. **A.** Holes are drilled with a Kirschner wire on each side of the fracture. **B.** Interfragmentary wires are passed through the holes. **C.** After the fracture is reduced and an intramedullary pin is driven, the wires are tightened. (From Straw RC, Withrow SJ. Cerclage wiring. In: Bojrab MJ, ed. Current techniques in small animal surgery. 3rd ed. Philadelphia: Lea & Febiger, 1990.)

pin is driven, and each strand of the wire is tightened according to the configuration chosen. Increasing the overall length of the cruciate pattern decreases the antirotational effects (11). Placing a single strand wire through the entire configuration and tightening the wire with only one knot compromises the ability to tighten the wire uniformly.

Simple interrupted interfragmentary wire placement is not as effective in counteracting shear and rotational forces as the other patterns. A hole is drilled on each side of the fracture such that the wire is placed perpendicular to the fracture line. The wire may be placed around the intramedullary pin, if desired, for an added fixation point (see Fig. 58.18**C**). More than one interfragmentary wire can be placed if indicated on the opposite cortex. Interfragmentary wires should be placed on the tension side of the bone if possible.

Cerclage wiring offers an effective means to provide stable fixation of fractures when applied properly. Cerclage wires should not be used as a primary mode of fixation. Depending on the nature of the fracture and the forces acting on the bone, various combinations of cerclage wiring can be used. Loosening and shifting of cerclage wire noted at the time of radiographic assessment of fracture healing indicate that the principles of cerclage wiring were not properly followed. Not all patients are ideal candidates for the use of cerclage wiring and pinning, but the principles of cerclage wiring still apply if other methods of fixation are used in conjunction with this technique.

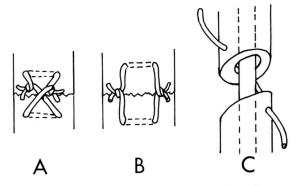

Fig. 50.18. Common patterns for placement of interfragmentary (hemicerclage) wires. **A.** Cruciate pattern with two twists. **B.** Horizontal mattress pattern with two twists. **C.** Simple interrupted pattern with one twist. (From Straw RC, Withrow SJ. Cerclage wiring. In: Bojrab MJ, ed. Current techniques in small animal surgery. 3rd ed. Philadelphia: Lea & Febiger, 1990.)

References

1. Withrow SJ. Use and misuse of full cerclage wires in fracture repair. Vet Clin North Am 1978;8:201.
2. Rhinelander FW. Tibial blood supply in relation to fracture healing. Clin Orthop 1974;105:34.
3. Straw RC, Withrow SJ. Cerclage wiring. In: Bojrab MJ, ed. Current techniques in small animal surgery. 3rd ed. Philadelphia: Lea & Febiger, 1990.
4. Wilson JW. Effect of cerclage wires on periosteal bone in growing dogs. Vet Surg 1987;16:299.
5. Blass CE, Piermattei DL, Withrow SJ, et al. Static and dynamic cerclage wire analysis. Vet Surg 1986;15:181.
6. Rooks RL, Tarvin GB, Pijanowski GJ, et al. In vitro cerclage wiring analysis. Vet Surg 1982;11:39.
7. Pardo AD. Cerclage wiring and tension band fixation. In: Slatter DH, ed. Textbook of small animal surgery. 3rd ed. Philadelphia: WB Saunders, 1993.
8. Egger EL, Whittick WG. Principles of fracture management. In: Whittick WG, ed. Canine orthopedics. Philadelphia: Lea & Febiger, 1990.
9. Nunamaker DM, Hayes WC, Schei, S, et al. Mechanical properties of healing fractures following removal of compression plate fixation. In: Transactions of the 28th annual meeting of the Orthopedic Research Society.: Orthopedic Research Society, 1982.
10. Willer RL, Schwarz PD, Powers BE, et al. Comparison of cerclage wire placement in relation to a neutralization plate: a mechanical and histological study. Vet Comp Orthop Traumatol 1990;3:90.
11. Blass CE, Caldarise SG, Torzilli PA, et al. Mechanical properties of three orthopedic wire configurations. Am J Vet Res 1985;46:1725.

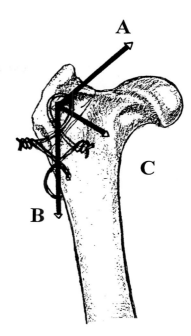

Fig. 50.20. The pull of a muscle, tendon or ligament (*A*), when countered with the opposing pull of a tension band device (*B*), results in a compressive force across the fracture or osteotomy (*C*).

Tension Band Wiring

Karl H. Kraus

Tension banding is an engineering technique by which tensile forces are converted into compressive forces (1). This principle can be applied to the repair of fractures in which a fragment is distracted from its original position by the pull of a muscle, tendon, or ligament. The area of fracture opposite the pull under tension is termed the tension side of the fracture. If the tension side of the fracture is fixed with a tension device, the force of the distractive pull is redirected to a resulting vectorial force across the fracture line (Fig. 50.20).

Indications

In tension band wiring, orthopedic wire and Kirschner wires (intramedullary pins) are used to fix and apply compression to the tension side of a fracture. Indications for use of this technique include repair of fractures or osteotomies of the acromion of the scapula, supraglenoid tubercle, greater tubercle of the humerus, olecranon, greater trochanter of the femur, supracondylar epiphysis of the femur, medial malleolus of the tibia, tuber calcis, tibial tuberosity, and attachments of collateral ligaments (2). Because these are frequent sites of fracture and osteotomies for surgical exposure, tension band wiring is a common technique. A tension band wire can be successfully applied in many situations, if principles of application are followed and proper technique is used.

Technique

Before a tension band wire is applied, the direction of the distractive forces should be estimated. Because forces can change through the range of motion of a joint, the "average" distractive force should be estimated. The tension band should be applied to the side opposite the distractive forces, the tension side of the fracture.

After the fracture or osteotomy is reduced, two Kirschner wires (intramedullary pins) are inserted from the distracted fragment across the fracture line and into the attaching bone (Fig. 50.21**A**). Two pins are used whenever possible to provide rotational stability. The pins should be applied parallel to the direction of desired compression and in such a way that an orthopedic wire placed over them applies even, undeterred pressure to the tension side of the fracture. These pins should be seated in cortical bone in the opposite cortex to prevent migration.

With a Steinmann pin or drill, a hole is drilled through the cortex to accommodate the tension band wire. The distance of this hole from the fracture line

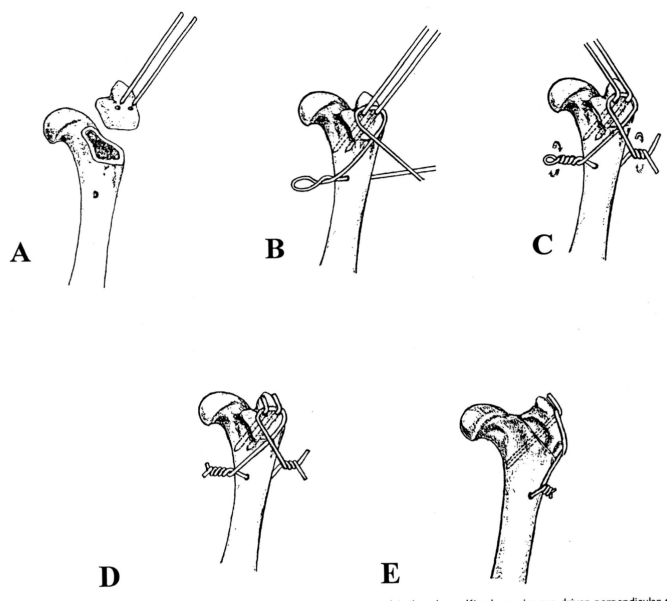

Fig. 50.21. Application of a tension band wire. **A.** First the fragment is replaced, and two Kirschner pins are driven perpendicular to the fracture line. **B.** A figure-of-eight wire is placed over the pins and through a hole in the cortex. **C.** The wires are twisted and tightened alternatively. **D** and **E.** The pins and wires are bent, cut, and seated next to bone.

should be at least as great as the length of the fragment. A piece of 18- to 20-gauge orthopedic wire is looped one-third of the distance from one end. The short end is inserted through the hole in the cortical bone, and the long end with the loop is brought over the Kirschner wire in a figure-of-eight pattern and is twisted to the other loose end (Fig 50.21**B**). The pre-placed loop and twisted ends are tightened alternatively or with the help of an assistant so the wire is evenly tightened (Fig. 50.21**C**). The orthopedic wire should be cut, leaving two to four twists, and bent toward the bone. The Kirschner wires are bent over the tension band wire and are cut to secure it (Fig.

50.21**D** and **E**). The ends of the wires are seated in soft tissue. Soft tissues are closed in routine fashion.

Aftercare of the tension band wire itself is minimal, because weightbearing aids in the healing by providing fracture line compression. General postoperative care depends on the specific repair undertaken.

Complications

Complications are uncommon and are usually the result of improper technique. The six most common technical errors resulting in failure are depicted in Figure 50.22. The first error is having too small a fragment

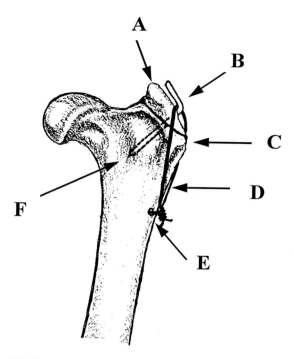

Fig. 50.22. Six common errors in placing a tension band wire: *A*, fragment is too small; *B*, only one pin is used. *C*, the wire forms a loop and not a figure-of-eight; *D*, too small a gauge of wire is used; *E*, the hole in the cortex does not engage enough bone; *F*, the pins are not seated in the opposite cortex.

to accommodate an appropriately sized tension band device. Fractures and avulsions can be small, and applying a proper tension band may be a challenge. More commonly, however, this error occurs when performing an osteotomy for a surgical exposure, such as an osteotomy of the greater trochanter of the femur or greater tubercle of the humerus. One usually avoidable technical error is the placement of only one pin. Because the vector of the distracting muscle, tendon, or ligament pull may change through a range of motion, there may be a torsional force across the fracture. Two pins prevent rotation. Small avulsion fragments may only accommodate a single pin. However, placing two smaller pins should be used before one larger pin whenever possible. Use of a loop instead of a figure-of-eight wire is a completely avoidable technical error. A loop tends to center the compression more toward the pin and allows the fracture line (see Fig. 50.22, *C*) on the tension side to open up. Heavy-gauge wire should be used. Although 18- or 20-gauge wire is difficult to manipulate and twist, 22-gauge or smaller wire is rarely appropriate. The hole in the bone anchoring the tension band wire should engage enough material to counter the force of the tension device. These forces can be substantial. The pins should be anchored into the opposite cortex. Failure to do so can allow the pin to migrate.

References

1. Schatzker J. Screws and plates and their application. In: Muller ME, Allgower M, Scheider R, et al, eds. Manual of internal fixation. 3rd ed. Berlin: Springer-Verlag, 1995:179–290.
2. Kraus KH. Tension band wiring. In: Bojrab MJ, ed. Current techniques in small animal surgery. 3rd ed. Philadelphia: Lea & Febiger, 1990:815–816.

Intramedullary Fracture Stabilization: Interlocking Nail and Intramedullary Pin Fixation

Tass Dueland

Indications

Fractures of the diaphyseal region of certain long bones (femur, tibia, and humerus) are suitable for fixation with either an intramedullary (IM) pin or interlocking nail (IN) type of fixation; less suitable cases are metaphyseal or epiphyseal fractures. In our unreliable canine patients, the IN system, with locking screws placed above and below the fracture site (static mode) or screws placed only above or only below the fracture (dynamic mode), gives more reliable fixation than an IM pin, which is unlocked.

Surgical Description

The approach to the humeral and femoral diaphysis is generally lateral, whereas the tibia is usually approached medially (1). Both IM and IN devices may be introduced into the proximal IM canal either in a normograde manner or by retrograde insertion from the fracture site. With tibial fractures, to visualize and thereby to avoid important stifle structures, a medial parapatellar approach to the stifle is advised, with normograde insertion of the IN or IM pin. Preoperative radiographs of the opposite normal bone are helpful to estimate the proper length and diameter of the device to be used. In the IN system, once bone length, fracture reduction, and rotational alignment of the fracture are achieved and held with bone reduction forceps, the IM device is driven the appropriate distance into the distal segment, and the drill jig is then attached to the proximal end of the IN (Fig. 50.23). The jig has holes aligned with the holes in the IN, and, using drill guide sleeves, holes are then sequentially drilled, and screws are inserted proximally and distally in the bone. The screws are inserted in the drilled near

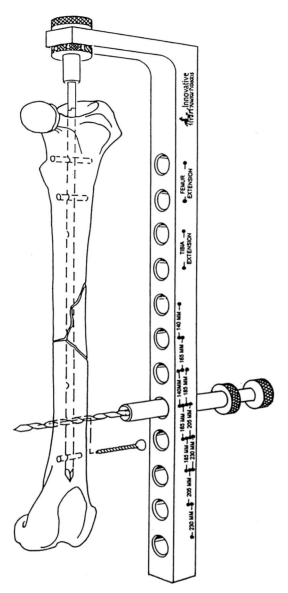

Fig. 50.23. Drill jig attached to the proximal end of the interlocking nail.

ning include adding a supplementary type I external fixator or using an external fixator "tied-in" to an IM pin that has been left protruding from the bone. Other IM devices and techniques used for fracture treatment include Rush rods and stacked IM pins or stacked Kirschner wires. My experience with these implants has been minimal.

IM stabilization of canine long bone fractures has been used since the introduction of IM pins in the 1930s. Many cases have been successfully treated with this technique. However, serious deficiencies have also been noted, including rotational instability, collapse of comminuted fractures with weightbearing, and migration of the pin, often leading to secondary complications of infection, nerve damage, and erosion of joint cartilage (3–6).

A refinement of the IM pin, the IN, has been reported clinically in veterinary surgery (7–9). This technique has been successful in treatment of human fractures (10). With this system, the IM device is locked in position by screws placed through both bone and device above and below the fracture site. This technique overcomes the previously mentioned deficiencies of an unlocked IM pin. The IN has good biomechanical properties for fracture stabilization and is stronger and stiffer than many IM pins and plates (2). An additional advantage is limited surgical exposure, thereby minimizing disruption of the fracture hematoma with its pluripotential milieu. In addition, the soft tissue vascularization of fracture fragments can be minimally disturbed; individual fragments do not need to be manipulated because rigid fixation of fragments is generally not necessary. However, cerclage wires (18 to 20 gauge) may be indicated if severe displacement of large fragments has occurred.

Occasionally, to facilitate IN insertion, I prefer to ream the IM canal gently using a hand reamer (Synthes, Paoli, PA) that is 1 mm larger than the IN. The reamed material obtained is also useful as an autogenous graft. Perioperative care consists of systemic antibiotics and appropriate analgesics continued as needed. Postoperatively, I prefer to use encircling ice packs of the injured area for 10 to 15 minutes, four times daily, followed by gentle passive flexion and extension of the limb (20 repetitions), so all joints of the affected limb are put through an adequate range of motion. After 3 days, warm compresses are substituted for the ice packs, with the physical therapy continued as before. Restricted leash exercise is advised until the 2-month follow-up radiographs confirm adequate progression of bone healing.

Approximately 150 to 200 cases have been successfully treated to date in the United States, in addition to other cases in Europe and Asia. Most of these fractures were comminuted (7–9, 11). The IN system appears to be as successful in dogs as in human patients. Currently, the diameters available in the small animal IN

cortex, in the IN, and in the drilled far cortex of each screw hole. The IN is thereby secured in its IM position. The IN instrumentation allows the surgeon to insert the IN to the proper position in the IM canal so the device does not protrude from the canal, thereby preventing any soft tissue or joint irritation. Pretapped or self-tapping screws may be used. The drill jig is then removed, and wound closure is routine, as with IM pinning. A large-diameter IN, snugly fitting the IM canal, is used whenever possible. The surgeon also should avoid placing an IN screw hole near a fracture site; both these measures help to prevent fatigue failure of the implant. Biomechanical tests have indicated that IN removal is optional after fracture healing (2).

Methods to improve fracture stability with IM pin-

system are 4, 6, and 8 mm, in various lengths (Innovative Animal Products, Rochester, MN).

References

1. Piermattei DL, Greeley RG. An atlas of surgical approaches to the bone of the dog and cat. 2nd ed. Philadelphia: WB Saunders, 1979:132–133.
2. Dueland RT, Berglund L, Vanderby R Jr, et al. Structural properties of interlocking nails, canine femora, and femur-interlocking nail constructs. Vet Surg (in press).
3. Cechner PE, Knecht CD, Chaffee VW, et al. Fracture repair failure in the dog: a review in 20 dogs. J Am Anim Hosp Assoc 1977;13:613–615.
4. Hunt JM, Aitken ML, Denny HR, et al. The complications of diaphyseal fractures in dogs: a review of 100 cases. J Small Anim Pract 1980;21:103–119.
5. Withrow SJ, Amis TC. Sciatic nerve injury associated with intramedullary fixation of femoral fractures. J Am Anim Hosp Assoc 1977;74:562–568.
6. Schraeder SC. Complications associated with the use of Steinmann intramedullary pins and cerclage wires for fixation of long bone fractures. Vet Clin North Am 1991;21:687–704.
7. Dueland RT, Johnson KA. Interlocking nail fixation of diaphyseal fractures in the dog: a multi-center study of 1991–92 cases. Vet Surg 1993;22:377.
8. Durall I, Diaz MC, Morales I. Interlocking nail stabilization of humeral fractures: initial experience in seven clinical cases. Vet Comp Orthop Traumatol 1994;7:3–8.
9. Duhautois B. L'encloure verrouille veterinaire: étude clinique retrospective sur 45 cas. Prat Med Chir Anim Comp 1995; 30:613–630.
10. Brumback RJ. The rationales of interlocking nailing of the femur, tibia, and humerus: an overview. Clin Orthop 1996; 324:292–320.
11. Muir P, Parker RB, Goldsmid SE, et al. Interlocking intramedullary nail stabilization of a diaphyseal tibial fracture. J Small Anim Pract 1993;34:26–30.

Stack-Pinning Techniques

Paul W. Dean

The primary goal of internal fracture fixation is stability of the fracture site with an early return to function. Intramedullary pinning of fractures is the most common form of internal fixation used. Properly applied, an intramedullary pin should nearly fill the medullary cavity of the bone to achieve its greatest stabilizing effect. Because of the degree of curvature of the various long bones and the variability in size of the medullary cavity, to achieve adequate fixation of fractures using a single intramedullary pin is frequently impossible. The use of multiple intramedullary pins, in an effort to increase stability by increasing the area of contact between the pins and bone, is termed stack-pinning.

The five basic forces acting on a fracture site are bending, rotation, shear, compression, and distraction. Single intramedullary pins are effective in primarily counteracting bending forces acting at the fracture site. Unless the medullary cavity is filled completely by the pin, the other forces acting on the fracture are not neutralized. The use of stack-pinning allows for neutralization of bending forces as well as shear and rotational forces by achieving multiple points of contact with the cortex and multiple sites of fixation in the proximal and distal metaphyses.

Indications

Stack-pinning is particularly suitable for transverse as well as short oblique fractures of the middle humerus and femur. When used in conjunction with another form of fixation such as cerclage or hemicerclage wires, stack-pinning may also be suitable for long oblique and comminuted fractures of the humerus and femur. Occasionally, stack-pin fixation of midshaft humeral fractures causes the pins to converge at the fracture site and allows rotational instability to occur. In these cases, rotational stability can be achieved using a type I Kirschner–Ehmer apparatus in conjunction with the stack-pinning technique, with the proximal pin of the Kirschner–Ehmer apparatus placed caudal to the intramedullary pins and the distal pin seated across the humeral condyles (Fig. 50.24) (1). A Kirschner–Ehmer apparatus may also be used to provide addi-

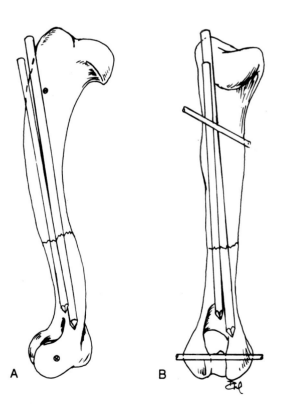

Fig. 50.24. Placement of pins for a Kirschner–Ehmer apparatus in a stack-pinned humerus. **A.** Lateral view; pin locations are indicated by circled Xs. **B.** Craniocaudal view. (From Chaffee VW. Stack-pin technique in the humerus and femur. In: Bojrab MJ, ed. Current techniques in small animal surgery. 2nd ed. Philadelphia: Lea & Febiger, 1983:734–737.)

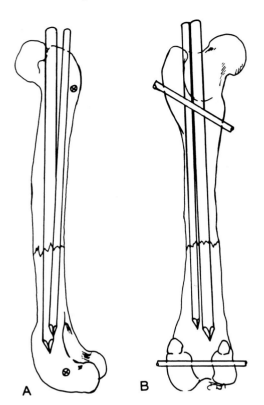

Fig. 50.25. Placement of pins for a Kirschner–Ehmer apparatus in a stack-pinned femur. **A.** Lateral view; pin locations are indicated by circled Xs. **B.** Craniocaudal view. (From Chaffee VW. Stack-pin technique in the humerus and femur. In: Bojrab MJ, ed. Current techniques in small animal surgery. 2nd ed. Philadelphia: Lea & Febiger, 1983:734–737.)

tional rotational stability for fractures of the midshaft of the femur by placing the proximal pin of the Kirschner–Ehmer device caudal to the intramedullary pins and the distal Kirschner–Ehmer pin through the femoral condyles (Fig. 50.25) (1).

Surgical Techniques

Humeral Fractures

Before anesthesia is induced, the function of the radial nerve must be determined. A lateral approach to the shaft of the humerus is made (2), and the fracture ends are inspected and debrided. Trial reduction of the fracture should be attempted and any fragments located. The medullary canal of the humerus is not symmetric; therefore, the number of intramedullary pins used to fill the canal must be determined at its narrowest point (Fig. 50.26**A**). (3). Minimally two, and preferably three, suitably sized intramedullary pins are selected. Pin placement is done in retrograde fashion, with the largest pin placed against the caudomedial cortex of the proximal fragment and driven proximally to emerge from the crest of the greater tubercle (Fig. 50.26**B**). The smaller pin is then driven in retrograde manner into the proximal fragment in a similar fashion until the ends of the pins are flush with the distal edge of the proximal fragment (Fig. 50.26**C**). The fracture is then reduced and is held in position with bone-holding forceps. If hemicerclage wires are

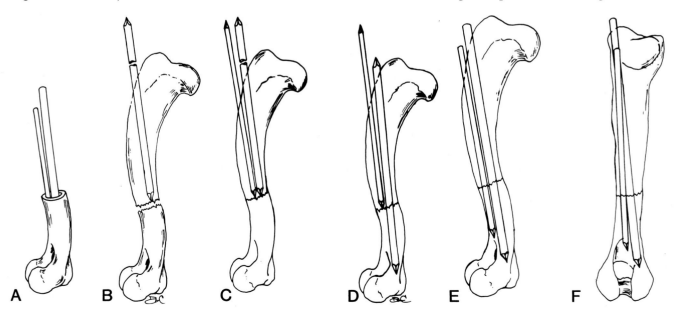

Fig. 50.26. Placement of multiple pins in the intermedullary canal of a fractured humerus. **A.** The number of pins to use is determined by the diameter of the canal at its narrowest point. **B.** The largest pin is driven in retrograde fashion from the caudomedial cortex to exit from the crest of the greater tubercle. **C.** The smaller pin is driven in a similar fashion until the end is flush with the distal edge of the proximal fragment. **D.** After fracture reduction, the largest pin is driven into the distal fragment and is seated in the medial condyle. **E** and **F.** Lateral and craniocaudal views after seating of all pins in the distal humerus. (From Chaffee VW. Stack-pin technique in the humerus and femur. In: Bojrab MJ, ed. Current techniques in small animal surgery. 2nd ed. Philadelphia: Lea & Febiger, 1983:734–737.)

to be used, they are left untwisted until final reduction of the fracture. The largest pin is then driven into the distal fragment with a hand chuck and is seated at the level of the medial condyle or just proximal to the supratrochlear foramen, depending on the size of the pin (Fig. 50.26**D**). The smaller pin is then seated in the distal fragment, with care taken not to distract the fracture site as the pins are being seated (Fig. 50.16**E** and **F**). If hemicerclage wires are used, they are now tightened, and final reduction of the fracture is inspected. Radiographs are taken to document pin location and reduction, and the pins are then cut off below the level of the skin. Bandaging is unnecessary, and the animal's activity is restricted to leash walking during bone healing. Radiographs are taken at 4 weeks and every 3 to 4 weeks thereafter to monitor fracture healing and to check for possible pin migration. The pins are removed when union is evident.

Femoral Fractures

The stack-pinning technique is well suited for repair of midshaft fractures of the femur as well as for fractures involving the proximal third of the femur. After exposing the fracture through an approach to the midshaft of the femur (2), the fracture ends are debrided, and trial reduction is performed. The medullary cavity of the femur is straight, as compared with the humerus, allowing for more complete filling of the canal with intramedullary pins. Appropriately sized pins are selected based on the size of the canal. Pins are inserted in either a retrograde or a normograde fashion. Retrograde insertion of IM pins is most common. To avoid the sciatic nerve as the pins exit the trochanteric fossa, the proximal fracture segment should be held in neutral or slight internal rotation, adduction, and with the femur at a 90° angle to the spine or in slight extension as the pins are driven. The pins are directed so they exit the trochanteric fossa or the greater trochanter. Pin placement within the greater trochanter may provide greater stability for fractures involving the proximal third of the femur (4). The pins are driven until they are flush with the distal edge of the proximal fragment.

Normograde insertion of multiple pins requires blind insertion of pins from the trochanteric fossa and greater trochanter, through the metaphyseal region, and down the shaft of the femur. Although technically more difficult, this technique allows for greater protection of the sciatic nerve because the site for pin insertion can be chosen to avoid impingement on this nerve. Pins are driven until flush with the distal edge of the proximal fragment, as with the retrograde insertion technique. The fracture is then reduced, and reduction is maintained with bone-holding forceps as the pins are driven into the distal fragment and are

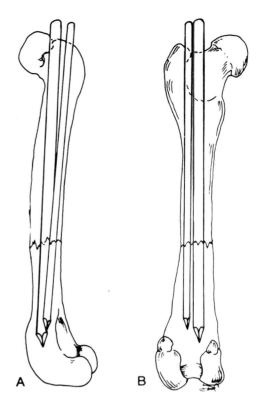

Fig. 50.27. Stack-pinned femoral fracture. **A.** Lateral view. **B.** Craniocaudal view. (From Chaffee VW. Stack-pin technique in the humerus and femur. In: Bojrab MJ, ed. Current techniques in small animal surgery. 2nd ed. Philadelphia: Lea & Febiger, 1983:734–737.)

seated in the distal metaphysis (Fig. 50.27). The surgeon should use multiple (three to four) small pins rather than two larger pins because it is easier to seat smaller pins more securely in the caudal distal aspect of the condyles. Larger pins have a tendency to contact the cranial cortex beneath the trochlear groove and are not seated as firmly. After final pin placement, any wires are tightened, and the final reduction is checked. Follow-up care is the same as described for fractures of the humerus.

Few complications are associated with proper use of stack-pinning in fracture repair. Failure to identify fissures within the cortex of the bone may lead to splitting of the cortex as the medullary canal is filled with pins. Fissures should be identified before insertion of the pins and cerclage wires used to stabilize the fissures or an alternate method of fixation used (1, 5).

After retrograde insertion of pins into the proximal fragment, it may be difficult to drive the pins into the distal fragment with a hand chuck because of the close proximity of the pins. Use of a mallet to drive the smaller pins may be necessary to avoid bending the pins with the hand chuck. Alternatively, the first pin may be placed in retrograde fashion out the proximal fragment, the fracture may be reduced, and the pin may be seated in the distal segment. Subsequent pins may be normograded from the crest of the greater tubercle in the humerus or from the greater trochanter and trochanteric fossa in the femur. This technique is especially applicable in the femur, where the pins tend to converge at the exit point in the trochanteric fossa if all pins are placed in a retrograde manner.

Migration of the pins may be a potential problem, particularly if the pins are not seated adequately in the distal metaphysis (5). Should migration of one or more pins occur, the pin should be removed and ancillary fixation applied, such as a Kirschner–Ehmer apparatus, until fracture union is complete. Reinsertion of the pin should not be attempted (5).

References

1. Chaffee VW. Stack-pin technique in the humerus and femur. In: Bojrab MJ, ed. Current techniques in small animal surgery. 2nd ed. Philadelphia: Lea & Febiger, 1983:734–737.
2. Piermattei DL. An atlas of surgical approaches to the bones and joints of the dog and cat. 3rd ed. Philadelphia: WB Saunders, 1993:128–131, 270–271.
3. Chaffee VW. Multiple (stacked) intramedullary pin fixation of humeral and femoral fractures. J Am Anim Hosp Assoc 1977; 13:599–601.
4. DeAngelis MP. Fractures of the femur. In: Bojrab MJ, ed. Current techniques in small animal surgery. Philadelphia: Lea & Febiger, 1975:453–461.
5. Nunamaker DM. Methods of internal fixation. In: Newton CD, Nunamaker DM, eds. Textbook of small animal orthopedics. Philadelphia: JB Lippincott, 1985:261–270.

Suggested Readings

McCurnin DM, Jones RL. Principles of surgical asepsis. In: Slatter DH, ed. Textbook of small animal surgery. vol. 1. Philadelphia: WB Saunders, 1985:250–261.
Rudy RL. Principles of intramedullary pinning. Vet Clin North Am 1975;5:209–228.

Screw Fixation: Cortical, Cancellous, Lag, and Gliding

Brian Beale

Cortical and cancellous screws are commonly used for fracture repair in small animals. Cortical screws are fully threaded and are designed for use in cortical bone (Fig. 50.28). Cancellous screws are fully or partially threaded and are used where cortical bone is thin and cancellous bone predominates (Fig. 50.28). Cancellous screws have a steeper thread pitch, deeper threads, and a thinner core as compared with cortical screws.

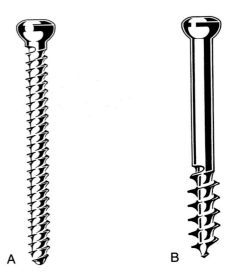

Fig. 50.28. Cortical and cancellous screws. **A.** Cortical screws are fully threaded. The thread pitch is less steep as compared with cancellous screws to increase holding power in cortical bone. **B.** Cancellous screws can be fully or partially threaded and are used where cortical bone is thin and cancellous bone predominates. Cancellous screws have a steeper thread pitch and thinner core as compared with cortical screws.

Partially threaded cancellous screws are generally not used in cortical bone because removal of the screw is difficult as bone grows around the unthreaded shank. Both types of screws can be used for different purposes, including lag screws, positional screws, and plate fixation screws.

Lag screws are used for interfragmentary compression of fracture fragments (Fig. 50.29). Compression occurs if the screw engages the far cortex and glides

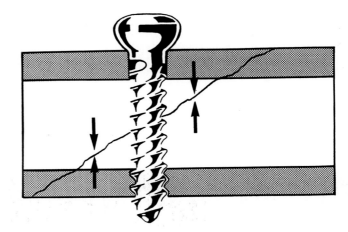

Fig. 50.29. Screws can be used to provide interfragmentary compression. When using a fully threaded screw for this purpose, a glide hole must be drilled in the near cortex equal in size to the thread diameter of the screw.

in the near cortex adjacent to the screw head. Cortical screws are selected for stabilization of cortical fragments in the diaphyseal region of the bone. The fragments are reduced and are secured temporarily with an appropriate bone clamp. Predrilling of the guide hole or thread hole before reduction and temporary stabilization is sometimes advantageous because it allows accurate placement of the hole in narrow segments of the bone fragment. If predrilling is done, a pointed drill guide is used to align the predrilled hole with the opposite hole to be drilled. The use of cortical screws requires drilling of a glide hole in the near cortex, equal in size to the thread diameter of the screw, to prevent the screw from making purchase. Screw holes should be drilled in the center of the fragment to prevent shifting during tightening. The hole should be drilled in a direction that bisects the angle formed by perpendicular lines to the fracture line and the longitudinal axis of the bone in fragments having less than 40° inclination. If inclination of the fracture is greater than 40°, the hole should be drilled perpendicular to the fracture line. The holes should also be placed an adequate distance away from the edge and tip of the fragment to prevent fracture of the fragment at the screw hole. A countersink tool is optimally used in the near cortex to distribute loads transferred by the screw head to the bone more evenly, thus making fracture less likely. A drill sleeve (outer diameter equal in size to the glide hole, inner diameter equal in size to the thread hole) is inserted in the glide hole until it meets the opposite cortex. A thread hole equal in size to the core of the screw is drilled in the far cortex. A depth gauge is used to measure the length of screw needed. The selected screw should be 1 to 2 mm longer than the measured hole depth to ensure adequate thread purchase in the far cortex. The hole is carefully threaded with the appropriate tap. The surgeon must insert the tap at the same angle as the drill bit and must avoid excessive wobble during tapping to prevent stripping or microfracture of the screw hole. The appropriate screw is then inserted and tightened. Overtightening can lead to stripping of the screw threads or fracture of the bone fragment; appropriate tightness can usually be attained by grasping the screwdriver with the thumb and the first two fingers, instead of the entire hand, when tightening.

Cancellous screws are often used to stabilize fragments in the metaphyseal or epiphyseal regions (Fig. 50.30). When using cancellous screws in lag fashion, a glide hole is not needed if partially threaded screws are used. The smooth shaft should traverse the near fragment completely. Compression does not occur if screw threads engage the near fragment. The diameter of the hole in both cortices should be equal to the diameter of the core of the screw. Predrilling one frag-

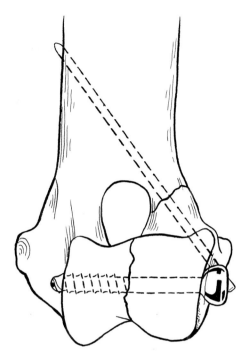

Fig. 50.30. A cancellous screw and Kirschner wire are used for repair of a lateral condylar fracture of the distal humerus. When using cancellous screws in lag fashion, a glide hole is not needed if partially threaded screws are used. The smooth shaft must traverse the near fragment completely.

ment is often helpful for alignment of the hole in the center of the fragment. The fragments are reduced and temporarily are stabilized with a bone clamp. The hole is drilled, measured and tapped. Tapping of the hole is optional; it is often helpful to tap only the first few millimeters of the hole to assist with insertion of the screw. Pullout strength of these screws is enhanced if the entire length of the hole is not tapped. The screw is inserted and is tightened as described earlier for cortical screws.

Positional screws can be placed to hold fragments in alignment while a method of primary stabilization is applied. Small cortical fragments can be secured to the diaphysis with a screw that engages the cortices of both fragments. A glide hole is not used; therefore, compression of the fragment does not occur. This type of application is useful when compression of the fragment is likely to lead to its collapse into the medullary cavity or shifting of the fragment out of reduction.

Plate fixation screws are used to fasten a plate to bone. Glide holes are not used unless compression of fragments beneath the plate is desired. Both cortical and cancellous screws can be used, depending on the region of bone. The screws glide in the holes of the plate, thereby compressing the plate against the bone.

Practical Techniques for Fractures

Dennis N. Aron

Principles and Terminology

An *osteosynthesis* is the contribution of both the implant and the bone to the stability of the fixed fracture. A *compression osteosynthesis,* which is used with a transverse fracture, is stable because the bone ends are tightly compressed and are held in this manner by the major stabilizing implant. The bone ends are stable and resist disruptive forces as a result of friction. The bone carries most of the load, whereas the implant holds the bone ends in compression. With this situation, the patient can bear weight on the operated limb for a prolonged period without the risk of failure. A *neutralization osteosynthesis* is less stable than a compression osteosynthesis. The major stabilizing implant protects the bone ends from many of the disruptive forces, whereas the bone shares some of the loading with the implant. A *lengthening osteosynthesis* is less stable than either a compression or a neutralization osteosynthesis. In this situation, the bone ends are held apart by the major stabilizing implant. The implant bears all the loads, whereas the bone ends contribute nothing to the stability of the fracture. A lengthening osteosynthesis is at risk for premature failure of the fixation and an increase in patient morbidity.

Patient morbidity refers to the experience of the animal or human patient with the fixation system and fracture healing. For example, premature loosening of the implants causes pain, decreased usage of the limb, attenuation of blood supply, and delayed healing, all leading to an increase in patient morbidity. All too frequently, the end result (whether the fractured healed or not) is the single concern. This is not sufficient. As veterinary orthopedic surgeons, we need to make sure that patient morbidity is as low as possible. This goal is realized only when the veterinarian is equally concerned with achieving the shortest healing period, maximum patient comfort, and least cost to the owner.

The *orthopedic race* is the race between implant failure and bone healing. When the implant begins to fail, it starts a negative chain of events leading to an increase in patient morbidity. Conversely, when the fracture begins to heal, it starts a positive chain of events leading to a decrease in patient morbidity.

Fracture disease is the irreversible situation of atrophied soft tissues, stiff joints, and less than adequate use of the limb. This complication is usually the result of premature loosening and failure of implants or post-operative coaptation and immobilization of the operated limb. Premature loosening of implants causes pain and decreased use of the limb leading to fracture disease. The only effective method of preventing fracture disease in small animal orthopedic practice is early postoperative voluntary weightbearing of the limb. Therefore, initial fixation of the fracture must be stable enough, and this stability must be maintained for a sufficient period to allow early weightbearing without implant loosening until a positive cycle of healing (callus formation) supplements the osteosynthesis.

Mechanical method of fracture fixation is when the surgeon's emphasis is on a maximum load-sharing osteosynthesis. This is achieved by careful reduction of fracture segments and reconstruction of butterfly fragments. This method features mechanical stability, but it sacrifices biology of healing.

Biologic method of fracture fixation is when the surgeon's emphasis is on a rapid orthopedic race. This is achieved by a "hands off" philosophy with minimal to no manipulation of fracture segments and reconstruction of butterfly fragments. This method features biology of healing, but it sacrifices mechanical stability.

Plate fixation system includes integrating bone plates, bone screws, and orthopedic wire for fracture management. With this system, the pivotal implant is the bone plate.

External skeletal fixation system includes integrating external skeletal fixators, pins, orthopedic wire, and possibly bone screws for fracture management. With this system, the pivotal implant is the external skeletal fixator. Neither the plate fixation system nor the external skeletal fixation system is preferred. Each has unique strengths and weaknesses. The plate fixation system's fundamental strengths are high mechanical stability and low maintenance. Weaknesses are problems with the remodeling stage of healing and biologic considerations. The external skeletal fixation system's principal strengths are with biologic considerations, progressive disassembly, and versatility, whereas weaknesses are high maintenance and the potential for the development of high stresses at the implant bone interface. Both systems give predictable and consistent results.

Progressive staged disassembly is a powerful technique unique to the external skeletal fixation system. With most fracture repairs, rigid stability is beneficial to healing for the first 4 to 6 weeks after fixation. After this time (or when the fracture first shows signs of bony union), one should allow a progressive but controlled increased loading of the fracture. This is easily accomplished with the external skeletal fixation system by the progressive disassembly of the component hardware. This method enhances remodeling of the healing fracture and leads to rapid maturation of the callus.

Table 50.1.
Patient Fracture Assessment Scale

Difficult	Middle	Easy
Lengthening osteosynthesis	Neutralization osteosynthesis	Compression osteosynthesis
Highly comminuted fx, segmental fx, missing bone	Three-piece fx, oblique fx	Transverse fx, spiral fx
Large patient	Middle-sized patient	Small patient
Multiple limb injury	Multiple same limb injury	Single injury
Hyperactive patient; poor client compliance		Calm, careful patient; conscientious owner
Healing		
Highly comminuted fx, segmental fx, missing bone	Three-piece fx, oblique fx	Transverse fx, spiral fx
Much hardware at fx site		Minimal hardware at fx site
Prolonged open reduction and fixation		Closed reduction and fixation
Type III open fx		Closed fx
Old age	Types II and I open fx	Puppy or kitten
High energy	Middle age	Low energy
Sick patient		Healthy patient

fx, fracture.

Animals are animals, and unlike human patients, they do not consistently limit the loads on their fractured limbs. Thus, the fixation must be such that it does not fail, despite our patients' periodic escape from their confinement. The veterinary surgeon must avoid directing the blame to the owner or animal for high morbidity and implant failures; to do so hinders one from learning from mistakes and impedes individual growth with fracture orthopedics.

The patient fracture assessment scale (modified from DN Aron and Palmer teaching notes) is given in Table 50.1. Based on this scale from 1 to 10, the surgeon can be guided into the most correct fracture management regimen. The patient needs to be assessed using the treatment scale. The lower the preoperative score, the more difficult is the treatment. Unless the surgeon is highly skilled and experienced in orthopedics, he or she should seriously consider referral of these cases (open fractures are only referred after debridement and wound dressing). These osteosyntheses are unstable, and the race is prolonged. Higher scores suggest a more stable osteosynthesis, a shorter race, and a more predictable satisfactory outcome. Based on the foregoing, the guidelines shown in Table 50.2 are suggested. This scoring scheme is to be used only as a *guide* to choose referral or treatment options. These guidelines have many exceptions; however, they should help as a starting point for the surgeon with limited experience in fracture orthopedics.

The *question* that must always be asked is this: Do I have the proper fixation for this particular patient and fracture to win the race?

Fracture Location

Epiphyseal and Metaphyseal Fractures

Epiphyseal and metaphyseal fractures are predisposed to fracture disease and losing the orthopedic race. The bone fragment is small (extremely small in many epiphyseal fractures). This limitation prevents the surgeon from using bone plates and rigid configurations of the external skeletal fixator system, thus sacrificing the inherent stability provided by these methods. Often the fracture, directly or closely, involves the associated joint surface requiring perfect anatomic alignment and rigid stability to avoid fracture disease. These fractures are in close vicinity to a high-motion area (the joint) and are predisposed to loss of anatomic reduction. These fractures have strong tensile disruptive forces because of direct tendon and ligament insertion on the fracture fragment. This feature is challenging to the maintenance of fracture fixation and predisposes the patient to losing anatomic reduction and developing fracture disease. On the positive side, fractures in this location heal quickly as a result of the profuse metaphyseal blood supply (the race is short). Epiphyseal fractures lend themselves best to being stabilized with Kirschner pins, tension band techniques, and lag screws. Whenever possible, lag screws and tension band techniques are preferred to improve stability and to lessen the chance of fracture disease. Metaphyseal fractures are best treated with Rush pins or stress-pin and cross-pin techniques. Rush pins or stress-pin techniques are preferred because they counteract the disruptive tensile forces directly. When the fracture

Table 50.2.
Fracture Assessment Scale Scoring

Score	Fixation
1–3	Biologic method; bone plate, complex configuration of external skeletal fixation system
4–7	Biologic or mechanical method; bone plate, moderately complex configuration of external skeletal fixation system
8–10	Biologic or mechanical method; closed coaptation; simple configuration of external skeletal fixation system

directly involves the growth plate and when the animal has yet to undergo considerable long bone growth (up to 5 to 6 months with small and medium breeds; 6 to 9 months with large and giant breeds), lag screw and tension band techniques are avoided. Early implant removal may be necessary in extremely young patients.

Diaphyseal Fractures

Diaphyseal fractures are treated using either a plate fixation system or an external skeletal fixation system. Rush pins, stress-pin techniques, and cross-pin techniques are not used with these fractures. The biggest problem with diaphyseal fractures is they often have prolonged healing times resulting in a lengthy orthopedic race. This slow healing is the result of the decreased blood supply to diaphyseal bone because of the fracture. Healing times and the race can be shortened by using autogenous cancellous bone grafts with fracture repair.

Application of the External Skeletal Fixation System to Shaft Fractures

Fractures of the Shaft of the Femur and Humerus

Fractures of the shaft of the femur and humerus in small animals are common; thus, fixation of these fractures is widespread in practice. Unfortunately, fixation of these fractures has been reported to cause high patient morbidity. The application techniques of external skeletal fixation presented here dramatically lower patient morbidity and give predictable and consistent success for managing shaft fractures of the femur and humerus.

APPROACH TO THE SHAFT OF THE FEMUR
The extent of exposure may be dictated by the location of the fracture. A craniolateral incision is made from just above the greater trochanter to the patella. The tensor fasciae latae and its associated muscle proximally are incised along the cranial border of the biceps femoris muscle for the length of the skin incision. The biceps femoris muscle is retracted caudally, and the vastus lateralis and intermedius muscles are retracted cranially to visualize the shaft of the bone.

APPROACH TO THE SHAFT OF THE HUMERUS
The extent of exposure may be dictated by the location of the fracture. A craniolateral incision is made from the level of the greater tubercle to the lateral epicondyle. The cephalic vein and branches can be avoided or ligated and incised. The brachial fascia is incised to allow retraction of the triceps muscle caudally and the

superficial pectoral and brachiocephalicus muscles cranially. The most dangerous and important aspect of the approach to the humerus is to avoid damaging the radial nerve. Branches of this nerve are present just under the fascia at the level of the distal third of the diaphysis (especially superficial in the cat). One must identify the radial nerve before proceeding with the exposure. The cranial and caudal borders of the brachialis muscle are dissected to allow retraction caudally with proximal and midshaft fractures and cranially with distal fractures. The radial nerve is best protected by placing a Penrose drain or umbilical tape around the entire belly of the brachialis muscle so the nerve is retracted with the muscle.

REPAIR OF SIMPLE FEMORAL OR HUMERAL FRACTURES
Simple femoral or humeral fractures can be repaired using an intramedullary (IM) pin tied in to a unilateral–uniplanar (type I) configuration (Fig. 50.31). This configuration is used in patients with high (uncomplicated) fracture assessment scores. Fracture configurations include transverse, oblique, spiral, and simple (one to two large fragments) comminuted patterns. One needs to reconstruct these fractures in an anatomic manner with negligible missing bone. The long oblique and spiral fractures are supplemented with cerclage wiring techniques in addition to the fixator and the tied-in IM pin. Comminuted fragments can

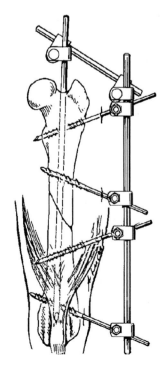

Fig. 50.31. Repair of simple femoral or humeral fractures using an intramedullary pin tied in to a unilateral–uniplanar (type I) configuration.

be anatomically reconstructed with interfragmentary wiring techniques before application of the fixator and IM pin.

A $\frac{1}{8}$-inch IM pin is used for small dogs and cats, and a $\frac{3}{16}$-inch pin is used for medium and large dogs. Applying an IM pin for fractures of the femur and humerus in the dog and cat provides moderated stabilization against disruptive bend at the fracture site. The IM pin, as used in small animal practice, gives poor stabilization for disruptive shear with oblique fractures and poor stabilization for disruptive torsion with almost all fracture patterns. The fixator complements the IM pin, giving good stabilization against shear and torsion but poor stabilization for bend. In situations with good apposition of the bone segments and slight soft tissue damage, allowing rapid formation of periosteal callus (high patient fracture assessment score), an IM pin tied in to a simple fixator design (24-pin unilateral–uniplanar frame) works well. With spiral fractures of these bones, IM pinning and supplementary cerclage wiring, without a fixator, can succeed because the wires can adequately reduce shear and torsion at the fracture site. Yet, the oblique fracture pattern (different from spiral pattern) is inherently unstable. These fractures need to be stabilized with the simple fixator design besides the IM pin and cerclage wires. Wires become loose when applied to short oblique or transverse fractures and lead to nonunion by hindering the ingrowth of blood vessels for periosteal callus formation. When a fracture pattern does not lend itself to cerclage wiring, the surgeon should not apply "suture wire patterns" for control of the demanding disruptive forces at the fracture site. If the wiring pattern should prove insufficient and become loose, it acts as a deterrent to the ingrowth of blood supply. With short oblique and transverse fractures, the fixator tied in to the IM pin provides stability against shear, torsion, and bend, while having no metal to interfere with the healing process at the fracture site. The advantage of a tied-in fixator and IM pin is that more strength is added, and implant loosening and migration is decreased. To gain even more strength, one can easily add a second ("stacked") connector rod to the lateral frame, increase fixator pins in the lateral frame, or convert the fixator to a modified unilateral–biplanar configuration (see later).

REPAIR OF DIFFICULT FEMORAL OR HUMERAL FRACTURES WITH A FIXATOR TIED IN TO AN INTRAMEDULLARY PIN

Difficult femoral and humeral fractures can be repaired using a modified unilateral–biplanar (double frame) fixator configuration tied in to an IM pin (Fig. 50.32). The fracture patterns included in this application are those with moderate to high comminution (intermediate to low patient fracture assessment score). Crucial

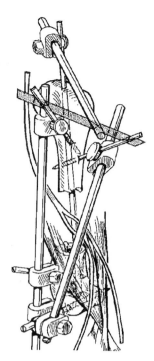

Fig. 50.32. Repair of difficult femoral and humeral fractures using a modified unilateral–biplanar (double frame) fixator configuration "tied in" to an intramedullary pin.

to success with this fixation is providing sufficient stability with the fixator and IM pin while disrupting minimal soft tissue and blood supply in the application process (biologic application). In most instances, the butterfly fragments are left completely undisturbed. The surgeon passes the appropriately sized IM pin and exposes the fracture only enough to identify and reduce the distal bone segment to receive the IM pin. A four-pin unilateral–uniplanar configuration is constructed. The proximal bone segment is pulled out to length with a grasping instrument before securing the fixator. Fixation is enhanced for the difficult biomechanical demand and healing period by creating a second frame by first inserting a fixator pin craniolaterally to caudomedially. This pin is positioned 60 to 90° from the plane of the lateral pins. The second frame is assembled by joining the cranial pin with the distal most lateral pin. The two frames are linked by constructing a proximal articulation. The IM pin is tied in to the articulation. This double frame biplanar configuration adds significant strength to the fracture fixation. Added strength should not be attained by building a biplanar configuration that uses a cranial fixator pin to penetrate the quadriceps or biceps muscles and tendons of the distal femur or humerus. The pin placed in this manner increases patient morbidity and leads to stiffness of the stifle or elbow.

The application of fixator and IM pin for stabilization of fractures of the femur and humerus has several potential problems. This has prompted many small animal surgeons to avoid completely the use of a fixator and IM pin for fracture repair of the femur and humerus and to favor only bone plate applications. The fixator and IM pin can be used successfully in the femur and humerus, even for difficult fracture repairs, when certain application principles are understood. In fact, this repair method has advantages over bone plate repair. Examples include the ability to progressively disassemble or to dynamize the fixation easily and to attain less disruption of soft tissues (biologic application). The negative is that this repair does not provide as much absolute fracture stability as a plate repair. Yet, the amount of absolute stability is less important than the ability to provide sufficient stability for the biomechanical demand and anticipated healing process (one should think about the patient fracture assessment score). Even so, to use the fixator and IM pin method successfully with difficult fractures of the femur and humerus, several specific problems must be understood. First, the anatomy of the femur and humerus does not allow the surgeon to use the strong bilateral (type II) fixator configuration. Second, bulky muscles and tendons surrounding these bones must be penetrated by the fixator pins, a factor that increases pin-track problems and patient morbidity. Third, the bulky muscle mass results in a high bending moment on the fixator, leading to poor resistance of the strong disruptive forces of bend and disruptive axial compression. Fourth, the cut end of the IM pin can dramatically increase patient morbidity. Fifth, adequate seating of the IM pin can be difficult to achieve. This method and the one described previously are designed to reduce these problems. The tied-in IM pin complements the fixator by resisting disruptive bend and compression, whereas the previously described biplanar arrangement helps to resist disruptive bend and compression and avoids the muscles and tendon on the craniodistal femur. One only needs four to six fixator pins, even when repairing unstable and difficult fractures, thus avoiding the use of multiple pins that penetrate the bulky muscles of the femur. The application of the fixator and IM pin readily lends itself to progressive staged disassembly of the fixation hardware to allow gradual, yet protected, loading of the healing bone. Progressive disassembly is begun by removing the cranial or lateral fixator frame (or both) 6 weeks postoperatively or when immature bridging callus is noted radiographically (whichever occurs first). Once the fixator is removed completely, the surgeon leaves the IM pin protruding to be tied in to a fixator pin left in the proximal bone segment. This maneuver prevents discomfort created by cutting the IM pin so it rests under the skin and prevents the IM pin from migrating after it is detached from the fixator. If appropriate, any time after surgery, the fracture can be dynamized by removing the fixator and leaving only the IM pin to allow load sharing at the fracture. Sometimes, the IM pin is removed before the fixator if the surgeon thinks that the IM pin is hindering healing at the fracture site.

REPAIR OF DIFFICULT FEMORAL OR HUMERAL FRACTURES WITH ONLY A FIXATOR

Difficult femoral and humeral fractures can be repaired using only a modified unilateral–biplanar (double or triple frame) fixator configuration (Fig. 50.33). The fixator can be applied to the femur and humerus without the IM pin. Yet, with difficult fracture situations, not using the IM pin can make the configuration dangerously weak and can predispose the patient to high morbidity. Therefore, one needs to be especially knowledgeable when stabilizing fractures of these bones with only a fixator. Common indications for application of only a fixator to the femur and humerus are severely comminuted fractures and open (compound) fractures. With open fractures, an IM pin may help to create chronic suppurative osteomyelitis by spreading microorganisms throughout the medullary canal and by providing foreign material to interfere with the medullary blood supply. With highly comminuted fractures, the IM pin may be harmful by slowing the healing process across the fracture gap.

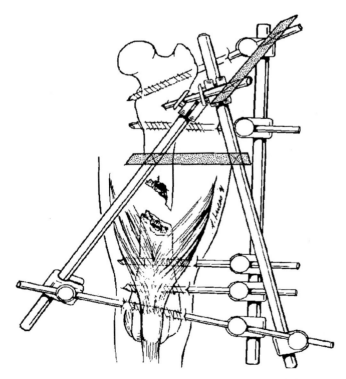

Fig. 50.33. Repair of difficult femoral and humeral fractures using only a modified unilateral–biplanar (double or triple frame) fixator configuration.

The fixator can be built as described previously, but without the IM pin. Again, critical to success is a biologic application, which can be facilitated by temporarily inserting a small IM pin to hold the bone reduced. The surgeon removes the IM pin after achieving stability with the first two lateral fixator pins and connector rod and then continues with the construction. Strength of the double-frame modified unilateral–biplanar configuration, without the IM pin, can be insufficient for many fractures involving the femur and humerus. However, a third frame can easily be added to increase the strength of the fixation dramatically. To add the third frame, the surgeon makes one of the pins in the distal bone segment a full pin and uses a third connector rod to join the medial pin with the cranial pin (the connector rod may need to be bent slightly to conform to the cranial thigh). This triple-frame configuration gives excellent stability without exploiting the negatives of an IM pin or additional fixator pins. However, the presence of the full pin near the highly mobile stifle joint can potentially increase patient morbidity, so one must be careful with the application of this pin.

GENERAL COMMENTS

All the techniques presented use the Kirschner external skeletal fixator method as an example; however, all techniques are just as easily applied to an acrylic external skeletal fixator method. The following ancillary techniques are also essential for low patient morbidity and consistent success. The surgeon must perform progressive disassembly in a thoughtful and timely manner. One must also use autogenous bone grafts with all repairs, insert closed-suction drainage systems in the presence of excessive "dead space" and contamination, manage open fractures properly, and use a 90–90 flexion sling for all patients with femoral fractures less than 1 year old and all those sustaining high-energy fractures. Last, proper postoperative management of the patient, fixator, and tied-in IM pin must be performed.

Fractures of the Shaft of the Radius or Ulna and Tibia

Fractures of the shaft of the radius or ulna and tibia occur commonly and often are open (compound) and complex (comminuted), the result of an anatomic scarcity of soft tissues surrounding these bones. However, because of the lack of soft tissues, with the use of the external skeletal fixation system, it is easier for the surgeon to gain mechanical stability with the radius or ulna and tibia than it is with the femur and humerus. Mechanical advantages include the ability to place connector rods close to the bone and the capa-

bility to use the strong bilateral and biplanar frame configurations. Conversely, the radius or ulna and tibia can have a problem with healing (biology) because the production of periosteal callus correlates closely with the amount of surrounding soft tissue. As with the femur and humerus, the application techniques discussed here lower patient morbidity and give predictable and consistent success for managing shaft fractures of the radius or ulna and tibia.

BIOLOGIC METHOD USING THE HANGING LIMB PREPARATION

The biologic method using the hanging limb preparation is a technique my colleagues and I frequently use for fractures (especially difficult fractures) of the radius or ulna and tibia. The forelimb or hind limb is secured at the paw and is suspended from the ceiling or to an intravenous infusion stand. The limb is pulled up sufficiently tight to allow the limb to be suspended by a portion of the animal's weight. This helps to reduce the fracture and maintain alignment as the surgeon is applying the fixation frames. This method allows the fixation to be applied in a closed manner or by only a small "miniapproach." With fractures of the radius–ulna and tibia, the elbow–carpus and stifle–ankle joints, respectively, must not be hidden from view with the sterile draping to allow fine-tuning of torsional alignment before securing the fixation. With this technique, the surgeon can emphasize a biologic repair, to encourage rapid healing. This technique is advantageous with fractures involving the radius or ulna and tibia because these particular bones have an anatomic deficiency of soft tissues.

REPAIR OF SIMPLE TIBIAL, RADIAL, OR ULNAR FRACTURES WITH FIXATION AND WITH OR WITHOUT AN INTRAMEDULLARY PIN

Simple tibial fractures can be repaired using an IM pin and unilateral (type I) configuration, and simple tibial and radial or ulnar fractures can be repaired using a unilateral–biplanar (type Ib) configuration without an IM pin (Figs. 50.34 and 50.35). The surgeon applies the IM pin and unilateral frame or unilateral–biplanar configuration without an IM pin to transverse, oblique, spiral, and simple comminuted (one to two large fragments) fractures. It should be possible to reconstruct these fractures in an anatomic manner with negligible missing bone. When using open reduction, long oblique and spiral fractures are supplemented with cerclage wiring techniques, and comminuted fragments are reconstructed anatomically with interfragmentary wires or lag screws. Autogenous bone grafts are inserted to any fractures repaired with an open technique.

The surgeon uses an IM pin with a diameter that measures approximately 50 to 60% of the diameter of

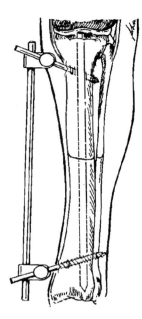

Fig. 50.34. Repair of simple tibial fractures using an intramedullary pin and a unilateral (type I) configuration.

the medullary canal of the tibia at the narrowest point. The pin is placed in the standard way from the craniomedial tibial plateau and is seated well into trabecular bone of the distal bone segment. The IM pin is cut short so it does not interfere with movement of the stifle joint, yet, it is allowed to protrude from the bone

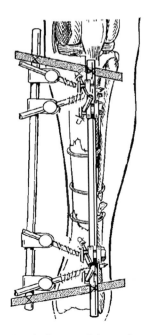

Fig. 50.35. Simple tibial or radial or ulnar fractures using a unilateral–biplanar (type Ib) configuration without an intramedullary pin.

for removal. A two-pin unilateral frame is constructed to complement the IM pin and is applied to the medial side of the tibia.

The unilateral–biplanar configuration is applied without using an IM pin because the presence of the IM pin makes it difficult to insert more than two fixator pins. A two- to four-pin unilateral frame is applied to both the medial and cranial tibia. The medial and cranial frames are articulated (tied in) at both the proximal and distal ends. This design allows the surgeon to construct a four-pin (minimum) to eight-pin (maximum) biplanar configuration, depending on the stability required (determined by patient fracture assessment score). The advantage of the IM pin and unilateral two-pin configuration is that fewer fixator pins are required. This configuration is used only on the tibia, and it works best with transverse fractures and for patents with a high fracture assessment score. The unilateral–biplanar configuration is applied to the radius or ulna and the tibia and allows the surgeon more versatility of design for stiffness and strength, a feature that is especially useful with the oblique and slightly comminuted fractures. The biologic method hanging limb preparation is more easily performed with the unilateral–biplanar configuration, because passing the IM pin can be technically challenging with this method.

REPAIR OF DIFFICULT RADIAL, ULNAR, OR TIBIAL FRACTURES WITH FIXATION

Difficult radial or ulnar or tibial fractures can be repaired using a bilateral–biplanar (type III) configuration (Fig. 50.36). Common indications for application of a bilateral–biplanar configuration to the tibia and radius or ulna are for high comminution and open (compound) fractures. Open fractures are frequently concurrent with severe soft tissue damage and contamination. These patients require proper wound management, the exceedingly rigid stabilization provided by this configuration, and careful postoperative management. When these open fractures are comminuted, two approaches are possible: open and closed. It is preferable to apply the fixator and reduce the fracture closed (or with only a minimal approach for fracture reduction) using a hanging limb preparation. This biologic method conserves significantly more blood supply than an open reduction, which can potentially jeopardize viable soft tissue.

The bilateral–biplanar configuration is constructed by placing a fixator pin through the proximal segment of the bone positioned 2 to 3 cm proximal to the fracture site. The surgeon starts the pin from the medial aspect of the bone and exits it from the contralateral side, with at least 3.0 cm of pin extending out the bone. The procedure is repeated for the distal segment,

to the bilateral frame. The bilateral frame is articulated to the unilateral frame to make a bilateral–biplanar (type III) configuration. This is done with four pin grippers and two short connector rods. A pin gripper is stacked on the first medial half-pin and another is stacked on the first cranial pin. These pin grippers are joined with a short connector rod. The process is repeated on the lateral aspect of the distal configuration.

GENERAL COMMENTS

All the techniques presented in this discussion use the Kirschner external skeletal fixator method as an example; however, all techniques are just as easily applied to an acrylic external skeletal fixator method. Once again, the ancillary techniques are critical to decreasing patient morbidity. Progressive staged disassembly should be done by 6 weeks or when evidence first shows bony union. Initially, the surgeon removes either frame with the unilateral–biplanar configuration or the mediolateral frame with the bilateral–biplanar configuration. The rest of the configuration is removed after healing has matured further. The surgeon must perform an autogenous cancellous bone graft on all repairs that are opened, diligent wound management in patients with open fractures, and proper postoperative management of the patient and fixator.

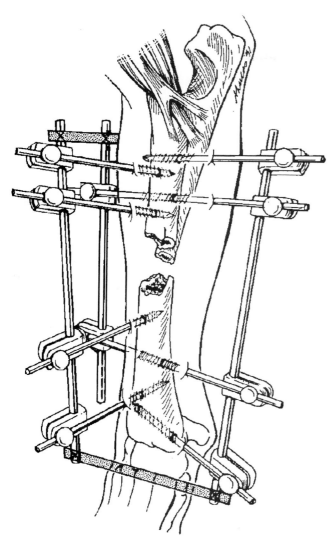

Fig. 50.36. Repair of difficult radial, ulnar, or tibial fractures using a bilateral–biplanar (type III) configuration.

but this pin is positioned near the hock or carpal joint. Both pins must be parallel to their respective joint surfaces and 90° perpendicular to the plane of joint motion. A long connector rod with four pin grippers is placed on the medial side of the bone, and the pin grippers are fit to the pins. A second long connector rod is applied with two pin grippers on the lateral side. The fracture is aligned by holding the fixator pins parallel to each other and tightening the pin grippers onto the pins. The alignment of the joints is checked above and below the fractured bone. The connector rods are secured a sufficient distance from the bone to allow for intervening soft tissues. Half-pins are placed into the two empty pin grippers on the medial connector rod. The surgeon constructs a four-pin unilateral frame on the cranial aspect of the bone positioned 90°

External Skeletal Fixation

Erick L. Egger

External skeletal fixation is a means of stabilizing fractures or joints using percutaneous fixation pins that penetrate the bone cortices internally and are connected externally to form a rigid frame or bridge. The basic components of an external fixator are these pins and the connecting bars or columns and clamps necessary to complete the frame (Fig. 50.37**A**). This device, commonly called a Kirschner–Ehmer splint, provides stable fixation of bone fragments without implants in the fracture site, with no or minimal damage to soft tissue vascularity and without immobilizing adjacent joints. Consequently, it is particularly useful for open or highly comminuted fractures with vascular compromise that require prolonged fixation. In addition, the low initial cost of fixators and the reusability of many of their components make them economically realistic for most practices and clients. Finally, the ease of application and the wide spectrum of indications make the fixator particularly useful for the veterinarian in general practice.

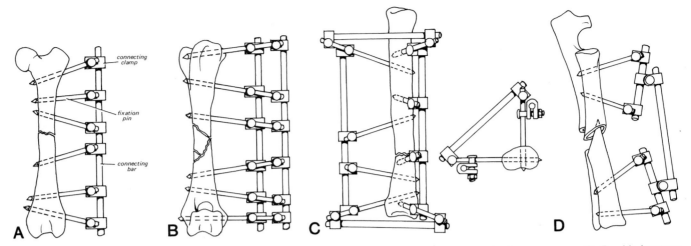

Fig. 50.37. Variations of type I (half-pin) Kirschner–Ehmer splints. **A.** Uniplanar splint showing basic components. **B.** Double-bar type I splint. **C.** Biplanar type I splint. **D.** Double-clamp type I splint.

Fixator Types and Characteristics

Basic Configurations

Fixation pins that pass through only one side of the limb and both bone cortices are called half-pins. They can be connected with a bar to form a type I (half-pin) splint. Type I splints can be used on the humerus or femur to avoid interfering with the body wall; they can also be positioned to avoid soft tissue injuries on the lower limbs. With proper application techniques, all the fixation pins can be attached to a single connecting bar (Fig. 50.37**A**). The resulting uniplanar type I single-bar splint provides adequate stability for treating most stable simple fractures in smaller animals (1). For larger animals or less stable fractures, a second connecting bar can be added to the same fixation pins (Fig. 50.37**B**). This arrangement nearly doubles the splint's resistance to compressive forces (2). Two single connecting bar splints can be applied parallel to and at 90° axial rotation to each other. The ends of the splints are connected, to form a triangular cross section. The resulting biplanar type I splint (Fig. 50.37**C**) is more resistant to bending forces than uniplanar splints (even full pin). In addition, the device can be applied to short fragments and yet obtain adequate pin–bone fixation (3). Double connecting clamps can be used to hold an additional connecting bar that connects two pin splints placed in each fragment. Such a double-clamp type I splint (Fig. 50.37**D**) is highly adjustable after placement. However, the double clamp itself is weak, resulting in minimal resistance to compressive forces (1). Consequently, its usefulness is limited to rapidly healing situations such as corrective osteotomies.

Fixation pins that pass through both sides of the limb and the bone are called full pins. The pins can be connected to form a type II (full-pin) splint (Fig. 50.38). Because type II configurations are resistant to compressive forces (1), they can be used on unstable fractures. However, to avoid interference with the body wall, they are limited to use below the elbow and the stifle.

A type I and a type II splint can be combined to form a type III (trilateral) frame (Fig. 50.39). Type III splints are the most rigid of currently used splints

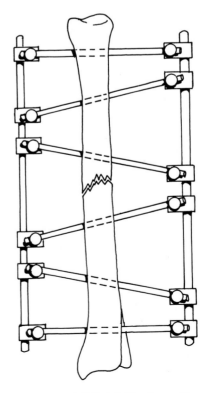

Fig. 50.38. Type II (full-pin) Kirschner–Ehmer splint.

external fixator systems can certainly be successfully applied on veterinary patients (4), but their expense precludes wide clinical usage.

Another form of external skeletal fixation, which has been described for managing maxillary fractures and is increasingly used for mandibular and long bone fractures, is that of pins and methylmethacrylate. Construction of this type of fixator is described later.

Fracture Healing With External Skeletal Fixation

The process of fracture healing varies depending on the nature of the fracture itself, the age of the animal, and the rigidity of fracture fixation. An unstable fracture in a young animal with a flexible fixator heals with much periosteal callus proliferation. On the other hand, a fracture in a mature animal stabilized with rigid fixation often heals with direct bone formation and little periosteal callus formation. The "best" method of fracture healing has not been conclusively determined (and may vary with different fractures). However, the ease with which the rigidity of external skeletal fixation can be adjusted allows the clinician to manipulate this healing process. Another exciting prospect currently being investigated is the manipulation of fixation rigidity as a fracture heals to enhance either callus formation or remodeling stages of the healing process.

Indications

External skeletal fixation was originally described in 1897 as being appropriate for highly unstable, comminuted, or open fractures with significant soft tissue injury (5). Whereas these situations remain the primary indication for use of an external fixator in human patients, the veterinary profession has expanded the fixator's use. Its ability to control rotation makes it useful as an adjunctive device to intramedullary pinning of transverse fractures. Traditionally, a type 1 splint with two pins has been used for this purpose, although experience suggests that use of at least three pins (two in one fragment) significantly decreases the incidence of premature pin loosening and loss of fixation (Fig. 50.40). Usually, the fixator can be removed after 3 to 5 weeks when the callus has become "sticky" enough to prevent rotation. The intramedullary pin is removed at a later time, after fracture healing is complete.

External skeletal fixation can be used for transarticular stabilization either to provide support while soft tissue structures such as ligaments and tendons heal or to provide the long-term fixation necessary for arthrodesis (6). Again, it is especially useful in those

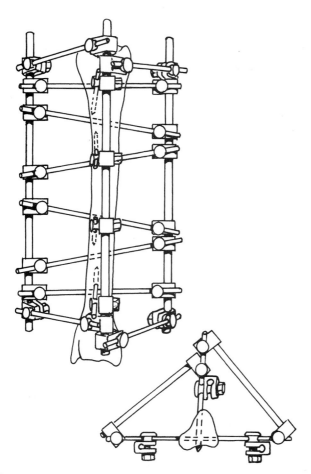

Fig. 50.39. Type III (trilateral) Kirschner–Ehmer splint formed by the combination of a type I and a type II splint.

(roughly 10 times as resistant to axial compression as type I splints) (1). Consequently, they are used for highly unstable fractures and arthrodesis in larger animals.

Available Fixation Devices

The most common external skeletal fixation device used in veterinary orthopedics is manufactured by the Kirschner Company (Timonium, MD). Three sizes are produced. The small apparatus is appropriate for use on cats, dogs up to approximately 20 lb, some exotic pets, and raptors. The medium-size apparatus is the most commonly used and is appropriate for most dogs. The large apparatus has recently been redesigned to be the same size as the human tibial frame. It should be most useful for giant breed dogs and other larger animals. With the small and medium-size devices, standard Steinmann pins can be used for both fixation pins and connecting bars. This requires only the addition of a few clamps to make most existing orthopedic packs applicable to external skeletal fixation. Human

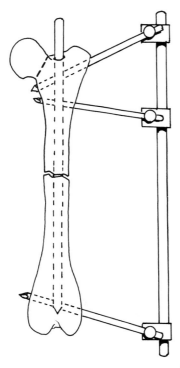

Fig. 50.40. A three-pin type I fixator can be added to intramedullary pin fixation to control rotation with transverse fractures.

cases of open soft tissue trauma or infection in which internal fixation would be less desirable. The postoperative adjustability of an external skeletal fixator makes it suitable for use with corrective osteotomies in the treatment of growth deformities in mature animals or as a lengthening device in the dynamic treatment of progressive deformities in immature patients (7).

Finally, many practitioners find the external fixator to be a practical means of treating many simple fractures that could be managed in several ways. The reduced incidence of decubital sores and cast changes associated with external coaptation, without the need for a major investment in the specialty equipment and supplies necessary for plate and screw fixation, makes external skeletal fixation economically advantageous for both the clinician and the client.

Application of Kirschner–Ehmer Splints

General Principles

Although the application and use of external fixators are easy, close adherence to several principles improves results and reduces the incidence of postoperative problems.

One of the most important advantages of external skeletal fixation is that it causes minimal damage to vascularity and hence the healing process. Closed re-

duction of a fracture minimizes such damage, but it may not result in adequate fracture reduction, particularly with complex fractures or fractures located proximal to the elbow or stifle joint. Consequently, I prefer a limited open reduction to achieve better overall fracture alignment. A limited open reduction also allows the incorporation of an autogenous cancellous bone graft into any persistent fracture defects (8). This graft usually is collected from the fractured limb; the craniolateral humeral greater tubercle is the common donor site for forelimb fractures and the medial aspect of the tibial crest for hind limb fractures.

The method of fixation pin insertion is important. In the past (9), hand chuck placement was advocated to avoid thermal necrosis of bone from frictional heat. However, wobbling of a hand chuck causes oversized pin holes, which lead to pin loosening. Furthermore, manual pin placement in cortical bone is hard work, commonly resulting in use of less than the optimal number of pins. Current research has shown that low-speed (150 rpm or less) power drill placement results in no significant temperature elevation or premature pin loosening (10). I prefer a $\frac{3}{8}$-inch electric drill that has been gas-sterilized or wrapped in a sterile shroud for pin placement because it possesses high torque at low speeds. Excess pressure and high speed should be avoided. Predrilling the pinhole with a twist bit is a commonly accepted technique in human orthopedics (11), but it has not shown any significant advantage in canine bone (10).

Threaded pins provide much better grip on bone than nonthreaded pins. However, the traditional threaded pins used in veterinary medicine are manufactured by cutting threads into the shaft, resulting in a decreased core diameter; consequently, these pins have a tendency to break or bend at the junction of the threaded and nonthreaded shaft. A new half-pin design, which is threaded only far enough to engage the far cortex (Fig. 50.41**A**), offers five to seven times the resistance to pullout of nonthreaded pins while maintaining all their resistance to bending (12). Alternatively, pins with rolled-on threads (Turner half-pins, Zimmer Co., Warsaw, IN; Bonner full pins, Kirschner Co.) (Fig. 50.41**B**) have excellent pullout resistance and bending strength, but they are expensive, costing seven to ten times as much as nonthreaded pins. Consequently, I often use one of these pins in each fragment, with the balance nonthreaded to reduce costs. Nonthreaded pins must be placed at a divergent angle to each other to maintain a mechanical grip on the bone. An angle of 30 to 40° between the outermost pins placed in each fragment (Fig. 50.42) has been suggested as offering the best compromise between pin strength and bone grip (9).

The number of pins placed in each fragment affects the stiffness of the fixator. More important, increasing

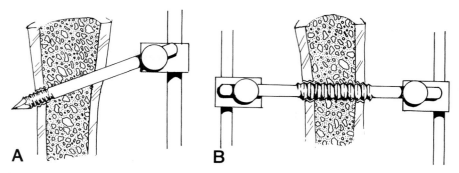

Fig. 50.41. Partially threaded half-pins (**A**) and rolled-on threaded pins (**B**) have greater resistance to pullout than nonthreaded fixation pins but the same resistance to bending.

the number of pins avoids overloading the bone surrounding each pin. Such overloading apparently causes microfractures, and the subsequent bone resorption results in premature pin loosening (13). Consequently, I use a minimum of three, preferably four, pins on each side of a fracture. These pins are best spread over the length of the fractured bone to distribute the disruptive forces and to maintain maximum fixator strength.

Half-pins need to be driven so the tip completely penetrates the far cortex because the triangular shape of the pin tip tends to make incompletely penetrated pins back up and consequently loosen. When pins are inserted, they should be driven through small, separate skin incisions. This precludes the skin's tendency to wrap up around the rotating pin. The pin should not be driven through the approach incisions because doing so makes closure difficult. In general, fixation pins should not penetrate large muscle masses and

areas of high skin motion because such penetrations often cause poor postoperative limb use and serum drainage from the pin tract. Likewise, the fracture should be roughly reduced after the first two pins are placed, so excessive skin tension does not develop against the pin when final reduction is achieved.

General Application Procedures

The following procedure applies to the placement of most common external fixation splints:

1. The fracture is roughly reduced by closed manipulation or through a limited open approach that minimizes soft tissue damage.

2. The most proximal and distal fixation pins are driven through small skin incisions into the two fragments at appropriate angles (Fig. 50.43**A**).

3. A connecting bar with clamps is slid onto the end pins with the anticipated number of "open" clamps in the middle (Fig. 50.43**B**).

4. After final fracture reduction is achieved, the end clamps are tightened (Fig. 50.43**C**). The connecting bar should be positioned far enough from the body to allow for swelling and callus formation without encroachment of the skin on the clamps.

5. A second connecting bar can now be added to create either a double-bar type I half-pin splint (Fig. 50.43**D**) or a type II full-pin splint (Fig. 50.43**E**).

6. The remaining fixation pins are driven through the open clamps at appropriate angles. The clamps are tightened as each pin is placed (Fig. 50.43**F**).

7. If desired, a second half-pin splint is applied at a roughly 90° axial rotation to the first to create a biplanar configuration (see Fig. 50.37**C**).

8. With an open approach, the incision is thoroughly lavaged. If indicated, an autogenous cancellous bone graft is inserted in any remaining fracture deficits, and the approach incision is closed.

9. Excessive fixation pin length is removed with a pin cutter.

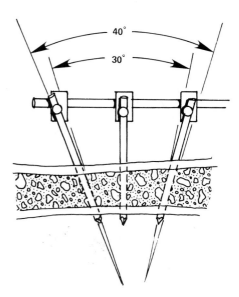

Fig. 50.42. Angle of divergence between nonthreaded half-pins required to maintain mechanical grip on bone.

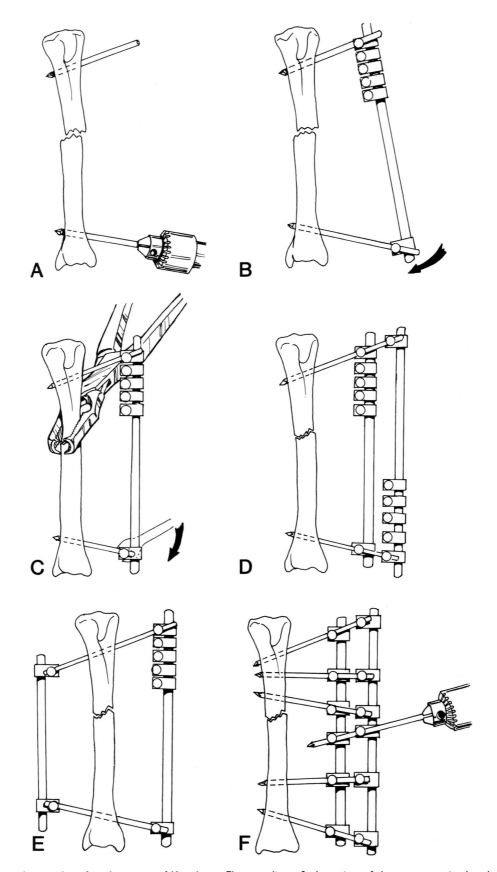

Fig. 50.43. General procedure for placement of Kirschner–Ehmer splints. **A.** Insertion of the most proximal and distal fixation pins. **B.** Placement of a connecting bar with an anticipated number of open connecting clamps. **C.** Tightening of the end clamps after final fracture reduction. **D.** Placement of a second connecting bar to give a double-bar type I configuration. **E.** Alternative placement of a second connecting bar to give a type II configuration. **F.** Insertion of the remaining fixation pins at appropriate angles through the open connecting clamps. See text for details.

Fixator Placement on Specific Long Bones

HUMERUS

Application of an external skeletal fixator to the humerus usually requires a minimal open approach to achieve adequate reduction. Type I splints usually are oriented laterally with the proximal pins placed cranial to the deltoid muscle; the distal pins can be placed through the condyle, but they must avoid the supracondylar foramen and the radial nerve. Biplanar type I splints are oriented cranially and laterally.

RADIUS

The radius can be stabilized with external skeletal fixation after either open or closed reduction. Uniplanar type I splints usually are oriented laterally for proximal fractures, cranially for small bones, and medially for distal fractures, although any of these orientations are acceptable in terms of avoiding penetration of and interference with soft tissue injuries. Biplanar type I splints are oriented cranially and laterally for proximal fractures or cranially and medially for distal fractures. Type II splints usually are applied medially to laterally.

FEMUR

Femoral fractures require an open approach to obtain reduction. To avoid muscle entrapment and subsequent stifle joint stiffening, type I uniplanar splints applied from the lateral aspect should be used. A second connecting bar can be applied to the half-pins if needed for fixator strength.

TIBIA

Either open or closed reduction of tibial fractures can be achieved. Uniplanar type I splints are best applied from the medial aspect to minimize soft tissue penetration, but they can be applied either cranially or laterally if necessary to avoid soft tissue wounds. Type II splints are placed medially to laterally. Biplanar type I splints are usually placed cranially and medially. The proximal pins should be placed in the wider and stronger caudal aspect of the tibia.

Application of Pins and Methylmethacrylate Splint

With the pins and methylmethacrylate method of external skeletal fixation, connecting bars are used only temporarily; permanent stabilization of a fracture is achieved by the hardening of methylmethacrylate around fixation pins inserted into the fracture fragments.

The procedure for applying this type of splint starts by insertion of the appropriate number of fixation pins (Fig. 50.44A), as described previously for pin placement with Kirschner–Ehmer splints. One or more of the pins are bent to lie parallel to the bone an appropriate distance (usually 2 to 4 cm) from the skin (Fig. 50.44B). The fracture is reduced and temporarily is stabilized with connecting clamps and bars placed farther away from the skin on a few of the pins (Fig. 50.44C). The approach incision is then closed. Nonsterile methylmethacrylate is mixed until it becomes doughy (3 to 4 minutes) and then is molded around the bent pins to form a connecting column that incorporates all the pins (Fig. 50.44D). This material is commonly available as dental molding acrylic and generally costs around $10 per pound (enough to do at least 10 fractures). Once the methacrylate has set (8 to 10 minutes), the connecting clamps and bars are removed, and excessive fixation pin length is cut off (Fig. 50.44E). Alternatively, sterile methylmethacrylate (bone cement) can be used with an open approach, thus negating the need for the temporary connecting clamps and bars. Sterile bone cement is used for implanting total joint replacements and costs around $35 per pack. Two or three packs may be needed for some fractures.

Postoperative Management and Home Care

Postoperatively, long bone fractures are placed in a compressive (Robert Jones) bandage to protect the incision and to minimize swelling. Any open wounds or incisions are covered with a sterile nonadherent dressing, and roll cotton or cast padding is packed around the pins and under connecting bars. Additional cotton or padding is rolled on the leg from the toes to above the injury. The padding is then compressed with elastic gauze and is fixed with tape (Fig. 50.45A). In most cases, this bandage is removed after 2 to 5 days. With open fractures or with severe soft tissue injury, the wound is often debrided, lavaged, and rebandaged every 2 to 3 days until it is covered with granulation tissue. Because of the stability the fixator provides, such frequent bandage changes can be performed without traumatizing early vascular proliferation and callus formation.

When the compressive bandage is no longer necessary, it is replaced with a gauze and tape cover that envelops the connecting clamps and bars of the fixator (Fig. 50.45B). This cover protects the animal and the owner from the sharp ends of the fixation pins and decreases the incidence of catching the apparatus on fixed objects. The cover should be applied so it does not contact the skin and allows air circulation around the skin–pin interface.

The use of antibiotic therapy with external skeletal fixation is still controversial. Certainly, the use of a broad-spectrum antibiotic is indicated for contami-

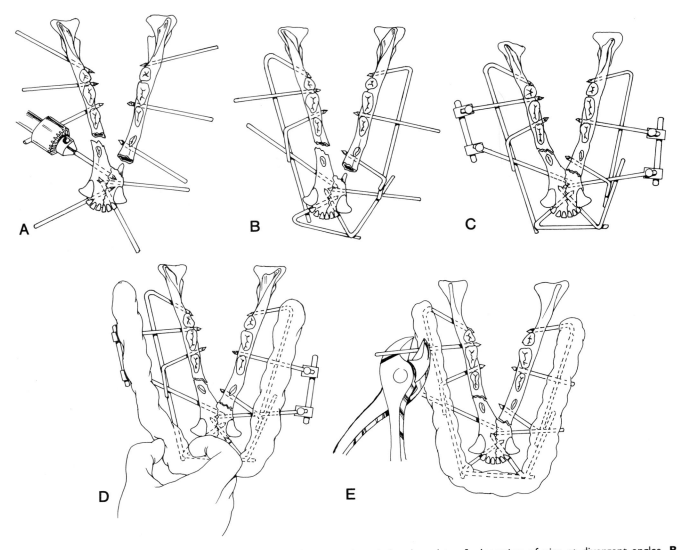

Fig. 50.44. Application of external skeletal fixation with pins and methylmethacrylate. **A.** Insertion of pins at divergent angles. **B.** Bending of several pins parallel to bone. **C.** Reduced fracture temporarily stabilized with connecting bars and clamps. **D.** Placement of methylmethacrylate around the bent pins to form a connecting column. **E.** Completed device after removal of connecting clamps and bars and trimming of pins. See text for details.

nated open or infected fractures until culture and sensitivity testing can direct more specific therapy. Furthermore, because of the soft tissue trauma attending even most closed fractures, and the use of the pins that extend from the environment to bone, I tend to use a broad-spectrum antibiotic for 4 to 7 days after the surgical procedure until the body's defenses are mobilized.

Most animals with an external fixator can be released to their owners within 2 to 4 days after surgery. Owners should be instructed to limit exercise to leash walking and to take particular care to avoid fences or similar open structures that could catch the splint. The fixator should be covered with tape until the device is removed, and the owner should inspect the apparatus daily. A small amount of dry crust is likely to develop at the skin–pin interface. Although opinions vary concerning proper pin care, I advise not removing this material or cleaning the pin sites. Significant serous or serosanguineous discharge, which may indicate a serious problem, is discussed in the next section on complications. The patient should return after 10 to 14 days for suture removal and evaluation for loose clamps. Further rechecks are performed at 3- to 4-week intervals, depending on the anticipated rate of healing.

A simple fracture in a young dog commonly heals completely in 6 weeks, whereas a comminuted fracture in a mature dog may require much longer (up to 6 months). Loss of sharpness in detail of the fracture edges is the earliest sign of fracture healing. External callus production is often minimal, particularly with

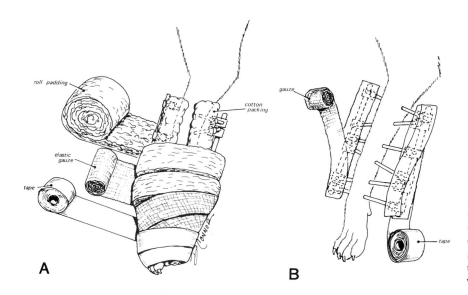

Fig. 50.45. **A.** A Robert Jones compressive wrap is initially applied over additional padding to prevent excessive swelling of the limb on which an external fixator is placed. **B.** After removal of the compressive wrap, gauze and tape are used to protect the splint and the environment.

the more rigid fixator configurations. However, young animals may produce a large callus because of the presence of an active periosteum. Clinical healing is determined by the loss of discernible fracture lines and the development of bony continuity in at least three of four cortices, as seen on two radiographic views.

In fractures treated initially with a rigid form of external fixation, healing appears to benefit from destabilization of the fixator, which allows increasing amounts of weightbearing stress to enhance remodeling and strengthening of the fracture while providing some protection from excessive stress. Preliminary research has indicated that around 6 weeks postoperatively is the optimal time for destabilization of simple fractures. This can be achieved by removing the connecting bars and pins from one side of a type II or type III splint or by removing alternate fixation pins from a type I splint.

When fracture healing is deemed clinically complete, the fixator can usually be removed with no or minimal sedation. The connecting clamps and bars are removed, and the fixation pins are pulled using a hand chuck or pin puller in a twisting motion. If threaded pins were used, they must be "unscrewed." After pin removal, a small amount of serosanguineous fluid often drains from the pin site, and a soft padded bandage may be appropriate for a day. The pin hole should not be sutured closed. Continued activity restriction for 6 to 8 weeks is usually indicated while the fracture remodels and the bone hypertrophies.

Complications

The most common complication of external skeletal fixation of a fracture is drainage around the fixation pins. This is often caused by excessive skin and soft tissue movement or tension against the pins. Careful placement of the pins through nondisplaced tissue and away from large muscle masses minimizes this problem in most cases. In some locations such as the distal femur, soft tissue movement against the pins is unavoidable, and some drainage is common. I recommend restriction of activity and periodic cleansing of the pin site with 2% hydrogen peroxide in such cases.

Loosening of the fixation pin at the pin–bone interface, which is indicated by a lucency surrounding the pin on radiographs, commonly results in drainage and infection of the pin tract. Once a pin becomes loose, the only effective treatment is removal. The pin tract drainage usually clears up rapidly. Aside from the nuisance of drainage, loosening of pins may cause a late-developing decrease in leg use. If too many pins loosen too quickly, adequate stability for osseous healing may be lost, and nonunion may develop. In my experience, the use of three or four pins per fracture segment and the use of threaded pins greatly reduce the likelihood of premature pin loosening and subsequent pin tract infection or drainage.

References

1. Egger EL. Static strength evaluation of six skeletal fixation configurations. Vet Surg 1983;12:130.
2. Egger EL, Runyon CL, Rigg DL. Use of the type 1 double connecting bar configuration of external skeletal fixation on long bone fractures in dogs: a review of 10 cases. J Am Anim Hosp Assoc 1986;22:57.
3. Egger EL, et al. Type I biplanar configurations of external skeletal fixation: application technique in nine dogs and one cat. J Am Vet Med Assoc 1985;187:262.
4. Olds R, Green SA. Hoffman's external fixation for arthrodesis and infected nonunions in the dog. J Am Anim Hosp Assoc 1983;19:705.
5. Parkhill C. A new apparatus for the fixation of bones after resection and in fractures with a tendency to displacement. Trans Am Surg Assoc 1897;15:251.

6. Bjorling DE, Toombs JP. Transarticular application of the Kirschner–Ehmer splint. Vet Surg 1982;11:34.

7. Robertson JJ. Application of a modified Kirschner device in the distraction mode as a prevention of antebrachial deformities in early physeal closure. J Am Anim Hosp Assoc 1983;19:345.

8. Johnson KA. Cancellous bone graft collection from the tibia in dogs. Vet Surg 1986;15:334.

9. Brinker WO, Flo GL. Principles and application of external skeletal fixation. Vet Clin North Am 1975;2:197.

10. Egger EL, Histand MB, Blass CB, et al. Effect of fixation pin insertion on the bone-pin interface. Vet Surg 1985;15:246.

11. Matthews LS, Green CA, Goldstein SA. The thermal effects of skeletal fixation-pin insertion in bone. J Bone Joint Surg Am 1984;66:1077.

12. Bennett RA, Egger EL, Histand MB, et al. Comparison of the strength and holding power of 4 pin designs for use with half-pin (type 1) external skeletal fixation. Vet Surg 1987;16:207.

13. Wu JJ, Shyr HS, Chao EYS, et al. Comparison of osteotomy healing under external fixation devices with different stiffness characteristics. J Bone Joint Surg Am 1984;66:1258.

Ilizarov Technique

Arnold S. Lesser

Forty-five years ago, the Russian physician Gavriil Ilizarov developed a technique for the regeneration of bone through the stretching of an osteotomy. The technique, called distraction osteogenesis, was only introduced to Western European medicine in 1981, when an Italian explorer had his infected tibial pseudarthrosis treated and healed by Ilizarov and introduced the method to Italian surgeons. The method did not reach the United States until 5 years later. Ilizarov's technique has greatly expanded our ability to treat deformities in length and angulation as well as bone defects and infected pseudarthrosis. As veterinary orthopedic surgeons, we now have the ability to treat severe bone defects effectively that would have previously led to almost certain amputation or euthanasia of the patient.

Ilizarov developed an external fixator made up of rings, threaded connecting bars, cannulated bolts, and thin transosseus wires. Supposedly, one of his patients turned the nuts on the threaded bars in the wrong direction, distracting the fracture instead of compressing it, and Ilizarov observed the formation of bone between the fracture ends. From this finding, he discovered that bone could be mechanically induced or regenerated by distracting bone ends. This phenomenon is explained thus: "discontinuity of a skeletal segment necessarily triggers the repair process which will continue as long as the integrity of both the osteogenic tissue and its vascular supply is maintained" (1). We can manipulate this process by applying tension by gradually pulling apart the bone ends. New bone or callus is laid down between the ends along the lines of tension and continues to do so as long as the foregoing criteria are met. Factors restricting the amount of new bone formation are the soft tissues surrounding the bone, especially tendons and nerves. Investigators have also reported that lengthening of more than 20% of a bone adversely affects the cartilage of the adjacent joint (2). Ilizarov likened this process to the natural growth of the physis in immature individuals. He believed that the tension created in the limb from the growth of a physis stimulates the growth of muscles, tendons, vessels, and nerves in the young, and that distraction osteogenesis is merely creating a new physis in a patient. He also believed that distraction osteogenesis stimulated the growth of these soft tissues along with the regeneration of bone. This concept, however, has not been proved, and we do not know whether nerves and muscle actually regenerate or merely stretch in response to this slow distraction in limb lengthening.

Pathophysiology

The biology of distraction osteogenesis begins with an osteotomy. Ilizarov described a specialized osteotomy, called a corticotomy, in which the cortex is cut two-thirds of the way around, and the last segment is fractured manually by twisting the limb gently to preserve the medullary blood supply (Fig. 50.46). He also attempted to preserve the periosteal envelope. More recently, experiments have shown that the medullary blood supply quickly reforms after a conventional osteotomy, and the method works just as well with a routine osteotomy or corticotomy. The periosteum should be protected as much as possible with both procedures. The second stage is a lag or latency period in which nothing is done to the bone while the neovascularization and osteogenic precursor cells form at the site. In one study, the volume of mineralized callus was greater after delaying distraction than after immediate distraction (3). Various recommendations have been made for the length of this latency period. A study performed in skeletally mature dogs showed that a latency period of 0 to 14 days successfully produced bone (1). The recommendation based on this study was that, if the medullary blood supply and the periosteum are preserved, then distraction can begin immediately, but if the medullary canal is damaged, a 14-day latency period optimizes osteogenesis (1). The latency period recommended by this investigator is 5 to 7 days when dealing with lengthening or bone defects in older patients. My experience has been that, in correcting growth deformities in young dogs less than 1 year of age, no lag or latency period is needed because the biggest problem is early consolidation of the dis-

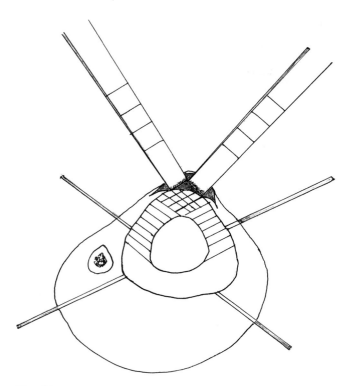

Fig. 50.46. In a corticotomy, two-thirds of the cortex is cut with an osteotome through a stab incision, and the remaining caudal cortex is broken by twisting the limb. The idea is to preserve both the periosteum and medullary blood supply.

traction callus. Admittedly, this finding is based on a small number of cases. Factors such as the age of the patient, the site of the osteotomy, and the degree of soft tissue trauma should be considered in making this decision (3). When one has a choice, making the osteotomy through metaphyseal bone enhances callus production.

After the osteotomy, fibrovascular tissue forms between the bone ends, and the third stage of controlled, gradual distraction causes this tissue to align parallel to the direction of distraction. Bone forms from both cut surfaces and eventually forms into microcolumns along those same lines of tension (Fig. 50.47). In an experimental study of mature dogs, this bone was first seen at 14 days of distraction after a 7-day latency period and formed into microcolumns 7 days later. New fibrous tissue is laid down in the center of the distraction callus, aligned parallel to the tension forces, and mineral is laid down around the strands of fibrous tissue, forming the microcolumns of bone originating at the cut ends and continuing to form at the edge of this fibrous interzone (Fig 50.47). If the fibrous interzone becomes too wide, a risk of nonunion exists, and if the interzone becomes too narrow, a risk of early bridging exists, preventing further lengthening. Therefore, clinically one must follow the case radio-

graphically at least every 2 to 3 weeks to be sure to maintain a 3- to 4-mm wide fibrous interzone.

Much concern and discussion of the ideal rate and rhythm of distraction have taken place because these elements are key to the process. Everything from once a day to mechanized distracters that perform constant slow distraction has been used at a rate of 0.5 to 2 mm a day. At this point, a rate of 1 mm a day at a rhythm of every 6 hours (1 mm split four times daily) is recommended (1), but this rate can vary according to the clinical situation. I usually recommend 0.5 mm twice a day. One study showed that osteogenesis was significantly inhibited at a distraction rate of 1 mm once a day when compared with 0.5 mm twice a day (1). I have gone to 2 mm a day split to 1 mm twice a day for angular limb corrections on young, giant breed dogs.

Once the desired amount of bone is formed, whether to gain length or to fill a gap, the distraction is terminated, and the consolidation period is begun. The fixator is locked, allowing the fibrous interzone to bridge and bone to form throughout the distraction callus. These effects were seen 42 days after distraction was ceased in the foregoing study, at which time the external fixator was removed (1). Eventually, lamellar bone, haversian systems, and hematopoietic marrow form in the remodeled callus.

Equipment

Some confusion exists between the equipment Ilizarov developed and the biologic technique, which allows for the regeneration of bone through distraction of two bone ends. Ilizarov developed an external fixator using thin transosseus wires attached to external rings connected by threaded rods. The threaded rods allow either compression or distraction of the bone ends. This equipment is also used for fracture fixation. Any internal or external fixator that allows for gradual, measured distraction also can use Ilizarov's biologic technique. Therefore, these are two separate concepts, one biologic and one mechanical, that can be used together or can stand on their own.

The Ilizarov ring fixator may have started out as a simple frame, but today it is sophisticated and complex, with numerous attachments, such as hinges, extensions, angulation motors, and adapters, that allow a wide selection of constructs to handle various clinical problems (Fig. 50.48). The use of rings allows these connecting rods to be placed on all sides of the lower limb to provide even support. This fixator is similar to a type III external skeletal fixator (ESF), which we know from experimental work is much stronger in bending in all planes than a type I or II. Partial rings allow the use of the ring fixator in the upper limb. Another innovation of this system is the use of thin wires, 1.5 to 1.8 mm in diameter, to attach the bone

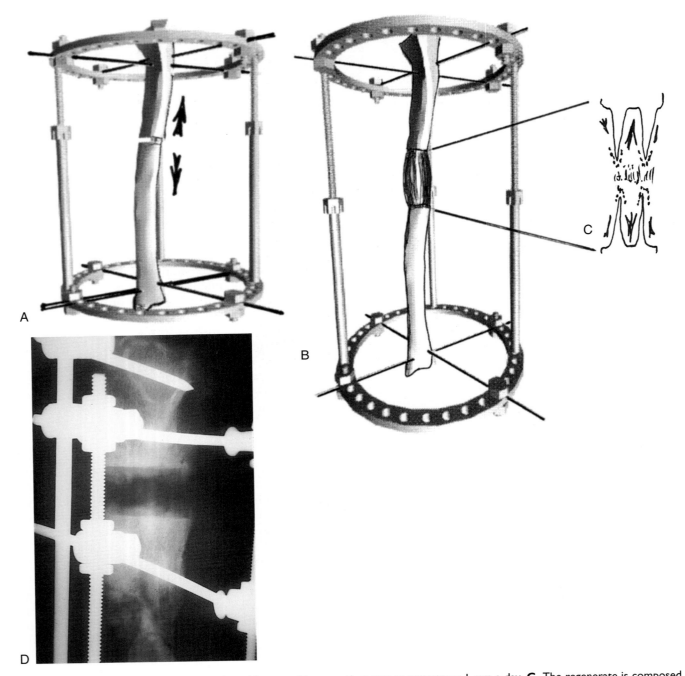

Fig. 50.47. **A** and **B.** Bones can be lengthened by stretching a corticotomy or osteotomy 1 mm a day. **C.** The regenerate is composed of microcolumns (*MIC*), originating from both bone ends (*BE*), a primary mineralization front (*PMF*), and a central fibrous interzone (*CFI*). **D.** Radiograph of distraction callus at 3 weeks. (**C** from Maiocchi A, Aronson J, eds. Operative principles of Ilizarov. Milan: Medi Surgical, 1991.)

to the rings. These thin wires appear to be less traumatic to the soft tissues than the larger pins often used. The wires, however, must be tensioned to provide stability, and a tensioner is included with the equipment. Recommended tension varies from author to author, from 50 to 150 kg (1, 3). When lengthening bone, the process itself adds tension to the wires as distraction progresses, so less initial tension is necessary than in

fracture fixation, in which tension does not increase. A safe range to use is 50 to 90 kg, but few veterinary ring fixators have expensive tensioners that record the tension. The wires can also be tensioned by twisting the cannulated bolts, but this causes some translation of the bone (Fig. 50.49). These bolts fit into holes drilled all along the ring to allow various positions for the wires. In addition, grooves in the top of the bolt

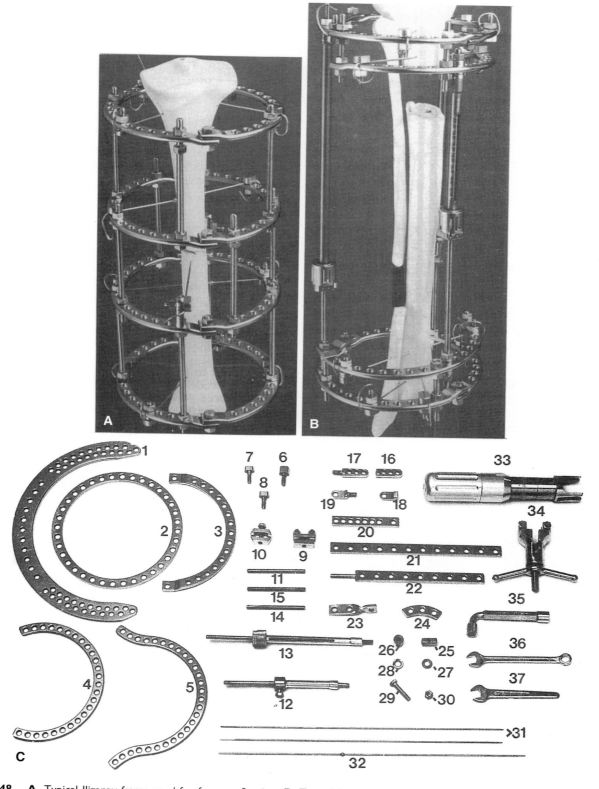

Fig. 50.48. **A.** Typical Ilizarov frame used for fracture fixation. **B.** Typical Ilizarov frame used for leg lengthening. **C.** This system has many adaptations and modifications to conform to various clinical situations: *1*, arch with holes; *2*, full ring; *3*, half-ring; *4*, ⅝ half-ring; *5*, half-ring with curved extremities; *6*, wire fixation bolt cannulated; *7*, wire fixation bolt cannulated with threaded head; *8*, wire fixation bolt slotted; *9*, detachable wire fixation buckle; *10*, dual-sided wire fixation buckle; *11*, threaded rod; *12*, telescopic rod and partial threaded rod (assembled); *13*, graduated telescopic rod; *14*, slotted threaded rod; *15*, threaded rod with hole; *16*, postfeminine end; *17*, support (masculine end); *18*, hinge (feminine end); *19*, hinge (masculine end); *20*, short connection plate; *21*, long connection plate; *22*, connection plate with threaded end; *23*, twisted plate; *24*, curved plate; *25*, threaded socket; *26*, bushing; *27*, washer; *28*, slotted washer; *29*, bolt; *30*, nut; *31*, Ilizarov wire; *32*, Ilizarov wire with stopper; *33*, dynamometric wire tensioner; *34*, wire tensioner; *35*, tubular angulated wrench; *36*, wrench; *37*, wrench for telescopic rod. (From Maiocchi A, Aronson J, eds. Operative principles of Ilizarov. Milan: Medi Surgical, 1991:9, 12, 18.)

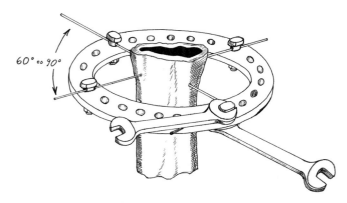

Fig. 50.49. **A.** The transfixation wires should be placed between 60 and 90° to each other. Less than 60° is unstable. **B.** A simple way to tension these wires is to twist the cannulated bolts as they are tightened.

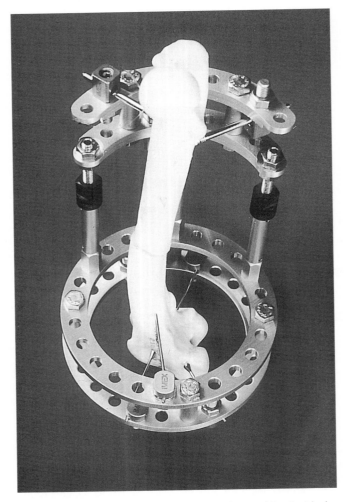

Fig. 50.50. Larger transfixation pins can be combined with the use of rings and wires in hybrid frames.

accept a wire that is slightly off center. Larger transfixation pins have been combined with the use of wires in hybrid frames, especially in the proximal femur and humerus, and are more comfortable and better tolerated by human patients (4) (Fig. 50.50). Specialized wires, called olive wires, were developed with a stop molded on the shaft. These wires allow tensioning of the bone or fragments by pulling on the opposite end of the wire as the stop pulls against the bone. This maneuver allows adjustment of fragments and even compression of oblique fracture lines by using opposing olive wires (Fig 50.51). Many of these innovations are currently available in a veterinary ring fixator (Imex ring fixator, Imex Veterinary, Longview, TX).

The ring fixator using transfixation wires has different mechanical properties than a stiff pin fixator. The ring fixator is strong in bending and torsion, but it does allow motion in the axial direction because of the flexibility of the wires. This feature is considered an advantage by proponents of this equipment because axial motion, especially if cyclic, enhances healing of a fracture compared with rigid fixation (1).

Various companies in the United States and Europe produce veterinary ring fixators. However, the clinician can also create a ring fixator from the Kirschner–Ehmer external fixator equipment. Threaded $\frac{3}{16}$-inch Steinmann pins along with stainless steel nuts can be used to connect rings fabricated from $\frac{1}{8}$-inch connecting bars (Fig. 50.52). The small clamps connect the transfixation wires to the ring, and the medium clamps connect the threaded rods to the rings. Nuts lock the

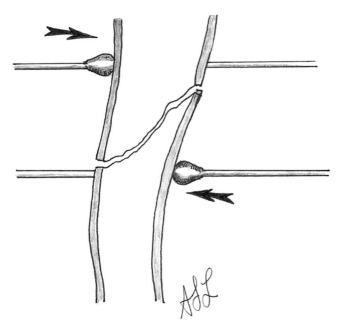

Fig. 50.51. Special wires with stops attached called olive wires allow for manipulation of the fragments for reduction and compression.

in their use in the proximal humerus and femur. An intermedullary nail can be combined with a type I ESF in the femur or humerus.

Clinical Uses

Fracture Fixation

The Ilizarov method has been used in veterinary medicine in the United States for almost a decade, mostly for the treatment of angular limb deformities. However, the apparatus or ring fixator is just recently finding use in the treatment of fresh fractures. Ring fixators have several advantages. Smaller-diameter transfixation wires tend to create less soft tissue damage, especially in high-risk areas such as those in which the surgeon must penetrate thick muscle. The use of rings and crossed wires also allows the placement of two to four wires in short distal or proximal fragments that would not be possible with conventional fixators. The use of olive wires allows the positioning of fragments without opening the fracture, as long as a ring is nearby. More rigid conventional fixators tend to show plastic deformation in a gap situation, whereas the tensioned wires of a ring fixator usually show elastic deformation providing cyclic, axial motion conducive to healing (1).

The disadvantages of ring fixators are their complexity and more exacting nature. A simple construct restricts the angle between the connecting bars and the rings to 90°. This means that everything must be placed precisely at 90° or the components start to bind. If the transfixation wires wander off 90° to the bone, then the rings will not be at a 90° angle, and either the connecting bars will bind or the fracture will be malaligned (Fig. 50.53). Some of the modifications incorporated in the Ilizarov equipment allow the attachment of wires and connecting bars that are slightly offset. Some of the veterinary rings also use short connectors, spheric washers, and the like to allow the rings to be set at angles other than 90°. Without these attachments, trying to reduce and stabilize fractures closed requires careful planning and accurate placement of both wires and rings. The alternative is to open the fracture, reduce it, and hold it reduced while applying the frame. This negates one of the big advantages of ESF, which is its adaptability to the biologic approach to fracture treatment. In this approach, the reduction is carried out closed or with minimal exposure and fragment manipulation. The addition of all these attachments makes the equipment adaptable but more demanding to use.

Preplanning is critical, and it is helpful to construct the frame first, place it over the limb, and then drive the transfixation wires through the cannulated bolts into the bone. The bolts can be placed in many loca-

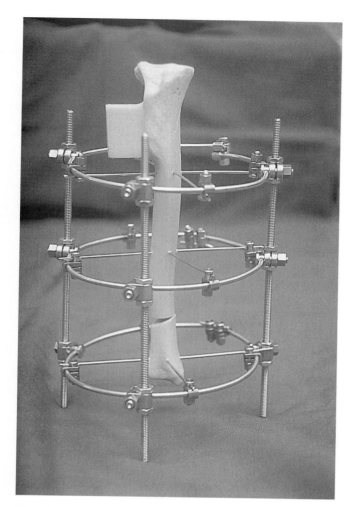

Fig. 50.52. A ring fixator can be created from equipment routinely used in veterinary practice. A round bar used for the rings allows various angles for pins and rods to articulate, but it is not as stiff as flat rings.

medium clamps and allow distraction. The Ilizarov equipment, designed for use in human medicine, is expensive, but used components are sometimes available.

As mentioned previously, one does not need to use a ring fixator to regenerate bone. Manufacturers of other unilateral external fixators have modified their equipment to allow both distraction and bone transport. All that is necessary is to be able to move one section of bone independently in measured increments of 0.5 to 1 mm while supporting the rest of the bones and limb. Distraction osteogenesis can be performed with a simple type I Kirschner–Ehmer ESF on a threaded connecting bar. The problem with a unilateral frame is that it is not strong enough to resist angulation deformities that develop from soft tissue resistance to lengthening. Type II and type III fixators are better at resisting these forces, but they are limited

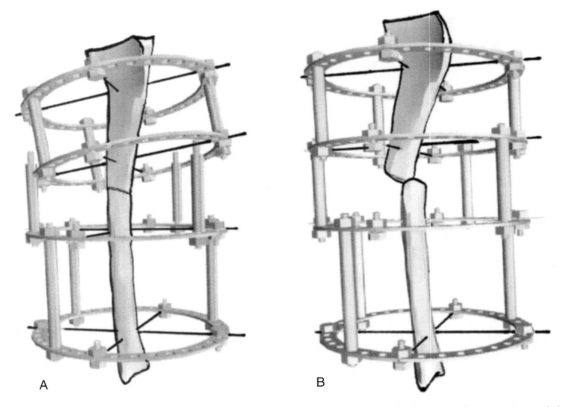

A   B

Fig. 50.53. Many frames require the pins and connecting rods to attach to the ring at 90°. If the transfixation wires and therefore the rings are not 90° to the bone, then either the connecting rods will bind (**A**) or the alignment of the fracture will be incorrect (**B**).

tions on the ring to allow placement of the wires through safe areas, and the two wires on one level should be placed between 60 and 90° to each other. A 90° angle is best, and anything less than 60° causes instability (see Fig. 50.49). Just as with any ESF, one ring and set of wires should be placed at either end of the bone, and one set should be placed close to the fracture ends. Therefore, four rings are ideal for fracture fixation, although in special situations the combination with conventional transfixation pins or sets of wires on either side of a ring can allow the use of fewer rings. The top and bottom rings are attached to the bone, with care taken first that they are set parallel to the adjacent joint surface. Then the fracture is aligned. If the fragments are overriding, then the threaded bars allow distraction, which should tend to align the fracture if the rings are properly aligned. The fracture can be further aligned with olive wires and fixed to the middle rings. When this device is used properly, the patient should be able to bear weight early because the physiologic use of the leg is important in the healing process. Tensioning of the wires is important, especially in larger patients, to prevent excessive motion from an unstable frame. Excessive motion can lead to loosening of the wires, which can cause the patient significant pain and lameness. In small patients, the smaller rings mean shorter wires, which are inherently stiffer even without tensioning. The goal is to have the wires taut.

Lengthening and Angular Correction

The most common indication for the use of distraction osteogenesis is the treatment of growth deformities. Occasionally, a mature animal is presented with a shortened limb or angular deformity from an old physeal injury or malunion. Usually, the veterinary surgeon is presented with a young, large or giant breed dog with an arrested or closed distal radial or ulnar physis. These limbs have craniocaudal and mediolateral angular deformities, as well as rotational and length deformities. Occasionally, one sees subluxation of the adjacent joints as well. These patients are often presented at 7 to 8 months of age when further growth is negligible and a single correction is possible. In these cases, a ring fixator allows multiple wires to be placed in a short distal segment, and in severe deformities, a gradual correction can be made. These young, fast-growing dogs heal so well that a single-step correction works as long as the soft tissues are not compromised and no length discrepancy exists. The 3- to 4-month-old dog benefits most from distraction. If the surgeon performs an immediate correction and release of the slow-growing bone, the risk of early bridging and recurrence of the deformity exists. If one waits until growth stops, one risks permanent damage to the adjacent joints. With distraction osteogenesis, one can make angular corrections and then lengthen the leg to prevent shortening and recurrence of deformity. In essence, a new physis is created. The physis itself can be stretched (epiphysiolysis), but it is always injured and closes prematurely, so it is more practical to distract a new osteotomy or corticotomy. When planning repair in these young animals, the surgeon first must identify the cause of the deformity, the nature of all components of the deformity, and any possible future deformity that may occur after surgical correction. Once these factors are determined, the procedure can be planned to manage them all. When dealing with a two-bone system, the surgeon must cut the slow-growing bone creating the deformity and lengthen, derotate, and straighten the deformed bone or bones. If the limb must be lengthened, both bones should be cut because distracting one bone tends to injure the physis of the other. This injury can then create a new deformity during lengthening.

If a progressive angular correction is planned, the surgeon must know the plane of correction. This plane can be calculated from the ventrodorsal and lateral radiographs. A simpler method is to place a pin parallel to the distal radial joint line in an exact medial-to-lateral plane and a second and third pin parallel to the proximal radial joint line and along the axis of the radius proximal to the deformity. When these three pins are lined up and are parallel, all three deformities are corrected. The same procedure can be applied with a ring fixator. The distal and two proximal rings are placed parallel to the plane of their adjacent joints. If possible, any rotational deformity is corrected in one step. Then the rings are gradually aligned until they are parallel to each other (Fig. 50.54). If a large rotational deformity exists, a single acute correction may compromise the vasculature, leading to ischemia. An alternate approach is to derotate about 15% initially and then wait until the angular and length deformities are corrected before completing the rotational correction. Angular corrections require a hinge in the apparatus, and the placement of the hinge is important. The axis of the hinge must be parallel to the plane of correction, but, just as important, the placement of the hinge dictates the effects at the osteotomy site. If the hinge is placed in the center of the bone at the point of curvature, then the convex cortex will be corrected and compressed. If the hinge is placed at the outside cortex of the curvature, one will see filling in of the angular correction, and if the hinge is placed lateral to the

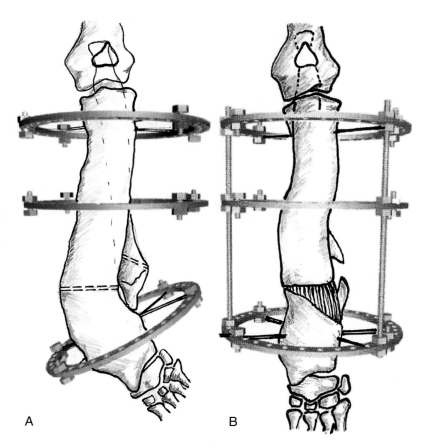

A   B

Fig. 50.54. **A.** The rings are placed parallel to the plane of the adjacent joints, and any rotational deformity is corrected in one step. **B.** Then the rings are gradually aligned until they are parallel to each other.

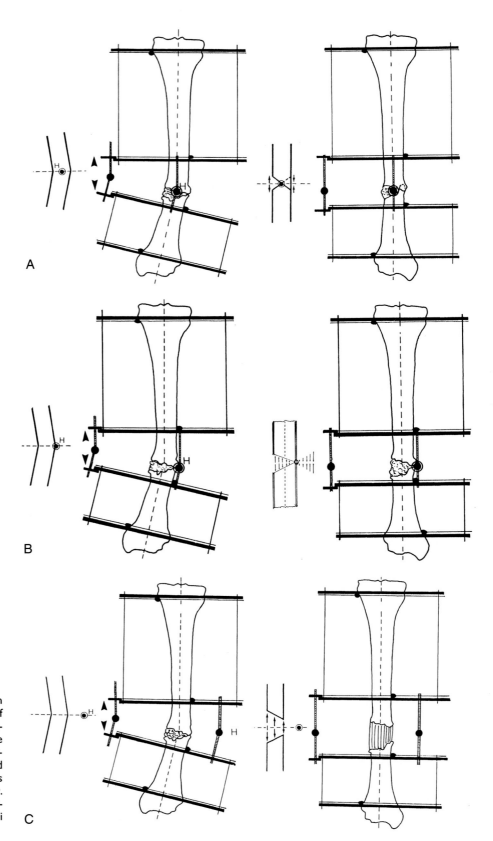

Fig. 50.55. **A.** If the hinge is placed in the center of the bone at the point of curvature, then correction alone will occur. **B.** If the hinge is at the outside cortex of the curvature, the angular correction will fill in. **C.** If the hinge is placed lateral to the convexity, lengthening as well as angular correction will occur. (From Maiocchi A, Aronson J, eds. Operative principles of Ilizarov. Milan: Medi Surgical, 1991:74–76.)

convexity, lengthening and angular correction will occur (Fig. 50.55). By moving the hinge proximally or distally, one can create translation of the bone ends (Fig. 50.56). Placement of the hinges on the ring is determined by drawing a cross section of the bone and then drawing lines proportional in length to the angles of deformity as measured on the ventrodorsal and lateral radiographs. These lines are at 90° to each other, and a resultant diagonal is proportional to the degrees of correction and represents the angle of correction. A line drawn perpendicular to this diagonal and tangent to the bone intersects the ring at the points where the hinges should be placed (Fig. 50.57) (5). Besides the

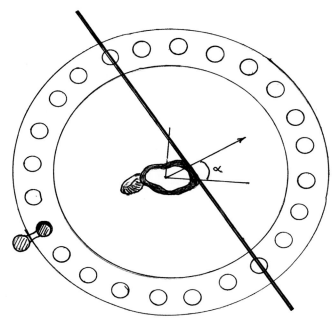

Fig. 50.57. The placement of the hinge on the ring is determined by drawing a cross section of the bone and then drawing lines proportional in length to the angles of deformity (*a* and *b*), as measured on the ventrodorsal and lateral radiographs. The resultant diagonal (*c*) is be proportional to the degree of correction and represents the angle of correction. A line drawn perpendicular to this diagonal and tangent to the bone intersects the ring at the points where the hinges should be placed (*d* and *d1*). The distraction motor is placed at (*e*). (From Marcellin-Little, Denis J. In: Fifth American College of Veterinary Surgeons Symposium. Chicago, IL: American College of Veterinary Surgeons, 1995:312.)

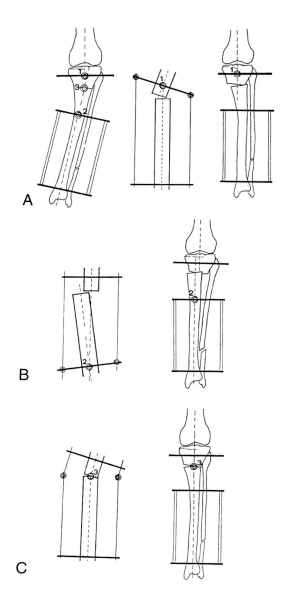

Fig. 50.56. By moving the hinge proximally or distally, the surgeon can create translation of the bone ends. (From Maiocchi A, Aronson J, eds. Operative principles of Ilizarov. Milan: Medi Surgical, 1991:73.)

hinges, an extra threaded bar, called a distraction motor, is placed on the rings to provide the angulation correction.

These young dogs heal so quickly that, in my experience, no latency period is necessary, although other investigators have recommended 1 to 2 days. Lengthening should be started at the same time as angular correction. I have also gone to a rate of 2 mm, at a rhythm of 1 mm twice daily. Otherwise, these dogs tend to bridge their distraction callus before the lengthening is complete. The surgeon must monitor the limb for joint contracture when distracting at this rate. When doing angular corrections using a hinge, 1 mm of movement on the bar may not translate to 1 mm of movement of the bone. The theory of similar triangles is used to determine how much movement must occur on the threaded bar to create 1 mm of movement at the bone (Fig. 50.58) (3). Limb lengthening can be accomplished with only two rings, but because most clinical cases entail a distal osteotomy, I usually use one ring on the distal fragment and two rings on the proximal fragment.

When lengthening the femur or humerus, the surgeon has the added difficulty of working around large

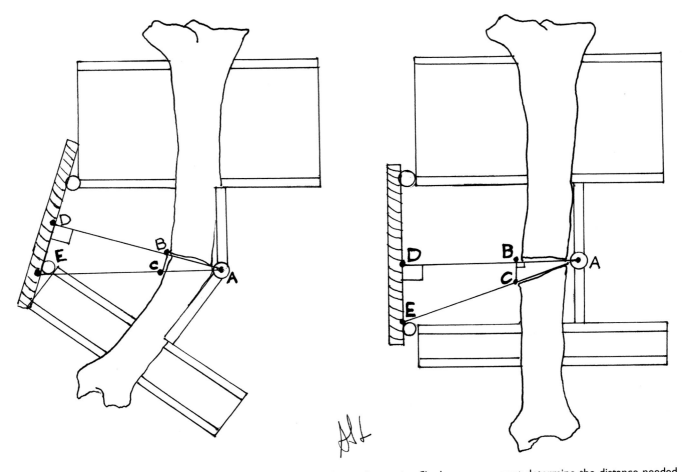

Fig. 50.58. If I mm of movement at the osteotomy is desired (point B to point C), the surgeon must determine the distance needed to move the distraction motor (point D to point E). This problem is solved with the equation BC/DE = AB/AD where BC = I and AB and AD are measured from the frame and radiograph.

muscle mass and the body wall medially. This configuration makes it difficult to support the proximal fragment medially. This large muscle resistance and reduced support can lead to angular deformation as the bone is distracted. A unilateral frame does not prevent this complication. Some of the newer veterinary frames have half-rings to help overcome this problem. Another solution is to combine an intermedullary interlocking nail (Innovative Animal Products, Rochester, MN) with a unilateral Kirschner–Ehmer-type apparatus using positive profile threaded transfixation pins catching the holes in the nail in the proximal fragment and lying next to the nail in the distal fragment. As distraction is produced in the lateral bar, the distal cortex slides along the nail. This process, in turn, prevents the caudal bending that would otherwise occur from the pull of the hamstring muscles (Fig. 50.59).

Complications of limb lengthening are joint contractures, neurapraxia, ischemia, malalignment, nonunion or premature bridging of the callus, and lack of client compliance. Joint contractures are best prevented by encouraging full function to stretch the muscles with exercise during the distraction period. In Russia, children are encouraged to play ball and ride bikes while wearing the apparatus. At the first sign of any stiffness or pain, the surgeon should stop distraction, back off if necessary, and encourage limb use to stretch the muscles. An elastic band can be placed from the apparatus to the foot in apposition to the contracture to encourage stretching further. In animals, we veterinary surgeons must look for vascular and nerve problems because our patients cannot talk. Temperature or color change and sudden chewing of the limb are important signs of impending neurovascular problems. Malalignment is a big problem in the femur, which cannot be supported evenly on the medial side proximally. Care must be taken not to place a wire through both the radius and the ulna proximal to the osteotomy, creating a synostosis. If this occurs, then the open proximal radial physis will create a subluxation of the elbow joint. Ischemia of the distraction

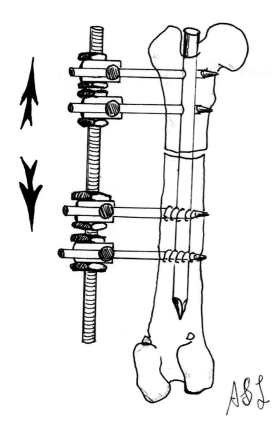

Fig. 50.59. To overcome the problem of placing a support medially with the proximal humerus or femur, an intermedullary nail can be combined with a type I external skeletal fixation to prevent angular deformity from occurring during limb lengthening.

callus can occur from too rapid stretching of the neovascular tissue leading to a nonunion, and stretching too slowly can lead to premature bridging of the distraction callus. Keeping the fibrous interzone between 2 and 4 mm prevents early bridging and nonunions. Therefore, frequent radiographic rechecks 2 to 3 weeks apart maximum are necessary to monitor these patients. Even with close monitoring, young, rapidly growing dogs can bridge between rechecks, leading to a decision whether to refracture the callus or to accept the present amount of correction. Many clients choose the latter over another procedure. The improvements tend to be dramatic even when not 100% (Fig. 50.60).

Bone Transport for Bone Defects

Maybe the most dramatic use of the Ilizarov method in veterinary surgery is the treatment of bone defects. These defects are usually secondary to infected nonunions previously treated with a sequestrectomy. In the past, massive cancellous grafts were necessary because cortical grafts are contraindicated when infection is present. When the gap was too long, amputation was often performed. Bone transport can also be used in limb-salvage procedures in which the defect is created by excising a bone tumor. The advent of bone regeneration by distraction osteogenesis has allowed the filling of these gaps with the use of bone segment transport. In this technique, a segment of bone is created with a corticotomy or osteotomy made 2 to 3 cm from one end of one of the main fragments. After an appropriate latency period (4 to 7 days), the newly created bone segment is transported at 1 mm a day down to the opposite end of the gap, where it is compressed against the opposing bone end (1, 3, 6). This procedure is accomplished by placing a pin through this bone segment and attaching both ends to clamps placed on two threaded bars (motors) or a separate ring. The pin can be placed parallel to the transfixation pins or angled distally in a V shape to reduce trauma to the skin as the segment is advanced. The ring or motors are advanced along the bars and pull the bone segment toward the opposite end. The gap is indirectly filled with regenerate bone created in the expanding osteotomy (Fig. 50.61). In the final stage, the bone segment is compressed against the opposite cortex until union occurs. If necessary, a cancellous graft can be placed in this site to enhance healing of the bone segment to the opposite fragment.

This technique has been performed by Ilizarov without the use of any antibiotics or sequestrectomy (1, 7). In my cases, I have not been so bold and have followed more routine preparation and ancillary culture and sensitivity testing with the use of appropriate

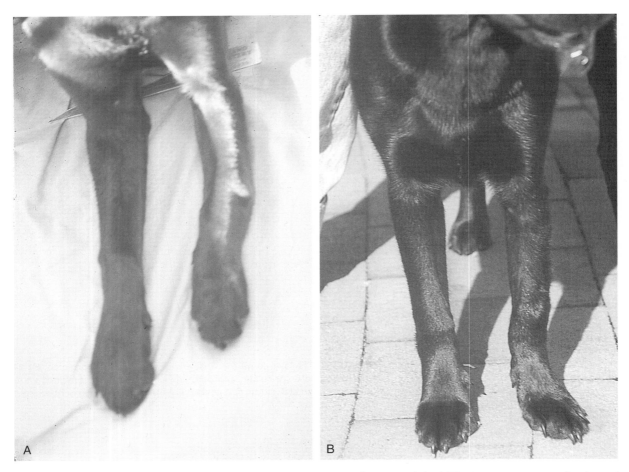

Fig. 50.60. **A** and **B.** Young dogs often bridge before full lengthening can be accomplished. The improvements can be dramatic even when not 100%.

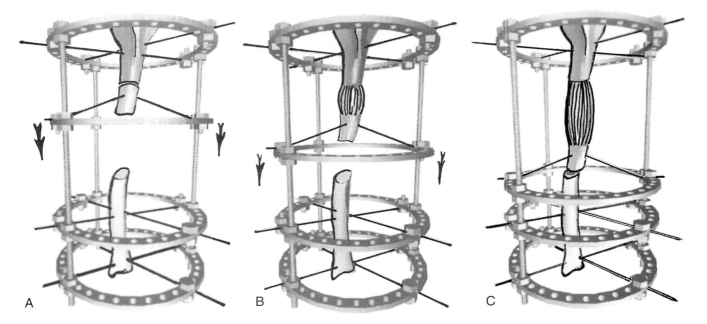

Fig. 50.61. A large bone gap can be filled by creating a bone segment with an osteotomy (**A**), by moving this segment 1 mm a day toward the opposite end (**B**), and by filling the gap indirectly with regenerate callus while compressing the segment onto the opposite fragment (**C**).

antibiotics along with the bone transport (6). As with limb lengthening, one does need to use ring fixators exclusively to accomplish this technique, but they have the advantage of being designed with this use in mind. Type II or type III ESF can be used with threaded connecting bars to move the bone segment and to stabilize the fracture. This technique is successful and greatly expands the treatment of osteomyelitis and limb salvage.

Acknowledgment

I would like to thank Peter Wadsworth, DVM, for his assistance in the computer drawings.

References

1. Maiocchi A, Aronson J, eds. Operative principles of Ilizaro. Milan: Medi Surgical, 1991.
2. Nakamura E, Mizuta H, Akira S, et al. Knee articular cartilage injury in leg lengthening. Acta Orthop Scand 1993;64:437–440.
3. Green S, ed. Limb lengthening, Orthop Clin North Am 1991; 22:4.
4. Maiocchi A, ed. Advances in Ilizarov apparatus assembly. Milan: Medicalplastic, 1994.
5. Marcellin-Little, Denis J. In: Fifth American College of Veterinary Surgeons Veterinary Symposium.: American College of Veterinary Surgeons, 1995:312.
6. Lesser A. Segmental bone transport for the treatment of bone deficits. J Am Anim Hosp Assoc 1994;30:322–330.
7. Dagher F, Roukoz S. Compound tibial fractures with bone loss treated by the Ilizarov technique. J Bone Joint Surg Br 1991; 73:316–331.

51

POSTOPERATIVE MANAGEMENT

Implant Removal

Charles M. Pullen

Over the course of my practice career, I have developed the philosophy of removing all plates from patients with routine extremity fractures in which motion and weightbearing are factors. Exceptions include nonunions or delayed unions, distal radial fractures in toy breeds, and geriatric patients. Primary factors motivating this philosophy are problems encountered when plates are left in extremities. The reasons for this protocol include the following:

1. Removal of implants prevents the formation of draining tracts from micromovement secondary to screw or plate loosening, a complication that often occurs 4 to 6 years after placement of the implant.

2. Implant removal avoids discomfort to the patient during cold weather caused by the implant and resulting in intermittent lameness.

3. Implant removal prevents weakening or decalcification of the bone secondary to assumption by the plate of a large portion of the normal stresses. This assumption prevents the bone from returning completely to its prefracture strength because it relies partly on the plate.

4. Removal of the implant returns the bone and its surrounding soft tissue structures to their normal integrity (i.e., tendons do not have to glide over a metal implant), and the marrow cavity and trabecular structures can resume their normal pattern. Removal thus leaves the healed bone in a more natural state.

5. Once fracture healing is complete, the only disadvantage to plate removal is the need for a second minor surgical procedure. The advantages far outweigh this concern.

6. Finally, and most important reason, I have never encountered a problem after removal of a plate from a healed fracture. On the other hand, significant problems have been encountered when plates have been left in place.

In my experience, the time for plate removal, as dictated by clinical and radiographic evidence of healing, is 8 to 10 months after placement of the implant in immature patients and 12 to 18 months after placement of the implant in mature patients.

Postoperative Instructions

Edward Leeds

How often as a surgeon have you spent hours repairing a fracture to your satisfaction only to have the animal go home and return on recheck with the repair compromised? On questioning the client, one often hears "I thought the animal would limit its own activity and would not do anything that would disrupt the repair." Oral postoperative instructions, although better than none at all, may be misunderstood or not properly communicated to other family members. Thus, precise written instructions and frequent rechecks are important.

Veterinary surgeons are usually not afforded the luxury of being able to limit or restrict weightbearing on a repaired limb until healing is complete. When complete immobilization is attempted, the results are often severe muscle atrophy or joint ankylosis ("fracture disease"). Most veterinary surgeons have experienced the frustration of attempting physical therapy to reverse ankylosed joints secondary to prolonged im-

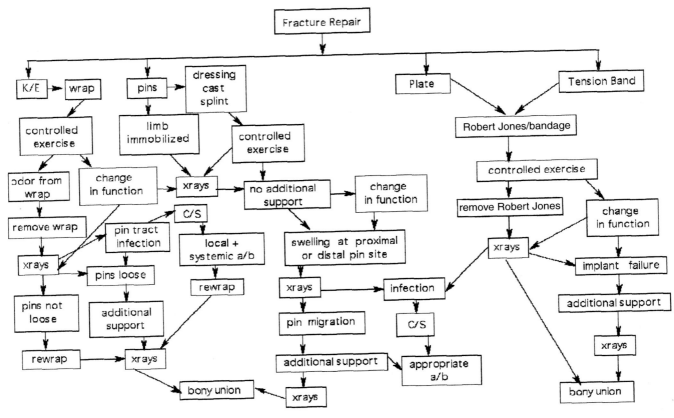

Fig. 51.1. Postoperative algorithm of fracture repair.

mobilization. For this reason, veterinary patients are immobilized for shorter periods and are in a race between fracture healing and implant failure (Fig. 51.1).

As surgeons, we must realize that postoperative instructions and follow-up care are as important to the successful outcome of surgery as the actual surgical procedure itself. Postoperative instructions should be reviewed *before* performing the surgical procedure, to prepare the client for the altered lifestyle required by the patient.

The type of fixation or fracture stabilization (Kirschner–Ehmer apparatus, plate, intramedullary pin, or tension band) or the type of splint, cast, or bandage alters the postoperative instructions. I use the following as general guidelines:

Home Care for Veterinary Patients*

Pet's name:
Diagnosis/surgery performed:

Home care is usually where most healing occurs; therefore, the care you provide is vital to your pet's

recovery. Our staff will assist you in any way possible to ensure success in your efforts.

Vomiting may occur if your pet is allowed to gorge itself with food or water as soon as it arrives home. Pets tend to do this even though they received proper nutrition while hospitalized.

Instructions and Information: Please Note the Items Checked

_____ Your pet has received (some) (all) of its medication today. Begin giving the medication at home (today) (tomorrow) as directed.

_____ Begin giving the medication today as follows:

_____ Give all of today's dose according to the label.

_____ Give only half of today's doses this first day.

_____ Special instructions: 1) No lying in grass or dirt. 2) No doggy-doors. 3) No stairs. 4) No jumping on or off furniture. 5) Walk slowly on a leash when outside, and only to urinate and defecate. 6) If your pet is wearing an Elizabethan collar, do NOT remove it; your pet can eat and sleep with the collar on.

_____ No changes in the diet or water are required at this time.

_____ Feed the following special diet: _____

_____ Keep your pet's splint, cast, or bandage as clean

*Erlewein DL, et al. Instructions for veterinary clients. 2nd ed. Philadelphia: W.B. Saunders Co. 1975.

and dry as possible (see separate instructions). If surgery was performed, inspect the site daily.

_____ Restrict activity. Do not allow any playing.

_____ Do not allow your pet to play with or be with other pets until released from our care. Other pets may irritate your pet's surgical site, disrupt the surgical procedure, or lick out the sutures.

_____ Please set up a recheck appointment for next week

_____ Additional information and instructions are attached.

Notify the Doctor If Any of the Following Occur

Your pet's illness worsens or vomiting or bleeding occurs.

Your pet chews at its dressing, splint, cast, or bandage.

Bandages or splints become wet, or sutures are out.

You cannot give the medication as directed.

Home Care for Splints, Casts, and Bandages

Splints, casts, and bandages (dressings) are designed to protect and immobilize injured body parts. A splint or cast actually bears the animal's weight. These devices also prevent self-mutilation from licking or chewing.

Your pet cannot understand the function of a splint, cast, or bandage and therefore may want only to remove the device in any manner possible. Your pet may shake, bite, pull, and push on the dressing in an effort to remove it. Fortunately, most pets accept the dressings. An Elizabethan collar is usually provided as protection for the dressing.

Important Points

Keep the device dry. If your pet goes outside in wet weather, place a plastic bag or baggy over the dressing to keep it dry. Do not allow the bag to remain on for long periods. As a rule, remove the bag after 1 hour or less.

Inform the doctor of any loosening or loss of the dressing.

Discourage your pet from licking or chewing at the dressing. An Elizabethan collar is provided in most cases and should not be removed. Call us if your pet is still able to lick or chew at the dressing.

Call us if you see any signs of pain, discomfort, or swelling.

Your pet's dressing will be (removed) (changed) in _____ (days) (weeks).

Kirschner–Ehmer Apparatus

Wraps are placed over the pins and bar to protect the pins from damaging or catching on furniture. The wrap also protects the patient when it is placed on the medial aspect of the bone. The owner is advised about discharge from the pin sites and about care of the pin tracts after pin removal. Controlled exercise is maintained to ensure joint mobility. Any change in function alerts the surgeon to a problem, such as pin tract infection and implant loosening. Follow-up radiographs are taken as needed.

Intramedullary Pins

Weightbearing is a stimulus to fracture healing, but uncontrolled exercise can cause pin migration and fracture collapse. Controlled exercise is essential, as well as placement of an appropriate dressing or sling. Any change in function or swellings at the proximal or distal pin sites alerts the surgeon to a potential problem. Radiographs are taken as needed.

Plates

Because healing with a plate and screws is meant to occur by primary bone healing, a true race occurs between fracture healing and metal fatigue with subsequent implant failure. Because primary bone healing (endosteal callus) is slower than with those forms of fixation that rely on the production of a periosteal callus, the implants must be protected with controlled exercise and an appropriate dressing. Exercise is limited, but it is controlled to maintain joint mobility and to prevent "fracture disease." Exercise is not required for fracture healing. Once again, any change in function alerts the surgeon to a problem. Radiographs are taken as needed.

Tension Bands

Weightbearing converts distraction to compression. Controlled exercise with an appropriate dressing is maintained. After removal of the dressing, controlled exercise is maintained. Any swelling or change in function is an indication for radiography.

Osteomyelitis

Peter K. Shires

Periostitis, osteitis, and myelitis refer to inflammation of the periosteum, cortical bone, and medullary tissues, respectively. Osteomyelitis has become generally accepted to mean an infection of all portions of a bone. Infection of bone is an ever present risk associated with orthopedic practice and deserves constant alertness on the part of emergency clinicians, primary care practitioners, and referral orthopedists to mute its effects on fracture management.

Pathogens and Route of Infection

Infection of the bone can be caused by bacteria or fungi. The most common bacterial pathogens are *Staphylococcus aureus, Escherichia coli,* and *Proteus* species. About 40% of cases have mixed populations of bacteria; previous surgical intervention increases the incidence of *E. coli* and *Proteus* contamination from hospital sources. Fungal infection usually is systemic, but localization in the bone has been frequently described in cryptococcosis and blastomycosis.

The presence of bacteria or fungi in a bone does not inevitably lead to osteomyelitis. On the contrary, significant abuse is required to precipitate an active infection. Defects in the immune system, massive contamination, virulent strains of bacteria, tissue trauma and ischemia, and foreign material in the tissue are a few of the potentiating factors.

The route of infection in adult animals is invariably exogenous contamination. Open fractures, open reductions of fractures, puncture wounds, extensive bone exposure, and gunshot wounds account for most cases of osteomyelitis in dogs and cats. A hematogenous route of infection is seen in calves and foals. In dogs, the only osteomyelitis that frequently has a hematogenous route is spondylitis or discospondylitis, although epiphysitis has been described as well.

Pathogenesis

Contamination is followed by inflammation. The induced hyperemia is accompanied by vascular permeability, phagocytic migration, and leakage of plasma that contains protein, antibody, complement, fibrin, and kinins, all of which localize and contain the contaminant. In most situations, these and other inherent defenses subdue the invasion, and the inflammation subsides. In isolated instances, pockets of material are walled off in cavities lined by connective tissues. Some of these filled spaces contain organisms, and others are sterile. Often called Brodie's abscesses, these cavities can be a source of chronic reinfection if contaminated. Although described in dogs and cats, they are most commonly found in cattle and horses.

Osteomyelitis develops when a segment of devitalized bone or some foreign material serves as a focus of persistent infection. The growing volume of exudate confined within a rigid framework results in increased pressure. Pressurized exudate is forced into the medullary canal and through the cortex. In young animals, holes called cloacae form through the tightly adherent periosteum; fistulous tracts connect them to the skin (Fig. 51.2).

The foreign material or dead bone provides a protective haven for the contaminant to linger despite efforts by the body or exogenous antimicrobials to eradicate it. The ensuing cyclic buildup and release of purulent

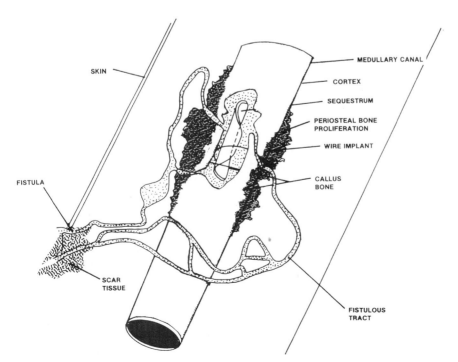

SKIN

MEDULLARY CANAL

CORTEX

SEQUESTRUM

PERIOSTEAL BONE PROLIFERATION

WIRE IMPLANT

CALLUS BONE

FISTULA

SCAR TISSUE

FISTULOUS TRACT

Fig. 51.2. A chronic osteomyelitic bone with draining fistulous tracts originating from a sequestered bone fragment that can be surrounded by an involucrum of proliferating bone.

discharge are little affected by medical therapy because of the avascular wall of connective tissue and sclerotic bone that develops around the sequestrum. Bone proliferates in a futile attempt to contain the focus of infection, but the involucrum that develops is seldom successful in walling off the source of infection completely.

The predisposing factors that lead to most cases of osteomyelitis are frequently preventable. Because trauma is the primary influencing factor, practitioners should be aware of and take measures to avoid or counteract the following:

1. Vascular compromise (blood loss, shock, avascular bone fragments, soft tissue trauma)

2. Iatrogenic contamination (hospital and operative)

3. Dead space hematoma at the fracture site (injury and surgery related)

4. Destructive fixation devices or techniques (intramedullary pins, which destroy medullary blood supply; excessive soft tissue dissection, which isolates bone fragments from their vascular supply)

5. Immunosuppression by corticosteroids (exogenous or endogenous), shock, anesthesia, and surgery

At least 15 to 30% of cases of acute osteomyelitis become chronic because of all or one of the foregoing factors. Because diagnosis and treatment of established osteomyelitis are arduous, one should make every effort to reduce the incidence of chronic osteomyelitis by preventive measures.

Clinical Signs and Diagnosis

Acute exogenous osteomyelitis is characterized by local heat, pain, and swelling. Lameness is accompanied by anorexia and depression, which occurs 5 to 21 days after the insult. A purulent exudate often is seen through the wound, and leukocytosis with a degenerative left shift may be documented. Radiographs taken 10 to 14 days after the onset of infection show bone destruction and new bone formation in varying proportions, depending on bacterial activity. Because periosteal new bone formation secondary to exuberant surgical manipulations is radiographically similar to early osteomyelitis, serial radiographs should be taken to document the active progression that occurs with osteomyelitis. The bone lysis seen in unstable fractures can also be mistaken for the bone resorption associated with infection.

A definitive diagnosis can be made with a positive culture taken directly from the involved bone by needle aspiration or surgical exposure of the area. Blood cultures are less rewarding because they require circulating bacteremia for a positive culture, and bacteremia may be intermittent even in acute osteomyelitis.

Chronic osteomyelitis is most frequently marked by intermittent or persistent lameness, which may be partially weightbearing or nonweightbearing. Intermittently or constantly draining fistulas are the most consistent clinical finding in these cases. Associated secondary observations include atrophy, induration, local pain, fluctuant swellings, periodic febrile reactions, and inappetence. Circulating leukocytosis is sporadic, and the hemogram depends on when the sample was taken.

Radiographs show extensive bone remodeling. Although the radiographic findings are similar to those seen with unstable fractures, surgical manipulations, and neoplasias, the extent, progression, and level of activity usually are distinct enough to suggest a diagnosis. The presence of a foreign body or sequestrum should always be presumed and carefully looked for, because this confirms the diagnosis of chronic osteomyelitis. Final confirmation can be secured by a direct culture from the bone. The mixed infections obtained from cultures of the fistulous tract can be confusing because of the overgrowth of contaminants.

Treatment

Therapy for osteomyelitis should be applied both locally and systemically. Aerobic cultures must be taken before instituting antimicrobial therapy. Anaerobic cultures should be considered, especially in chronic situations. Antimicrobial sensitivity is a valuable aid in selecting appropriate systemic antibiotic therapy. Before culture and sensitivity results are available, a short-term course of a parenteral bactericidal, penicillinase-resistant antibiotic should be started. Because most infections involve *Staphylococcus aureus*, first-generation cephalosporins, dicloxacillin, and clindamycin are all appropriate choices before culture results are available; clindamycin is also effective against gram-negative isolates. Three recommended regimens are as follows: cefalozin, 15 to 20 mg/kg intravenously three times daily; oxacillin, 20 mg/kg intravenously four times daily; and Antirobe, 11 mg/kg intravenously twice daily.

Oral therapy can be used after the first 24 hours, but the appropriate alternative form of antibiotic must be used. When culture and sensitivity results are available, prolonged antibiotic therapy is adjusted according to the results. Therapy should continue for 6 weeks in all patients with osteomyelitis. At the end of 6 weeks, a second culture can be taken by needle aspiration from the site after waiting 3 to 5 days for serum antibiotic levels to subside. If this culture is positive, therapy will have to be changed, and aggressive surgical exploration may be necessary to determine and remove the source of infection. Infection is unlikely to persist in the face of appropriate antibiotic therapy unless a protected focus exists within the bone. Radiographic reevaluation at this time may help to localize the source.

Local therapy frequently is not pursued because of economic and aesthetic considerations. The resulting prolonged, even permanent infection ultimately has far more of an impact on the patient and client than an aggressive initial approach would have had. This finding supports the use of early, aggressive intervention in osteomyelitis.

In acute osteomyelitis, drainage should be used if local swelling, heat, and pain have not subsided within 2 to 3 days of starting appropriate antibiotic therapy. A skin incision is made over the area, the periosteum is exposed, and ⅛-inch or similar-sized holes are drilled in several directions through the infected bone. If frank exudate is present in pockets, it may be necessary to remove the segments of affected bone.

Mechanical lavage of the site with sterile saline effectively reduces the sheer bulk of necrotic material, debris, and bacteria. Lavage is performed at the time of surgery and should be continued for a few days or until the irrigating solution remains clear. Prolonged irrigation can be accomplished either when the wound is left open to heal by granulation or after a drainage system is implanted.

One suitable drainage system is an ingress–egress drain consisting of rigid polypropylene or rubber catheters (Fig. 51.3). The ingress catheter is placed through normal tissue above the site and ends in the infected bony defect. The catheter is secured with retention sutures and is sealed when not in use. The egress catheter is multifenestrated and can be of the "sump drain" type. The drain should pass ventrally through a dependent area of the limb to the outside. This, too, is secured but not sealed unless a closed vacuum system is used.

Large volumes of sterile saline (500 to 1000 mL) are infused through the ingress drain on a daily basis. Negative pressure can be applied to the egress drain to help draw the flush solution through the site. Some investigators suggest a final injection of antibiotic or antiseptic into the ingress drain on a daily basis. If antibiotics are used, the dose should be the appropriate daily dose of that drug and must not compromise the serum levels of any parenteral drugs used simultaneously. The concentration of antiseptic solutions should be low enough to cause no tissue damage.

The drains should be covered by a protective bandage when not in use. When no longer necessary, the ingress drain is removed, and 24 hours later the egress drain is pulled. This same drainage system can be used in patients with chronic osteomyelitis.

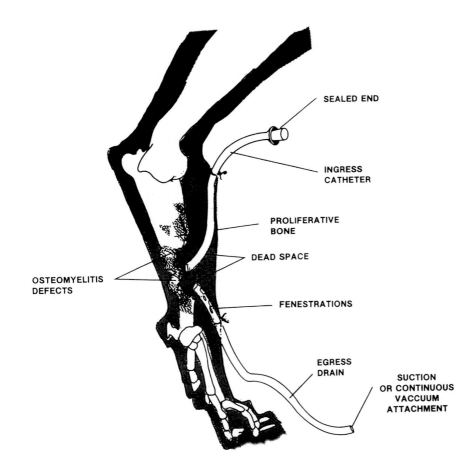

SEALED END

INGRESS CATHETER

PROLIFERATIVE BONE

DEAD SPACE

OSTEOMYELITIS DEFECTS

FENESTRATIONS

EGRESS DRAIN

SUCTION OR CONTINUOUS VACCUUM ATTACHMENT

Fig. 51.3. Ingress–egress drain placed in osteomyelitic lesion. The ingress catheter is sealed and can be used to deliver large volumes of sterile fluid, which drains through the fenestrated, dependently placed, egress drain. A negative pressure can be applied to the egress drain to improve the collection of fluids and to "close" the system.

Any acute or chronic osteomyelitic lesion that involves a fracture or bone fragmentation must be approached surgically if the fragments are unstable or dead. Rigid stabilization of bone is essential to the successful treatment of concurrent infections. The negative effects of an inert foreign object (e.g., plate, screw, wire, pin) are far outweighed by the positive effects of a stable fracture. All avascular fragments of bone should be discarded if infection is present.

In more chronic cases, usually one must remove the avascular proliferative tissue and bone that surround infected areas and often cover the ends of unhealed bony fragments. The bone is rongeured until interosseous bleeding is observed. If healing has already taken place, all implants should be removed whenever possible. If the implant is not adding to the stability, it should be removed. When all necrotic and avascular tissue has been removed from the infected site, the bone as a whole must be evaluated for strength and fracture potential. When necessary, additional support

should be applied externally or internally to protect the bone during this weakened phase.

To reduce the dead space and to promote healing, a fresh autogenous cancellous bone graft is recommended. The graft is collected from a sterile site with separate instruments and gloves to avoid cross-contamination. The graft is placed in the defect, and the wound is closed routinely. Lavage drainage is contraindicated when a graft is used. In some cases, the infection may require lavage instead of a bone graft in the early stages; in such cases, a second procedure is required to place the graft at an appropriate time. To decrease dead space further, coaptation bandages can be used to increase tissue pressure, provided no vascular compromise is precipitated in the process.

Treatment of osteomyelitis is prolonged, intensive, and expensive. Most cases of osteomyelitis could have been avoided by application of the preventive measures already mentioned.

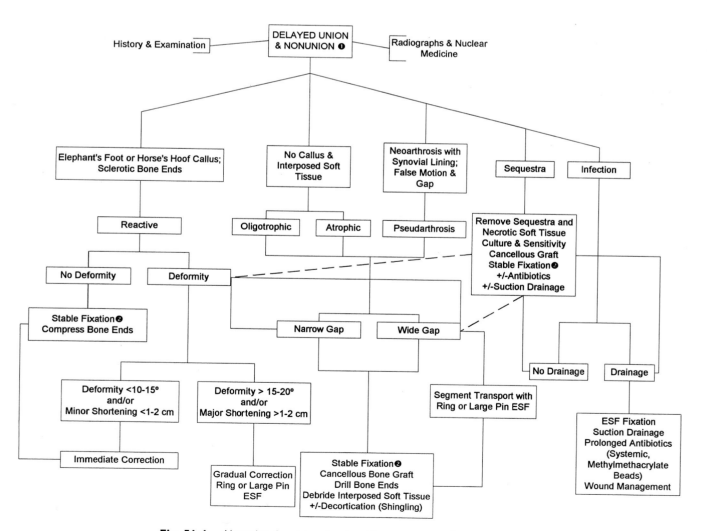

Fig. 51.4. Algorithm for delayed union (*1*) or nonunion. 2, stable fixation.

Suggested Readings

Caywood DD, et al. Osteomyelitis in the dog: a review of 67 cases. J Am Vet Med Assoc 1978;172:943.

Harari J. Osteomyelitis. J Am Vet Med Assoc 1984;184:101.

Herron MR. Osteomyelitis. In: Bojrab MJ, ed. Pathophysiology in small animal surgery. Philadelphia: Lea & Febiger, 1981.

Johnson KA. Localized osteomyelitis in cats and dogs. Aust Vet Pract 1983;13:27.

Mader JT. Animal modes of osteomyelitis. Am J Med 1985;78:213.

Smith CW, et al. Osteomyelitis in the dog: a retrospective study. J Am Anim Hosp Assoc 1978;14:589.

Stead AC. Osteomyelitis in the dog and cat. J Small Anim Pract 1984;25:1.

Algorithm for Delayed Union and Nonunion

Dennis N. Aron

Delayed Union

Healing has not advanced at the average rate, given the patient profile, location and type of fracture, and the stabilization method used (Fig. 51.4). The fracture may go on to union if the surgeon waits longer. However, surgery may be justified when compared with the risk of prolonging recovery and patient morbidity.

Nonunion

Clinical and radiographic evidence indicates that healing has ended and union is not going to occur without surgical intervention.

Stable Fixation

The fixation method chosen is stable enough to allow the patient to be comfortable and to lead to weight-bearing of the injured limb with each step at a walking pace. Joints on either side of the fractured bone need to be freely mobile and able to function normally. Fundamental to treatment of delayed union and nonunion is active use of the limb, to allow soft tissues to recover and become healthy, thereby enabling bone healing.

References

Aron DN. Delayed union and nonunion. In: Bojrab MJ, ed. Current techniques in small animal surgery. 3rd ed. Philadelphia: Lea & Febiger 1990:895.

Connolly JF, ed. Tibial nonunion: diagnosis and treatment.: American Academy of Orthopaedic Surgeons, 1991.

Pseudarthroses. In: Muller ME, Allgower M, Schneider R, et al., eds. Manual of internal fixation. 3rd ed. Berlin: Springer-Verlag, 1991:713.

Taylor JC. Delayed union and nonunion of fractures. In: Crenshaw AH, ed. Campbell's operative orthopaedics. 8th ed. St. Louis: Mosby–Year Book, 1992:1287.

— 52 —

FRACTURES OF THE SKULL AND MANDIBLE

Surgical Repair of Maxillary Fractures

Bradford C. Dixon & David L. Bone

Although not commonly encountered in small animal patients, maxillary fractures can result in significant morbidity and are often challenging to treat. Tremendous anatomic variation exists between dogs and cats and among various breeds of dogs with respect to the area of the muzzle. A thorough understanding of the local anatomy is important for proper treatment of maxillary fractures. Because of variation in anatomy and fracture location and configuration, all the techniques described here may not be appropriate for a given patient. Furthermore, the most effective treatment may often be a combination of two or more of the described techniques. In addition to fractures of the maxilla, fractures of the incisive, nasal, and palatine bones are also considered.

Preoperative Considerations

Most animals with fractures of the upper jaw have undergone significant trauma. Initial efforts should be directed toward identifying and treating life-threatening trauma to major organ systems. Specifically, the central nervous system should be carefully assessed and monitored, because brain injury from concussion or contusion or additional skull fractures may often be present in patients that have received a blow to the head sufficient to cause a maxillary fracture. Prompt medical or surgical treatment of central nervous system trauma may be lifesaving and takes priority over specific treatment of jaw fractures.

Partial or complete upper airway obstruction may result from hemorrhage, edema, and fragment displacement with maxillary fractures. Emergency oxygen therapy and tracheotomy may be necessary. Shock and other cardiopulmonary injuries are treated appropriately as with any traumatized patient.

If, because of the planned treatment or the animal's condition, prolonged inability or reluctance to masticate normally is anticipated, then a feeding tube should be included in the treatment plan. Pharyngostomy, esophagostomy, and gastrostomy tubes can all be used successfully for enteral nutritional support. Nasal feeding tubes are not as well tolerated because of the local nasal trauma and are not practical for long-term use.

Not all maxillary fractures require surgical treatment. Simple fractures with minimal displacement and adequate soft tissue support often heal adequately without specific stabilization. Indications for surgical intervention include malocclusion, oronasal communication, facial deformity, and airway obstruction. As with mandibular fractures, maintenance of normal occlusion takes precedence over anatomic reduction in upper jaw fractures.

Fractures of the maxilla are usually open, often having direct communication with the oral cavity. Because of the potential for osteomyelitis, prophylactic use of antibiotics is justified. Broad-spectrum antibiotics should be chosen because of the variety of potential pathogens in the oral cavity. Antibiotic treatment can usually be discontinued 24 to 48 hours postoperatively in the absence of a confirmed infection.

Surgical Approaches

Fractures of the maxilla and associated bones of the upper jaw can be accessed through either an oral or a dorsal approach, depending on the fracture location and the proposed method of fixation. Because most fractures involve the hard palate or the dental arcade, an intraoral approach is used most commonly. The mucoperiosteum of the palate or the gingival mucosa is usually traumatically lacerated along the fracture line, resulting in an open fracture. However, the mucoperiosteum can be incised and elevated as necessary to expose the underlying fracture line and to apply the implants. Hemorrhage is controlled with digital pressure and judicious use of electrocoagulation. Excessive use of electrocoagulation may lead to delayed healing or dehiscence of the mucoperiosteal incisions. The major palatine arteries are avoided in elevating palatal mucoperiosteal flaps. Gingival and mucoperiosteal incisions are closed in two layers, when possible, with synthetic absorbable suture material.

Fractures of the nasal bones and dorsal maxilla can be approached through a dorsal midline incision. A midline skin incision is extended through the underlying subcutaneous tissue and periosteum. The periosteum then is elevated and is reflected laterally to expose the bone adequately for fracture reduction and fixation. The periosteum is closed securely to minimize air leakage and subcutaneous emphysema. Subcutaneous tissues and skin are closed separately.

External Coaptation (Tape Muzzle)

Fractures of the upper jaw can occasionally be stabilized effectively using a tape muzzle alone. Tape muzzles may also be useful to protect a surgical repair postoperatively. Since tape muzzling relies on interdigitation of the teeth (especially the canines) to maintain fracture alignment and dental occlusion, it is only effective in dogs with intact dentition. This method is best suited for minimally displaced fractures and is not possible in cats or brachycephalic dogs. Commercial nylon muzzles are available and may be easier to clean and maintain than tape muzzles. Muzzles must be kept clean and changed frequently to prevent dermatitis and rub sores on the skin and lips. Muzzles are contraindicated in animals at high risk of vomiting, because of the possibility of aspiration. The muzzle is usually maintained for approximately 4 weeks or until a grossly stable fibrous union is present (see the next section of this chapter, on mandibular fractures, for details of tape muzzle application).

External Fixation

Interdental Wiring

Interdental wiring may be used to stabilize intraoral fractures, either by itself or as an adjunct to other fixation methods. Interdental wiring relies on solid anchoring of the tooth–bone interface and is not applicable if teeth are loose. Interdental wiring as a sole method of fixation is rarely used because canine and feline dental anatomy does not lend itself to this technique. The short or absent supragingival neck of teeth in small animals makes seating the wires difficult. Undercutting the tooth with a dental bur prevents slippage of the wire when tightened, but it results in periodontal disease.

Various wiring configurations have been described, but for most fractures a simple figure-of-eight pattern is easiest to apply and provides adequate stabilization. Twenty- to 24-gauge orthopedic wire is appropriate for most dogs and cats. At least two teeth rostral and two caudal to the fracture are incorporated. The wire is passed between teeth through small holes created in the gingiva at the level of the neck of the tooth. Holes can be created using a hypodermic needle or a Kirschner wire. Undercutting the teeth is performed only if necessary. With the wire in place and the fracture held in reduction, the wire is twisted to tighten and stabilize the fracture. Both rostral and caudal ends of the wire loop should be twisted individually to ensure uniform tightness (Fig. 52.1). Overtightening of

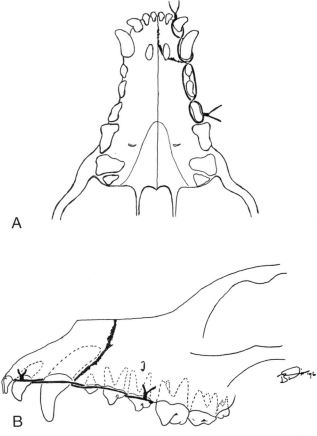

Fig. 52.1. A and **B.** Figure-of-eight interdental wire used to stabilize a transverse maxillary fracture. Wire loop is twisted from both ends to ensure uniform tension.

interdental wires should be avoided, to prevent distraction of the fracture line dorsally.

Acrylic Dental Splinting

Acrylic dental splints, like interdental wires, require intact solid teeth on both sides of the fracture. Interdental wires can be used in conjunction with acrylic splints to increase the surface area for cohesion of the acrylic and to increase the mechanical strength of the splint. Acrylic splints are particularly useful for incisive bone and rostral maxillary fractures (Fig. 52.2).

The teeth to be incorporated in the splint are first polished, rinsed, and dried. Acid etching of the teeth with orthophosphoric acid gel or paste demineralizes the tooth surface and increases adherence of the acrylic. The dental acrylic is applied to the teeth, while fracture reduction is maintained, either by applying the acrylic powder and liquid sequentially to the dental surface and thus building the splint in "layers" or by premixing the powder and liquid to a putty consistency, applying a layer of liquid directly to the teeth, and molding the acrylic putty onto the dental surface.

The fracture is held in reduction with proper occlu-

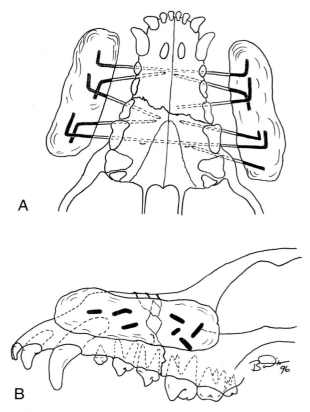

Fig. 52.3. A and **B.** Comminuted maxillary fracture stabilized with a modified type II acrylic external fixator. Tooth roots and neurovascular structures are avoided when placing pins.

sion while the acrylic polymerizes. Once it has hardened, the splint can be shaped and smoothed further with a dental bur. Care should be taken to ensure that no rough edges that may irritate soft tissues are present and that nothing interferes with the opposite dental arcade.

Home care includes daily flushing of the area with dental chlorhexidine solution. Brushing also helps to dislodge food that accumulates under the splint. Once the fracture has healed (usually 4 to 6 weeks), the splint is removed by sectioning it with a dental bur and prying the sections free. The teeth should be polished and treated with topical fluoride after splint removal.

Pins and Acrylic

External skeletal fixation using multiple pins and methylmethacrylate acrylic can be an effective technique in certain fractures of the upper jaw. The technique may be particularly useful in highly comminuted fractures in which anatomic reduction is not possible. The application of external skeletal fixation to the maxilla has several unique technical considera-

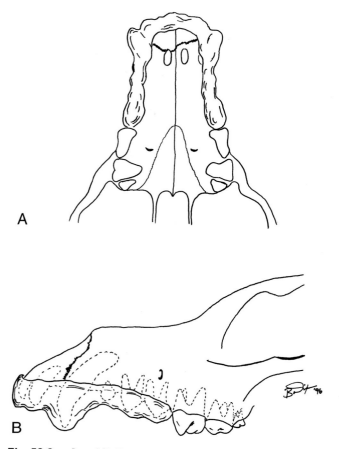

Fig. 52.2. A and **B.** Rostral maxillary and incisive bone fracture stabilized with an acrylic dental splint.

tions. Because of the thin bone, the tendency for pin loosening is greater; therefore, more smaller pins or Kirschner wires are used per fragment. Care should be taken to avoid tooth roots and the infraorbital foramina. Pins are preplaced in the major fracture fragments parallel to the hard palate and at 30 to 40° divergent angles from one another (Fig. 52.3). Pin placement and fracture reduction are generally accomplished by closed technique. Either a type I (half-pins) or type II (full pins across the muzzle) configuration can be used. The exposed portion of the pins can be bent to increase contact with the methylmethacrylate. Once the pins have all been preplaced, the fracture is reduced by aligning teeth into proper occlusion. The pins are then connected with cylindric columns of acrylic on both sides of the maxilla (Fig. 52.3).

Internal Fixation

Interfragmentary Wiring

One of the more versatile techniques for repair of fractures of the upper jaw is interfragmentary wiring. Interfragmentary wires are used primarily as wire sutures securing two flat bone fragments. Using either a small dental bur or a Kirschner wire, holes are drilled at an angle toward the fracture line to facilitate passing the wires (Fig. 52.4). At least two 22- to 24-gauge orthopedic wires are used in each fracture. For oblique fractures, a triangulated wiring technique may be used (Fig. 52.5). All wires should be preplaced before tightening.

Longitudinal splits of the hard palate are a common type of maxillary fracture and are often amenable to interfragmentary wire repair. The mucoperiosteum is elevated laterally to expose the maxillary and palatine bones sufficiently to place several wires. Three to four wires are usually sufficient, depending on the size of the animal (Fig. 52.6). Once the wires have been tightened, the mucoperiosteum is closed over the fracture with synthetic absorbable sutures.

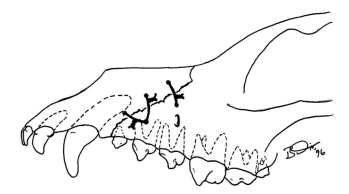

Fig. 52.5. Oblique fracture repaired with three interfragmentary wires. The rostral two wires demonstrate the triangulated wiring technique.

Interfragmentary Pins

An alternative technique for longitudinal splits of the hard palate is use of an interfragmentary pin. A small Steinmann pin or Kirschner wire is driven transversely across the fracture just dorsal to the hard palate, avoiding tooth roots. Orthopedic wire is then passed between the bone and the mucoperiosteum to loop around the pin ends; a large hypodermic needle is helpful in passing the orthopedic wire. When the wire is tightened, it compresses the fracture line, whereas the pin provides protection against bending and shear stresses (Fig. 52.7).

Avulsion fractures of the teeth and surrounding alveolar bone can sometimes be repaired using divergent Kirschner wires (Fig. 52.8). Technically, however, performing this technique without penetrating tooth roots is often difficult or impossible. For rostral avulsion fractures, other techniques, such as acrylic dental splinting, may be more appropriate.

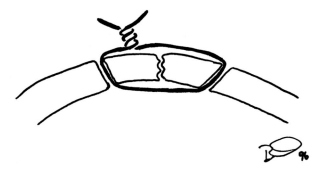

Fig. 52.4. Holes for interfragmentary wires are drilled at a slight angle toward the fracture to facilitate passing the wire.

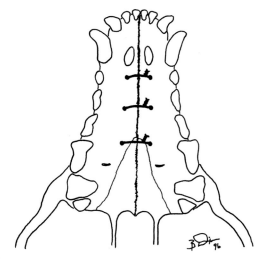

Fig. 52.6. Interfragmentary wires used to stabilize a longitudinal split of the hard palate.

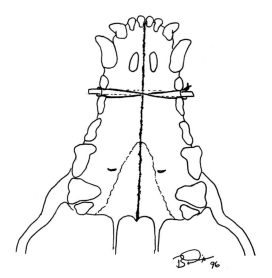

Fig. 52.7. Longitudinal palatal split stabilized with a small Steinmann pin and a figure-of-eight wire. The orthopedic wire is passed between the bone and the mucoperiosteum.

Plates and Screws

Because of the thin bone in the upper jaw and the usual effectiveness of other techniques, bone plates are rarely used in fractures of the maxilla. If used, bone plates must be applied such that adequate soft tissue covers the implant, and the implant is not exposed to the oral cavity. At least two screws must be used on either side of the fracture; three or more screws are preferable because of the poor holding power of each individual screw in the thin bone. Tooth roots and the infraorbital vessels and nerves emerging from the

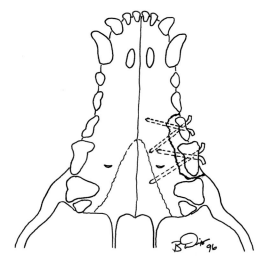

Fig. 52.8. Avulsion-type fracture of the third and fourth upper premolars repaired with divergent Kirschner wires. The pins pass through the area of the dental furcation, thus avoiding the tooth roots.

infraorbital foramen should be avoided when placing screws.

Suggested Readings

Bone DL. Maxillary fractures. In: Bojrab MJ, ed. Current techniques in small animal surgery. 3rd ed. Philadelphia: Lea & Febiger, 1990:883–890.

Brinker WO, Hohn RB, Prieur WD, eds. Manual of internal fixation in small animals. New York: Springer-Verlag, 1984:215–218.

Brinker WO, Piermattei DL, Flo GL, eds. Handbook of small animal orthopedics and fracture treatment. 2nd ed. Philadelphia: WB Saunders, 1990:241–243.

Egger EL. Skull and mandibular fractures. In: Slatter DH, ed. Textbook of small animal surgery. 2nd ed. Philadelphia: WB Saunders, 1993:1910–1921.

Harvey CE, Emily PP, eds. Small animal dentistry. St. Louis: CV Mosby, 1993.

Surgical Repair of Mandibular Fractures

Robert A. Taylor

Mandibular fractures are common. The use of the mandible for prehension, its exposed location, and the presence of the symphyseal joint probably account for its frequent fractures.

Animals presenting with facial trauma should be carefully examined. Injuries to the respiratory system, central nervous system, or cardiovascular system can be immediately life-threatening. The patient should be carefully assessed and its injuries prioritized.

Mandibular fractures have been repaired in many ways (1–6). The type of repair possible is often limited only by the surgeon's imagination; however, certain principles should be followed carefully, whichever repair method is used. Accurate anatomic reduction and rigid fixation optimize fracture healing. Equally important is proper occlusion. During the repair, the patient's mouth should be closed and the upper and lower dental arcade carefully checked for proper occlusion. Fractures extending through the alveoli may heal poorly, and the affected tooth may be devitalized. Gum or soft tissue lacerations that communicate with the mandible can serve as portals of contamination. Although mandibular osteomyelitis is rare, its effects can be devastating.

Anatomic Review

The mandible consists of two flat bones united at their rostral extremity by a symphyseal joint. All the teeth of the lower arcade are imbedded in alveoli found in the body of the mandible. The ramus (vertical) is thin but protected by the zygomatic arch. The condyloid process articulates with the temporal bone to form the temporomandibular joint.

The temporomandibular joint is a condylar articulation. A small articular disc is interposed between the two bones. The joint is strengthened laterally by the lateral ligament.

The mandibular alveolar artery enters the mandibular foramen on the medial caudal surface of the body and runs along the ventral surface of the mandibular canal. The mandibular alveolar artery, in combination with its three terminal branches (caudal, middle, rostral mental arteries), supplies nourishment to the entire lower jaw. The mandibular alveolar nerve (a branch of the trigeminal nerve) supplies sensory and motor innervations to the jaw (7). The mandible houses 14 deciduous teeth and 19 permanent teeth. The lower arcade contains one more molar than the upper arcade.

General Considerations

The ideal method of mandibular fracture repair is quick, atraumatic, and inexpensive and follows the principles of anatomic reduction, rigid fixation, and proper occlusion. Knowledge of the location and number of tooth roots, and of nerve and blood supply, is essential to successful repair of mandibular fractures. Economic factors and the willingness and ability of the owner to provide postoperative care must all be considered in the selection of a repair method. With unilateral fractures, the contralateral mandible serves as a splint. With the exception of some symphyseal fractures, most mandibular fractures are open. Nevertheless, the resistance of mandibular fractures to infection makes internal fixation an option (2). Placement of an endotracheal tube through a pharyngotomy can be of great benefit in monitoring intraoperative occlusion of the jaw.

Surgical Techniques

Mandibular Symphyseal Fractures

Fractures of the mandibular symphysis are common and can be repaired easily with a loop cerclage wire (Fig. 52.9). With a wire passer, curved hypodermic needle, or large suture needle, the wire is introduced just caudal to the canine teeth and is passed ventral to the mandibular halves and brought out on the opposite side. The mandibular halves are held in opposition manually, and the jaws are apposed to check for proper occlusion. The loop cerclage is tightened and cut, and the short end is bent down. Once the fracture has healed, the wire can be cut and removed, usually

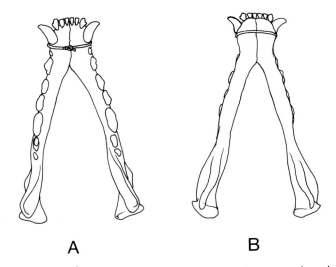

Fig. 52.9. Loop cerclage wire used to stabilize a symphyseal separation. **A.** Dorsoventral view. **B.** Ventrodorsal view.

without anesthesia. I recommend that the wire be left in place for 4 to 6 weeks.

Mandibular Body Fractures

Many devices have been used for fixation of mandibular body fractures. These include cerclage wires, hemicerclage wires, intramedullary pins, bone plates, acrylic splints (both intraoral and extraoral), external fixators, and tape (1–6). Fractures through dental alveoli can be troublesome because bone does not heal when in opposition with enamel (2). In some cases,

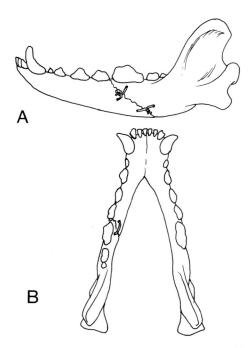

Fig. 52.10. Hemicerclage wires used to repair an oblique mandibular fracture. **A.** Lateral view. **B.** Dorsoventral view.

the exposed tooth must be removed to allow for proper healing.

Tape muzzling has been reported to work well in mandibular body fractures (5). Minimally displaced fractures, as well as severely comminuted fractures, can be treated in this manner. An intact opposite hemimandible acts as a splint to help stabilization. The surgeon must allow enough space rostrally so the animal can lap water and eat food. Problems with this technique include patient intolerance, severe tape burns, and prolonged fracture healing.

The curved nature of the mandibular medullary canal makes intramedullary pin fixation difficult. Malocclusion may result from this technique (8).

Hemicerclage wiring can provide stable fixation of mandibular body fractures. Comminuted fractures in small mandibles can be repaired with this technique. Although this technique does not provide adequate fixation in long bone fractures, the opposite hemimandible affords further stability and makes this an effective, easily applied treatment option for mandibular fractures (Fig. 52.10).

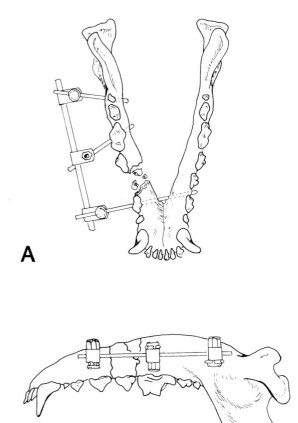

Fig. 52.11. A Kirschner–Ehmer apparatus used to repair a comminuted mandibular fracture. **A.** Lateral view. **B.** Dorsoventral view.

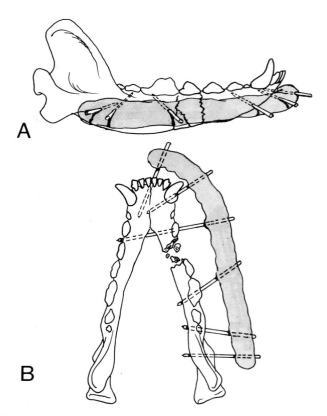

Fig. 52.12. An acrylic external fixator applied to a comminuted mandibular fracture. **A.** Lateral view. **B.** Dorsoventral view.

Body fractures can be repaired with external skeletal fixators such as the Kirschner–Ehmer splint (Fig. 52.11). An alternative technique is placement of multiple Steinmann pins, or Kirschner wires that are wired together, onto which dental acrylic is molded. Silastic tubing can be impaled over the pins, and acrylic can be injected into the tubing (Fig. 52.12). These methods are well suited for severely comminuted fractures, open fractures, or gunshot injuries. Pin placement is important with this technique. Ideally, the pins should avoid the mandibular alveolar artery and the roots of adjacent teeth. This technique is economical in both time and money; furthermore, it is technically easy, and most offices have the equipment. Dental acrylic is inexpensive and is obtained easily from local dental supply houses.

Plate fixation of mandibular body fractures allows for accurate and rigid reduction. This method is beneficial in patients with bilateral fractures (Fig. 52.13).

Fractures of the Ramus and Articular Fractures

The vertical ramus consists of thin, weak bone and is difficult to approach surgically. In many cases, tape muzzling or interarcade wiring (5, 6) is the most appropriate way to treat fractures of the ramus. These

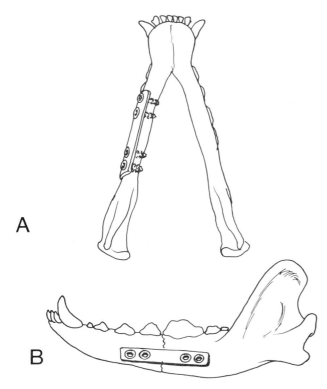

Fig. 52.13. Bone plate used to stabilize a transverse mandibular fracture. **A.** Dorsoventral view. **B.** Lateral view.

techniques also work well for fractures of the mandibular condyle.

Postoperative Care

The types of postoperative care after repair of a mandibular fracture are dictated by the repair procedure. In general, a soft diet is recommended. The client should be instructed concerning wound care, daily management, and follow-up visits. When possible, radiographic confirmation of fracture healing is advisable; it should be obtained before implant removal.

References

1. Dulish ML. Skull and mandibular fractures. In: Slatter DH, ed. Skull and mandibular fractures in veterinary surgery. 2nd ed. Philadelphia: WB Saunders, 1979.
2. Nunamaker DM. Fractures and dislocation of the mandible. In: Small animal orthopedics. Philadelphia: JB Lippincott, 1985.
3. Greenwood KW, Creach GB. Biphasic external skeletal splint fixation of mandibular fractures in dogs. Vet Surg 1980;9:128.
4. Nibley W. Treatment of caudal mandibular fractures. J Am Anim Hosp Assoc 1981;17:555.
5. Withrow SJ. Taping of the mandible in treatment of mandibular fractures. J Am Anim Hosp Assoc 1981;17:27.
6. Lantz GC. Interarcade wiring as a method of fixation for selected mandibular injuries. J Am Anim Hosp Assoc 1981;17:599.
7. Evans H, Christensen G. Miller's anatomy of the dog. 2nd ed. Philadelphia: WB Saunders, 1979.
8. Cechner PE. Malocclusion in the dog caused by intramedullary pin fixation of mandibular fractures: two cases. J Am Anim Hosp Assoc 1980;16:79.

Editor's Note

As mentioned previously, tape muzzling can be used as primary or adjunctive fixation of certain mandibular fractures. Minimally or nondisplaced fractures, highly comminuted fractures with an intact opposite hemimandible, and vertical ramus fractures can be repaired by this method. Depending on the size of the animal, half-inch to 2-inch white medical tape is used. The sticky side of the tape is kept away from the skin. The first piece of tape is placed as far caudally around the nose as possible, with the sticky side out (Fig. 52.14**A**). A second piece of tape is then placed from the front of the nose, behind and below the ears (the ears should be held up and out of the way), and back to the nose with the sticky side out. This piece of tape should stick out far past the nose (Fig. 52.14**B**). A third piece of tape is then passed around the caudal aspect of the nose, but with the sticky side down, on top of the first piece of tape that went around the nose. The extra tape that was left sticking out in front of the nose from the second piece of tape placed is now folded back over onto itself so the two sticky sides are touching (Fig. 52.14**C**). Thus, when application of the tape is completed, no sticky side is left exposed. Additional layers of tape can be applied to provide more strength. A narrow strip of tape can be added ventrally or running between the eyes as a chin strap to prevent removal of the muzzle (Fig. 52.14**D**). A small gap is left between the teeth to allow the animal to eat and drink. The animal should not be able to open the mouth enough to disarticulate the canine teeth. If the muzzle must be completely closed, a pharyngostomy tube must be placed.

Acrylic Pin Splint External Skeletal Fixators for Mandibular Fractures

Dennis N. Aron

Acrylic pin splints are external skeletal fixators that use acrylic as both the connector rod and linkage. This fixation method can be accomplished in numerous ways, using either homemade materials or commercial kits (Acrylic Pin External Fixation System, Innovative Animal Products, Rochester, MN). Use of an acrylic pin splint has several advantages over standard metal

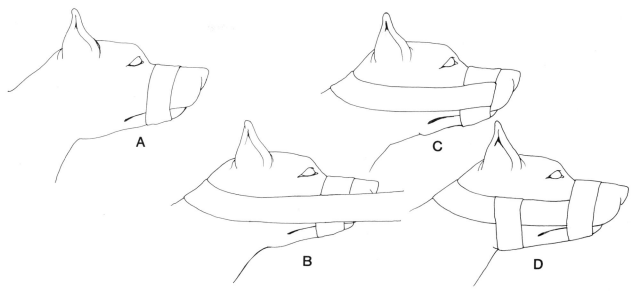

Fig. 52.14. Application of a tape muzzle. **A.** The first piece of tape is placed around the nose with sticky side out. **B.** The second piece of tape is placed behind the back of the head and along both sides of the muzzle, again with sticky side out. The ends of the tape on both sides should extend past the nose for a distance equal to that from the nose to the middle of the back. **C.** The third piece of tape with the sticky side down is placed around the nose, and then the long ends of the second piece are folded back onto itself. **D.** A chin strap can be added.

external skeletal fixators for the mandible. The acrylic pin splint is lightweight, radiolucent, and versatile. The acrylic pin splint enables the surgeon to position pins to avoid tooth roots and vital structures easily and to combine pins of various sizes in a singular frame (Fig. 52.15). The acrylic pin splint is easy to contour to the shape of the mandible (Fig. 52.15). The advantage of using a homemade acrylic pin splint is that the surgeon can purchase specifically needed components from different sources. The commercial kit provides convenience of application because it contains all materials in a single package.

The homemade splint consists of methylmethacrylate, which can be obtained as either hoof repair (Technovit Hoof Acrylic, Jorgensen Laboratories, Loveland, CO) or dental molding acrylic (Orthodontic Resin, L.B. Caulk Co., Milford, DE). The acrylic column can be free-formed or injected into a tube to serve as a mold. When free-formed, the acrylic is molded by hand to the required shape. The free-form method is easiest with most applications to the mandible, especially for smaller dogs and cats. The tube method may be best for larger dogs. The commercial kit uses a tube method. Research has shown that a $\frac{3}{4}$-inch acrylic column diameter provides fixation strength comparable with or greater than that of the medium Kirschner $\frac{3}{16}$-inch connector rod. Given this guideline, the surgeon can extrapolate the needed width of the acrylic column to various sizes of animals.

Two considerations are important to predictable and consistent success when using acrylic pin splints for

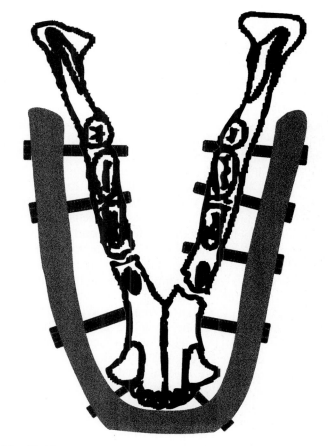

Fig. 52.15. Acrylic pin splint is easy to contour. Normal occlusion is a high priority in splinting.

mandibular fractures. First, the surgeon needs to establish normal occlusion and mastication for the patient. Failure to accomplish this goal predisposes the patient to abnormalities of the temporomandibular joint and pain, with the possibility of negative consequences on nutritional balance. Normal occlusion in the dog is seen when the mandibular canine teeth are positioned between the maxillary incisors and canine teeth and the mandibular fourth premolar is situated between the maxillary third and fourth premolars. Achieving normal occlusion is always a higher priority than accomplishing accurate reduction at the fracture site (see Fig. 52.15). When performing surgical correction of mandibular fractures, placement of the endotracheal tube through a pharyngostomy enables the surgeon to assess occlusion during the operative procedure. When the endotracheal tube is positioned routinely, it interferes with normal closure of the mouth and prevents the surgeon from assessing accurate occlusion.

The second important consideration is the need to use screws or positive profile end-threaded pins (fasteners) for attachment of the acrylic column to the mandible. The mandible is a relatively flat bone without two nicely separated dense cortices. This configuration predisposes nonthreaded pins to premature loosening, which leads to discomfort and, possibly, to delayed healing with the fixation of mandibular fractures. Because of this situation, screws or threaded pins, which provide a screwed-in anchorage, are advantageous when used for treating fractures of the mandible with external skeletal fixation. Bone screws work well for this purpose because they can be obtained in varied sizes corresponding to patient size. The head of the screw and exposed thread provide a secure linkage to the acrylic column. For use in particularly small animals is a small-diameter (0.9, 1.1, 1.6, 2.0, and 2.4 mm) positive-profile end-threaded pin (Miniature Interface Fixation Half Pins. IMEX Veterinary, Inc., Longview, TX) that is an excellent fastener designed to be used with acrylic. One end is intended to provide screwed-in fixation with the bone, and the opposite end is a roughened thread to allow for strong linkage with the acrylic column. The pin is remarkably stiff, given its diminutive size, a positive mechanical property not found in most small-diameter pins. Fully threaded Steinmann pins or negative-profile threaded pins should not be used with the acrylic pin splint because they are mechanically weak and are predisposed to loosening or breakage. The threaded pins and screws should be inserted by first drilling a hole with a sharp drill bit sized to approximate the core diameter of the fastener. This gives maximum stability to the fastener–bone interface. The tip of the threaded pin must exit the transcortex completely to engage thread throughout the bone.

Often, a combination of threaded and smooth fasteners is used together. When this method is used, at least one threaded fastener needs to be positioned in each bone segment on either side of the fracture. By combining smooth and threaded fasteners, the surgeon gains both stability and ease of application, especially when using a biphase technique (see later). At least two fasteners need to be positioned in each bone segment on either side of the fracture. Frequently, more fasteners are placed in each individual bone segment, a maneuver that enhances the strength of the construct. It is possible, and advantageous, with the acrylic pin splint to stabilize fractures involving both hemimandibles with a singular acrylic column (see Fig. 52.15). The vertical ramus of the mandible is a poor location for securing fasteners because this soft, flat bone does not hold a fastener well. Because of this limitation, caudal mandibular fractures do not lend themselves well to fixation with the acrylic pin splint.

Free-Form Acrylic Pin Splint

The patient is administered a perioperative antibiotic regimen. The appropriate number of fasteners is placed into each bone segment. Aseptic technique is always used when applying the fasteners and during fracture manipulation and closure of the soft tissues, when using an open reduction technique. Aseptic technique is not necessary for application of the acrylic connector when this procedure is done after closure of the wound. Fasteners can be wedged between tooth roots, but they should not be drilled through these roots, and mandibular vessels and nerves need to be avoided. If smooth pins are used in the configuration, they need to be bent to lie parallel to but elevated from the skin, to allow secure adherence to the column and room to accommodate the acrylic mass (Fig. 52.16). Fasteners should be positioned so, after the acrylic column is in place, distance of 1 to 2 cm will be present between the acrylic column and the skin. This distance is necessary to avoid thermal damage to the soft tissues and bone while the acrylic sets. Moistened gauze sponges can be placed to protect the skin and to cool the pins, thereby impeding conduction of excessive heat to the bone. All methylmethacrylate products use two components, a liquid (monomer) and a powder (polymer). For the Caulk orthodontic dental resin, three parts powder are mixed with one part liquid. For Technovit Hoof Acrylic, two parts powder are mixed with one part liquid. A disposable cup and wooden tongue depressor can be used to mix the acrylic. These two portions are mixed until they become doughy (3 to 4 minutes). The acrylic is hand molded to form a column long enough to incorporate all the preplaced fasteners and wide enough to provide adequate strength for the particular size of the animal. Approximate occlusional

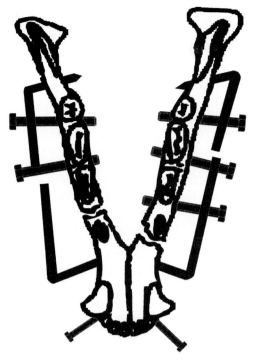

Fig. 52.16. Free-form acrylic pin splint.

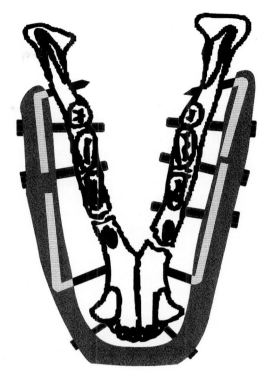

Fig. 52.18. Long pins cut short and bent to lie flush with acrylic.

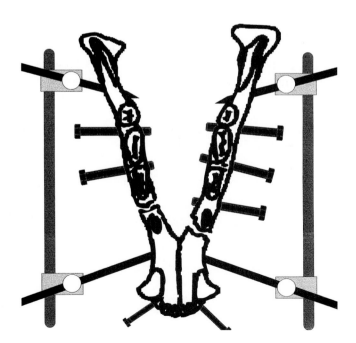

Fig. 52.17. Biphase technique using Kirschner clamps and connector rods.

alignment and fracture reduction are achieved. The acrylic column is placed on the fasteners and is conformed to the appropriate shape; then final occlusional alignment and fracture reduction are completed and held. The acrylic is adequately hardened 8 to 12 minutes after mixing, to enable the surgeon to abandon temporary holding of occlusion and reduction.

A biphase technique can be used to facilitate application of the acrylic pin splint. With this technique, the surgeon applies a temporary adjustable reduction device such as Kirschner clamps and connector rods (phase 1) separate and external to the acrylic column, to hold occlusional alignment and fracture reduction temporarily (Fig. 52.17). The acrylic is mixed and molded to all fasteners and is allowed to set (phase 2); then the external device is removed. The long pins are cut short once the acrylic has hardened; alternatively, the long pins can be bent over to lie flush with the acrylic column, and more acrylic can be mixed and added to the column to incorporate the bent pins (Fig. 52.18). This technique enhances the stability of the smooth pin acrylic linkage. The surgeon must bend the pins over using one pair of pliers as a lever positioned at the point of bend and another pair of pliers or hand chuck to exert bending of the pin. This prevents the formation of high stresses at the fastener–bone interface when bending over the pin.

Tube Acrylic Pin Splint

For this splint, either a commercial device or a home-made tube can be used. A homemade method is described here. The patient is administered a perioperative antibiotic regimen. The appropriate number of fasteners is placed into each bone segment using sterile technique, and surgical wounds are closed. Plastic tubing is pressed over the ends of the fasteners and is positioned 1 to 2 cm from the skin. Corrugated plastic anesthetic tubing (anesthesia breathing circuit, $\frac{1}{2}$-inch for small frames and $\frac{3}{4}$-inch for large frames, King Systems Corp., Nobelsville, IN) or Silastic tubing works well, serving as an injection mold for the acrylic. The most dependent end of each tube is plugged with cotton, and modeling clay is used at each junction of the tube and fastener to prevent excessive leakage of acrylic at these sites. Approximate occlusional alignment and fracture reduction are achieved. The powder and liquid components of the acrylic are mixed and are poured into the top end of the plastic tube. This maneuver can be facilitated by using a large-dose syringe to inject the acrylic into the plastic tube. Accurate occlusional alignment and fracture reduction are maintained until the acrylic sets. The acrylic must fill the tube completely, and no air bubbles can be present to weaken the acrylic column. If large air bubbles are noted, holes can be made in the plastic tube and more acrylic can be injected into the area before or after the acrylic sets. The biphase technique can easily be adapted to the tube acrylic pin splint, with considerations and technique similar to that described for the free-form method. A frame alignment kit (Innovative Animal Products, Rochester, MN) is available and is advantageous because it allows phase 1 reduction equipment to be placed either above or below the plastic tubes.

The fracture reduction or the splint can be adjusted after the acrylic has set by removing a short segment of the acrylic column with a hacksaw blade, obstetric or Gigli wire, or a cast cutter. A portion of the tubing is peeled back, and several channels are drilled into a portion of acrylic on either end of the cut column to provide an anchor for the new acrylic patch. A small amount of acrylic is mixed and hand molded to fill the gap and to overlap a portion of the exposed acrylic containing the channels. Occlusional alignment or fracture reduction is then manipulated, while the acrylic is still soft, and is held until the acrylic hardens. New fasteners can be placed to add additional strength to the configuration or to replace fasteners that are loose. Fasteners are placed adjacent to the existing acrylic column using aseptic technique. The fasteners are then incorporated into the column with the addition of a new patch of acrylic.

Suggested Readings

Egger EL. Management of mandibular fractures with external fixation. In: Proceedings of the 5th annual Complete Course in External Skeletal Fixation. Athens, GA:, 1996:113–115.

Toombs JP. Nomenclature and Instrumentation of external skeletal fixation systems. In: Proceedings of the 5th annual Complete Course in External Skeletal Fixation. Athens, GA:, 1996:2–9.

53

FRACTURES OF THE SPINE

Surgical Treatment of Fractures of the Dens

Kurt Schulz & Don R. Waldron

Preoperative corticosteroids (Solu-medrol 15 to 30 mg/kg intravenously) should be administered to diminish spinal cord inflammation subsequent to manipulations.

Surgical Technique

The animal is placed in dorsal recumbency with the head extended and the neck elevated by padding. The skin incision begins at the level of the larynx and extends to the manubrium. The paired sternomastoideus and sternohyoideus muscles are separated on the midline and are lateralized with self-retaining retractors. The trachea and esophagus are bluntly dissected from the loose deep fascia with finger dissection and are retracted to the left temporarily by an assistant. The carotid sheath should be identified and protected. Proper location of the C1–2 interspace is confirmed by palpation of the wings of the atlas laterally, the large transverse processes of C6 caudally, and palpation and counting of the ventral processes of the cervical vertebrae. The paired longus colli muscles are separated on midline and are retracted laterally from C1 through C3. Excessive lateral retraction should be avoided, to prevent bleeding from branches of the vertebral arteries. Self-retaining retractors are used to lateralize the longus colli muscles and retract more superficial structures simultaneously, so all other retractors may be removed.

The joint capsule of the two lateral atlantoaxial articulations and the fascia between C1 and C2 covering the dens should be identified. If the fracture involves the body of C2 or if atlantoaxial luxation has occurred, as is found in most cases, then arthrodesis of the atlantoaxial joint is recommended. When only the dens is fractured, the membranes covering the foramen magnum and between C1 and C2 are opened with a No. 11 or 12 Bard–Parker blade. The alar and apical ligaments of the dens are transected through the ventral occipitoatlantal space, and the dens is removed through the ventral atlantoaxial space. The stability of the atlantoaxial joint without the dens in a previously normal animal is unknown; therefore, prophylactic stabilization of the joint is recommended.

In most reported cases, fractures of the dens also involve a portion of the body of C2 (Fig. 53.1). Stabilization of a small cranial fragment may be difficult, and arthrodesis of the atlantoaxial joint may be indicated in these cases. The joint capsule should be opened bilaterally with a No. 11 Bard–Parker blade to aid in visualization for fracture reduction and to facilitate removal of the articular cartilage with rongeurs or an air drill. Reduction of the fracture is aided by caudal traction on small, pointed reduction forceps placed on the caudal body of C2 or by caudal traction on a small threaded pin placed in the caudal body of C2. Cranial traction on the head may also be necessary. Caution is indicated to avoid damaging the vertebral sinuses, particularly in patients with chronic cases.

Removal of the dens from the C2 fracture fragment is unnecessary if adequate stabilization of the fracture and atlantoaxial joint can be achieved, because the ligaments of the dens are unlikely to have been damaged in combination with the fracture. The dens may, however, be removed if necessary as described previously. The cranial fracture fragment may be exteriorized in some cases, so the dens can be removed with an air drill, rongeurs, or bone-cutting forceps. Once adequate reduction has been achieved and the opera-

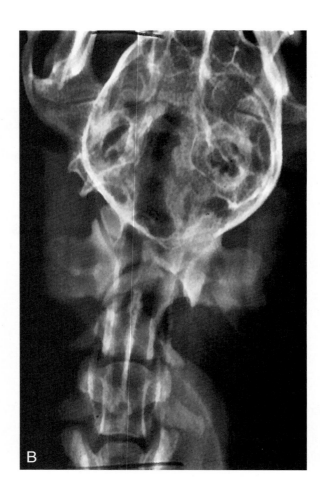

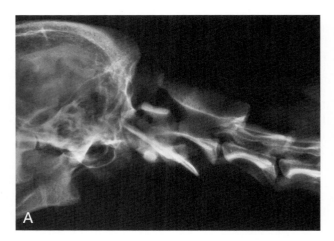

Fig. 53.1. Lateral (**A**) and ventrodorsal (**B**) radiographs of a 6-year-old cocker spaniel with a 1-month-old fracture of the body of C2.

tive area has been lavaged, cancellous bone graft collected from the proximal humerus should be packed around the fracture site and in the articular spaces to promote arthrodesis.

The choice of stabilization technique depends on the nature of the fracture, the size of the patient, and the surgeon's preference. Techniques that have been used include pins, lag screws, pins and polymethylmethacrylate, and plates (1, 2). If the dens only was fractured and has been removed, the joint is stabilized as for atlantoaxial instability with lag screws or pins with or without polymethylmethacrylate (see Chap. 45). In cases involving fracture of the body of C2, pins and polymethylmethacrylate or bone plates are recommended (Fig. 53.2). In larger dogs, lag screw fixation of the fracture fragment may be possible; however, pins or screws with polymethylmethacrylate or bone plating can permit simultaneous fracture fixation and arthrodesis of the atlantoaxial joint (Fig. 53.3).

Bone plates are placed on the ventrolateral surface of C1 and C2. T plates and veterinary cuttable plates may be well suited for this application. Particular attention must be paid to screw length and direction.

Gentle caudal retraction of C2 allows visualization of the spinal canal to aid in screw placement in the atlas. The small size of many patients may limit the practicality of the use of bone plates for stabilization.

Pins or screws and polymethylmethacrylate are placed as in the procedure for atlantoaxial instability (see Chap. 45). At least one pin should engage the cranial fragment of C2. Two pins should engage the atlas, and two should engage the caudal fragment of the axis. Pins are first placed in the axis, a procedure facilitated by gentle dorsiflexion of the atlantoaxial joint for visualization of the spinal canal. Kirschner wires or small threaded pins are directed perpendicular to the long axis of the spine, from ventral to dorsal, into each of the pedicles of the atlas. The atlantoaxial joint is then reduced, and pins are driven from the center of the caudal surface of each caudal articular region across the atlantoaxial joints and are seated in the atlas just medial to the alar notches. One of these pins should engage the cranial fragment of C2. Two pins are then placed into the caudal body of the axis. In some cases, this placement necessitates penetration of muscle and other soft tissue to obtain the correct

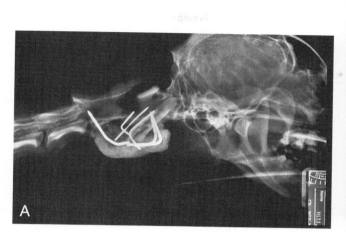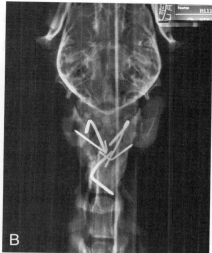

Fig. 53.2. Lateral (**A**) and ventrodorsal (**B**) radiographs of a 6-year-old cocker spaniel after C2 fracture stabilization with ventral pins and polymethylmethacrylate.

angulation. All pins are cut short, crimped, and bent, leaving enough pin length to engage a small mass of polymethylmethacrylate. Antibiotic powder is added to the monomer before mixing, and the cement is applied at a doughy consistency to cover and encompass the pins. The cement mass should not be so large that it causes significant ventral deviation of the trachea. Cool saline flush should be applied to the operative area to dissipate heat associated with polymerization.

Closure of the longus colli muscles is neither possible nor necessary after many of the stabilization techniques. The sternohyoideus muscles are reapposed gently with absorbable suture in a simple continuous pattern. Subcutaneous and skin closures are routine. Postoperative radiographs are indicated to demonstrate appropriate reduction and adequate stabilization, and a ventral neck brace and cage rest are indicated for 3 to 4 weeks.

Complications

Potential complications of these techniques include tracheal necrosis from devascularization or thermal injury and laryngeal paralysis secondary to damage to the recurrent laryngeal nerve. These problems may be avoided by careful, gentle dissection and retraction. Hemorrhage from the vertebral sinuses or branches of the vertebral arteries is a frequent complication that may obscure the surgical field and cause life-threatening blood loss. Concern for infection is heightened when polymethylmethacrylate is implanted; therefore, strict attention to asepsis is imperative. The surgeon may elect to culture the surgical site before closure and to maintain prophylactic antibiotics until a negative culture result is obtained. The fixation may fail because of inadequate or inappropriate application. Prognosis depends on the severity of the initial spinal cord injury. If fracture stabilization is successful and spinal cord manipulation is minimal at the time of surgery, the overall prognosis is favorable.

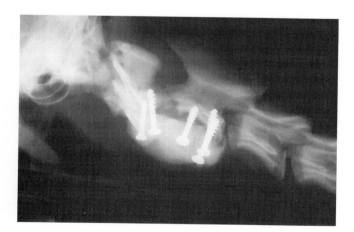

Fig. 53.3. Lateral radiograph of an 8-month-old rottweiler after C2 fracture stabilization with ventral screws and polymethylmethacrylate.

Suggested Readings

Blass CE, Waldron DR, Van Ee RT. Cervical stabilization in three dogs using Steinmann pins and methylmethacrylate. J Am Anim Hosp Assoc 1988;24:61–68.

Stone EA, Betts CW, Chambers JN. Cervical fractures in the dog: a literature and case review. J Am Anim Hosp Assoc 1979; 15:463–471.

Surgical Treatment of Spinal Fractures, Luxations, and Subluxations

Kenneth A. Bruecker

When considering treatment options for a patient with a spinal fracture, luxation, or subluxation, several factors should be considered: 1) results of the neurologic examination; 2) whether the fracture is pathologic or traumatic; and 3) whether the fracture is stable or unstable.

The neurologic examination is critical in determining prognosis. If the patient has lost all sensory and motor function caudal to the lesion, the prognosis is unfavorable, and treatment is generally supportive. Surgery in this situation may be indicated for prognostic purposes only (i.e., exploratory laminectomy). If deep pain perception is still present, the prognosis is guarded to favorable (depending on the degree of neurologic dysfunction), and surgical decompression and stabilization are performed with curative intent.

Patients with pathologic fractures have an underlying localized or generalized disorder. The cause of the underlying disorder must be determined, and therapy instituted before the spinal fracture or luxation is repaired. Once the underlying disorder is controlled, the spinal fracture or luxation can be treated as described for traumatic fracture or luxation.

Physical examination findings and radiographic assessment may be helpful in determining the inherent stability of the fracture or luxation (1). In small animal patients, traumatic disruption of the spinal column can be divided into dorsal compartment injuries, ventral compartment injuries, and combined compartment injuries. Combined compartment injuries are more devastating and more common than injuries isolated to one compartment. Most spinal injuries are flexional injuries, but occasionally hyperextension or direct compression injuries occur. Rotation is a common force associated with these injuries.

Fractures may be classified as stable or unstable by the radiographic appearance and by the force causing the injury. Forces that damage the dorsal compartment generally result in an unstable injury. Examples include laminar or pedicle fracture, dorsal spinous process fracture, articular process fracture, and supraspinous or interspinous ligament rupture (2).

If surgical treatment is deemed necessary, the surgeon should select a technique that will not further destabilize the spine. Herniated disc material or osseous fragments within the spinal canal may be anticipated in flexion or bursting-type injuries. Concussive and contusive forces can cause spinal cord swelling even without evidence of an extradural mass. Infolding of the ligamentum flavum during hyperextension injuries may also result in spinal cord injury.

Generally, stable fractures in patients with good voluntary motor movements to the limbs are successfully managed by conservative means, including the use of anti-inflammatory agents, body splints, and strict cage confinement (3). Serial neurologic examinations are performed (twice daily) to determine the response to treatment.

Surgical management is indicated 1) if the fracture or luxation is considered unstable, 2) if the patient presents nonambulatory paraparetic or tetraparetic with no voluntary motor movements, or 3) if with conservative therapy, the patient remains unacceptably static or deteriorates neurologically.

Several factors must be considered when selecting a stabilizing technique: 1) location of the fracture or luxation (cervical, thoracic, lumbar, sacral); 2) presence of a compressive lesion within the spinal canal (i.e., osseous fragment, disc material); 3) size of the patient; 4) age of the patient; 5) equipment available; 6) experience of the surgeon; and 7) physical and emotional capability of the owner to provide postoperative nursing care.

Surgical Principles

The two objectives of any surgical technique used to repair spinal fracture or luxation are decompression and stabilization. Many techniques have been used successfully to stabilize spinal fracture or luxation in small animals. In the following discussion, techniques commonly used to repair fractures and luxations of the spine are described as they are indicated in various regions of the vertebral column.

Fractures of the Cervical Spine

Cervical spinal fractures are uncommon (4, 5). Most fractures of the cervical spine involve C1 (axis), particularly the dens and body (5). Generally, surgical techniques used to repair cervical fractures or luxations are dictated by the type and location of the lesion.

Fractures of the dorsal spine of the axis should be approached dorsally and stabilized with orthopedic wire to reestablish the continuity of displaced fragments. A decompressive hemilaminectomy can be performed if fragments of bone are present in the spinal canal or if a displaced body fracture cannot be reduced. Atlantoaxial subluxation can be repaired from a dorsal approach using either a double-wiring or single-wiring or suturing technique (6).

C1–C2 body fractures or luxations, traumatic cervical disc extrusions, and atlantoaxial subluxation can be approached ventrally. Ventral cross-pin techniques may be used for stabilization of atlantoaxial subluxation (7) (Fig. 53.4).

Fractures and luxations rarely occur from C3 to C7; however, a predisposition to luxations at C5–6 may exist (5, 8). Fractures or luxations of C3–C7 may be approached dorsally or ventrally. Dorsal techniques include articular facet wiring or screwing, dorsal spinous process plating, and multiple Steinmann pins and polymethylmethacrylate (see the next section of this discussion). Ventral techniques include pins and polymethylmethacrylate and ventral body plating, either plastic (Lubra plate, Lubra Co., Fort Collins, CO) or metal (Auburn spinal plate, Richard Manufacturing Co., Memphis, TN). One advantage to the ventral approach is that a ventral slot can be performed if disc fragments have extruded into the spinal canal.

The use of pins and polymethylmethacrylate should be considered for cervical spinal fractures involving the vertebral bodies of C2–7. The ventral aspect of the involved vertebra is exposed (9). Once the fracture is reduced, a minimum of two trocar tip pins should be placed in the cranial fragment, and a minimum of two pins should be placed in the caudal fragment. Alternatively, the fractured vertebral body can be bridged by insertion of pins into the vertebra cranial and caudal to the fracture. Two cortices must be engaged with each pin. The pins are inserted on the ventral midline of the vertebral body and are directed 30 to 35° dorsolaterally to avoid entering the spinal canal. In addition, the pins can be angled cranially and caudally to enhance stability of the implant. The pins are cut, leaving 1 to 1.5 cm exposed. The exposed pins are notched with pin cutters and are covered with sterile polymeth-

ylmethacrylate (10) (Fig. 53.5). The heat of polymerization is dissipated with 5 to 10 minutes of cool saline irrigation. A neck brace may be used for 4 to 6 weeks postoperatively. The limiting factor of this technique is the purchasing ability of the pins in small fragments.

Reduction of cervical fractures or luxations can be facilitated by gently distracting the affected vertebral bodies. Fenestration of the adjacent intervertebral discs or slots drilled into the vertebral bodies cranial and caudal to the fracture or luxation can be created to accommodate a vertebral distractor. A Gelpi retractor, modified by blunting the tips, is a useful vertebral distractor.

Fractures of the Thoracolumbar and Lumbar Spine

The thoracolumbar and lumbar spine is a common location for spinal fractures in the dog and cat. As previously mentioned, the higher incidence of fractures or luxations at certain sites along the vertebral canal may not correlate with differences in muscular or ligamentous attachments, but rather with areas of the vertebral column with a static–kinetic relationship (i.e., thoracolumbar and lumbosacral junction) (1, 4).

Technique Selection

Numerous techniques have been developed to stabilize thoracolumbar and lumbar spinal fractures in dogs (11–18). The technique chosen is dictated by the location of the fracture, size, age, and disposition of the

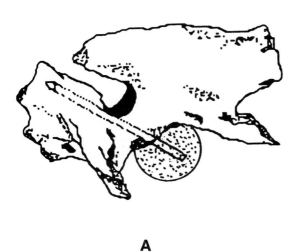

A

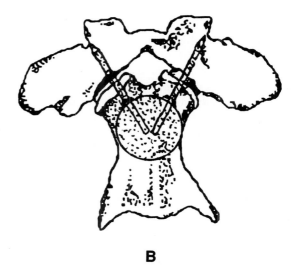

B

Fig. 53.4. **A** and **B.** Pin placement for arthrodesis of atlantoaxial joints in treating atlantoaxial subluxation by the ventral approach. The exposed portions of the pins (depicted within the *dotted circle*) can be notched and covered with methyl methacrylate to prevent pin migration. (From Sorjonen DC, Shires PK. Atlantoaxial instability: a ventral surgical technique for decompression, fixation, and fusion. Vet Surg 1981;10:22–29.)

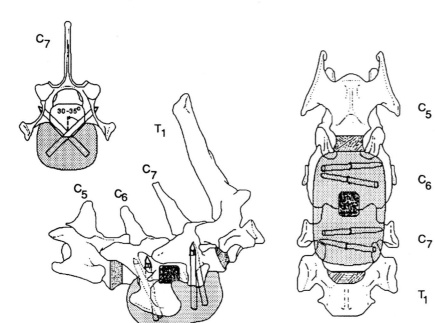

Fig. 53.5. Stabilization with ventrally placed Steinmann pins and methylmethacrylate of cervical fracture or luxation. Ventral slot can be performed to remove herniated disc material. (From Blass CE, Waldron DR, van Ee RT. Cervical stabilization in three dogs using Steinmann pins and methylmethacrylate. J Am Anim Hosp Assoc 1988;24:61–68.)

patient, equipment available, and experience of the surgeon.

Surgical Techniques

Dorsal spinous process plating requires exposure of the dorsal spinous processes and articular facets (9). The supraspinous and interspinous ligaments should be preserved if possible. A minimum of three spinous processes on each side of the fracture or luxation should be exposed. Metal or plastic plates are available for dorsal spinous process plating. When using plastic plates, a plate is used on each side of the exposed dorsal spinous processes (two plates total) (11, 12) (Fig. 53.6). The roughened side of the plate is placed against the dorsal spinous processes. The plates are attached with nuts and bolts of appropriate size placed between the dorsal spinous processes. The plates should be kept as close to the base of the dorsal spinous processes as possible. Grooves can be created in the lamina at the base of the spine using a high-speed bone bur or rongeurs to help keep the plates low on the spine. This procedure allows maximal purchase of the spinal plates to the dorsal spinous processes. Metal plates are used in a similar fashion; however, the nuts and bolts are placed through the dorsal spinous processes (Fig. 53.7). The advantage of dorsal spinous process plating is preservation of the inherent stability provided by the articular facets and the supraspinous and interspinous ligament.

The major limiting factors of dorsal spinous process plating are the age and size of the patient. The dorsal spinous processes must be large enough and the bone compact enough to support the stresses on an unstable spine. This technique is commonly used in combination with other stabilization techniques (i.e., pins and polymethylmethacrylate, vertebral body plating). The most common postoperative complications are fracture of the spinous processes and plate slippage.

Spinal stapling also requires exposure of the dorsal spinous processes and facet joints. An intramedullary pin is placed through a dorsal spinous process, bent 90°, laid along the lamina between the base of the spinous processes and articular processes, and secured to the base of the dorsal spinous processes with orthopedic wire (Fig. 53.8). Added security can be accom-

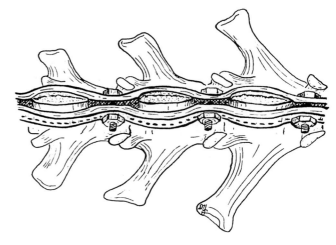

Fig. 53.6. Dorsal spinal plating using plastic plates. (Redrawn from Walker TL, Tomlinson J, Sorjonen DC, et al. Diseases of the spinal column. In: Slatter DH, ed. Textbook of small animal surgery. Philadelphia: WB Saunders, 1985.)

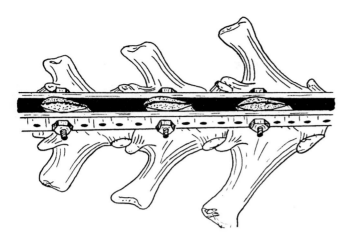

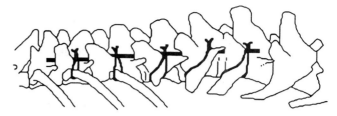

Fig. 53.9. Added stability can be achieved to the spinal stapling if rib heads or transverse processes are incorporated into the repair. (From Helphrey M, Seim HB. Spinal trauma. In: Bojrab MJ, ed. Current techniques in small animal surgery. 3rd ed. Philadelphia: Lea & Febiger, 1990.)

Fig. 53.7. Dorsal spinal plating using metal plates. (Redrawn from Walker TL, Tomlinson J, Sorjonen DC, et al. Diseases of the spinal column. In: Slatter DH, ed. Textbook of small animal surgery. Philadelphia: WB Saunders, 1985.)

plished by wiring the pin around the base of the transverse processes in the lumbar spine or around the rib heads in the thoracic spine (Fig. 53.9) or by incorporating multiple pins and wires in a modified segmental spinal instrumentation technique (Fig. 53.10) (13). At least two interspaces on each side of the fracture or luxation should be included in the repair. This technique should be reserved for patients that weigh less than 10 kg.

Vertebral body plating (dorsal body plating) requires dorsolateral exposure of the articular facet, vertebral body and transverse process of the lumbar vertebra or the articular facet, and vertebral body and rib head of the thoracic vertebra (14) (Fig. 53.11). Care should be taken to protect the spinal nerve roots encountered cranial and caudal to the fracture or luxa-

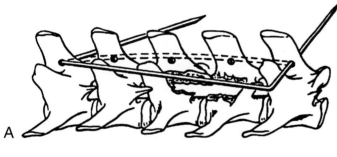

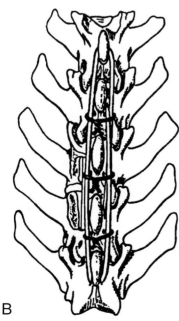

Fig. 53.8. A and **B.** Spinal stapling using single pin, doubled on the contralateral side of the dorsal spinous processes. (Redrawn from Walker TL, Tomlinson J, Sorjonen DC, et al. Diseases of the spinal column. In: Slatter DH, ed. Textbook of small animal surgery. Philadelphia: WB Saunders, 1985.)

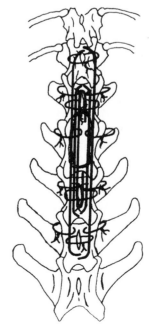

Fig. 53.10. Modified segmental spinal instrumentation using multiple Steinmann pins and orthopedic wire. (From McNaulty JF, Lenehan TM, Maletz LM. Modified segmental spinal instrumentation in repair of spinal fractures and luxations in dogs. Vet Surg 1986;15:143–149.)

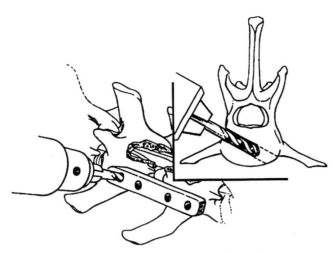

Fig. 53.11. Application of a vertebral body plate. (From Swaim SF. Vertebral body plating for spinal stabilization. J Am Vet Med Assoc 1971;158:1653–1695.)

tion. The spinal nerve and vessels at the involved space must be severed. The proper length and size plate is selected and is placed on the dorsolateral aspect of the vertebral bodies. At least four cortices should be engaged cranial and caudal to the involved fracture or luxation. If a luxation, subluxation, or fracture close to the interspace exists, stabilization of the two adjacent vertebrae is adequate; however, if a midbody fracture exists, three vertebral bodies should be spanned. The holes are drilled, and screws are placed in a ventral and medial direction, with care taken to avoid entering the spinal canal dorsally or the abdominal cavity ventrally. Placement of the plate on the thoracic vertebrae is more difficult because of the presence of the rib heads. The rib heads must be removed and the transverse process contoured so the plate lies flat against the vertebral body. An anatomic specimen should be available for visualization during placement of plates and screws. The need for rhizotomy precludes the use of vertebral body plating caudal to the fourth lumbar vertebra (14).

Stabilization techniques using pins and polymethylmethacrylate require exposure of the dorsal spinous processes, articular facets, and transverse processes bilaterally (15, 16). A minimum of two trocar-tip pins of appropriate size should be placed into the vertebral bodies on each side of the fracture or luxation. In the thoracic vertebrae, the pins are inserted into the pedicle and are driven into the vertebral bodies, using the tubercle of the ribs and the base of the accessory processes as landmarks. In the lumbar vertebrae, pins are inserted directly into the vertebral bodies using the accessory processes and transverse processes as landmarks. Because pin placement is critical and landmarks vary depending on the level of the spine, a skeleton should be available for reference. The pins are directed

cranioventrally and laterally to medially in the vertebral body cranial to the fracture or luxation and caudoventrally and laterally to medially in the vertebral body caudal to the fracture or luxation. Steinmann pins are driven so they exit 2 to 3 mm from the ventral aspect of the vertebral body, are cut leaving 1.5 to 2 cm exposed dorsally, and are notched with a pin cutter. The polymethylmethacrylate forms around the notched pin and helps to prevent pin migration. The surgical field is lavaged and dried in preparation for application of polymethylmethacrylate. If a laminectomy is not performed, polymethylmethacrylate is simply applied as a spheric mass, incorporating the Steinmann pins as well as the articular facets and adjacent dorsal spinous processes (Fig. 53.12). If a laminectomy is performed, the exposed spinal cord is covered with an autogenous fat graft, and the polymethylmethacrylate is molded into the shape of a donut (Fig. 53.13). Care is taken not to allow the polymethylmethacrylate to contact the spinal cord. The polymeth-

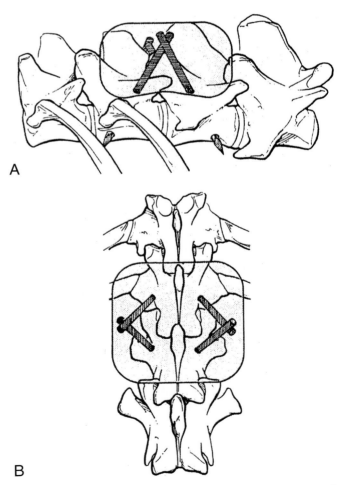

A

B

Fig. 53.12. **A** and **B.** Dorsal placement of Steinmann pins and polymethylmethacrylate to stabilize lumbar fractures or luxations. (From Blass CE, Seim HB. Spinal fixation in dogs using Steinmann pins and methylmethacrylate. Vet Surg 1984;13:203–210.)

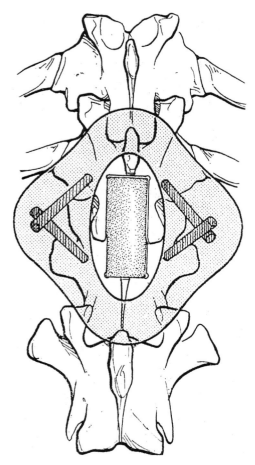

Fig. 53.13. Dorsal placement of Steinmann pins and polymethylmethacrylate to stabilize lumbar fractures or luxations after laminectomy. The polymethylmethacrylate is not placed over the laminectomy site. (From Blass CE, Seim HB. Spinal fixation in dogs using Steinmann pins and methylmethacrylate. Vet Surg 1984; 13:203–210.)

ylmethacrylate is lavaged with cool saline to dissipate the heat of polymerization. Portions of the epaxial muscles adjacent to the polymethylmethacrylate may have to be excised to facilitate closure. Rarely, relief incisions in the lumbodorsal fascia lateral to the polymethylmethacrylate are necessary to allow closure of the primary incision (15, 16).

The major disadvantage of this technique is the exposure necessary for pin placement; however, in a series of dogs treated with this technique, no failures were associated with stress fatigue (15). The technique is straightforward and requires minimal special equipment, although a thorough knowledge of anatomy and constant reference to an appropriate anatomic specimen are recommended.

In some instances (generally, thoracolumbar fractures or luxations in large breed dogs with hyperactive personalities), a combination of the foregoing techniques should be considered. Combinations such as

pins and polymethylmethacrylate with dorsal spinous process plating, cross pins with dorsal spinous process plating, or body plating with dorsal spinous process plating have proved successful.

Fractures of L6, L7, and S1

Fractures and luxations of the caudal lumbar and sacral vertebrae are common because of the static–kinetic relationship of the sacral and lumbar segments, respectively. Neurologic signs secondary to trauma of the cauda equina result in varying degrees of femoral, sciatic, and sacral nerve dysfunction. Because the spinal cord ends cranial to L7, patients with 60 to 70% displacement of the spinal canal may still have a favorable prognosis (1).

Because of the increased shearing forces present in the lumbosacral region, caudal lumbar and lumbosacral fractures or luxations are difficult to stabilize. Techniques used to treat L7–S1 fractures or luxations successfully include transilial pinning, transilial pinning with Lubra plate support, pins and polymethylmethacrylate, transilial pinning with external skeletal fixation, and spinal stapling (11, 13, 17–21).

Surgical Techniques

Transilial pinning requires exposure of the dorsal L7–S1 region (21). The caudal segment is most often displaced ventrally and cranially. Bone forceps are placed on each ilial wing to help elevate the ilium and sacrum dorsally, to align the articular processes of L7 with the cranial articular surface of the sacrum. A trocar-tip pin of appropriate size ($\frac{1}{8}$-inch or smaller) is driven through the wing of the ilium, across the laminae of L7, and through the opposite wing of the ilium (Fig. 53.14). The most common problem associated with this technique is migration of the Steinmann pin. A more stable technique is generally recommended.

The use of plastic dorsal spinous process plates and transilial pins has been reported (11, 17). This procedure requires a similar approach and reduction as previously described. Plastic dorsal spinous process plates are placed on each side of the three dorsal spinous processes cranial to the fracture or luxation and are secured with nuts and bolts, as previously described for plastic dorsal spinous process plating. The plastic plates extend caudad to S2–3. A $\frac{3}{32}$-inch or $\frac{1}{8}$-inch trocar-tip pin is driven through one ilial wing, through the plastic plate at the level of L7–S1, and through the opposite ilial wing. A second pin is placed caudal to the first pin. The ends of the pins are bent craniad at a 90° angle and are cut to leave 5 mm protruding (Fig. 53.15). Postsurgical complications include fracture of the dorsal spinous processes or migration of the transi-

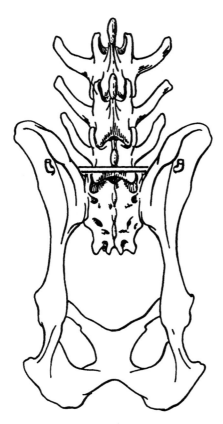

Fig. 53.14. Transilial pin used to stabilize a fracture of the body of L7 or lumbosacral luxation. (Redrawn from Walker TL, Tomlinson J, Sorjonen DC, et al. Diseases of the spinal column. In: Slatter DH, ed. Textbook of small animal surgery. Philadelphia: WB Saunders, 1985.)

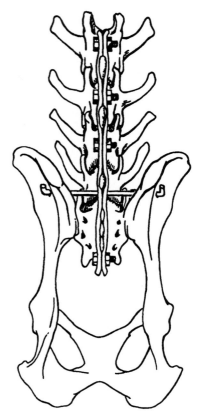

Fig. 53.15. A transilial pin used in conjunction with plastic dorsal spinal plates provides additional support for lumbar or lumbosacral fractures. (Redrawn from Walker TL, Tomlinson J, Sorjonen DC, et al. Diseases of the spinal column. In: Slatter DH, ed. Textbook of small animal surgery. Philadelphia: WB Saunders, 1985.)

lial pins. Pin migration may be decreased by application of polymethylmethacrylate to notched pins.

Transilial pinning and external skeletal fixation with a Kirschner–Ehmer (Kirschner Co., Timonium, MD) apparatus have been described (19, 20). In this technique, the transilial pins are placed percutaneously. In addition, one pin is inserted percutaneously through the vertebral body cranial to the fracture or luxation. Kirschner clamps attach the pins to a connecting bar on each side of the spine (Fig. 53.16).

Pins and polymethylmethacrylate can also be used to stabilize lumbosacral fractures or luxations. The approach and reduction are as previously described. Two pins are placed in the vertebral body cranial to the fracture or luxation, and two pins are placed in the wings of the ilium. The pins are incorporated with polymethylmethacrylate as previously described. The disadvantage of this technique is the large amount of polymethylmethacrylate needed for adequate stabilization, making closure difficult.

Modified segmental spinal instrumentation has been used successfully to stabilize lumbosacral fractures. Pins are prebent 90°, placed through holes drilled in the wings of the ilium, laid alongside the

dorsal spinous processes of at least two vertebra cranial to the fracture or luxation, and wired in place to the adjacent articular facets, dorsal spinous processes, and lamina (Fig. 53.17). Combinations of the foregoing techniques may be used in large breed dogs with hyperactive personalities.

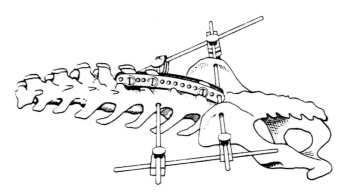

Fig. 53.16. A transilial pin with external skeletal fixation also provides additional support for lumbar or lumbosacral fractures. (From Shores A, Nichols C, Rochat M, et al. Combined Kirschner–Ehmer device and dorsal spinal plate fixation technique for caudal lumbar vertebral fractures in dogs. J Am Vet Med Assoc 1989; 195:335–339.)

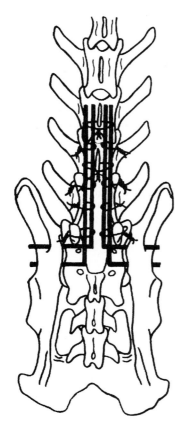

Fig. 53.17. The use of modified segmental spinal instrumentation for the repair of lumbosacral and caudal lumbar fracture or luxation. (From McNaulty JF, Lenehan TM, Maletz LM. Modified segmental spinal instrumentation in repair of spinal fractures and luxations in dogs. Vet Surg 1986;15:143–149.)

Sacral and Sacrococcygeal Fractures

Special attention to the S2–3 dermatomes and evaluation of bowel and bladder function should be considered when performing a neurologic examination on patients with sacral and sacrococcygeal fractures or luxations. Fracture of the sacral wings generally occurs through the sacral foramina, damaging the S1, S2, and S3 nerve roots. Sacroiliac luxation, however, rarely affects the nerve roots.

A dorsal approach to the sacroiliac junction can be used to expose fractures of the sacral wing. Careful periosteal elevation of the paraspinal musculature allows visualization of the fracture fragments. Once reduced, the fracture can be stabilized with a lag screw inserted through the ilium and sacral fragment and into the sacral body (22). A parallel trocar-tip pin or wire may be inserted to provide rotational stability (Fig. 53.18). If the neurologic examination reveals severe nerve root damage (shearing of the S1–3 nerve roots), laminectomy and exploration of the cauda equina should be considered.

Patients sustaining a sacral or sacrococcygeal frac-

ture or luxation may present with an anesthetic tail. If the tail remains anesthetic at 2 to 3 weeks after the injury, amputation may be necessary to eliminate associated fecal matting, urine scalding (cats), and self-mutilation (18).

Traumatic injury of the sacrococcygeal area frequently occurs in cats (4, 23). Avulsion of the nerve roots of the cauda equina is a frequent sequela of injuries causing sacrococcygeal fractures or luxations. The prognosis is good for return of normal urinary function in cats that have anal tone and perineal sensation at the time of initial examination (23). Cats that are unable to urinate normally within 4 to 6 weeks after the injury are not expected to recover normal urination habits (23).

Coccygeal Fractures

Coccygeal fractures may result in various neurologic deficits to the tail. Rarely should they be treated surgically. If anesthesia of the tail persists, amputation may be the only feasible alternative.

Postoperative Management

Postoperative management of spinal fracture patients generally is divided into ambulatory and nonambulatory convalescence. Patients with an ambulatory status postoperatively are generally managed in the following manner: cage confinement, brief exercise 2 to 3 times a day for 2 to 3 weeks, serial neurologic and radiographic examinations, and home on restricted exercise or passive range-of-motion exercises until radio-

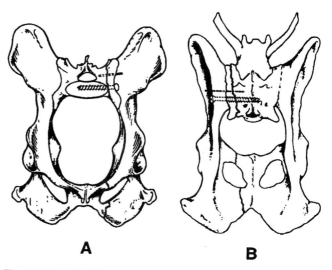

A   **B**

Fig. 53.18. Stabilization of sacral fracture using lag screw and Kirschner wire; cranial (**A**) and dorsal (**B**) views. (From Bruecker KA, Seim HB. Spinal fractures and luxations. In: Slatter DH, ed. Textbook of small animal surgery. 2nd ed. Philadelphia: WB Saunders, 1993.)

graphic evidence of healing is present. Nonambulatory patients are managed in the following manner: elevated padded cage rack or waterbed, turning every 2 to 4 hours, bladder expressions four to five times a day, passive range-of-motion exercises, serial neurologic and radiographic evaluations, and frequent hydrotherapy until return to an ambulatory status is achieved.

The use of back braces or splints is controversial. Braces that are comfortable, lightweight, and tolerated by the patient are helpful; however, most braces are heavy, nonconforming, result in rub sores, and are not well tolerated by the patient (3). The surgeon should not rely heavily on the help of a back brace, especially in large breed, hyperactive dogs.

References

1. Feeney DA, Oliver JE. Blunt spinal trauma in the dog and cat: neurologic, radiologic and therapeutic correlations. J Am Anim Hosp Assoc 1980;16:664–668.
2. Swaim SF. Biomechanics of cranial fractures, spinal fractures, and luxations. In: Bojrab MJ, ed. Pathophysiology in small animal surgery. Philadelphia: Lea & Febiger, 1981:774–778.
3. Carberry CA, Flanders JA, Dietze AK, et al. Nonsurgical management of thoracic and lumbar spinal fractures and fracture/luxations in the dog and cat: a review of 17 cases. J Am Anim Hosp Assoc 1989;25:43–54.
4. Feeney DA, Oliver JE. Blunt spinal trauma in the dog and cat: insight into radiographic lesions. J Am Anim Hosp Assoc 1980;16:885–890.
5. Stone EA, Betts CW, Chambers JN. Cervical fractures in the dog: a literature and case review. J Am Anim Hosp Assoc 1979;15:463–471.
6. Oliver JE, Lewis RE. Lesions of the atlas and axis in dogs. J Am Anim Hosp Assoc 1973;9:304–313.
7. Sorjonen DC, Shires PK. Atlantoaxial instability: a ventral surgical technique for decompression, fixation, and fusion. Vet Surg 1981;10:22–29.
8. Basinger RR, Bjorling DE, Chambers JN. Cervical spinal luxation in two dogs with entrapment of the cranial articular process of C6 over the caudal articular process of C5. J Am Vet Med Assoc 1986;188:865–867.
9. Piermattei DL. An atlas of surgical approaches to the bones and joints of the dog and cat. 3rd ed. Philadelphia: WB Saunders, 1993:45–89.
10. Blass CE, Waldron DR, van Ee RT. Cervical stabilization in three dogs using Steinmann pins and methylmethacrylate. J Am Anim Hosp Assoc 1988;24:61–68.
11. Dulisch ML, Nichols JB. A surgical technique for management of lower lumbar fractures: case report. Vet Surg 1981;10:90–93.
12. Lumb WV, Brasmer TH. Improved spinal plates and hypothermia as adjuncts to spinal surgery. J Am Vet Med Assoc 1970;157:338–342.
13. McNaulty JF, Lenehan TM, Maletz LM. Modified segmental spinal instrumentation in repair of spinal fractures and luxations in dogs. Vet Surg 1986;15:143–149.
14. Swaim SF. Vertebral body plating for spinal stabilization. J Am Vet Med Assoc 1971;158:1653–1695.
15. Blass CE, Seim HB. Spinal fixation in dogs using Steinmann pins and methylmethacrylate. Vet Surg 1984;13:203–210.
16. Rouse GP, Miller JI. The use of methylmethacrylate for spinal stabilization. J Am Anim Hosp Assoc 1975;11:418–425.
17. Lewis DD, Stampley A, Bellah JR, et al. Repair of sixth lumbar vertebral fracture-luxations, using transilial pins and plastic spinous-process plates in six dogs. J Am Vet Med Assoc 1989;194:538–542.
18. Matthiesen DT. Thoracolumbar spinal fractures/luxations: surgical management. Compend Contin Educ Pract Vet 1983;5:867–878.
19. Shores A, Nichols C, Koelling HA. Combined Kirschner–Ehmer apparatus and dorsal spinal plate fixation technique of caudal lumbar vertebral fractures in dogs: biomechanical properties. Am J Vet Res 1988;49:1979–1982.
20. Shores A, Nichols C, Rochat M, et al. Combined Kirschner–Ehmer device and dorsal spinal plate fixation technique for caudal lumbar vertebral fractures in dogs. J Am Vet Med Assoc 1989;195:335–339.
21. Slocum B, Rudy RL. Fractures of the seventh lumbar vertebral in the dog. J Am Anim Hosp Assoc 1975;11:167–174.
22. Taylor RA. Treatment of fractures of the sacrum and sacrococcygeal region. Vet Surg 1981;10:119–124.
23. Smeak DD, Olmstead ML. Fracture/luxations of the sacrococcygeal are in the cat: a retrospective study of 51 cases. Vet Surg 1985;14:319–324.

Fracture of the Seventh Lumbar Vertebra

Barclay Slocum & Theresa Devine Slocum

Fracture of the caudal half of the body of the seventh lumbar vertebra has special anatomic features that allow good fixation and healing. This fracture has a distinctive oblique appearance on the lateral radiograph that extends from the ventral midbody of the seventh lumbar vertebra to the L7–S1 intervertebral foramina. The caudal segment of the fracture is pulled ventrally and forward by the powerful longissimus lumborum, psoas, and abdominal muscles (Fig. 53.19). The dramatic displacement gives the appearance of spinal trauma so massive that no neurologic structure

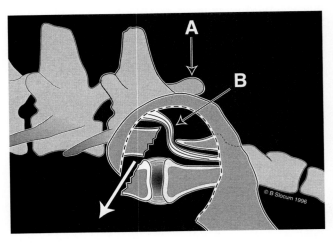

Fig. 53.19. Fracture of the seventh lumbar vertebral body is characteristically oblique with a cranioventral displacement of the caudal portion (*white arrow*). The joint capsule of the articular process (*A*) is torn. The spinal nerves of the cauda equina at L7–S1 are distorted but seldom are crushed (*B*).

could survive the insult. Fortunately, the spinal cord stops at the midbody of L5, leaving the spinal nerves of the cauda equina to traverse this area. That these nerves move within the spinal canal, within the foramina, and within soft tissues helps to prevent nerve damage. Rarely do dogs have permanent loss of sciatic nerve function or control of the anal and urinary sphincters. The strong articular facets of L7 and the wings of the ilium allow for good fixation. Fractures through the body have excellent blood supply and heal rapidly. Although care must be taken to remove any fracture fragments from within the canal, most dogs have a complete return of function.

Surgical Procedure

The patient is positioned in sternal recumbency with the hips and stifles flexed in the DAR position. A dorsal skin incision is made from L6 to S3. The right and left sacrocaudalis dorsalis medialis muscles are separated on the midline. The dorsal spinal musculature is elevated off the lateral aspect of the dorsal spinous process and dorsal lamina laterally to the mammillary process. Gelpi retractors are used to expose the dorsal lamina of L7 and the sacrum.

The dorsal lamina of the sacrum is removed to assess the nerves of the cauda equina at L7–S1. The articular processes of L7 are moved dorsally with respect to the sacrum. A vertebral spreader is used to separate L7 and the sacrum. The nerves of the cauda equina are moved to the side so the fracture site can be evaluated. A small midline laminectomy of the caudal L7 may assist in visualization.

Once adequate visualization of the fracture site is obtained and the bone fragments are identified, a small instrument similar to a carpenter's nailset is used to force the bone fragments into the fracture site. The surgeon must avoid damaging the nerves by carefully placing the tip of the nailset between the nerves and delivering only one rap with a mallet before reassessing placement of the fragment. L7 should be moved to determine whether any fragments protrude into the spinal canal. If necessary, the surgeon should repeat repelling the fragments until they are apparently stable.

The L7–S1 articular facets are reduced by directly visualizing the matching of the articular cartilage (Fig. 53.20). A transarticular screw is placed through the articular process of L7 into the S1 segment on both the right and left sides. A 2.0-mm cortical screw is generally used. It is placed equidistant from the medial, lateral, and caudal margins of the L7 articular process. The screw is directed caudally 30° from the transverse plane and 20° laterally to the sagittal plane. The purpose of these screws is to prevent the overrid-

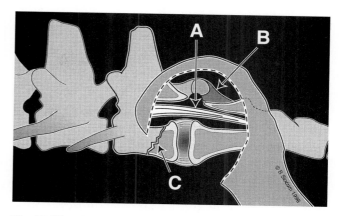

Fig. 53.20. Reduction of the fracture of the L7 body fracture relieves the stretching on the spinal nerves of the cauda equina at L7–S1 (*A*) by aligning the articular facets between L7–S1 (*B*) and by reducing the fractured L7 body (*C*).

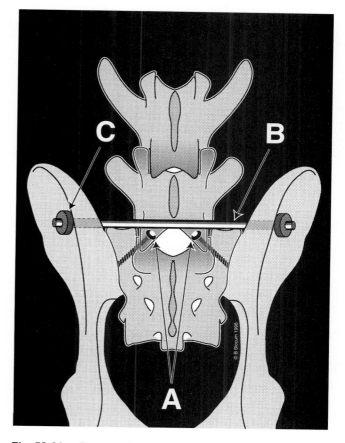

Fig. 53.21. Fixation of the fracture L7 vertebral body is accomplished by debridement of articular cartilage and lag screw fixation of the L7 articular facets (*A*) or a transilial pin (*B*), which is secured by a Pin Stop (*C*) on each end. Both methods of fixation prevent ventral and cranial displacement of the caudal fragments. Healing of the vertebral body is usually rapid.

ing of the L7 body fragments in the cranial to caudal direction.

A transilial pin is placed through the wings of the ilium and over the caudal articular process of L7. In a small dog, a 3.5-mm ($\frac{1}{8}$-inch) nonthreaded pin is usually sufficiently strong. Large dogs may require a 5-mm ($\frac{3}{16}$-inch) nonthreaded pin. The pin may be placed freehand or with an aiming device. The target point of the aiming device is placed on the dorsal aspect of the articular facet, and the pin is inserted through the skin incision, the middle gluteal muscle, and the wing of the ilium at 10° of inclination. The pin is advanced over the dorsum of the L7 articular processes, and the tip of the pin is depressed horizontally. The pin is advanced horizontally in the frontal plane through the opposite wing of the ilium to bulge the skin. A stab incision allows access to the end of the pin. A Pin Stop (Slocum Enterprises, Eugene, OR) or polymethylmethacrylate is attached to the end of the pin, and the point is removed. The pin is retracted until the Pin Stop is in contact with the lateral wing of the ilium. A Pin Stop is attached to the other end of pin adjacent to the wing of the ilium. The remainder of the pin is removed lateral to the Pin Stop (Fig. 53.21). The purpose of the transilial pin is to prevent dorsal migration of the L7 segment.

A free fat graft is applied directly over the exposed cauda equina. Direct closure of the superficial lumbosacral fascia, subcutaneous tissue, and skin is routine.

Patients generally recover well from L7 fractures. The strong articular facets of L7 and the wings of the ilium allow for good fixation. Fractures through the body of the seventh vertebra have excellent blood supply and heal rapidly. Care must be taken to remove fracture fragments from the area of the nerves of the cauda equina. Accurate assessment of transection of the nerves at the fracture site is difficult preoperatively because clinical signs are the same as for compression of those nerves. Fortunately, the results of healing are far better than the radiographic displacement of fracture fragments would deem possible.

Suggested Reading

Slocum B, Rudy R. Fractures of the seventh lumbar vertebra in the dog. J Am Anim Hosp Assoc 1975;11:167.

54

FRACTURES OF THE FORELIMB

Repair of Scapular Fractures

Randy Willer

The scapula is a large, flat bone of the shoulder that serves as support for the thoracic limb and is attached to the trunk by several large muscle masses. The scapula is located adjacent to the chest wall with extensive muscle masses surrounding it, a configuration that helps to prevent the occurrence of fractures. In one study, the incidence of scapular fractures was reported to be 2.4% of fracture cases treated, with most resulting from vehicular trauma (1). Because of the increased forces necessary to create such a fracture in this location, a thorough physical, neurologic, and orthopedic examination is necessary to detect other possible concurrent problems such as spinal, skull, and brachial plexus injuries and other musculoskeletal injuries that may influence prognosis. In patients with scapular fractures, approximately two-thirds have concurrent thoracic cavity lesions, which include pneumothorax, pneumomediastinum, pulmonary contusions, cardiac arrhythmias, and fractured ribs (1). Prognosis and treatment options depend on the anatomic location of the fracture, classified as the body, spine, acromion, neck, supraglenoid tubercle, and glenoid of the scapula (1, 2).

Diagnosis and Cinical History

Clinical signs on presentation of a scapular fracture vary depending on the location and the severity of the fracture. Signs range from a mild weightbearing lameness to a severely dysfunctional nonweightbearing lameness of the limb. The latter is usually associated with intra-articular fractures of the glenoid and neck fractures that cause the animal to carry the injured leg lower than the opposite limb, with the carpus held in a flexed position or the paw dragging (3). Localized pain, swelling, and crepitus on palpation may be present. Comparing findings of palpation of the opposite normal limb with those of the injured limb is valuable when attempting to localize the source of the problem. A thorough history, physical examination, and radiographs are necessary to make a diagnosis.

Radiographs are necessary to confirm the anatomic location and extent of the fracture. Heavy sedation or general anesthesia may be required to position the scapula accurately while also maintaining comfort for the animal. Four views may be necessary to maximize visualization of the entire scapula. Caudocranial views are taken with the animal positioned in dorsal recumbency and the affected limb drawn forward, but with the sagittal plane of the thorax rotated 30° away from the affected limb to prevent superimposition of bony densities (4) (Fig. 54.1). The mediolateral view is taken with the animal in lateral recumbency, the affected limb against the film and extended approximately 45° craniad with the opposite limb pulled caudad. The positioning prevents superimposition of the ribs and sternum (4). The scapular neck, glenoid, and supraglenoid tubercle are best visualized radiographically with this position, but to view the body of the scapula with the mediolateral view, the affected limb should be superimposed over the cranial thorax with the opposite limb pulled craniad instead of caudad (4–6). The distoproximal (axial) radiographic view may be helpful in visualizing and diagnosing scapular fractures when other views do not. The dog is placed in dorsal recumbency with the elbows extended and the limb pulled caudad and parallel to the table surface. The humerus is at a 90° angle to the scapular spine, and the scapula is perpendicular to the table top. The thickness of the tissues is measured at the level of the greater tubercle

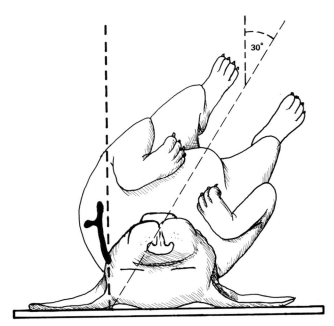

Fig. 54.1. A caudocranial radiograph of the scapula is taken with the sagittal plane rotated 30° away from the affected side.

of the humerus, and the beam is centered over the shoulder joint (7).

Treatment Options

Recommended treatment options have not changed significantly over the past 15 years. The healing potential of the scapula is excellent because of the abundance of cancellous bone, the intrinsic support from the musculature, and the abundant contribution of blood supply from the musculature and surrounding soft tissues (8). Fractures of the scapula can be managed either conservatively or with internal fixation. The method chosen depends on the anatomic location and type of fracture. In general, fractures of the scapula can be managed conservatively except when they involve the articular surface (glenoid), when the fracture results in a distinct change in the angulation of the shoulder joint articulation (displaced scapular neck and body fractures), and when the injury is an avulsion fracture of the acromion and supraglenoid tubercle. Conservatively managed fractures require only limited activity for 3 to 4 weeks, whereas others may benefit from a modified Velpeau sling or spica splint (2). Support bandages add to the comfort of the animal during the healing period.

Surgical Techniques

Approaches to the scapula, which vary and depend on the anatomic location of the fracture, have been well described and illustrated (9). Approaches to the scapu-

lar neck, glenoid, and supraglenoid tubercle are more difficult and require more advanced surgical skills than approaches to the scapular body. Anatomically, the suprascapular nerve, artery, and vein course across the lateral aspect of the scapular neck distal to the acromial process and should be avoided and protected. Damage to the nerve can lead to atrophy of the supraspinatus and infraspinatus muscles.

Scapular Body and Spine Fractures

Fractures that involve the body and spine of the scapula are most often managed conservatively. Limited activity should be advised until clinical union of the fracture is determined. Because of the abundance of cancellous bone and the inherent support of the fracture by the surrounding musculature along with the presence of an abundant blood supply, healing progresses rapidly, and many animals are clinically normal within 4 weeks, although others may require a longer healing period (1). Limitation in activity should be dictated by clinical progression of the animal. The fracture may not be completely healed when clinical function first appears normal; therefore, activity is limited for an additional few weeks. If a modified Velpeau sling is used for immobilization or to provide comfort for the animal, the bandage should be monitored closely and removed in 2 to 3 weeks to allow for return to normal shoulder joint function and to prevent unwanted contracture of soft tissues and limitations in joint motion (3). Fractures that are severely displaced or comminuted or those that change the angle of the normal joint articulation should be repaired with internal fixation. Internal fixation improves the cosmetic result, especially in short-haired dogs, and provides the support necessary for early return to ambulation and better function.

Internal fixation of scapular body and spine fractures consists primarily of the use of wires, plates, or a combination of both (Fig. 54.2). When placing interfragmentary wires, predrilling the holes and preplacing wires (18-, 20-, or 22-gauge wire) simplify the procedure. The fractures are then reduced, and the wires are tightened. If the spine of the scapula is fractured, tension band wiring may be used. The scapula lacks an abundance of harder cortical bone, and care should be taken when tightening the wires so they do not cut through the bone. Minimal fixation can be combined with a Velpeau sling. Interfragmentary wires may be adequate for small dogs and cats, whereas a plate may be required in larger dogs or when angulation displacement is not controlled by wire alone. For plate fixation, the surgeon should place a plate in the angle formed between the junction of the body and the spine and place the screws at an angle for maximum screw purchase in the thickest portion of the bone (Fig.

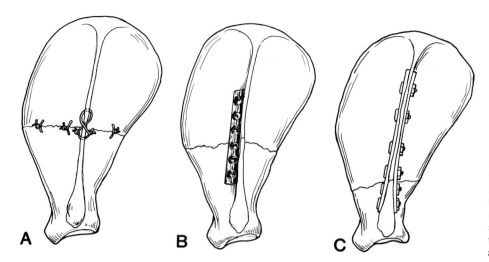

Fig. 54.2. Repair of scapular body fractures. **A.** Interfragmentary wires with a tension band in the scapular spine. **B.** Inverted semitubular steel plate with screws directed at an angle into the thickest bone at the junction of the scapular spine and body. **C.** Plastic plate secured to the spine of the scapula with screws and nuts.

54.2**B**). Inverting a semitubular plate and placing it in this location may enhance the fit of the plate to the bone in this area. Cerclage wires placed around the plate may be used in conjunction with the screws for added fixation support of the plate if the screws do not purchase the bone well. Plastic plates may also be placed on both sides of the spine and secured with nuts and screws, to provide the support and fixation necessary for preventing angulation and overriding displacement of the fractures (Fig. 54.2**C**). Perfect fracture alignment and anatomic reconstruction may not be consistently achieved, but the goal of preventing overriding and angulation of the fracture segments with internal fixation methods is adequate to allow good functional and cosmetic results.

Acromial Fractures

The bony prominence of the distal end of the spine of the scapula, the acromion, is the site at which the acromial head of the deltoid muscle arises and runs distally. The acromion is easily palpable under the skin and can be compared with the opposite limb for asymmetry and identification of a fracture. Fracture of the acromion results in distal displacement created from the pull of the acromial head of the deltoid muscle. The diagnosis can be made with palpation and radiographic findings. The animal typically has a weightbearing lameness, and pain is elicited on palpation. With constant pull from the acromial head of the deltoid, all forms of closed reduction and fixation are inadequate, and internal fixation is required (3). Typically, one of two methods are used to stabilize the fragment. Either two small pins and a tension band wire can be applied, or two twisted stainless steel interfragmentary wires are placed, depending on the size of the animal and the fragment (Fig. 54.3). If the fixation is secure, no additional support is required, limited activity is ad-

vised for 6 to 8 weeks, and the prognosis for a complete recovery is good.

Scapular Neck Fractures

Animals with scapular neck fractures often present with severe lameness and dysfunction of the limb. If the fracture is not displaced, a spica splint may be applied for immobilization to prevent further displacement. The placement of a Velpeau sling may create stress on the fracture site by creating internal rotation and flexion of the shoulder (3). The distal segment often displaces medially and proximally, and closed reduction is difficult. The risk of suprascapular nerve damage is present, and the client should be warned of the possibility. In addition, the supraspinatus and infraspinatus muscles may atrophy, leaving a cosmetically altered appearance and impaired function. Internal fixation is recommended to achieve the best result. The suprascapular nerve should be retracted and protected during repair. Many combinations of methods

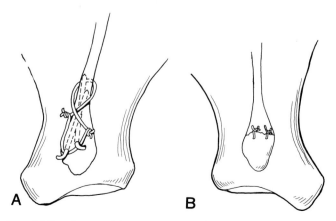

Fig. 54.3. Acromial features repaired with Kirschner wires and a tension band (**A**) or with wire sutures (**B**).

can be used to repair fractures of the scapular neck. Cross-pinning the fracture with Steinmann pins or Kirschner wires inserted from the body into the neck is often adequate stabilization for these fast-healing fractures (Fig. 54.4**A** and **B**). The cross-pins alternatively can be placed from the supraglenoid tubercle across the neck fracture into the body, and the other pin can be inserted from the caudal aspect of the glenoid across the fracture in a similar fashion. In larger breeds, the use of a screw placed in lag fashion or T or L plates can be used to provide more rigid fixation (Fig. 54.4**C**). The technique depends on the size of the animal, the nature of the fracture, and the level of exposure created by the surgeon, who should be willing to expose as much as necessary to achieve adequate anatomic reduction and stable fixation. Because these methods of fixation are stable, further support is usually not necessary, and with adequate limitation of activity for 6 to 8 weeks, return to normal function is expected.

Glenoid Fractures

Fractures of the glenoid are intra-articular (Fig. 54.5**A**). The animal presents with severe lameness and a dysfunctional limb. Palpation reveals an unstable shoulder, with crepitus demonstrated when the joint is manipulated. Radiographs are necessary to assess the extent of the fracture. The fracture may involve the cranial half of the glenoid, as is most common (10), or the caudal half of the glenoid; alternatively, both portions may be fractured involving a neck fracture as well (T or Y fracture). The degree of comminution may vary. This fracture requires great external forces, and the possibility of other injuries should be

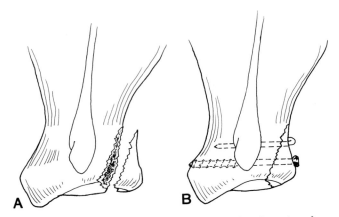

Fig. 54.5. Glenoid fracture (**A**) compressed with an interfragmentary lag screw and derotational Kirschner wire (**B**). Anatomic alignment of the joint surface is important.

explored. Most patients have concurrent injury to another body region (10). Brachial plexus injuries and thoracic trauma should be considered. Unless the fracture is so severely comminuted that it cannot be repaired, internal fixation is required. Closed methods of repair are not adequate and should only be considered if the goal is to allow the fractures to heal and later to perform an arthrodesis or excision of the humeral head and glenoid as a salvage procedure. A spica splint should be placed with the leg in a more natural functional angle if this option is pursued. The goal of surgery is to expose the surgical site adequately and perfectly reconstruct the alignment of the articular surface of the glenoid to minimize secondary osteoarthritis as a result of incongruence of the articular surface. A combination of pins and screws is used to repair the glenoid first, and if the scapular neck is also frac-

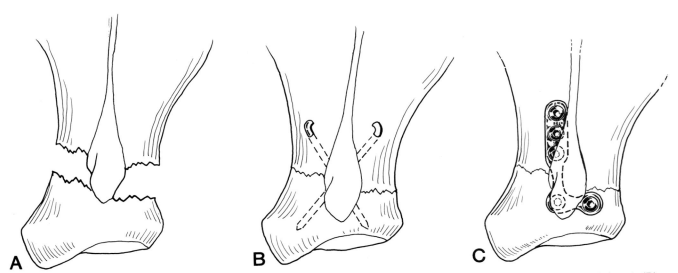

Fig. 54.4. Scapular neck fracture (**A**) repaired by cross-pinning with Kirschner wires introduced from the body into the neck (**B**) or with an L-shaped bone plate in large dogs (**C**).

tured, it is repaired with one of the techniques described previously. Depending on the type and location of the fracture segments, various methods of cross-pinning, lag screws, and plating may all be used to achieve a congruent and stable fracture repair (Fig. 54.5). The prognosis for regaining function of the limb is good, but an extended convalescent period can be expected, and most patients continue to have some degree of lameness after fracture repair (10).

Supraglenoid Tubercle Fractures

The supraglenoid tubercle is the point of origin of the tendon of the biceps brachii muscle on the cranial portion of the glenoid. The supraglenoid tubercle develops as a separate center of ossification, and through endochondral ossification, it should fuse to the glenoid by 5 months of age (11). In the skeletally immature dog, before endochondral ossification is complete, an avulsion fracture may develop through the growth plate, and the pull of the biceps brachii muscle distracts the fragment. This type of fracture can occur in the mature animal as well. A pin and tension band technique or lag screw fixation can be used successfully to repair the fracture (Fig. 54.6). The surgical exposure to accomplish this repair can be challenging. If the fragment is too small, removal may be necessary, and the biceps tendon is secured to the proximal humerus creating a tenodesis.

All animals identified as having scapular fractures should be examined carefully for concurrent body injuries, specifically cardiopulmonary, neurologic, and other musculoskeletal injuries. Scapular fractures tend to heal rapidly. In general, fractures of the body and spine of the scapula do not require repair if the dis-placement is minimal and if the angulation of the shoulder articulation is not impaired, whereas intra-articular fractures must be properly aligned and stabilized to achieve good long-term functional results. Velpeau slings or spica splints can be used to immobilize the fracture and to provide comfort for the animal during the early healing period. Fractures of the glenoid, supraglenoid tubercle, acromion, and most scapular neck fractures require internal fixation for best results. Inadequate anatomic reconstruction and instability can result in malalignment of the fractures, nonunion, secondary degenerative joint disease, an unsatisfactory cosmetic appearance, and poor limb function. The suprascapular nerve should be retracted and protected during repair of scapular fractures to prevent iatrogenic injury, resulting in muscle atrophy and impaired function. The surgeon should be familiar with scapular anatomy and with different surgical approaches and should be willing to achieve the exposure necessary to reconstruct the fractures in a stable and anatomic fashion. Pins, wires, screws, and plates provide adequate means for stabilizing scapular fractures.

References

1. Harari J, Dunning D. Fractures of the scapula in dogs: a retrospective review of 12 cases. Vet Comp Orthop Traumatol 1993;6:105–108.
2. Brinker WO, Piermattei DL, Flo GL, eds. Handbook of small animal orthopedics and fracture treatment. Philadelphia: WB Saunders, 1990.
3. Newton CD. Fractures of the scapula. In: Newton CD, Nunamaker DM, eds. Textbook of small animal orthopedics. Philadelphia: JB Lippincott, 1985.
4. Parker RB. Musculoskeletal system: scapula. In: Slatter DH, ed. Textbook of small animal surgery. 2nd ed. Philadelphia: WB Saunders, 1993.

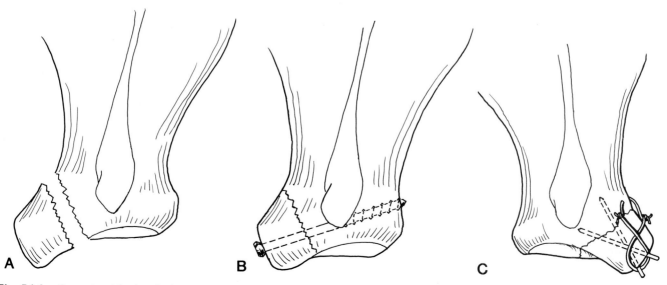

Fig. 54.6. Supraglenoid tubercle fracture (**A**) repaired with a lag screw (**B**) or with Kirschner wires and a tension band (**C**).

5. Ticer JW. Radiographic technique in veterinary practice. Philadelphia: WB Saunders, 1984.
6. Straw RC. Thoracic limb: repair of scapular fractures. In: Bojrab MJ, ed. Current techniques in small animal surgery. Philadelphia: Lea & Febiger, 1990.
7. Roush JK, Lord PF. Clinical application of a distoproximal (axial) radiographic view of the scapula. J Am Anim Hosp Assoc 1990;26:129–132.
8. Brinker WO, Hohn RB, Prieur WD, eds. Manual of internal fixation in small animals. New York: Springer-Verlag, 1984.
9. Piermattei DL. An atlas of surgical approaches to the bones and joints of the dog and cat. 3rd ed. Philadelphia: WB Saunders, 1993.
10. Johnston SA. Articular fractures of the scapula in the dog: a clinical retrospective study of 26 cases. J Am Anim Hosp Assoc 1993;29:157–164.
11. Denny HR. Pectoral limb fractures. In: Whittick WG, ed. Canine orthopedics. Philadelphia: Lea & Febiger, 1990.

Repair of Fractures of the Humerus

Dennis A. Jackson

Proximal Fractures

Greater Tubercle

Fractures involving the greater tubercle of the humerus are rare. In young animals, these fractures are stabilized with two Kirschner wires or small Steinmann pins. In mature animals, a tension band wire technique is recommended. In both cases, open reduction is required through a craniolateral approach to the proximal humerus. External coaptation is not required, but restricted weightbearing is recommended until bone healing is confirmed by radiographic evaluation.

Humeral Head

Most fractures of the humeral head are caused by gunshot injuries and are highly comminuted. Reconstruction of the articular surface must be exact and is paramount to the successful return of joint function. Exposure of the articular surface of the humeral head can be difficult. A craniolateral approach to the shoulder joint is combined with an osteotomy of the acromion process and tenotomy of the infraspinatus and teres minor muscles as required to obtain surgical exposure. A supraspinatous tenotomy may be necessary to provide adequate visualization of the joint.

The fracture is reduced, and large articular fragments are compressed with lag screw fixation. Small fragments are reduced and are stabilized with multiple Kirschner wires or Stille nails placed at divergent angles. All pins and screws should be countersunk be-

low the articular cartilage. Small Kirschner wires may be used to immobilize articular fragments temporarily while lag screws are placed. The Kirschner wires can be removed once lag screw fixation is completed. Autogenous cancellous bone grafts are used to fill large bone defects. After placement of each implant, the joint should be palpated in all planes to evaluate range of motion and crepitus. If crepitus is detected, the fixation is adjusted before the placement of the remaining implants. The fracture is stabilized, and the joint is lavaged thoroughly before joint capsule closure. Osteotomy of the acromion process is repaired with a tension band wire. The tenotomies and remaining soft tissues are sutured routinely.

For patients with fractures with severe comminution of the articular surface, surgical arthrodesis should be considered as a salvage procedure. Arthrodesis is especially indicated in medium to large breed dogs with severe joint comminution. For small dogs and cats with irreparable joint damage, the humeral head may be excised, or a Velpeau bandage or spica splint may provide adequate coaptation for functional healing. The goal of external coaptation or excision of the humeral head is to produce a functional, pain-free joint or pseudoarthrosis. Failure to obtain functional use of the limb or persistent pain in these patients is an indication for arthrodesis of the joint.

Growth Plate Injuries

Growth plate injuries, which occur in young animals with an open epiphyseal plate, are usually secondary to direct trauma or avulsion injuries. Physeal or epiphyseal plate injuries are classified by the Salter system. This clarifies the site of injury and is useful when selecting treatment and for predicting outcome. A Salter I fracture extends across the epiphyseal plate parallel to the joint surface. A Salter II fracture extends through the epiphyseal plate and includes a small portion of the metaphysis. These fractures are the most common growth plate injuries of the proximal humerus, and both carry a good prognosis if they are repaired early and accurately.

Most Salter I and II fractures require open reduction and internal fixation. The exception is selected Salter I fractures of less than 24 hours' duration in small dogs and cats. These fractures may be managed by closed reduction with the animal under general anesthesia. Manual traction of the distal limb is performed to fatigue the muscle contraction and to achieve reduction and alignment. The proximal physeal fragment is immobilized by grasping the acromion process of the scapula while the distal segment is gently reduced by abduction and adduction of the elbow. Care must be taken to avoid splitting the proximal physis at the thin junction between the humeral head and greater tubercle. Once reduction is achieved, closed normograde pinning using Kirschner wires or Steinmann pins is performed. The pins or wires are passed from the craniolateral aspect of the greater tubercle at a 20 to 30° angle to the long axis of the humeral shaft (Fig. 54.7). Alignment and fixation are evaluated with anteroposterior and lateral postreduction radiographs.

Failure to obtain closed reduction or fracture duration of more than 24 to 36 hours is an indication for an open craniolateral approach to the proximal humerus. The fracture should be reduced carefully by gentle levering and distraction to ensure that soft tissues do not become interposed in the fracture site. A small Adson periosteal elevator or a Hohmann retractor facilitates levering and reduction of the fragment. Small Kirschner wires, Steinmann pins, or double Rush pins are the preferred methods for internal fixation. Tension band wires, screws, and bone plates are not used because they cross the epiphyseal plate, create compression, and may lead to premature physeal arrest and growth deformity. Double Rush pinning, with the pins placed craniomedially and craniolaterally through the greater tubercle, is the preferred method of repair. Prebending the pins and using a Rush awl to create

guide holes facilitate their insertion. Rush pins of appropriate size are driven in normograde fashion at an angle of approximately 20° to the long axis of the bone. While placing the pins, the lateral pin is directed toward the caudomedial cortex and the medial pin is directed toward the caudolateral cortex of the shaft

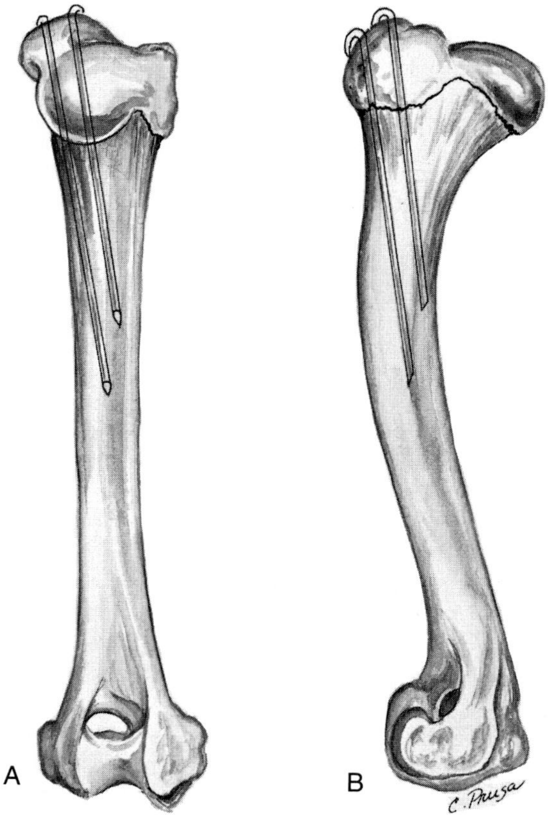

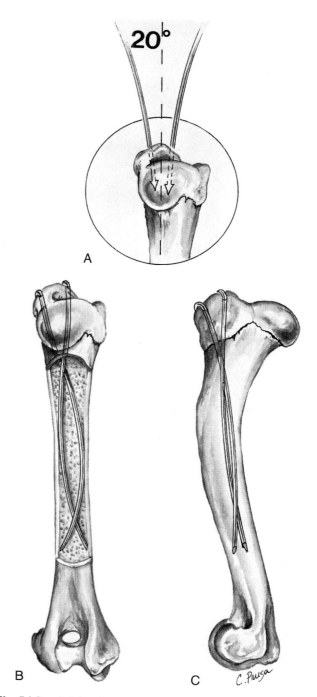

Fig. 54.7. A Salter I proximal epiphyseal fracture repaired with two pins or Kirschner wires passed in a normograde fashion from the greater tubercle into the metaphysis after closed or open reduction. **A.** Caudocranial view. **B.** Lateral view.

Fig. 54.8. A Salter I proximal epiphyseal fracture stabilized with double Rush pins. Prebent pins are placed craniolaterally and craniomedially through the greater tubercle at an angle of approximately 20° to the long axis of the bone. **A** and **B.** Craniocaudal views. **C.** Lateral view.

(Fig. 54.8). The pins should cross distal to the fracture site and should seat firmly against the cortex to provide rigid three-point fixation. For small dogs and cats, Kirschner wires can be substituted for Rush pins by a similar technique. No additional fixation is required, and early restricted weightbearing is encouraged post-operatively.

Infrequently, Salter injuries of the physis may occur simultaneously with fractures of the greater tubercle and humeral head. In young, growing animals, the repair involves pin fixation of the greater tubercle and humeral head through a craniolateral approach to the shoulder joint combined with tenotomy of the infra-spinatous and teres minor muscles. Pin fixation technique is selected in these animals to avoid interfering with future growth potential of the physis (Fig. 54.9).

In mature animals, these fractures are repaired using tension band wire fixation of the greater tubercle combined with lag screw and Kirschner wire stabilization of the humeral head (Fig. 54.10). Surgical exposure is through a craniolateral approach, with tenotomy of the infraspinatus and teres minor muscles, as described for a young, growing animal.

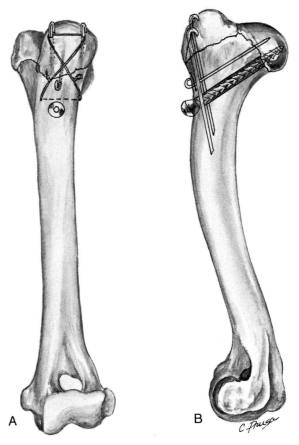

Fig. 54.10. Capital and greater tubercle fractures in a mature animal. The greater tubercle is repaired with tension band wire. The capital fracture is stabilized with a Kirschner wire, and a cortical lag screw is placed in the neck of the humerus. **A.** Caudocranial view. **B.** Lateral view.

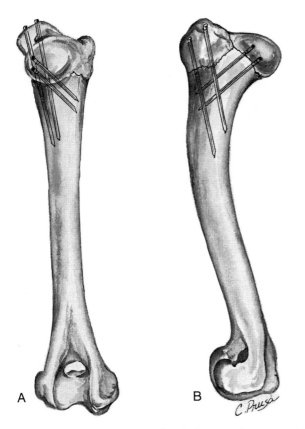

Fig. 54.9. Capital and greater tubercle fractures in a young animal. The greater tubercle is repaired with Kirschner wires. The caput is stabilized with Kirschner wires or Stille nails driven through the lateral surface of the humeral head and countersunk below the article cartilage. **A.** Caudocranial view. **B.** Lateral view.

General Comments on Treating Proximal Fractures

For surgery, the animal is positioned in lateral recumbency, and the site is aseptically prepared from the proximal scapula to the level of the elbow. The limb is positioned through the body drape to facilitate surgical manipulation of the fragments. When exposing the proximal humerus by osteomy of the acromion process, the surgeon should be careful to preserve the suprascapular nerve, which courses deep to the infraspinatus muscle. The nerve lies lateral to the joint and medial and deep to the acromion process. In cats, a small metacromion protuberance is encountered just proximal to the acromion process. Its presence has no clinical significance and does not alter the surgical approach. The acromion process frequently is not ossified in young animals, and tenotomy of the acromion deltoid, rather than osteotomy, is recommended for exposure. For most proximal fractures, external support is usually not required, and an early return to weightbearing is encouraged after surgery. The exception is a questionable repair of a comminuted articular fracture. Unstable articular repairs should be immobilized with a Velpeau bandage or a spica splint for 2 to 4 weeks postoperatively. Active physical therapy of the shoulder joint combined with swimming is recommended to obtain the best functional results. For patient comfort, appropriate analgesics should be used in the postoperative period to control pain and to facilitate physical therapy sessions. Early limb use is encouraged by slow, controlled leash walking. Activity during the third through eighth postoperative week should be confined to house and leash. For cases of articular fractures, the client should be advised of the possibility for developing secondary degenerative joint disease and the potential need for anti-inflammatory therapy.

Healing time with epiphyseal injuries can be as short as 3 to 4 weeks. Articular fractures may take several weeks to obtain clinical union. Depending on the age of the animal and the type of fracture, follow-up radiographs are scheduled for 3 to 6 weeks postoperatively. Serial radiographs are obtained at 3 to 4 months postoperatively to evaluate bone healing further. Unless contraindicated, all implants should be removed once radiographic union is complete.

Shaft Fractures

Proximal Metaphysis

The proximal metaphysis of the humerus is broad and strong relative to the rest of the bone. Proximal fractures may be described as transverse, short or long oblique, spiral, segmental, or comminuted. Fractures of this area are rare and usually result from a gunshot injury, vehicle injury, or other direct force or from a pathologic condition. Most cases occur in medium to large breed dogs. When animals are presented with pathologic fractures, nutritional, metabolic, or neoplastic causes should be considered and managed appropriately.

Simple transverse metaphyseal fractures of short duration in immature dogs and cats can be managed by closed reduction and normograde intramedullary pinning. A single intramedullary pin of appropriate size is placed normograde from the greater tubercle and is passed toward the medial epicondyle and seated at that site. A smaller-diameter pin placed in similar fashion often exits through the medial epicondyle in close proximity to the ulnar nerve. Stack-pinning with two or more smaller pins may be used to increase resistance to rotational forces. Application of an external half- or full Kirschner splint in combination with intramedullary pinning may also be used to neutralize rotational forces.

Open reduction is required if the fracture is of long duration or if soft tissue swelling is significant. Fixation can be achieved with two Rush pins placed as described for repair of a proximal Salter epiphyseal fracture (see Fig. 54.8). Alternatively, pins and tension band wire may be applied using appropriately sized Kirschner wires or Steinmann pins and orthopedic wire. With the tension band technique, pins are placed parallel and penetrate the midpoint of the greater tubercle. The wire is positioned in figure-of-eight fashion over the pins and is anchored in the distal fragment through a hole drilled in the bone (Fig. 54.11).

Proximal Shaft

Proximal shaft fractures usually occur at or just distal to the deltoid tuberosity. Contraction of the deltoideus and latissimus dorsi muscles produces caudal displacement of the proximal fragment. Closed reduction with normograde intramedullary pinning or application of a Kirschner splint may be difficult because of fragment distraction and soft tissue swelling.

For oblique, segmental, and comminuted fractures of this area, open reduction is the preferred method of repair. A craniolateral approach to the proximal

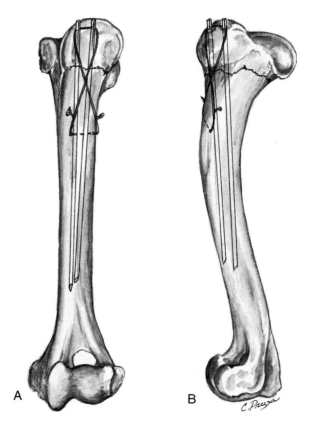

Fig. 54.11. A proximal metaphyseal fracture stabilized with a tension band wire and two Kirschner wires or small Steinmann pins passed in normograde fashion from the greater tubercle into the shaft. **A.** Craniocaudal view. **B.** Lateral view.

shaft with subperiosteal elevation of the deltoideus muscle is used to gain exposure. Several options are available for fixation, including single intramedullary pinning, stack-pins, Rush pinning, pin and tension band wire, hemicerclage wire, half- or full Kirschner splint, and bone plating.

Intramedullary pinning combined with half- or full Kirschner splinting usually provides good fixation for transverse fractures. Shear forces that occur with oblique fractures may be neutralized by the addition of full-cerclage or hemicerclage wire, Kirschner pins, or interfragmentary screws. Secure placement of cerclage wires is enhanced by creating grooves in the cortex or by placing transverse Kirschner pins to prevent the wires from migrating distal on the shaft and becoming loose. The use of single cerclage wires is avoided because it may create a fulcrum effect.

In large to giant breed dogs, or in animals with segmental and comminuted fractures of the proximal shaft, bone plating is the preferred method of repair. Evaluation of preoperative radiographs should ensure that sufficient bone is present to allow placement of two and preferably three bone screws on either side of the fracture site. Subperiosteal elevation of the insertion of the deltoid muscle is performed to provide exposure for reduction of the fracture, and the limb is held in external rotation to facilitate application of the bone plate. The bone plate is conformed to the cranial aspect of the proximal shaft and is applied to the bone.

Comminuted proximal fractures with loss of bone, as occurs with gunshot injuries, result in an unstable fracture and slow bone healing. These fractures are subjected to considerable rotational, compression, and bending forces and are susceptible to infection. Such fractures require rigid internal bone plate fixation combined with an autogenous cancellous bone graft. Alternatively, intramedullary pinning (single or stack) combined with autogenous cancellous bone grafting and Kirschner splint may be used. With open fractures of this type, Penrose drains should be placed at the surgical site. The Penrose drains are removed 3 to 5 days postoperatively.

Middle and Distal Shaft

Most humeral fractures involve the middle or distal diaphyseal regions of the bone. They present as transverse, oblique, spiral, comminuted, or multiple fractures. Overriding of bone fragments is common with midshaft to distal shaft fractures, and most cases require open reduction for repair. Select transverse midshaft fractures can be managed by closed reduction and intramedullary pinning.

Open intramedullary pinning is most applicable to transverse and short oblique shaft fractures in cats and small to medium breed dogs. This type of fixation can also be used for long oblique, spiral, comminuted, or multiple fractures in combination with cerclage wires, stack-pins, and Kirschner splints. Kirschner splints alone are most frequently used to stabilize open or closed, multiple, or comminuted shaft fractures. Bone plates are used most commonly for midshaft to distal shaft fractures in large and giant breed dogs.

INTRAMEDULLARY PIN FIXATION

Closed Reduction and Pinning

Closed reduction may be possible in small breed dogs and cats with recent transverse or short oblique midshaft to distal shaft fractures; closed reduction may be possible if the fracture site can be readily palpated. In medium to large breed dogs, closed reduction can be difficult because of the large muscle mass, soft tissue swelling, and fragment distraction. Open reduction is usually required for repair of shaft fractures in these breeds of dogs. When closed reduction is possible, an intramedullary pin is placed by inserting the pin in normograde fashion from the midpoint of the greater tubercle into the shaft. An intramedullary pin is selected that fills 70 to 75% of the medullary cavity at the fracture site. The size of the medullary cavity can be readily estimated and used to select the pin size based on the preoperative craniocaudal radiograph.

The pin is passed down the medullary cavity to a point just distal to the fracture site. The fracture is reduced by toggling the distal fragment onto the exposed pin. The pin is advanced to the distal fragment and is seated at a point just proximal to the supratrochlear foramen. Care is taken at this point to avoid penetrating the olecranon fossa (Fig. 54.12). The joint should be palpated to ensure a full range of crepitus-free motion after pin placement. For closed intramedullary pinning of fractures at the junction of the middle and distal third of the shaft, a smaller pin is selected to allow for placement into the medial epicondyle. The pin should be of sufficient size to fill the medial epicondyle, based on the preoperative craniocaudal radiograph. The pin is inserted at the midpoint of the greater tubercle, is passed in normograde fashion down the medullary cavity, and is seated in the medial epicondyle. The pin is advanced until the tip is felt to penetrate the distal surface of the medial epicondyle. To ensure that the pin does not penetrate the medial olecranon fossa, the joint should be palpated repeatedly for crepitus and limited range of motion during pin placement. After insertion of an intramedullary pin for stabilizing either middle or distal diaphyseal fractures, persistent rotational instability can be controlled by closed application of a half-Kirschner splint.

Open Reduction and Pinning

Although closed reduction is possible, open reduction is preferred for repair of midshaft and distal shaft frac-

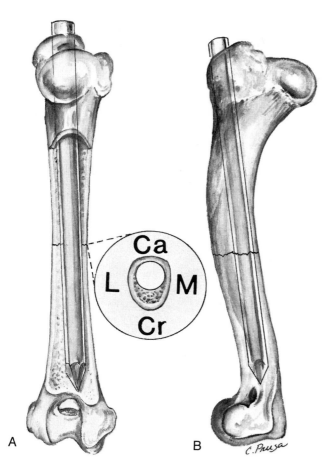

Reduction of shaft fractures often requires considerable traction with bone-holding forceps or the use of a bone distractor in large breed dogs to correct overriding from muscle contraction. In small dogs and in cats, open reduction and fixation may be achieved with a single intramedullary Steinmann pin. A pin of appropriate size is passed in retrograde fashion from the fracture site to the greater tubercle, the fracture is reduced, and the pin is seated in the distal fragment. To ensure proper pin placement, the pin is directed to accentuate placement either in the distal medullary cavity just proximal to the supratrochlear foramen or in the medial epicondyle. For midshaft fractures repaired by intramedullary pinning, the pin is started against the caudal cortex of the proximal fragment and is directed toward the greater tubercle (see Fig. 54.12). For distal shaft fractures in which pin placement is desired in the medial epicondyle, the pin is started against the caudomedial cortex of the proximal fragment and is directed toward the midpoint of the greater tubercle (Fig. 54.13). If the fracture remains unstable after single intramedullary pinning, addi-

Fig. 54.12. A transverse midshaft fracture demonstrating pin placement at the fracture site. The pin, which fills approximately 70 to 75% of the medullary cavity and contacts the caudal cortex of the bone at the fracture site, is inserted into the medullary cavity to a point just proximal to the supratrochlear foramen. **A.** Caudocranial view. *Ca*, caudal cortex; *L*, Lateral cortex; *M*, medial cortex; *Cr*, cranial cortex. **B.** Lateral view.

tures in all breeds of dogs and cats. The animal is placed in dorsal recumbency to allow for a lateral or medial approach to the shaft. Although the medial approach avoids muscle mass, it does encounter extensive neurovascular structures; for this reason, most fractures are handled by a lateral approach. The lateral approach provides exposure of the proximal three-fourths of the humeral shaft. The superficial cephalic vein and radial nerve lying between the brachialis muscle and the lateral head of the triceps brachii muscle should be identified and preserved. Proximal exposure of the shaft, when necessary, can be obtained by subperiosteal elevation of the deltoideus muscle. Distal exposure can be gained by extending the incision to the lateral epicondyle and by dissecting the brachialis muscle to allow cranial and caudal retraction of the muscle and radial nerve as a unit. Gelpi retractors placed at either end of the wound facilitate muscle retraction and surgical exposure.

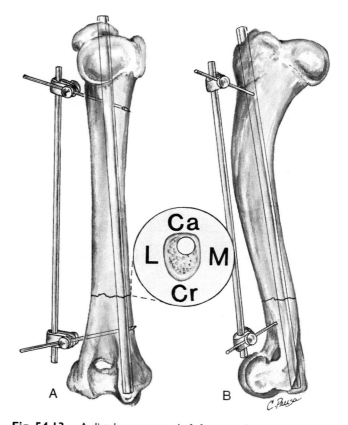

Fig. 54.13. A distal transverse shaft fracture showing pin placement at the fracture site and application of a half-Kirschner splint. The intramedullary pin can be directed in a retrograde fashion against the caudomedial cortex of the proximal fragment to accentuate placement in the medial epicondyle. **A.** Caudocranial view. *Ca*, caudal cortex; *L*, lateral cortex; *M*, medial cortex; *Cr*, cranial cortex. **B.** Lateral view.

tional fixation by cerclage wire, stack-pins, or a half-Kirschner splint is added. The intramedullary pin can be included within a hemicerclage wire to gain additional stability by compressing the pin against the cortex of the bone. Fractures most applicable to full-cerclage wire technique include fissure fractures, long oblique fractures, and spiral fractures of the shaft. For cerclage techniques, monofilament wire of sufficient size and strength should be used. Twenty- to 22-gauge wire is usually sufficient for small dogs and cats. Eighteen-gauge wire should be used for medium to large breed dogs. When using cerclage, a minimum of two wires is recommended to avoid creating a fulcrum effect.

In large dogs with spacious medullary cavities, stack-pins provide more points of bone contact and improve rotational stability. Two pins or more of appropriate size are placed by directing the first pin in retrograde fashion into the proximal fragment and then seating it in the medial epicondyle. Alternatively, the second or subsequent pins are started at a point cranial and distal to the greater tubercle and are passed in a normograde direction down the medullary cavity to a point just proximal to the supratrochlear foramen. The second and subsequent pins can also be passed in a retrograde direction into the proximal fragment and then seated distally (Fig. 54.14).

Half-Kirschner splints may be used with intramedullary pinning to provide rotational stability. A single intramedullary pin is seated in the medial epicondyle, allowing sufficient room between the pin and the cranial cortex of the shaft for placement of two Kirschner pins. Estimation of the combined Kirschner and intramedullary pin diameters can be obtained by studying the preoperative lateral radiograph. A Kirschner pin is placed in each fragment at 35 to 40° to the long axis of the bone and should penetrate both cortices. Both pins enter the bone through separate stab wounds away from the primary incision site. The pins are joined by a connecting bar and two single Kirschner clamps (Fig. 54.13). The half-Kirschner splint is usually removed in 3 to 6 weeks after development of a bridging callus, as demonstrated by radiographic examination.

Full Kirschner Splint Fixation
A full Kirschner splint can be used as the sole means of fixation for shaft fractures in cats and in small to medium breed dogs (Fig. 54.15). Kirschner splints, when used alone, are placed by closed reduction or by a limited approach to the fracture site to facilitate reduction and fixation. They cause minimal disruption of blood supply and allow for free joint movement and the nursing care of open wounds during the healing period. When deciding on pin placement for a full Kirschner splint, preoperative radiographs should be

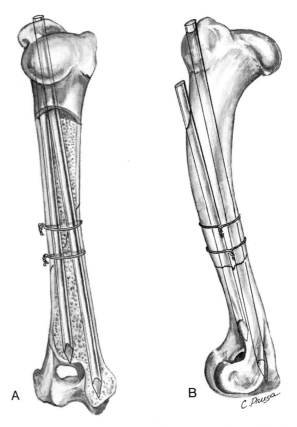

Fig. 54.14. An oblique midshaft fracture repaired with stack-pins and full-cerclage wires. The first pin is passed in a retrograde direction from the caudomedial cortex of the fracture site and is placed in the medial epicondyle. The second pin is inserted in a normograde fashion from craniodistal to the greater tubercle to a point proximal to the supratrochlear foramen. **A.** Caudocranial view. **B.** Lateral view.

evaluated carefully for the presence and location of fissure fractures. The presence of fissures may necessitate altering pin placement or may contraindicate the application of a Kirschner splint.

When placing a full Kirschner splint, two pins are positioned craniolaterally in each major fragment. When possible, all pins are placed at 35 to 40° to the long axis of the bone and should penetrate both proximal and distal cortices. The proximal pin is placed just distal to the greater tubercle, and the distal pin is placed just proximal to the supratrochlear foramen or in transcondylar fashion using the epicondyles as landmarks. The two pins are joined with a connecting bar containing empty Kirschner clamps for placement of the two middle pins. The deltoid tuberosity is used as a landmark for placement of the second pin in the proximal fragment. The second pin in the distal fragment is placed just proximal to the epicondylar ridges. The surgeon must be careful to avoid striking the radial nerve when placing this pin. For Kirschner splinting, a limited lateral approach can be useful to facilitate

plating the humeral shaft, the surgeon should use as broad a plate as possible. In cases with oblique, spiral, or multiple fractures, lag screws or cerclage wires can be combined with plate fixation as indicated to provide additional fixation.

Exposure is through a craniolateral approach to the proximal shaft, with subperiosteal elevation of the superficial pectoral and deltoideus muscles and caudal retraction of the brachialis and triceps brachii muscles. For midshaft fractures, the plate is conformed to the bone and is placed on the cranial surface of the shaft (Fig. 54.16).

For distal shaft fractures, the plate is positioned laterally along the musculospiral groove, the lateral epicondyle, and the lateral epicondylar crest (Fig. 54.17). The plate is conformed to the surface of the distal musculospiral groove and lateral epicondyle and is positioned under the brachialis muscle. Exposure is obtained using a lateral approach to the shaft, and the incision is extended proximally and distally as required.

For distal-third shaft fractures with a comminuted medial cortex, the plate can be applied to the caudal

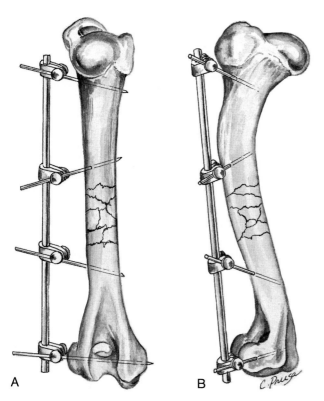

Fig. 54.15. A comminuted midshaft fracture repaired with a full Kirschner splint. The splint is positioned on the craniolateral surface of the humerus, with the pins driven through both cortices at approximately 35° to the long axis of the bone. **A.** Caudocranial view. **B.** Lateral view.

fracture reduction. For both closed and open repairs, a half-Kirschner splint is initially positioned as described, and traction is applied to obtain axial alignment of the proximal and distal fragments. The two end Kirschner clamps are tightened to maintain reduction while the two middle pins are placed and seated in the bone through clamps previously positioned on the connecting bar. When inserting the two middle pins, medial support should be provided with the surgeon's free hand to prevent medial collapse of the fragments and loss of reduction. When open reduction is performed through a limited surgical approach, lag screws or cerclage wires can be combined with the Kirschner splint as needed to provide additional fixation. Cortical defects should be packed with autogenous cancellous bone grafts harvested from the iliac crest, proximal tibia, or proximal humerus.

BONE PLATE FIXATION

Bone plates can be applied to most shaft fractures, but they are especially indicated in large and giant breed dogs and for multiple and comminuted fractures. A dynamic compression plate is recommended, with three screws placed on each side of the fracture. When

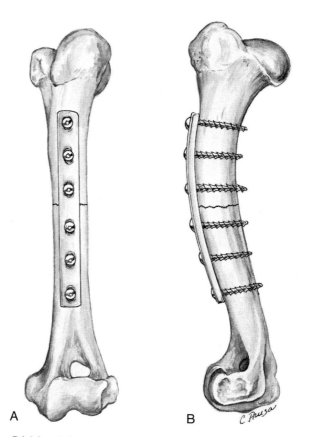

Fig. 54.16. A bone plate applied to the cranial surface of the humerus for fixation of midshaft fracture. Three screws should be placed in the plate on each side of the fracture site. **A.** Craniocaudal view. **B.** Lateral view.

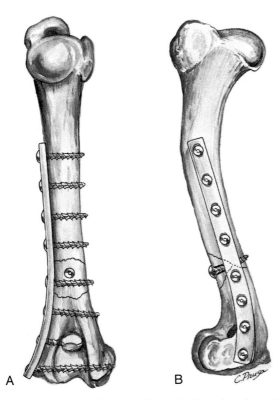

Fig. 54.17. A bone plate placed on the lateral surface of the humerus for repair of a distal shaft fracture. The plate is conformed to the musculospiral groove, the lateral epicondyle, and the lateral epicondylar crest. Lag screw compression of a butterfly fragment is combined with plate fixation. **A.** Caudocranial view. **B.** Lateral view.

medial surface of the medial shaft and epicondyle (Fig. 54.18). Surgical exposure can be achieved using a medial approach to the distal shaft. Care must be taken to preserve the brachial and collateral ulnar vessels and the ulnar and median nerves. The nutrient artery located on the caudal surface of the bone should also be preserved. A transolecranon osteotomy can be performed if additional distal exposure is required.

General Comments for Managing Shaft Fractures

For repair of shaft fractures, the animal is positioned in lateral recumbency with the injured limb suspended and aseptically prepared from the midradius to the proximal scapula. Placing the affected limb outside the body drape facilitates fracture manipulation and reduction.

Midshaft fractures frequently occur where the radial nerve crosses the musculospiral groove medially to laterally. These patients often have considerable overriding of sharp bone fragments, especially with oblique or spiral fractures. Radial nerve function

should be evaluated carefully in these animals because of the close proximity of the nerve to the fracture site. The radial nerve courses over the musculospiral groove of the distal humerus in association with the brachialis muscle. During the surgical procedure, the nerve should be identified, tagged, and assessed for damage. A large-diameter Penrose drain is passed around the brachialis muscle and radial nerve and is used to retract these structures cranially and caudally during the reduction process.

Autogenous cancellous bone grafts enhance healing of severely comminuted or multiple shaft fractures repaired with open reduction and internal fixation. Indications include middle-aged and older patients or patients with large bone defects at the fracture site. Cancellous bone is taken from surgically prepared sites at the greater tubercle, the tibial crest, or the wing of the ilium. Once the graft is harvested, it is immediately placed in the fracture site before closure of the soft tissues.

Severely comminuted shaft fractures with large bone defects may require full-cylinder cortical bone grafting. Suitably prepared cortical bone allografts can be used for this purpose. Bone grafts of this type are usually reserved for comminuted shaft fractures that

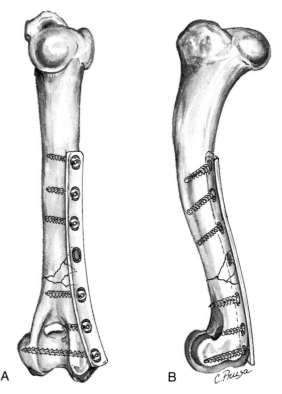

Fig. 54.18. A bone plate positioned on the caudomedial surface of the shaft and the medial epicondyle for repair of distal shaft fractures with a comminuted medial cortex. **A.** Caudocranial view. **B.** Lateral view.

cannot be repaired by conventional reconstructive techniques.

Postreduction radiographs are obtained to evaluate reduction and fixation. Appropriate analgesics are provided to ensure patient comfort. Most patients with shaft fractures benefit from a Robert Jones bandage applied to the limb for 3 to 5 days postoperatively to control swelling. Twice-daily hydrotherapy is recommended to clean pin sites when a Kirschner splint is used. For patients with these fractures, activity is restricted to house and leash for 6 to 8 weeks or until bone healing is demonstrated by radiograph examination.

Supracondylar and Condylar Fractures

Supracondylar Fractures

Most supracondylar fractures pass through the supratrochlear foramen. In young animals, an epiphyseal separation may occur in association with a supracondylar fracture. Metaphyseal fractures with no involvement of the supratrochlear foramen can also be seen. Closed reduction is not advisable with this type of fracture. Open reduction with internal fixation provides early joint motion and weightbearing and produces the best results. Surgical exposure is through a medial or lateral approach to the distal shaft, or, if necessary, the two approaches are combined to facilitate reduction. A transolecranon approach provides the best exposure for large breed dogs requiring double bone plating for multiple or comminuted supracondylar fractures.

TRANSVERSE FRACTURES

The preferred method for repair of transverse supracondylar fractures involving the foramen is open intramedullary pinning combined with cross-pinning of the lateral epicondyle (Fig. 54.19). This technique provides rigid internal fixation for most transverse supracondylar fractures and is applicable to all sizes of dogs and cats. The fracture is reduced, and the proximal fragment is immobilized with bone-holding forceps. With the patient's elbow flexed, a pin of sufficient size to fill the medial epicondyle is passed in normograde fashion from the medial epicondyle to the greater tubercle. The pin is advanced parallel to the caudomedial cortex of the medial epicondyle and penetrates the greater tubercle. During pin placement, reduction is maintained by counterforce applied through Kern bone-holding forceps attached to the proximal fragment. Rotation of the distal fragment is controlled by bone-holding forceps placed over the fracture site of the lateral epicondyle. The fracture site is inspected repeatedly during pin placement to ensure that reduction

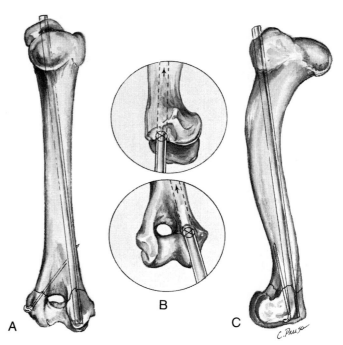

Fig. 54.19. A–C. A transverse supracondylar fracture showing normograde placement of an intramedullary pin parallel to the caudal cortex of the medial epicondyle. A Kirschner wire or a small Steinmann pin is passed through the lateral epicondyle to penetrate the medial cortex and to provide rotational stability. **A.** Caudocranial view. **C.** Lateral view.

is maintained. When the pin penetrates the greater tubercle, the bone chuck is removed, and the distal point of the pin is cut off. The bone chuck is reapplied to the proximal portion, the distal part of the pin is drawn into the medial epicondyle, and the proximal pin is cut off at the greater tubercle.

An alternate method advances the pin in a retrograde direction up the caudomedial cortex of the proximal fragment from the fractured site. The fracture is reduced and the pin is passed into the distal fragment and is seated in the medial epicondyle. With both methods, a Kirschner wire or a small Steinmann pin is passed from distal and caudal to the lateral epicondyle to penetrate the medial cortex of the humeral shaft. The pin in the lateral epicondyle should pass between the intramedullary pin and cranial cortex of the shaft (Fig. 54.19**C**).

Double Rush pinning provides an alternative technique for repair of transverse supracondylar fractures. Rush pins of appropriate size are prebent to facilitate their insertion and are placed slightly distal and caudal to the medial and lateral epicondyles. During pin placement, reduction is maintained with bone-holding forceps. Guide holes are made with an intramedullary pin or a Rush awl to allow introduction of the pins at approximately 20 to 30° to the long axis of the bone. The pins should be placed so they cross above the

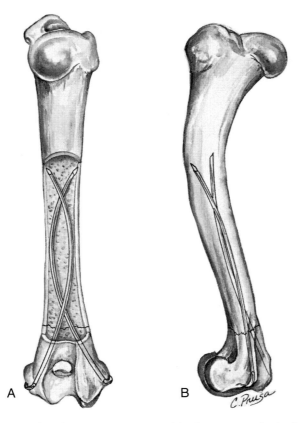

Fig. 54.20. A transverse supracondylar fracture repaired using a double Rush pin technique. The pins are placed in the bone slightly distal and caudal to the epicondyles and at an angle of approximately 20 to 30° to the shaft of the humerus. **A.** Caudocranial view. **B.** Lateral view.

fracture site and provide rigid three-point fixation (Fig. 54.20). In small dogs and in cats, Kirschner wires or small Steinmann pins can be substituted for Rush pins and placed in similar fashion.

OBLIQUE FRACTURES

Oblique supracondylar fractures in cats and small to medium breed dogs can be repaired with intramedullary pinning and hemicerclage wires. The intramedullary pin is directed from the fracture site in a retrograde fashion into the proximal fragment, the fracture is reduced, and the pin is seated in the medial epicondyle. Hemicerclage wire, preplaced through the bone and around the pin, is tightened to provide additional stability and rotational control. To control rotational forces unstable fractures may require addition of a half-Kirschner splint.

MULTIPLE AND COMMINUTED FRACTURES

Fixation of multiple and comminuted supracondylar fractures in cats and small to medium breed dogs can be achieved by intramedullary pinning of the medial

epicondyle combined with cerclage wire and a full Kirschner splint (Fig. 54.21). Surgical exposure for repair of these fractures requires a combined medial and lateral or transolecranon approach. Reduction and repair are first attempted through a combined lateral and medial approach. If surgical exposure is inadequate, a transolecranon osteotomy can be performed. A Steinmann pin is placed in the medial epicondyle in retrograde fashion, and the fracture site is reduced. The pin is advanced in normograde fashion into the proximal fragment and exits at the greater tubercle. For additional fixation, a full-Kirschner splint is applied to the craniolateral aspect of the bone. The proximal Kirschner pin is inserted below the greater tubercle and passes between the intramedullary pin and the cranial cortex of the bone. The distal pin is placed in transcondylar fashion from the lateral epicondyle and angles toward the medial epicondyle. A connector bar containing two single Kirschner clamps for placement of the middle pins is connected between the proximal and distal pins. Traction is applied, and the fragments are placed in axial alignment and are immobilized temporarily by tightening the proximal and distal

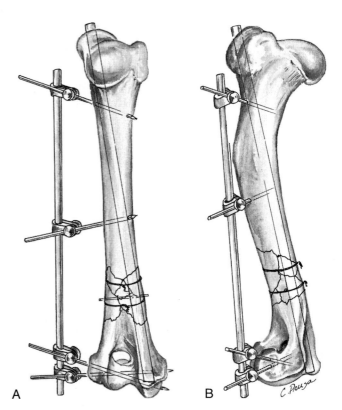

Fig. 54.21. A comminuted supracondylar fracture stabilized with an intramedullary pin placed in the medial epicondyle and application of a full Kirschner splint. The intramedullary pin is directed in a retrograde fashion into the medial epicondyle and then is advanced into the proximal fragment. Full-cerclage wires are used to stabilize the multiple bone fragments. **A.** Caudocranial view. **B.** Lateral view.

Kirschner clamps. The Kirschner splint can be adjusted as required to provide for surgical manipulation and reduction. The proximal and distal clamps are tightened once reduction is achieved. Cerclage wires or lag screws are used to stabilize any comminuted or multiple bone fragments. The cortex of the bone is grooved to accept the cerclage wire and to prevent it from becoming loose. At this point, the second Kirschner pin in the proximal fragment is seated in the shaft between the intramedullary pin and the cranial cortex. The second pin in the distal fragment is placed in transcondylar fashion from the lateral to the medial epicondyle. The result is two Kirschner pins placed in cross-pin fashion within the condylar bone. Care is taken to support the fracture site during placement of the two middle Kirschner pins to prevent medial collapse and loss of fracture reduction (Fig. 54.21).

In large dogs, double bone plating is usually required to provide fixation for comminuted or multiple supracondylar fractures (Fig. 54.22). A transolecranon approach creates the best exposure for application of the plates. To use the bone plating technique, the condylar fragment must be large enough to allow place-

ment of at least two screws distal to the fracture site. The larger plate is positioned on the caudomedial surface of the medial epicondyle. The second, smaller plate is placed on the caudal surface of the lateral epicondyle and the lateral epicondylar crest. Consideration is given to placement of all screws in both plates before drilling the holes to allow interdigitation of the screws. Compression of large bone fragments by lag screws placed through the plates should be performed whenever possible. Inadvertent placement of screws into the joint or olecranon fossa must be avoided to ensure an unrestricted, crepitus-free range of motion and a functional joint.

Condylar Fractures

Fractures of the lateral condyle of the humerus occur more frequently than medial condyle fractures. Forces transmitted along the radius largely affect the lateral condyle, creating shear forces and predisposing it to fracture. Radiographs of lateral condyle fractures usually reveal a subluxated elbow joint with cranial and lateral rotation of the fragment secondary to contraction of the extensor muscles. Fracture of the medial condyle causes caudal and medial displacement of the fragment.

Closed reduction of lateral condyle fractures is possible if soft tissue swelling is minimal and if the fracture is not of more than 24 to 36 hours' duration. Closed reduction requires considerable surgical expertise and is not generally recommended.

Lateral and medial condyle fractures are best managed by open reduction. A transolecranon approach provides the best exposure, although a medial or lateral approach may be adequate in selected cases. Subperiosteal elevation of the extensor carpi radialis muscle provides better visualization for reduction of lateral condyle fractures. Accurate anatomic reduction is paramount to a successful repair of the articular surface. Gentle curettage of the fracture site removes fibrin clots and interposed soft tissue that facilitates reduction. The fragment is reduced by digital manipulation and is stabilized temporarily with a condyle or bone clamp placed over the epicondyles. The clamp is positioned to allow access to an area slightly distal and cranial to the epicondyles for placement of a transcondylar screw. Reduction is evaluated by palpating the caudal surface of the lateral epicondyle, by assessing joint motion and by direct articular visualization. In cats and small breed dogs, a C-clamp placed across the condyles maintains reduction and provides a guide for drilling the condylar hole. The hole is measured with a depth gauge and is tapped to receive a cortical bone screw. The fracture is separated, the condyle fragment is overdrilled to create a glide hole, and the fracture is reduced. A transcondylar cortical screw of appropriate

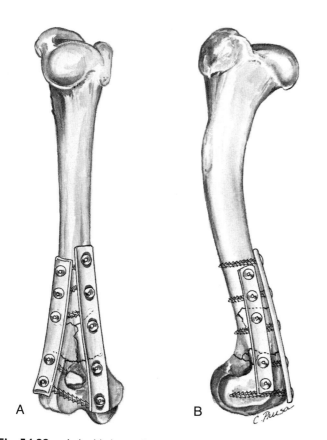

Fig. 54.22. A double bone plate repair of a multiple supracondylar fracture. The plates are positioned on the caudomedial surface of the medial epicondyle and the caudal surface of the lateral epicondyle. A minimum of two screws should be placed distal to the fracture site in each plate. **A.** Caudocranial view. **B.** Lateral view.

length is inserted and is tightened to provide lag screw compression.

An alternate technique predrills the lateral or medial condyle fragment from the fracture site and uses the hole as a guide to drill the opposite condyle. With both techniques, a Kirschner wire is placed caudal to the screw head and is driven up the lateral or medial epicondyle to the opposite cortex to prevent rotation (Fig. 54.23). The transolecranon approach is repaired and is stabilized using a tension band wire technique. The joint is palpated to ensure a crepitus-free and unrestricted range of motion before closure. Postreduction radiographs are taken to assess implant placement, fracture reduction, and alignment of the articular surface.

General Comments For Management of Supracondylar and Condylar Fractures

For repairs of this type, the animal is positioned on its back, and the affected limb is aseptically prepared from the scapula to the carpus. A lateral approach is made, and the skin and subcutaneous layer are undermined and reflected as required to expose both sides of the elbow joint and distal shaft. When approaching the supracondylar area in cats, special care should be taken to preserve the median nerve, which passes through the supratrochlear foramen, and the ulnar nerve, which is located under the medial head of the triceps brachii muscle. Comminuted or multiple supracondylar fractures may require autogenous cancellous bone grafting, as described for comminuted shaft fractures. When bone grafting is anticipated, one or more donor sites are prepared preoperatively. After reduction and fixation, the graft is harvested and is placed in the fracture site immediately before closure.

A Robert Jones bandage is placed on the limb for 2 to 3 days postoperatively to control soft tissue swelling. Early physical therapy and restricted weightbearing are encouraged for the first 6 to 8 weeks. Unless contraindicated, removal of implants is recommended when the bone has healed, as demonstrated by radiograph examination. Appropriate analgesics are administered postoperatively to provide for patient comfort.

Intercondylar Fractures

Supracondylar fractures of the humerus occurring simultaneously with a condyle fracture are referred to as T or Y fractures. They are usually seen in mature animals in which the epiphysis has fused. Closed reduction with external fixation is not advisable. These

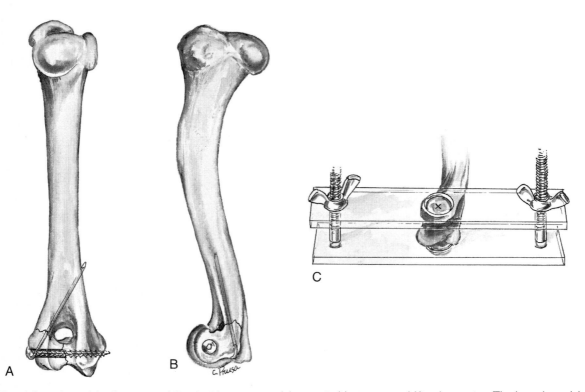

Fig. 54.23. A lateral condylar fracture stabilized with a transcondylar cortical lag screw and Kirschner wire. The lateral condyle can be reduced temporarily with a condyle clamp (C) during placement of the transcondylar screw. Overdrilling the lateral condyle provides lag screw compression at the fracture site. The Kirschner wire placed in the condyle prevents rotation of the fragment. **A.** Caudocranial view. **B.** Lateral view.

fractures involve articular surface, and open reduction with internal fixation should be recommended as early as possible.

A transolecranon approach provides good visualization and facilitates anatomic reduction of the articular surface. The fracture site is exposed and is curetted to remove fibrin clots and interposed soft tissue. Reduction is performed and evaluated by observing the articular surface of the condyles and the alignment of the humeral shaft with the epicondylar ridges. The multiple fracture is converted to a single supracondylar injury by first repairing the intercondylar fracture. The condyles are immobilized with a condyle clamp or bone forceps, and two small Kirschner wires are passed in a transcondylar fashion to provide temporary fixation. A guide hole for a drill bit is placed distal and cranial to the lateral epicondyle using a small intramedullary pin. The drill site is located on a line 45° cranial and distal to a line passing through the lateral epicondyle and shaft of the humerus (Fig. 54.24). The drill is directed toward a similar point cranial and distal to the medial epicondyle. Placement of the screw should be in the center of the condyles and parallel to the joint surface. In small breed dogs and cats, a C-clamp can be used to immobilize the condyles and to provide a guide for screw placement. A depth gauge is used to determine the screw length, and the hole

is threaded with a bone tap. The lateral fragment is overdrilled to create a glide hole, and a cortical screw is inserted to create lag screw compression. Care must be taken to avoid over-compressing the fracture when tightening the screw and collapsing the soft cancellous bone of the condyle.

An alternative method for drilling the condyle is to predrill the proximal hole from the fracture site to a point cranial and distal to the lateral epicondyle. The hole is carefully centered in the lateral condyle. The fracture is reduced and is immobilized with a condyle clamp or small Kirschner wire. The medial condyle is drilled using the hole in the lateral condyle as a guide. The depth of the hole is measured, and the entire length is threaded with a bone tap. The lateral condyle is overdrilled, and a cortical screw is selected and inserted to provide lag screw compression. The transcondylar Kirschner wires are removed, except when additional fixation may be desirable. In cats and extremely small dogs, threaded pins or Kirschner wires can be substituted for screws to provide fixation.

Before repairing the supracondylar fracture, the condyles are palpated to ensure a crepitus-free, unrestricted range of motion. The condyles are attached to the shaft using the intramedullary pinning technique described for supracondylar fractures. After reduction of the supracondylar fracture, a pin of suffi-

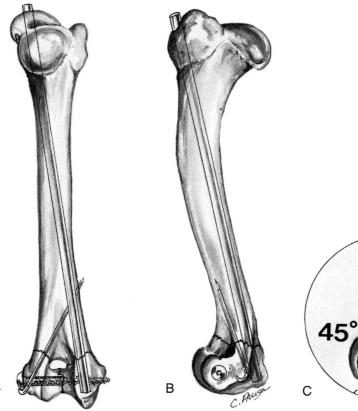

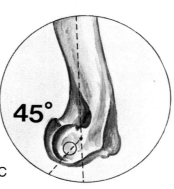

Fig. 54.24. An intercondylar T fracture repaired with a transcondylar cortical lag screw, pinning of the medial epicondyle, and a Kirschner wire placed in the lateral epicondyle. The site for screw placement (C) is located on a line 45° cranial and distal to a line drawn through the shaft of the humerus and lateral epicondyle. **A.** Caudocranial view. **B.** Lateral view.

cient size to fill the medial epicondyle is selected, based on assessment of the preoperative craniocaudal radiograph. The pin is passed parallel to the caudal cortex of the medial epicondyle and is advanced in normograde fashion to penetrate the greater tubercle. The distal pin is cut off, and the bone chuck is applied to the proximal pin. The distal pin is drawn into the medial epicondyle, and the proximal portion is cut off at the greater tubercle. During placement of the intramedullary pin, the supracondylar and condylar fracture sites are checked repeatedly to ensure that reduction is maintained.

An alternative method of intramedullary pin placement passes the pin in retrograde fashion through the medial epicondyle. The fracture is reduced, and the pin is passed in normograde fashion up the humeral shaft, penetrating the greater tubercle. The pin is cut off as described in the previous technique. A Kirschner wire or a small Steinmann pin of appropriate size is directed up the lateral epicondyle to provide rotational stability. This pin enters the epicondyle immediately caudal to the transcondylar screw head, passes between the intramedullary pin and the cranial cortex of the humeral shaft, and penetrates the medial cortex (see Fig. 54.24**B**). The combination of transcondylar screw fixation with pinning of the supracondylar fracture is applicable to all sizes of dogs and cats and provides an excellent method of fixation for this type of fracture.

A third technique for repair of these fractures uses double Rush pinning or cross-pinning of the supracondylar fracture combined with transcondylar lag screw fixation of the condylar fracture. This technique is more challenging, and maintaining anatomic reduction between the condyles and the shaft during pin placement can be more difficult (Fig. 54.25).

Comminuted T or Y condylar fractures are unstable and usually require double bone plating for repair. These challenging fractures require exact anatomic reduction to achieve the best functional results. A transolecranon approach provides good exposure for reducing and stabilizing the fracture. A transcondylar lag screw is used to stabilize the condyles, and two bone plates are applied. One plate is positioned over the medial epicondyle and humeral shaft, and the other is placed over the lateral epicondyle and lateral epicondylar crest. For each plate, two screws are placed in the condylar fragment, and three screws are positioned in the humeral shaft. An autogenous cancellous bone graft is harvested and is placed in the fracture site before closure. The transolecranon osteotomy is repaired with a tension band wire technique.

Postreduction radiographs are obtained to assess articular reduction and implant placement. Analgesics are administered to ensure patient comfort in the postoperative period. A Robert Jones bandage is applied

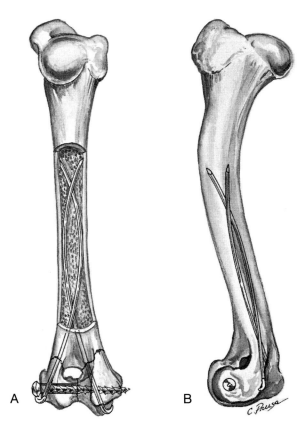

Fig. 54.25. An intercondylar T fracture is stabilized with a transcondylar cortical lag screw and double Rush pins. **A.** Caudocranial view. **B.** Lateral view.

to the limb for 3 to 5 days, followed by swimming physical therapy and range-of-motion exercises with controlled weightbearing for 6 to 8 weeks. The intramedullary pin should be removed when the bone has healed. The transcondylar screw, Kirschner wires, Steinmann pin, and bone plates are usually not removed unless they loosen or cause soft tissue irritation.

Suggested Readings

Brinker WO, Piermattei DL, Flo GL. Handbook of small animal orthopedics and fracture treatment. Philadelphia: WB Saunders, 1983.

Egger EL. Complications of external fixation: a problem-oriented approach. Vet Clin North Am 1991;21:705.

Evans HE, Christensen GC. Miller's anatomy of the dog. 2nd ed. Philadelphia: WB Saunders, 1979.

Hulse D, Hyman B. Biomechanics of fracture fixation failure. Vet Clin North Am 1991;21:647.

Lipowitz AJ, Caywood DD, Newton CD, et al. Complications in small animal surgery: diagnosis, management, prevention. Baltimore: Williams & Wilkins, 1996.

Newton CD, Nunamaker DM. Textbook of small animal orthopaedics. Philadelphia: JB Lippincott, 1985.

Olmstead ML. Complications of fracture repaired with plates and screws. Vet Clin North Am 1991;21:669.

Piermattei DL, Greely RG. An atlas of surgical approaches to the bones of the dog and cat. 2nd ed. Philadelphia: WB Saunders, 1979.

Rudy RL. Principles of intramedullary pinning. Vet Clin North Am 1975;5:209.

Rush LV. Atlas of Rush pin techniques. Meridian, MS: Berivon, 1955.

Schrader SC. Complications associated with the use of Steinmann intramedullary pins and cerclage wires for fixation of long bone fractures. Vet Clin North Am 1991;21:687.

Sherding RG. The cat: diseases and clinical management. 2nd ed. New York: Churchill Livingstone, 1994.

Fixation of Lateral Humeral Condylar Fractures with Multiple Kirschner Wires

*James L. Tomlinson, Jr. &
Gheorghe M. Constantinescu*

Lateral condylar fractures of the humerus are commonly encountered in small animal practice. Although these fractures can occur in any age or size of dog, they seem to occur most frequently in young small breed dogs. Spaniel breeds, in particular, seem to have a high incidence of this type of fracture.

Compression fixation of lateral condylar fractures with a lag screw technique is generally the preferred method of repair (see Fig. 54.23 and accompanying text by Jackson for description of this technique). Because of the small size and soft bones of some of these patients, however, repair with a bone screw may not be the best choice. The goals of repair for this type of fracture are anatomic alignment and excellent stability. Excellent alignment of these fractures is needed to allow good postoperative use of the limb and to prevent degenerative joint disease from developing. Maximal stabilization of the fracture is needed to allow early return to function with minimal callus formation. A simple and effective way to repair these fractures in small dogs is with Kirschner wires (1). This technique should only be used for animals that weigh 5 kg or less.

Surgical Technique

The first step is to reduce the fracture anatomically. Generally, reduction of the fracture is the most difficult part of the procedure. Either an open or closed reduction can be performed. If the fracture can be aligned with closed digital manipulation, a condylar clamp (Kirschner Co., Timonium, MD) is used to maintain reduction (see Fig. 54.23**C**). If open reduction of the fracture is undertaken, we recommend use of a craniolateral approach (2).

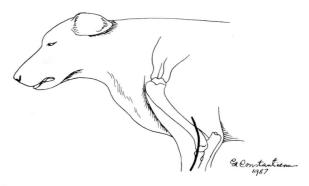

Fig. 54.26. Lateral view of the elbow showing the location of the incision for the craniolateral approach to the elbow joint. The incision is slightly cranial to the lateral epicondyle of the humerus.

The craniolateral approach to the elbow is started by making a curvilinear incision that begins at the epicondyloid crest, passes cranial to the lateral epicondyle, and ends slightly distal to the radial head (Fig. 54.26). After retraction of the skin and subcutaneous tissue, the brachial fascia is incised along the same line. The superficial and deep branches of the radial nerve should be identified as they emerge from beneath the lateral head of the triceps brachii and pass over the brachialis muscle (Fig. 54.27). The distal half of the extensor carpi radialis and the proximal portion of the common digital extensor muscles are elevated from the lateral epicondyloid crest to the level of the lateral epicondyle and are retracted distomedially along with the radial nerve (Fig. 54.28). The joint cap-

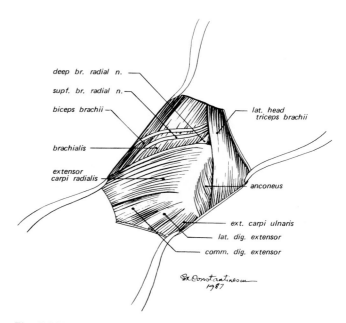

deep br. radial n.
supf. br. radial n.
biceps brachii
brachialis
extensor carpi radialis
lat. head triceps brachii
anconeus
ext. carpi ulnaris
lat. dig. extensor
comm. dig. extensor

Fig. 54.27. Exposure of underlying musculature after the skin and subcutaneous tissue have been retracted and the brachial fascia has been incised along the same line and reflected. Note the location of the superficial and deep branches of the radial nerve as they emerge from beneath the lateral head of the triceps muscle.

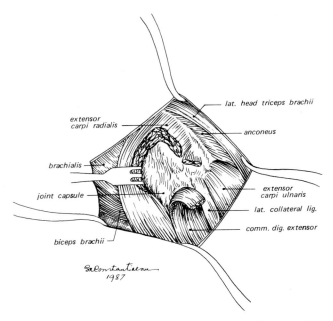

Fig. 54.28. View of surgical site after the attachments of the distal half of the extensor carpi radialis muscle and the common digital extensor muscle have been detached from lateral epicondyloid crest and lateral epicondyle and retracted distomedially to protect the radial nerve.

sule is incised in an inverted L shape. The first incision in the joint capsule is made proximally to distally along the cranial edge of the lateral collateral ligament. The second incision runs from the first incision medially as far as needed to expose the medial condyle of the

humerus (Fig. 54.29). On the extreme medial side of the joint, the brachial vessels and the median nerve must be protected.

After removal of blood clots, a procedure that aids in fracture reduction, it is easiest to align the supracondylar portion of the fracture first and then squeeze the condyles back together. AO bone-reduction forceps (reduction forceps with points for small fragments, No. 399.07, Synthes, Paoli, PA) work well for this procedure; a towel clamp also is effective, however. The bone clamp (towel clamp) is used to compress the fracture together and to hold the alignment until the Kirschner wires are in place.

Once the fracture is reduced and is held in place with the clamp, the first Kirschner wire is started in the area of the lateral epicondyle and is driven across the fracture line and into the medial condyle. The second wire is also started in the area of the lateral epicondyle. The goal is to have the two wires cross in the medial condyle (Fig. 54.30). The Kirschner wires must not be driven parallel to each other or cross at the fracture line. The crossing of the wires helps to maintain the reduction and compression achieved by the bone clamp. A third Kirschner wire can be driven from the lateral epicondyle, up the supracondylar ridge, and into the far cortex of the humerus for additional support if needed (Fig. 54.31). After fracture fixation, closure proceeds in reverse order. The extensor carpi radialis is sutured to the anconeus, and the common digital extensor is sutured to the adjacent tissue.

Postoperative Care

A light padded bandage is placed on the limb for the first 2 days after surgery and then is removed. Restricted activity is recommended for the first 4 weeks postoperatively. Passive range-of-motion exercise is

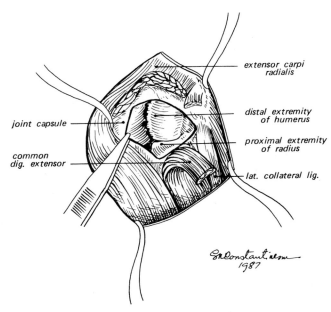

Fig. 54.29. Exposure of medial condyle after the joint capsule has been incised in an inverted L shape and retracted.

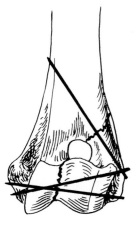

Fig. 54.30. Placement of Kirschner wires to stabilize reduced lateral condylar fracture.

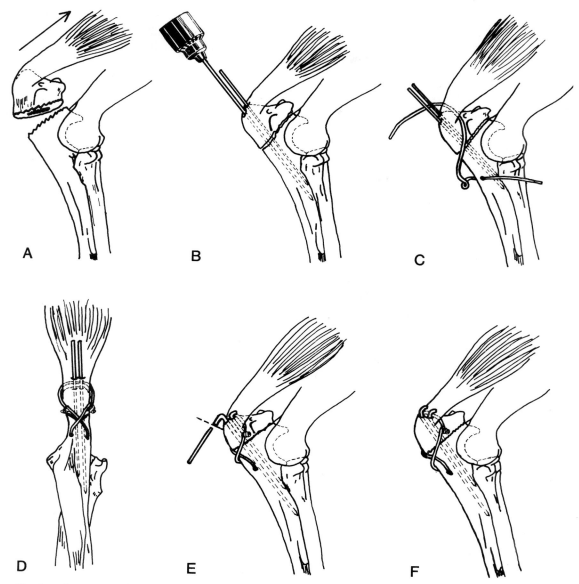

Fig. 54.31. Fixation of extra-articular olecranon fracture with a tension band wire. **A.** Typical fracture location proximal to the trochlear notch. **B.** Placement of two Kinchner wires or Steinmann pins across the reduced fracture in a normograde fashion. **C.** Insertion of orthopedic wire through a hole in the distal fragment. **D.** Figure-of-eight tension wire in place. **E.** Trimming of bent pin ends. **F.** Completed repair with pin ends lying flat against triceps tendon. See text for details.

also encouraged to reduce joint stiffness. The Kirschner wires are removed only if they migrate or if the animal shows persistent lameness after healing is confirmed radiographically.

References

1. Morshead D, Stambaugh JE. Kirschner wire fixation of lateral humeral condylar fractures in small dogs. Vet Surg 1984;13:1.
2. Turner TM, Hohn RB. Craniolateral approach to the canine elbow for repair of condylar fractures or joint exploration. J Am Vet Med Assoc 1980;176:1264.

Stabilization of Fractures of the Radius and Ulna

Curtis W. Probst

Radial and ulnar fractures are seen frequently in small animal practice. These fractures often, but not always, involve both the radius and the ulna. Most fractures are the result of automobile trauma; however, fractures in toy breeds often result from jumps or falls.

As with all traumatized animals, the first step in managing patients with radial and ulnar fractures is to perform a complete physical examination. The surgeon should pay particular attention to the cardiovascular and respiratory systems. Approximately 40% of animals that have been hit by a car have some type of respiratory system damage; therefore, thoracic radiographs are advisable. One should also carefully assess the patient for the presence of cardiac arrhythmias that may result from traumatic myocarditis. Once the patient's condition has been stabilized, the surgeon can attend to the fracture.

Radiographs (at least two views) of the radius and ulna are essential to define the fracture properly. The fractured limb should be protected by applying a Robert Jones bandage until definitive treatment can be performed. This bandage should extend from the toes to well above the elbow. Mason metasplints are ineffective in immobilizing radial and ulnar fractures.

Radial and ulnar fractures may be associated with a higher complication rate than fractures of other long bones. Because of the potential complications, which include delayed union, nonunion, joint stiffness, and growth deformities, one should not dismiss these fractures lightly.

I prefer to group radial and ulnar fractures into several categories because of the difference in principles of treatment. These categories include olecranon fractures, Monteggia fractures, isolated ulnar or radial diaphyseal fractures, radial or ulnar styloid fractures, radial head fractures, combined radial–ulnar diaphyseal fractures, and radial physeal fracture–separations.

Olecranon Fractures

The olecranon—the proximal portion of the ulna—serves as a fulcrum for the extensor muscles of the elbow joint. Fractures of the olecranon can occur proximal to the trochlear notch (i.e., extra-articular fractures) or through the trochlear notch (i.e., intra-articular fractures). These fractures can be simple two-piece fractures or complex comminuted fractures. Regardless of the type of fracture, the proximal fragment usually is severely displaced because of the pull of the triceps muscle (Fig. 54.31**A**). Open reduction and internal fixation of these fractures are required because external coaptation is unable to counteract the distractive force of the triceps muscle.

Generally, olecranon fractures are exposed through a caudal approach in which the extensor carpi ulnaris and flexor carpi ulnaris muscles are subperiosteally elevated, thus exposing the ulnar diaphysis and olecranon. The skin incision is made slightly lateral to rather than directly over the caudal surface of the olecranon.

With an intra-articular fracture, the anconeus muscle and joint capsule must be incised so the surgeon can see the articular surface. Perfect reduction of articular fractures is essential to minimize the development of secondary degenerative joint disease. Extension of the elbow relaxes the triceps pull, thus facilitating fracture reduction. After reduction, olecranon fractures can be stabilized with pins and tension band wire, lag screws, or bone plates.

Tension Band Fixation

The preferred technique for repairing extra-articular olecranon fractures and transverse or short oblique intra-articular fractures involves pinning and placement of a tension band wire. After exposure of the fracture and removal of blood clots and fibrous tissue, the elbow is extended, and the fracture fragments are reduced. Reduction usually can be maintained with digital pressure or a bone clamp.

The reduced fracture is initially stabilized by driving two Kirschner wires or Steinmann pins across the fracture. The pins are driven in a normograde fashion into the proximal fragment with a Jacob's pin chuck. The pins should be parallel to each other to allow compression of the fracture with the tension band wire. The pins should be directed so they engage the cranial cortex of the distal ulnar fragment, rather than extending directly down the medullary cavity, because the latter placement may not counteract rotation effectively (Fig. 54.31**B**); similarly, a single pin does not counteract rotation. A hole is then drilled transversely in the caudal aspect of the distal fragment. The hole should be large enough to accept 18-gauge orthopedic wire (20-gauge wire in small dogs and cats) and should be placed roughly the same distance distal to the fracture as the length of the proximal fragment. A single tightening twist is made in the center of an appropriate length of wire, and one end is then passed through the hole. The other end of the wire is then passed underneath the triceps tendon and cranial to the pins (Fig. 54.31**C**). The free ends of the wire are twisted together, thus forming a figure-of-eight (Fig. 54.31**D**). The two ends are alternately tightened until the fracture is compressed. The wire should not be overtightened because this may cause a gap to form in the cranial aspect of the fracture. The excess wire is cut off, leaving three or four twists, and the two ends of the wire are bent so they lie flat against the bone. The pins are bent in a caudal direction and are cut to leave 4 to 5 mm of pin; the ends are then turned cranially so they lie flat against the triceps tendon (Fig. 54.31**E** and **F**). If the pins are initially bent in a cranial rather than a caudal direction, the cut ends will not lie flat against the triceps tendon.

If properly applied, the tension band wire is strong

enough that no postoperative support is needed. The wound is covered with a sterile dressing, and the limb is placed in a light support wrap for 48 hours postoperatively. The animal's activity should be limited to leash walks for 6 to 8 weeks after surgery. The implants usually are not removed unless they loosen, break, or cause soft tissue irritation.

Bone Plating

I prefer to use a bone plate to repair comminuted olecranon fractures and olecranon fractures in large and giant breed dogs. A plate applied to the caudal aspect of the ulna acts as a tension band, provided cortical fragments are missing in the cranial cortex. Screws can be applied through the plate using the lag principle, thus achieving interfragmentary compression in comminuted fractures (Fig. 54.32**A** and **B**). Screws must not be placed through the articular surface of the trochlear notch. With fractures that are sufficiently proximal to require plating up to the most proximal aspect of the ulna, pressure sores frequently develop over the olecranon if the plate is applied caudally. The plate should be applied to the lateral aspect of the ulna (Fig. 54.32**C**).

Monteggia Fractures

Fractures of the proximal half of the ulna with luxation of the radial head are known as Monteggia fractures. The radial head usually luxates cranially, and the ulna may be fractured anywhere from the middle of the diaphysis to the trochlear notch. The proximal annular ligament can be torn (Fig. 54.33**A**) or can remain intact, as is common when the ulnar fracture is at the base of or into the trochlear notch (Fig. 54.33**D**). Early treatment is helpful for ease of reduction of the luxation and fracture.

A caudal approach usually provides adequate exposure to allow reduction of both the radial head luxation and the ulnar fracture. A craniolateral approach can be used in addition to the caudal approach if the luxation cannot be reduced.

If the proximal annular ligament is torn, as occurs when the ulnar fracture is distal to the annular ligament, one must not only stabilize the ulnar fracture but also secure the radial head in its normal relationship with the ulna. Although suture repair of the annular ligament has been described, this is seldom possible. I prefer to secure the radial head to the ulna with lag screws alone or in conjunction with a bone plate. If the ulnar fracture is oblique enough, lag screws alone are sufficient to repair the fracture (Fig. 54.33**A** and **B**). If the ulnar fracture is comminuted, I prefer to use a bone plate and place one or two screws through the plate into the proximal radius (Fig. 54.33**C**).

If the proximal annular ligament is intact, reduction of the ulnar fracture results in reduction of the radial head luxation. Because the intact annular ligament maintains the normal relationship between the radial head and the ulna, the surgeon only needs to stabilize the ulnar fracture. I prefer to use a bone plate and screws to stabilize this type of ulnar fracture (Fig. 54.33**D** and **E**), although repair with pins and tension wire has been described.

Postoperatively, the incision is covered with a sterile dressing, and the limb is placed in a modified Robert Jones bandage. The bandage helps to minimize postoperative swelling and is left in place for several days. The animal's activity should be limited to leash walks only for 10 to 12 weeks after surgery, but early movement of the elbow is encouraged to minimize stiffness.

Isolated Ulnar or Radial Diaphyseal Fractures

Isolated radial or ulnar fractures generally are the result of falls, gunshot wounds, or horse kicks, for example, rather than automobile accidents. Isolated ulnar

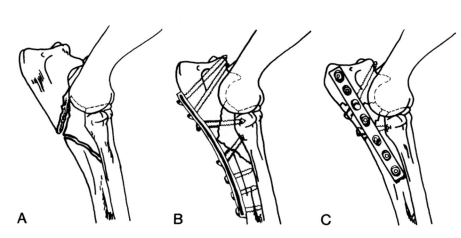

A **B** **C**

Fig. 54.32. A comminuted intra-articular olecranon fracture (**A**) repaired with a bone plate applied to the caudal aspect of the ulna (**B**). Screws have been applied through the plate in lag fashion, thus achieving interfragmentary compression. With more proximal fractures (**C**) that must be plated to the most proximal end of the ulna, the plate is applied on the lateral surface. Lag screws can be applied in a caudal to cranial direction if necessary.

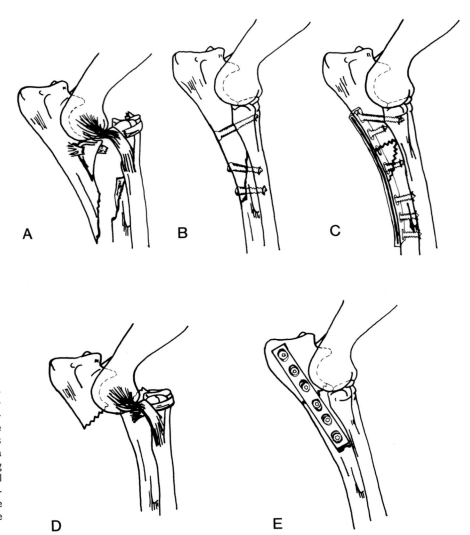

Fig. 54.33. Stabilization of Monteggia fractures. An oblique fracture with ruptured proximal ligament (**A**) can be repaired with three lag screws (**B**); if the fracture is comminuted, a bone plate is applied to the caudal aspect of the ulna (**C**). In both cases, the most proximal lag screw holds the radial head in its normal position. A Monteggia fracture with an intact proximal annular ligament (**D**) can be repaired with a bone plate applied to the lateral aspect of the ulna (**E**).

diaphyseal fractures occur more frequently than isolated radial diaphyseal fractures. These fractures usually are minimally displaced because the intact companion bone acts as an internal splint. Radiographic diagnosis of these fractures may be difficult because of the minimal displacement; therefore, one should obtain two radiographic views of diagnostic quality.

Most isolated radial or ulnar fractures can be stabilized with a fiberglass cast, although a Schroeder–Thomas splint is acceptable if properly applied. The joints proximal and distal to the fracture must be immobilized to stabilize a fracture properly with external coaptation. Mason metasplints, although used frequently, are an unacceptable means of stabilizing radial or ulnar fractures because they do not immobilize the elbow joint.

The cast is applied with the patient under general anesthesia. The fracture is manually reduced. The reduced fracture should have at least 50% purchase (i.e., contact between fracture ends) before the reduction is considered adequate. One should avoid casting the limb with a varus or valgus angulation at the fracture. This type of angulation can lead to secondary arthritis because of abnormal stresses placed on the joints during weightbearing. The cast should extend from the midshaft of the humerus to the digits, with only the distal phalanx of the third and fourth digits left exposed distal to the cast.

External coaptation is not without complications, but many problems can be avoided by applying the cast properly. Pressure sores over the accessory carpal bone and olecranon are common. They can be avoided by applying "donuts"—layers of cast padding with a hole cut in the center—over these pressure points (Fig. 54.34**A**). Donut pads placed around a pressure point alleviate the pressure directly on the bone. Simply adding more padding directly over a pressure point actually increases the pressure and should be avoided. The distal end of the cast can cause severe erosions to the dorsal aspect of the protruding toes as the animal

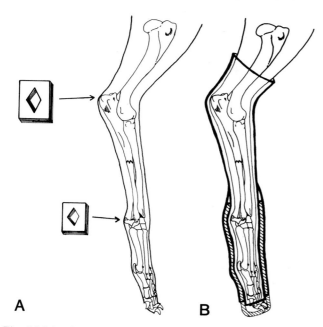

Fig. 54.34. Isolated ulnar and radial diaphyseal fractures can be treated with external coaptation. **A.** Cut-out "donut"" pads are applied over accessory carpal bone and the olecranon to relieve pressure from the cast. **B.** A walking bar incorporated into the distal aspect of the cast prevents damage to the dorsal surface of the protruding toes.

walks. Applying a walking bar (i.e., aluminum rod) to the distal end of the cast prevents damage to the dorsum of the protruding toes (Fig. 54.34**B**). The walking bar can be incorporated into the cast or can be secured to the dried cast with adhesive tape. A cast also may not immobilize the elbow joint properly. This problem usually occurs because the cast is not applied as far proximal to the elbow as it should be or because the cast is applied too loosely proximal to the elbow.

Fractures of the radial or ulnar diaphysis that are the result of gunshot wounds may not be amenable to treatment by external coaptation. Because such fractures frequently are severely comminuted, restoration of cortical continuity may be difficult, if not impossible. Fractures involving only the radial diaphysis are best treated with an external fixator (Fig. 54.35). The external fixator provides direct skeletal fixation and allows treatment of open wounds. Generally, the major segments of the radius are not severely displaced; therefore, the external fixator can be applied after closed reduction. This technique minimizes further disruptions of the blood supply to the fracture fragments. If the major fracture segments are displaced, or if one chooses to use a cancellous bone graft, then open reduction is required. The application of external fixators is described later, in the discussion of combined radioulnar diaphyseal fractures.

Isolated ulnar diaphyseal fractures resulting from gunshot wounds can be treated with a cast, provided

no extensive open wounds are present. Such fractures usually do not require rigid fixation because the radius is the major weightbearing bone. The limb can be immobilized temporarily in a Robert Jones bandage until any swelling subsides or the open wounds begin to heal.

Radial and Ulnar Styloid Fractures

The radial and ulnar styloid processes serve as the origins of the collateral ligaments of the antebrachiocarpal joint. The styloid processes also extend distal to the proximal row of carpal bones, thus providing a buttress for medial and lateral stability. Because carpal instability results from fracture of one or both styloid processes, internal fixation of these fractures is required.

The styloid processes are exposed by incising directly over the process. Fixation of radial styloid fractures usually is accomplished with tension band wire or lag screws (Fig. 54.36**A–C**). It may not be possible to place two pins into the distal ulna in small dogs; therefore, ulnar styloid fractures may not be completely rotationally stable (Fig. 54.36**D** and **E**).

Because uncomplicated healing of these fractures is

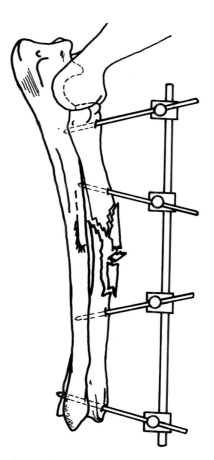

Fig. 54.35. A severely comminuted isolated radial fracture stabilized with a four-pin, single-bar external fixator.

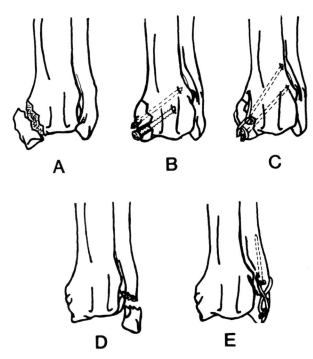

Fig. 54.36. A radial styloid fracture (**A**) can be repaired with a lag screw and Kirschner wire (to prevent rotation of the fragment) if the fragment is large enough (**B**) or with two Kirschner wires and a tension band wire (**C**). An ulnar styloid fracture (**D**) can be repaired with a pin and tension band wire (**E**).

necessary to prevent carpal instability, supplemental external coaptation is necessary. A fiberglass half-cast or Mason metasplint provides satisfactory support. External coaptation can be discontinued after 6 to 8 weeks. The animal's exercise should be restricted until fracture healing is complete.

Radial Head Fractures

Radial head fractures, which are uncommon, may or may not involve the articular surface. If the articular surface is involved, perfect reduction and rigid fixation are required to minimize secondary arthritis and joint stiffness.

The radial head is most easily approached through a lateral skin incision. A fascial incision is made between the common and lateral digital extensor muscles near their origin. These muscles are separated to expose the supinator muscle, deep branch of the radial nerve, branches of the dorsal interosseous artery, and part of the radius. One should protect the radial nerve during the surgical procedure. Incision of the supinator muscle along its insertion on the radius exposes the lateral collateral ligament, annular ligament, and joint capsule. The annular ligament and joint capsule are incised along the cranial border of the collateral ligament, thus exposing the radial head. After the fracture is repaired, the joint capsule and annular ligament are

reapposed. The supinator muscle may be sutured to the radial periosteum. The remainder of the closure is routine.

Extra-articular radial head fractures can be repaired with a T-plate or crossed Kirschner wires (Fig. 54.37**A** and **B**). The latter method is used in cats and small dogs in which T-plate fixation often is not feasible. Intra-articular radial head fractures can be repaired with lag screws or divergent Kirschner wires, depending on the size of the fragment. Lag screw fixation is ideal because it provides interfragmentary compression. A small Kirschner wire should be used in conjunction with the lag screw to counteract rotation of the fragment around the screw (Fig. 54.37**C**). If the fragment is too small for lag screw fixation, then multiple divergent Kirschner wires can be used. Because interfragmentary compression is not achieved with Kirschner wires, the fracture should be reduced and compressed as much as possible with a bone clamp before the Kirschner wires are placed. At least two, and preferably more, Kirschner wires should be driven at maximally divergent angles across the fracture and through the opposite cortex (Fig. 54.37**D**). The divergence of the wires prevents the fragment from loosening and sliding along the wires.

Preventing the animal from bearing weight on the radial head for several weeks postoperatively may be advisable, depending on the stability of the repair. This goal may be accomplished by placing the limb in a carpal flexion bandage, Velpeau bandage, or cast.

Salvage procedures such as elbow joint arthrodesis or excision of the radial head can be considered for treatment of severely comminuted radial head fractures.

Combined Radioulnar Diaphyseal Fractures

Most fractures of the antebrachium involve both the radius and ulna, and many of these fractures occur in the middle or distal third of the diaphysis. These fractures can be managed in several ways, depending on the fracture type, patient, client cooperation, facilities available, and the surgeon's capabilities. The methods of managing these fractures include closed reduction and external coaptation, open reduction and bone plating, open reduction and pinning, and closed or open reduction and external skeletal fixation. Each method is described here.

Closed Reduction and External Coaptation

Some combined fractures of the radius and ulna can be managed adequately with external coaptation after closed reduction. This method should be reserved for treatment of incomplete or transverse midshaft frac-

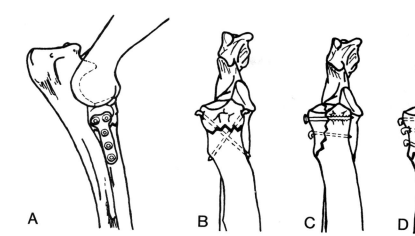

Fig. 54.37. After reduction, an extra-articular radial head fracture can be stabilized with a small T-plate (**A**) or crossed Kirschner wires (**B**) in the case of small animals. Intra-articular radial head fractures are stabilized with a cancellous screw placed in lag fashion and a Kirschner wire to counteract rotation (**C**) or with multiple Kirschner wires placed at divergent angles (**D**).

tures in young, medium-sized dogs and in cats. External coaptation of radial and ulnar fractures should be avoided in toy breeds and in large, active dogs. The incidence of delayed union or nonunion in distal radial and ulnar fractures seems to be high in toy breeds treated with external coaptation. With these fractures, reduction is considered adequate only when a 50% or more purchase is achieved. The limb should not have a varus or valgus angulation when it is cast. (See the earlier discussion of isolated ulnar or radial diaphyseal fractures for guidelines and complications of external coaptation.)

Open Reduction and Bone Plating

The radius is an ideal bone to plate because the approach to it is simple, its cranial surface is the tension side of the bone, and little bending is required to contour the plate properly to the bone. Open reduction and bone plating are the treatments of choice for combined radioulnar fractures in toy breeds, in large or giant breeds, and in animals with multiple limb fractures. In toy breeds, distal radial and ulnar fractures seem to have an unusually high incidence of delayed or nonunion when treated conservatively; plating these fractures provides the rigid fixation necessary for healing. Properly applied bone plates are better than are other methods of fracture repair to withstand the tremendous stress placed on fracture repairs by active large and giant breed dogs. Similarly, the rigid fixation provided by bone plates permits earlier return to function in the patient with multiple limb fractures than when more conservative treatment methods are used.

Usually, only the radius needs to be plated, although plating both the radius and ulna may be advisable in large or active dogs. The radius is exposed through a craniomedial approach; the ulna can be exposed through a caudal or caudolateral approach if it is to be plated also. The most proximal and distal aspects of the radius are more difficult to expose than

the diaphysis because of proximal muscular insertions and tightly adherent extensor tendons distally. The plate is applied to the cranial surface of the radius and, if necessary, the caudolateral surface of the ulna (Fig. 54.38). One must be certain that a plate applied to the radius is beneath the extensor tendons. Failure to do so results in limited function of the carpus or digits.

With proximal radial fractures, screws can be placed through the radial plate into the ulna. This procedure may increase fracture stability, but it prevents supina-

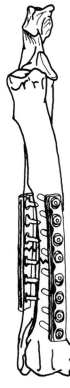

Fig. 54.38. Combined radioulnar shaft fracture repaired with bone plates. Usually, only the radius needs to be plated except in extremely large dogs or in dogs with multiple limb fractures.

tion and pronation of the antebrachium. Screws should never be placed through the radius into the ulna in a growing animal because doing so causes the animal to develop an angular limb deformity.

A cancellous bone graft is recommended for comminuted fractures and for fractures in older animals. The proximal humerus is a convenient site to harvest cancellous bone for radial and ulnar fractures. The cancellous graft can be placed around the fracture site as it is removed from the humerus, or the graft can be put into a stainless steel bowl until enough cancellous bone has been harvested. The fracture site should not be lavaged after the graft has been placed.

A light padded bandage is applied to the limb after wound closure. The bandage is applied snugly from the toes to the midshaft of the humerus. The bandage minimizes postoperative swelling of the limb and keeps the incision clean. The bandage can be removed in 48 hours. The dog's activity should be restricted to leash walks only for 10 to 14 weeks postoperatively. The plate can be removed 10 to 12 months after the fracture has healed.

Open Reduction and Intramedullary Pinning

The radius is not as amenable to intramedullary pinning as the other major long bones for several reasons. Because the radius is relatively straight and both ends are completely covered with articular cartilage, retrograde pin placement causes the pin to enter either the elbow or the carpal joint. The oval cross-sectional shape of the medullary cavity limits the size of the pin that can be used. Furthermore, many toy breed dogs do not have a distinct medullary cavity in the radius, making it difficult or even impossible to pin. A single medullary pin does not provide stable fixation of a radial fracture even if the ulna is also pinned. An intramedullary pin only provides alignment; therefore, supplemental fixation (e.g., cast, external fixator) must also be used to achieve fixation (Fig. 54.39**A**).

The radius should be pinned in a normograde fashion. The pin is inserted starting on the dorsal surface of the radius (near the distal physeal scar) between the extensor carpi radialis and the common digital extensor tendons. A flexible pin is necessary because it must glance off the caudal cortex and slide proximally in the medullary canal. A large pin is inflexible and penetrates the caudal cortex rather than bending and sliding proximally in the medullary canal. Rush pins can be used in the radius, but their use should be reserved for distal metaphyseal fractures (Fig. 54.39**B**). The use of Rush pins is limited in small and medium-sized dogs because the smallest pin manufactured is $\frac{3}{32}$-inch in diameter. The ulna may be pinned in retrograde (i.e., toward the proximal fragment) or normograde (i.e., from the olecranon toward the distal end)

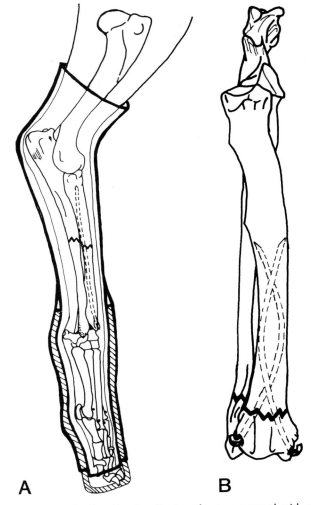

Fig. 54.39. **A.** Combined radioulnar fracture treated with an intramedullary pin and a fiberglass cast. **B.** Distal metaphyseal radial fracture stabilized with double Rush pins. These pins are prebent and driven in a normograde fashion. Rush pins provide stable three-point fixation of metaphyseal fractures but should not be used for diaphyseal fractures.

fashion. The size of the distal ulna limits the pin size that can be used.

Intramedullary pinning is the least desirable method of managing radial and ulnar fractures. Some type of secondary fixation is needed in conjunction with the pin. If external coaptation is chosen, one advantage of internal fixation (i.e., early return to function) is lost. The main advantages of external coaptation (i.e., decreased incidence of infection and minimal tissue trauma) are also lost.

Closed or Open Reduction and External Skeletal Fixation

External skeletal fixation is a versatile and useful method of managing many combined radioulnar fractures. An external fixator can be applied after open or closed fracture reduction. If open reduction is chosen, the approach should be limited in length to what is necessary to see the fracture site. I prefer to use a limited craniomedial approach. The open approach offers the advantages of seeing the fracture during reduction and allowing application of a cancellous bone graft.

Many configurations of external fixators are available. Stable transverse or short oblique fractures in medium-sized dogs can be treated with a type 1 half-pin splintage applied to the radius with four pins and a single connecting bar (Fig. 54.40**C**). A similar configuration with six pins and a single connecting bar is used for similar fractures in larger dogs (Fig. 54.40**D**). The fixator is applied on the cranial or craniomedial aspect of the radius. Driving the pins in a true medial to lateral direction across the radius is difficult and may result in iatrogenic fracture because of the oval shape of the radius.

The pins must be inserted in a particular order during application of an external fixator with only one connecting bar. The fracture is reduced, and the most proximal and distal pins are inserted first. These pins should be inserted as far away from the fracture as possible and at a 45 to 60° angle to the long axis of the bone (Fig. 54.40**A**). A connecting bar with four clamps is attached, and the two outermost clamps are tightened on the pins. The middle two pins are placed through the clamps and then are driven into the bone (Fig. 54.40**B**). These pins should be 1 to 2 cm from the fracture. The greatest biomechanical stability is achieved when there is maximal distance between the two pins on each side of the fracture (Fig. 54.40**C**). All clamps are then completely tightened, and postoperative radiographs are obtained. Minor adjustments in fracture reduction can be made if the clamps are loosened. Because use of a single connecting bar precludes major adjustments in fracture reduction once all the pins have been placed, one should reduce the fracture properly before applying the external fixator.

A six-pin, single-connecting-bar fixator is applied similarly to a four-pin, single-bar fixator. Six clamps are placed on the bar instead of four. The middle pins on either side of the fracture are placed last (Fig. 54.40**D**).

A quadrilateral frame external fixator is useful for unstable comminuted fractures and open fractures

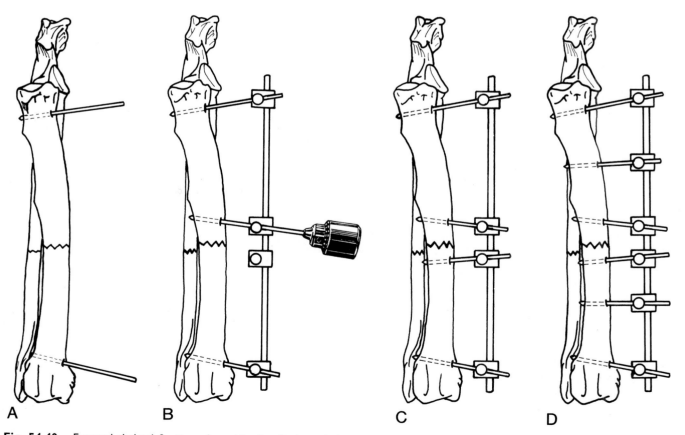

Fig. 54.40. External skeletal fixation of combined radioulnar shaft fractures. **A.** Insertion of most distal and most proximal pins. **B.** Attachment of connecting bar with clamps and placement of middle two pins. **C.** Completed four-pin, single-bar fixator in place. **D.** Six-pin single-bar fixator in place.

with missing bone fragments (Fig. 54.41). This configuration is also particularly useful for proximal or distal fractures in which one segment is short. A quadrilateral frame allows pin fixation in two planes, thus providing stable fixation of short fragments that would not be possible with other configurations. A quadrilateral frame, like other external fixators, can be applied after open or closed reduction. If reduction is not possible (i.e., if cortical fragments are missing), the bone is anatomically aligned before the fixator is applied. The first row of pins is applied from the craniomedial aspect of the radius toward the caudolateral aspect in the same way as described for a four-pin, single-bar fixator. Once the first row of pins is placed and the connecting bar is applied, the second row of pins is placed. The second row of pins is placed identically to the first, except it is applied from the craniolateral aspect of the radius toward the caudomedial aspect. The second connecting bar is then applied. The two rows of pins are connected to each other by applying a connecting bar to the two most proximal and distal pins (Fig. 54.41).

Regardless of the configuration chosen, the points of the pins should protrude slightly beyond the second cortex. The pins should be driven by hand or with a

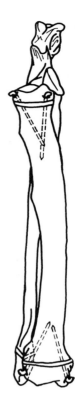

Fig. 54.42. Proximal and distal radial physeal fractures can be stabilized with two small Kirschner wires. External coaptation may also be necessary, especially with distal physeal fractures.

low-speed power drill. The clamps should not touch the skin; rather, they should be approximately 1 cm above the skin. The pins are cut off near the clamps after any necessary adjustments have been made. Postoperative placement of the limb in a light compression bandage is helpful. The bandage helps to minimize postoperative swelling and is left on for 48 hours. The fixator is wrapped with cotton and elastic tape after the compression bandage has been removed. This wrap covers any sharp pins and prevents the fixator from catching on carpet and similar objects. The client should limit the animal's exercise to leash walks until the fracture has healed.

Fixation pins may loosen before a fracture has healed. The likelihood of this complication depends on the type of fracture, the configuration of the fixator, the animal's age, and the amount of activity the animal is allowed. One may choose to replace the loose pins or to remove the fixator and use external coaptation for the remainder of fracture healing. In certain cases, one may be able to remove only the loose pins and leave the rest of the fixator undisturbed. This can only be done if at least two pins remain fixed on each side of the fracture.

Generally, an external fixator can be removed without anesthesia or even sedation. The clamps and connecting bars are loosened and removed. The pins can

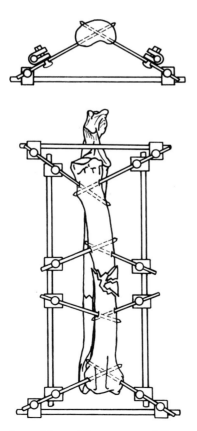

Fig. 54.41. A quadrilateral frame external fixator is useful for unstable comminuted radial and ulnar fractures, especially those that occur in the distal third of the shaft.

be pulled out by hand or with a pair of pliers. The small amount of hemorrhage that usually occurs from the pin holes can be controlled with a light pressure bandage. The animal's activity should be restricted for several weeks after removal of the fixator while remodeling of the holes in the bone begins.

Radial Physeal Fracture–Separations

Fracture-separation through either radial physis is uncommon. Such fractures occur through the zone of hypertrophied cartilage. The animal's owner should always be warned that premature physeal closure and angular limb deformity may follow such a fracture. If premature physeal closure does occur, it usually happens within 2 weeks of the fracture.

Closed reduction of a radial physeal fracture and external coaptation should be attempted first. If closed reduction fails, open reduction should be performed. The fracture can be stabilized with small Kirschner wires (Fig. 54.42). The wires are driven from the epiphysis across the physis and into the metaphysis. To minimize premature physeal closure, the wires should be as parallel to one another as possible and as perpendicular to the physis as possible. Some form of

external coaptation is advisable for 2 weeks, especially for distal physeal fractures. These fractures usually heal within 3 weeks. The pins should be removed if possible.

Suggested Readings

Boltz WH, Chiguet C, Niederer PG. Der fixateur externe (Rohrsystem) Stabilitatsprüfung. AO Bulletin, Frühling, 1978.

Brinker WO, Hohn RB, Prieur WD. Manual of internal fixation in small animals. New York: Springer-Verlag, 1984.

Brinker WO, Piermattei DL, Flo GL. Handbook of small animal orthopedics and fracture treatment. Philadelphia: WB Saunders, 1983.

Brinker WO, Verstraete MC, Soutas-Little RW. Stiffness studies on various configurations and types of external fixators. J Am Anim Hosp Assoc 1985;21:801.

Dieterich HF. Repair of a lateral radial head luxation by radial head ostectomy. Vet Med Small Anim Clin 1973;68:671.

Egger EL. Radius and ulna. In: Slatter DH, ed. Textbook of small animal surgery. Philadelphia: WB Saunders, 1985.

Egger EL. Static strength of six external skeletal fixation configurations. Vet Surg 1983;12:130.

Phillips IR. A survey of bone fractures in the dog and cat. J Small Anim Pract 1979;20:661.

Piermattei DL, Greeley RG. An atlas of surgical approaches to the bones of the dog and cat. Philadelphia: WB Saunders, 1979.

Putnam RW, Archibald J. Excision of canine radial head. Mod Vet Pract 1968;49:32.

— 55 —

FRACTURES OF THE HIND LIMB

Repair of Ilial Shaft Fractures

Timothy M. Lenehan & Guy B. Tarvin

For most ilial shaft fractures, a lateral approach (1) allows optimal visualization of all portions of the ilium (Fig.55.1**A**). The patient is placed in lateral recumbency with the affected side up, and the limb is prepared for aseptic surgery. A skin incision is made starting cranially at the ventral aspect of the rostralmost portion of the wing of the ilium. It is continued caudally in a straight line to the greater trochanter. The fat and fascia are dissected until the intermuscular septum between the tensor fasciae latae and middle gluteal muscles are found and incised. This plane is developed from the ventral iliac spine to the biceps femoris muscle caudally. The tensor fasciae latae is incised along the cranial border of the biceps femoris muscle creating a T-shaped incision. Retraction of the middle and deep gluteal muscles and the tensor fasciae latae muscles with one or two Gelpi retractors allows for palpation of the ventral ilium and fracture components. Often, the gluteal musculature can be elevated off the lateral face of the ilium using a periosteal elevator. Sharp dissection of the ventral origin of the gluteal muscles on the wing of the ilium allows greater retraction and better exposure of the fracture site. Ilial fractures can be repaired by several fixation procedures including bone plating and pinning.

Bone Plating

When the ilial fragments are of sufficient length to allow at least two bone screws proximally and distally, bone plating is preferred. Because the ilium is a wide, flat bone, it lends itself readily to this technique. Re-

duction sometimes can be accomplished by grasping the fragment ends with Verbrugge forceps and bringing the ends into proper alignment; however, further manipulation is often needed. One technique that can be used when the hip joint is intact but the ischium is broken is to grasp the greater trochanter with Lewin forceps and then manipulate the distal ilial fragment into reduction (see Fig. 55.1**B**). Alternatively, if the hemipelvis is intact, forceps (Kern bone-holding forceps or an intramedullary pin) can be placed in the tuber ischiadicum to provide caudal traction or pelvic rotation. Once the fracture has been reduced, bone-holding forceps are applied, or an assistant maintains reduction while the plate is contoured and applied (Fig. 55.2**A**).

In some cases, the aforementioned reduction techniques are insufficient because of muscle contracture. In these patients, the following procedure may be used. The plate is contoured, using the radiograph of the intact opposite side as a guide when possible, and is applied only to the distal fragment. The fragment ends are brought as close to reduction as possible. A Verbrugge clamp then is used to complete reduction, and the plate is secured to the proximal segment (2) (Fig. 55.2**B** and **C**).

During drilling, gauging, and tapping of the screw holes, care must be taken not to injure medial structures such as the rectum and sciatic nerve. Optimally, at least one screw in the proximal segment should engage the wing or body of the sacrum. Although this maneuver results in greater holding power, care should be taken, just as in repair of the sacroiliac dislocation, to avoid penetrating the spinal canal in this area.

Fractures of the ilium near the acetabulum also can be repaired with bone plates. If further exposure is needed, a trochanteric osteotomy can be used to reflect the gluteal mass dorsally (Fig. 55.3).

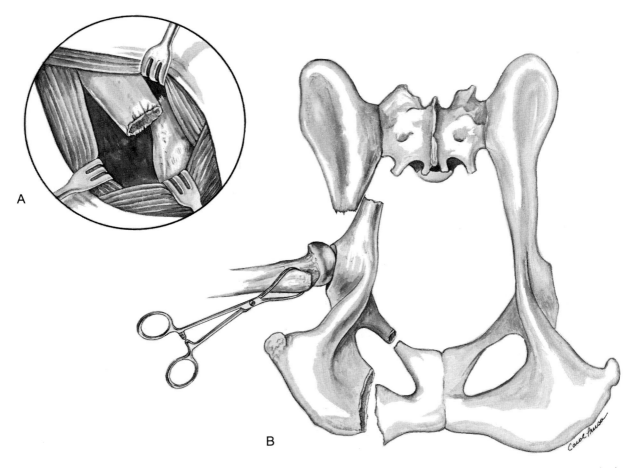

Figure 55.1. A. Lateral approach and exposure of fractured ilial shaft. **B.** Reduction with aid of a Lewin clamp attached to the greater trochanter.

Fractures of the ilium with concurrent sacroiliac luxations are best treated with plate fixation. The approach is a modification of the lateral approach to the ilium (3). Once the ilium is exposed, the attachment of the iliacus muscle to the ventral border of the ilium is incised. Blunt dissection, preferably with the finger, is directed along the medial face of the ilium until the articular surfaces of the sacral wing and ilium are palpated (Fig. 55.4A). Once the sacroiliac luxation has been reduced, a small Kirschner wire is inserted through the ilium and into the sacral wing to maintain reduction. The plate is applied as previously described for ilial fractures. The screws over the sacroiliac joint are purposely applied to engage the wing of the sacrum and to afford compression of the ilium to the sacrum (Fig. 55.4**B**).

Pinning

Some fractures of the ilium are amenable to pinning. The technique seems to be most successful in fractures involving the proximal or midbody area of the ilium in small dogs and cats. Fractures distal to the midbody of the ilium do not often permit sufficient length of insertion of the pins to provide adequate stability.

Insertion of each pin is started in the proximal fragment near the cranial dorsomedial aspect of the wing of the ilium. The pin is driven down the shaft of the ilium and into the distal segment (Fig. 55.5). A pin of identical length is used to check the distance traversed. The hip joint should also be palpated to determine whether the implant has entered the joint. If so, the pin is retracted until no palpable evidence of joint invasion is noted. At least two pins should be driven in a similar manner to improve rotational stability.

Ilial pinning is technically difficult because the medullary cavity of the ilium is narrow, and the cortex is often penetrated during pin insertion. Although the stability achieved with pins is rarely as satisfactory as that with bone plates, pinning may be a suitable alternative when bone-plating equipment is not available. Hemicerclage wiring also can be used in smaller dogs and cats to aid in stability in fractures of the ilial midbody.

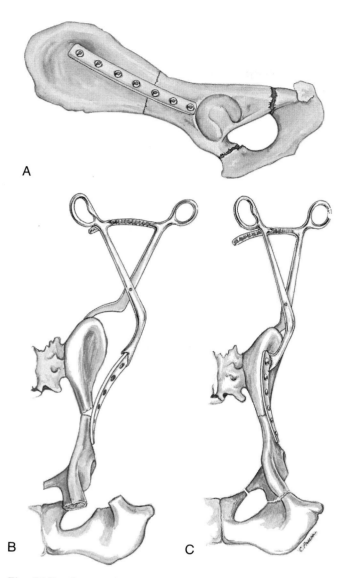

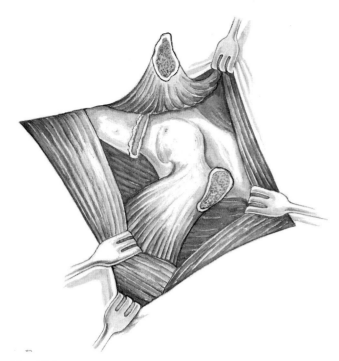

Fig. 55.3. Trochanteric osteotomy sometimes is necessary to expose fractures near the acetabulum for repair.

Fig. 55.2. Repair of ilial fracture with bone plate. **A.** Reduced fracture with bone plate in place. **B** and **C.** Reduction by precontouring a plate, attaching it to one fragment, and then levering the other fragment in place with a Verbrugge clamp.

Postoperative Care

Postoperative radiographs (ventrodorsal, lateral, and oblique hemipelvic) are indicated to evaluate the implant and reduction. Appropriate steps should be taken if errors in reduction have occurred. If adequate fixation is accomplished, no special aftercare is required. Appropriate bedding and nursing care, along with confinement for 3 to 4 weeks, are advised. In 3 to 4 weeks, physical and radiographic assessments are necessary to determine whether further confinement is needed.

Fractures involving both sides of the pelvis are dealt with individually. Surgical procedures can be staged approximately 2 days apart if the animal's condition disallows simultaneous fixation of both sides.

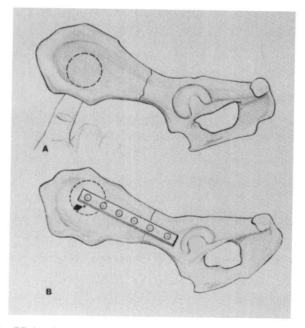

Fig. 55.4. Repair of concurrent ilial fracture and sacroiliac luxation. **A.** The index finger is used to palpate the sacrum from a ventrolateral approach. This helps to reduce the sacroiliac luxation and in screw placement. **B.** After a small pin (*arrow*) is placed, the plate is applied to the ilium. The most rostral screw is placed through the ilium and into the sacrum.

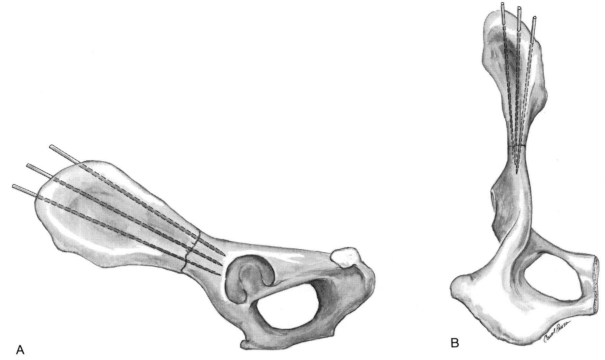

Fig. 55.5. Placement of pins for repair of ilial fractures.

Indications exist for both surgical and nonsurgical therapy. Although injuries in this area involve multiple fractures or dislocations within the pelvic girdle, surgical repair of the ilial fracture or the sacroiliac luxation usually is sufficient to achieve adequate stability of the weightbearing segment and to correct the compromise of the pelvic canal.

References

1. Hohn RB, Janes JM. Lateral approach to the canine ilium. Anim Hosp 1966;2:111.
2. Brown SG, Biggart JF. Plate fixation of ilial shaft fractures in the dog. J Am Vet Med Assoc 1975;167:472.
3. Montavoin PM, Bouchieau RJ, Hohn RB. Ventrolateral approach for repair of sacroiliac fracture–dislocation in the dog and cat. J Am Vet Med Assoc 1985;186:1198.

Surgical Repair of Acetabular Fractures

Marvin L. Olmstead

One of the principles of joint fracture repair is that the weightbearing articular surface must be reconstructed to be as anatomically correct as possible. This reduces the injured joint's risk of developing osteoarthritis. The acetabulum is one-half of the coxofemoral joint, and its cranial two-thirds are generally considered the primary weightbearing area. Optimal surgical repair should restore normal joint mechanics and gliding motion.

Surgical treatment of acetabular fractures involves four steps: exposure of the fracture site, reduction of the fracture, fracture stabilization, and closure. Several different approaches and surgical techniques have proved effective for completing these steps successfully.

Surgical Technique

Acetabular fractures are approached either by a trochanteric osteotomy or the caudal approach (1–3). In most cases, I prefer the caudal approach. This approach provides exposure of the acetabulum equal to a trochanteric osteotomy, it does not require creation of a femoral fracture, and it is more quickly closed than a trochanteric osteotomy.

With both approaches, the superficial gluteal muscle is first isolated, incised at its insertion, and reflected dorsally. If the surgeon is performing an osteotomy of the greater trochanter, it is started at the level of the third trochanter and is extended dorsally to the junction of the greater trochanter and the femoral neck. The middle and deep gluteal muscles are reflected dorsally with the greater trochanter. The caudal portion of the deep gluteal and the gemellus muscles are elevated with a periosteal elevator from their origin over the dorsal rim of the acetabulum. This maneuver exposes the fracture site. The sciatic nerve is identified and protected. After repair of the fracture, the greater trochanter is reattached to the proximal femur with the tension band technique (Fig. 55.6). The remaining layers are closed routinely.

In the caudal approach, after the superficial gluteal muscle is incised and retracted dorsally, the external and internal obturator and gemellus muscles are incised at their insertion in the trochanteric fossa, are tagged, and are retracted caudodorsally. Elevation of these muscles exposes the caudal acetabulum. The muscles can be used to protect the sciatic nerve. The caudal portions of the deep gluteal and gemellus muscles are elevated, exposing the dorsal aspect of the acetabular rim. The caudal ilium is exposed by inserting a Hohmann retractor under the middle and the deep gluteal muscles and hooking its tip just cranial to the ventral border of the ilium. Pushing the retractor's handle ventrally displaces the middle and deep gluteal muscles distally. Maintaining the hip in an extended and internally rotated position provides maximal ex-

posure to the acetabular rim (Fig. 55.7). After the fracture is stabilized, the external and internal obturator and gemellus muscles are sutured to fascial tissue over the lateral surface of the trochanter near the muscle's original insertion point. The remaining tissues are closed routinely.

The acetabulum must be anatomically reduced for the outcome to be successful. The caudal bone segment is often displaced cranially and medially. The fragment can be moved to a caudal position by one of two methods. An intramedullary pin is driven ventrally to dorsally through the ischium just cranial to the ischial rim while the hip joint is flexed. The pin should penetrate the skin dorsal and ventral to the ischium. Pin chucks are attached to exposed ends of the pin and are used as handles to pull the fracture segment caudally (Fig. 55.8). Limited rotation of the segment is provided with this method. Another method for providing caudal traction uses a large Kern bone-holding clamp. An incision wide enough to allow insertion of the end of the clamp is made parallel to the ischial rim. Because the fixation teeth of the Kern clamp provide four points of fixation, this instrument can be used for both caudal retraction and rotation of the segment (Fig.

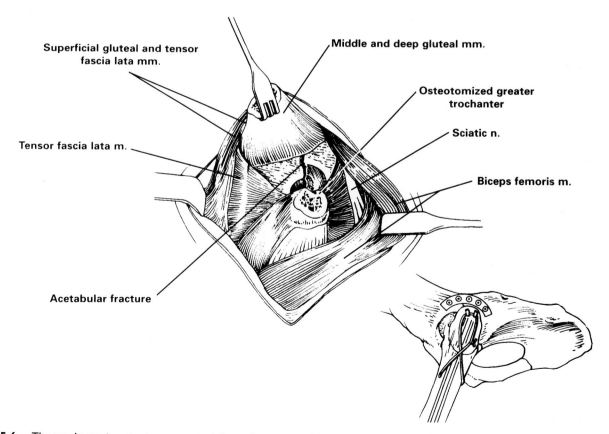

Fig. 55.6. The trochanteric osteotomy approach is used to expose fractures of the acetabulum. The sciatic nerve is isolated before the osteotomy is performed. Two pins and a tension band wire reattach the trochanter following fracture repair (*inset*). (From Olmstead, ML. Fractures of the bones of the hindlimb. In: Olmstead ML, ed. Small animal orthopedics. St. Louis: CV Mosby, 1995:223.)

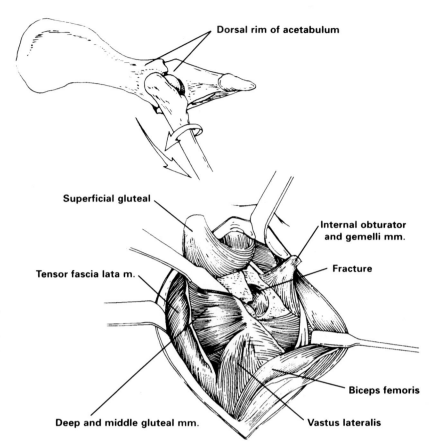

Dorsal rim of acetabulum

Superficial gluteal

Internal obturator
and gemelli mm.

Tensor fascia lata m.

Fracture

Biceps femoris

Deep and middle gluteal mm.

Vastus lateralis

Fig. 55.7. The external rotators of the hip are incised at their insertion in the trochanteric fossa during a caudal approach. These muscles are retracted caudally, protecting the sciatic nerve. Extension and internal rotation of the femur (*inset*) enhances fracture exposure. These muscles are retracted ventrally by a Hohmann retractor placed under the middle and deep gluteal muscles and hooked on the ventral edge of the ilium. (From Olmstead, ML. Fractures of the bones of the hind limb. In: Olmstead ML, ed. Small animal orthopedics. St. Louis: CV Mosby, 1995:222.)

55.9). If the fracture segments are collapsed medially, the Lahey retractor is helpful in repositioning the fragments laterally. A Lahey retractor, which is blunt, strong, and bent 90° at its end, is passed along the medial wall of the free segment. The retractor's tip is maintained on the bone's surface as it is passed along the medial wall to avoid compromising the sciatic nerve. Pulling laterally moves the fracture segments laterally.

Acetabular fracture reduction is maintained with pointed reduction bone forceps or by manually holding the fragments in place until the permanent stabilization procedure is completed. Reduction of an acetabular surface is checked by applying ventral traction on the greater trochanter. This maneuver pulls the femoral head out of the acetabulum enough so the articular rim of the acetabulum can be observed through an incision in the joint capsule or an existing capsular tear.

Nonplating surgical techniques for repair of acetabular fractures have not proved as effective as bone plates, nor have they provided the clinical results obtained with bone plates. Two different sizes of C-shaped acetabular plates, minifragment plates, and standard dynamic compression plates (Synthes, Paoli, PA) have been used successfully to stabilize acetabular fractures. Some surgeons use reconstruction plates for acetabular fractures because these devices can be bent easily in several different planes.

Bone plates must be anatomically contoured to the dorsal rim of the acetabulum. The bone fragments shift

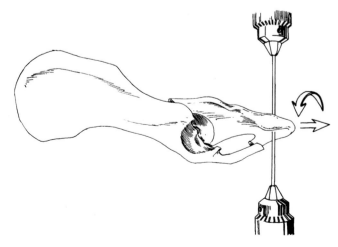

Fig. 55.8. An intramedullary pin driven through the ischium can be used for caudal traction and minimal rotation of the free pelvic segment. (From Olmstead, ML. Fractures of the bones of the hind limb. In: Olmstead ML, ed. Small animal orthopedics. St. Louis: CV Mosby, 1995:225.)

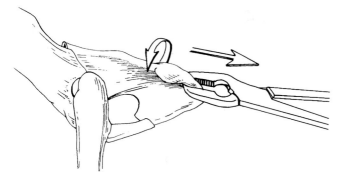

Fig. 55.9. A Kern bone-holding clamp applied to ischium through an incision over the tuber ischia is used to rotate and caudally retract the free segment. (From Olmstead, ML. Fractures of the bones of the hind limb. In: Olmstead ML, ed. Small animal orthopedics. St. Louis: CV Mosby, 1995:226.)

in position as the screws are tightened if the plate is not properly contoured. The C-shaped acetabular plates are easily contoured to the acetabulum's dorsal surface (Fig. 55.10). Miniplates are also easy to bend because they are thin. However, this characteristic makes them weak and limits the size of animal in which they can be used. The dorsal surface of the acetabulum is used for plate placement because adequate bone is present there and this is the tension surface of the bone. In all acetabular fractures, at least two screws should be located on either side of the fracture line, and they should be angled so they do not penetrate the articular cartilage surface (Fig. 55.11).

One of the most difficult fractures to stabilize is one involving the medial wall of the acetabulum. If a large section of this wall is involved, the femoral head is displaced medially into the pelvic canal. If the fracture segment containing the medial wall extends far enough cranially, lag screw or intramedullary pin fixation of the ilial segment is used to stabilize the fragment. When the fragment cannot be stabilized, a slight overbending of the plate, closing the diameter of the articular surface, makes it more difficult for the femo-

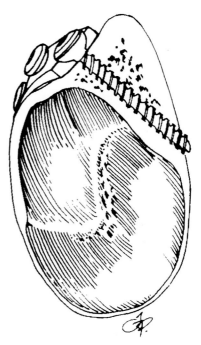

Fig. 55.11. This cut-away view of the acetabulum shows a bone screw directed through the plate in a direction that does not violate the articular surface. (From Olmstead, ML. Fractures of the bones of the hind limb. In: Olmstead ML, ed. Small animal orthopedics. St. Louis: CV Mosby, 1995:227.)

ral head to displace medially. When the femoral head cannot be prevented from displacing medially, a salvage procedure, excision arthroplasty, should be considered. For severe acetabular fractures in which reconstruction is not possible, excision arthroplasty may also be performed. This procedure is done only as a last resort because it sacrifices joint function, but it is intended to save limb function.

The weightbearing surface of the acetabulum, the cranial two-thirds, must be reconstructed if its integrity is to be maintained. Repair of fractures in the caudal one-third of the acetabulum is controversial. Although unrepaired fractures in this area result in coxofemoral osteoarthritis (4), research has not proved that repairing fractures in this area improves the patient's recovery. Although osteoarthritis may be present, limb function may be unaffected. Because of their small size, fractures of the caudal one-third of the acetabulum can be difficult to stabilize adequately. With a caudal fracture, the sciatic nerve is at greater risk of injury during surgery than when the fracture is located more cranially.

When both the ilium and the acetabulum are fractured, I prefer to repair the ilial shaft first. Repair of the ilium is often done with a stronger fixation system than that used in the acetabulum because more screws and a longer and stronger plate usually can be applied to the ilium. Reconstruction of the ilium does not have

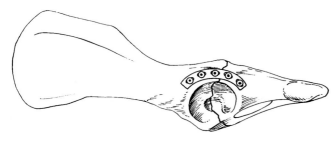

Fig. 55.10. Bone plates are placed over the dorsal rim of the acetabulum because it is the most accessible area and largest visible bone surface and tension surface of the acetabulum. (From Olmstead, ML. Fractures of the bones of the hind limb. In: Olmstead ML, ed. Small animal orthopedics. St. Louis: CV Mosby, 1995:227.)

to be as anatomically exact as reconstruction of the acetabulum. When the acetabulum is repaired last, it is fixed to a solidly stabilized ilial segment. In addition, its fixation is not subjected to additional loads that would be generated during manipulation of the ilial fragments if the ilium were fixed last.

References

1. Piermattei DL. The hind limb. In: Piermattei DL, ed. An atlas of surgical approaches of the bones of the dog and cat. 3rd ed. Philadelphia: WB Saunders, 1993:264.
2. Olmstead ML. Surgical repair of acetabular fractures. In: Bojrab MJ, ed. Current techniques in small animal surgery. 3rd ed. Philadelphia: Lea & Febiger, 1990:656–659.
3. Slocum B, Hohn RB. A surgical approach to the caudal aspect of the acetabulum and body of the ischium in the dog. J Am Vet Med Assoc 1975;65:167–170.
4. Boudrieau RJ, Kleine LJ. Nonsurgically managed caudal acetabular fractures in dogs: 15 cases (1979–1984). J Am Vet Med Assoc 1988;193:701–705.

Suggested Readings

Betts CW. Pelvic fractures. In: Slatter DH, ed. Textbook of small animal surgery. 2nd ed. Philadelphia: WB Saunders, 1993: 1769–1780.
Brinker WO, Piermattei DL, Flo GL. Fractures of the pelvis. In: Handbook of small animal orthopedics and fracture treatment. 2nd ed. Philadelphia: WB Saunders, 1990:76–104.
Brinker WO, Braden TD. Pelvic fractures. In: Brinker WO, Hohn RB, Prieur WD, eds. Manual of internal fixation in small animals. Berlin: Springer–Verlag, 1984:152–165.
Denny, HR. Pelvic fractures in the dog: a review of 123 cases. J Small Anim Pract 1978;19:151–156.
Olmstead ML. Fractures of the bones of the hindlimb. In: Olmstead ML, ed. Small animal orthopedics. St. Louis: CV Mosby, 1995: 219–243.

Internal Fixation of Femoral Fractures

Dougald R. Gilmore

Fractures of the Femoral Head and Neck

Pelvic limb lameness with vehicular trauma often is caused by a fracture of the acetabulum or proximal femur. In the immature animal, fracture through the physis of the femoral head is encountered most commonly. This fracture is due to the weak area at the zone of hypertrophy at the growth plate. Other, less common fractures involve the base of the neck or the trochanteric region (Fig. 55.12).

When examination of a dog less than 12 months of age reveals pain on manipulation of the hip joint, one should suspect either a fracture of the proximal femur

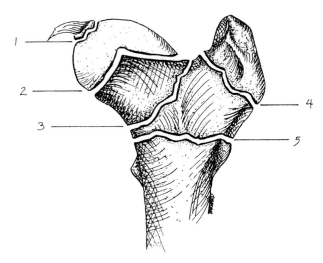

Fig. 55.12. Sites of common fractures of the femoral head and neck and of the proximal femur: *1*, capital epiphysis (avulsion fractures); *2*, capital (proximal) physis; *3*, femoral neck; *4*, greater trochanteric physis; and *5*, intertrochanteric region.

or acetabulum or a coxofemoral luxation. The exact diagnosis requires radiographic evaluation including ventrodorsal (normal hip dysplasia position) and lateral views. Occasionally, a "frog leg" view assists in the diagnosis. This view requires the animal to be in dorsal recumbency with the pelvic limbs held in a flexed and slightly abducted position. An awake animal is more likely to cooperate for this view than for the normal ventrodorsal view.

Anatomic Considerations

In the extremely young animal, the proximal growth plate extends from the greater trochanter to the femoral head. As the animal matures, separation into a capital femoral growth plate and a greater trochanteric growth plate occurs. Investigators have estimated that the capital physeal growth plate contributes up to 25% of the femoral length, whereas the greater trochanteric physis contributes little to the length. The ligament of the femoral head, which extends from the femoral fovea to the acetabular fossa, provides significant support to the hip joint.

The vascular supply to the femoral head continues to be of concern to most veterinary surgeons. If precise, delicate surgical intervention with appropriate stabilization is practiced, few complications should be encountered. Important aspects of the vascular supply include the lateral and medial circumflex femoral arteries, which are branches of the femoral and deep femoral arteries. The lateral branch provides most of the supply to the femoral head and the dorsal aspect of the femoral neck. The medial branch supplies the ventral aspect of the joint capsule, and a branch of the caudal gluteal artery supplies a small portion of the dorsal aspect. Dorsal and ventral ascending branches from the lateral and medial circumflex femoral arteries anastomose and form a rich interosseous arch within the epiphysis. Metaphyseal branches of the lateral and medial circumflex vessels do not communicate with the epiphyseal branches in the immature animal. No evidence suggests that a blood supply enters the epiphysis from the ligament of the femoral head.

Presurgical Considerations

Avascular necrosis of the femoral head secondary to a fracture is not a significant problem if appropriate surgical treatment is followed. Most reports of repair list few cases of avascular necrosis. Although the femoral head completely loses its vascular supply at the time of the initial trauma, revascularization is rapid after stabilization. The time interval to surgery is important because more damage is sustained if the repair is delayed. Attempts by the animal to walk on the affected limb may damage the soft metaphyseal bone of the neck as it rubs on the acetabular rim. Loss of bone results in the inability to reduce and stabilize the fracture components correctly. The degree of damage is most often ascertained at the time of surgery. Occasionally, radiographic evaluation reveals the damage.

Surgical Approach

The craniolateral approach is most often recommended for femoral head and neck fractures because of the preservation of vascular supply. The dorsal approach, including greater trochanteric osteotomy, may be used if increased exposure is required, but it damages the branches of the lateral circumflex femoral artery. In addition, damage to the physis of the greater trochanter may lead to a valgus deformity in a young animal. Successful use of the dorsal approach has been reported, but research also shows that the vascular damage may not be significant.

In the craniolateral approach, the skin incision is curved in a cranial direction starting 3 to 4 cm proximal to the greater trochanter and extending distally to include the proximal one-quarter of the femoral shaft. An incision is made into the fascia lata just cranial to the greater trochanter and is extended to allow retraction of the biceps femoris muscle caudally and the fascia cranially. The muscular tensor fasciae latae is then dissected from the fascia of the vastus lateralis and the middle gluteal muscles. The gluteal muscles are retracted dorsally and the tensor fasciae latae cranially to allow visualization of the cranial aspect of the joint capsule. The joint capsule is incised perpendicular

to the acetabular rim, extending to the origin of the vastus intermedius and lateralis. The exposure can be increased by performing a partial tenotomy of the deep gluteal muscle. If difficulty is encountered in visualization and reduction of the fracture, trochanteric osteotomy may be performed. With either approach, the location of the sciatic nerve should be noted.

Fixation Techniques

CAPITAL PHYSEAL FRACTURES
Reduction of a capital physeal fracture may be difficult. Handling of the femoral head with a retractor or bone-holding forceps should be minimized to lessen damage to the articular cartilage. One or several Kirschner wires are placed to stabilize the fracture after reduction. These pins are placed in retrograde fashion from the fracture site laterally or in a normograde manner from the lateral surface of the proximal femur (Fig. 55.13**A**). After fracture reduction, the pins are seated in the femoral head.

If a lag screw is to be used, the gliding hole through the proximal femur may be drilled before reduction to ensure placement into the center of the neck. A small threaded hole is drilled into the femoral head before measuring and tapping the hole (Fig. 55.13**B**). As the head is encountered, tapping becomes more difficult. Care is taken to ensure that the articular surface is not penetrated. A screw that is 2 to 4 mm shorter than the measured length should be used because of the shortening obtained during lag screw fixation (Fig. 55.13**C**).

Use of measurements taken from the radiographs can help to ensure that implants of appropriate size are used. The articular surface should be inspected after implant placement to check for implant penetration. Areas not visualized may be inspected using a curved instrument to check for any irregularities. Any articular damage fills with fibrocartilage, which permits satisfactory recovery of most animals.

Interfragmentary compression alone should be adequate for most animals. Kirschner wires may be left in place to increase rotational stability if necessary. After the joint is flushed, the joint capsule is closed with a nonreactive suture material before anatomic closure of the other layers.

OTHER ARTICULAR FRACTURES
Occasionally, an avulsion fracture of the ligament of the femoral head occurs in association with a coxofemoral luxation. Removal of this fragment and the ligament is recommended if surgical intervention is necessary for stabilization of the hip joint. Closed reduction of this type of coxofemoral luxation may result in degenerative joint disease because the interposed avulsed fragment produces cartilaginous damage.

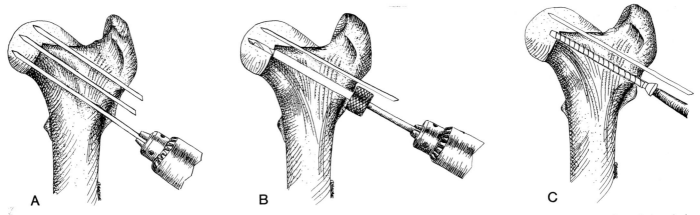

Fig. 55.13. A capital physeal fracture can be stabilized by multiple Kirschner wires placed from the lateral surface into the subchondral bone (**A**), or by lag screw fixation. In the latter method, after normograde or retrograde drilling of the glide hole, a drill guide is inserted and a thread hole drilled (**B**); a screw is then inserted to compress the fracture (**C**). The Kirschner wire can be left in place to provide further stabilization.

Fractures involving the dorsal articular surface require stabilization to lessen degenerative joint disease. Femoral head and neck excision is an alternative if the articular cartilage is severely damaged or if reduction is too difficult. Fracture fragments involving the non-articular surfaces may be removed.

EXTRACAPSULAR FRACTURES

Fractures through the base of the femoral neck are most often encountered in mature animals. Repair is performed as described previously for femoral head fractures (see Fig. 55.13). Osteonecrosis is not a problem because of the extracapsular nature of the fracture.

Fractures through the apophysis of the greater trochanter sometimes occur in association with a capital physis fracture. Careful evaluation of the radiographs may be necessary because of the superimposition of the greater trochanter on the femoral shaft. Stabilization is performed through a craniolateral approach with retraction of the greater trochanter. After stabilization of the femoral head with a Kirschner wire and lag screw, the greater trochanter is reattached by tension band fixation (Fig. 55.14). Care is necessary to ensure complete reduction and realignment before stabilization.

Proximal Femoral Fractures

Greater Trochanteric Fractures

Fractures of the greater trochanter are commonly associated with fractures involving the femoral head in young animals and with comminuted proximal femoral fractures in mature animals. The traction physis associated with the greater trochanter is believed to provide no significant contribution to longitudinal bone growth.

Repair of a greater trochanteric fracture is necessary because the distraction forces applied by the gluteal muscles do not allow for normal union. Approach is made just cranial to the greater trochanter, allowing separation of the fascia lata from the biceps femoris muscle. Incision into the origin of the vastus lateralis may be necessary to allow visualization of the fracture.

Of the repair methods available, tension band fixa-

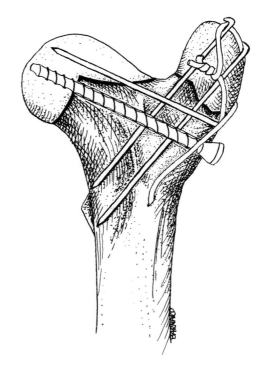

Fig. 55.14. Fractures involving both the greater trochanteric and capital physis are stabilized by a lag screw, Kirschner wire, and tension band fixation. This type of fixation also is used when a trochanteric osteotomy is performed to approach the coxofemoral joint.

tion is probably the easiest and most satisfactory. This method converts distracting forces into compressive forces at the fracture site. Two Kirschner wires are inserted at right angles to the fracture line (see Fig. 55.14). Care is taken to gain maximum purchase proximally in the greater trochanter and to ensure purchase into the medial cortex at or below the lesser trochanter. Orthopedic wire (18 to 20 gauge) is placed through a hole drilled in a craniocaudal direction 3 to 4 cm distal to the fracture line. This wire is placed around the proximal ends of the Kirschner wires in a figure-of-eight configuration and then is tightened to counteract the distracting forces of the gluteal muscles.

Intertrochanteric and Subtrochanteric Fractures

Either stack-pinning or plate fixation can be used to neutralize both bending and rotational forces acting on the intertrochanteric and subtrochanteric fractures. Approach to the area requires transection of the origins of both the vastus lateralis and intermedius muscles. Pin placement should originate from the proximal point of the greater trochanter and should extend distally, gaining maximal purchase in the femur. A common mistake is to exit the pins within 3 to 4 cm of the fracture line. This technique provides less than satisfactory stabilization. A figure-of-eight wire may be placed in association with the pins to provide increased rotational stability for subtrochanteric fractures (Fig. 55.15).

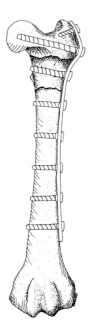

Fig. 55.16. Intertrochanteric and subtrochanteric fractures can be stabilized with a bone plate applied to the lateral surface of the femur. A cortical or cancellous screw is placed through the femoral neck for increased purchase.

Application of a bone plate to the lateral surface is indicated in large dog breeds for repair of these fractures. Careful contouring of the bone plate allows for the placement of at least two screws in the short proximal segment in most cases. One screw (usually cancellous) should extend into the femoral neck for increased purchase, and at least four screws should be placed in the distal segment (Fig. 55.16).

Comminuted Fractures

Highly comminuted fractures of the proximal femur require aggressive fixation, usually with a bone plate and lag screws. Care must be taken to ensure adequate stabilization of the calcar region (lesser trochanter) because it is an important medial buttress. Early fixation failure can be expected if stabilization is inadequate. The fracture segments are reduced and stabilized with both lag screws and Kirschner wires. The plate is then contoured and is attached to the proximal segment with one screw placed through the second hole into the femoral neck and head. The proximal screw is placed into the greater trochanter. Use of a dynamic compression plate permits angling of the screws up to 30° from center. The plate acts as a neutralization or buttress plate for this type of fracture. The plate should be attached to the distal segment with at least three screws penetrating six cortices (Fig. 55.17**A**). A cancellous bone graft should be placed into any areas that lack cortical bone.

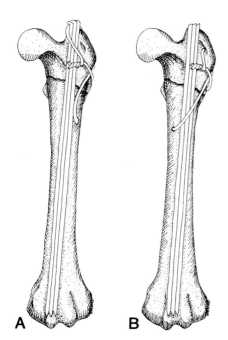

Fig. 55.15. **A** and **B.** An intertrochanteric fracture of the femur is repaired with multiple intramedullary pins and a figure-of-eight tension band wire. Two different methods of attaching the wire are shown.

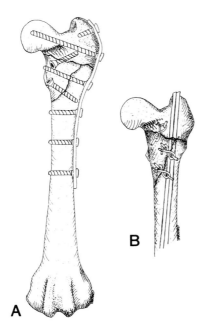

Fig. 55.17. A comminuted proximal femoral fracture can be stabilized by a bone plate applied to the lateral surface and lag screw fixation of the butterfly fragment (**A**) or by intramedullary pins with the butterfly fragment attached by transcortical pins and figure-of-eight wires (**B**).

Intramedullary fixation of comminuted proximal fractures is more applicable to small and medium-sized dogs than to large ones, especially if the fracture has only three or four segments. By use of hemicerclage wire and transcortical pins, a comminuted fracture can be reduced to a two-piece fracture, which then is fixed by normograde or retrograde stack-pinning (Fig. 55.17**B**). Care must be taken to ensure that the transcortical pins do not enter to the medullary canal to allow for the introduction of a maximum number of stack pins. Lag screws are more difficult to incorporate into fractures stabilized with intramedullary pins.

Diaphyseal Fractures of the Femur

Transverse Fractures

Transverse diaphyseal fractures are most commonly repaired with one intramedullary pin. Although success is often reported with this method, so too is failure, mainly because of the lack of rotational stability provided by one pin. This method is most likely to succeed with immature animals in which healing is rapid and with small to medium-sized adult animals in which the single pin tends to fill a significant part of the medullary canal. Failure occurs most often in large dogs, when a small pin that does not fill a significant portion of the canal is used. Use of a Kirschner–Ehmer external fixation device (two-pin half-pin splint) in association with the intramedullary pin increases rotational stability.

Stack-pinning of transverse fracture is an easy procedure that results in few complications in most cases. The curved skin incision should be just cranial to the femoral shaft. The biceps femoris muscle belly is encountered if the incision is directly over the shaft; incision through this muscle belly is not the approach of choice. After approaching the fracture by incising the fascia lata cranial to the biceps muscle, the vastus lateralis muscle is retracted cranially, and the biceps femoris muscle is retracted caudally to allow visualization of the fracture site. Minimal stripping of the periosteum is done to check for any fissure lines in the fracture segments. The pins are placed in retrograde fashion, exiting proximally through the trochanteric fossa (Fig. 55.18**A**). The surgeon must extend the animal's hip joint and adduct the femur when passing the pin proximally to avoid the sciatic nerve as it passes over the greater trochanteric notch. All pins are placed proximally before reduction of the fracture segment. Enough pins are used to fill the medullary canal at its narrowest point. The pins are then driven distally into cortical bone. Because of the cranial curvature of the femoral shaft, the pins usually seat distally in the cranial metaphyseal area near the proximal end of the trochlea (Fig. 55.18**B**). Overreduction of the distal segment allows seating of the pins further distally, but usually this leads to malalignment and instability. Because the feline femur has less curvature, the pins can be seated farther distally in the intercondylar region in cats (Fig. 55.18**C**).

Several methods are available to add rotational support to pin fixation of transverse diaphyseal fractures. A two-pin half-pin Kirschner–Ehmer splint in association with a single intramedullary pin is one method. Use of hemicerclage or figure-of-eight orthopedic wire also can increase rotational stability. The figure-of-eight wire can be passed through holes drilled proximal and distal to the fracture line, or two can be placed around transverse Kirschner wires and tightened to form a cruciate pattern (Fig. 55.19). The distance from the holes or Kirschner wires to the fracture should be at least equal to the width of the femur at the fracture site.

Application of a bone plate to the lateral or cranial surface is indicated for stabilization of transverse fractures in large breeds or in any animal requiring rigid internal fixation. Compression of the fracture line allows for rapid primary bone healing. Screw fixation in at least six cortices above and below the fracture should be obtained.

Oblique and Spiral Fractures

Oblique and spiral fractures are most successfully repaired with intramedullary pins, with additional stability provided by transcortical pins and hemicerclage wire or by full-cerclage orthopedic wire. The fracture

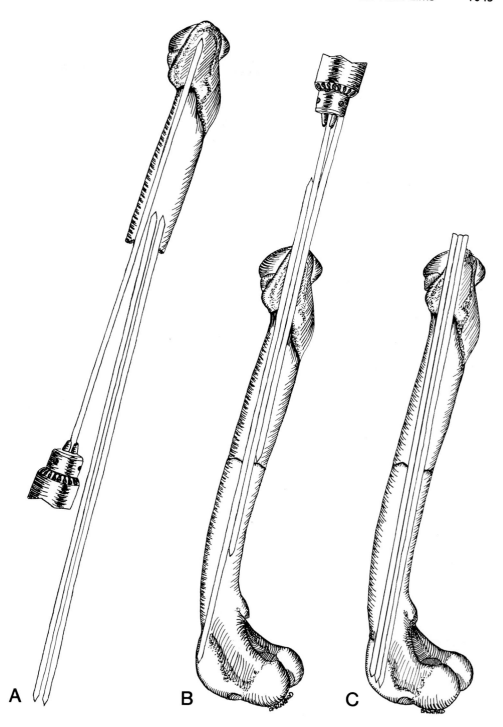

Fig. 55.18. Retrograde stack-pinning of a transverse midshaft femoral fracture. **A.** The hip is extended and the femur is adducted before retrograde placement of all pins through the trochanteric fossa. **B.** The pins are driven distally to engage cortical bone. **C.** The pins are placed into but not through the distal cortex beneath the trochlear groove.

is first stabilized with intramedullary pins, as discussed in the section on transverse fractures. Wire can be placed around transcortical pins in a figure-of-eight pattern to provide increased rotational stability (Fig. 55.20A). Alternatively, full-cerclage wires can be used (Fig. 55.20B).

Although investigators initially thought that full-cerclage wires interfered with the new periosteal blood supply needed for fracture healing, more recent studies have shown that this may not occur. Problems only arise when the wire is improperly applied. Common mistakes include inappropriate wire diameter (18 to 20 gauge is appropriate for most animals), placement too close to the fracture ends (a minimum of 5 mm is appropriate), and use of insufficient number of wires (a minimum of two wires placed 1 cm apart is appro-

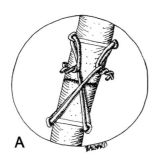

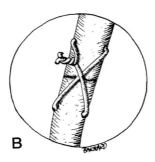

Fig. 55.19. Increased rotational stability of transverse femoral fractures is achieved by use of two figure-of-eight wires placed around transversely placed Kirschner wires (**A**), or by orthopedic wire placed in a figure-of-eight fashion through two holes drilled proximal and distal to the fracture line (**B**).

priate). As with any technique, failure is more likely to occur when wires are applied in less than ideal fashion. Most complications occur when the wire slips into the fracture site, producing a nonunion.

Comminuted Fractures

Reduction of the fracture segments into two main segments before primary fixation with intramedullary pins provides successful stabilization of most comminuted fractures. Pin fixation is less effective with highly comminuted fractures because of the inability to neutralize compressive forces. Collapse of the fracture is more likely in these cases. Midshaft fractures with one or two butterfly fragments can be stabilized with techniques similar to those discussed in the section on oblique fractures.

Application of a bone plate to the lateral or cranial surface as a neutralization plate (no compression at the fracture site) or a buttress plate (a cortical gap is present) can stabilize most comminuted diaphyseal fractures. The large fragments are attached with Kirschner wires, orthopedic wire, or lag screws before plate attachment. Care must be taken to ensure that

these implants do not interfere with placement of the plate. If possible, the plate is positioned to allow for placement of screws in all holes. Occasionally, the number of fissure lines necessitates leaving one or more holes vacant. This situation is to be avoided, especially with a buttress plate, because fatigue failure is more likely to occur at this site. Use of a leg-lengthening plate that lacks holes in the central one-third of the plate may be indicated in these cases (Fig. 55.21). Contouring of the plate is made easier if a radiograph of the contralateral femur is available for comparison. By using the greater trochanter, stifle, and linea aspera (the caudal rough surface where the adductor magnus muscle attaches) as reference points, normal anatomic alignment can be obtained in these comminuted fractures.

Occasionally, highly comminuted diaphyseal fractures cannot be pieced together with pins or lag screws. Both removing these fragments and leaving them in place while spanning the gap with a bone plate have been reported. The gap is filled with autogenous can-

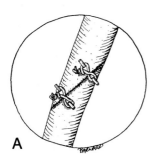

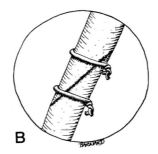

Fig. 55.20. Long oblique fractures of the femur can be stabilized by transcortical pins with figure-of-eight wires (**A**) or by full-cerclage wires (**B**). The transcortical pins should not enter into the medullary canal, to avoid interference with intramedullary pin placement.

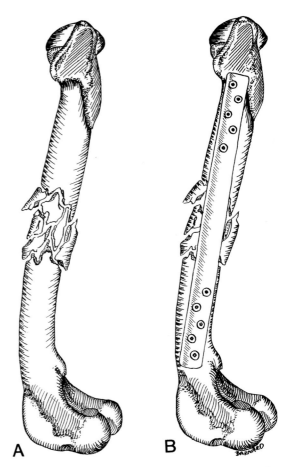

Fig. 55.21. A comminuted midshaft femoral fracture (**A**) can be stabilized by a buttress plate applied to the lateral surface (**B**). A leg-lengthening place is used so no vacant holes are positioned over the comminuted segments.

cellous bone to stimulate healing. Leg-lengthening plates are ideally suited, because they allow the closer placement of screws in the proximal and distal fragments without leaving several vacant holes over the gap. Success has been reported with the use of dynamic or standard plates with vacant holes. The plate used must be as large as possible in such cases.

Distal Femoral Fractures

Metaphyseal (Supracondylar) Fractures

Although encountered infrequently, distal metaphyseal fractures provide a challenge for repair. Fortunately, the rich blood supply to this trabecular bone promotes rapid bone healing in most cases. This type of fracture occurs most often in mature animals and is often associated with comminution.

The approach to this region is an extension of the approach used for stifle arthrotomy. The incision in the fascia lata cranial to the biceps femoris muscle is extended distally to include the lateral fascia of the stifle. Incision into the joint capsule is extended proximally, lateral to the vastus lateralis muscle to allow medial retraction of the quadriceps group and the patella. A large muscular branch of the popliteal artery must be ligated as this incision is made. Flexion of the stifle with medial retraction of the muscles allows visualization of the medial surface of the distal femur.

Bone plating of the lateral surface is recommended for stabilization of metaphyseal fractures in larger dogs, especially if comminution is present. Use of cancellous screws in the distal segment increases holding power, which is often needed because of the short length of the distal segment. Intramedullary pinning is more appropriate for stabilization in small and medium-sized animals (Fig. 55.22). The techniques discussed in the following sections on physeal and epiphyseal fractures are used.

Physeal Fractures

Most distal physeal fractures occur in immature animals (4 to 12 months old) because the zone of hypertrophy is structurally much weaker than the surrounding bone, tendons, and ligaments. The most common fractures are Salter I (involvement of the growth plate only) and Salter II (involvement of the growth plate and metaphysis), which fortunately do not involve the germinative or growth layer of the physis. Few complications associated with premature closure of the physis have been noted. Rapid healing can be expected because of the adjacent rich blood supply.

External support alone infrequently allows for nor-

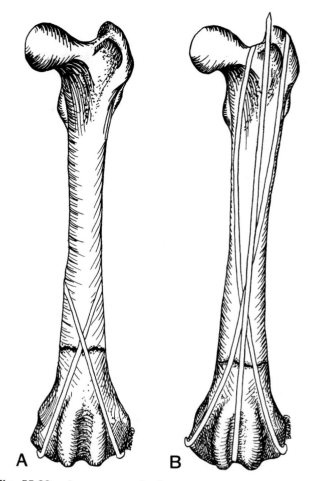

Fig. 55.22. A transverse distal metaphyseal femoral fracture can be stabilized by cross-pins driven from the condyles (**A**) or by double intramedullary pins driven in a Rush pin technique from the condyles and one intramedullary pin driven from the trochlea (**B**).

mal reduction and bone union and subsequent normal functional use. As with any joint, immobilization of the stifle may lead to adhesion formation and loss of joint motion. Most distal physeal fractures, however, require internal fixation by some type of pinning procedure.

Antegrade introduction of a single Steinmann pin from the trochlea just cranial to the origin of the cruciate ligaments provides maximum purchase in the small distal segment. Reduction of the fracture before pin placement is ideal. Careful handling of the distal segment is important because of the softness of the bone and the presence of articular cartilage. Overzealous use of bone forceps may result in significant damage. Placement of the pin in the distal segment before reduction, using the pin as a lever, is possible if done carefully (Fig. 55.23**A**). The pin may pull out of the bone, resulting in enlargement of the hole, if the veterinary surgeon is not careful. The pin is driven

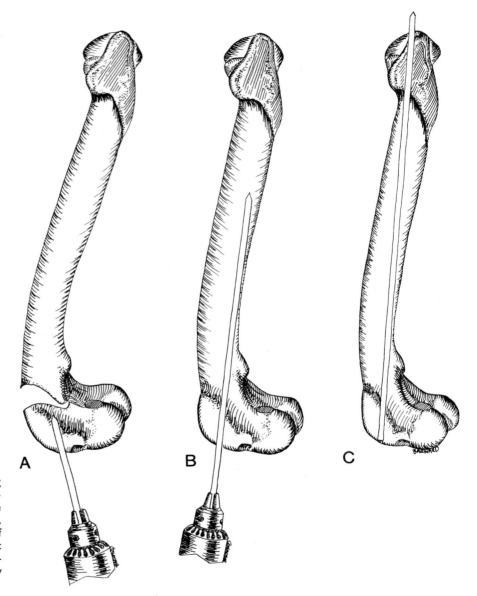

Fig. 55.23. Single intramedullary pinning of a Salter I or II fracture of the distal femoral physis. **A.** The pin is placed through the epiphysis. **B.** After the fracture is reduced, the pin is driven up the caudal surface of the shaft, exiting through the trochanteric fossa. **C.** The pin is cut distally and retracted proximally until embedded below the articular surface.

proximally, exiting through the trochanteric fossa (Fig. 55.23**B**). After the distal end is cut, the pin is retracted proximally until the blunt end is seated just below the cartilaginous surface of the trochlea (Fig. 55.23**C**). Stabilization of these fractures is aided by the interlocking of metaphyseal protuberances in epiphyseal fossae, providing rotational stability.

Retrograde placement of the pin avoids damage to the articular cartilage, but it may not always provide adequate purchase in the distal segment. If this method is used, the pin is placed along the caudal aspect of the femur to allow for maximum purchase in the distal segment.

Other methods of fixation include double pinning, modified Rush pinning, and cross-pinning (see Fig. 55.22). With all methods, the pins are started just lat-eral and medial to the trochlear ridges and cranial to the collateral ligaments (Fig. 55.24). Larger, less flexible pins are used with cross-pinning fixation. The pins must cross above the fracture line. Exiting of the pins too close to the fracture may lead to failure with weightbearing. Placement of the pins in retrograde fashion results in less than maximum purchase in the distal segment.

Epiphyseal Fractures

Excellent radiographic technique is required to demonstrate distal epiphyseal fractures because displacement is often minimal. If not stabilized, these fractures result in degenerative joint disease because of the articular involvement.

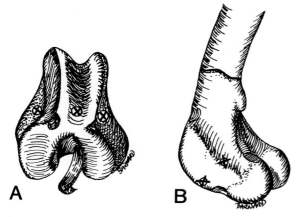

Fig. 55.24. Craniocaudal (**A**) and lateral views (**B**) of the placement of intramedullary pins into the distal femoral segment. The lateral and medial pins are placed cranial to the collateral ligaments on either side of the trochlear ridges. The pin placed through the trochlea is just cranial to the origin of the cranial cruciate ligament. Normograde placement of these pins provides maximum purchase in the distal segment.

The medial condyle is most often involved. Exploration of the joint is required to remove any cartilage and bone fragments and to inspect the menisci and cruciate ligaments. Lag screw fixation, the recommended repair technique, achieves accurate realignment of the articular surfaces and compresses the fracture. In small dogs and cats, multiple Kirschner wires or a single wire and lag screw can provide good fixation (Fig. 55.25).

Postoperative Management and Complications

Physical therapy is an important part of the total treatment regimen in all animals with femoral fractures.

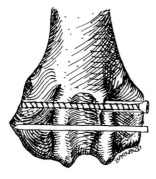

Fig. 55.25. Condylar or epiphyseal fractures of the distal femur usually involve the articular surface. Lag screws and Kirschner wire fixation provide rigid fixation.

The soft tissue structures around a fracture also sustain trauma, and the bruised and swollen muscles require appropriate therapy after fracture fixation.

Fractures of the Femoral Head and Neck

All animals require strict confinement for the first 4 to 6 weeks after repair of a femoral head and neck fracture. The owner should be instructed on the method of physical therapy of the hip joint to help to restore early limb function.

Radiographic evaluation at 4 to 6 weeks usually reveals thinning of the femoral neck. In most cases, this thinning is normal, but if pronounced lameness is still apparent at this time, these findings suggest avascular necrosis and possible failure of the fixation. If the animal is recovering use of the limb, radiographic evaluation usually is delayed until 6 to 8 weeks after stabilization. Radiographic evaluation after complete healing has occurred usually reveals a thickening of the femoral neck and some evidence of degenerative joint disease. Removal of the implants is not recommended unless complications occur.

Other Femoral Fractures

Physical therapy should be instituted within 2 to 3 days of the surgical procedure. Gentle flexion and extension of the hip and stifle joints for 3 to 5 minutes, a minimum of three times daily, assist in the early return of limb function. This is especially important in an immature dog with a fractured femur, which is prone to quadriceps muscle contraction and tie-down. If this syndrome is allowed to progress to the stage of severe stifle hyperextension, the prognosis for return of limb function is poor. Walking the animal on a leash during the first 4 weeks postoperatively also encourages use of the limb and a return of the normal range of motion in all joints.

Pin migration into the stifle results in damage to the trochlear groove and the patella and, ultimately, in degenerative joint disease. Migration proximally may cause open wounds and possibly osteomyelitis. Sciatic nerve entrapment may result from pin migration or formation of fibrous tissue at the proximal end of adequately seated pins. Clinical signs include acute onset of lameness, pain in the hip region, and eventual knuckling of the paw and hypalgesia over the area of nerve distribution. Exploration and freeing of the nerve from the fibrous tissue are required to allow recovery; in addition, the pins should be shortened or removed if complete fracture healing has occurred. Return of normal limb function depends on the degree of nerve damage sustained in such cases.

Suggested Readings

Aron DN, et al. A review of reduction and internal fixation of proximal femoral fractures in the dog and man. J Am Anim Hosp Assoc 1979;15:455.

Daly WR. Femoral head and neck fractures in the dog and cat: a review of 115 cases. Vet Surg 1978;7:29.

Frey AJ, Olds R. A new technique for repair of comminuted diaphyseal fractures. Vet Surg 1981;10:51.

Gambardella PC. Full cerclage wires for fixation of long bone fractures. Compend Contin Educ Pract Vet 1980;11:665.

Gilmore DR. Application of the lag screw. Compend Contin Educ Pract Vet 1983;5:217.

Grauer GF, Banks WJ, Ellison GW, et al. Incidence and mechanisms of distal femoral physeal fractures in the dog and cat. J Am Anim Hosp Assoc 1981;17:579.

Hauptman J, Butler HC. Effect of osteotomy of the greater trochanter with tension band fixation on femoral conformation in beagle dogs. Vet Surg 1979;8:13.

Hulse DA, Abdelbaki YZ, Wilson J. Revascularization of femoral capital physeal fractures following surgical fixation. J Vet Orthop 1981;2:50.

Hulse DA, et al. Use of the lag screw principle for stabilization of femoral neck and femoral capital epiphyseal fractures. J Am Anim Hosp Assoc 1974;10:29.

Kaderly RE, Anderson WD, Anderson BG. Extraosseous vascular supply to the mature dog's coxofemoral joint. Am J Vet Res 1982;43:1208.

Kagan KG. Multiple intramedullary pin fixation of the femur of dogs and cats. J Am Vet Med Assoc, 182:1251, 1983.

Milton JL, Horne RD, Goldstein GM. Crosspinning: a simple technique for treatment of certain metaphyseal and physeal fractures of the long bones. J Am Anim Hosp Assoc 1980;16:891.

Milton JL, Newman ME. Fractures of the femur. In : Slatter DH, ed. Textbook of small animal surgery. Philadelphia: WB Saunders, 1985.

Nunamaker DM. Repair of femoral head and neck fractures by interfragmentary compression. J Am Vet Med Assoc 1973;162:569.

Renegar WR, Leeds EB, Olds RB. The use of the Kirschner–Ehmer splint in clinical orthopedics. Compend Contin Educ Pract Vet 1982;4:381.

Rhinelander FW, Wilson JW. The blood supply of developing mature and healing bone. In: Sumner-Smith G, ed. Bone in clinical orthopedics. Philadelphia: WB Saunders, 1982.

Rivera LA, Aldelbaki YZ, Hulse DA. Arterial supply to the canine hip joint. J Vet Orthop 1979;1:20.

Shires PK, Hulse DA. Internal fixation of physeal fractures using the distal femur as an example. Compend Contin Educ Pract Vet 1980;11:854.

Stone EA, Betts CW, Rowland GN. Effect of Rush pins on the distal femoral growth plate of young dogs. Am J Vet Res 1981;42:261.

Fixation of Tibial Fractures

Eric R. Pope

Fractures of the tibia are common in small animals, accounting for 14.8% of long bone fractures in one study. Because of the unusual anatomic structure of the tibia, complex shaft fractures are common. In addition, the tibia is predisposed to open fractures because of the minimal soft tissue surrounding the bone. Concurrent fracture of the fibula almost always occurs. Repair of the fibula is generally not indicated unless the proximal fibula or the lateral malleolus is involved.

Fractures of these segments should be repaired because of the important ligamentous structures attached to them.

Fractures of the distal diaphysis, particularly oblique fractures, commonly are open because of the minimal soft tissue coverage. Care should be taken during palpation and manipulation of these fractures to avoid creating open fractures. For this reason and also to prevent excessive swelling of the limb, all tibial fractures should be immobilized with a Robert Jones or similar bandage until definitive repair is performed.

As with any fracture patient, a thorough physical examination should be performed to rule out life-threatening injuries. The integrity of the blood supply and nervous innervation of the limb should be assessed before repairing the fracture. Thoracic radiographs are indicated to rule out the possibility of a diaphragmatic hernia or pulmonary parenchymal damage if anesthesia is anticipated. At least two views (craniocaudal and lateral) of the limb, including the stifle and hock joints, should be taken. The radiographs should be closely examined for the presence of free gas, which indicates that the fracture is open.

Selection of a repair procedure for tibial fractures depends on the type and location of the fracture, the age of the animal, the presence of associated soft tissue defects or infection, and economic considerations. Closed reduction with the application of a cast or coaptation bandage, Kirschner–Ehmer apparatus, intramedullary pinning, and plating can all be used successfully in properly selected cases. The procedure chosen should neutralize the forces acting on the fracture (i.e., bending, rotation, shear, and compression forces).

Proximal Fractures

Fractures of the proximal tibia generally involve the physis in young animals and the metaphysis in mature animals. Physeal injuries (Salter–Harris fractures) and avulsion fractures occur most commonly.

Avulsion Fractures

The tibial tuberosity and the insertions of the cruciate ligaments and collateral ligaments are subject to avulsion fractures in the immature animal. Avulsion of the tibial tuberosity occurs with hyperflexion of the stifle and causes pain and swelling of the stifle and a reluctance or inability to bear weight. This type of fracture is best demonstrated on a lateral radiograph, especially when the leg is flexed. Care should be taken not to mistake the normally wide growth plate in the immature animal for a fracture. With an avulsion fracture, the smooth contour of the cranial tibia is disrupted, and the patella may be displaced proximally (Fig. 55.26A). If any doubt exists about the diagnosis, radio-

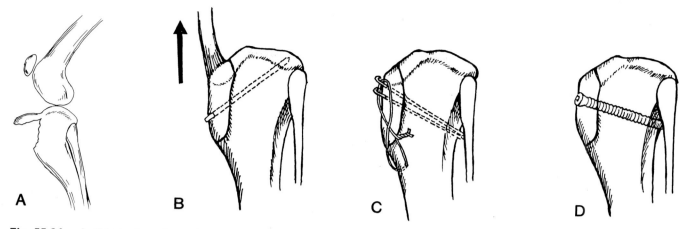

Fig. 55.26. **A.** Tibial tuberosity avulsions alter the normal contour of the cranial tibia. Avulsions can be repaired with pins (**B**), pins and tension band wires (**C**), or lag screws (**D**). Note the direction of pin insertion in **B** to counteract the pull of the quadriceps mechanism. (**B–D** from Sinibaldi KR. Fractures of the tibia. In: Bojrab MJ, ed. Current techniques in small animal surgery. 2nd ed. Philadelphia: Lea & Febiger, 1983.)

graphs of the opposite limb should be taken for comparison.

Avulsion fractures of the proximal tibia are repaired through a lateral parapatellar approach. Extending the leg makes reduction easier by relieving the pull of the quadriceps mechanisms. AO reduction forceps or a similar instrument is helpful for maintaining reduction while the fracture is repaired with pins (or Kirschner wires, depending on the size of the animal), pins and tension band wire, or a lag screw (Fig. 55.26**B–D**). The choice of technique should take into account the size of the animal and the remaining growth potential. If pins are used as the sole method of repair, they should be inserted in a dorsocaudal direction to counteract the considerable pull of the quadriceps mechanism (Fig. 55.26**B**).

The stifle joint should be evaluated carefully for concurrent ligamentous or meniscal damage. Avulsion of the cruciate ligament insertions and collateral ligament avulsions are discussed in Chapter 62.

Physeal Fractures

Fractures of the proximal growth plate (Salter–Harris fractures) occur in immature animals, in which the physis is weaker than the ligaments supporting the stifle. Salter I and II fractures are most commonly seen. Because the contour of the proximal tibia is irregular and the fracture segments interdigitate, these fractures can be managed by closed reduction and application of a cast or coaptation bandage for 3 to 4 weeks if they are treated soon after injury. The owner should be warned of the possibility of premature closure of the physis and deformity if significant growth potential remains. Premature closure usually is visible radiographically by 2 to 3 weeks after injury.

Fractures that cannot be reduced in a closed manner, unstable Salter I and II fractures, and Salter III and IV fractures (articular surface involved) should be managed by open reduction. The type of implant chosen for stabilization depends in part on the remaining potential for growth. Single or multiple parallel smooth Steinmann pins (smaller than $\frac{5}{32}$ inches) cause minimal damage to the physis and retardation of growth if they are removed as soon as the fracture is healed (generally by 4 weeks). Screw fixation generally is avoided unless little growth remains. Pins should be inserted from the proximal fragment (near the insertion of the collateral ligaments) and directed into the opposite cortex distally (Fig. 55.27). The pins should not interfere with the motion of the stifle joint.

If an intra-articular fragment is present (Salter III

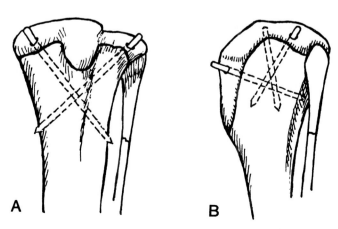

Fig. 55.27. Proximal tibial physeal fractures can be repaired with cross-pins (**A**) or multiple pins if the tibial tuberosity is also avulsed (**B**). (From Sinibaldi KR. Fractures of the tibia. In: Bojrab MJ, ed. Current techniques in small animal surgery. 2nd ed. Philadelphia: Lea & Febiger, 1983.)

or IV fracture), accurate anatomic reduction is required, and the fragment usually is stabilized with one or more lag screws (Fig. 55.28). The screws should be inserted so the physis is not crossed. Additional fixation to the distal segment is accomplished as previously described. Fractures of the proximal fibula, if present, should be repaired because of the attachment of the lateral collateral ligament and potential instability of the stifle joint.

Postoperatively, a padded bandage is applied for 7 to 10 days. After bandage removal, the animal should be kept confined until the fracture is healed, and physical therapy should be recommended.

Diaphyseal Fractures

The unusual anatomic structure of the tibia leads to a high frequency of oblique, spiral, and comminuted shaft fractures, any of which may be open. Stable closed shaft fractures in young animals can be treated by close reduction and casting. The surgeon must immobilize the joint above and below the fracture whenever casts are used. The use of casts with comminuted fractures or in older animals frequently is associated with prolonged fracture healing.

Pins and Wires

Oblique and spiral fractures with minimal comminution (e.g., butterfly fragment) are amenable to intramedullary pin fixation and cerclage wiring. Cerclage wires effectively counteract angular, shear, and rotational forces and also provide compression of the fracture segments. Because of the stresses produced by early weightbearing, cerclage wires should not be used as the sole means of fixation for tibial shaft fractures; wires usually are used in conjunction with intramedullary pins. The obliquity of the fracture line should be at least twice the diameter of the diaphysis; a minimum of two wires (18- to 20-gauge orthopedic wire)

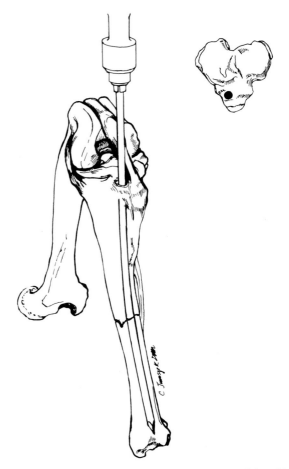

Fig. 55.29. Pin insertion in normograde pinning of the tibia for repair of transverse shaft fracture. The pin is inserted on the medial side midway between the straight patellar tendon and the medial collateral ligament. (From DeYoung DJ, Probst CW. Methods of internal fracture fixation. In: Slatter DH, ed. Textbook of small animal surgery. Philadelphia: WB Saunders, 1985.)

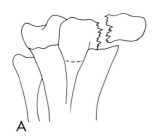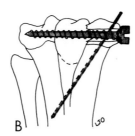

Fig. 55.28. A proximal tibial physeal fracture with an intra-articular component (**A**) is repaired by anatomic reduction of the intra-articular portion followed by insertion of lag screws and fixation to the distal segment with cross-pins (**B**). (From Gofton N. Fractures of the tibia and fibula. In: Slatter DH, ed. Textbook of small animal surgery. Philadelphia: WB Saunders, 1985.)

should be used. Looped wires work well because the wire ends can be bent against the bone without causing loosening.

Intramedullary pins should always be inserted in normograde fashion from the medial side of the proximal tibia (Fig. 55.29). The point of pin insertion is approximately midway between the straight patellar tendon and the medial collateral ligament. Because large pins are stiff, the opposite cortex often is penetrated as the pin is advanced down the S-shaped medullary canal. Penetration can be avoided by using a small pin to create a guide hole. The smaller pins deflect off the opposite cortex and continue down the medullary canal. As progressively larger pins are inserted, the guide hole is generally followed. Pins placed in retrograde fashion invariably enter the joint and may interfere with normal joint motion or may damage the menisci, patella, or femoral condyles, with consequent degenerative joint disease. Multiple small pins

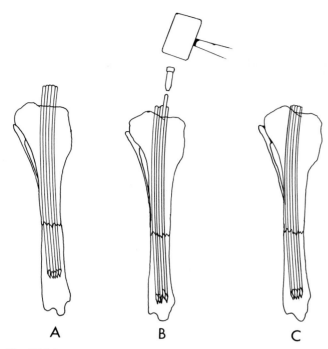

Fig. 55.30. Pinning of transverse tibial shaft fracture. After filling the medullary canal with pins (**A**), a pin setter is used to seat the pins distally (**B**). The pins can be bent and cut close to the bone (**C**).

conform to the shape of the tibia, providing a dynamic fixation and increased rotational stability. After insertion, the pins are seated with a pin setter (Fig. 55.30).

Kirschner–Ehmer Splints

A Kirschner–Ehmer (K–E) apparatus is suitable for repair of many tibial fractures. This device is particularly useful in the management of contaminated or infected open fractures or when skin loss has occurred and the wound cannot be closed. If the proper configuration is selected, a stable fixation can be achieved. Highly comminuted midshaft fractures can be stabilized without open reduction with a K–E splint. As a result, the fracture hematoma is not disturbed, and further soft-tissue trauma is not produced.

A type I K–E splint (half-pin) using a single or double connecting bar provides adequate stability for simple fractures or mildly comminuted fractures in small dogs and cats. At least two pins should be used in each fracture segment; greater stability is achieved by the addition of more pins in each segment. The greatest strength and stability are obtained when the pins are spread out over the length of the bone. All pins should engage both cortices of the bone. If only two pins are used in each segment, they are placed at diverging angles of 20 to 30° from a line perpendicular to the long axis of the bone. The most proximal and distal pins are inserted first (Fig. 55.31**A**). A connecting bar

is selected, and the clamps for all the pins are placed on the connecting bar before it is attached to the end pins (Fig. 55.31**B** and **C**). The remaining pins are inserted through the connecting clamps and into the bone (Fig. 55.31**D** and **E**). The pins are inserted through small stab incisions made with the skin in a relaxed position. The pins may be inserted with a hand chuck or power drill. Excessive wobbling of the hand chuck and high-speed insertion with power equipment causing thermal necrosis of the bone result in premature loosening of the pins.

A type II K–E splint (full-pin, through-and-through) is stronger than a type I splint and may be desired for more comminuted fractures. Although insertion of all pins parallel to each other provides a biomechanically stronger support, the pins are less likely to slide back and forth if they are inserted at slight angles (Fig. 55.32**A**). Application of a type II splint using two single connecting bars is difficult because all the pins must be inserted in the same plane if both bars are to be contacted. This technique may be modified by use of full pins on the ends and half-pins in between (Fig. 55.32**B**). This configuration is easier to apply, and because the half-pins can be inserted at various angles, the pins cannot slide back and forth.

Three-dimensional configurations provide the greatest stability (Fig. 55.33). This type of fixation generally is reserved for highly comminuted fractures, particularly in larger dogs.

Bone Plates

Plate fixation is stable and is recommended for comminuted shaft fractures as long as the proximal and distal fragments are long enough to allow at least two and preferably three screws in each end. In addition, sufficient soft tissue should be present to allow the plate to be covered. Plates usually are applied to the medial side of the tibia because of the ease of exposure. The plate should extend from metaphysis to metaphysis. Comminuted fractures are first reconstructed with lag screws or cerclage wires before plating. Fractures near the proximal metaphysis can be repaired with T plates (Fig. 55.34**A**). Fractures near the distal metaphysis can be repaired with hook plates if the distal fragment is not long enough for normal plate application (Fig. 55.34**B**). If fracture gaps exist, the use of cancellous bone grafts should be considered in conjunction with the reconstruction.

Distal Fractures

Distal fractures consist of Salter–Harris fractures (in immature animals) and malleolar fractures. Type I and II Salter–Harris fractures that can be reduced closed

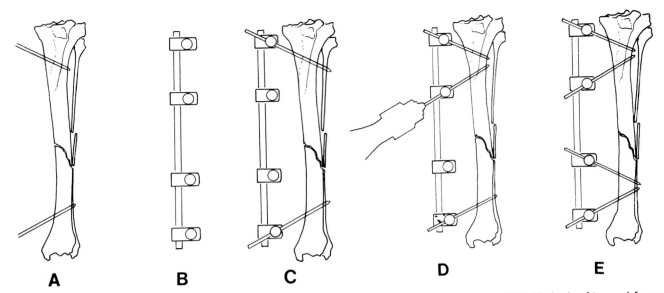

Fig. 55.31. A-E. Application of a type I Kirschner–Ehmer apparatus. (From DeYoung DJ, Probst CW. Methods of internal fracture fixation. In: Slatter DH, ed. Textbook of small animal surgery. Philadelphia: WB Saunders, 1985.)

may be treated by cast fixation if stable. Unstable fractures or fractures that require open reduction respond well to fixation by cross-pinning (Fig. 55.35**A** and **B**). The easiest method of pin insertion is through bilateral skin incisions made over the malleoli. Care must be

taken to angle the pins correctly to avoid entering the joint because the malleoli extend farther distally than the articular surface. If the distal segment is too small for cross-pinning, a single transarticular pin may be placed to stabilize the fracture. This is achieved by plac-

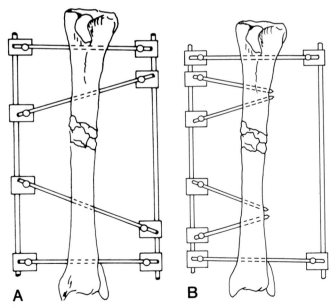

Fig. 55.32. A. Type II Kirschner–Ehmer splint with all pins connected to both bars. **B.** Modified Type II Kirschner–Ehmer splint with full pins placed at each end and half-pins placed in between. (**A,** from Egger EL. Static strength evaluation of six external skeletal fixation configurations. Vet Surg 1983;12:130; **B,** from Egger EL, Greenwood KM. External skeletal fixation. In: Slatter DH, ed. Textbook of small animal surgery. Philadelphia: WB Saunders, 1985.)

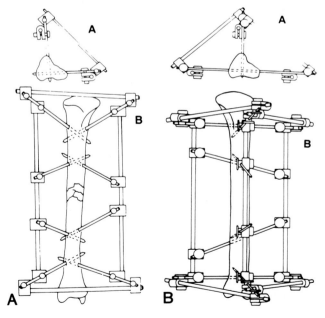

Fig. 55.33. Three-dimensional Kirschner–Ehmer splints produced by joining two type I Kirschner–Ehmer splints placed at a 90° angle (*left*) and by combining a full-pin and half-pin splint (*right*). **A.** View along long axis of shaft. **B.** Lateral view. (From Egger EL. Static strength evaluation of six external skeletal fixation configurations. Vet Surg 1983;12:130.)

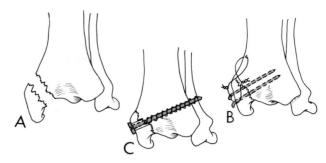

Fig. 55.36. An avulsion fracture of the medial malleolus (**A**) can be repaired with Kirschner wires and tension band wires (**B**) or with lag screws (**C**). (From Gofton N. Fractures of the tibia and fibula. In: Slatter DH, ed. Textbook of small animal surgery. Philadelphia: WB Saunders, 1985.)

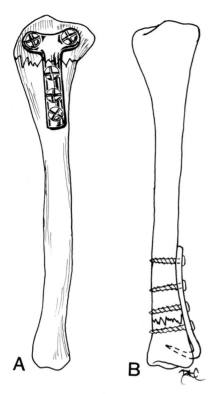

Fig. 55.34. **A.** Repair of a proximal metaphyseal fracture with a T plate. **B.** Repair of a distal metaphyseal fracture with a hook plate.

ing the animal's hock in a normal walking angle (115 to 125° for the cat; 125 to 145° for the dog) and then driving a Steinmann pin from the talus into the medullary cavity of the tibia (Fig. 55.35**C**). This technique is less desirable than cross-pinning because of the possibility of development of degenerative joint disease. This fixation must be supported with a cast, or the pin will break.

Malleolar fractures should be repaired because of the collateral ligaments that attach to them. If these fractures are difficult to diagnose from plain films, stress films are helpful. Accurate reduction and stable fixation are necessary to reduce the occurrence of degenerative joint disease. Stabilization with Kirschner wires and a figure-of-eight tension band wire is effective for medial and lateral malleolar fractures; a lag screw also may be used (Fig. 55.36). Care must be taken to avoid the joint when inserting the implants.

Distal tibial fractures should be supported with a coaptation bandage for 3 to 4 weeks postoperatively. A soft padded bandage can be used for an additional 1 to 2 weeks to limit use of the limb if desired. The bandages should be changed at 5- to 7-day intervals, and physical therapy should be given at that time to decrease joint stiffness.

Suggested Readings

Campbell CJ, Grisola A, Zanconato G. The effects produced in the cartilagenous epiphyseal plate of immature dogs by experimental surgical traumata. J Bone Joint Surg 1959;4:1221.

DeYoung DJ, Probst CW. Methods of fracture fixation. In: Slatter DH, ed. Textbook of small animal surgery. Philadelphia: WB Saunders, 1985.

Egger EL. Static strength evaluation of six external skeletal fixation configurations. Vet Surg 1983;12:130.

Gofton N. Fractures of the tibia and fibula. In: Slatter DH, ed. Textbook of small animal surgery. Philadelphia: WB Saunders, 1985.

Phillips IR. A survey of long bone fractures in the dog and cat. J Small Anim Pract 1979;20:661.

Sinibaldi KR. Fractures of the tibia. In: Bojrab MJ, ed. Current techniques in small animal surgery. 2nd ed. Philadelphia: Lea & Febiger, 1983.

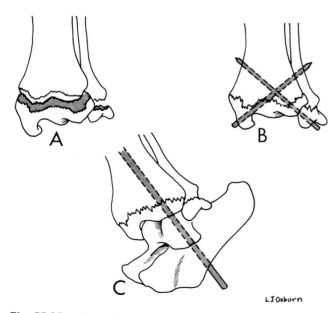

Fig. 55.35. A distal tibial physeal fracture (**A**) can be repaired with cross-pins (**B**) or a single transarticular pin (**C**). (From Gofton N. Fractures of the tibia and fibula. In: Slatter DH, ed. Textbook of small animal surgery. Philadelphia: WB Saunders, 1985.)

—•56•—

ARTHROCENTESIS AND SYNOVIAL FLUID ANALYSIS

Scott M. Lozier & Michele Menard

Arthrocentesis

Normal synovial fluid is a plasma dialysate (1). The synovium acts as a filter preventing plasma proteins of high molecular weight from entering the joint fluid while hyaluronic acid is secreted by type II synoviocytes (1). Pathologic joint conditions may interfere with these processes, resulting in altered synovial fluid composition. Examination of the fluid can provide clues to the nature of the joint disorder. With the exception of readily detectable sepsis, synovial fluid analysis does not usually yield a specific diagnosis. Rather, the value of synovial fluid analysis lies in classifying arthropathies as inflammatory or noninflammatory (2–5). In so doing, this information, combined with the historical, physical, and radiographic findings, helps to narrow the list of differential diagnoses and directs subsequent diagnostic testing.

Synovial fluid collection is minimally invasive. In most cases, successful aspiration can be performed easily, quickly, and with minor expense. Arthrocentesis should therefore be a standard skill and a routine part of a thorough diagnostic joint evaluation. Indications for performing arthrocentesis include painful or effusive joint conditions of unknown origin.

Collection Method

Synovial fluid potentially can be harvested from any diarthrodial joint. The most commonly aspirated joints include the tarsus, carpus, stifle, shoulder, elbow, and hip. A 1-inch, 22-gauge needle and a 3-mL syringe are used most commonly. A 2- to 3-inch, 22-gauge spinal needle may be required for the hip joint in large or obese dogs. A 23- or 25-gauge needle with a 1-mL syringe may be used for distal joints of cats and small dogs.

Minimizing patient motion during collection aids in preventing sample contamination by peripheral blood. The degree of manual and chemical restraint should correspond to the temperament of the patient and the degree of difficulty of the aspiration site. Arthrocentesis of severely effusive, distal limb joints with palpable joint capsule distension seldom requires sedation or anesthesia. A minimal hair clip and thorough surgical preparation of the target site should be performed. When possible, digital pressure placed over portions of the joint adjacent to the target site causes the joint capsule to bulge and facilitates aspiration. Less effusive and more proximal joints often require a more extensive hair clip and surgical preparation to allow palpation of the anatomic landmarks without contaminating the target site. Sterile gloves should be worn during these procedures. Draping of the site is not necessary. Sedation or anesthesia may be required when a more difficult aspiration is to be attempted. Neuroleptanalgesia produced by the combination of 0.05 mg/kg acepromazine (acepromazine maleate injection, Fermenta Animal Health Co., Kansas City, MO) and 0.05 mg/kg oxymorphone (Numorphan) administered intravenously generally provides a profound state of relaxation suitable for most aspirations. The opiate can be reversed quickly with the pure antagonist naloxone, administered intravenously at a dose of 0.015 mg/kg. The mildly sedated patient may then be returned to the owners within minutes of completing the procedure. If needed, 2 to 6 mg/kg of propofol (Diprivan), administered intravenously to effect, may be added to the regimen to induce short-term general anesthesia. Anesthesia may be prolonged by readministering propofol or administering isoflurane (IsoFlo, Solvay Animal Health, Inc., Mendota Heights, MN) by endotracheal tube or mask. Recovery is rapid from these protocols, and patients still can be discharged early.

Aspiration Sites

Joint disease may be classified as monarticular, pauciarticular, or polyarticular. Immunologic joint disease is more frequently polyarticular or pauciarticular and often follows a distal joint distribution (6). Septic joints are frequently pauciarticular or monarticular (6). When multiple joint involvement is clinically evident or suspected, diagnostic information is enhanced by multiple joint aspiration. Knowledge of the local anatomy surrounding the target joint is important to minimize blood contamination of the sample, which can severely compromise the diagnostic quality of the joint fluid. If blood is seen within the hub of the needle before entering the joint, the needle should be changed. The needle should be aimed carefully toward the joint space such that minimal or no redirection is necessary. Needle redirection and wobble may lacerate blood vessels or articular cartilage. Ideally, the syringe plunger should not be withdrawn until the joint space has been penetrated. Minimal suction is needed to withdraw fluid. If redirection is required, all suction should be released. Once an adequate amount of fluid is obtained, the syringe plunger is released before the needle is withdrawn.

CARPUS

Carpal joint fluid is most commonly accessed through a dorsomedial site over the radiocarpal joint. The carpus is partially flexed to allow palpation of the joint space, and the needle is placed just distal to the radius, roughly parallel to the radial articular surface (Fig. 56.1). Synovial fluid collection from intercarpal and carpometacarpal joints is occasionally required. These joints interconnect but do not communicate with the radiocarpal joint. Fluid is most readily obtained from the space between the second and third carpal bones. Access is gained through the dorsal surface directly over the space (Fig. 56.1). Slight flexion facilitates aspiration.

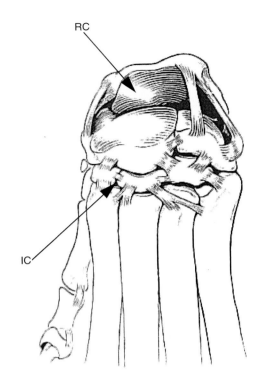

Fig. 56.1. View of the dorsal aspect of the left carpus in a flexed position showing sites for arthrocentesis. *RC,* radiocarpal; *IC,* intercarpal joint.

ELBOW

With severe joint effusions of the elbow, the caudomedial and caudolateral pouches can be detected. Direct puncture of either pouch is easily accomplished. When minimal effusions are present, joint fluid retrieval from the elbow can be difficult. Sedation or anesthesia is often necessary. With the joint in a partially flexed position, the needle is inserted from a proximal caudal position along the lateral surface of the joint between the lateral humeral epicondyle and the apex of the anconeal process of the ulna. The needle is directed medially toward the olecranon fossa (Fig. 56.2).

SHOULDER

The greater tubercle of the humerus and the acromion process of the scapula are included in the skin preparation and are used as palpation landmarks. Flexion and extension of the joint help to define the joint space. The needle is inserted proximal to the greater tubercle and craniodistal to the acromion. The needle is directed slightly distally and caudally. Sedation is recommended for arthrocentesis of this joint (Fig. 56.3).

TARSUS

Tarsal joint fluid is most easily collected from the tarsocrural joint. With effusive joints, dorsolateral, planterolateral, dorsomedial, and planteromedial joint dis-

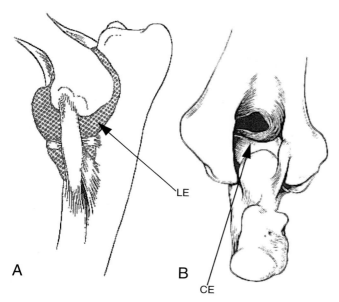

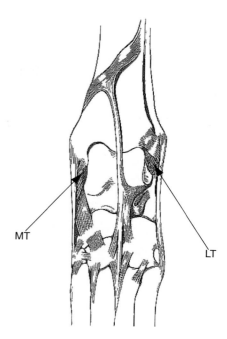

Fig. 56.2. **A.** Lateral view of the left elbow. *LE*, arthrocentesis site for the lateral aspect of the elbow joint. **B.** Caudal view of the left elbow. *CE*, arthrocentesis site for the caudal aspect of the elbow joint.

Fig. 56.4. Dorsal view of the left tarsus: arthrocentesis sites for the tarsus. *LT*, lateral aspect of the talocrural joint; *MT*, medial aspect of the talocrural joint.

tension can be appreciated. Any of these sites is suitable for aspiration. In less effusive joints, the dorsolateral joint pouch is the site from which a "clean" sample is most easily obtained. From a cranial approach, the needle is aimed toward the joint space between the lateral malleolus of the fibula and the

talus (Fig. 56.4). Similar craniomedial and caudolateral approaches may also be attempted.

STIFLE

The stifle is clipped to allow palpation of the patella, tibial tuberosity, and medial or lateral femoral condyle. Flexion of the joint favors fluid distension of the cranial aspect of the joint capsule. Pressure medial or lateral to the patellar ligament may cause the joint capsule to bulge on the opposite side of the joint. The needle is placed two-thirds of the distance from the patella to the tibial tuberosity and just lateral or medial to the patellar ligament. The needle is directed slightly proximally and centrally toward the intercondylar region (Fig. 56.5). Sedation is recommended for patients undergoing stifle aspiration unless an effusion is obvious.

HIP

The hip may be difficult to aspirate. Sedation or anesthesia is usually required. Lateral and ventral approaches have been described (5). For lateral aspiration, the region around the greater tubercle is clipped and scrubbed. With the patient in lateral recumbency and the limb slightly abducted, the needle is placed just proximal to the greater trochanter and is directed medially and slightly distally toward the dorsal rim of the acetabulum. Slight distal limb traction may aid in allowing entrance into the joint in minimally effusive conditions (Fig. 56.6). Ventral aspiration of the hip is

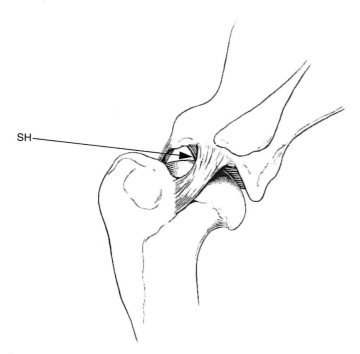

Fig. 56.3. Lateral view of the left shoulder. *SH*, site for arthrocentesis from scapulohumeral joint.

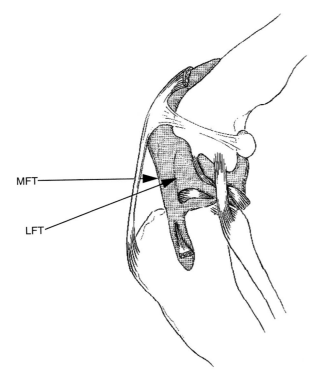

Fig. 56.5. Lateral view of the left stifle: sites for arthrocentesis from the femorotibial joint. *LFT,* lateral aspect of the femorotibial joint; *MFT,* medial aspect of the femorotibial joint.

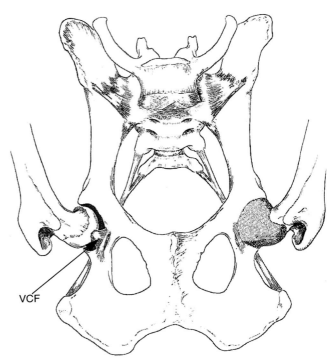

Fig. 56.7. Ventral view of the pelvis and coxofemoral joints. *VCF,* site for arthrocentesis from the ventral aspect of the coxofemoral joint.

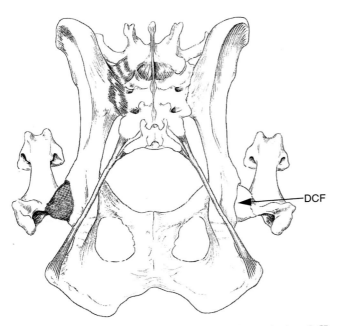

Fig. 56.6. Dorsal view of the pelvis and coxofemoral joints. *DCF,* site for arthrocentesis from the dorsal aspect of the coxofemoral joint.

achieved with the patient in dorsal recumbency. The femur is abducted and is held perpendicular to the ventral midline. The origin of the pectineus can be palpated on the iliopectineal eminence of the pelvis. The acetabular fossa lies just caudal and medial to the origin of the pectineus. The needle is directed caudal to cranial into the joint space and may encounter some resistance as it passes through the ligament of the head of the femur (Fig. 56.7). With either approach, care should be taken to avoid the caudal aspect of the joint because of the proximity of the sciatic nerve.

Sample Handling

Normal joints yield little joint fluid. The amount of fluid collected varies with the dog's size, the joint aspirated, the degree and type of joint disease present, and technique of the sampler. The average amount of joint fluid collected from stifles of normal dogs in one study was 0.24 mL (2). Large quantities of fluid are not needed for synovial fluid evaluation. Harvesting a small but adequate amount of "clean" joint fluid is better than risking blood contamination of the sample by probing with the needle for more fluid. If a small amount of fluid is obtained, one or two smears are made for cytologic evaluation. The syringe may then be swabbed or capped for bacterial culture and sensitivity testing. Air in the syringe should be expelled if the sample is also submitted for anaerobic bacterial culture. If a larger amount of fluid is obtained, some fluid should be placed in an ethylenediaminetetra-acetic acid tube and submitted along with a direct smear for a complete fluid analysis.

Synovial Fluid Analysis

Routine synovial fluid analysis includes a nucleated cell count and a concentrated and direct smear evaluation. If volume is sufficient, a mucin clot test and total protein evaluation can also be performed. If a single drop of fluid is obtained, a smear is made for an estimated nucleated cell count, nucleated cell differential, and screening for infectious organisms. The volume of the sample, appearance, blood contamination during sample collection, and viscosity should also be noted when the sample is collected.

Appearance

Normal synovial fluid is clear and colorless. Swirling blood in the fluid indicates contamination from a traumatic tap. A homogeneous pink-to-reddish fluid or turbid fluid is found with hemorrhage, including blood contamination during sample collection and noninflammatory and inflammatory arthropathies. Xanthochromia, a yellowish color imparted to the fluid by erythrocyte degradation, indicates previous hemorrhage.

Viscosity

The viscosity of synovial fluid is imparted by hyaluronic acid, a mucopolysaccharide secreted by synovial cells. Viscosity can be evaluated by slowly expressing a drop of synovial fluid from a needle attached to a syringe held horizontally or by placing a drop of fluid between the thumb and forefinger and spreading them apart. A string longer than 2.5 cm before breaking is seen with normal viscosity. Degradation of hyaluronic acid by bacterial hyaluronidase or by neutrophilic lysosomal enzymes and dilutional effect of increased synovial fluid production can decrease the viscosity of synovial fluid.

Nucleated Cell Count

The nucleated cell count is done by the unipette technique (unipette No. 58550 for platelet or leukocyte counts, Becton–Dickinson, Rutherford, NJ) and with a hemacytometer. Diluents with acetic acid should be avoided because they clot the sample. Normal synovial fluid in dogs usually contains less than 1500 cells/μL,

although a value of up to 3000 cells/μL is considered normal.

Cytologic Evaluation

This evaluation is the most important aspect of synovial fluid analysis. Normal synovial fluid is composed of more than 90% poorly vacuolated mononuclear cells. Occasional neutrophils and large vacuolated mononuclear cells can be observed. The background has a fine eosinophilic granular proteinaceous texture caused by hyaluronic acid precipitation and should not be confused with bacteria.

Total Protein

The protein content is only measured after the other tests have been performed and a sufficient amount of sample is still available. This count is usually made with a refractometer. The protein content of synovial fluid can be increased with hemorrhage and inflammation.

Mucin Clot Test

This acid precipitation test evaluates the quality of the synovial fluid hyaluronic acid polymerization. This test is also affected, although to a lesser degree, by the quantity of hyaluronic acid in the synovial fluid. It is usually affected by the same causes that decrease the viscosity of synovial fluid, and it is only performed if a sufficient sample remains after fluid analysis.

Synovial Fluid Analysis Interpretation

Synovial fluid analysis is usually classified in two main categories: noninflammatory and inflammatory arthropathies.

NONINFLAMMATORY ARTHROPATHIES

These conditions include degenerative joint disease, traumatic arthropathies, and hemarthrosis. Neoplasia involving the joint cavity usually causes a noninflammatory arthropathy, although it occasionally is associated with an inflammatory arthropathy. The volume of fluid may vary from normal to increased. The color, turbidity, and viscosity are usually normal. The viscosity is occasionally decreased if a large amount of effusion is present with dilution of hyaluronic acid (hydrarthrosis). The nucleated cell count is normal to slightly increased (usually less than 10,000/μL), with a predominance of mononuclear cells. Large vacuolated mononuclear cells can be increased (more than 10% of the mononuclear cells). Neutrophils and erythrocytes may be slightly increased. Cartilage fragments, osteoblasts, and osteoclasts are occasionally seen in severe cases. Synovial fluid analysis is within normal limits in a many animals with degenerative joint disease and traumatic arthropathies.

True hemarthrosis is rare and must be distinguished from iatrogenic blood contamination during sample collection. Iatrogenic blood contamination is usually associated with fluid free of blood at the beginning of sample collection with subsequent blood contamination during the collection procedure. After centrifugation, the supernatant of iatrogenically contaminated samples is clear. In true hemarthrosis, the supernatant is yellow or reddish because of erythrocyte degradation. The nucleated cell count is similar or mildly increased compared with peripheral blood, and leukocytes can be hypersegmented. Platelets are decreased or absent, and macrophages show evidence of phagocytosis of erythrocytes and contain hemosiderin pigments. The viscosity is decreased from the dilution effect, and the mucin clot quality is variable. Hemarthrosis can be caused by trauma or coagulopathies, especially hemophilia A or hemophilia B. Hemorrhage associated with degenerative and inflammatory arthropathy is usually mild when compared with that in true hemarthrosis.

INFLAMMATORY ARTHROPATHIES

These disorders can be divided into two groups: infectious and immune-mediated. The differentiation between these two groups is usually not possible by cytologic study unless infectious organisms are seen on the smears, as only applies to a small portion of inflammatory arthropathies. Inflammatory arthropathies are associated with a moderate to marked increase of nucleated cells (usually greater than 10,000/L), which are predominantly neutrophils in good morphologic condition. Mild to moderate hemorrhage may also be present. The fluid is often creamy or pink and turbid because of the large number of neutrophils. The viscosity and mucin clot are variable but often poor, and the protein content is often elevated.

Immune-mediated polyarthropathies are usually a diagnosis of exclusion, after having ruled out an infectious polyarthropathy. Bacterial culture should be performed for all inflammatory arthropathies. The most common infectious organisms isolated from synovial fluid are *Staphylococcus* spp., *Streptococcus* spp., and coliform bacteria. A negative culture does not rule out an infectious arthropathy. Serologic examination for canine ehrlichiosis and Lyme disease and fungal cultures are indicated if the animal has been in an area where these disorders are endemic. Blood cultures should be performed when a systemic infection is suspected. A thorough evaluation for an underlying infection, including bacterial endocarditis, discospondylitis, sublumbar abscess, and respiratory or urinary tract infection should also be performed. Positive antinuclear antibody (ANA) testing can further support an immune-mediated arthropathy, although a large proportion of these patients are ANA negative. The rheumatoid factor test is not specific for rheumatoid arthritis and can be affected by several infectious and immune-mediated disorders. The diagnosis of rheumatoid arthritis is usually based on synovial fluid analysis and radiographic abnormalities. LE cells are rarely seen in synovial fluid from patients with systemic lupus erythematosus. Most cases of immune-mediated polyarthropathies are idiopathic, and the diagnosis is usually based on negative cultures, negative serologic findings and no exposure, lack of response to antibiotic therapy, and marked improvement with immunosuppressive therapy.

References

1. Parry BW. Synovial fluid. In: Cowell RL, Tyler RD, eds. Diagnostic cytology of the dog and cat. Goleta, CA: American Veterinary Publications, 1989:121–136.
2. Wallace LJ. Invasive diagnostic techniques. In: Whittick WG, ed. Canine orthopedics. 2nd ed. Philadelphia: Lea & Febiger 1990: 104–120.
3. Pedersen, NC. Synovial fluid collection and analysis. Vet Clin North Am 1978;8:495–499.
4. French TW. Basic synovial fluid analysis. In: Proceedings of the 8th American College of Veterinary Internal Medicine Forum.: American College of Veterinary Internal Medicine, 1990:29–32.
5. Hardy RM, Wallace LJ. Arthrocentesis and synovial membrane biopsy. Vet Clin North Am 1974;4:449–459.
6. Breitschwerdt EB. Infectious polyarthritis. In: North American Veterinary Conference Proceedings., 1994:305–306.

Suggested Readings

Bennett D. Immune-based erosive inflammatory joint disease of the dog: canine rheumatoid arthritis. J Small Anim Pract 1987; 28:779–797.
Bennett D, May C. Joint diseases of dogs and cats. In: Ettinger SJ, Feldman EC, eds. Textbook of veterinary internal medicine. 4th ed. Philadelphia: WB Saunders, 1995:2032–2077.
Bennett D, Taylor DJ. Bacterial infective arthritis in the dog. J Small Anim Pract 1988;29:207–230.
Montgomery RD, Long IR, Milton JL, et al. Comparison of aerobic culturette, synovial membrane biopsy, and blood culture medium in detection of canine bacterial arthritis. Vet Surg 1989;18:300–303.
Pedersen NC. Collection and analysis of canine synovial fluid. Pamphlet No. GP 5553B 80011. St. Louis: Ralston Purina, 1981: 1–10.

— 57 —

SHOULDER

Algorithms for Diagnosis and Treatment of Shoulder Disorders

R. Jeffrey Todoroff

Figures 57.1 through 57.5 are algorithms for the diagnosis and management of disorders of the shoulder.

Specific Diagnostic Tests of the Shoulder

Sharon Ullman & R. Jeffrey Todoroff

Specific diagnostic tests of the shoulder joint can be divided into four major categories: physical examination tests, radiographic views, arthrographic views, and joint tap evaluations. Each of these tests, when

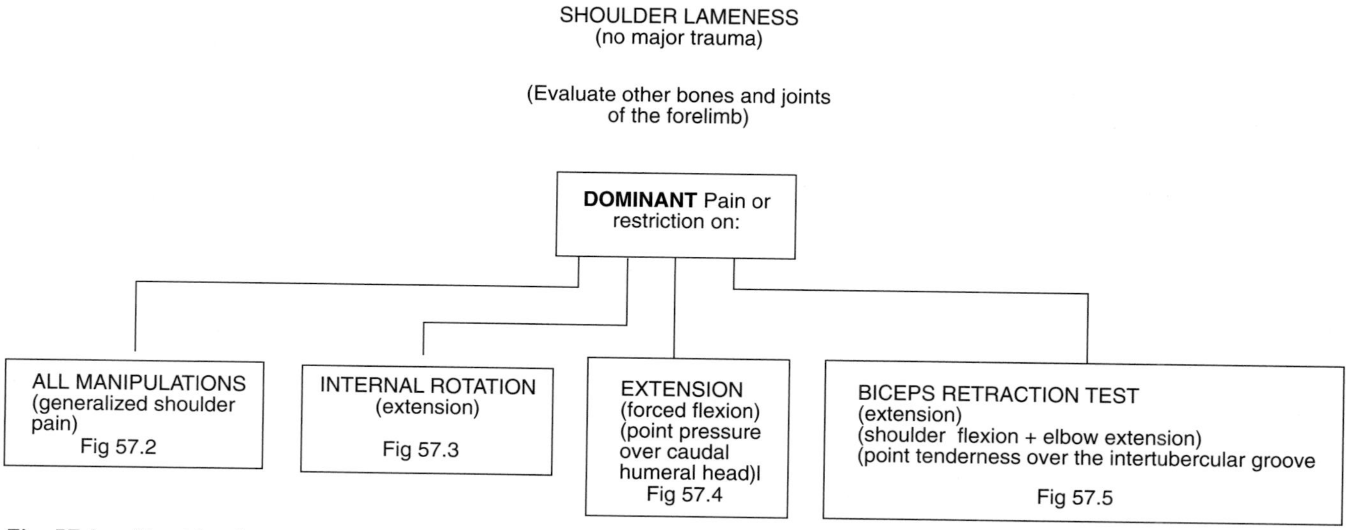

SHOULDER LAMENESS
(no major trauma)

(Evaluate other bones and joints
of the forelimb)

DOMINANT Pain or
restriction on:

| ALL MANIPULATIONS (generalized shoulder pain) Fig 57.2 | INTERNAL ROTATION (extension) Fig 57.3 | EXTENSION (forced flexion) (point pressure over caudal humeral head)l Fig 57.4 | BICEPS RETRACTION TEST (extension) (shoulder flexion + elbow extension) (point tenderness over the intertubercular groove Fig 57.5 |

Fig. 57.1. Algorithm for management of shoulder lameness. Shoulder lameness is typified by general signs of forelimb lameness (head-bobbing with lifting of the head as the affected limb strikes the ground, shortened stride, and variable atrophy of the supraspinatus and infraspinatus muscles), with point tenderness, pain, or restriction to manipulation of the shoulder itself. Muscle injuries such as tearing of the deltoideus, deep pectoral, or long head of the triceps bracii muscle occur in racing greyhounds and are associated with a palpable defect, swelling, and tenderness. An occasional dog or cat may tear the serratus ventralis muscle, resulting in upward displacement of the scapula. The uncommon injuries are usually repaired primarily to maintain optimal function and are not discussed in this algorithm.

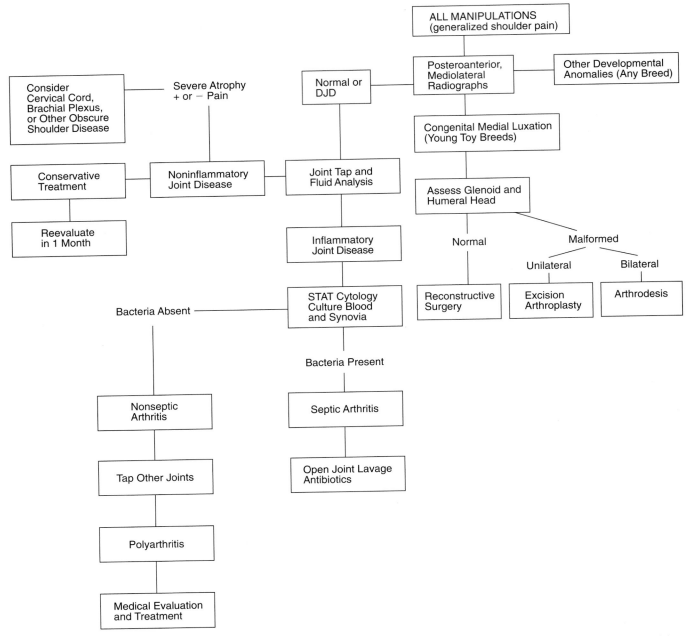

Fig. 57.2. Specific lesions in the differential diagnosis include cervical intervertebral disc extrusion with root signature, discospondylitis, and neoplasia of the vertebrae, spinal cord, or nerve roots; neoplasia of the brachial plexus or other axillary soft tissues; infection or neoplasia of the proximal humerus or scapula; and synovial cell sarcoma of the shoulder joint. Anesthesia or deep sedation is required for animals undergoing radiography. *DJD*, degenerative joint disease.

performed in an appropriate sequence, can aid in the diagnosis of all shoulder abnormalities.

Gait Analysis

Injury to the shoulder or biceps mechanism typically causes a weightbearing lameness with a shortened an-terior stride and resultant "head-bob." Severe injury to the shoulder, including fractures, may cause a non-weightbearing lameness of the affected limb.

The first step in diagnosing the cause of lameness is to determine which limb is affected and specifically which joint is involved. By watching an animal move, before physical examination, one can gather informa-

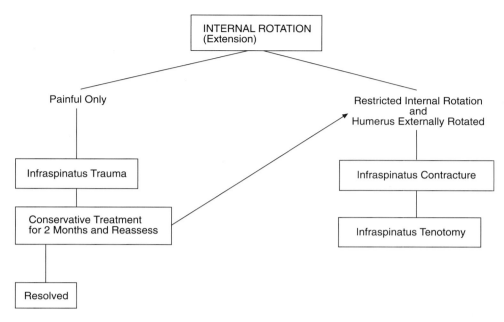

Fig. 57.3. Internal rotation algorithm.

tion on the range of motion of each joint in the limb. Contracture of the infraspinatus tendon is a diagnosis made by physical examination. When standing, an affected dog holds the elbow in adduction and the shoulder in abduction with the antebrachium outwardly rotated. During walking, the affected limb is advanced with lateral circumduction.

Point Tenderness Over the Biceps Tendon of Origin

Pressure over the intertubercular groove can elicit a pain response in dogs with inflammation or injury of the biceps mechanism or bicipital tenosynovitis. The test is best performed with the examiner standing alongside the dog on the side to be tested. The dog's left elbow is flexed and held in the examiner's left hand, which lightly can rotate the shoulder externally. The tip of the index finger of the examiner's right hand can then be pressed medial to the greater tubercle of the humerus and can also be pressed in the direction of the supraglenoid tubercle. The right side is tested similarly (with the examiner's hands reversed). A positive test is evidence of discomfort when point pressure is applied. The dog may retract the limb, stop panting, or vocalize.

The biceps tendon and its associated structures lie deep to the pectoral and brachiocephalicus muscles. Pressure on these structures may also yield a pain response (false-positive test). The presence of these mus-

cles may also shield the biceps tendon from the direct pressure (false-negative test).

Biceps Retraction Test

This test consists of traction on the tendon of insertion of the biceps and is performed with the dog in a standing position. The examiner stands just behind or to the side of the dog and reaches underneath the dog's chest to curl the fingers of the right hand around the left biceps tendon of insertion just medial to the elbow (and vice versa).

This most specific test of the biceps mechanism consists of the supraglenoid tubercle, the biceps brachii tendon or origin, the synovium adjacent to the tendon ("biceps bursa"), the intertubercular ligament, the muscle itself, and its tendon of insertion. The tendon of insertion is normally a tense cord; retracting it with the curled fingers permits the examiner to test for tenderness and laxity without otherwise moving the shoulder joint itself. A positive test merely indicates the presence of pain of the biceps mechanism. It does not define source or location. A snap or a click may be elicited in luxation of the tendon of origin with this test.

Biceps Stretch Test

The examiner stands next to the dog on the side to be tested. The shoulder is slowly flexed to maximum flexion with the dog's elbow held 90° to the humerus.

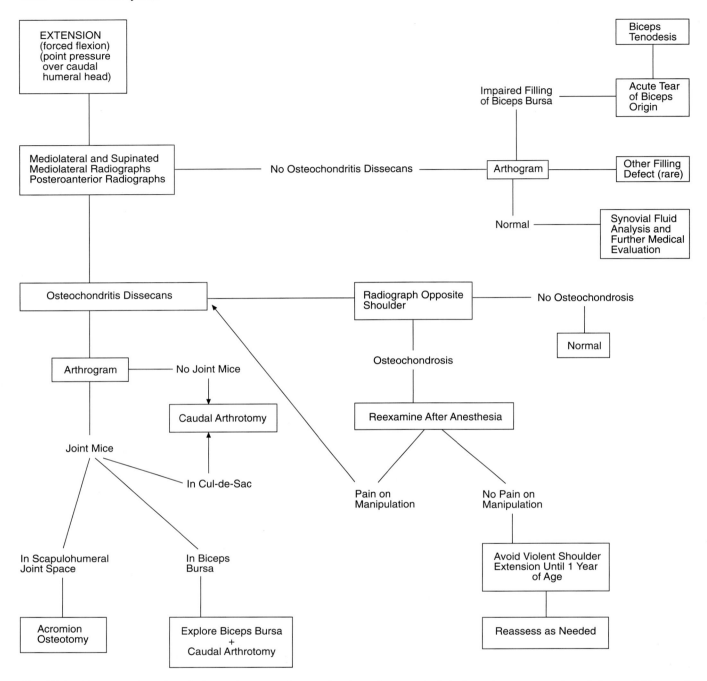

Fig. 57.4. Extension algorithm. Radiographic signs of osteochondritis dissecans include flattening or excavation of the caudal humeral head, subchondral sclerosis under the cartilage flap, mineralization of the cartilage flap itself, and occasionally mineralization of joint mice. Anesthesia or deep sedation is required for animals undergoing radiography.

The elbow is then extended fully along the dog's side. A positive test is evidenced by reproducible tenderness as the elbow is repeatedly extended and flexed. Retraction of the biceps tendon of insertion can be added to stress the biceps apparatus further.

This test stretches the biceps to its greatest length, revealing tenderness in many dogs with abnormalities of the biceps mechanism. The elbow must be tested for pain on extension before performing this test. Otherwise, elbow pain may be confused with a positive biceps stretch test. Dogs with severe elbow arthrosis and restricted elbow extension cannot be tested in this manner. Supraspinatus tendon pain may also be elicited as the shoulder is flexed.

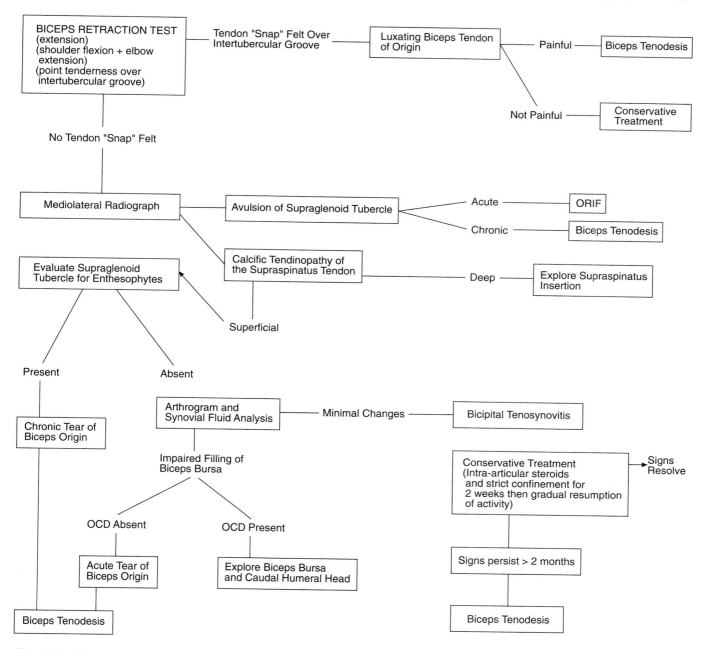

Fig. 57.5. Biceps retraction test algorithm. Deep mineralizations of the supraspinatus tendon are superimposed on the greater tubercle in the area of the intertubercular groove and impinge on the biceps tendon. Superficial mineralization is seen near the margin of the greater tubercle and is of no known significance. (See Krieglander H. Mineralization of the supraspinatus tendon: clinical observations in seven dogs. Vet Comparative Orthop Traumatology 1995;8:91–97.) *OCD,* osteochondritis dissecans; *ORIF,* open reduction with internal fixation.

Caudocranial and Mediolateral Shoulder Radiography

Standard radiographic views are made to evaluate the shoulder for many common abnormalities. Sedation or anesthesia is strongly recommended for adequate positioning. The caudocranial view is helpful in evalu-

ating luxations and fractures, but it is rarely helpful in the diagnosis of abnormalities of the biceps mechanism or the humeral head. The diagnosis of osteochondritis dissecans can usually be made on the basis of a good-quality plain mediolateral radiograph. A second lateral radiograph, underexposed by 5 kVp, is helpful in defining the presence of osteophytes, osteochondral fragments, or mineralizations about the intertubercular groove. Other abnormalities easily diagnosed by plain radiographs include avulsion of the supraglenoid tubercle and calcific tendinopathy of the supraspinatus.

Cranioproximal–Craniodistal Radiography

This view is obtained with a sedated animal positioned in sternal recumbency. The shoulder and elbow are hyperflexed while the radius and ulna are positioned along the thoracic wall. A radiographic cassette is placed parallel to the radiographic table on the cranial surface of the radius and ulna. The olecranon must be positioned directly beneath the humerus to prevent obliquity of the humeral head and distortion of the groove.

This test was introduced by Flo and Middleton (1) for better localization of mineralizations of the supraspinatus tendon in relation to the biceps tendon sheath. It can aid in the differentiation between loose joint mice and osteoarthritic spurs within the intertubercular groove from mineralization of the supraspinatus tendon.

Craniodistal–Cranioproximal (Flexed) Radiography

This view is obtained with the dog in dorsal recumbency, with the affected shoulder joint hyperflexed and the limb rotated externally approximately 30°. This test was introduced by Stobie and associates (2) for better evaluation of bicipital tenosynovitis. This view isolates the intertubercular groove, making it easy to identify subtle irregularities and biceps tendon mineralization.

Shoulder Arthrography

The animal is anesthetized, and the caudal aspect of the shoulder joint is clipped and surgically prepared. The site for insertion of a 20-gauge, 1.5-inch needle is approximately 1 cm caudal and 1 cm distal to the acromion in an average-sized Labrador retriever. This is the area of the caudal edge of the acromial head of the deltoid. The needle is advanced until joint fluid is aspirated. The needle is held steady, and the syringe is changed to a diluted contrast agent solution. The hub of the needle is filled with solution to avoid air bubbles before the rest of the injection is made. Any myelographic or intravenous contrast agent can be used if it is diluted to less than 100 mg iodine/mL diluent (3). For an 80-lb dog, the use of 1.25 mL of diatrizoate (Hypaque) with 1.75 mL bacteriostatic wa-

ter to a total volume of 3.0 mL works well. Depending on the size of the dog, between 2 and 4 mL diluted contrast agent should be used for an arthrogram of the shoulder joint. The most helpful radiographic view for an arthrogram is the mediolateral view with the shoulder in a neutral position. The contralateral shoulder may be used as a normal control to aid in interpretation, assuming that the disease is unilateral.

Positive-contrast scapulohumeral arthrography is critical in the evaluation of shoulder problems. This test is accurate, with a low rate of false-positive and false-negative results. One study rated the accuracy of positive-contrast shoulder arthrograms at 88% (4). A lower contrast is used to enable visualization of filling defects. The status of the articular cartilage, the presence of joint mice, and the entire joint can be evaluated with this technique. Abnormalities include impaired filling of the biceps tendon sheath, extravasation of the dye through a tear in the biceps tendon, and irregularity or filling defects within the biceps tendon sheath. Filling defects along the tendon correspond to proliferative synovium, adhesions between the tendon and its sheath, or joint mice. Arthrography is also helpful in the diagnosis of osteochondritis dissecans. The presence or absence of a radiolucent flap of cartilage over a defect and the extent of the caudal humeral head defect can only be determined with an arthrogram.

Joint Tap

A joint tap of the shoulder is described earlier in the discussion of arthrography. An adequate amount of fluid can usually be retrieved for clinicopathologic evaluation. The synovial sheath surrounding the biceps tendon is continuous with the shoulder joint capsule. Therefore, most shoulders with bicipital tenosynovitis have corresponding synovial fluid abnormalities consistent with degenerative joint disease. Inflammatory joint disease of the shoulder may be due to a specific disease of that joint or a component of polyarthritis. Synovial analysis is critical for evaluation of septic arthritis and other inflammatory joint diseases.

References

1. Flo GL, Middleton D. Mineralization of the supraspinatus tendon in dogs. J Am Vet Med Assoc 1990;197:95–97.
2. Stobie D, Wallace LJ, Lipowitz AJ, et al. Chronic bicipital tenosynovitis in dogs: 29 cases (1985–1992). J Am Vet Med Assoc 1995;207:201–207.
3. Brinker WO, Piermattei DL, Flo GL. Handbook of small animal orthopedics and fracture treatment. Philadelphia: WB Saunders, 1990:472–496.
4. van Bree H. Comparison of the diagnostic accuracy of positive-contrast arthrography and arthrotomy in evaluation of osteochondrosis lesions in the scapulohumeral joint in dogs. J Am Vet Med Assoc 1993;203:84–88.

Surgical Treatment of Osteochondritis Dissecans of the Shoulder

Dean R. Gahring

Treatment of osteochondritis dissecans of the shoulder is the removal of loose fragments of cartilage and bone from all aspects of the joint. This technique decreases inflammation and pain resulting from impingement and irritation of the joint capsule. Loose bone and cartilage fragments can enlarge over time and can move to other segments of the joint. Removal of loose cartilage also includes any cartilage of the humeral head that is still attached but has been undermined from subchondral bone. If the undermined loose cartilage is not removed, it may not reattach and may eventually break loose to become free-floating fragments. The exposed subchondral bone is curetted to "bleeding bone" so the resultant defect may be resurfaced with new fibrocartilage. Unless the vessels in the bone are ex-

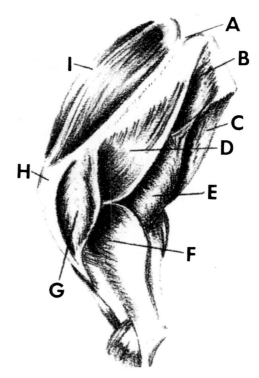

Fig. 57.7. The landmark to look for is the fascial raphe between the spinous head of the deltoid and the long head of the triceps muscles: *A*, spine of scapula; *B*, infraspinatus muscle; *C*, teres major muscle; *D*, spinous head of the deltoid muscle; *E*, long head of the triceps muscle; *F*, lateral head of the triceps muscle; *G*, acromial head of the triceps muscle; *H*, greater tubercle of the humerus; *I*, supraspinatus muscle. (From Gahring DR. A modified caudal approach to the canine shoulder joint. J Am Anim Hosp Assoc 1985;21:613–617.)

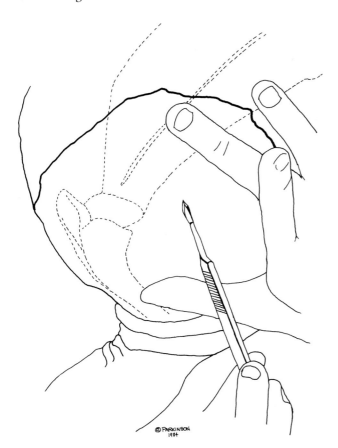

Fig. 57.6. The skin incision is made from the midpoint of the scapular spine to the midpoint of the humerus. (From Gahring DR. A modified caudal approach to the canine shoulder joint. J Am Anim Hosp Assoc 1985;21:613–617.)

posed, new fibrocartilage may not be produced or may be produced inconsistently.

This section describes the caudal approach to the shoulder joint. This muscle-separating approach provides excellent access to the caudal humeral head, where osteochondritis dissecans lesions are almost always found in the shoulder joint. It also provides access to all aspects of the caudal joint capsule cul-de-sacs, both caudolaterally and caudomedially, where loose fragments of cartilage are often found.

Surgical Technique

The patient is placed in lateral recumbency with the affected leg in an upward position. The location of the skin incision is identified by connecting the midpoint of the scapular spine with the midpoint of the humerus (Fig. 57.6). The skin, subcutaneous tissue, and superficial fascia are retracted to expose a whitish linear fascial raphe between the spinous (or scapular) head of the deltoid muscle and the long head of the triceps muscles (Figs. 57.7 and 57.8). This fibrous raphe is

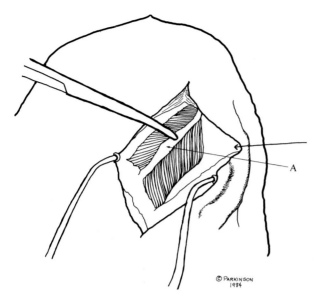

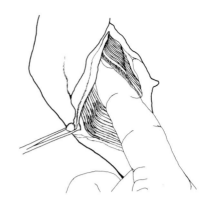

Fig. 57.10. Digital blunt dissection between the spinous head of the deltoid and long head of the triceps muscles is carried out to the caudal shoulder joint capsule. (From Gahring DR. A modified caudal approach to the canine shoulder joint. J Am Anim Hosp Assoc 1985;21:613–617.)

Fig. 57.8. Using the landmarks in Figure 57.6, the fascial raphe between the spinous head of the deltoid and the long head of the triceps muscles (A) should be immediately beneath the skin and subcutaneous tissue incision. The *large arrow* depicts retraction of subcutaneous areolar tissue. (From Gahring DR. A modified caudal approach to the canine shoulder joint. J Am Anim Hosp Assoc 1985;21:613–617.)

incised either sharply or bluntly. Blunt dissection between these two muscles is continued until the caudal shoulder joint capsule is identified (Figs. 57.9 and 57.10). It is easier to start the blunt separation digitally between the spinous (scapular) head of the deltoid and the long head of the triceps slightly above the level of the caudal shoulder joint and proceed in a cranioventral direction than to begin the blunt dissection from

below the caudal shoulder joint and proceed in a craniodorsal direction. Thus, the surgeon does not have to deal with the lateral head of the triceps (see Fig. 57.7). The few small muscular branch vessels encountered are either retracted or ligated. A self-retaining retractor is used to maintain separation of the spinous (or scapular) head of the deltoid and the long head of the triceps muscles (Fig. 57.11). The teres minor muscle is seen crossing the dorsal aspect of the caudal joint capsule (Figs. 57.12 and 57.13). The axillary nerve is identified as it crosses the ventral aspect of the caudal joint capsule (Figs. 57.14 and 57.15). An incision in the joint capsule is made transversely (perpendicular to the long axis of the humerus) between, and parallel to, the teres minor muscle and the axillary nerve (Fig. 57.16). This incision exposes the caudal glenoid, caudal humeral head, and caudal joint cul-de-sac (Fig. 57.17). Another self-retaining retractor may be used

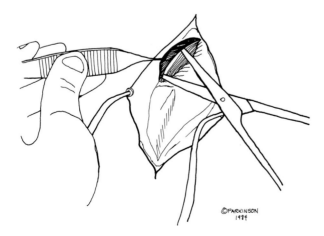

Fig. 57.9. Blunt or sharp separation of the fascial raphe between the spinous head of the deltoid and the long head of the triceps muscles is performed. (From Gahring DR. A modified caudal approach to the canine shoulder joint. J Am Anim Hosp Assoc 1985; 21:613–617.)

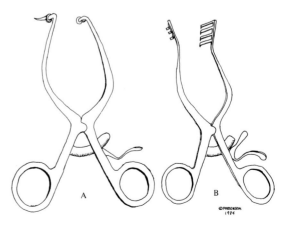

Fig. 57.11. Self-retaining Gelpi (**A**) or Weitlaner (**B**) retractors aid the exposure. (From Gahring DR. A modified caudal approach to the canine shoulder joint. J Am Anim Hosp Assoc 1985;21:613–617.)

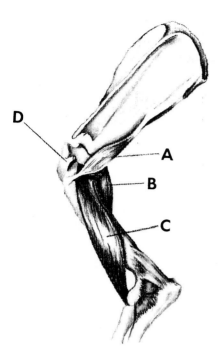

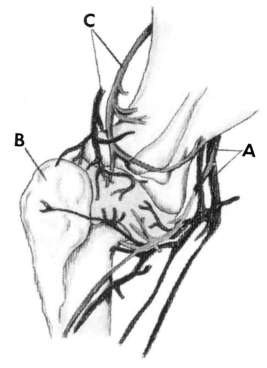

Fig. 57.12. The caudal shoulder joint capsule exposed by the muscle separation described in Figures 57.7 to 57.10 lies caudoventrally to the teres minor muscle belly (*A*). *B,* coracobrachialis muscle; *C,* brachialis muscle; *D,* tendon of insertion of the infraspinatus muscle. (From Gahring DR. A modified caudal approach to the canine shoulder joint. J Am Anim Hosp Assoc 1985;21:613–617.)

Fig. 57.14. The axillary nerve (*A*) exposed in this approach to the shoulder joint runs horizontally across the ventral border of the caudal shoulder joint capsule. *B,* greater tubercle of the humerus; *C,* suprascapular artery and nerve. (From Gahring DR. A modified caudal approach to the canine shoulder joint. J Am Anim Hosp Assoc 1985;21:613–617.)

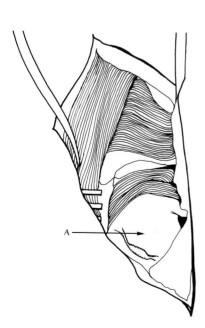

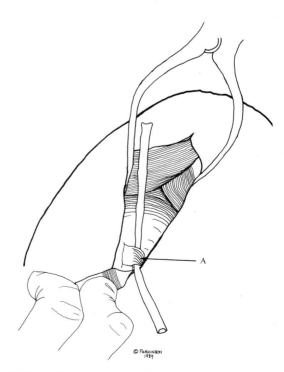

Fig. 57.13. Using self-retaining retractors described in Figure 57.11, the caudal shoulder joint capsule is identified easily (*A*). (From Gahring DR. A modified caudal approach to the canine shoulder joint. J Am Anim Hosp Assoc 1985;21:613–617.)

Fig. 57.15. The axillary nerve (*A*) is retracted with a soft rubber seton. (From Gahring DR. A modified caudal approach to the canine shoulder joint. J Am Anim Hosp Assoc 1985;21:613–617.)

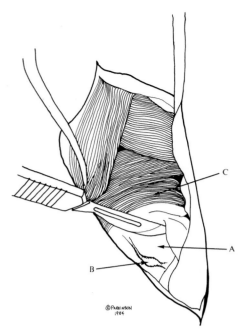

Fig. 57.16. The caudal shoulder joint capsule (A) is incised longitudinally parallel to, and between, the axillary nerve (B) ventrally, and the teres minor muscle dorsally (C). (From Gahring DR. A modified caudal approach to the canine shoulder joint. J Am Anim Hosp Assoc 1985;21:613–617.)

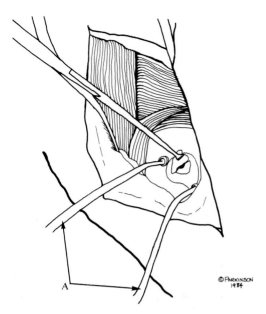

Fig. 57.18. Improved exposure for joint inspection is allowed by using a self-retaining retractor (A) to retract the incised edges of the joint capsule. (From Gahring DR. A modified caudal approach to the canine shoulder joint. J Am Anim Hosp Assoc 1985;21:613–617.)

here to retract the cut edges of the joint capsule if desired (see Fig. 57.11).

A lesion of osteochondritis dissecans can be identified and treated (Fig. 57.18). Manipulation of the leg by an assistant aids in identifying the full extent of the lesion (Fig. 57.19). The caudal cul-de-sac can be examined thoroughly and flushed (Fig. 57.20).

The caudal shoulder joint capsular incision is closed with a horizontal mattress absorbable suture (Fig. 57.21). The fasciae of the spinous (or scapular) head of the deltoid and the long head of the triceps muscles

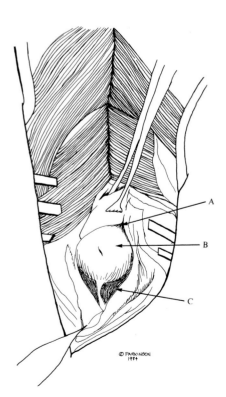

Fig. 57.17. Joint capsular incision exposes the caudal glenoid (A), caudal humeral head (B), and caudal joint capsule cul-de-sac (C). (From Gahring DR. A modified caudal approach to the canine shoulder joint. J Am Anim Hosp Assoc 1985;21:613–617.)

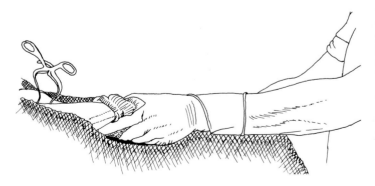

Fig. 57.19. An assistant usually is needed to manipulate the patient's leg to allow the surgeon full inspection of an osteochondritis dissecans lesion of the caudal humeral head. (From Gahring DR. A modified caudal approach to the canine shoulder joint. J Am Anim Hosp Assoc 1985;21:613–617.)

are reapposed with simple continuous absorbable suture (Fig. 57.22). The subcutaneous and skin closures are routine (Fig. 57.23). Restricted activity is allowed for the first 2 weeks postoperatively. Slings and splints are not necessary or advised.

This surgical approach to the shoulder joint for treatment of osteochondritis dissecans is a caudal, muscle-separating approach. This approach is surgically less traumatic, offers a faster recovery, and has fewer complications than any procedure requiring tenotomy or osteotomy. In addition, it causes no significant loss of range of motion. The caudal approach provides access for evaluation of the caudomedial aspect of the shoulder joint to search for loose fragments of cartilage, a feature not provided by caudolateral approaches. In addition, the vascular and neural plexuses are easier to retract and avoid in the caudal approach than in the caudolateral approaches. In the caudolateral approaches, the infraspinatus and teres minor muscles have to be identified, separated, and retracted once they have been reached by separating the deltoideus muscles. In the caudal approach, the teres minor muscle is of little concern, does not have to be specifically identified, and is retracted when the joint capsule is opened.

Some manipulation of the leg is necessary to identify the extent of an osteochondritis dissecans lesion completely, but this manipulation is required in all exposures. Significant advantages of the caudal ap-

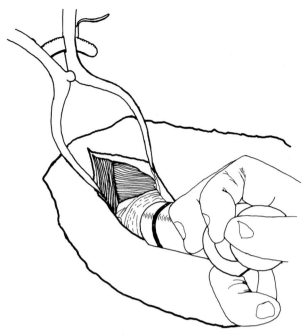

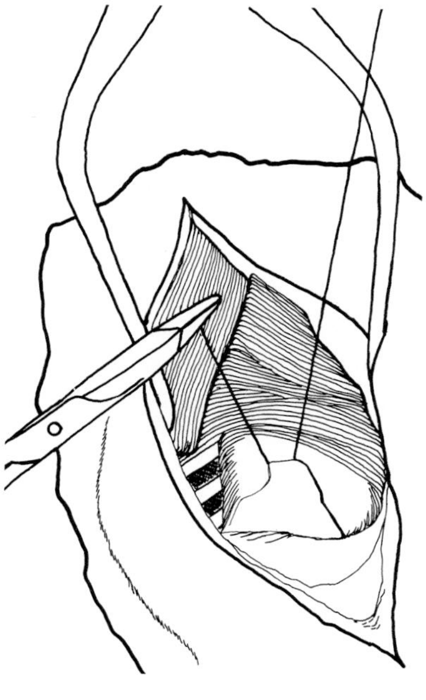

Fig. 57.20. The caudal shoulder joint is flushed to remove debris. (From Gahring DR. A modified caudal approach to the canine shoulder joint. J Am Anim Hosp Assoc 1985;21:613–617.)

Fig. 57.21. An absorbable mattress suture is placed to close the caudal shoulder joint capsular incision. (From Gahring DR. A modified caudal approach to the canine shoulder joint. J Am Anim Hosp Assoc 1985;21:613–617.)

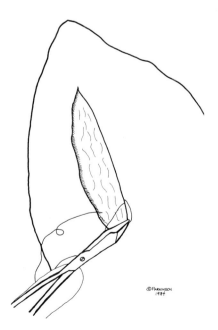

Fig. 57.22. A continuous absorbable suture is placed to reappose the spinous head of the deltoid and the long head of the triceps muscles. (From Gahring DR. A modified caudal approach to the canine shoulder joint. J Am Anim Hosp Assoc 1985;21:613–617.)

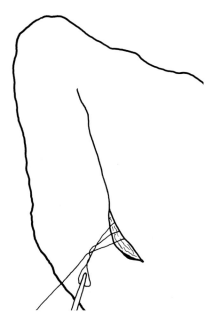

Fig. 57.23. Subcutaneous and skin closures are routine. (From Gahring DR. A modified caudal approach to the canine shoulder joint. J Am Anim Hosp Assoc 1985;21:613–617.)

proach to the shoulder are that all loose fragments of cartilage or bone that may become lodged in the caudal or caudomedial joint capsular cul-de-sacs can be identified and removed, and the approach only involves separating two muscles. Closure is simple, and return to activity is almost immediate, with minimal complications.

Surgical Treatment of Biceps Brachii Tendon Injury

R. Jeffrey Todoroff

Injury of the biceps brachii tendon of origin is usually chronic and is associated with degenerative changes of the associated bone, synovium, transverse humeral ligament, and the tendon itself, rendering primary tendon repair inappropriate. Tenodesis is the preferred treatment in these cases.

Surgical Technique

The dog is placed in dorsal recumbency, and the entire forelimb is prepared for aseptic surgery. A surgical assistant is helpful for manipulation of the limb. A modified craniomedial approach (1) is made to the shoulder through a skin incision that commences 5 cm proximal to the supraglenoid tubercle, curves lateral to the cra-

nial midline over the greater tubercle of the humerus, and ends medially over the proximal third of the biceps brachii. The lateral margin of the brachiocephalicus muscle is incised from the omobrachial vein proximad to the level of the supraglenoid tubercle, and the muscle is retracted medially, exposing the humeral insertions of the superficial and deep pectoral muscles, which are divided close to the humerus. Medial retraction of the pectoral muscles exposes the biceps brachii and the transverse humeral ligament. External rotation of the humerus by the assistant surgeon is helpful at this point. Further proximal separation of the deep pectoral muscle from the supraspinatus exposes the transverse humeral ligament and the cranial joint capsule of the scapulohumeral joint, which forms the biceps tendon sheath. The biceps tendon sheath is opened distal to the transverse humeral ligament, and the incision is carried through the ligament and is extended proximad to the level of the supraglenoid tubercle, exposing the biceps tendon of origin. The tendon can be further inspected by having the assistant flex the patient's elbow to 90° and extend the shoulder by lifting the limb with the antebrachium held parallel to the surgical table. This maneuver relieves tension from the biceps tendon and allows it to be luxated from the intertubercular groove and rolled for inspection of its deep surface, and it also permits exposure of its origin on the supraglenoid tubercle.

At this point, the remaining attachments of the injured tendon are severed from the supraglenoid tubercle, the tendon is retracted distally, and the joint capsule incision proximal to the greater tubercle is closed with 1–0 or 2–0 polydioxanone sutures. The limb is relaxed and externally rotated, and a hole is drilled through the humerus 5 to 10 mm distal to the lip of the bicipital groove, after excising a 1-cm patch of synovium to expose the bone. A 5-mm incision is made longitudinally in the middle of the biceps tendon about 1 cm proximal to its musculotendinous junction, and an appropriately sized cancellous bone screw and spiked washer are used to attach the tendon to the bone. The tendon proximal to the screw is removed and is used for biopsy, or it is discarded. Closure is completed by suturing the pectoral insertions to the deep brachial fascia and the brachiocephalicus to the brachial fascia with polydioxanone sutures. Subcutis and skin are closed in the usual fashion.

Postoperative radiographs are taken, and analgesics are administered during anesthetic recovery. Activity is strictly restricted for 2 weeks, and leash restriction is maintained for an additional 4 weeks.

The resection of the injured tendon of origin and the use of a spiked washer to anchor the remaining short segment of tendon to the humerus are important in relieving stresses on the chronically injured tendon and adjacent ligament and synovium. Dogs with biceps tendon injuries treated with tenodesis are often clinically improved within 2 weeks and are expected to regain all their muscle mass and clinically normal function within 2 months despite the chronicity of the problem.

Tenodesis of the biceps tendon of origin is also useful in the management of bicipital tenosynovitis unresponsive to medical treatment, fractures of the supraglenoid tubercle in which conventional repair is not possible, and treatment of luxation of the biceps tendon of origin.

Reference

1. Piermattei DL. An atlas of surgical approaches to the bones and joints of the dog and cat. 3rd ed. Philadelphia: WB Saunders, 1993:114.)

Surgical Treatment of Shoulder Luxations

Mark H. Engen

Shoulder luxations are an uncommon cause of lameness in small animals. Trauma is the most common cause of the luxation, and congenital malformation of the scapulohumeral joint is less frequent.

Congenital Shoulder Luxations

Small breeds are most commonly affected with congenital luxation. This condition is believed to be hereditary, and therefore owners should be informed not to use these animals for breeding. Congenital luxations are usually medial, are frequently bilateral, and are most common in the small breeds, such as toy poodles, Chihuahuas, and Pomeranians. Some of these small breed dogs with congenital luxations have only mild lameness with occasional exacerbations, and they learn to tolerate the condition and live with minimal symptoms. These dogs have essentially no glenoid cavity, and the flattened humeral head is supported by a fibrotic joint capsule and surrounding "cuff muscles." Surgery may not be necessary in these patients unless their lameness is severe and causes significant disability.

Surgical stabilization of congenital shoulder luxations is frequently unrewarding because of the shallow glenoid and flattened humeral head. Should surgery be necessary, these patients are best treated by arthrodesis of the shoulder. In my experience, the dogs regain good functional use of their legs, and the pain is resolved after an arthrodesis. Resection of the glen-oid rim and humeral head has also been described as an alternative to arthrodesis or amputation. Good functional results in small breeds have been described for nonathletic function (1).

Techique for Scapulohumeral Arthrodesis

The shoulder should be fused in a functional standing position of approximately 150°. The angle can be determined with a goniometer on the opposite leg when the dog is bearing weight. A craniolateral approach (2) combined with an osteotomy of the greater tubercle is performed to expose the articular cartilage of the shoulder. The cartilage is debrided from the glenoid and humeral head. A cancellous graft from the proximal humerus is taken through the greater tubercle osteotomy with a bone curette and is packed in and around the joint. The joint is temporarily immobilized in a standing angle of approximately 150° with one or two small pins or Kirschner wires driven from the proximal humerus across the joint into the scapula. A lag screw is then placed across the joint for compression and additional stabilization. Alternatively, a plate is conformed to the craniolateral aspect of the joint for stabilization (four screws in the scapula and four screws in the humerus); however, plate fixation is usually not necessary in small breeds for arthrodesis. If an arthrodesis is necessary in a large breed dog, plate immobilization is recommended for its rigid fixation. The greater tubercle is immobilized with one or two Kirschner wires and a figure-of-eight tension band wire. Supporting the leg with a bandage postoperatively for 1 to 2 weeks and strict confinement to a crate are recommended. Follow-up radiographs are taken at 4-week intervals until the fusion is complete (Fig. 57.24).

Traumatic Shoulder Luxations

Traumatic shoulder luxations are usually medial, but they can also be lateral or cranial. Because of the high potential for concurrent trauma to the chest area, all patients should have thoracic radiographs, electrocardiograms, and blood tests as part of their preoperative workup. If any thoracic or cardiac abnormalities are found, these should be treated and should be under control before anesthesia for closed reduction or surgery.

Diagnosis and Treatment

Severe lameness, pain and reluctance to move the limb, and crepitation in the shoulder area on manipulation are physical abnormalities noted in shoulder luxations. Radiographs are necessary to confirm the

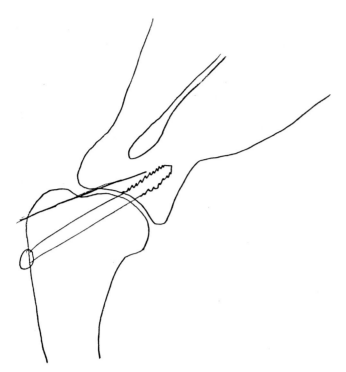

Fig. 57.24. Scapulohumeral arthrodesis.

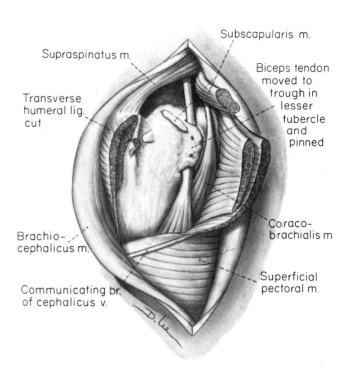

Fig. 57.25. Craniomedial view of the shoulder showing the bicipital tendon fixed in place beneath the bone flap on the lesser tubercle. (From Hohn RB, Rosen H, Bohning RH Jr, et al. Surgical stabilization of recurrent shoulder luxation. Vet Clin North Am 1971;1:537.)

luxation and to determine the direction of luxation. The radiographic views should be lateral and ventrodorsal or dorsoventral.

Early closed reduction under anesthesia or heavy sedation should be attempted before surgical intervention, and, in my experience, this technique is successful in 50 to 60% of patients. After closed reduction, the limb should be immobilized in a nonweightbearing sling for 2 to 3 weeks. A modified Velpeau sling is used for medial luxations because it directs the humeral head laterally. A nonweightbearing sling that abducts the shoulder is used for lateral luxations. A nonweightbearing sling should be used for 2 to 3 weeks to allow healing of supporting soft tissues, that is, the joint capsule and glenohumeral ligaments and surrounding muscles. A radiograph should be taken to confirm shoulder reduction after sling immobilization. If the shoulder cannot be maintained in reduction or if it reluxates after sling removal, then open reduction and surgical stabilization will be necessary.

Surgical Stabilization

The techniques for surgical stabilization using local anatomic structures (bicipital tendon transfer, supraspinatus tendon transfer) are described in the literature (2–4).

MEDIAL LUXATIONS

Medial luxations are stabilized by transferring the biceps tendon medially and immobilizing it beneath a bone flap on the lesser tubercle of the humerus (4) (Fig. 57.25). Alternatively, the supraspinatus tendon can be transferred medially to the area of the lesser tubercle of the humerus and immobilized in this location (5) (Fig. 57.26). If additional medial support is needed, a combined technique using both the biceps and supraspinatus tendons can be performed. The limb

Fig. 57.26. Supraspinatus tendon technique for repair of medial luxation of the shoulder joint. **A.** View of the shoulder joint after parahumeral incision (*inset*); retraction of the skin, subcutaneous tissues, and brachiocephalicus muscle; and transection and medial retraction of the proximal insertion of the superficial pectoral muscle. **B.** View of the shoulder with deep pectoral muscle separated from its fascial attachment to the medial fleshy border of the supraspinatus muscle and from its insertion on the greater and lesser tubercle. **C.** Position of the osteotome on the greater tubercle of the humerus. The lateral view is shown in the *inset*. **D.** View after splitting of the supraspinatus tendon, with about half of the insertion left attached to the humerus, and removal of outer cortex of the lesser tubercle. **E.** Attachment of the severed portion of the greater tubercle to the prepared area on the lesser tubercle with Kirschner pins and a tension band wire. (From Craig E, Hohn RB, Anderson WD. Surgical stabilization of traumatic medial shoulder dislocation. J Am Anim Hosp Assoc 1980;16:93.)

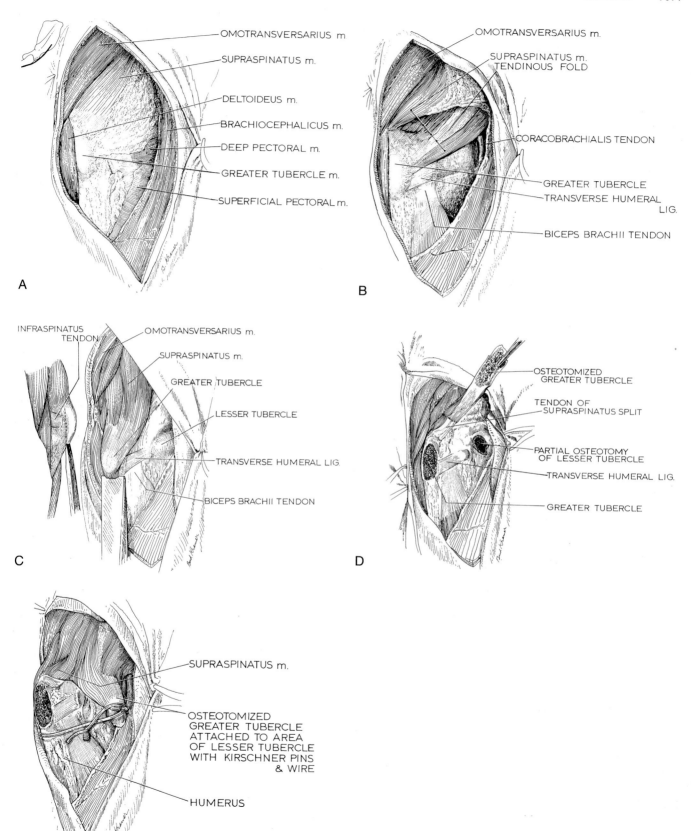

A

OMOTRANSVERSARIUS m.
SUPRASPINATUS m.
DELTOIDEUS m.
BRACHIOCEPHALICUS m.
DEEP PECTORAL m.
GREATER TUBERCLE m.
SUPERFICIAL PECTORAL m.

B

OMOTRANSVERSARIUS m.
SUPRASPINATUS m.
TENDINOUS FOLD
CORACOBRACHIALIS TENDON
GREATER TUBERCLE
TRANSVERSE HUMERAL LIG.
BICEPS BRACHII TENDON

C

INFRASPINATUS TENDON
OMOTRANSVERSARIUS m.
SUPRASPINATUS m.
GREATER TUBERCLE
LESSER TUBERCLE
TRANSVERSE HUMERAL LIG.
BICEPS BRACHII TENDON

D

OSTEOTOMIZED GREATER TUBERCLE
TENDON OF SUPRASPINATUS SPLIT
PARTIAL OSTEOTOMY OF LESSER TUBERCLE
TRANSVERSE HUMERAL LIG.
GREATER TUBERCLE

E

SUPRASPINATUS m.
OSTEOTOMIZED GREATER TUBERCLE ATTACHED TO AREA OF LESSER TUBERCLE WITH KIRSCHNER PINS & WIRE
HUMERUS

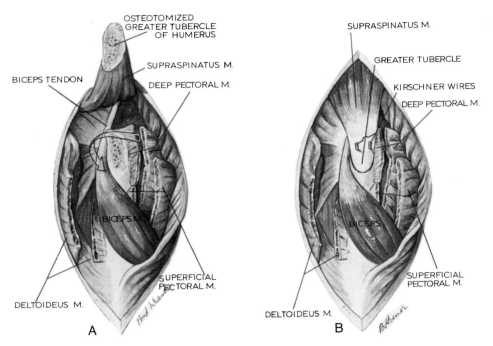

Fig. 57.27. A. Craniomedial view of the shoulder after osteotomy and dorsal reflection of the greater tubercle and supraspinatus muscle and lateral transposition of the bicipital tendon (*arrow*). **B.** Cranial view of the shoulder showing the lateral transposition of the bicipital tendon and the repositioning of the greater tubercle. (From Hohn RB, Rosen H, Bohning RH Jr, et al. Surgical stabilization of recurrent shoulder luxation. Vet Clin North Am 1971;1:537.)

must be immobilized in a modified Velpeau sling for 2 to 3 weeks postoperatively. The use of synthetic materials for medial shoulder luxations is not practical because of the anatomic difficulty of adequate exposure for placement of anchor screws for prosthetic materials.

LATERAL LUXATIONS

Lateral luxations can also be stabilized by transferring the biceps tendon laterally after greater tubercle osteotomy and subsequent immobilization of the greater tubercle (4) (Fig. 57.27). Prosthetics can be used to stabilize lateral luxations by placing large suture or polypropylene mesh strips through a transverse hole drilled in the distal spine of the scapula and around a screw with a washer placed in the proximal lateral humerus. The humerus screw is positioned as close as possible to the center of the arc of rotation of the joint, to avoid interfering with joint range of motion and to provide maximum stability. Wire (0.8 to 1.0 mm) can also be used, with the knowledge that it will later break and may have to be removed if it causes pain or lameness (Fig. 57.28). The limb should be immobilized in a nonweightbearing sling postoperatively for 2 to 3 weeks.

Cranial Luxations

Cranial luxations are rare, but they can be stabilized by transferring the biceps tendon cranially (3). An osteotomy of the greater tubercle is performed, and a groove is cut into the bed of the osteotomy site into

which the biceps tendon is placed. The greater tubercle is then replaced to its original location and immobilized with Kirschner wires and a figure-of-eight tension band wire. The limb is immobilized in extension using a coaptation splint or modified Thomas splint for 2 weeks (Fig 57.29).

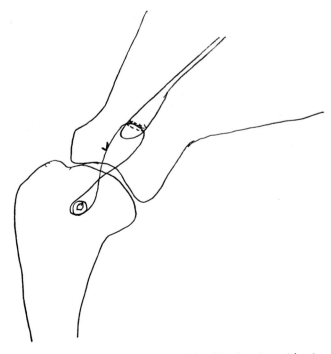

Fig. 57.28. Stabilization of lateral shoulder luxation with wire.

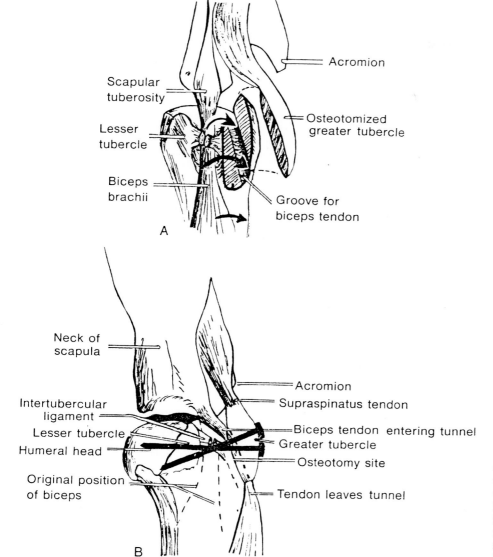

Fig. 57.29. Repair of cranial luxation of the shoulder joint. **A.** Cranial view of the shoulder showing the groove that has been prepared for the bicipital tendon beneath the osteotomized greater tubercle. **B.** Stabilization of the shoulder by luxation of the bicipital tendon beneath the greater tubercle. (From DeAngelis M, Schwartz A. Surgical connection of cranial dislocation of the scapulohumeral joint in a dog. J Am Vet Med Assoc 1970;156:435.)

Approximately one-half of closed reductions fail and require surgical stabilization. Results with the foregoing techniques, combined with postoperative limb immobilization to protect the repair, are good to excellent. Most patients regain full functional use of the limb and retain excellent use of the limb throughout their remaining life.

References

1. Piermattei DL, Blass DH. Resection of the glenoid rim and humeral head. In: Bojrab MJ, ed. Current techniques in small animal surgery. 3rd ed. Philadelphia: Lea & Febiger, 1990:748–749.
2. Piermattei DL, Greeley RG. An atlas of surgical approaches to the bones of the dog and cat. 3rd ed. Philadelphia: WB Saunders, 1993:114–121.
3. Craig E, Holm RB, Anderson WD. Surgical stabilization of traumatic medial shoulder dislocation. J Am Anim Hosp Assoc 1980; 16:93.
4. De Angelis M, Schwartz A. Surgical correction of cranial dislocation of the scapulohumeral joint in a dog. J Am Vet Med Assoc 1970;156:435.
5. Hohn RB, Rosen H, Bohning RH, et al. Surgical stabilization of recurrent shoulder luxation. Vet Clin North Am 1971;1:537.

Suture Stabilization for Luxations of the Shoulder

Barclay Slocum & Theresa Devine Slocum

The purpose of stabilizing the luxating shoulder by suture is to maintain a normal shoulder motion without luxation until the torn structures can heal. The indications for using suture stabilization of the shoulder are limited to acute or recent injuries of the medial or lateral collateral ligaments of the shoulder and their associated joint capsule. Congenital or chronic luxations of the shoulder have deformed osseous components and permanent contracture of the soft tissues that preclude healing to normal anatomic relationships. Malunions and chronic traumatic lesions have improper alignment of the structures and cannot support the forces of weightbearing.

Surgical Procedure

The size of the surgical exposure to the lateral shoulder is determined by the surgeon's preference. Minimal exposure is provided by incision of the humeral attachment of the deltoideus muscle and by caudal and ventral retraction of the infraspinatus muscle after en bloc osteotomy of the humeral insertion of the tendon from the greater tubercle. Maximal exposure is provided by osteotomy and caudal retraction of the acromion process with the attached deltoideus muscle and by caudal and ventral retraction of the infraspinatus muscle after en bloc osteotomy of the humeral insertion of the tendon from the greater tubercle. This technique exposes the lateral shoulder joint capsule and distal scapula. The teres minor and the lateral and accessory head of the triceps muscles are elevated from tricipital line and are retracted distally to expose the humeral neck.

Two holes are drilled laterally to medially in the distal scapula just proximal to the subchondral bone of the glenoid. The first hole is placed cranial to the scapular spine, and the second is placed caudal to the spine. A single lateral-to-medial hole is drilled through the center of motion of the humeral head, which is located at the ventral margin of the lateral joint capsule half-way between the proximal tricipital line and the caudal limit of the humeral neck.

Suture Stabilization of the Medial Shoulder Joint

The stabilization suture for a medial luxation of the humeral head is passed in the following sequence (Fig. 57.30). The first end of the suture is passed through the cranial hole in the scapula and is retrieved by using Mixter forceps, passed caudal to the humeral neck. The second end of the suture is passed through the caudal hole in the scapula and retrieved by using Mixter forceps passed caudal to the humeral neck, a maneuver that leaves the bite of the suture on the lateral cortex just proximal to the glenoid. An 18-inch length of 20-gauge stainless steel wire is doubled back on itself to form an acute angle in the bite. The bite of the wire is passed laterally to medially through the hole in the humerus and is retrieved by using Mixter

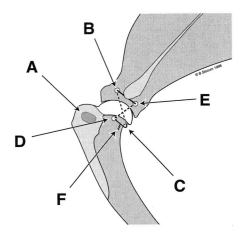

Fig. 57.30. Medial luxation of the humeral head is approached by en bloc osteotomy of the infraspinatus tendon insertion (*A*). The first end of the suture is passed through a cranial scapular hole (*B*) and is retrieved by the caudal humerus (*C*). A retrieval wire is passed through the humeral hole (*D*). The second end of the suture is passed through the caudal scapular hole (*E*) and is pulled through the humeral hole with the retrieval wire. The two free ends of the suture are tightened and are tied (*F*).

forceps passed caudal to the humeral neck. The two portions of the wire adjacent to the bite are separated, and the second end of the suture is passed through the opening. As the wire is withdrawn from the humeral hole by simultaneously pulling on the two free wire ends, the second end of the suture passes the hole medially to laterally. The first suture end, which passes around the humeral neck, and the second suture end, which emerges from the humeral hole, are tightened to stabilize the shoulder and are tied.

Suture Stabilization of the Lateral Shoulder Joint

The stabilization suture for a lateral luxation of the humeral head is passed in the following sequence (Fig. 57.31). The first end of the suture is passed through the cranial hole in the scapula and is retrieved by using Mixter forceps passed caudal to the humeral neck. An 18-inch length of 20-gauge stainless steel wire is doubled back on itself to form an acute angle in the bite. The bite of the wire is passed laterally to medially through the caudal hole in the scapula and is retrieved by using Mixter forceps passed caudal to the humeral neck. The two portions of the wire adjacent to the bite are separated, and the first end of the suture is passed through the opening. As the wire is withdrawn from the humeral hole by simultaneously pulling on the two free wire ends, the first end of the suture passes the caudal scapular hole medially to laterally. Again, the bite of the wire is passed laterally to medially through the humeral hole and is retrieved caudal to the humeral neck. The second end of the suture is withdrawn from the humeral hole medially to later-

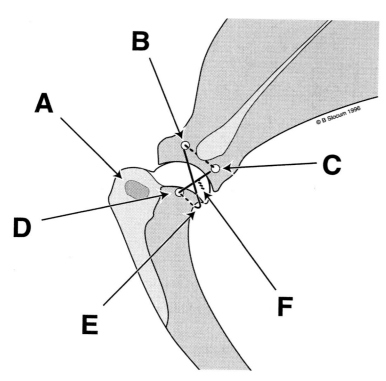

Fig. 57.31. Lateral luxation of the humeral head is approached by en bloc osteotomy of the infraspinatus tendon insertion (*A*). The first end of the suture is passed through a cranial scapular hole (*B*) and is retrieved by the caudal humerus (*E*). A retrieval wire is passed through the caudal scapular hole (*C*), and the first end is placed in the retrieval wire and pulled through the caudal scapular hole (*C*). A retrieval wire is passed through the humeral hole (*D*), and the second end is place in the retrieval wire and is pulled through the humeral hole (*C*) medially to laterally. The two free ends of the suture are tightened and are tied (*F*).

ally. The first suture end, which emerges from the caudal scapular hole, and the second suture end, which emerges from the lateral humeral hole, are tightened to stabilize the shoulder and are tied.

Closure

The teres minor and the lateral and accessory head of the triceps muscles are sutured to the tricipital line and joint capsule. The infraspinatus muscle is reattached to the greater tubercle at the humeral insertion of the tendon by a lag screw. The humeral attachment of the deltoideus muscle is sutured to its humeral attachment, or the acromion process with the attached deltoideus muscle is reattached to the scapular spine by tension band wire. The skin closure is routine.

The appropriate size suture for an 8-kg poodle is size 2 monofilament polypropylene, whereas a 40-kg Labrador retriever may require the strength of 1-mm braided polyester suture or large nylon monofilament suture. Monofilament suture is preferred to braided suture.

The torn collateral ligament and joint capsule of the shoulder can be repaired by placing a temporary suture that limits motion to a normal range. By maintaining a normal range of motion and providing strict rest conditions, the joint capsule and ligament heal over 6 to 8 weeks. Maturation of the newly healed joint capsule is encouraged by a gradual return to normal function and is controlled by leash walking between the eighth and sixteenth weeks. Normal activities are resumed after 16 weeks.

58

ELBOW

Algorithms for Diagnosis and Treatment of Elbow Disorders

James Boulay & Peter D. Schwarz

Figures 58.1 through 58.3 are algorithms for the evaluation and management of disorders of the elbow.

Surgical Treatment of Ununited Anconeal Process of the Elbow

K. Ron Presnell

In the dog, the anconeal process usually is united to the dorsocranial border of the proximal ulnar metaphysis and is intimately associated with the trochlea of the olecranon fossa of the humerus. An ununited anconeal process is a developmental entity in the young, growing dog in which the anconeal process is partially or completely separated from the rest of the diaphysis of the ulna or in which the anconeal process is fused to the ulna in an abnormal location (Fig. 58.4A). This disorder initially causes a mild forelimb lameness, which becomes more severe as degenerative joint disease progresses. Ununited anconeal process in dogs sometimes occurs concurrently with fragmented coronoid process, osteochondrosis of the distal humerus, or growth defects of the radius and ulna (espe-

cially in dogs that have had a cessation of growth in the radius resulting in a valgus deformity and radius curvus syndrome).

Ununited anconeal process is primarily a condition affecting young dogs between 5 and 9 months of age. It usually occurs in medium to large breeds of dog, most notably the German shepherd. It has also been reported in St. Bernards, Great Danes, Labrador retrievers, pointers, bloodhounds, Great Pyrenees, rottweilers, weimaraners, and Newfoundlands (1, 2). The disorder also occurs in basset hounds and dachshunds, two chondrodystrophoid breeds with a marked incidence of dissimilar growth rates of the radius and ulna. This dissimilar growth results in shearing stress on the anconeal process, which fractures it off or prevents its normal attachment. Ununited anconeal process occasionally is seen in older dogs, from 3 to 9 years of age, that present with an acute episode of severe forelimb lameness localized to the elbow joint.

Pathogenesis

The pathogenesis of ununited anconeal process has not been established definitively. The disorder is thought to be an inherited developmental anomaly in which the anconeal process, which develops from a separate ossification center, fails to fuse to the ulna. It may result from a growth rate defect such that the ulna's growth rate is decreased relative to the radius. This decreased growth pushes the humerus proximally and produces shearing stress on the anconeal process (Fig. 58.4B). Breeding of affected animals is not recommended.

The ossification of the anconeal process usually is first apparent between 11 and 12 weeks of age, when it is seen as several centers of ossification (3). These centers tend to coalesce to form a large center of ossification within the anconeal process, which then goes

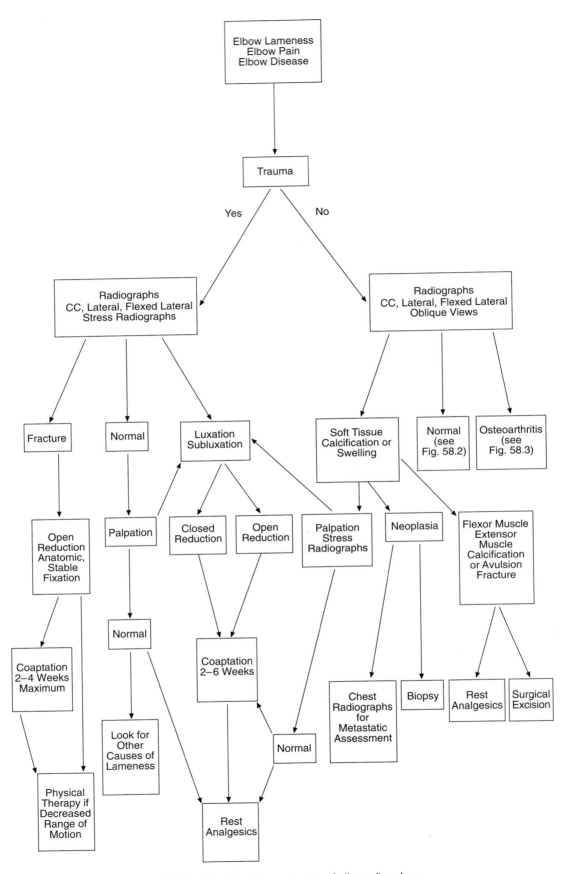

Fig. 58.1. Algorithm for evaluation of elbow disorders.

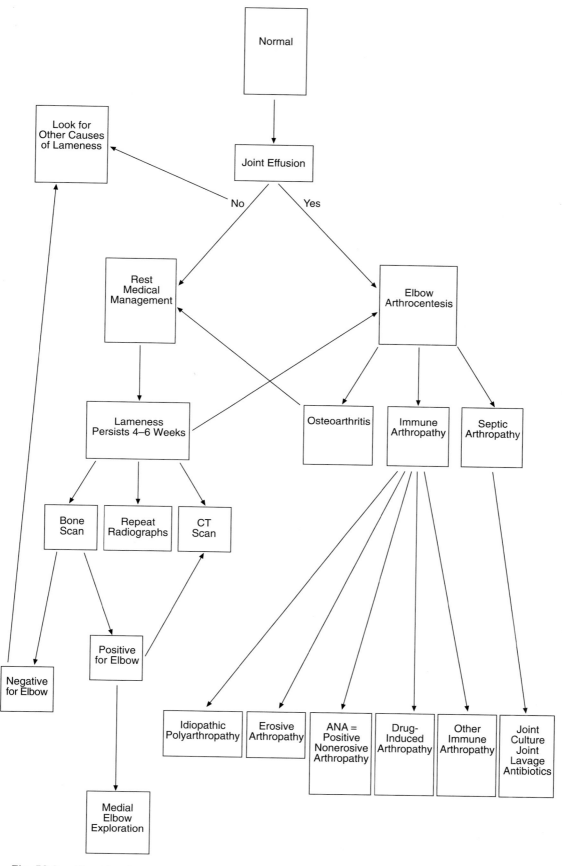

Fig. 58.2. Algorithm for management of patients with elbow disorders and normal radiographic findings.

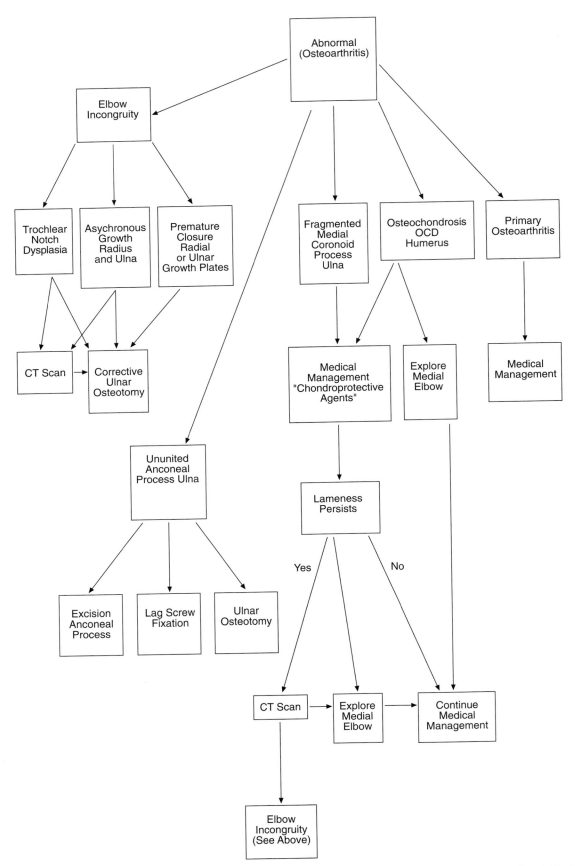

Fig. 58.3. Algorithms for management of patients with radiographic evidence of osteoarthritis. *OCD,* osteochondritis dissecans.

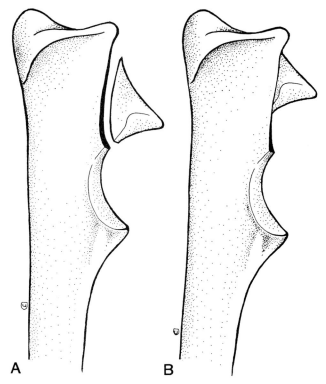

Fig. 58.4. **A.** Typical line of cleavage of an ununited anconeal process. **B.** Proximally displaced anconeal process resulting from shearing effect caused by dissimilar ulnar and radial growth rates.

on to fuse to the ulna. Osseus union of the anconeal process to the metaphysis of the ulna usually occurs first between the anconeal process and the ulnar metaphysis adjacent to the articular cartilage of the trochlear notch. The time for complete ossification of this site and for fusion between the anconeal process and the ulna varies with the breed. In the greyhound, it may be as late as 18 weeks of age. A diagnosis of ununited anconeal process should not be made until an animal is at least 5 months of age.

An ununited anconeal process interferes with joint function and also acts as a loose body within the joint. It leads to erosion of the articular cartilage in the trochlear notch distal to the line of cleavage. Bony proliferative changes occur on both sides of the cleavage line at its proximal end and on the rim of the articular surface of the lateral condyle of the humerus. The joint capsule usually is inflamed and thickened, and one sees an increase in joint fluid, which produces overall joint swelling and enlargement.

Clinical Presentations

As noted previously, three groups of dogs present with ununited anconeal process. The most prevalent group consists of medium to large breed dogs that present between 6 and 9 months of age with varying degrees of lameness. Initially, the dog has mild lameness. Often, this lameness is first noticed in purebred dogs after they have been to a show and the judge suggests that they are not moving correctly on their front end. The condition can progress so the animal is nonweightbearing if the disorder only involves one leg. The lameness is usually worse after exercise, and the dogs are stiff after their postexercise rest, but they warm out of the lameness.

The second group of patients comprises chondrodystrophoid dogs that have a relative shortening of the ulna compared with the radius. This configuration produces a shearing effect of the humerus on the anconeal process, which is pushed proximally on the ulnar shaft, resulting in either a shearing fracture or a failure to unite. The third group of affected dogs are 3 to 9 years of age and have no history of previous lameness. They present with a sudden severe lameness of the forelimb, which can be localized to the elbow. On radiographic examination, these animals have ununited anconeal processes and severely degenerative elbows.

Radiographic Examination

Radiographs are necessary for confirmation of the diagnosis of ununited anconeal process. Because the dog experiences pain on flexion of the elbow, sedation or general anesthesia often is required to allow the elbow to be flexed sufficiently for a lateral radiograph. This position helps to expose the anconeal process without overshadowing of the humerus. Both elbows should be radiographed, because ununited anconeal process may be bilateral. In addition to a lateral view, a craniocaudal radiographic view[1] is required to help evaluate the degenerative joint disease and to rule out other problems.

Radiographically, the anconeal process is separated from the proximal ulnar metaphysis by a line of cleavage of varying width (Fig. 58.5). The fragment can appear normal in size, shape, and density, or it can be sclerotic or osteoporotic and show various degenerative changes. The degree of degenerative joint disease often depends on the chronicity of the disease. The other feature often noted on radiographic evaluation is that the anconeal process often sits proximally on the olecranon. In this situation, the most proximal end of the anconeus is in line with the proximal line of the olecranon. The relation of the radial head to the coronoid process of the ulna and the relation of the humerus to the trochlear notch of the ulna should be

---

[1] Editor's note. I have seen a significant number of German shepherds with fragmented coronoid process concurrent with ununited anconeal process.

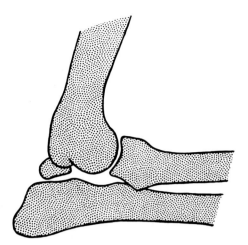

Fig. 58.5. Typical radiographic appearance of an ununited anconeal process. Lateral view.

evaluated for evidence of abnormal growth defects or changes in the joint.

Treatment Options and Indications for Surgery

Dogs older than 15 months of age that have had a short, acute onset of lameness should be treated conservatively and given salicylates to help ease the pain and inflammation for a minimum of 2 weeks. This treatment does nothing for an ununited anconeal process and degenerative joint disease; however, most of these dogs have been normal up to this time, and most go back to being normal within a short period. In my experience, a strain, a sprain, or a secondary injury has caused the elbow pain in most such cases. If the animal is not normal within 2 weeks, then further therapy is initiated.

Younger dogs with a clinical presentation similar to that described earlier and with radiographic signs of ununited anconeal process should be treated surgically, either by reattachment of the anconeal process or by its removal. With young animals, a period of conservative therapy usually simply allows the degenerative joint disease to progress.

In some young dogs, the anconeal process can be salvaged by reattaching it to the ulna, thus returning the elbow to as near-normal function as possible. This procedure does not produce the instability that results from removal of the anconeal process. Reattachment is indicated only when the anconeal process appears normal in size, shape, and density on both the radiographs and surgical evaluation and when the animal has limited secondary degenerative joint disease and osteophyte production. Second, the anconeal process must fit or be made to fit the site on the ulna from which it was removed and thus must be capable of articulating normally with the humerus to allow full

flexion and extension of the joint. Third, the anconeus must be able to be attached in the exact location where it would normally be, so the joint can function properly. Thus, anconeal processes that are sclerotic or deformed or have moved or slid proximally on the ulna are not candidates for this type of repair.

The anconeal process should be removed in all young dogs when it is osteolytic, malformed, sclerotic, or difficult to return to its normal anatomic position. The decision to remove the anconeal process is based on radiographic and visual evaluation of the process and the joint itself. In older dogs, the anconeal process may be removed if the surgeon is sure that it is causing a problem; however, the results of removal in older dogs (i.e., over 3 years of age) have been much less rewarding than in younger dogs.

In a normal dog, the anconeal process locks into the olecranon fossa of the humerus when the elbow is in moderate to full extension. This locking tends to stop the medial and lateral motion of the elbow during weightbearing. Hence, removal of the anconeus may allow a "wobbling" of the elbow, especially when the dog lands with the leg extended. The elbow instability resulting from removal of the anconeal process usually makes operated animals unfit for showing or performance work, because they usually have an abnormal gait. Moreover, degenerative joint disease still progresses after removal, although at a much slower rate than when surgical treatment is not performed.

Surgical Techniques

Surgical repair of an ununited anconeal process, either by reattachment or by removal, is begun with a lateral approach to the caudolateral compartment of the elbow joint and evaluation of the anconeal process. A lateral skin incision is made just caudal to the humerus, curved over the olecranon, and continued distally along the lateral side of the ulna (Fig. 58.6**A**). The incision for reattachment of the anconeal process needs to be somewhat longer than the incision for removal of the anconeal process.

After dissection through the subcutaneous tissue, the lateral head of the triceps is elevated to expose the anconeus muscle. The anconeus muscle and attached joint capsule are incised across their caudal attachment on the lateral epicondyle of the humerus (Fig. 58.6**B**). A stab incision is made through the anconeus muscle, which then is extended dorsally and ventrally to allow visualization of the joint and hence the anconeal process (Fig. 58.6**C**).

Reattachment of the Anconeal Process

After the anconeal process and elbow joint are exposed, they are evaluated carefully to determine whether the prerequisites for reattachment are met. If

through the anconeal process. The screw head must be placed on the caudodorsal aspect of the anconeal process so the screw head cannot contact the articular cartilage or interfere with the extension of the joint. The screw should pass in a 45° angle down the shaft of the ulna. The anconeal process is drilled at the appropriate angle and then is overdrilled to form the gliding hole (Fig. 58.7**A**). The drill insert sleeve is placed into the glide hole, and the anconeal process is positioned on the precise spot of fixation. The thread hole is drilled into the ulna. A screw of the required length is measured, and the hole in the ulna is tapped. The head of the screw may need to be countersunk gently into the anconeal process. This is done, if necessary, before the screw is inserted. The screw is inserted and is tightened down into position (Fig. 58.7**B**).

Care must be taken that the anconeal process is in the correct location and that it is not allowed to rotate as the screw is tightened. Rigid compression must be achieved to hold the anconeus securely in place and to allow it to heal. At this stage, the joint should be moved through its full range of motion to see that the anconeal process is in the right position and is not interfering with joint function. The joint is inspected for any loose fragments or fibrous tissue and then is flushed with Ringer's solution.

The anconeal muscle and the joint capsule are reattached with an absorbable suture material in a simple interrupted pattern. Subcutaneous tissue and skin are closed in routine fashion.

Postoperatively, the leg is supported in a moderately heavy padded bandage running from the nails to above the elbow. The bandage is kept in place for 7 to 10 days

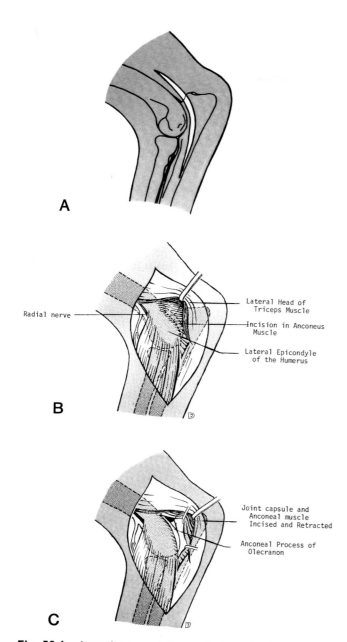

Fig. 58.6. Lateral approach for surgical repair of an ununited anconeal process. **A.** Skin incision. **B.** Exposure of anconeal muscle and site of incision into the joint capsule. **C.** Exposure of anconeal process after incision and retraction of anconeal muscle and joint capsule.

the anconeus can be reattached, the two surfaces to be apposed are curetted and are trimmed free of fibrous tissue, which usually covers them, to provide bleeding bone. The surfaces also are shaped to allow a precise fit of the anconeal process onto the ulna. To increase visualization at this stage, the elbow is placed in a flexed position, and the radius and ulna are rotated laterally as much as possible.

An interfragmentary compression technique must be used to hold the anconeal process firmly in place. Because of its size, only one screw can be placed

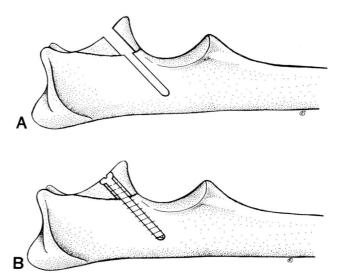

Fig. 58.7. Reattachment of the anconeal process with a lag screw. **A.** Schematic illustration showing glide hole in the anconeal process and the olecranon drilled at a 45° angle to its axis. **B.** Schematic illustration showing the screw in place with its head off the articular surface and countersunk flush with the surface.

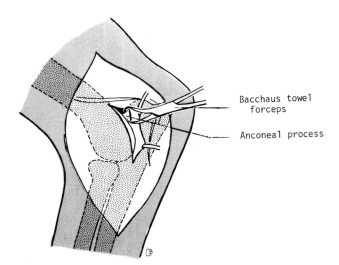

Fig. 58.8. Removal of the anconeal process. The anconeal fragment is grasped with Backhaus towel forceps, freed from any fibrous attachments to the ulna, and lifted from the joint.

to reduce swelling and to prevent seroma formation. Exercise is restricted to leash walks for 6 weeks to allow the anconeal process to heal. Healing usually requires 6 to 8 weeks.

Removal of the Anconeal Process

The surgical approach when removal of the anconeal process is anticipated is the same as described previously, although the incision may be shorter than for the reattachment procedure. If removal is indicated after exposure and evaluation of the anconeal process and elbow joint, the anconeal fragment is grasped with bone-holding forceps, Allis tissue forceps, or a large pair of old Backhaus towel forceps, and mild traction is applied (Fig. 58.8). A scalpel is used to free the anconeal process from its fibrous attachments, which usually join the proximal aspect of the anconeal process to the ulna. Once the anconeal process is freed from its attachments, it is lifted from the joint. The joint again is inspected carefully for any loose pieces or fragments of bone, cartilage, or fibrous tissue. If present, they should be removed, and the joint should be flushed with Ringer's solution. The joint is closed as described for the reattachment procedure.

Postoperatively, a padded bandage is applied to the leg from the toes to above the elbow for 7 to 10 days. During the first 2 weeks after surgery, the animal needs to be encouraged to use the leg for gentle exercise (e.g., walking on a leash, physical therapy, or swimming) to speed the return to function. After an additional 2-week period, the animal often can be returned to normal activity.

References

1. Herron MR. Canine ununited anconeal process. Vet Clin North Am 1971;1:417.
2. Mason TA, Lavelle RB, Skipper SC, et al. Osteochondrosis of the elbow joint in young dogs. J Small Anim Pract 1981;21:641.
3. Van Sickle DC. The relationship of ossification to elbow dysplasia. J Am Anim Hosp Assoc 1966;2:24.

Surgical Treatment of Fragmented Medial Coronoid Process

K. Ron Presnell

The coronoid process of the ulna is that portion of the distal ulnar trochlear notch that flares into a prominent medial projection and a much less prominent lateral projection. These projections are articular and help to increase the surface area of the joint (Fig. 58.9). The narrow medial condyle of the humerus articulates with the coronoid process of the ulna. The lateral condyle of the humerus articulates with the radial head. In the normal animal, the coronoid process is estimated to provide about 20 to 25% of the total articular weightbearing surface, whereas the remaining 75 to 80% of weightbearing surface is through the radial head.

Fragmented coronoid process (FCP) was first recognized in the mid–1970s and initially was called ununited coronoid process because it was thought to be similar to ununited anconeal process (UAP). This usage was later disputed, and the term FCP is now considered more appropriate, because the lesion is not truly an ununited process. This condition is often seen in conjunction with osteochondritis dissecans (OCD) of the medial condyle of the humerus. The lesion on the medial condyle leads to a cartilage flap or loose joint mouse. The FCP is an ossified fragment that has fractured off or that has a deep fissure and cleft separating it from the rest of the coronoid process. The fragmented medial coronoid process can involve up to 50% of the coronoid itself (Fig. 58.10).

Pathogenesis and Associated Osteochondrosis

The cause of FCP is not clear, but the disorder appears to be a manifestation of osteochondrosis. The cartilage and bone weakness, combined with mechanical overloading, lead to fragmentation of the coronoid process itself. It is easy to anticipate that if radial growth slows

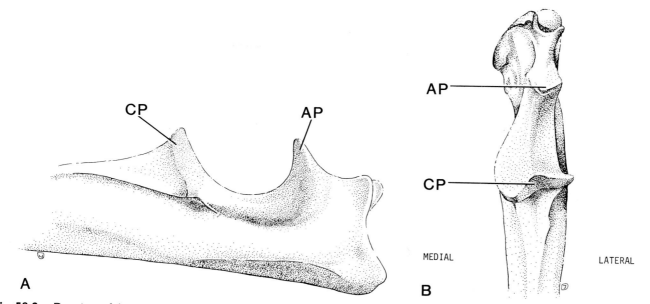

Fig. 58.9. Drawings of the ulna showing the anconeal process (*AP*) and the coronoid process (*CP*). **A.** Lateral view. **B.** Craniocaudal view.

even mildly compared with ulnar growth, more weight is borne on the coronoid process of the ulna. If the animal walks with an abnormal gait or posture, it could produce greater weightbearing on the medial condyle of the humerus. FCP usually originates at 4 to 6 months of age when the pup is in a rapid growing phase and is awkward in its gait and when the bones are more subject to injury than they are once they mature.

Some patients with FCP have a distinct OCD lesion and a flap on the humerus. Other patients have just a wear-and-tear ("kiss") lesion of the articular cartilage opposite the primary FCP lesion. An OCD lesion usually is an ulcerated area with a cartilage flap; a wear-and-tear lesion is simply an abrasion or wearing off of the cartilage and appears different from an OCD-type lesion. A wear-and-tear lesion usually does not involve a defect in the bone, and the injury is primarily on the surface. Conversely, an OCD lesion on the humerus can result in a wear-and-tear lesion on the radius and ulna.

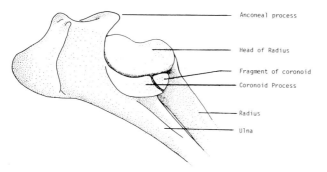

Fig. 58.10. A fragmented medial coronoid process.

FCP occurs most commonly in Newfoundlands, Labrador retrievers, golden retrievers, and German shepherds, but it can be seen in most large breeds of dogs. Affected dogs usually are presented with the problem between 6 and 12 months of age. A few cases have been reported in older dogs.

Clinical Signs and Diagnosis

All three disorders of the elbow joint—FCP, UAP, and OCD—have similar early clinical signs and are often difficult to separate from shoulder lameness. The owner usually describes the dog as first showing mild lameness at 4 to 5 months of age. This may appear as mild stiffness, which occurs most commonly when the dog first gets up in the morning or after a period of rest, especially if the rest period was preceded by a period of vigorous exercise. The dog often walks with a shortened stride; because FCP is often bilateral, the dog may not show obvious lameness. The progress of this disease is slow and may be so mild that the dog may not be presented to the veterinarian until it is 7 to 9 months of age (while the condition starts at 4 to 5 months). At a later stage, the dog usually has a bilaterally stiff gait, with the elbows carried more widely apart than normal. The dog may have a mild rolling gait with the elbows rotated slightly inward with forward advancement of the leg. The dog usually has a shortened forward stride and tends to walk as though its front end were tender. Some dogs with FCP are presented for evaluation of the hips because of an awkward rear leg gait, which results from shifting of weight to the rear legs. Usually, the hips are found to be normal.

Physical examination usually reveals a mild muscle atrophy of the forelimbs. Pain can often be elicited by maximal extension or flexion of the elbow joint or deep palpation over the medial aspect of the joint in the area of the coronoid. The joint often feels thickened, especially medially. This feature is more evident as the disease progresses.

Radiographic examination is indicated in all suspected cases of elbow lameness. Only the highest-quality radiographs are suitable, because FCP and OCD lesions are difficult to see at the best of times. A craniocaudal and two oblique craniocaudal views (one rotated slightly medially and the other rotated slightly laterally with the leg in about 30° of flexion) are desirable. Oblique views help to project the coronoid process free of the radius and also help to hit the medial humeral condyle tangentially to show the OCD lesion better. A lateral view taken in moderate flexion is essential to help expose the anconeal process, which is usually the first area of the elbow joint to show osteophyte production or degenerative joint disease. Radiographically, an OCD lesion is seen as a small defect on the medial condyle of the humerus (Fig. 58.11). It can vary from narrow to wide and may involve only a small portion or most of the humeral condyle.

Because a FCP rarely is visualized on radiographs, one looks for the secondary changes that occur after 7 to 8 months of age. These changes include osteophyte production on the medial coronoid process and the anconeal process (see Fig. 58.11) and osteophytes on the lateral and medial epicondyles of the humerus. In more advanced cases, osteophyte production is seen on the craniodorsal portion of the radius at the joint margin and under the semilunar notch of the ulna.

Diagnosis of FCP in a younger dog usually is based on history, the gait of the animal, and the clinical impression if radiographic signs are not present. If the diagnosis is still in doubt with a 4- to 5-month-old animal, one can wait and reevaluate the dog radiographically at 7 to 8 months of age when the secondary changes are more obvious, or one can perform an exploratory operation of the joint at this stage. In the young dog (4 to 6 months of age), some clinicians recommend ruling out all other tentative diagnoses. If they are left with a patient of a susceptible breed with a characteristic gait, they perform an exploratory operation to confirm the diagnosis of FCP.[2]

Indications for Surgery

Early surgical exploration and removal of an FCP or curettage of OCD lesions in dogs suspected of having FCP disorder have been advocated by some surgeons. This approach appears to be most effective if the operation is done before severe degenerative joint disease is evident. The efficacy of surgical therapy after a dog is 18 to 20 months of age and has severe secondary changes is debatable.

The decision to operate is not easy in a 4- to 7-month-old dog because radiographic confirmation of the diagnosis usually is absent. Generally, one has to rely on the history, the clinical signs, and elimination of all other causes of forelimb lameness in the large breed, rapidly growing dog. Dogs under 16 months of age who are operated on before they have severe secondary changes usually improve clinically. The rate of progress and the development of osteoarthritis appear to be reduced in these dogs. Surgical treatment in dogs older than 16 months or in those with severe osteoarthritis usually has been clinically unrewarding.

Surgical Technique

The surgical procedure for treatment of FCP disorder is not difficult if one is familiar with the anatomy of the elbow. The aim is to open the joint medially, to remove the FCP and the OCD flap, and to curette out the OCD lesion. One must evaluate the joint critically for fissures and cracks in the cartilage and secondary

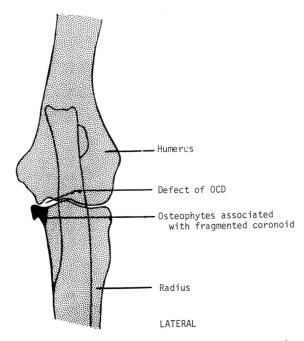

Humerus

Defect of OCD

Osteophytes associated with fragmented coronoid

Radius

MEDIAL   LATERAL

Fig. 58.11. A fragmented coronoid process with an associated osteochondritis dissecans lesion.

---

[2] Editor's note: Another useful method for diagnosing fragmented coronoid process is tomography, which can demonstrate the actual fragmented piece of the coronoid process. I have found tomography especially helpful in diagnosis of fragmented coronoid process in the young dog before secondary degenerative joint disease is readily apparent.

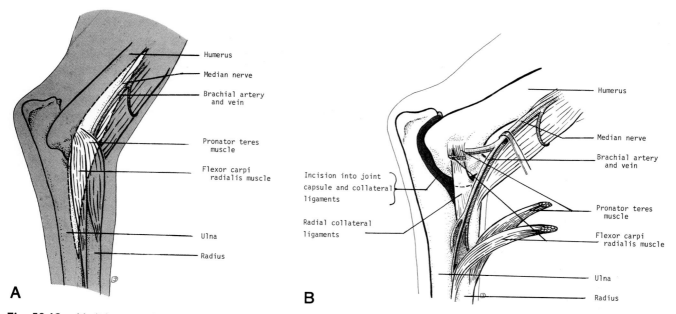

Fig. 58.12. Medial approach to the elbow joint through tenotomy of the pronator teres and the flexor carpi radialis tendons. **A.** Location of the skin incision. **B.** Exposure of the joint after tenotomy and retraction of muscles.

arthritic changes. Two techniques[3] for approaching the medial aspect of the joint are available: tenotomy of the pronator teres and flexor carpi radialis tendons, and osteotomy of the medial epicondyle of the humerus. The tenotomy technique is described here.

After the animal is placed in lateral recumbency with the affected limb down and lying flat on the table, and after the drapes are applied, a skin incision is made over the craniomedial aspect of the elbow. The fascia is dissected to reveal the distal humerus and the pronator teres muscle (Fig. 58.12**A**). Care must be taken at this stage to identify the median nerve and artery and its several branches, which run in different directions around the elbow joint itself. These branches are usually deep to the pronator, with one large branch curving between the tendons of the pronator teres and the flexor carpi radialis. After all the branches of the median nerve are identified, the tendon of the pronator teres is carefully transected near its origin on the humerus. The flexor carpi radialis tendon is transected at the tendon–muscle interface, leaving enough ten-

don attached to the humerus to reattach it. These two muscles are elevated and are retracted distally (Fig. 58.12**B**), a maneuver that exposes the joint capsule, the distal humeral condyle, and the collateral ligament.

The joint capsule is identified, and the capsule and the collateral ligament are cut to allow adequate opening of the joint (i.e., 20 to 25°). The opening of the joint is best achieved by lateral rotation. One can flex the elbow laterally over the edge of the table or over towel pads if operating on one leg. If the dog is bilaterally affected, both legs can be operated on simultaneously by two surgical teams if the dog is placed in dorsal recumbency. In this case, the assistant has to flex the leg laterally and externally rotate the radius to open the joint. A simultaneous bilateral operation with the dog positioned on its back is slightly more difficult to perform than a unilateral operation; however, the time saving is beneficial.

A liberal incision into the joint capsule is necessary to allow adequate opening of the joint so proper visualization and inspection of the coronoid area, the radial head, the trochlear notch, and the distal humerus can be performed. When the joint capsule is opened, a small fragment about 2 mm in diameter may come floating out with the joint fluid. The coronoid area must be inspected carefully for loose pieces or fissure lines through the cartilage. In about half these patients, a piece of FCP is still loosely attached to the remainder of the coronoid. In such cases, inspection of the articular surface reveals a fissure line running across the articular surface. By sliding a periosteal elevator into the fissure and gently rotating it, one usually can re-

---

[3] Editor's note: A modified approach to the joint has been reported (Probst CW, Flo GL, McLoughlin MA, et al. A simple medial approach for treatment of fragmented medial coronoid process and osteochondritis dissecans. J Am Anim Hosp Assoc 1989;25:331) in which the tendons of the pronator teres and flexor carpi radialis are not cut. The approach involves dissecting between the two muscles to expose the joint capsule. The capsule and lateral collateral ligament are incised to expose the articular surfaces. Adduction of the lower limb gives good exposure to the coronoid and medial condyle areas. I prefer this approach for coronoid and OCD removal.

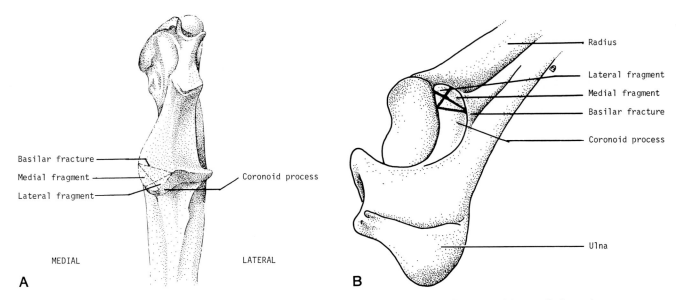

Fig. 58.13. Coronoid area of the ulna showing various types of fragment. **A.** Craniocaudal view. **B.** Lateral view.

move the FCP readily. The portion of the coronoid process that is removed may be cranial, medial, or lateral (Fig. 58.13). Any bone or cartilage that is abnormal must be removed. Any osteophytes that are readily visible are removed as well.

The humerus is checked for OCD lesions. If one sees a flap and a soft underlying area of bone on the medial condyle of the humerus, it is curetted down to bleeding bone. If the lesion is a small wear-and-tear lesion and it is only partially through the cartilage, the lesion is not curetted. This sign of chronicity of the disease most often is seen in older patients. The prognosis for this type of case is guarded, and curetting these wear-and-tear lesions does not help.

After a thorough inspection of the joint, the joint is flushed liberally with Ringer's solution and is reinspected. The joint capsule is closed with size 0 absorbable suture in a simple interrupted pattern. The collateral ligament, flexor carpi radialis, and pronator teres muscle are reapposed with large mattress sutures of nonabsorbable material or polydioxanone. The subcutaneous tissue and skin are closed in a normal manner.

Postoperative Care

The animal is kept in a well-padded bandage from the toes to above the elbows until the sutures are removed in 10 to 14 days. Because dogs can easily reach the elbow joint with their mouths, they can often pull the sutures out by licking or chewing if they are not kept bandaged. Activity is restricted for at least 3 to 4 weeks to give the muscles and tendons a chance to heal. The dog is slowly returned to regular activity.

Suggested Readings

Berzon JL, Quick CB. Fragmented coronoid process: anatomic, clinical and radiographic consideration with case analysis. J Am Anim Hosp Assoc 1980;16:241.

Denny HR, Gibbs C. The surgical treatment of osteochondritis dessicans and ununited coronoid process in the canine elbow joint. J Small Anim Pract 1980;21:323.

Evans HE, Christensen GC. Miller's anatomy of the dog. Philadelphia: WB Saunders, 1979.

Fox SM, Bloomberg MS, Bright RM. Developmental anomalies of the canine elbow. J Am Anim Hosp Assoc 1983;19:605.

Grondalen J. Arthrosis in the elbow joint of young rapidly growing dogs. Part III. Ununited medial coronoid process of the ulna and osteochondritis dessicans of the humeral condyle. Surgical procedures for the correction and postoperative investigation. Nord Vet Med 1979;31:520.

Grondalen J, Grondalen T. Arthrosis in the elbow joint of rapidly growing dogs. Part V. A pathoanatomical investigation. Nord Vet Med 1981;33:1.

McCurnin DM, Slusher R, Grier RL. A medial approach to the canine elbow joint. J Am Anim Hosp Assoc 1976;12:475.

Correction of Radial and Ulnar Growth Deformities Resulting from Premature Physeal Closure

Ann L. Johnson

Ulnar Ostectomy and Insertion of a Free Autogenous Fat Graft

The purpose of this technique is to release the constraint of the ulna on the growth of the radius, and it is coupled with the placement of a free autogenous fat

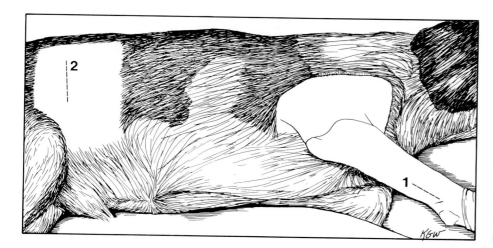

Fig. 58.14. The affected fore-limb and the ipsilateral flank are prepared for aseptic surgery. The incision for exposure of the distal ulna is labeled *1*. The incision for harvesting the fat graft is labeled *2*.

graft to prevent union of the ulnar segments. If the radial physes have sufficient growth potential, an increase in radial length and, in some cases, correction of the angular deformity are the desired outcomes.

Both the affected forelimb and the ipsilateral flank are prepared for aseptic surgery (Fig. 58.14). The distal ulna is approached from the lateral side through a skin incision extending over the mid-distal to distal ulnar area. The subcutaneous tissue is incised, and the lateral digital extensor muscle is separated from the extensor carpi ulnaris muscle, exposing the distal metaphyseal portion of the ulna (Fig. 58.15**A**). The area for the ostectomy is isolated by elevating the surrounding musculature and fascia, carefully ensuring that all periosteum, with its osteogenic potential, remains with the segment of bone to be resected. A 1- to 2-cm segment of the ulna is resected using bone cutters or an oscillating bone saw cooled with a saline flush. The segment of bone and its associated periosteum are removed (Fig.58.15**B**). The interosseous artery may be encountered at this time, and hemostasis should be achieved.

A 2- to 3-cm skin incision is made in the ipsilateral flank area, exposing the subcutaneous fat. A large single piece of fat is sharply dissected free and is placed in the ostectomy gap (Fig. 58.15**C** and **D**). Hemostasis is achieved at the donor site, and the subcutaneous tissue and skin are sutured. The transplanted fat is secured in the ostectomy gap by suturing the adjacent soft tissues. The subcutaneous tissues and skin are sutured.

Postoperative radiographs are made to document the location and length of the ostectomy gap. A soft padded bandage or splint may be used to protect the limb for 2 weeks if bilateral procedures are done. The dog is released to the owners with instructions to limit activity and to return for monthly reexaminations. Radiographs are made monthly and are compared with the postoperative radiographs for growth of the radius,

correction of the angular deformity and patency of the ostectomy gap. The release of the proximal ulna may restore the normal configuration of the elbow. Reevaluations are discontinued when the animal is skeletally mature. Union of the ulna while the animal is still growing is an indication for reoperation. A corrective osteotomy of the radius may be indicated if the angular deformity has not corrected when the dog has reached maturity.

The ostectomy should be performed in the distal ulna just proximal to the physis. In this location, the discontinuity of the ulna does not appear to affect the stability of the elbow or carpus. Failure to remove all the periosteum at the ostectomy site results in premature bone bridging of the ostectomy gap. The surgeon must securely close the soft tissues over the fat graft. Herniation of the graft can lead to dehiscence of the wound and loss of the graft. Careful closure of the donor site is also important to decrease the incidence of seroma formation. Postoperative splint support for 2 weeks is important with bilateral ostectomies to prevent motion at the ostectomy gap and displacement of the fat graft. However, splinting an immature dog often leads to laxity of the flexor tendons and hyperextension of the carpus. Therefore, careful attention must be paid to removing the splint at the appropriate time.

Technique for Bone Bridge Resection and Free Autogenous Fat Graft for Treatment of Partial Premature Closure of the Distal Radial Physis in the Immature Dog

The purpose of this technique is to remove the bone bridging the physis to allow unrestricted growth of the normal portion of the distal radial physis. A free

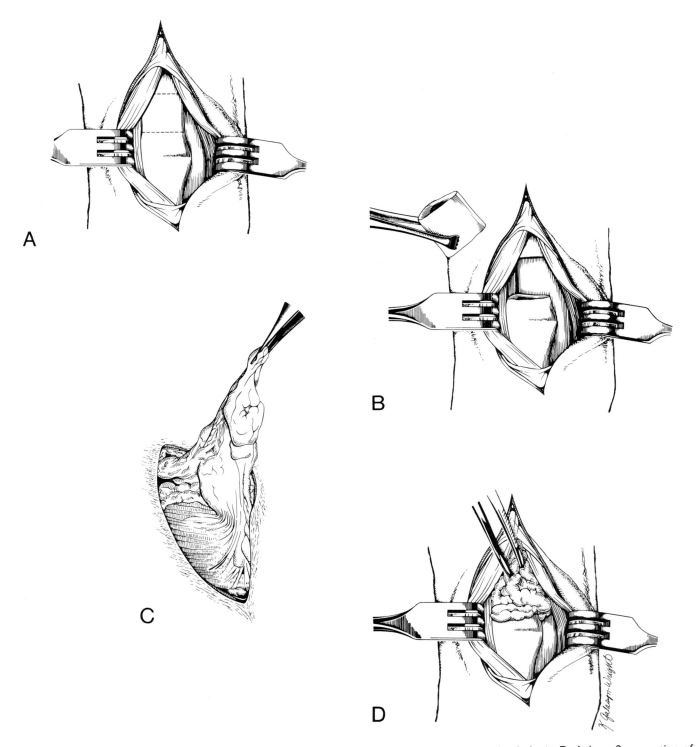

Fig. 58.15. **A.** The distal ulna is exposed. The ostectomy is performed just proximal to the distal physis. **B.** A 1- to 2-cm section of bone and surrounding periosteum is removed. **C.** A large piece of fat is atraumatically harvested from the flank. **D.** The fat is placed in the ostectomy gap.

autogenous fat graft is placed in the defect to prevent reestablishment of the bone bridge. Tomographic examination of the distal radial physis may be indicated to define the area of the physis bridged by bone accurately.

Both the affected forelimb and the ipsilateral flank are prepared for aseptic surgery. The bridged portion of the distal radial physis is surgically exposed. The limitations of the bone bridge are determined by exploring the area with a hypodermic needle (Fig.

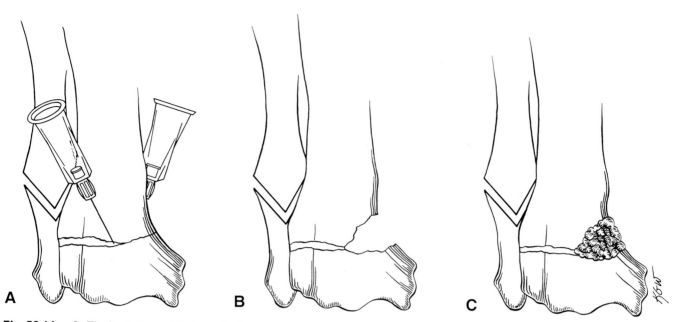

Fig. 58.16. **A.** The limitations of the bone bridge are determined using a hypodermic needle. The cartilage of the normal physis is easily penetrated by the needle. **B.** The bone bridge is removed using a curette or a high-speed bur. **C.** Free autogenous fat is placed within the physeal defect.

58.16**A**). The cartilage of the normal physis is easily penetrated by the needle, as opposed to the resistance felt when the bone bridge or adjacent metaphyseal or epiphyseal bone is probed. The bone bridge is removed using a curette or a high-speed bur. Curettage is complete when normal physeal cartilage is observed or probed with the needle (Fig. 58.16**B**). Free autogenous fat is harvested as described for ulnar ostectomy and is placed within the physeal defect (Fig. 58.16**C**). The soft tissues and skin are sutured over the transplanted fat. Postoperative radiographs are made to document complete resection of the bone bridge and placement of the fat graft. A soft padded bandage is used to protect the limb postoperatively. The dog is released to the owners with instructions to limit exercise and to return in 2 weeks for suture removal and every 4 to 6 weeks for reevaluation. Radiographs are made and compared with the postoperative radiographs for length of the radius, correction of angular deformity, and patency of the resected area. The goniometer is used to determine angular limb deformity, and results are compared with preoperative results for changes in severity of the deformity. Reevaluations are discontinued when the animal reaches skeletal maturity. Reestablishment of the bone bridge or worsening of the angular deformity may be an indication for reoperation. A corrective osteotomy of the radius may be indicated if the angular deformity is not corrected when the dog reaches maturity.

Animals rarely present early enough in the development of asymmetric physeal closure for this procedure to be indicated. Most animals present with evidence of early closure of one side of the physis followed by closure of the rest of the physis. However, if early diagnosis of a problem can be made, this procedure can allow continued function of the physis.

Oblique Corrective Osteotomy of the Radius and Transverse Osteotomy of the Ulna Stabilized With Type II External Fixation

The purpose of this procedure is to correct angular and rotational forelimb deformities while preserving as much length of the limb as possible. External fixation is a versatile method of stabilizing the osteotomy that allows postoperative correction. This technique can be converted to a distraction procedure to gain additional limb length by using connecting bars that permit daily distraction.

Preoperative radiographs are made of the affected and contralateral radius and ulna, including the adjacent joints. The radiographs of the affected radius are studied to determine the location of the point of greatest curvature of the radius and to evaluate the anatomy of the adjacent elbow and carpus. The affected radius or ulna is compared with the contralateral radius or ulna to determine the discrepancy in length.

The dog is anesthetized, and the affected forelimb and a donor site for cancellous bone (usually the proximal humerus of the affected forelimb) are prepared for aseptic surgery. The limb is securely suspended from the ceiling and draped for the procedure.

The lateral aspect of the head of the radius is palpated, the overlying skin is incised, and the bone is exposed by blunt dissection of the subcutaneous tissues and grid dissection of the muscle. Using a predrilling technique, a centrally threaded positive profile fixation pin is placed through the proximal radius from the lateral aspect. The pin should parallel the proximal radial articular surface and should be within the lateral transverse plane of the proximal radius. The lateral aspect of the distal radius is palpated, and the ulnar styloid process is identified. After a limited exposure of the bone and predrilling the hole, a centrally threaded positive profile fixation is placed through the distal radius, starting cranially to the ulnar styloid process, from the lateral aspect. The pin should parallel the distal radial articular surface and should be within the lateral transverse plane of the distal radius (Fig. 58.17). A lateral approach is made to the distal ulna (see the discussion of ulnar ostectomy), and a transverse osteotomy is performed with an osteotome or oscillating saw. A skin incision is made over the craniomedial aspect of the distal radius at its point of greatest curvature. Dissection through the subcutaneous tissues ex-

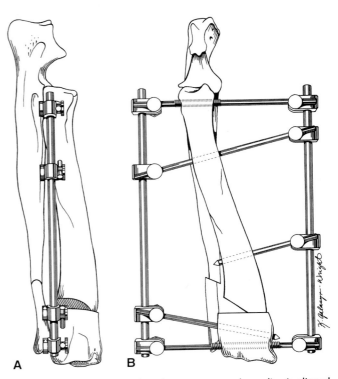

Fig. 58.18. **A** and **B.** After the osteotomy, the radius is aligned so the proximal and distal transfixation pins parallel each other and are in the same transverse plane. The rest of the type II external fixator frame is constructed.

poses the radial diaphysis. An oblique osteotomy of the radius is made at the point of greatest curvature with an osteotome or an oscillating bone saw, directing the osteotomy line parallel to the distal radial articular surface (see Fig. 58.17). The operating table is lowered until the animal's shoulder is no longer contacting the table. The weight of the animal distracts the distal radius and helps to align the proximal and distal joint surfaces parallel. The proximal and distal transfixation pins are aligned parallel to each other and in the same transverse plane, to eliminate any angular or rotational deformity. Connecting bars with two to six single fixation clamps are joined to the transfixation pins on the lateral and medial aspect of the limb. Additional fixation pins are driven through the unused single clamps and into the radius, penetrating both cortices. One to two additional pins should be placed in each radial segment (Fig. 58.18). Autogenous cancellous bone graft is harvested from the proximal humerus and is placed at the radial osteotomy site. The wounds are closed by suturing the subcutaneous tissue and skin separately.

Postoperative radiographs are made to document radial alignment and implant position. Correction of residual angular deformity can be made by loosening the clamps on the distal fixation pins and realigning the distal bone segment. Correction of residual rotational deformity can be made by removing one con-

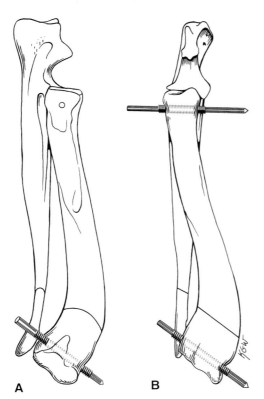

Fig. 58.17. **A** and **B.** The proximal pin should parallel the proximal radial articular surface and should be within the lateral transverse plane of the proximal radius. The distal pin should parallel the distal radial articular surface and should be within the lateral transverse plane of the distal radius. An oblique osteotomy of the radius is made at the point of greatest curvature with an osteotome or an oscillating bone saw, directing the osteotomy line parallel to the distal radial articular surface. An osteotomy of the ulna is performed.

necting bar and rotating the single clamps so the pins in the distal segment are positioned on the opposite side of the connecting bar. Finally, all clamps are checked for tightness, and the fixation pins are cut to the desired length.

Postoperatively, the limb may be bandaged to minimize soft tissue swelling. Gauze sponges should be wedged between the connecting bars and the skin, and the entire limb is bandaged in a soft padded wrap. As postoperative swelling decreases, the limb may be left unbandaged. The animal is released to the owner with instructions for the animal's confinement, to limit limb use and to avoid catching the fixation on surrounding objects; the owner is also advised to administer daily hydrotherapy to keep pin tracts clean. Rechecks should be scheduled at 2 weeks for suture removal and fixator evaluation and every 4 to 6 weeks for radiographic evaluation of healing of the osteotomy. The fixator is removed when the osteotomy site is bridged with bone.

Suspending the limb from the ceiling during the osteotomy aids the surgeon in aligning the limb and decreases the amount of postoperative swelling because of the minimal manipulation needed to support the limb during correction and fixation. The surgeon must make the radial osteotomy cut parallel to the distal radial joint surface, not only in the lateromedial plane but also in the craniocaudal plane, to make correction of a severe cranial bowing deformity possible. External fixation of the osteotomy is useful for several reasons. The proximal and distal transfixation pins serve as external landmarks to help align the bone after osteotomy. Additional manipulations can be made easily after the surgical procedure if the surgeon is not satisfied with the corrections. The rigidity of the fixator can be altered to suit the animal and the stage of bone healing. Finally, removal of the fixation after bone healing is simple and generally requires only sedation. The disadvantages of external fixation lie in the aftercare that the owner must perform and in the damage that the external fixator can do to the dog's surrounding environment.

Technique for Radial Ostectomy and Insertion of a Free Autogenous Fat Graft for Treatment of Complete Premature Closure of the Proximal or Distal Radial Physis in the Immature Dog

The purposes of this technique are to release the constraint of the radius on the growth of the ulna and to prevent distraction of the radial head from its articulation with the humerus. If the distal ulnar physis has

sufficient growth potential, the animal will achieve additional limb length.

Both the affected forelimb and the ipsilateral flank are prepared for aseptic surgery. The animal is positioned in lateral recumbency, and the forelimb and flank are draped. A skin incision is made over the craniomedial aspect of the mid-diaphysis of the radius. The subcutaneous tissue is incised, and the extensor carpi radialis muscle is elevated and is retracted laterally to expose the mid-diaphysis of the radius. The area for the ostectomy is isolated by elevating the surrounding musculature and fascia, carefully ensuring that all periosteum remains with the segment of bone to be resected. A 1- to 2-cm segment of the radius is resected using bone cutters or an oscillating bone saw cooled with a saline flush. The segment of bone and its associated periosteum are removed (Fig. 58.19**A**). The interosseous artery may be encountered at this time, and hemostasis should be achieved.

A 2- to 3-cm skin incision is made in the ipsilateral flank area, exposing the subcutaneous fat. A large single piece of fat is sharply dissected free and is placed in the ostectomy gap (Fig. 58.19**B**). Hemostasis is achieved at the donor site, and the subcutaneous tissue and skin are sutured. The transplanted fat is secured

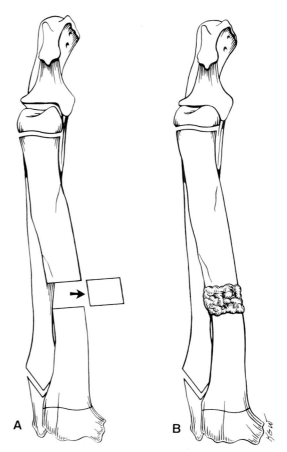

Figure 58.19. **A.** A 1- to 2-cm segment of the radius is resected. **B.** A large single piece of fat is placed in the ostectomy gap.

in the ostectomy gap by suturing the adjacent soft tissues. The subcutaneous tissues and skin are sutured.

Postoperative radiographs are made to document the location and length of the ostectomy gap. A soft padded bandage or splint may be used to protect the limb and to provide additional support to the ulna. The dog is released to the owners with instructions to limit the animal's activity and to return for monthly reexaminations. Radiographs are made monthly and are compared with the postoperative radiographs for growth of the ulna and patency of the ostectomy gap. The release of the radius may restore the normal configuration of the elbow. Reevaluations are discontinued when the animal is skeletally mature. Union of the radius while the animal is still growing is an indication for reoperation. A lengthening osteotomy of the radius may be indicated if the radial head does not articulate with the humerus. If the limb is substantially shorter when the ulnar physis closes, a lengthening osteotomy of the radius and ulna may be indicated.

Failure to remove all of the periosteum at the ostectomy site results in premature bone bridging of the ostectomy gap. The surgeon must close the soft tissues securely over the fat graft. Herniation of the graft can lead to dehiscence of the wound and loss of the graft. Careful closure of the donor site is also important to decrease the incidence of seroma formation. Bandage or splint support is usually provided for 2 to 3 weeks because the radius is the primary weightbearing bone in the distal forelimb. For the same reasons, a second surgical procedure to reunite the radial segments by bridging the ostectomy gap with autogenous cancellous bone graft may be indicated when the dog has reached maturity.

Technique for Transverse Lengthening Osteotomy for Treatment of Premature Closure of the Proximal or Distal Radial Physis in the Mature Dog

The purpose of this technique is to reestablish normal length to the radius and to reestablish a congruent elbow to improve function of the limb. The indications for this procedure are animals with a normal length of the forelimb but decreased length of the radius, resulting in distraction of the radial head from its articulation with the humerus.

The dog is anesthetized, and the affected forelimb and a donor site for cancellous bone (usually the proximal humerus of the affected forelimb) are prepared for aseptic surgery. The dog is positioned in lateral or dorsal recumbency, and the forelimb is draped for the procedure.

The lateral head of the radius is identified, the skin is incised, and the bone is exposed by blunt dissection of the subcutaneous tissues and grid dissection of the muscle. Using a predrilling technique, a centrally threaded positive-profile cortical fixation pin is placed through the proximal radius from the lateral aspect. The pin should parallel the proximal radial articular surface and should be within the lateral transverse plane of the proximal radius. The lateral aspect of the distal radius is palpated, and the ulnar styloid process is identified. Using a predrilling technique, a centrally threaded positive-profile cancellous fixation pin is placed through the distal radius, starting cranially to the ulnar styloid process, from the lateral aspect. The pin should parallel the distal radial articular surface and should be within the lateral transverse plane of the distal radius (Fig. 58.20A). A skin incision is made over the cranial medial aspect of the mid-diaphysis of the radius. The subcutaneous tissue is incised, and the extensor carpi radialis muscle is elevated and retracted laterally to expose the mid-diaphysis of the radius. A transverse osteotomy is made with an osteotome or oscillating saw. The proximal and distal segments of the radius are distracted until the head of the radius has contracted the capitulum of the humerus. Con-

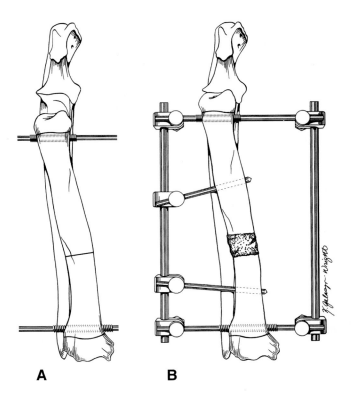

A   **B**

Fig. 58.20. **A.** Proximal and distal transfixation pins are placed, and a transverse radial osteotomy is performed. **B.** The proximal radial segment is distracted until the radial head contacts the capitulum of the humerus. The type II external fixation frame is constructed to stabilize the osteotomy.

necting bars with two to six single fixation clamps are connected to the transfixation pins on the lateral and medial aspect of the limb. Additional fixation pins are driven through the unused single clamps and into the radius, penetrating both cortices. One to two additional pins should be placed in each radial segment (Fig. 58.20**B**). Autogenous cancellous bone graft is harvested from the proximal humerus and is placed at the radial osteotomy site. The wounds are closed by suturing the subcutaneous tissue and skin separately.

Postoperative radiographs are made to document the position of the radial head and the locations of the fixation pins. Some correction of the radial segment location can be made at this time by adjusting the external fixator. If the head of the radius does not appear to contact the capitulum of the humerus, a transverse bilateral fixation pin is placed through the olecranon proximally to the most proximal transverse pin through the radius. The external fixator clamps proximal to the radial osteotomy are loosened. The ulnar pin and the proximal radial pin are connected bilaterally with elastic bands, placing tension on the proximal radius and pulling it toward the humerus. The limb is radiographed in 24 to 48 hours, and when the articulation is correct, the elastic bands and the ulnar pin are removed and the are clamps tightened.

Postoperatively, the limb may be bandaged to minimize soft tissue swelling. Gauze sponges should be wedged between the connecting bars and the skin, and the entire limb should be bandaged in a soft padded wrap. As postoperative swelling decreases, the limb may be left unbandaged. The animal is released to the owner with instructions for the animal's confinement to limit limb use and to avoid catching the fixation on surrounding objects; the owner is also advised to administer daily hydrotherapy to keep pin tracts clean. Rechecks should be scheduled at 2 weeks for radiographic evaluation of healing of the osteotomy. The fixator is removed when the osteotomy site is bridged with bone.

The critical part of this technique is to reestablish articulation of the radial head with the capitulum of the humerus accurately. A lateral approach to the elbow may be used to visualize the reduction of the radial head. However, using the external fixator in the manner described previously allows additional reduction of the radial head after the procedure is complete without the trauma of approaching the elbow. In some cases, after reduction of the radial head, angulation of the proximal radial segment is noted. Fracture healing is rapid in these young dogs, and removal of the fixation after bone healing is simple and generally requires only sedation. The disadvantages of external fixation lie in the aftercare that the owner must perform and in the damage that the external fixator can do to the dog's surrounding environment.

Treatment of Elbow Luxations

Robert A. Taylor

Elbow luxation refers to the disruption of the articular congruity of the three bones that constitute the elbow joint. Luxation can be traumatic or congenital, with the former more common. Most acute traumatic luxations can be reduced by closed methods; chronic luxations sometimes require open reduction. Surgical repair of congenital elbow luxation is directed at the underlying defect.

The elbow joint is a compound joint formed by the articulation of the humeral condyle, the radial head, and the semilunar notch of the ulna. It is classified as a hinge joint; that is, its major motion is confined to swinging in one plane. The humeral radial articulation allows for 90° supination of the distal extremity (1). The unique configuration of the articulation with the anconeal process located deep in the olecranon fossa, the prominent medial epicondyle of the humerus, and the ligaments of this joint creates a stable articulation. The medial and lateral collateral ligaments connect all three bones; in addition, the oblique ligament, olecranon ligament, and annular ligament further enhance the stability of the elbow.

Congenital Luxations

Congenital elbow luxation is most common in small breed dogs and is thought to have a hereditary basis (2). Agenesis or hypoplasia of the medial collateral ligament allows for rotation of the proximal radius and ulna with subsequent subluxation. The humeral trochlea and anconeal process usually are underdeveloped, and other secondary joint changes may exist in affected animals. This disorder has been reported to occur in combination with ectrodactyly (3).

Closed and open methods of reduction of congenital elbow luxation have been reported (4). Limb salvage and function, rather than complete articular reconstruction, should be the main objectives of surgical correction. Closed reduction has been recommended for dogs under 4 months of age. In older animals with long-standing luxation, open reduction is necessary.

Surgical repair of congenital elbow luxation may involve capsulorrhaphy, reconstruction of the humeral trochlea, reconstruction of the semilunar notch, partial removal of the anconeal process, and capsular imbrication. One should be aware of possible iatrogenic injury to the physis associated with elbow development during surgical reduction. In some cases, owners may elect conservative treatment or euthanasia.

Owners should be counseled with regard to the probable hereditary nature of this problem (2).

Traumatic Luxations

In the absence of fractures, traumatic elbow luxation results in caudolateral or lateral displacement of the radius and ulna. The larger size of the medial condylar surface of the humerus compared with the lateral condyle partly explains the motion of luxation. In addition, the orientation of the oblique ligament and the olecranon ligament is such that lateral luxation is more likely than medial luxation.

Animals with acute traumatic elbow luxation present with a nonweightbearing lameness of the affected limb. The limb usually is flexed, abducted, and pronated. Pain is evident on manipulation, and crepitus and articular incongruity are present. The elbow usually is twice its normal width.

Radiographs taken in two planes are needed to confirm the diagnosis (Fig. 58.21). The surgeon must rule out articular fractures before attempting closed reduction of a luxated elbow.

Closed Reduction

General anesthesia is required for closed reduction of elbow luxations. Because the animal has sustained a recent trauma, a careful physical examination and assessment of associated injury must be performed before anesthesia is induced.

The animal is positioned in lateral recumbency with the affected limb uppermost. In long-haired patients, clipping the hair may be helpful to aid in the manual reduction of the luxation. Radiographs should be examined to determine the location of the anconeal process. If the anconeal process is laterally luxated, the elbow is flexed and the forepaw is rotated internally to force the anconeal process into the olecranon fossa.

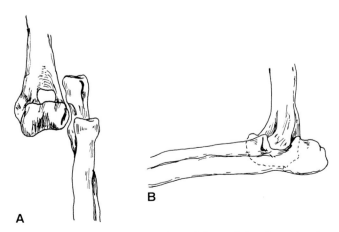

Fig. 58.21. Craniocaudal and lateral views of the elbow showing the typical position of the radius and ulna after lateral luxation of the elbow.

With digital pressure on the radial head, the elbow is held flexed and the radius is pushed onto the humeral capitulum; the leg is then extended and flexed several times to ensure joint congruity. With the elbow flexed 90°, the forepaw can be rotated medially and laterally to check for collateral ligament integrity. If marked postreduction instability is present, surgical repair of the ligaments is indicated.

A soft padded bandage is used to support the limb and to limit swelling. Because early mobilization of the joint surfaces is necessary, the duration of immobilization is limited to 5 to 7 days. During this time, passive range-of-motion exercise should be encouraged.

The trauma necessary to produce luxation in a joint as stable as the elbow invariably results in damage to the articular cartilage, joint capsule, and collateral ligamentous support. Given time, some degree of degenerative joint disease usually results, and owners should be made aware of this possibility.

Open Reduction

Open reduction rarely is required in patients with acute elbow luxations; however, those with chronic luxations with associated capsular adhesions and contractures may require open reduction. In general, a lateral approach to the elbow is satisfactory, although in long-standing cases, a transolecranon approach gives greater exposure (5). It is helpful to lever the radius and ulna (6) into place with a smooth periosteal elevator. Caution is necessary to avoid undue articular cartilage damage. Once reduced, the joint is worked through a normal range of motion, and any fibrin tags and debris are removed. If the lateral collateral ligament has been ruptured, the surgeon must decide to select primary repair or use screw and suture augmentation of the ligament.

Postreduction support is similar both with surgically reduced elbow luxations and with manually reduced luxations. Early activity, range-of-motion exercise, and weightbearing are important for proper rehabilitation.

References

1. Evans H, Christensen G. Miller's anatomy of the dog. 2nd ed. Philadelphia: WB Saunders, 1979.
2. Bingel SA, Rizer, WH. Congenital elbow luxation in the dog. J Small Anim Pract 1977;18:45.
3. Montgomery M, Tomlinson J. Two cases of ectrodactyly and congenital elbow luxation in the dog. J Am Anim Hosp Assoc 1985;21:781.
4. Nunamaker DW. Fracture and dislocation of the elbow. In: Small animal orthopedics. Philadelphia: JB Lippincott, 1985.
5. Piermattei DL, Greeley RG. Atlas of surgical approaches to the bones of the dog and cat. Philadelphia: WB Saunders, 1979.
6. Stayak JW. Elbow luxations. In: Bojrab MJ, ed. Current techniques in small animal surgery. Philadelphia: Lea & Febiger, 1975.

59

CARPUS

Diagnostic Tests for Fractures, Luxations, and Radial Carpal Injuries

Christopher M. Boemo

The carpus is a complex and critical structure with the bones arranged in proximal and distal rows and three joint levels (antebrachiocarpal, middle carpal, and carpometacarpal). Ligaments of the carpus are generally short, spanning usually only one joint connecting adjacent carpal bones, radius, ulna, or metacarpal bones (Fig. 59.1). On the palmar aspect, the joint capsule is well developed and merges with the palmar carpal ligaments and carpal fibrocartilage.

Algorithm for Diagnosis and Treatment of Carpal Injuries

Carpal injuries sustained in falls, from jumping from heights, or as a result of motor vehicle accidents may be severe and extensive. The prognosis for return to adequate function depends on the degree of damage to the region, together with the adequacy of repair procedures instituted.

Many veterinary practices treat ligamentous injuries of the carpus conservatively with cast immobilization and cage confinement, relying on the production of sufficient fibrous tissue to stabilize the affected joints. Although this approach may be adequate for small and inactive breeds, it is rarely successful in larger and athletic breeds or in overweight animals; the randomly arranged collagen in scar tissue cannot resist cyclic tensile stress and ultimately fails, resulting

in joint instability and the development of degenerative joint disease.

Figure 59.2 depicts a systematic approach to the diagnosis and treatment of carpal injuries. Although not intended as an exhaustive regimen, it does depict the methods most commonly used to repair the respective injuries successfully.

Specific Diagnostic Tests

Carpal injuries may consist of fractures, ligamentous damage, or various combinations. Many such injuries are accompanied by lameness, instability, and swelling. A thorough understanding of the anatomy and physiologic functioning of the carpus is imperative to proper diagnosis, treatment, and return to function.

The physical examination should be thorough and systematic to ensure diagnosis of all significant injuries. The examination in the conscious patient may be hindered by the extent of swelling and pain. Sedation or anesthesia may be necessary to examine the area fully by both manipulating the joint through its range of motion (flexion, extension, and rotation), and stress loading of suspect ligaments. Clinical signs of carpal injuries are discussed here under their respective headings.

Carpal Injuries

Styloid Fractures: Radial, Ulnar, and Combined

The origins of the short radial and short ulnar collateral ligaments of the antebrachiocarpal joint arise from the radial and ulnar styloid processes, respectively, and the processes also provide lateral and medial stability because of their protrusion distal to the proximal row of carpal bones. Styloid fractures are avulsion sprain fractures; they affect joint surfaces and result in insta-

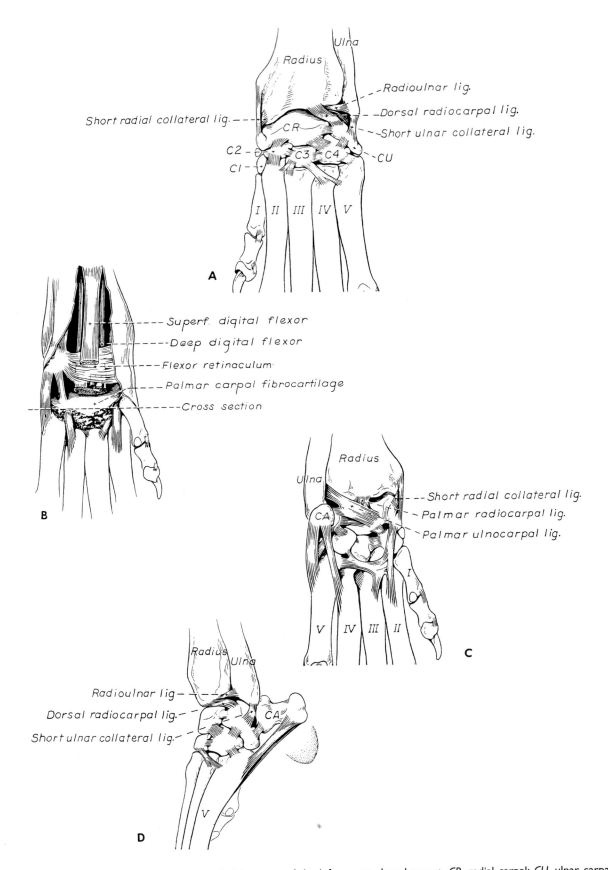

Fig. 59.1. Bones and ligaments of the carpus. **A.** Ligaments of the left carpus, dorsal aspect. *CR,* radial carpal; *CU,* ulnar carpal; *CI* to *C4,* first through to fourth carpals; *I* to *V,* first through to fifth metacarpals. **B.** Superficial ligaments of the left carpus, palmar aspect. **C.** Deep ligaments of the left carpus, palmar aspect. *CA,* accessory carpal; *I* to *V,* first through to fifth metacarpals. **D.** Ligaments of the left carpus, lateral aspect. *CA,* accessory carpal; *V,* fifth metacarpal. (From Evans HE, Christensen GC. Miller's anatomy of the dog. 2nd ed. Philadelphia: WB Saunders, 1979.)

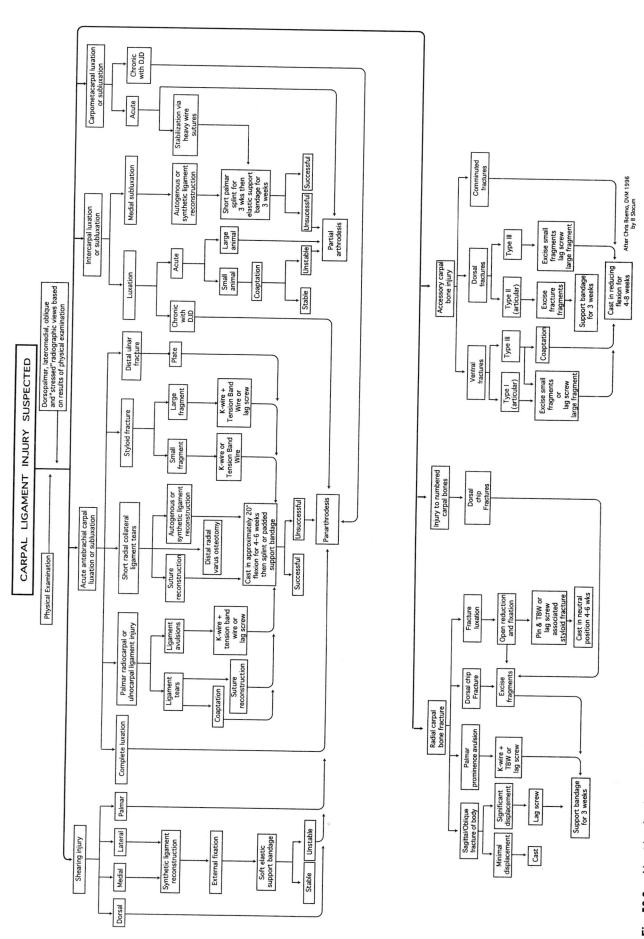

Fig. 59.2. Algorithm for diagnosis and treatment of carpal injuries. Although not exhaustive, it represents a systematic approach to the diagnosis and treatment of carpal injuries. *TBW,* tension band wire; *DJD,* degenerative joint disease.

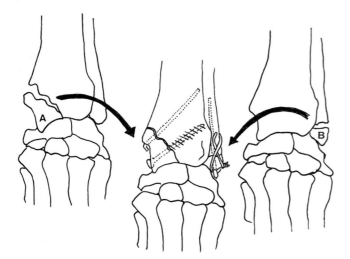

Fig. 59.3. Radial and ulnar styloid fractures. Fractures of the radial styloid process (A) may be stabilized with a K-wire and a lag screw. Fractures of the ulnar styloid (B) are more commonly repaired by the use of a K-wire and figure-of-eight tension band wire as can smaller fractures of the radial styloid.

bility of the antebrachiocarpal joint. Lameness, soft tissue swelling, crepitus, instability, and altered range of motion are commonly observed on clinical examination. The amount of swelling and subluxation depends on the severity and extent of other injuries involving the distal radius, carpus, or metacarpus. Anteroposterior and lateromedial radiographs aid in the assessment of the severity and number of fractures. Open reduction and internal fixation are indicated, and, depending on the adequacy of the fixation, some form of external support may be required during the healing period.

The styloid processes are exposed by a medial or lateral approach directly over the affected areas. After reduction, fixation of radial styloid fractures is usually achieved by placement of either two lag screws, one lag screw and a single Kirschner wire for rotational stability, or a Kirschner wire and tension band wire in the case of small fragments incapable of lag screw fixation. Ulnar styloid process fractures are best repaired by means of a Kirschner wire and tension band wire (Fig. 59.3), although, depending on the type of fracture, this may not achieve rotational stability. Supplementary external support may take the form of a fiberglass cast, half-cast, or metasplint, and coaptation should be continued through to the sixth to eighth postoperative week.

Acute Antebrachiocarpal Luxation or Subluxation

Antebrachiocarpal subluxation or luxation usually results from an excessive load applied to the affected limb in a hyperextended (dorsiflexed) position. The palmar radial carpal (ulnocarpal) ligaments or radial (ulnar) collateral ligaments are commonly affected, sustaining tears or avulsions. Ligament injury may be concurrent with styloid fractures or fractures of the distal radius or ulna. The radial collateral ligament is most commonly affected at this joint level, and rupture or avulsion results in medial instability and valgus deformation of the forepaw.

The joint must be examined fully and stressed through its full range of motion (flexion, extension, rotation). Frequently, the acute antebrachiocarpal subluxation or luxation is accompanied by lameness and extensive soft tissue swelling, the latter potentially hindering a thorough physical examination. In these instances, a combination of rest, ice, and compression is followed by reexamination in 24 to 48 hours, after some of the swelling has been reduced. Radiographic evaluation should include standard dorsopalmar and lateromedial projections, as well as "stressed" and oblique views. If one is in doubt, these radiographs should be compared with similar views of the opposite limb.

ANTEBRACHIOCARPAL LUXATION

Complete luxation of the antebrachiocarpal joint is a rare injury, and fortunately so, because total disruption of the ligamentous support of this joint carries a poor prognosis for primary repair and return to function. Most surgeons suggest panarthrodesis as the most applicable method of treatment.

ANTEBRACHIOCARPAL SUBLUXATION

Subluxation resulting from rupture of the palmar radial carpal or ulnocarpal ligaments has been managed principally by coaptation in decreasing degrees of flexion over a 6- to 8-week period. Although access is limited, lag screw fixation may be contemplated in patients with avulsion injury in which the bone fragments are of sufficient size. Countersunk Kirschner wires may be used for fixation of smaller fragments.

Antebrachiocarpal subluxation resulting from injury to the medial collateral support is more common. The short radial collateral ligament has straight and oblique components: the straight component is under tension during extension, the oblique component is stressed during flexion, and together they limit the degree of dorsopalmar movement. Adequate return to function after subluxation requires that the tendency for distraction of the joint surfaces of the radio-radial carpal joint after ligament rupture or avulsion be limited. The ligaments are exposed by a medial incision directly over the area, with incision and retraction of the antebrachial fascia. Primary reconstruction of the ligaments is difficult because of their size, and autoge-

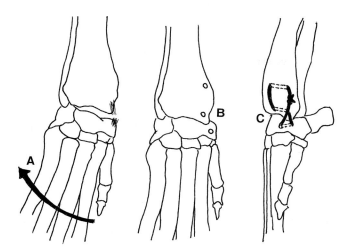

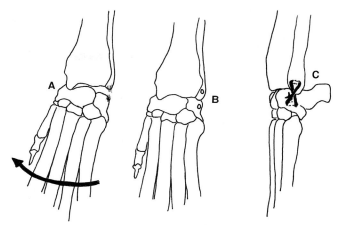

Fig. 59.4. Radial collateral ligament rupture. **A.** Valgus deformity of the paw results from medial instability. **B.** Bone tunnels drilled through both the distal radius and the radial carpal bone are threaded with a synthetic braided suture to simulate the action of both the long and the short collateral ligaments (**C**).

Fig. 59.5. Ulnar collateral ligament rupture. **A.** Varus deformity of the paw results from the lateral instability. **B.** Bone tunnels drilled through the ulnar styloid and the lateral prominence of the ulnar carpal bone are threaded with a synthetic nonabsorbable suture to simulate the ulnar collateral ligament (**C**).

nous or synthetic reconstruction is advisable as the principal repair or as a means of protection for primary ligament reconstruction. Autogenous reconstruction using a portion of the tendon of insertion of the flexor carpi radialis has been described by Earley (1). Synthetic reconstruction involves drilling three bone tunnels (one in the medial prominence of the radial carpal bone and two in the distal radius) (Fig. 59.4) through synthetic nonabsorbable suture material (size 0 to 2) is passed in a manner that simulates the oblique and straight components of the ligament. The suture is tightened to the point where the joint is stable but still able to move, and then it is tied.

Injury to the lateral collateral ligament is less common and less serious because the lateral aspect of the carpus is subject to less tensile stress than the medial side. Short lateral (ulnoulnar carpal) collateral ligaments are similarly repaired either by using a portion of the tendon of insertion of the ulnaris lateralis muscle (2) or by drilling bone tunnels at the origin and insertion of the ligament and threading nonabsorbable suture material to replicate the ligament or to protect a primary ligament reconstruction (Fig. 59.5).

Styloid avulsion fractures or fractures of the distal ulnar shaft occurring in conjunction with palmar or collateral ligament rupture should be repaired with lag screws, Kirschner wires, and tension band wires, or, in the case of ulnar shaft fractures, with bone plating.

Postoperatively, the repair is protected by splinting or casting the carpus in approximately 20° of palmar flexion for 4 to 6 weeks, followed by a further 3 to 4 weeks of either an elastic support bandage or a splint with progressive reduction of the degree of flexion.

Radial Carpal Bone Injuries

Radial carpal bone fractures and luxations are uncommon injuries, but they may occur after a jump or fall from a height or from a moving vehicle. These are hyperextension injuries. In racing greyhounds with hairline oblique fractures of the body of the radial carpal bone, the only clinical signs may be a decreased range of, and slight pain on, carpal flexion. Lameness, pain, crepitus, and variable soft tissue swelling accompany more severe fractures with fragment displacement or radial carpal bone luxation. Luxation is often seen in association with fracture of the radial styloid process or the palmar prominence of the radial carpal bone.

Dorsopalmar, lateromedial, and often oblique views are indicated to reveal the extent of the fracture or luxation. Although the radiographic diagnosis of fractures with significant fragment displacement or bone luxations is straightforward, nondisplaced oblique fractures of the body of the radial carpal bone require careful examination of radiographs.

FRACTURES

Oblique fractures of the body of the radial carpal bone have their axially oriented fracture plane originating on the dorsal surface of the radial carpal bone above the second carpal bone and extend obliquely in a palmarolateral direction to emerge on the palmar surface of the bone below the middle of the distal radius (Fig. 59.6).

When these fractures do not extend through both cortices, coaptation in a neutral cast or splint may produce a satisfactory result. When fracture fragments are

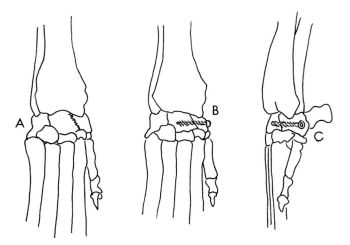

Fig. 59.6. Oblique fracture of the body of the radial carpal bone. **A–C.** Dorsal and medial views of fracture repair using lag screw fixation from the palmaromedial aspect of the bone (through the insertions of the radial collateral ligaments), directed to emerge on the dorsal surface of the bone above the middle of the third carpal bone.

displaced, open reduction and fixation are indicated. Access is through a medial skin incision and incision through the flexor retinaculum directly over the palmar prominence. Reduction of the fracture is followed by the placement of a lag screw directed dorsolaterally from the palmar prominence to emerge on the dorsal

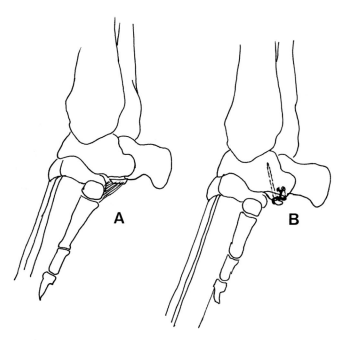

Fig. 59.7. Fracture of the palmar prominence of the radial carpal bone. **A** and **B.** Avulsion of the palmar radial carpometacarpal ligament usually results in a bone fragment suitable for reattachment with a fine Kirschner wire and tension band wire.

surface (see Fig. 59.6). Postoperatively, the limb is supported in a padded bandage for approximately 3 weeks with minimal activity.

Fractures of the palmar prominence of the radial carpal bone are avulsions of the palmar radial carpometacarpal ligaments or the insertion of the oblique component of the short radial collateral ligament, or both. These fragments are repaired by either lag screw placement or pin and tension band wire fixation (Fig. 59.7). Surgical treatment is followed by the placement of a support bandage or a splint for 3 to 4 weeks and minimal exercise. Exercise is slowly resumed over a further 3 to 4 weeks.

Small dorsal chip fractures of the radial carpal bone can occur in isolation. These fractures are best viewed on lateral or rotated lateral radiographs, and they are removed through a dorsal approach by antebrachiocarpal or intercarpal arthrotomy.

LUXATION

Luxation of the radial carpal bone coincides with disruption of its attachment to the ulnar carpal, second carpal and fourth carpal bones, the palmar radial and ulnar carpal ligaments, and the short radial collateral ligaments. The luxated bone often rests palmaromedially in a rotated position (Fig. 59.8). Palpation reveals crepitus, displacement of the bone, and usually a depression in the bone's normal position. Closed reduction of the luxation may be possible if the animal is seen soon after the injury occurs. Splint or cast support for 3 to 4 weeks may then be adequate in small or toy breeds, but open reduction and surgical stabilization are usually necessary in most breeds.

After a dorsal midline approach to the joint, the bone is derotated and reduced. A Kirschner wire is

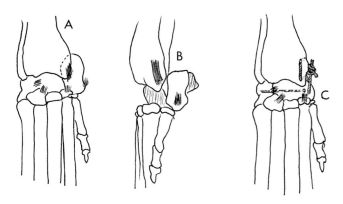

Fig. 59.8. Luxation of the radial carpal bone. **A** and **B.** Dorsal and medial views of the luxation, with the bone rotated through 90° both medially and dorsopalmarly. **C.** After derotation and reduction, the bone is secured with a Kirschner wire to the ulnar carpal bone, and the torn radial collateral ligaments are repaired as described in Figure 59.4.

then driven from the dorsomedial nonarticulating surface of the bone into the ulnar carpal bone. The pin is cut off and is countersunk. Reconstruction of the short radial collateral ligament using synthetic nonabsorbable material is then performed as detailed previously in the section on acute antebrachiocarpal subluxation (see Fig. 59.4). Ligament and joint capsular remnants are sutured when possible, and small bone fragments are excised. The carpus is supported postoperatively in a cast or palmar splint molded into a neutral position for 3 weeks, with a further 3 weeks in a support bandage before gradual reintroduction of exercise.

References

1. Earley T. Canine carpal ligament injuries. Vet Clin North Am 1978;8:183.
2. Roe SC, Dee JF. Lateral ligamentous injury to the carpus of a racing greyhound. J Am Vet Med Assoc 1986;1189:453.

Classification and Treatment of Injuries to the Accessory Carpal Bone

Kenneth A. Johnson

The accessory carpal bone seems more prone to injury than the other carpal bones, perhaps because it is such an integral component of the palmar support structures that prevent hyperextension during full weightbearing. Fractures of this bone are commonly in the region of ligamentous insertions (sprain avulsion fractures), and frequently they involve the articular cartilage surface on the dorsal end of the bone that forms part of the accessory–ulnar carpal joint. Most fractures of this bone occur in racing greyhounds. Similar types of fractures are seen occasionally in dogs of other breeds, and these fractures may be due to trauma, landing awkwardly on the limb, stepping in a hole while running, and falling from heights. Swelling, instability, and pain are common features of carpal injuries, but the diagnosis and classification of fractures are made from radiographs. Fractures can usually be visualized in mediolateral radiographic views with the carpus in full extension or slight flexion. Additional information about the type and extent of the fracture can be obtained from the dorsopalmar radiographic view.

Fracture Classification

These fractures have been classified into five types, on the basis of their radiologic and pathologic features (Fig. 59.9) (1).

Type I injuries are avulsion fractures of bone in the region of the insertion of the accessory–ulnar ligament. Fracture fragments may be large slabs or multiply comminuted chips that are best appreciated on the mediolateral radiographic views. These fractures involve the distal margin of the articular surface, and this feature, combined with disruption of the ligamentous support, leads to instability, subluxation, cartilage damage, and secondary osteoarthritis. Chronic fractures often do not proceed to bony union, and the bone fragments become surrounded by proliferative bone and fibrous tissue.

A variation of the typical type I fracture is an avulsion fracture of the lateral articular prominence of the accessory carpal bone (2). This fracture of the lateral prominence is visualized on a dorsolateral palmarodorsal oblique radiographic view.

Type II injuries are avulsion fractures of the proximal margin of the articular surface and involve bone at the insertion of the palmar ulnocarpal and radial carpal ligaments that connect to the caudomedial surface of distal ulna and the caudal surface of the distal radius. They are often associated with a type I injury. Like type I injuries, they allow subluxation, and articular cartilage damage and secondary osteoarthritis are sequelae.

Type III injuries are avulsion fractures of the distal surface of the palmar end of the bone, at the origin of the two large accessory–metacarpal ligaments that connect to metacarpal bones IV and V. Such injuries disrupt the stay apparatus provided by the accessory–metacarpal ligaments that normally counteract carpal hyperextension during full weightbearing.

Type IV injuries are strain–avulsion fractures of bone from the proximal surface of the palmar end of the bone, at the tendon of insertion of the flexor carpi ulnaris muscle. Bone fragments are distracted proximally by the flexor tendon. The fracture may be an epiphyseal avulsion in dogs up to 5 months of age.

Type V injuries include all other fractures of the carpal body, and these fractures may be comminuted or intra-articular. Fractures may be in a longitudinal, sagittal, or transverse plane, dividing the bone into halves.

Treatment and Prognosis of Fractures

Screw Fixation

Open reduction and internal fixation with screws are indicated in certain type I, II, and III injuries with large, noncomminuted bone fragments (Fig. 59.10) (3). The aims of treatment are restoration of ligamentous integrity and the prevention of subluxation and secondary

Accessory Carpal Bone Fractures

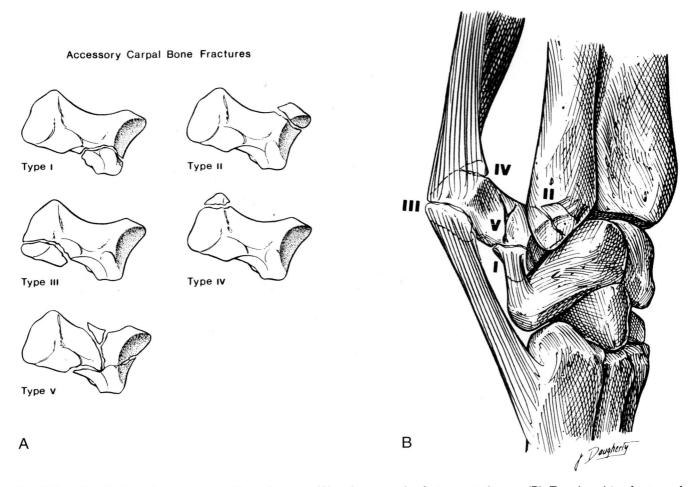

Fig. 59.9. Classification of accessory carpal bone fractures (**A**) and associated soft tissue attachments (**B**). Type I: avulsion fracture of the distal margin of the articular surface at the origin of the accessory–ulnar ligament. Type II: avulsion fracture of the proximal margin of the articular surface at the insertions of the palmar radial carpal and ulnocarpal ligaments. Type III: avulsion fracture at proximal insertions of accessory–metacarpal IV and V ligaments. Type IV: avulsion fracture at the insertion of flexor carpi ulnaris tendon. Type V: comminuted fracture. (From Johnson KA, et al. Characteristics of accessory carpal bone fractures in 50 racing greyhounds. Vet Comp Orthop Traumatol 1988;2:104–107; and Johnson KA, Dee JF, Piermattei DL. Screw fixation of accessory carpal bone fractures in racing greyhounds: 12 cases (1981–1986). J Am Vet Med Assoc 1989;194:1618–1625.)

osteoarthritis. Dogs are positioned in lateral recumbency with the affected limb uppermost for surgery. A skin incision, 5 cm long, is made palmarolateral to the carpus. The palmar carpal retinacular fascia is incised to expose the accessory carpal bone and supporting ligaments. The abductor digiti quinti muscle is elevated and is retracted medially from the accessory–metacarpal IV and V ligaments. A lateral arthrotomy of the accessory–ulnar joint is performed to allow inspection of the articular cartilage surface and accurate reduction in type I and II injuries. Small pointed AO/ASIF forceps are used to maintain reduction (Fig. 59.11). Lag screw fixation is with 1.5- or 2.0-mm cortical screws (Fig. 59.12). If the fragment is thin, countersinking is not performed. The drill hole should be measured and tapped completely to minimize the risk of

screw breakage, an occasional problem with 1.5-mm screws.

The internal fixation is protected with a palmar fiberglass slab splint for 4 to 6 weeks after surgery. Initially, the carpus is immobilized in slight flexion, but then it is moved progressively to a more extended position. Radiographs are taken at 6 and 12 weeks postoperatively to monitor fracture healing.

One study of 12 greyhounds with fractures treated by internal fixation found that 10 returned to racing, and 5 of those won 1 or more races (3). Animals with type I and II fractures are expected to have a worse prognosis because these fractures are intra-articular, but further studies are needed. Although internal fixation of these fractures seems more logical, this operation is technically demanding, and some fracture frag-

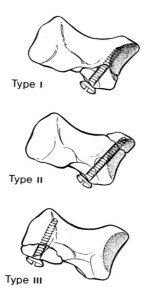

Type I

Type II

Type III

Fig. 59.10. Screw fixation of fracture types I, II, and III. (From Johnson KA, Dee JF, Piermattei DL. Screw fixation of accessory carpal bone fractures in racing greyhounds: 12 cases (1981–1986). J Am Vet Med Assoc 1989;194:1618–1625.)

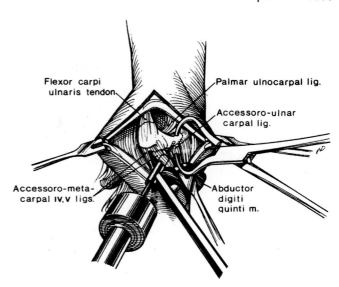

Flexor carpi ulnaris tendon

Palmar ulnocarpal lig.

Accessoro-ulnar carpal lig.

Accessoro-meta-carpal IV,V ligs.

Abductor digiti quinti m.

Fig. 59.12. Fixation of a type I fracture with a 1.5-mm cortical screw. (From Johnson KA, Dee JF, Piermattei DL. Screw fixation of accessory carpal bone fractures in racing greyhounds: 12 cases (1981–1986). J Am Vet Med Assoc 1989;194:1618–1625.)

ments are simply too small to permit screw fixation, so excision becomes unavoidable.

Fragment Excision

Removal of avulsed fracture fragments is an alternative treatment for type I and II fractures. Access for fragment excision is a limited lateral approach, similar

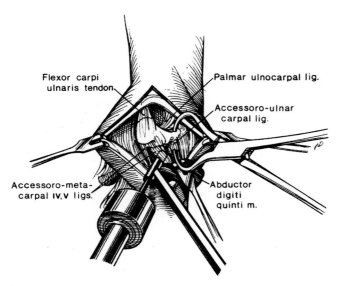

Flexor carpi ulnaris tendon

Palmar ulnocarpal lig.

Accessoro-ulnar carpal lig.

Accessoro-meta-carpal IV,V ligs.

Abductor digiti quinti m.

Fig. 59.11. Reduction of a type I fracture with pointed reduction forceps and drilling a 1.1 hole for screw fixation. (From Johnson KA, Dee JF, Piermattei DL. Screw fixation of accessory carpal bone fractures in racing greyhounds: 12 cases (1981–1986). J Am Vet Med Assoc 1989;194:1618–1625.)

to that used for lag screw fixation. Fragments are usually found attached to the accessory–ulnar ligament or joint capsule, and they are excised with a No. 11 or 15 scalpel blade.

No attempt is made to suture the damaged ligament or capsule after fragment excision, and healing proceeds by fibroplasia. Without surgical treatment, type I and II fractures do not naturally heal by bony union, and often they damage the articular cartilage on the ulnar carpal bone. When internal fixation is not possible, fragment excision perhaps may be preferable to nonsurgical management, but further studies are needed. One study in Scotland found that, of 19 racing greyhounds that had type I fragments removed, 13 returned to race, and 9 won races. Of the other 6, 3 became sound but were unable to race, whereas the other 3 remained lame (4).

External Coaptation

For comminuted fractures that are not amenable to internal fixation and for minimally displaced fractures in young dogs, immobilization of the carpus in flexion is indicated. Malunion of the fracture may be well tolerated unless the fracture is intra-articular.

Partial Arthrodesis

Animals with hyperextension injuries confined to the accessory–ulnar joint frequently have concurrent type I and II fractures of the accessory carpal bone. A partial carpal arthrodesis of this joint stabilizes the carpus while preserving motion in the antebrachiocarpal joint (5). The surgical approach is similar to that used for fracture repair by internal fixation. After the joint is opened, articular cartilage is removed, the space is bone grafted, and a lag screw is placed in a palmarodorsal direction from the accessory carpal bone into the ulnar carpal bone. Additional support is provided by a cerclage wire from the palmar pole of the bone, down to the fifth metacarpal bone.

References

1. Johnson KA. Accessory carpal bone fractures in the racing greyhound: classification and pathology. J Vet Surg 1987;17:60–64.
2. Boemo CM. Fracture of the accessory carpal lateral articular prominence in a racing greyhound. Aust Vet Pract 1994;24: 70–73.
3. Johnson KA, Dee JF, Piermattei DL. Screw fixation of accessory carpal bone fractures in racing greyhounds: 12 cases (1981–1986). J Am Vet Med Assoc 1989;194:1618–1625.
4. Chico AC. Accessory carpal bone fracture in greyhounds: assessment of prognostic indicators and outcome following surgical management by fragment removal. M Vet Med thesis, University of Glasgow, 1992.
5. Lenehan TM, Tarvin GB. Carpal accessorioulnar joint fusion in a dog. J Am Vet Med Assoc 1989;194:1598–1600.

Distal Radial Osteotomy for Treatment of Carpal Collateral Ligament Damage

Barclay Slocum & Theresa Devine Slocum

Injury to the medial collateral ligament of the radial carpal joint often is refractory to immediate reconstruction. Small fragments at the origin or insertion of the medial collateral ligament do not offer a good point of fixation for reattachment of the damaged ligament. Sometimes, damage to the superficial or straight part of the medial collateral ligament is minimal, whereas the deeper oblique portion of the ligament is severely torn, so access to the deeper portion of the ligament requires disruption of the superficial portion of the ligament. Unless the joint is grossly unstable to the surgeon or the patient, surgical repair of the ligament may be possible by relieving the stresses on the ligament by a medial closing wedge osteotomy of the distal radius rather than by direct reconstruction.

In patients with complete disruption of both straight and oblique portions of the medial collateral ligament, other more subtle injuries to the caudal joint capsule and palmar fibrocartilage may have occurred. Treatment by coaptation or pancarpal fusion may be contemplated, but these injuries frequently can heal if the stress is removed from them by medial closing wedge osteotomy of the distal radius.

Chronic short medial collateral ligament instability can occur for various reasons. A dog may run away after an accident and may become lost. Automobile trauma may cause multiple injuries, and the carpus may be the last priority for treatment in the general health of the patient. Patients may be injured in remote areas that cause considerable delay in treatment. Financial restraints may affect the type of treatment chosen. These chronic injuries are another indication for this technique to remove the ligament stress by a medial closing wedge osteotomy of the distal radius.

Surgical Procedure

The preoperative craniocaudal radiograph is taken with the carpus in an extended position that locks the carpus in the weightbearing position. Preoperatively, valgus deviation is determined by first constructing the antebrachial axis (Fig. 59.13, *F*). This line is drawn from the sulcus of the trochlea humeri through a point

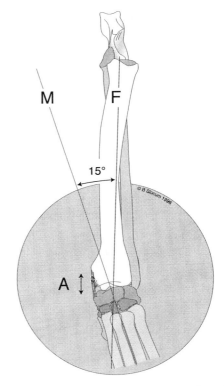

Fig. 59.13. Method for determining angle of medial closing wedge osteotomy. The axis of the antebrachium (*F*) is drawn from the sulcus of the trochlea humeri and is centered between the cortices of lateral and medial distal radius. The metatarsal axis (*M*) is drawn parallel and is centered between the third and fourth metatarsal bones. The angle between these axes is the angle of the medial closing wedge osteotomy, 15° in this example. The purpose of the surgery is to relieve the stresses on the medial collateral ligament (*A*).

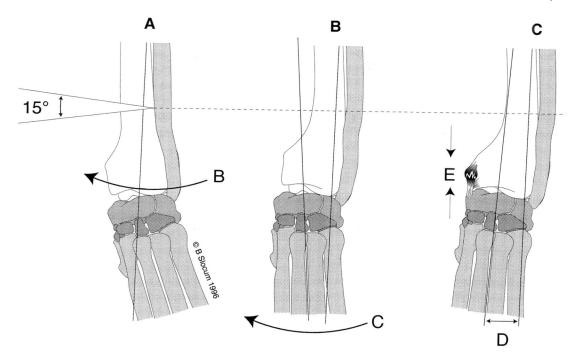

Fig. 59.14. **A.** With the medial closing wedge osteotomy, the distal radius is moved medially (*B*). **B.** The varus of the radius increases compression on the medial aspect of the carpus that causes the metacarpal bones to deviate toward varus (*C*). **C.** The stress is removed from the medial collateral ligament (*E*) as the axis shifts medially (*D*).

centered between the medial and lateral cortices of the distal radius and is extended past the digits. A second line, the metatarsal axis (Fig. 59.13, *M*), is drawn parallel and is centered between the third and fourth metatarsal bones. These two axes intersect with valgus deviation. The angle between the first and second line is the angle for the apex of the medial closing wedge at the lateral distal radial cortex. In our example of Figure 59.13, a 15° medial closing wedge osteotomy of the distal radius is planned. The wedge to be removed from the distal radius is drawn on the radiograph (Fig. 59.14**A**). The base of the wedge is measured as a linear distance from the radiograph.

The patient's forelimb below the midbrachium is prepared for aseptic surgery. The patient is positioned in dorsal recumbency for draping and is rolled toward the affected limb, so the medial aspect of the distal radius is most accessible. Placement of a sterile pad under the limb for stability is helpful.

A skin incision is made over the medial aspect of the distal antebrachium. The cephalic and accessory cephalic veins and nerves are identified and are left intact. Subperiosteal elevation of the extensor carpi radialis tendon and the abductor pollicis longus muscle exposes the cranial portion of the distal radius. Using care to protect the integrity of the radial artery, subperiosteal elevation of the pronator quadratus muscle exposes the caudal portion of the distal radius. An appropriately sized five-hole plate is bent to match

the caudomedial aspect of the radius, with two holes placed distally and three holes proximally. The plate is positioned on the bone, and the location of the distal cut of the wedge osteotomy is marked on the medial aspect of the distal radius with an osteotome. The predetermined distance of the base of the wedge is measured in the proximal direction from the first mark and is scored with an osteotome. Sponges are used to pack all soft tissues away from the distal radius. A saw is used to cut and remove the wedge of bone from the distal radius.

The removed osteotomy wedge is measured to confirm that the desired angle of wedge was achieved. The prebent plate is applied to the distal medial radius, and a cancellous bone graft from the proximal humerus is applied to the caudal radius. Skin closure is routine. A coaptation splint is applied for support during the healing process.

The conformation of the patient is of great importance in considering the use of a medial closing wedge osteotomy of the distal radius. This technique is contraindicated in the patient with a bowlegged and pronated conformation of the forelimb demonstrating a "winging" foot flight.

The patient with normal alignment of the antebrachium and a valgus deviation at the antebrachial carpal joint, demonstrating a paddling foot flight, benefits from this surgical procedure. The patient with normal alignment of the radius and ulna but an external tor-

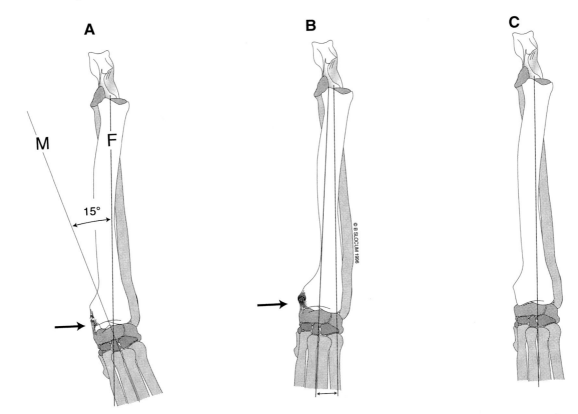

Fig. 59.15. A. The alignment axis of the antebrachium (*F*) is medial to the paw when the medial collateral ligament (*arrow*) is under stress. **B.** The alignment axis of the antebrachium is lateral to the paw (*arrow*) when stress on the medial collateral ligament (*arrow*) is relieved. **C.** In normal alignment, the axes of the antebrachium and the metacarpals are superimposed.

sion or supination of the antebrachium and a valgus deviation at the antebrachial carpal joint showing a paddling foot flight also benefits from a medial closing wedge osteotomy of the distal radius.

The varus osteotomy of the radius moves the distal radius medially (*B* in Fig. 59.14**A**). The varus of the radius increases the compression on the medial aspect of the carpus and causes the metacarpal bones to deviate further toward varus (*C* in Fig. 59.14**B**). This stabilizes the medial antebrachial carpal joint and thus relieves the stress on the medial collateral ligament (*E* in Fig. 59.14**C**), promoting the healing process. The medial closing wedge osteotomy of the distal radius does not reestablish the normal ligamentous structure, but rather takes the stress off the damaged structure so natural healing of the medial collateral ligament by secondary scar formation can occur. This allows the return of collagen integrity, reduces inflammation, and restores function.

The alignment axis of the forearm (*F* in Fig. 59.15**A**) begins medial to the paw when the medial collateral ligament (*arrow* in Fig. 59.15**A**) is under stress. This axis becomes lateral to the paw when stress on the medial collateral ligament (*arrow* in Fig. 59.15**B**) is relieved. The alignment axes of the antebrachium and the metacarpus in normal dogs (Fig. 59.15**C**) are usually superimposed.

Carpal Shearing Injuries: Algorithm and Treatment

Thomas Van Gundy

Carpal shearing injuries usually occur as a result of automobile injury. The obvious severity of this type of wound should not overshadow the search for concurrent injuries. However, as soon as the animal's condition is stable, early evaluation and cleansing of the carpal wound allow formulation of a treatment plan to incorporate all aspects of the traumatic injury.

Early evaluation and treatment include evaluation of circulatory and neurologic damage. Circulatory evaluation may be performed with pulse and temperature evaluation of the extremity. A toenail may be

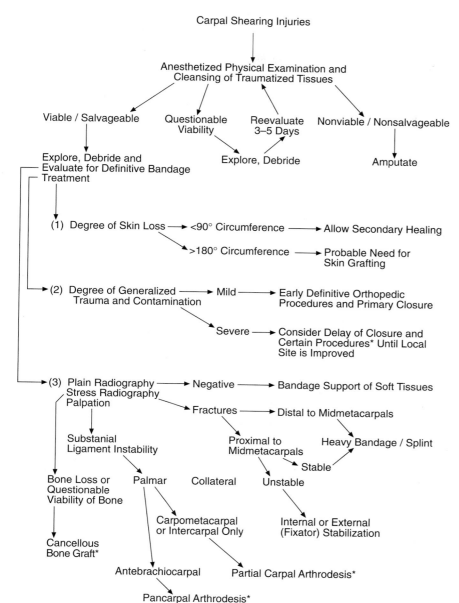

Fig. 59.16. Algorithm shows the decision-making processes for carpal shearing injuries. After evaluation of viability, three concurrent evaluations determine the courses of treatment. Some procedures (*) may be delayed if indicated.

closely trimmed, or distal extremity skin may be nicked by a scalpel to evaluate for bleeding. Early circulatory and neurologic evaluations may be falsely pessimistic if local or systemic vasoconstriction is substantial from trauma and shock. As pulse oximetry and Doppler equipment become more readily available, these techniques may become useful in evaluating wound or limb vascularity. Neurologic evaluation is usually performed by response to deep pain stimulation. However, loss of sensory response in the lower forelimb alone does not necessarily indicate a nonsalvageable limb. If the ability to extend the elbow is still present (radial nerve), long-term lower nerve injury may be tolerated by the animal. The prognosis, however, is more guarded.

With the animal under anesthesia, physical examination and cleansing of the traumatized tissue are performed as soon as feasible after the initial overall patient evaluation (Fig. 59.16). The purpose of surgical intervention is fourfold: 1) injury evaluation and cleansing; 2) debridement of devitalized tissue; 3) stabilization of fractures and ligamentous injury; 4) closure or preparation for healing of skin defects. Initial palpation and radiographs (plain and stressed) allow evaluation of bone and ligament damage. Shearing of the extensor carpi radialis tendon and joint surface does not necessarily imply a poor prognosis. Periarticular scar tissue or eventual arthrodesis often results in satisfactory function. Thorough exploration, meticulous debridement, and copious lavage are essential to remove the often deep-seated foreign material or hair. If viability of tissue or limb is questionable, thorough reevaluation in 3 to 5 days with interim daily bandage management is warranted. Daily or more frequent rebandaging, lavage, and debridement are performed as necessary. A common mistake is changing bandages too infrequently. In addition, strict adherence to aseptic technique minimizes nosocomial infections.

After evaluation, cleansing, and debridement, definitive surgical treatment may be indicated. Surgical stabilization of fractures or torn or sheared ligamentous structures may be necessary. Bone screws, washers, pins, wires, and external fixtures may be used. Substantial healing of all but palmar ligament injuries may be possible with careful external fixator (or coaptation) applications. Delay of certain surgical procedures and closure may be prudent in the presence of severe trauma or contamination (see Fig. 59.16). Sterile bandaging and splint support are adequate for the interim. Loosely placed skin sutures or delayed closure may be helpful to encourage drainage of exudate and to avoid skin tension. Often only partial, if any, closure is prudent, and the exposed tissues may need to be allowed to develop granulation tissue. Cortical bone, fascia, ligaments, and tendons do not support a bed of granulation tissue well and may be covered only as developing granulation tissue envelops these structures. Fascia may be debrided and cortical bone drilled (1-mm drill bit) to the medullary canal to allow granulation tissue "buds" to develop, coalesce, and hasten coverage of these structures. Second-intention healing or delayed skin grafting is then pursued. Generally speaking, wet-to-dry bandaging is used when necrotic tissue is present to be debrided. Otherwise, a nonadherent bandage primary layer best encourages granulation tissue growth. As healing progresses, bandages are changed less frequently. Overall, 2 to 8 weeks of bandaging may be necessary, with restricted activity of the animal depending on the severity of the injuries.

Prognosis is based on the severity of the injuries and the potential for complications. Nonresolvable osteomyelitis is rare, and functional use is usually achievable if no substantial neurologic or circulatory impairment is present. Predicting treatment needs early in the evaluation process prepares the client for the expense and aftercare required. The estimated expenses and aftercare associated with bandaging and debridement may be comparable to those associated with surgery in some cases.

Suggested Reading

Brinker WO, et al. Handbook of small animal orthopedics and fracture treatment. Philadelphia: WB Saunders, 1990.

Treatment of Carpal Hyperextension Injuries

Thomas D. Earley

Hyperextension injuries can result in loss of palmar support to any of the three carpal joints. Often, this type of injury is misdiagnosed because abnormalities are not always seen in the two normal radiographic positions. The mild-to-moderate swelling in the carpal region that accompanies these injuries is often regarded as "just a sprain," and either no treatment or short-term support is offered. The dog invariably walks on the palmar aspect of its metacarpal bones if proper surgical treatment is not accomplished. Most of these injuries occur when the dog jumps or falls from a high place, and the owner often sees the injury take place. A lateral-to-medial hyperextension radiograph, with the dog under heavy sedation, demonstrates which joint is subluxated or luxated. In my experience, the percentage of joint involvement is as follows: antebrachiocarpal, 5 to 10%; middle carpal 65 to 70%; and carpometacarpal, 15 to 20%.

Surgical Correction

The surgical correction of hyperextension injuries demands a thorough knowledge of the palmar region of the carpus. Treatment of hyperextension of the antebrachiocarpal joint with long-term coaptation splints succeeds only occasionally. Reconstruction of the oblique part of the short radial collateral ligament with the tendon of the abductor pollicis longus muscle or the tendon of the flexor carpi radialis muscle, in addition to coaptation, has been advocated (Fig. 59.17).

Successful surgical treatment of the hyperextension injury of the middle carpal joint has been achieved by use of orthopedic wire and screws to maintain a proper bone and joint relationship during the ligament healing process (Fig. 59.18). The ruptured ligaments, which normally attach to the free end of the accessory carpal bone to the fourth and fifth metacarpal bones, should be sutured once the orthopedic wire is secured. Coaptation support for 6 to 8 weeks is recommended. The phalanges should be left free for the last 3 to 4 weeks. The wire that attaches the free end of the accessory carpal bone to the metacarpal bones should be removed at approximately 4 months. The wire from the ulnar carpal bone to the fifth metacarpal bone is not removed.

A unique avulsion fracture of the base of the fifth metacarpal bone, which occurs in hyperextension injuries, is the result of the pull of the lateral palmar accessory carpometacarpal ligament. This fracture can

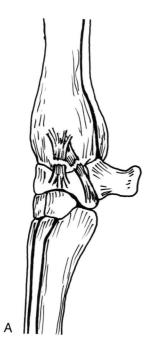 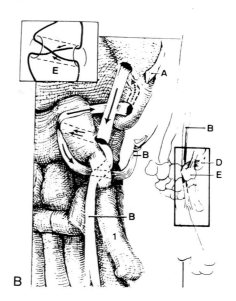

Fig. 59.17. **A.** Damaged radial collateral ligament resulting from hyperextension injury. **B.** Reconstruction of the radial collateral ligament with the tendon of the flexor carpi radialis: *A,* ends of excised abductor pollicis longus tendon; *B,* tendon of the flexor carpus radialis; *D,* medial styloid process; *E,* radial carpal bone; and *I,* first metacarpal bone. *Upper left inset* shows the direction of the tendon of the flexor carpi radialis as it passes through the radial carpal bone twice. (**B** from Earley T. Canine carpal ligament injuries. Vet Clin North Am 1978;8:183.)

be repaired with either a compression screw or a tension band wire (Fig. 59.19).

Fracture of the radial carpal bone involves the palmar medial process. This avulsion fracture of the attachment of the palmar radial carpometacarpal liga-

ment should be repaired with a tension band wire (Fig. 59.20). Fractures of the radial carpal bone often involve the body, which constitutes the articular surface; repair of these fractures with a compression screw should strive for anatomic reduction (Fig. 59.21). Lux-

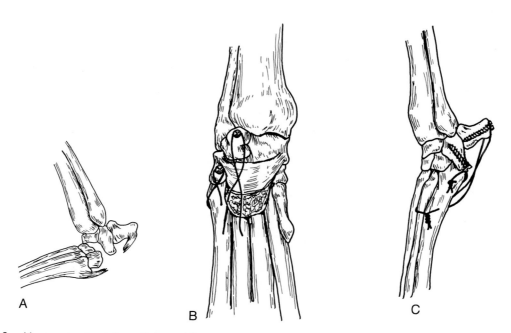

Fig. 59.18. Hyperextension injury of the middle carpal joint (**A**) stabilized with screws and orthopedic wire (**B** and **C**).

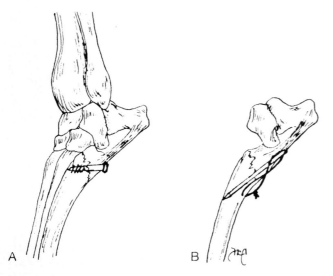

Fig. 59.19. Avulsion fracture of the base of the fifth metacarpal bone repaired with a compression screw (**A**) or a tension band wire (**B**).

ation of the radial carpal bone is a rare injury that results in detachment of the radial carpal bone from the ulnar carpal bone, the palmar ulnar carpal ligament, the palmar radial carpal ligament, and the short radial collateral ligament (Fig. 59.22). Open reduction, with ligament reconstruction of the short radial collateral ligament, and splinting for 6 weeks are curative.

Carpometacarpal hyperextension generally ruptures the palmar carpal fibrocartilage's attachment to the base of the metacarpal bones. Often, the ligaments

that support the middle carpal joint are also ruptured. The middle carpal joint reconstruction technique is recommended, in addition to wiring of the fibrocartilage to the metacarpal bones (Fig. 59.23).

Occasionally, carpometacarpal luxation occurs unrelated to hyperextension. Closed reduction results in a stable realignment that, when combined with coaptation splint support for 6 weeks, is satisfactory. If stability is not satisfactory after closed reduction, two or three Kirschner wires are driven, in a Rush-pin fashion, from the third and fourth metacarpal bones into the distal row of carpal bones (Fig. 59.24). These pins are removed in 6 to 8 weeks.

If either the middle carpal or the carpometacarpal joint is severely damaged or diseased, a partial arthrodesis of both distal joints is indicated. Two surgical techniques are commonly used, both accomplished through a dorsal approach separating the tendons of the common digital extensor and the extensor carpi radialis muscles. The first technique uses a small, T-shaped bone plate secured to the dorsum of the radial carpal bone with two screws, which should not exit the opposite side of the bone. Another screw is inserted into the third carpal bone and two screws are placed in the third metacarpal bone (Fig. 59.25). The plate generally is removed once radiographic evidence of arthrodesis is observed, usually in 6 to 9 months.

The second technique uses three small pins or Kirschner wires introduced into the second, third, and fourth metacarpal bones, driven proximally through the second, third, and fourth carpal bones, and seated into the radial and ulnar carpal bones, respectively (Fig. 59.26).

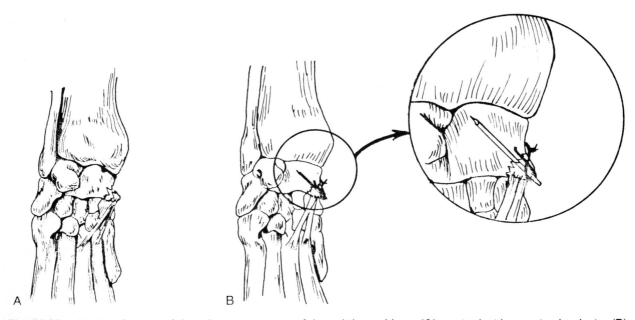

Fig. 59.20. Avulsion fracture of the palmar prominence of the radial carpal bone (**A**) repaired with a tension band wire (**B**).

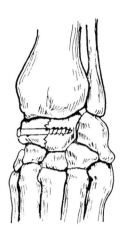

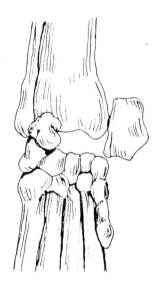

Fig. 59.21. Intra-articular fracture of the radial carpal bone repaired with a compression screw.

Fig. 59.22. Palmar medial luxation of the radial carpal bone. See Figure 59.17**B** for reconstruction of radial collateral ligament.

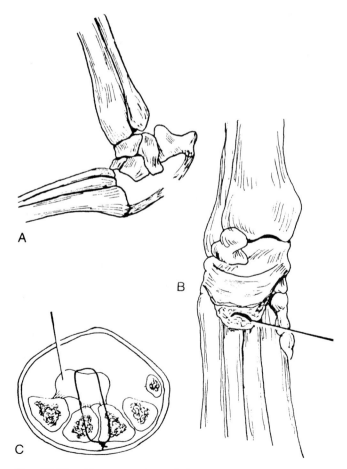

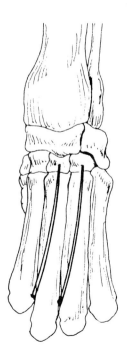

Fig. 59.23. Hyperextension of the carpometacarpal joint (**A**) repaired with wire to secure the palmar carpal fibrocartilage to the third metacarpal bones (**B** and **C**). A leader line is shown.

Fig. 59.24. Carpometacarpal luxation stabilized with Kirschner wires.

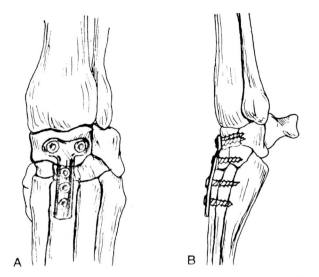

Fig. 59.25. **A** and **B.** Partial arthrodesis of the carpus with a bone plate.

Suggested Readings

Dee JF. Fractures in the racing greyhound. In: Bojrab MJ, ed. Pathophysiology in small animal surgery. Philadelphia: Lea & Febiger, 1981.

Dee JF, Earley TD. Fractures of the carpus and tarsus and paw. In: Veterinary manual of internal fixation (in press).

Dietrich HF. Arthrodesis of the proximal intertarsal joint for repair of rupture of the proximal plantar intertarsal ligaments. Vet Med Small Anim Clin 1974;69:995.

Earley TD. Canine carpal ligament injuries. Vet Clin North Am 1978;8:183.

Earley TD. Hyperextension injuries of the canine carpal joint. Georgia Vet 1976;29:24.

Earley TD, Dee JF. Trauma to the carpus, tarsus, and phalanges of dogs and cats. Vet Clin North Am 1980;107:717.

Farrow CS. Carpal sprain injury in the dog. J Am Vet Radiol Soc 1977;18:38.

Punzet G. Fixation of the os carpi radialis in the dog: pathogenesis, symptoms and treatment. J Small Anim Pract 1974;15:751.

Slocum B, Devine T. Partial carpal fusion in the dog. J Am Vet Med Assoc 1982;180:1204–1208.

Treatment of the carpus for injuries resulting from hyperextension requires accurate identification of the pathologic lesions. This requires high-detail stress radiography to demonstrate abnormal limits of motion secondary to ligamentous disruption and identification of fractures resulting from hyperextension. Early anatomic reconstruction is necessary for optimal results. If early reconstruction must be delayed, then partial arthrodesis usually provides the necessary stability, but flexibility of the metacarpal region is lost.

***

Treatment of Hyperextension and Hyperflexion in Puppies

Mary Lynn E. Stanton

Hyperextension

Treatment of carpal hyperextension in juvenile dogs varies with the age at presentation and the degree of severity (Fig. 59.27). In young (2- to 4-month-old)

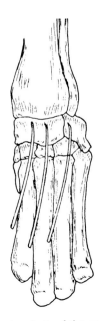

Fig. 59.26. Partial arthrodesis of the carpus with small pins.

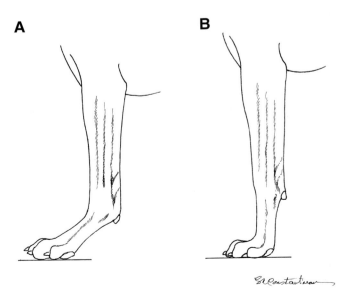

Fig. 59.27. Diagram of a carpal hyperextension (**A**) in comparison with a normal standing position (**B**).

puppies, initial conservative recommendations of regulated exercise (1), nonslip footing, and restricted caloric intake are indicated. Any concurrent orthopedic abnormalities such as panosteitis or premature closure of the distal ulnar growth plate should be addressed. Many cases resolve with this approach.

Use of metasplints is not recommended. This technique promotes further laxity of the flexor tendons and decreased muscle tone, thus aggravating the problem. A reverse metasplint may be used in patients nonresponsive to conservative measures, to maintain carpal alignment and to limit degenerative changes. However, these hyperextensions often break down again once splinting is discontinued. If an arthrodesis is indicated, splinting may be useful while waiting for skeletal maturity.

Cases involving one limb only in puppies 3 to 6 months old may benefit from short-term application of a carpal sling. This sling may be applied for 5- to 7-day intervals, and these patients must be monitored closely. This technique is most useful in patients that have sustained mild trauma to the palmar carpal supporting structures. Use of this sling may be followed by a period of flexion splinting. The duration of immobilization depends on the degree of hyperextension and the growth rate of the patient.

Patients with hyperextension that does not resolve conservatively may require carpal arthrodesis to relieve pain resulting from degenerative joint disease. Patients must achieve physeal closure before this operation can be performed. Pancarpal arthrodesis is necessary when the radial carpal joint is involved and can be accomplished by dorsal (2) or palmar (3) plating techniques. Regardless of technique, the normal standing position must be determined for the individual animal and the plate contoured accordingly. All joint surfaces must be debrided of cartilage and packed with cancellous graft, and one screw should be set in the radial carpal bone. A period of at least 4 to 6 weeks of coaptation follows arthrodesis.

Hyperflexion

The earlier this condition is addressed, the better the response is to treatment. The affected limb should be placed in a full-length padded metasplint. This device should be maintained for 3 days and the effect evaluated. A metasplint may be reapplied for a few days at a time if sufficient lengthening of the flexor mechanism has not been achieved. The puppy should be maintained on good footing and adequate nutrition.

References

1. Shires PK, Hulse PA, Kearney MT. Carpal hyperextension in two-month-old pups. J Am Vet Med Assoc 1980;186:49–52.
2. Brinker WO, Piermattei DL, Flo GL. Handbook of small animal orthopedics and fracture treatment. Philadelphia: WB Saunders, 1983:398–400.
3. Chambers JN, Bjorling PE. Palmar surface plating for arthrodesis of the canine carpus. J Am Anim Hosp Assoc 1982;98:875–882.

Partial Carpal Arthrodesis

Thomas Van Gundy

The purpose of partial carpal arthrodesis is to provide a bony union across the carpometacarpal, middle carpal, and intercarpal joints. Indications for this procedure include luxation, subluxation (e.g., hyperextension injury), chronic instability resulting in degenerative joint disease, intra-articular nonunion, and arthritis (septic or immune-mediated) not responsive to medical treatment. The antebrachiocarpal joint must be stable and pain free. Stability is assessed by palpation and stress radiography. Instability and subluxation of the accessory–ulnar carpal joint complicate partial carpal arthrodesis, making pancarpal arthrodesis the procedure of choice.

The animal is placed in dorsal recumbency. The limb is prepared for surgery. Proper use of a temporary tourniquet fashioned of wide Penrose drain or elastic bandage material facilitates the surgical procedure. Ac-

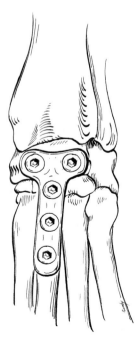

Fig. 59.28. A T plate is applied to the dorsal aspect of the left carpus with two bone screws seated in the radial carpal bone, one in carpal bone III and two in the proximal aspect of metacarpal III.

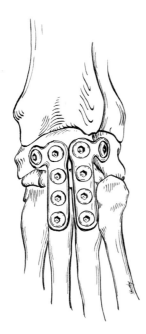

Fig. 59.29. Paired 2.7-mm L plates are applied to the dorsal aspect of the left carpus. With this technique, two carpal bones are secured with screws, and the lateral plate spans the radial and ulna carpal bones. A total of four screws may purchase in metacarpal bone.

cess to the joints involved is gained through a cranial approach. The skin incision is offset, to avoid overlying bone plates directly. The middle carpal, intercarpal, and carpometacarpal joints are opened with full carpal flexion, and the cartilage surfaces removed using an air-powered bur and rongeurs. The joints are then lavaged thoroughly and are placed in extension (neutral alignment of carpal and metacarpal bones) and stabilized. Preferred stabilization uses a cranially applied T or L plate with screws in the radial carpal, intercarpal (if possible), and metacarpal bones. A single plate overlies the proximal third or fourth metacarpal bone (Fig. 59.28). Larger dogs may have two opposite-angle L plates applied, allowing screw purchase in the radial and ulnar carpal bones and both central metacarpal bones (Fig. 59.29). Proper plate and screw placement is crucial to avoid impingement of screws or plates on the antebrachiocarpal joint. Cancellous bone graft harvested from the ipsilateral humerus is liberally packed into all joints to be fused, and overlying tissues are closed in a routine manner. An alternative method of fixation uses intramedullary Kirschner wires placed in retrograde fashion from the distal dorsal surfaces of the second, third, fourth, and fifth metacarpal bones,

seating into the radial and ulnar carpal bones (Fig. 59.30).

Postoperative radiographs (including stress views) determine implant placement and the need for further implant removal if antebrachiocarpal joint impingement is noted. Postoperative management includes 6 weeks in a cast or splint and implant removal at the time of bony fusion if clinically indicated.

Proper patient selection and procedure are paramount for success. Insufficient evaluation of a pathologic antebrachiocarpal joint may allow progressive hyperextension and may require subsequent pancarpal arthrodesis. Careful radiographic comparison of the accessory–ulnar carpal bone articulation with normal stress radiographs is helpful. Proper placement of implants can be facilitated by careful antebrachiocarpal joint arthrotomy to visualize radial and ulnar carpal bone geometry. Persistent lameness may require re-evaluation of implant placement or of antebrachiocarpal joint disease.

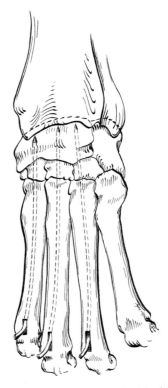

Fig. 59.30. Kirschner wires are used with this technique by retrograde placement. The wires are started from an extra-articular position just proximal to the metacarpophalangeal joint. The points of the Kirschner wires extend to just below radial carpal bone articular cartilege.

• 60 •

SACROILIAC DISLOCATIONS

Timothy M. Lenehan & Guy B. Tarvin

The purpose of surgery for sacroiliac dislocation is to recreate a firm attachment between the appendicular and the axial skeleton, thus facilitating pain-free and normally aligned force transmission though them. Accurate alignment also minimizes osteoarthritic symptoms and lessens the likelihood of nerve root entrapment. Two surgical approaches to the sacroiliac joint are popular, depending on the surgeon's preference and schooling and on the existence of any accompanying pelvic or sacroiliac damage.

Lateral Approach to the Sacroiliac Joint

The animal is placed in lateral recumbency, and the entire limb is prepared for an aseptic surgical procedure. A lateral approach to the ilial wing is performed (1). The origin of the iliacus muscle is reflected ventrally from the ilium to gain digital access to the pelvic inlet, the medial ilium, and the sacroiliac junction. Using Kern bone-holding forceps placed on the iliac crest, accompanied either by Lewin bone-holding forceps placed in the greater trochanter (hemipelvis not intact) or Kern bone-holding forceps placed on the tuber ischiadicum (hemipelvis intact), the sacroiliac dislocation is reduced. The reduction is confirmed by feeling the sacrum and ilium interlock and by digitally palpating a smooth craniomedial and ventromedial junction between the sacral wing and medial ilium. Downward (medial) pressure on the ilium easily maintains the reduction a Kirschner wire is driven through

the wing of the ilium into the sacrum to maintain the reduction temporarily. The sacral wing notch is palpated digitally (Fig. 60.1), and a drill hole is placed through the ilial wing and into the sacrum just caudal to the notch. One interfragmentary lag screw is placed across the sacroiliac junction, and compression is confirmed by digital palpation as the final turns on the screw are applied. The temporary Kirschner wire is then removed, and a second interfragmentary lag screw may be placed, depending on the size of the patient, accompanying pelvic trauma, and purchase of the first screw. One should use the largest screw possible and place it into the body of the sacrum to maximize pullout strength. A cumulative measurement of screw depth to sacral width of 60% or more seems necessary to maximize holding strength and to minimize loosening of the fixation before union (2). Care should be taken to avoid screw placement either in the L7–S1 intervertebral disc space or through the articular process of the sacrum into the spinal canal.

Should the surgeon prefer to visualize drill hole placement directly, then before reduction, further dissection is necessary to expose the medial aspect of the ilial wing further. The superficial fascia and aponeurosis of the sacrospinalis muscle are dissected from the craniodorsal iliac spine, and then the origin of the sacrospinalis and quadratus lumborum muscles are elevated to expose the iliac surface. The surgeon must be careful not to dissect caudal to the dorsal iliac spine, thereby injuring the cranial gluteal vessels and nerve. Ventrolateral retraction of the ilium then allows exposure of the sacrum (Fig. 60.2). A drill hole may then

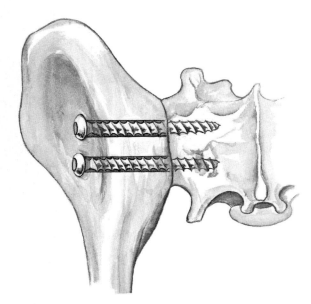

Fig. 60.1. Lag screw fixation of the sacroiliac luxation.

be placed accurately into the sacral body, and the overlying ilial hole may be drilled in approximately the same location by palpating the articular prominence of the ilium on the medial surface of the ilial wing that fits into the sacral wing notch. The sacral hole is tapped, the screw is advanced through the ilial hole until visualized on the medial surface, and the separation is reduced and lagged together. A second screw may be placed as described previously.

Muscle groups are approximated with horizontal mattress sutures, and subcutaneous tissues and skin are closed routinely. No postoperative bandaging is necessary. Strict confinement to a small area is necessary for 3 to 4 weeks to minimize implant failure. If 4-week follow-up radiography reveals good healing and minimal to no implant failure, then more activity can be allowed.

Dorsal Approach to the Sacroiliac Junction

The animal is placed to ventral recumbency, and the dorsal lumbosacral area is prepared for aseptic surgery. The hind limbs are placed either in a frogleg or a moderately extended position. A separate dorsal approach is made to each sacroiliac joint (3). If a single transsacral screw is to be used, then one sacroiliac joint is reduced (side 1) and is held with a Speedlock or pointed reduction forceps while a Kirschner wire is temporarily placed to maintain the reduction. A drill hole is then made starting from the center of the auricular surface of the opposite sacrum (side 2) and is advanced through the sacrum and out the reduced ilium on the opposite side. The hole is tapped, a guide

hole is drilled in the nonreduced ilial wing, and an appropriately long lag screw is started through the ilial wing across the newly reduced sacroiliac joint (side 2), through the body of the sacrum and out the opposite sacroiliac joint (side 1). Hence, the one screw reduces both luxations (Fig. 60.3) (4).

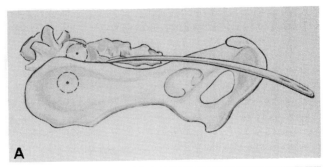

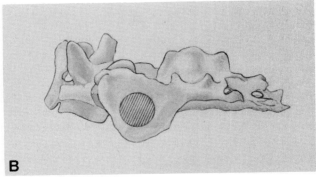

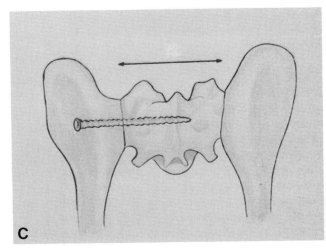

Fig. 60.2. Fixation of unstable sacroiliac dislocation. **A.** A Hohmann retractor is used to lever the sacrum dorsally (or the ilium ventrally) to expose the articular surfaces of the sacrum (*dotted circles*). *Solid dots* within the circles indicate location of the drill holes. **B.** The *shaded area* in this lateral projection indicates the location of the screw or pin placement. This area avoids the spinal canal and offers good implant purchase. **C.** The *double-headed arrow* indicates the width of the sacrum. Screw or implant purchase should be at least 60% of the sacral width to provide adequate holding power.

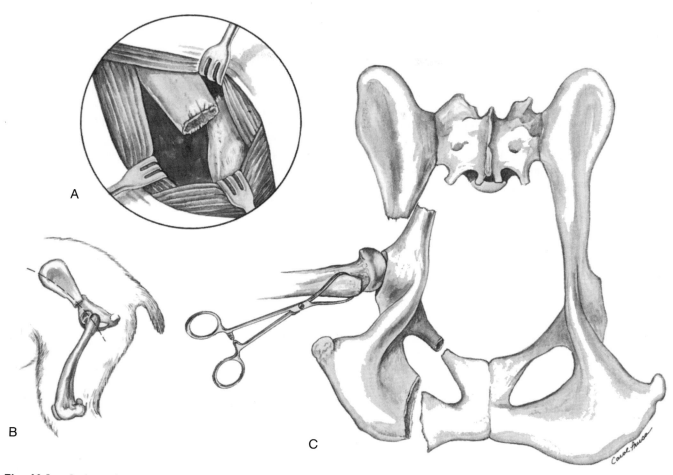

Fig. 60.3. **A.** Lateral approach and exposure of fractured ilial shaft. **B.** Pelvic fracture with an unstable weightbearing segment. **C.** Reduction with aid of a Lewin clamp attached to the greater trochanter.

Alternatively, each sacroiliac joint can be reduced separately, with drill hole placement either preceding or following sacroiliac reduction, depending on the surgeon's comfort level with either technique.

Some comments on technique are appropriate to sacroiliac reduction. Overdrilling the ilium is rarely necessary to achieve a lag effect because of the inherent weakness of the bone. The drill hole in the sacrum must be longer than the screw placed therein, to ensure a lag effect at the sacroiliac junction; otherwise, the end of the screw will hit the end of the hole before lag reduction of the sacroliac joint. If concerns exist about drilling into the spinal canal, then one can measure the distance from the lateral ilium to the lateral extent of the spinal canal on a preoperative ventrodorsal pelvic radiograph and only drill and place screws that are shorter than the measured distance. Placement of the surgeon's digit medial to the sacral wing at the level of the body of S1 helps to orient placement of the drill hole on the ventrolateral approach. These

procedures should be performed within 3 to 5 days of injury, because rapid callus formation can make it difficult to reduce sacroiliac dislocations if one waits too long following injury. Although the adhesions can be broken down, nerve injury may result.

The advantage of the dorsal surgical approach is that it allows direct visualization of the sacroiliac joint and permits bilateral procedures to be performed without changing the position of the animal on the surgical table. The lateral approach is particularly useful for sacroiliac dislocations accompanied by ipsilateral ilial shaft, acetabular, or ischial fractures that require repair.

Typically, the ilial wing is displaced cranially and dorsally in relation to the sacrum. A blunt Hohmann retractor or curved Carmalt forceps placed dorsal to the dorsal ilial wing and ventral to the sacrum can provide excellent leverage to expose the sacrum for drilling, should it be necessary to visualize the sacral drill site.

Postoperative Care

Postoperative radiographs (lateral and ventrodorsal) should be taken to assess screw placement and depth. Appropriate steps should be taken if screws are suspected of impinging on spinal nerves or if reduction is inadequate. Minimal postoperative care should include 4 weeks of strict confinement to a small area with only necessary leash walking outside. More activity can be allowed if 4 week follow-up radiographs reveal adequate healing.

References

1. Piermattei DL, Greeley RG. Atlas of surgical approaches to the bones of the dog and cat. 3rd ed. Philadelphia: WB Saunders, 1993:224–227.
2. DeCamp CE, Braden TD. Sacroiliac fracture—separation in the dog: a study of 9 cases. Vet Surg 1985;14:127–130.
3. Piermattei DL, Greeley RG. Atlas of surgical approaches to the bones of the dog and cat. 3rd ed. Philadelphia: WB Saunders, 1993:222–223.
4. Kaderly RE. Stabilization of bilateral sacroiliac fracture–luxations on small animals with a single transsacral screw. Vet Surg 1991;20:91–96.

— 61 —

HIP

Algorithms for Treatment

Barclay Slocum & Theresa Devine Slocum

Figures 61.1 through 61.5 are algorithms for treatment of hip disorders.

Diagnostic Tests

Barclay Slocum & Theresa Devine Slocum

Clinical Observations

"Boxy" Hips

The observation of gait is important to distinguish between functional abnormalities such as ataxia, and conformational abnormalities. "Boxy" hips are a change in shape of the rump from smooth and rounded to that of a rounded square (Fig. 61.6), caused by a luxated hip.

OBSERVATION PROCEDURE

The patient is observed from behind during walking. The examiner notes the width between the animal's feet in the transverse plane. The normal patient places the foot beneath the hip joint, which is 7 to 10 cm apart on a dog the size of a Labrador retriever. This is called base normal. On the same dog with boxy hips, the feet will be 2 to 5 cm apart, which is called base narrow. Some patients walk base narrow, convert to base wide (feet are 12 to 15 cm apart), and oscillate between the two (Fig. 61.7).

The second characteristic to notice is the contour of the rump from behind. The rump of the normal dog is smooth and rounded, sloping ventrally from the caudal vertebrae, as the contour is traced laterally. The dog with "boxy" hips has minimal or no slope from the caudal vertebrae as the contour of the rump is traced laterally, and then it is round (with a smaller radius of curvature) as the contour curves around the greater trochanter to continue along the lateral thigh. Occasionally, the trochanter intermittently protrudes, causing the shape to change between the two contours (Fig. 61.8).

The difference between normal and "boxy" hips is the difference between a normally reduced femoral head and a luxated femoral head. In the luxated hip, the femoral head has translated laterally and dorsally. This projects the greater trochanter laterally and dorsally and gives the contour of the rump the "boxy" appearance of a rounded square. The luxated hip is supported by the joint capsule, rather than by the acetabulum. Abduction is limited because the adductor muscles, especially the pectineus, are excessively lengthened by the amount of displacement of the femoral head when abduction occurs. This abduction of the luxated femoral head creates extra forces on the already stretched and inflamed joint capsule, which causes the patient pain. The dog limits the amount of this abduction by walking base narrow (see Fig. 61.7).

The reduced or normal position of the hip in the acetabulum is nonpainful. Because the increased slope of the acetabulum in the dysplastic hip allows the femoral head to drift into the luxated position, the patient has two means of reducing the femoral head into the acetabulum. The combined muscle forces of the hip abductors and rotators can create sufficient pull to reduce the femoral head, but this force must be sustained to maintain reduction. These muscles are not created

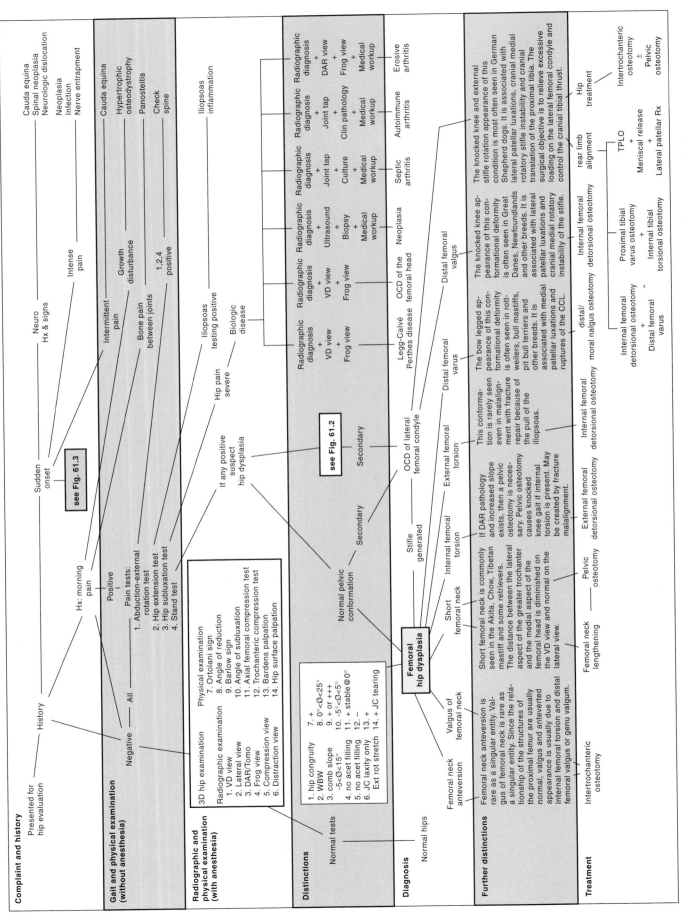

Fig. 61.1. General hip algorithm. *CCL*, cranial cruciate ligament; *DAR*, dorsal acetabular rim; *JC*, joint capsule; *OCD*, osteochondritis dissecans; *TPLO*, tibial plateau leveling osteotomy; *VD*, ventrodorsal; *WBW*, white, black, white on lateral radiograph.

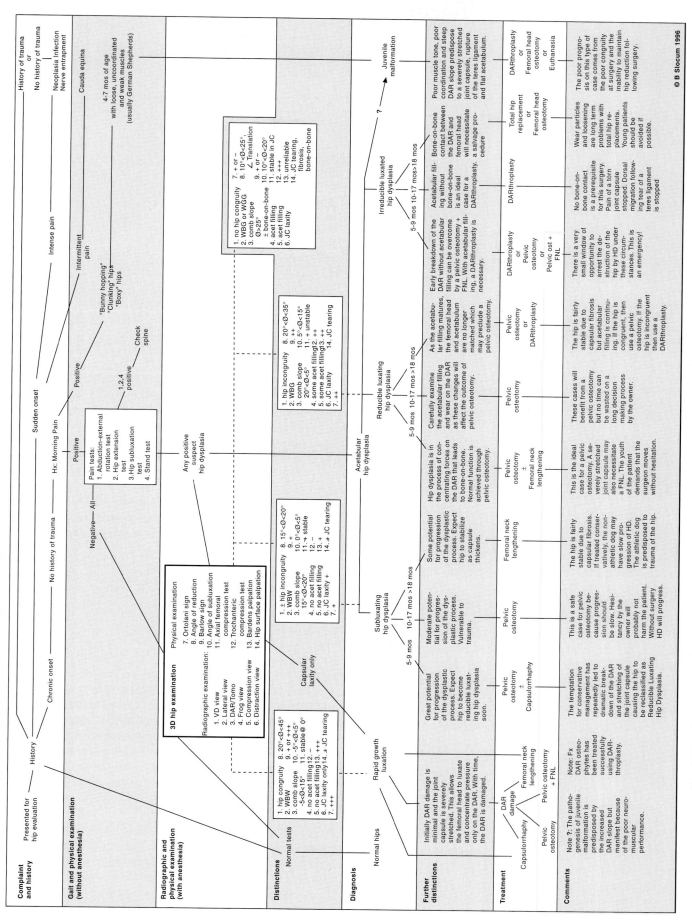

Fig. 61.2. Acetabular hip dysplasia algorithm. *DAR*, dorsal acetabular rim; *FNL*, femoral neck lengthening; *JC*, joint capsule; *VD*, ventrodorsal; *WBG*, white, black, black, gray; *WBW*, white, black, white.

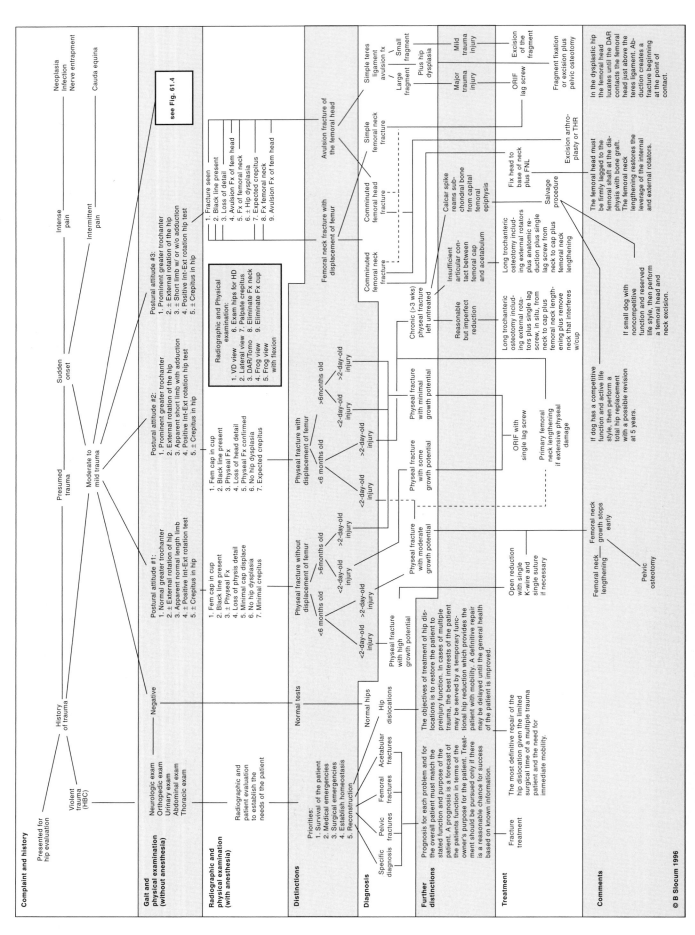

Fig. 61.3. Algorithm for trauma to the hip. *DAR,* dorsal acetabular rim; *FNL,* femoral neck lengthening; *HBC,* hit by car; *HD,* hip dysplasia; *ORIF,* open reduction with internal fixation; *THR,* total hip replacement; *VD,* ventrodorsal.

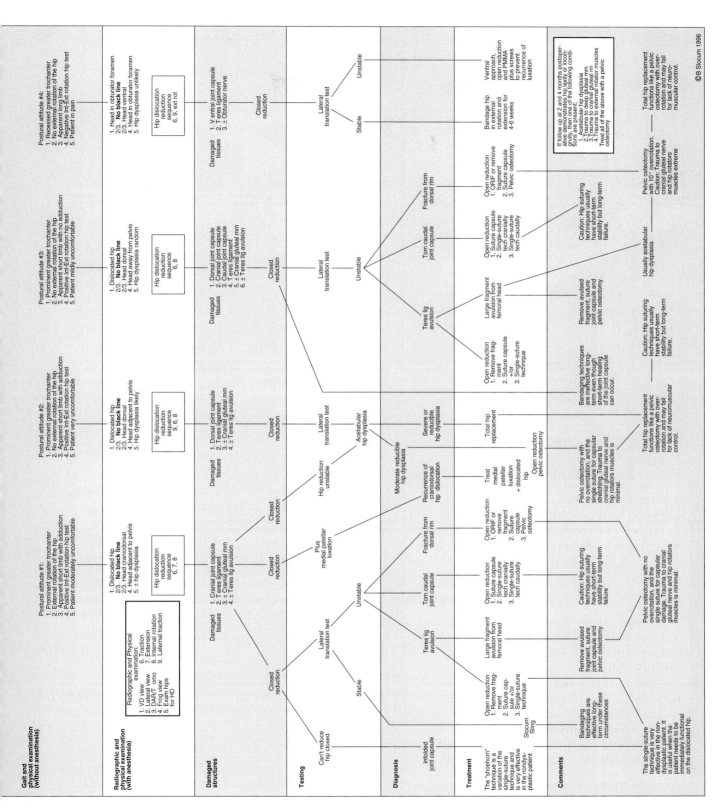

Fig. 61.4. Hip dislocation algorithm. *DAR,* dorsal acetabular rim; *HD,* hip dysplasia; *ORIF,* open reduction with internal fixation; *PMMA,* polymethylmethacrylate; *VD,* ventrodorsal.

1131

Normal Hip

V-D Rads	congruent
Frog	thin cartilage
Cupping	none
Lat Rads	WBW
DAR	<7.5°
Dors Osteo	none
Distract Index	<0.30
Red/Sub	none/none
Cartilage	ok
Joint Caps	ok
Acetabulum	no filling
ROM	ok
AM Pain	ok
Activity	ok
Abd-Ext Rot	no pain
Jumping	ok
Stand Test	ok
Treatment 1	none
Treatment 2	
Treatment 3	

Subluxating Hip Dysplasia

V-D Rads	congruent + cup
Frog	thin cartilage
Cupping	±
Lat Rads	WBW
DAR	8° to 10°
Dors Osteo	none
Distract Index	0.30>DI>0.40
Red/Sub	20°/5°
Cartilage	ok
Joint Caps	stretched (or torn)
Acetabulum	no filling
ROM	ok
AM Pain	ok
Activity	ok
Abd-Ext Rot	occasional pain
Jumping	ok
Stand Test	ok
Treatment 1	reevaluation 6 mo
Treatment 2	FNL
Treatment 3	

Mild Reducible Hip Dysplasia

V-D Rads	incongruity + cup
Frog	usually thin cart
Cupping	+
Lat Rads	WB ± G
DAR	10°<slope<20°
Dors Osteo	slight
Distract Index	0.40>DI>0.75
Red/Sub	>25°/<15°
Cartilage	ok or fibrillation
Joint Caps	torn or fx labrum
Acetabulum	maybe some filling
ROM	abduction ok
AM Pain	slow to rise
Activity	bursts, quits early
Abd-Ext Rot	pain
Jumping	some difficulty
Stand Test	some positive
Treatment 1	PO 20°
Treatment 2	PO 20°+FNL
Treatment 3	

Severe Reducible Hip Dysplasia

V-D Rads	incongruent
Frog	incr cartilage space
Cupping	cupping or deform
Lat Rads	WGG
DAR	15°<slope<30°
Dors Osteo	significant
Distract Index	0.30>DI>1.0
Red/Sub	25°-35° / 20°-25°
Cartilage	worn or eburnation
Joint Caps	torn, fx labrum & fibrosis
Acetabulum	almost filled
ROM	restricted abduction
AM Pain	slow to rise
Activity	+ handstands / sleeps lots
Abd-Ext Rot	restricted
Jumping	difficult or refuse
Stand Test	positive
Treatment 1	DARthroplasty
Treatment 2	THR
Treatment 3	

Rapid Growth Hip

V-D Rads	congruent or not
Frog	thin cartilage
Cupping	none
Lat Rads	WBW or G
DAR	<7.5°
Dors Osteo	none
Distract Index	0.30>DI>0.75
Red/Sub	15° to 45°/-7° to 5°
Cartilage	ok
Joint Caps	stretched (or torn)
Acetabulum	no filling
ROM	ok
AM Pain	ok
Activity	ok
Abd-Ext Rot	occasional pain
Jumping	ok
Stand Test	ok
Treatment 1	FNL
Treatment 2	abduction brace
Treatment 3	reevaluation

Intermittent Hip Dysplasia

V-D Rads	± congruent + cup
Frog	thin cartilage
Cupping	+
Lat Rads	WB ± W
DAR	>10°
Dors Osteo	none
Distract Index	0.40>DI>0.50
Red/Sub	>20°/<10°
Cartilage	ok
Joint Caps	stretched or torn
Acetabulum	little or no filling
ROM	ok
AM Pain	occ slow to rise
Activity	may quit early
Abd-Ext Rot	some pain
Jumping	usually ok
Stand Test	ok, some positive
Treatment 1	PO 20°
Treatment 2	FNL
Treatment 3	

Moderate Reducible Hip Dysplasia

V-D Rads	incongruent
Frog	incr cartilage space
Cupping	+
Lat Rads	W ± BG
DAR	15°<slope<30°
Dors Osteo	moderate
Distract Index	0.40>DI>0.75
Red/Sub	25°-30°/15°-20°
Cartilage	fibrillation or worn
Joint Caps	torn, fx labrum & fibrosis
Acetabulum	incomplete filling
ROM	abduction reduced
AM Pain	slow to rise
Activity	sleeps more, burst of activity
Abd-Ext Rot	pain
Jumping	usually difficult
Stand Test	usually positive
Treatment 1	PO 20°
Treatment 2	PO 20°+FNL
Treatment 3	PO 30°

Irreducible Hip Dysplasia

V-D Rads	incongruent
Frog	thick cart space
Cupping	cupping or deform
Lat Rads	WGG
DAR	25°<slope<40°
Dors Osteo	large
Distract Index	0.30>DI>1.0
Red/Sub	25°-40°/20°-30°
Cartilage	eburnation
Joint Caps	fibrosis
Acetabulum	filled
ROM	restricted abduction
AM Pain	slow to rise
Activity	+ handstands / sleeps lots
Abd-Ext Rot	restricted
Jumping	difficult or refuse
Stand Test	positive
Treatment 1	THR
Treatment 2	DARthroplasty
Treatment 3	excision / arthroplasty

Fig. 61.5. Summary of examination findings (*left column*) for clinical classification of hip dysplasia. The *right column* indicates the radiographic features corresponding to the clinical findings. *Abd-Ext Rot*, abduction with external rotation; *DAR*, dorsal acetabular rim; *FNL*, femoral neck lengthening; *PO*, pelvic osteotomy; *Red/Sub*, reduction/subluxation; *ROM*, range of motion; *THR*, total hip replacement; *VD*, ventrodorsal;

the reduced position, but the foot is not under the femoral head. The patient must walk base wide to maintain reduction of the luxated hip (see Fig. 61.7). This base wide effect has been observed in several circumstances. Some dogs shift from a base narrow gait to a base wide gait and back, as the discomfort of luxation dictates a base wide configuration for comfort. Some dogs shift to base wide to go up stairs. Some dogs hesitate slightly before jumping into a car or the bed of a pickup truck, to go base wide and relocate the hip before jumping.

The presence of "boxy" hips indicates that the hips are luxated and are in a severe and rapid stage of degeneration. If the dog is young, these hips may be saved and made functional by a pelvic osteotomy. Most frequently, dogs are presented beyond this stage.

"Bunny Hopping" Gait

The observation of gait is important in the determination of functional abnormalities such as ataxia and conformational abnormalities. "Bunny hopping" gait is a running gait in which the patient runs with both feet in adduction, simultaneously.

OBSERVATION PROCEDURE

The patient is observed from behind during running. The examiner notes the width between the feet in the transverse plane. The normal patient places the foot beneath the hip joint, which is 7 to 10 cm apart on a dog the size of a Labrador retriever. On the same dog

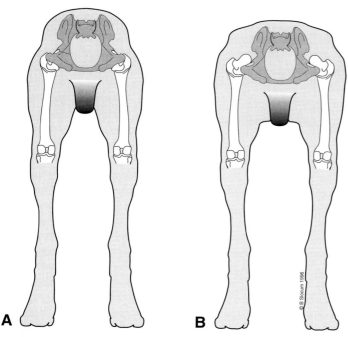

Fig. 61.6. **A.** The contour of the normal rump is like a beautifully arched doorway. **B.** The contour of the rump of a dysplastic dog with luxated hips is like a rectangular doorway.

with the purpose of maintaining the reduced hip. As these muscles fatigue, the hip again luxates.

The second means of creating hip reduction is to abduct the hip, a maneuver that redirects the axial muscle forces of the femur into the acetabulum. This requires minimal abductor forces to hold the hip in

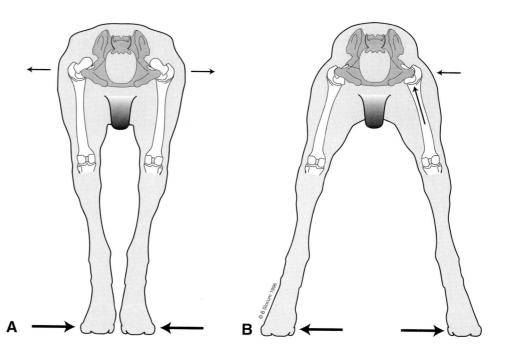

Fig. 61.7. **A.** The dysplastic dog with luxated hips is likely to stand with the feet together, base narrow. **B.** The dysplastic dog with reduced hips stands with the feet apart, base wide, to direct the axial femoral force into the acetabulum and ease hip reduction.

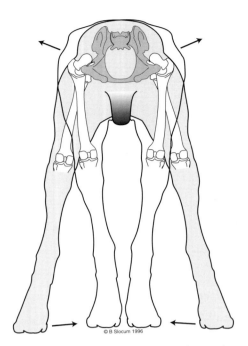

Fig. 61.8. As the dog goes from a base wide to a base narrow stance, the width of the rump may increase as the hips luxate. As the dog goes from a base narrow to a base wide stance, the width of the rump may decrease as the hips reduce. This is called a base shift.

with a "bunny hopping" gait, the feet are 2 to 5 cm apart, and use of the hind limbs is simultaneous (Fig. 61.9).

The difference between the normal running and "bunny hopping" gait is that, in the normal gait, the feet are apart by approximately the width of the hip joints, and one hind foot is used slightly before the other. In the "bunny hopping" gait, the feet are placed close together and are used together, with the back performing the greater part of extension. The difference between the hips in the normal and "bunny hopping" gait is the difference between a normally reduced femoral head and a luxated femoral head. The luxated hip is supported by the joint capsule rather than by the acetabulum and is therefore limited in its abduction. When the femoral head is laterally displaced, the adductor muscles are excessively lengthened. Abduction of the luxated femoral head creates large forces on the already inflamed joint capsule. This causes the patient pain and a base narrow gait. The patient seems to be incapable of reducing the femoral head into the acetabulum by either abductor and rotator muscle forces or abduction of the hip. By using both limbs together, the forces are greatly reduced in each hip.

The presence of a "bunny hopping" gait indicates that the hips are luxated and are in a severe and rapid stage of degeneration. These hips are usually beyond reconstruction by means of a pelvic osteotomy unless the patient is young and the severe luxation is a recent occurrence.

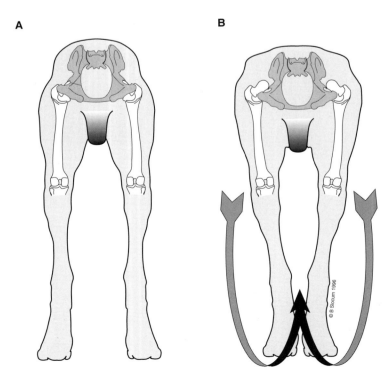

Fig. 61.9. **A.** Normal. **B.** "Bunny hopping" is an abnormality of gait that occurs when hips are luxated. Both rear limbs are used simultaneously during extension to limit hip pain. The back is hyperextended, to assist in lengthening the stride.

"Clunking" Hips

The observation of gait is important in the determination of functional abnormalities. "Clunking" hips are a result of the hip relocating from the luxated position to the reduced position during ambulation.

OBSERVATION PROCEDURE

The client often brings the "clunking" of the hips to the attention of the orthopedist. The patient is observed during walking. The examiner's hand can be placed on the animal's rump to feel the hip being reduced during ambulation. One can also hear the "clunk" of reduction (Fig. 61.10). A positive observation of "clunking" hips is to experience the feel of the "clunk" and to hear the "clunking" sound.

The presence of a "clunk" in a hip means that the hip begins in a luxated position, and the femoral head falls into an acetabulum of some depth. The combined muscle force of the hip abductors and rotators can create sufficient pull to reduce the femoral head, but this force must be sustained to maintain reduction. Because these muscles are not created with the purpose of maintaining hip reduction, they soon fatigue, and the hip again luxates. The reduced or normal position of the hip in the acetabulum is nonpainful, but the increased slope of the acetabulum in the dysplastic hip allows the femoral head to drift into the luxated position.

The presence of a "clunking" hip, whether by direct observation or by client observation, clearly indicates an orthopedic emergency in which the patient should be placed under absolute rest conditions until the hips can be evaluated and treated. If the hips are "clunking," then usually enough acetabulum is left to reseat the femoral head. A pelvic osteotomy will be successful if the acetabulum has not filled with osteophytes and the dorsal acetabular rim (DAR) still has sufficient integrity and depth to maintain the femoral head in the acetabulum after pelvic osteotomy.

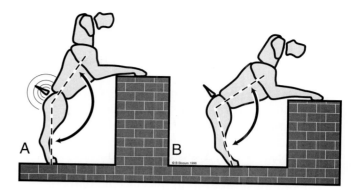

Fig. 61.11. The stand test is performed by picking up the front legs of a standing dog. **A.** A normal dog extends the hips and back to relish the attention of the owner. **B.** The abnormal dog protrudes the rump in an attempt to maintain flexion of the hip and back. The abnormal dog usually attempts to return to the standing on all four legs and may even mock bite the hands holding the dog.

The DAR is under immediate trauma by the femoral head because the femoral head just proximal to the ligament of the femoral head is incongruent with the acetabulum and is concentrating forces on the DAR and the adjacent joint capsule. If the DAR breaks down, then the "clunk" will cease. The femoral head remains permanently in the luxated position in the dorsal joint capsule. Acetabular filling follows breakdown of the DAR because it is secondary to the inflammation generated by the breakdown process at the DAR. The hip will stop "clunking" if the hip is neglected because acetabular filling occurs. The window of opportunity to correct this patient's acetabular hip dysplasia by pelvic osteotomy is lost if dorsal acetabular breakdown or acetabular filling occurs. Under these circumstances, the attending veterinarian has lost the chance to reconstruct the patient's hip.

The presence of "clunking" hips indicates that the hips are luxated and are in a severe and rapid stage of degeneration. If the dog is young, these hips may be saved and made functional by a pelvic osteotomy; however, immediate action must be taken to identify the source of damage accurately and to correct the incongruity.

Stand Test

The stand test creates extension of the hip and lordosis of the spine (Fig. 61.11). This test is a functional exercise that stresses the spine (especially the L7–S1 with cauda equina impingement) and hip in extension. Because the interaction to perform this test is between the owner and the patient, resistance to the test is minimal, and the results are reliable. If the owner is unable to handle the patient, or if the patient intimidates the owner, then the test should be bypassed to avoid injury.

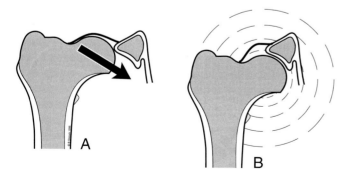

Fig. 61.10. **A.** The "clunking" sound emanating from the hip is generated by the luxated hip, rapidly returning to the acetabulum (*arrow*) during ambulation. **B.** When the femoral head seats in the bottom of the acetabulum, a "clunking" sound is heard, and this corresponds to the vibration felt as the medial translation of the greater trochanter is palpated during ambulation.

TESTING PROCEDURE

Clear and specific instructions to the owner are the basis of this test:

1. "Allow your dog to stand on all four legs and face you."

2. "Pick up your dog by the front legs as if you are going to dance with him or her. All the way up."

The patient and owner are observed from the side. Some patients (but few) refuse to stand facing the owner because they have been disciplined for jumping up on the owner.

The normal dog stands in this position without discomfort and enjoys the attention. The dog does not attempt to get down. The dog extends to be closer to the owner. The dog's back and hips are extended and flat as the dog stretches to reach the owner's face.

The abnormal dog stands in this position with discomfort and does not enjoy the test. The dog attempts to get down. The dog does not extend to be closer to the owner and shifts body weight to the side to return to the ground. The dog's back and hips are maintained in flexion, and the dog attempts to disengage from this activity. The dog may even mock bite at the owner's hand as the owner holds the dog's forelimbs.

The stand test stresses the hips and spine of the patient by forced extension. Dogs with abnormal hips respond differently, depending on the degree of inflammation and fibrosis. Young dogs with stretched joint capsules that have little inflammation give the response of a normal dog. The young dog with highly inflamed joints and joint capsules adamantly resists the test. Older dogs with capsular fibrosis of chronic hip dysplasia simply cannot flex at the hips and stand with their rump sticking out.

Dogs with an abnormal spine also vary in their response, depending on the degree of inflammation. The patient with a highly inflamed spine from a disease such as discospondylitis fights this test violently. Dogs with cauda equina syndrome resist to a lesser degree. Patients with mild spondylosis do not fight the test, but they prefer to stand with their rump sticking out.

Even though the stand test is not pathognomonic for a disease, it consistently regionalizes the problem to the back or hip. It is an easy test to perform to demonstrate a problem in these regions.

Physical Examination in an Awake Patient

Abduction External Rotation Test

The physical examination is the primary means of demonstrating that a patient's lameness or soreness is coming from the hip, lower lumbar spine, or lumbosacral disc. The abduction external rotation test is not specific to hip dysplasia, but it suggests dorsal joint capsule inflammation. Because this test creates dis-

comfort in the hip, the owner should be forewarned of the patient's possible pain response. Only enough external rotation to elicit a response is necessary. This should be the last test performed on the caudal portion of the dog if patient cooperation is expected.

TESTING PROCEDURE

The orthopedist is caudal to the patient while an animal health technician restrains the patient's head. The right and left hips are tested independently. The examiner's right hand holds the patient's right stifle. The stifle is used to flex and externally rotate the right hip. The hip is abducted, externally rotated, and extended simultaneously. A negative response from the patient is indifference. A positive response from the patient varies, depending on the dog's personality, from guarding the hip against manipulation, to vocalization, to attempting to bite the operator.

The abduction external rotation test stresses the attachment of the joint capsule at the DAR, to stimulate a pain response in the inflamed hip. The hip inflammation is caused by repeated tearing of the joint capsule as the femoral head translates laterally and dorsally. The final dorsal migration of the femoral head creates the capsular tearing. After the repeated tearing of the capsule dorsally, the capsule thickens and attempts to heal by fibrosis. The normal joint capsule at the DAR is thin and almost transparent, but it is stout cranially and caudally.

A positive response from the patient indicates that inflammation is present. This test does not quantify the amount of inflammation. The acute tearing of the young patient is usually painful, because it is complete and creates a tremendous stretching on the cranial and caudal capsule. The tearing of the older patient's joint capsule is usually not so extensive. The joint capsule with a more chronic disorder supports the femoral head by hypertrophy and fibrosis. This test is also positive if the lower lumbar spine or lumbosacral disc is inflamed by causing a torsion of the affected inflamed disc.

Hip Extension Test

This physical examination is a primary means of demonstrating that lameness is emanating from the hip or back. This test is not specific to the hip because it tests the dog's response not only to the inflamed and thickened joint capsule, but also to the contracted iliopsoas and lower back inflammation. Because the hip extension test creates discomfort, the owner should be forewarned of the possibility of aggressive or painful behavior.

TESTING PROCEDURE

The orthopedist is caudal to the patient while an animal health technician restrains the patient's head. The right and left hips are tested independently. For testing a small dog's right hip, the operator places his or her fingers around the cranial thigh and the thumb on the dorsal ischial table. The patient's hip is extended by pulling the examiner's fingers to the thumb. For large dogs, the fingers of the right hand are placed around the cranial right thigh at the stifle, and the left hand is placed over the dog's rump. The operator extends the dog's hip by pulling the femur caudally, while the left hand prevents the dog moving away from the doctor. The left hip is similarly tested. A negative response from the patient is indifference. A positive response from the patient varies, depending on the dog's personality, from guarding the hip against manipulation, to vocalization, to attempting to bite the operator.

The hip extension test tightens the joint capsule around the neck of the femur. This stretches an inflamed joint capsule like wringing a mop. The hip inflammation is present because of repeated tearing of the joint capsule as the femoral head translates laterally and dorsally. After the repeated tearing of the capsule dorsally, the inflamed capsule thickens and attempts to heal by fibrosis. A positive response from the patient indicates that hip joint capsule inflammation is present. This test does not quantify how much inflammation is present, only that it is present. This test may show discomfort of the lower lumbar spine or lumbosacral disc inflammation by extending the lower back.

The stand test creates similar conditions of hip extension and lordosis (back extension), but in the stand test, the patient extends only as far as comfort allows. Interpretation of the hip extension test and the stand test is similar.

Hip Subluxation Test

This physical examination is a primary means of demonstrating that a patient's lameness or soreness is coming from the hip. This test is specific to the dysplastic hip because it tests the dog's response to the inflamed dorsal joint capsule. The owner should be forewarned that the patient may create its own discomfort by contracting the muscles that force the femoral head against the irritated joint capsule. This should be the last test performed on the caudal portion of the dog, if patient cooperation is expected.

TESTING PROCEDURE

The orthopedist is on the side of the hip to be tested, while an animal health technician restrains the patient's head. The right and left hips are tested independently. For the right hip, the fingers of the examiner's right hand are placed medial to the proximal femur from cranially, and the right thumb is placed on the right ilium. For large dogs, it may be helpful to prevent

the hip from abducting by placing the left hand on the lateral stifle. The examiner pulls laterally on the femur and pushes medially on the ilium with the thumb at the same time. A negative response from the patient is indifference. A positive response from the patient varies from guarding the hip against further manipulation, to vocalization, to attempting to bite, depending on the dog's personality. The left hip is similarly tested.

The hip subluxation test stresses the attachment of the joint capsule at the DAR. As the hip subluxates laterally by the examiner's lateral pressure on the proximal femur, the patient contracts the thigh muscles to protect the hip against the anticipated pain. This muscular contraction causes the hip to translate dorsally into the inflamed dorsal joint capsule. This causes a positive pain response. The hip inflammation is present because of repeated stretching of the joint capsule as the femoral head translates laterally. The dorsal migration of the femoral head after lateral translation creates the capsular tearing and high inflammation in the diseased hip.

The normal joint capsule at the DAR is thin and almost transparent, but it is stout cranially and caudally. After repeated stretching and tearing of the capsule dorsally, the capsule thickens and attempts to heal by fibrosis. A positive response from the patient indicates that inflammation is present. This test does not quantitate the amount of inflammation. The acute stretching in the young patient is usually painful because it creates a tremendous stretching on the cranial and caudal capsules. The acute tearing of the dorsal joint capsule resulting from dorsal translation in the young patient is usually painful because it lacks capsular support of the more chronic cases. The per incident tearing of the older patient joint capsule is usually not so extensive, and the joint capsule with a more chronic disorder has the support of hypertrophy and fibrosis cranially and caudally.

The hip subluxation test is useful in distinguishing between hip and back pain because it is specific to the hip and independent of the lower lumbar spine or lumbosacral disc inflammation.

Iliopsoas Testing

This physical examination is a primary means of demonstrating that lameness is emanating from the iliopsoas muscle. This test is specific to the iliopsoas because it tests the dog's response to the inflamed iliopsoas muscle. Because iliopsoas testing creates discomfort, the owner should be forewarned of the possibility of aggressive or painful behavior.

TESTING PROCEDURE

The orthopedist is lateral to the patient while an animal health technician restrains the patient's head. The right and left hips are tested independently. For testing a dog's right iliopsoas muscle, the operator places his or her fingers around the patient's cranial thigh and applies digital pressure over the iliopsoas just caudal to the origin of the pectineus muscle. The iliopsoas muscle is further tested by extending the hip and digital palpation. In addition, the iliopsoas muscle is tested further by extending the hip plus digital palpation of the muscle with internal rotation of the hip. The left hip is similarly tested. A negative response from the patient is indifference. A positive response from the patient varies, depending on the dog's personality, from guarding the hip against manipulation, to vocalization, to attempting to bite the operator.

The direct digital palpation of the iliopsoas muscle causes pain in the inflamed muscle. Extension of the hip causes pain by stretching the inflamed muscle. The internal rotation of the hip also lengthens the inflamed iliopsoas muscle. The pain experienced by the patient is in direct proportion to the amount of inflammation, digital pressure, and stretching of the muscle. This test does not quantify the degree of inflammation. The digital test and internal rotation test are specific to the iliopsoas muscle.

Physical Examination in an Anesthetized Patient

Angles of Reduction and Subluxation

The meaning of hip palpation has been incompletely understood because of imprecise definition and measurement. The Ortolani sign occurs during hip abduction and is created when the femoral head is reduced into the acetabulum from a luxated position with a "shift" or "clunk." The angle of reduction is the measurement of the angle of abduction from the sagittal plane to the physical position at which hip reduction occurs.

The Barlow sign is a palpation event during which the femoral head is luxated from the acetabulum. The Barlow sign occurs during hip adduction and is created when the femoral head is luxated from the acetabulum into a position of joint capsular support with a "shift." The angle of subluxation is the angle between the sagittal plane and the physical event of hip luxation at which the hip first begins to luxate. By definition, the angle of subluxation is measured as positive if the hip is lateral to the sagittal plane when subluxation occurs (Fig. 61.12) and negative if the hip is medial to the sagittal plane when subluxation occurs.

TECHNIQUES OF MEASUREMENT
The patient is anesthetized and is placed in dorsal recumbency.

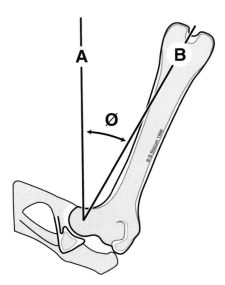

Fig. 61.12. Measuring hip angle (∅) is done in dorsal recumbency with the sagittal plane (A) as vertical. The femoral axis (B) is between the center of the femoral head and the center of the intercondylar notch where it meets the articular surface of the trochlear sulcus. ∅ is positive when the hip is abducted; that is, the distal femur is lateral to the sagittal plane as shown; ∅ is negative when the hip is adducted, and the distal femur is medial to the sagittal plane.

Angle of Reduction
The stifle is brought to the starting position of vertical, without hip flexion or extension, by using a medially directed force of the operator's hand on the lateral stifle. Axial femoral compression by the operator is not necessary in the immature patient, although it may clarify the angle at which reduction occurs in a patient with a chronic case. The hip is then abducted slowly by reducing the medially directed force at the stifle. When hip reduction occurs, abduction is stopped. Reduction of the hip is detected in three possible ways: a "clunk" is heard; a shift of the patient's limb is seen or palpated; or the event can be recorded by cineradiography. In chronic hip dysplasia, a "fast spot" or rapid abduction is palpated, instead of a "clunk," as the hip reduces under the influence of abduction.

The angle of reduction is measured by the Canine Electronic Goniometer (Slocum Enterprises, Eugene, OR), which was designed for this purpose. The probe is placed just caudal to the attachment of the pectineus on the iliopectineal eminence. The side of the goniometer is touched to the medial side of the stifle (Figs. 61.13 and 61.14). The angle of reduction is read directly from the digital readout with accuracy to 0.1° (Fig. 61.15).

Angle of Subluxation
To obtain the angle of subluxation, the stifle is slowly returned to vertical from the abducted position at which the angle of reduction was taken. The hip is

adducted slowly by increasing the medially directed force at the stifle. When the hip begins to luxate (subluxate), adduction is stopped. Here again, axial femoral compression by the operator is not necessary, but it may clarify the angle at which subluxation occurs in patients with a chronic disorder.

Luxation of the hip is detected in three ways: a "shift" is palpated; a "shift" is seen; or the event can be recorded by cineradiography. In cases of chronic hip dysplasia, a "fast spot" or rapid abduction is palpated, instead of a "shift," as the hip luxates under the influence of adduction. The angle of subluxation is measured by the Canine Electronic Goniometer. The probe is placed just caudal to the attachment of the pectineus on the iliopectineal eminence. The side of the goniometer is touched to the medial side of the stifle (Fig. 61.16), and the measurements are recorded. The measurements of the angles of reduction and subluxation are repeated on the other hip.

Two angles are measured for each hip, the angle of reduction and the angle of subluxation. The format for recording this information is (angle of reduction/the angle of subluxation), that is, AR/AS = 29.9°/14.5°. The angle of reduction is always greater than the angle of subluxation.

The angle of reduction represents joint laxity, that is, the stretching of the joint capsule and its tearing from the DAR. The greater the angle of reduction, the greater is the stretching of the joint capsule dorsally. The stretching of the joint capsule dorsally determines

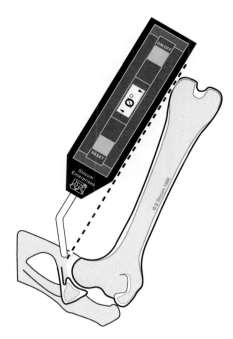

Fig. 61.14. The Canine Electronic Goniometer measures the angle with respect to gravity, the sagittal plane is 0°, obtained in dorsal recumbency of the patient. The probe is placed just caudal to the iliopectineal eminence; the body of the goniometer is touched to the medial femoral condyle, and the angle ∅ is recorded from the digital readout.

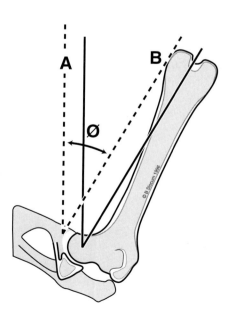

Fig. 61.13. The axis of measurement for the Canine Electronic Goniometer (*dotted line, B*) is parallel to the defined axis (*solid line*). Because the sagittal plane (*A*) is defined by gravity, the angle ∅ remains the same.

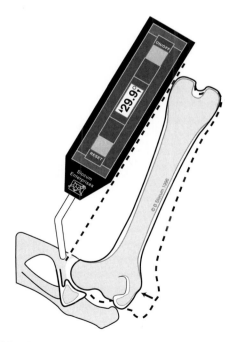

Fig. 61.15. The angle of reduction is measured, 29.9° in this example, immediately after the abduction event of hip reduction (*arrow*).

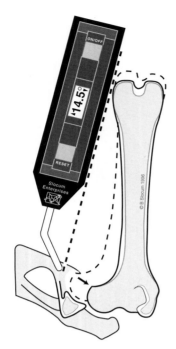

Fig. 61.16. The angle of subluxation is measured, 14.5° in this example, immediately after the adduction event of hip luxation (*arrow*).

where the DAR will contact the femoral head. The physical contact point between the rim and the femoral head determines the amount of abduction necessary before the axial force of the femur (the direction not the magnitude) is directed medial to that contact point. The femoral head falls into the acetabulum when that condition exists (Fig. 61.17). For this reason, abduction is necessary to create hip reduction.

When the stretching of the joint capsule is small, the contact point is almost dorsal on the femoral head when the limb is in the sagittal plane. As the joint capsule stretches, the femoral head is allowed to translate laterally and then dorsally, and the point of contact between the DAR and the head moves further medially on the femoral head. The lateral and dorsal translation of the femoral head is limited by the ligament of the femoral head. This causes the contact point of the DAR and the femoral head to be just dorsal to the fovea capitis. This is the outer limit of capsular stretching without damage to the teres ligament. When the femoral head rests in this position, all the forces transmitted to the DAR from the femoral head have to do so through a reduced area of contact. This extreme force per unit area of contact between the femoral head and the DAR damages the cartilage of the femoral head just above the fovea capitis. This

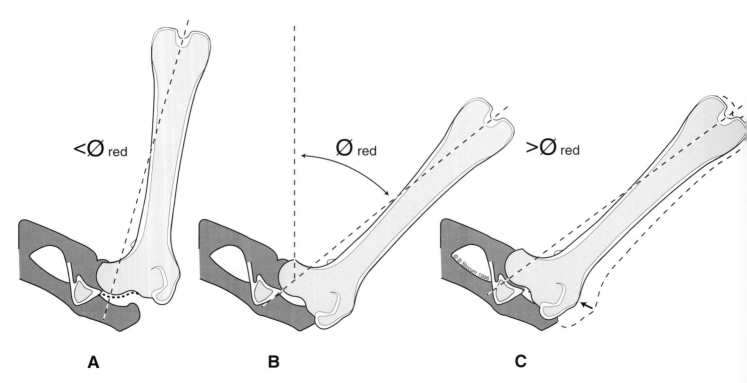

$<\varnothing_{red}$ $\varnothing_{red}$ $>\varnothing_{red}$

A   **B**   **C**

Fig. 61.17. **A.** Hip reduction by abduction begins (less than $\varnothing^{red}$) with the femoral head resting and stable in the dorsal joint capsule (*dotted line*) (hip luxated) and the acetabulum contacting the femoral head medial to the axial line of femoral force between the joints (*dashed line*). **B.** As the hip is abducted, the joint capsule supporting the femoral neck through the cranial and caudal ligaments causes the femoral head and the dorsal acetabular rim to contact along the axial line at angle $\varnothing^{red}$, which makes the hip unstable. **C.** Any further abduction (greater than $\varnothing^{red}$) causes the femoral head to contact the dorsal acetabular rim lateral to the axial line of force, and the femoral head shifts into the acetabulum (*arrow*). The femoral head is now stable within the confines of the acetabulum when greater than $\varnothing^{red}$.

damage begins with fibrillation of the cartilage and ends with bone rubbing on bone and distortion of both the femoral head and acetabulum as end-stage events. The angle of reduction increases further only with stretching of the teres ligament or breakdown of the dorsal acetabulum. The angle of reduction decreases with capsular fibrosis and osteophyte production on the DAR that initiates capsular stabilization by resisting further dorsal translation.

The angle of subluxation represents the functional slope of the acetabulum beneath the dorsal rim. The actual slope of the DAR may be less than the angle of subluxation, if the ligament of the femoral head is redundant or the acetabulum is filling with osteophytes. For subluxation of the hip to occur, the femoral head and the acetabulum must interact, but not the joint capsule (Fig. 61.18). The direction of the axial femoral force is into the acetabulum following the measurement of the angle of reduction. As the hip is adducted, the axial femoral force becomes normal to the DAR slope that was the last position of stability. Any further adduction of the hip directs the axial femoral force lateral to the perpendicular of the DAR surface, and so the femoral head translates laterally to rest in the joint capsule. In the normal hip, no significant joint capsule laxity exists to allow enough lateral translation of the femoral head for subluxation. All hips have some laxity, as clearly established by Penn-Hip. PennHip is a commercial registry which reads dis-

traction and compression hip radiographs for hip laxity. The laxity is normalized to the femoral head and expressed as the Compression Index, C.I. (C.I. = displacement of the femoral head divided by the radius of the femoral head.) C.I. < 0.30 is normal for most breeds.

As some normal puppies undergo rapid growth between 4 and 6 months of age, the adductor muscle mass (and moment) overpowers the abductor muscles because of the temporary lack of adductor muscle length. As a consequence, the relative hip adduction directs the axial femoral force lateral to the DAR, and the femoral head is contained in its lateral translation by the joint capsule. The joint capsule is stretched, producing joint laxity. The result is an increased angle of reduction and distractive index of PennHip. In such patients, the angle of reduction is high because of the lax joint capsule, but the DAR angle is normal. The angle of subluxation may be 0° or negative because the DAR slope is normal. Such laxity is not hip dysplasia, because the conformation of the hip is normal and the stretched capsule is temporary, whereas hip laxity, caused by capsular stretching that accompanies acetabular hip dysplasia, is secondary to an increased slope of the DAR (the cause of stretching) and remain until the slope of the DAR is normalized by a pelvic osteotomy. This example of rapid growth syndrome in puppies with lax capsules that allow hip luxation confirms our clinical experience that hip joints can be lax with-

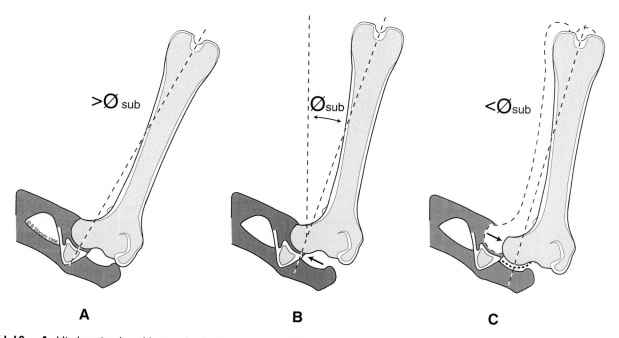

A   **B**   **C**

Fig. 61.18. **A.** Hip luxation by adduction begins (greater than $\emptyset^{sub}$) with the femoral head resting and stable in the acetabulum and the femoral head contacting the dorsal acetabular rim lateral to the axial line of femoral force between joints (*dashed line*). **B.** As the hip is adducted, the femoral head contacts the dorsal acetabular rim at $\emptyset^{sub}$ along the axial line, and the hip is unstable. **C.** Any further adduction (less than $\emptyset^{sub}$) causes the femoral head to contact the dorsal acetabular rim medial to the axial line of force, and the femoral head luxates (*arrow*) into the joint capsule (*dotted line*).

out being pathologic. In addition, these puppies have become certified by OFA as normal when trauma to the hip is prevented by conservative management during 5 to 12 months of age. The angle of subluxation may even be a negative number in the nonpathologic hip or after a pelvic osteotomy.

In the pathologic hip, the angle of reduction is easily palpated in the young patient (6 months), but it may be difficult to palpate in the older patient (often by 2 years). The angle of reduction usually increases until the patient reaches the limit of stretching of the teres ligament and the joint capsule. Once the femoral head rests in the luxated position, the acetabulum fills with osteophytes, even though the femoral head may occasionally reduce. The joint capsule becomes fibrotic and thickened. As this dysplastic process progresses, the angle of reduction begins to decrease and finally becomes difficult to palpate.

In the pathologic hip, the angle of subluxation is greater than 0° and slowly increases, but it never decreases. This increasing angle is caused by the increased DAR slope because of acetabular filling and teres ligament redundancy. As the angle of reduction decreases and the angle of subluxation increases, one sees a single angle at which the femoral head shifts between capsular support and acetabular support. This is called the angle of translation (Fig. 61.19).

Simply stated, a great difference between the angle of reduction and the angle of subluxation (i.e., 40/5) indicates a healthy hip with a stretched joint capsule, or a young dog's hip in the early stages of hip dysplasia that can be readily repaired with good results and no arthritis. A moderate difference between the angle of reduction and the angle of subluxation (i.e., 30/15) indicates a hip in immediate need of a pelvic osteotomy, but the status of the articular cartilage and acetabular filling needs to be assessed. A small difference between the angle of reduction and the angle of sub-

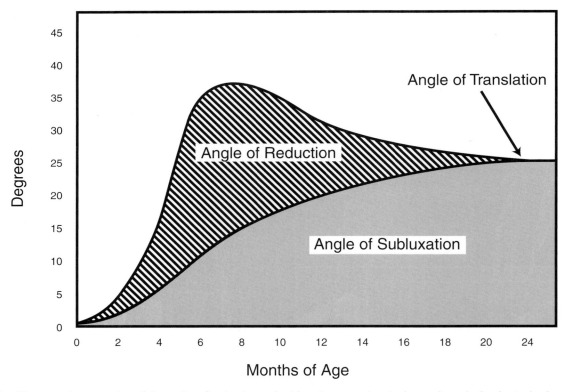

Hip Palpation Angles

Fig. 61.19. The natural progression of the angles of reduction and subluxation over time in the moderately dysplastic dog has repeatable characteristics. Early (0 to 7 months) joint capsular stretching is accompanied by a rapid increase in the angle of reduction. As time passes, the capsule becomes thickened and stabilizes the hip. The angle of subluxation, which is a function of femoral head and acetabular interaction, represents dorsal acetabular damage, acetabular filling, and ligamentum teres redundancy. The angle of subluxation increases most rapidly in the early adolescent period (5 to 8 months), when the acetabulum is subjected to high force per unit area by the luxating femoral head in the lax joint capsule. As filling of the acetabulum occurs by osteophytes forming under the influence of inflammation within the joint and the joint capsule thickens, the rate of increase of the angle of subluxation slows. The angle of subluxation continues to increase until the angle of reduction equals the angle of subluxation, called the angle of translation (AT). At the AT, the femoral head is supported by the capsule when ∅ is less than AT, and the femoral head is supported by the acetabulum when ∅ is greater than AT.

luxation (i.e., 25/22) indicates a hip that is filling with osteophytes and is no longer a candidate for a pelvic osteotomy. A small difference between the angle of reduction and the angle of subluxation in the near-0° range (i.e., 10/0) indicates a normal hip with some capsular stretching with no need for surgical intervention.

The angle of reduction and the angle of subluxation are critical parts of the hip evaluation and are excellent indicators of status of hip health, especially at 6 months of age. Hip palpation at the time of neutering is a perfect opportunity to assess the patient for future hip problems, because it gives the owners information about whether their pet is at risk for hip dysplasia.

Suggested Readings

Bardens JW. Palpation for the detection of joint laxity. In: Proceedings of the Canine Hip Dysplasia Symposium and Workshop. St Louis: Orthopedic Foundation for Animals, 1972:105–109.

Bardens JW, Hardwick H. New observations in the diagnosis and cause of hip dysplasia. Vet Med Small Anim Clin 1968;63:238.

Belkoff SM, Padgett G, Soutas-Little RW. Development of a device to measure canine coxofemoral joint laxity. VCOT 1989;1:31–36.

Slocum B, AVORE. Pelvic osteotomy: the results of 285 pelvic osteotomies (abstract). Vet Surg 1986;15:134.

Slocum B, Devine T. Pelvic osteotomy in the dog as treatment for hip dysplasia. Semin Vet Med Surg 1987;2:107.

Slocum B, Devine T. Femoral neck lengthening for hip dysplasia in the dog. Vet Surg 1989;18:81.

Slocum B, Devine T. Pelvic osteotomy. In: Whittock W, ed. Canine orthopedics. 2nd ed. Philadelphia: Lea & Febiger, 1990:471.

Slocum B, Devine T. Pelvic osteotomy for axial rotation of the acetabular segment. Vet Clin North Am 1992;22:645.

Slocum B, Slocum TD. Slope of the dorsal acetabular rim for hip evaluation in the dog. In: 17th annual conference of the Veterinary Orthopedic Society. Jackson Hole, WY: Veterinary Orthopedic Society, 1990:12.

Smith G, Biery D, Gregor T. New concepts of coxofemoral joint stability and the development of a clinical stress-radiographic method for quantitiating hip joint laxity in the dog. J Am Vet Med Assoc 1990;196:59–70.

Wright PJ, Masson TA. The usefulness of palpation of joint laxity in puppies as a predictor of hip dysplasia in a guide dog breeding programme. J Small Anim Pract 1977;18:513.

Ortolani Sign

The Ortolani sign is a palpation finding which was originally used in human medicine as an indicator of hip dysplasia. This sign occurs when the luxated hip enters the acetabulum with a "clunk."

TESTING PROCEDURE

The anesthetized patient is placed in dorsal recumbency. The palm of the operator's left hand is lightly placed on the lateral side of the patient's flexed right stifle. The left thumb is placed over the medial femoral condyle adjacent to the patella. The starting position is hip adduction without flexion or extension. In this position, the hip luxates from the acetabulum. The hip is slowly abducted.

If a "shift" or "clunk" in the hip is palpated, then the Ortolani sign is positive. If no "shift" or "clunk" in the hip is palpated, then the Ortolani sign is negative. The process is also repeated for the left hip by using the operator's right hand on the patient's left stifle.

The "shift" or "clunk" palpated in the hip is the reduction of the femoral head. Reduction of the femoral head into the acetabulum can only occur if the joint capsule has been stretched. A positive Ortolani sign means that the joint capsule is stretched. A negative Ortolani sign means either that the joint capsule is not stretched or that the hip is not reducible into the acetabulum. Chronic fibrosis of the joint capsule often makes the transition from luxation to reduction so subtle as to go undetected.

The Ortolani sign does not represent hip dysplasia, but it indicates joint capsule stretching, which often accompanies hip dysplasia. Joint laxity is not hip dysplasia, but it is one secondary manifestation of the hip dysplastic process. Joint laxity occurs when the joint capsule is stretched. Joint capsule stretching has many causes, the most common being hip dysplasia.

To reduce the hip, the femoral head must enter the acetabulum. The angle of abduction at which the head begins to enter the acetabulum during hip abduction is the angle of reduction. This angle is the angle at which the femoral head becomes stable and relocates because of the axial compressive force direction. The angle of reduction depends on the amount of stretching of the joint capsule.

Barlow Sign

The Barlow sign is a palpation finding originally used in human medicine as an indicator of hip dysplasia. This sign occurs when the reduced hip leaves the acetabulum.

TESTING PROCEDURE

The anesthetized patient is placed in dorsal recumbency. The palm of the operator's left hand is placed lightly on the lateral side of the patient's flexed right stifle. The left thumb is placed over the medial femoral condyle adjacent to the patella. The starting position is hip abduction without flexion or extension. This position reduces the hip into the acetabulum. The hip is slowly adducted.

If a "shift" of the femoral head is palpated, then the Barlow sign is positive. If no "shift" of the femoral head is palpated, then the Barlow sign is negative. The process is also repeated for the left hip by using the operator's right hand on the patient's left stifle.

The "shift" palpated with the Barlow sign is luxation of the femoral head. Luxation of the femoral head from the acetabulum can only occur if the joint capsule has been stretched. A positive Barlow sign means that the joint capsule is stretched. A negative Barlow sign means either the joint capsule is not stretched or the hip will not reduce into the acetabulum. If the hip has chronic disease with a thickened joint capsule, the shift may be so subtle that it is missed by the operator.

The Barlow sign does not represent hip dysplasia, but it indicates joint capsule stretching, which often accompanies hip dysplasia. Joint laxity is not hip dysplasia, but it is a secondary manifestation of the hip dysplastic process. Joint laxity occurs when the joint capsule is stretched. Joint capsule stretching has many causes, and the most common cause of joint laxity is hip dysplasia.

To luxate the hip, the femoral head must leave the acetabulum. The angle of *ab*duction at which the head begins to leave the acetabulum during hip *ad*duction is the angle of subluxation. This angle is the angle at which the femoral head becomes unstable because of the axial compressive force direction and luxates. The angle of subluxation depends on the functional slope of the DAR.

Bardens Palpation

Bardens recognized laxity in the hip joints of 8-week-old puppies and discovered that those puppies were dysplastic as adults. Later, Brown studied the laxity of hips in rottweiler puppies by the Bardens method and confirmed that laxity and hip dysplasia were associated. Recently, laxity testing has been addressed by radiography and statistical analysis and has been shown to be present in hip dysplasia.

BARDENS PALPATION

The anesthetized 6- to 8-week-old puppy is placed in right lateral recumbency for testing of the left (up) hip (Fig. 61.20). The operator's right hand is the measuring hand and the left hand is the testing hand. The thumb of the operator's right hand is placed on the left lateral prominence of the patient's tuber ischiadicum. The middle finger of the operator's right hand is placed on the left wing of the ilium. The index finger of the operator's left hand is placed on the left greater trochanter. The patient's left femur is grasped just below the greater trochanter by the left hand of the operator. A medial to lateral force is exerted on the proximal femur by the left hand that translates the greater trochanter laterally. This translation is recorded and measured.

For testing of the right hip, the operator's left hand is the measuring hand and the right hand is the testing hand. The experienced operator can distinguish

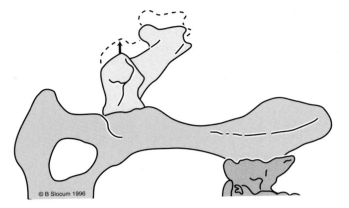

Fig. 61.20. Bardens palpation of the left hip (up) requires the patient to be in right lateral recumbency. The left proximal trochanter is translated laterally (*dotted femur*) by a medial-to-lateral force on the proximal femur with the left hand. The right hand calibrates the amount of translation (*arrow*).

among four groups of lateral hip translation: 1 to 2 mm; 3 to 4 mm; 5 to 6 mm; and greater than 6 mm:

Normal hip: 1 to 2 mm
Borderline hip: 3 to 4 mm
Dysplastic hip: 5 to 6 mm
Severely dysplastic hip: more than 6 mm

Although the Bardens palpation has never been well accepted as a definitive index of hip dysplasia, it is useful as a general indicator of hip dysplasia. The Bardens palpation has four main objectives. First, the method requires a skilled operator who can detect and measure the lateral laxity accurately. This makes the test difficult to generalize to all veterinarians. Second, the patient must be between 6 and 8 weeks of age to achieve uniformity in the population and the dysplastic process. Third, the scientific correlation of confirmation between the Bardens palpation and degree of hip dysplasia in the mature patient has not been clearly established. Fourth, hip laxity is not hip dysplasia but rather one measurable aspect of hip dysplasia and is dependent on joint capsule stretching. As we develop better means of measuring the lateral translation with accuracy and repeatability, this test may become the basis for future decisions about hip dysplasia.

Suggested Readings

Bardens JW. Palpation for the detection of joint laxity. In: Proceedings of the Canine Hip Dysplasia Symposium and Workshop. St. Louis: Orthopedic Foundation for Animals, 1972:105–109.
Bardens JW, Hardwick H. New observations in the diagnosis and cause of hip dysplasia. Vet Med Small Anim Clin 1968;63:238.
Belkoff SM, Padgett G, Soutas-Little RW. Development of a device to measure canine coxofemoral joint laxity. VCOT 1989;1:31–36.
Smith G, Biery D, Gregor T. New concepts of coxofemoral joint

stability and the development of a clinical stress-radiographic method for quantitiating hip joint laxity in the dog. J Am Vet Med Assoc 1990;196:59–70.

Wright PJ, Masson TA. The usefulness of palpation of joint laxity in puppies as a predictor of hip dysplasia in a guide dog breeding programme. J Small Anim Pract 1977;18:513.

Axial Compression Test of the Hip

The axial compression test is an intraoperative test for hip stability. Hip stability is achieved when the reduced hip remains in the acetabulum on axial compression of the femur in the sagittal plane.

TESTING PROCEDURE

To test the left hip, the patient is placed in right lateral recumbency. The examiner's right hand is placed on the dorsal rump of the patient. The left hand gently grasps the stifle and applies axial compression of the femur in the sagittal plane to the reduced hip (Fig. 61.21).

If a "shift" of the femoral head is palpated as the hip luxates from the acetabulum, then the axial compression test is positive and the hip is unstable. If no "shift" of the femoral head is palpated, then the axial compression test is negative and the hip is stable. When the test is applied to the right hip, the operator's right hand is on the patient's stifle, and the left hand is on the rump.

The palpated "shift" is luxation of the femoral head. Luxation of the femoral head from the acetabulum can only occur if the slope of the DAR is too great to contain the head, if acetabular filling is present, or if the femoral head has a redundant ligament. No "shift" means that the DAR is able to contain the femoral head. Surgically, it means the axial rotation of the acetabular segment by pelvic osteotomy is sufficient. A hip joint is either stable or unstable to axial compression in the sagittal plane. If a hip is stable in the sagittal plane, additional rotation of the acetabular segment by pelvic osteotomy will only limit abduction of the hip and cause hip degeneration.

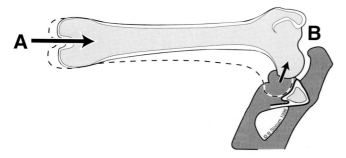

Fig. 61.21. The axial compression test (A) is positive and the hip is unstable if a dorsolateral translation of the femoral head (*small arrow*) is detected by a lateral movement of the greater trochanter (B). The test is negative, and the hip is stable, if no translation is noted.

Radiographic Characteristics of Hip Dysplasia

Theresa Devine Slocum & Barclay Slocum

Evaluation of the canine hip for hip dysplasia involves gathering information on the history and attitude of the dog from the owner, performing a series of hip function assessment tests on the awake and anesthetized dog, and obtaining a three-dimensional view of the hip joint by radiographs. Examination of the dog for hip dysplasia is an important service to predict the physical ability of the young dog (6 months of age and older) to meet the owners' expectations for function and to provide the appropriate treatment for a dysplastic dog. Although hip dysplasia is defined by many authors as a congenital, bilateral, degenerative joint disease, or as hip laxity, limitations of these definitions are recognized clinically as we expand our knowledge of the disease and separate acetabular hip dysplasia from femoral hip dysplasia. The most important aspect of any definition is to acknowledge that hip dysplasia is a dynamic process, and any view of the disease is a window at one point in its progression.

Most cases of dysplasia involve acetabular hip dysplasia, which is characterized by excessive slope of the dorsal rim of the acetabulum, and its secondary osteoarthritic changes. Because the major forces of the hip run parallel to the long axis of the femur, the contact between the femoral head and the acetabulum should be perpendicular to the axial femoral forces for a stable hip joint. In the young puppy, the femoral head presses into the pliable acetabulum to form a deep socket. After 4 months, the formation of the acetabulum is becoming complete. If the acetabulum is shallow because of insufficient magnitude or direction of forces pushing the femoral head into the developing acetabulum, the joint capsule becomes stretched or, worse, the cartilaginous labrum becomes fractured. With insufficient dorsal support to the femoral head, muscular forces must be relied on to stabilize the joint by forcing the head into the acetabulum. As the muscles become fatigued, the joint capsule becomes stretched, and the dorsal rim becomes damaged. The femoral head resides in an incongruent subluxated position. As the restraints to subluxation, the joint capsule and teres ligament, stretch and tear, the vicious cycle of osteoarthritis becomes evident. When the hip cannot be maintained in the acetabulum, yet is within the joint capsule, the hip is considered luxated. When the acetabulum fills with osteophytes and the femoral head cannot be congruent with the acetabulum, the hip has irreducible luxating hip dysplasia. A dislocated

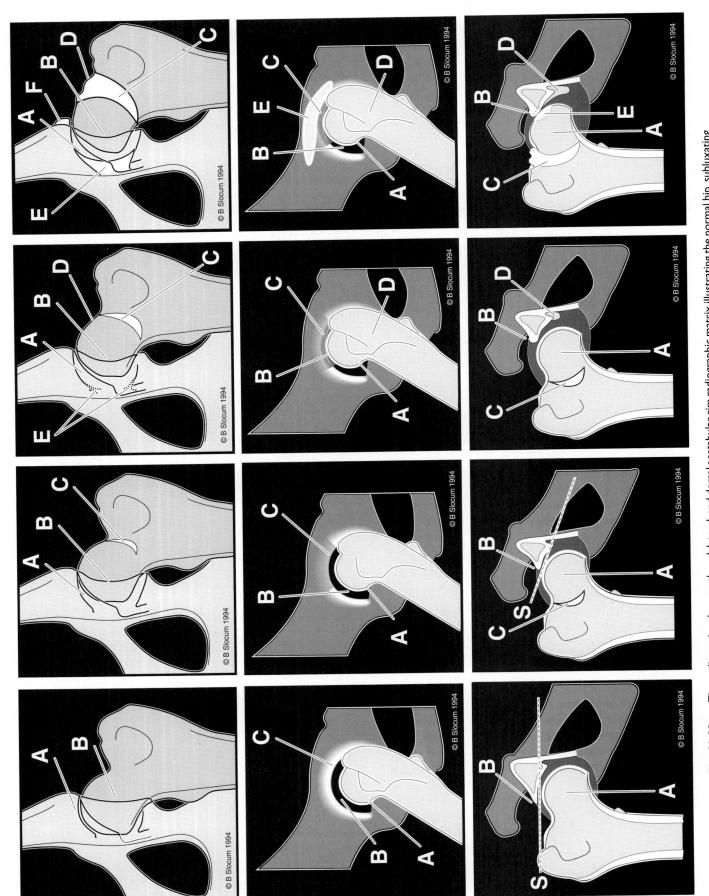

Fig. 61.22a. Three-dimensional ventrodorsal, lateral, and dorsal acetabular rim radiographic matrix illustrating the normal hip, subluxating hip dysplasia, reducible luxating hip dysplasia, and irreducible hip dysplasia.

Normal Hip

A. Congruity between subchondral bone of cranial acetabulum and head
B. DAR almost linear

Subluxating Hip Dysplasia

A. Congruity variable with capsule stretching and lateral distraction
B. DAR cupping (curvature due to repeated subluxation)
C. Small osteophyte at the margin of the caudal articular surface

Reducible Luxating Hip Dysplasia

A. Hip consistently incongruent
B. DAR cupping loses crisp margin
C. Osteophyte at the margin of the caudal articular surface
D. Neck thickened by osteophyte production
E. Acetabular filling prevents deep seating of femoral head

Irreducible Luxating Hip Dysplasia

A. Permanent incongruity
B. DAR deformed and indistinct
C. Osteophytes at margins of all articular surfaces
D. Neck and head deformed by osteophyte production
E. Acetabular filling prevents reduction of femoral head
F. Acetabular osteophyte indicative of severe DJD

Normal Hip

A. White subchondral bone
B. Black articular cartilage
C. White subchondral bone

Subluxating Hip Dysplasia

A. White subchondral bone
B. Black articular cartilage
C. Gray subchondral bone

Reducible Luxating Hip Dysplasia

A. White subchondral bone
B. Gray articular cartilage dorsally
C. Gray subchondral bone
D. Femur may translate dorsally

Irreducible Luxating Hip Dysplasia

A. White subchondral bone
B. Acetabular filling prevents reduction of femoral head
C. Gray subchondral bone
D. Femur may translate dorsally
E. Acetabular osteophyte indicative of severe DJD

Normal Hip

A. Center of femoral head lies medial to the lateral margin of the DAR
B. DAR is pointed
C. Slope of the DAR is less than 7.5°

Subluxating Hip Dysplasia

A. Center of the femoral head is at the lateral margin of the DAR
B. DAR is rounded
C. A fine osteophyte at the margin of the caudal articular surface
D. Slope of DAR is greater than 7.5°

Reducible Luxating Hip Dysplasia

A. Center of femoral head is lateral to the margin of the DAR
B. Osteophytes or beveling evident
C. Mature osteophyte at the margin of the caudal articular surface
D. Small acetabular osteophyte developing

Irreducible Luxating Hip Dysplasia

A. Center of femoral head lateral to DAR
B. Well-developed osteophytes dorsally within a deformed DAR
C. Femoral neck osteophytes deformed neck
D. Acetabular filling prevents reduction of femoral head
E. Loss of articular cartilage seen by narrowing of joint space

Fig. 61.22b. Three-dimensional radiographic matrix findings for normal hip, subluxating hip dysplasia, reducible luxating hip dysplasia, and irreducible hip dysplasia.

hip occurs when the hip is outside the traumatically torn joint capsule. As the stages of acetabular dysplasia progress, the treatment and prognosis for the hip must also match the degenerative process. Physical and radiographic information must be combined to provide the best evaluation of the canine hip.

The hip is a three degree of freedom joint, which means that it allows rotation about three orthogonal axes but no translation along those axes. Normal movements are flexion–extension, internal rotation–external rotation, and adduction–abduction. The dog is examined at a walk, trot, and run. Leg alignment, stride length, and movement in the sagittal plane are all noted. With the dog standing, the hip is slowly flexed and extended. A thickened and inflamed joint capsule causes the patient discomfort, and extension is resisted. Similarly, dysplastic patients usually refuse to stand erect with the hip in an extended position. The leg is abducted and externally rotated. Any apprehension indicates irritation to the inflamed tissue between the femoral neck and the dorsal rim of the acetabulum. Inability to abduct the leg indicates a contracted pectineus muscle. With the patient under anesthesia, the hip is palpated to reveal the viability of the cartilage of the femoral head and the acetabulum. With the dog in dorsal recumbency, the angle of reduction (the angle from vertical when reduction occurs during abduction) is measured; this angle is an indicator of joint capsule laxity. The greater the angle of reduction, the greater is the stretching or tearing from the dorsal acetabular rim (DAR) that has occurred to the joint capsule. The angle of subluxation (the angle from vertical when the luxation occurs during adduction) is measured. This angle increases proportionally to the damage to the dorsal rim of the acetabulum and acetabular filling. The trochanteric compression test reveals the preferred position of the femoral head with respect to the acetabulum; normally, it is within the acetabulum. A normal dog shows no apprehension or pain during the physical examination and enjoys the attention. Under anesthesia, a dog with normal hips demonstrates no angle of reduction or subluxation and has a negative trochanteric compression test.

Clinically, our radiographic examination uses six radiographic views: ventrodorsal, lateral, DAR, frog, compressed ventrodorsal, and distracted ventrodorsal views. The ventrodorsal, lateral, and DAR views are orthogonal and therefore give a "three-dimensional" study of the hip (Fig. 61.22**A** and **B**). Because positioning is essential in evaluating these radiographs, the dog is anesthetized for this portion of the examination. In the normal hip, the ventrodorsal view shows the femoral head to be deeply seated under the acetabulum with at least 50% coverage by the dorsal rim. Congruence exists between the subchondral bone of the

femoral head and the cranial acetabulum. Any torsion of the femur or anteversion of the femoral head is readily recognized with this view. The ventrodorsal view is useful for determining pelvic torsion, which often mimics unilateral hip dysplasia and is usually associated with a transitional vertebra. In the subluxated hip, the femoral head is partially covered by the dorsal rim of the acetabulum. One sees incomplete congruence of the joint and cupping of the acetabulum. In the luxated hip, the femoral head resides outside the acetabulum, and there is no congruence of the hip joint. As the disease process worsens, one can see a thickening of the neck of the femur and, occasionally, dorsal acetabular osteophytes forming.

The frog view is useful to determine acetabular filling with osteophytes (Fig. 61.23). The examiner must not lever the femoral head out of the acetabulum by abduction beyond 45°. The normal hip joint rests easily in the socket, whereas in the dysplastic hip, the femoral head is unable to seat fully in the acetabulum. This is indicative of filling of the acetabulum with osteophytes or a redundant teres ligament. As the dysplastic process progresses, the frog view demonstrates this condition.

The lateral radiograph of the pelvis and lower lumbar spine is useful for differentiating hip dysplasia from spondylitic bridging at L7–S1, which is often associated with the painful cauda equina syndrome. A normal hip shows congruence and concentricity of the femoral head within the acetabulum. In the dysplastic hip, the concentricity of the femoral head becomes less visible, and rather than a "white-black-white" description of normal congruence, a "white-gray-gray" description is common. Dorsal acetabular osteophytes are often seen as a white line over the femoral head.

Perhaps the most informative radiographic view is the DAR view. The dog is placed in a sternal recumbency with the hind legs pulled cranially to rest along the side of the thorax. A circumferential belt holds the stifles against the torso. Four-inch elevation of the hocks provides hamstring tension that causes enough rotation on most dogs to allow the x-ray beam to pass through the longitudinal axis of the pelvis. This view enables us to see the weightbearing portion of the acetabulum in cross section. In normal dogs, the DAR view shows the dorsal rim of the acetabulum to be sharply pointed. The femoral head is well seated and is covered by the acetabulum. When measured, the DAR angle is 7.5° or less, from a line perpendicular to the long axis of the pelvis. Normal hips have a combined left and right DAR measurement of 15° or less. Congruence of the hip joint is apparent with this view. A dog with normal hips continues to have a normal DAR angle throughout its lifetime.

As the hip is damaged by dysplasia, sclerosis of the rim can be seen on the DAR radiograph. The shape of

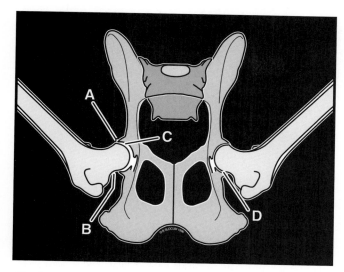

Fig. 61.23. A frog view is taken with the hips in 45° of abduction. The normal hip has a narrow cartilage line (*D*) and no osteophytes, whereas the dysplastic hip may have a dorsal acetabular osteophyte (*A*), a femoral neck osteophyte (*B*), and a wide cartilage space (*C*), indicating acetabular filling by osteophytes or redundant ligamentum teres.

the rim progresses from slightly rounded to blunted and broken off. Concurrently, the slope of the rim becomes increased. The dorsal acetabular osteophytes, so difficult to visualize on the ventrodorsal radiograph, are obvious with the DAR view. The femoral head moves dorsally and laterally, and filling of the acetabulum occurs. As the process of dysplasia progresses, the osteoarthritic changes can be seen clearly with this view. Lack of congruity and loss of cartilage are easily noted. When measured on the DAR view, dogs with hip dysplasia have a combined DAR slope of 20° or more. The slope continues to increase as the dysplastic changes occur.

The importance of the DAR view is that it corresponds to hip palpation under anesthesia and provides the information necessary to determine the treatment of choice for the individual dog. As stress is placed on the DAR with the early stages of dysplasia, the rim shows slight rounding. On palpation, the hip makes a smooth transition from the subluxated position into the acetabulum, indicating integrity of articular cartilage of the head and acetabulum and minimal stretching of the joint capsule. As frequent intermittent subluxation occurs, palpation reveals smooth cartilage and a stretched joint capsule, noted by a "clunk" as the hip moves from subluxation to reduction. The acutely luxating femoral head causes a bevel to the rim, characteristic of a torn joint capsule and a worn labrum. With palpation, this correlates to a fine granular crepitus of articular cartilage fibrillation and abrupt dorsal translation of the femoral head. In chronic conditions, no distinct transition between reduction and subluxa-

tion is palpated because of acetabular filling and capsular fibrosis. The DAR radiograph measurement provides the amount of pelvic rotation for a triple pelvic osteotomy in patients that still have cartilage on the femoral head. This measurement is the amount of rotation necessary for support of the femoral head by the acetabulum. If the DAR measurement shows a 20° slope, then a 20° Canine Pelvic Osteotomy Plate (Slocum Enterprises, Eugene, OR) is necessary for corrective surgery. Postsurgically, a tomogram of the DAR allows visualization of the amount of rotation performed with pelvic osteotomy. Overrotation can be prevented as a result of this radiographic technique.

Femoral dysplasia on physical examination has the same characteristics as acetabular dysplasia; however, it is most easily differentiated radiographically, and with palpation under anesthesia. The ventrodorsal radiograph shows a shortened femoral neck and a lack of coverage and congruity in the hip joint. In the early stages of femoral dysplasia, the hip may have an angle of reduction of less than 10° and an angle of subluxation of less than 0° on palpation. The lateral radiograph shows femoral head anteversion. The DAR view may appear normal if damage to the rim has not yet occurred. As the hip degenerates because of lack of support from the acetabulum, the dorsal rim becomes blunted. As a result, we then observe radiographically the same characteristics as acetabular dysplasia. Correct diagnosis of early femoral dysplasia is critical to

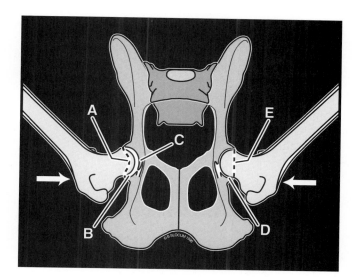

Fig. 61.24. A compression view is a ventrodorsal view with the hips in 0° of abduction, no flexion, and a medial force on both greater trochanters (*white arrows*). The normal hip has a narrow cartilage line (*D*), no osteophytes, and a linear dorsal acetabular rim (*E*) viewed through the femoral head, whereas the dysplastic hip may have a cupped dorsal acetabular rim (*A*), a wide cartilage space (*B*), which indicates acetabular filling by osteophytes or redundant ligamentum teres, and ventral acetabular filling osteophytes (*C*).

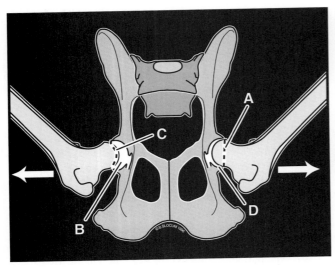

Fig. 61.25. A distraction view is a ventrodorsal view with the hips in 0° of abduction, no flexion, and a lateral force on both proximal femurs (*white arrows*). The normal hip has a narrow cartilage line (*D*), no osteophytes, and linear dorsal a acetabular rim (*A*) viewed through the femoral head, whereas the abnormal hip may have a cupped dorsal acetabular rim (*C*) and a wide cartilage space (*B*), which indicates a stretched joint capsule but not necessarily hip dysplasia.

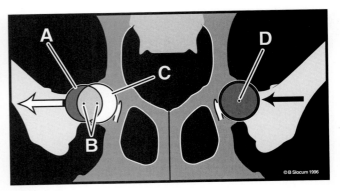

Fig. 61.26. Lateral distraction of the femur (*white arrow*) causes lateral translation of the femoral head. The circle that overlies the acetabular subchondral bone (*C*) is larger than the circle that overlies the femoral head subchondral bone (*A*). The centers of the two circles (*B*) are displaced by *d*. The distraction displacement index is equal to the displacement divided by the radius of A, r: (DDI = d ÷ r). Medial compression of the greater trochanter (*black arrow*) causes the circles overlying the acetabular and femoral head subchondral bone of the hip to be concentric and the centers superimposed (*D*), indicating that this hip is not abnormal. The compression displacement index is equal to the displacement (*d*) divided by the radius of A, r: (CDI = d ÷ r). In the normal hip, d = 0; therefore, CDI = d ÷ r = 0.

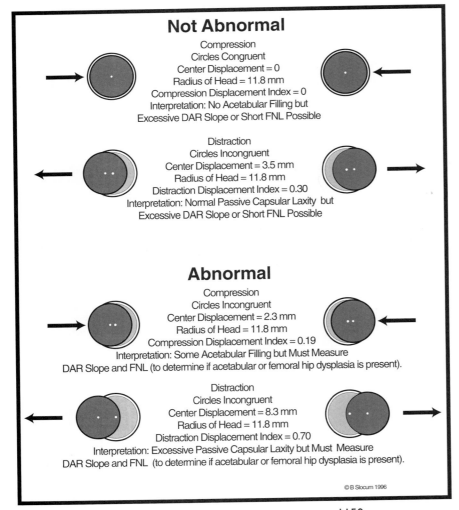

Not Abnormal

Compression
Circles Congruent
Center Displacement = 0
Radius of Head = 11.8 mm
Compression Displacement Index = 0
Interpretation: No Acetabular Filling but
Excessive DAR Slope or Short FNL Possible

Distraction
Circles Incongruent
Center Displacement = 3.5 mm
Radius of Head = 11.8 mm
Distraction Displacement Index = 0.30
Interpretation: Normal Passive Capsular Laxity but
Excessive DAR Slope or Short FNL Possible

Abnormal

Compression
Circles Incongruent
Center Displacement = 2.3 mm
Radius of Head = 11.8 mm
Compression Displacement Index = 0.19
Interpretation: Some Acetabular Filling but Must Measure
DAR Slope and FNL (to determine if acetabular or femoral hip dysplasia is present).

Distraction
Circles Incongruent
Center Displacement = 8.3 mm
Radius of Head = 11.8 mm
Distraction Displacement Index = 0.70
Interpretation: Excessive Passive Capsular Laxity but Must Measure
DAR Slope and FNL (to determine if acetabular or femoral hip dysplasia is present).

Fig. 61.27. Schematic illustration of interpretation of the compression and distraction radiography. *DAR*, dorsal acetabular rim; *FNL*, femoral neck lengthening.

the success of surgical treatment. If medially directed muscle force is insufficient to hold the hip in the acetabulum, an excessive amount of pelvic rotation will correct the situation but will lead to femoral neck impingement and reduced abduction. Femoral neck lengthening is the surgical treatment of choice. As the disease process continues, both femoral neck lengthening and pelvic osteotomy are necessary to obtain return of normal function. When both operations are necessary, a much lower rotation of the pelvis is adequate for correct coverage of the femoral head with acetabular stability.

Radiographic views taken using compression (Fig. 61.24) and distraction (Fig. 61.25) provide information on hip laxity. Bardens (1) first proposed a wedge technique to demonstrate radiographic joint laxity in the early 1960s, along with palpation. Radiographic techniques were further defined by Belkoff and associates in 1989 (2), using a distraction device. Although this device allows passive laxity to be seen radiographically, this has been used by Stoll (3) as a measure of the amount of femoral neck lengthening necessary when the dorsal acetabular slope has been reduced to 0°. Because passive capsular laxity is present in both dysplastic and nondysplastic hips, it should be considered a secondary indicator of hip dysplasia (Figs. 61.26 and 61.27). The distraction displacement index is an indicator of passive joint laxity. Smith and colleagues (4) determined that a distraction index of 0.30 is the dividing line between normal hips and hips predisposed to hip dysplasia. Some dysplastic hips, however, have a distraction index less than 0.30, and some hips with a distraction index greater than 0.30 fail to show other dysplastic characteristics. The compression displacement index is an indicator of acetabular filling. In the clinical situation, laxity of the joint capsule is palpated and measured as the angle of reduction. The angle of subluxation is a measure of the functional slope of the dorsal acetabulum because it is the result of interaction between the acetabulum and the femoral head.

In summary, correct evaluation of the hip joint is essential to understand the progression of hip dysplasia and to recognize the choice points of intervention. Physical and radiographic examination of dogs 6 months of age and older can provide accurate assessment of the hips. The patient can be treated appropriately to provide for the enjoyment and functioning of the dog for the rest of its lifetime.

References

1. Bardens J. Joint laxity as hip dysplasia. In: Canine Hip Dysplasia Symposium. St. Louis: , 1972:71.
2. Belkoff SM, Padgett G, Soutas-Little RW. Development of a device to measure canine coxofemoral joint laxity. Vet Compar Orthop Traumatol 1989;1:31–36.
3. Stoll S. Femoral neck lengthening using distraction measurements. In: American College of Veterinary Surgeons Surgical Forum.: American College of Veterinary Surgeons, 1996.
4. Smith G, Biery D, Gregor T. New concepts of coxofemoral joint stability and the development of a clinical stress-radiographic method for quantitating hip joint laxity in the dog. J Am Vet Med Assoc 1990;196:59–70.

Suggested Readings

Corley EA. Hip dysplasia: a report from the Orthopedic Foundation for Animals. Semin Vet Med Surg 1987;2:141.
Henry J, Park R. Wedge technique for demonstration of coxofemoral joint laxity in the canine. In: Canine Hip Dysplasia Symposium. St. Louis: Arthur Freeman, 1972:117.
Lanting F. Canine hip dysplasia and other orthopedic problems. Loveland, CO: Alpine Publications, 1981.
Morgan JP, Stephens M. Radiographic diagnosis and control of canine hip dysplasia. Davis, CA: Venture Press, 1985.
Pappas AM. Congenital hip dysplasia. In: Tronzo R, ed. Surgery of the hip joint. Philadelphia: Lea & Febiger, 1973.
Rendano V, Ryan G. Canine hip dysplasia evaluation: a positioning and labeling guide for radiographs to be submitted to the Orthopedic Foundation for Animals. Vet Radiol 1985;26:170.
Rettenmaier J, Constantinescu G. Canine hip dysplasia. Compend Contin Educ Pract Vet 1991;13:643.
Riser WH. The dog as model for the study of hip dysplasia. Vet Pathol 1975;12:229.
Riser WH, Shirer JF. Hip dysplasia: coxofemoral abnormalities in neonatal German shepherd dogs. J Small Anim Pract 1966;7:7.
Riser WH, Rhodes WH, Newton CD. Hip dysplasia. In: Newton CD, Nunamaker DM, eds. Textbook of small animal orthopedics. Philadelphia: JB Lippincott, 1985.
Sage FP. Campbell's operative orthopedics 4th ed. St. Louis: CV Mosby, 1963:1708–1709.
Slocum B, AVORE. Pelvic osteotomy: the results of 285 pelvic osteotomies (abstract). Vet Surg 1986;15:134.
Slocum B, Devine TM. Dorsal acetabular rim radiographic view for evaluation of the canine hip. J Am Anim Hosp Assoc 1990;26:289–296.
Slocum B, Devine T. Pelvic osteotomy in the dog as treatment for hip dysplasia. Semin Vet Med Surg 1987;2:107.
Slocum B, Devine T. Femoral neck lengthening for hip dysplasia in the dog. Vet Surg 1989;18:81.
Slocum B, Devine T. Pelvic osteotomy. In: Whittick W, ed. Canine orthopedics. 2nd ed. Philadelphia: Lea & Febiger, 1990:471.
Slocum B, Slocum TD. Slope of the dorsal acetabular rim for hip evaluation in the dog. In: 17th annual conference of the Veterinary Orthopedic Society. Salt Lake City, UT: Veterinary Orthopedic Society, 1990:12.
Slocum B, Slocum TD. Examination of the canine hip. Canine Pract 1991;15:5–10.
Slocum B, Slocum TD. Pelvic osteotomy for axial rotation of the acetabular segment in dogs with hip dysplasia. Vet Clin North Am Small Anim Pract 1992;22:645–682.
Snavely JG. The genetic aspects of hip dysplasia in dogs. J Am Vet Med Assoc 1959;135:201.
Wallace L. Canine hip dysplasia: past and present. Semin Vet Med Surg 1987;2:92.

Definitions of Hip Terms

Barclay Slocum & Theresa Devine Slocum

ACETABULAR HIP DYSPLASIA: Acetabular hip dysplasia is the malorientation of the acetabulum in the presence of normal depth. A slope of the dorsal acetabular rim (DAR) greater than 10.0° is considered to be acetabular hip dysplasia. The slope is usually reported as the sum of both the right and left DAR slopes, so a combined slope greater than 20.0° would be dysplastic. (A combined slope of 15.0 to 20.0° is suspect, whereas a combined slope of 15.0° or less is considered normal.) The minimum depth of the normal hip is 50% coverage of the femoral head by the DAR under ideal circumstances.

ANGLE OF REDUCTION: The angle of reduction is the angle between the sagittal plane and the longitudinal axis of the femur when a "clunk" or shift is palpated as the femoral head enters the acetabulum during abduction of the hip in the anesthetized patient.

ANGLE OF SUBLUXATION: The angle between the sagittal plane and the longitudinal axis of the femur when a "clunk" or shift is palpated as the femoral head leaves the acetabulum during adduction of the hip in the anesthetized patient.

BARDEN PALPATION: Barden palpation is a test for lateral translation of the hip. The lateral translation is a sign of joint capsule stretching: 1 to 2 mm is normal; 3 to 4 mm is suspicious; 4 mm or more is considered dysplastic.

BARLOW SIGN: The Barlow sign is the "clunk" or shift palpated as the femoral head leaves the acetabulum during adduction of the hip.

COXARTHROSIS: Coxarthrosis is a general term for hip degeneration from nondysplastic sources that include, but are not limited to, rapid growth syndrome, osteochondritis dissecans of the lateral femoral condyle and transitional vertebra at the seventh lumbar vertebra or first sacral vertebral segment, osteochondritis dissecans of the femoral head, neurologic or neuromuscular insufficiency, degenerative myelopathy, intervertebral disc disease, autoimmune arthritis of the hip, infection of the hip joint, and neoplasia of the hip. Secondary manifestations of coxarthrosis are joint capsule laxity, tearing of the joint capsule, increase of synovial fluid, acetabular osteophytes, femoral osteophytes, acetabular filling, destruction of the dorsal acetabular rim, teres ligament hypertrophy or degeneration, and articular cartilage fibrillation or eburnation.

DARTHROPLASTY: A DARrthroplasty is a dorsal acetabular rim arthroplasty. The dorsal rim of the acetabulum is augmented by bone graft that supports the joint capsule in cases that have a luxated hip. In essence, a new acetabulum is created to support the luxated hip.

DISLOCATION: The femoral head is unsupported by and resting outside the torn joint capsule, the ligament of the femoral head is torn, and the femoral head is outside the acetabulum.

DISTRACTION INDEX: The distraction index is a ratio of the linear distance between the center of the femoral head and the center of the acetabulum with the hip in distraction, to the radius of the femoral head.

In most breeds, normal hips have a distraction index up to and including 0.30.

DORSAL ACETABULAR RIM (DAR): The DAR rim is that portion of the lateral rim of the acetabulum of about 30° that is crossed by a line through the centers of motion of the hip and stifle in the normal standing patient as viewed in the sagittal plane (lateral radiograph). This portion of acetabular rim is subjected to trauma by the femoral head during the dysplastic process.

FEMORAL ANTEVERSION: Femoral anteversion is the cranial position of the femoral head when compared with normal. The femoral neck often has a valgus conformation. However, the relationships of other components of the femur are normal. Femoral anteversion alone is considered one form of hip dysplasia. Femoral anteversion in the presence of osteochondritis dissecans (OCD) of the lateral femoral condyle is considered a growth disturbance secondary to the OCD.

FEMORAL HIP DYSPLASIA: Femoral hip dysplasia is malorientation of the femoral head with respect to the greater trochanter when the limb is in the sagittal plane.

FEMORAL NECK LENGTH: Femoral neck length is the distance from the lateral aspect of the greater trochanter to the medial aspect of the femoral head. A short femoral neck is considered one form of hip dysplasia.

FEMORAL TORSION: Femoral torsion is malorientation of the proximal femur with respect to the distal femur. However, the relationships of the components of the ends of the femur are normal. Femoral torsion is considered one form of hip dysplasia.

HIP DYSPLASIA: Hip dysplasia is an inherited condition of the hip that leads to the degeneration of the joint. Several anatomic variations from normal provide the biomechanical prerequisites for predictable and progressive degeneration of the hip. Acetabular hip dysplasia is caused by malorientation or shallowness of the acetabulum. Femoral hip dysplasia is caused by a short femoral neck, anteversion of the femoral neck, or femoral torsion. Secondary manifestations of hip dysplasia are joint capsule laxity, tearing of the joint capsule, increase of synovial fluid, acetabular osteophytes, femoral osteophytes, acetabular filling, destruction of the dorsal acetabular rim, teres ligament hypertrophy or degeneration, and articular cartilage fibrillation or eburnation. These secondary changes are not hip dysplasia, but rather result from hip disorders. Nondysplastic conditions can cause the same secondary manifestations as hip dysplasia.

JUVENILE HIP MALFORMATION: Juvenile hip malformation is the hip deformity in which an extraordinarily shallow acetabulum is elongated and fails to match the femoral head. The pathogenesis of this condition is thought to be of neuromuscular origin because these patients usually have poor muscular tone, muscular weakness, and an uncoordinated movement. The condition is usually seen in young German shepherd dogs. Because of the pathogenesis, one could term the problem "neuromuscular hip dysplasia" or developmental coxarthrosis of neuromuscular origin.

LUXATION: The femoral head is supported by and resting in the intact joint capsule and is incongruent with and not supported directly by the acetabulum.

NORMAL HIP: A normal hip has no appreciable laxity of the hip joint capsule, with a distraction index less than or equal to 0.30, and no angle of reduction is palpated. The hip has normal acetabular orientation (combined dorsal acetabular rim slope of up to 15°), normal acetabular depth (at least 50%), normal sacral conformation, normal femoral neck length, normal white-black-white articular line on the lateral radiograph, and no palpable angle of subluxation. The determination of normal hips can be made at 6 months of age.

ORTOLANI SIGN: The Ortolani sign is the "clunk" or shift palpated as the femoral head enters the acetabulum during abduction of the hip.

PELVIC OSTEOTOMY: A pelvic osteotomy is a surgical procedure in which a triple osteotomy of the pelvis (pubis, ischium, and ilium) frees the acetabular segment for rotation about an axis parallel to a line tangent to the dorsal acetabular rim (DAR). The amount of axial rotation brings the slope of the DAR to 0°. Excessive rotation of the pelvic osteotomy causes interference between the DAR and the femoral neck. If the acetabulum is filled with osteophytes, then the articular cartilage of the femoral head will erode, and congruity of the femoral head and acetabulum is improbable.

PELVIC TORSION: Pelvic torsion is a spiral deformity of the entire pelvis around its median axis. It can be identified in the ventrodorsal, lateral, and dorsal acetabular rim radiographs. Pelvic torsion is associated with transitional vertebrae of the first sacral segment and is considered a secondary manifestation of the vertebral abnormality. One hip is usually considered normal, whereas the other is "dysplastic." Because the origin of the problem is the sacral deformity, one should term the problem "sacral hip dysplasia" or coxarthrosis of sacral origin.

RAPID GROWTH SYNDROME: Rapid growth syndrome is laxity of the hip joint capsule in the presence of normal acetabular orientation (combined dorsal acetabular rim slope up to and including 15°), normal acetabular depth (at least 50%), normal sacral conformation, normal femoral neck length, normal white-black-white articular line on the lateral radiograph, and normal angle of subluxation (up to and

including 0°). The distraction index is greater than normal (greater than 0.30), and the angle of reduction is present (none is normal). The pathogenesis of this condition is the maldirection of the axial femoral force during a rapid growth spurt at 4 to 6 months of age. This maldirection of the axial femoral force stretches the hip joint capsule, but it is otherwise harmless to the hip. Restricted nutrition reduces the excessively rapid rate of growth and should have a preventive influence on capsular laxity. If the patient applies excessive axial load to the hip in the luxated position, the joint capsule can tear, the dorsal acetabular rim (DAR) can fracture, or the DAR can deform over time. If caught at the joint capsule stretching stage, strict confinement and elimination of play for 4 to 6 weeks allow the stretched joint capsule to contract. Normal hips are obtained on OFA examination at 2 years of age. A femoral neck lengthening is curative if performed before increase of the DAR slope into the pathologic range. If the affected patient is allowed to damage the DAR, then traumatic coxarthrosis will result and secondary manifestations of trauma will later be misdiagnosed as hip dysplasia. Because the origin of the problem is the rapid growth of the distal femur (12 to 15 mm per week for 6 to 8 weeks), one should term the problem "rapid femoral growth hip dysplasia" or coxarthrosis of rapid growth of distal femur origin.

SLOPE OF THE DORSAL ACETABULAR RIM (DAR): The slope of the DAR is defined as the angle formed by a line normal to the sagittal plane (horizontal line) and a line created by the intersection of the acetabular subchondral bone at the DAR, and a plane defined by the intersection of the horizontal line and line through the centers of motion of the hip and stifle in the normal standing patient as viewed in the sagittal plane. The slope of acetabular subchondral bone at the DAR is linear, based on a study of 25 normal pelves. Clinically, the slope of the DAR is the angle between the tangent to the reduced femoral head at its first point of contact with the acetabulum and the horizontal line as seen on the DAR radiographic view.

SUBLUXATION: The femoral head is incongruent and supported directly by the acetabulum, and it is allowed some lateral translation, but it is prevented from dorsal translation by the intact joint capsule.

TOTAL HIP REPLACEMENT: A total hip replacement is a salvage procedure in which the worn acetabulum is replaced by a high-molecular-weight polyethylene acetabular cup, and the worn femoral head is replaced by a molybdenum–chromium–stainless steel alloy femoral prosthesis. The components are maintained in position by polymethylmethacrylate. The replaced components are devoid of nerve endings and therefore are pain free. This surgical procedure is best used when the femoral head rubs bone on bone with the acetabulum.

Femoral Neck Lengthening

Barclay Slocum & Theresa Devine Slocum

In the biomechanical sense, the femoral neck length is defined as the distance between the lateral limit of the greater trochanter and the medial limit of the femoral head. Both the internal and external rotator muscles attach to the greater trochanter and exert equal moments about the femoral head. The moment is defined as force times distance. By lengthening the femoral neck, the moments become greater, yet internal and external moments are still equal. This creates a greater medially directed resultant force more capable of holding the hip in the acetabulum.

The primary indication for a femoral neck lengthening is a short femoral neck. Short femoral necks are common in some breeds such as the akita, chow, and Tibetan mastiff. These hips are frequently diagnosed as dysplastic (Fig. 61.28). Short femoral necks can also occur secondary to trauma to the growing capital physis (Salter type IV), as well as secondary to the surgical manipulation and fixation of a fracture of the capital physis. In dogs less than 6 months of age, rigid internal fixation of a fractured capital physis is likely to result in degeneration of the hip from a shortened femoral neck. Similar patients have no arthritis if the femoral neck is lengthened. If a nondisplaced capital physeal fracture is left undiagnosed or unattended, the femoral neck often resorbs, and a short femoral neck results.

Surgical Technique

The lateral approach to the femur is used to gain access to the lateral, cranial, and medial aspects of the femur. The vastus lateralis is detached from its origin just distal to the greater trochanter and is elevated from the femur as far as the distal lateral circumflex femoral vessels. A small Hohmann retractor is placed beneath the deep gluteal muscle and over the web between the greater trochanter and the femoral head. Two Gelpi retractors are used to separate the biceps femoris and vastus lateralis muscles. External rotation of the hip exposes the proximal femur and the femoral diaphysis for osteotomy.

The greater trochanter is freed from the femoral head by an osteotomy cut in the sagittal plane for two-thirds the length of the femur (Fig. 61.29). The cranial cortex of the femur is penetrated by an oscillating saw beginning just proximal to the distal lateral circumflex femoral vessels. The cranial cortical cut is carried proximally in the sagittal plane to the Hohmann retractor between the greater trochanter and the femoral head. The cranial cortex is used as a saw guide to direct the osteotomy of the caudal cortex. Because the osteotomy is medial to the external rotator muscle group, little danger exists of traumatizing the sciatic nerve, which lies lateral to these muscles. Considerable hemorrhage is sometimes encountered at the level of the nutrient foramen, but this soon stops with minimal blood loss. If the patient's profile indicates the potential for hemophilia, coagulation potential and von Willebrand factor should be tested before the operation.

Lateralization of the greater trochanter is accomplished by placing a 40-mm cortical screw in only the lateral cortex of the femur at the level of the third trochanter, perpendicular to the sagittal plane. With the limb held in the sagittal plane, the proximal femur is manually moved laterally (Bardens test). The laxity

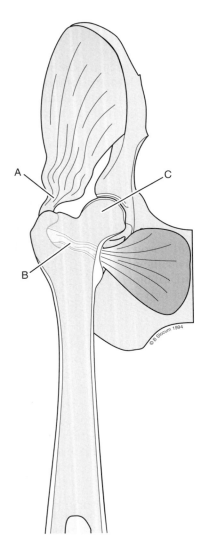

Fig. 61.28. In the dysplastic hip, the internal hip rotator group (A), external hip rotator group (B), and joint capsule are lax when the femoral head (C) is reduced.

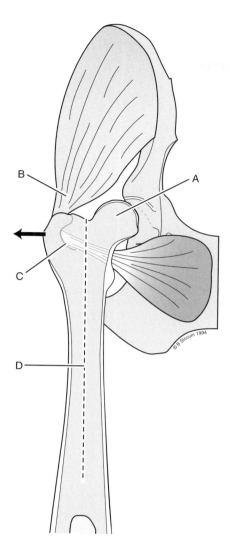

Fig. 61.29. When the greater trochanter is moved laterally (*arrow*), the femoral head (*A*) luxates. The internal (*B*) and external (*C*) hip rotators are no longer lax. A sagittal plane osteotomy (*D*) is made in the femur.

wire passer is used to pass a heavy (1.25-mm or 18-gauge) wire around proximal femur. The wire should be proximal to the lesser trochanter. The point of the pin keeps it from migrating distally. After directly observing the sciatic nerve to ensure that it not entrapped, the wire is securely tightened. The screw is removed.

Another wedge is placed halfway down the osteotomy and is secured in a like manner. Care is taken to avoid driving the wedge distally because this splits the femur. The cerclage wire is proximal to the pin on the lateral cortex and is distal to the pin on the medial cortex, to prevent the pin from migrating. A third pin and cerclage wire are placed at the distal end of the osteotomy (Fig. 61.30). No bone graft is necessary because healing takes approximately 5 weeks.

Closure is direct. The vastus lateralis can be re-

of the Bardens test is decreased by advancement of the screw through the lateral cortex, but not into the medial cortex. Interference of the cancellous surface of the medial segment separates the medial from the lateral cortex, which tightens the rotators as the femoral neck is lengthened. When laxity by Bardens palpation becomes zero, the advancement of the screw is sufficient.

The appropriate Femoral Neck Lengthening Wedge (US Patent No. 4,759,351, Slocum Enterprises, Eugene, OR) is inserted just proximal to the screw to maintain the femoral neck length. A towel clamp or small fragment reduction forceps is used to grasp and manipulate the wedge. The wedge is held in place by predrilling a 2.7-mm ($\frac{7}{64}$-inch) hole through the lateral cortex, wedge, and medial cortex and then placing a 3.2-mm ($\frac{1}{8}$-inch) threaded pin into the hole such that the point completely penetrates the medial cortex. A

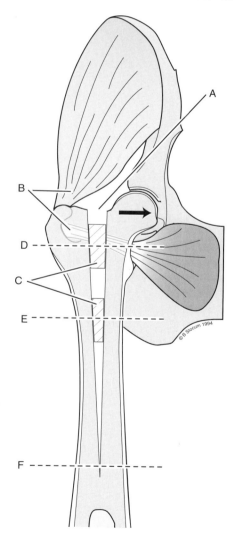

Fig. 61.30. The proximal portion of the femoral osteotomy is spread apart (*A*), which moves the femoral head into the reduced position (*arrow*). This tightens the hip rotators (*B*). Femoral Neck Lengthening Wedges are placed into the osteotomy (*C*) to maintain the femoral neck length. Internal fixation is first placed at the level of the third trochanter (*D*), followed by additional fixation (*E* and *F*).

attached with horizontal mattress sutures. Holes can be drilled in the greater trochanter if greater purchase is necessary. The vastus lateralis is usually attached to the tendon of the deep gluteal muscle cranially.

Procedure for Capital Physeal Fracture

Femoral neck lengthening is indicated for a capital physeal fracture when growth potential has been lost, when chronic capital physeal nonunion has occurred because of the trauma of delayed treatment, or when the young patient has only one opportunity for surgical correction permitted by the owner. In the last circumstance, failure of the capital physis to grow after smooth pin fixation leads to a short femoral neck and degeneration of the hip without opportunity to compensate for this lack of growth surgically. The femoral

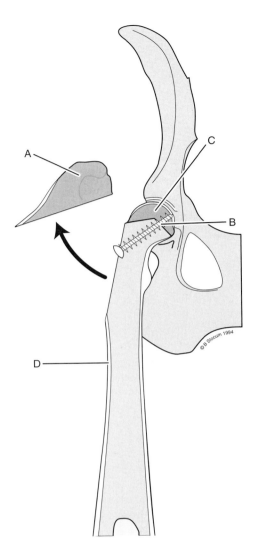

Fig. 61.32. After osteotomy, the greater trochanter (*A*), with the internal and external rotators attached, is retracted dorsally (*arrow*). A small opening in the cranial joint capsule gives access for assessment of the reduction and placement of the screw. Respecting the blood supply to the epiphysis, which enters dorsally, a lag screw (*B*) is used to fix the epiphysis (*C*) to the femur (*D*).

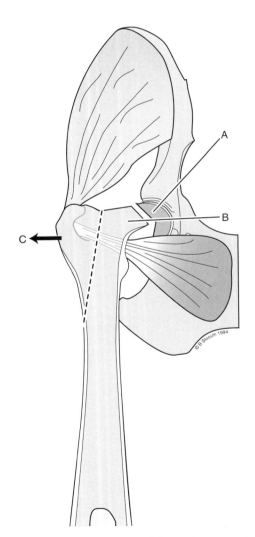

Fig. 61.31. Fracture of the capital femoral physis and displacement of the epiphysis (*A*) and the femoral neck (*B*) are often accompanied by lateral movement of the proximal femur (*arrow*) and visual prominence of the greater trochanter (*C*). A long trochanteric osteotomy (*dashed line*) provides good access for surgical repair.

neck length deficiency may be anticipated, and compensation by fusing the capital physis and adding the anticipated femoral neck deficit may be undertaken at the initial surgical procedure.

A lateral approach to the proximal half of the femur is achieved by unwrapping the origin of the vastus lateralis muscle from the femur as previously described, while leaving the femoral insertion of the deep gluteal intact. A 7.5-cm (3-inch) osteotomy of the greater trochanter in the craniocaudal direction from the web between the greater trochanter and the femoral head to the lateral cortex is made (Fig. 61.31). The internal hip rotators (superficial, middle, and deep gluteal muscles) and the external hip rotators (gemelli, internal and external obturator, and quadratus femoris muscles) remain attached to the greater trochanter.

osteotomy kerf; overtightening the screw causes the end of the screw to protrude from the surface of the femoral head (see Fig. 61.32). The cranial joint capsule is closed by cranial capsulorrhaphy.

Femoral neck lengthening is performed to establish the adult femoral neck length (Fig. 61.33). This length is determined by measuring the neck length in the parent of the same sex (if the patient resembles that parent) or by measuring neck length in another dog of the same breed and body type. A Femoral Neck Lengthening Wedge of the appropriate thickness is placed at the level of the third trochanter. A lag screw is placed in the distal end of the trochanteric segment. The glide hole should be large enough to accommodate lateralization of the greater trochanter. The lag screw is tightened while taking care not to split the cortex of the trochanteric fragment. The Femoral Neck Lengthening Wedge can be fixed by a screw through the lateral cortex, wedge and medial cortex, but a pin and cerclage wire, as previously described, are more secure. Closure is similar to that described for classic femoral neck lengthening.

Modified Technique

A lateral approach to the proximal half of the femur is achieved by unwrapping the origin of the vastus lateralis muscle from the femur as previously described while leaving the femoral insertion of the deep gluteal intact. An osteotomy of the femur is made in the sagittal plane from the depression in the web between the greater trochanter and the femoral head to a point 6.5-cm (2.5-inch) distal. A small biradial or cylindric saw blade is used to complete the osteotomy between the kerf generated and the lateral cortex. The internal hip rotators (superficial, middle, and deep gluteal muscles) and the external hip rotators (gemelli, internal, and external obturator, and quadratus femoris muscles) remain attached to the greater trochanteric segment (Fig. 61.34).

A 3.5-mm hole is drilled through the distal end of the trochanteric segment and also through the medial cortex. The depth of the hole is measured with a depth gauge, and a screw 2 to 4 mm longer is selected. The lateral cortex is overdrilled using a 4.5-mm drill bit and is countersunk. The medial cortex is tapped with a 3.5-mm tap. A 3.5-mm cortical lag screw is placed through the lateral cortex and loosely engaged in the medial cortex. A second hole is drilled through the lateral cortex at the level of the third trochanter, is countersunk, and is tapped. The depth of the hole is measured to the medial cortex. The screw selected is equal to the depth of the hole plus the displacement of the femoral head obtained by comparing the compression and distraction radiographic views. When the screw is placed in the second hole, the greater trochanter is lateralized the appropriate amount. Third and

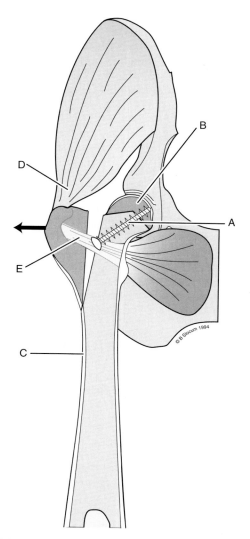

Fig. 61.33. The screw (A) that holds the capital femoral epiphysis (B) to the femur (C) is hidden by the replacement of the greater trochanter. Femoral neck lengthening moves the trochanter laterally (*arrow*) to establish the adult femoral neck length in anticipation of the capital femoral physeal fusion because of the trauma and screw fixation. The internal (D) and external (E) rotators of the hip are placed under tension. Trochanteric fixation is not shown.

The distal end of the trochanteric section is reflected dorsally to expose the hip joint capsule (Fig. 61.32).

Subperiosteal elevation of the vastus lateralis from the cranial femoral neck to the joint capsule exposes the femoral side of the capital physis or the capital epiphysis if it is displaced cranially. The joint capsule is minimally opened cranially, to observe the articular surface of the femoral head. The capital epiphysis is anatomically reduced, if possible. If anatomic reduction is not possible because of trauma, then the capital epiphysis is positioned over the femoral neck to be functional for weightbearing. A lag screw is placed up the femoral neck or remnant of the femoral neck from the surface of the osteotomy to secure the relationship between the head and the neck. The screw head is countersunk only enough to avoid protrusion into the

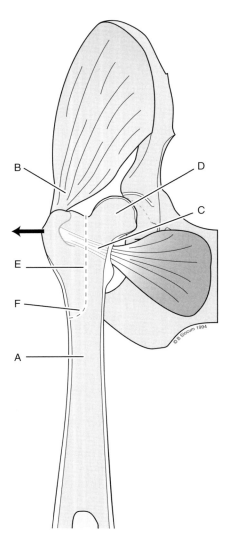

Fig. 61.34. The femur (*A*) is moved laterally (*arrow*) to tension the internal hip rotator group (*B*) and external hip rotator group (*C*). The femoral head (*D*) is in the luxated position. A linear portion (*E*) and a cylindric portion (*F*) of the modified femoral neck lengthening osteotomy are shown by the *dashed line*.

fourth screws are placed proximal and distal to the second screw, engaging both the lateral and medial cortices (Fig. 61.35). The first screw is then firmly tightened. Closure is routine.

A more stable configuration is the application of an appropriately sized wedge placed at the second screw hole. The wedge size is determined from the displacement of the femoral head obtained by comparing the compression and distraction radiographic views. This configuration prevents the femoral neck lengthening from relying on the threads of the screws alone.

Although the primary indication for femoral neck lengthening is hip dysplasia, this technique can also be used with a pelvic osteotomy in patients with an excessively stretched joint capsule. The excessive slope of the dorsal acetabular rim is corrected before the femoral neck lengthening. A dorsal acetabular rim

slope greater than 7.5° is addressed by a pelvic osteotomy because that surgical procedure deals with the axial compressive forces of the femur; the femoral neck lengthening technique increases the medial directed forces created by the rotators. Bone graft has not been necessary for augmenting bone healing, because bone marrow elements promote extraordinarily rapid bone healing, usually within 5 to 6 weeks.

The postoperative instructions are strict for femoral neck lengthening surgery. The patient must be kept under direct control of the owner while in the house, on good footing, with no playing, and with no other dogs or other excitable activities. The patient is allowed outside only to perform bodily functions on a leash

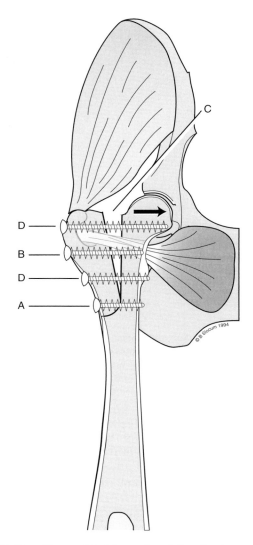

Fig. 61.35. The modified femoral neck lengthening osteotomy is fixed by four screws. The distal screw (*A*) is a lag screw, which is initially loosely applied. Only the lateral cortex is drilled and tapped for femoral neck lengthening screw (*B*), which is equal in length to the depth plus displacement measured from the compression and distraction radiographs. The first screw (*A*) is firmly tightened to complete the creation of the femoral neck lengthening gap (*C*). Both the lateral and medial cortices are drilled and tapped for neutral screws (*D*) used to maintain fixation.

with a bellyband. The patient is kept in a traveling kennel when the owner is not present, to prevent the patient from injuring itself. Tranquilizers may be necessary to maintain this confinement until the femoral neck lengthening is healed.

Femoral neck anteversion can also be corrected using the femoral neck lengthening procedure. In addition to lateralizing the greater trochanter, the lateral cortex is moved cranially to detorse the femur and to provide the appropriate relationship between the greater trochanter and the femoral head. The Femoral Neck Lengthening Wedge and internal fixation are applied with routine closure.

The femoral neck lengthening technique is powerful when used according to the proper indications. Overlengthening the femoral neck can cause the femoral head to move ventral to the acetabulum, particularly if performed concurrently with a pelvic osteotomy technique. The advantage of the femoral neck lengthening technique is that it provides an increase in the medially resultant force holding the hip in the acetabulum. This reestablishes stable hip biomechanics without the necessity for overrotating the acetabular segment in patients with excessive joint capsule laxity. In addition, this procedure is gentle on the patient, the owner, and the surgeon.

Acknowledgments

Kenneth Sinibaldi, DVM, Steven Stoll, DVM, and Gary Brown, DVM, have made contributions to the modification of the femoral neck lengthening technique.

Suggested Readings

Slocum B, Devine T. Pelvic osteotomy in the dog as treatment for hip dysplasia. Semin Vet Med Surg 1987;2:107.
Slocum B, Devine T. Femoral neck lengthening for hip dysplasia in the dog. Vet Surg 1989;18:81.
Slocum B, Devine T. Pelvic osteotomy. In: Whittick W, ed. Canine orthopedics. 2nd ed. Philadelphia: Lea & Febiger, 1990:471.
Slocum B, Slocum TD. Pelvic osteotomy for axial rotation of the acetabular segment. Vet Clin North Am 1992;22:645.
Slocum B, Slocum TD. Femoral neck lengthening: the cutting edge. 1988.
Stoll S. Femoral neck lengthening. San Francisco, CA: American College of Veterinary Surgeons, 1996.

Pelvic Osteotomy

Barclay Slocum & Theresa Devine Slocum

The first principle in treating acetabular hip dysplasia is to neutralize any luxating force created by a slope of the dorsal acetabular rim (DAR) or adduction of the femur. This requires an axial rotation of the acetabular segment by pelvic osteotomy. The second principle is the establishment of a greater trochanteric muscle force moment for creating dynamic stability of the femoral head by femoral neck lengthening, when the femoral neck is short or the joint capsule is excessively lax. The third principle is to reduce the redundancy of the joint capsule by capsulorrhaphy, which adds static stability to the hip when the femoral neck is normal and excessive laxity of the joint capsule is greater than 6 mm. This discussion addresses the first principle, the surgical technique of pelvic osteotomy.

Pelvic osteotomy is a triple osteotomy of the pelvis that frees the acetabular segment for axial rotation to reduce the DAR angle to 0° (Fig. 61.36). The primary indication for pelvic osteotomy is excessive slope to the DAR. By far the most common circumstance for this condition is acetabular hip dysplasia, which is an excessive slope of the DAR by definition. Occasionally, pelvic torsion, secondary to a transitional vertebra of the sacrum, causes a unilateral excessive slope of the DAR that is also treated by pelvic osteotomy. Dislocation of a dysplastic hip is an immediate indication for pelvic osteotomy, as long as the articular surfaces can be replaced with congruity. Reduction of a dislocated dysplastic hip fails unless pelvic osteotomy is performed. Reduction of a dislocated hip without treating the underlying hip dysplasia is unacceptable. A short femoral neck as in an akita, chow, or Tibetan mastiff, or secondary to premature closure of the capital femoral physis, requires femoral neck lengthening if found primarily, but damage to the DAR by the head of the femur with the shortened neck reduces the coverage of the DAR and requires a pelvic osteotomy to stabilize the hip.

The degree of correction for rotation of the pelvic osteotomy is determined by looking at the abnormalities in specific structures. Joint capsule laxity can be

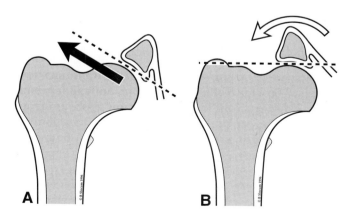

Fig. 61.36. **A.** The excessive slope (*dotted line*) of the Dorsal Acetabular Rim (DAR) causes the femur under axial load to luxate (*solid arrow*). **B.** After pelvic osteotomy (*white arrow*), the DAR slope is 0°, and the hip is functionally stable.

calibrated by the angle of reduction, stress radiography, and the Bardens palpation. Damage to the articular cartilage can be assessed by palpation, with the patient under anesthesia, to distinguish joint capsule distraction from tearing. The characteristics of the articular cartilage can also be distinguished by hip palpation as normal, fibrillated, or eburnated. The DAR radiographic view and linear tomography create a visual representation of articular cartilage thickness and damage to the weightbearing portion of the acetabulum. Acetabular depth can be evaluated radiographically using the frog view at 45° of abduction, the compression view in the ventrodorsal position, and the DAR view. Acetabular depth can also be assessed by the angle of subluxation and the combined interpretation of actual DAR slope and ligament of femoral head redundancy.

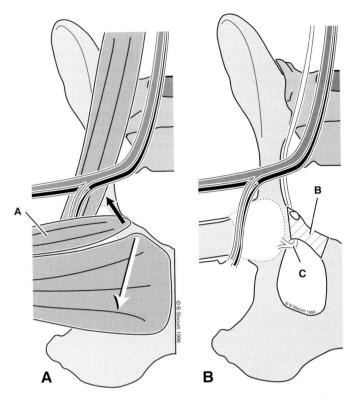

Fig. 61.38. A. The pubic osteotomy is performed through a 3-cm incision centered on the inguinal crease and just caudal to the pectineus muscle (*A*). The gracilis and adductor magnus are elevated and retracted caudally (*white arrow*). The pectineus is elevated from the pubis and retracted cranially (*black arrow*). **B.** With the elevation of the musculature, the pubis is exposed completely (*B*). The obturator nerve (*C*) is retracted from the pubis. The pubic ramus (*striped area*) is cut medially and laterally and removed. It is reduced to 3-mm fragments and used as bone graft for the ilial osteotomy.

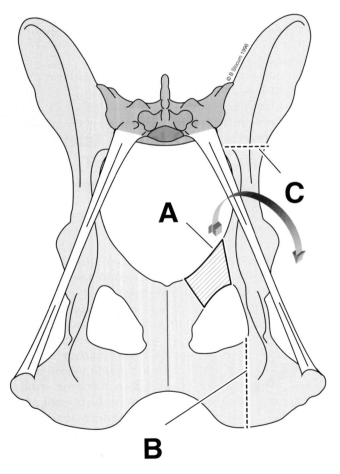

Fig. 61.37. Three osteotomies of the pelvis are necessary to free the pelvis for axial rotation of the acetabular segment (*arrow*). The pubic osteotomy (*A*) is performed first and includes removal of the pubic ramus (*shaded area*). The ischial osteotomy (*B*) is performed in the sagittal plane through the table of the ischium at the lateral margin of the obturator foramen. The ilial osteotomy (*C*) is performed perpendicular to a line in the sagittal plane that is tangent to the portion of the acetabulum to be rotated.

The slope of the DAR is measured directly from the DAR radiograph. The subchondral surface of the dorsal acetabulum is linear unless distorted by acetabular filling or chronic luxation of the femoral head. The angle of subluxation provides a good assessment of the functional slope of the DAR.

Surgical Procedures

The acetabular segment of the pelvis is freed for axial rotation by osteotomies of the pubis, ischium, and ilium and is fixed with just enough rotation by a Canine Pelvic Osteotomy Plate (Slocum Enterprises, Eugene, OR) to stabilize the femoral head in the acetabulum (Fig. 61.37). The patient is anesthetized, the limb is prepared for surgery with the dog in lateral recumbency, and the limb is hung by a foot wrap. The entire hindquarter is draped free to allow for access to the pubis, tuber ischiadicum, and ilium.

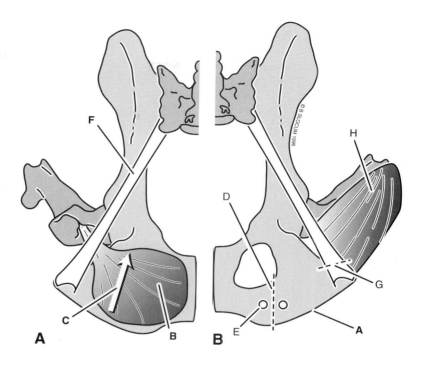

Fig. 61.39. A. The ischial osteotomy is made through a 3-cm incision in the sagittal plane over the midtuber ischiadicum. The internal obturator muscle (B) is elevated from the ischial table, parallel and medial to the body of the ischium (C). The sacrotuberous ligament (F) extends between the sacrum and the lateral prominence of the tuber ischiadicum. **B.** With the table of the ischium freed from muscle (A), a reciprocating saw is used to make a sagittal plane osteotomy in the tuber ischiadicum, as far laterally in the obturator foramen as possible (D). A wire hole is placed on either side of the osteotomy (E). The sacrotuberous ligament is incised just proximal to the lateral prominence (G). The ligament is held loosely in relative position by the biceps femoris muscle (H).

Pubic Osteotomy

The skin is incised over the proximal one-fourth of the pectineus muscle and inguinal crease. The gracilis and adductor muscles are elevated from the ventral pubis. The prepubic tendon and pectineus are elevated from the cranial pubis (Fig. 61.38). The obturator nerve is retracted caudomedially. An osteotomy is made in the sagittal plane at both the medial and lateral limits of the pubis. The entire pubis along the cranial margin of the obturator foramen is removed and is saved for an ilial osteotomy bone graft. The gracilis muscle is closed to the prepubic tendon to prevent an inguinal hernia. Subdermal sutures are used to preclude difficult suture removal.

Ischial Osteotomy

A sagittal incision is made over the midtuber ischiadicum and is carried to bone of the dorsal ischial plateau. The internal obturator muscle is elevated from the dorsal table of the tuber ischiadicum. The sacrotuberous ligament is elevated from the lateral prominence of the tuber ischiadicum medially to laterally. An osteotomy of the tuber ischiadicum at the lateral limit of the obturator foramen (Fig. 61.39) is performed in the sagittal plane. A 20-gauge fixation wire is preplaced through two holes on either side of the osteotomy site. Closure is delayed until after the ilial osteotomy and plate application is completed. Once the ilial osteot-

omy is plated, then the ischial wire is tightened. The perineal fascia is closed using a cruciate suture pattern. The skin of the ischial incision is closed with a simple interrupted pattern.

Ilial Osteotomy

A skin incision is made from the midcranial wing of the ilium to the base of the cranial aspect of the greater trochanter (Fig. 61.40). The gluteal fascia is incised parallel to the skin incision. The separation between the middle gluteal muscle and the tensor fasciae latae is made. En masse, the deep and middle gluteal muscles are elevated from the body and wing of the ilium cranially, but they are left intact dorsally on the tuber sacrale (Fig. 61.41). The cranial circumflex iliac artery is cauterized, but the cranial gluteal nerve to the tensor fasciae latae is preserved. A Langenbeck periosteal elevator is placed dorsal to the body of the ilium in the greater ischiatic notch and is moved cranially until contact is made between both the ilium and the sacrum. A relaxing incision in the tensor fasciae latae tendon provides the extra exposure to the greater ischiatic notch. A guide pin is placed dorsal to the lateral prominence of the tuber ischiadicum, beneath the internal obturator muscle. The pin is pushed cranially to the junction between the ventral and middle third of the cranial margin of the wing of the ilium (Fig. 61.42). The ilial osteotomy is made perpendicular to the axis

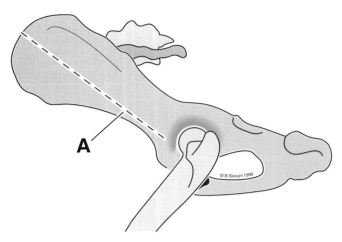

Fig. 61.40. For the ilial osteotomy, a linear skin incision (A) is made from the cranial border of the wing of the ilium, halfway between the tuber sacrale and the tuber coxae, to the cervical tubercle of the femur.

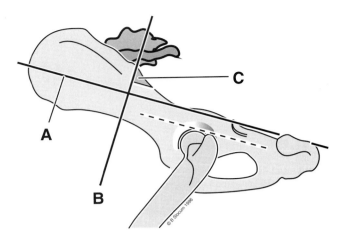

Fig. 61.42. The tangent to the acetabulum (*broken line*) contacts the acetabulum at the singular point at which the femoral head leaves during subluxation. The guide pin (A) is placed parallel to the tangent to the acetabulum. The ilial osteotomy (B) is made perpendicular to the guide pin at the junction of the sacrum and the pelvis. The pointed piece of bone (C) is removed.

of the guide pin, just cranial to the Langenbeck elevator. The free acetabular segment is moved cranially into the operative field.

The caudal half of the Canine Pelvic Osteotomy Plate is applied to the body of the ilium (Fig. 61.43) 3 mm dorsal to the ventral margin of the ilium using a spheric drill guide and 4.0-mm fixation screws. A 1.25-mm hemicerclage wire is placed through the wire hole in the caudal half of the plate, encircling the ilial body ventrally. The spike of ilial bone dorsal to the plate is removed.

The ilial osteotomy is reduced, and a 4.0-mm screw is placed in the ventral compression hole of the cranial portion of the Canine Pelvic Osteotomy Plate using a 1.0-mm compressive drill guide. The hip is tested for stability by axial compression of the femur in the sagittal plane (Fig. 61.44). If the hip is unstable (the femoral head luxates), then the next larger angle of plate needs to be used. The screw holes of all Canine Pelvic Osteotomy Plates are in the same relative position. When applying the remaining two screws, care should be taken to place the screws perpendicular to the plate.

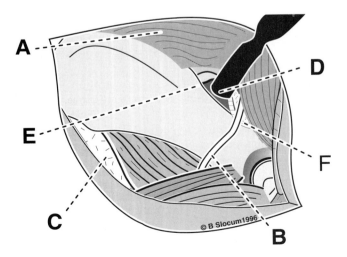

Fig. 61.41. The ilial approach is made by rolling up the middle and deep gluteal muscles (A). The cranial gluteal nerve to the tensor fasciae latae muscle (B) can be preserved by a relaxing incision in the tensor fascia origin (C). A Langenbeck retractor (D) is placed dorsal to the body of the ilium and is moved cranially to contact the sacrum (E). This protects the cranial gluteal neurovascular bundle to the gluteals (F), and the cranial margin of the retractor is a guide for the osteotomy.

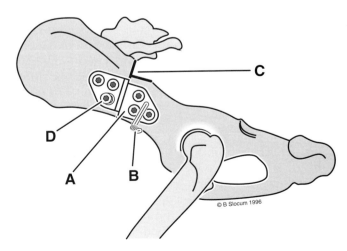

Fig. 61.43. The Canine Pelvic Osteotomy Plate (A) is applied to the acetabular segment, and a hemicerclage wire (B) is added. The point (C) is removed. The compression screw (D) is applied, and the hip is checked for stability by the femoral axial compression test. If the hip is unstable, a capsulorrhaphy, femoral neck lengthening or the next larger angle of osteotomy plate should be considered.

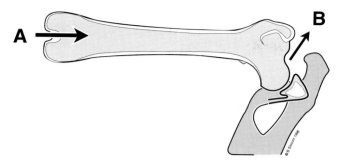

Fig. 61.44. The axial compression test of the femur is performed by applying a force (*A*) to the distal femur in the sagittal plane and witnessing the response of the femoral head (*B*). A positive test is when the femoral head leaves the acetabulum and represents hip instability. A negative test is when the hip remains within the acetabulum.

tween the sacrum and the acetabular segment. Closure of ilial approach is routine.

The objective of the pelvic osteotomy technique is to provide acetabular support and stability for the femoral head by increasing the acetabular coverage. Reducing the acetabular slope to 0° is optimal. The preoperative examination of the patient determines the angle for the Canine Pelvic Osteotomy Plate to be used. Although the angle of subluxation is theoretically the ideal angle for pelvic osteotomy, it is usually insufficient to provide hip stability unless the DAR is undamaged. The angle of reduction, which indicates joint capsule stretching, is the absolute maximum angle for pelvic osteotomy and is excessive, especially if a great difference exists between the angles of reduction and subluxation. The slope of the rim as determined from the DAR radiograph is an accurate reference for the amount of axial rotation for the acetabular segment.

If joint capsule laxity is excessive, femoral neck lengthening or capsulorrhaphy should be used to achieve hip stability while maintaining an optimum range of motion rather than overrotation of the acetabular segment. Overrotation causes impingement of

On small patients, these screws may have to be directed caudally to drill into the body of the sacrum. A bone graft of the pubis, fragmented to 3 mm or less, is placed caudal to the wing portion of the ilium be-

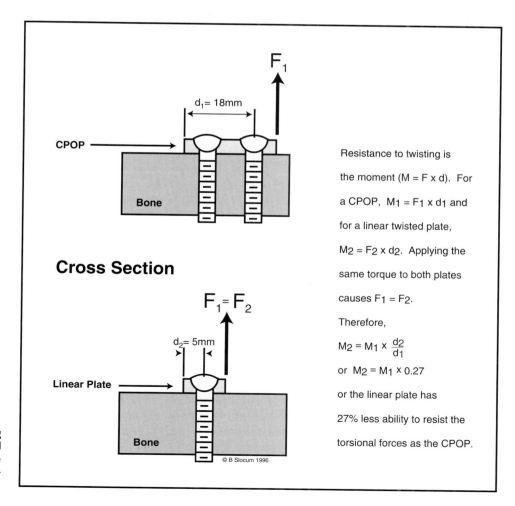

Cross Section

Resistance to twisting is the moment ($M = F \times d$). For a CPOP, $M_1 = F_1 \times d_1$ and for a linear twisted plate, $M_2 = F_2 \times d_2$. Applying the same torque to both plates causes $F_1 = F_2$.

Therefore,

$$M_2 = M_1 \times \frac{d_2}{d_1}$$

or $M_2 = M_1 \times 0.27$

or the linear plate has 27% less ability to resist the torsional forces as the CPOP.

Fig. 61.45. Diagram comparing the resistance of a torsional load of a Canine Pelvic Osteotomy Plate (CPOP) with that of a standard 10-mm wide linear plate.

the femoral neck, the advancement of degenerative joint disease, and pain.

Several aspects of the pelvic osteotomy need to be observed to ensure consistently good results from the procedure. Most important, only enough axial rotation of the acetabular segment to provide hip stability should be performed. The slope of the DAR should be brought to 0° and not beyond, for the benefit of the function of the patient. When the ilial osteotomy is placed as described, the ilial osteotomy overlies the sacrum about 3 mm cranial to its caudal margin. This prevents the saw from penetrating the ilium, to damage the pelvic plexus and cause dysuria, as may occur when the osteotomy is made caudal to the sacrum. Using the guide pin properly orients the osteotomy and prevents excessive angulation of the caudal portion of the acetabular segment, as occurs when the osteotomy is made perpendicular to the long axis of the ilium, rather than the long axis of the pelvis. Rotation of the acetabular segment and internal fixation are much more difficult when the cut is incorrect. A Hohmann retractor should not be used dorsal to the body of the ilium. The sciatic nerve, which lies medial to the body of the ilium, is easily crushed between the tip of the retractor and the bone during retraction. The well-intentioned assistant often replaces a displaced Hohmann retractor into a position of danger.

If the S1 nerve root is encountered when drilling the dorsal holes in the cranial portion of the plate, then the screw applied to that hole should be short enough to avoid contact with the nerve or the hole should be redirected to avoid the nerve root.

The Canine Pelvic Osteotomy Plate has two characteristics which makes it superior to twisted linear plates. The width of this plate and the placement of screws more efficiently resist the torsional moments of the acetabular segment than the linear plates, which tend to pry the screws from the bone (Fig. 61.45).

The sacrotuberous ligament release prevents elevation of the caudal acetabular segment during axial rotation that would otherwise malalign the ilial osteotomy and place static tension on the sacrotuberous ligament, leading to a gradual release of tension in the elongating ligament and subsequent loss of compression at the ilial osteotomy as the sacrotuberous ligament lengthens (Fig. 61.46). The loss of compression by yielding of the sacrotuberous ligament causes cyclic forces on the screws with premature loss of fixation. This same effect is noted when the angle of the osteotomy is not perpendicular to the axis of the pelvis. The greater the angle of the osteotomy from the perpendicular to the guide pin, the greater is the ventralization of the tuber ischiadicum (Fig. 61.47). With the release of the sacrotuberous ligament at surgery, the fixation relies on compression of the bone that statically loads the screws only in one direction and prevents cycling.

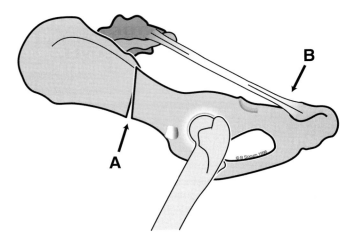

Fig. 61.46. The sacrotuberous ligament maintains a fixed length between the sacrum and the lateral prominence of the tuber ischiadicum. Unrestricted rotation of the acetabular segment around the guide pin axis lengthens the distance between the sacrum and the tuber ischiadicum. As a result, a gap will occur (A) unless the ligament is released (B).

The results of pelvic osteotomy are predictably good if meticulous attention is paid to case selection, surgical technique, and aftercare. The technique provides for the return of normal function and activity for dogs with hip dysplasia and prevents the progression of degenerative osteoarthritis. The ideal candidate for this procedure has minimal filling of the acetabulum, an intact DAR, and an increased slope of the DAR of 10 to 20° on the dysplastic hip. The amount of joint capsule laxity (angle of reduction or distraction index) is smaller after healing of the pelvic osteotomy because the joint capsule tightens when the capsule-stretching

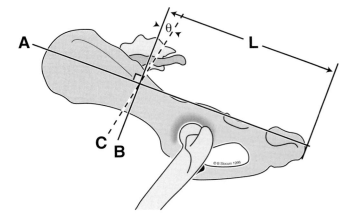

Fig. 61.47. The direction of the ilial osteotomy (B) is ideally made perpendicular to the guide pin (A). If the osteotomy were made parallel to the guide pin, then the tuber ischiadicum would be lateralized by the distance from the osteotomy to the tuber ischiadicum, L, times the sine of the angle, θ, of the plate used. If the osteotomy (C) is made at angle θ to the perpendicular to the guide pin, then lateralization of the tuber ischiadicum, T, can be expressed as: $T = L \times \sin \varnothing \times \sin \theta$.

forces created by the increased slope of the DAR are treated by the pelvic osteotomy. The most advanced stage of acetabular hip dysplasia that has a good functional result for the patient depends on the amount of acetabular filling and trauma to the DAR.

Suggested Readings

Slocum B, AVORE. Pelvic osteotomy: the results of 285 pelvic osteotomies (abstract). Vet Surg 1986;15:134.

Slocum B, Devine T. Pelvic osteotomy in the dog as treatment for hip dysplasia. Semin Vet Med Surg 1987;2:107.

Slocum B, Devine T. Femoral neck lengthening for hip dysplasia in the dog. Vet Surg 1989;18:81.

Slocum B, Devine T. Dorsal acetabular rim radiographic view for evaluation of the canine hip. J Am Anim Hosp Assoc 1990;26:289.

Slocum B, Devine T. Pelvic osteotomy. In: Whittock W, ed. Canine orthopedics. 2nd ed. Philadelphia: Lea & Febiger, 1990:471.

Slocum B, Slocum TD. Slope of the dorsal acetabular rim for hip evaluation in the dog. In: 17th annual conference of Veterinary Orthopedic Society. Jackson Hole, WY: Veterinary Orthopedic Society, 1990:12.

Intertrochanteric Osteotomy

Wolff-Dieter Prieur

In canine hip dysplasia, the femoral head and the acetabulum may exhibit different degrees of anomaly. The proximal femur, ilium, and ischium also may show deformities, although these generally are not so readily apparent. The acetabulum and the proximal end of the femur, which form one functional unit, depend on each other for proper growth and shape. Malformation of one component induces deformation of the other, but the extent of the malformation is different and individual in each affected dog. Radiographs of dysplastic hips may show any of the following combinations of deformities: 1) a flat acetabulum and a nearly normal proximal femur; 2) a normal acetabulum and a proximal femur with increased anteversion and valgus deviation of the neck; or 3) a flat acetabulum and a deformed proximal femur.

In dogs with hip dysplasia, the severity of the clinical signs does not necessarily correlate with the severity of the radiographic alterations. In some dysplastic animals, clinical signs occur before skeletal growth is completed, whereas in others they occur after the appearance of severe degenerative joint disease in the second or third year of life. Degenerative joint disease is caused by joint instability and joint incongruence, which results in an increased amount of force placed on a decreased amount of joint surface. If the stress to the joint cartilage and subchondral bone surpasses the normal mechanical resistance of these tissues, degen-

eration of the articular cartilage and sclerosis of the subchondral bone occur. The joint instability induces fibrotic thickening of the joint capsule and painful contraction of the periarticular muscles, especially the pectineus and iliopsoas muscle.

In human hip diseases, hip pain is caused by tearing of the joint capsule, contracture of the periarticular muscles, and venous stasis in the femoral head and neck. No pain receptors are present within the cartilage or the bone. Canine hip dysplasia also produces pain, which causes affected dogs to decrease motion in the hip. Pain, decreased joint mobility resulting from a thickened joint capsule, and muscle contracture are the main reasons for the gait abnormalities and lameness that prompt owners to seek veterinary help. The aim of any surgical intervention in hip dysplasia is to reduce pain and to improve hip biomechanics, to avoid or to diminish the development of osteoarthritis.

Rigid internal fixation of a femoral osteotomy near the hip joint is more difficult in dogs than in human patients because of the small size of the femoral head and neck and the complicated shape of the proximal femur owing to the trochanteric fossa and the bony ridge between the greater trochanter and femoral head. The proximal femur also is loaded in a different way in dogs, because the hind limbs do not carry the whole body weight as in human beings, but instead propel the body forward.

Preoperative Considerations

Intertrochanteric osteotomy is best done at the level of the lesser trochanter for two reasons: 1) malformation of the proximal femur can be corrected optimally in all three planes in this area without changing the shape of the femoral shaft; and 2) bone healing in cancellous bone is faster. The difficult problem of fixing the small proximal bone segment to the shaft is accomplished by use of a double-hook plate that allows compression of the osteotomy gap. The following corrections can be achieved singularly or in combination with an intertrochanteric osteotomy:

1. Alteration of the angle of the femoral neck by removal of a bony wedge from the medial side of the proximal femur

2. Reduction of anteversion by derotation

3. Lateralization by shifting the distal segment more lateral in order to biomechanically increase the length of the femoral neck (Fig. 61.48).

By use of a special instrument set, the osteotomy can be accomplished precisely in the correct planes and angles. With a special drill guide, holes for the double-hook plate can be seated in the proximal segment using a drill bit with a stop that allows one to drill holes the length of the hooks. A saw guide is used to direct the oscillating saw precisely. Removal of a

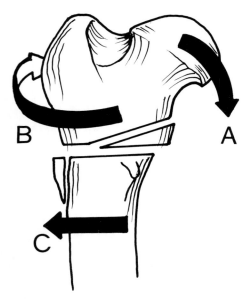

Fig. 61.48. Abnormalities in three planes of the femur can be changed with the intertrochanteric osteotomy. An increased angle of inclination of the femoral head and neck can be decreased (*A*), abnormal anteversion can be corrected (*B*), and the length of the femoral neck can be lengthened by lateralization of the distal femur (*C*).

bony wedge with a predetermined angle is possible by use of a goniometer adapted to the saw guide.

The surgical procedure should be carefully planned with the help of a ventrodorsal radiograph of the pelvis that shows both femurs parallel to the film plane, parallel to each other, and rotated inward until the patella is projected between both femoral condyles. The pelvis should not be tilted. The inclination angle of the neck is measured, and the angle of the wedge to be removed is determined from the radiograph. Anteversion causes the projected inclination angle to be slightly more obtuse than the real inclination angle. Because it is impossible to measure the extent of anteversion on the radiograph, increased anteversion is assumed to be present if the whole outline of the lesser trochanter is projected on the radiograph. In dogs with normal anteversion angles, only the point of the lesser trochanter is visible on a correctly positioned radiograph. If an increased anteversion angle is suspected, the surgeon deducts about 5 to 8° from the projected inclination angle to obtain the real inclination angle of the femoral neck. For best results, any valgus deformity of the femoral neck is corrected to a slight varus position of about 135°. To calculate the angle of the bony wedge to be removed, the surgeon deducts 135° from the inclination angle. In animals with a short femoral neck, shifting the distal segment 3 to 5 mm more laterally biomechanically elongates the femoral neck. This shifting is done by removing a small wedge from the lateral aspect of the distal segment.

Surgical Technique

A lateral approach to the proximal femur is used. After the skin is incised and the biceps muscle is reflected caudally, the deep layer of the fascia lata is cut along the caudal border of the vastus lateralis and superficial gluteal muscles. The tendon of insertion of the superficial gluteal muscle to the third trochanter is cut. The proximal insertion of the vastus lateralis is incised along the third trochanter, and the muscle is subperiosteally detached from the bone. A Hohmann retractor inserted with its tip under the cranial edge of the proximal femur is used to retract the superficial gluteal and vastus lateralis muscles cranially. A second Hohmann retractor is used to retract the biceps femoris caudally. This maneuver exposes the whole proximal third of the bone. The sciatic nerve should always be identified and protected.

A 2.0-mm Kirschner wire is passed under the vastus intermedius muscle along the cranial aspect of the femoral neck and is inserted into the femoral head (Fig. 61.49**A**). If correctly placed, the wire will move when the femur is rotated. The direction of the wire corresponds to the axis of the femoral neck, and its deviation from the transverse plane corresponds with the anteversion angle, which is normally about 15°. The lesser trochanter can be palpated on the caudomedial surface after inward rotation of the femur, and the level of its point is marked on the lateral aspect of the femur with a chisel. In dogs with a short distance between the intertrochanteric crest and the point of the lesser trochanter, the osteotomy line runs through the point of the lesser trochanter or slightly distal to it, but it may run slightly proximal to it. The osteotomy must always preserve the intertrochanteric crest.

The drill guide is placed on the caudolateral aspect of the trochanter with the plate perpendicular to the anteversion plane defined by the Kirschner wire. The line marked on the instrument must be over the planned osteotomy line. The tail of the instrument must be parallel to the cranial border of the femur; the plate is adjusted with the screw so it is parallel to the femoral axis (Fig. 61.49**B**). Correct placement of the drill guide is the most important step because all other procedures depend on it. With a 2-mm drill bit inserted through the 2-mm sleeve in the guide head, a hole is drilled into the greater trochanter; a 2-mm locking pin then is inserted to fix the drill guide to the bone. All adjustments are rechecked now and are corrected if necessary. With a 3.2-mm drill bit with a stop, a hole is drilled in the bone through the cranial 3.2-mm drill sleeve (Fig. 61.49**C**); after removal of the drill bit, a 3.2-mm locking pin is inserted. A second 3.2-mm hole is drilled through the caudal 3.2-mm sleeve, and a locking pin is inserted. With a 2.0-mm drill bit, a hole is drilled through both cortices of the

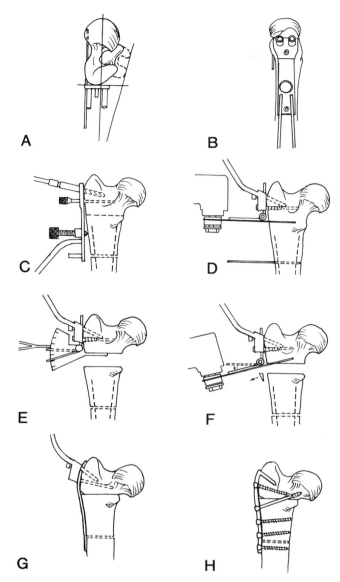

contacts the saw blade and the set screw is tightened. With the saw blade in touch with the wing, the first cut is made (Fig. 61.49**D**). Care must be taken to avoid tilting or bending the saw blade and to protect the soft tissue with the two Hohmann retractors.

The short proximal fragment can be manipulated easily with the handle of the saw guide. After the hinge screw is loosened slightly, the goniometer is placed with its tip in the socket of the hinge screw and its blade touching the osteotomy surface of the proximal segment (Fig. 61.49**E**). The direction of the wing of the saw guide is changed according to the planned osteotomy angle, and the hinge screw is tightened. In the osteotomy surface of the proximal segment, about 8 to 12 mm from the lateral cortex, a small rim is cut with the saw parallel to the plate of the saw guide as a support for the blade. The wing is shifted until it is touching the saw blade and the second cut is made (Fig. 61.49**F**). The wedge is freed from soft tissue with scissors or a periosteal elevator and is removed. If lateralization is planned, a bony wedge about 2 to 3 mm wide is removed from the third trochanter of the distal segment.

The set screw is loosened, and the wing is removed from the saw guide. A template is inserted into the saw guide and is fixed with the set screw. After both segments are reduced, the template is molded to the lateral surface of the distal segment (Fig. 61.49**G**). The saw guide is carefully removed without bending the template by dragging its pin out of the holes in the trochanter. Double-hook plates are sold overbent near the hooks because it is easy to straighten them but difficult to bend them at this point without damaging the hooks. A double-hook plate is contoured to the shape of the template with the hooks in the direction of the pins of the saw guide. After contouring the plate, the hooks are pressed into the 3.2-mm holes of the proximal segment, and the plate is fixed by inserting a 3.5-mm cancellous screw in the predrilled and pretapped hole in the greater trochanter (Fig. 61.49**H**).

The distal segment is fixed to the plate with bone-holding forceps. The Kirschner wire is reinserted into the femoral head for defining anteversion. With the tibia aligned parallel to the table, the Kirschner wire should be perpendicular to the table or show a slight anteversion of up to 5°. For correction, the distal segment is rotated inward or outward until the wire is in the right position. The osteotomy gap is compressed with one or two pointed reduction forceps. Using the 3.5-mm load guide in two holes and the neutral one in one hole, the plate is fixed to the distal segment with 3.5-mm screws. A 4.0-mm cancellous screw that is 40 to 50 mm long is inserted in the direction of the femoral head through the hole near the fracture gap (Fig. 61.49**H**). This lag screw achieves additional compression of the osteotomy gap.

Fig. 61.49. A–H. Intertrochanteric osteotomy. See text for details. (From Brinker WO, Hohn RB, Prieur W-D. Manual of internal fixation in small animals. Heidelberg: Springer-Verlag, 1984.)

femoral shaft using the middle hole of the distal three 2-mm sleeves in the tail of the guide.

After the drill guide is removed, the saw guide is fixed to the femur by inserting its two pins into the 3.2-mm holes within the greater trochanter (Fig. 61.49**D**). Through the opening of the saw guide, the 2-mm drill hole in the trochanter is tapped with a 3.5-mm cancellous tap. A 2-mm Kirschner wire is inserted into the 2-mm drill hole in the shaft; the wing of the saw guide is then adjusted parallel to it, and the wing screw is tightened. After the saw blade of the oscillating saw is positioned on the marked osteotomy line, the wing of the saw guide is shifted distally until it

The vastus lateralis muscle is fixed to the proximal segment by a 2–0 absorbable suture winding around the cranial hook. The deep layer of the fascia lata is closed, bringing the superficial gluteal muscle into its normal position. The biceps muscle is fixed to the superficial layer of fascia lata, and the skin is closed routinely.

Postoperative Care

Starting the day after the surgical procedure, the dog is exercised on a leash for about 10 minutes each day. After the first 2 weeks, the exercise time is slowly increased daily for 2 months. While the dog is walking, its head is lifted by the owner, a maneuver that causes the dog to put more weight on the hind limbs. In the second week after surgery, the owner should start lifting the dog's forelimbs several times a day to encourage the dog to stand on its hind limbs for several minutes. Starting 4 weeks postoperatively, the owner should lift up the dog's forelimbs and force the dog to walk on the hind limbs for several steps. This physical therapy is important to improve joint motion and to increase the strength of the atrophied muscles. Running and jumping must be avoided in the first 3 months after surgery because the femoral neck is remodeling at this time.

The results of intertrochanteric osteotomy usually are gratifying. The pain should decrease and the gait of the dog should improve within a few months. In some cases, the progression of osteoarthritis has been stopped, and in others, it has decreased after this surgical procedure.

Suggested Readings

Muller ME. Die Huftnahen Femurosteotomien. Stuttgart: Georg Thieme, Stuttgart, 1971.
Nunamaker DM. Surgical correction of large femoral anteversion angles in the dog. J Am Vet Med Assoc 1974;165:1061.
Paatsama S. Healing process after intertrochanteric osteotomy in canine hip dysplasia: an experimental study. J Am Vet Radiol Soc 1974;15:61–65.
Prieur WD. Intertrochanteric osteotomy in the dog: theoretical consideration and operative technique. J Small Anim Pract 1987;28:3–20.
Prieur WD, Scartazzini R. Grundlagen und Ergenbnisse der Intertrocantaren Variationsostoeotomie bei Huftdysplasie. Kleintierpraxis 1980;25:393.

DARthroplasty

Barclay Slocum & Theresa Devine Slocum

The dysplastic hip before acetabular filling is well treated by pelvic osteotomy for acetabular hip dysplasia. Total hip replacement is used in patients with advanced degenerative joint disease including the destruction of joint cartilage. The treatment algorithm has lacked a procedure for dysplastic hips that are too far advanced for pelvic osteotomy but are not yet candidates for end-stage salvage procedures. The DARthroplasty is a surgical procedure for hips that have acetabular filling and yet still have an intact articular cartilage.

DARthroplasty provides dorsal support for the femoral head and prevents the pain associated with joint capsule tears from the dorsal acetabular rim (DAR). A bone graft from the wing of the ilium is placed over the joint capsule at the DAR. As the bone graft forms an extracapsular DAR, the capsule becomes a weight-bearing surface for the hip.

Bone Graft Source

Bone is harvested from the wing of the ilium. If the need for additional bone is anticipated because of dramatic dorsal displacement of the femoral head, as in juvenile hip dysplasia, then a rib graft is also used. Bone bank graft (Veterinary Transplant Services, Seattle, WA) can be used if insufficient graft is anticipated because of previous autogenous bone graft harvests or when surgical time is a factor.

Surgical Procedure

The hair is clipped and shaved over the affected hip dorsally to the midline, to 2.5 cm cranial to the wing of the ilium, ventrally 5 cm below the greater trochanter, and caudally to the medial limit of the tuber ischiadicum. After appropriate sterile preparation and draping with the patient in lateral recumbency, bone graft is harvested from the wing of the ilium. A bone gouge is used to obtain appropriately sized graft curls.

A linear incision is made in the skin, parallel to the cranial margin of the biceps femoris muscle from the level of the third trochanter to level of the sacrotuberous ligament. The fascia along the cranial margin of the biceps femoris is incised from the level of the third trochanter to the sacrotuberous ligament. The biceps femoris muscle is retracted caudally, and the superficial and middle gluteal muscles are retracted cranially. The joint capsule can be palpated between the deep gluteal muscle and the cranial belly of the gemellus muscles. Beginning from this reference point, the caudal joint capsule is freed from the external rotators, and the bone of the caudal acetabulum is exposed. The deep gluteal muscle is elevated from the joint capsule and pelvis to expose the bone of the acetabulum dorsally and cranially.

A protected $\frac{1}{8}$-inch (3.2-mm) Steinmann pin is used to perforate the lateral cortex with multiple holes (approximately 10) around the acetabulum (Fig. 61.50).

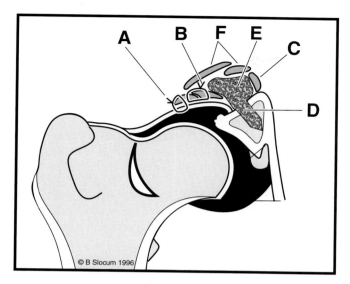

Fig. 61.50. The DARthroplasty is formed from a bone graft. A corticocancellous strip is contoured to the joint capsule at the dorsal apex of the femoral head, and it is held in place by a capsular suture (*A*). A second strip is contoured to the joint capsule and sutured to the first (*B*). Barrier strips are placed dorsally, cranially, and caudally (*C*). The lateral cortex of the pelvis is perforated with multiple holes (*D*), which are packed with cancellous bone (*E*) and are covered with additional corticocancellous strips (*F*).

The dorsal apex of the femoral head is palpated through the joint capsule. A strip of corticocancellous bone from the ilium is contoured (cortical side to the joint capsule) and is sutured to the joint capsule dorsally, cranially, and caudally so the high point of the femoral head in its luxated position is covered dorsally. A second corticocancellous strip is placed medial to the first strip and is sutured to it. Additional strips are placed against the pelvis to limit the dorsal, cranial, and caudal extents to which additional bone graft can be placed. Cancellous bone graft is placed among the dorsal, cranial, and caudal limiting strips and the joint capsule. This cancellous bone graft is in direct contact with the holes in the acetabulum, so blood supply and the conditions for healing directly between the graft and acetabulum are established. Additional corticocancellous strips are contoured and placed over the remaining exposed joint capsule parallel and medial to the sutured lateralmost strip. The partial strips of corticocancellous and cancellous bone are packed obliquely over the new graft and future DAR.

The deep gluteal muscle is sutured to the cranial margin of the internal obturator tendon, which stabilizes the graft and protects it from migration. Closure is completed by reapposing the biceps femoris muscle to the gluteal fascia. Skin closure is routine.

Results

The description of this surgical procedure is the result of experience with more than 300 hips. The primary indication for this surgical procedure is hip dysplasia with acetabular filling while the joint cartilage is intact. The status of the hip joint cartilage can be determined from the DAR radiographic view, linear tomography, and hip palpation. The procedure allows for immediate weightbearing in all but the most painful cases. Bilateral hip surgery is the rule rather than the exception.

Frequently, pelvic osteotomy and DARthroplasty are both done on the same day, and the patient is sent home to the care of the owner on the following day. Immediately after the operation, the limb that underwent DARthroplasty is the dominant hind limb. After long-term follow-up, the limb that underwent pelvic osteotomy is the dominant hind limb, as evidenced by greater thigh diameter. Both limbs demonstrate pain-free function.

Results at 2 months postoperatively show performance that is normal, although no propulsive activity is permitted until after fusion is radiographically visible. Function is pain free, and no further subluxation or luxation of the femoral head from its surgical position is evident. All patients experience a reduction in abduction as a result of the additional DAR. Radiographically on the DAR view, independent strips of bone graft can be seen. Linear tomography confirms connected and unconnected strips of bone in the process of fusing. An indentation is often seen where the joint capsule attaches to the DAR.

Four months postoperatively, the dogs are fully functional and playing and jumping without pain. After activity, they have no morning soreness. Limited abduction of 35 to 40° is typical, although the range of hip extension does increase. Radiographically, the DARthroplasty has fused completely to itself and to the DAR (Fig. 61.51). The femoral head may have migrated medially back into the acetabulum.

Annual follow-up examinations clearly demonstrate continued pain-free function without discomfort after a full day of high activity. Extension of the hips is increased and allows the patient to stand on the hind limbs to investigate counter tops, to run after a ball, and to jump into a pickup truck or up after a Frisbee. A history of 4 to 8 hours of bird hunting without pain or soreness the next day is common. Medial migration of the femoral head occurs as the DARthroplasty process matures. This makes prediction of the amount of femoral head coverage by the DARthroplasty difficult. The early presence of the joint capsule over the original DAR gives way to remodeling, which makes the old and new DAR continuous (Fig. 61.52).

Several complications have been encountered in the development of the technique. One patient had a temporary sciatic dysfunction that returned to normal by 6 months postoperatively. Several patients with luxated head displacement twice the femoral head diameter had the sciatic nerve trapped between the bone

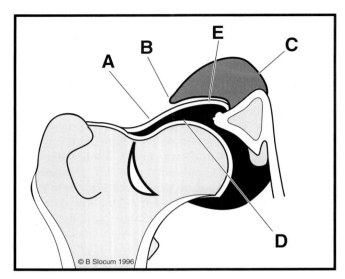

Fig. 61.51. Four months after bone grafting, the joint capsule (A) is covered by the new dorsal acetabular rim (DAR) (B). The DARthroplasty (C) is maturing into a solid bone continuous with the pelvis. The dorsal apex of the femoral head (D) lies beneath the new DAR (B). Usually, one sees a concavity for the joint capsule (E), and the femoral head does not subluxate.

graft and the sacrotuberous ligament. The entrapment was reduced by severing the sacrotuberous ligament. Direct trauma to the sciatic nerve can be avoided by directing all forceful manipulations, such as periosteal elevation, away from the nerve. No case of infection has been seen.

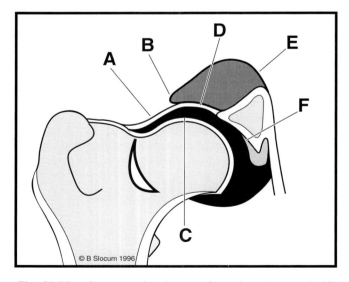

Fig. 61.52. One year after bone grafting, the joint capsule (A) is covered by the new dorsal acetabular rim (DAR) (B). The dorsal apex of the femoral head (C) lies beneath the new DAR (B). The concavity for the head beneath the DARthroplasty (D) is often continuous with the old DAR. The DARthroplasty (E) is mature bone that is continuous with the pelvis. Acetabular osteophytes (F) continue slow and progressive filling of the acetabulum until the femoral head is stable in the "new acetabulum."

The single example of DARthroplasty with early evidence of cartilage eburnation was in a 6-month-old Old English sheepdog with permanently subluxated hips, acetabular filling, and fresh tearing of the joint capsule at the DAR. This patient was deemed too hyperactive for a total hip replacement. Six-year follow-up showed this patient to be fully active for all functions, although the dog experienced occasional mild soreness on resting after a daily 3-mile jog with the owner. The patient was not on medication.

Long-term follow-up on four hips on which autopsy was performed showed stable hip joints in which no subluxation was present. The joint capsule had lost its fully collagenous appearance, with the presumption of metaplasia to fibrocartilage. These patients had been 100% functional before they died.

Usually, an owner can perceive no difference between pelvic osteotomy and DARthroplasty when these procedures are done simultaneously in the same patient. However, clinical examination clearly demonstrates that the thigh circumference 1 inch above the patella is always greater on the side of the pelvic osteotomy. This result is anticipated because the indications for pelvic osteotomy require a hip without acetabular filling, whereas the indications for DARthroplasty require both acetabular filling and distortion of the DAR. In addition, weightbearing is on the joint capsule instead of on the articular cartilage.

The DARthroplasty technique fills the indication between pelvic osteotomy and total hip replacement. Although previous DARthroplasty does not preclude total hip replacement, in our 6-year experience, none of the patients that have undergone DARthroplasty have begun to demonstrate painful signs that would remotely suggest the necessity for a total hip replacement.

Femoral Head and Neck Ostectomy

Philip B. Vasseur

The purpose of femoral head and neck ostectomy (FHO), in dogs, is to eliminate physical contact between the bone surfaces of the femur and the acetabulum. Dysplasia involving the hip joints is the most frequent reason for considering this operation. Dysplastic hips are incongruent and develop various degrees of degenerative joint disease with associated pain. FHO is a surgical option for dogs with advanced degenerative joint disease in which reconstructive osteotomies would not be effective. In mature dogs with severe degenerative joint disease involving the hip joints, total hip replacement restores hip function more consistently, and much more rapidly, than FHO.

If both hip joints are affected, I usually recommend that the operations be done sequentially, with the second hip operated on when reasonable function has been regained in the first hip (usually 1 to 2 months). Young, ectomorphic dogs can undergo bilateral FHO during one anesthetic period, and it saves considerable expense and time. The owner should be prepared for a 3- to 7-day period, after surgery, in which more intensive nursing care is necessary.

Surgical Technique

The animal is placed in lateral recumbency, and the surgical site is aseptically prepared to give wide exposure of the hip and to permit manipulation of the limb during the operation. A pursestring suture in the anus is advised to prevent contamination during the operation. The joint is visualized using a craniolateral approach (Fig. 61.53) (1). The skin incision is started dorsal and slightly cranial to the greater trochanter and extends distally one-third to one-half the length of the femur. The subcutaneous tissues are carefully dissected from the superficial fascia, which is incised to permit caudal retraction of the biceps femoris muscle. The deep fascia is then incised, freeing the tensor fasciae latae muscle. The incision in the deep fascia is extended proximally between the tensor fasciae latae and the superficial gluteal muscle. The superficial gluteal muscle is retracted dorsally and caudally, and the tensor fasciae latae muscle is retracted cranially. A self-retaining retractor is useful to maintain this exposure. The middle gluteal muscle is retracted dorsally, exposing the tendon of the deep gluteal muscle, and the latter tendon is separated from the underlying joint capsule with a periosteal elevator or blunt scissors. Annoying hemorrhage may be encountered at this point, and electrocautery is useful. A partial tenotomy of the deep gluteal tendon permits continued dissection and elevation of the deep gluteal muscle from the joint capsule. The muscle is closely attached to the dorsal joint capsule, especially in arthritic joints, and the dissection causes considerable hemorrhage. When dorsal exposure has been obtained and hemorrhage is controlled, a radial capsulotomy is started at the

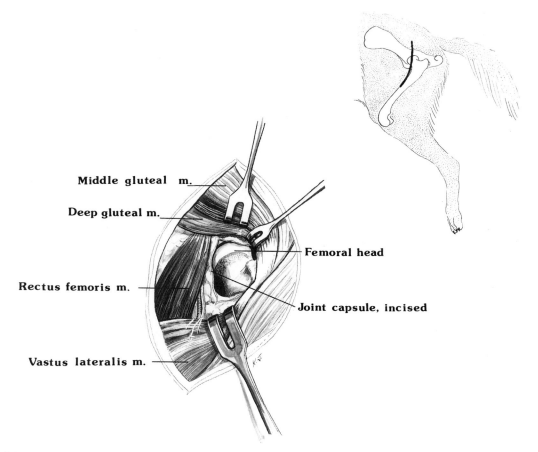

Fig. 61.53.   Schematic illustration of the craniolateral approach to the hip joint. Note the dorsal and caudal retraction of the gluteal muscles and the orientation of the radial capsulotomy. Wide exposure of the neck is necessary to perform an adequate resection arthroplasty.

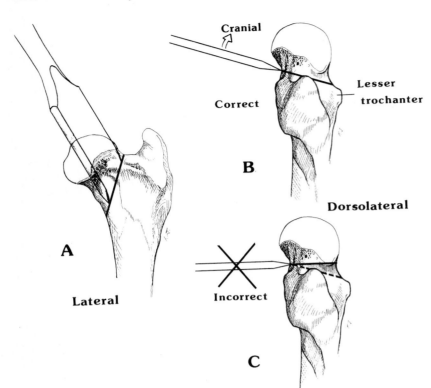

Fig. 61.54. Schematic illustration showing the correct placement of an osteotome for ostectomy of the femoral head and neck. With the limb in a neutral position, the surgeon must direct the osteotome cranially to excise the femoral neck completely.

acetabular margin and is extended along the femoral neck, incising a portion of the origin of the vastus muscle group. The capsular attachments and muscle origins are then elevated from the femoral neck using a periosteal elevator.

Luxation of the hip is helpful before ostectomy, if the hip is not already luxated. The luxated position places the bone in a more superficial position, thus improving exposure and permitting more accurate osteotomy. The hip can be luxated by severing the ligament of the femoral head with Mayo scissors or a Hatt spoon. The surgeon must be aware of the location of the sciatic nerve to protect it throughout the procedure. A hand-held retractor can be placed under the luxated femoral head and neck to provide stabilization and to protect the surrounding soft tissues. The cut in the femoral neck can be made using a power saw, an osteotome, a Gigli saw, or obstetric wire. The last two methods are relatively safe in that the cutting motion is directed outward, thus preventing damage to nerves and other soft tissues. A power saw, if available, is preferred because of the speed, ease, and accuracy of the osteotomy. An osteotome is effective, but care must be taken not to damage surrounding soft tissues or to split the femoral shaft. In small dogs and cats, a large rongeur can be used to excise the femoral head and neck.

Positioning of the osteotome or saw blade is im-

portant. The osteotome or saw blade is placed on the lateral surface of the femoral neck, and the instrument is held cranially, directing the cut caudally and medially (Fig. 61.54). A common error is to make the cut directly medially, that is, perpendicular to the table. This usually results in incomplete excision of a portion of the caudal femoral neck, depending on the position of the femur during the ostectomy. The goal is to remove as much of the femoral neck as possible, to prevent subsequent contact with the acetabular rim. The lesser trochanter is preserved to retain function of the iliopsoas muscle (Fig. 61.55).

After the femoral neck is cut, the femoral head is grasped with a Lewin bone clamp or a towel clamp, and any remaining capsular attachments are cut, allowing removal of the femoral head and neck. Any bony projections or irregularities that remain on the cut surface of the femur are removed with a rongeur or bone rasp. If hemorrhage from the medullary surface is persistent, bone wax is used to achieve hemostasis. The wound is irrigated thoroughly with saline solution, and any remaining hemorrhage is controlled. The deep gluteal tendon is repaired with one or two mattress sutures using polydioxanone. The vastus muscles are sutured to remaining capsule and, if necessary, to the tendon of insertion of the deep gluteal muscle using horizontal mattress sutures. The deep and superficial layers of the fascia lata are apposed as independent

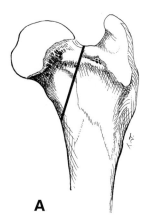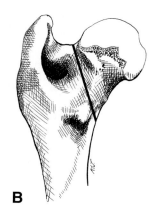

Fig. 61.55. Schematic illustration showing the correct location for osteotomy of the femoral head and neck. **A.** Lateral view. **B.** Medial view.

layers, using continuous patterns of fine absorbable suture material. The subcutaneous tissues and the skin are apposed in a routine manner. Objective, controlled studies have failed to document any benefit associated with placement of soft tissues between the cut surface of the femur and the acetabulum.

Postoperative Rehabilitation, Complications, and Prognosis

Vigorous exercise in the postoperative period is essential for restoration of muscle strength and function in the affected limbs. As soon as the stitches are removed, an organized program of physical activity should be initiated. Swimming is the best activity, because it forces use of the limb without the need for weightbearing; however, lack of facilities or inclement weather may preclude swimming, and the owner may need to walk or run the dog to provide the necessary exercise. During the first week, the activity should only last for 5 to 10 minutes, three times daily. As the animal gains strength, the duration of exercise is gradually increased. Passive range-of-motion exercise is also of value and should be carried out for at least 10 minutes, three to four times daily. Anti-inflammatory medication is useful during this rehabilitation period to facilitate early use of the limb. Carprofen (2.2 mg/kg every 12 hours orally) or aspirin (20 mg/kg every 12 hours orally) is recommended. Frequent rechecks by the veterinarian are of considerable value to encourage the client and to ensure that the animal is progressing in terms of limb use, resolution of atrophy, and restoration of joint motion. Anti-inflammatory medication is discontinued when limb use is consistent and is steadily improving.

Complications of this operation can include shortening of the operated limb, with prominence of the greater trochanter, decreased range of motion in the pseudoarthrosis as compared with the normal hip, muscle atrophy, and impaired function. Occasional lameness is not unusual in larger dogs, and they may have difficulty in jumping or climbing stairs. The physical therapy described previously, including the use of anti-inflammatory drugs and maintenance of normal body weight, can minimize the severity of the aforementioned problems.

Although FHO is generally successful in relieving pain and many patients are active after recovery, owners of hunting dogs or dogs expected to perform other challenging physical tasks should not anticipate a complete return to normal function. The prognosis is best if the animal is lean and active, has no concurrent orthopedic disorders, and has an owner willing to pursue the necessary aftercare. It may take as long as 6 to 12 months for the animal to achieve an optimal result after FHO, and the client must be made aware of the prolonged recovery time. I find the results in dogs to be basically the same as those reported in human patients, that is, good pain relief and only fair return of function (2). For dogs that do not do well after FHO, total hip replacement is an option. If reasonable bone stock remains, the surgeon usually can perform a successful hip replacement in dogs with a failed FHO.

References

1. Piermattei DL. Atlas of surgical approaches to the bones and joints of the dog and cat. 3rd ed. Philadelphia: WB Saunders, 1993:230–235.
2. Bohler M; Salzer M. Girdlestone's modified resection arthroplasty. Orthopedics 1991;14:661–666.

Total Hip Replacement

Marvin L. Olmstead

Surgical Technique

Total hip replacement is a the most effective way to provide a canine patient with a mechanically sound, pain-free, ball and socket hip joint, once osteoarthritis is present. Both cemented and uncemented prostheses have been successfully used to treat noninfectious, nonneoplastic disabling conditions of the canine coxofemoral joint (1–10). The uncemented hip is not commercially available and thus has limited use. The most commonly implanted prosthesis is a cemented modular prosthesis (BioMedtrix, Inc., Allendale, NJ). Dogs with clinical signs related to hip dysplasia or other disabling hip conditions are candidates for surgery, once their physes have closed at 9 to 10 months of age and they have a skeletal size that will accommodate the available prosthesis, which generally starts at 14 kg (5, 7, 8).

Special care must be taken to ensure that the surgery is done under strict aseptic conditions. The dog's hind limb is clipped the day before the surgical procedure. The skin is evaluated for bacterial dermatitis, which, if present, delays the procedure until the condition is resolved. If the skin is dirty, the dog is bathed. Intravenous antibiotics are administered immediately before the operation. Draping of the patient with sterile paper and plastic drapes provides a barrier at the surgical site that is impermeable to bacteria. Special instrumentation has been developed to facilitate the implantation of the modular prosthesis (BioMedtrix, Inc., Allendale, NJ). Radiographic templates are used preoperatively to estimate the size of acetabular cup and femoral stem that will be implanted.

The coxofemoral joint is exposed through a craniolateral approach. The skin incision starts dorsal and caudal to the greater trochanter and curves along the front edge of the femur. The tensor fasciae latae is reflected cranially. The deep gluteal muscle is exposed

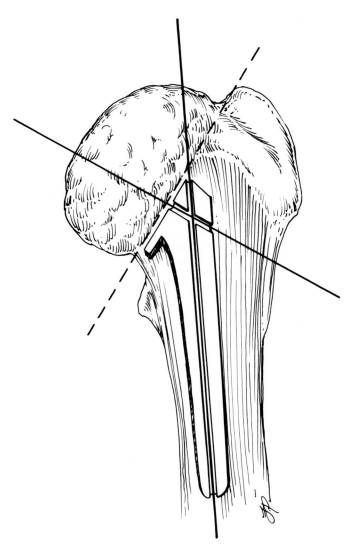

Fig. 61.57. A template is used to ensure that the osteotomy of the femur is properly positioned. The line running the long axis of the template should parallel the long axis of the femur. The short line on the template is aligned parallel to the axis of the femoral neck. The medial edge of the trochanter is the landmark for the origin of osteotomy. The cut should parallel the collar of the prosthesis. (Courtesy of BioMedtrix, Inc., Allendale, NJ.)

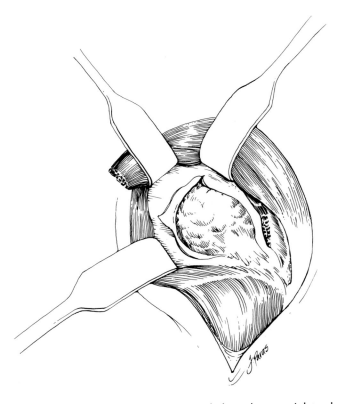

Fig. 61.56. The hip joint is exposed through a craniolateral approach. The deep gluteal muscle is partially incised at its origin, is divided longitudinally, and is retracted cranially. The joint capsule is incised parallel to the axis of the femoral neck and along its insertion on the femur. (Courtesy of BioMedtrix, Inc., Allendale, NJ.)

by reflecting the middle and superficial muscles dorsally. The deep gluteal muscle is incised at its origin and is split into two segments. The joint capsule is incised along with the vastus medialis and lateralis (Fig. 61.56).

At various points in the surgical procedure, the femur is rotated in position. All references in the following discussion to the lateral, medial, cranial, or caudal surface of the femur refer to that surface when the femur is in normal position. To perform femoral osteotomy properly, the femur is rotated externally so the patella is oriented 90° lateral to its normal position.

The medial edge of the greater trochanter is identified. The femoral osteotomy originates at this point. A template of the femoral prosthesis is aligned parallel to the long axis of the femur and the axis of the femoral neck (Fig. 61.57). The template acts as a guide for performing the osteotomy. The diseased femoral head is removed. Instrumentation developed specifically for the modular prosthesis allows power-driven reaming of the femur and acetabulum. Although the reaming can be done by hand, it is easier and more accurately done with a power-driven instrument.

The acetabular bed is prepared first using the acetabular reamer (Fig. 61.58). No flush is used during the acetabular reaming so the cancellous bone shavings can be collected and saved for possible use later. The shavings can be packed into areas of deficit in the acetabulum or along fissures in the femoral neck, should either of these be present. The acetabulum is reamed until the medial cortical wall is exposed. Remnants of the ligament of the head of the femur may need to be removed to expose the medial wall fully. Three or more holes are drilled around the rim of the acetabulum using a drill bit from the modular system and the tissue guard that protects soft tissues (Fig. 61.59). The holes are connected with a curette. This undercut provides anchor sites for the bone cement or polymethylmethacrylate (PMMA).

The femoral shaft is rotated laterally 90°. A wide-tipped Hohmann retractor is used to elevate its proximal end lateral to the tissues that lie dorsal to it. The femoral shaft is first drilled with a drill bit that matches the size of the femoral stem selected for insertion (Fig.

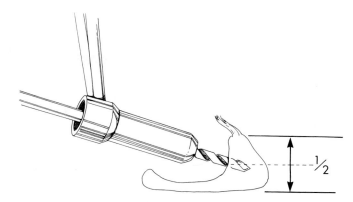

Fig. 61.59. Multiple holes in the acetabular bed provide anchor points for the polymethylmethacrylate (PMMA) or "bone cement." A tissue guard is used with the drill bit. The holes should be located in the cancellous bone halfway between the medial cortical wall and the lateral most edge of the acetabular rim. (Courtesy of BioMedtrix, Inc., Allendale, NJ.)

61.60). The surgeon may need to start drilling with the bit oriented perpendicular to the osteotomy line. As soon as the proximal cancellous bone is penetrated, the drill bit should be reoriented so it is parallel with

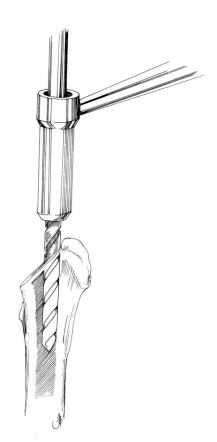

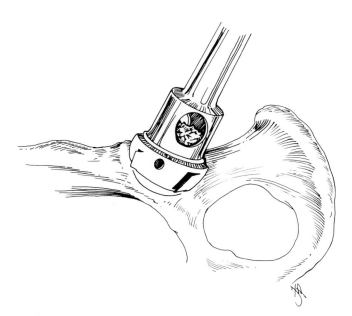

Fig. 61.58. An acetabular reamer is used to remove degenerative bone and cartilage to the level of the medial cortical wall of the acetabulum. (Courtesy of BioMedtrix, Inc., Allendale, NJ.)

Fig. 61.60. The opening into the femoral canal is started with a drill bit the same size as the femoral stem selected for implantation. (Courtesy of BioMedtrix, Inc., Allendale, NJ.)

ular bed first. Specific landmarks and the acetabular cup positioner are used to achieve proper position of the acetabular cup (Fig. 61.63). All excess PMMA is removed. A second batch of PMMA is mixed for the femoral shaft injection. The shaft is cleared of blood and debris, and PMMA is injected into the femoral canal using a 60-mL catheter-tip syringe. The cobalt chrome femoral stem is aligned with the long axis of the femur and is inserted down the shaft until the prosthesis collar rests flush with the osteotomy line. The stem is held solidly in place with the stem impactor. Excess PMMA is removed while the cement in the femoral canal hardens.

A trial plastic head is placed on the femoral stem so neck length can be assessed (Fig. 61.64). The prosthesis with the trial head is reduced, and the tightness of fit is tested. Once the proper neck length has been determined, the cobalt chrome head is placed on the stem and is tapped securely into position. The head is reduced into the acetabular cup. Cultures are taken, and the joint capsule is tightly closed. The surgical site is closed in layers.

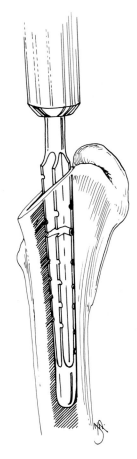

Fig. 61.61. The femoral canal is opened further with a power-driven fluted reamer. (Courtesy of BioMedtrix, Inc., Allendale, NJ.)

the long axis of the femur. The fluted reamer that is the same number as the drill bit used widens the hole in the femoral shaft (Fig. 61.61). The final preparation of the femoral shaft is done by hand with a finishing file and sometimes a broach (Fig. 61.62). The femoral shaft should be reamed along the medial edge of the trochanter to permit complete access to the femoral canal. In some cases, the wall of the trochanteric fossa must be removed to ensure that the femoral canal is opened adequately. Reaming along the endosteal surface of the femoral neck accommodates the curved portion of the femoral prosthesis. A trial prosthesis, the same size as the one to be implanted, is inserted to ensure that the prosthesis will fit properly and that the cement mantel around the prosthesis will be adequate.

Thorough cleaning of the acetabular bed and the femoral shaft is necessary before the cement is injected. The PMMA should be mixed according to the manufacturer's specifications. Only PMMA with a liquid phase of 3 to 7 minutes can be injected. PMMA is injected through a catheter-tip syringe into the acetab-

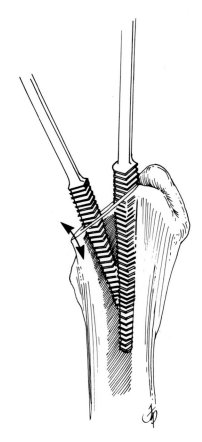

Fig. 61.62. After power-driven reamers are used to make holes in the femoral shaft, a finishing file and sometimes a broach (not shown) are used to make the hole in the shaft of an adequate size to accept the femoral stem. (Courtesy of BioMedtrix, Inc., Allendale, NJ.)

in prosthesis implantation. The modular system allows the size of prosthesis to match the size of the dog's femoral canal and acetabular cup. The clinical results achieved with the modular system are equal to or better than those of the fixed-head system. Experience obtained with the fixed-head system has shortened the learning curve for the modular system.

Dogs with total hip replacements achieve normal or near-normal hind limb function 95% or more of the time (7–9). Pain-free function, a full-range hip motion, increased exercise tolerance, increased muscle mass, and an improved quality of life are standard findings. Working dogs returned to field or police work and pets have been exercised more without pain. Investigators have found that 80% of the dogs do not need the other unoperated hip replaced. These animals obtain enough relief from one total hip replacement that operating on the other side is not necessary. Often, on reevaluation, neither hip is painful when both had hurt before surgery. The thigh circumference of the side with total hip replacement is routinely 1 to 4 cm larger than the unoperated side. Because the

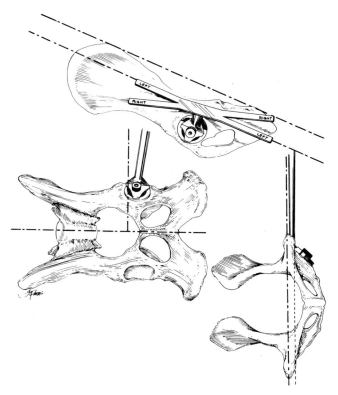

Fig. 61.63. To position the acetabular cup correctly, the positioner must be aligned in three planes relative to specific anatomic landmarks. In the *top drawing*, the bar of the positioner is aligned parallel with the top of the ilium and the ischium. In the *middle left drawing*, the bar of the positioner is tilted caudally, positioning the cup in retroversion. In the *bottom right drawing*, the shaft of the positioner is aligned parallel with the tuber ischiadicum. (Courtesy of BioMedtrix, Inc., Allendale, NJ.)

Lateral and ventrodorsal pelvic radiographs are taken immediately postoperatively so the position of the acetabular and femoral components and the fill of the PMMA can be assessed. Antibiotic therapy is continued until the culture results are known. If the results are negative, as is almost always the case, antibiotics are discontinued. On the rare occasion when results are positive, antibiotics based on sensitivity patterns should be continued for at least 4 weeks. The dogs are maintained on limited activity for 2 months postoperatively. No activity more strenuous than a walk is allowed, and the dog is allowed outside only on a leash. After that period, the dog can return to normal activity gradually.

The modular system has improved the technique of total hip replacement in the dog over the previously used fixed-head prosthesis. It gives the surgeon excellent instrumentation, a wider choice of neck lengths, and increased implant sizes. Thus, the veterinary surgeon can offer better care for the dog with disabling hip conditions. Smaller dogs can be treated because a wider range of prosthesis sizes is available. The size of the femoral canal and acetabulum are limiting factors

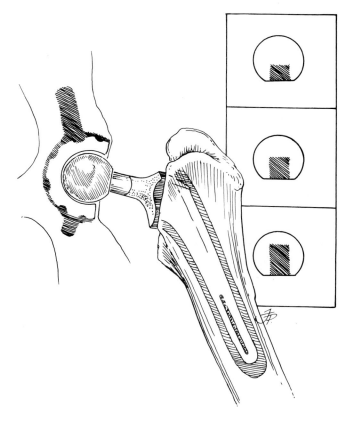

Fig. 61.64. Cross-sectional cuts of the femoral head show the three different depths of holes that are found in the femoral head. Placing a head with the shallow hole on the stem results in a long femoral neck, whereas placing a head with the deep hole on the stem gives a short femoral neck. Femoral neck lengths are determined with trial heads after the femoral stem and acetabular cup are cemented. (Courtesy of BioMedtrix, Inc., Allendale, NJ.)

prosthesis provides the normal ball and socket arrangement of the hip joint, the femur maintains its normal position relative to the pelvis, and the hind limb is able to generate maximal propulsive forces during locomotion. This is not the case if the ball and socket joint configuration is not present.

Total hip replacement in the dog is an effective way of treating disabling conditions of the hip joint. To be proficient at this procedure, a surgeon must be well trained in the technique and must do it routinely. Not every veterinarian should perform this operation. However, every veterinarian should know enough about the procedure to be able to discuss it as a treatment option when indicated.

Total hip replacement is well known by the general public as a treatment for people with hip problems. Because of this, more owners are demanding this operation for their pets, and more referral centers are offering it as part of their service. The future of total hip replacement in veterinary medicine is bright and will continue to be so as long as the latest information and technical developments are incorporated into the treatment protocol.

References

1. Hoefle WD. A surgical procedure for prosthetic total hip replacement in the dog. J Am Animal Hosp Assoc, 1974, 10:269–276.
2. Leighton RL. The Richard's II canine hip prosthesis. J Am Anim Hosp Assoc 1979;15:73–76.
3. Lewis RG, Jones JP. A clinical study of canine total hip arthroplasty. Vet Surg 1980;9:20–23.
4. Olmstead ML, Hohn RB. Ergbisse mt der hufltoltal-Prostheses bei 103 klinischen fallen an der Ohio State University. Klin Prox 1980;25:407–415.
5. Olmstead ML, Hohn, RB, Turner TM. A five year study of 221 total hip replacements in the dog. J Am Vet Med Assoc 1983;183:191–194.
6. Parker RB, Bloomberg MS, Bitetto W, et al. Canine total hip arthroplasty: a clinical review of 20 cases. J Am Anim Hosp Assoc 1984;20:97–104.
7. Olmstead ML. Total hip replacement. Vet Clin North Am 1987;17:943–955.
8. Olmstead ML. The canine cemented modular total hip prosthesis: surgical technique and preliminary clinical results. J Am Anim Hosp Assoc 1995;109–123.
9. DeYoung DJ, DeYoung BA, Aberman HA, et al. Implantation of an uncemented total hip prosthesis: technique and initial results of 100 arthroplasties. Vet Surg 1992;21:168–177.
10. Paul HA, Bargar WL. A modified technique for canine total hip replacement. J Am Anim Hosp Assoc 1987;23:13–18.

Reduction of Coxofemoral Luxations

James L. Tomlinson, Jr.

Coxofemoral luxation is a common injury suffered by both dogs and cats after various forms of trauma to the pelvis. The hip joint is the most commonly luxated joint in dogs and cats. In most coxofemoral luxations, the femoral head is displaced cranial and dorsal to the acetabulum. In about 10% of hip luxations, the femoral head is displaced either ventrally or caudodorsally.

The severity of tissue damage associated with hip luxations varies. In all luxations, the round ligament and part of the joint capsule are torn. In more severe cases, part of the gluteal musculature also may be torn. Small avulsion fractures of the femoral head where the round ligament attaches are common. Erosion of the cartilage of the femoral head sometimes results from the femoral head's rubbing on the ilium, especially in more chronic cases. On rare occasions, portions of the dorsal rim of the acetabulum are fractured off.

Diagnosis of a coxofemoral luxation usually is simple. Most animals have a history of trauma such as having been hit by a car. The animal does not bear weight on the leg; with a craniodorsal luxation, the leg is adducted and externally rotated. On physical examination, a greater than normal distance can be palpated between the greater trochanter of the femur and the tuber ischiadicum. The "thumb test" also is useful in diagnosing a craniodorsal luxation. To perform this test, the animal is placed in lateral recumbency with the affected leg up. The examiner stands behind the animal and places the thumb of the hand closest to the spine in the depression between the greater trochanter of the femur and the tuber ischiadicum while the other hand is grasping the stifle joint. The leg then is externally rotated. In a normal animal, the greater trochanter of the femur should pinch or displace the thumb from the depression between the greater trochanter of the femur and the tuber ischiadicum during rotation, whereas in an animal with a dislocated hip, the thumb is not pinched or displaced. A third way to evaluate a patient for a luxated hip is to extend the animal's legs out caudally while the animal is in either dorsal or lateral recumbency. With a craniodorsal luxation, the affected limb appears shorter than the normal leg; with a ventral luxation, the leg appears longer. Radiographs are needed to confirm the diagnosis, because animals with fractures of the femoral head or neck present with clinical signs similar to those of animals with luxations. The radiographs should be evaluated for direction of luxation, avulsion fractures of the femoral head, other pelvic fractures, and hip dysplasia.

Surgical Options

Closed reduction with application of a nonweightbearing sling is the method of choice for most acute luxations. The application of an Ehmer sling after closed reduction is described in Chapter 50. Failure rates for coxofemoral luxations treated by closed reduction have been reported to be as high as 50 to 70% (1, 2).

Open reduction is indicated for acute luxations that will not remain reduced closed, irreducible acute luxations, chronic luxations, luxations associated with avulsion fractures of the femoral head, and luxations associated with other fractures (ipsilateral pelvis, femur, or tibia). Animals with moderate-to-severe degenerative changes of the hip are not candidates for open or closed reduction. Other methods of treatment should be used with such animals.

Numerous methods for open reduction of coxofemoral luxations have been devised including DeVita pinning, Yarbough pinning, use of Knowles toggle pin, joint capsule imbrication with trochanteric transposition, acetabular rim extension, transacetabular pinning, and retention suturing with joint capsule imbrication. The goal of open reduction of a coxofemoral luxation is to reestablish normal function and conformation of the hip. Once healing is complete, the anatomic shape of the hip joint and fibrosis of the joint capsule hold the hip in place.

Surgical Techniques

The techniques for performing transacetabular pinning and retention suturing with joint capsule imbrication are described in this section. Both procedures are easy to perform, do not require special equipment, and have a high success rate.

Open reduction of coxofemoral luxations can be performed by one of two surgical approaches to the joint. Transacetabular pinning is best performed through a craniolateral approach (3), except in patients with chronic luxations. Retention suturing with joint capsule imbrication is best performed through a dorsal approach by osteotomy of the greater trochanter of the femur (3). With acute craniodorsal luxations, the femoral head is easily identified during the approach. If the luxation is chronic, the femoral head is surrounded by a fibrous pseudojoint capsule. With craniodorsal luxations, the acetabulum is caudoventral to the femoral head and may be difficult to find, espe-

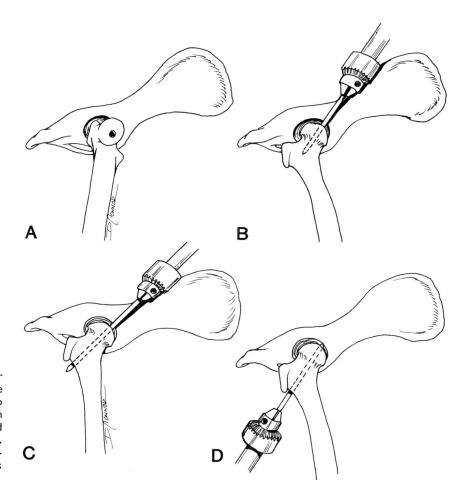

Fig. 61.65. Placement of transacetabular pin. After exposure of the femoral head, the leg is rotated to bring the fovea capitis into view. **A.** An intramedullary pin is placed on the fovea capitis. **B.** The pin is advanced through the head and neck of the femur. **C.** The pin exits at the level of the third trochanter. **D.** The pin is adjusted until the end is flush with the fovea capitis.

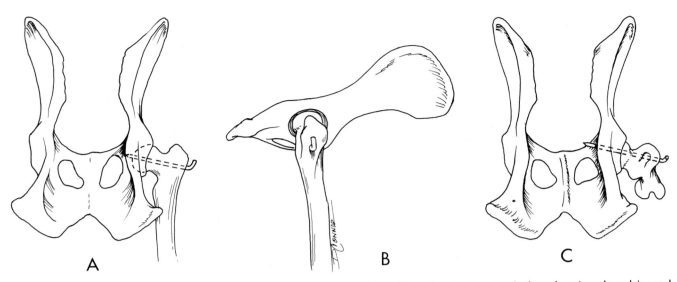

Fig. 61.66. **A–C.** Final placement of transacetabular pin after reduction of joint. Note that the pin extends about 1 cm into the pelvic canal.

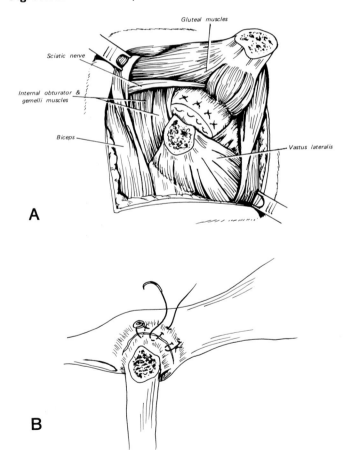

Fig. 61.67. Imbrication of coxofemoral joint capsule. **A.** When sufficient joint capsule is present, nonabsorbable sutures are placed in a horizontal mattress pattern. **B.** When insufficient joint capsule is present on the acetabular side for suturing, small tunnels can be drilled through the acetabular rim and the sutures passed through them and tied. (From Brinker WO, Piermattei DL, Flo GL, eds. Handbook of small animal orthopedics and fracture treatment. Philadelphia: WB Saunders, 1983:272.)

cially in chronic luxations. The acetabulum may have joint capsule, blood, or fibrin clots, remnants of the round ligament, avulsed pieces of the femoral head, and fibrous tissue (chronic luxations) within the joint. The joint must be cleaned out before the femoral head can be reduced into the acetabulum. The joint capsule should be preserved for later suturing. The femoral head can be retracted caudal to the acetabulum with a Hohmann retractor by hooking the tip of the retractor on the caudal edge of the acetabulum and prying caudally against the proximal metaphysis of the femur. Care must be taken not to entrap the sciatic nerve under the retractor.

Transacetabular Pinning

Transacetabular pinning is a practical and successful procedure for repair of coxofemoral luxations. The best results are obtained when this procedure is used for acute luxations in nondysplastic patients, although I have used this procedure successfully for chronic luxations. The only equipment needed are standard operating instruments, Jacob's pin chuck, and intramedullary pins.

The animal is placed in lateral recumbency on the operating table with the affected leg suspended from an intravenous pole. The leg is scrubbed and draped for aseptic surgery. For acute luxations, the hip is exposed through a craniolateral approach (3). For chronic luxations, a dorsal approach to the hip by osteotomy of the greater trochanter of the femur (3) is preferred. Once the femoral head is exposed and the acetabulum is cleaned of debris, the luxation is reduced temporarily. The hip is reluxated, and the femur is rotated externally until the fovea capitis of the femoral head is visible (Fig. 61.65**A**).

An intramedullary pin with a diameter that is two-thirds to three-fourths that of the fovea capitis is selected. The pin is advanced from the fovea capitis, down the femoral neck, and out the cortex of the third trochanter of the femur (Fig. 561.65**B** and **C**). The pin is adjusted until the tip is flush with fovea capitis (Fig. 61.65**D**). After the luxation is reduced, the femur is placed parallel to the table top and at a 90° angle to the spine. The pin is driven across the acetabulum while firm downward pressure is applied to the greater trochanter of the femur. If inadequate pressure is applied to the greater trochanter, the femoral head will back part way out of the acetabulum. The pin is driven approximately 1 cm into the pelvic canal for the average-size dog. An assistant can palpate the pin rectally to determine whether it has been driven the correct distance. Care must be taken not to puncture the colon. Once the pin has been driven the correct

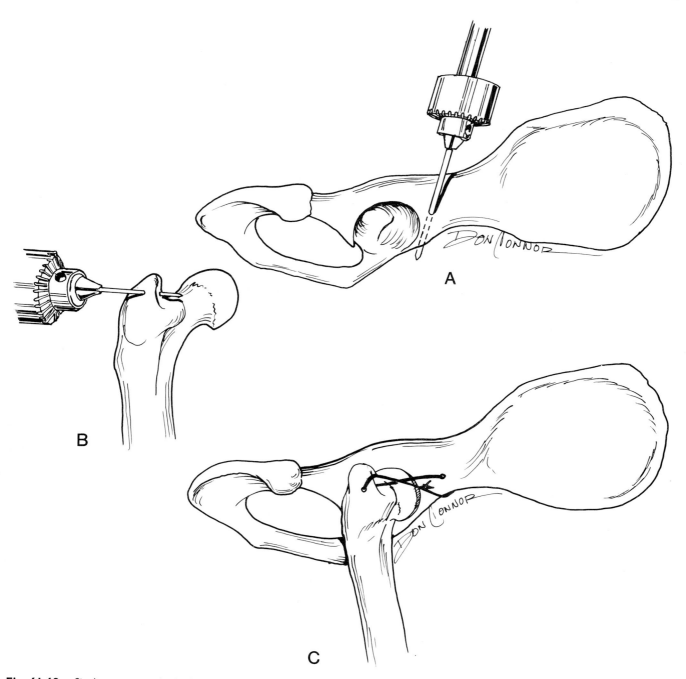

Fig. 61.68. Single-suture method of retention suturing. One hole is drilled through the ilium (**A**), and a second hole is drilled through the greater trochanter (**B**). **C.** Heavy nonabsorbable suture is passed through the holes and is tied. See text for details.

distance, the end of the pin is bent over and cut off (Fig. 61.66).

Postoperatively, the hip is radiographed to check for proper pin placement and reduction of the luxation. The leg is placed in a nonweightbearing sling (Ehmer or Robinson), and the animal is discharged with instructions for limited exercise until the pin is removed. The pin should be removed in 14 to 21 days; the animal's activity is restricted for 3 weeks after pin removal.

Complications associated with transacetabular pinning include pin migration and breakage and reluxation of the hip. Pin migration and breakage generally result from failure of the owner to keep a sling on the animal. The owner should be instructed to return the animal immediately if the sling comes off.

Joint Capsule Imbrication With Retention Suturing

Joint capsule imbrication with retention suturing is a useful method for treating patients with acute luxations, chronic luxations, and luxations with concurrent lesions such as acetabular fractures that require an approach to the hip by osteotomy of the greater trochanter of the femur. Retention suturing can be a valuable technique by itself when the joint capsule is missing or traumatized to such an extent that it will not effectively hold sutures.

The animal is placed in lateral recumbency with the affected hip up and is prepared for aseptic surgery. The luxated joint is exposed through a dorsal approach by osteotomy of the greater trochanter of the femur (3).

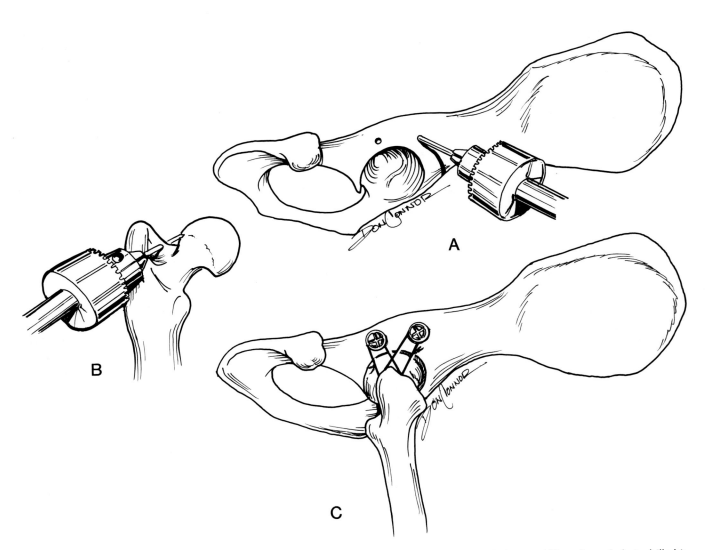

Fig. 61.69. Double-suture method of retention suturing. Two holes are drilled into the acetabular rim (**A**), and one hole is drilled in the greater trochanter (**B**). **C.** Screws are inserted into the acetabular holes; then two suture strands are passed through the femoral tunnel and around the screws. See text for details.

Great care must be taken during this approach to preserve the joint capsule for later suturing.

After the femoral head has been identified and the acetabulum cleared of debris, the luxation is reduced. If adequate joint capsule is present on both sides of the joint, a simple horizontal mattress pattern of 3–0 or 2–0 polypropylene is used to imbricate the joint (Fig. 61.67**A**). Placement of sterile towels on the medial side of the leg is beneficial, to hold the leg in abduction during the imbrication to relieve the pressure on the joint capsule. If insufficient joint capsule is present on the acetabular side of the joint, the joint capsule can still be attached by using tunnels or screws to secure the suture on the acetabular side (Fig. 61.67**B**). The bone tunnels can be drilled with either Kirschner wires or drill bits. If holes are used, they must originate as close to the acetabular rim as possible so they do not interfere with the femoral head.

Two methods for retention suturing have been described. The single-suture method (4) is started by drilling a hole dorsally to ventrally at the attachment of the rectus femoris to the ventral aspect of the ilium (Fig. 61.68**A**). A second hole is drilled cranially to caudally through the greater trochanter of the femur (after the trochanter is reattached) at about the level of attachment of the deep gluteal tendon (Fig. 61.68**B**). Heavy nonabsorbable suture material (No. 5 Ethibond or 5-mm Mersilene [Ethicon, Inc., Somerville, NJ]) is threaded through the holes, and the suture material is tightened (Fig. 61.68**C**). The suture should not be tightened to the extent that flexion and extension of the hip are restricted, or the suture will break.

In the double-suture method, two sutures are passed from the greater trochanter to the dorsal rim of the acetabulum (5). Two holes are drilled in the dorsal acetabular rim at the 11 and 1 o'clock positions (Fig. 61.69**A**); a third hole is drilled cranially to caudally through the greater trochanter of the femur (Fig. 61.69**B**). After screws are inserted into the holes in the acetabular rim, two strands of heavy nonabsorbable suture material are passed through the femoral tunnel. One strand is passed around the cranial acetabular screw and the other around the caudal screw; the screws are then tightened (Fig. 61.69**C**). Spiked washers (Synthes, Paoli, PA) may be needed to hold the sutures in place. The greater trochanter is reattached with two Kirschner wires and a tension band wire.

With either retention suture technique, the animal is placed in a nonweightbearing sling for 2 to 3 weeks postoperatively with exercise restriction. Once the sling is removed, the animal is slowly returned to normal exercise over the next month.

References

1. Bone DL, Walker M, Cantwell HD. Traumatic coxofemoral luxation in the dog. Vet Surg 1984;13:263.
2. Dobbelaar MJ. Dislocation of the hip in dogs. J Small Anim Pract 1963;4:101.
3. Piermattei DL, Greeley RG. An atlas of surgical approaches to the bones of the dog and cat. Philadelphia: WB Saunders, 1979.
4. Slocum B, Devine T. Dislocation of the canine hip: treatment of the normal and dysplastic hip. Am Anim Hosp Proc 1987;372.
5. Allen SW, Chambers JN. Extracapsular suture stabilization of canine coxofemoral luxation. Compend Contin Educ Pract Vet 1986;8:457.

Single-Suture Technique for a Dislocated Hip

Barclay Slocum & Theresa Devine Slocum

The single-suture technique is primarily indicated in trauma patients in which the hip is dislocated craniodorsally, but immediate use of the leg is important because of the severity of multiple trauma to the other limbs. For this technique to be successful, the hip must be normal and must have a normal slope to the dorsal acetabular rim. This procedure is contraindicated in the dysplastic hip or the hip with a deficit in the external rotator muscle group or caudal joint capsule.

Surgical Technique

Preoperatively, the dog is anesthetized and radiographed. The position of the femoral head as revealed from the lateral and ventrodorsal radiographs is dorsoventral. The hip should be reduced into the acetabulum, by externally rotating the hip, applying distal traction on the limb, moving the greater trochanter caudally, and internally rotating the femur. Axial compression should be applied to the hip while internally rotating the femur, to ensure the success of this surgical procedure. If the hip remains stable with this test, the single-suture technique is a viable option for the patient. If the hip does not remain stable with axial compressive forces, a pelvic osteotomy is recommended. Any reduction of a dislocated hip by a suture is not meant to be a long-term solution, because the suture is expected to break as soon as normal activity is resumed. The single-suture technique is designed to provide time for the cranial and dorsal joint capsule to heal, while enabling the patient to bear weight on the limb.

The anesthetized patient is placed in lateral recumbency and is prepared for surgery. After draping of the proximal half of the lateral thigh, a skin incision is made along the cranial border of the biceps femoris muscle from the greater trochanter to 10 cm distally. The fascia of the biceps femoris muscle is incised, and the biceps muscle is retracted caudally. The sheet of fascia containing the superficial gluteal and the tensor fasciae latae muscles is incised, beginning just proximal to the third trochanter, continuing distally to the limit of the skin incision. The cranial portion of this fascia containing the tensor fasciae latae muscle is retracted cranially. This maneuver exposes the middle and deep gluteal muscles as they insert on the greater trochanter. The cervical tubercle is identified as the osseous knob lying just beneath the deep gluteal tendon. A bursa is present beneath the deep gluteal tendon at this location on the craniolateral aspect of the greater trochanter.

The hip is reduced by external rotation, distal traction on the limb, caudal transposition of the greater trochanter, and internal rotation. With the hip held in mild internal rotation, the proximal femur is moved laterally using the caudal joint capsule as the stabilizing joint structure. The entire caudal half of the dog should be able to be elevated off the table during this test, to ensure the success of the single-suture procedure. Any chips of bone in the depth of the acetabulum attached to the teres ligament should be removed. If the joint capsule is still attached to the rim of the acetabulum, and torn free from the femoral neck, it may have become infolded in the acetabulum, preventing reduction. A modification of the single-suture technique, called the shoehorn technique, is described later in this discussion.

A hole is drilled in the greater trochanter, beginning just caudal to the insertion of the deep gluteal and exiting on the cranial aspect of the femoral neck (Fig. 61.70). For large dogs, a $\frac{1}{8}$-inch Steinmann pin may be used. A hole is drilled in the pelvis, just cranial to the acetabulum, laterally to medially. A slight ventral direction of the Steinmann pin used to drill this hole eases the suture through it. A 10-inch piece of 20-gauge stainless steel wire is folded back on itself to form an acute bend. This acute bend is passed through the pelvic hole laterally to medially. Placing the index finger just caudal to the rectus femoris assists in locating the tip of this wire as it protrudes from the hole. Curved forceps or a needle holder such as a Stratte instrument will allow a firm grasp on the tip of the wire, which is partially withdrawn into the incision opening. Two strands of the wire are spread apart to allow a large suture, such as 5-mm polyester (Merseline), to be placed between the two wires. The wire is pulled out of the lateral hole, to lock the suture in the apex of the acute bend. It is withdrawn into the incision. The wire is removed from the suture. The wire is now passed caudally to cranially through the greater trochanter hole. The medial portion of the suture that passes through the pelvic hole is placed through the wire loop as it exits the hole in the femoral neck. The wire is withdrawn through the caudal trochanteric hole. The free ends of the suture are tied with a double half-hitch, which is slid down the suture until the sin-

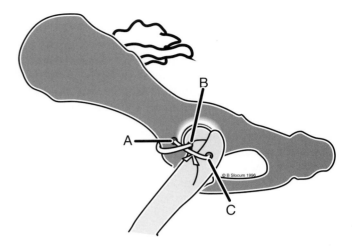

Fig. 61.70. The single figure-of-eight suture enters the pelvic hole (A), turns under the ventral pelvis, and enters the cranial cervical opening (B) of the trochanteric hole. The suture exits the lateral aspect of the greater trochanter (C) and is tied on itself.

gle suture is tight between the greater trochanter and the pelvis when the limb is in the sagittal plane. The double half-hitch is converted into a square knot, and a third knot is applied to secure the suture. The hip is tested, and the femur should not be able to be luxated. Reapposition of the sheet of fascia containing the tensor fasciae latae and superficial gluteal muscles is performed. The incision along the cranial edge of the biceps femoris is reapposed, followed by routine skin closure.

The single-suture technique relies on the strength of the single suture to provide stability to the hip in the neutral position. By preventing external rotation with an intact caudal joint capsule, the hip is maintained in a reduced position. Because rapid healing of the joint capsule is necessary, corticosteroids are contraindicated. The race is between healing and failure of the single suture. Once it has served its purpose, the suture should be removed; a neoplasm did form around one suture in a clinical case.

Although resuturing the torn joint capsule is appealing, to provide continuity to the hip enclosure, anatomic reconstruction of the capsule has not been necessary as long as the components of the joint capsule are somewhere near each other.

The patient must be confined to a rug while indoors, to a leash while outside, and to a traveling kennel when the owner is not in attendance. This regimen must be maintained for 6 to 8 weeks, a reasonable healing time for collagen.

Failure of the single-suture technique results from premature excessive stress by the patient or from applying the suture too tightly at the time of surgery. Overtightening the suture causes the limb to be in an internally rotated position, rather than in a neutral position in the sagittal plane.

The single-suture technique can be used for a deficit in the caudal joint capsule when the cranial joint capsule is intact. Unfortunately, the external rotators are more prone to permanent damage during caudal dislocation of the hip. The single-suture technique can be used to hold a craniodorsal dislocation of the hip in conjunction with a medial patellar luxation, but the medial patellar luxation must be repaired or the dislocation will recur along with breakage of the suture.

After the removal of the teres ligament in a patient with a chronic case, or a chip fracture, the reduced hip must be tested for stability before application of the single suture. Testing is performed by reduction, followed by internal rotation and axial compression. The entire hindquarters should be capable of being elevated off the table with the hip in this position. This test checks the integrity of the caudal joint capsule in maintaining its portion of hip reduction.

Follow-up on this procedure at 3 to 4 months postoperatively is imperative because healing of the joint capsule and maintenance of reduction of the femoral head within the confines of the joint capsule represent success of the technique. However, if damage of the internal rotators is too great, the hip may drift laterally without continued input from the gluteal muscles. In such a case, a pelvic osteotomy is curative, because slight overrotation by a pelvic osteotomy causes the hip to fall into the socket even in the absence of a strong gluteal muscle force.

Shoehorn Modification

The shoehorn technique is a modification of the single suture technique. It is used whenever the joint capsule is torn free of the femoral neck cranially, without tearing the main substance of the joint capsule, in much the same manner as pulling a foot from a sock.

Exposure of the femoral head is performed as previously described. Testing the stability of the hip reveals incomplete reduction. The source of the problem is an infolded joint capsule that is torn from the femoral neck and remains intact at the rim of the acetabulum. Once the head has slipped from within the joint capsule, it is impossible to replace it without open reduction.

In preparation for reduction and fixation, a trochanteric hole is drilled as previously described. The margins of the lateral joint capsule are carefully identified, and the joint capsule is maintained intact. Grasping the cranial portion of the joint capsule with forceps or a temporary retention suture, the opening through which the femoral head had exited is expanded. Using an instrument as a hip skid, the hip is reduced into the joint capsule as one uses a shoehorn when putting on a shoe. A long, curved needle attached to No. 2 polypropylene (Prolene) suture is passed from lateral to medial through the $\frac{1}{8}$-inch trochanteric hole. The tip of the needle is passed inside the joint capsule and exits the cranial joint capsule, traverses the gluteal musculature, and penetrates the skin cranially. The needle is grasped external to the skin and is withdrawn only far enough to allow the juncture of needle and suture to clear the cranial limit of the joint capsule. The blunt end of the needle is passed out the incision and is tagged with a mosquito hemostat. A similar suture is passed through the $\frac{1}{8}$-inch hole in the trochanter and into the craniodorsal joint capsule, and again it is tagged. A third suture is placed through the $\frac{1}{8}$-inch trochanteric hole to the cranioventral joint capsule. The sutures are drawn tight, and the hip is tested for stability before the sutures are tied. The hip should be reduced and stable. Once this is confirmed, the knots are secured to allow the hip to be weight-bearing immediately. Closure is routine.

The shoehorn technique provides immediate stability for the hip, and weightbearing is usually excellent and immediate. The animal's owners must be cautioned to adhere to a confinement regimen for the patient until healing has been ascertained at the 2-month recheck examination. Client compliance is often difficult because of the superb response of the patient. This technique is meant to be used on normal hips only or in conjunction with a pelvic osteotomy on dysplastic hips.

A variation of this technique can be used for capsulorrhaphy with a pelvic osteotomy technique. The craniolateral approach to the hip is made by leaving the deep and middle gluteal muscles intact. The vastus lateralis muscle is elevated from the cervical tubercle and cranial femoral neck. The elevation is carried through the joint capsule until joint fluid and the articular cartilage can be identified. The three sutures are passed as previously described through an $\frac{1}{8}$-inch trochanteric hole and through the joint capsule. The entire joint capsule is tightened as a single sheet, which includes and is attached to the vastus lateralis muscle. After the capsulorrhaphy, the vastus lateralis is sutured to the deep gluteal tendon with mattress sutures. Routine closure follows.

— 62 —

KNEE

Algorithm for Diagnosis and Treatment of the Stifle for Cranial Cruciate Ligament Rupture

Barclay Slocum & Theresa Devine Slocum

Figure 62.1 is an algorithm for the evaluation and management of the stifle for rupture of the cranial cruciate ligament.

Diagnostic Tests

Barclay Slocum & Theresa Devine Slocum

General Conformation

The stifle joint is affected by local pathologic processes and by alignment of the limb owing to its strategic location midway between the hip and the foot. It is a two degree of freedom joint that includes rotation about the long axis of the tibia, traversing the tibial plateau just medial to the intercondylar eminences on the medial tibial plateau. The second motion allowed in the stifle is flexion–extension about a transverse axis through the center of the femoral condyles. Translation is an abnormal motion of the stifle joint. Because the stifle is basically a cylinder, two condyles, lying on a flat surface, tibial plateaus, the motions allowed by the joint are controlled by the ligaments and not by the osseous structures. The joint is ligament dependent.

Cranial motion of the tibia with respect to the femur is called cranial drawer motion and is restricted by an intact cranial band of the cranial cruciate ligament. Internal rotation is controlled by the posterior band of the cranial cruciate ligament. A secondary restraint of the tibia with respect to the femur is the caudal horn of the medial meniscus. Additional limitations are provided by the lateral collateral ligament and the caudomedial joint capsule. Caudal translation of the tibia with regard to the femur is controlled by the caudal cruciate ligament. Medial and lateral translations are rarely affected by ruptures of the cranial cruciate ligament, but they are noted when a history of trauma is present. Medial translation of the tibia with respect to the femur occurs with damage to the lateral joint capsule and the femoral meniscal ligament. Lateral translation of the tibia with respect to the femur occurs with damage to the caudomedial joint capsule and fibrous extensions in the caudal intercondylar region. Varus and valgus deviations at the stifle occur when the distractive side of the joint has a torn joint capsule or a torn collateral ligament.

The second major influence in the stifle is the overall limb alignment of the joint. This is under the control of the structure of the hip, femur, tibia, hock, and foot. Anteversion and valgus of the femoral neck contribute to a knock-kneed cow-hocked conformation, as does osteochondritis dissecans (OCD) of the lateral femoral condyle. Torsion in the diaphysis between the proximal and distal femur may have a similar effect. Varus of the distal femur is common with a bowlegged patient and medial patellar luxations. Valgus of the distal femur is common with a knock-kneed appearance and lateral patellar luxations.

A varus deformity of the distal tibia is often, but not necessarily, accompanied by a medial position of the tibial tubercle that favors medial patellar luxations. A

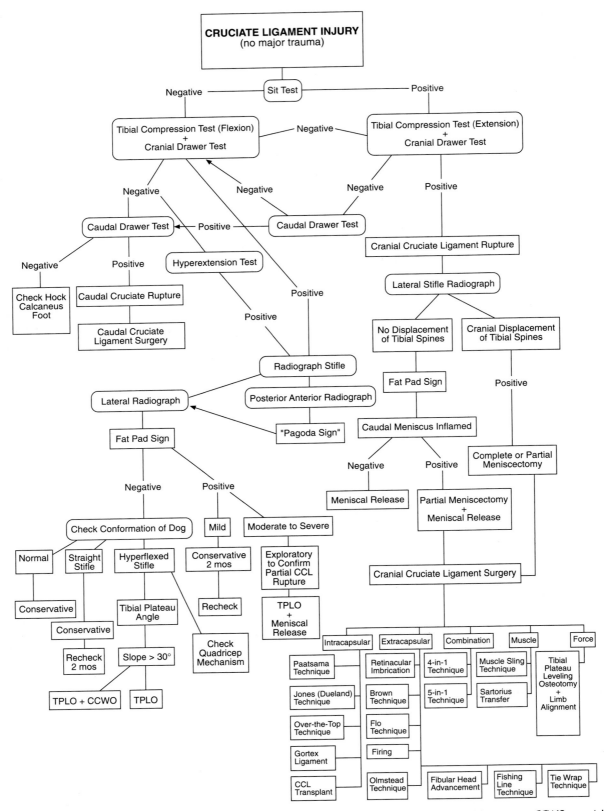

Fig. 62.1. Algorithm for the diagnosis and treatment of the stifle for cranial cruciate ligament (CCL) rupture. CCWO, cranial closing wedge osteotomy; TPLO, tibial plateau leveling osteotomy.

valgus deformity of the proximal tibia favors lateral patellar luxation. Internal torsion of the tibial diaphysis is also a component of the bowlegged conformation and directly contributes to medial patellar luxation, partial and complete rupture of the cranial cruciate ligament, and medial compartment arthrosis in older patients. External torsion of the tibia contributes to the discomfort experienced by dogs with OCD and anteromedial rotary instability of the stifle. Varus and valgus deformities of the distal tibia affect a small segment of dogs, most notably such chondrodystrophic dogs as the dachshund.

Valgus of the midfoot, frequently seen in breeds such as the rottweiler, partially compensates for the bowlegged conformation of the upper limb. Normally, patients have a cranial silhouette of the hind limb, including a patellar deviation and a tibial tubercle deviation. In patients with dramatic and excessive tibial plateau slopes, 35 to 60°, the conformation creates a cranial translation of the tibia and loss of the patellar silhouette. These patients appear to have a long thigh and a short crus. Angulation of the stifle is flexed, yet the stifle is straight.

Patients whose owners report a recent change in stifle conformation from normal flexion to straight or post-leggedness often have stretching of the cranial cruciate ligament. When viewed from behind, patients with ruptures of the cranial cruciate ligament often show a prominent knob in the region of the caudomedial aspect of the stifle, which appears even more prominent as the muscles of the hamstrings atrophy. Direct observation of bilateral muscle atrophy, especially from the hind limbs, and excessive development of the forelimbs, often accompanies bilateral cranial cruciate ligament ruptures. Any patient with ruptures of the cranial cruciate ligament has a positive sit test.

Specific Tests

Sit Test

The sit test is valuable for localizing hind limb pathology to the stifle primarily and the hock secondarily. The owner is asked to have the dog sit. The normal dog sits with full knee flexion that allows the tuber calcanei to come in close proximity to the tuber ischiadicum. The hock is in sufficient flexion so the patient rests on its haunches. The abnormal test shows the patient to sit in a raised position with an increased distance between the calcaneus and the tuber ischiadicum. This is particularly evident in well-disciplined dogs as field trial dogs with stifle disease. Less well-disciplined dogs simply rock to one side or the other and sit on the side of the hip, holding the affected leg extended in both the stifle and hock. Dogs with chronic disease may extend the stifle almost completely when sitting. Patients with mildly affected stifles may appear to sit on their haunches but allow their hips to externally rotate. Patients with partial or early ruptures of the cranial cruciate ligament often sit fully on the initial command, but soon rock to one side to extend the stifle. Arising from the flexed knee position often causes a cantilevering of the patient over the forelimbs rather than a simple extension of the hind limbs. Cantilevering is a sign of forward weight transfer, which decreases the quadriceps force and relieves discomfort in the inflamed knee. The hock joint is normally flexible, and in some patients (most notably rottweilers), the hock does not flex sufficiently to allow the patient to sit on its haunches. Lack of flexion in the hock may also be due to an OCD lesion or other pathologic process in the joint. Whenever the patient initially sits on its haunches and then rocks on the tuber ischiadicum, one must distinguish between disorders of the hock and those of the stifle.

Although most show dogs and some pets are not taught to sit, most patients sit as a matter of lifelong training. This test has been useful in creating a high level of suspicion in determining stifle pathology. The sit test becomes accentuated as the meniscal disorder increases, a finding indicating that stifle flexion creates compression on the inflamed tissues of the meniscus and caudal stifle. When the sit test is positive, the patient usually has radiographic evidence of inflammation in the caudomedial stifle.

Cranial Drawer Sign

Cranial drawer sign is a manipulation of the stifle created by the operator. The surgeon places an index finger on the patella and the thumb of the same hand on the fabella. With the other hand, the index finger is placed on the tibial tubercle and the thumb is placed on the head of the fibula. Cranial translation of the tibia with respect to the femur is attempted by operator force. Tranquilization or anesthesia is sometimes necessary for patients in great pain or for aggressive patients, because many dogs are apprehensive or feel discomfort associated with cranial translation of the tibia. Any cranial translation of the tibia is considered a cranial drawer sign, and a positive drawer sign is pathognomonic for rupture of the cranial cruciate ligament. In some patients, the cranial drawer sign is absent in the presence of stifle disease; most of these patients have damage to the caudal horn of the medial meniscus in which a portion of the caudal horn resides cranial to the femoral condyle. Often, the lateral radiograph shows cranial displacement of the tibia as the intercondylar eminences are seen cranial to the ventral apex of the condylar curvature. Some patients have cranial translation only with the leg in flexion. These dogs usually have morning pain.

The anterior drawer sign is due to rupture of the cranial cruciate ligament. This ligament is the only structure in the body that restricts cranial translation of the femur with respect to the tibia. A clear-cut drawer sign is unmistakable and is pathognomonic for rupture of the cranial cruciate ligament. Once the cranial cruciate ligament is ruptured, the tibia translates cranially, and the femoral condyle crushes the medial meniscus. This damage to the caudal horn of the medial meniscus is secondary to rupture of the cranial cruciate ligament. As damage progresses to the caudal horn of the medial meniscus, it splits into a bucket handle tear; the free portion is moved cranially and locks the condyle in that position, in which case a drawer sign is not palpated. Most of these patients have a cranial translation of the femur with respect to the tibia on the lateral radiograph. After recent rupture of the cranial cruciate ligament, one often hears a popping sound as the patient bears weight on the foot. This sound is due to the cranial tibial thrust, which is a patient-generated thrust that draws the meniscus between the femoral condyles. In cases of chronic rupture of the cranial cruciate ligament, the drawer sign may be difficult to palpate or may be absent because of the large amount of fibrosis of the capsule and a severely damaged caudal horn of the medial meniscus wedged between the femoral condyle and the tibial plateau.

The anterior drawer sign may demonstrate only 1 to 2 mm of cranial translation in patients with partial rupture of the cranial cruciate ligament. This sign is seldom palpated with the leg in extension and requires flexion of the stifle to at least 60° to appreciate this motion. This physical finding, combined with a history of morning pain and nonweightbearing after usage, is a sign of a partial rupture of the cranial cruciate ligament. A partial rupture of the cranial cruciate ligament can be treated by a tibial plateau leveling osteotomy without invasion of the joint in the early and intermediate stages of injury. In the early stage of cranial cruciate ligament rupture, cranial translation may be dramatic, but when the leg is tested for caudal translation, the examiner can feel an abrupt stop to the posterior translation of the tibia, because of the intact caudal cruciate ligament.

Caudal Drawer Sign

The caudal drawer sign is elicited by placing the hands as for the cranial drawer sign but moving the tibial caudally. The sign is positive when the tibia moves caudally with no firm end point, but it moves cranially with a firm hitting of the limit of the cranial cruciate ligament.

The presence of a caudal drawer sign indicates rupture of the caudal cruciate ligament. The hamstring musculature often pulls the proximal tibia posteriorly in the apprehensive patient, and therefore, the operator experiences cranially movement of the tibia with respect to the femur. Most posterior drawer signs are misinterpreted as cranial drawer signs until a posterior sag to the tibia is noted, or until the joint is opened and the ligaments are inspected. If the femur is placed vertically while the anesthetized patient is placed in dorsal recumbency with the stifle flexed to 90°, the silhouette normally has two protrusions, one at the patella and the other at the tibial tubercle. With the patient in this position, the patellar silhouette is accentuated, and the tibial tubercle silhouette is absent. A conclusive distinction between a cranial drawer sign and a caudal drawer sign can be made: a caudal drawer sign is obtained if the cranial translation of the tibia meets abrupt resistance as the intact cranial cruciate ligament reaches the limit of the ligament length, whereas the cranial drawer sign reaches an abrupt stop with posterior movement of the proximal tibia as the intact caudal cruciate ligament reaches the limit of its length.

Tibial Compression Test

The tibial compression test is a test of the cranial cruciate ligament. With the patient in a standing position for testing the right hind limb, the operator's right hand is positioned so that digits 3, 4, and 5 are placed on the tibial crest and are pulled in a caudal direction. The index finger is passed medial to the straight patellar tendon and is placed at the juncture of the distal femoral condyle and the tibia plateau. The left hand is placed on the metatarsus, and the animal's hock is flexed. Cranial translation of the tibia with respect to the femur is appreciated by the index finger of the examiner's right hand. No translation is a negative test. The test is performed with the leg in moderate extension and the leg in flexion.

Interpretation is as for the cranial drawer sign. The presence of a caudal drawer sign indicates rupture of the caudal cruciate ligament. The hamstring musculature often pulls the proximal tibia posteriorly in the apprehensive patient, and therefore the operator experiences cranially movement of the tibia with respect to the femur. Most posterior drawer signs are misinterpreted as cranial drawer signs until a posterior sag to the tibia is noted, or until the joint is opened and the ligaments are inspected. If the femur is placed vertically while the anesthetized patient is placed in dorsal recumbency with the stifle flexed to 90°, the silhouette normally has two protrusions, one at the patella and the other at the tibial tubercle. With the patient in this position, the patellar silhouette is accentuated, and the tibial tubercle silhouette is absent. A conclusive distinction between a cranial drawer sign and a caudal drawer sign can be made: a caudal drawer sign is obtained if the cranial translation of the tibia meets abrupt resistance as the intact cranial cruciate ligament reaches the limit of the ligament length, whereas the cranial drawer sign reaches an abrupt stop with posterior movement of the proximal tibia as the intact caudal cruciate ligament reaches the limit of its length.

Meniscal Examination

The caudal horn of the medial meniscus lies at the caudomedial limit of the tibial plateau and can be observed or palpated caudal to the medial collateral ligament. Direct observation of a severely damaged caudal horn of the medial meniscus can be made when viewing the patient from behind, as a swelling at the level of the medial stifle, and this becomes partially evident as the muscles atrophy. This severe form of meniscal damage causes an enlargement and changes the attachment of the joint capsule to the tibial plateau and osteophyte formation of the subepicondylar portion of the medial femoral condyle. The medial collateral ligament becomes buried within the inflamed scar tissue and cannot be palpated. In cases of moderate duration, damage to the caudal horn of the medial meniscus is less severe, and the medial collateral ligament can be palpated or noted as a dimple in the inflammation of the medial portion of the medial meniscus. In cases of early rupture, the joint capsule is inflamed as it attaches to the tibia, the meniscus is inflamed, and the femoral condyle is not discretely palpated caudal to the medial collateral ligament. If the patient is seen at the time of an acute rupture, or when the animal has an advanced partial rupture, discrete palpation reveals the femoral condyle and tibial plateau caudal to the medial collateral ligament, but the meniscus is protruding; this is termed bone–swelling–bone. In subtle cases of lameness associated with early and intermediate partial ruptures of the cranial cruciate ligament, the medial meniscus has a dimple or recess compared with the level of the tibial plateau and femoral condyle caudal to the medial collateral ligament; this is termed bone–meniscus–bone.

This distinction in the palpation findings is important to determine whether a meniscal release will be appropriate surgical treatment. When the palpation findings are bone–meniscus–bone with not much translation, and all clinical signs of fat pat inflammation, but no meniscal swelling, then no meniscal release is necessary. When bone–swelling–bone is palpated, a meniscal release is warranted.

Medial Translation

Patients that receive trauma to the stifle need to be tested for lateral translation of the tibia with respect to the femur. For the right stifle, the examiner's left thumb and forefinger are placed on the lateral and medial epicondyles of the femur, respectively. The thumb of the right hand is placed on the patient's fibular head, and the right index finger is placed on the medial collateral ligament at the tibial plateau joint line. With the tibia displaced caudally to tense the caudal cruciate ligament, the tibia is moved laterally with respect to the femur. Normally, one notes no medial or lateral translation to the tibia when the caudal cruciate ligament is brought under tension. A positive test consists of lateral translation of the proximal tibia with respect to the femoral condyles.

The meniscofemoral ligament arises from the medial wall of the posterior intercondylar notch. This powerful ligament attaches to the caudal horn of the lateral meniscus and inserts on the posterior aspect of the lateral tibial plateau. Traumatic disruption of this ligament allows lateral translation of the tibia. A weaker but corresponding structure from the posterior medial joint capsule to the posterior intercondylar wall allows medial translation if it is disrupted The accompanying joint capsule must also be stretched to allow these abnormal motions to occur. The presence of either medial or lateral translation with the tibia locked posteriorly against the caudal cruciate ligament diminishes the prognosis for surgical repair because it is a major instability not addressed by routine cranial cruciate ligament procedures.

Craniomedial Rotary Instability

Craniomedial rotary instability is tested when a cranial drawer test is applied to the medial aspect of the stifle joint. A negative craniomedial rotary instability test is indicated when the cranial portion of the tibial plateau maintains a stable relationship with respect to the femoral condyle as cranial tibial pressure is applied. A positive test occurs when the cranial aspect of the tibial plateau moves cranially and laterally with rotation.

A negative craniomedial rotary instability test indicates that the medial capsular structures and short portion of the medial collateral ligament are integral. A positive test indicates stretching or laxity to the same structures. Laxity of these structures causes a lateral shift of the axial rotation axis of the tibia from the medial slope of the medial intercondylar eminence laterally. This test is usually negative in all patients with genu varum, distal femoral varus, or internal tibial torsion and is the domain of dogs with genu valgum, external tibial torsion, and distal femoral valgus. In its mildest form, craniomedial rotary instability causes a mild lameness secondary to impingement of the caudal horn of the medial meniscus. Severe craniomedial rotary instability may occur in conformationally susceptible patients that may also have OCD of the lateral femoral condyle and lateral patellar luxations.

Pivot Shift

A pivot shift is observed in patients with rupture of the cranial cruciate ligament and internal tibial torsion. As these patients bear weight during walking, an internal rotation occurs simultaneous with a craniotibial shift of the proximal tibia. This is termed a pivot shift.

When a pivot shift is observed, the patient is unable to contain the internal rotation and cranial translation of the proximal tibia with respect to the tibia. The biceps femoris muscle has inadequate strength to resist the pivot shift and to provide dynamic stability to the knee. An external torsion osteotomy with valgus correction of the proximal tibia is usually necessary to neutralize the internal rotatory forces that create this shift.

Fat Pad Palpation

The examiner's index and forefinger are used to palpate the fat pad on either side of the straight patellar tendon. Normally, the fat pad is quiescent and soft and has no tendency to protrude beyond the triangle formed by the tibial tubercle, the distal pole of the patella, and the cranial limit of the meniscus. Swelling of the fat pad beyond the limits of this triangle indicates inflammation of the fat pad or increased interarticular synovial fluid pressure.

A positive fat pad palpation is a nonspecific indicator of inflammation within the stifle. The cause can be traumatic, autoimmune, infectious, or ligamentous instability. Dramatic fat pad inflammation as seen on the lateral radiograph is necessary before palpation findings are present.

Palpation for Interarticular Fluid

Increase in interarticular fluid pressure and volume is seen by a bulging of the sheath around the long digital extensor, which gives the external appearance of a subcutaneous lump that distorts the normal smooth hair pattern overlying it. On direct digital palpation, a lump on the lateral side of the stifle, distal and cranial to the meniscus, is caused by excessive fluid or a tumor tissue within the long digital extensor sheath. A second prominence on the lateral aspect of the stifle below the meniscus is the fibular head. Palpation on either side of the rectus femoris tendon at the proximal pole of the patella may indicate fluid within the suprapatellar pouch. Increase in suprapatellar fluid pressure by stifle flexion may increase the prominence of the fluid-filled long digital extensor tendon synovial-filled sheath.

Increased synovial fluid and pressure are indicators of stifle inflammation and usually occur with dramatic increases in pressure and volume. If the prominent long digital extensor sheath expansion is accompanied by severe pain and the distension does not disappear on digital compression, then synovial cell sarcoma should be suspected.

Medial Patellar Luxations

Testing for medial patellar luxation is performed by extension of the stifle, internal rotation of the stifle, and medially directed digital pressure on the patella. While the examiner maintains patellar pressure, the patient's knee is flexed, and the patellar luxation and behavior are noted, as follows:

Grade I medial patellar luxation: The patella returns to the trochlear sulcus immediately on stifle flexion.

Grade II medial patellar luxation: The patella remains medial to the medial trochlea throughout flexion and extension, but it returns to the sulcus on the release of digital pressure.

Grade III medial patellar luxation: The patella begins medial to the medial trochlea throughout flexion and extension and returns to the sulcus on the application of lateral digital pressure on the patella.

Grade IV medial patellar luxation: The patella begins medial to the medial trochlea throughout flexion and extension and may or may not return to the sulcus on the application of lateral digital pressure on the patella, and it is accompanied by medial retinacular contraction.

In chronic medial patellar luxation in which the patella rides on the medial trochlear ridge, eburnation of joint cartilage may occur, with the effect of leveling the trochlear ridge. If severe fibrosis has occurred, no appreciable medial movement of the patella may be palpated. This malalignment of the patella is usually accompanied by medial tibial tubercle malposition, genu varum, or distal femoral varus. In a severe grade IV medial patellar luxation, the patella may be located on or caudal to the flexion–extension axis of the stifle. In this case, the quadriceps will be ineffective in extension of the stifle or actually may cause flexion of the stifle. This is accompanied by severe medial tibial tubercle malposition, genu varum, or distal femoral varus.

Patients with a straight standing angle of the stifle, such as chows or akitas, are predisposed to medial patellar luxation by a reduction in femoropatellar compression. Normal femoropatellar compression maintains the patella in the trochlear sulcus. Medial patellar luxation is often accompanied by complete or partial rupture of the cranial cruciate ligament, and the cranial drawer sign and tibial compression test must be used. If rupture or incompetence of the cranial cruciate ligament is not addressed, treatment of the medial patellar luxation may fail.

Patients with a luxated or dislocated hip are predisposed to medial patellar luxation because the rectus femoris muscle has a linear pull from its origin just cranial to its insertion on the tibial tubercle. A functional medial pull can be created by the patient that ambulates with an external rotation of the hip and internal rotation of the tibia. This finding is not uncommon in field springer spaniels.

Lateral Patellar Luxations

Testing for lateral patellar luxation is performed by extension of the stifle, external rotation of the stifle, and laterally directed digital pressure on the patella. While the examiner maintains patellar pressure, the patient's knee is flexed, and the patellar luxation and behavior are noted, as follows:

Grade I lateral patellar luxation: The patella returns to the trochlear sulcus immediately on stifle flexion.
Grade II lateral patellar luxation: The patella remains lateral to the lateral trochlea throughout flexion and extension, but it returns to the sulcus on the release of digital pressure.
Grade III lateral patellar luxation: The patella begins lateral to the lateral trochlea throughout flexion and extension and returns to the sulcus on the application of medial digital pressure on the patella.
Grade IV lateral patellar luxation: The patella begins lateral to the lateral trochlea throughout flexion and extension and may or may not return to the sulcus on the application of medial digital pressure on the patella, and it is accompanied by lateral retinacular contraction.

Overall limb alignment assessment is of primary importance because patellar reduction can only be accomplished and maintained when the foot, hock, stifle, and hip are in the sagittal plane. External tibial torsion, genu valgum, OCD of the lateral condyle, and anteversion and valgus of the femoral neck frequently accompany this condition when the stifle is medial to a line between the foot and the hip. Lateral patellar luxation is likely. This condition is often accompanied by a craniomedial rotary instability. Treatment must be directed toward achieving sagittal plane alignment of the foot, hock, tibial tubercle, patella in the trochlear sulcus, and hip. A submissive posture may cause the patient to rotate the stifle externally and may predispose the animal to a lateral patellar luxation.

Meniscectomy

Susan L. Schaefer & Gretchen L. Flo

In the dog, meniscal damage is most commonly seen secondary to disruption of the cranial cruciate ligament. The medial meniscus is injured more often than the lateral because of its tight synovial attachments and subsequent lack of mobility in the unstable stifle. Secondary meniscal damage is also occasionally seen beneath old femoral osteochondritis dissecans lesions or as the result of violent trauma. The purpose of a meniscectomy is to remove torn, crushed, or otherwise damaged meniscal tissue. Two types of meniscectomy procedures are available: total and partial. Total meniscectomy involves removal of 80 to 90% of the meniscal fibrocartilage, including material peripheral to any visible disease. Partial meniscectomy involves the removal of the inner axial "bucket handle" strip of the torn meniscus.

Total Meniscectomy

To perform a total medial meniscectomy, the limb is clipped and prepared in the standard surgical fashion, and the dog is positioned in dorsal recumbency. After a medial parapatellar skin and deep fascia incision, a medial arthrotomy is made, and the patella is luxated laterally (Fig. 62.2). The medial meniscus is best visualized and removed through a medial arthrotomy. If medial meniscal damage is identified through a lateral arthrotomy, it may be beneficial to perform a second, medial arthrotomy for easier removal.

Both menisci are examined directly by "drawering" the tibia forward and moving the stifle through mild extension and flexion to enhance visualization. This drawering motion can be accomplished by placing a small Hohmann retractor in back of the tibia and levering against the nonarticular femoral trochlea. Alternatively, the concave side of a small curved hemostat can be placed under the cranial intermeniscal ligament and levered against the femoral trochlea. A 2-cm plastic sleeve (ethylene oxide sterilized, soft plastic suction tubing) can be placed over the hemostat to protect the femoral articular cartilage from pressure damage.

With moderate to severe instability, the cranial one-half to two-thirds of the C-shaped meniscus can be visualized directly with the tibia in "cranial drawer." In dogs with minimal joint instability from partial cranial cruciate ligament tears or chronic osteoarthritis, meniscal visualization can be more difficult. If necessary, the central portion of the patellar fat pad can be resected to aid visualization (Fig. 62.3). The articular surface of the femoral trochlea and condyles should

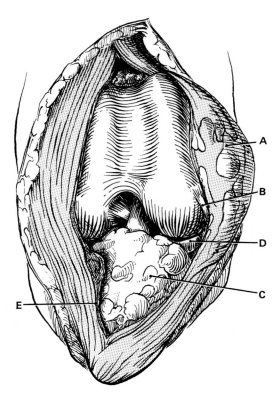

Fig. 62.2. Medial parapatellar arthrotomy: *A,* patella; *B,* long digital extensor tendon; *C,* fat pad; *D,* lateral meniscus; *E,* cut edge of fibrous joint capsule. (From Flo GL, DeYoung D. Meniscal injuries and medial meniscectomy of the canine stifle. J Am Anim Hosp Assoc 1978;14:683.)

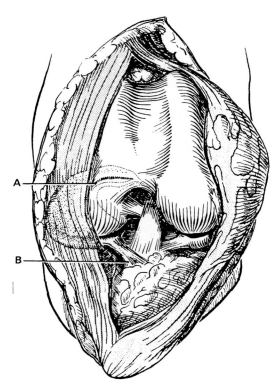

Fig. 62.4. Position of undisplaced torn meniscus in relation to the femoral condyles: *A,* longitudinal tear of the medial meniscus in a reduced position; *B,* cranial ligamentous attachment of the medial meniscus. (The cranial cruciate ligament is left intact for orientation purposes.) (From Flo GL, DeYoung D. Meniscal injuries and medial meniscectomy of the canine stifle. J Am Anim Hosp Assoc 1978;14:683.)

also be examined for evidence of erosive lesions. The presence of such erosive lesions on the weightbearing surface should increase the suspicion of meniscal damage. Common types of meniscal damage include large longitudinal axial "bucket handle" tears and crushing

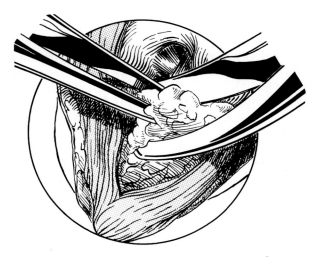

Fig. 62.3. Partial excision of fat pad for exposure if necessary. (From Flo GL, DeYoung D. Meniscal injuries and medial meniscectomy of the canine stifle. J Am Anim Hosp Assoc 1978;14:683.)

parenchymal lesions identified by persistent blood-stained tissue. Less commonly seen are transverse parenchymal tears and extensive peripheral detachments.

A total medial meniscectomy is initiated by transecting the cranial intermeniscal and tibial ligaments that anchor the meniscus to the cranial tibia (Figs. 62.4 and 62.5). This is achieved by placing a hemostat under the ligaments to protect the underlying tibial articular cartilage, while severing them with a scalpel blade. The joint capsule and synovial lining are then retracted medially (abaxially) with a Senn retractor or Kocher's forceps, exposing the cut end of the medial meniscus. The meniscus adheres tightly to the synovium at this position and must be carefully dissected away. A vertical incision is made just peripheral to the cut end of the meniscus close to the division between the meniscus and synovial tissue. A small amount of meniscal tissue may be left attached to the synovium. The meniscus is then grasped with either Kocher's forceps or a meniscal clamp and is drawn laterally (axially) across the joint. With the free portion of the meniscus pulled laterally (axially) and the joint capsule pulled me-

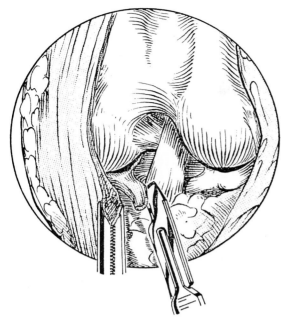

dially (abaxially), sharp vertical dissection separating the meniscus from the joint capsule is continued with either a No. 15 Bard–Parker scalpel blade (Becton–Dickinson, Franklin Lakes, NJ) or a No. 64 Beaver miniblade (Becton–Dickinson) (Fig. 62.6). The syno-

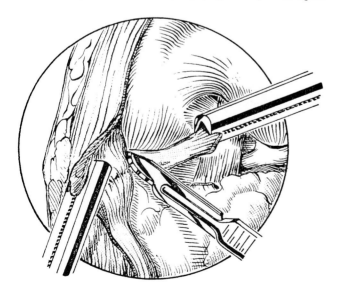

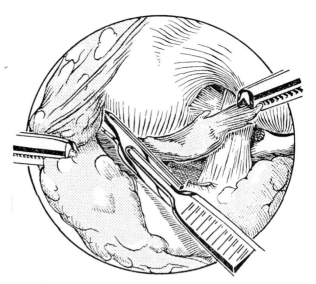

vial–meniscal junction may become visible cranially. If indiscernible, the guideline for the plane of dissection is to "aim" just inside (axial) of the abaxial border of the medial femoral condyle. This dissection must not go medial (abaxial) to the visible edge of the femoral condyle, or damage to the medial collateral ligament may occur. The surgeon may need to use a horizontal cutting angle to resect small femoral–synovial attachments. Vertical dissection continues blindly past the medial collateral ligament. The synovium is continually regrasped close to the undissected meniscus and is retracted for greater exposure (Fig. 62.7). The caudal peripheral synovial attachments are often stretched, torn, or atrophied. Once the dissection has been carried around two-thirds of the meniscus, these atrophied attachments can often be detached by firm axial traction on the meniscus. If not, a valgus stress applied to the stifle opens the joint enough to accommodate continued dissection. Care should be taken to avoid the popliteal vessels immediately caudal to the capsule.

Once detached from the synovium, the meniscus lies in the interior of the joint attached solely by the caudal tibial meniscal ligament. The entire meniscus should be visible if the tibia is "drawered" forward at this time. The resection is completed by placing a scalpel blade under the meniscus at the level of the caudal tibial ligament and slowly pulling the tissue past the cutting edge. This maneuver avoids iatrogenic scalpel blade damage to the caudal cruciate and articular cartilage (Fig. 62.8). The joint is then reexamined to ensure that sufficient meniscal tissue and all cruciate rem-

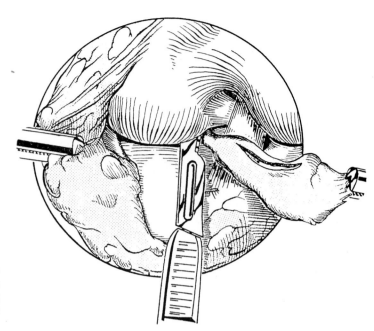

Fig. 62.8. Careful severance of the caudal ligamentous attachment of the medial meniscus. (The cranial cruciate ligament is left intact for orientation purposes.) (From Flo GL, DeYoung D. Meniscal injuries and medial meniscectomy of the canine stifle. J Am Anim Hosp Assoc 1978;14:683.)

nants have been removed. The arthrotomy is closed with absorbable suture in a simple interrupted pattern.

Removal of the lateral meniscus is rarely indicated and is more difficult to perform. The lateral meniscus is most commonly damaged from severe stifle trauma, from contact with an overlying femoral condylar osteochrondritis dissecans lesion, or as the result of a congenital disc-shaped meniscus. In rare instances, lateral meniscal damage may be seen accompanying spontaneous cranial cruciate rupture. The approach to resect a lateral meniscus is easier through a lateral parapatellar arthrotomy. If a lateral meniscal injury is identified from a medial arthrotomy a second, lateral arthrotomy aids in its removal. The resection technique is similar to that for the medial meniscus, except for two important points. The tendon of the long digital extensor obscures access and makes it vulnerable to iatrogenic laceration, and, unlike the medial meniscus, the lateral meniscus has an additional caudal femoromeniscal ligament that must be transected.

Partial Meniscectomy

Localized longitudinal bucket handle tears of the free edge of the meniscus can be removed by partial menisectomy. The torn strip may be grasped with forceps while the peripheral attachments both cranial and caudally are dissected free with a No. 11 or 15 Bard–Parker blade or a No. 64 Beaver miniblade. However, with partial menisectomy, only normal meniscal tissue must remain in the joint. If one has any question about the extent of the damage or tear, the entire meniscus should be removed.

We prefer total meniscectomy because it ensures the removal of damaged fibrocartilage, which may not have been fully detected on visual examination. It also decreases the risk of articular cartilage or caudal cruciate damage, which may occur during partial meniscectomy. Finally, with total meniscectomy, the fibrocartilage is excised to the level of its vascular blood supply. The meniscal vascular supply lies in the outer 25% and must be invaded for regeneration to occur (1, 2). In some human patients undergoing total menisectomy, severe unicompartmental osteoarthritis has been reported later in life, necessitating partial arthroplasty (3–7). We have not seen dogs that have undergone total meniscectomy return later in life with clinical problems. This difference between the human and the dog may be attributed to the shorter life span of the dog.

In animals with trauma-induced multiple ligamentous damage to the stifle, one or both menisci may become partially detached peripherally. If the inner 75% of the meniscal parenchyma is not damaged, the meniscus may be sutured to the synovium.

Postoperative care after meniscectomy should be dictated by the joint stabilization technique. Generally, the stifle should be bandaged for 2 weeks, with activity restricted for a minimum of 6 to 8 weeks. Longer periods of activity restriction may be required for some animals.

References

1. Arnoczky SP, Warren RF. The microvasculature of the meniscus and its response to injury: an experimental study in the dog. Am J Sports Med 1983;11:131–141.

2. DeYoung D, Flo GL, Tvedten HW. Experimental medial meniscectomy in dogs undergoing cranial cruciate ligament repair. J Am Anim Hosp Assoc 1980;16:639–645.
3. Appel H. Late results after meniscectomy in the knee joint: a clinical and roentgenologic follow-up investigation. Acta Orthop Scand Suppl 1970;133:1–111.
4. Lauttamus L, Haikara J, Korkala O. Late results of meniscectomy of the knee: a follow-up study of 41 patients. Ann Chir Gynaecol 1979;68:169–171.
5. Tapper EM, Hoover NW. Late results after meniscectomy. J Bone Joint Surg Am 1969;51:517–526.
6. Kozinn SC, Scott RD. Surgical treatment of unicompartmental degenerative arthritis of the knee. Rheum Dis Clin North Am 1988;14:545–564.
7. Scott RD, Santore RF. Unicondylar unicompartmental replacement for osteoarthritis of the knee. J Bone Joint Surg Am 1981;63:536–544.

Meniscal Release

Barclay Slocum & Theresa Devine Slocum

The meniscal release is an original surgical procedure designed for use with the tibial plateau leveling osteotomy, an operation for rupture of the cranial cruciate ligament (CCL) that reduces the effects of the cranial tibial thrust to inconsequential levels. The meniscal release is the incision of the lateral attachment of the caudal horn of the medial meniscus or an incision of the caudal horn of the medial meniscus. The purpose of the meniscal release is to allow the caudal horn of the medial meniscus to move away from the medial femoral condyle during cranial translation of the tibia.

Surgical Procedure

Complete Cranial Cruciate Ligament Ruptures

Meniscal release of the caudal horn of the medial meniscus can be performed through a medial parapatellar arthrotomy. Complete rupture of the CCL is necessary to obtain access to the caudal horn of the medial meniscus. After debridement of the remnants of the CCL, a stifle retractor is placed in the void lateral to the caudal cruciate ligament where the CCL had been attached before rupture. The retractor is hooked over the caudal aspect of the tibial plateau, and leverage on the cranial aspect of the intercondylar notch causes cranial translation of the tibia. A headlight may be necessary in stifles with chronic degenerative joint disease to allow adequate visualization of the caudal horn of the medial meniscus. The damaged portion of the caudal horn of the medial meniscus is excised. A sagittal incision is made completely through the caudal horn of the medial meniscus just medial to its lateral attachment on the intercondyloid eminence (Fig. 62.9). The arthrotomy is closed routinely.

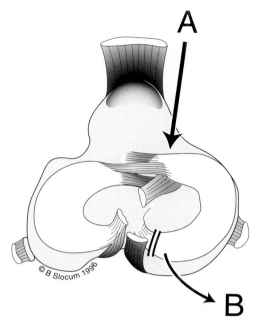

Fig. 62.9. Meniscal release for complete cranial cruciate ligament ruptures. Access to the joint is made through a craniomedial incision (A). After cranially luxating the tibia using a stifle retractor, a sagittal incision is made completely through the caudal horn of the medial meniscus just medial to its lateral attachment on the intercondyloid eminence. This gives the caudal horn of the medial meniscus the freedom to move (B).

Advanced Partial Cranial Cruciate Ligament Ruptures

Meniscal release of the caudal horn of the medial meniscus can be performed through a medial arthrotomy just caudal to the medial collateral ligament. This form of meniscal release is used when the meniscus is first impinged but before the caudal horn of the medial meniscus is crushed, because access is limited through this approach. The CCL is at the stage of advanced partial rupture. An incision is made parallel and caudal to the medial collateral ligament from the level of the medial fabella to just proximal to the insertion of the tibial head of the semimembranosus muscle. The stifle is extended, a maneuver that moves the medial collateral ligament cranially. A small Gelpi retractor is helpful to hold the caudal joint capsule open. A Senn retractor is used to pull the tibial head of the semimembranosus distally, to expose the caudomedial border of the medial meniscus. A transecting incision of the medial meniscus begins at the caudal margin of the medial collateral ligament and is directed 30° cranial to the frontal plane (Fig. 62.10). Three sutures are necessary to close the incision in the joint capsule.

Rupture of the CCL is a common injury in the canine stifle. In a CCL–deficient stifle, the cranial tibial thrust causes cranial translation of the tibia. Because

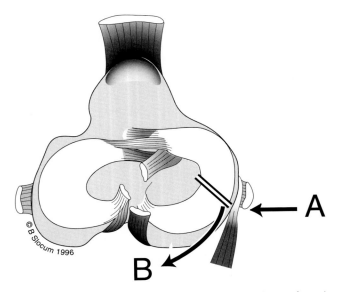

Fig. 62.10. Meniscal release with advanced partial cruciate ligament ruptures. An incision (A) is made caudal to the medial collateral ligament. Using retraction to hold the joint capsule open, a transecting incision of the medial meniscus is made 30° cranial to the frontal plane. The caudal horn of the medial meniscus is given freedom to move caudolaterally (B).

the CCL is the primary passive restraint to cranial translation, without an intact CCL, the cranial tibial motion is opposed by the caudal horn of the menisci.

The caudal horn of the lateral meniscus is mobile and rarely becomes impinged between the femoral condyle and the tibial plateau, because the axis of rotation of the stifle is located on the medial tibial plateau under the medial femoral condyle. The lateral condyle translates caudally on the tibial plateau as a natural part of internal rotation. The attachments of the lateral meniscus to the tibia are located so the lateral meniscus can accommodate cranial translation whether through rotation or translation.

The caudal horn of the medial meniscus is attached to the medial aspect of the medial intercondyloid eminence and to the short portion of the medial collateral ligament. These two points of meniscal attachment form a firm medial and lateral anchor for the caudal horn of the medial meniscus that prevents the caudal horn of the medial meniscus from moving caudally. The triangular cross section of the caudal horn of the medial meniscus and the nature of its tibial attachments create a firmly anchored chock caudal to the medial femoral condyle. This is the second passive restraint to cranial tibial thrust and opposes the cranial translation of the tibia with respect to the femur. If the tibia is prevented from translating cranially by the caudal horn of the medial meniscus, that structure is excessively and repeatedly compressed between the tibial plateau and the femoral condyle, causing it to

undergo metaplasia from a supple three-dimensional weave of collagen to a woody-textured meniscus of fibrocartilage. Such alteration in the structure creates a painful yet intact-appearing meniscus that is predisposed to calcification. If the tibia does translate cranially with the rupture of the CCL, the caudal horn of the medial meniscus is crushed between the tibial plateau and the femoral condyle.

A crushed meniscus has several forms in gross appearance. The caudal horn may have a "bucket handle" tear that has split free from the caudal vascular portion and projects cranial to the femoral condyle at the time of the medial parapatellar arthrotomy. The caudal horn may be crushed without being split from the caudal vascular portion, and may appear as flattened tissue when the tibia is pulled cranially at the time of arthrotomy. The more subtle form of damage is the split of the caudal horn of the medial meniscus on the ventral surface that cannot be seen without removing the meniscus. This type of injury allows slip beneath the femoral condyle during cranial tibial translation, yet the dorsal surface of the caudal horn of the medial meniscus appears intact.

A patient with a partial rupture of the CCL usually has no damage to the caudal horn of the medial meniscus, but just pain after vigorous exercise from meniscal pinching. As a partial rupture of the CCL progresses under the influence of cranial tibial thrust, the CCL becomes incompetent before it ruptures completely. At the stage of incompetence the meniscus first becomes acutely damaged. If the CCL has been ruptured completely, the caudal horn of the medial meniscus usually is damaged.

The traditional means of addressing a damaged caudal horn of the medial meniscus is to remove any damaged portion of the meniscus. Because healing of the avascular portion of the meniscus is unlikely, removal of any damaged portion of the meniscus is appropriate surgical therapy. Many menisci are apparently uninjured at the time of surgical correction, and they become injured subsequent to surgical intervention for CCL deficiency. The cause is the inability of traditional cruciate surgical techniques to stabilize the stifle in function, a situation that allows the cranial tibial thrust to create impingement of the caudal horn of the medial meniscus.

A meniscal release alters the function of the medial meniscus. The immediate stabilizing function of the caudal horn of the medial meniscus is lost if this surgical procedure is performed, but more important, the meniscus-crushing effect by the femoral condyle is avoided. The effectiveness of the meniscal release was demonstrated in a clinical evaluation of 212 stifles over a 4-year period, in conjunction with the tibial plateau leveling osteotomy for CCL rupture. No reinjury of the meniscus occurred with the meniscal release. The long-term effects on healing of the meniscal release site, the integrity of the tension band ring, and the effect on degenerative joint disease have not yet been determined. What can be stated truly with regard to the meniscal release, however, is that this surgical procedure is successful in preventing injury to the caudal horn of the medial meniscus when the operation is combined with a tibial plateau leveling osteotomy.

"Over-the-Top" Patellar Tendon Graft for Cranial Cruciate Ligament Repair

Steven P. Arnoczky

The cranial cruciate ligament constrains joint motion. It prevents cranial subluxation of the tibia on the femur (cranial drawer sign), hyperextension of the stifle joint, and, along with the caudal cruciate ligament, excessive internal rotation of the tibia on the femur (1). Excessive forces during extremes of any of these movements damage this ligament (2). Although excessive trauma causes acute rupture of the cranial cruciate ligament, most cruciate ligament lesions are thought to result from chronic degenerative changes within the ligaments themselves (2, 3). Variations in conformation, valgus (knock-knee) and varus (bowleg) deformities of the stifle, and repeated minor stresses can result in progressive degenerative joint disease. As these joint changes develop, the cruciate ligaments undergo alterations in their microstructure and may be more susceptible to damage from minor trauma (4).

Because rupture of the cranial cruciate ligament results in progressive degenerative joint changes within the joint (3, 5, 6), most such injuries should be repaired. Some chronic cases of cranial cruciate ligament rupture, however, may have an unfavorable prognosis after surgical repair because severe degenerative joint changes are present. In these patients, conservative management with anti-inflammatory drugs and somatic pain relievers may provide adequate palliative care. Moreover, concurrent joint diseases, such as rheumatoid arthritis and systemic lupus erythematosus, may obviate the repair of the ligament insufficiently.

Whereas extra-articular repairs stabilize the joint by tightening or altering the position of extra-articular structures, intra-articular repairs anatomically replace the cranial cruciate ligament with some type of graft. The over-the-top procedure (7) is an intra-articular

repair that uses a patellar tendon graft to replace the cranial cruciate ligament. This procedure was designed for use in dogs weighing more than 15 kg. In my experience, most extra-articular repairs do not produce long-term joint stability in larger dogs. The over-the-top patellar tendon graft provides a functional replacement for the cranial cruciate ligament and thereby limits any abnormal joint motion.

Surgical Technique

The animal is placed in lateral recumbency, and the affected limb is prepared for an aseptic surgical procedure. A lateral parapatellar skin incision is made extending from the midshaft of the femur to the proximal tibia. The subcutaneous and fascial tissues are dissected free, and the patellar ligament is clearly defined. The patellar ligament is incised longitudinally between the junction of the middle and medial thirds of its width. The incision is extended over the patella and into the patellar tendon, where it is directed in a proximolateral direction to incorporate the fascia lata (Fig. 62.11**A**). The incision proximal to the patella should be made 1 to 1.5 times the distance from the patella to the tibial tuberosity; this incision ensures an adequate length of graft in dogs of all sizes.

An osteotome is placed in the groove of the patella created by the scalpel blade, and a craniomedial wedge of bone is removed with the medial third of the patellar tendon and ligament attached (Fig. 62.11**B**). Extreme care should be taken during the osteotomy to preserve the entire articular surface of the patella. The medial third of the patellar ligament is then dissected free to the level of the tibial tuberosity. An incision through the infrapatellar fat pad is necessary to mobilize the graft, but the fat pad should not be stripped from its ligamentous attachments because it provides much of the blood supply to the patellar ligament. To free the proximal fascial portion of the graft, an incision extending proximal and parallel to the initial incision is made in the joint capsule at the medial border of the patellar ligament. An autogenous graft consisting of fascia, patellar tendon, a patellar bone wedge, and patellar ligament with a distal attachment to the tibial tuberosity is thus created (Fig. 62.11**C**).

The remnants of the ruptured cranial cruciate ligament are then removed through the medial arthrotomy, and the joint is inspected for further pathologic features. The patella, joint capsule, and soft tissues are retracted laterally to expose the lateral femoral condyle and fabella (Fig. 62.11**D**). The lateral fabella is located by palpation, and a small vertical incision is made in the femorofabellar ligament. With the joint in extreme flexion, curved hemostatic forceps are inserted into the incision and are passed over the top of the lateral femoral condyle and into the intercondylar

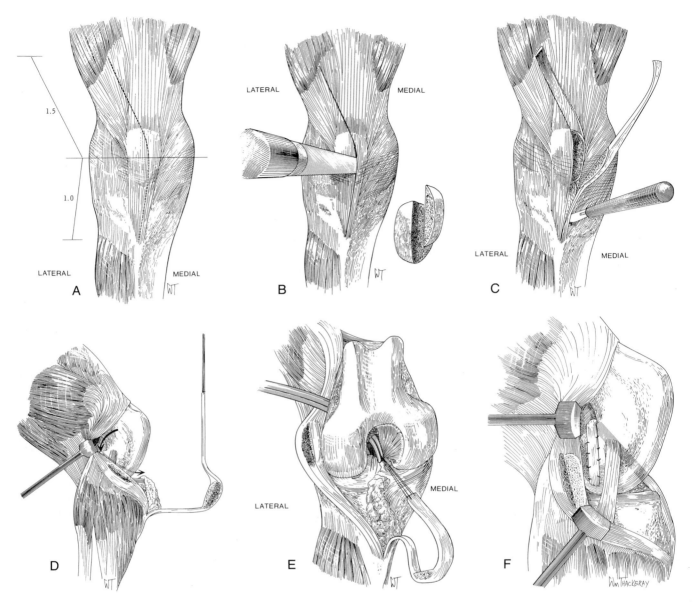

Fig. 62.11. Over-the-top patellar tendon graft. **A.** Cranial view of the stifle showing the location of the initial incision for the proposed graft. The proximal portion of the incision is directed laterally to incorporate the fascia lata. **B.** Placement of osteotome to remove craniomedial wedge of patella with accompanying soft tissue. The *inset* shows cranial view of the patella indicating the extent of the osteotomy, which does not extend to the caudal articular surface of the patella. **C.** The graft is completed by incising the joint capsule, patellar tendon, and fascia lata parallel to the initial incision and by freeing the graft at its proximal end. **D.** Lateral view of the stifle showing retraction of the patella and soft tissues of the joint laterally to expose the lateral femoral condyle and fabella. *Arrows* indicate the path of the hemostatic forceps over the top of the lateral femoral condyle and into the joint. **E.** Cranial view of flexed stifle showing tips of the hemostatic forceps emerging lateral to the caudal cruciate ligament and grasping the sutures in the free end of the graft. **F.** Lateral view of the stifle showing the graft passing through the joint and over the top of the lateral femoral condyle. The graft is then sutured to the soft tissues of the lateral femoral condyle. (From Arnoczky SP, Tarvin GB, Marshall JL, et al. The over-the-top procedure: a technique for anterior cruciate ligament substitution in the dog. J Am Anim Hosp Assoc 1979;15:283.)

notch; one must take care to preserve the caudal joint structures by staying close to the bone. The tips of the hemostatic forceps are gently manipulated until they can be seen within the joint (Fig. 62.11**D** and **E**). After a suture is placed in the free end of the graft, the suture is grasped with the hemostat. The graft is gently pulled

through the joint and over the top of the lateral condyle by gentle traction on the hemostat. Flexing and extending the joint during this maneuver facilitate passage of the graft.

After the graft has been pulled through the joint, it is held under gentle traction, and the joint is tested for craniocaudal stability. Once cranial drawer motion has been eliminated, the graft is attached to the lateral femoral condyle. With traction maintained and the leg in a functional position (approximately 35 to 40° of flexion), the graft is sutured to the tissues of the lateral femoral condyle with simple interrupted sutures of nonabsorbable suture material (Fig. 62.11F). Alternatively, a screw and spiked washer can be used to secure the tissue to the lateral femoral condyle. The incision in the femorofabellar ligament then is closed with simple interrupted sutures.

The arthrotomy is closed in a routine manner. During closure of the medial arthrotomy, care should be taken to avoid excessive tension on the patella and patellar ligament, which may predispose the joint to a medial luxation of the patella. If tension is a problem, loose approximation sutures should be placed in the joint capsule, and the subcutaneous soft tissues should be used to cover the arthrotomy defect.

Postoperatively, the limb is placed in a modified Robert Jones dressing for 2 weeks, and the animal's activity is restricted for a total of 4 weeks. In larger dogs (over 30 kg), a lateral splint is added for the first 2 postoperative weeks, and activity is restricted for a total of 4 to 6 weeks.

The biologic fate of the patellar tendon graft within the joint was investigated in an experimental study (8). The results of this study demonstrate that if the blood supply of the graft is disrupted at the time of surgery, approximately 20 weeks are needed for the graft to become completely revascularized. During this period, the graft undergoes ischemic necrosis, and its strength may be at risk. In an effort to minimize this revascularization process, my colleagues and I proposed a modification of the over-the-top technique in which the medial vascular supply of the patellar tendon graft is carefully preserved and maintained (9). We suggested that if a "vascularized" patellar tendon graft were used to reconstruct the cranial cruciate ligament, the revascularization and remodeling process would be eliminated, or at least minimized. Furthermore, the use of a vascularized patellar tendon graft would prevent, or at least minimize, any changes in the material strength of the graft secondary to the ischemic changes or revascularization process. However, a subsequent study evaluating the strength of vascularized and nonvascularized patellar tendon grafts with time failed to demonstrate any significant differences in any of their biomechanical parameters with time (10). It thus appears that there is no inherent advantage of preserving the blood supply to the graft at the time of surgery.

Several other modifications of the over-the-top graft technique have been proposed and have produced good results (7, 9, 11). Although these techniques use other tissues for the graft (fascia lata, lateral

aspect of the patellar tendon) and may include the addition of other ancillary stabilization procedures (lateral imbrication suture), they all incorporate the over-the-top femoral positioning of the intra-articular graft. The over-the-top positioning allows the most consistent placement of the graft in the most biomechanically and anatomically correct position (Fig. 62.12). In my opinion, this positioning may be the most important consideration in intra-articular reconstructions of the cranial cruciate ligament. Indeed, an evaluation of two over-the-top techniques by Denny and Barr suggests that this biomechanically correct placement of the graft, and not the type of graft used, is responsible for the success of this repair technique (12).

In summary, successful repair of insufficiency of the cranial cruciate ligament depends on the reestablishment of joint stability. Although this end can be accomplished by the aforementioned techniques, other components of the stifle (patella, menisci, collateral ligaments) must not be overlooked when evaluating the joint. These structures work in concert to allow normal joint motion, and failure to recognize concurrent patellar malalignment or meniscal injury in cra-

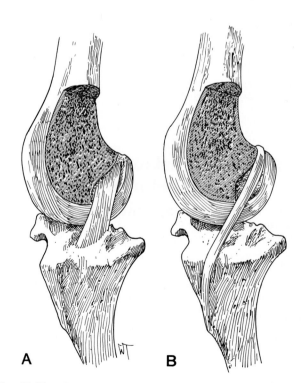

Fig. 62.12. Schematic illustration of the normal anatomy and spatial orientation of the cranial cruciate ligament (**A**) and the orientation of the patellar tendon graft within the joint that is achieved with the over-the-top technique (**B**). (From Arnoczky SP, Tarvin GB, Marshall JL, et al. The over-the-top procedure: a technique for anterior cruciate ligament substitution in the dog. J Am Anim Hosp Assoc 1979;15:283.)

nial cruciate ligament insufficiency may result in less than optimal postoperative function.

References

1. Arnoczky SP, Marshall JL. The cruciate ligaments of the canine stifle: an anatomical and functional analysis. Am J Vet Res 1977;38:1807.
2. Arnoczky SP, Marshall JL. Pathomechanics of cruciate and meniscal injuries. In: Bojrab MJ, ed. Pathophysiology of small animal surgery. Philadelphia: Lea & Febiger, 1981.
3. Arnoczky SP. Surgery of the stifle: the cruciate ligaments. Compend Contin Educ Pract Vet 1980;2:106.
4. Vasseur PB, Pool RR, Arnoczky SP, et al. Correlative biomechanical and histologic study of the cranial cruciate ligament in dogs. Am J Vet Res 1985;46:1842.
5. Hulse DA, Michaelson F, Johnson C, et al. A technique for reconstruction of the anterior cruciate ligament in the dog: preliminary report. Vet Surg 1980;9:135.
6. Strande A. Repair of the ruptured cranial cruciate ligament in the dog. Baltimore: Williams & Wilkins, 1967.
7. Arnoczky SP, Tarvin GB, Marshall JL, et al. The over-the-top procedure: a technique for anterior cruciate ligament substitution in the dog. J Am Anim Hosp Assoc 1979;15:283.
8. Arnoczky SP, Tarvin GB, Marshall JL. Anterior cruciate ligament replacement using patellar tendon: an evaluation of graft revascularization in the dog. J Bone Joint Surg Am 1982;64:217.
9. Boudrieau RJ, et al. Vascularized patellar tendon graft technique for cranial cruciate ligament substitution in the dog: vascular evaluation. Vet Surg 1985;14:196.
10. Butler DL, et al. Mechanical properties of primate vascularized vs. nonvascularized patellar tendon grafts: changes over time. J Orthop Res 1989;7:68–79.
11. Shires PK, Hulse DA, Liu W. The under-and-over fascial replacement technique for anterior cruciate ligament rupture in dogs: a retrospective study. J Am Anim Hosp Assoc 1984;20:69.
12. Denny HR, Barr ARS. An evaluation of two "over the top" techniques for anterior cruciate ligament replacement in the dog. J Small Anim Pract 1984;25:759.

Cranial Cruciate Ligament Repair by Fibular Head Transposition

Gail K. Smith

Fibular head transposition (FHT) is an extracapsular surgical technique to stabilize the cranial cruciate ligament–deficient stifle (1). Cranial advancement of the fibular head with its attached insertion of the lateral collateral ligament (LCL) fixes the stifle in external rotation. Cranial drawer motion is prevented by the combined tensioning of the medial and LCLs. Biomechanical testing has shown the resistance to drawer occasioned by FHT to be superior to other popular methods of stifle reconstruction (2). As in other forms of lateral extracapsular stifle reconstruction techniques, elimination of cranial drawer is achieved through sacrifice of normal tibial rotation about its

central axis. Knee motion, therefore, is not kinematically normal, but rather it is more like a pure "hinge-type" joint. This factor notwithstanding, clinical trials have reported the efficacy of this method (1, 3, 4) to be equal or superior to other forms of stifle reconstruction.

Surgical Technique

The anesthetized patient is placed in lateral recumbency, the affected extremity is prepared aseptically, and a sterile impervious stockinette is used to cover the leg completely (1). A craniolateral, parapatellar skin incision is made beginning at the distal one-third of the femur and extended distally to the proximal one-third of the tibia. The edges of the stockinette are sutured to the skin to establish a skin barrier. A routine stifle arthrotomy and joint exploratory and debridement are performed. After thorough joint lavage with isotonic saline, the joint capsule is closed using simple interrupted absorbable sutures.

Using Metzenbaum scissors, the lateral retinaculum is freed from the underlying capsule. The distal end of the incision in the retinaculum is extended through the tough fibrous iliotibial band at its attachment to Gerdy's tubercle (human nomenclature) and then is continued 2 to 3 cm distal to the level of the fibular head. The retinaculum is retracted caudally to reveal the underlying fibular and cranial tibial musculature. The peroneal nerve must be identified, although it is not commonly visible because of its investment in fat. It courses proximocaudally to distocranially over the lateral head of the gastrocnemius muscle before going out of view under the fibularis longus muscle (Fig. 62.13). If not visible, the nerve can be palpated by gently strumming across its fibers with one's index finger. The location of the fibular head and LCL is determined by palpating through the thin overlying fascia and soft tissue. Identification of the LCL is facilitated by manipulating or rotating the tibia relative to the femur causing the ligament to become taut and therefore more easily palpable. An incision is made into the deep fascia cranial to the femoral origin of the LCL and is continued distally parallel to the LCL, crossing the femorotibial joint line and extending through the thin fascia overlying the separation between the fibularis longus muscle and the tibialis cranialis muscle (see Fig. 62.13). The natural separation between these two muscle bellies is developed in a craniomedial direction to the level of the bony sulcus muscularis of the proximal tibia. A sharp periosteal elevator is used to cut the periosteum parallel to the tibial axis and to elevate it and its overlying muscles (cranial tibial and long digital extensor) from the tibia. The periosteum is elevated cranially toward the tibial tuberosity and crest. Caudal to the periosteal incision,

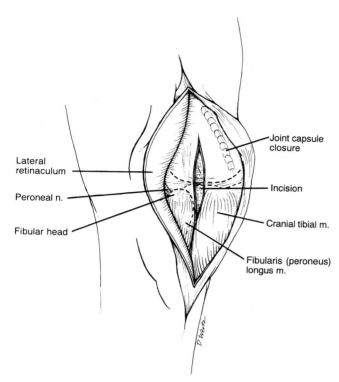

Fig. 62.13. Illustration showing the incision into the deep fascia cranial to the fibular head–lateral collateral ligament (LCL) complex. Note the reflection of the lateral retinaculum and the position of the peroneal nerve. Neither the LCL nor the fibular head is visualized directly in this exposure, however, both are readily palpable.

the fibularis longus is sharply excised from its origin on the proximal tibia. The fibular origin of this muscle is left intact. The proximal lateral portion of the tibia (sulcus muscularis) is now exposed.

The cut edge of the deep fascia at the level of the proximal fibular head is picked up with forceps. This maneuver tenses the fibrous attachments securing the fibula to the tibia. A scalpel (No. 15 or 10 blade) is used to incise these fibrous attachments, dissecting along the bony contour of the proximal tibia and joint line from cranial to caudal. The dissection proceeds until the small syndesmotic attachment of the fibula to the tibia is visualized at the caudolateral corner of the tibial plateau. *At no point in the dissection is the fibular head itself exposed other than the actual tibiofibular articulation. The lateral surface of the fibular head remains covered by muscle and ligamentous attachments.* The scalpel blade is directed along the planar surface between the fibula and tibia, and the cranial and caudal fibular ligaments are cut (Fig. 62.14). In large dogs or those with chronic stifle arthrosis, a sharp, broad periosteal elevator aids in performing this part of the procedure. *Caution should be used because the fibular head is a small, flat bone that can be overpowered easily and fractured when one tries to free it from the tibia by injudicious use of the periosteal*

elevator. Fibular head fracture is most commonly associated with the learning process. The recommendation is to cut (rather than bluntly tear) the fibers holding the fibula to the tibia.

With the attachments of the fibular head cut, the LCL is separated from its underlying attachments proximal to the level of its femoral origin. Once freed, the fibular head–LCL complex should move easily both cranially and caudomedially relative to its original attachment. The fibular head is retracted caudally to provide wide exposure to the bony surface of the proximal tibia to receive the fibular head. The area is prepared

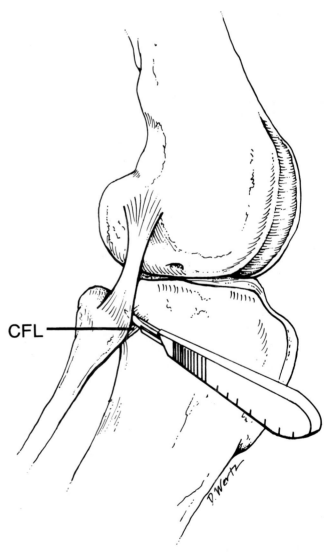

Fig. 62.14. The syndesmotic attachment of the fibular head to the proximal tibia is incised sharply using a No. 15 or No. 10 scalpel blade, depending on the size of the dog. The scalpel should be positioned so as to follow the plane of the fibulotibial articulation. Complete separation of the fibular head–lateral collateral ligament complex from underlying attachments is required to facilitate cranial transposition of the fibular head. *CFL*, cranial fibular ligament.

by scraping with an elevator or curette down to bone, and, if necessary, a rongeur is used to smooth any rough bony irregularities. The ultimate position at which the LCL crosses the joint line should be anticipated, and this area, particularly, should be smooth and free of protrusions or osteophytes.

To preplace the orthopedic wire, two holes are drilled in the tibial crest under the craniolateral tibial musculature using a 0.0625-inch (1.59-mm) Steinmann pin (Fig. 62.15). The proximal hole starts cranial to the fibular head and is directed caudolaterally to craniomedially exiting on the proximomedial surface of the tibial crest. A 20-cm length of straight 18-gauge orthopedic wire (20-gauge for dogs under 16 kg) is inserted through the hole. A second hole is drilled in the same direction but approximately 0.5 to 1.0 cm distal to the first. As the pin is backed out of the hole, the free end of wire on the medial side is made to follow the pin through the hole to exit on the lateral side of the tibial crest. The two ends of the wire are pulled firmly to seat the wire loop securely (see Fig. 62.15). To secure the fibular head to the tibia, a Steinmann pin (1.1 to 3.2 mm, depending on size of

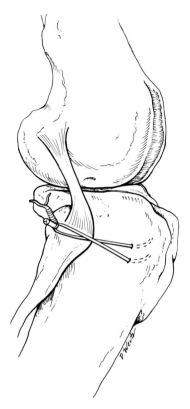

Fig. 62.16. Illustration showing the lateral-to-medial pin orientation and the tightening of the figure-of-eight wire to adjust and secure pin position. Note the new orientation of the lateral collateral ligament *CFL, cranial fibular ligament.*

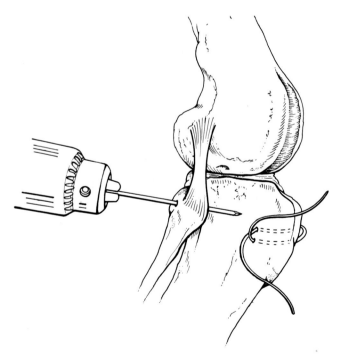

Fig. 62.15. Two holes are drilled into the tibial crest cranial to the proposed site of fibular head attachment, and a wire (18- or 20-gauge) is preplaced. A Steinmann pin is drilled through the caudal half of the proximal fibular head, and the pin tip is advanced onto the proximal tibia in preparation for levering the fibular head craniad. To aid in pin placement, the tibia is put into hard external rotation with the knee in a neutral position. The tip of the pin is placed at the appropriate location on the flare of the proximal tibia cranial to the fibular head. The pin is gently levered with Jacob's chuck until it can be fully seated into the tibia in a lateral-to-medial direction.

dog) is drilled through the proximal and caudal third of the fibular head perpendicular to the plane of the fibular head. *Care is taken to avoid the cranial half of the fibular head, where the LCL attaches.* After passing through the thin fibular head, the pin tip is brought into the area previously prepared to receive the fibula (see Fig. 62.15). To seat the pin optimally, the tibia is first placed into hard external rotation (for big dogs an assistant is helpful) with the stifle in a neutral position. The surgeon then inserts the tip of the pin cranial to the fibular head on the cortical flare of the proximal tibia and gently levers the pin with Jacob's chuck until the pin can be seated into the tibia in a lateral-to-medial direction (Fig. 62.16). *The pin is much stronger than the fibular head, and the surgeon has great mechanical advantage during the levering procedure, so care must be exercised to avoid fracturing the fibular head.* Some surgeons prefer to use a self-retaining retractor to pull and hold the fibular head into a craniad position on the proximal tibia. Here again, care must be exercised not to overpower the strength of the fibular head. After the pin is seated firmly into the tibia, drawer movement should be retested. If drawer movement is not markedly reduced after pin placement, the pin should be withdrawn and placed into a more craniad position on the proximal tibia.

To maintain pin position or, if necessary, as a means to advance the fibular head further craniad, the two wire ends are crossed in figure-of-eight fashion and are twisted caudal to the pin (see Fig. 62.16). With the stifle in a neutral position (approximately 120°) the wire is tightened to eliminate all cranial drawer and to minimize internal tibial rotation. *The wire may fracture the fibular head as overtightening occurs.* When sufficient stability is achieved, the twisted end of wire is cut approximately three turns from the pin and is tucked under the superficial tissue plane onto the surface of the flexor hallucis longus muscle in a caudomedial direction from the pin. The pin is then driven (mallet and impactor) down to the level of the wire so both pin and wire are in a tissue plane medial to that of the peroneal nerve (see Fig. 62.16).

Closure begins with a vertical vest-over-pants imbrication of the lateral retinaculum in an effort to derotate the tibia externally dynamically when the biceps femoris muscle contracts during gait. Particular attention should be directed to overlap and suture the fibrous part of the lateral retinaculum (iliotibial band) that formerly inserted on the bony prominence (Gerdy's tubercle) immediately lateral to the tibial tuberosity. Subcutaneous tissues and skin are closed in routine fashion. Postoperative pain management is achieved by intra-articular injection of 0.5% bupivacaine HCl (Marcaine) at 0.5 mL/kg (5).

Postoperative care consists of a soft, padded, Robert Jones–type bandage for 2 weeks accompanied by 8 full weeks of activity restricted to leash walking only. Thereafter, the dog gradually can be eased back into normal activity. Large or obese dogs may require supplemental aluminum or lateral plaster coaptation to add support and to keep the bandage positioned proximally on the femur. For the occasional dog presenting with acute bilateral cranial cruciate ligament tears, both stifles may be repaired at the same time. If so, no padded bandages are applied to facilitate early, but controlled, ambulation.

The method of FHT has been considered by many surgeons to be technically difficult. Reported technical complications include accidental transection of the LCL, iatrogenic injury to the peroneal nerve, laceration of the caudal geniculate artery, and fracture of the fibular head (3). These complications are rare in the hands of the experienced surgeon. Accordingly, ample practice on cadavers is recommended to acquire expertise in performing the method before use on client-owned animals. Mechanically, the technique of FHT has superior stability immediately postoperatively when compared with other popular methods of stifle reconstruction (2). Unfortunately, the long-term stabilities of stifle reconstruction methods have been

poorly studied. Clinically, surgeons have long been aware that cranial drawer in some dogs increases with time irrespective of surgical method used. Experimentally, a report by Dupuis and associates showed that the LCL hypertrophies approximately 300% after FHT, increasing in strength and stiffness 33 and 36%, respectively, yet elongating only 7% by 10 months postoperatively (6). A companion study, however, concluded that FHT did not control cranial drawer and permitted meniscal degeneration in 50% of experimental dogs at 10 months postoperatively (7). This study was criticized for deficiencies in experimental design, the most noteworthy inadequate experimental control; that is, the protocol was not applied to other popular methods of stifle reconstruction (8). To add perspective, Smith and associates reported on the long-term (1 year) functional and biomechanical evaluation of experimental dogs treated with the fascial strip and patellar tendon intra-articular repairs (9). The intra-articular methods of cranial cruciate ligament repair were associated with higher frequencies of meniscal damage (determined at necropsy) and greater cranial drawer (mechanically measured) than those reported for FHT in the study by Dupuis and colleagues (7). In further support of this position, a clinical report comparing FHT, lateral retinacular imbrication, and the "four in one" intra-articular method found FHT to be associated with a significantly lower rate of return for second arthrotomy because of poor clinical outcome and secondary meniscal injury (4).

From this discussion, it is clear that although FHT may yield better clinical outcomes, none of the popular methods of stifle reconstruction consistently achieve the desired surgical objectives of long-term stability and prevention of progressive degenerative joint disease. To foster good client communication, the surgeon must convey this clinical reality to the patient's owners at the time of original orthopedic examination and diagnosis. Until the many stifle reconstruction methods are directly compared using standardized experimental protocols (including histopathology, mechanical testing, and force plate analysis), selection of surgical technique should be based on the skill level of the surgeon and what empirically works best in his or her hands.

References

1. Smith GK, Torg JS. Fibular head transposition for repair of the cruciate–deficient stifle in the dog. J Am Vet Med Assoc 1985;187:375–383.
2. Patterson RH, Smith GK, Gregor TP, et al. Biomechanical stability of four cranial cruciate ligament repair techniques in the dog. Vet Surg 1991;20:85–90.
3. Mullen HS, Matthiesen DT. Complications of transposition of the fibular head for stabilization of the cranial cruciate–deficient stifle in dogs: 80 cases (1982–1986). J Am Vet Med Assoc 1989;195:1267–1271.

4. Metelman LA, Schwarz PD, Salman M, et al. An evaluation of three different cranial cruciate ligament surgical stabilization procedures as they relate to postoperative meniscal injuries. Vet Comp Orthop Traumatol 1994;8:118–123.
5. Sammarco JL, Conzemius MG, Perkowski SZ, et al. Postoperative analgesia for stifle surgery: a comparison of intra-articular bupivicaine, morphine, or saline. Vet Surg 1996;25:59–69.
6. Dupuis J, Harari J, Blackletter DM, et al. Evaluation of lateral collateral ligament after fibular head transposition in dogs. Vet Surg 1994;23:456–465.
7. Dupuis J, Harari J, Papageorges M, et al. Evaluation of fibular head transposition for repair of experimental cranial cruciate ligament injury in dogs. Vet Surg 1994;23:1–12.
8. Smith GK. Perspective missing in fibular head transposition study. Vet Surg 23:286–288,1994.
9. Smith GK, Chen EH, Clemow AJT. Long-term functional and biomechanical evaluation of fascial strip substitution for repair of the cruciate–deficient stifle in dogs. In: Proceedings of the 21st annual meeting of the Veterinary Orthopedic Society.: Veterinary Orthopedic Society, 1994:3.

Cranial Cruciate Ligament Repair by Modified Retinacular Imbrication Technique

Susan L. Schaefer & Gretchen L. Flo

The purpose of the modified retinacular imbrication technique (MRIT) is to provide extracapsular stabilization of the stifle after partial or full rupture of the cranial cruciate ligament. The technique described here is a slight modification of Flo's original procedure because the fabellar–patella stabilizing suture is now rarely incorporated. The overall objective is to place stabilizing sutures from both the medial and lateral fabella to the tibial tuberosity. The intention is for these sutures to mimic the activity of the cranial cruciate ligament in the sagittal plane, eliminating cranial drawer movement when tightened. Although these sutures stabilize the stifle on a short-term basis, it is theorized that fibrous tissue laid along the suture track maintains long-term stability. Suture size and the number of sutures used vary by case and are reviewed in the discussion.

Before extra-articular stabilization of the stifle, an arthrotomy always should be performed and the joint thoroughly examined. Any remaining tags of the cranial cruciate ligament are removed, and both menisci are examined. If necessary, a meniscectomy should be performed and any large, rough osteophytes may be removed. The joint capsule is then closed with a synthetic absorbable suture in a simple interrupted pattern.

The MRIT is begun by identifying both fabellae. The fabellae are located caudomedial and caudolateral to the joint. In surgery, their position can be approximated by moving either medially or laterally at the level of the distal third of the patella. A cutdown should be performed through the insertions of the sartorius medially and the biceps femoris laterally to aid in suture placement. Medially, a longitudinal incision is made in the fibrous insertion of the caudal head of the sartorius muscle at the level of the patella (Fig. 62.17). With the caudal sartorius muscle retracted caudally, the medial fabella should be palpable under the medial head of the gastrocnemius muscle (Fig. 62.18). Laterally, a slightly curved longitudinal incision is made in the fibrous insertion of the biceps femoris muscle (Fig. 62.19). With this muscle retracted caudally, the lateral fabella should be palpable under the lateral head of the gastrocnemius muscle (Fig. 62.20). The peroneal nerve should then be identified. This nerve lies underneath the biceps femoris muscle and runs in a caudoproximal–craniodistal direction. Locating this nerve is essential to avoid damaging it during suture placement. The advantages of performing a cutdown procedure include easy identification of the fabellae, visualization of the peroneal nerve, and the use

Medial

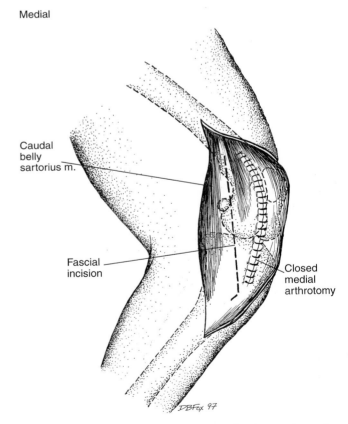

Fig. 62.17. Medial aspect of the left stifle. Approach to the medial fabella is made through an incision in the fascia along the cranial border of the caudal belly of the sartorius muscle. Joint arthrotomy has been performed and closed medially.

Caudal belly sartorius m.

Fascial incision

Closed medial arthrotomy

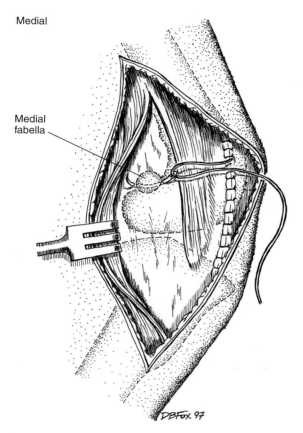

Fig. 62.18. Medial aspect of left stifle. Retraction of the caudal head of the sartorius muscle allows palpation of the medial fabella and medial suture placement. The needle should be passed in a cranial-to-caudal direction. The suture should anchor around the proximal aspect of the fabella to avoid suture pullout into the soft tissue distally.

ture is cut behind the eye of the needle, resulting in two independent strands. Heavy, nonabsorbable suture should be used. We prefer ethylene oxide sterilized, monofilament nylon fishing leader (20- to 80-lb test, hard hylon leader, Mason Tackle Co., Otisville, MI) with a heavy, half-curved Martin's uterine needle.

A hole is then drilled in the tibial tuberosity for fabellar suture anchoring. This hole is placed just caudal and distal to the patellar tendon insertion (Fig. 62.21). For a 60-lb dog, this hole is made with a $\frac{5}{64}$-inch pin and is placed 8 to 10 mm caudal and 8 to 10 mm distal to the point of insertion of the patellar tendon (Fig. 62.22). If the hole is too close to the insertion of the patellar tendon, the fabellar sutures may impinge on the tendon or may pull through the bone when tightened. If the hole is too distal, the suture will not approximate the original angle of the cranial cruciate ligament and will be less effective. The caudodistal strand of each suture is then passed through this hole. Two sutures can be passed through the same hole. If more than two sutures are used, a larger hole or two smaller holes should be drilled.

The lateral suture is tied first because it alone should eliminate most drawer movement. The medial suture

of a smaller needle to avoid peroneal nerve entrapment. The cutdown procedure also avoids suture compression on top of the biceps femoris. Compression of the thick biceps femoris may lead to focal necrosis and subsequent suture loosening.

To place the fabellar sutures, the stifle is held in moderate flexion with the overlying muscle (sartorius or biceps femoris) retracted. The fabellofemoral junction is identified by placing a curved hemostat around the caudal aspect of the fabella and pulling it up or outward, away from the femur. The needle is placed at this junction and is passed around the proximal third of the fabella in a craniocaudal direction (see Figs. 62.19 and 62.20). Care must be taken on the lateral side to avoid the peroneal nerve. Correct suture placement is confirmed by lifting up on both ends of the suture and palpating the fabella to ensure that the suture is well locked behind the bone. If two sutures are to be placed on a side, a double length of the suture material is threaded through the needle to the midpoint. After needle passage around the fabella, the su-

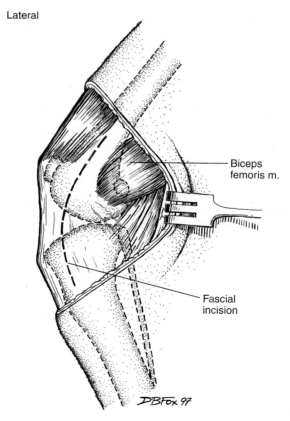

Fig. 62.19. Lateral aspect of left stifle. Exposure to the lateral fabella is made through an incision in the fibrous insertion of the biceps femoris muscle.

Lateral

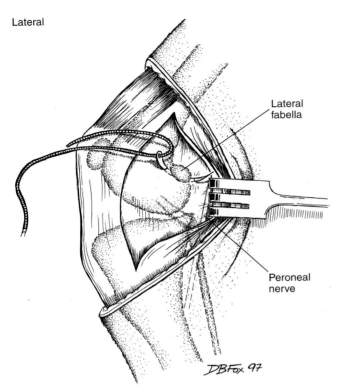

Fig. 62.20. Lateral aspect of left stifle. Retraction of the biceps femoris muscle allows palpation of the lateral fabella and lateral suture placement. The peroneal nerve, running in a craniodistal direction from behind the joint, should be avoided during suture placement.

plays a more secondary role in stifle stabilization. To tie the suture, the limb is held at the angle of flexion that produces the most cranial drawer while an assistant externally rotates the tibia and pushes it in "caudal drawer." This manipulation removes any instability while the sutures are being tied. The suture can be tightened by using either two interlocking slip knots or a surgeon's throw. If monofilament nylon is used, a smooth-faced needle holder may be used to grasp and lightly hold the first throw while the second throw is being prepared. No fewer than four throws should be used. The knots for all sutures should be placed within a few centimeters of the tibial tuberosity, either next to the patella tendon or adjacent to the hole in the tibial tuberosity (Fig. 62.23). Knots should be placed in the same location each time the procedure is performed to aid in postoperative suture location, should future removal be indicated. Knots placed back by the fabella are difficult to find postoperatively.

After suture placement, both the sartorius fascia and the biceps femoris fascia are closed in an imbricating fashion. The subcuticular tissue and skin are closed in a routine fashion. The limb is bandaged with a soft padded bandage for 2 weeks. The animal's activity should be restricted for 6 to 8 weeks, with no running

or jumping and short leash walks only. After this 6- to 8-week period, the dog is slowly reintroduced to normal levels of activity over a 4-week period. If animals are overactive during the recovery period, immature fibrotic tissue can be stretched, resulting in joint instability. Adequate exercise restriction is essential for clinical success. Weight loss should be recommended if indicated, and owners should also be advised that contralateral cranial cruciate ligament rupture occurs in 30 to 40% of patients.

Although some surgeons reserve this technique for smaller dogs, we have had consistent success over a wide range of weights. The number of sutures placed is determined by the weight of the animal, body condition, activity level, and degree of joint instability. The following are only general guidelines for the number of sutures placed. Dogs weighing less than 50 lb receive two fabellotibial sutures (one lateral, one medial). Dogs weighing 50 to 80 lb receive three sutures (two lateral, one medial). In dogs weighing more than 80 lb with severe instability, four sutures are placed (two lateral, two medial). Dogs with chronic cruciate ligament rupture and minimal instability may only receive one or two sutures (one lateral or one lateral and one

Cranial

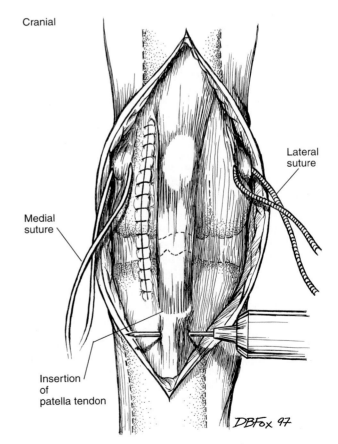

Fig. 62.21. Cranial aspect of left stifle. The hole in the tibial tuberosity is placed caudal and distal to the insertion of the patella tendon.

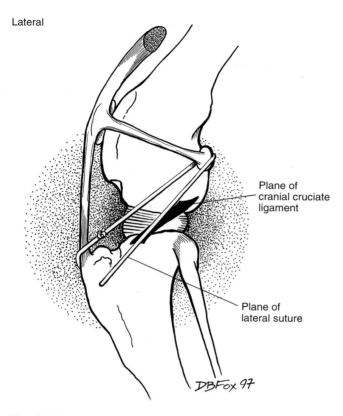

Fig. 62.22. Lateral aspect of left stifle. Correct placement of the tibial hole ensures that the plane of the fabellar suture approximates the plane of the cranial cruciate ligament.

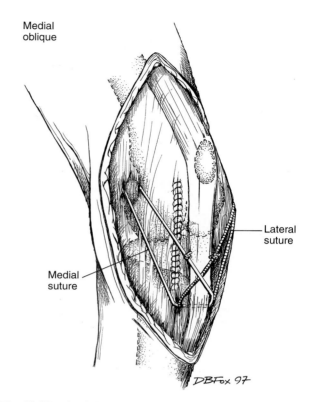

Fig. 62.23. Medial oblique aspect of left stifle. Both sutures have been tied. Suture knots are placed near the patella tendon. This placement facilitates suture identification should removal be required postoperatively.

medial). If monofilament nylon (fishing leader) is used, the strength of the material selected should roughly correspond to the weight of the animal (40-lb test for a 40-lb animal, 60-lb test for a 60-lb animal); 80-lb test, although "unwieldy," can be used in animals 80 lb and over. On rare occasions, in patients with chronic cruciate injury with no "drawer" movement, fabellotibial stabilization sutures are unnecessary after arthrotomy. The primary cause of lameness in these animals is often chronic inflammation, meniscal damage, or osteophyte formation.

Complications are uncommon (less than 10%) but include suture rupture, meniscal damage, and seroma formation because of suture irritation. Suture rupture and meniscal damage are the most common causes of poor recovery. Clinically, these patients may show either lack of full recovery or full recovery followed by return of lameness. Meniscal damage should be suspected if a popping or clicking noise is heard on ambulation or is palpated on examination. If a total meniscectomy has already been performed adequately, suture rupture should be suspected. If poor recovery is seen with the formation of large seromas over the suture knots, suture irritation should be suspected. In dealing with animals with poor or inade-

quate recovery from the MRIT, if meniscal damage is not suspected or if a meniscectomy has been previously performed, simple MRIT suture removal should be attempted first. Lameness usually resolves within 2 weeks if it resulted from suture problems. Suture replacement is rarely required and only in cases of gross stifle instability. Suture removal as early as 12 weeks postoperatively should not increase drawer movement. If lameness persists after suture removal and a meniscectomy has not been previously performed, a repeat arthrotomy and medial meniscectomy are advised.

Tibial Plateau Leveling Osteotomy for Cranial Cruciate Ligament Rupture

Barclay Slocum & Theresa Devine Slocum

The cranial cruciate ligament is the main stabilizing structure of the canine stifle. This ligament limits both cranial translation between the tibia and the femur

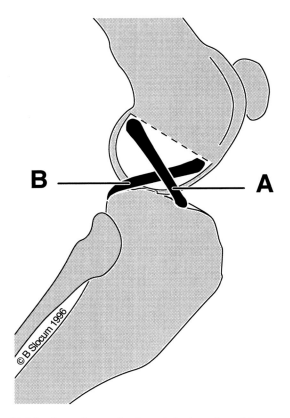

Fig. 62.24. Lateral view of stifle with the lateral condyle removed showing cranial cruciate ligament (A) and posterior cruciate ligament (B).

(Fig. 62.31). Unilateral cruciate ruptures progress to bilateral ruptures of the cranial cruciate ligament in 30% of clinical cases.

Many attempts have been made to compensate for a lack of a cranial cruciate ligament. Traditional surgical methods have tried to overpower cranial translation and to control the stifle motion by sutures and replacement ligaments. These procedures have failed to return dogs to normal function and activity. The tibial plateau leveling osteotomy reduces the cranial tibial thrust and enhances the effectiveness of the hamstring muscles. This technique has had excellent success in returning active working dogs to their preinjury function on a long-term basis.

Surgical Technique

The tibial plateau leveling osteotomy is a patented surgical technique for restoration of stifle function in the cranial cruciate ligament-deficient stifle (US Patent No. 4,677,973, Slocum Enterprises, Eugene, OR). The objective of the surgery is to neutralize the detrimental effects of the cranial tibial thrust. The operation makes no attempt to reconstruct the cranial cruciate ligament or caudal horn of the medial meniscus, which restrains the cranial tibial thrust. The cranial tibial thrust is controlled by leveling the tibial plateau, to increase the

and internal rotation of the tibia (Fig. 62.24). The cause of the ligament rupture is excessive force applied to the cranial cruciate ligament by the cranial tibial thrust (Fig. 62.25), excessive internal rotation of the stifle, or hyperextension of the stifle (Fig. 62.26). Occasionally, direct external trauma to the stifle causes rupture of the cranial cruciate ligament.

In 1978, the tibial compression test (Fig. 62.27) was described and led directly to the clinical recognition of the cranial tibial thrust (Fig. 62.28). The cranial tibial thrust is an internally generated force that causes the proximal tibia to translate cranially (Fig. 62.29); it is opposed by the cranial cruciate ligament. The cranial tibial thrust in the normal stifle is primarily controlled by the caudally directed forces of the hamstring muscles (Fig. 62.30). When the hamstring muscles are weak, their neuromuscular timing is out of sequence, or if the hamstring muscles are overpowered by the quadriceps, then the burden for the prevention of cranial translation of the tibial with respect to the femur finally falls on the cranial cruciate ligament. Secondary to cranial cruciate ligament rupture, the tibia translates forward and the caudal horn of the medial meniscus is trapped between the femoral condyle and the tibial plateau. The result is a crushed portion of meniscus

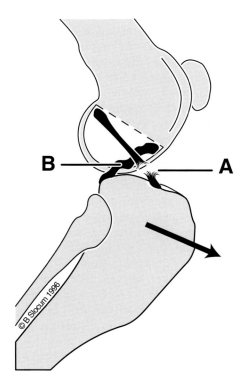

Fig. 62.25. Rupture of the cranial cruciate ligament (A) under the effect of the cranial tibial thrust results in cranial translation of the tibia and laxity of the caudal cruciate ligament (B).

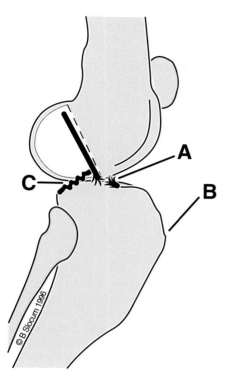

Fig. 62.26. Some breeds such as the akita, mastiff, and chow have a hyperextension conformation, and the cranial cruciate ligament (*A*) is ruptured or plastically elongated. The reason is that the shape of the condyle acts as a cam and causes the distance between the femoral and tibial attachment to become greater than the length of the ligament. As the tibia (*B*) moves cranially, the caudal cruciate ligament (*C*) becomes lax.

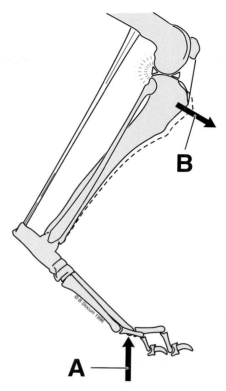

Fig. 62.28. As the dog walks, weightbearing force (*A*) creates a cranial tibial thrust (*B*). This results in cranial translation of the tibia (*dotted tibia*) when the cranial cruciate ligament is ruptured. In some cases, an audible click is heard as the caudal horn of the medial meniscus becomes impinged between the femur and the tibia.

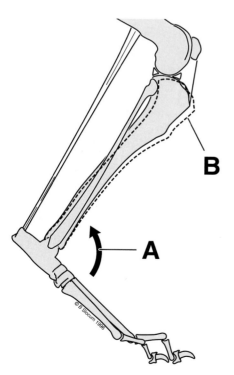

Fig. 62.27. A tibial compression test is positive when, after flexion of the hock (*A*) by the examiner, the proximal tibia translates cranially (*B*).

effectiveness of the hamstring and biceps femoris muscles (Fig. 62.32).

The diagnosis of rupture or partial rupture of the cranial cruciate ligament is outlined in the first section of this chapter. The history of a subtle hind limb lameness that does not overtly affect performance, but is seen after exercise and disappears with rest, indicates a partial rupture of the cranial cruciate ligament (Fig. 62.33). A history of a continuing lameness in which the dog is marginally functional usually indicates a rupture of the cranial cruciate ligament without crushing of the caudal horn of the medial meniscus. Often, the patient who was lame and now is nonweightbearing had a previous rupture of the cranial cruciate ligament that has impinged on the caudal horn of the medial meniscus.

The anesthetized patient is prepared for surgery from the midmetatarsal region to the level of the proximal thigh, is placed in dorsal recumbency, and is draped for sterile surgery. A craniomedial skin incision is made from just above the level of the patella to the proximal third of the tibia. An arthotomy is made by a medial parapatellar approach. The incision is ended on the proximal tibia just cranial to the medial menis-

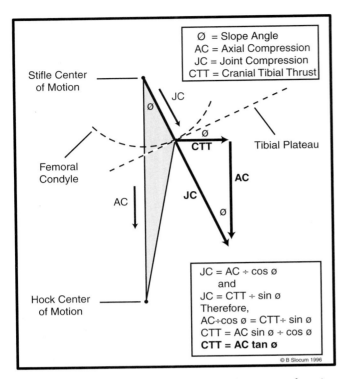

Fig. 62.29. Because the moments about the center of motion in the stifle and hock are zero, compression acts along a line (AC) between the centers. The slope of the tibial plateau (∅) determines the point of contact between the femoral condyle and the tibial plateau. Because the stifle is stable, the joint compression (JC) is perpendicular to the tibial slope. The joint compression can be expressed as vector AC, parallel to the line between the centers, and cranial tibial thrust (CTT) perpendicular to that line.

cus, at the caudal limit of the fat pad. The patella is luxated laterally.

The stifle is explored to confirm the preoperative diagnosis. The frayed ends of the cranial cruciate ligament and a "bucket handle" tear of the caudal horn of the medial meniscus are debrided. A meniscal release of the remaining caudal horn of the medial meniscus is performed, as described in an earlier section of this chapter.

The insertions of the gracilis and semitendinosus muscles and the caudal belly of the sartorius are elevated from the proximal medial tibia, with care taken to leave the medial collateral ligament intact. A tibial plateau leveling osteotomy is performed and may contain variations, depending on the alignment and structure of the patient. A jig (US Patent No. 5,578,038, Slocum Enterprises) is applied to the medial tibia to guide the osteotomy in the sagittal plane and parallel to the straight patellar tendon. A biradial saw blade (US Patent No. 4,955,888, Slocum Enterprises) is used to create a cylindric cut in the proximal tibia. The blade design must have the same radius for matching both portions of the tibial plateau osteotomy. The proximal

fragment is rotated until the tibial plateau is level. The two portions of the osteotomy are held in position with a Tibial Plateau Leveling Osteotomy Plate (US Patent No. 5,304,180, Slocum Enterprises) (Fig. 62.34). Routine closure is performed.

Postoperative Care

After surgery, the patients are strictly confined indoors, on a leash or in a kennel if unattended, until radiographic evidence indicates osseous union. At 2 weeks, the soft tissues are examined. The patient is usually toe touching by 10 days (range 3 days to 3 weeks) postoperatively. Between the 2-week and 6-week examinations, the owners may find it difficult to maintain control of the patient, because the dog feels good. Tranquilization may be necessary.

Once the tibial plateau leveling osteotomy is healed, a rehabilitation regimen is initiated within a comfortable range of controlled activity for the patient. First, unlimited swimming is permitted, but the patient must avoid an explosive water entry. The patient is permitted to be active on a 6-foot lead for 3 weeks and on a

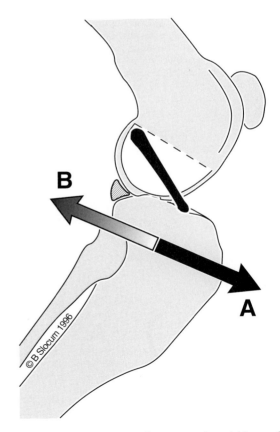

Fig. 62.30. The cranial cruciate ligament and caudal horn of the medial meniscus experience no stress when the cranial tibial thrust (A) is neutralized by the pull of the hamstrings and biceps femoris muscles (B).

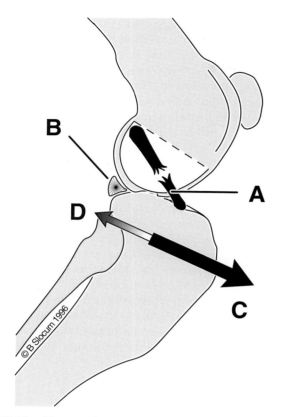

Fig. 62.31. The cranial cruciate ligament is ruptured (A) and the caudal horn of the medial meniscus (B) is impinged on when the cranial tibial thrust (C) is not neutralized by the pull of the hamstrings and biceps femoris muscles (D).

20-foot lead for another 3 weeks, which brings the time from surgery to 12 weeks. From the third to the fourth month postoperatively, the patient may run moderately off leash with random sniffing and investigation while the owner is walking. No excitable activity, including interaction with a second dog, is permitted. If during the rehabilitation the patient appears sore or excessively tired, the owner is to revert to the last distance and activity at which the patient was comfortable.

At 4 months postoperatively, the patient is ready to resume normal activities cautiously until the musculature attains normal size. The biceps femoris muscle atrophies immediately after surgery and regains full size by 4 to 6 months.

The singular criterion used to evaluate the success of surgery of the cruciate ligament–deficient stifle after traditional stabilization techniques is the cranial drawer sign. This passive test is performed by the operator to determine cranial drawer motion. The drawer sign is of no value in evaluating the success of the tibial plateau leveling osteotomy. Cranial drawer motion is not eliminated by this surgery (Fig. 62.35). However, cranial translation during functional loading and activity is neutralized by this surgical procedure, as evidenced by the return of normal function to clinical cases.

Five observations after tibial plateau leveling osteotomy surgery demonstrate its success. First, full flexibility of the stifle returns, as demonstrated by the patient's sitting symmetrically in a full squat. This usually

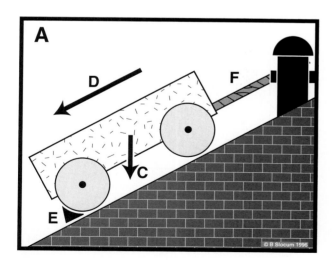 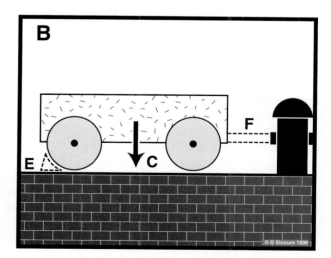

Fig. 62.32. An analogy is helpful to understanding the process of tibial plateau leveling osteotomy. Consider a wagon parked on a hill. **A.** The weight of the wagon (C, axial compression), pulls downward because of gravity and creates a force (D) because of the slope. If a rope (F, cranial cruciate ligament), is tied from the wagon to a fire hydrant and a chock (E, meniscus), is placed behind the tire (condyle), then the wagon is prevented from rolling down hill (cranial tibial translation). If the rope breaks, the wagon rolls downhill and crushes the chock. **B.** Force (D) can be eliminated by parking the wagon on a level surface and the rope (F) and chock (E) are not needed. The joint compression force is reduced to the weight of the wagon (C). Although the weight of the wagon (C) is not eliminated, its destructive effects are overcome.

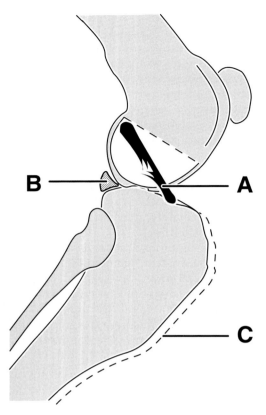

Fig. 62.33. A partial tear of the cranial cruciate ligament first occurs in the caudal fibers of the ligament (*A*). In the early stages, the animal has subtle lameness after hard exercise, slight soreness on arising, and no soreness of the meniscus (*B*). The intermediate stage of partial rupture has subtle lameness after all exercise, soreness on arising, subtle cranial translation of the tibia on palpation of the stifle in flexion (*C*), subtle swelling over the caudal medial meniscus, and an intermittently positive sit test. The advanced stage of partial rupture produces lameness after all exercise, consistent soreness on arising, cranial translation of the tibia on palpation of the stifle, swelling over the caudal medial meniscus, and a positive sit test.

occurs within 3 months of surgery in patients with an acute disorder, but it may take longer in those with chronic disorders. Chronically disordered stifles with established caudal tibial plateau osteophytes dramatically improve but may lack full flexion because of physical interference. Second, full muscular development of the affected limb returns 3 to 4 months postoperatively. Third, the stifle becomes calm and free of inflammation by the third month postoperatively. Palpating the structures of the stifle, the surgeon notices that the spongy texture of the joint capsule is lost and is replaced by firm collagen. Fourth, radiographs show no progression of osteoarthritis. Fifth and most important, full function returns by the fourth postoperative month.

Partial and complete ruptures of the cranial cruciate ligament precede the impingement of the caudal horn

of the medial meniscus, and this is a direct effect of the cranial tibial thrust. When a partial rupture of the cranial cruciate ligament is present and the caudal horn of the medial meniscus is intact, the joint is usually calm, and arthritic changes are minimal. A tibial plateau leveling osteotomy without arthotomy protects the partial rupture from the abusive effects of the cranial tibial thrust. The remaining cruciate ligament and the medial meniscus maintain their integrity. The protection of the remaining cruciate ligament and the caudal horn of the medial meniscus by the tibial plateau leveling osteotomy is direct evidence that the cranial tibial thrust is the causative factor behind the cruciate rupture and meniscal damage, because no other changes have occurred to the joint. Overzealous rotation of the tibial plateau places extra force on the caudal cruciate ligament, causing it to stretch. Consequently, more rotation is not better.

Genu varum with internal tibial torsion of the tibia occurs in more than 50% of rottweilers and is considered a normal, desirable conformation for the breed. Corrections of this deformity through tibial plateau

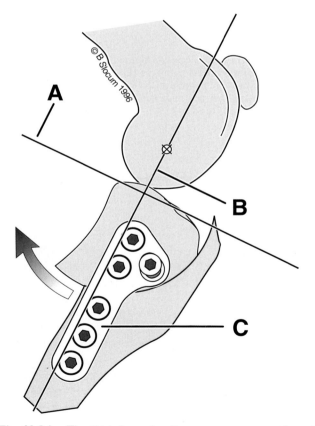

Fig. 62.34. The tibial plateau leveling osteotomy rotates (*arrow*) the sloped tibial plateau segment (*A*) until it is 5° more than perpendicular to the line between the stifle and hock joint centers (*B*). A Tibial Plateau Leveling Osteotomy Plate (*C*) compresses the proximal portion of the tibia against the distal portion by means of radially aligned compression holes and secures the rigid internal fixation for optimum bone healing.

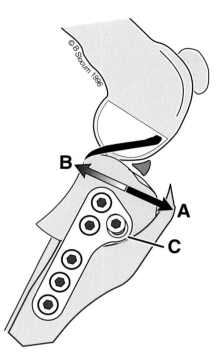

Fig. 62.35. The cranial tibial thrust (*A*) is reduced by the tibial plateau leveling osteotomy until it is in balance with the pull of the hamstrings and biceps femoris muscles (*B*). The tibia is functionally stabilized by the caudal pull (*B*) that is passively opposed by the caudal cruciate ligament. The Tibial Plateau Leveling Osteotomy Plate (*C*) maintains bone relationship during the healing process.

leveling osteotomy have controlled not only the cranial tibial thrust, but also the internal rotation forces of the stifle that are responsible for failure of the fibular head transposition, lateral imbrication, and lateral fabella to tibial tubercle techniques.

In older dogs, although external trauma can cause disruption of the cranial cruciate ligament, an observation more consistent with our experience is that the hamstring and biceps femoris muscle forces diminish as the patient ages. As a consequence, the active muscle force that protects the cranial cruciate ligament from the damaging effects of the cranial tibial thrust decreases, as patients become older or obese. With a small protective muscle force, the cranial tibial thrust exceeds the strength of the cranial cruciate ligament, and rupture occurs from an internally generated force (cranial tibial thrust) by a series of incremental or whole ligament ruptures. The tibial plateau leveling osteotomy is successful in neutralizing the effects of the cranial tibial thrust and in returning dogs to normal function and activity.

Suggested Readings

Arnoczky SP. Cranial cruciate ligament repair. In: Bojrab MJ, ed. Current techniques in small animal surgery. 3rd ed. Philadelphia: Lea & Febiger, 1990:708.

Arnoczky SP, Marshall JL. The cruciate ligaments of the canine stifle: an anatomical and functional analysis. Am J Vet Res 1977; 38:1807.

Arnoczky SP, Torzilli PA, Marshall JL. Biomechanical evaluation of anterior cruciate ligament repair in the dog: an analysis of the instant center of motion. J Am Anim Hosp Assoc 1977;13:553.

Arnoczky SP, Tarvin GB, Marshall JL, et al. The over-the-top procedure: a technique for anterior cruciate ligament substitution in the dog. J Am Anim Hosp Assoc 1979;15:283.

Daniel D. Principle of knee ligament surgery. In: Daniel, Akeson, O'Connor, eds. Knee ligaments: structure, function, injury, and repair. New York: Raven Press, 1990:11.

DeAngelis M, Lau R. A lateral retinacular imbrication technique for the surgical correction of anterior cruciate ligament rupture in the dog. J Am Vet Med Assoc 1970;157:79.

DePalma AF. Diseases of the knee. Philadelphia: JB Lippincott, 1954.

Dueland R. Recent techniques for reconstruction of the anterior cruciate ligament. J Am Anim Hosp Assoc 1966;2:2.

Eriksson E. Reconstruction of the anterior cruciate ligament. Orthop Clin North Am 1976;7:167.

Flo GL. Modification of the lateral retinacular imbrication technique for stabilizing cruciate ligament injuries. J Am Anim Hosp Assoc 1975;11:570.

Henderson R, Milton J. The tibial compression mechanism: a diagnostic aid in stifle injuries. J Am Anim Hosp Assoc 1978;14:474.

Hey Groves EWH. Operation for the repair of the cruciate ligaments. Lancet 1917;2:674.

Hohn B, Newton C. Surgical repair of ligamentous structures of the stifle joint. In: Bojrab MJ, ed. Current techniques in small animal surgery. Philadephia: Lea & Febiger, 1975:470.

Jones KG. Reconstruction of the anterior cruciate ligament using the central one-third of the patellar ligament. J Bone Joint Surg 1970;52:1302.

Müller W. The primary repair of special injuries. In: The knee. New York: Springer-Verlag, 1983:223.

Paatsama S. Ligament injuries in the canine stifle joint: a clinical and experimental study. Helsinki: Kauppakirjapaino OY, 1952.

Read RA, Robins GM. Deformity of the proximal tibia in dogs. Vet Rec 1982;111:295.

Rudy RL. Stifle joint. In: Archibald J, ed. Canine surgery. 2nd ed. Santa Barbara, CA: American Veterinary Publications, 1974: 1104.

Slocum B, Devine T. Cranial tibial thrust: a primary force in the canine stifle. J Am Vet Med Assoc 1983;183:456.

Slocum B, Devine T. Cranial tibial wedge osteotomy: a technique for eliminating cranial tibial thrust in cranial cruciate ligament repair. J Am Vet Med Assoc 1984;184:564.

Slocum B, Slocum TD. Tibial plateau leveling osteotomy for repair of cranial cruciate ligament rupture in the canine. Vet Clin North Am 1993;23:777.

Smith GK, Torg JS. Fibular head transposition for repair of cruciate-deficient stifle in the dog. J Am Vet Med Assoc 1985;187:375.

Strande A. Repair of the ruptured cranial cruciate ligament in the dog. Baltimore: Williams & Wilkins, 1967.

Thorson, E, Rodrigo J, Vasseur P, et al. Replacement of the anterior cruciate ligament: a comparison of autografts and allografts in dogs. Acta Orthop Scand 1989;60:555.

Treatment of Collateral Ligament Injuries

Erick L. Egger

The collateral ligaments are important stabilizing elements in the stifle joint. Injury to the collateral ligaments usually is caused by trauma and often is associated with disruption of either the cranial or caudal cruciate ligament.

Anatomic Features

The medial collateral ligament originates on the medial epicondyle of the femur and passes distally in the joint capsule. It passes over the medial lip of the tibial plateau, where an underlying bursa allows the ligament to slip back and forth as the joint moves. The ligament attaches to the medial shaft of the tibia with a long, narrow insertion (1). The medial collateral ligament is positioned over the central axis of the stifle to remain tight throughout flexion and extension of the joint (2).

The lateral collateral ligament originates on the lateral epicondyle of the femur and passes distally in the joint capsule to insert on the fibular head (1). The lateral collateral ligament is caudal to the central axis of the joint (2). This results in a tight ligament in extension, which limits internal rotation and contributes to craniocaudal stability. The ligament loosens as the joint flexes, allowing the tibia to rotate internally.

Diagnosis and Treatment Options

The clinical diagnosis of isolated collateral injuries can be difficult. With the joint held in full extension, varus and valgus forces occasionally result in angulation away from the side with ruptured ligament. However, if both cruciate ligaments are intact, they will greatly reduce or prevent this instability. Some increase in rotational movement may occur. Evidence of a widened joint space on one side on radiographs taken while the joint is stressed may aid in the diagnosis. Collateral rupture in the presence of a cruciate disruption is readily revealed by the presence of varus or valgus angulation of the joint when stress is applied and a dramatic increase in rotational instability with the stifle extended.

Management of collateral ligament injuries varies with the severity of injury and resultant instability. A stretched or isolated torn collateral ligament without gross instability can often be managed with external coaptation. A contoured lateral splint fashioned of plaster or Hexcelite (Hexcel Medical Products, Dublin, CA) in a padded bandage is used to stress the joint toward the injured collateral ligament. This coaptation must be maintained for at least 3 to 4 weeks. Collateral ligament injuries resulting in gross instability are repaired by suturing or other internal fixation procedures.

Surgical Technique

Because the collateral ligaments are extrasynovial, blood supply is adequate to allow simple ruptures to heal if the ends are adequately apposed. A three-loop pulley pattern of monofilament nonabsorbable material such as nylon or polypropylene can be used to

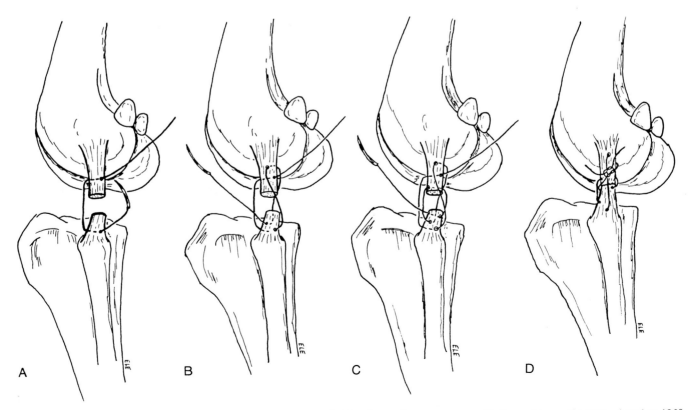

Fig. 62.36. Primary suturing of a collateral ligament rupture. **A.** First loop of suture pattern. **B.** Second loop of suture placed at 120° rotation to the first. **C.** Third loop of suture again rotated. **D.** Suture pulled tight and tied.

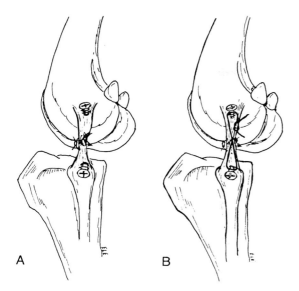

Fig. 62.37. Figure-of-eight support of weak collateral ligament repair. **A.** Collateral ligament repaired as well as possible and bone screws placed at both attachments of the ligament. **B.** Figure-of-eight suture placed around the screw head.

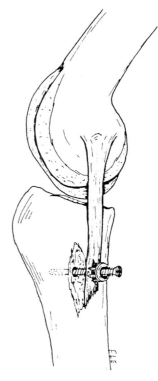

Fig. 62.38. Reattachment of an avulsed ligament with a spiked washer and a bone screw.

suture collateral ligaments (3) (Fig. 62.36). Each pass of the suture is a different distance from the torn ends and axially at a 120° rotation from the previous passage. In one study, this three-loop pulley pattern tolerated approximately 25% more tensile load and allowed only 34% as much distraction before failure under tension as the locking-loop pattern in canine collateral ligaments (4).

Suturing of severely traumatized ligaments may not provide adequate support. For these cases, a large

figure-of-eight suture of nylon or polypropylene can be placed between bone screws seated at the collateral ligament's attachments to provide additional support while the tissues heal (Fig. 62.37).

Care must be taken to tighten a lateral collateral

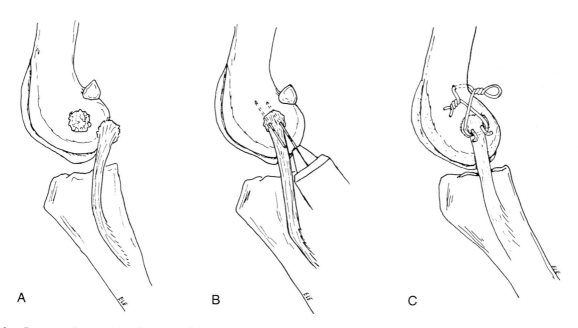

Fig. 62.39. Fixation of an avulsion fracture of the attachment of a collateral ligament. **A.** Avulsion of the proximal attachment of the medial collateral ligament. **B.** Fixation of the fragment with two Kirschner wires. **C.** Placement of a figure-of-eight wire to counteract the ligament pull.

ligament repair only in moderate extension because overtightening of this area prevents normal range of motion. Cases in which the ligament has been torn away from the bone are best managed by fixation with bone screws. A spiked washer (Synthes, Paoli, PA) can be used to trap the ligament without compromising its vascularity (Fig. 62.38). Any concurrent injury (e.g., a torn meniscus or cruciate ligament rupture) should be dealt with, and then the joint should be externally supported with a lateral splint for 3 to 4 weeks while the collateral ligament heals.

Avulsion fractures of the ligament's bony attachments are best handled by surgical reduction and fixation (Fig. 62.39). One or two Kirschner wires are driven through the fragment to hold reduction. A figure-of-eight tension band wire is then passed behind the Kirschner wires and through a transverse hole in the bone. This wire is tightened to counteract the pull of the ligament. The Kirschner wires should be cut off and bent back to reduce soft tissue irritation. Alternatively, a bone screw can be used if the avulsion fragment is large enough. Because internal fixation of a fracture should result in a stable repair, extended external coaptation is usually not indicated. However, a soft, padded bandage may be used for several days postoperatively to control soft tissue swelling.

References

1. Evans HE, Christensen CG. Miller's anatomy of the dog. 2nd ed. Philadelphia: WB Saunders, 1979.
2. Arnoczky SP, Tarvin GB, Vasseur P. Surgery of the stifle: the menisci and collateral ligaments. Compend Contin Educ Pract Vet 1980;2:395.
3. Griffiths RC. Collateral ligament injuries. In: Proceedings of the 7th annual surgical forum.: American College of Veterinary Surgeons, 1979.
4. Berg RJ, Egger EL. In vitro comparison of the three loop pulley and locking loop suture patterns for repair of canine weightbearing tendons and collateral ligaments. Vet Surg 1985;15:107.

Treatment of Caudal Cruciate Ligament Rupture by Lateral and Medial Imbrication

Joseph Harari

Surgical Technique

The primary purpose of these extracapsular procedures is to reduce caudal displacement of the tibial plateau relative to the femoral condyles, and the secondary purpose is to reduce excessive internal tibial rotation.

The animal is placed in dorsal recumbency, and a lateral parapatellar approach is used for a stifle joint arthrotomy. The joint is examined for concurrent ligamentous or meniscal injuries, which are treated accordingly. The remnants of the caudal cruciate ligament (CaCL) are resected, and the joint is lavaged with sterile saline or lactated Ringer's solution. Joint capsule closure is performed using 2–0 or 3–0 monofilament nylon, polypropylene, or polydioxanone suture material placed in a continuous pattern while a cranially directed force on the tibia is used to reduce caudal drawer motion.

Extracapsular imbrication is performed by placing a single mattress suture of size 1 or 2 nonabsorbable suture (polypropylene or nylon) on the lateral and medial aspects of the joint between the head of the fibula (laterally) or proximal tibial (medially) and just proximal or distal to the patellar (Fig. 62.40). The direction of these sutures mimics the orientation of the CaCL to reduce abnormal caudal displacement and internal rotation of the proximal aspect of the tibia. To perform lateral imbrication, the suture is passed into the quadriceps tendon above or below the patella, is directed caudodistally under or through the head of the fibula, and then is directed cranioproximally to be tied along the lateral aspect of the stifle joint while caudal drawer motion and internal tibial rotation are reduced and the normal standing angle of the joint is maintained. To place the medial imbrication suture, the skin incision is displaced medially, and subcutaneous tissues are dissected to reveal the medial retinaculum of the stifle joint. The mattress suture is placed in the quadriceps tendon above or below the patella and is oriented caudodistally through the caudal aspect of the proximal tibia. The suture is then directed cranioproximally and is tied along the medial aspect of the stifle joint. Placement of medial and lateral sutures in the quadriceps tendon prevents unilateral displacement of the patella or tendon.

The lateral retinaculum opened during the arthrotomy can be closed with 0 or 2–0 nonabsorbable sutures placed in a mattress pattern resembling the direction of the lateral imbrication suture. The subcutaneous tissues and skin are closed in a routine manner. Postoperatively, a soft, padded limb bandage is used for 2 weeks, and exercise is restricted for 1 month to protect soft tissue healing.

Lateral and medial imbrications are recommended for midsubstance ligamentous tears. Bone avulsion injuries involving the origin or insertion of the CaCL can be repaired by stabilization of bone fragments with a small bone screw or with Kirschner or orthopedic wires (Fig. 62.41) (1). Small unattachable fragments can be removed (along with the CaCl), and extracapsular imbrication can be performed.

Surgical stabilization of a CaCL-deficient stifle joint

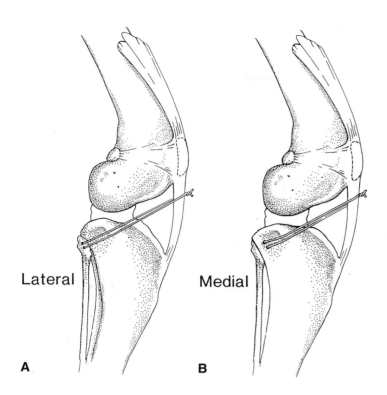

Lateral

Medial

A

B

Fig. 62.40. Extracapsular imbrication of a caudal cruciate ligament-deficient stifle joint using nonabsorbable mattress sutures. **A.** Lateral view. **B.** Medial view. (From Harari J. Caudal cruciate ligament injury. Vet Clin North Am Small Anim Pract 1993;23:826.)

is controversial for human and veterinary patients. In human patients, unidirectional (anteroposterior) instability is treated conservatively along with physical therapy designed to strengthen the quadriceps muscles of the CaCL (2, 3). In animals, persistent caudal drawer motion in experimental and clinical patients after resection with or without surgical stabilization has not

been consistently associated with lameness or lack of limb function (4–6). This finding has been attributed to the lack of importance in stabilization of the canine stifle joint by the CaCL at normal angles of the limb. At our clinic, therefore, surgical stabilization of tears of this ligament is not routinely performed. An arthrotomy is performed to remove proliferative ends

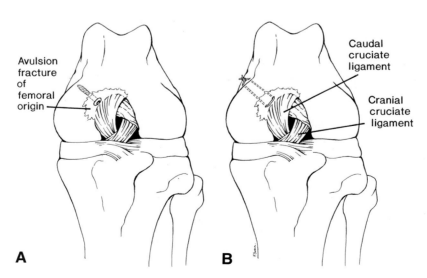

Avulsion fracture of femoral origin

Caudal cruciate ligament

Cranial cruciate ligament

A

B

Fig. 62.41. Repair of a femoral avulsion fracture in a caudal cruciate ligament-deficient stifle joint using a bone screw (**A**) or orthopedic wire (**B**). (From Harari J. Caudal cruciate ligament injury. Vet Clin North Am Small Anim Pract 1993;23:826.)

of the damaged ligament and to inspect the joint for concurrent meniscal or cranial cruciate ligament lesion (6). Bone avulsions are reattached if technically feasible. A caudomedial stifle joint arthrotomy is necessary to attach or resect avulsion of the CaCL tibial insertion (1). Long-term, objective clinical evaluations of affected stifle joints, therefore, are warranted to delineate the natural progression of CaCL–deficient canine stifle joints.

References

1. Reinke JD. Cruciate ligament avulsion injury in the dog. J Am Anim Hosp Assoc 1982;18:257–264.
2. Torg JS, Barton TM, Pavlov H. Natural history of the posterior cruciate ligament-deficient knee: Clin Orthop 1989;246:209–217.
3. Shino K, Nakata K, Maeda A. Conservative treatment of isolated injuries to the posterior cruciate ligament in athletes. J Bone Joint Surg Br 1995;77:895–900.
4. Pournaras J, Symeonides PP, Karkavales G. The significance of the posterior cruciate ligament in the stability of the dog's knee. J Bone Joint Surg Br 1983;65:204–209.
5. Harari J, Johnson AL, Stein LE. Evaluation of experimental transection of the caudal cruciate ligament in dogs. Vet Surg 1987;16:151–154.
6. Johnson AL, Olmstead ML. Caudal cruciate ligament rupture: a retrospective analysis of 14 dogs. Vet Surg 1987;16:202–206.

Tibial Tubercle Recession for the Caudal Cruciate Ligament–Deficient Stifle

Barclay Slocum & Theresa Devine Slocum

The caudal cruciate ligament (CaCL) prevents caudal translation of the tibia with respect to the femur. Rupture of this ligament as a solitary injury occurs infrequently, in about 1 per 150 cases. The injury usually occurs by a craniocaudal blow to the tibial tubercle by a stationary object such as a post or log as the dog runs at high speed. The patient usually has a mild but persistent limp if left untreated. Successful treatment involves increasing the cranial tibial thrust (CTT), which maintains the tibia in its normal relationship with the femur during function.

Surgical Procedure

The anesthetized patient is prepared for surgery from the midmetatarsal region to the level of the proximal thigh, is placed in dorsal recumbency, and is draped for sterile surgery. A craniomedial skin incision is made from the level of the patella to the proximal third of the tibia. An arthrotomy is made by a medial parapatellar approach. The incision is terminated on the proximal tibia just caudal to the patellar tendon. The patella is luxated laterally. The stifle is explored to confirm the preoperative diagnosis. The frayed ends of the CaCL are debrided and removed.

The arthrotomy incision is extended distally a distance equal to the length of the tibial crest in the fascia along the craniomedial margin of the cranial tibial muscle, approximately 10 mm medial to the tibial crest. The insertions of the gracilis and semitendinosus muscles and the caudal belly of the sartorius are elevated from the proximal medial tibia, with care taken to leave the medial collateral ligament intact. Sponges are packed between the cranial tibial muscles and the proximal lateral tibia. A V-shaped wedge is removed from the proximal tibia as seen from the medial aspect. The cranial cut of the V is made perpendicular to the sagittal plane from the caudal margin of the bursa between the distal patellar tendon and the tibial tubercle moving distally and parallel to the entire tibial crest (Fig. 62.42). The caudal cut of the V is made perpendicular to the sagittal plane from just cranial to the meniscus, extending distally to join the cranial portion of the V cut. The V wedge is removed. The bottom of the V is extended distally by a single cut perpendicular to the sagittal plane just caudal to the cranial cortex of the tibia for approximately 2.5 cm. This maneuver allows the tibial tubercle to be sprung caudally without breaking. Bone-holding forceps between the tibial crest and the caudal cortex of the proximal tibia hold the position for fixation. A single screw is placed through the tibial tubercle and proximal tibia to maintain reduction (Fig. 62.43). The soft tissues are closed in a routine manner.

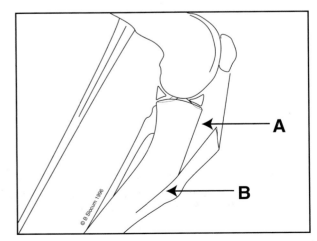

Fig. 62.42. A V-shaped wedge perpendicular to the sagittal plane is removed (A) and a stress-relief kerf is made caudal to the cranial cortex (B).

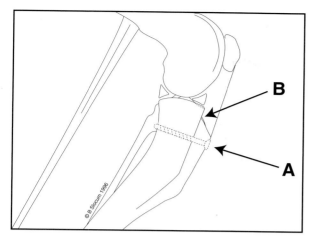

Fig. 62.43. A lag screw (*A*) collapses the wedge (*B*), thus recessing the tibial tubercle.

In the CaCL-deficient stifle, the tibia moves caudally with respect to the femur. Because the CTT drives the proximal tibia cranially, this force can be used to counteract the lack of an intact CaCL. By enhancing the

CTT in the CaCL-deficient stifle, the balance of forces can be maintained.

The CTT force vector can be increased by changing the magnitude or direction of the input force of tibial compression. For example, by increasing the slope of the tibial plateau, a change in direction, CTT can be increased. Unfortunately, this places the cranial cruciate ligament at greater risk and requires more hamstring and biceps femoris muscular participation. To maintain the equilibrium of the flexion and extension moments of the stifle when the tibial tubercle is recessed, the patellar tendon force must be increased. This results in an increase in force of compression across the joint. Because moment equals force times distance, as the distance between the quadriceps attachment and the point of contact between the femur and tibial plateau is decreased, the compressive force must be increased (Fig. 62.44). In addition, the tibial tubercle recession causes the angle of the straight patellar tendon to incline more cranially with respect to the proximal tibia, thereby pulling the tibia in a more cranial direction. The combination of these two

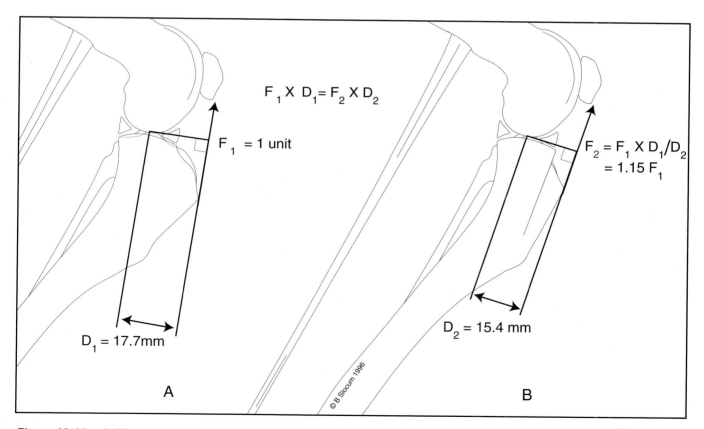

Figure 62.44. **A.** The moment created by the straight patellar tendon before the tibial tubercle recession is the product of the tension in the tendon (F_1) and the perpendicular distance (D_1) between the contact point of the femur and tibia and the straight patellar tendon. **B.** The moment created by the straight patellar tendon after the tibial tubercle recession is the product of the tension in the tendon (F_2) and the perpendicular distance (D_2) between the contact point of the femur and tibia and the straight patellar tendon because F_1 equals F_2, $F_2 = F_1 \times D_1/D_2$. This enhances the cranial tibial thrust (*CTT*). In this example, F_2 is 15% greater than F_1 and the direction of F_2 is inclined 11° cranially compared to F_1. This creates an increase in joint compression and therefore an increase in CTT. These two effects, an increase in CTT and the increased inclination of F_2, functionally stabilize the stifle in the absence of a caudal cruciate ligament.

changes, direction and magnitude of force, creates a subtle cranially directed force during weightbearing that functionally stabilizes the stifle. The passive test for caudal drawer motion is able to be elicited by the veterinarian, but the stifle is stable in function.

Patellar Luxation Algorithm

Barclay Slocum & Theresa Devine Slocum

The patella is a sesamoid bone within the tendon of the quadriceps muscles. It is located on the cranial aspect of the distal femur and is normally pressed into the trochlear sulcus of the femur. The quadriceps muscle bellies all arise from the proximal femur, except the rectus femoris, which originates from the pelvis cranial to the acetabulum. The quadriceps muscles end in the patellar tendon that inserts on the tibial tubercle. Because a muscle can only pull, the powerful quadriceps muscle group is attempting to align its origin, the patella, and its insertion.

The deviation of the patella around the distal femur creates femoropatellar compression, which results in a trochlear sulcus. Once formed, the trochlear ridges maintain the patella in the trochlear sulcus under many laterally and medially directed forces. To support the patella further, the joint capsule, fabellopatellar ligaments, and retinaculum guide the path of the patella during stifle flexion and extension. Finally, the overall alignment of the limb dictates the manner in which the muscular forces are exerted through the limb.

The patella and its alignment are a result of limb growth and use. The orthopedist must determine these factors before surgery, because muscle forces acting on bones determine the behavior of the patella. Forcible containment of the patella in the trochlear sulcus is

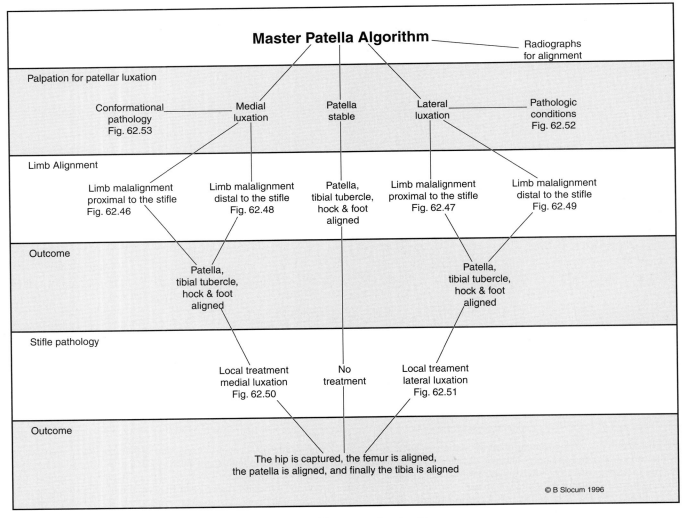

Fig. 62.45. Master patellar algorithm.

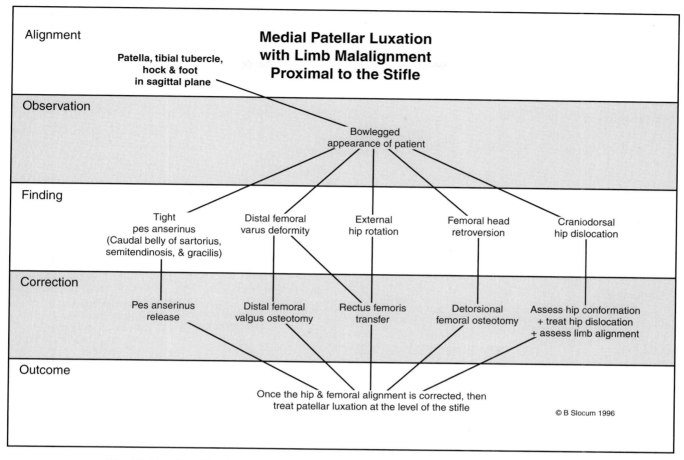

Fig. 62.46. Algorithm for medial patellar luxation with limb malalignment proximal to the stifle.

doomed to failure. Only realignment of the bones and of the origin and insertion of the quadriceps restores the alignment and balance of muscular forces.

The algorithms of the patella set forth a logical sequence for diagnosis and treatment of patellar luxations to restore balance to the patella. If, for example, local treatment for medial patellar luxation is insti-

tuted without limb alignment, the muscular forces cause medial patellar luxation to recur. If the patella is overpowered to maintain reduction, the results will be poor, and the patient will be predisposed to additional injury such as rupture of the cranial cruciate ligament. The patient is best served by our understanding of the limb as a whole and the effect of the quadriceps on its function (Figs. 62.45 to 62.54).

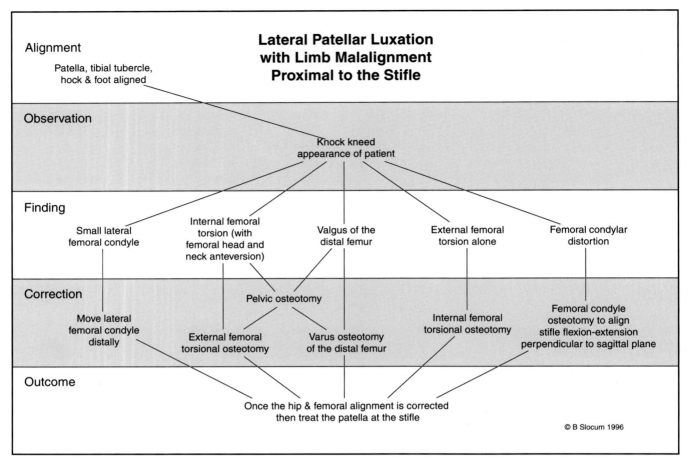

Fig. 62.47. Algorithm for lateral patellar luxation with limb malalignment proximal to the stifle.

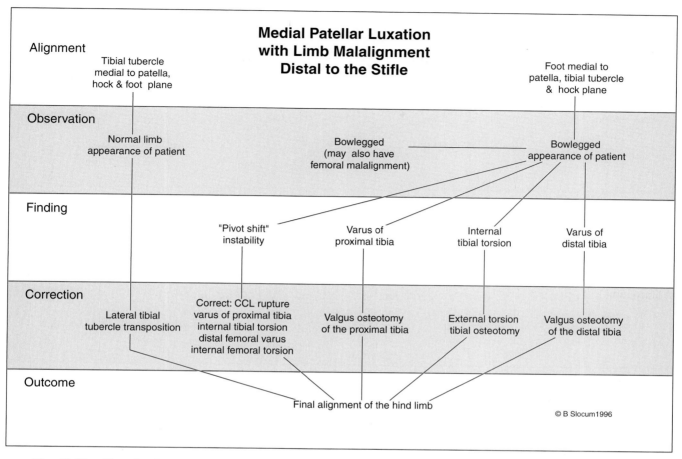

Fig. 62.48. Algorithm for medial patellar luxation with limb malalignment distal to the stifle. *CCL*, cranial cruciate ligament.

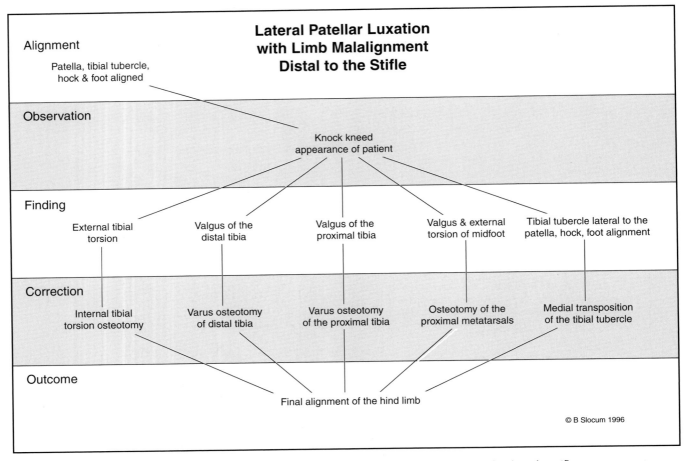

Fig. 62.49. Algorithm for lateral patellar luxation with limb malalignment distal to the stifle.

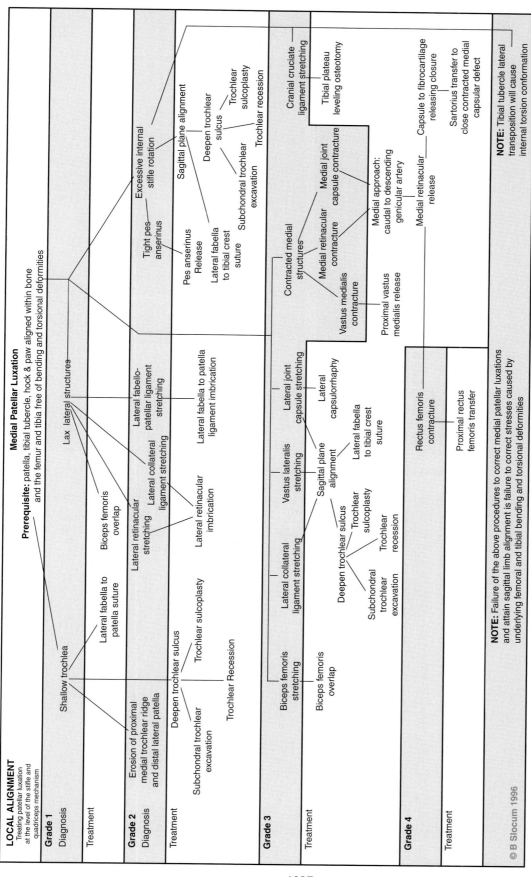

Fig. 62.50. Medial patellar luxation algorithm.

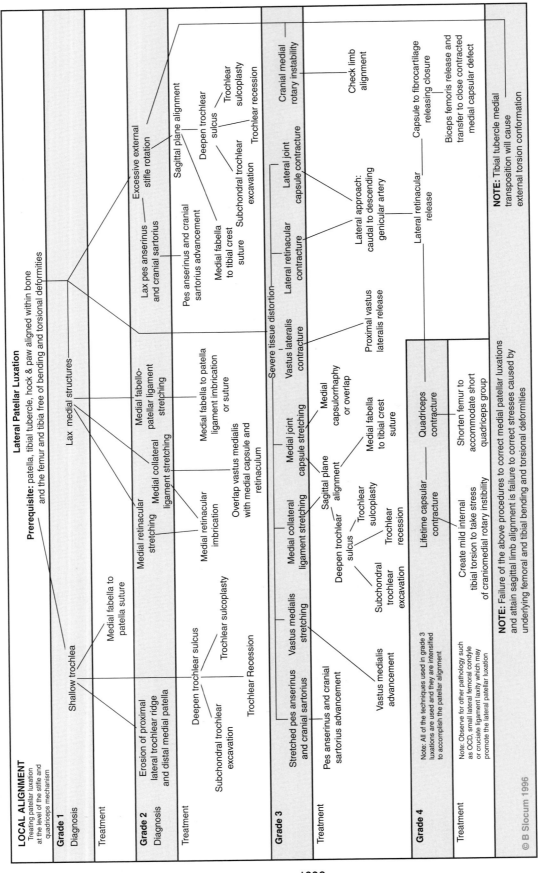

Fig. 62.51. Lateral patellar luxation algorithm.

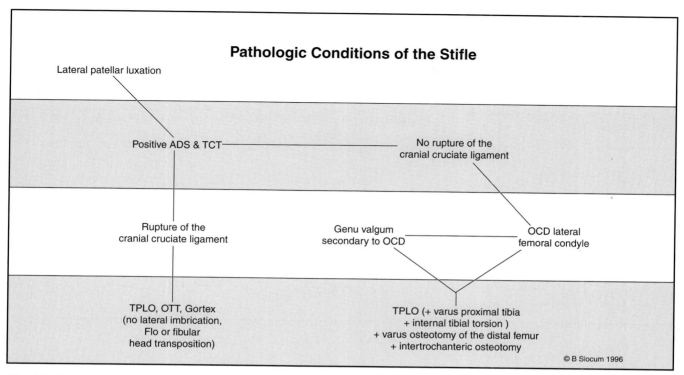

Fig. 62.52. Pathologic conditions of the stifle. *ADS,* anterior drawer sign; *OCD,* osteochondritis dissecans; *OTT,* over-the-top technique; *TCT,* tibial compression tent; *TPLO,* tibial plateau leveling osteotomy.

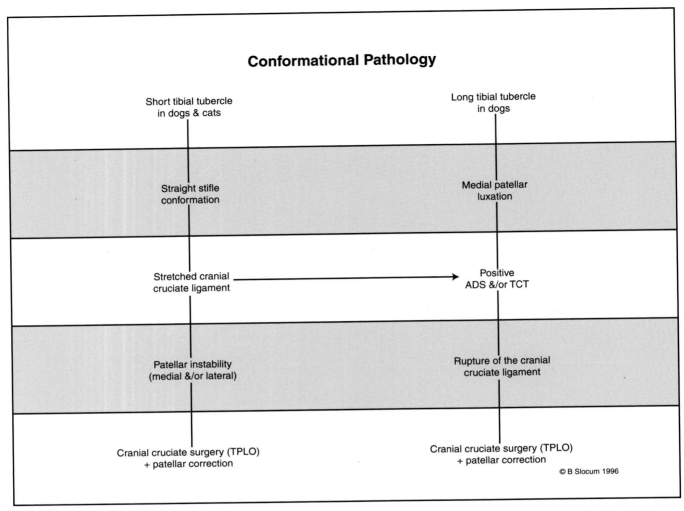

Fig. 62.53. Conformational pathology algorithm. *ADS,* Anterior Drawer Sign; *TCT,* Tibial Compression Test; *TPLO,* tibial plateau leveling osteotomy.

Radiographs for Hind Limb Alignment

Valgus Hind limb, incongruity alignment (left) — **Valgus Hind limb, incongruity alignment** (right)

PA radiographic signs	Finding	Lateral radiographic signs
Mass, distortion or lysis	Tumor or infection	Mass, distortion or lysis
Apparent short femoral neck length	Short femoral neck	Apparent short femoral neck length
Apparent short femoral neck length	Valgus and anteversion of the femoral neck	Apparent long femoral neck length
Incongruity of the hip	Femoral head luxation	White, black, grey or white, grey, grey
Cancellous lesser trochanter	Internal femoral torsion	No lesser trochanter outline
A perpendicular to femoral condyles lateral to femoral shaft	Varus of the distal femur	Proximal-distal condylar offset
	OCD of medial femoral condyle uncommon	
Femoral condyle overlap tibial plateau	Excessive tibial plateau slope	Measure excessive tibial slope
See radiographic evaluation of the CCL	Cranial cruciate ligament pathology	See radiographic evaluation of the CCL
PA of distal femur & tibial crest outline medial to tibial shaft	Stifle distortion by chronic forced internal stifle rotation	Cranial-caudal condylar offset
A perpendicular to tibial plateau lateral to sagittal sulcus of talus	Varus of the proximal tibia	Proximal-distal condylar offset
Femoral condyle aligned & calcaneus lateral to sulcus of the talus	Internal tibial torsion	Cranial-caudal condylar offset
A perpendicular to talar ridges lateral to tibial shaft	Varus of distal tibia	Proximal-distal condylar offset
Calcaneus in line with talar sulcus & metatarsus at angle to calcaneus	Valgus & external torsion of the midfoot	Lateral of tarsus but oblique of metatarsus

Finding	PA radiographic signs	Lateral radiographic signs
Tumor or infection	Mass, distortion or lysis	Mass, distortion or lysis
Short femoral neck	Apparent short femoral neck length	Apparent short femoral neck length
Valgus and anteversion of the femoral neck	Apparent short femoral neck length	Apparent long femoral neck length
Femoral head luxation	Incongruity of the hip	White, black, grey or white, grey, grey
External femoral torsion	Cortical bone at lesser trochanter	Lesser trochanter outline
Valgus of the distal femur	A perpendicular to femoral condyles medial to femoral shaft	Proximal-distal condylar offset
OCD lateral femoral condyle	Defect in lateral condyle	Defect in lateral condyle
Excessive tibial plateau slope	Femoral condyle overlap tibial plateau	Measure excessive tibial slope
Cranial cruciate ligament pathology	See radiographic evaluation of the CCL	See radiographic evaluation of the CCL
Stifle distortion by chronic forced external stifle rotation	PA of distal femur & tibial crest outline lateral to tibial shaft	Cranial-caudal condylar offset
Valgus of the proximal tibia	A perpendicular to tibial plateau medial to sagittal sulcus of talus	Proximal-distal condylar offset
External tibial torsion	Femoral condyle aligned & calcaneus medial sulcus of the talus	Cranial-caudal condylar offset
Valgus of distal tibia	A perpendicular to talar ridges medial to tibial shaft	Proximal-distal condylar offset
Valgus & external torsion of the midfoot	Calcaneus in line with talar sulcus & metatarsus at angle to calcaneus	Lateral of tarsus but oblique of metatarsus

© B Slocum 1996

Fig. 62.54. Radiographs for hind limb alignment. *CCL*, cranial cruciate ligament; *OCD*, osteochondritis dissecans; *PA*, posteroanterior.

Trochlear Wedge Recession for Medial Patellar Luxation

Barclay Slocum & Theresa Devine Slocum

The purpose of the trochlear wedge recession is to deepen the trochlear sulcus of the patellofemoral articulation while maintaining both a viable articular cartilage of the sulcus and the integrity of the medial trochlear ridge. The medial trochlear ridge acts as a buttress to prevent the patella from luxating medially.

Surgical Technique

A medial approach to the stifle is used so any contracture of the medial stifle structures can be released. The incision follows the medial border of the vastus medialis and transects the medial fabellopatellar ligament, retinaculum, and joint capsule just cranial to the medial descending genicular artery. The incision ends just medial to the insertion of the straight patellar tendon on the tibial tubercle. The entire quadriceps mechanism is luxated laterally, and this situation may necessitate excision of the contracted joint capsule of the suprapatellar pouch. If the vastus medialis is contracted, it is released by subperiosteal elevation of the entire muscle from its origin on the proximal femur. The distal femur containing the trochlear exposure is maintained by placing Kern bone-holding forceps on the cranial midshaft femur in the sagittal plane and keeping the stifle flexed.

A wedge containing the distal femoral trochlear sulcus is formed by two intersecting saw cuts that create an apex angle of 30 to 40° (approximately 15 to 20° medial and lateral to the sagittal plane) (Fig. 62.55). The first saw cut is made in the plane formed by three points: distally, the cranial limit of the intercondylar

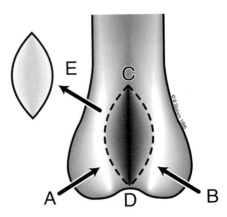

Fig. 62.56. The medial trochlear ridge (*A*) the proximal midfemoral extent of the suprapatellar pouch (*C*), and the cranial midfemoral limit of the intercondylar notch (*D*) are three points that form the plane for the medial osteotomy. The lateral trochlear ridge (*B*) and *C* and *D* are the three points that form the plane for the lateral osteotomy. The two osteotomy cuts meet at the midline of the femoral condyle to form an osteochondral wedge (*E*) that will be recessed.

notch halfway between the trochlear ridges; proximally, the suprapatellar pouch at the proximal limit of the articular cartilage halfway between the trochlear ridges; the third point is just lateral to the medial trochlear ridge. The second saw cut uses the same proximal and distal points, but the third point is just medial to the lateral trochlear ridge (Fig. 62.56). The width of

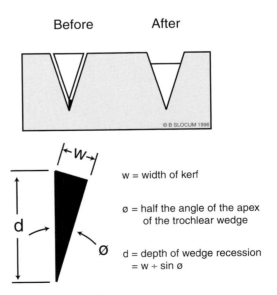

Fig. 62.57. The schematic diagram of the trochlear recession wedge, *white triangle*, is seen before and after its recession. The apex of the intersecting kerfs form the *black triangle* that is enlarged. The geometry of the *black triangle* demonstrates that the surgeon can control the width of the kerf (*W*) by the choice of saw blade. The angle formed by the intersecting osteotomy planes, two times ∅, is also under control of the surgeon. Therefore, the depth of the wedge recession, *d*, is predictable and controllable.

In the schematic:

w = width of kerf

ø = half the angle of the apex of the trochlear wedge

d = depth of wedge recession
= w ÷ sin ø

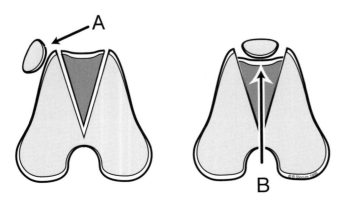

Fig. 62.55. A medial patellar luxation (*A*) can be stabilized by removing bone at the kerf that allows the trochlear wedge to be recessed (*B*).

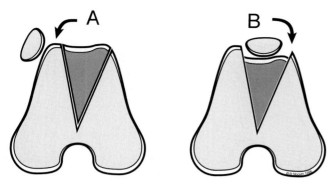

Fig. 62.58. A thick medial trochlear ridge (*A*) and a diminished lateral trochlear ridge (*B*) can be created to reinforce the strength of the medial trochlear bone that opposes the patellar luxation without stressing the lateral ridge.

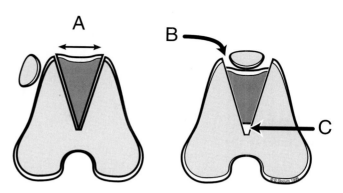

Fig. 62.60. If the trochlear wedge rocks, medial and lateral (*A*) resection of the wedge apex (*C*) allows the wedge to be in contact with the walls of the V-shaped osteotomy groove and the wedge to be recessed (*B*).

the kerf and the angle of the wedge apex determine the depth of the trochlear wedge recession (Fig. 62.57).

To prevent the medial trochlear ridge from being weak or to avoid creating an abrupt apex in the wedge, the trochlear wedge cuts can be shifted laterally (Fig. 62.58). Regardless of the variation of forming the trochlear wedge, the proximal trochlear sulcus must be flared to receive and guide the patella into the trochlea as flexion of the stifle begins. A round rasp is used to open a trough proximal to the wedge in the femur (Fig. 62.59).

The wedge and the V-shaped cavity must allow recession of the patella to one-half its thickness into the depth of the new trochlea and must also allow the patella sufficient width to prevent it from binding on the trochlear ridges. If the apex of the wedge interferes and causes rocking in the depth of the V, the surgeon simply should cut off a slight amount of the apex so the wedge contacts the sides of the V (Fig. 62.60). If the sides of the wedge bind on the sides of the V with

no contact of the wedge in the depth of the V, then the apex angle of the wedge and V are different. The surgeon presses the wedge into the condyle and passes the saw blade between the wedge and the lateral condyle to match the surfaces. This prevents the wedge from tilting in the V.

If the medial trochlear ridge is too thin, the trochlea is deepened by removing bone from the lateral wall of the V. If the saw blade is too thin, the trochlear recession will be too shallow. The surgeon presses the wedge into the condyle and passes the saw blade lateral to the wedge, thus deepening the trochlea by removing bone from the lateral wall of the V (Fig. 62.61). A thicker saw blade during the original procedure eliminates this extra step.

If the sulcus is too narrow for the patella, then the angle of the wedge apex is too small. The sulcus is widened by rasping additional cancellous bone from the lateral trochlear ridge above the level of the wedge (Fig. 62.62). The patella is reduced into the newly formed sulcus, and the stifle is tested for patellar stability.

Before closure, the joint is lavaged with saline to remove all debris created by the trochlear recession. If additional alignment procedures of the quadriceps mechanism are necessary, they should be performed. If mild stretching of the retinaculum has occurred, a lateral fabella-to-patella suture allows the affected collagen to contract spontaneously. If severe stretching of the retinaculum has occurred, the lateral parapatellar fibrocartilage and retinaculum are overlapped cranially on the rectus femoris muscle, the patella, and the patellar tendon. If the medial retinaculum and quadriceps mechanism are insufficient to close without tension on the sutures, no sutures are placed medially. The opening is closed by transferring either belly of the sartorius muscle to cover the gap without tension.

Although the wedge is a free osteochondral graft,

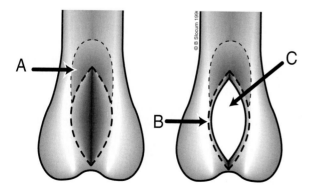

Fig. 62.59. The suprapatellar region of the midline femur (*A*) is rasped so the patella is guided onto the trochlear wedge (*C*) that lies in a recessed bed, lateral to the medial trochlear ridge (*B*).

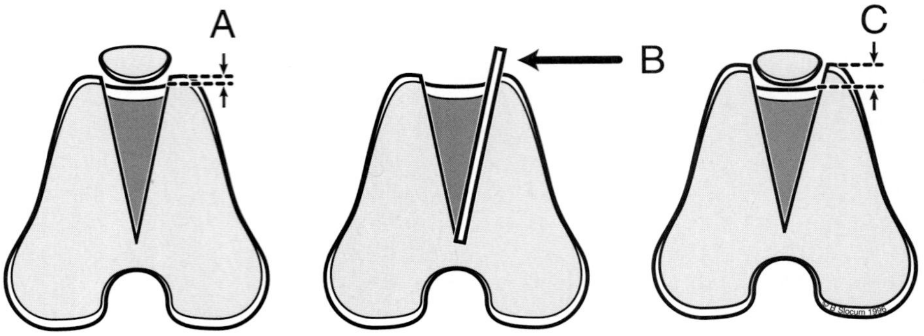

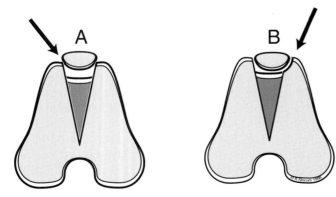

Fig. 62.61. If the trochlear recession is shallow (A), more bone can be removed from the lateral wall of the condylar V with a saw blade (B), to deepen the trochlear sulcus (C).

blood supply to the osseous portion of the wedge is provided by the adjacent bone of the femoral condyle. The articular cartilage receives nutrients from the joint fluid.

Stability of the wedge and its proper orientation prevent wedge migration without additional fixation. In our clinical experience, no properly seated trochlear wedge has migrated. An excessively deep trochlear recession decreases the femoropatellar compression. This situation can be used to advantage to relieve excessive compression when the articular cartilage is damaged or missing from the patella or trochlea.

Suggested Readings

Arnoczky S, Tarvin G. Surgical repair of patellar luxations and fractures. In: Bojrab MJ, ed. Current techniques in small animal surgery. 3rd ed. Philadelphia: Lea & Febiger, 1990:716.

Boone E, Hohn B, Weisbrode S. Trochlear recession wedge technique for patellar luxation: an experimental study. J Am Anim Hosp Assoc 1983;19:735.

Brinker W, Piermattei D, Flo G. Diagnosis and treatment of orthopedic conditions of the hindlimb. In: Handbook of small animal orthopedics and fracture treatment. Philadelphia: WB Saunders, 1990:388.

Robins G. The canine stifle joint. In: Whittick W, ed. Canine orthopedics. 2nd ed. Philadelphia: Lea & Febiger, 1990:715.

Roush J. Canine patellar luxation. Vet Clin North Am 1993;23:855.

Slocum B, Devine T. Trochlear recession for correction of luxating patella in the dog. J Am Vet Med Assoc 1985;186:365.

Slocum B, Slocum TD. Trochlear wedge recession for medial patellar luxation. Vet Clin North Am 1993;23:869.

Slocum B, Slocum D, Devine T, et al. Wedge recession for treatment of recurrent luxation of the patella. Clin Orthop 1982;164:48.

Rectus Femoris Transposition for Medial Patellar Luxation

Barclay Slocum & Theresa Devine Slocum

Treatment of medial patellar luxation has traditionally used three techniques. Trochlear chondroplasty or trochlear recession has been successfully used to control medial patellar luxation, if the patient has a shallow trochlear sulcus, but medial luxation often recurs even if the sulcus was initially deep enough. Lateral transposition of the tibial tubercle has been successful in restoring leg alignment and patellar relocation if the tubercle is medially located. If patellotubercular alignment was initially normal, then lateral transposition of the patella will produce internal rotation of the tibia with respect to the femur and will cause the dog to be bowlegged. The lateral fabella-to-patella suture has been used to prevent medial patellar luxation. The success of this technique is limited to grade I medial patellar luxations and to use with adjunct techniques in more advanced luxations.

The common thread in failures of all the foregoing techniques is a bowlegged conformation of the patient, whether preexisting or created by the surgeon by performing a lateral tibial tubercle transposition when this conformation is present, thereby accentuating the problem. In a patient with a bowlegged conformation and medial patellar luxation, a rectus femoris transfer, used in concert with a medial retinacular release and release of the vastus medialis muscle, alleviates most luxations without an osteotomy.

Fig. 62.62. If the trochlear wedge is too narrow because the apex angle of the wedge is too acute, the patella will bind between the medial and lateral trochlear ridges (A). Removal of bone on the lateral trochlear ridge above the level of the wedge (B) reestablishes an effective trochlear recession.

Surgical Procedure

A medial retinacular release is first performed. A medial arthrotomy of the stifle is performed by incising the medial retinaculum and joint capsule (not the parapatellar fibrocartilage) just cranial to the descending genicular artery. The patella should be luxated laterally during exploration of the stifle. This maneuver requires incising the contracted joint capsule both distally in the retinaculum and proximally in the suprapatellar pouch. At closure, this release is left unsutured. The caudal belly of the sartorius muscle is transferred from its original insertion on the craniomedial aspect of the tibia to bridge the retinacular release deficit by suturing its cranial border to the parapatellar fibrocartilage cranially and to the retinaculum adjacent to the descending genicular artery caudally.

The vastus medialis muscle is usually contracted in cases of chronic medial patellar luxation. After medial retinacular release, the vastus medialis muscle is freed from the femur by subperiosteal elevation as far proximally as the femoral neck, to allow the entire quadriceps mechanism to be moved laterally. No suturing of

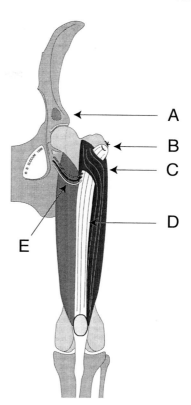

Fig. 62.64. The rectus femoris muscle (*D*) is transferred from its origin on the pelvis (*A*) by tunneling under the vastus lateralis (*C*) to attach to the cervical tubercle (*B*) or the third trochanter. The femoral artery, vein, and nerve (*E*) move with the rectus femoris.

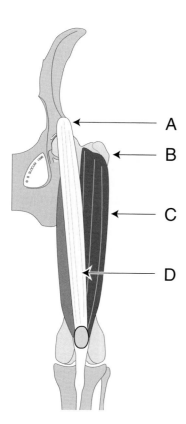

Fig. 62.63. The rectus femoris muscle (*D*) originates just cranial to the acetabulum (*A*) and inserts on the patella. It is the only member of the quadriceps group to cross both the hip and stifle. The vastus lateralis muscle (*C*) originates on the cranial and lateral femur just distal to the greater trochanter (*B*) and inserts on the patella.

this structure at closure is necessary. The rectus femoris transfer is the last component of the proximal quadriceps realignment.

Rectus Femoris Transfer

To expose the rectus femoris muscle at its origin on the pelvis, a 4-cm incision is made through the skin and fascia parallel to the cranial edge of the biceps femoris muscle, from 2 cm proximal to the insertion of the deep gluteal muscle on the greater trochanter to 2 cm distal to the deep gluteal insertion. The tendon of the deep gluteal muscle is retracted proximally. The biceps femoris muscle is retracted caudally, and the tensor fasciae latae muscle is retracted cranially to expose the rectus femoris muscle as it originates cranial to the acetabulum (Fig. 62.63).

The attachment of the rectus femoris to the pelvis is isolated for good visualization to prevent damage to the cranial circumflex iliac vessels. A gouge is used to excise the origin of the rectus femoris muscle, including a small piece of bone at its pelvic attachment. A tunnel for the rectus femoris is made between the

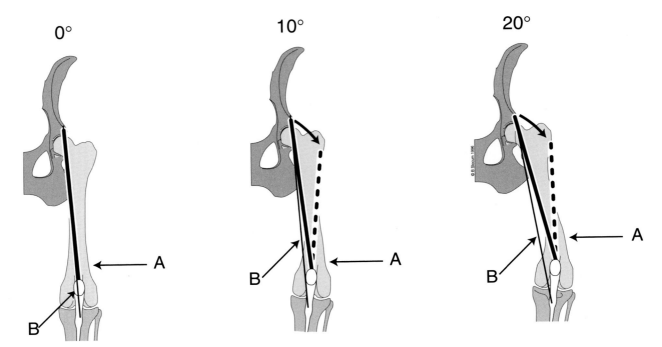

Fig. 62.65. As the varus of the distal femur (A) increases from 0 to 20,° the displacement of the line between the origin of the rectus femoris and the tibial tubercle is more lateral. If the patella luxates medially, the patella and quadriceps alignment will be along this line (B). If the origin of the rectus femoris is transferred to the cervical tubercle of the greater trochanter (*curved arrow*), depending on the degree of the femoral varus, then the quadriceps will be restored to a straight line pull in alignment with the sulcus of the distal femoral trochlea (*broken line*). In addition, the patellar position is made independent of external hip rotation, which would otherwise accentuate the medial patellar luxation.

proximal vastus lateralis and the femur, from the cervical tubercle of the greater trochanter medially to the interval between the rectus femoris and the vastus lateralis muscles. The origin of the rectus femoris is brought through this tunnel. The origin of the rectus femoris is secured to the cervical tubercle by wires that penetrate the cervical tubercle and provide rigid fixation to the small bone at the origin of the rectus (Fig. 62.64). If the bone is not present, a locking loop suture is passed similarly through the cervical tubercle to secure the tendinous origin of the rectus femoris muscle. Direct closure of the fascia and skin using subcutaneous absorbable suture is routine.

The rectus femoris is the primary alignment muscle of the quadriceps muscle group. Its origin on the pelvis is unique to the muscles of the quadriceps (Fig. 62.65, *left*), because the rectus femoris spans two joints (the hip and the stifle); it originates on the pelvis and inserts on the tibial tubercle. Because the line of force of the rectus femoris is between the pelvis (cranial to the acetabulum) and the tibial tubercle, external rotation at the hip predisposes animals to medial patellar luxation. The transfer of the rectus femoris origin to the cervical tubercle eliminates the effects of the hip rotation on the medial patella and reduces the luxation problem from a two-joint problem to a one-joint prob-

lem. If the patient has a varus bowing to the distal femur (Fig. 62.65, *middle*), in addition to the external rotation at the hip, the transposition of the rectus femoris may be as far lateral as the third trochanter (Fig. 62.65, *right*). This conformation is most prevalent in the pitbull, bull terrier, bullmastiff, and rottweiler.

The femoral causes of medial patellar luxation, such as varus of the distal femur and external femoral torsion, as well as the tibial causes of medial patellar luxation, such as medial placement of the tibial tubercle, varus of the proximal tibia, and internal torsion of the tibia, must be addressed separately.

Some field trial springer spaniels have medially luxating patellae, but they have normal conformation and extraordinarily well developed biceps femoris muscles. The apparent cause of the medial patellar luxation lies in the functional usage of the limb by the patient and the promotion of that usage by the field trial judges. These dogs run for miles in a low, crouched position with the hip in external rotation and abduction, but with the stifle in internal rotation. This deviation from sagittal plane alignment causes a large, medially directed force on the patella that must be contained by the lateral patellofabellar ligament and the biceps femoris, which supports the stifle in internal rotation. Trauma to the lateral patellofabellar ligament and temporary weakness of the biceps femoris muscles are the probable events that precipitate medially luxating patellae. Once established, luxating patellae are self-perpetuating.

Surgical Repair of Patellar Luxations and Fractures

Steven P. Arnoczky & Guy B. Tarvin

Injuries and dysfunctions of the patella are frequent causes of rear limb lameness in small animals. Although medial patellar luxation and, to a lesser extent, lateral patellar luxation constitute the majority of patella-associated lesions, fractures of the patella also must be considered in any discussion of patellar surgery.

Functional Anatomy

The patella can be described as the ossified portion of the quadriceps tendon. Although the patella itself is a passive structure in the body, it plays an important role in a dynamic system referred to as the extensor mechanism of the stifle. Movement of the patella is under direct influence of this mechanism, and knowledge of the mechanics of this system is essential in the treatment of patellar dysfunctions.

The primary extensor group of muscles of the stifle is the quadriceps femoris. Three of the four muscles in this group—the vastus lateralis, the vastus medialis, and the vastus intermedius—originate from the proximal femur, whereas the fourth—the rectus femoris—originates from the ilium; all four converge to form the quadriceps tendon (1). This tendon primarily attaches to the proximal portion of the patella; however, a thin portion crosses over the cranial surface of the patella to blend with the patellar ligament.

The patellar ligament is a strong band of fibrous connective tissue that courses from the patella to the tibial tuberosity. When the quadriceps muscle group contracts, the resulting force pulls on the patella, the patellar ligament, and the tibial tuberosity, causing extension of the stifle. During this motion, the patella rides in the trochlear groove. A cross section of the patella reveals a convex articular surface. The corresponding trochlear groove is concave and therefore allows for an intimate articulation between the femur and the patella. On both sides of the patella and attached to the joint capsule are the parapatellar fibrocartilages. These structures articulate with the trochlear ridges and increase the surface area and thus disperse the force of the quadriceps muscles.

Normal alignment of the extensor mechanism is necessary for stability of the stifle joint. Dysfunction of this mechanism results in abnormal joint mechanics and joint instability (2). Such instability not only causes degenerative joint disease but also places increased stress on other supporting structures, such as the cranial cruciate ligament, the collateral ligaments, and the menisci (3).

Repair of Patellar Luxations

Medial Patellar Luxations

Medial patellar luxation is one of the most common patellar problems presented to the veterinary practitioner (3–5). This disorder can be either congenital or traumatic. The congenital form, which is more common, usually is observed in small breed dogs (6) and may cause minimal to severe gait abnormalities. The clinical picture often is one of an obese animal with a varus (bowlegged) deformity of the rear limbs. The animal often crouches, owing to the inability to extend the stifles fully, with its toes pointed inward. Often, the owner describes a skipping or hopping type of gait in which the animal skips one or more steps on the involved limb. This gait, which generally is transient, is caused by the patella's riding up and over the medial trochlear ridge and being "trapped" on the medial aspect of the joint. Medial patellar luxations, unless traumatic, rarely cause acute lameness. Although medial patellar luxations sometimes coexist with acute lameness, these luxations usually are chronic; thus, other causes of acute lameness should be pursued. Those dogs with a history of patellar luxation and a sudden onset of pain in the stifle should be examined carefully to rule out cruciate ligament injury.

Various causes of congenital medial patellar luxation have been proposed (5, 7–9). Its pathogenesis, however, probably involves a combination of underlying bony abnormalities, any of which may be a cause or an effect of the disorder. Any of the following abnormalities can result in congenital medial patellar luxation; coxa vara, medial displacement of the quadriceps tendon, external femoral torsion, medial deviation of the distal femur, shallow trochlear groove, and internal rotation and medial deviation of the proximal tibia (5, 9). Some degree of each deformity probably is present in all cases.

Because the presenting symptoms and signs of medial patellar luxation vary in severity, each patient should be handled individually. Numerous methods exist for the repair of medial patellar luxation (3–5, 10–14), and a single technique does not work or is not indicated for all degrees of medial patellar luxation. The following discussion presents our treatment approach, which is based on the grading system of Putnam (9).

GRADE I LUXATIONS

In a grade I medial patellar luxation, the stifle joint is almost normal, and the patella luxates only when the joint is extended and digital pressure is applied. Animals with grade I medial patellar luxation often have no clinical signs when presented. Indications for surgical treatment should be weighed carefully because it is difficult to suggest operating on a clinically normal animal. That these asymptomatic animals may be prone to future ligamentous or bony abnormalities (15), owing to the abnormal pull across the joint, may justify them as surgical candidates. We recommend, however, that these animals not be operated on until they become clinically symptomatic for the disease.

The bony structures of the joint in grade I luxation are nearly normal; that is, the tibial tuberosity and the femoral trochlea are properly formed and have proper anatomic relationships within the joint. When surgical treatment is considered necessary, these two structures should be checked at the time of operation.

Surgical Approach and Assessment

A lateral parapatellar incision is made, and the extensor mechanism is visualized. Before opening the joint capsule, one should examine the alignment of the tibial tuberosity and the patella. These structures should be in a straight line parallel to the long axis of the limb when viewed from a craniocaudal direction. In grade I medial patellar luxation, these structures usually line up well. The joint capsule is then opened, and the patella is retracted medially to permit visualization of the trochlear groove. The groove is examined for depth and any degenerative changes. If the groove is normal in appearance, no reconstructive procedures are needed.

Creation of Lateral Restraint

In most cases of grade I medial patellar luxation, the only repair required is the creation of a lateral restraint to prevent medial displacement of the patella. This can be accomplished by imbricating the lateral joint capsule with an interrupted Lembert suture pattern. In smaller animals (15 kg or less), 2–0 chromic gut is used; in larger animals, 1–0 chromic gut usually suffices. Another technique that has worked well is the use of a single suture of 1–0 or 2–0 nylon passed around the lateral fabella and through the quadriceps tendon just proximal to the patella. The suture is then directed distally along the medial border of the patella and is passed through the patellar ligament immediately distal to the patella. The structure then is tied

on the lateral aspect of the joint and restricts medial displacement of the patella. This technique works especially well in large dogs (2).

The patella is now examined by placing a varus stress on the stifle and by internally rotating the tibia. If the patella does not luxate through a range of motion with the limb in this position and with digital pressure applied to the patella, the repair is sufficient. If the patella still has a tendency to luxate, a medial releasing incision is created by making a longitudinal parapatellar incision through the fibrous portion of the joint capsule; this incision is not closed. These procedures work well if the tibial tuberosity and femoral trochlea are normal. If these structures are abnormal, soft tissue procedures alone are not capable of overcoming the problem.

GRADE II LUXATIONS

The patella usually lies in its normal position in grade II luxation, but it luxates with flexion of the joint and remains luxated until relocated by manual pressure or extension of the joint. Animals with grade II medial patellar luxation usually have some form of gait disturbance. They also are more likely to develop degenerative changes than are animals with grade I luxation because of the greater degree of malarticulation.

Trochleoplasty

The tibial tuberosity and trochlear groove are evaluated as described for grade I luxations. If the trochlear groove is shallow, it is corrected first. A trochleoplasty is performed by first making two parallel incisions into the trochlear cartilage with a scalpel blade. These incisions delineate the medial and lateral boundaries of the new trochlear groove. The groove should be wide enough to permit proper seating of the patella while maintaining an adequate lateral and, especially, medial trochlear ridge. The cartilage between the incisions is removed with a bone rongeur or a high-speed drill (5). In younger dogs, the cartilage can easily be removed with a No. 15 scalpel blade. The groove must be deepened uniformly to the level of bleeding subchondral bone to ensure the regeneration of fibrocartilage (14). The new groove should be of sufficient width to accommodate the patella, it should have a well-developed medial ridge, and it should be of sufficient depth to discourage luxation (Fig. 62.66).

After this type of trochleoplasty, fibrocartilaginous tissue forms over the articulating surface of the deepened trochlear groove (14). Although this newly regenerated fibrocartilage surface does not possess the same physical properties of articular (hyaline) cartilage, it was thought to be sufficiently similar to be clinically effective, and indeed this technique has given good results over the years. Nonetheless, preservation of the normal hyaline cartilage surface of the trochlear

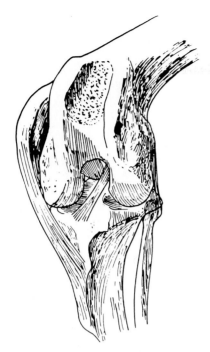

Fig. 62.66. Trochleoplasty is performed to widen and deepen the femoral trochlear groove. (From Arnoczky SP, Tarvin GB. Surgery of the stifle: the patella. Compend Contin Educ Pract Vet 1980;2:200.)

groove would be expected to enhance the results of the deepening procedure (16). To that end, a newer procedure—the trochlear wedge recession technique—was developed to deepen the trochlear groove without destroying the cartilage present (16, 17).

Trochlear Wedge Recession Technique
In this technique, an osteochondral wedge is removed from the trochlear groove with a fine-tooth bone saw. As in the previously described trochleoplasty, an adequate trochlear ridge must be maintained on the medial and lateral aspect of the trochlear groove. To do this, the saw cuts are started at the highest point on the medial and lateral trochlear ridges (Fig. 62.67**A**). The cuts are then directed to intersect at a point just proximal to the femoral origin of the caudal cruciate ligament. Care is taken not to extend the osteochondral wedge into the intercondylar notch. The osteochondral wedge is then removed to reveal a V-shaped trochlear bed (Fig. 62.67**B**). Owing to the width of the saw blade used to remove the wedge, the wedge of bone is actually smaller than the created bed. Therefore, when the osteochondral wedge is replaced into the groove, the wedge is naturally recessed, resulting in a deepened trochlear groove. If additional depth is required (at least 50% of the patellar depth should be seated in the groove), approximately 1 to 1.5 mm of additional bone can be removed by making another

set of saw cuts parallel to the first (Fig. 62.67**C**). The wedge is then replaced in the bed, so the original cartilage surface is recessed (Fig. 62.67**D**). The friction of the cancellous bone surfaces (plus the compressive force of the articulating patella) keeps the wedge in place, and no fixation appliances are needed.

Transposition of Tibial Tuberosity, Lateral Imbrication, and Medial Releasing Incision
If the tibial tuberosity is deviated medially, this deviation is corrected by transplanting the attachment of the patellar ligament to a more lateral position. This transplantation is done by osteotomy of the tibial tuberosity and lateral placement of the tuberosity under the cranial tibialis muscle (3, 4, 10, 12, 13). The tibial tuberosity is then fixed in place by one or two small Kirschner wires (Fig. 62.68). The patella is then tested in the previously described manner. Little, if any, tendency for luxation should be noted. If some tendency for medial luxation still exists, the tibial tuberosity can be moved farther laterally, or the joint capsule can be imbricated laterally; a medial releasing incision can be added if necessary (Fig. 62.69).

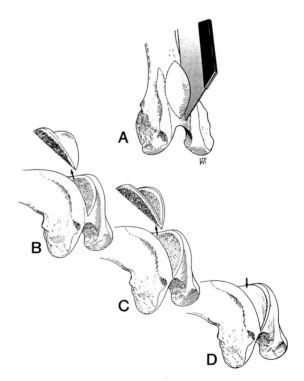

Fig. 62.67. Trochlear wedge recession technique. **A.** Location of medial and lateral saw cuts. **B.** Removal of osteochondral wedge. **C.** Deepening of trochlear bed by removal of a second wedge. **D.** Replacement of osteochondral wedge with original cartilage surface into the trochlear bed. See text for details. (Adapted from Boone EG Jr, Hohn RB, Weisbrode SE. Trochlear recession wedge technique for patellar luxation: an experimental study. J Am Anim Hosp Assoc 1983;19:735.)

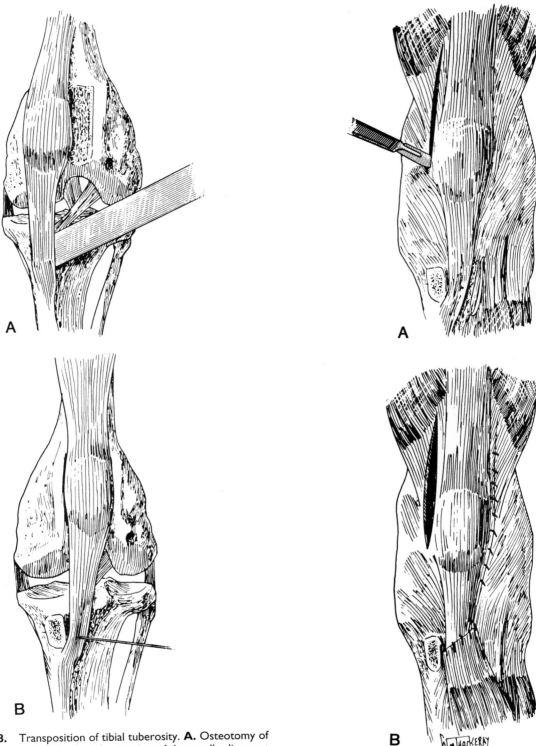

Fig. 62.68. Transposition of tibial tuberosity. **A.** Osteotomy of the tibial tuberosity. The fascial extension of the patellar ligament onto the tibial crest is left intact. **B.** Lateral transplantation and fixation of the tibial tuberosity with a Kirschner wire. (From Arnoczky SP, Tarvin GB. Surgery of the stifle: the patella. Compend Contin Educ Pract Vet 1980;2:200.)

Fig. 62.69. **A.** Medial releasing incision. **B.** Lateral imbrication of the joint capsule. (From Arnoczky SP, Tarvin GB. Surgery of the stifle: the patella. Compend Contin Educ Pract Vet 1980;2:200.)

GRADE III LUXATIONS

The patella is luxated most of the time, but it may be reduced with the limb in the extended position in grade III medial patellar luxation. All the techniques used in treating grade II medial patellar luxations probably are needed to correct grade III luxations. The same format for examining the structures should be followed to assess the necessity of each procedure, however.

If the tendency for luxation remains after correction with these techniques, the medial releasing incision may be inadequate, or a medial rotatory instability of the tibia may be present. The medial releasing incision can be extended proximally to incise a portion of the sartorius and vastus medialis muscles. Rotational instability can be corrected with a lateral suture of heavy nonabsorbable material placed around the lateral fabella and through a drill hole in the tibial crest (Fig. 62.70). Usually, a combination of the aforementioned techniques corrects a grade III medial patellar luxation.

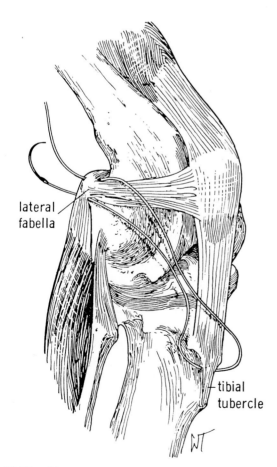

lateral fabella

tibial tubercle

Fig. 62.70. Placement of lateral derotational suture. (From Arnoczky SP, Tarvin GB. Surgery of the stifle: the patella. Compend Contin Educ Pract Vet 1980;2:200.)

GRADE IV LUXATIONS

The patella is dislocated and cannot be reduced without surgical intervention in grade IV medial patellar luxation. This least common type of luxation should be corrected at an early age to prevent the resulting bony deformities of the femur and tibia. In most cases, the previously discussed techniques are inadequate to correct the disorder because of the severe bony deformities. These patients usually require osteotomies (derotational, cuneiform) of the tibia or femur to correct the anatomic structures and thereby the mechanics of the patella (3, 4).

Lateral Patellar Luxations

Lateral patellar luxations, which are not as common as medial patellar luxations, occur most often in large breed dogs (3, 4). The disorder can be congenital or traumatic. In the congenital form, this condition is often associated with hip dysplasia, and thus simple correction of the resulting patellar alignment may eliminate the signs and symptoms but may not correct the underlying problem. Isolated deformities, such as genu valgum, also may cause lateral patellar luxations. The deformities causing lateral malalignment of the extensor mechanism are coxa valga, lateral displacement of the quadriceps tendon, internal femoral torsion, laxity of medial fascia and contraction of lateral fascia, and external rotation and lateral deviation of the proximal tibia. These disorders are, for the most part, the opposite of those causing medial luxations.

As in medial patellar luxations, the severity of the lesion varies widely. Affected animals usually have a valgus (knock-knee) deformity of the rear limbs and are first seen in a crouched stance with the toes pointing outward. Correction of this disorder is based on the grading system described for medial luxations. In each case, the structures of the stifle are assessed and are corrected in the same stepwise manner as for medial patellar luxation with the following obvious modifications to the procedures: 1) *medial* (not lateral) imbrication; 2) *lateral* (not medial) releasing incision; 3) *medial* (not lateral) transposition of the tibial tuberosity; and 4) *medial* (not lateral) derotational suture.

Postoperative Care

After surgical repair of both medial and lateral patellar luxations, patients should be fitted with a soft, padded bandage for 2 weeks and have restricted exercise for a minimum of 3 weeks. In the case of bilateral patellar luxations, the most severely affected limb is usually operated on first, and at least a 4-week healing period is observed before the second limb is treated.

Repair of Patellar Fractures

Patellar fractures are uncommon in veterinary practice and are associated with severe trauma to the stifle (2). It is therefore imperative that all structures of the stifle be carefully evaluated when patellar fractures are encountered.

As noted previously, the patella plays an intricate role in the extensor mechanism of the stifle. Removal of the patella consistently results in degenerative lesions within the stifle (2). Therefore, in the treatment of patellar fractures, the patella should be preserved whenever possible. Patellectomy should be performed only as a salvage procedure and only when the patella is destroyed so completely that no fragment is large enough to contribute effectively to the extensor mechanism.

Tension Band Fixation

Because the patella is under great tensile force from the pull of the quadriceps muscles, fracture fragments often distract. Internal fixation is the treatment of choice to restore normal anatomic structure and function. Fracture repair consists of reduction of the fragments, reestablishment of a smooth articular surface, preservation of the extensor mechanism, and fixation.

The greatest chance for successful surgical treatment is with a simple transverse fracture through the patella that leaves two fragments of equal size (Fig. 62.71**A**). Fixation can be accomplished with a tension band wire to neutralize the distractive forces of the quadriceps muscles. The patella is approached through a lateral arthrotomy, and the articular surface is examined as the fracture is reduced.

Orthopedic wire (18- or 20-gauge wire) is passed laterally to medially through the quadriceps tendon just proximal to the patella; the wire is brought across the cranial surface of the patella and is reinserted into the patellar ligament just distal to the patella in a lateral-to-medial direction (Fig. 62.71**B**). With the stifle in extension, the free ends of the wire are twisted on each other until the fracture is reduced (Fig. 62.71**C** and **D**). The wire is cut, and the twisted portion is folded on itself. Another technique is to loop two wires around the patella, tightening one from the medial aspect and one from the lateral aspect of the patella. After the surgical procedure, the animal is placed in a soft, padded bandage and is allowed only limited weightbearing for 2 to 3 weeks.

Partial Patellectomy

In some patellar fractures, only the proximal portion of the patella can be salvaged. In such cases, the fracture fragments of the distal portion are resected. After this

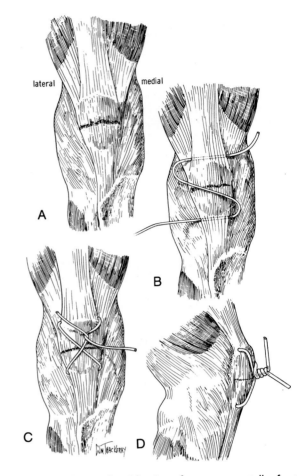

Fig. 62.71. Tension band fixation of transverse patellar fracture. **A.** Simple transverse patellar fracture. **B.** Placement of orthopedic wire. **C.** Tightening of wire. **D.** Lateral view of properly placed wire. See text for details. (From Arnoczky SP, Tarvin GB. Surgery of the stifle: the patella. Compend Contin Educ Pract Vet 1980;2:200.)

resection, the proximal portion of the patellar ligament is weakened or may actually be ruptured. Horizontal mattress sutures of 4–0 stainless steel are used to reinforce this attachment. If the tendon is torn, simple interrupted sutures can be used to approximate the torn ends (Fig. 62.72).

The tensile forces across this compromised portion of the patellar ligament must be neutralized to allow for adequate healing. This is accomplished by passing 18- or 20-gauge orthopedic wire through the quadriceps tendon proximal to the patella and continuing it distally, where it is passed through a drill hole in the tibial crest (see Fig. 62.72). With the limb in extension, the wire is tightened until the stress on the patellar ligament is relieved. Thus, the wire transmits the force of the quadriceps tendon to the tibia and puts the patellar ligament at rest.

The animal is placed in a soft, padded bandage and is allowed only limited exercise for 2 to 3 weeks. The

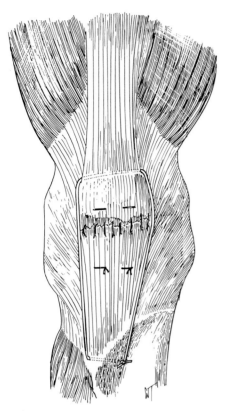

Fig. 62.72. Placement of mattress sutures and tension band wire in partial patellectomy. (From Arnoczky SP, Tarvin GB. Surgery of the stifle: the patella. Compend Contin Educ Pract Vet 1980;2:200.)

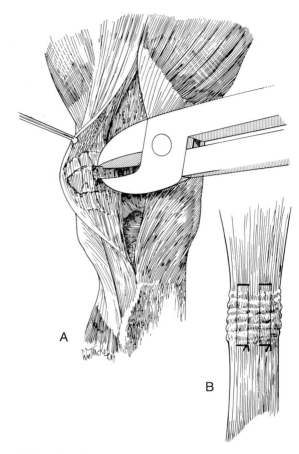

Fig. 62.73. Patellectomy. **A.** Removal of fractured patellar fragments from the articular surface of the patella with a rongeur. **B.** "Snugged-up" patellar ligament after patellectomy. (From Arnoczky SP, Tarvin GB. Surgery of the stifle: the patella. Compend Contin Educ Pract Vet 1980;2:200.)

orthopedic wire can be removed in 4 to 6 weeks (18). These wires often break by the fourth postoperative week because of fatigue (2).

In cases of patellar ligament rupture, a similar technique can be used. After repair with mattress or Bunnell sutures of 4–0 stainless steel, a tension band of orthopedic wire is similarly placed around the patella and through a drill hole in the tibial crest. Postoperative considerations are as previously described.

PATELLECTOMY

As previously noted, the patellofemoral articulation plays an important role in the biomechanics of stifle motion. Removal of the patella alters this function, and severe degenerative changes result. Patellectomy is therefore indicated *only* when patellar damage is so severe that repair is impossible.

Patellectomy is most easily performed through a standard lateral arthrotomy. The fractured patella is retracted medially and is everted to expose its fragmented articular surface. The fracture fragments are then removed with a ronguer or a periosteal elevator and scalpel (Fig. 62.73**A**). Removal of the patella alters the biomechanics of the quadriceps pull and also

weakens that portion of the patellar ligament. Hence, mattress sutures of 4–0 stainless steel are used to reinforce and tighten the patellar ligament (Fig. 62.73**B**). This maneuver accommodates for the laxity in the extensor mechanism caused by the absence of the patella and also reinforces the weakened patellar tendon. The sutures are placed with the limb in extension. The animal is placed in a soft, padded bandage and is allowed only restricted exercise for 2 to 3 weeks.

References

1. Evans HE, Christensen GC. Miller's anatomy of the dog. 2nd ed. Philadelphia: WB Saunders, 1979.
2. Arnoczky SP, Tarvin GB. Surgery of the stifle: the patella. Compend Contin Educ Pract Vet 1980;2:200.
3. Rudy RL. Stifle joint. In: Archibald J, ed. Canine surgery. 2nd ed. Santa Barbara, CA: American Veterinary Publications, 1974.
4. Harrison JW. Patellar dislocation. In: Bojrab MJ, ed. Current techniques in small animal surgery. Philadelphia: Lea & Febiger, 1975.
5. Trotter E. Medical patellar luxation in the dog. Compend Contin Educ Pract Vet 1980;2:58.

6. Priester WA. Sex, size, and breed as risk factors in canine patellar dislocation. J Am Vet Med Assoc 1972;160:740.
7. Hobday F. Congenital malformation and displacement of the patella. Vet J 1905;60:216.
8. Lacroix JV. Recurrent luxation of the patella in dogs. North Am Vet 1930;2:47.
9. Putman RW. Patellar luxation in the dog. Master's thesis, University of Guelph, Ontario, Canada, 1968.
10. Brinker WO, Keller WE. Rotation of the tibial tuberosity for correction of luxation of the patella. Mich State Univ Vet 1962;22:92.
11. DeAngelis MP. Patellar luxations in dogs. Vet Clin North Am 1971;1:403.
12. Flo G, Brinker WO. Fascia lata overlap procedure for surgical correction of recurrent medial luxation of the patella in the dog. J Am Vet Med Assoc 1970;156:595.
13. Singleton WB. Transplantation of the tibial crest for treatment of congenital patellar luxation. In: Proceedings of the 27th Annual Meeting of the American Animal Hospital Association. Denver, CO: American Animal Hospital Association, 1960.
14. Vierhelle, RC. Grooving the femoral trochlea. In: Proceedings of the 34th Annual Meeting of the American Animal Hospital Association.: American Animal Hospital Association, 1967.
15. O'Brien TR. Developmental deformities due to arrested epiphyseal growth. Vet Clin North Am 1971;1:441.
16. Slocum B, Slocum DB, Devine T, et al. Wedge recession for treatment of recurrent luxations of the patella. Clin Orthop 1982;164:48.
17. Boone EG Jr, Hohn RB, Weisbrode SE. Trochlear recession wedge technique for patellar luxation: an experimental study. J Am Anim Hosp Assoc 1983;19:735.
18. Carb A. A partial patellectomy procedure for transverse patellar fractures in the dog and cat. J Am Anim Hosp Assoc 1975;11:659.

Treatment of Osteochondritis Dissecans of the Stifle

Ron K. Fallon

The purpose of surgical intervention of osteochondritis dissecans lesions of the stifle is to remove large or free cartilaginous flaps in exploring the acutely lame patient.

Surgical Technique

The animal is best placed in dorsal recumbency, and the limb is prepared aseptically. A standard medial or lateral parapatellar arthrotomy is performed (1). Complete visualization of the articular surfaces is necessary, and a medial approach seems to provide a slightly better exposure for lateral condylar lesions. The use of a Gelpi self-retaining retractor aids in the exposure for the surgeon who is working alone.

The offending osteochondral flap and any "joint mice" are removed until a healthy bed of cartilage remains and subchondral bone is present. The margins are curetted perpendicular to the articular surfaces (2). A 0.045 Kirschner wire is inserted into the defect in multiple areas to aid in revascularization. The joint is thoroughly lavaged of any loose debris. The arthrotomy, subcutaneous tissues, and skin are closed with monofilament absorbable suture in a routine manner.

A modified Robert Jones bandage is applied to the limb for up to 2 weeks. Daily physical therapy consisting of swimming or leash walking is indicated for an additional 2 weeks, after which no exercise restrictions are necessary.

History and signalment of osteochondritis dissecans of the stifle are similar to those of both hip dysplasia and cranial cruciate ligament injury and may often be associated with concomitant disorders. Surgical management is indicated both as a diagnostic tool and as a therapeutic procedure when arthroscopy is not available or when a high suspicion of a large osteochondral fragment exists. In many patients with osteochondritis dissecans of the stifle, lameness has been relieved by removal of a joint mouse (3, 4). Nonsurgical management may be appropriate for dogs without cartilage flaps or free joint mice (5).

Once osteoarthrosis develops, one can do little to improve joint function. Dogs with an early onset of clinical signs, advanced degenerative joint disease, and large lesions have the worst prognosis (4).

References

1. Piermattei DL. An atlas of surgical approaches to the bones and joints of the dog and cat. 3rd ed. Philadelphia: WB Saunders, 1993:276–281.
2. Rudd RG, Visco DM, Kincaid SA, et al. The effects of beveling the margins of articular cartilage defects in immature dogs. Vet Surg 1987;16:378–383.
3. Berzoin JL. Osteochondritis dissecans in the dog: diagnosis and therapy. J Am Vet Med Assoc 1979;175:796–799.
4. Montgomery RD, Milton JL, Henderson RA, et al. Osteochondritis dissecans of the canine stifle. Compend Contin Educ Pract Vet 1989;11:1199–1205.
5. Olsson SE. Osteochondrosis in the dog. In: Kirk RW, ed. Current veterinary therapy VI. Philadelphia: WB Saunders, 1977: 880–886.

63

TARSUS

Algorithm for Treatment of Tarsal Injuries

Jon F. Dee

Figure 63.1 is an algorithm for the management of injuries of the tarsus.

Suggested Readings

Dee JF, Dee LG. In: Sumner-Smith G, ed. Decision making in small animal orthopedic surgery. Philadelphia: BC Decker, 1987.

Dee JF. In: Refresher course for veterinarians. Proceedings No. 22: greyhound medicine and surgery. Sydney, Australia: University of Sydney Postgraduate Committee in Veterinary Science, 1989:469–632.

Collinson R. A problem-oriented approach to individual joints. In: Holton J, Collinson R, eds. Manual of small animal arthrology. Gloucestershire, UK: British Small Animal Veterinary Association (BSAVA), 1994:51.

Specific Tests for Tarsal Injury

Christopher M. Boemo

Tarsal Anatomy

The tarsus is a complex structure, and its bony and ligamentous anatomic features are worthy of review by the reader (Fig. 63.2). The joint between the tibia and fibula and the talus and calcaneus is termed the tarsocrural joint, also often referred to as the tibiotarsal joint. Certain intertarsal joints refer to the articulations between adjacent tarsal bones, with four joints specifically named:

Talocalcaneal: the joint between the talus and the calcaneus

Calcaneoquartile: the joint between the calcaneus and the fourth tarsal bone

Talocalcaneocentral: the joint with articulation principally between the talus and central tarsal bone but with the joint capsule extending to have some communication with the calcaneus

Centrodistal: the joint between the central tarsal bone and the more distal numbered tarsal bones

The joints between the numbered tarsal bones and the metatarsal bones are termed the tarsometatarsal joints. As in the carpus, the most proximal joint is supported by both short and long collateral ligaments. The long components of the ligaments provide hock stability during extension, whereas the short components act in flexion. Further sideways stability is provided by the presence of the tibial and fibular malleoli. The plantar ligaments and tarsal fibrocartilage are well developed and limit dorsal hyperextension of the intertarsal and tarsometatarsal joints. The dorsal ligaments are much smaller and shorter, and they connect adjacent tarsal bones.

Specific Tests

The tarsus is subject to both osseous and ligamentous injury, especially in athletic animals. Fractures, ligamentous tears, and avulsions occur commonly as a result of propulsive effort rather than external trauma, and these injuries are accompanied by lameness, soft tissue swelling, joint instability, tarsal deformation,

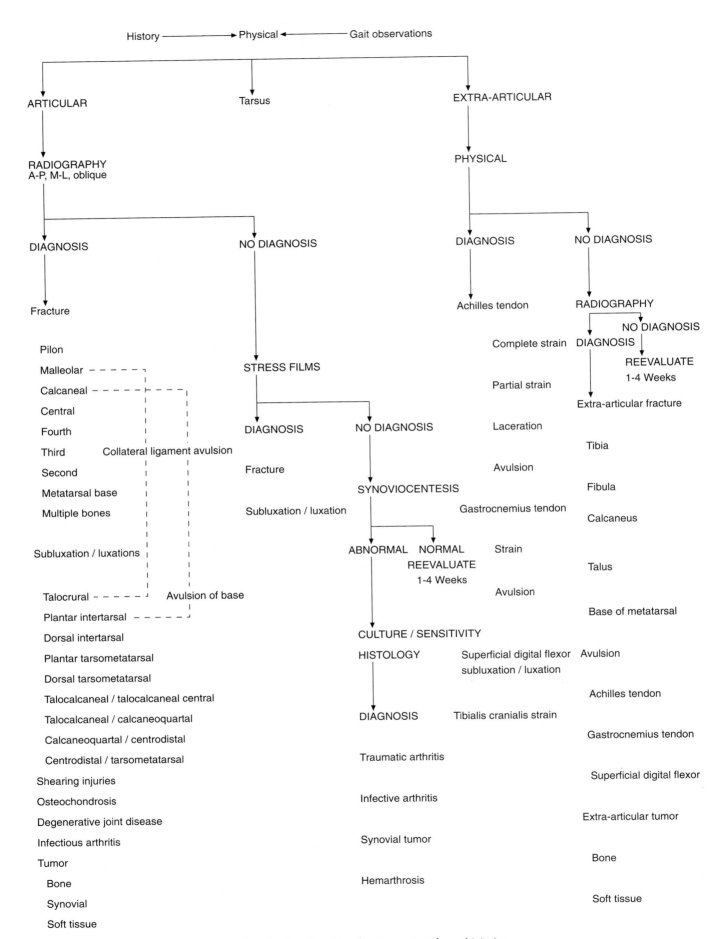

Fig. 63.1. Algorithm for treatment of tarsal injuries.

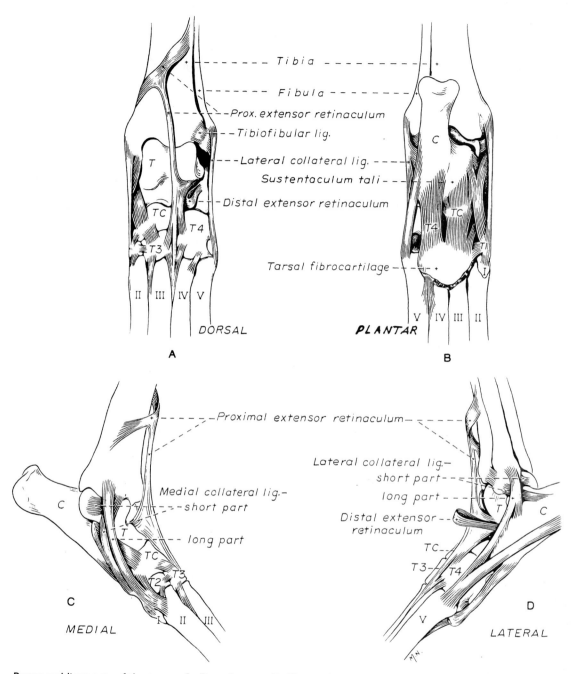

Fig. 63.2. Bones and ligaments of the tarsus. **A.** Dorsal aspect. **B.** Plantar aspect. **C.** Medial aspect. **D.** Lateral aspect. *C,* calcaneus; *T1,* *T3, T4,* first, third, and fourth tarsals; *T,* talus; *I* through *V,* first to fifth metatarsals; *TC,* central tarsal. (From Evans HE, Christensen GC. Miller's anatomy of the dog. 2nd ed. Philadelphia: WB Saunders, 1979.)

and crepitus. A good working knowledge of the region is necessary for proper diagnosis and treatment.

Physical Examination

The physical examination needs to be thorough and systematic in order that all the injuries of significance are diagnosed. The examination of the conscious ani-

mal may be restricted by swelling and the patient's response to pain. Sedation or anesthesia may facilitate a more comprehensive evaluation of the tarsal injuries. The tarsus should be examined visually for deformation, as is seen with plantar ligament rupture or calcaneus fracture, and it should be palpated carefully for crepitus and bone or bone fragment luxation. The affected tarsus should be flexed, and the degree of flexion should be compared with that of the contralateral limb because hock flexion is reduced with tarsal osteochondrosis dissecans. Because the tibiotarsal joint is ostensibly a hinge joint, it should be examined for any valgus or varus deformations of the joint, which occur with rupture of the medial and lateral collateral ligaments, respectively.

Tarsal Injuries

Plantar Proximal Intertarsal Subluxation and Luxation

Proximal intertarsal subluxation with plantar instability results from rupture or avulsion of the plantar ligament and fibrocartilage and is the most common ligamentous injury affecting the tarsus in small animals. Although both proximal intertarsal joints are involved, the calcaneoquartile joint is more significant because compromise of the plantar ligament between the calcaneus and the fourth tarsal bone results in the subluxation. It is a hyperextension injury, often occurring without a history of known trauma, and although it is seen in all breeds of dogs, the collie and Shetland sheepdog are overrepresented. Highly athletic breeds and obese, poorly conditioned animals are more commonly affected.

The affected limb presents with a plantigrade stance varying in severity from little more than a slight bowing to the worst cases, in which the animal is walking on the plantar aspect of the metatarsus. Pain and soft tissue swelling are variable, but usually not severe, and flexion of the hock may elicit only a mild reaction from the patient.

Complete luxation of the tarsus at the level of the proximal intertarsal joint is much less common than plantar subluxation, usually results from severe trauma, and may be complicated by tarsal fractures. Pain, swelling, and lameness are much more pronounced.

Radiography, using routine and stress views, reveals hinging at the dorsal surface. with or without avulsed bone fragments from the base of the calcaneus or the fourth tarsal bone in cases of subluxation. These signs must be differentiated from the dorsal displacement of the distal tarsal structures observed radiographically in cases of luxation.

Most patients with plantar subluxations require pri-

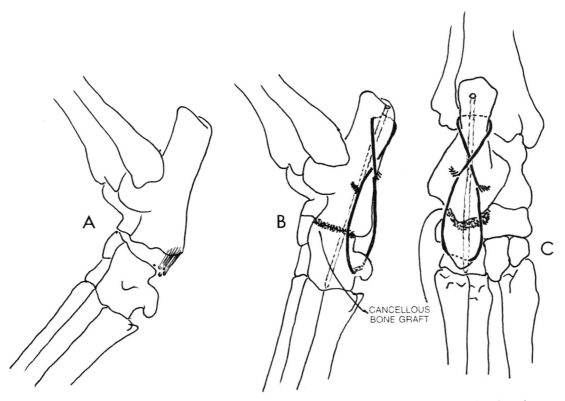

Fig. 63.3. Plantar proximal intertarsal subluxation. **A.** Tearing or avulsion of the plantar ligament supporting the calcaneoquartile joint results in dorsiflexion of the proximal intertarsal joint and a plantigrade stance. Arthrodesis of the calcaneoquartile joint is indicated. **B** and **C.** The joint is exposed through a plantarolateral approach, and the superficial digital flexor tendon is retracted medially after incision of the deep fascia and the tendon's lateral attachments to the tuber calcanei. The joint cartilage is removed, and a cancellous bone graft is incorporated into the joint space. A figure-of-eight tension band wire is placed between the tuber calcanei and the plantar tubercle of the fourth tarsal, and a 2- to 3.5-mm pin is driven along a predrilled pilot hole down the calcaneus into the distal fourth tarsal bone and is countersunk below the articular cartilage. The wire is then tightened.

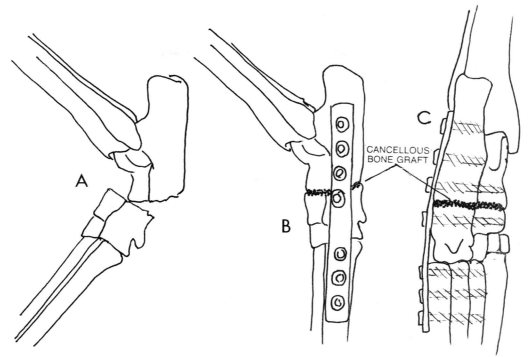

Fig. 63.4. Proximal intertarsal luxation. **A.** Complete luxation of the proximal intertarsal joint occurs after severe trauma and soft tissue injury. Arthrodesis of the entire intertarsal joint is indicated. **B** and **C.** The joints are exposed through a lateral approach, joint cartilage is removed, and a cancellous bone graft incorporated. The lateral surfaces of the fibular tarsal and fifth metatarsal are flattened to allow proper seating of the plate. Typically, a seven-hole plate is used with three screws in the calcaneus, one through the fourth tarsal into the central tarsal and three into the metatarsals.

mary arthrodesis of the calcaneoquartile joint (Fig. 63.3). The joint is exposed through a plantarolateral incision extending from the proximal end of the tuber calcanei to the distal fourth tarsal bone, with the superficial digital flexor tendon retracted medially. Ligament remnants and avulsed bone chips are excised to expose the joint. The articular cartilage is removed by manual curettage or with the aid of an air bur. A lateromedial hole is drilled through the proximal middle third of the calcaneus and the plantar tubercle of the fourth tarsal bone. A figure-of-eight stainless steel tension band wire is threaded through the holes but left loose.

A pilot hole for a single intramedullary pin is drilled the length of the calcaneus, preferably with a bone drill because of the significant hardness of the bone. Autogenous cancellous bone harvested from the surgeon's preferred site is packed into the joint space while the joint is flexed to open it. The intramedullary pin is directed and driven from the tuber calcanei to the distal end of the fourth tarsal bone. The pin is retracted, cut off, and countersunk below the articular cartilage of the tuber calcanei to prevent trauma to the superficial digital flexor tendon.

The tension band wire is then tightened, with the wire twists cut short and folded flat against the bone. The superficial flexor tendon is relocated, and the lat-

eral retinaculum is sutured to prevent its displacement postoperatively. A padded support bandage is applied for 7 to 10 days, and the patient is confined with restricted exercise (small pen or leash controlled walking) for approximately 8 weeks postoperatively.

In patients with complete luxation of the proximal intertarsal joint, arthrodesis is again the preferred method of repair. Bone plate fixation or medial and lateral placement of lag screws provides a more stable fixation than does placement of an intramedullary pin and tension band wire.

If using bone plate fixation, the joint is exposed laterally with an incision extending from the tuber calcanei to the distal proximal third of the metatarsus. An air bur, bone rasp, or curette is used to remove the cartilage from the joint surfaces, and the lateral surfaces of the fibular tarsal bone and proximal metatarsal V are flattened to allow proper placement of the plate. Cancellous bone grafting is performed.

Typically, a seven-hole 2.7- or 3.5-mm plate is used with three screws placed in the calcaneus, one through the fourth and central tarsal bones, and three in the proximal aspect of metatarsals IV and V (Fig. 63.4). Because the plate is not placed on the tension side of the injury, the repair is supported postoperatively in a splint or cast until one sees radiographic signs of fusion, usually in 6 to 8 weeks. The plate should be left in situ for at least 4 months, but, because of movement at the tarsometatarsal joint, the screws placed into the metatarsals loosen and may have to be removed before this time. Occasionally, skin necrosis occurs over the plate. This should be treated as an open wound with the plate left in situ until removed at approximately 4 months postoperatively.

The intertarsal luxation may also be stabilized by the placement of two lag screws, one directed distolaterally from the medial side of the head of the tibiotarsal bone into the central tarsal and more distal third tarsal bones and the other screw directed distomedially from the body of the calcaneus into the fourth tarsal bone (Fig. 63.5). The surgical sites are accessed through both medial and lateral incisions directly over the joint. The articular cartilage of the proximal intertarsal joint is debrided before screw or pin placement, and cancellous bone grafting is performed. Two Kirschner wires may be substituted for the screws in smaller animals. The repair needs to be protected from cyclic loading of the screws while fusion is progressing, so the limb must be supported in a splint or cast until radiographic evidence indicates bone fusion.

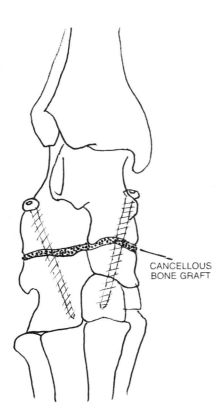

CANCELLOUS
BONE GRAFT

Fig. 63.5. Proximal intertarsal luxation. In smaller animals, the proximal intertarsal joint may undergo arthrodesis through placement of two lag screws. Lateral and medial approaches are required, the joint cartilage is debrided, and a cancellous bone graft is incorporated. One screw is directed distolaterally from the medial side of the talus into the central and third tarsals, and the other is directed distomedially from the lateral aspect of the calcaneus into the fourth tarsal.

Dorsal Proximal Intertarsal Subluxation

Proximal intertarsal subluxation with dorsal instability is much less common than plantar subluxation of the proximal intertarsal joint. The dorsal ligament rupture is often accompanied by either medial or, more commonly, lateral collateral ligament injury and resultant instability. It is a self-compressing injury, relatively stable during the weightbearing phase of the gait and less stable during the swing phase. The patient stands normally because the plantar ligaments are intact, but subtle lameness and soft tissue swelling are present. The lameness is more severe if medial or lateral collateral ligament injury is present.

Diagnosis is based on palpation of the tarsus with hyperextension of the tarsal joint resulting in an angular deformity to the plantar surface. Stress lateromedial radiographic projections confirm the affected joint level. Varus deformity of the foot during weightbearing occurs when the patient has concurrent lateral collateral ligament damage.

Coaptation in a plantar splint or half-cast for 4 to 6 weeks may well be satisfactory in cases not complicated by lateral or medial instability. Primary surgical repair is indicated when coaptation is unsuccessful or when the patient has concurrent collateral ligament damage and resultant instability. Commonly, both medial and lateral sides need to be repaired, and the areas are approached through incisions directly over the respective sites. Dorsal and medial instability can be corrected by the placement of a lag screw directed distolaterally from the medial side of the head of the tibiotarsal bone into the central tarsal and more distal third tarsal bones (Fig. 63.6). One or two Kirschner wires may be substituted for screws in smaller animals. The articular cartilage of the proximal intertarsal joint is debrided before screw or pin placement, and cancellous bone grafting is performed. Any ligament remnants suitable for suturing are repaired. When instability is present laterally, the same lag screw technique may be performed with the screw directed distomedially from the body of the talus into the fourth tarsal bone (see Fig. 63.5), or a tension band wire may be placed through dorsoplantarly directed bone tunnels in the lateral bony projections of the distal calcaneus and proximal fourth tarsal bones (see Fig. 63.6).

Postoperatively, a plantar splint or half-cast is applied for approximately 3 weeks, with restricted exercise for 3 to 4 more weeks.

Intertarsal Subluxation Distal to the Talocalcaneocentral and Calcaneoquartile Joints

Intertarsal subluxation involving the centrodistal joint, with or without involvement of the proximal intertarsal (calcaneoquartile) or tarsometatarsal joint, occurs

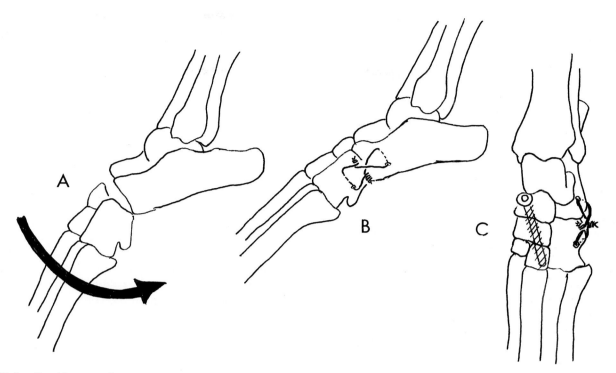

Fig. 63.6. Dorsal proximal intertarsal subluxation. **A.** Rupture of the dorsal ligaments results in hyperextension of the tarsus and angular deformity of the plantar surface. **B.** Lateral instability is corrected by the placement of a figure-of-eight wire through dorsoplantarly directed drill holes in the lateral bony prominences of the calcaneus and the fourth tarsal bone. **C.** Dorsal and medial instability is corrected by a neutralization screw directed distolaterally from the medial base of the talus into the central and third tarsals.

less commonly than proximal intertarsal subluxation. Fourth tarsal bone fracture is a frequent complication of the injury.

Swelling is usually minimal, and careful palpation reveals valgus deformation resulting from the dorsomedial ligamentous rupture. Further instability may be detected when either the calcaneoquartile or tarsometatarsal joint is involved as well. Commonly, the plantar support is intact. Stress view radiographs are important to determine which joints are involved.

Repair is by arthrodesis of the involved joints. When only the centrodistal intertarsal joint is affected, the area is exposed by a medial incision directly over the site. The articular cartilage is removed from the joint by means of an air bur, bone rasp, or curette. A cancellous bone graft is incorporated into the joint space, and bone screws are directed laterally from the medial aspect of the central and second tarsal bones into the fourth tarsal bone. Stainless steel orthopedic wire (0.8 to 1.0 mm) is looped around the screw shanks in a figure-of-eight pattern and is tightened (Fig. 63.7).

When both the centrodistal and the calcaneoquartile joints are involved, arthrodesis of all the affected joints, including the vertical intertarsal joint, is indicated. Both lateral and medial aspects of the tarsus need to be exposed. The articular cartilage of all affected joints is removed, and a cancellous bone graft is incorporated. The joint spaces are stabilized and

compressed by the placement of a seven-hole 2.7- or 3.5-mm dynamic compression plate laterally, as described in the section of this discussion on plantar proximal intertarsal luxation (see Fig. 63.4), and medially either by two screws and the figure-of-eight wire, as described for centrodistal intertarsal subluxation in isolation (see Fig. 63.7), or by a two-hole dynamic compression plate.

With subluxation of the centrodistal and tarsometatarsal joints, the joints involved are those between the central and second or third tarsal bones and those between the fourth tarsal and the third and fourth metatarsal bones. These joints and the vertical intertarsal joint between the third and fourth tarsal bones undergo arthrodesis. The affected joints are approached through dorsal midline incision, with retraction of soft tissues to expose the dorsal surfaces of the central, third, and fourth tarsal bones and the proximodorsal surfaces of the third and fourth metatarsal bones. The articular cartilage is removed, and cancellous bone is incorporated as a graft. Two four- or five-hole dynamic compression bone plates are placed dorsally, with one located over the central tarsal, third tarsal, and third metatarsal bones and the other placed over the fourth tarsal and fourth metatarsal bones (Fig. 63.8).

Because the implants are not placed on the tension side of the injury, the repair of centrodistal subluxation, with or without involvement of the calcaneo-

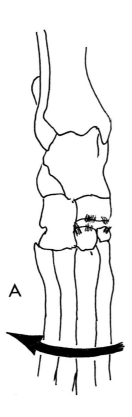

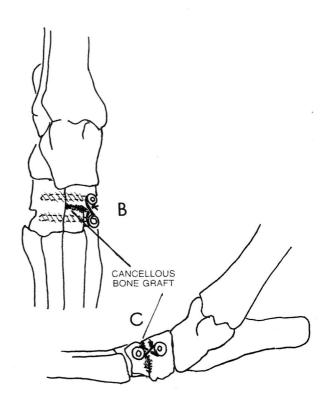

CANCELLOUS
BONE GRAFT

Fig. 63.7. Centrodistal subluxation. **A.** Rupture of the supporting ligaments results in valgus deformation of the foot. **B** and **C.** Repair is through arthrodesis of the joint. A medial approach is followed by curettage of the joint cartilage and the incorporation of a cancellous bone graft into the joint space. Bone screws directed laterally through the central and numbered tarsals into the fourth tarsal are tied together by a figure-of-eight wire, which is then tightened.

quartile or tarsometatarsal joint, must be protected during bone fusion. A plantar splint or cast is applied until radiographic evidence indicates osseous union, usually in 6 to 8 weeks. Bone plates extending over a joint that has not undergone arthrodesis eventually have screws loosen, necessitating their removal. Plate removal should be delayed, if possible, for at least 4 months postoperatively.

Central Tarsal Bone Fractures

Fractures of the central tarsal bone occur almost exclusively in racing greyhounds, with the right leg showing the highest incidence. Luxation of the central tarsal bone occurs sporadically in most breeds.

The high compression forces experienced by the bone during racing often result in explosive fractures with displacement of fragments. Fractures of the fibular tarsal or fourth tarsal bone may occur with central tarsal bone fractures. The more extensive the fracture pattern, and the greater is the involvement of other tarsal bones, and the poorer the prognosis is for return to racing.

Central tarsal bone fractures have been classified into five types, based on the number and type of displaced fragments seen radiographically or surgically:

Type 1: dorsal slab fracture without displacement
Type 2: dorsal slab fracture with displacement

Type 3: fracture in a sagittal plane with displacement of the medial fragment medially or dorsally
Type 4: dorsal displaced slab fragment in conjunction with a (usually) larger medial displaced fragment
Type 5: severely comminuted fractures with displacement of fragments

Type 1 and type 2 central tarsal bone fractures are usually associated with minimal swelling, and subtle, weightbearing lameness. In the case of racing greyhounds, the animal usually performs satisfactorily, and lameness becomes obvious only after the animal has cooled down. Hock flexion and point pressure over the dorsomedial or dorsal aspect of the bone cause discomfort and a reluctance to return to weightbearing. No crepitus or angular deformity is noted. Type 1 fractures heal with coaptation in a splint for 4 to 6 weeks, although during the healing phase, some dorsal displacement of the fragment may result in a slight incongruity at the talocalcaneocentral joint. For this reason, type 1 fractures are commonly repaired by the placement of a lag screw, as are type 2 fractures. The dorsal surface of the bone is approached through a dorsomedial incision directly over the bone, and the lag screw is centered in the middle of the fragment and is directed dorsoplantarly (Fig. 63.9).

Type 3 fractures are rare and usually present surgically with a small dorsal fragment not apparent radiographically; in reality, these are type 4 fractures. True

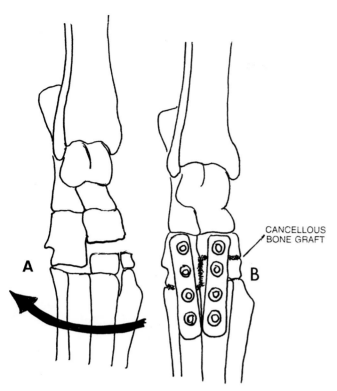

Fig. 63.8. Centrodistal–tarsometatarsal subluxation. **A.** Rupture of the ligaments between the fourth tarsal and metatarsals may occur in conjunction with rupture of the centrodistal ligaments and subsequent medial instability. **B.** Repair is achieved by arthrodesis of all affected joints. A dorsal approach is followed by removal of the joint cartilage in the centrodistal, tarsometatarsal, and vertical intertarsal joints, the incorporation of a cancellous bone graft, and the placement of dynamic compression plates to maintain the reduction.

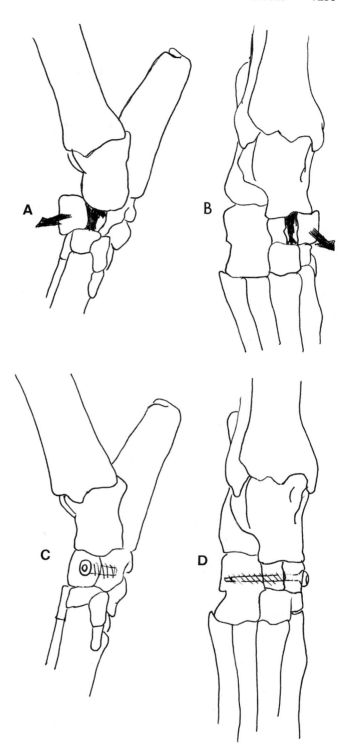

Fig. 63.10. Type 3 central tarsal fracture. **A** and **B.** Medial and dorsal views of a type 3 central tarsal bone fracture with dorsomedial displacement of the medial fracture fragment. **C** and **D.** After a medial approach, the fragment is reduced and fixed by placement of a mediolaterally directed lag screw.

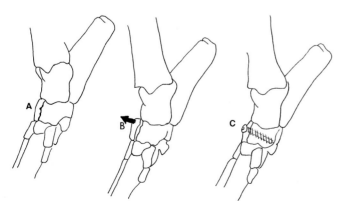

Fig. 63.9. Type 1 and type 2 central tarsal fractures. **A.** Type 1 central tarsal bone fracture. **B.** Type 2 central tarsal bone fracture. **C.** Repair is through a dorsomedial approach to the bone and involves placement of a lag screw in a dorsoplantar direction.

type 3 fractures are approached through a dorsomedial incision over the bone and are repaired with a single mediolaterally directed lag screw extending into the fourth tarsal bone with the screw centered just proximal to the origin of the ligament between the central and third tarsal bones (Fig. 63.10).

Type 4 fractures are the most frequently encountered type of central tarsal bone fracture, and they are essentially a combined type 2 and type 3 fracture. The size of the dorsal and medially displaced fragments can vary. A slight varus deformity of the foot is increased when the more lateral, nondisplaced fragment becomes comminuted (type 5 fracture). Repair is achieved by the placement of two lag screws, with accurate placement required to allow both screws to be placed in bone of its size. The bone is approached through a dorsomedial incision, and the mediolateral screw is placed first, centered on the junction between the middle and distal thirds of the bone. The second screw is a dorsoplantarly directed screw centered on the junction between the proximal and middle thirds of the bone (Fig. 63.11). The angle of the screw hole must be placed carefully to allow the screw to pass proximal to the mediolateral screw but not enter the talocalcaneocentral joint.

Type 5 fractures carry the poorest prognosis of the five types of central tarsal bone fracture for return to a competitive career. Radiographically, the joint space is narrowed because of comminution of the nondisplaced, lateral fragment. Type 5 fractures are commonly accompanied by fracture of the fourth tarsal bone, with varus and plantigrade deformation of the paw. If fragments are large enough, lag screw fixation similar to that described for type 4 fractures may be contemplated, although anchorage in the fourth tarsal bone may be difficult because of fractures within it. When fragments are sufficiently small to preclude screw fixation, a 2.7-mm finger plate may be used as a buttress plate. The site is exposed through a dorsomedial incision, the plate is fixed to the body of the talus and to the third tarsal bone (Fig. 63.12), and bone fragments are packed back loosely. A cancellous bone graft is incorporated into the repair. This repair results in a dog sound for kennel duties, but the length of time required for adequate bone strength to be achieved probably precludes a return to a competitive career.

Lag screw fixation does not provide adequate fixation of these fractures to allow early, nonprotected weightbearing, especially in the pain-tolerant greyhound. The limb tends to be excessively loaded even with strict kennel confinement. A splint or half-cast should be applied for approximately 3 to 4 weeks postoperatively, with kennel confinement for a further 2 weeks, followed by a gradual return to work. Screws need not be removed unless, as may occur with the dorsoplantarly directed screw in the repair of type 4 central tarsal bone fractures, the screw enters the calcaneotalocentral joint space.

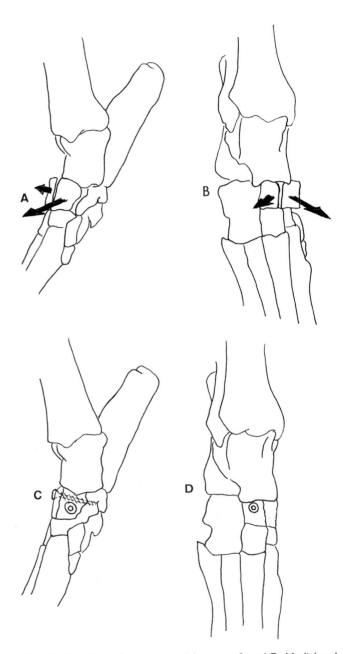

Fig. 63.11. Type 4 central tarsal fracture. **A** and **B.** Medial and dorsal views of a type 4 fracture showing dorsomedial displacement of the medial fragment and dorsal displacement of the dorsolateral fragment. **C** and **D.** After a dorsomedial approach and reduction of the fracture fragments, a mediolateral screw centered on the junction between the middle and distal thirds of the bone is placed through the fragment into the fourth tarsal. This is followed by placement of a dorsoplantar or dorsoplantaromedial screw through the dorsal fragment so as not to interfere with either the first screw or the talocentral joint space.

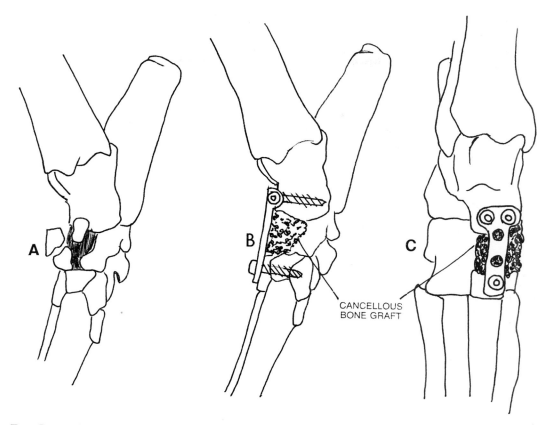

CANCELLOUS
BONE GRAFT

Fig. 63.12. Type 5 central tarsal fracture. **A.** Type 5 central tarsal fracture with high comminution of the bone. **B** and **C.** Medial and dorsal views of repair approached dorsomedially with incorporation of cancellous bone graft into the fracture site and stabilization by placement of a dorsal finger plate.

Treatment of Lateral Luxation of the Superficial Digital Flexor Tendon

Jerome Reinke

Surgical Stabilization

The animal is placed in lateral recumbency with the affected leg prepared for surgery. A curvilinear skin incision is made over the plantaromedial aspect of the calcaneus. The incision is made 4 cm proximally from the point of the hock extending distally along one-half the length of the calcaneus. The skin is reflected, and an incision is made parallel to the superficial digital flexor (SDF) tendon into the fluid distended calcanean bursa. The proximal part of the SDF tendon is separated from the other calcanean tendons. This allows the SDF tendon to be everted, providing visualization

of the medial collateral attachment. The SDF tendon is centered in the intertubercular groove, and surgical stabilization is attempted. Collateral stability is accomplished by suturing the stretched and torn retinacular tissue along the medial aspect of the SDF tendon to the paratendinous and periosteal tissue along the calcaneus. Eight to 10 well-placed simple interrupted monofilament nonabsorbable 2–0 sutures are used to stabilize the tendon. The hock joint is manipulated through all ranges of motion to ensure proper function of the SDF tendon (Fig. 63.13).

A semirigid cotton-padded bandage is applied from the toes to just distal to the stifle. The bandage is made from several layers of thick rolled cotton covered by gauze and tape. Recheck examinations are performed at 2, 4, and 6 weeks postoperatively. The bandage is changed and sutures are removed at 2 weeks, and a bandage is applied for an additional 2 weeks. The bandage is removed at 1 month, and restricted exercise is encouraged for an additional 2 weeks.

Repair of the luxated SDF tendon is not a demanding surgical procedure. The goal of the surgery

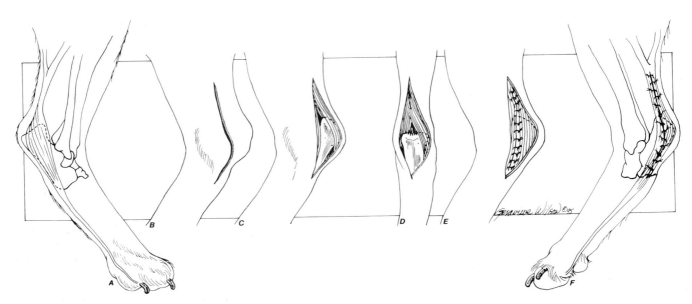

Fig. 63.13. **A.** Drawing of lateral aspect of the right hock depicting lateral displacement of the superficial digital flexor (SDF) tendon. **B.** Medial aspect of the right hock; a curvilinear incision is made over the plantaromedial aspect of the calcaneus. Medial (**C**) and plantar (**D**) aspects of the right hock showing the edge of the SDF tendon exposed by surgical incision. **E.** Medial aspect of the right hock; depicted is closure of medial retinacular tissue to the periosteal tissue along the caudomedial calcaneus. **F.** Medial aspect of the right hock. Skin closure is shown. (From Reinke JD, Mugbannam AJ. Lateral luxation of the superficial digital flexor tendon in 12 dogs. J Am Anim Hosp Assoc 1993;29:303.)

is to stabilize the tendon in the center of the intertubercular groove of the calcaneus, to allow free flexion and extension of the tibiotarsal joint.

All dogs should be walking normally 3 months postoperatively. Surgical failure is possible if nonabsorbable suture is not used or if an inadequate period of postoperative bandaging is not provided, thereby allowing too much movement in the healing period.

Previous reports of this condition suggest that the SDF tendon usually luxates laterally. Shetland sheep-

Fig. 63.14. **A.** Drawing taken from radiograph of a clinical case with a deformed calcaneus. The superficial digital flexor (SDF) tendon cap is shown to luxate laterally. The calcaneal groove is shallow, and the tip slants distolaterally. **B.** The opposite, more normal-appearing calcaneal tuber. The groove is deeper and lacks a significant slant. (From Reinke JD, Mugbannam AJ. Lateral luxation of the superficial digital flexor tendon in 12 dogs. J Am Anim Hosp Assoc 1993;29:303.)

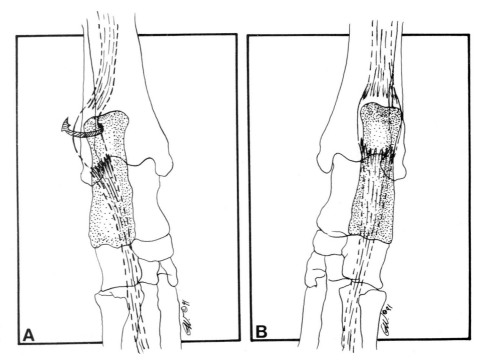

dogs and collies appear to be predisposed to the disorder. These two breeds compose 8 of 12 cases in my study and 4 of 9 in another study (1, 2). The two predisposed breeds appear to have an unusually narrow, delicate calcaneal tuber with a shallow intertubercular groove. The conformational abnormality may decrease the stability of the SDF tendon and may allow it to luxate. A deformity of the calcaneus has been seen radiographically and during surgical stabilization. This deformity consisted of a shallow groove and an indistinct lateral process of the tip of the calcaneal tuber (Fig. 63.14) (1). A study suggested that the tendon insertion on the medial aspect of the calcaneal tuber was weaker than the lateral component (2). The exact mechanism of tendon luxation is unknown. However, injury is suspected to be a factor because lameness associated with this condition has been seen frequently after vigorous exercise.

Five cases were studied in which nonsurgical methods were attempted for up to 6 weeks before surgical intervention. These patients were managed with padded bandages and, in some cases, anti-inflammatory drugs. Four of five patients had minimal or no response to either method of conservative treatment (2).

I managed a dog with bilateral simultaneous lateral tendon luxation. Only the most severely affected limb underwent operation. The opposite side was managed conservatively. Two years postoperatively, both limbs were examined and radiographed. The unoperated limb healed with a great deal of periosteal new bone deposited along the edges of the calcaneal tuber. The operated limb had fewer proliferative changes and resulted in a stronger limb when compared with the conservatively managed opposite leg.

References

1. Reinke JD, Mugbannam AJ. Lateral luxation of the superficial digital flexor tendon in 12 dogs. J Am Anim Hosp Assoc 1993;29:303.
2. Mauterer JV, et al. Displacement of the tendon to the superficial digital flexor muscle in dogs. J Am Vet Med Assoc 1993; 203:1162.

Treatment of Avulsion of the Gastrocnemius Tendon

Jerome Reinke

Surgical Technique

The animal is placed in sternal recumbency with the affected leg extending beyond the end of the surgical table. A medial curvilinear incision 6 to 8 cm proximal and 6 cm distal to the tip of the calcaneal tuber is made. The distal half of the common calcanean tendon is dissected from the surrounding soft tissue. A longitudinal incision is made through the paratenon and fibrous tissues. The superficial digital flexor tendon (SDF) at this level partially encircles the gastrocnemius tendon (GT) and the much smaller combined tendon of the gracilis, biceps femoris, and semitendinosus (CT). The latter two components of the common calcanean tendon are generally both torn free together from the tip of the calcaneus. The three components of the common tendon are exposed by blunt and sharp dissection. Cautery is needed to control bleeding in the surgical field. The SDF is rolled laterally, and the other two tendons can be identified. The proliferative ends of the tendons are debrided and approximated at the attachment site, with care taken not to remove excessive tissue, resulting in a significantly shortened tendon. Flexion of the stifle and extension of the tibiotarsal joint allow easier apposition of the tendons at the calcaneal tuber.

The CT and GT are secured to the calcaneal tuber by using a "locking loop" suture pattern of polypropylene (0 to 2) secured in the CT and GT (1). A small transverse bone tunnel is drilled medially to laterally in the tip of the calcaneal tuber. One free end of the suture through the two tendons is passed through the bone tunnel and then is tied together with the other loose end of tendon suture. This apposes the avulsed tendon to the calcaneal tuber (Fig. 63.15). Both the GT and CT are sutured as one in this procedure. The suture knots should be tied at the side of the tendons and not at the site of the bone tunnel.

After tendon repair, the tarsocrural joint is immobilized in extension between 135 and 150° by the use of a large, self-tapping bone screw passed from the caudal border of the calcaneus cranially into the distal caudal tibia. The paratenon, subcutaneous tissues, and skin are closed in a routine manner using a simple interrupted suture pattern. Occasionally, a large, avulsed piece of bone may be present at the distal end of the avulsed tendon. If this piece is large enough, tension band fixation of the tendon and bone fragment to the calcaneus may be used instead of the suture and bone tunnel method (see Fig. 63.15). An alternative technique of anchoring tendon to bone is with a spiked washer and long cortical bone screw (see Fig. 63.15).

A resin–epoxy half-cast is applied to the rear limb for 6 to 8 weeks. The cast should extend from just below the stifle to the digits. Follow-up examinations are conducted at 2, 4, 6, and 8 weeks postoperatively. At 2 weeks, the cast is changed and the sutures are removed. At 4 weeks, the cast is examined and changed if needed. At 6 weeks, the cast and bone screw are removed with the patient under general anesthe-

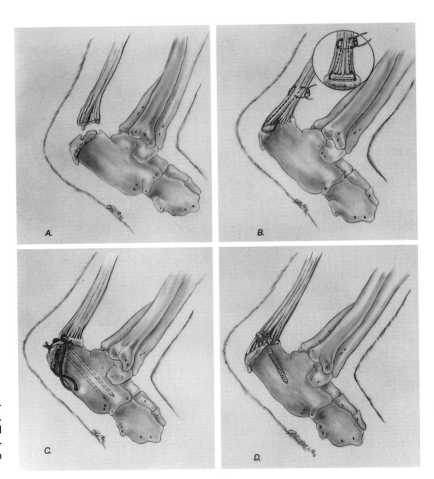

Fig. 63.15. **A.** Drawing of affected hock. **B.** Locking loop suture pattern placed through bone tunnel. **C.** Figure-of-eight tension band fixation. **D.** Spiked washer fixation technique. (From Reinke JD, Mughannam AJ. Avulsion of the gastrocnemius tendon in 11 dogs. J Am Anim Hosp Assoc 1993;29:410.)

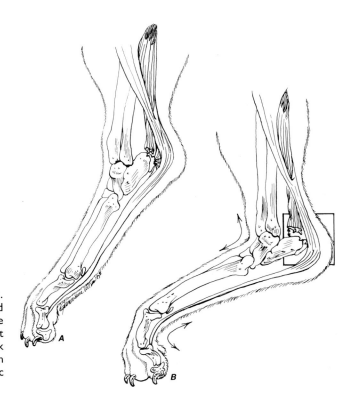

Fig. 63.16. **A.** Drawing of the limb in a nonweightbearing position. The superficial digital flexor (SDF) tendon is relaxed, and the avulsed tendon is minimally displaced. As a result, no postural changes are noted. **B.** Limb in a weightbearing position. Because of displacement of the avulsed tendon and tension on the SDF tendon, both the hock joint and digits are flexed. (From Reinke JD, Mughannam AJ. Avulsion of the gastrocnemius tendon in 11 dogs. J Am Anim Hosp Assoc 1993;29:410.)

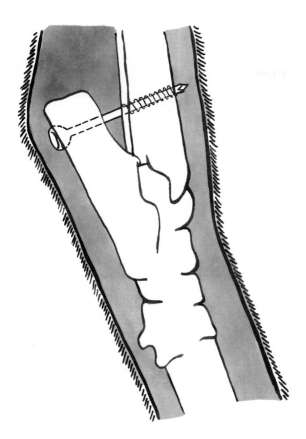

Fig. 63.17. Drawing showing placement of a self-tapping cortical bone screw from the calcaneal tuber into the tibia that maintains the hock joint in a weightbearing position.

after surgical stabilization is essential. A malleolar screw, 55 to 60 mm by 4.5 mm in diameter, from the caudal calcaneus into the tibia to stabilize the hock works well in Labrador retrievers and Doberman pinschers (Fig. 63.17). Most dogs reported with this condition have been of these two breeds (2, 3). External fixators also provide good stabilization of the tibio-tarsal joint and are another option to prevent distraction of the tendon repair during healing.

If this injury is diagnosed before complete tendon avulsion, conservative treatment with external support may be attempted. However, long-term splintage has failed in dogs with complete tendon avulsion.

Cats also have been reported with this injury (4). External splintage has been successful in some cases, but surgery may be necessary in active animals or in

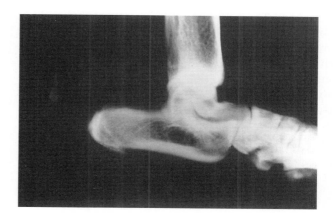

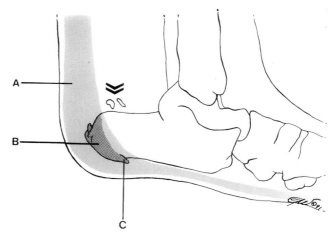

Fig. 63.18. **A.** Lateral radiograph of an affected hock. **B.** Line drawing of the same radiograph. The light gray shading (A) denotes the superficial digital flexor (SDF) tendon. The dark gray shading (B) denotes the attachment of the SDF tendon (cap appearance) as it courses over the tip of the calcaneal tuber. The characteristic beaklike projection (C) of the plantar aspect of the cap also is seen. The *arrow* shows two bone chips in the end of the avulsed gastrocnemius tendon. (From Reinke JD, Mughannam AJ. Avulsion of the gastrocnemius tendon in 11 dogs. J Am Anim Hosp Assoc 1993;29:410.)

sia, and another cast or a heavy padded bandage is applied. At 8 weeks, the external support is removed, and gradually increasing exercise is allowed.

Surgical stabilization should be performed when any increased flexion is detected in the tarsocrural joint. When the "claw" effect of the toes and "dropped hock" are observed in this unique form of lameness, the GT and CT have pulled from the calcaneus (Fig. 63.16). Swelling, lameness, and tendon tenderness on palpation but without postural changes indicate a severe strain injury or a partial tendon avulsion. The accurate apposition of tendon to bone is important because the blood supply to the distal one-third of the tendon is from the tendinosseus junction. Increased contact between tendon and bone aids in revascularization and healing of the tendinosseus junction. Drilling tiny holes at the site of attachment may allow ingrowth of tendinous tissue into bone and may strengthen and hasten the surgical repair.

This injury occurs primarily in large breed dogs that place severe forces at the site of tendon attachment. Immobilization of the tibiotarsal joint for 6 to 8 weeks

animals with a widely distracted avulsion fracture at the tip of the calcaneus.

Radiographic deformity of the calcaneus secondary to this injury has a specific appearance. On lateral radiographs, a beaklike projection, "enthesophyte formation," is seen at the cranial tip of the calcaneal tuber. This bony deposition is at the site of the SDF tendon insertion. Extra stress is placed on this tendon insertion when the GT is avulsed. Craniocaudal radiographs reveal bony proliferation of the medial and lateral margins of the tip of the calcaneal tuber giving a widened, ragged appearance. In this area, the SDF tendon attaches along the proximal edges of the calcaneus. In addition, an avulsion fragment from the calcaneus may be seen distracted proximally in a thickened common calcanean tendon (Fig. 63.18).

This clinical entity and its associated radiographic changes must be recognized for proper diagnosis and treatment. The body responds to stress at the tendon–bone junction with bone deposition or "enthesophyte" formation. The radiographic changes are chronic, yet the clinical symptoms are often acute. This situation is similar to that seen with an apparent acute anterior cruciate ligament injury associated with chronic radiographic changes.

References

1. Tomlinson J, Moore R. Looking loop tendon suture use in repair of five calcanean tendons. Vet Surg 1982;11:105.
2. Bonneau NH, Olivieri M, Breton L. Avulsion of the gastrocnemius tendon causing flexion of the hock and digits. J Am Anim Hosp Assoc 1983;19:410.
3. Reinke JD, Mughannam AJ. Avulsion of the gastrocnemius tendon in 11 dogs. J Am Anim Hosp Assoc 1993;29:410.
4. Mughannam A, Reinke J. Avulsion of the gastrocnemius tendon in three cats. J Am Anim Hosp Assoc 1994;30:550.

Treatment of Joint Mice in the Deep Digital Flexor Tendon Sheath

Jerome Reinke

Surgical Exploration

A routine dorsomedial incision is made to expose the tibiotarsal joint. The hock is extended, and the medial trochlear ridge of the talus is examined. The joint is then flexed, and a plantaromedial incision is made to explore the plantar aspect of the joint space. Investigators have shown that 96% of the medial trochlear ridge can be visualized with both a dorsomedial and a plantaromedial surgical approach (1). A swelling may

be noted in the plantaromedial area of the tibiotarsal joint. This swelling may be partially a result of distension of the tendon sheath of the flexor hallucis longus (lateral head of the deep digital flexor [DDF]), which communicates with the tibiotarsal joint. The DDF tendon sheath can be opened by extending the plantar incision proximally. The tissues in this area are thickened and extremely vascular. A bony fragment may be found adherent to or free in the tendon sheath. The arthrotomies are closed routinely, and a padded bandage is applied to the hock joint for 2 weeks.

Osteochondritis dissecans (OCD) of the tibiotarsal joint commonly accompanies enlargement of the plantaromedial aspect of the joint. Some of the enlargement may be from distension of the tendon sheath of the DDF tendon because of a cartilage fragment that has migrated proximally from the tibiotarsal joint as a consequence of OCD. I have observed this condition, as have others (2). Joint mice in the distal tendon sheath have not been reported. Arthrograms in clinically normal animals show the communication be-

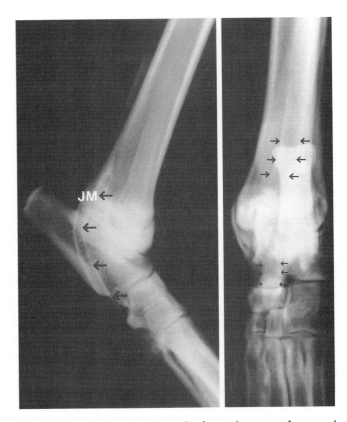

Fig. 63.19. A. Lateral radiograph of an arthrogram of a normal hock joint. A dye column can be visualized (*arrows*) coursing in the tendon sheath of the flexor hallucis longus(lateral head of the deep digital flexor) muscle. The area of joint mice migration is identified (*JM*). **B.** Craniocaudal arthrogram showing dye in the tarsocrural joint and extending proximally (*large arrows*) and distally (*small arrows*) in a small linear column in the tendon sheath of the deep digital flexor tendon.

tween the tibiotarsal joint and the DDF tendon sheath. The tendon can be seen to run on the plantaromedial aspect of the hock. (Fig. 63.19). Dye studies of the tibiotarsal joint in clinically affected animals have proved disappointing because inflammation and swelling appear to alter dye flow through the joint and into the tendon sheath. I have seen four dogs less than 24 months of age (two Labrador retrievers, a golden retriever, and a rottweiler) with joint mice in the tendon sheath associated with OCD of the medial trochlear ridge. This condition is probably similar to entrapment of joint mice in the bicipital tendon sheath as a consequence to OCD in the shoulder joint (3). OCD of the lateral trochlear ridge of the talus has been seen and can be expected to produce joint mice that may also migrate to the DDF tendon sheath (4).

References

1. Beale BS, Goring RL. Exposure of the medial and lateral trochlear ridges of the talus in the dog. Part 1. Dorsomedial and plantaromedial surgical approaches to the medial trochlear ridge. J Am Anim Hosp Assoc 1990;26:13.
2. Todroff J. Tips, quips, and pearls. The Avore File, Eugene, OR, June 1990.
3. LaHue TR, et al. Entrapment of joint mice in the bicipital tendon sheath as a sequela to osteochondritis dissecans of the proximal humerus in dogs: a report of six cases. J Am Anim Hosp Assoc 1988;24:99.
4. Goring RL, Beale BS. Exposure of the medial and lateral trochlear ridges of the talus in the dog. Part 2. Dorsolateral and plantarolateral surgical approaches to the lateral trochlear ridge. J Am Anim Hosp Assoc 1990;26:19.

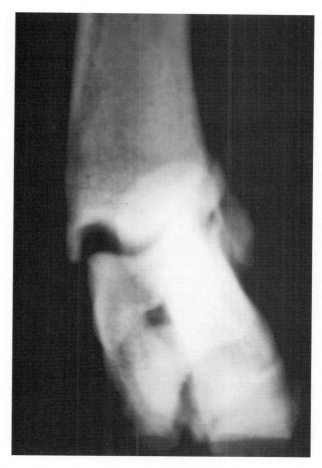

Fig. 63.20. Craniocaudal radiographic view of the left tarsocrural joint of a 4-year old German shepherd dog with a medial shearing injury. The distal extremity has been pulled laterally to demonstrate the medial instability.

Malleolar Shearing Injuries Treated by Double Ligament Replacement

Geoffrey N. Clark

Shearing injuries of the distal tibia and fibula are often associated with severe damage to the collateral ligaments of the tarsocrural joint (Fig. 63.20). Replacement of the damaged ligaments is necessary to stabilize the joint and to minimize secondary degenerative changes in the affected joint. The purpose of the double ligament replacement technique for repair of malleolar shearing injuries is to provide joint stability while maintaining near normal joint motion.

The animal is placed in lateral recumbency with the injured limb up for lateral ligament replacement and the injured limb down for medial ligament replacement. The limb is prepared for aseptic surgery. Minimal dissection is needed in patients with extensive shearing injuries. The surgical approach should be lim-

ited to that necessary to identify landmarks for screw insertion. Debridement of nonviable tissue and lavage of the joint should be performed. The double ligament replacement technique uses three bone screws and two figure-of-eight sutures. Screws are placed close to the sites of origin and the insertion of the injured ligaments (Fig. 63.21). In cases of medial shearing injuries, the origin screw is placed in the distal tibia to the cranial side of midline. Care must be taken to avoid entering the joint with the drill bit, tap, or screw. The insertion screw for the short component of the collateral ligament complex is placed in the proximoplantar quadrant of the medial aspect of the trochlea of the talus. This screw should appear to be slightly distal and plantar to the origin screw. The insertion screw for the long component of the collateral ligament complex is placed through a tubercle located at the plantar base of the talus. This screw is directed in a slightly proximodorsal direction to achieve maximum bone purchase and to avoid penetrating articular cartilage. On the lateral side, the origin screw is placed through the

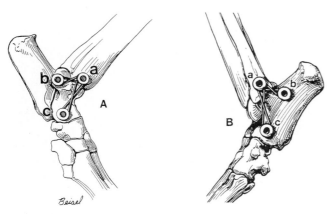

Fig. 63.21. Diagram of the medial (**A**) and lateral (**B**) aspects of the canine tarsocrural joint demonstrating placement of the origin (*a*) and insertion (*b, c*) screws. (From Aron DN, Purinton PT. Replacement of the collateral ligaments of the canine tarsocrural joint: a proposed technique. Vet Surg 1985;14:178–184.)

distal fibula into the distal tibia. The location is more caudal than that of the corresponding screw on the medial side. The insertion screw for the short component of the lateral collateral ligament complex is placed in the calcaneus in a position proximal and plantar to the lateral articular facies. The insertion screw for the long ligament is placed through a tubercle located at the dorsal extent of the base of the calcaneus. This screw is directed in a slightly proximoplantar direction (Figs. 63.22 and 63.23). Screw size varies with the size of the patient. In medium to large dogs, 3.5-mm cortical bone screws or 4.0-mm cancellous screws are most appropriate. In smaller dogs and cats, 2.7-mm cortical screws are used.

Two separate sutures are used to recreate the long and short portions of the collateral ligament complex. Braided polyester (Ethibond, Ethicon, Inc., Somerville, NJ) suture is recommended over monofilament nylon or polypropylene sutures because it tends to resist stretching. Suture size varies with patient size. Larger dogs require No. 5 suture, and smaller patients use No. 1 or 2 suture. The short component sutures are tied with the tarsocrural joint held in approximately 90° flexion. The medial long or lateral long suture

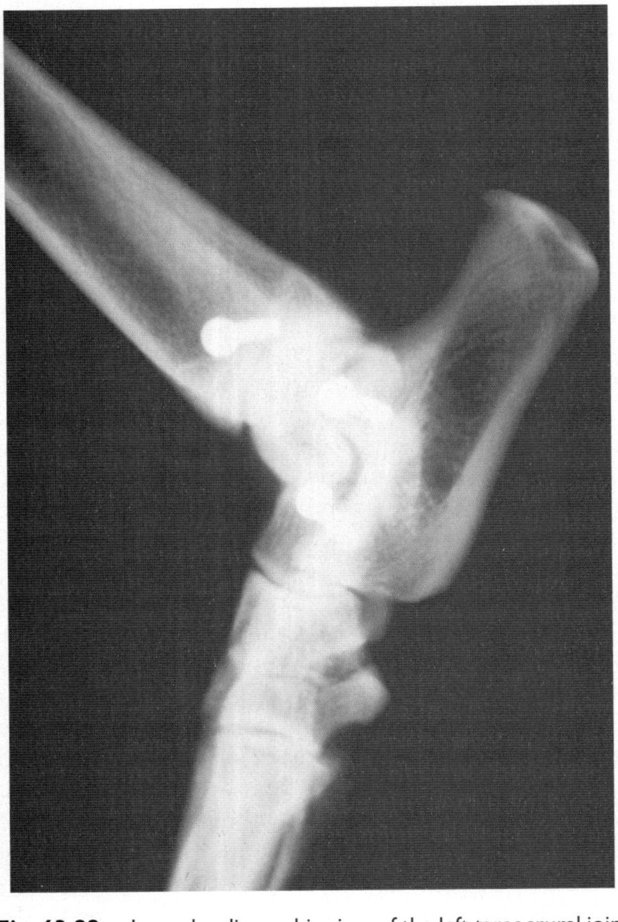

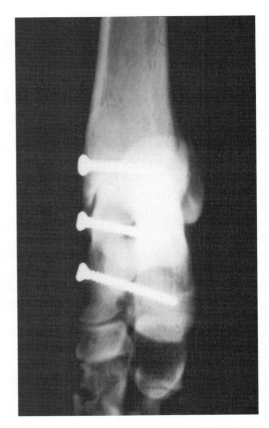

Fig. 63.22. Lateral radiographic view of the left tarsocrural joint of the dog in Figure 63.20 after surgical stabilization using the double ligament replacement technique.

Fig. 63.23. Craniocaudal radiographic view of the left tarsocrural joint after surgical stabilization using the double ligament replacement technique.

prosthesis is tied with the joint held in the functional standing angle. This angle is 135° for the dog and 120° for the cat. All screws are tightened against the bone after the sutures are tied.

Closure of the wound may not be possible if soft tissue loss is significant. Partial closure is attempted when possible. Second-intention healing of the wound followed by delayed closure is often necessary in patients with extensive shearing injuries. Delayed closure of the wound should only be attempted after all surfaces are covered with healthy granulation tissue. Granulation tissue formation over exposed bone can be accelerated by penetrating through the remaining cortex multiple times with a small Kirschner wire (0.035 or 0.045 inch). This maneuver creates bleeding that should not be blotted or wiped. The blood clot that forms serves as a source of additional granulation tissue. I have used this technique effectively in some clinical cases.

The tarsocrural joint must be immobilized for a minimum of 4 weeks after surgical stabilization. If the remaining wound is small and wound dressings do not require frequent changes, then a soft, padded bandage with a fiberglass or plastic splint may be effective. When daily wound management is necessary, then transarticular external skeletal fixation may be necessary to maintain support when dressings are changed. After 4 weeks or removal of the external fixator, controlled progressive weightbearing is allowed with the aid of soft wraps. No unrestricted activity should be allowed before 8 weeks postoperatively.

The double ligament replacement technique has provided better clinical results than single prosthetic ligament replacement in tarsocrural shearing injuries (1). Formation of fibrous tissue is necessary to provide stability additional to that supplied by the prosthetic ligaments. Delayed development of fibrous tissue may lead to cyclic stress on the repair and failure of the prosthesis. Transarticular external skeletal fixation has been reported to provide more stability in the joint than when coaptation splints are used (1). The exact duration of postoperative immobilization varies with the degree of injury, but the use of transarticular fixation for a minimum of 3 weeks is recommended. After removal of the external fixator, splints and soft, padded bandages allow gradual use of the affected limb.

Reference

1. Aron DN. Prosthetic ligament replacement for severe tarsocrural joint instability. J Am Anim Hosp Assoc 1987;23:41–55.

Suggested Reading

Aron DN, Purinton PT. Replacement of the collateral ligaments of the canine tarsocrural joint: a proposed technique. Vet Surg 1985;14:178–184.

Surgical Treatment of Malleolar Fractures

Brian Beale

Fractures of the medial or lateral malleolus of the tibia result in instability of the tarsus because of disruption of the origin of the collateral ligament complex. Subluxation or dislocation may occur if instability is severe. Occasionally, both the medial and lateral malleoli are fractured concurrently. The fractures may be simple and closed, or they may involve loss of bone and soft tissue in cases of shear wounds. External coaptation is usually inadequate because accurate anatomic reduction and rigid stabilization are necessary to decrease the chance of developing degenerative joint disease. Most fractures are best repaired using open reduction and internal fixation. Bone screws and pins and tension bands are the most common implants used to stabilize these fractures (Fig. 63.24).

Pin and tension band fixation provides good stability and anatomic reduction in most cases. An approach to the fractured malleolus is performed by incising skin and subcutaneous tissues directly over the fragment. A periosteal elevator is used to expose the distal aspect of the tibia or fibula and the fracture site. The fracture site is cleaned of hematoma and fibrinous debris, to allow better visualization of the articular surface and the edges of the fracture fragments. The fracture is reduced anatomically; this is extremely important because of the intra-articular nature of the fracture. Bone-reduction forceps can be used to provide temporary stability. Two pins are driven in normograde fashion sequentially through the fractured malleolar fragment perpendicularly across the fracture site into the main fragment, with care taken to avoid the articular surface of the tibiotarsal joint. In small fragments, a single pin may be used. The pin size varies, depending on the size of patient and the size of malleolar fragment. Most cats and small dogs can accommodate 0.035- or 0.045-inch Kirschner wires, whereas medium-size and large dogs may accommodate 0.062-inch Kirschner wires or $\frac{5}{64}$-inch pins. The tension band wire used is 20 or 22 gauge in cats and small dogs and 16 or 18 gauge in medium and large breed dogs. A hole, large enough to pass the selected wire, is drilled from cranial to caudal in the main fragment approximately 1 cm proximal to the fracture line. A small loop is created in the wire to permit tightening of the wire on the opposite side of the knot formed by twisting the ends of the wire. The wire is passed through the hole and around the Kirschner wires in figure-of-eight fashion. The wire is tightened by simultaneously twist-

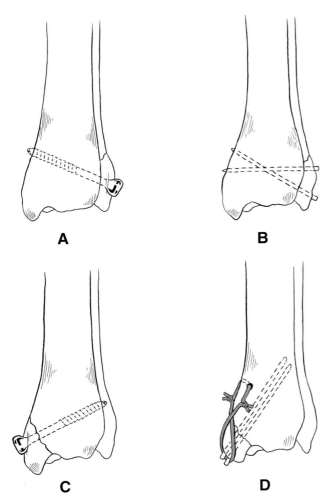

A   **B**

C   **D**

Fig. 63.24. Repair of malleolar fractures. **A.** Lateral malleolar fracture stabilized with a partially threaded cancellous screw. **B.** Lateral malleolar fracture stabilized with two divergent Kirschner wires. **C.** Medial malleolar fracture stabilized with a partially threaded cancellous screw. **D.** Medial malleolar fracture stabilized with pins and tension band.

fibial diaphysis. The screws should be placed in lag fashion, by either using partially threaded cancellous screws or overdrilling the near cortex when using cortical screws. The size of screw (1.5 to 4.5 mm) selected depends on the size of the fragment size and the patient. One or two screws can be placed; placement of two screws may help to prevent rotation of the fragment. The fracture can be reduced and temporarily stabilized with bone-reduction forceps. The appropriate thread hole and gliding hole (if using a cortical screw) are drilled perpendicularly across the fracture line, with care taken to avoid the articular surface of the tibiotarsal joint. Alternatively, a hole can be predrilled in the small fragment to allow more precise centering. The fragment is reduced and temporarily stabilized. The far hole is drilled. After drilling, the hole is measured and tapped, and the screw is inserted and tightened.

External coaptation is recommended for 4 weeks after internal stabilization. A lateral fiberglass splint is inexpensive and easily applied. The splint is applied while placing the tarsus at a functional angle. The bandage is changed if it becomes soiled or wet. After 4 weeks, the splint is removed, and physical therapy is performed several times daily until range of motion is improved. Exercise should be limited to leash walks only for 2 months postoperatively or until radiographic healing is evident. Running and jumping should be prevented. Implant removal is not necessary unless the implant migrates or loosens.

Surgical Treatment of Talus Fractures

Brian Beale

ing the loop and ends of the wire while applying moderate traction. This forms a knot on each side of the loop that allows greater and more even wire tension after tightening. The knots should be centered if possible. The wires are tightened onto the surface of the bone, they are cut leaving a minimum of three twists, and they are bent over if irritation of the soft tissues is likely.

Lag screw fixation of the medial malleolus provides excellent stability if the distal fragment is large enough to accommodate a screw. Lag screw fixation of the medial malleolus may be preferred to pin and tension band fixation, especially if the fracture involves a large articular segment. Lag screw fixation of the lateral malleolus usually requires its attachment to the tibia, rather than to the fibula, because of the thin distal

Fractures of the talus can be intra-articular or extra-articular. Intra-articular fractures include those involving the medial or lateral trochlear ridge proximally or the head of the talus distally. Extra-articular fractures involve the neck, body, or head of the talus. External coaptation is inadequate because accurate anatomic reduction and rigid stabilization are necessary to decrease the chance of developing degenerative joint disease. Most fractures are best repaired using open reduction and internal fixation. Bone screws and Kirschner wires are the most common implants used to stabilize these fractures. Highly comminuted fractures, especially those involving articular surfaces, may be more amenable to arthrodesis than to primary repair.

Fractures of the medial trochlear ridge are approached through an osteotomy of the medial malleolus. Fractures of the lateral trochlear ridge are approached through an osteotomy of the distal fibula, just above the lateral malleolus (Fig. 63.25). The fracture site is cleaned of hematoma and fibrinous debris, to allow better visualization of the articular surface and edges of the fracture fragments. The fracture is reduced anatomically; this is extremely important because of the intra-articular nature of the fracture. Bone-reduction clamps can be used to provide temporary stability; however, digital pressure can also suffice. The fracture can be stabilized using multiple Kirschner wires or lag screw fixation. Lag screw fixation is preferable, but the small size of the fragment often precludes its use. Two or three Kirschner wires are driven sequentially in normograde fashion through the fractured talar fragment perpendicularly across the fracture site into the main fragment. The surgeon should countersink the wires to avoid damage to the tibial trochlea. Most fractures can be repaired adequately using 0.035- or 0.045-inch Kirschner wires. If screw fixation is used, the screws should be placed in lag fashion, by either using partially threaded cancellous screws or overdrilling the near cortex when using cortical screws. The size of screw (1.5 to 4.0 mm) selected depends on the size of the fragment and the patient. One or two screws can be placed; however, one screw is usually sufficient. The fracture can be reduced and temporarily stabilized with bone-reduction forceps. The appropriate thread hole and gliding hole (if using a cortical screw) are drilled per-

pendicularly across the fracture line, with care taken to avoid the articular surface of the tibiotarsal joint. Alternatively, a hole can be predrilled in the small fragment to allow more precise centering. The fragment is reduced and temporarily stabilized. The far hole is drilled. Countersinking of the near hole should be performed to ensure that the head of the screw is completely below the articular surface. After drilling, the hole is measured and tapped, and the screw is inserted and tightened. The malleolar osteotomy is reduced and is stabilized by pin and tension band or lag screw fixation (see the section of this chapter on malleolar fractures).

Fractures of the neck of the talus usually are associated with a concurrent luxation of the fragment at the proximal intertarsal joint. A medial approach to the talus is performed. The fracture site is cleaned of hematoma and fibrinous debris to allow better visualization of the edges of the fracture fragments. The fracture is reduced anatomically, and vulsellum reduction forceps can be used to provide temporary stability. Reduction is often helped by flexing the tarsus while applying pressure to the lateral surface to open the medial aspect of the joint. The fracture is best stabilized by screw fixation (Fig. 63.26). Cortical or cancellous screws can be used. The size of screw (1.5 to 4.0 mm) selected depends on the fragment size and patient size. One or two screws can be placed; however, one screw is usually sufficient. If fixation can be accomplished by placement of a lag screw into the trochlea of the talus, a hole is drilled from the mediodistal aspect of the distal

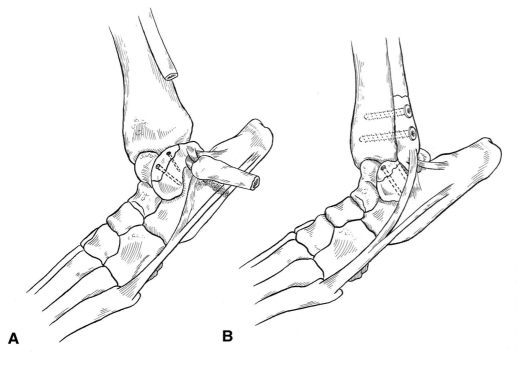

A　　　　　**B**

Fig. 63.25. **A.** A lateral malleolar osteotomy allows access for repair of a lateral trochlear ridge fracture with countersunk, divergent Kirschner wires. **B.** The osteotomy is stabilized with two positional screws.

talar fragment, in a proximolateral direction into the talar trochlea. Stabilizing the fragment by fixation to the calcaneus is often necessary because of insufficient obliquity of the fracture. The screws do not need to be placed in lag fashion in this application. A hole is drilled from the craniomedial aspect of the distal talar fragment, in a caudolateral direction, into the body of the calcaneus. The near hole is overdrilled if lag screw fixation is desired when using cortical screws. The hole is measured and tapped, and the screw is inserted and tightened.

Fractures of the body and head of the talus are accessed by a medial approach. Mild subluxation of the talocalcaneal articulation is usually present. The fracture site is cleaned of hematoma and fibrinous debris to allow better visualization of the edges of the fracture fragments. The fracture is reduced and temporarily stabilized digitally or with bone-reduction forceps. The cranial aspect of the distal talus can be visualized by periosteal elevation, to aid reduction. Placing the joint in extension may help to maintain reduction. The fracture is stabilized with crossed Kirschner wires or a modified T plate (Fig. 63.27). A Kirschner wire is placed from the caudomedial aspect of the distal talar fragment, in a proximal direction, into the craniolateral aspect of the talar trochlea. A second Kirschner wire is placed from the proximal, caudomedial as-

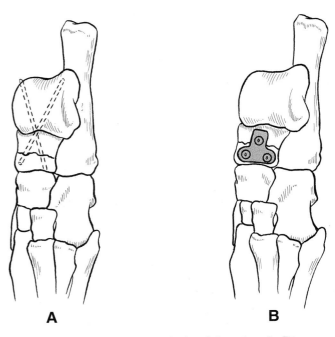

Fig. 63.27. Fractures of the body of the talus. **A.** Divergent Kirschner wires are placed from a medial approach to stabilize a fracture of the talar body. **B.** A modified T plate is placed through a craniomedial approach to stabilize a talar body fracture.

pect of the talar trochlea, in a distal direction, into the craniolateral aspect of the distal talar fragment. Lag screw fixation can be substituted for Kirschner wires, but the fragment size and fracture orientation usually prevent their use. In medium-size and large dogs, these fractures can sometimes be repaired with a modified T plate placed on the cranial surface of the body of the talus. A 1.5-, 2.0-, or 2.7-mm T plate is modified by cutting the long arm to the appropriate length to allow placement of the plate distal to the trochlea (usually only one hole remains). The plate is applied and secured in routine fashion. External coaptation is essential because of the presence of a single screw in the proximal fragment. Intra-articular fractures of the head should be reduced with anatomic precision, or degenerative joint disease is likely to ensue. Partial arthrodesis of the tarsus can be considered in these patients.

Adjunctive external coaptation is recommended for 4 to 6 weeks after internal reduction and fixation of fractures of the talus. Lateral fiberglass splints are easy to apply, inexpensive, and effective. The splint is applied while placing the tarsus at a functional angle. The bandage is changed if it becomes soiled or wet. After 4 weeks, the splint is removed, and physical therapy is performed several times daily until range of motion is improved. Exercise should be limited to leash walk only for 2 months postoperatively or until radiographic healing is evident. Running and jumping

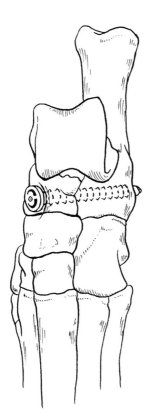

Fig. 63.26. A fracture of the neck of the talus is repaired through a medial approach using a positional cortical screw.

should be prevented. Implant removal is not necessary unless implant migration or loosening occurs.

Surgical Treatment of Calcaneal Fractures

Brian Beale

Fractures of the calcaneus may involve the tuber calcanei, shaft, or base. These fractures may be associated with other tarsal fractures (central or fourth tarsal bone fractures) or subluxation of the proximal intertarsal joint (calcaneoquartel joint). Subluxation associated with distal fractures occurs because of the pull of the plantar ligament, which attaches to the plantarodistal aspect of the calcaneus. Repair by external coaptation is inadequate in most cases because of the

presence of significant bending forces generated through the common calcaneal tendon that occur during weightbearing. Most fractures are best repaired using open reduction and internal fixation. Simple fractures can be treated effectively with a pin and tension band. Comminuted fractures may be stabilized with a pin and tension band or a bone plate placed on the lateral surface of the calcaneus. A tension band is also useful in combination with plate fixation. Adjunctive lag screws are often helpful in rebuilding the shaft in comminuted fractures or for stabilizing distal avulsion fractures of the base.

Fractures of the calcaneus are accessed through a plantarolateral approach. The lateral retinaculum of the superficial digital flexor tendon is incised to allow elevation of the tendon off the calcaneus. The fracture site is cleaned of hematoma and fibrinous debris, to allow better visualization of the edges of the fracture fragments. The fracture is reduced anatomically and temporarily stabilized with bone-reduction forceps. For pin and tension band repair, two Kirschner wires

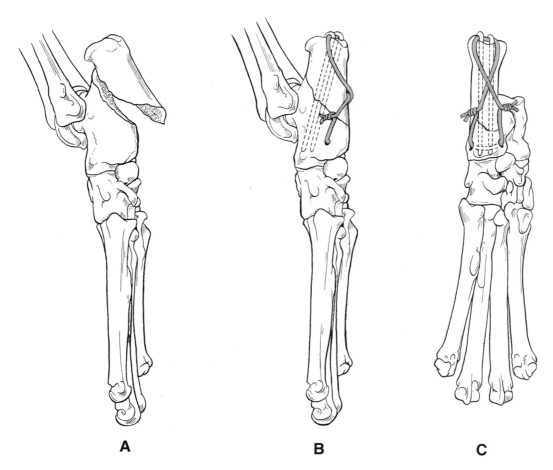

A   **B**   **C**

Fig. 63.28. Fracture of the shaft of the calcaneus. **A.** An oblique fracture of the calcaneal shaft is accessed through a plantarolateral approach. **B.** Lateral view showing normograde placement of two Kirschner wires after reduction of the fracture. A tension band is applied to counteract distractive forces created by the common calcaneal tendon. **C.** Plantar view of pin and tension band repair. Both knots of the tension band are tightened simultaneously to provide even compression across the fracture line.

are driven sequentially in normograde fashion from the proximal aspect of the tuber calcanei through the shaft of the calcaneus (Fig. 63.28). In distal fractures of the base of the calcaneus, the Kirschner wires can be seated across the calcaneoquartel joint into the fourth tarsal bone. Most fractures can be repaired using 0.045- to 0.062-inch Kirschner wires or small Steinmann pins. Insertion of the pins in the dense cortical bone of the calcaneus must not generate excessive heat, which could result in thermal bone necrosis and pin loosening. Predrilling the shaft of the calcaneus with a drill bit having a smaller diameter than the intended pin makes placement of the pin easier and decreases the chance of premature pin loosening. Proximally, the tension band can be placed around the Kirschner wires, or alternatively, a hole can be drilled laterally to medially through the proximoplantar aspect or the calcaneus. The latter method probably is less irritating to the overlying superficial digital flexor tendon. The tension band wire used is 20 or 22 gauge in cats and small dogs and 16 or 18 gauge in medium and large breed dogs. The tension band is placed between the bone and flexor tendons. A hole, large enough to pass the selected wire, is drilled from lateral to medial in the calcaneus in the distal half of the calcaneus (at least 1 cm distal to the fracture line). If the fracture is extremely distal, the hole can be drilled through the plantar tubercle of the fourth tarsal bone. A small loop is created in the wire to permit tightening of the wire on the opposite side of the knot formed by twisting the ends of the wire. The wire is passed through the hole and around the Kirschner wires or through the proximal hole in figure-of-eight fashion. The wire is tightened by simultaneously twisting the loop and ends of the wire while applying moderate traction. This forms a knot on each side of the loop that allows greater and more even wire tension after tightening. The knots should be centered if possible. The wires are tightened onto the surface of the bone, they are cut leaving a minimum of three twists, and they are bent over if irritation of the soft tissues is likely. The Kirschner wires should be bent over in a plantar direction, cut short, and rotated cranially to minimize trauma to the flexor tendons. If the tension band is not anchored by the Kirschner wires, the wires can be countersunk below the surface of the bone.

Bone plates can be placed on the lateral surface of the calcaneus to stabilize comminuted fractures not amenable to repair with a pin and tension band (Fig. 63.29). If possible, the shaft of the calcaneus should be reconstructed using lag screws. The plate should be applied as a neutralization or buttress plate. The size of plate selected varies with patient size, but typically it is a 2.0- or 2.7-mm dynamic compression plate. The plate can be applied across the calcaneoquartel joint if necessary in distal calcaneal fractures. A tension band

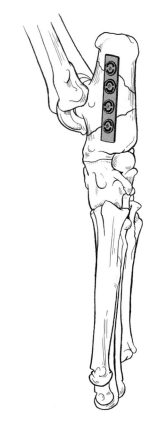

Fig. 63.29. Neutralization plates placed on the lateral surface can be used to repair comminuted calcaneal fractures.

should be used in combination with plate fixation to counteract bending forces. The figure-of-eight band should span the fracture lines and should be placed through proximal and distal holes drilled from lateral to medial in the calcaneus.

Adjunctive screw fixation is useful to provide supplemental stability for slab fractures, comminuted fragments, or avulsion fractures of the base of the calcaneus. The screws should be placed in lag fashion if possible, by either using partially threaded cancellous screws or overdrilling the near cortex when using cortical screws. The size of screw (1.5 to 4.0 mm) selected depends on the fragment size and patient size. One or two screws can be placed, depending on the fragment size. The fracture can be reduced and temporarily stabilized with bone-reduction forceps. The appropriate thread hole and gliding hole (if using a cortical screw) are drilled perpendicularly across the fracture line. After drilling, the hole is measured and tapped, and the screw is inserted and tightened

Adjunctive external coaptation is recommended for 4 to 6 weeks after internal reduction and fixation of comminuted fractures of the calcaneus. Coaptation is usually not needed for simple fractures of the tuber calcanei or shaft of the calcaneus. Lateral fiberglass splints are easy to apply, inexpensive, and effective. The splint is applied while placing the tarsus in moderate extension. The bandage is changed if it becomes soiled or wet. After 4 weeks, the splint is removed, and physical therapy is performed several times daily until range of motion is improved. Exercise should be limited to leash walks only for 2 months postoperatively or until radiographic healing is evident. Running and jumping should be prevented. Implant removal is not necessary unless implant migration or irritation of the flexor tendons occurs.

Joint Hinge for Shearing Injuries

Barclay Slocum & Theresa Devine Slocum

Traumatic injuries to the hock and elbow often result in open shearing wounds or dislocation of the joint. Both these joints have one degree of freedom, which means that they hinge around a single axis. Currently, only the Slocum Joint Hinge (Slocum Enterprises, Eugene, OR) preserves physiologic motion of joints during healing.

The Slocum Joint Hinge is an external fixator hinge specifically designed for use on canine hock and elbow subluxations, dislocations, and shearing injuries. Besides the long-term return of the injured joint to function, this hinge has several advantages. Immediate usage in the physiologic range of joint motion prevents further joint damage. Patients with multiple limb trauma can walk on the joint hinge immediately while the other injured limbs are treated. Early return of the physiologic range of motion reduces the morbidity of long-term joint stiffness. The key to success is stabilization of the joint while allowing normal range of motion.

Application

The same principles for application of the Slocum Joint Hinge pertain to the elbow, hock, and stifle joint. Because the hock is most commonly affected, the steps are detailed for use in that joint.

Once the injured hock joint has been evaluated and medial joint instability has been established, then a Slocum Joint Hinge is indicated on the medial aspect of the hock joint. If the hock has a closed injury, then the joint hinge is applied after standard surgical preparation. If the hock has an open wound, debridement of the wound and thorough joint lavage are followed

by reasonable surgical reconstruction of the injured ligament. Fresh wounds are sutured; however, if 8 to 12 hours have elapsed from the time of injury, the precaution of treating the wound as infected is advised.

The first step in hinge application is location of the center of motion (Fig. 63.30). The surgeon places a $\frac{1}{8}$-inch pin ($\frac{3}{32}$-inch pin on a small dog or cat) perpendicular to the sagittal plane and through both cortices of the tibia just distal to the insertion of the semitendinosus muscle (Fig. 63.30, *A*). The hinge is placed over the medial hock in the sagittal plane with the center of the hinge at the estimated center of motion of the hock. To determine the center of joint motion, a $\frac{3}{32}$-inch pin is placed through the hinge, embedding just the tip of the pin in the center of the talus (Fig. 63.30, *B*). The surgeon flexes and extends the hock. If no movement occurs between the proximal tibial pin and the proximal bar on the hinge, then the hinge is located at the hock center of motion. If movement occurs, the $\frac{3}{32}$-inch pin is relocated as described previously, and the patient is retested until the center of hock motion is located.

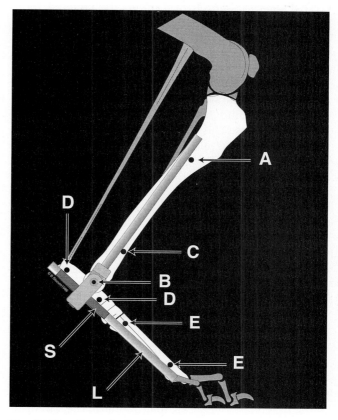

Fig. 63.30. To apply the Slocum Joint Hinge to the medial hock of a large dog for medial collateral ligament damage, a $\frac{1}{8}$-inch pin is placed in the proximal tibia (*A*); then a $\frac{3}{32}$-inch pin is placed through the hinge center into the joint center (*B*) and is tested. The distal tibial pin (*C*) and two calcaneal pins (*D*) are applied on a short bar (*S*). A long bar (*L*) and pins (*E*) can be applied if additional metatarsal support is desired.

The appropriate ($\frac{1}{8}$- × $\frac{3}{16}$-inch or $\frac{3}{32}$- × $\frac{3}{16}$-inch) CLAMp Shell is applied proximally to secure the bar to the proximal tibial pin. Enough distance is allowed between the bar and the skin for swelling and wound treatment. The distal tibial pin is placed by "touching" a $\frac{1}{8}$- or $\frac{3}{32}$-inch pin to the fixation hinge bar in the distal tibia and drilling the pin though both cortices of the bone. The appropriate ($\frac{1}{8}$- or $\frac{3}{32}$-inch × $\frac{3}{16}$-inch) CLAMp Shell is applied in the distal tibia to secure the bar to the distal tibial pin (Fig. 63.30, C). CLAMp Shells are only available from Slocum Enterprises, Inc., Eugene, OR.

Two pins (Fig. 63.30, D), are inserted into the calcaneus with a short distal bar using the "touch method" (Fig. 63.30, S). If the calcaneus is damaged, a long distal bar can be used to span from the calcaneus to the metatarsal bones (Fig. 63.30, L). Pins of appropriate number and size ($\frac{1}{8}$- or $\frac{3}{32}$- inch) are applied by the "touch method" to the calcaneus and metatarsus (Fig. 63.30, E). Appropriate CLAMp Shells are applied to secure the pins to the distal bar of the Slocum Joint Hinge. The $\frac{3}{32}$-inch guide pin is removed from the hinge center of hock motion (Fig. 63.30, B).

The Slocum Joint Hinge should be covered by a protective bandage to keep the skin clean, dry, and stable. The first step in application of the protective bandage is to be sure that no tension exists between the skin and the pins. If necessary, the skin is incised around the pin to relax any tension. Once the skin is clean and dry, the skin–pin interface is wrapped with cotton, and liquid benzoin is applied to the cotton around the pins. This technique stops movement between the skin and pin and thus reduces irritation and infection. The sharp edges of the joint hinge bar and pins are padded with cotton, balls of polymethylmethacrylate, or rubber pin covers, and the two sections of external fixator apparatus are padded with cotton. Vetwrap is applied over the padding while making sure that the joint is able to move.

A functionally stable, pain-free joint with a normal range of motion is the desired outcome of any joint surgery. Stability can be controlled by the way in which the surgeon uses the Slocum Joint Hinge. Although most hocks are stable with the described application, the degree of rigidity can be adapted easily for additional stability. The hinge can be made rigid by attaching a connecting bar between the proximal and distal ends of the rods to form a triangular fixator that has maximum stiffness. This configuration can be used in the first phase of healing to immobilize the damaged tissues, so injured structures can begin the fragile first stages of capillary development with no motion. Once healing is underway with blood supply established, the rigid connecting bar can be removed, and mild flexibility of the joint (only in the physiologic range of motion) can be permitted by a Robert Jones–type

bandage over the joint and hinge. This bandage can be reduced in rigidity to match the need of the patient. A full physiologic range of motion is beneficial for final orientation and strength of the collagen fibers during the later stages of healing. This can be accomplished by applying little or no wrap.

If the injury has not caused disruption of the skin, then application of the Slocum Joint Hinge will allow the damaged tissue to heal without invasion of the traumatized joint. The external fixator pins penetrate the skin in the adjacent areas.

If the joint injury is an open wound, access to the joint for wound treatment is maintained even though the external fixator is in place. Soaking the limb and joint without removal of the fixator is easily performed. This technique is also compatible with delayed closure after treatment of severe contamination or infection of the joint.

The joint hinge is not ideally suited to the treatment of stifle trauma. The stifle is basically a two degree of freedom joint. The first freedom is rotation about an axis perpendicular to the sagittal plane (the center of motion for flexion and extension). The second freedom is the rotation about an axis in the sagittal plane that passes through the centers of motion of both the stifle and hock (the center of motion for internal and external rotation of the stifle). All other motions are abnormal.

Complete stifle derangement resulting from trauma requires reconstruction of both the cranial and caudal cruciate ligaments, the medial and lateral menisci, the medial collateral ligament, and the medial and caudal joint capsule. The Slocum Joint Hinge can be applied to the stifle medially or both medially and laterally to neutralize cranial tibial thrust. A $\frac{3}{32}$-inch Steinmann centering pin is placed through the axis of stifle flexion and extension in the femur. Transfemoral and tibial pins attach to the medial and lateral joint hinges, which are centered on the $\frac{3}{32}$-inch centering pin. The centering pin is then removed. The joint hinges allow only flexion and extension of the stifle. This configuration controls the cranial tibial thrust and is of primary importance in allowing the soft tissues (substitute cranial cruciate ligament and joint capsule) to heal.

The Slocum Joint Hinge also controls internal and external axial rotation of the stifle during healing. The return of this motion, after removal of the joint hinge, stretches lateral capsular imbrications or fibular head transpositions in all but the sturdiest of repairs. Stretching of lateral joint capsule or lateral collateral ligament after fibular head transposition allows normal internal rotation to return to the stifle, but this indicates failure of those procedures by definition of their intended purpose.

A tibial plateau leveling osteotomy has proved effective in protecting the stifle joint from the destructive effects of the cranial tibial thrust after the Slocum Joint Hinge has been removed. Dogs with complete derangement of the stifle have returned to preinjury function without physical limitations with both the tibial plateau leveling osteotomy and the joint hinge.

The purpose of the Slocum Joint Hinge is to support the soft tissues during healing, while maintaining the physiologic motion of the joint in patients with traumatic injuries to the hock, elbow, and stifle. The hinge is applied to the side of the ligament deficit in the hock or the elbow. If both the medial and lateral collateral ligaments are damaged, then hinges are applied both medially and laterally with the hinge axes coaxial. If the hinge is used on the two degree of freedom stifle joint because of severe trauma and stifle derangement, a tibial plateau leveling osteotomy may be needed to control the effects of the cranial tibial thrust.

Surgical Treatment of Osteochondritis Dissecans of the Hock

Brian Beale

Lesions associated with osteochondritis dissecans (OCD) of the hock occur on the medial or lateral troch-lear ridge of the talus. The lesions may be characterized as small, cartilage flaps or large, osteochondral fragments. Early diagnosis and prompt surgical removal of these fragments are recommended, before the onset of significant degenerative joint disease (DJD). Several approaches have been described to gain access to the flaps. Severance of either collateral ligament allows subluxation of the joint and excellent visualization of the trochlear ridges; however, this approach should be avoided because of the probability of causing iatrogenic joint instability, predisposing the dog to greater DJD. Osteotomy of the medial or lateral malleolus also gives excellent surgical exposure; however, this approach can also be associated with increased morbidity. Medial malleolar osteotomy is technically demanding and requires iatrogenic formation of an articular fracture of the distal tibia. Precise reduction and rigid stabilization is necessary to prevent DJD. Lateral malleolar osteotomy is preferred, but precise reduction and rigid stabilization are necessary to prevent joint instability or nonunion of the osteotomy site. The preferred approaches are the dorsolateral and plantarolateral approaches to the lateral trochlear ridge and the dorsomedial and plantaromedial approaches to the medial trochlear ridge. Accurate radiographic assessment of the location of the OCD lesion is necessary to select the appropriate surgical approach. Most OCD lesions can be accessed through a single approach; however, a combination of the dorsal and plantar approaches is necessary to gain access to some large le-

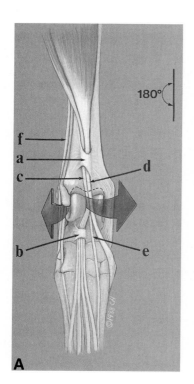 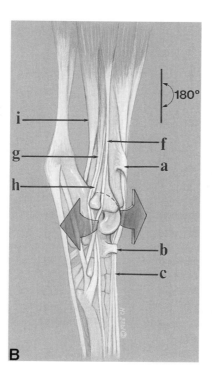

Fig. 63.31. Dorsolateral approach to the hock. **A.** Dorsal view of the lateral trochlear ridge showing medial retraction of the tendons of the extensor digitorum longus, extensor hallucis longus, and tibialis cranialis muscles. **B.** Lateral view of the lateral trochlear ridge showing plantar retraction of the tendons of the peroneus longus, extensor digitorum lateralis, and peroneus brevis muscles. The lateral collateral ligament (not shown) is preserved. *a*, proximal extensor retinaculum; *b*, distal extensor retinaculum; *c*, extensor digitorum longus muscle; *d*, tibialis cranialis muscle; *e*, extensor hallucis longus muscle; *f*, peroneus longus muscle; *g*, peroneus brevis muscle; *h*, extensor digitorum lateralis muscle; *l*, flexor hallucis longus muscle.

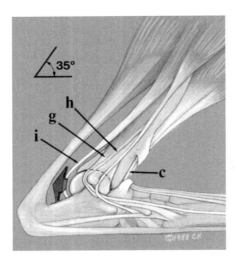

Fig. 63.32. Plantarolateral approach to the hock. Flexion of the hock to 35° results in passive dorsal movement of the tendons of the peroneus brevis, extensor digitorum lateralis, and peroneus longus muscles. The tendon of the flexor hallucis longus muscle is retracted medially, resulting in exposure of the lateral trochlear ridge. The lateral collateral ligament (not shown) is preserved. *c*, extensor digitorum longus muscle; *g*, peroneus brevis muscle; *h*, extensor digitorum lateralis muscle; *I*, flexor hallucis longus muscle.

sions or lesions located on the midportion of the trochlear ridges. A combined approach to the medial trochlear ridge allows access to all but approximately 5% of the ridge (the midportion). A combined ap-

proach to the lateral trochlear ridge allows access to the entire ridge. The advantage of using the combined approaches is the preservation of the collateral ligaments without the need for a technically demanding, time-consuming osteotomy. If these approaches fail to provide sufficient surgical exposure, a malleolar osteotomy can then be performed. Because of the low morbidity associated with these procedures, bilateral lesions can be operated on at the same time.

All four approaches are performed by making a curvilinear skin incision centered over the appropriate region of the trochlear ridge. Subcutaneous tissues are incised and are retracted. Certain anatomic structures should be avoided during each approach. The dorsolateral approach requires lateral retraction of the tendons of the extensor digitorum longus, tibialis cranialis, and extensor hallucis longus muscles, the dorsal branch of the lateral saphenous vein, and the superficial peroneal nerve (Fig 63.31). This approach also requires plantar retraction of the tendons of the peroneus longus, extensor digitorum lateralis, and peroneus brevis muscles. In the plantarolateral approach, the tendons of the peroneus brevis, extensor digitorum lateralis, and peroneus longus muscles must be avoided dorsally (Fig. 63.32). The plantar branch of the lateral saphenous vein and branch of the caudal cutaneous sural nerve are retracted in a plantar direction, and the flexor hallucis longus tendon is retracted medially. The dorsomedial approach requires lateral retraction of the

Fig. 63.33. Dorsomedial approach to the hock. **A.** Dorsal view of the medial trochlear ridge showing lateral retraction of the tendons of the extensor digitorum longus, extensor hallucis longus, and tibialis cranialis muscles. **B.** Medial view of the medial trochlear ridge showing dorsolateral retraction of the tendons of the tibialis cranialis, extensor hallucis longus, and extensor digitorum longus muscles. The medial collateral ligament is preserved. *b*, distal extensor retinaculum; *c*, extensor digitorum longus muscle; *d*, tibialis cranialis muscle; *e*, extensor hallucis longus muscle; *k*, long part of the medial collateral ligament.

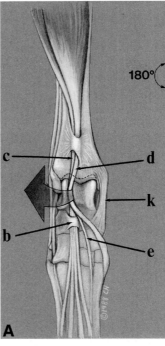

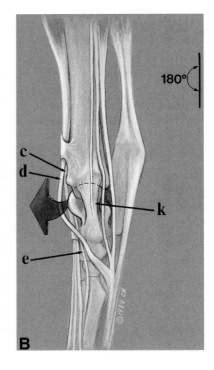

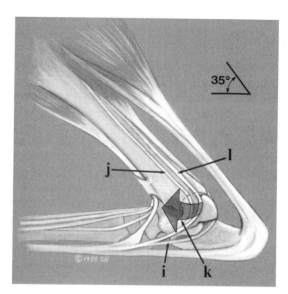

Fig. 63.34. Plantaromedial approach to the hock. The tendons of the flexor digitorum longus and tibialis caudalis are retracted dorsally resulting in exposure of the medial trochlear ridge. The tendon of the flexor hallucis longus muscle and the medial collateral ligament are avoided. *l*, flexor hallucis longus muscle; *j*, tibialis caudalis muscle; *k*, long part of the medial collateral ligament; *l*, flexor digitorum longus muscle.

tibialis cranialis tendon, saphenous nerve, cranial tibial artery and vein, and dorsal branches of the saphenous artery and vein (Fig. 63.33). In the plantaromedial approach, the tendon of the flexor digitorum longus muscle and the distal attachment of the tibialis caudalis tendon are retracted dorsally, and the flexor hallucis longus tendon, tibial nerve, and medial saphenous vein and artery are retracted laterally (Fig. 63.34). The collateral ligament complex is preserved in all four approaches. The joint capsule is incised longitudinally, directly over the palpable trochlear ridge, and is retracted. Extension and flexion of the joint allow access to the trochlear ridge for removal of the OCD fragment. Removal is usually simple using a Freer elevator or similar instrument. If present, synovial attachments to the fragment are sharply incised. Reattachment of the fragment with Kirschner wires or lag screws is not recommended because of the typical remodeling of the fragment present at the time of surgery, the technical difficulty of the procedure, and the possibility of implant failure. Gentle curettage of the subchondral lesion can be performed to remove loose debris and undermined edges at the periphery of the lesion. Fibrocartilaginous repair tissue within the defect should be left undisturbed. Forage (drilling of several small holes into the subchondral bone) of the defect to encourage vascular ingrowth has been proposed, but its efficacy is unknown. The joint capsule and subcutaneous tissues are closed in two layers using synthetic absorbable suture. The skin is closed using synthetic nonabsorbable suture. A soft, padded bandage is recommended for 7 to 10 days. Exercise should be restricted to leash walks only for 6 weeks.

64

END-STAGE PROCEDURES

Arthrodesis

Thomas M. Turner & Alan J. Lipowitz

Arthrodesis is the conversion of two or more articulating surfaces into bony union by use of a surgical procedure. Although arthrodesis may restore function to an otherwise nonfunctional limb, it should be used only when restoration of a healthy functional joint cannot be achieved.

Several prerequisites must be met if an arthrodesis is to be successful (1). The remainder of the involved limb and the adjacent joints must be functional and capable of compensating for the increased stresses that will be transmitted to them as a result of the arthrodesis. Second, the desired position in which the joint is to be fused must be determined preoperatively by evaluating the normal as well as the abnormal limb during gait and in the standing position. This position should obviously be the most functional for that particular animal. The surgeon must consider all three planes: the angle of extension or flexion, the degree of varus or valgus, and the proper rotational or axial alignment. These positions and angles are determined precisely with a goniometer. A sterile goniometer is used at the time of the surgical procedure to determine the precise angles required to maintain proper leg angulation and length. The third prerequisite is a method of rigid fixation, either an external or internal device, that maintains the desired joint position, using the principle of compression wherever possible. Some commonly used fixation devices are compression plates, lag screws, cross-pins, tension band wires, and external skeletal fixators.

Successful arthrodesis also depends on proper preparation of the joint before application of the fixation device and bone graft. The cartilage, adjacent synovium, and soft tissue must be removed to expose healthy, bleeding subchondral bone while preserving the contour of the articular surface. However, the surgeon should strive to oppose flat surfaces when possible to ensure a more even contact of the bone surfaces and also to add stability. Cartilage and subchondral bone can be removed with a power-driven bur, osteotome, curettes, or rongeurs. Any areas of cartilage or soft tissue not excised may delay the fusion. The joint should be liberally packed with autogenous cancellous bone to fill all defects at the fusion site. The limb is then placed in the proper degree of angulation and axial alignment, as determined preoperatively, and the fixation device is applied. Attention to aseptic technique and proper soft tissue handling throughout the surgical procedure are necessary to avoid secondary wound complications.

Indications

Arthrodesis of a joint is generally indicated for conditions that result in pain, instability, and loss of joint function. The indications can also be classified as neurologic or orthopedic. The primary neurologic indication is an irreparable peripheral nerve injury resulting in loss of function in the extremity joint (e.g., the carpus or hock) that is not amenable to a tendon transfer procedure (2). The proximal aspect of the limb must be completely functional. Function of the limb should be determined preoperatively by neurologic examination of the limb and evaluation of the animal's use of the limb with the affected joint in a temporary splint.

Orthopedic indications for arthrodesis include chronic instability or subluxation not amenable to reconstructive procedures and painful arthritis not responsive to medical therapy, such as septic arthritis, immune-mediated arthritis, and degenerative joint diseases (3–6). A primary arthrodesis may be necessary in cases of severe joint derangement or luxation, irreparable articular fractures, or severe open avulsion injury of the joint with extensive loss of soft tissue and bone. A painful intra-articular nonunion, failure of a previous joint reconstruction, and severe growth deformity may also require arthrodesis of the involved joint.

Carpal Arthrodesis

Arthrodesis of the carpus can be performed as either a partial or a total joint fusion (panarthrodesis), depending on the level of instability (4, 5, 7–9). Preoperative stress radiographs of the involved joint reveal the area of instability. The intraoperative use of an Esmarch bandage or a tourniquet reduces hemorrhage and thus facilitates the surgical procedure. Moreover, the use of plastic adherent drapes allows the entire limb to be visualized during the operation and aids in maintenance of an aseptic technique. A cranial approach is preferable; however, the skin incision should be placed so closure is not directly over the implant.

Partial Carpal Arthrodesis

Partial carpal arthrodesis involves only the carpometacarpal, middle carpal, and intercarpal joints. This procedure is indicated only when the antebrachiocarpal joint is functional, stable, and pain free.

A cranial approach is used to expose the affected joints (10). The angular relation of the metacarpal bones to the radial carpal and ulnar carpal bones is neutral. A Kirschner wire or a small Steinmann pin is inserted into the distal aspect of the medullary canal of each of the second, third, and fourth metacarpal bones (or only the third and fourth metacarpal bones) and is embedded into the radial carpal and ulnar carpal bones (Fig. 64.1). Cancellous bone graft is then liberally packed into all defects. If additional stability is desirable, an appropriate bone screw is inserted into the medial aspect of the radial carpal bone, and another is placed in the second metacarpal base. A figure-of-eight, heavy-gauge wire is passed around the screws and is tightened to achieve compression and stability. A preferred technique is to insert pins only in the third and fourth metacarpals and to direct a lag screw obliquely across the base of the second metacarpal into the radial carpal bone.

Postoperatively, the limb is protected for 6 weeks in a caudal splint. When the arthrodesis has healed, the pins are removed. The animal should have approximately a 90° range of motion of the antebrachiocarpal joint.

An alternative method of fixation is the use of a finger T or L plate. The plate is applied to the cranial aspect of either the third or fourth proximal metacarpal bone, with the T or L portion attached to the radial carpal bone (Fig. 64.2). The plate must be positioned

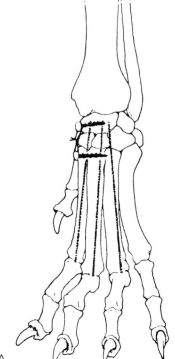
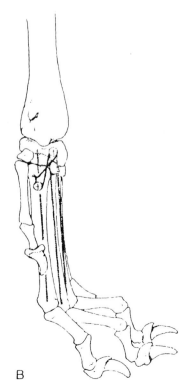

Fig. 64.1. Partial carpal arthrodesis using intramedullary pins in the second, third, and fourth metacarpal bones. Additional stability is gained by use of a figure-of-eight wire around screws placed in the radial carpal bone and the second metacarpal bone. A cancellous bone graft is packed in the fusion site. **A.** Craniocaudal view. **B.** Medial view.

A

B

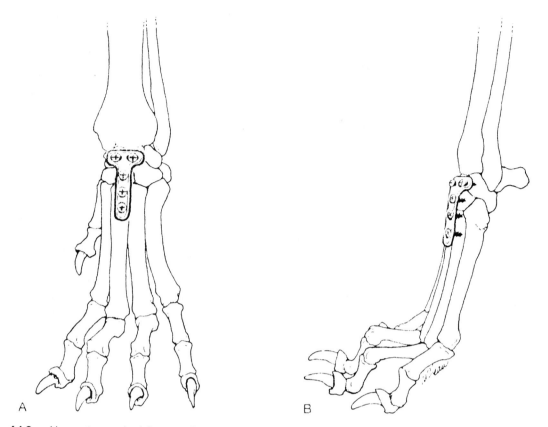

Fig. 64.2. Alternative method for partial carpal arthrodesis using a T plate. **A.** Craniocaudal view. **B.** Lateral view.

carefully so it does not impinge on the distal dorsal radial articular surface during normal extension of the joint.

Fusion of the antebrachial joint only is not recommended because it places excessive stress on the remaining joint and may lead to further degenerative joint disease and subluxation (11).

Carpal Panarthrodesis

Panarthrodesis is necessary when the entire carpus is involved in the disease process or is unstable. The fixation device of choice is a bone plate to achieve compression and stability. An external fixation device should be used only for cases involving extensive bone and soft tissue damage.

All carpal joints are prepared for arthrodesis through a cranial approach. Three locations are possible for plate application—cranial, medial, and caudomedial—each of which has advantages and disadvantages. The joint normally is fused in about 10° of hyperextension; however, the most desirable angle must be determined before the surgical procedure, as described previously. During application of a bone plate, strict attention must be given to maintaining

neutral valgus–varus angulation and axial alignment.

Medial application of one narrow plate allows excellent purchase for the distal screws. The screws are inserted transversely through the proximal aspect of two or more metacarpal bones and the radial carpal bone. For best results, at least three screws should obtain purchase distally in the metacarpal bones, and three or more screws should obtain purchase proximally in the distal radius (Fig. 64.3). A craniomedial approach to the carpus is used with this placement. In addition, excision of the first phalanx may be necessary for placement of the bone plate. The degree of hyperextension is obtained by adjusting the position and the contour of the proximal aspect of the bone plate along the medial aspect of the distal radius.

More commonly, the bone plate is applied to the cranial surface of the joint. Although the plate is more easily contoured to this surface, it is placed on the compression rather than the tension aspect of the joint. A straight bone plate can be applied along the cranial surface of the radius to the third or fourth metacarpal and radial carpal bones (5, 6, 8, 9) (Fig. 64.4). The disadvantage of this method is the necessity of relying on purchase in only one metacarpal bone. Therefore, in larger breeds of dogs, two cranial plates

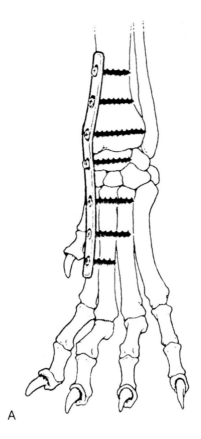

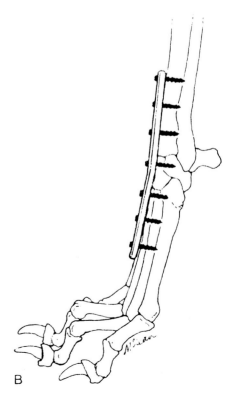

Fig. 64.3. Carpal panarthrodesis using a medially applied plate. The plate is contoured to the desired fusion angle, and cancellous bone is packed within the fusion site. **A.** Craniocaudal view. **B.** Lateral view.

A

B

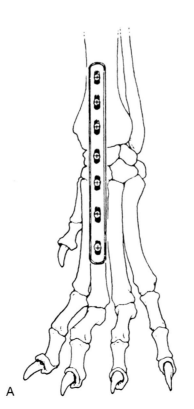

Fig. 64.4. Carpal panarthrodesis using a cranially applied compression plate secured to the radius, radial carpal bone, and third metacarpal bone. The plate is contoured for desired angulation. A cancellous bone graft is applied to the fusion site. **A.** Craniocaudal view. **B.** Lateral view.

A

B

can be applied, one along the cranial aspect of the radius to the cranial surface of the second or third metacarpal bone and the other along the cranial surface of the radius to the cranial aspect of the fourth metacarpal bone (Fig. 64.5). Special bone plates, such as a T plate, can be applied cranially to allow purchase in more than one metacarpal bone (Fig. 64.6). However, a plate of sufficient strength is imperative to avoid implant breakage.

Biomechanically, a caudomedially positioned plate is the most desirable; however, contouring and applying a plate in this position to obtain the necessary angulation and alignment may be technically difficult (Fig. 64.7).

An external fixation device also may be useful for arthrodesis, particularly for procedures in the carpus and hock in patients that have sustained severe trauma and bone loss. The joint is placed in the desired position for fusion, and two Kirschner wires or small Steinmann pins are inserted in crossed position to stabilize the carpus. Additional Kirschner wires are inserted to obtain purchase in the bone proximal and distal to the joint. These wires are connected medially and laterally in cement bars (methylmethacrylate). The precise angle of arthrodesis must be rigidly held while the cement cures (Fig. 64.8). This device allows treatment of an open wound while providing rigid external fixation with minimal metal implantation.

Postoperatively, all limbs undergoing carpal arthrodesis are protected by a padded bandage with a caudal splint (except when an external device is used) for 6 weeks. Because carpal arthrodesis procedures can cause moderate postoperative swelling of the limb, frequent examinations of the limb and bandage are necessary in the early postoperative period.

Elbow Arthrodesis

Arthrodesis of the elbow creates a long biomechanical lever from the shoulder to the carpus. The result is an altered, awkward gait, although the limb is functional. An elbow fusion therefore predisposes the limb to fracture because of the excessively long bone length created. Regardless of these disadvantages, some conditions necessitate elbow arthrodesis. Conditions that specifically may require arthrodesis are severe growth abnormalities of the proximal radius and ulna, painful intra-articular nonunions, and severe degenerative joint disease (4, 8).

A transolecranon approach is used to expose the caudal surfaces of the humerus and ulna and to prepare the joints for arthrodesis (8). The radial and ulnar nerves are isolated and retracted. Additional exposure of the joint can be gained through a craniolateral approach to the elbow (12) or by incision of the ulnar collateral ligament. The joint is prepared for arthrodesis as previously described. The plate is contoured to the predetermined angle and is secured to the caudal aspect of the humerus and ulna to achieve compression of the ulnohumeral joint. The plate should have

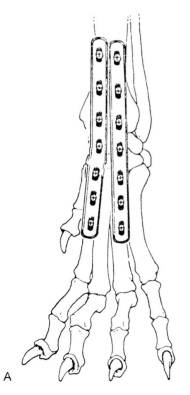

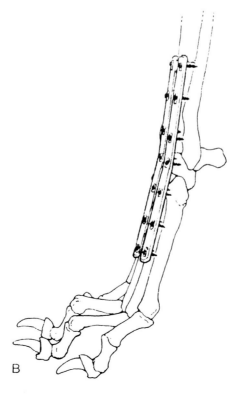

Fig. 64.5. Carpal panarthrodesis using double plates applied cranially to the radius, radial carpal bone, and second and fourth metacarpal bones. The plates are contoured for desired angulation, and a cancellous bone graft is applied to the fusion site. **A.** Craniocaudal view. **B.** Lateral view.

A

B

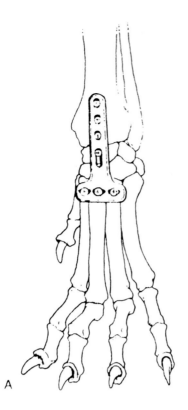

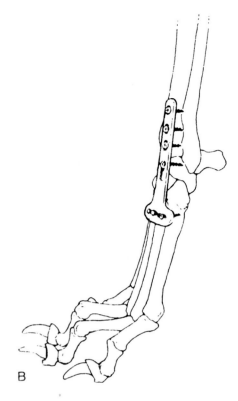

Fig. 64.6. Carpal panarthrodesis using a cranially applied T plate. The plate is secured to the radius, the radial carpal bone, and the second, third, and fourth metacarpal bones. **A.** Craniocaudal view. **B.** Lateral view.

A

B

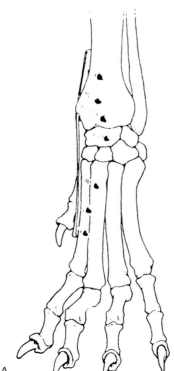

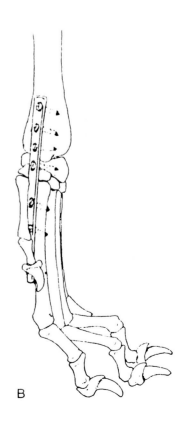

Fig. 64.7. Carpal panarthrodesis using a plate applied to the caudomedial aspect of the carpus. **A.** Craniocaudal view. **B.** Lateral view.

A

B

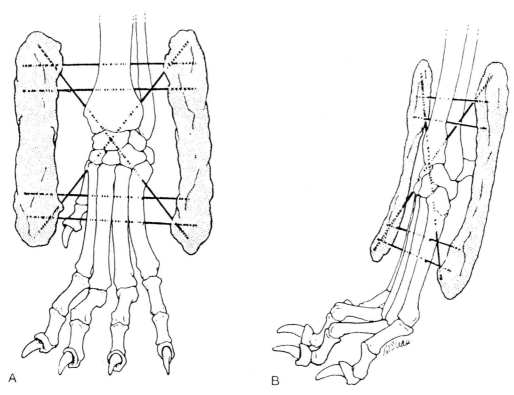

Fig. 64.8. Carpal panarthrodesis using an external fixation device. Methylmethacrylate bars connect the pins medially and laterally. A cancellous bone graft is applied to the fusion site. **A.** Craniocaudal view. **B.** Lateral view.

a minimum of eight holes, four proximally and four distally (8) (Fig. 64.9). When feasible, a lag screw should be inserted through the lateral humeral condyle into the radial head for compression of the radiohumeral joint. A lag screw also should be inserted though the ulnohumeral joint to provide additional compression of the joint. The olecranon is reattached lateral to the plate with a lag screw or a figure-of-eight tension band wire.

After the surgical procedure, the limb is maintained in a padded bandage for 2 weeks. The animal is then allowed limited activity until it has adapted to the limb and the arthrodesis has healed completely, as determined by periodic radiographic evaluations.

Shoulder Arthrodesis

Scapulohumeral arthrodesis is rarely indicated. Functionally, animals with a fused shoulder joint have a circumducting type of gait, similar to that of animals with a fused elbow or stifle, but these animals do not seem to be as incapacitated. The musculature sling that supports the scapula to the thoracic cage allows for some compensation for the loss of joint motion resulting from arthrodesis of the scapulohumeral joint.

A craniolateral approach to the shoulder is performed as well as osteotomy of the humeral greater tubercle (10). Because the proximal humerus is an area with a high density of cancellous bone, grafting of this area frequently is not required. After removal of the articular cartilage and positioning of the shoulder in the desired fusion position, the fixation device is applied. Preferably, stabilization of the shoulder is achieved by contouring a bone plate over the cranial surface of the proximal humerus to lie along the cranial and lateral aspects of the scapula neck, body, and spine (8). Four screws of purchase are preferable on either side of the joint. Once stability is ensured, the greater tubercle is reattached either lateral or cranial to the plate, and the remainder of the wound is closed in a routine manner.

After the surgical procedure, the animal's activity is limited until healing of the arthrodesis is evident radiographically.

Stifle Arthrodesis

Arthrodesis of the stifle is recommended for animals that have the previously discussed conditions resulting in severe pain or instability to the stifle. The most frequent indications appear to be severe derangement of the stifle and irreparable fractures or nonunion. Although this procedure can be used to salvage an otherwise nonfunctional limb, the animal will have an awk-

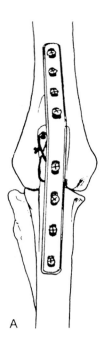

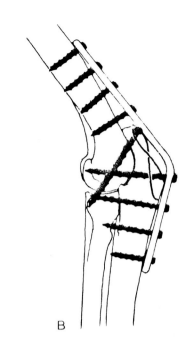

Fig. 64.9. Elbow joint arthrodesis using a plate applied to the caudal aspect of the humerus and ulna. A cancellous bone graft is applied to the fusion site. The olecranon is reattached lateral to the plate with a screw and a figure-of-eight wire. **A.** Craniocaudal view. **B.** Lateral view.

ward, debilitating gait. As with arthrodesis of the elbow, this gait occurs because of the long biomechanical lever created from the hip to the hock. The animal is then required to abduct and internally rotate the limb when bringing it forward during walking or running, referred to as a circumducting gait. Therefore, in addition to the routine preoperative considerations, particular attention should be focused on the function of the hip and the hock, which must compensate for the loss of function incurred in the stifle arthrodesis. Regardless of the abnormal gait incurred, this procedure can allow an animal to resume functional use of the limb.

Fixation devices used for stifle arthrodesis are a compression bone plate, lag screws, crossed Steinmann pins, and external fixator. The preferable fixation method is application of a compression plate to the cranial surface of the distal femur and proximal tibia. This technique allows application of the plate over the tension aspect of the joint and provides greater stability and compression than is achieved with cross-pinning techniques. The determination of the desired angle of flexion for arthrodesis of the stifle must be determined preoperatively, as previously discussed. However, the intra-articular resection of cartilage and subchondral bone along with internal joint structures will result in some loss of leg length. Therefore, fixation of the joint at an angle 5 to 10° greater than the measured flexion angle may be advantageous.

The surgical procedure is performed through a lateral parapatellar approach to the femur, stifle, and proximal tibia (10). The incision should extend from midfemur to midtibia. An osteotomy of the tibial crest

is performed to provide a site for application of the plate and to allow for the medial retraction of the quadriceps musculature and patellar tendon. The cruciate ligaments, menisci, and fat pad are resected, but the collateral ligaments are preserved. The proximal tibial articulating surface and subchondral bone are resected parallel to the transverse plane of the tibia to provide a healthy, bleeding surface of cancellous bone. After the limb is placed in the desired flexion angle for arthrodesis, the femoral condyles are resected parallel to the incised tibial surface (8). Overzealous resection of the femoral condyle results in considerable loss of limb length and should be avoided. If properly performed, the two opposed incised surfaces should place the limb in neutral version without varus or valgus angulation. The trochlear ridges and sulcus are resected as well as the cranial aspect of the proximal tibia to provide a bed for application of the plate (Fig. 64.10). The tendon of origin of the long digital extensor muscle generally needs to be resected. This tendon may be reattached to the proximal tibia by passing the tendon through a drill hole and suturing it to the adjacent tissues. The two incised surfaces are placed in apposition and are fixed temporarily either with reduction forceps or with two crossed Kirschner wires. In addition to avoiding any varus or valgus angulation, the limb should also be placed in neutral axial alignment.

Once the desired position for arthrodesis is achieved, a properly contoured plate is applied to the cranial aspect of the distal femur and proximal tibia. Preferably, the plate should cover the distal half of the femur and proximal half of the tibia. Therefore, a

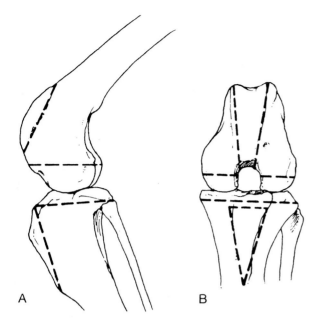

Fig. 64.10. Lateral (**A**) and craniocaudal (**B**) views of the stifle. *Dashed lines* indicate the approximate line for removal of the articular surfaces of the distal femur, proximal tibia, femoral trochlea, and tibial tuberosity in preparing the joint for arthrodesis.

minimum of three screws, preferably four to five screws, on both sides of the arthrodesis site should be inserted (Fig. 64.11). This application uses the principles of compression and thus achieves rigid stability of the arthrodesis site.

Because the two apposed surfaces have a high den-

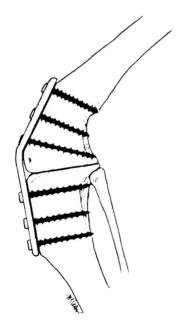

Fig. 64.11. Lateral view of the stifle illustrating plate application to cranial surfaces of the femur and tibia for arthrodesis. A cancellous bone graft is packed in the fusion site to fill any gaps between bone surfaces.

sity of cancellous bone, a bone graft may not be required in arthrodesis of the stifle. However, defects present in the joint should be filled with autogenous cancellous bone. The osteotomized tibial crest is re-attached lateral to the plate with either a screw or pin and figure-of-eight tension band wire. The remainder of the wound is closed in a routine fashion.

The limb is placed in padded supportive bandage for approximately 2 weeks after the procedure. The activity of the animal is limited to leash walking until radiographic evidence indicates that the arthrodesis has healed. After healing is complete, the plate is removed, and the limb is placed in a padded supportive bandage for 4 to 6 weeks. During this period, the screw holes fill with cancellous bone, thus decreasing the probability of fracture through a screw hole.

Hock Arthrodesis

Ligamentous injuries of the hock and shearing injuries result in instability that can usually be reconstructed and stabilized with conventional wiring or suturing techniques. However, severe articular fractures, degenerative joint disease, and irreparable ligamentous injuries may necessitate arthrodesis of the tibial tarsal joints or intertarsal joints (3, 4, 6, 11, 13, 14).

Similar to the carpus, the tarsal joints are composite articulations (15). The tibiotarsal articulation occurs between the talus or tibiotarsal bone and the distal end of the tibia. This joint has the greatest degree of motion of all the tarsal articulations. The proximal intertarsal articulations occur between the talus and central tarsal bone and between the calcaneus and the fourth tarsal bone. The distal intertarsal articulations are between the central tarsal bone and the second and third tarsal bones. Between the numbered tarsal bones and the metatarsal bones are the tarsometatarsal joints. Between the individual bones of the tarsus are the rigid, vertical intratarsal articulations.

Tibiotarsal Arthrodesis

Tibiotarsal arthrodesis can be done with crossed Steinmann pins or lag screws or with a single large compression screw across the joint and a tension band wire placed through the caudal cortex of the distal tibia and the calcaneus (3, 8). The preferred method is the use of a large compression screw.

The tibiotarsal joint can be approached through a curved incision that is begun several centimeters above the medial malleolus, crosses the cranial surface of the joint, and ends below the fifth metatarsal head; a lateral curvilinear incision also can be used. The subcutaneous tissues are incised in a similar line, and the long digital extensor tendon on the cranial aspect of the joint is identified. An arthrotomy is performed medial to the tendon, and the joint capsule is retracted sufficiently to expose the articular surfaces (10). The articular cartilage of both the distal tibia and the tibiotarsal bone is removed, exposing the bleeding subchondral bone.

After the joint is placed in the preoperatively determined fusion angle (proximally, 125 to 135° for dogs and 115 to 125° for cats), a small incision is made on the caudal aspect of the calcaneus. A small Kirschner wire is inserted through the calcaneus into the distal tibia for temporary stabilization of the tibiotarsal joint in the desired angle of arthrodesis. A screw hole is then prepared by drilling from the distal plantar aspect of the calcaneus through the tibia tarsal bone into the distal medullary canal of the tibia (Fig. 64.12**A**). Either a partially threaded cancellous screw or a fully threaded cortical screw is inserted in a lag screw technique through the guide hole. When a partially threaded cancellous screw is used, all screw threads must be in the distal tibia and fully cross the tibiotarsal joint. Screw threads must purchase well in the distal tibial medullary canal to achieve maximum compression of the tibiotarsal joint (3, 13) (Fig. 64.12**B**). In large dogs, two or more screws can be inserted at various angles, with one inserted from the distal tibia into the calcaneus in a cranial-to-caudal direction to achieve additional stabilization of the joint. If a single screw is used, a tension band orthopedic wire is placed through the tuber calcanei and through the caudal cortex of the distal tibia proximal to the level of the screw (3, 14). This wire neutralizes the flexion forces acting on the tibiotarsal joint and the screw during weightbearing (Fig. 64.13). After cancellous bone, obtained from a previously prepared site, is packed into any gaps or defects between the apposing surfaces of the fusion site, the compression screw and wire are tightened. The wound is closed in a routine manner.

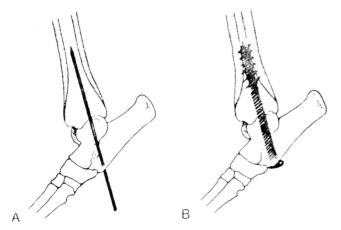

Fig. 64.12. A. Guide pin placement, traversing the tibiotarsal bone and penetrating the medullary cavity of the tibia, before placement of a compression screw for tibiotarsal arthrodesis. **B.** Placement of a cancellous bone screw for tibiotarsal arthrodesis.

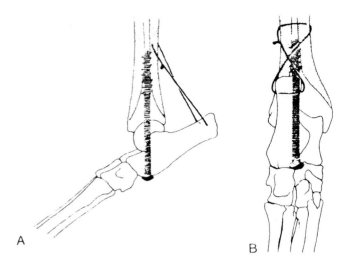

Fig. 64.13. Lateral (**A**) and caudocranial (**B**) views showing placement of a tension band wire through the fibular tarsal bone and the caudal cortex of the distal tibia for tibiotarsal arthrodesis.

The limb is placed in a padded supportive bandage with a splint along the caudal aspect. Radiographic evaluation is performed at periodic intervals of 4 to 6 weeks. The padded supportive bandage is changed as needed, but it should be maintained for 6 to 8 weeks until healing of the tibiotarsal arthrodesis is sufficient. Once healing of the arthrodesis is complete and a solid union has been achieved, the lag screw and tension band wire should be removed.

Intertarsal Arthrodesis

Arthrodesis of the intertarsal joints is indicated when injury has disrupted the plantar support resulting in gross instability and excessive dorsiflexion of the tarsus (3, 6, 16). The surgical approach is performed to the plantar surface of the tarsus with medial retraction of the flexor tendon (10). Stabilization of the arthrodesis is achieved with a pin and tension band wire. Once the articular cartilage is removed from the proximal aspect of the fourth tarsal and the calcaneus, cancellous bone graft is packed into the joint space. A heavy-gauge wire is passed through the plantar portion of the fourth tarsal bone. The joint is placed in anatomic position for the remainder of the procedure.

Because the calcaneus consists of dense compact bone, it is preferable to predrill a guide hole from the tuber calcanei along the long axis of the calcaneus into the fourth tarsal bone before placing a pin. A Steinmann pin slightly larger than that of the drill used is passed along the prepared site and is seated into the fourth tarsal bone. A heavy-gauge wire is passed in a figure-of-eight fashion over the end of the Steinmann pin, but beneath the superficial digital flexor tendon and crossed over the plantar surface of the calcaneus.

The wire is tightened, and the wound is closed in a routine manner (3, 11, 16). If a single Steinmann pin is used, it should be of large diameter and must be gauged by the width of the calcaneus and tarsal bones. However, insertion of a pin of too large a diameter may result in iatrogenic fractures. Alternatively, a cortical bone screw can be inserted as a lag screw. The tension band figure-of-eight wire should still be used; however, the proximal portion of the wire should be passed through a drill hole in the proximal calcaneus and subsequently tightened.

If disruption has occurred in additional intertarsal joints (e.g., the distal intertarsal joint) or if concomitant fractures are present in the tarsal bone, an alternative stabilization procedure may be necessary. Application of a bone plate to the lateral aspect of the calcaneus, passing over the lateral aspect of the tarsus to lie along the lateral aspect of the fifth metatarsal, allows for excellent purchase of the screws and provides rigid stabilization to the arthrodesis site (3).

After either surgical procedure, the limb is placed in a padded supportive bandage that incorporates either a cranial or caudal splint. Radiographic evaluations are performed at 4- to 6-week intervals. The limb is maintained in the bandage until a solid arthrodesis is obtained. The metallic implant may be removed once fusion is complete.

Tarsometatarsal Arthrodesis

The severe injury that results from disruption of the plantar support to the tarsometatarsal level of the joint, as well as irreparable fractures of the tarsal bones, necessitates arthrodesis of the involved joint levels. The surgical approach and surgical techniques are similar to those used for intertarsal arthrodesis. If a pin and tension band wire is used, the wire is passed through the base of the metatarsals, and a large Steinmann pin is inserted into the base of the fourth or fifth metatarsal (3, 6). The surgeon should make sure that the pin traverses all tarsal joints and is well seated into the metatarsals. A heavy-gauge figure-of-eight wire is crossed over the plantar surface of the tarsus and calcaneus with the proximal portion of the wire passing beneath the superficial digital flexor tendon and over the end of the protruding pin (Fig. 64.14). Before insertion of the pin, anatomic alignment without any dorsal or ventral flexion must be achieved.

Severe instability of the tarsus and comminution of the tarsal bones generally necessitate the use of a bone plate (3). The lateral application of a plate, as previously described for intertarsal arthrodesis, provides excellent screw purchase distally by insertion of the screws transversely through two or more of the metatarsals.

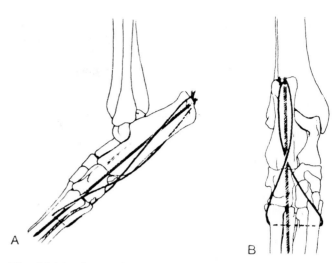

Fig. 64.14. Lateral (**A**) and caudocranial (**B**) views showing placement of a Steinmann pin and tension band wire for intertarsal arthrodesis.

In patients with severe open joint injury with loss of bone and soft tissue, an external fixation device may be preferable to internal fixation for arthrodesis of the hock.

Complications

The complications associated with arthrodesis on any joint include a delay in union, loosening or breakage of the metallic implant, and malalignment. These generally result from lack of attention to technical details or the use of implants of insufficient strength to maintain stability during the healing period. The complete removal of articular cartilage and subchondral bone and the subsequent packing of cancellous bone into and around the joint space are of utmost importance to the success of any arthrodesis. Likewise, maintenance of rigid stability during healing of the arthrodesis is fundamental.

The development of iatrogenic fractures after the insertion of implants that are too large must be treated immediately. If initial implant stability is not achieved, additional devices should be used to achieve stability, or alternative methods of fixation should be applied. If instability occurs during the healing process, additional external immobilization such as cast coaptation may still achieve a successful arthrodesis.

Malalignment of the arthrodesed joint should not occur if proper planning and technique are used. However, if the joint undergoes arthrodesis in a malaligned position, an anatomic position can still be achieved by performing a corrective osteotomy. Similarly, if the fusion angle has resulted in excessive limb shortening or limb lengthening, a corrective osteotomy can achieve a more functional position.

Complications of arthrodesis of the stifle or elbow include development of nonunion at the arthrodesis site, as a result of loosening or breakage of the orthopedic implant, and fractures of the adjacent long bones proximal or distal to the ends of the plate. Loosening of the screws and plate is related to technical errors in screw placement, infection surrounding the screw, poor quality of bone, and selection of an inadequate size of screw. Breakage of the implant usually indicates that a device of inadequate strength was used or that proper contouring principles were not followed.

Fractures occurring proximal or distal to the ends of the plate may indicate that a plate of insufficient length was applied or that postoperative care was not properly followed. Because the plate is more rigid than the bone, the end of the plate acts as a stress concentrator for the bone. Therefore, a plate of insufficient length allows the excessive bone length to concentrate movement at the end of the plate, which can then result in a fatigue fracture. However, the patient's owners must realize that arthrodesis of the stifle or elbow creates a long bone lever, which is predisposed to fracture even with successful arthrodesis.

In general, arthrodesis of a painful or unstable joint can preserve a functional limb. A normal or close-to-normal gait can be achieved in animals that have a fusion of the carpus or hock, even if fusion is bilateral. Although animals with an elbow or stifle arthrodesis have an awkward gait, without surgical treatment these animals would have a nonfunctional limb.

References

1. Crenshaw AH, ed. Campbell's operative orthopedics. 5th ed. St. Louis: CV Mosby, 1971.
2. Frost WW, Lumb WV. Radiocarpal arthrodesis: a surgical approach to brachial paralysis. J Am Vet Med Assoc 1966; 149:1073.
3. Dee JF, Dee LG, Early TD. Tarsal fractures, luxations and subluxations. In: Brinker WO, Hohn RB, Prieur WD. Small animal manual of internal fixation. New York: Springer-Verlag, 1984.
4. Olds RB. Arthrodesis of elbow, carpus, stifle and hock. In: Bojrab MJ, ed. Current techniques in small animal surgery. Philadelphia: Lea & Febiger, 1975.
5. Wind A. Surgical diseases of the carpal joint and methods of treatment. In: Bojrab MJ, ed. Current techniques in small animal surgery. Philadelphia: Lea & Febiger, 1975.
6. Early TD, Dee JF. Trauma to the carpus, tarsus and phalanges of dogs and cats. Vet Clin North Am 1980;10:717.
7. Moore RW, Withrow SJ. Arthrodesis. Compend Contin Educ Pract Vet 1966;3:319.
8. Newton CD, Nunamaker DM. Arthrodesis. In: Brinker WO, Hohn RB, Prieur WD. Small animal manual of internal fixation. New York: Springer-Verlag, 1984.
9. Parker RB, Brown GS, Wind AP. Pancarpal arthrodesis in the dog: a review of forty-five cases. Vet Surg 1981;10:35.
10. Piermattei DL, Greeley RC. An atlas of surgical approaches to the bones of the dog and cat. 2nd ed. Philadelphia: WB Saunders, 1979.
11. Early TD. Canine carpal ligament injuries. Vet Clin North Am 1978;8:183.
12. Turner TM, Hohn RB. Craniolateral approach to the canine elbow for repair of condylar fractures or joint exploration. J Am Vet Med Assoc 1980;176:1264.
13. Holt PE. Treatment of tibio-tarsal instability in small animals. J Small Anim Pract 1977;18:415.
14. Stoll SG, Sinibaldi KR, DeAngelis MP, et al. A technique for tibiotarsal arthrodesis utilizing cancellous bone screws in small animals. J Am Anim Hosp Assoc 1975;11:185.
15. Evans HE, Christensen GC. Miller's anatomy of the dog. 2nd ed. Philadelphia: WB Saunders, 1979.
16. Dieterich HF. Arthrodesis of the proximal intertarsal joint for repair of rupture of proximal plantar intertarsal ligaments. Vet Med Small Anim Clin 1974;69:995.

Amputation of the Forelimb

William R. Daly

Amputation of the forelimb is occasionally indicated as a primary treatment for severe traumatic injuries resulting in irreparable fractures and soft tissue injuries. Other indications are severe neurologic lesions such as brachial plexus avulsion, irreparable vascular occlusion, and severe congenital or acquired deformities. Amputation may also be considered an adjunct to the treatment of neoplasia or severe infections involving the limb. With the possible exception of neoplastic disease, amputation should be considered as a last-resort "salvage" procedure, indicated only when no alternative exists that would allow the retention of a useful limb.

Preoperative Considerations

Amputation performed at the shoulder joint or above is preferable because a stump below this level serves no useful function and is prone to abrasions and infections from frequent trauma. Small animals invariably adapt well to forelimb amputation; however, some giant breeds of dogs have difficulty. If the patient is able to ambulate while carrying the affected limb, usually it does well with forelimb amputation.

Forelimb amputation can be performed through or directly below the scapulohumeral joint, or the scapula can be removed with the limb. Forequarter amputation with removal of the scapula is advantageous because major vessels and nerves are easily visualized, bone-cutting instruments are not required, and no prominent scapular spine remains behind. The procedure of choice, however, is the one that works best for each individual veterinary surgeon.

Forelimb amputation is a major procedure that should be performed only with a thorough knowledge of the patient's physical status. Because blood loss is likely to be greater than in most major operations, the surgeon must evaluate both hematocrit and plasma proteins preoperatively. Anemic or hypoproteinemic patients should be treated medically, if time allows, or provisions should be made for transfusion of whole blood or plasma as the situation dictates. Balanced electrolyte solutions should be given intravenously continuously during the surgical procedure and until the patient has recovered from anesthesia. The intravenous catheter should be large enough to allow blood transfusion, should the need arise. In cases of amputation because of neoplasia or infection, a tourniquet may be used between the disease site and the amputation site to limit metastasis of infection or neoplasia to the general circulation.

Regardless of the amputation method used, preliminary preparations for the surgical procedure are identical. The affected limb is clipped with a No. 40 clipper blade from the carpus to the dorsal and ventral midlines. Clipping should extend well cranially and caudally to allow adequate draping. The paw is usually covered with a gauze wrap or a plastic bag before the patient is transported to the operating room, where final surgical skin preparation is done.

Forequarter Amputation

The objective of forequarter amputation is to remove the entire pectoral limb, including the scapula, from the thorax. This procedure involves the division of all muscles, nerves, and vessels that normally join the two parts. The muscles are the trapezius, rhomboideus, omotransversarius, serratus ventralis, brachiocephalicus, superficial and deep pectorals, and the latissimus dorsi.

After adequate preoperative evaluation and preparation, the patient is anesthetized and is placed in lateral recumbency with the affected limb uppermost. After draping, a skin incision is made over the scapular spine beginning at the dorsal rim of the scapula and proceeding downward to the acromion. At the acromion, the incision is curved cranially to cross the cranial aspect of the forelimb at the level of the greater tubercle. This incision eventually is extended to cross the medial surface of the forelimb in the axilla and to curve around the caudal aspect of the limb at the axillary fold, finally to join the lateral incision at the level of the acromion (Fig. 64.15**A,** *inset*). The entire skin incision does not need to be completed at the beginning of the operation. The lateral incision alone allows sufficient exposure to remove all muscle insertions, and the remainder of the incision can be delayed as the final act of amputating the limb.

After the lateral incision to the level of the greater tubercle is completed, subcutaneous dissection exposes the trapezius muscle. An incision is made in this muscle at its attachment to the scapular spine. The omotransversarius muscle is also divided at its attachment to the scapular spine (Fig. 64.15**A**). Retraction of

the trapezius muscle reveals the rhomboideus muscle, which is severed as close to its attachment to the scapula as possible (Fig. 64.15**B,** *inset*). Several blood vessels that require ligation are generally encountered in the muscle bellies as they are cut. Further lateral retraction of the scapula reveals the insertion of the serratus ventralis muscle on the medial face of the scapula. This insertion is easily elevated with a sharp periosteal elevator, and thus the detachment of all muscles connecting the scapula to the trunk is completed (Fig. 64.15**B**).

At this point, the vessels and nerves of the brachial plexus are easily visualized and are transected. The axillary artery and vein should be doubly ligated using the three-clamp technique. Use of a transfixation suture is recommended on the axillary artery (Fig. 64.15**C**). Nerves may be divided with a scalpel or scissors without special treatment of the proximal severed ends. Neuroma formation is not a common problem in the dog.

After division of the brachial plexus, attention is turned to the cranial portion of the limb. The brachiocephalicus muscle is transected near the greater tubercle of the humerus. At this point, the omocervical artery and vein are encountered and should be ligated. The superficial and deep pectoral muscles are transected near their insertions on the greater and lesser tubercles, respectively (Fig. 64.15**D**). The cephalic vein can also be ligated and divided at this point. The last remaining muscular attachment, the latissimus dorsi, is severed from its insertion on the teres tuberosity and the medial brachial fascia. The axillary lymph node and the accessory axillary lymph node are located just under the latissimus dorsi muscle near its attachment to the humerus and can be conveniently removed, if indicated, once this muscle has been cut (Fig. 64.15**E**).

The amputation is completed by incising the skin of the medial surface of the brachium. A flap must be made that is sufficiently large to cover the defect caused by removal of the limb. The base of this flap must be in the axillary space, and as much skin as possible must be taken from the medial brachium. It is always desirable to take extra skin because trimming is easily accomplished if necessary.

Once the limb has been removed, the muscle bellies are pulled together over the stumps of the severed nerves and vessels of the brachial plexus. This maneuver is accomplished by inverting the severed ends of the omotransversarius, trapezius, rhomboideus, and latissimus dorsi muscles over the serratus ventralis muscle with a continuous Lembert suture pattern (Fig. 64.15**F,** *inset*). The superficial and deep pectoral muscles are then similarly inverted by suturing them to the ventral margins of the more dorsal muscles. Closure of subcutaneous tissues and skin is routine (Fig. 64.15**F**).

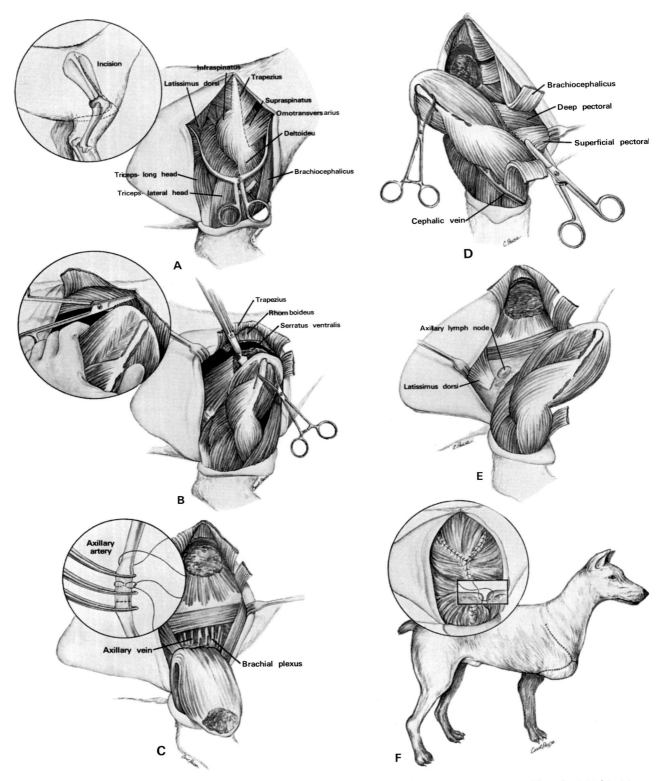

Fig. 64.15. **A.** The *inset* demonstrates the location of the skin incision used for forequarter amputation. After the initial incision over the scapular spine, subcutaneous dissection exposes the trapezius and omotransversarius muscles, which are severed at their insertions (*broken line*). **B.** The *inset* demonstrates the rhomboideus muscle as it is severed at its insertion on the scapula. Lateral retraction of the scapula then reveals the serratus ventralis muscle, which is sharply elevated from its insertion on the medial face of the scapula. **C.** Complete lateral retraction of the scapula exposes the entire brachial plexus. The axillary artery and vein are ligated and are severed using the three-clamp technique (*inset*). **D.** After transection of the brachial plexus, the brachiocephalicus muscle is divided, and the superficial and deep pectoral muscles are transected near their insertions on the humerus. **E.** The final muscular attachment, the latissimus dorsi, is severed at its insertion on the humerus. The axillary lymph node may be removed at this time if indicated. **F.** After removal of the limb, the muscle bellies are inverted over the severed nerves and vessels of the brachial plexus. A Lembert suture pattern works well for this purpose (*inset*). Subcutaneous tissues and skin are closed routinely.

If excessive skin is present, trimming should be done on the medial skin flap to preserve the thicker skin and hair coat present on the lateral surface of the limb.

Some veterinary surgeons place several Penrose drains into the wound before beginning closure. If placed, the drains should perforate the skin as ventrally as possible. If adequate attention is paid to the hemostasis and atraumatic operative technique, drains are not required. In all cases, a light-pressure bandage is used for 2 to 3 days to help prevent swelling, hematoma, and seroma formation. Dogs experiencing severe postoperative pain usually respond well to morphine at a dosage of 0.25 mg/kg subcutaneously or intramuscularly every 2 hours as needed.

Forelimb Amputation by Scapulohumeral Disarticulation

Scapulohumeral disarticulation is preferred by some veterinary surgeons for forelimb amputation. Preoperative evaluation, preparation, and positioning are identical to those described for forequarter amputation.

In this procedure, the initial skin incision is made as a semilunar incision that begins at the point of the shoulder, extends across the midpoint of the humerus, and curves back to the axillary fold. This incision produces a large flap that is used later to cover the wound. A similar flap is then made on the medial side of the limb to ensure adequate surgical exposure for the procedure and a generous supply of skin for closure (Fig. 64.16A, *inset*).

The brachiocephalicus muscle is transected first just below the clavicular tendon. The cephalic vein lies in this region and must also be ligated. External rotation of the limb exposes the superficial and deep pectoral muscles; these muscles are divided close to their insertions on the humerus (Fig. 64.16A). Retraction of the muscles exposes the nerves and vessels of the brachial plexus, which are then separated. The nerves may be cut with scissors or a scalpel, and the axillary artery and vein should each be doubly ligated. The axillary artery is divided distal to the point of origin of the external thoracic and lateral thoracic arteries, which arise close to the first rib.

After division of the brachial plexus, the acromial head of the deltoideus muscle is removed from its ori-

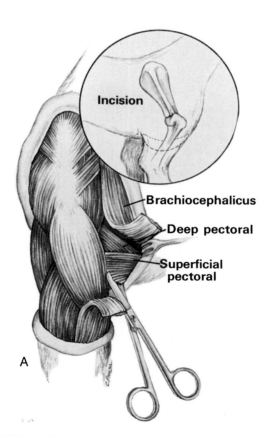

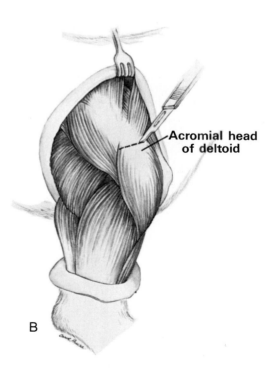

Fig. 64.16. **A.** The *inset* demonstrates the location of the incision for the scapulohumeral disarticulation technique of forelimb amputation. The brachiocephalicus muscle is transected, and then the insertions of the superficial and deep pectoral muscles are exposed and divided. Retraction of these muscles exposes the brachial plexus. **B.** The acromial head of the deltoideus muscle is severed at its origin on the scapula.

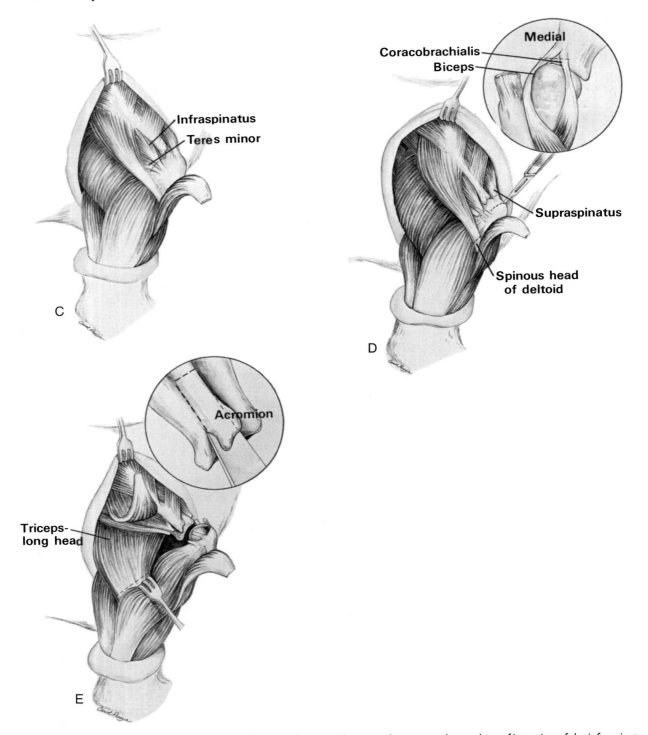

Fig. 64.16 (continued). C. Retraction of the acromial head of the deltoideus muscle exposes the tendons of insertion of the infraspinatus and teres minor muscles, which are severed. **D.** The supraspinatus muscle and the spinous head of the deltoid muscle are severed at their insertions. The joint capsule is then opened, and the humerus is totally dislocated after transection of the tendons of the biceps brachii, subscapularis, and the coracobrachialis muscles (*inset*). **E.** After division of the latissimus dorsi muscle, the long head of the triceps brachii muscle is divided as distally as possible to complete the amputation. The prominent scapular spine is removed with an osteotome (*inset*) for a better cosmetic effect.

gin on the acromion (Fig. 64.16). Distal retraction of this muscle exposes the insertions of the supraspinatus, infraspinatus, and teres minor muscles, which should be transected (Fig. 64.16**C**). The insertions of the latissimus dorsi, teres major, and cutaneous trunci muscles are next divided close to the humerus. The scapulohumeral joint capsule is then opened; total dislocation of the joint is easily accomplished once the tendons of the biceps brachii, coracobrachialis, and subscapularis muscles are severed over the joint space (Fig. 64.16**D,** *inset*). The spinous head of the deltoideus muscle is elevated from its insertion on the humerus (Fig. 64.16**D**). The long head of the triceps brachii muscle is then divided as distally as possible to complete the amputation (Fig. 64.16**E**).

The infraspinatus and supraspinatus muscles soon atrophy from disuse and loss of their nerve supply and expose the acromion and spine of the scapula. A better cosmetic effect is obtained if an osteotome is used to remove the scapular spine, or at least the prominent acromion (Fig. 64.16**E,** *inset*).

Closure of the wound involves suturing the superficial and deep pectoral muscles to the latissimus dorsi, teres major, infraspinatus, supraspinatus, and brachiocephalicus muscles. During closure of the subcutaneous tissues and skin, an attempt is made to preserve as much of the lateral skin flap as possible because this skin is thicker and has a denser hair coat that produces a more cosmetic final result. Postoperative bandaging for 2 to 3 days may be desirable to prevent seroma formation.

Suggested Readings

Evans HE, Christensen GC. Miller's anatomy of the dog. 2nd ed. Philadelphia: WB Saunders, 1979.

Harvey CE. Forequarter amputation in the dog and cat. J Am Anim Hosp Assoc 1974;10:25.

Hulland TJ, Pennock PW. Amputation of the forelimb. In: Archibald J, ed. Canine surgery. 2nd ed. Santa Barbara, CA: American Veterinary Publications, 1974.

Amputation and Disarticulation of the Hind Limb

*David W. Knapp &
Gheorghe M. Constantinescu*

Midshaft Femoral Amputation

The patient is placed in lateral recumbency with the affected leg up and suspended. The area is properly scrubbed, and the quadrant is draped and released into a sterile towel and wrapped. Curvilinear skin incisions are made on the lateral and medial aspects of the proximal thigh beginning at the fold of the flank and extending caudal and distal to a point just proximal to the stifle and continuing proximal and caudal to just distal to the tuber ischiadicum. The incisions should connect at each end, and the lateral flap should be slightly longer than its medial counterpart.

The skin distal to the incisions is undermined to expose the muscular insertions in the region of the stifle. The biceps femoris muscle is transected at its lateral insertion on the fascia lata and fascia cruris. The biceps femoris is reflected proximally to expose the combined insertions of the semitendinosus and semimembranosus muscles at the caudal aspect of the stifle. Both muscles are transected at the level of the crural fascia and caudal tibia. If present, the abductor cruris caudalis muscle is transected at its crural fascial insertion (Fig. 64.17**A**).

The quadriceps group makes up the muscles of the cranial thigh. The combined tendon of the vastus lateralis, vastus intermedius, vastus medialis, and rectus femoris muscles is transected just proximal to the patella. Proximal reflection of this muscle group exposes the lateral surface of the distal femur (Fig. 64.17**B**).

Access to the medial thigh is gained by abduction of the leg. Major blood vessels are identified, isolated and double ligated, transfixed, and divided individually. Monofilament nonabsorbable suture material is preferred. The saphenous vessels, branches of the femoral artery and vein, are located between the bellies of the caudal sartorius and gracilis muscles. The descending geniculate artery and vein lie deep to the semimembranosus muscle. The most distal ligation is at the bifurcation of the femoral artery and vein into the popliteal vessels and the caudal femoral vessels (Fig 64.17**B**). The sciatic nerve is also sharply transected at this level. Three thin, straplike muscles, the cranial and caudal bellies of the sartorius muscle and the gracilis muscle, are transected at their insertions near the cranial tibia and medial fascial area of the rectus femoris. The entire shaft of the distal femur is now exposed.

The more proximal femoral shaft is exposed by subperiosteally elevating the caudally located adductor magnus et brevis muscle. An osteotomy at the level of the proximal one-third of the femur may be performed using bone wire, an oscillating bone saw, or a small orthopedic hand saw. In patients with comminuted fractures, all that may be necessary is to remove free bone fragments and square off the remaining fracture site. Hemorrhage from the exposed marrow cavity can be controlled with bone wax or a cellulose fiber product.

Closure is accomplished by covering the exposed cut femoral shaft with the remaining muscle bellies. The combined tendon of the quadriceps muscle group

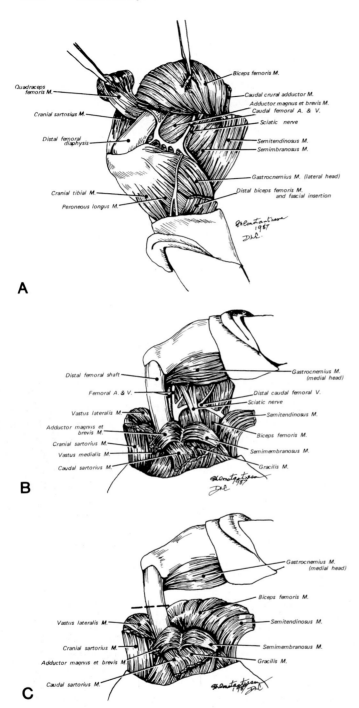

Quadraceps femoris M.

Cranial sartosius M.

Distal femoral diaphysis

Cranial tibial M.

Peroneous longus M.

Biceps femoris M.

Caudal crural adductor M.
Adductor magnus et brevis M.
Caudal femoral A. & V.

Sciatic nerve

Semitendinosus M.
Semimembranosus M.

Gastrocnemius M. (lateral head)

Distal biceps femoris M.
and fascial insertion

A

Distal femoral shaft

Femoral A. & V.

Vastus lateralis M.

Adductor magnus et brevis M.
Cranial sartorius M.
Vastus medialis M.
Caudal sartorius M.

Gastrocnemius M.
(medial head)

Distal caudal femoral V.
Sciatic nerve

Semitendinosus M.

Biceps femoris M.

Semimembranosus M.

Gracilis M.

B

Vastus lateralis M.

Cranial sartorius M.

Adductor magnus et brevis M

Caudal sartorius M.

Gastrocnemius M.
(medial head)

Biceps femoris M.

Semitendinosus M.

Semimembranosus M.

Gracilis M.

C

Fig. 64.17. Midshaft femoral amputation. **A.** Proximal and distal skin margins have been reflected. The biceps femoris and patellar tendons have been freed at their insertions and reflected proximally. Lateral view. **B.** The gracilis, semitendinosus, semimembranosus, and cranial and caudal bellies of the sartorius muscles are freed at their insertions on the medial aspect of the stifle and reflected proximally. The femoral artery and vein, as well as their distal branches, are ligated and divided. The sciatic nerve is also transected. Medial view. **C.** With the distal femoral shaft exposed, the adductor muscle is elevated subperiosteally, and the osteotomy is performed. The *dotted line* indicates the level of the osteotomy. Medial view.

is brought caudally and is sutured to the semitendinosus and semimembranosus muscles. The biceps femoris muscle is brought medially and is sutured to the sartorius and gracilis muscles. Subcutaneous and skin closure are routine. Muscle bellies are sutured with absorbable suture material in a horizontal mattress pattern, and the remaining layers are sutured with an absorbable suture material in a continuous pattern.

The combination of less hemorrhage resulting from transection at muscular insertions and the compact nature of the sutured muscle mass results in an infrequent need for drains. Postoperative care of the surgical wound is routine in most cases.

Coxofemoral Disarticulation

The patient is placed in lateral recumbency with the affected limb up and suspended. The leg is scrubbed, standard four-quadrant draping is completed, the limb is released, and a sterile distal wrap is placed.

The lateral skin incision starts at the fold of the flank, curving caudodistally to the midthigh and continuing proximally and caudally to the point of the tuber ischiadicum. The medial skin incision follows the lateral, except it is not carried as far distally; it meets the lateral incision at its cranial and caudal extents. Distal skin is undermined freely to expose muscle bellies. The proximal skin margins are undermined laterally to expose the greater trochanter and medially to the level of the femoral triangle.

Early ligation of the femoral artery and vein decreases bleeding later. These vessels are located at their exit from the abdomen within the femoral triangle, an anatomic area defined by the sartorius muscle cranially, the pectineus muscle caudally, and the iliopsoas muscle deeply (Fig. 64.18**A**). If neoplasia is the reason for limb removal and emboli are a concern, the femoral vein is double ligated, transfixed, and divided first. The femoral artery is isolated, double ligated, transfixed, and divided at a point proximal to the superficial circumflex iliac artery and lateral circumflex iliac artery branches. Monofilament nonabsorbable suture material is preferred.

Grouping muscles according to anatomic origins simplifies disarticulation. Abduction of the leg exposes the muscles of the medial and caudal area of the thigh. The pectineus muscle is elevated at its origin on the iliopectineal eminence, located at the ventral aspect of the lateral portion of the ilial body. The gracilis, adductor longus, and adductor magnus et brevis muscles share a common origin at the pelvic symphysis, at which point all three are sharply elevated and are reflected distally. Next, the semimembranosus muscle is sharply elevated from its origin on the roughened portion of the ischial tuberosity. Elevation of the semitendinosus muscle is at its origin just lateral to the

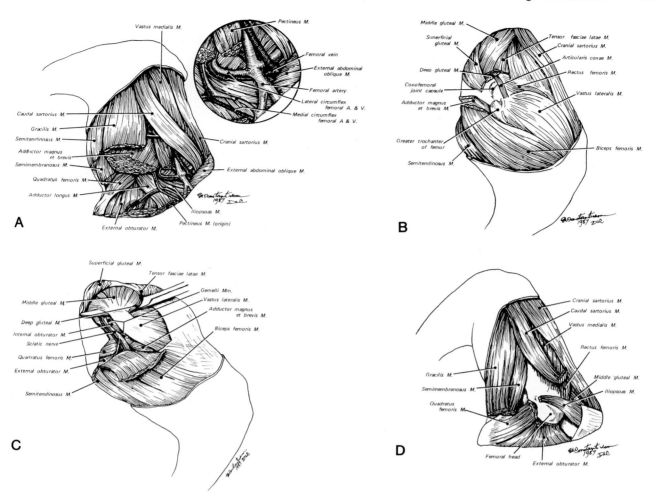

Fig. 64.18. Coxofemoral disarticulation. **A.** The proximal and distal skin margins are reflected. The femoral artery and vein are isolated and ligated proximal to the lateral circumflex femoral branches. The pectineus, gracilis, semitendinosus, semimembranosus, and adductor magnus et brevis muscles are elevated at their origins on the pubis. Medial view. **B.** The biceps femoris muscle is elevated from its origin on the sacrotuberous ligament and the tuber ischiadicum. The superficial gluteal and tensor fasciae latae muscles are elevated from their insertions on the proximal femur. The tendons of the middle and deep gluteal muscles are isolated at their insertions on the greater trochanter. Lateral view. **C.** The tendons of the middle and deep gluteal muscles are transected. The origin of the rectus femoris muscle is isolated and elevated from the body of the ilium. Lateral view. **D.** The cranial and caudal bellies of the sartorius muscle have been isolated, elevated, and reflected from their origins on the wing of the ilium. The iliopsoas, quadratus femoris, and external rotator muscles are isolated and elevated from their insertions on the proximal femur. The coxofemoral joint capsule is exposed and is incised along with the round ligament. Medial view.

semimembranosus muscle, on the lateral angle of the tuber ischiadicum. Both muscles are reflected distally (Fig. 64.18**A**).

Caudolateral thigh muscles are approached by adducting the limb. The biceps femoris muscle is transected at its combined origin on the sacrotuberous ligament and the lateral aspect of the ischial tuberosity (Fig. 64.18**B**). Reflection of the biceps distally exposes the sciatic nerve as it passes over the ischial body. The nerve is sharply transected at this level (Fig. 64.18**C**).

The muscles surrounding the femoral neck and greater trochanter are elevated next. The superficial

gluteal muscle is tenotomized at its insertion on the third trochanter and is reflected craniodorsally to expose the middle and deep gluteal muscles. These muscles are tenotomized at their insertions on the greater trochanter and are retracted cranially and dorsally. The tendons of insertion of the external obturator, internal obturator, gemelli, and quadratus femoris muscles are elevated from the trochanteric fossa (Fig. 64.18**C**).

Muscles originating on the wing and body of the ilium are identified and are isolated. The thin triangular tensor fasciae latae muscle is transected at its combined origin on the tuber coxae and aponeurosis with the gluteal muscles and is retracted distally. Both cranial and caudal bellies of the sartorius muscle are freed from the iliac crest and lumbodorsal fascia and are reflected distally. The rectus femoris muscle is subperiosteally elevated from its origin on the iliopubic eminence. Elevation of the iliopsoas muscle from its insertion on the lesser trochanter completes the muscular dissection and transections (Fig. 64.18**D**). The coxofemoral joint capsule and round ligament are sharply transected, completely freeing the limb from its pelvic attachments.

The surgical procedure is completed by apposing the remaining muscle bellies. The combined tendons of the gluteal muscles are sutured to the external rotator muscles. The iliopsoas muscle is pulled caudally and is sutured to the external obturator muscle. Horizontal mattress sutures of monofilament absorbable material are used. If one is successful in suturing these muscles together, the acetabulum will be covered by a layer of muscle. Subcutaneous and skin closures are routine.

The extensive undermining of skin combined with the removal of a large amount of muscle may lead to problems with dead space. The use of drains is left to the discretion of the surgeon. With this procedure, either Penrose drains or a closed-suction drainage system may be used. To avoid perianal contamination, drains should exit at the cranial aspect of the surgical site. The surgical incision and any drains exiting the area should be covered with a sterile nonadherent dressing immediately postoperatively; the dressing should be continued for several days after drain removal. if the wound is closed without drains, a pressure bandage will aid in the reduction of dead space and possible seroma formation.

With advancements in fracture repair, management of soft tissue injuries, and treatments for neoplastic disease, the need for amputation or disarticulation has lessened. However, when such procedures are indicated, convincing the owner to proceed may be the most difficult task. Removal of the hind leg more distal than the midfemur may result in complications. A limb that is too long may allow the animal to attempt weightbearing, resulting in chronic pressure sores at the distal end of the stump. If cosmetics are a concern, leaving the proximal femur with its associated muscles allows for more satisfactory results, especially in the male dog, in which the stump covers the scrotum and prepuce as well as protecting the external genitalia. Careful evaluation of the three other legs should be completed before the removal of the fourth. Severely dysplastic dogs and dogs with other debilitating conditions leading to severe degenerative joint disease involving any joint of the remaining legs may result in difficulties in ambulating after amputation or disarticulation.

A surgical assistant for holding the limb and retracting is of benefit during either of these procedures. Suction and cautery aid in maintaining a less bloody surgical field. Minimal undermining of skin is recommended, to help decrease dead space and potential seroma formation. Initial skin incisions should be liberal to ensure ease of closure, because any redundant skin may be excised at the time of closure. Nerves are sharply transected at their proximal limits, and a long-acting local anesthetic may be injected at that time. As a rule, owner satisfaction with these procedures is good.

65

BANDAGE TECHNIQUES

Application of a Robert Jones Bandage

David W. Knapp

The materials necessary to apply a Robert Jones bandage include one to three 1-lb rolls of absorbent cotton, 1- or 2-inch white adhesive tape, several rolls of 3- or 4-inch stretch gauze, one to three rolls of 3- or 4-inch elastic tape or self-adherent stretch tape, and a nonadherent dressing when indicated.

Application is begun by placing adhesive tape stirrups medially and laterally from the carpal or tarsal area distally (Fig. 65.1**A**). Dog-earing each end or placing a tongue depressor between the tape ends aids in separating the stirrups later. Placement of a nonadherent dressing on any open wound or surgical incision is done at this time.

The next portion of the bandage is the application of the cotton. One begins distally and wraps proximally, high into the axillary or inguinal regions (Fig. 65.1**B**). The ends of digits 3 and 4 should be left exposed, and the cotton should be wrapped with enough tension to make the bandage tight, but not tense enough to cause the cotton to tear. The final bandage should convert an irregularly shaped leg into a uniform-diameter or stovepipe configuration, thereby allowing the bandage to apply even pressure over the entire length of the leg (Fig 65.1**C**).

After application of the cotton, even pressure is accomplished by wrapping from distal to proximal with 3- or 4-inch stretch gauze (Fig. 65.1**D**). Each wrap should overlap the previous by about 50% its width, avoiding any formation of ridges and valleys, indications of uneven pressure. When wrapping the stretch gauze, one should apply enough tension to compress or reduce the size of the bandage adequately. In most cases, the final diameter of the bandage after the stretch gauze is applied is 40 to 50% of the original diameter.

To complete the bandage, the tape stirrups are separated and are placed along the appropriate medial and lateral sides. Using either elastic tape or self-adherent stretch tape, the final layer is started, again distally, wrapping proximally and continuing to overlap each layer by 50% while taking care to maintain even compression. When this layer is completed, only the distal ends of digits 3 and 4 should be exposed (Fig. 65.1**E**). If the toes are not visible, adequate amounts of the surrounding cotton should be removed to allow exposure of the digits.

The goal of the Robert Jones bandage is to provide immobilization while maintaining even compression over the length of the limb. Compression can be evaluated by tapping over the length of the bandage; a properly applied bandage sounds like a ripe watermelon when it is thumped. To obtain even compression may require several applications of the stretch gauze, beginning each wrap distally and continuing proximally to either the axillary or inguinal region. In smaller dogs and cats, cotton cast padding may be substituted for the roll cotton, thereby achieving a more uniform fit to the leg. A more uniform fit may also be accomplished by removing the paper insert in the cotton roll, tearing the roll in half, and wrapping with 6-inch widths rather than 12-inch widths of cotton strips. All layers of the bandage are wrapped in a lateral-to-medial rotation to allow for a neutral to slightly internally rotated position of the limb.

Postbandaging care should include keeping the bandage clean and dry and observing the exposed digits for swelling or coolness to the touch. If problems are noted, the bandage may have been improperly applied and should be removed and the leg reevaluated. If no

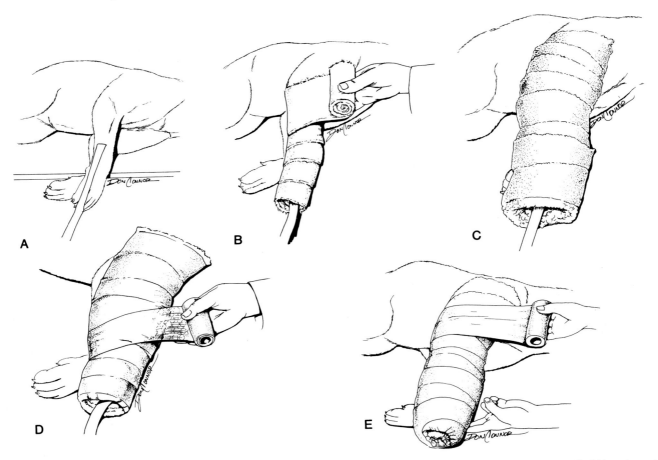

Fig. 65.1. Application of a Robert Jones bandage. **A.** Placement of stirrups on medial and lateral aspects of paw. **B.** Wrapping with rolled cotton starting at distal end. **C.** Cotton padding in place. **D.** Application of stretch gauze, compressing cotton. **E.** Application of elastic tape or self-adherent stretch tape after stirrups are folded up, leaving only digits 3 and 4 exposed.

signs of problems are evident, the Robert Jones bandage may be left in place for up to 3 weeks.

Ehmer Sling (Figure-of-Eight Sling)

Paul W. Dean

The Ehmer or figure-of-eight sling is a nonweightbearing sling for the pelvic limb. A properly applied Ehmer sling maintains the leg in a flexed position with the coxofemoral joint abducted and inwardly rotated.

The Ehmer sling is used primarily to maintain the coxofemoral joint in a stable position after closed reduction of craniodorsal coxofemoral luxations. Maintenance of the coxofemoral joint in an inwardly rotated and abducted position provides maximal cov-

erage of the head of the femur by the acetabulum while periarticular fibrosis stabilizes the coxofemoral joint. Use of an Ehmer sling may also be beneficial in maintaining stability of the hip joint in the immediate postoperative period after certain surgical procedures such as repair of fractures of the femoral head and neck and acetabular fractures and to provide stability after open reduction of coxofemoral joint luxations.

The only material necessary to apply an Ehmer sling is a roll of an elastic tape such as Elastikon (Johnson & Johnson, New Brunswick, NJ) or Conform (Kendall Co., Boston, MA). In the absence of elastic tape, white porous adhesive tape (Zonas porous tape, Johnson & Johnson, New Brunswick, NJ) may be substituted.

To begin placement of an Ehmer sling, the tape is first anchored to the metatarsal region of the foot by wrapping the tape loosely around the metatarsals. The tape is begun on the dorsal metatarsus and proceeds to the lateral and then plantar aspects of the metatarsus. The limb is then flexed, taking care not to hyperflex the hock joint, and the tape is continued up the

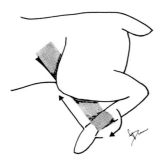

Fig. 65.2. Tape is placed loosely around lateral metatarsus and is brought up the medial side of the leg—adhesive surface of tape facing skin.

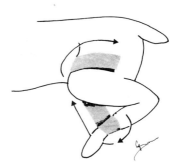

Fig. 65.4. Tape is continued from medial-to-lateral over the cranial quadriceps muscles to pass caudal to the stifle.

medial aspect of the tibia, medial to the stifle joint and medially over the thigh muscles (Fig. 65.2). The tape *should not* be passed up the medial aspect of the tibia, caudal to the stifle joint and over the lateral side of the thigh muscles because this predisposes the tape to slipping off the cranial thigh muscles (Fig. 65.3). After the tape is passed up the medial aspect of the thigh muscles, it is brought over the cranial thigh muscles to the lateral side of the thigh and continues distally caudal to the stifle joint, medial to the distal tibia and hock, and passes under the plantar aspect of the metatarsals medially to laterally (Figs. 65.4 and 65.5). Two or three wraps of tape are continued in a manner similar to that previously described. When the tape is properly applied, the toes should point slightly inward, the hock joint should be rotated outward, and the stifle and coxofemoral joint should be rotated internally. To provide maximal coverage of the femoral head by the acetabulum, abduction of the limb is provided by passing a length of tape from the plantar metatarsal region over the lateral aspect of the flexed limb and around the abdomen, where it is attached to a preplaced

bellyband (Fig. 65.6). Care should be taken to stay cranial to the prepuce with the bellyband in male dogs. Postreduction abduction of the leg is contraindicated when an Ehmer sling is used to stabilize ventral coxofemoral luxations because abduction may predispose to reluxation. A properly applied Ehmer sling is well tolerated by most dogs. The sling should be left in place for 2 to 3 weeks after closed reduction of coxofemoral luxations and after open reduction of coxofemoral luxations using the transacetabular pinning technique (1). Immobilization of joints beyond 3 weeks should be avoided because potentially irreversible changes such as capsular and pericapsular contracture, proliferation of intracapsular connective tissue, and major cartilage alterations may occur (2). Owners should be instructed to check the sling daily for slippage and to observe the toes daily for potential swelling. Should swelling of the toes be observed, the owner should be instructed to return the animal immediately to have the sling removed and reapplied correctly. Some irritation of the skin may result from contact with the tape, and it usually resolves spontaneously after removal of the sling.

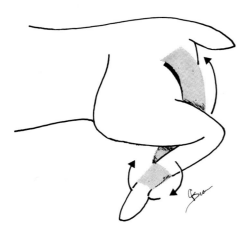

Fig. 65.3. Incorrect placement of tape predisposes the sling to slippage off the cranial aspect of the stifle.

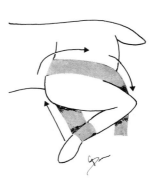

Fig. 65.5. Tape is continued from lateral aspect to pass medial to the hock and metatarsus and is then brought around the plantar surface of the metatarsus to the lateral side.

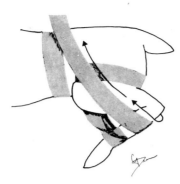

Fig. 65.6. After completion of two to three wraps of the tape as previously described, the tape is brought up the lateral side of the leg and attached to the preplaced bellyband to maintain abduction of the hip joint.

References

1. Wallace LJ. Pinning techniques for repairing coxofemoral luxations. In: Bojrab MJ, ed. Current techniques in small animal surgery. 2nd ed. Philadelphia: Lea & Febiger, 1983:611–616.
2. Herron AJ. Fracture disease. In: Bojrab MJ, ed. Pathophysiology in small animal surgery. Philadelphia: Lea & Febiger, 1981: 550–552.

Robinson Sling (Pelvic Limb Sling)

Paul W. Dean

The Robinson pelvic limb sling is a nonweightbearing sling that is useful in maintaining additional postoperative immobilization of the pelvic limb while still allowing limited flexion and extension of the leg. A Robinson sling produces less flexion of the hock and stifle joints than an Ehmer sling, or 90:90 flexion bandage, and should be considered when prolonged nonweightbearing is desired to minimize the occurrence of fracture disease. The Robinson sling is particularly useful in fractures involving the femur in which fixation may be less than optimum and a period of nonweightbearing on the limb is desired during the immediate postoperative period. The Robinson sling can also be used to prevent weightbearing in animals when poor owner compliance with postoperative instructions is suspected or when excessive early weightbearing on the limb by an overactive animal could compromise fracture healing.

To begin application of the Robinson sling, a circular bellyband of 2- or 3-inch adhesive tape is first applied around the abdomen of the dog, staying cranial to the prepuce in males. The foot on the affected side is bandaged with two to three light wraps of cast padding

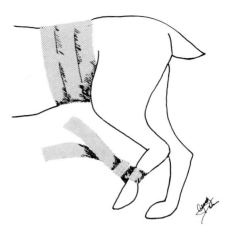

Fig. 65.7. The middle of the doubled over tape strip is passed around the plantar metatarsus and secured together over the dorsal surface using additional tape. A preplaced bellyband is shown in position.

and is covered with a wrap of adhesive tape. Next, a 10-foot-long strip of 2-inch porous adhesive tape is doubled on itself so the adhesive sides are together, creating one 5-foot-long piece of tape. The center of this tape is passed around the plantar surface of the bandaged metatarsus and is secured over the cranial surface of the metatarsus with a strip of 1-inch tape (Fig. 65.7). This should leave two ends of tape free, each approximately 2 feet long, extending toward the front of the dog. The tape ends are then attached to the bellyband, so when the dog is in a normal standing position, the leg is held off the ground slightly (Fig. 65.8). Another piece of 2-inch adhesive tape is used to maintain the tape medial and lateral to the leg by attaching one end of the tape to the lateral strip, passing the tape adhesive side–out caudal to the stifle joint, inside the medial strip, and back to the lateral side so

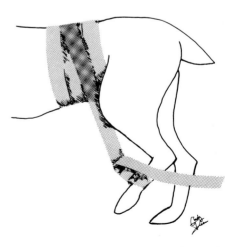

Fig. 65.8. The medial strip is brought up the inside surface of the leg.

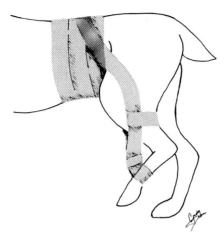

Fig. 65.9. The lateral strip is brought up the outside surface of the leg, and the length of the trips is adjusted to prevent weightbearing before securing the strips to the bellyband. The medial and lateral strips are maintained in position by a piece of 2-inch tape doubled on itself behind the stifle.

the two adhesive surfaces are together (Fig. 65.9). This prevents the leg from rotating excessively medially or laterally (1).

An alternative method of applying a pelvic limb sling that allows dynamic flexion and extension of the leg can be used in dogs with distal femoral fractures in which quadriceps contracture is a concern during the postoperative period (ER Pope, unpublished data, 1986). A rubber dog boot is used to protect the foot. A 5-foot length of $\frac{1}{4}$-inch latex tubing is doubled on itself, and the looped end is secured to the plantar aspect of the dog boot. One side of the tubing is brought up the medial side, and the other end is brought up the lateral side of the leg. One-inch adhesive tape is used to tape the tubing together in front of the hock, behind the tibia distal to the stifle and in

front of the femur proximal to the patella. The tubing is then secured to the bellyband in a position that maintains the leg in slight flexion (Fig. 65.10).

Complications can occur with the use of a Robinson sling, and close monitoring of the animal by the owner is necessary. An improperly adjusted sling allows the pet to bear weight or toe touch with the limb. During application, it is safer to err on the side of too much flexion of the limb rather than too little. If the bellyband should slip or rotate, the animal will bear weight; lightly spraying the bellyband tape with ether or other material that increases its adhesive properties minimizes this complication. Daily monitoring by the owner is essential to check for either of these complications.

Reference

1. Robinson GW, McCoy L. A pelvic limb sling for dogs. In: Bojrab MJ, ed. Current techniques in small animal surgery. Philadelphia: Lea & Febiger, 1975:567–569.

Slocum Sling for Dislocation of the Hip

Barclay Slocum & Theresa Devine Slocum

The Slocum sling is a bandaging technique used for closed reduction of dislocations of the hip. By understanding the principles of hip stability and the pathologic features of the injuries, the sling can be adapted for both craniodorsal and caudoventral dislocations. Open reduction and surgical repair should be used, however, if immediate weightbearing is needed to spare a traumatized contralateral limb.

Craniodorsal Dislocation

Most dislocations presented clinically are craniodorsal, as confirmed by ventrodorsal and lateral radiographs. This injury is an external rotation injury involving tearing of the craniodorsal hip joint capsule, as well as the ligament of the femoral head. For the sling method of closed reduction to be successful, the hip must be normal and have a normal slope to the dorsal acetabular rim. The caudal joint capsule and external hip rotators must be intact, to hold the hip in the acetabulum, permitting the cranial and dorsal joint capsule to heal.

Reduction of Craniodorsal Dislocation

The patient is anesthetized and is placed in lateral recumbency on a gurney with the dislocated hip upper-

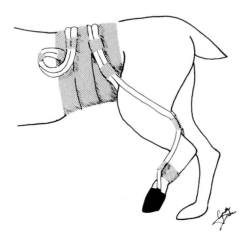

Fig. 65.10. Modified pelvic limb sling in position using a rubber dog boot and latex intravenous tubing to produce dynamic flexion of the limb.

most. The pelvis is supported so ventral traction will not move the patient. In a large dog, this is done by placing the middle of a towel under the affected leg in the pubic symphyseal region with the ends pulled dorsally by an assistant. Ventral traction of the affected limb is done simultaneously by the veterinarian. In a small dog, the veterinarian's hand is placed under the ventral midline of the dog's pubis, while the other hand is used to provide ventral traction to the affected limb.

The femur is then externally rotated at the hip to minimize the difficulty in lateralizing the femoral head, to clear the acetabular rim during reduction. Caudal traction on the greater trochanter moves the femoral head over the dorsal rim and brings it within the confines of the torn joint capsule. Finally, internal rotation of the femur forces the femoral head into the acetabulum by using the caudal joint capsule and external rotators as the restraint to this rotatory force.

Hip reduction is confirmed with a lateral radiograph of the hips, which should show a black articular cartilage line around both femoral heads. Lack of this cartilage line indicates that the femoral head is not yet in the acetabulum.

Testing the hip for stability is necessary to predict the success of this bandage. The reduced hip is internally rotated so the femoral head is forced into the acetabulum by creating tension in the external rotator muscles and the caudal joint capsule. Maintaining this internally rotated position of the hip, the femur is axially compressed against the supported pelvis. If the internally rotated hip does not dislocate with this test, then the hip will be maintained in reduction by the sling. The internally rotated hip should remain reduced, even if the pelvis is lifted off the gurney by the femur. Gradual external rotation of the internally rotated hip allows the hip to redislocate, giving the minimal amount of internal rotation necessary to maintain hip reduction.

If the internally rotated hip dislocates when tested by axial compression of the femur, then the hip will not be maintained in reduction by this sling. If the external rotators and caudal joint capsule have been damaged, open reduction and surgical stabilization by a pelvic osteotomy are required. The dorsal acetabular rim is used to capture and stabilize the hip, rather than the muscular forces of the traumatized internal and external rotators of the hip.

Slocum Sling Application for Craniodorsal Dislocation

The Slocum sling application for a craniodorsal hip dislocation requires the following steps:

1. The stifle and hock are comfortably (but not forcible) flexed, and 2-inch white (nonelastic) adhesive tape is circumferentially wrapped around the cranial thigh, plantar tarsus and metatarsus to encompass the entire limb in the flexed position (Fig. 65.11).

2. In the female, a bellyband of 4-inch Elastikon (elastic bandage with strong adhesive, Johnson & Johnson, Inc., New Brunswick, NJ) is wrapped around the abdomen twice by beginning dorsally, down the lateral abdomen on the up side of the dog, across the ventral abdomen, up the opposite lateral abdomen, which is against the gurney, and finally over the back. The roll end of Elastikon is not cut at this time.

3. In the male, a chest harness of 4-inch Elastikon is used to enclose the entire chest. Sheepskin or felt insoles can be used to pad the thoracic inlet.

4. A 6-inch web (multiple strips of 2-inch white nonelastic adhesive tape) is made by beginning on the flexed cranial thigh, then to the medial thigh, over the plantar metatarsus, the lateral thigh, and finally over the back. The strips of the web are secured temporarily on the edge of the gurney.

5. A 4-inch-thick pad of terry cloth is made of toweling and adhesive tape. The web is lifted off the edge of the gurney, and the pad is placed on the lateral stifle between the web and the stifle (Fig. 65.12).

6. The web is drawn over the pad and back with enough tension to internally rotate and stabilize the dislocated hip. The web is secured to the bellyband in the female or the chest harness in the male (Figs. 65.13 and 65.14).

7. A lateral radiograph is taken, and a black cartilage line around the femoral head confirms hip reduction.

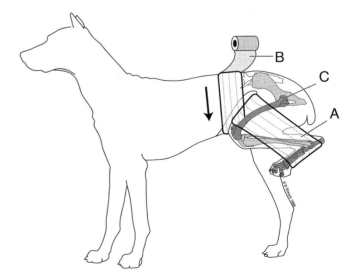

Fig. 65.11. The stifle and hock are comfortably flexed. White nonelastic, 2-inch porous tape (A) is circumferentially wrapped around the cranial thigh, plantar tarsus, and metatarsus. A bellyband of 4-inch tape (Elastikon) is wrapped around the abdomen twice (B), in the direction of the *arrow*. The position of the greater trochanter is caudal to the femoral head (C).

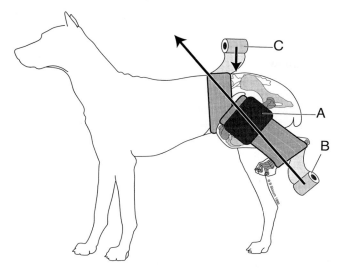

Fig. 65.12. A 4-inch pad of terry cloth (*A*) is placed on the lateral stifle to cause internal rotation of the femur. The metatarsal tape starts medially (*B*), crosses the metatarsus, and is drawn laterally over the pad and secured dorsally over the spine as shown (*black arrow*). The body wrap (*C*) captures the metatarsal tape to stabilize the limb and to create internal rotation and flexion of the hip.

Internal rotation of the hip is confirmed by the location of the greater trochanter cranial to the femoral head.

8. Additional tape is applied as necessary to secure the sling.

The sling should be adjusted once the patient is awake and has full muscular control. If a portion is too tight, it can be cut to relax the tension, and new adhesive tape can be applied over the original tape in the more relaxed position. Special attention should be

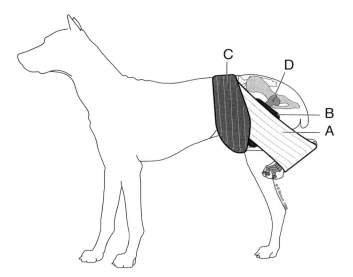

Fig. 65.13. The completed sling incorporates the metatarsal tape (*A*) over the internal rotation pad (*B*) and is secured by the torso bandage (*C*). The effect is to cause internal rotation of the hip in flexion (*D*).

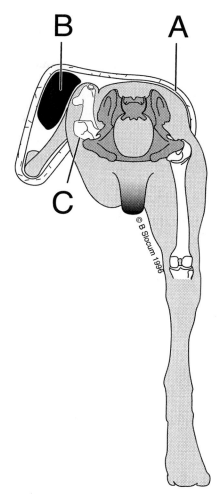

Fig. 65.14. The caudocranial view of the patient shows the torso bandage (*A*) putting a medial force on the stifle through the internal rotation pad (*B*) while creating an internal rotation of the hip by lateralizing the metatarsus.

directed to the tape over the Achilles tendon, the cranial thigh just proximal to the patella, and the ventral abdomen.

Managing a patient with a sling is more problematic than treating a patient with open reduction of a dislocated hip, but success is just a matter of good nursing care. Talcum powder should be used liberally to avoid chaffing. Follow-up adjustments should be made immediately after the patient is awake from anesthesia, in 24 hours, and at weekly intervals until the bandage is irreparable or has served its useful purpose. The owner should be encouraged to take an active role in management of the patient and sling by cutting out irritating portions of the sling, relaxing excessively tight portions of the sling, and inspecting the patient and sling frequently. If the owner is worried about the sling, the hip, or the patient, then the patient should be seen. If that is not possible, the bandage should be removed by the owner to ensure that no damage is done to the patient by the bandage, because the sling can always be replaced. Appropriate medications should be administered for fly strike or flea infestation.

Caudoventral Dislocation

Although the caudoventral dislocation is seen less frequently clinically, it is an internal rotation injury with a pathologic tearing of the ventral joint capsule and ligament of the femoral head. The dislocated femoral head is usually located in the obturator foramen. Extension of the hip with the femoral head in the acetabulum relaxes contracted cranial thigh muscles.

Reduction of the Caudoventral Dislocation

The patient is anesthetized and is placed in lateral recumbency on a gurney with the dislocated hip uppermost. With the hip in neutral to 45° of hip flexion, the femur is internally rotated at the hip to minimize the difficulty in lateralizing the femoral head, to clear the ventral acetabular rim during reduction. Cranial traction on the limb moves the femoral head into line with the ventral acetabulum. Firm medial-to-lateral pressure on the proximal femur lateralizes the femoral head to clear the ventral acetabulum. Simultaneous dorsal translation of the greater trochanter and external rotation of the femur force the femoral head into the acetabulum by using the cranial joint capsule and internal rotators as the restraint to these forces.

Hip reduction is confirmed with a lateral radiograph of the hips that shows a black articular cartilage line around both femoral heads. Lack of this cartilage line indicates that the femoral head is not in the acetabulum.

The hip should be tested for stability to ensure that the bandaging technique will be successful. The hip is externally rotated, which forces the femoral head into the acetabulum and prevents caudoventral dislocation of the hip on axial compression of the femur against the supported pelvis. If the externally rotated hip dislocates, then the hip will not be maintained in reduction by this sling. An open reduction with surgical stabilization is necessary in these cases. If the externally rotated hip does not dislocate, then the hip will be maintained in reduction by this sling. The external rotated hip should remain reduced even if the pelvis and hindquarters of the patient are lifted off the gurney by the limb. Gradual internal rotation of the externally rotated hip allows the hip to redislocate. This amount of external rotation will be necessary to maintain hip reduction.

Slocum Sling Application for Caudoventral Hip Dislocation

The Slocum Bandage application for a caudoventral hip dislocation requires the following steps, with the dog in lateral recumbency.

1. A chest band of 4-inch Elastikon is wrapped around the chest twice, just caudal to the forelimbs. The direction of the tape is dorsal to ventral on the up side of the thorax. The roll end of Elastikon is not cut at this time.

2. The stifle and hock are comfortably (but not forcibly) extended cranially, and the metatarsus is secured to the chest band at the level of the shoulder with tape.

3. A 4-inch-thick wedge shaped pad of terry cloth is made of toweling and adhesive tape.

4. The pad is placed between the caudal thorax and the medial stifle to maintain external hip rotation.

5. A circumferential wrap 8 inches wide around the lateral stifle, pad, and torso secures the bandage (Figs. 65.15 and 65.16).

6. A lateral radiograph confirms hip reduction with external rotation by showing the femoral head cranial to the greater trochanter.

Follow-up adjustments should be done immediately after the patient is awake from anesthesia, in 24 hours, and at weekly intervals until the bandage is irreparable or has served its useful purpose. Because any bandage can cause severe damage to the patient, the owner

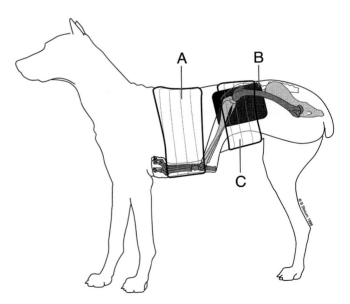

Fig. 65.15. The reduced caudoventral dislocation is held firmly in position by securing the metatarsus to the ventral thorax by a circumferential bandage (A) while externally rotating the hip by a pad (B) between the stifle and dorsolateral flank. A circumferential bandage around the abdominal torso of the affected limb (C) stabilizes the externally rotated hip.

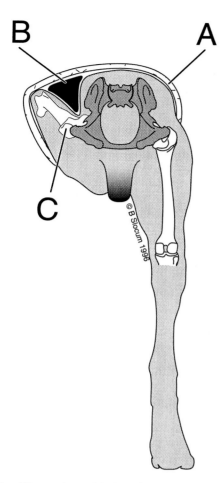

Fig. 65.16. The caudocranial view shows the abdominal torso bandage (*A*) stabilizing the pad (*B*) between the stifle and flank. The hip is rotated externally.

should be advised to remove the bandage if any concerns exist, and the patient should be seen. The bandage can always be reapplied. Appropriate medications should be administered for fly strike or flea infestation.

After the application of a Slocum sling for craniodorsal or caudoventral dislocation of the hip, the patient should be monitored closely so any compromise to circulation or discomfort from the sling can be adjusted or modified appropriately. The sling looks uncomfortable, but the patients seem to accept it well. Weekly examinations allow the bandage to be adjusted or modified in areas of irritation. Talcum powder liberally applied under the bandage dramatically reduces or eliminates chaffing. Often the hair is clipped, if it becomes soiled. Urine irritation or compromise to urination must be addressed immediately. As with all bandages, if the owner believes that the bandage may be causing harm to the dog, then the bandage should be removed immediately because healing can resume

as soon as the problem is solved. Although the bandages may look disgraceful because of patient abuse and client neglect, the outcome is usually good.

Failure of closed reduction of dislocated hips is a failure to recognize trauma to crucial structures necessary for maintaining hip stability. Craniodorsal dislocations fail in the long term if the hip is dysplastic and has an increased slope to the dorsal acetabular rim. This technique, and all other closed techniques, do not provide normal hip congruence, and the hip dysplasia progresses. If the caudal joint capsule and the external rotators of the hip are absent or deficient, no structures will be present to brace against during internal hip rotation to pull the femoral head into the acetabulum and allow the cranial joint capsule to heal. If the cranial gluteal nerve or the sciatic nerve is damaged, the internal hip rotator muscles will be unable to pull the hip into the socket. If the deep gluteal muscle or its tendon is damaged, it cannot pull the femoral head into the socket and long-term stability of the hip is questionable. Closed reduction of caudoventral dislocations fails in the long term if obturator nerve function is absent.

The Slocum sling is a powerful method of maintaining the reduced position of a hip, but follow-up at 1 and 2 months after sling removal is necessary to ensure proper maintenance of the femoral head in the acetabulum. Immediately after removing the Slocum sling, the scarred joint capsule tissue around the hip causes limited external rotation. Within 2 weeks of sling removal, the scarring is usually stretched to maintain a normally reduced hip and limb appearance. If the hip begins to demonstrate laxity, then the integrity of the cranial gluteal nerve and the deep gluteal muscle must be questioned. The appearance of degenerative joint disease indicates preexisting hip dysplasia or loss of hip rotator competence and not necessarily poor performance by the attending veterinarian, effects of the traumatic hip dislocation, or poor results of closed management of the dislocated hip. A pelvic osteotomy can be used to capture the femoral head, under these circumstances of hip rotator muscle force deficiency, by a 5 to 10° overrotation of the acetabular segment. When the acetabulum is overrotated (slightly), the femoral head is reduced into the acetabulum by the axial femoral forces that cause the femoral head to fall into the acetabulum instead of out of the acetabulum. Overrotation of the pelvic osteotomy gains hip stability at the expense of the abduction. Excessive overrotation causes rubbing of the dorsal acetabular rim on the femoral neck and discomfort.

With proper case selection, the Slocum sling is removed in 4 to 6 weeks, and a gradual progressive rehabilitation to normal activity is anticipated 12 weeks after injury.

Splinting Techniques

Douglas N. Lange & Kenneth E. Bartels

External fixation by coaptation implies the use of casts, splints, or bandages to provide immobilization of an injured limb. These devices approximate the shape of the limb to which they are applied, and they provide stable fixation of bone fragments without the need for surgical implants at the fracture site.

External fixation for orthopedic injuries in veterinary medicine offers distinct advantages over open reduction and internal fixation. In most instances, tissue and vascular trauma is reduced, the risk of infection is decreased, and the cost of application can be much lower than that of surgery (1). Careful case selection is required to achieve successful treatment of fractures with external coaptation. In general, these devices are best used in young patients (less than 1 year of age) that tend to heal rapidly with transverse or incomplete fractures distal to the elbow or stifle. External coaptation best neutralizes bending forces on fractures away from joints, rather than near joints, and requires stabilization of the joint above and the joint below the fracture (2). Therefore, coaptation does have disadvantages resulting from long-term limb immobilization that can cause severe disuse atrophy and possible "fracture disease." The use of a below-the-knee cast bracing (Sarmiento-type) system has been advocated; if properly used for certain tibial fractures, this type of system may reduce problems associated with total immobilization of the hind limb (3, 4). If a coaptation device is incorrectly applied, loosens, or becomes wet, skin necrosis and even gangrene can result. Certain cases of multiple or severely comminuted fractures are best managed by internal fixation techniques, because precise anatomic reduction and adequate neutralization of forces acting on the fractures cannot be achieved with external coaptation.

Indications

Coaptation splints are commonly used for immobilization of simple transverse fractures of the radius, ulna, fibula, metacarpals, metatarsals, and phalanges. They can also be useful for immobilization of certain joints, such as the stifle, after traumatic injuries or surgical stabilization (2, 5). With most fractures, however, use of both internal fixation and external coaptation combines the disadvantages of both and, in general, should be avoided whenever possible (1).

Temporary coaptation devices usually are indicated in the acutely traumatized animal for prevention of edema, relief of pain, reduction of subsequent damage to soft tissue, wound protection from further contami-

nation, prevention of development of closed fractures into open fractures, and fracture stabilization. Robert Jones bandages, coaptation splints of various materials, Schroeder–Thomas splints, tape hobbles, Ehmer slings, Velpeau slings, and nonweightbearing slings have been described for temporary immobilization as well as for definitive immobilization of certain orthopedic injuries.

The choice of coaptation device depends on each individual case and circumstance. The coaptation device may serve as a temporary splint for traumatic injuries while waiting for definitive internal fixation, as a primary treatment of certain fractures, or as an adjunct to internal fixation or ligament repair (1, 2). Cost is another important aspect that must be considered as well as the availability of materials required for different coaptation devices.

General Application Guidelines

A few general guidelines are relevant to application of all types of coaptation splints and casts. Depending on the animal's physical condition and the severity of the orthopedic problem, application of coaptation splints or casts is best performed with the patient sedated or under general anesthesia. When the patient's physical status precludes the use of chemical restraint, traction and excessive manipulation of the limb must be kept to a minimum.

Use of Stirrups

Application of adhesive tape on the cranial and caudal surfaces of the foot to form "stirrups" is usually necessary so the limb can be attached to the splint or cast securely (Fig. 65.17**A**). In some instances, one should

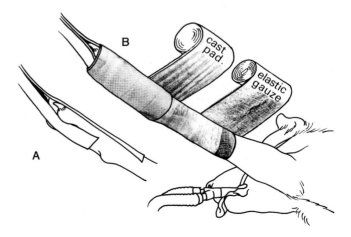

Fig. 65.17.   A. Application of adhesive tape stirrups on the cranial and caudal surfaces of the foot. **B.** Application of elastic gauze over the adhesive tape stirrups followed by overlapping layers of cast padding.

fix the strips of adhesive tape medially and laterally on the limb; this has been recommended for application of a full-encircling cast (6). When lateral and medial stirrups are used, they must be incorporated into the lateral and medial sides of the cast, respectively, to avoid excessive pressure and possible skin necrosis over the outer distal metatarsal or metacarpal epiphyseal areas (7). Encircling bands of tape should *never* be used on an animal's foot because they can cause irreparable vascular damage and skin necrosis.

If problems are encountered in attaching the tape to the foot, the skin can be dried with alcohol to increase the holding capacity on the foot. Some veterinarians spiral a piece of adhesive tape around the cranial and caudal tape pieces to increase fixation of stirrups to the skin (8). Two to three overlapping layers of elastic gauze (Kling or Sof-Kling, Johnson & Johnson Medical, Inc., Arlington, TX) applied snugly and evenly over the stirrups has also been used without problems to prevent the tape stirrups from slipping (Fig. 65.17**B**). Good judgment must be used during application of these gauze layers to prevent vascular compromise. Tape application over the carpal pad can cause mild irritation to this structure at the time of tape removal, but it is usually not severe.

A technique described specifically for cats uses longitudinal "anchor" strips of adhesive tape applied medially and laterally on the leg, with the tape ends extending *proximal and distal* to the bandage or splint. The exposed ends of the tape anchor strips are reflected back on the bandage and then are covered with a second layer of bandaging material, which locks the anchor strips on the bandage (9).

Use of Padding

The padding layer of the bandage provides protection, absorbency, and minimal support to the limb, depending on the thickness of the padding layer. The use of padding before cast or splint application may ensure patient comfort, but when used inappropriately or in excess, it may actually decrease a device's ability to provide adequate immobilization. Excessive padding, hair, and soft tissue structures increase the distance between the rigid part of the coaptation device and the rigid part of the limb (bone), and this can decrease the stiffness and effectiveness of the cast or splint. Therefore, long hair should be clipped, but not shaved, before bandage placement, and adequate cast padding should be applied to provide comfort and to prevent skin irritation. Hohn has stated that properly applied cast padding actually enhances fracture fixation by compensating for slight tissue shrinkage after cast application (6).

One or two layers of orthopedic stockinette often are adequate; in some cases, incorporation of hair with the encircling plaster during the cast application may provide enough padding to prevent chafing and pressure sores as well as slippage. Removal of a plaster cast in which hair is securely incorporated can be difficult, however. Although some veterinarians apply small pieces of cotton between the toes before cast or splint application, an excess of padding can lead to additional vascular compromise.

Cast padding is applied, beginning at the toes, by overlapping half of the roll's width as it is unrolled; it should be wrapped snugly but not tightly (see Fig. 65.17**B**). Cast padding applied in this manner provides two layers of padding, which is normally adequate. Pressure points over humeral or femoral condyles, olecranon, tuber calcis, or carpal pad may be padded with an extra piece or two of padding, although Swaim and colleagues noted that applying full-length cast padding provided the best form of protection from dermal pressure injury (10).

Limb Positioning

During application of any coaptation—in particular plaster, fiberglass, and thermolabile plastic casts—for immobilization of a front or rear leg, the limb should be placed in a functional position while the material is still moldable. The rear leg should be kept in a normal position with the hock slightly flexed. When the casting material is conformed to the shape of the front leg, the carpus should be placed in slight flexion (15°) and deviated medially by 15° (Fig. 65.18). This positioning helps to prevent a valgus deformity, which otherwise could occur during manipulation because of the normal laxity of the radial carpal joint or as a result of eccentric growth of the radius and ulna in the immature patient. External rotation of the metacarpus should be avoided, and the foot should be kept in a neutral position (4, 11). The old adage expressed by

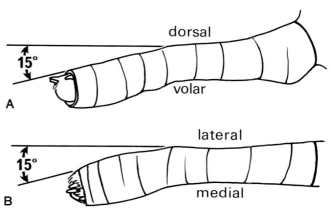

Fig. 65.18. Proper positioning of the front leg for application of a fully encircling cast. The carpus is flexed slightly and is deviated medially.

some experienced clinicians, "crooked leg in, straight leg out; straight leg in, crooked leg out," succinctly summarizes the preceding guidelines concerning proper limb position during cast application.

Coaptation Splints

Coaptation splints consisting of various rigid materials are used to approximate the shape of the limb to which they may be applied. In general, they should not be used for immobilization of the humerus or femur. Premade commercial splints consisting of plastic or aluminum are known as Mason metasplints or spoon splints. They are applied over padding on the caudal aspect of the limb. Because the limb is curved and the splint is straight, adequate padding is necessary to avoid soft tissue problems, but it may result in poor immobilization. Molded splints of plaster, water-activated fiberglass, or thermolabile plastic can be fitted to the limb almost perfectly. For this reason, they seem to be tolerated better by the patient and cause fewer soft tissue problems during long-term use than Mason metasplints.

Preformed Splints

INDICATIONS
Metasplints for the front or rear leg are primarily indicated for fractures of the distal radius and ulna, fracture–dislocations of the carpus or tarsus, and fractures of the metacarpal or metatarsal bones or phalanges. Stabilization of proximal radial or ulnar fractures usually is not adequate with these devices. Generally, the elbow joint cannot easily be immobilized without using a spica configuration over the shoulder.

APPLICATION TECHNIQUE
Adhesive tape stirrups are applied on the cranial and caudal aspects of the paw, with the cranial tape extending beyond the paw 2 to 3 inches farther than the caudal tape. The tape ends are then pressed together. A piece of precut cotton is applied to the back of the paw and antebrachium, or the leg is wrapped with at least two layers of cast padding, even if the splint is foam padded. The splint is snugly secured to the limb with elastic gauze by wrapping the leg with firm conforming pressure beginning at the toes and extending proximally up the limb. The stirrups are reflected up the caudal aspect of the splint and are secured with tape or another layer of elastic gauze (Fig. 65.19**A**). The "gauze-covered" splint is covered with adhesive tape, elastic tape (Elastikon, Johnson & Johnson, Medical, Inc.), or conforming elasticized tape (Vetwrap bandaging tape, Animal Care Products/3M, St. Paul, MN) (Fig. 65.19**B**). If the splint extends only to the elbow joint, a V-shaped section can be cut from the

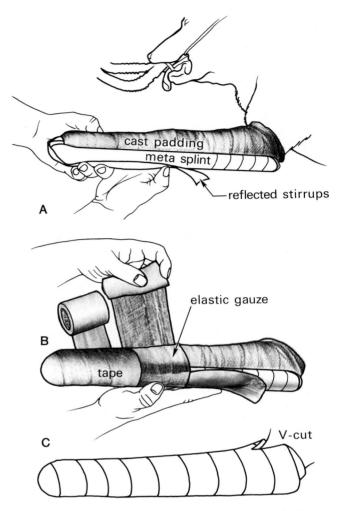

Fig. 65.19. Application of a foreleg Mason metasplint. **A.** Stirrups are reflected proximally and are secured to caudal aspect of metasplint. **B.** Metasplint is secured to the limb with overlapping layers of elastic gauze followed by application of adhesive or elastic tape. **C.** A V-shaped section is cut from the cranial aspect of bandage material at the elbow joint to prevent pressure necrosis.

cranial aspect of the bandage material just below the joint to prevent pressure necrosis in that area (Fig. 65.19**C**).

Some clinicians apply metasplints by an alternative method that does not involve use of tape stirrups. With this method, slippage of the splint is prevented by wrapping tape proximally around the elbow to prevent flexion (Fig. 65.20). The toes are left exposed, so circulation can be assessed.

Molded Lateral Splints

INDICATIONS
A molded splint applied laterally on either the forelimb or the rear leg can provide immobilization of the elbow joint or stifle, respectively. It can also stabilize less se-

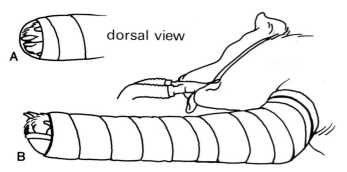

Fig. 65.20. **A** and **B.** Application of a foreleg Mason metasplint without the use of adhesive tape stirrups.

vere fractures of the radius, ulna, tibia, and fibula. This type of coaptation can be particularly helpful in providing protection from bending forces after internal fixation or joint stabilization. The casting material can be extended over the shoulder or hip as a modified spica to provide partial joint immobilization.

APPLICATION TECHNIQUE

Adhesive tape stirrups may not be necessary for application of this type of splint, especially if it extends proximally to include the shoulder or hip. The patient is placed in lateral recumbency with the injured limb positioned uppermost. The limb is padded with two layers of cast padding beginning at the toes and ending at the axilla or inguinal area.

If the shoulder or hip is to be immobilized through the use of a modified spica splint, the layers of padding should encircle the chest wall or pelvis, respectively. For splint application on the front leg, the padding creates a figure-of-eight pattern around the thorax and the affected limb, but the padding and the next layer of conforming gauze are carried behind the opposite axilla (Fig. 65.21**A**). For a hip spica, the cast padding and conforming gauze applied to the affected leg and the opposite limb create a figure-of-eight pattern and can incorporate the proximal half of the opposite leg. When this configuration is used, the resulting coaptation device is called a "one-and-a-half leg" spica (4). Care must be taken when applying a hip spica on a male dog so the prepuce is not included in the bandage. Spica splints are also restrictive, and some animals may not be able to stand without assistance.

Cast materials that can be molded to form a lateral splint are plaster, water-activated fiberglass, thermolabile plastic, or yucca board. Rolls of plaster, water-activated fiberglass materials, or thermolabile plastic can be cut to proper length or shape before application on the lateral aspect of the limb after activation. Elastic gauze is used to conform the softened splint material to the limb and to attach the splint to the shoulder

and chest wall or the hip and thigh area. The gauze-covered splint is then bandaged with elastic tape applied in a pattern similar to that of the gauze (Figs. 65.21**B** and 65.22).

Conformable materials used for molded lateral splints should be applied according to the manufacturer's directions and as each individual case dictates. A splint thickness of four to five layers of fiberglass or plaster casting material is usually adequate for the small animal patient. Prepackaged fiberglass splints are commercially available (Ortho-Glass Splinting System, Parker Medical Associates, Charlotte, NC) as well as unitized plaster splints (Specialist J-Splint plaster roll immobilizer, Johnson & Johnson Orthopaedics, Raynham, MA). These products consist of multiple layers (8

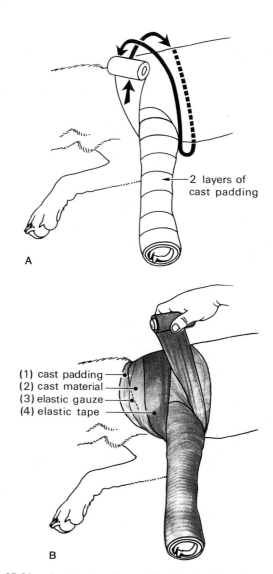

2 layers of cast padding

A

(1) cast padding
(2) cast material
(3) elastic gauze
(4) elastic tape

B

Fig. 65.21. Application of a molded foreleg lateral splint. **A.** Cast padding encircles the affected limb and thorax. **B.** Molded conformable material is secured to limb with elastic gauze and elastic tape.

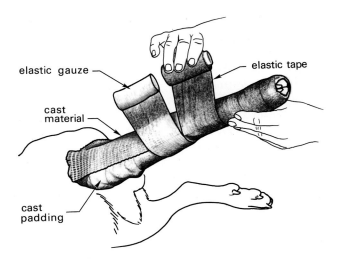

elastic gauze

elastic tape

cast
material

cast
padding

Fig. 65.22. Application of a molded lateral splint to the rear leg.

to 15) of casting tape enclosed in a stockinette, which is packaged in a roll and can be cut to any length. Sheets of fabric impregnated with a thermolabile plastic (Orthoplast Splint, Johnson & Johnson Orthopaedics) can be shaped according to a paper pattern of the affected limb and then softened in hot water (170°F) before application. Rolls of casting material composed of loosely knitted fabric impregnated with thermolabile plastic (Hexalite, Kirschner All Orthopedic Appliances, Marlow, OK) can be cut into splints as described earlier. The rigidity of this material requires that a five- to six-layer splint be used to immobilize a limb adequately. To provide as much strength as possible, splint width of each coaptation material should be approximately one-third to one-half the outside circumference of the affected limb. In other words, the splint configuration is similar to a full-encircling cast cut in half in a cranial-to-caudal direction, with the lateral half of the cast used as the coaptation device.

Schroeder–Thomas Splints

Probably the most misused and misunderstood coaptation device today is the Schroeder–Thomas splint. When correctly applied, this splint can be an excellent means for immobilizing joints postoperatively surgery and for immobilizing certain fractures. This *traction device* can provide accurate and continued fixation of bone fragments by counteracting muscle forces and immobilizing parts of the skeleton. Under certain circumstances, skeletal traction can be provided when transfixation pins located in the areas of the femoral or humeral condyles are incorporated into the splint so traction from the splint on the distal end of the affected limb controls the distal fracture fragment.

Indications and Possible Complications

The use of Schroeder–Thomas splints may be indicated for some fractures of the radius, ulna, and tibia; avulsion fractures of the tibial tuberosity and distal malleolar fractures are exceptions. These splints have been used for fractures of the distal humerus (distal one-third), although not for condylar fractures, which require precise reduction of the joint surface to avoid degenerative joint disease. Nonarticular fractures of the distal femur (distal one-third) are considered by some clinicians to be amenable to reduction and immobilization with a Schroeder–Thomas splint, although supracondylar or condylar fractures must receive superb postreduction care because immobilization can be difficult to maintain. The splint has been used for temporary immobilization of the stifle and elbow joints postsurgically.

Although a Schroeder–Thomas splint can be used successfully for more orthopedic conditions than are mentioned here, its inappropriate use can have disastrous consequences.

Application to a fracture of the proximal humerus or femur is definitely contraindicated because the ring of the splint must support and rest on the proximal fracture fragment. If the splint is used for proximal femoral and humeral fractures, the ring rests in the fracture site and acts as a fulcrum point, whereas the limb serves as the lever resulting in movement at the fracture site. In these circumstances, fracture disease (nonunion, quadriceps tiedown, joint stiffness) results. The splint often loosens with time because of the dynamic nature of its application. Circulatory problems causing tissue necrosis can develop as a result of loosening, swelling of the limb, or improper application. Pressure necrosis under the ring of the splint, edema of the scrotum, severe limb edema, and strangulation of the foot can occur.

Application Technique

Schroeder–Thomas splints should be custom-made for every individual case. Obviously, splint rods can be reused if they are the appropriate length for an individual patient. Because this type of splint is a dynamic traction device, it requires careful attention by the owner and periodic adjustment by the clinician. A Schroeder–Thomas splint is constructed of aluminum rods ($\frac{1}{8}$-, $\frac{3}{16}$-, or $\frac{3}{8}$-inch diameter) available in 6-foot lengths or 12-foot coils. For small dogs or cats, regular coat-hanger wire has been used. An average-size dog (30 to 40 lb) requires the $\frac{3}{8}$-inch diameter aluminum rod. Commercially available plastic or wooden ''ring'' blocks usually are used to form the elliptic ring at the

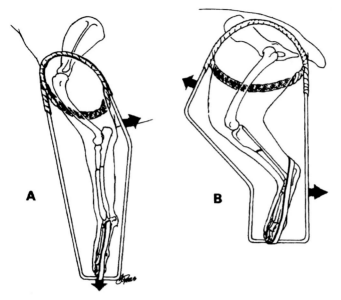

Fig. 65.23. Configurations of a foreleg and hind leg Schroeder–Thomas splint and traction application for radioulnar fractures (**A**) and tibial fractures (**B**). (From Tobias TA. Slings, padded bandages, splinted bandages, and casts. In: Olmstead ML, ed. Small animal orthopedics. St. Louis: CV Mosby, 1995:108.

proximal end of the splint. Adhesive tape and combine roll or elastic gauze are used for application of the stirrups and the traction slings, respectively. A vise is helpful in shaping the rod, and bolt cutters or a hacksaw are necessary for cutting the rod. The shape of the splint is modified in relation to the specific leg injured, the bone that is fractured, or the joint that is involved. Traction application also varies according to the fracture, so the fragments can be separated and aligned (Figs. 65.23).

The first step in construction of a Schroeder–Thomas splint is the formation of the upper ring at the proximal end of the splint. For the rear leg, the diameter of the ring is determined by measuring the distance between the cranial aspect of the wing of the ilium and the caudal point of the ischium; for the foreleg, the ring diameter can be determined by measuring the length of the scapular spine (4). The bottom of the ring should be flattened to conform to the animal's axillary area or thigh. The bottom of the ring must bend medial to the vertical bars at a 45° angle at the middle of the ring. The ring can be bent, or the vertical bars can be bent to accommodate this angle. The lower half of the ring should be padded; however, excessive padding may cause irritation and circulatory problems and should be avoided. Applying tape to the ring with the adhesive side facing outward and then wrapping the lower half of the ring with thin strips of cotton or cast padding work well. The tape with the adhesive

side inward is applied over the cotton loosely so the padding is soft and conforms to the inguinal or axillary region.

The vertical bars of the splint are sometimes left straight to accommodate certain fractures. However, each case should be considered on an individual basis and the splint configuration varied accordingly. For the rear leg, the front bar is bent to conform to the normal angulation of the stifle and hock; the rear bar is left straight. The angles of the front bar are varied according to the injury (see Fig. 65.23). For the forelimb, both bars are bent to conform to the angulation of the elbow. Although various configurations for humeral and radioulnar fractures have been described (4, 8, 12), the configuration illustrated in Figure 65.23**A** has been used successfully and seems to be well tolerated by most animals.

The vertical bars are bent and connected with adhesive tape at the bottom of the splint. The length of the splint is determined by gently extending the limb so the end of the splint coincides with the end of the toes. The limb should not be stretched taut in a Schroeder–Thomas splint. The middle of the horizontal bar formed by connecting the vertical bars can be bent into an inverse-V shape so the adhesive tape stirrups fastened there will not be worn away by walking. A separate piece of aluminum rod can also be added to the bottom of the splint to protect the tape. The width of the distal end of the splint should be approximately three times the width of the paw. The finished splint should be completely wrapped as smoothly as possible with adhesive tape for cosmetic purposes. More important, this procedure prevents slippage of traction slings. The completed splint is applied to the leg carefully, with the ring snugly placed in the axillary or inguinal area. The splint is secured initially to the distal end of the foot by means of an adhesive tape stirrup. For additional support, a spiral of tape ("barber pole") can be applied over the foot to help secure the vertical stirrups. Wrapping tape circumferentially around the foot usually causes swelling and should be avoided. Cotton can be used to pad between the toes. The adhesive tape stirrups should not be used to apply traction.

Traction is applied by means of the combine roll or wide elastic gauze used to secure the leg to the vertical bars of the splint. Both products, but especially the elastic gauze, must be used with caution, because the application of excessive tension can cause necrosis or edema. Positioning of the traction slings depends on the nature of the fracture. For fractures of the tibia, the traction slings are placed around the hock joint first and then in the femoral area to provide traction on the tibia (see Fig. 65.23**B**). For distal femoral fractures, the first traction sling is applied around the hock joint, and then one is applied around the proximal tibia to provide traction on the femur. Traction slings should be applied in such a manner that they provide adequate medial support to both the tibia and femur and avoid a valgus deformity of the limb (4). For fractures of the front leg, a traction sling is first applied at the level of the elbow, pulling the humerus caudally. The second sling is applied at the level of the carpus, pulling it cranially, which increases the traction on the radius, ulna, or humerus. As Figure 65.23**A** illustrates, tension can be applied caudally on the radius and ulna; a support sling placed in the area of the distal humerus maintains even pressure on the limb and reduces motion.

The entire Schroeder–Thomas splint can be covered with orthopedic stockinette to protect the device.

Postapplication Care

Excellent client and professional care is essential in maintaining a Schroeder–Thomas splint after application. The limb must be kept dry and clean, and the animal must be confined. Scheduled rechecks should be performed on a weekly basis, and clients must be diligent in evaluating the device for loosening, irritation, or swelling of the limb. If mild edema does occur, the animal must be monitored carefully for the next 24 to 48 hours; the splint may have to be adjusted or removed if this swelling persists or becomes more severe. Clients must be informed that reevaluation of the device whenever one suspects a problem is essential for proper splint management.

Tape Hobbles

Tape hobbles have been advocated as a method of protecting an injured limb and preventing additional trauma. This device can limit rotational stress on the limb and can aid in preventing stresses to proximal humeral or femoral fractures. It can also prevent excessive adduction or abduction of limbs with scapular or pelvic fractures. Hobbles must be used with caution when any possibility of vascular impairment or swelling in the areas of the metatarsus or metacarpus exists.

The first step in application of tape hobbles is wrapping of two or three layers of cast padding around the metatarsal or metacarpal areas. Adhesive tape, 1 or 2 inches in width (depending on the size of the dog), is carefully wrapped around the paw to form a sling. One must not wrap the tape tightly around the paws. Overlapping the tape ends unevenly to form a "tab" from each foot should be the desired goal. The two tape tabs are joined with additional stirrups of tape. Usually, the distance between the feet is about that of a normal standing position for that animal, which should allow for proper freedom of movement (Fig. 65.24).

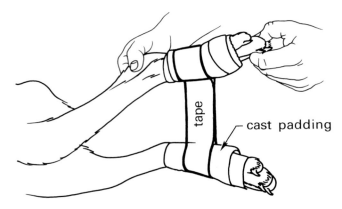

Fig. 65.24. Application of hind leg tape hobbles.

Animals should be confined after application of tape hobbles, and clients must be informed to evaluate the limbs for swelling at least twice a day. Hobbles can be left in place for prolonged periods if indicated and if adequate professional and client care is provided.

Velpeau Sling

The Velpeau sling is used for immobilization of the shoulder joint postsurgically, for stabilization of the shoulder joint after closed reduction of luxations, for immobilization of scapular fractures, and for other conditions that require a front leg to be non-weightbearing. A Velpeau sling should not be used on animals with oblique fractures of the distal humerus because compression by the sling may result in overriding of the fractured fragments and damage to the radial nerve. Olecranon fractures are also not amenable to this type of sling. A Velpeau sling is made of elastic gauze (2, 3, or 4 inches wide, depending on the size of the animal) or combine roll. It is started by loosely wrapping the conforming material around the paw in a lateral-to-medial direction. The wrap is continued laterally over the affected limb and shoulder and is placed around the thorax and behind the opposite axilla (Fig. 65.25**A**). With the elbow, carpus, and shoulder joints flexed, the wrap is continued to the starting point. Several more layers of conforming material are applied in a similar pattern, but these layers enclose the elbow and paw (Fig. 65.25**B**). Covering the entire limb prevents the lower limb or elbow from being forced out of the bandage if the animal tries to extend or flex the leg. The entire bandage is then covered with elastic tape in a similar manner.

The clinician must make the client aware that if the sling loosens and slips, besides the loss of immobilization, disastrous vascular impairment can occur. The animal should be strictly confined for the duration of the bandage's application. Animals usually tolerate the sling well, but it should be checked on a weekly basis. If it is used more than 2 weeks for immobilization,

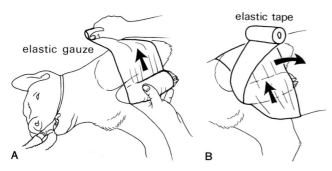

Fig. 65.25. Application of a Velpeau shoulder sling. **A.** Elastic gauze is wrapped around the paw and is continued laterally over affected limb with flexed elbow, carpus, and paw. **B.** Several additional layers of elastic gauze are applied and enclose the elbow and paw; the sling is then covered in a similar manner with elastic tape.

joint contracture can occur because the shoulder, elbow, and carpal joints are held in severe flexion.

Postapplication Management of Splints, Casts, and Slings

After application of any splint, cast, or sling, the limb should be observed every 4 to 6 hours to be certain that the device has been applied correctly. If it is constricting vasculature or lymphatic drainage and causing the proximal or distal aspects of the limb to swell, the device should be removed immediately and reapplied. At the time of discharge, clients must be educated in the proper care of the coaptation device. The splint or cast should be kept dry at all times. Cornstarch or talcum powder can be used to prevent chafing and pressure sores where the device irritates the axillary or inguinal areas.

Clients must feel free to seek professional advice concerning the coaptation device. If any of the following problems should develop, the animal must be examined as soon as possible (4):

1. Any sign of excessive discomfort
2. Any changes in position or shape of the splint or cast on the leg
3. Any unusual foul odors coming from the splint or cast
4. Any unexplained soiling of the splint or cast that was not present previously
5. Any sores that develop at the top of the splint or cast that do not respond to talcum powder or cornstarch application
6. Swelling of the toes or the leg above the coaptation device
7. Inappetence, depression, or fever in the animal
8. Any excessive chewing of the splint or cast

No splint or cast can be worn in complete comfort by an animal. Minor licking and chewing can be expected; however, when an animal continues to muti-

late the device, the device should be rechecked. If it has been properly applied and the animal continues to chew the splint or cast excessively, properly applied chemical or mechanical restraint devices may be needed separately or in combination (13).

References

1. Tomlinson J. Complications of fractures repaired with casts and splints. Vet Clin North Am 1991;21:735–744.
2. Leighton RL. Principles of conservative fracture management: splints and casts. Semin Vet Med Surg 1991;6:39–51.
3. Manziaro CF, Manziaro JR. Walking plaster cast for repair of tibial fractures in dogs. J Am Vet Med Assoc 1970;156:581.
4. Nunamaker DM. Methods of closed fixation. In: Newton CD, Nunamaker DM, eds. Textbook of small animal orthopedics. Philadelphia: JB Lippincott, 1985.
5. DeCamp CE. External coaptation. In: Slatter D, ed. Textbook of small animal surgery. 2nd ed. Philadelphia: WB Saunders, 1993.
6. Hohn RB. Principles and application of plaster casts. Vet Clin North Am 1975;5:291–303.
7. Leighton RL. Complications from mismanagement of fixation devices. Vet Clin North Am 1975;5:273.
8. Knecht CD, Allen AR, Williams DJ, et al. Casts and splints for small animals. In: Fundamental techniques in veterinary surgery. 2nd ed. Philadelphia: WB Saunders, 1981.
9. Robinson GW, McCoy L, Gili M. Feline bandaging and splinting. Feline Pract 1977;7:41.
10. Swaim SF, Vaughn DM, Spalding PJ, et al. Evaluation of the dermal effects of cast padding in coaptation casts on dogs. Am J Vet Res 1992;53:1266–1272.
11. Tobias TA. Slings, padded bandages, splinted bandages, and casts. In: Olmstead ML, ed. Small animal orthopedics. St. Louis: CV Mosby, 1995.
12. Knecht CD. Principles and applications of traction and coaptation splints. Vet Clin North Am 1975;5:177.
13. Seim HB, Creed JE, Smith KW. Restraint techniques for prevention of self-trauma. In: Bojrab MJ, ed. Current techniques in small animal surgery. 2nd ed. Philadelphia: Lea & Febiger, 1983.

Suggested Readings

Arnoszky SP, Blass CE, McCoy L. External coaptation and bandaging. In: Slatter DH, ed. Textbook of small animal surgery. Philadelphia: WB Saunders, 1985.
Brinker WO, Piermattei DL, Flo GL, eds. Principles of joint surgery. In: Handbook of small animal orthopedics and fracture treatment. Philadelphia: WB Saunders, 1983.
Leighton RL. Principles of conservative fracture management: splints and casts. Semin Vet Med Surg 1991;6:39–51.
Tobias TA. Slings, padded bandages, splinted bandages, and casts. In: Olmstead ML, ed. Small animal orthopedics. St. Louis: CV Mosby, 1995.

Principles and Application of Synthetic and Plaster Casts in Small Animals

Douglas N. Lange & Kenneth E. Bartels

The purpose of a cast is to provide rigid external coaptation to a reduced fracture or tenuous ligament repair so proper alignment and support are maintained during healing. Since 1851, the traditional plaster of Paris cast has been used when rigid external coaptation is required. Plaster casts provide an inexpensive means of providing molded external support, but they have the disadvantages of prolonged drying time, relative heaviness, decreased porosity, deterioration if exposed to moisture, and brittleness (1). Synthetic casting materials have been developed and are available to veterinarians. The newer synthetic materials include polyurethane resin–impregnated fiberglass or polyester–cotton knit, and thermolabile plastic. These materials have the advantages of being lightweight, less bulky, immersible, radiolucent, and quickly "set," but they are more expensive and can be difficult to mold. Although newer methods of internal fixation (bone plates and screws) are indicated for most complicated orthopedic problems, closed reduction and external coaptation can be the treatment of choice for selected fractures and ligamentous injuries. Long leg casts are most appropriate for fractures below the elbow and stifle that only require bending and rotational stability, such as incomplete or transverse fractures. The joint should be immobilized above and below the fracture in most cases, although functional below-the-knee casts have been used successfully (2). Fractures of the humerus and femur require a cast in a "spica" configuration that immobilizes the shoulder or hip, respectively.

Plaster Casting Material

Characteristics

Plaster of Paris can be shaped and molded with ease and should usually be chosen for immobilizing severely displaced or unstable fractures that require a closer fit when coaptation is indicated. Because plaster is less expensive than the newer synthetic materials, it is indicated if frequent changes of casts are required. It is suitable for an initial or primary cast after fracture reduction when mild edema or swelling of a limb can be expected, because a change of cast is usually necessary after the edema subsides *or* becomes more severe (3). Synthetic casts should be used with small patients requiring a lighter cast, with patients likely to abuse or moisten the cast, or when a plaster cast is likely to fail within the required time of immobilization.

Plaster of Paris is made of calcium sulfate crystals that have been reduced to powder and subjected to intense heat to expel the water. The resulting chalky white powder is then incorporated into gauze bandages. When water is added to the plaster, a crystallization process occurs, and the material hardens in an exothermic reaction. The time from which water is added to the plaster bandage until the material becomes hard is called its *setting time*. Plaster sets in 3 to 8 minutes, depending on whether it is fast or extrafast setting, the temperature of the water used, and the amount of water left in a roll after immersion. As the cast dries, the interlocking of the calcium sulfate crystals gives the plaster its strength. Further molding after a plaster cast has begun to set can prevent this interlocking of the crystals and may weaken the cast.

After the cast sets, the excess water must evaporate from the surface before the cast attains maximal strength. This period (*curing time*) while the cast is still "green" varies from 8 to 48 hours, depending on how large and thick a cast is, the type of plaster used, humidity, and air temperature. Excessive weightbearing during drying of the cast should be avoided. A plaster cast is heavy at first, but it becomes lighter as the water in the plaster evaporates. The strength of a plaster cast is proportional to its thickness, but the smallest possible amount of plaster should be used. Placement of plaster "splints" or reinforcing strips of cast material along one surface strengthens a cast without increasing its entire mass; this technique is especially useful over areas where angulation occurs and the cast is susceptible to stress and fracture.

Application Technique

No special equipment is required for preparation and application of a plaster cast, and a standard cast cutter can be used for removal. Gloves should be worn during application, because plaster can be irritating to the hands. The patient and casting area in the hospital should be protected from dripping plaster by the liberal use of newspaper or a plastic drop cloth.

Preparation of plaster bandages involves immersing them in tepid water (70 to 75°F) for a few seconds until the bubbling from the roll has stopped; the plaster rolls then are squeezed to remove excess water. A plaster bandage should be unrolled on the leg, as it is applied, in an encircling manner with overlapping of half of the roll's width; it should never be stretched or tightened around the limb. It should be applied in a smooth, conforming manner so no thick or thin spots result. Tucks can be made in the rolls to change directions or to contour the plaster smoothly. Molding the cast by rubbing each section with wet hands before the plaster is set is essential for proper lamination, to produce a smooth surface, and for conforming the material to the proper configuration of the affected limb. During application, the cast should be supported by the palms of the hands and not indented with the fingers, because the "dimples" that result could produce pressure points on the interior, which can lead to skin excoriation.

Once the cast is dry, any rough edges should be covered with adhesive tape. The cast should not be washed, although a damp cloth can be used to remove excessive dirt if the residual moisture is wiped away afterward. Immersion of the plaster cast can cause deterioration of the plaster, resulting in skin irritation and maceration.

Some manufacturers (Duracast, Duraflex, Carapace, Caraflex, Cellona, Carapace, Inc.. Tulsa, OK; Gypsona, IMEX Veterinary, Inc., Longview, TX) supply plaster casting material in various widths (2, 3, 4, and 6 inches) and setting times (slow, medium, fast, and extrafast). For small animals, the 2- and 4-inch widths are the most versatile; fast or extrafast setting times are more appropriate for veterinary patients. Various setting times can be achieved by adjusting the temperature of the water in which the plaster bandages are immersed before application. Use of colder water increases setting times, and use of warmer water decreases it. Because plaster of Paris products are significantly less expensive than the newer synthetic materials, they will continue to be an essential moldable coaptation material.

Synthetic Casting Materials

Characteristics

Several newer synthetic cast materials are available as alternatives to plaster of Paris. These newer materials are recommended for use as primary casts for nondisplaced fractures with minimal swelling or for long-term wear when multiple cast changes are not required (1, 3–7). They can be divided into three classifications according to their composition: polyester–cotton knit, fiberglass, and thermolabile plastic. Manufacturers are introducing new materials every year, and each product obviously is recommended over a competitor's for many different reasons. Clinicians should be aware of the advantages and disadvantages of several of the materials and should choose the one with the characteristics they regard as the most important.

Polyester–cotton casting material consist of a polyester and cotton, knitted, open-weave fabric impregnated with a water-activated polyurethane resin (Delta-Lite Fabric Casting Tape, Johnson & Johnson Orthopaedics, Inc., Raynham, MA). After immersion in cool tap water, this material is applied as casts or protective bandages. Casts formed from these products are lightweight, immersible, porous (permeable to water vapor), and fairly strong. Their biggest advantage is that they are virtually radiolucent (4).

Fiberglass casting tapes consist of a knitted fiberglass fabric impregnated with a polyurethane resin that is activated by water (Delta-Lite Conformable Casting Tape and Delta-Lite "S" Fiberglass Casting Tape, Johnson & Johnson Orthopaedics, Inc.; Synthocast, Kirschner All Orthopedic Appliances, Marlow, OK; Scotchcast II, Orthopedic Products, Surgical Products Division/3M, St. Paul, MN; and Vet Cast and Vet Cast II, Animal Care Products/3M) The water-activated fiberglass casting tapes have met with success in veterinary medicine despite their expense. Differences among the products involve mainly their "handling" ability during application and the final "finish" or smoothness of the cast after it has set. Both these characteristics are primarily influenced by the knitted weave of a product; closely knitted materials generally are more conformable and easier to apply. Casts made from the fiberglass products are strong, lightweight, radiolucent, permeable to water vapor, and immersible in water.

The third type of synthetic casting material is an open-weave cotton fabric coated with high-density thermoplastic resin (Hexcelite, Kirschner All Orthopedic Appliances). A roll is immersed in hot water (65.5°C) for approximately 30 seconds until soft, it is drained of water, and it is applied when comfortable to the touch. The material begins to harden in approximately 3 minutes and achieves rigidity in 10 minutes. Specific areas can be remolded by application of heat with a 1000-watt portable hair dryer until the material is pliable. Thermolabile casting material is permeable to water vapor because of its open weave and does not exhibit an exothermic reaction while curing; it has a rough finish after application.

Bartels and associates evaluated some synthetic casting materials for their tensile strength, fatigue strength, exothermicity (evolution of heat during polymerization), permeability, radiolucency, and cost (4). Although statistically significant differences were found for some of the criteria, no one material was best in all categories tested. Other "clinical" studies have revealed similar results (8, 9). They confirm that no one material is best in all areas because the newer synthetic casting materials, although easier to handle, are not as strong as the previous, tackier synthetic cast materials.

Packages of water-activated casting tape should be opened one at a time and used within 2 to 3 minutes because exposure to humidity in the air hardens the tape. Because unused packages can deteriorate on the shelf, sealed, unused rolls should be stored in a refrigerator to retard premature hardening. Most manufacturers date their products and recommend that the rolls of dated cast material be used within 6 months.

Application Technique

Water-activated synthetic casting products should be immersed in cool water (21 to 27°C), because warmer water temperatures greatly decrease setting time, and the heat produced during polymerization can be uncomfortable to the patient during cast application. Immersion in water can vary from 5 to 15 seconds, and the cast rolls should be drained of excess water. Gloves should be worn when handling any of the water-activated materials to protect the hands from any residue, which is difficult to remove. Four to five layers of material should be used, according to manufacturer's recommendations for weightbearing casts in small animals (4).

Techniques for applying synthetic casting materials differ from those usually recommended for plaster casting material. To change directions during application, tucks are made in plaster and thermolabile materials while fiberglass material is twisted. Synthetic materials are molded only in a horizontal motion to ensure lamination. Maximum bonding of the cast layers can be achieved by firmly blotting the exterior of the cast with the open palms in a rolling motion. Molding is achieved by maintaining a desired position for about 1 minute during the last few minutes of the setting period, which varies from 2 to 6 minutes, depending on the temperature of the water for activation. One manufacturer (Vet Cast, Vet Cast II, Animal Care Products/3M) supplies a hand cream to facilitate smoothing and molding of the cast, but water-soluble lubricating jelly (K-Y Lubricating Jelly, Johnson & Johnson Products, Inc., New Brunswick, NJ) can also be used for this purpose. Another manufacturer includes casting gloves that give the polyurethane resin–impregnated fiberglass substrate tack-free working properties (Johnson & Johnson Orthopaedics, Inc.).

Synthetic casts are lighter than their plaster counterparts and, when applied using polypropylene stockinette and polyester padding, they can be immersed in water. Synthetic casts are easier to keep clean because they can be washed with mild soaps, and hydrotherapy for postoperative orthopedic rehabilitation is possible with them. If inadequate drying of the cast occurs and the skin remains wet, irritation and possible skin maceration can occur. Hair dryers can be used to dry wet fiberglass casts.

Long Leg Cylinder Cast

Application Technique

If external coaptation is chosen for fracture repair, the fracture must be reduced before cast placement. Manipulation of the cast after placement causes creases and pressure points in the cast. General anesthesia facilitates fracture alignment and prevents the animal from disrupting reduction while the cast becomes rigid. At least 50% of the fracture ends should be in contact with each other to expect fracture healing, although perfect reduction is the goal for every fracture (1). In addition, the limb should be reduced in a

normal walking position to facilitate early usage of the casted limb and normal limb function after cast removal. The leg should be clipped and aseptically prepared as for surgery in case a closed fracture becomes an open fracture during manipulation. The animal should be placed in lateral recumbency with the affected limb down; this positioning helps to prevent a valgus deformity at the fracture site during cast application (2). The following description of application of a long leg cylinder cast to the front leg emphasizes points that can be recommended when using either plaster or synthetic casting materials:

Adhesive tape stirrups are applied to the cranial and caudal surfaces of the foot with the ends of the tape fixed to a tongue-depressor blade to facilitate separation later. The leg is elevated, and the stirrups can be fastened to an intravenous stand or held in an elevated position by an assistant. One or two layers of orthopedic stockinette are rolled up over the entire limb with no wrinkles and are snugly held by an assistant at the proximal end (Fig. 65.26). The stockinette should be long enough to extend distally beyond the toes and into the axillary or inguinal region proximally. Synthetic cast padding that repels moisture is wound around the leg from distal to proximal as snugly as possible. Wrapping the padding from cranial to caudal around the medial aspect of the limb helps to prevent supination when wrapping the forelimb (10). Two layers are usually adequate, although extra padding may be needed at the proximal and distal aspects of the cast. Uniform full-length padding provides the best protection against dermal injury (11). The cast material is rolled around the leg beginning at the distal

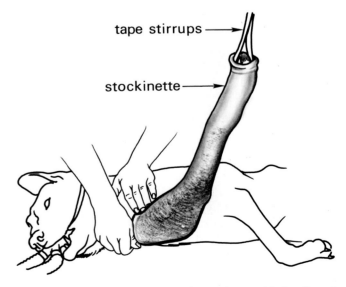

Fig. 65.26. Animal placed in lateral recumbency with the affected limb down. Adhesive tape stirrups are applied to cranial and caudal surfaces of the foot; an orthopedic stockinette is rolled over the entire limb.

end and overlapped by half the width of the roll. The material should be applied smoothly using even conforming pressure; smooth application is facilitated by rolling continuously around the limb in a spiral fashion and not raising the roll away from the skin (5). Regardless of the casting material used, a cast should be supported with the palms of the hands and not the fingertips because indentations from the fingers may result in pressure sores. If applied properly, four layers of material are usually adequate for the average-size dog. The pads and toenails of the two central toes may be left exposed if there is no weightbearing on the foot. If the animal is weightbearing on the limb, an aluminum rod walking bar can be applied to the end of the cast to prevent excoriation of toes and excessive wear to the cast (1, 2). Longitudinal splints of cast material can be applied medially and laterally or cranially and caudally to strengthen the cast before the final layer of casting material is applied (Fig. 65.27).

After application of the cast and while the material is still moldable, the leg must be positioned properly as described. The stockinette and padding at the ends of the cast and the tape stirrups are reflected over the ends of the cast. These are secured to the proximal and distal aspects of the cast with circular wraps of tape (Fig. 65.28).

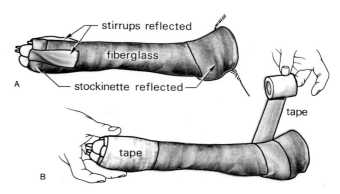

Fig. 65.28. Final steps in cast application. **A.** Tape stirrups and stockinette are reflected back over the completed cast. **B.** Reflected stirrups and stockinette are taped to the distal and proximal aspects of the cast.

Postapplication Care

For plaster casts, the animal should be hospitalized for at least 24 hours after application to allow for adequate drying. Synthetic materials such as fiberglass can bear weight in as little as 20 minutes, but the animal should be observed closely for at least 12 to 24 hours to be certain that cast application has been correct and is being tolerated well. While the animal is in the hospital, the cast can be covered with a piece of stockinette to prevent soiling before discharge. Care of a cast is similar to care provided for any splint. The cast should be kept dry and as clean as possible. Routine rechecks should be scheduled, and particular care should be taken to educate the owner on cast management. At removal, the cast should be split longitudinally using a cast saw with short bites made perpendicular to the long axis of the cast, rather than sliding the cast saw down the length of the cast. Cutting a cast in this manner helps to reduce chances of damaging the underlying structures. Cuts should be made on either side of the limb, and the two "half-casts" should be removed carefully. Cast spreaders widen the groove made by the cast saw to facilitate cutting the deeper bandage layers with scissors. Windowing of casts should be avoided because of the danger of edematous tissue herniating through the window (1, 12). If the cast loosens, it should be removed and replaced, because immobilization is lost and pressure necrosis occurs as the cast slips and moves.

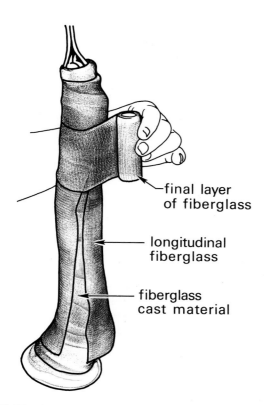

Fig. 65.27. Longitudinal splints of cast material are applied cranially and caudally to strengthen the cast before rolling final layer of material. Layers of cast material are applied as shown.

final layer
of fiberglass

longitudinal
fiberglass

fiberglass
cast material

References

1. DeCamp CE. External coaptation. In: Slatter D, ed. Textbook of small animal surgery. 2nd ed. Philadelphia: WB Saunders, 1993.
2. Nunamaker DM. Methods of closed fixation. In: Newton CD, Nunamaker DM, eds. Textbook of small animal orthopedics. Philadelphia: JB Lippincott, 1985.

3. Marshall PD, Dibble AK, Walters TH, et al. When should a synthetic casting material be used in preference to plaster of Paris? A cost analysis and guidance for casting departments. Injury 1991;23:542–544.
4. Bartels KE, Penwick RC, Freeman LJ, et al. Mechanical testing and evaluation of eight synthetic casting materials. Vet Surg 1985;14:310.
5. Brinker WO, Piermattei DL, Flo GL, eds. Principles of joint surgery. In: Handbook of small animal orthopedics and fracture treatment. Philadelphia: WB Saunders, 1983.
6. Vet Cast Veterinary Casting Tape: Comparative study of commonly used cast materials. St. Paul, MN: Animal Care Products/3M, 1984.
7. Lane PL, Lee MM. New synthetic casts: what nurses need to know. Orthop Nurs 1982;1:13.
8. Bowker P, Powell ES. A clinical evaluation of plaster of Paris and eight synthetic fracture splinting materials. Injury 1992;23:13–20.
9. Wilson DG, Vanderby R. An evaluation of six synthetic casting materials: strength of cylinders in bending. Vet Surg 1995;24:55–59.
10. Tobias TA. Slings, padded bandages, splinted bandages, and casts. In: Olmstead ML, ed. Small animal orthopedics. St. Louis: CV Mosby, 1995.
11. Swaim SF, Vaughn DM, Spalding PJ, et al. Evaluation of the dermal effects of cast padding in coaptation casts on dogs. Am J Vet Res 1992;53:1266–1272.
12. Hohn RB. Principles and application of plaster casts. Vet Clin North Am 1975;5:291.

Suggested Readings

DeCamp CE. External coaptation. In: Slatter D, ed. Textbook of small animal surgery. 2nd ed. Philadelphia: WB Saunders, 1993.
Leighton RL. Principles of conservative fracture management: splints and casts. Semin Vet Med Surg 1991;6:39–51.
Tobias TA. Slings, padded bandages, splinted bandages, and casts. In: Olmstead ML, ed. Small animal orthopedics. St. Louis: CV Mosby, 1995.

Bandages for Sciatic Nerve Deficit

Barclay Slocum & Theresa Devine Slocum

A sciatic nerve deficit can occur as the result of spinal disease, trauma to the skeleton or peripheral nerve, or iatrogenic trauma. The most subtle form of sciatic nerve deficit that represents reduced sensation is dragging of the toenails of the hind limb. This amount of sciatic loss can be expected to recover spontaneously; protection of the foot is usually not necessary.

The next level of sciatic nerve deficit is loss of sensation plus diminished or loss of conscious proprioception. This is manifested as knuckling or standing on the dorsum of the toes of the hind foot. Sensory input to the spinal cord from the lateral three digits is supplied by the sciatic nerve, whereas the medial digit is supplied by the femoral nerve. The skin of the foot may become abraded by the repeated walking on the top of the foot, but a bandage covering the foot alone does not prevent trauma to the dorsum of the foot. Repeated contusion of the end of the metatarsal bones and overlying soft tissues causes trauma ranging from bruising to sloughing of the skin. The sciatic toe bandage prevents flexion of the phalangeal metatarsal joints and causes the patient to weight bear on the foot pads.

The third level of sciatic nerve deficit is the temporary loss of sensation, proprioception, and motor function manifested by a knuckling or standing on the dorsum of the toes of the hind foot and a characteristic "drop foot" gait. In the "drop foot" gait, the foot liftoff is initiated by flexion of the stifle. During the cranial footflight, the hock is not flexed by the cranial tibial musculature, and relative extension of the hock is noted. Flexion of the hip is greater than normal. The stifle seems to lead the advancement of the hind limb. Just before footstrike, the quadriceps is contracted to cause extension of the stifle and to advance the tibia. The rapid extension of the stifle, followed by immediate extension of the hip, causes the foot to flip forward just before contacting the ground with a characteristic "goose step." Hock and toe flexion can be maintained by recovery phase of gait by a modified sciatic hock bandage (1).

The fourth level of sciatic nerve deficit is the permanent loss of sensation, proprioception, and motor function manifested as knuckling or standing on the dorsum of the toes of the hind foot, and a characteristic "drop foot" gait without any flexion of the hock or toes. The permanent loss of both sciatic sensory and motor function necessitates the transfer of skin with sensation from the femoral distribution on the second digit to the dorsum of the paw, and the transfer of the vastus lateralis with motor function to the origin of the long digital extensor tendon at the stifle.

Sciatic Toe Bandage

The purpose of the sciatic toe bandage (Fig. 65.29) is to maintain dorsiflexion of the toes during ambulation. Because a simple foot wrap does not cause the foot to be placed on the plantar surface, trauma is caused to the dorsal foot during knuckling. Nonadherent ointment–soaked gauze is placed over the traumatized tissue on the dorsal paw. A large cotton ball 3 to 6 cm in diameter is placed over the dorsum of the metatarsal phalangeal joints. Cotton adhesive tape is wrapped in a figure-of-eight pattern around the plantar aspect of the distal metatarsus, dorsal to the ball of cotton and plantar to the toe pads of the third and fourth digits. The remaining paw can be included to stabilize the bandage.

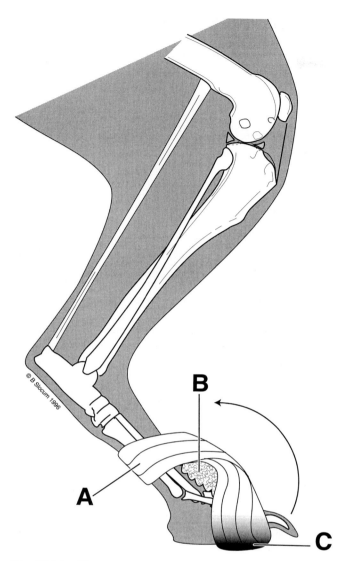

Fig. 65.29. The sciatic toe bandage is a figure-of-eight configuration that starts at the distal metatarsus (*A*) and crosses dorsally a large mass of cotton (*B*) and dorsiflexes (*arrow*) the third and fourth digits (*C*). The remainder of the foot is enclosed in the bandage to prevent slippage.

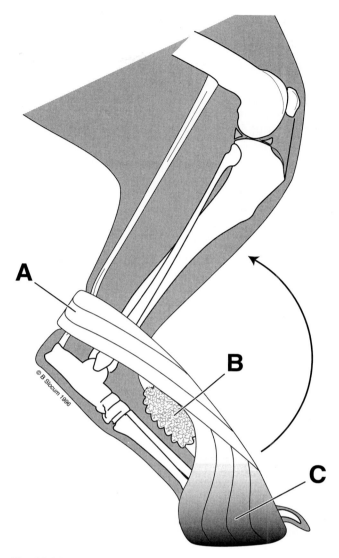

Fig. 65.30. The sciatic hock bandage is a figure-of-eight configuration that starts at the distal crus (*A*) and passes over a large piece of cotton (*B*) to elevate the third and fourth digits (*C*) and flex the hock simultaneously. Elastikon is used as the material of choice, applied with mild tension to prevent trauma to the Achilles tendon.

Modified Sciatic Hock Bandage

The purpose of the modified sciatic hock bandage (Fig. 65.30) is to maintain dorsiflexion of the hock and toes during walking. Nonadherent ointment–soaked gauze is placed over the traumatized tissue on the dorsal paw. A large cotton ball (5 to 7.5 cm in diameter) is placed over the dorsum of the metatarsus. A 2-inch Elastikon adhesive flexible tape is wrapped in a figure-of-eight pattern around the caudal aspect of the distal crus, dorsal to the ball of cotton on the metatarsus and plantar to the toe pads of the third and fourth digits.

The remaining metatarsus and paw can be included in a foot wrap to stabilize the bandage.

Patients with mild sensory and proprioceptive deficits usually return to proper paw placement in 2 to 4 weeks. The neurologic deficit is usually undetectable within to 2 to 4 months. Patients with temporary sensory and motor deficits may require bandaging for 1 to 4 months, depending on the severity of the injury to the nerve. The complete resolution of the sciatic may never be forthcoming. The patient should be kept under restricted activity to protect the tissues during the healing process. The bandage should be kept dry.

The bandages can be left on some patients for extended periods, but most patients require intermittent bandage application to prevent pressure sores between the toes. Excessive tension on the Elastikon or inflexible cotton tape may cause pressure necrosis on the calcaneal tendon with the potential of crippling the patient. The patient often chews or pay excessive attention to an irritating bandage. Both the described bandages should be examined frequently by both the owner and the veterinarian for abnormal odors, inflammation, or irritation. If a problem is suspected, then the bandage should be removed and reapplied.

Reference

1. Stoll S. Sciatic palsy bandage. AVORE file, Eugene, OR, 1986.

◆— INDEX

Page numbers in *italics* refer to illustrations; numbers followed by t indicate tables.